Primary Care
of **Children** with
Chronic Conditions

Primary Care of Children with Chronic Conditions

CHERI BARBER, DNP, RN, PPCNP-BC, FAANP

DNP Program Director, PNP Programs Coordinator
Department of Nursing
University of Missouri–Kansas City
Kansas City, Missouri

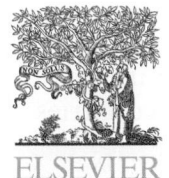

ELSEVIER

Elsevier
3251 Riverport Lane
Maryland Heights, Missouri 63043

PRIMARY CARE OF CHILDREN WITH CHRONIC CONDITIONS   ISBN: 978-0-443-10695-8

Senior Content Strategist: Sandra Clark
Content Development Specialist: Deborah Poulson
Publishing Services Manager: Catherine Jackson
Senior Project Manager/Specialist: Carrie Stetz
Book Design: Renee Duenow

Printed in India

Last digit is the print number: 9 8 7 6 5 4 3 2 1

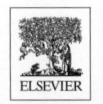 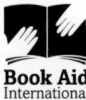

Working together to grow libraries in developing countries

www.elsevier.com • www.bookaid.org

Through the writing and gathering of this book, I have begun my own journey with a chronic condition and can personally appreciate the power of love, support, and education from family, friends, and healthcare providers. May this book inspire all who read it to be "that person" for anyone with a chronic condition.

To my family (Chris, Danielle, Megan, Emily, and my beautiful granddaughters Lilyann, Jocelyn, Brooklyn, and Zoey), thank you for supporting me through this book and on the new journey that we have found ourselves. May every rainbow be a reminder of my love for you.

And to the "little Leahs" and all the children and families with chronic conditions, may you feel blessed and supported by the care of your Pediatric Nurse Practitioners and healthcare providers.

Cheri Barber

Acknowledgments

I would like to thank Pat Jackson Allen, Judith Vessey, and Naomi Shapiro for entrusting me with this book and guiding me through the process, knowing that it would be a labor of love from start to finish. To all the chapter authors, past and present, thank you for sharing your time and expertise. The legacy of this book will live on to educate and support the next generation of pediatric healthcare providers.

Reviewers

Lori S. Anderson, PhD, RN, CPNP-PC, NCSN-E
Clinical Professor Emeritus
University of Wisconsin–Madison School of Nursing
Madison, Wisconsin

Elizabeth Burch, MSN, RN, CPNP-PC, APRN III
Clinical Coordinator
Boston Children's Hospital
President
Association of Pediatric Gastroenterology and Nutrition
    Nurses
Boston, Massachusetts

April V. Catlett, PhD
Dental Hygiene Instructor
Senior Clinical Coordinator
Central Georgia Technical College
Warner Robins, Georgia

**Brittany Christiansen, PhD, DNP, APRN, CPNP-PC/
    AC, FNP-C, AE-C, CNE**
Associate Professor of Health Sciences
Acute Care Pediatric Nurse Practitioner Specialty
    Coordinator
University of California San Francisco
San Francisco, California

Elizabeth DeSantis, MSN, RN, CPNP-AC
Pediatrics Department
Atlantic Health System
Morristown, New Jersey

Amy Donegan, MS, RN, APRN-CNP
Pediatric Certified Nurse Practitioner
Nationwide Children's Hospital
Columbus, Ohio

Sally Humphrey, DNP, APRN, CPNP-PC
Coordinator
Primary Care Pediatric Nurse Practitioner Program
University of Tennessee Health Sciences Center College
    of Nursing
Memphis, Tennessee

Rita Marie John, EdD, DNP, PNP-PC, PMHS, FAANP
Special Lecturer
Columbia University School of Nursing
New York, New York

**Michaela Lewis, DNP, ARNP, CPNP-PC, PMHS, CPN,
    CPEN, CNE, CNE-cl, VA-BC, CCRN**
Assistant Professor
College of Nursing
University of Colorado Anschutz Medical Campus
Aurora, Colorado

Marian Malone, DNP, APRN, CPNP-AC/PC
College of Nursing
University of Tennessee-Knoxville
Knoxville, Tennessee

Brittany Nelson, DNP, APRN, CPNP-PC
Director
Pediatric Nurse Practitioner-Primary Care Program
Vanderbilt University School of Nursing
Nashville, Tennessee

Margaret Quinn, DNP, CPNP-PC, CNE
School of Nursing
Rutgers University
Newark, New Jersey

Laura Roettger, PhD, MSN
College of Nursing
Thomas Jefferson University
Philadelphia, Pennsylvania

Dorothy Wyatt, PhD, MSN, NNP-BC, PPCPNP-BC
Lead Advance Neonatal Nurse Practitioner
Einstein Medical Center
Neonatology Department
Philadelphia, Pennsylvania

Contributors

Alison Ballard, MSN, RN, CPNP-PC
Neuromuscular Pediatric Nurse Practitioner
Physical Medicine and Rehabilitation
Children's Hospital Colorado
Aurora, Colorado

Cheri Barber, DNP, RN, PPCNP-BC, FAANP
DNP Program Director, PNP Programs Coordinator
Department of Nursing
University of Missouri–Kansas City
Kansas City, Missouri

Patricia A. Bierly, RN, MSN, CPNP
Advance Practice Nurse
Gastroenterology
Children's Hospital of Philadelphia
Philadelphia, Pennsylvania

Megan Bolch, PhD
Section Chief, Clinical Child Psychology
Division of Developmental and Behavioral Health
Children's Mercy Kansas City
Kansas City, Missouri

Pamela Harris Bryant, DNP, CRNP, PNP, AC/PC
Assistant Professor
School of Nursing
University of Alabama at Birmingham
Birmingham, Alabama

Melissa Campbell, PsyD
Psychologist
Division of Developmental and Behavioral Health
Children's Mercy Kansas City
Kansas City, Missouri

Megan Canavan, MSN, CPNP-PC
Nurse Practitioner
Pediatrics
Children's Hospital of Philadelphia
Philadelphia, Pennsylvania

Lucy Delaney Carter Reardon, MSN, RN, FNP-C
Department of Hemophilia Nurse Practitioner
Hematology/Oncology/BMT
Children's Mercy Kansas City
Kansas City, Missouri

Cathy C. Cartwright, DNP, RN-BC, PCNS, FAAN
Director of Advanced Practice Professional Development
Advanced Practice Programs
Children's Mercy Kansas City
Kansas City, Missouri

July Jean Cuevas, MD
Clinical Assistant Professor
School of Medicine
University of Missouri–Kansas City
Kansas City, Missouri

Renée L. Davis, DNP, APRN, CPNP-PC
Associate Professor, Traditional BSN Coordinator, Level II
Trudy Busch Valentine School of Nursing
Saint Louis University
St. Louis, Missouri

Elizabeth A. Doyle, DNP, APRN, PPCNP-BC, BC-ADM, CDCES
Assistant Professor
Primary Care Division
Yale University School of Nursing
Orange, Connecticut

Ragan DuBose-Morris, PhD, EdS
Associate Professor, Telehealth Education
Center for Telehealth
Medical University of South Carolina
Charleston, South Carolina

Julie Prasad Dunne, PhD, PMHNP-BC, RN, RYT
Clinical Assistant Professor
William F. Connell School of Nursing
Boston College
Chestnut Hill, Massachusetts

Hanein Edrees, MD, FAAP
Clinical Assistant Professor
Department of Pediatrics
Children's Mercy Kansas City
Kansas City, Missouri

Mindy Eldridge, MSN, RN, FNP-BC, CPN
APRN II
Kansas City Regional Hemophilia Treatment Center
Children's Mercy and University Health
Kansas City, Missouri

Erin Fecske, DNP, APRN, CNRN, CPNP-PC, FAES
Advance Practice Registered Nurse III
Neurology
Children's Mercy Kansas City
Kansas City, Missouri

Kelli Garber, DNP, APRN, PPCNP-BC
Clinical Assistant Professor
School of Nursing
Clemson University
Clemson, South Carolina

Elise M. Geithner, CPNP-AC, MSN, RN
Graduate
Pediatric Acute Care Nurse Practitioner Program
University of Pennsylvania
Philadelphia, Pennsylvania

Randi J. Hagerman, MD
Distinguished Professor of Pediatrics and Endowed
    Chair in Fragile X Research
Department of Pediatrics
University of California Davis Medical Center
Sacramento, California

**Donna Hallas, PhD, PPCNP-BC, CPNP, PMHS, FAANP,
    FAAN**
Clinical Professor
Meyers College of Nursing
New York University
New York, New York

Elizabeth Hastings, MD
Associate Director, Developmental and Behavioral
    Pediatrics Fellowship Program
Section Chief, Developmental Behavioral Pediatrics
Children's Mercy Kansas City
Kansas City, Missouri

**Stacia Marie Hays, DNP, APRN, CPNP-PC, CNE,
    CCTC, FAANP**
Clinical Associate Professor
Nursing
Louise Herrington School of Nursing
Baylor University
Dallas, Texas

Beth Heuer, DNP, CRNP, CPNP-PC, PMHS
Associate Professor of Clinical Instruction
Department of Nursing
College of Public Health
Temple University
Philadelphia, Pennsylvania

Jennifer Hill, MSN, CPNP-PC, PMHS
Lecturer, Pediatric Nurse Practitioner Specialty
Yale University School of Nursing
Orange, Connecticut

Paige Johnson, RN, DNP, MPH, CPHON, CPNP-PC
Nurse Practitioner
Department of Hematology/Oncology
Children's Mercy Kansas City
Kansas City, Missouri

Michelle M. Kelly, PhD, CRNP, CNE
Associate Professor
M. Louise Fitzpatrick College of Nursing
Villanova University
Villanova, Pennsylvania

Girwan Khadka, PhD
Assistant Professor of Pediatrics
Developmental and Behavioral Sciences, Section of
    Psychology
Children's Mercy Kansas City
Kansas City, Missouri

Nellie R. Lazar, MSN, MPH
Nurse Practitioner
Adolescent Medicine, Children's Hospital of
    Philadelphia
Philadelphia, Pennsylvania

**Jamie Neal Lewis, BSN, MSN, CPN, CPNP-PC,
    PMHNP-BC**
Pediatric Nurse Practitioner
Developmental and Behavioral Health
Children's Mercy Kansas City
Kansas City, Missouri

Wendy Lord Mackey, DNP, APRN, CORLN
Senior Lecturer
School of Nursing
Yale University
West Haven, Connecticut

**Kathleen F. Mallett, MSN, APRN, FNP-C, CNN-NP,
    FNKF**
APRN III
Department of Nephrology, Dialysis and Kidney
    Transplant
Children's Mercy Kansas City
Kansas City, Missouri

Julie Martin, RN, MSN, FNP-BC, PPCNP-BC
Advanced Practice Nurse
Heart Center
Children's Mercy Kansas City
Kansas City, Missouri

Lauren Mitchell, DNP, APRN, FNP-C
Neurosurgery Nurse Practitioner
Children's Mercy Kansas City
Kansas City, Missouri

Simone Moody, PhD
Clinical Psychologist, ADHD Specialty Clinic Director of
    Psychological Services
Division of Developmental & Behavioral Health
Children's Mercy Kansas City
Overland Park, Kansas

Amee Moreno, DNP, APRN, CPNP-PC/AC
Graduate Program Clinical Instructor
Louise Herrington School of Nursing
Baylor University
Dallas, Texas

Cy Nadler, PhD
Director of Autism Services
Developmental and Behavioral Health
Children's Mercy Kansas City
Kansas City, Missouri

Jessica Peck, DNP, APRN, CPNP-PC, CNE, CNL, FAANP
Clinical Professor
Louise Herrington School of Nursing
Baylor University
Dallas, Texas

Michele Polfuss, PhD, RN, APNP-AC/PC, FAAN
Associate Professor
College of Nursing
University of Wisconsin–Milwaukee
Milwaukee, Wisconsin

Neesha Ramchandani, PhD, PNP, CDCES
Lecturer
MSN Program
Yale School of Nursing
Orange, Connecticut

Kelsey Reilly, RN, MSN, FNP-BC, CPSN
Nurse Practitioner
Plastic and Reconstructive Surgery
Children's Hospital of Philadelphia
Philadelphia, Pennsylvania

Roni Lynn Robinson, MSN, RN, CRNP
Pediatric Nurse Practitioner
Trauma Program
Children's Hospital of Philadelphia
Philadelphia, Pennsylvania

Julia Sabrick, MPH
Clinical Research Coordinator
Department of Hematology
Children's Hospital of Philadelphia
Philadelphia, Pennsylvania

Nancy Shreve, RN, MS, APRN, BMTCN
Family Nurse Practitioner
Blood and Marrow Transplant
Children's Mercy Kansas City
Kansas City, Missouri

Jodi Shroba, MSN, APRN, CPNP-PC
Pediatric Nurse Practitioner
Allergy and Immunology
Children's Mercy Kansas City
Kansas City, Missouri

Tedra S. Smith, DNP, CRNP, CPNP-PC, CNE, CHSE
Assistant Dean for Graduate Clinical Education–MSN
Family and Community Health
University of Alabama at Birmingham School of Nursing
Birmingham, Alabama

Brenda Snyder, MSN, APRN, CPNP, CIgNS
Certified Pediatric Nurse Practitioner
Division of Asthma, Allergy, Immunology, Pulmonology and Sleep Medicine
Children's Mercy Hospital Kansas City
Kansas City, Missouri

Jamie Nicole Tabb, MSN, RN, CPNP-PC, CPSN
Pediatric Nurse Practitioner
Plastic, Reconstructive, and Oral Surgery
Children's Hospital of Philadelphia
Philadelphia, Pennsylvania

Heather Thomas, MD
Associate Professor
Department of Pediatrics
University of Nebraska Medical Center
Omaha, Nebraska

Devyn R. Thurber, MSN, MPH, PCPNP-BC
Type 1 Diabetes Program Coordinator
Pediatrics
Chiricahua Community Health Centers, Inc.
Douglas, Arizona

Gladesia Tolbert, DNP, MSN, CPNP, PMHS
Pediatric Nurse Practitioner
Children's Mercy Kansas City
Kansas City, Missouri

Laura White, PhD, RN, CPNP-PC, PMHNP-BC
Clinical Associate Professor
William F. Connell School of Nursing
Boston College
Chestnut Hill, Massachusetts

Teresa Whited, DNP, APRN, CPNP-PC
Associate Dean of Academic Programs, Clinical Associate Professor
College of Nursing
University of Arkansas for Medical Science Center
Little Rock, Arizona

Rachel Whitfield, MSN, APRN, FNP-C
Family Nurse Practitioner
Teen Primary Care
Children's Mercy Kansas City
Kansas City, Missouri

Amy K. Williams, DNP, APRN, CPNP-PC
Pediatric Otolaryngology
University of Arkansas for Medical Sciences
Little Rock, Arkansas

Jo Ann Youngblood, PhD
Assistant Professor of Pediatrics
School of Medicine
University of Missouri–Kansas City
Kansas City, Missouri

Preface

My desire in writing this text was to bring back a textbook about children with chronic conditions and to provide faculty who teach pediatric nurse practitioners and other pediatric healthcare providers with the information necessary to support children with chronic healthcare needs. The text is purposely formatted to give essential information to build a strong foundation for the primary care provider.

I have tried to provide a textbook that honors Patricia Jackson Allen, Judith Vessey, and Naomi Schapiro and is supportive of students and faculty. The chapters are written using a format that enhances specifics within each chapter. Part I addresses the issues that are common for children with chronic conditions. Part II identifies chronic conditions found in children, with each chapter written by pediatric healthcare professionals with expertise in caring for children with complex healthcare needs. The chronic conditions are described by their etiology, incidence and prevalence, diagnostic criteria, clinical manifestations, treatments, prognosis, and primary care management. The chapters end with resources and a detailed summary to assist students as they learn from the text.

As this book goes to press, we have witnessed within the past 4 years a pandemic that has forever changed how healthcare is provided. COVID-19 significantly impacted primary care in four main areas: changes in consultation style, provisions for the care of those with chronic illnesses, care impact on healthcare staff, and the future practice of primary care. COVID-19 demonstrated globally how a pandemic can drastically change how we provide primary healthcare, with the typical face-to-face mode moving to remote consultations. It also showed the impact on our healthcare workers both physically and mentally, reinforcing the importance of teamwork and the ability of our healthcare workers to prioritize self-care.

With the ever-changing landscape of chronic conditions seen in childhood and the continued advancement in medical knowledge, there has been an increase in children living longer with chronic conditions, necessitating a need for more knowledge from the primary care providers who follow children with chronic conditions. Information and chapters have been added to support what has been learned throughout the pandemic. Inclusive language has been used whenever possible to include nurse practitioners, physicians, and other healthcare providers who care for children with chronic conditions.

This text has been personally rewarding for me, and at the completion of its writing, I could not have done this without the help of numerous people. I would like to extend my gratitude to the many contributors for sharing their time and expertise and to all the past contributors whose work and early development have been important to the continued evolution of this book. To the Elsevier staff for their assistance and support throughout the development of this text and their continued commitment to excellence, I would like to give a heartfelt thank you to Sandra Clark, Deborah Poulson, and Carrie Stetz.

Cheri Barber

Contents

PART I CONCEPTS IN PEDIATRIC PRIMARY CARE

1 **The Primary Care Provider and Systems of Care, 1**
Cheri Barber

2 **Chronic Conditions and Child Development, 25**
Amee Moreno, Jessica Peck

3 **School and the Child With a Chronic Condition, 49**
Jennifer Hill, Wendy Lord Mackey, Neesha Ramchandani

4 **Transitions to Adulthood, 73**
Rachel Whitfield, Gladesia Tolbert

5 **Ethics and the Child With a Chronic Condition, 87**
Elise M. Geithner

6 **Managing Chronic Conditions via Telehealth, 103**
Kelli Garber, Ragan DuBose-Morris

PART II CHRONIC CONDITIONS

7 **Asthma and Allergies, 123**
Jodi Shroba, Brenda Snyder

8 **Anxiety Disorders and Obsessive-Compulsive Disorder, 163**
Girwan Khadka

9 **Attention-Deficit/Hyperactivity Disorder, 179**
Jamie Neal Lewis, Megan Bolch, Simone Moody, Hanein Edrees

10 **Autism Spectrum Disorder, 210**
Cy Nadler, Melissa Campbell, July Jean Cuevas, Elizabeth Hastings, Jamie Neal Lewis, Jo Ann Youngblood

11 **Bleeding Disorders, 237**
Lucy Delaney Carter Reardon, Mindy Eldridge

12 **Bone Marrow Transplantation, 269**
Nancy Shreve

13 **Cancer, 318**
Paige Johnson

14 **Celiac Disease, 341**
Patricia A. Bierly, Amy K. Williams

15 **Cerebral Palsy, 352**
Cheri Barber

16 **Cleft Lip and Palate, 372**
Jamie Nicole Tabb, Kelsey Reilly

17 **Congenital Adrenal Hyperplasia, 395**
Teresa Whited

18 **Congenital Heart Disease, 417**
Julie Martin

19 **Cystic Fibrosis, 463**
Heather Thomas

20 **Diabetes Mellitus (Types 1 and 2), 487**
Elizabeth A. Doyle, Devyn R. Thurber

21 **Down Syndrome, 510**
Teresa Whited

22 **Eating Disorders, 536**
Laura White, Julie Prasad Dunne

23 **Epilepsy, 560**
Erin Fecske

24 **Fragile X Syndrome, 581**
Randi J. Hagerman

25 **Human Immunodeficiency Virus Infections and Acquired Immunodeficiency Syndrome, 597**
Nellie R. Lazar

26 **Hydrocephalus, 619**
Cathy C. Cartwright

27 **Inflammatory Bowel Disease, 639**
Megan Canavan

28 **Juvenile Idiopathic Arthritis, 668**
Tedra S. Smith

29 Kidney Disease, Chronic, 683
Kathleen F. Mallett

30 Mood Disorders: Behavioral and Developmental Influences, 716
Beth Heuer, Donna Hallas

31 Muscular Dystrophy, Duchenne, 735
Alison Ballard

32 Obesity, 755
Renée L. Davis, Michele Polfuss

33 Organ Transplantation, 787
Stacia Marie Hays

34 Phenylketonuria, 818
Pamela Harris Bryant

35 Prematurity, 837
Michelle M. Kelly

36 Sickle Cell Disease, 855
Julia Sabrick, Cheri Barber

37 Spina Bifida, 886
Lauren Mitchell

38 Tourette Syndrome, 900
Cheri Barber

39 Traumatic Brain Injury, 914
Roni Lynn Robinson

INDEX, 941

The Primary Care Provider and Systems of Care

1

Cheri Barber

THE HEALTH OF AMERICA'S CHILDREN

Millions of children in the United States and around the world are alive and thriving due to medical research and advances that have led to prevention strategies, treatments, or cures for once common causes of childhood illness and death. Childhood infections have continued to decrease through better public health, immunizations, and the development of effective antibiotic and antiviral medications. Safety standards and regulations, such as the use of infant car seats, safety caps on medications, and the removal of lead from paint, have significantly reduced the number of children with unintentional injuries. Advanced pediatric medical knowledge, surgical techniques, diagnostic procedures for infants and children, pediatric intensive care centers, and trauma centers have improved the health outcomes of children requiring these services.

Children with complex health conditions or disabilities now survive with a multidisciplinary team of health care professionals to maximize their function and quality of life, allowing them to transition into adult care with proper support and preparation. Adolescents with chronic diseases must develop independent self-management practices and learn to communicate effectively with their health care team to have a smooth transition to adult-oriented health care systems. Care for these children with complex medical needs is now routinely provided by the multidisciplinary team, parents, and health care providers in the home, school, and community.

Child health is a state of the complex interplay of biologic, environmental, and societal factors. Children are cared for within the family unit; however, they are influenced by family culture, the family environment, socioeconomic status, educational level, and the current health care systems to meet their medical or health promotion needs. A review of current child health statistics is necessary to establish the context for primary care of children with chronic conditions and their families, along with understanding the changing demographics of America's children. The demographic composition helps to provide a context for understanding key indicators and the future of American families.

HEALTH STATISTICS FOR CHILDREN

The State of America's Children is an annual report from the Children's Defense Fund (2021). This report aims to ensure that all children have a healthy start, a head start, a fair start, a safe start, and a moral start to successfully pass to adulthood. The 2021 report includes a comprehensive overview of how the coronavirus (COVID-19) pandemic has impacted America's children. In addition to the statistics on COVID-19, it became apparent that the pandemic had a major impact on child and adolescent education and other facets of their well-being (Children's Defense Fund, 2021). The American Academy of Pediatrics (AAP) held a virtual parent-focus survey in April 2021 to look at the impact of the pandemic on households with children and youth with special health care needs (CYSHCN) (Cohen et al., 2022). Exacerbated by COVID-19, CYSHCN families met many challenges because of disruptions in care and services (Fig. 1.1).

CHILD POPULATION

In the United States, racial and ethnic diversity have grown dramatically over the past 3 decades. Nationwide the number of children under 18 years old in the United States in 2020 was 72.8 million, 22% of the population (Childstats.gov, n.d.). In 2020, 50% of the pediatric population were White, non-Hispanic; 14% Black, non-Hispanic; 26% Hispanic; 5% Asian, non-Hispanic; and 5% non-Hispanic "all other races" (Childstats.gov, n.d.). The US pediatric population is projected to become even more diverse over the next several decades, with the percentage of children who are White, non-Hispanic at 39% in 2050; 31% Hispanic; 14% Black, non-Hispanic; 7% Asian, non-Hispanic; and 9% non-Hispanic "all other races" (Childstats.gov, n.d.). The most current data analysis from the National Survey of Children's Health (NSCH, n.d.) shows the distribution by race/ethnicity for CYSHCN (Fig. 1.2).

CHILD POVERTY

The US Census Poverty Data showed that in 2021 the Supplemental Poverty Measure (SPM) for childhood poverty rates fell 9.7% in 2020 and 5.2% in 2021 (Fig. 1.3). This is the lowest SPM child poverty rate ever recorded,

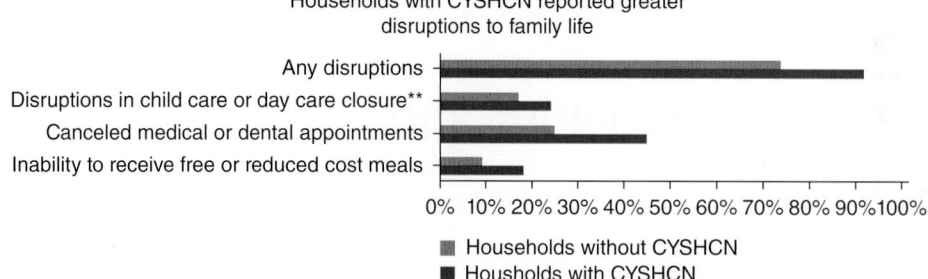

Fig. 1.1 **Households with children and youth with special health care needs** *(CYSHCN)* **reported greater disruptions to family life.** **Only respondents with at least one child <5. +Only respondents with one child ≥5. (From American Academy of Pediatrics [AAP]. Impact of the Pandemic on Households with CYSHCN. Copyright 2023 AAP.)

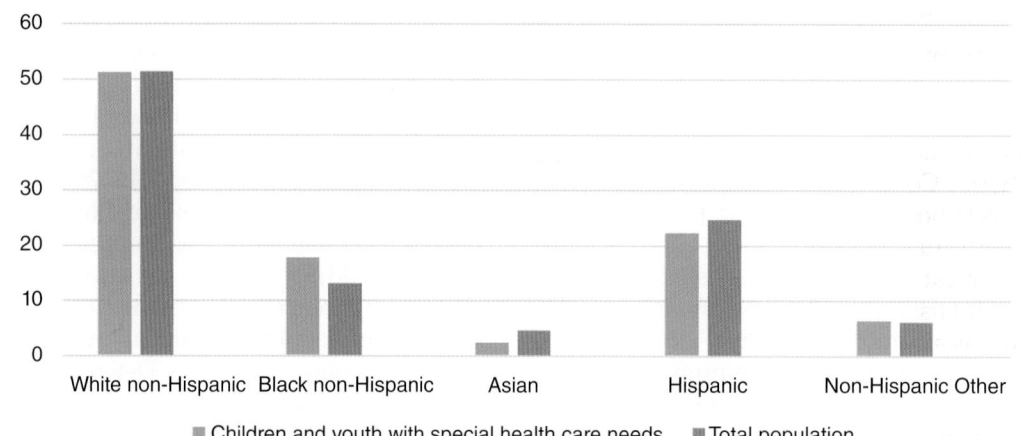

Fig. 1.2 **Distribution by race/ethnicity: total child population and children/youth with special health care needs (2016–2017) (weighted percentages).** (From: Child Trends analysis of data from the National Survey of Children's Health, 2016–2017.)

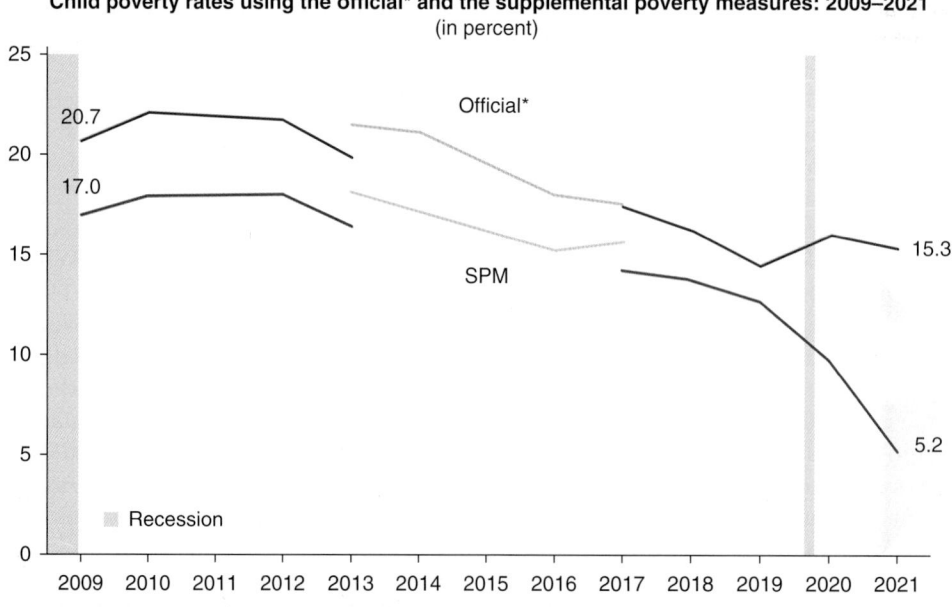

Fig. 1.3 **Child poverty rates using the official* and supplemental poverty measures** *(SPM)*: **2009–2021.** Notes: Population as of March of the following year. Official* includes unrelated individuals under age 15. SPM estimates for 2019 and beyond reflect the implementation of revised SPM methodology. More information is available in Poverty in the United States: 2021. The data for 2013 and beyond reflect the implementation of the redesigned income questions. The data points are placed at the midpoints of the respective years. More information on confidentiality protection, sampling error, nonsampling error, and definitions is available at https://www2.census.gov/programs-surveys/cps/techdocs/cpsmar22.pdf. (From: US Census Bureau, Current Population Survey, 2010–2022. Annual social and economic supplements. (Burns, 2022). https://www.census.gov/library/stories/2022/09/record-drop-in-child-poverty.html.)

Table 1.1	2022 Poverty Guidelines for the 48 Contiguous States and the District of Columbia	
PERSONS IN THE FAMILY HOUSEHOLD	**POVERTY GUIDELINE**	
1	$13.590	
2	$18.310	
3	$23.030	
4	$27.750	
5	$32.470	
6	$37.190	
7	$41.910	
8	$46.630	

For families/households with more than eight persons, add $4720 for each additional person.
From US Department of Health and Human Services. (2022). HHS poverty guidelines. https://aspe.hhs.gov/topics/poverty-economic-mobility/poverty-guidelines.

showing that more than 10 million children (14.4%) still live in poverty (US Census Bureau, 2021). Families are classified as "deep poverty" if their income falls below 50% of the poverty guidelines (Table 1.1). Hispanic children were the largest group of poor children in 2021 at 8.4%; White, non-Hispanic at 2.7%; and Black at 8.1%. The pandemic has exposed the unequal economy and the injustice of poverty among our pediatric population (Children's Defense Fund, 2021). Evidence shows that the benefits of government assistance programs help limit poverty's negative effects on our children. Investing in children and their healthy development supports the economy, helps reduce racial disparities, and improves future opportunities for this population. Child poverty and racial disparities will worsen if continued support relief for families and basic needs

programs, including rental and housing support, supplemental nutrition assistance program (SNAP), and unemployment insurance, are not supported. According to the most recent survey of families with children, racial income and wealth inequality in our nation has proven to be staggering, with the median income of Black ($43,900), Hispanic ($52,300), and American Indian ($48,000) about half the median income of White families with children ($95,700), in 2019 (Children's Defense Fund, 2021).

CHILD HUNGER AND NUTRITION

In 2020, at least one in seven children lived in food-insecure households in 24 states and the District of Columbia. Food-insecure households are defined as the inability to meet the basic food needs within the household for adults, children, or both (US Department of Agriculture [USDA], n.d.). Households with children experienced statistically significant increases in food insecurity during the COVID-19 pandemic even as overall food insecurity stayed the same. In 2020, 85.2% of households with children were food secure, whereas 14.8% were food insecure (Fig. 1.4), up from 13.6% in 2019 (CDF, 2020). More than 21.6 million children received free or reduced-price lunches during the 2018–2019 school year, but less than 3 million received meals in the summer of 2019. The food security status of a household is determined by parental reports of difficulty in obtaining enough food for each member, reduced food intake or food quality caused by the inability to secure food, or concerns about being able to provide sufficient food for all family members (Figs. 1.5 and 1.6).

Food insecurity in the early years is especially detrimental and can compound the effects of other risk

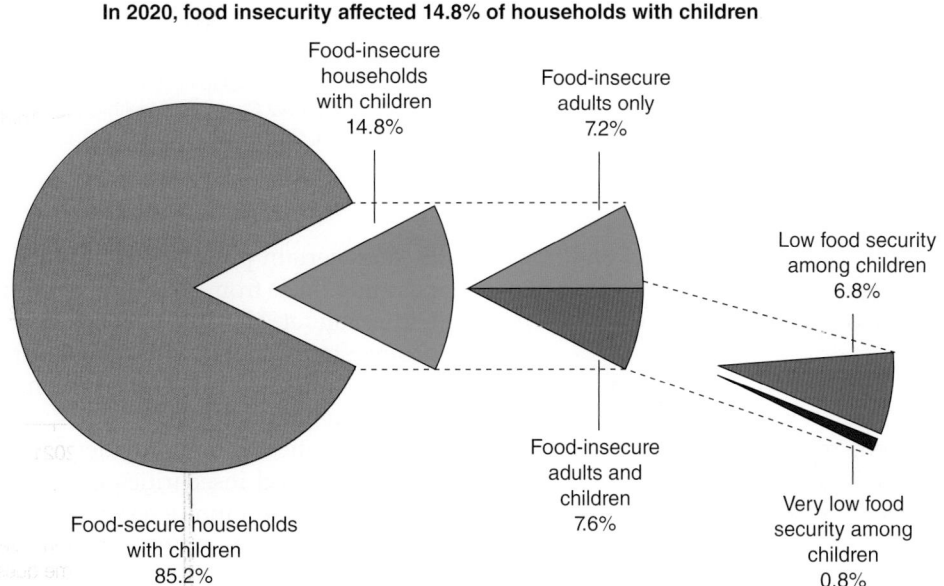

In 2020, food insecurity affected 14.8% of households with children

Food-insecure households with children 14.8%
Food-insecure adults only 7.2%
Low food security among children 6.8%
Food-insecure adults and children 7.6%
Very low food security among children 0.8%
Food-secure households with children 85.2%

Note: In most instances, when children are food insecure, the adults in the household are also food insecure.

Fig. 1.4 Food insecurity in households with children in 2020.

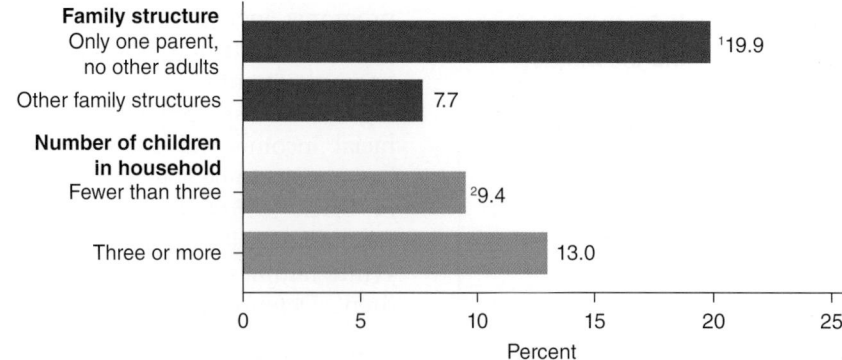

Fig. 1.5 **Family structure and food insecurity.** [1]**Significantly different from households with other family structures (*p* <0.05). [2]Significantly different from households with three or more children (p < 0.05).** (From US Department of Health and Human Services, Centers for Disease Control and Prevention, National Center for Health Statistics. [2022]. Children living in households that experienced food insecurity: United States, 2019–2020. NCHS Data Brief No. 432. https://www.cdc.gov/nchs/data/databriefs/db432.pdf.)

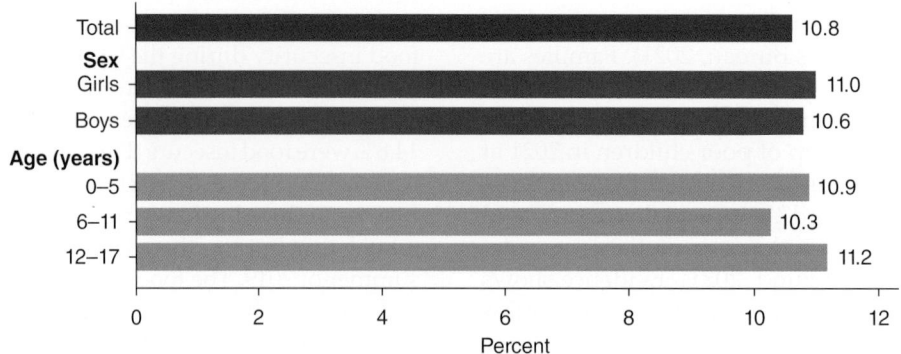

Fig. 1.6 **Percentage of children aged 0–17 years who live in households that experience food insecurity by sex and age: United States, 2019–2020.** Notes: Household food insecurity status was determined by responses to 10 questions: whether the respondent (1) worried that food would run out before there was money to buy more; (2) found food that was purchased did not last and did not have money to get more; (3) could not afford to eat balanced meals; (4) had to cut the size of meals or skip meals because there was not enough money for food and (5) the number of days this happened; (6) ate less than they should because there was not enough money for food; (7) was hungry but did not eat because there was not enough money for food; (8) lost weight because there was not enough money for food; (9) did not eat for a whole day because there was not enough money for food and (10) the number of days this happened. The questions measured the households' food situation based on the past 30 days. Based on the responses to these questions, households are categorized as being food secure, low food secure, or very low food secure. For this analysis, households that are categorized as low food secure or very low food secure are considered food insecure. Estimates are based on household interviews of a sample of the US civilian noninstitutionalized population. (From US Department of Health and Human Services, Centers for Disease Control and Prevention, National Center for Health Statistics. [2022]. Children living in households that experienced food insecurity: United States, 2019–2020. NCHS Data Brief No. 432. https://www.cdc.gov/nchs/data/databriefs/db432.pdf.)

factors associated with poverty and chronic conditions due to the importance of adequate nutrition for brain growth and early development (Hales & Coleman-Jensen, 2022).

Food insecurity is associated with many factors, including poverty. Children with food insecurity tend to be sick more often, recover from illnesses more slowly, and are hospitalized more frequently. The inability to consistently provide food creates additional stress on the family and contributes to depression, anxiety, and toxic stress; this can also lead to less positive parenting and behavior problems in children (Gitterman et al., 2015). Although food insecurity is not a direct cause of obesity, it can disproportionately

threaten certain populations at higher risk of obesity, including those from racial and ethnic minority groups (Gitterman et al., 2015). Food insecurity and low-income status, along with their health-compromising coping strategies, can exacerbate mental health and other chronic conditions.

Pediatric health care providers play a pivotal role in identifying food insecurities within families, facilitating access to community resources, and advocating for food and nutrition policies that address social determinants of health (SDH). Screening protocols vary widely without identified standards of practice. Still, the AAP recommends implementing a two-item screen designed by Hager et al. (2010) (Box 1.1), which uses

Box 1.1	Screening for Food Insecurity

1. Within the past 12 months, we worried whether our food would run out before we got money to buy more. (Yes or No)
2. Within the past 12 months, the food we bought just didn't last, and we didn't have money to get more. (Yes or No)

Although an affirmative response to both questions increases the likelihood of food insecurity existing in the household, a positive response to only 1 question is often an indication of food insecurity and should prompt additional questioning.

Modified from Hager, E. R., Quigg, A. M., Black, M. M., et al. (2010). Development and validity of a 2-item screen to identify families at risk for food insecurity. *Pediatrics, 126*(1).

a subset of two questions from the Household Food Security Scale. Positive answers to either of the two questions identify food insecurity with a sensitivity of 97% and a specificity of 83%. A team-based approach is necessary to address SDH in the health care setting. Knowing the relationship between the food environment, neighborhood factors, and health outcomes supports counseling patients at risk for obesity and other chronic conditions.

Food insecurity during the COVID-19 pandemic has illustrated the complexities of food inequity in the United States. Approximately 35 million US households rely on SNAP (Food and Nutrition Service, n.d.), with 7 million women relying on the Special Supplemental Nutrition Program for Women, Infants, and Children (WIC; https://www.nutrition.gov/topics/food-security-and-access/food-assistance-programs) (Thorn et al., 2018). Both are federally funded programs that help to meet the needs of children and families who are food insecure. These programs have dramatically increased since the COVID-19 pandemic began in the United States in early 2020. States have responded to the increasing needs in many ways, but food access and distribution have remained a central challenge to implementing program services across the country (Dunn et al., 2020).

CHILDREN AND YOUTH WITH SPECIAL HEALTH CARE NEEDS

CHRONIC AND DISABLING CONDITIONS IN CHILDREN

There are fundamental differences in the type and profile of chronic conditions in children and adults. Children are affected by a broad spectrum of rare and genetic or prenatal conditions (Table 1.2), whereas adults are affected by a relatively small number of common conditions (e.g., heart disease, emphysema, hypertension, diabetes) that increase morbidity with age. Children with chronic illnesses have unique health and social needs (Box 1.2). Chronic conditions in children are often not stable but subject to acute exacerbations and remissions that are superimposed on the child's growth and development, making them dependent on adults for care. Parent/family health, ethnicity,

Table 1.2	Most Prevalent Conditions Among CYSHCN: 2016–2017 (Weighted Percentages)
CONDITION	**PERCENTAGE**
Attention-deficit/hyperactivity disorder	33.5
Asthma	33.0
Externalizing disorders (behavioral or conduct problems)	30.4
Internalizing disorders (anxiety or depression)	28.2
Learning disability	25.3
Developmental delay	24.9
Speech disorder	22.5
Autism (autism spectrum disorder)	12.3
Genetic condition	11.7
Brain injury	6.2
Intellectual disability	5.4
Epilepsy	3.7
Diabetes	2.1
Blood disorder	1.6
Cerebral palsy	1.3
Down syndrome	0.8
Tourette syndrome	0.7
Cystic fibrosis	0.1

Note: Percentages sum to more than 100% because parents may report a child has more than one condition.
CYSHCN, Children and youth with special health care needs.
From National Survey of Children's Health. (2017). Child trends analysis. https://www.childhealthdata.org/learn-about-the-nsch/NSCH.

Box 1.2	Type of Special Health Care Needs Among CYSHCN, 2019–2020

25.5% Functional limitations
26.7% Elevated service and prescription medication(s)
20.6% Elevated service ONLY
27.2% Prescription medications(s) ONLY

From Health Resources and Services Administration, Maternal and Child Health Bureau. (2022). Children and youth with special health care needs. https://www.mchb.hrsa.gov.

culture, socioeconomic status, education, and source of health care insurance all affect the child's access to services, use of services, and adherence to management plans.

CHRONIC CONDITIONS IN CHILDREN

In 1981, President Ronald Reagan signed the Omnibus Budget and Reconciliation Act, which converted Title V into block grants programs, specifically the Maternal and Child Health (MCH) block grant for mothers and children (Warren et al., 2022), allowing state health agencies to allocate funding to a wider range of services and encourage a more hands-off approach from the federal government. This MCH block grant supports the infrastructure for MCH in every state and territory. Surgeon General C. Everett Koop coined the phrase "children with special health care needs"

(CSHCN) in 1985, amending the language in Title V from "crippled children's services" to CSHCN. In the early 2000s, CSHCN was updated to include youth: children and youth with special health care needs (CYSHCN) (Chief, Integrated Services Branch HRSA, personal communication, October 24, 2022). In 1987, the first CSHCN report was released as a call to action focusing on family-centered, community-based approaches to health care (Association of Maternal and Child Health Programs, n.d.), with the number of children who have chronic conditions, and the relative severity of the conditions is unknown.

The Maternal and Child Health Bureau (MCHB) defines children with special health care needs as those with chronic conditions or at an increased risk for chronic physical, developmental, behavioral, or emotional conditions who require health and related services or amount beyond that required by children generally. Within each state, the MCH and CYSHCN programs (known as Title V programs) are charged with providing family-centered, community-based coordinated care. These Title V programs support both private and public sectors in shaping and monitoring health-related services for women, children, and youth.

CSHCN SCREENER

The Child and Adolescent Health Measurement Initiative was established in 1998 by the Foundation for Accountability (FACCT) and the National Committee for Quality Assurance. A national collaborative coordinated by FACCT provides leadership and resources for measuring and communicating relevant, actionable information about the quality of health care for children and adolescents to consumers, pediatric health care providers, policymakers, researchers, and consumer groups to develop a method to identify children with special health care needs. The CSHCN Screener was developed by this task force as a short, five-question parent-report screening tool (Box 1.3) (Bethell et al., 2015, 2002; van Dyck et al., 2002). The screening tool identifies children based not on the diagnosis but on the functional limitation or service user needs that are the direct result of an ongoing physical, emotional, behavioral, developmental, or other health condition and has been used to determine more accurately the prevalence of CSHCN in studied populations (Bethell et al., 2008, 2015). The CSHCN Screener continues to be used in large-scale population-based surveys to estimate the prevalence of CSHCN (Bethell et al., 2015) and has not been updated to include youth in its title.

COLLECTING CYSHCN DATA

The State and Local Area Integrated Telephone Survey (SLAITS) of CSHCN began in 1997 as a pilot study in Iowa and Washington (Bramlett et al., 2014). In 2001, the Health Resources and Services Administration's MCHB (HRSA MCHB) sponsored the NSCH and companion survey, the National Survey of Children with Special Health Care Needs (NS-CSHCN). These surveys have provided critical data on key measures of child health; the presence and impact on special health care needs; health care access, utilization, and quality; and the family and community factors that impact children with special health care needs. From 2001 to 2015, the survey data was collected using SLAITS by the Centers for Disease Control and Prevention (CDC) and its National Center for Health Statistics (Kogan, 2022). With the SLAITS system, surveys utilized a random-digit-dial sample of landline telephone numbers, with cell phone supplementations in the last year of administration.

Through the years that SLAIT was being used, it gave a good geographic representation, sample size, and content range, but over time HRSA MCHB and its stakeholders came to realize that a redesign of the two surveys was needed due to the declining response rate and the proportion of US households with landline telephones. The decision was made to change from telephone numbers to household addresses for the NSCH and the NS-CSHCN. In 2015, HRSA MCHB redesigned the NSCH and NS-CSHCN into a single combined survey that utilizes an address-based sampling frame and incorporated questions from both surveys retaining the NSCH name. On behalf of the HRSA MCHB and the US Department of Health and Human Services (HHS) under Title 13, the US Census Bureau now conducts the NSCH to determine the prevalence and impact of special health care needs among children, using the definition of children with special health care needs (van Dyck et al., 2002, Bramlett et al., 2014). The use of SLAITS was discontinued in 2015, with the 2016 NSCH being the first production implementation following the redesign and merging of the previous NSCH and the NS-CSHCN. Data collection beginning in 2016 is completed through the mail and data capture methods for web, paper, and telephone questionnaire assistance operations. It is important to understand the history of data collection for CYSHCN and how it has changed over time to understand the importance of the data and how this data collection continues to improve outcomes for this population.

FINANCIAL BURDEN AND UNMET NEEDS

The financial burden experienced by families with CYSHCN is mainly determined by the degree of functional ability of the affected child, the time required by parents or caretakers to care for the child, and the impact this has on the employment of the caretakers, family income, and insurance coverage. Almost 34% of families caring for children whose daily activities were affected "usually," "always," or "a great deal" experienced financial burden as compared with 7.5% of families where the child's daily activities were never affected (Simpser et al., 2017). Time spent providing, arranging, or coordinating health care for CYSHCN varied significantly, with 47% of families spending less than 1 hour per week in these activities, 34% spending

Box 1.3   Children With Special Health Care Needs (CSHCN) Screening Tool (Mail or Telephone)

1. Does your child currently need or use medicine prescribed by a doctor (other than vitamins)?
   Yes → Go to Question 1a
   No → Go to Question 2

1a. Is this because of ANY medical, behavioral, or other health condition?
   Yes → Go to Question 1b
   No → Go to Question 2

1b. Is this a condition that has lasted or is expected to last for at least 12 months?
   Yes
   No

2. Does your child need or use more medical care, mental health, or educational services than are usual for most children of the same age?
   Yes → Go to Question 2a
   No → Go to Question 3

2a. Is this because of ANY medical, behavioral, or other health condition?
   Yes → Go to Question 2b
   No → Go to Question 3

2b. Is this a condition that has lasted or is expected to last for at least 12 months?
   Yes
   No

3. Is your child limited or prevented in any way in his or her ability to do the things most children of the same age can do?
   Yes → Go to Question 3a
   No → Go to Question 4

3a. Is this because of ANY medical, behavioral, or other health condition?
   Yes → Go to Question 3b
   No → Go to Question 4

3b. Is this a condition that has lasted or is expected to last for at least 12 months?
   Yes
   No

4. Does your child need or get special therapy, such as physical, occupational, or speech therapy?
   Yes → Go to Question 4a
   No → Go to Question 5

4a. Is this because of ANY medical, behavioral, or other health condition?
   Yes → Go to Question 4b
   No → Go to Question 5

4b. Is this a condition that has lasted or is expected to last for at least 12 months?
   Yes
   No

5. Does your child have any kind of emotional, developmental, or behavioral problem for which he or she needs or gets treatment or counseling?
   Yes → Go to Question 5a
   No

5a. Has this problem lasted or is it expected to last for at least 12 months?
   Yes
   No

SCORING THE CSHCN SCREENING TOOL
Conceptual Background

The CSHCN screener uses consequences-based criteria to screen for children with chronic or special health needs. To qualify as having chronic or special health needs, the following set of conditions must be met:

1. The child currently experiences a specific consequence.
2. The consequence is due to a medical or other health condition.
3. The duration or expected duration of the condition is 12 months or longer.

The first part of each screener question asks whether a child experiences one of five different health consequences:

1. Use or need of prescription medication
2. Above average use or need of medical, mental health, or educational services
3. Functional limitations compared with others of same age
4. Use or need of specialized therapies (occupational, physical, speech, etc.)
5. Treatment or counseling for emotional or developmental problems

The second and third parts* of each screener question ask those responding yes to the first part of the question whether the consequence is due to any kind of health condition and if so, whether that condition has lasted or is expected to last for at least 12 months.

All three parts* of at least one screener question (or in the case of question 5, the two parts) must be answered yes for a child to meet CSHCN screener criteria for having a chronic condition or special health care need.

The CSHCN screener has three definitional domains:

1. Dependency on prescription medications
2. Service use above that considered usual or routine
3. Functional limitations

Continued

1 to 4 hours per week, almost 9% spending 5 to 10 hours per week, and nearly 10% spending over 11 hours per week (Simpser et al., 2017). The time burden was greater on low-income families, with almost 19% of poor families spending at least 11 hours per week providing needed care as compared to only 4.3% of families living at or above 400% federal poverty level (FPL). Families with children whose activities were affected "usually," "always," or "a great deal" were also more likely (23.5%) to spend greater than 11 hours per week in the care of their children, and 47% reported having to cut back on work or stop altogether, affecting family income and sometimes insurance coverage. Only 3.2% of parents of children without limitations in daily activities reported spending more than 10 hours per week in time providing, arranging, or coordinating

Box **1.3**   **Children With Special Health Care Needs (CSHCN) Screening Tool (Mail or Telephone)—cont'd**

The definitional domains are not mutually exclusive categories. A child meeting the CSHCN screener criteria for having a chronic condition may qualify for one or more definitional domains (see diagram below).

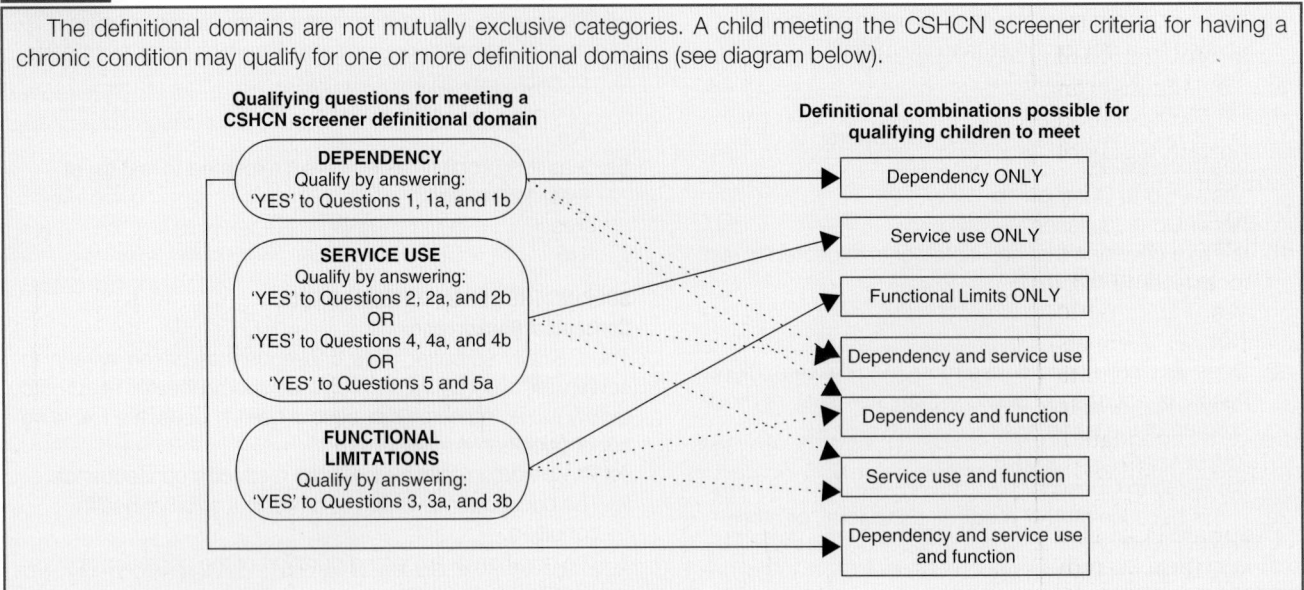

*Note: CSHCN screener question 5 is a two-part question. Both parts must be answered yes to qualify.
From Child and Adolescent Health Measurement Initiative. Children With Special Health Care Needs (CSHCN) Screening Tool, www.cahmi.org. Retrieved August 27, 2023.

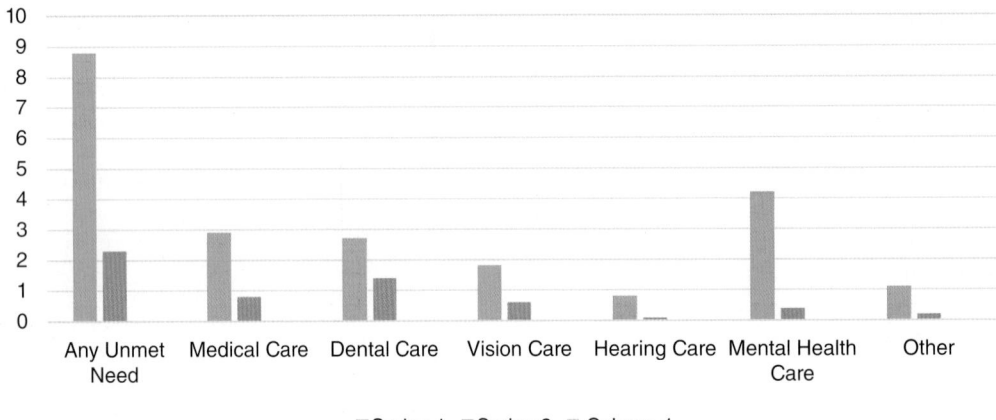

Fig. 1.7 Percent of children with unmet health care needs by CYSHCN status, 2019–2020. (From Health Resources and Services Administration, Maternal and Child Health Bureau. (2022). Children and youth with special health care needs. NSCH Data Brief. https://www.mchb.hrsa.gov.)

health care for their child, and only 9% reported cutting back on work to care for the child.

Families of uninsured children reported the highest financial burden (42%) as compared with those with public insurance (19.5%) and private insurance (15%); the financial burden is higher on families of children with public insurance even though out-of-pocket expenses are lower because family income is lower, so costs are proportionally higher than for higher-income families (Simpser et al., 2017). The percentage of unmet health care needs continues to rise as the financial burden increases (Fig. 1.7).

ORAL HEALTH CARE

Oral health care and dental caries are the most prevalent among CYSHCN. Data on dental caries and other oral health conditions for CYSHCN are based on parent- or caregiver-report measures. In 2016, the NCSH and the NS-CSHCN began collecting additional data on preventive NSCH services (including cleanings, prophylaxis, instruction on tooth brushing, fluoride treatments, and sealants). The findings revealed that CYSHCN supported by a medical home were more likely to receive preventative oral health (POH) services than those who do not have a medical home. Risk factors associated with dental caries among CYSHCN include frequent use of sugar-containing liquid medicines and dependence on their caregiver for regular oral hygiene. Children with chronic conditions often have special diets or eating patterns that can affect oral health. Medications may affect tooth or gum development, and dental hygiene may be very difficult in children with severe disabilities or oral aversion.

Financial barriers may interfere with good oral health care for CYSHCN and nonfinancial barriers such as language and psychosocial, structural, and cultural considerations. The structural barriers include transportation, school absence policies, discriminatory treatment, and difficulty with the location of providers that accept Medicaid (American Academy of Pediatric Dentistry [AAPD], 2021).

This population's most common oral diseases are gingivitis and periodontal disease (Lebrun-Harris et al., 2021). Dentists skilled in the care of children with complex conditions are often challenging to find but important in helping to maintain oral health and long-term adequate nutrition. Every health care provider needs skilled dentists in their local area as part of their toolkit to support this population. Ensuring that appropriate POH is available to the CYSHCN population is critical to reducing oral health problems. The AAP Bright Future Guidelines and the US Preventative Services Task Force recommend that pediatric primary care providers provide POH services to infants and children, including fluoride treatments, supplementation, and oral hygiene education.

The AAPD recommendations on the management of CYSHCN were originally adopted by the Council on Clinical Affairs in 2004 and revised in 2016. The latest revision in 2021 was based on a review of the current dental and medical literature on CYSHCN. The AAPD (2021) defines special health care needs as "any physical, developmental, mental, sensory, behavioral, cognitive, or emotional impairment or limiting condition that requires medical management, health care intervention, and/or use of specialized services or programs." Just as the medical home is important to this population, it is recommended by the AAPD (2021) to establish a dental home by 12 months of age. The dental home will provide an opportunity for individualized preventive oral health practice, establishing routine dental care and reducing the child's risk of preventable dental and oral disease (AAPD, 2021).

The goals for CYSHCN oral health care include (1) establishing a dental home at an early age; (2) obtaining thorough medical, dental, and social patient histories; (3) creating an environment conducive for the child to receive care; (4) providing comprehensive oral health education and anticipatory guidance to the child and caregiver; and (5) providing preventive and therapeutic services, including behavior guidance and a multidisciplinary approach when needed (AAPD, 2021). As CYSHCN approach adulthood, it is important to plan and coordinate the successful transition to an adult dental home to ensure the continuity of oral health care.

FOREIGN-BORN PERSONS

The US Census Bureau defines foreign-born as anyone who is not a US citizen at birth; one or both of the child's parents may be foreign-born (US Census Bureau, 2021). Foreign-born population in the United States has grown since 1970 mainly due to immigration from Latin America and Asia. This growth has led to the diversity of language and cultural backgrounds of children growing up in the United States. According to the US Census Bureau (2021), 22% of the US population in 2020 were children with one foreign-born parent, and 3% were foreign-born with at least one foreign-born parent. More than one in four (26%), or approximately 18 million, US children lived with at least one foreign-born parent in 2018. In 2019, more than one in four foreign-born children were without health coverage, and in July 2019 six states and the District of Columbia used state funds to provide Medicaid coverage to income-eligible children regardless of their immigration status (Children's Defense Fund, 2021). By January 2020, 35 states and the District of Columbia provided health care coverage to lawfully residing foreign-born children without a 5-year wait. Twenty-eight percent of families with foreign-born parents live below the FPL and have parents with less than a high school degree (42%), both factors contributing to increased health risks in children (Federal Interagency Forum on Child and Family Statistics, 2021).

HEALTHY PEOPLE 2030

The focus of Healthy People 2030 is to improve children's health, safety, and well-being directly and indirectly (HHS, 2022). One aim is to decrease the child mortality rate from 25% to 18.4% per 100,000 by 2030 (Box 1.4). Injuries continue to be the leading cause of death in children and adolescents. Primary care providers play an important role in preventable injuries, such as promoting the use of child restraints and proper car seats, encouraging the use of properly fitting helmets to reduce traumatic brain injuries, and creating interventions to change health care providers prescribing habits. The incidence of injuries among children, with their subsequent health problems or disabilities, is more prevalent in racial minority groups.

Box 1.4	Healthy People 2030 Action Plan for Children, Youth, and Families with Special Health Care Needs

Goal 1: Assure access of equitable and high-quality health care for children and adolescents to optimize health and well-being for all populations.
Goal 2: Achieve health equity for all child populations.
Goal 3: Strengthen public health capacity and workforce for children with special health care needs.
Goal 4: Maximize impact through leadership, partnership, and stewardship.

Modified from Maternal and Child Health Bureau. (2021). Maternal and Child Health Bureau strategic plan. https://mchb.hrsa.gov/sites/default/files/mchb/about-us/maternal-child-health-bureau-strategic-plan.pdf.

Although the incidence of congenital disabilities does not vary significantly across racial groups, chronic health conditions and the incidence of injuries, with their subsequent health problems or disabilities, are more prevalent in children of racial minority groups.

INFANT MORTALITY

Infant mortality rates are an important marker of the overall health of society. In 2020, the US infant mortality rate was 5.4 deaths per 1000 live births, which shows a large decline over the past 18 years. The latest CDC data for subpopulations at the time of this publication was the 2019 data showing infant mortality rates by race and ethnicity:

- Non-Hispanic Black: 10.6
- Non-Hispanic Native Hawaiian or other Pacific Islander: 8.2
- Non-Hispanic American Indian/Alaska Native: 7.9
- Hispanic: 5.0
- Non-Hispanic White: 4.5
- Non-Hispanic Asian: 3.4

There continues to be a racial disparity in characteristics of mothers known to be associated with poor outcomes for newborns; overall, minority mothers are younger, have lower levels of education, and are more frequently unmarried. The 10 leading causes of death in this population are listed in Fig. 1.8.

CULTURALLY SENSITIVE CARE FOR CHILDREN WITH CHRONIC CONDITIONS AND THEIR FAMILIES

Discussion of systems of care for children and families must include the cultural appropriateness of services. Critical to service design and delivery is the extent to which systems focus on family and community uniqueness, including the diversity of backgrounds of those seeking care within the systems. The seminal work of Cross and colleagues (1989) continues to be a well-cited model and is a good starting place for systems design and evaluation related to inclusivity and diversity. Cross et al. (1989) included congruent behaviors, attitudes, and policies as key components of systems, agencies, and professional practice. Their work has been expanded to include measures of inclusivity related to race, ethnicity, class, religion, gender, geography, and income. Linguistic services are key to quality care but are not sufficient.

Adapted from Cross et al. (1989) are the following five ideal organization characteristics:

1. Valuing diversity
2. Carrying out cultural self-assessment
3. Promoting awareness of cultural interaction dynamics
4. Building the organization's knowledge base about culture
5. Adapting services according to cultural knowledge

These five elements should be manifested at every level of an organization, including policymaking, administration, and practice. Creating climates of tolerance and safety with processes for addressing conflict must be intentional and constantly monitored. Integrity, authenticity, and legal protections must be modeled throughout systems, organizations, and professions, with clear expectations and sanctions when goals are not met. Weaving inclusivity into the fabric of organizations that care for children and families is mandated by the MCHB.

With growing awareness of the need to provide culturally sensitive care to all pediatric patients, health

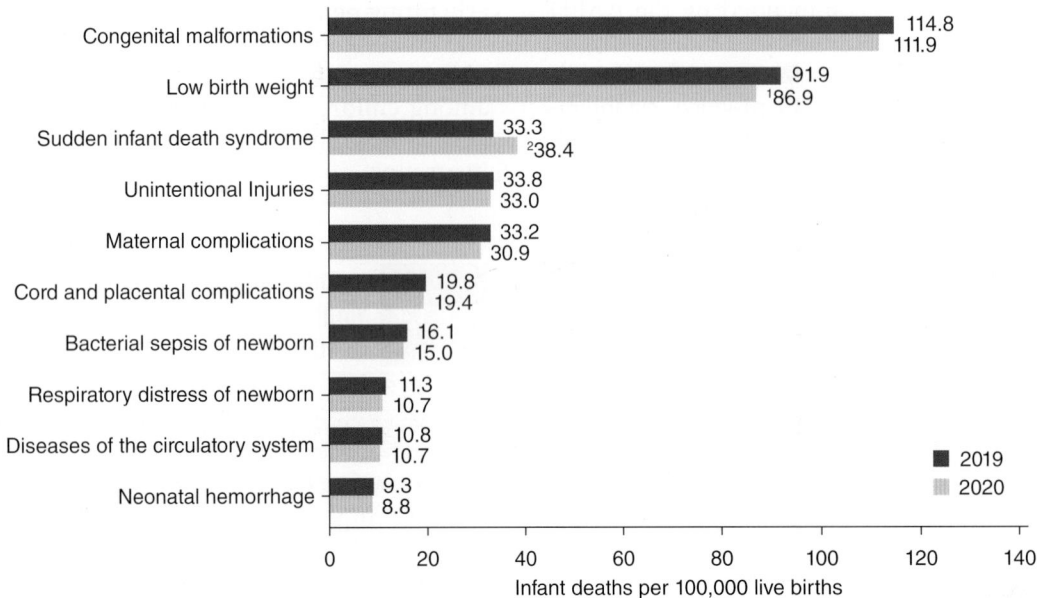

Fig. 1.8 Infant mortality rates for the 10 leading causes of infant death in 2020: United States, 2019 and 2020.
(From: National Center for Health Statistics, Centers for Disease Control and Prevention. [2019]. Mortality in the United States [fig 5]. NCHS Data Brief No. 395. https://www.cdc.gov/nchs/products/databriefs/db395.htm.)

care providers have recognized that cultural sensitivity is important to provide all children with high-quality, comprehensive care. Cultural sensitivity is a key component of the patient-centered medical home model, with parents reporting that culturally sensitive care in the primary care settings has been associated with higher-quality well-child care (Okoniewski et al., 2022). Over the past 2 decades culturally sensitive care interventions for the pediatric primary care setting have been developed to align with the call to action to address child health disparities. One example of a culturally sensitive intervention that is considered standard of care is ensuring language supports are available to all patients and families. Medical interpreters bridge the gap when patients and providers do not speak the same language and can be professional medical interpreters, health care providers, and online or tele-language services. Another key tenet of culturally sensitive care is addressing structural factors such as poverty and racism, which are both discussed in this chapter.

CAREGIVER STRAIN

Caregivers are an integral part of the medical care of CYSHCN and are affected physically, mentally, and financially. Caregivers are parents (55%) and grandparents (18%) but can also be other relatives (e.g., aunt or uncle, 13%), family friends (8%), or siblings (1%) (Pilapil et al., 2017). Many caregivers are negatively impacted by employment due to the time needed for medical visits, family functioning, and financial security. Caring for this population affects the whole family, making it important for the health care providers who maintain the medical home to be aware of potential challenges that caregivers face. The providers must screen for caregiver strain and be familiar with the resources available to support and reduce the burden on families of CYSHCN (Pilapil et al., 2017). Longer overall life expectancies and advances in medical technology have extended survival for medically complex children, increasing the strain on caregivers. Caregiver burden is the multifaceted strain the caregiver perceives from caring for a family member or loved one over time. When caring for a medically ill child, the impact on the parents' or caregivers' quality of life can be noted in their inability to complete daily activities, find time to complete household chores, greater family conflict, and less family support. The Modified Caregiver Strain Index (MCSI) is a brief and easy tool for caregiver strain with long-term family caregivers (Box 1.5). It

---

Box 1.5   Modified Caregiver Strain Index

Directions: Here is a list of things that other caregivers have found to be difficult. Please put a checkmark in the columns that apply to you. We have included some examples that are common caregiver experiences to help you think about each item. Your situation may be slightly different, but the item could still apply.

Key: Yes, on a regular basis = 2; Yes, sometimes = 1; No = 0.

1. My sleep is disturbed _____ _____ _____ (e.g., the person I care for is in and out of bed or wanders around at night).
2. Caregiving is inconvenient _____ _____ _____ (e.g., helping takes so much time or it's a long drive over to help).
3. Caregiving is a physical strain _____ _____ _____ (e.g., lifting in or out of a chair; effort or concentration is required).
4. Caregiving is confining _____ _____ _____ (e.g., helping restricts free time or I cannot go visiting).
5. There have been family adjustments _____ _____ _____ (e.g., helping has disrupted my routine; there is no privacy).
6. There have been changes in personal plans _____ _____ _____ (e.g., I had to turn down a job; I could not go on vacation).
7. There have been other demands on my time _____ _____ _____ (e.g., other family members need me).
8. There have been emotional adjustments _____ _____ _____ (e.g., severe arguments about caregiving).
9. Some behavior is upsetting _____ _____ _____ (e.g., incontinence; the person cared for has trouble remembering things, or the person I care for accuses people of taking things).
10. It is upsetting to find the person I care for has changed so much from his/her former self _____ _____ _____ (e.g., he/she is a different person than he/she used to be)
11. There have been work adjustments _____ _____ _____ (e.g., I have to take time off for caregiving duties).
12. Caregiving is a financial strain _____ _____ _____ (e.g., I live paycheck to paycheck).
13. I feel completely overwhelmed _____ _____ _____ (e.g., I worry about the person I care for; I have concerns about how I will manage).

Sum responses for "Yes, on a regular basis" (2 pts each) and "Yes, sometimes" (1 pt each).

Total score = _____

Modified from Thornton, M., & Travis, S.S. (2003). Analysis of the reliability of the Modified Caregiver Strain Index. *Journal of Gerontology, Series B, Psychological Sciences and Social Sciences, 58*(2), S129.

is a 13-question tool that measures strain related to care provision. This instrument can assess individuals of any age who have assumed the caregiving role with the original version, the Caregiver Strain Index, developed in 1983. The higher the score on the MCSI, the greater the need for more in-depth assessment to facilitate appropriate intervention.

INEQUALITIES IN CHILD HEALTH

DISPARITIES BASED ON RACE, ETHNICITY, AND FAMILY/SOCIAL COMPLEXITIES

Race, family structure (single parent vs. two parents), parent education, poverty, and culture/language are closely linked in the United States. In addition, disparities in access, quality, costs, health promotion, and early child development services have been found to have wide variation by state with strong regional patterns in the quality of child health care performance. Children with chronic conditions residing in regions with poorer access to health care and quality health services may not receive preventive care or early treatment of complications necessary to maintain optimal health and prevent complications from their chronic condition. Family/social complexities (i.e., poverty, mental health problems, competing family demands) or chronic condition complexities may overshadow the perceived need for certain treatments or routine health care, such as immunizations or vision and hearing screening. Transportation to appropriate health facilities may be difficult or expensive, or access to specialists may be restricted by a lack of availability in a geographic region.

BIRTH OF A NATIONAL FRAMEWORK

The HRSA MCHB has spent decades as the national locus of responsibility and leadership for CYSHCN and their families. MCHB, along with the Division of Services for Children with Special Health Needs, gathered self-advocates, families, doctors, advocacy groups, local and national organizations, state public health agencies, federal offices, academic institutions, and researchers through a 2-year process that included a summit, listening sessions, meetings, and a public request for information (Brown et al., 2022). A national framework for a system of supplement services for CYSHCN was introduced in 2022 by the AAP. The *Blueprint for Change: Guiding Principles for a System of Services for CYSHCN and Their Families* (hereafter referred to as *Blueprint for Change*) supports health equity as a key pillar in supporting the future of CYSHCN. The other three critical areas identified in the *Blueprint for Change* are family and child well-being and quality of life, access to services, and financing of services. To achieve these goals, several factors need to be considered that impact the outcome for this population, including but not limited to lack of resources, insufficient training, political will (the commitment

to undertake actions to achieve a set of objectives to achieve change), poverty, and discrimination even by health care professionals.

HEALTH EQUITY

"Health equity means that everyone has a fair and just opportunity to be as healthy as possible. This requires removing obstacles to health such as poverty, discrimination, and their consequences, including powerlessness and lack of access to good jobs with fair pay, quality education, housing, safe environments, and health care" (Braveman et al., 2018). Health equity is essential to population health, and research is required to achieve extensive monitoring beyond traditional disparities. Health equity among children increased gradually over the past 2 decades, guiding the work for the *Blueprint for Change* and consistent with the work of Healthy People 2030. The values for both include the following: All children should be equally valued; resources to promote health should be distributed fairly; commitment to health equity represents justice in health; a reduction in health disparities measures progress. Although equity in the pediatric population has also been threatened due to decreases in government spending on programs affecting children and the COVID-19 pandemic, progression in health equity requires accountability by everyone who has a stake in the end goal (Houtrow et al., 2022). The inequalities that must continue to be measured by different indicators show that these disparities persist.

FAMILY AND CHILD WELL-BEING AND QUALITY OF LIFE

Data must continue to be gathered on the quality of life and well-being to assist CYSHCN patients and their families to thrive. The CDC (2021) defines the health-related quality of life as "an individual's or group's perceived physical and mental health over time." Components that contribute to the quality of life and well-being, according to Coleman et al. (2022), include protective factors (socializing with friends, participating in accessible activities, etc.) and risk factors (missing school for medical appointments, experiencing bullying). For the health care system to address these issues, more focus must be placed on promoting dignity, autonomy, and independence for CYSHCN and their families (Coleman et al., 2022). This can be accomplished through gathering data on quality of life and well-being to develop services to promote rather than hinder their quality of life.

ACCESS TO SERVICES

Access to services for CYSHCN and their families has been described as fragmented, unaffordable, stressful, and untimely, with no available roadmap on how to access them, with further disparities existing by race and ethnicity (Kuo et al., 2022). Fragmentation of care may interfere with comprehensive care. Many children with chronic conditions receive most of their medical care in specialty clinics that do not provide routine health care management. When children are shuffled from specialist to specialist, they often miss the screenings, developmental assessments, anticipatory guidance, and immunizations that healthy children of the same age receive. The development of medical specialization has improved the disease control and life expectancy of CYSHCN but has also resulted in fragmentation of health care delivery and increased medical costs.

The families of CYSHCN must interact with multiple institutions and systems that provide care for their child (e.g., early intervention programs, equipment vendors, social services, special education programs, and federal, state, or private financial providers of care). In addition, there are often medical subspecialists whose expectations may or may not be realistic for the family or child. Demands are sometimes conflicting, uncoordinated, and incomprehensible to the family. Subspecialists rarely address primary health care needs, developmental concerns, or common illness management. Primary care providers, on the other hand, frequently cite a lack of specialty knowledge, lack of adequate time with children and families, lack of proper reimbursement for care of children with complex medical or behavioral conditions, and unavailability of subspecialists to collaborate within their community as barriers to their provision of comprehensive care to children with chronic conditions (Agrawal et al., 2011; Barclay, 2003). An integrated, proactive system of services that meets the needs of CYSHCN families requires partnership, flexibility, innovation of design, and creative thinking (Kuo et al., 2022).

FINANCING OF SERVICES

Policy opportunities exist to improve outcomes for CYSHCN through system transformation at the policy level. Financing requires coordinated efforts among federal and state agencies, the provider community, diverse racial and ethnic communities, as well as the families and CYSHCN (Schiff et al., 2022). The vision outlined in the *Blueprint for Change* is that health care and related services will be accessible, affordable, comprehensive, continuous, and prioritized for CYSHCN and their families. Barriers that currently exist for this population are racial disparities and societal risks, finding appropriate and knowledgeable provider care teams, and ensuring adequate and continuous coverage for services. Financing innovations must use new and up-to-date measures to assess value and provide evidence for improvement. Insurance coverage is insufficient to ensure that all services for CYSHCN are met. The most recent NSCH data revealed that one-third of CYSHCN parents and caregivers reported their child's coverage was inadequate (Ghandour et al., 2022).

CYSHCN often have numerous service sectors: primary care, multiple specialty providers, and prescription providers, as well as nonhealth-related services such as social services, education, and home and community-based services. Lack of these critical services is often seen more during adolescence and adulthood; consistent and adequate funding for care coordination and telehealth services has been more prominent during the pandemic (Schiff et al., 2022). To improve family-identified outcomes and well-being, state health officials are increasingly linking quality measures to alternative payment models, rewarding providers for delivering high-quality, cost-effective care (Fig. 1.9).

HEALTH INSURANCE COVERAGE

In the United States the majority of children and youth rely on insurance to access health care; although many families living in or near poverty may qualify for public coverage, families who lack insurance pay out of pocket, often delaying care for their children. Families with CYSHCN with low to middle income are particularly sensitive to insurance variations. Families' perceived adequacy of their children's health insurance varies substantially, with some families having inaccurate knowledge of the exact coverage offered by their insurance (Fig. 1.10). Berry et al. (2021) found that families with CYSHCN with greater health care needs reported more problems with their children's insurance, especially with direct coverage. Public insurance has proven to have better coverage and benefits than a commercial for CYSHCN.

In 2019, 1 in 18 US children were uninsured. Hispanic children were much more likely to be uninsured than White, Black, and Asian children. Children in families living below 100% of the poverty line were more likely to be uninsured than their counterparts. In 2019, Medicaid and the Children's Health Insurance Program (CHIP) provided comprehensive and affordable health and mental health coverage to more than 36 million children, but more than 4 million children remained uninsured. Unfortunately, children's access to health coverage and services across the United States remains a lottery of geography.

From a historical perspective, Medicare and Medicaid were established in 1965. Medicare lacked long-term care benefits due to the increased cost of those benefits (Berry et al., 2021). Medicaid served as a safety net for low-income families covering those with CSHCN (now CYSHCN). Early and periodic screening and diagnostic and treatment benefits were added to ensure the availability of health services and treatments for disabling conditions affecting growth and development (Berry et al., 2021).

CYSHCN remain a sizable and diverse population with distinct challenges and the greatest needs in accessing health care. According to the US Census Bureau's annual report, the number of children under 19 without insurance fell by 3.9 million in 2021—that is, 475,000

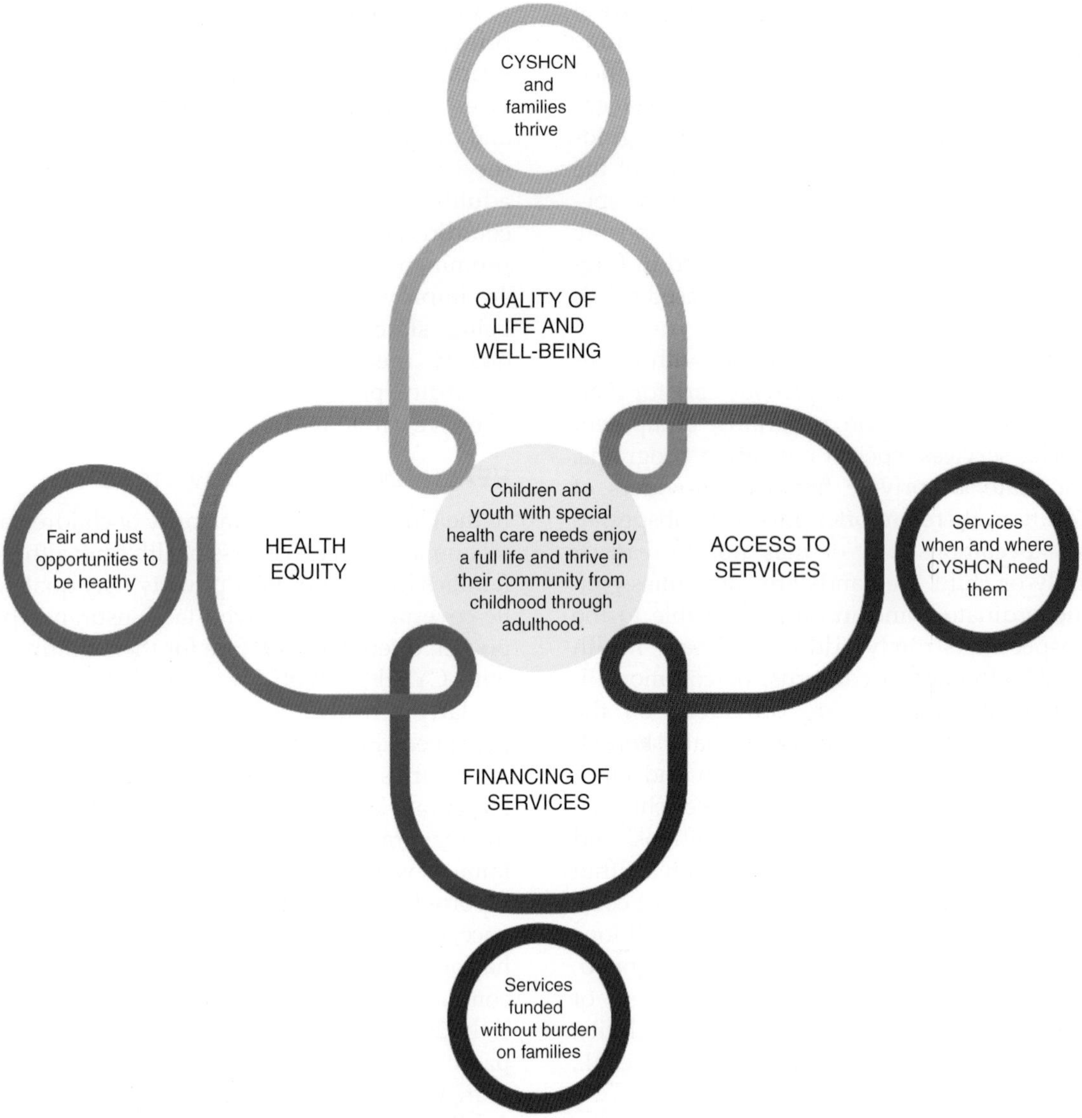

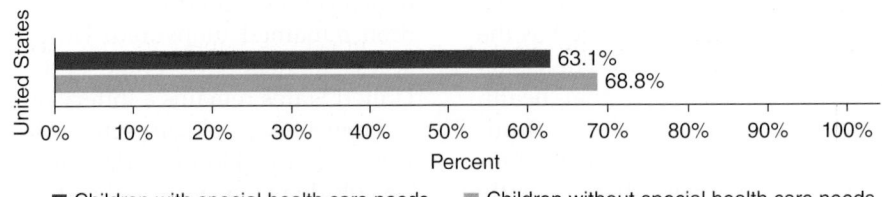

Fig. 1.9 Blueprint for change: guiding principles for a system of services for children and youth with special health care needs *(CYSHCN)* and their families. (From McLellan, S. E., Mann, M. Y., Scott, J. A., & Brown, T. W. [2022]. A blueprint for change: Guiding principles for a system of services for children and youth with special health care needs and their families. *Pediatrics, 149*[Suppl. 7].)

Fig. 1.10 Adequacy of health insurance coverage by special needs status, 2016–2019. Definition: Estimated percentage of children ages 0–17 with and without health insurance coverage that is consistent and meets their needs, by special health care needs status (e.g., in 2016–2019, among California children with special health care needs, both insured and uninsured, 61.2% had adequate health insurance coverage). (From Chidren with Special Health Care Needs: KidsData.org. Copyright 2023. All rights reserved.)

fewer children had coverage than in 2020. Most children (61.9%) had private coverage, with a growing number above the poverty level being covered by public programs (Fig. 1.11). Lower-income families benefited from Medicaid and CHIP. Although changes by Congress with increased funding for Medicaid and states enacting measures to make it easier to apply for health insurance through the Patient Protection and Affordable Care Act (ACA) have contributed to the increase in health coverage for all children, including those above the poverty

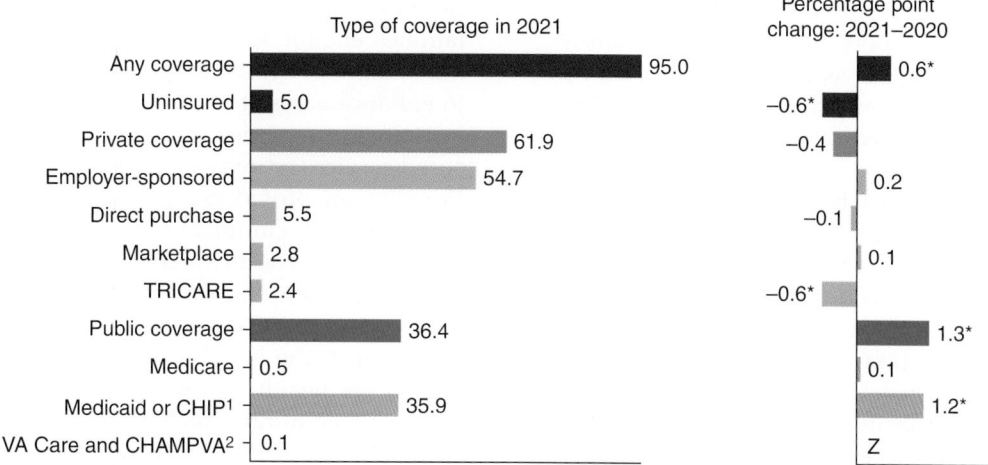

Fig. 1.11 Health insurance coverage status and type of coverage for children under 19: 2020 and 2021. Bunch L, Bandekar A. (2021). Changes in children's health coverage varied by poverty status from 2018–2020. (Available at https://www.census.gov/library/stories/2021/09/uninsured-rates-for-children-in-poverty-increased-2018-2020.html.)

level, many CYSHCN in the United States continue to be uncovered (Bunch & Bandekar, 2021).

In 2014, the MCHB, with support from the Lucile Packard Foundation for Children's Health, released a groundbreaking set of standards to build and improve systems of care for CYSHCN. These were the result of decades of work to establish and endorse a set of standards that are now used by national, state, and local stakeholder groups, including Title V CYSHCN programs, health plans, state Medicaid and CHIP agencies, as well as pediatric provider organizations, children's hospitals, insurers, and consumers.

National Standards: Core Domains for System Standards

1. Identification, Screening, Assessment, and Referral
2. Eligibility and Enrollment in Health Coverage
3. Access to Care
4. Medical Home
   - Pediatric Preventive and Primary Care
   - Medical Home Management
   - Care Coordination
   - Pediatric Specialty Care
5. Community-Based Services and Supports
   - Respite Care
   - Palliative and Hospice Care
   - Home-Based Services
6. Transition to Adulthood
7. Health Information Technology
8. Quality Assurance and Improvement

PRIMARY CARE MANAGEMENT

AAP RECOMMENDATIONS

- Screen and identify children at risk for food insecurity at each visit.
- Connect families to the necessary community resources (Table 1.3).
- Advocate with other key partners and stakeholders for federal, state, and local policies that will help support access to adequate and healthy food so that all children and their families can be nourished, active, and healthy.

ROLE OF THE PRIMARY CARE PROVIDER IN CARING FOR CHILDREN WITH CHRONIC CONDITIONS

The role of the primary care provider is an integral part of the interdisciplinary team of professionals caring for children with chronic conditions. The AAP encourages the medical home concept, where the primary care provider is the umbrella to the team. A medical home is a comprehensive approach to primary care, facilitating partnerships between patients, families, clinicians, and medical staff. This approach extends past the clinical practice and includes specialty care, educational services, and family support. Pediatric subspecialists with advanced training and skills gained from caring for children with similar conditions are the best professionals to deal with the medical complexities of many chronic conditions.

A comprehensive medical home is the foundation of quality primary care services for all children, especially those with special health care needs. The AAP introduced the medical home concept and terminology in 1967 to describe a central location for children's medical records. The focus was on CYSHCN and later defined by the AAP as an approach to providing comprehensive primary care that facilitates partnerships between patients, clinicians, medical staff, and families, extending beyond the four walls of clinical practice to include specialty care, educational services, family support, and more (Lichstein et al., 2018). Passage of the ACA in 2010 identified the medical home model as a standard of care for CYSHCN with the intent of improving systems of care and coverage for this population of children and youth. Although coverage gaps and system fragmentation continue, there have been great strides with implementing the medical home model.

To support the broader needs of the child and family (i.e., education on well care and safety, health promotion, support, advocacy, referral to community resources) with a focus on care, there continues to be a prominent role for the primary care provider, especially in a medical home. The primary care provider in caring for children with chronic conditions needs to have the ability to accomplish the following:

1. Holistic health care of children requires that they be viewed first and foremost as children, with any child's health care and developmental needs.
2. The family must be considered an integral part of the child's growth and development and recognized for its strengths and weaknesses. Developing partnerships with families in caring for their children is a fundamental tenet of pediatric primary care.
3. Health promotion, disease prevention, and anticipatory guidance have even greater significance when children already have a condition putting them at increased risk. Subspecialists are experts in disease management but often have limited knowledge of normal growth and development and standard health care practices for health maintenance.
4. Primary care providers most likely know a family's community resources better than subspecialists, who may have practices many miles from the family's home. This knowledge of community resources is essential in helping families receive optimal care and support for their children. Care coordination in partnership with families is critical, especially when the condition is complex or unstable or the child has functional limitations.
5. Primary providers are best positioned to advocate for families' health care needs and to interact with the health care system. They can ensure that all families eligible for insurance, particularly Medicaid or state CHIP, can successfully obtain insurance to enhance access to care. They can intercede with insurance companies to obtain coverage for uninsured services or items of medical necessity.
6. Primary care providers can evaluate the compounding effects of cumulative social disadvantages—poverty, food insecurity, language barriers, racial or cultural barriers, mental health problems, domestic or community violence—and how these social issues affect the health care of the child. Working with other health professionals or agencies in the family's community, such as social workers, mental health counselors, early parenting projects, and government and private agencies that assist the impoverished, foreign-born, or people with a particular chronic condition, the primary care provider can help reduce the stress on families caring for a child with special needs. Although no primary care provider can resolve all social disadvantages, seemingly small changes (e.g., having a special formula donated to a family by the formula company, finding a dentist willing and able to provide services to the child, or a mental health worker to meet with a depressed parent) can help parents of CYSHCN feel supported by their health care team.

LEVELS OF PRIMARY CARE INTERVENTION FOR CHILDREN WITH CHRONIC OR DISABLING CONDITIONS

Caring for children with chronic conditions is challenging, often complex, and time consuming, but rewarding. It requires a commitment to service beyond routine ambulatory pediatric care and increased knowledge about children, chronic conditions, community resources, health care systems, insurance, interpersonal communication, and organizational skills necessary to provide optimal child and family care.

Levels of intervention for primary care providers of children, along with the knowledge base and skills needed at each level, are outlined in Box 1.6. These levels of intervention are cumulative (i.e., level 3 intervention cannot be attained until the knowledge base and skills of levels 1 and 2 are mastered), and as the levels increase, so do the provider's commitment and the comprehensiveness of care for the child and family. This model of care is important for the new primary care provider and was inspired by work done in family-centered care by Doherty and Baird (1987), the Maternal and Child Health Leadership Competencies Workgroup (2007), and further developed by Drs. Patricia Jackson Allen, Judith Vessey, and Naomi Schapiro, prior editors of *Primary Care of the Child with a Chronic Condition*. The Hierarchic Intervention Framework for Practitioners is the most

| Box 1.6 | Hierarchic Intervention Framework for Practitioners Caring for Children With Chronic Conditions |

LEVEL 1

Ongoing health care and illness management for children without chronic conditions

Knowledge Base Needed

- Routine health care maintenance and common condition management for children and youth without chronic conditions and their families
- Biologic, environmental, economic, racial, cultural, and societal factors affecting health and access to care for children
- Health insurance coverage of children and families receiving care

Skills Needed

- The ability to collect and record subjective and objective data related to child health maintenance and common pediatric conditions
- The ability to elicit relevant data related to family structure, socioeconomic environment, medical history, and current health problems and concerns
- The ability to listen effectively
- The ability to assess and critically evaluate objective and subjective information obtained to formulate a differential diagnosis
- The ability to assess and critically evaluate growth and development of children from birth to young adulthood
- The ability to identify and implement a treatment plan consistent with scientific evidence for children without chronic conditions and families
- The ability to effectively communicate treatment plans to children and families and obtain their assent to the plan
- The ability to monitor children's and families' response to treatment plans and make modifications as needed
- The ability to identify children with more complex needs requiring additional services
- The ability to provide culturally sensitive care to children and families
- The ability to always provide care in an ethical and professional manner

LEVEL 2

Task-oriented care for children with chronic conditions; primary care needs and specialty care needs managed by other professionals

Additional Knowledge Base Needed

- Task-related knowledge

Additional Skill Needed

- Performance of tasks in efficient, correct manner, consistent with evidence-based practice

LEVEL 3

Management of routine health care needs for children with chronic conditions; collaboration or referral for care related to the chronic condition

Additional Knowledge Base Needed

- Pathophysiology of chronic conditions
- Common associated problems of chronic conditions
- Biologic, environmental, economic, racial, cultural, and societal factors affecting health and access to care for children with chronic conditions and their families
- Noncategorical effect of chronic conditions and treatment on child development

- Role functions of interdisciplinary team members and how to access their services
- Community subspecialists, health care and social agencies, school systems, and tertiary care centers for children and youth with special health care needs (CYSHCN)
- Common health services needed by CYSHCN and means of accessing these services

Additional Skills Needed

- The ability to teach/coach children and families regarding health care maintenance needs, management plans, and accessing chronic care services
- The ability to partner with families in their efforts to manage children's chronic condition, growth, and development
- The ability to monitor and critically assess children with chronic conditions, identifying changes requiring consultation or referral to a specialist
- The ability to identify family strengths and incorporate them into the plan of care and make effective referrals for families having difficulty managing children's health care needs or coping with the demands of care
- The ability to communicate physical or psychosocial changes in children or families to the appropriate professional
- The ability to access community and educational services for children with special needs
- The ability to provide culturally sensitive care to children and families experiencing chronic health conditions

LEVEL 4

Comprehensive primary care of children with chronic conditions and their families

Additional Knowledge Base Needed

- In-depth pathophysiology of chronic conditions
- Unique primary care needs of children with chronic conditions
- Effective management of common associated problems found in chronic conditions
- Differential diagnosis for common pediatric illnesses occurring in children with chronic conditions
- Specific stressors for children and families with chronic conditions
- Effects of specific chronic conditions on children's growth, development, and activities of daily living
- Community resources, including educational resources, available to assist children and families and mean of accessing these services
- Components of family-centered care in a medical home
- Insurance coverage for special services, equipment, or treatments for children and families
- Cost and scientific evidence of effectiveness of services provided to families

Additional Skills Needed

- The ability to systematically assess the medical condition and health care needs of children with chronic conditions
- The ability to plan and implement primary health care, including common illness management that is individualized for the child, the family, and the chronic condition

Continued

Box 1.6   Hierarchic Intervention Framework for Practitioners Caring for Children With Chronic Conditions—cont'd

- The ability to identify complications of chronic conditions requiring more complex care and to make appropriate referrals
- The ability to educate/counsel families on the special health care needs of children with chronic conditions, management plans, and accessing of services
- The ability to access services within the health care system and community, including the educational system to meet the child's health care needs
- The ability to work with families to plan short- and long-term care consistent with medical needs and family function
- The ability to assist parents and children in problem solving both medical and family issues
- The ability to help families recognize the needs of individual members and balance these needs
- The ability to assist families in planning services and activities to reduce stress
- The ability to make interdisciplinary referrals communicating children and family needs and expectations
- The ability to provide consistent, available, long-term care in partnership with families

LEVEL 5
Care coordination of families and children with chronic conditions
Additional Knowledge Base Needed
- Service networks involved with children with special health care needs
- Information systems available to collect and communicate health inform
- Cost of resources
- Quality outcomes measures
- Service planning and systems coordination
- Team building and coordination
- Eligibility requirements, referral process, and utilization measures for agencies or services that might benefit families and children

Additional Skills Needed
- The ability to identify outcome measures of quality care for children with chronic conditions
- The ability to develop an alliance with families and children to work in partnership to plan and provide optimum care
- The ability to make a comprehensive needs assessment for children and families
- The ability to plan and initiate appropriate and successful referrals for services within the health care system and community

- The ability to work effectively in teams with other interdisciplinary professionals
- The ability to analyze the cost/benefit ratio for services provided
- The ability to coordinate services and personnel working with the families and children
- The ability to use information systems to collect and evaluate outcome data and communicate health information
- The ability to measure and monitor progress in attaining identified goals in children and families
- The ability to make changes in management and service plans as necessary
- The ability to communicate findings from multiple interdisciplinary sources to families, children, and others involved in addressing the needs of children and families
- The willingness to function as the child and family advocate

LEVEL 6
Leadership in systems advocacy for children with chronic conditions and their families
Additional Knowledge Base Needed
- Institutional structures governing the care of children
- Health care systems and health economics
- Current rules, regulations, and laws at the institutional, local, state, and national levels regarding health care for children and families
- Legislative and regulatory process at the local, state, and national levels
- Community, state, and national policymakers
- Research on evidence-based practice and quality outcome indicators for children with chronic conditions and their families

Additional Skills Needed
- The ability to identify and articulate important children's health issues that are measurable and achievable
- The ability to communicate a vision of quality comprehensive, family-centered services for children with special health care needs and their families
- The ability to influence decision making with available data
- The ability to build coalitions of individuals/professionals around children's health issues
- The ability to negotiate, compromise, and formulate alternative proposals
- The ability to work within the political and legislative systems and with politicians

up to date, and the current author of this chapter believes it continues to be important information for the novice pediatric provider caring for children with chronic conditions.

SYSTEM LEVELS OF CARE FOR CHILDREN WITH CHRONIC CONDITIONS: MICROSYSTEMS, MESOSYSTEMS, AND MACROSYSTEMS

Comprehensive, coordinated systems of care for CYSHCN and their families require a holistic assessment.

The Model for Effective Chronic Illness Care, developed with support of the Robert Wood Johnson Foundation, addresses the need to move beyond the episodic provision of acute and chronic care by designing comprehensive systems for chronic condition care (Wagner, 1998) (Fig. 1.12). Productive interactions between informed, empowered families and prepared proactive practice teams of health care providers and a consistent, engaged medical home provider will improve the child's functional and clinical outcomes.

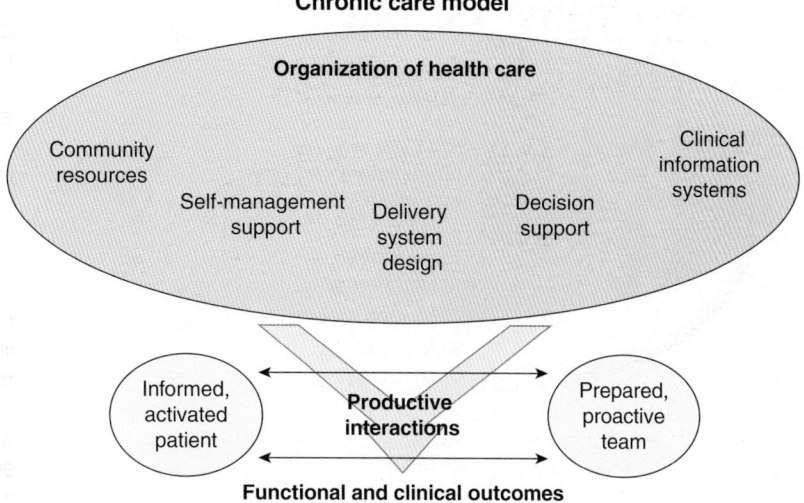

Fig. 1.12 Chronic care model. (From Wagner E. H. [1998]. Chronic disease management: What will it take to improve care for chronic illness? *Effective Clinical Practice, 1,* 2–4.)

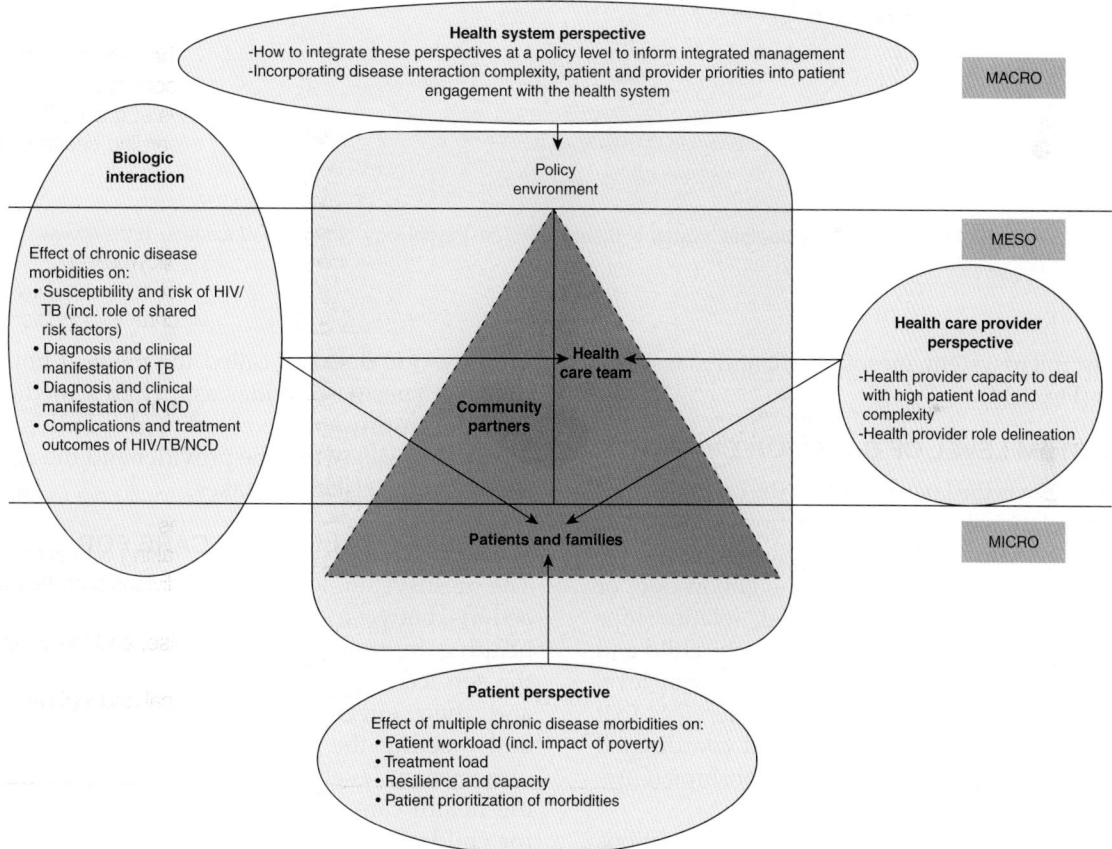

Fig. 1.13 Conceptual modification of the World Health Organization's Innovative Care for Chronic Conditions Framework represented within shaded square, and modification represented by arrows and text bubbles. *HIV,* Human immunodeficiency virus; *NCD,* noncommunicable disease; *TB,* tuberculosis.

The World Health Organization (WHO) further developed this model as the basis of the WHO Innovative Care for Chronic Conditions (ICCC) Framework (Fig. 1.13). The ICCC framework recognizes that optimal care for a child with a chronic health condition requires partnerships between families and health care providers, community agencies that provide resources needed for comprehensive care, and the broader system of health care organizations, funding sources, and government policies.

Providing comprehensive and coordinated systems of care, the care must be provided and evaluated at

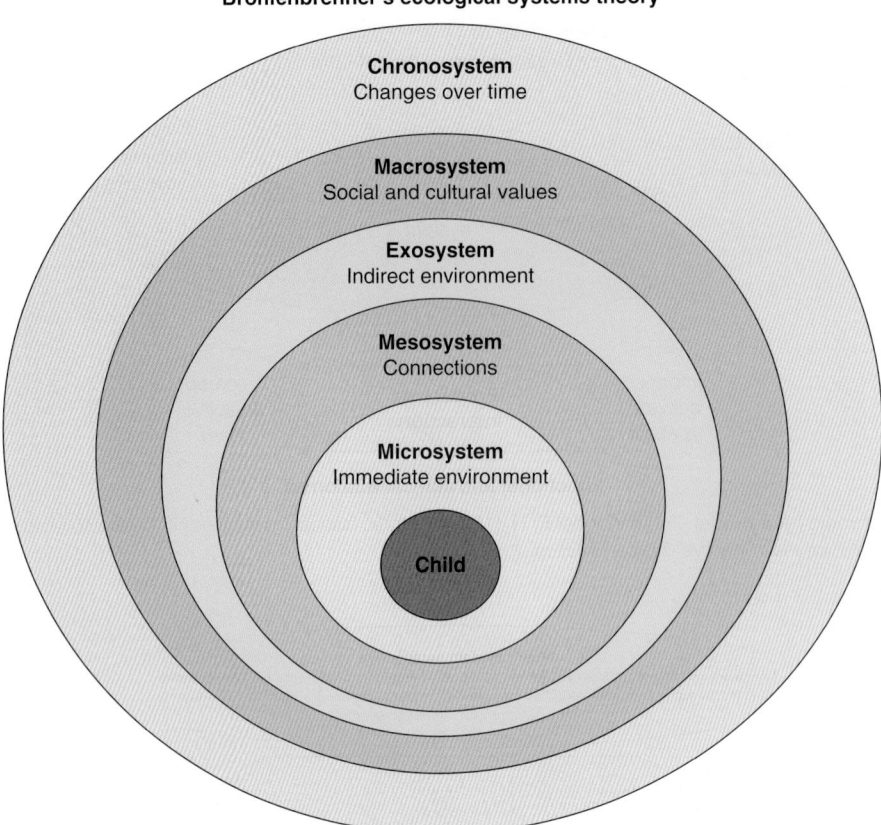

Fig. 1.14 Bronfenbrenner's ecological systems theory. (© The Psychology Notes Headquarters, https://www. PsychologyNotesHQ.com.)

three levels: microsystem, mesosystem, and macrosystem levels (Fig. 1.14).

MICROSYSTEM LEVEL OF CARE FOR CYSHCN

The microsystem is the layer closest to the child, encompassing the relationships and interactions a child has with the immediate surroundings. Structures in the microsystem include family, school, neighborhood, or child care environments. At this level, relationships impact in two directions: both away from the child and toward the child. The goal of the microsystem level of care is for families to receive needed services that are accessible, affordable, seamless, and coordinated through interagency collaborative relationships (Guy-Evans, 2020; Perrin et al., 2007).

Microsystem care refers to the direct interactions among children, families, and health care providers within complex care delivery systems and the coordination of those services. Several circumstances influence the development of models and financing mechanisms for care coordination for families of CYSHCN within primary care settings. Some of the factors discussed in this chapter are the historic advocacy of federal and state maternal and child health services under Title V and Healthy People 2030, family access to a myriad of fragmented services, and the ongoing, ever-changing health care system and a highly recognized model of primary care delivery called the medical home. Identifying a specific provider as a child's medical home provider improves care coordination, builds trust and relationships between the provider and the family, and decreases the risk of mistakes.

MESOSYSTEM LEVEL OF CARE FOR CYSHCN

The mesosystem level of care encompasses the interactions between the child's microsystems and the health care organizations, community organizations, the services provided, information systems in place, and their effectiveness in delivering quality care and meeting the needs of populations served. The mesosystem level looks at the systems of care affecting health care delivery to children. Systems of care for children with chronic conditions and their families will be most successful when they move from the provider-focused, deficit-based, crisis-oriented approaches to family-focused, strengths-based, and prevention-oriented approaches.

The values and principles of the medical home model specify that care is accessible, continuous, comprehensive, family centered, coordinated, compassionate, and culturally effective. The medical home has become the main care model proposed for CYSHCN and their families in many states through Title V programs and nationally in various demonstration projects.

MACROSYSTEM LEVEL OF CARE FOR CYSHCN

The macrosystem level includes policies and financing of health care systems, insurance programs, eligibility requirements, government (federal, state, and local) agencies, and legal protections for families and children with chronic health conditions (Guy-Evans, 2020; Perrin et al., 2007). This level focuses on how cultural elements such as socioeconomic status, wealth, poverty, and ethnicity affect a child's development. Entities at this level globally would include the WHO and United Nations; at the national level entities would include but are not limited to the MCHB, Social Security Administration, and Medicaid; state-level entities include CHIP, public schools, and social services. All three levels must function in partnership for care to be comprehensive, coordinated, and accessible to families. Developing services for CYSHCN at the macrosystem level requires the following:

1. Standardized eligibility protocols
2. Legal and accounting mechanisms for flexible funding streams
3. Development of cost-sharing mechanisms to allocate costs fairly among all payers, including families
4. Measures to eliminate duplication of effort based on resource allocation
5. A flexible point of entry such that a family need only apply once to access all needed services

Achieving these macrosystem-level services for CYSHCN requires major changes in legislation, interagency agreements, funding sources, and political commitment to health services for all people in need (Guy-Evans, 2020; Perrin et al., 2007). Health care professionals must be knowledgeable regarding the importance of restrictions created by the macrosystem level of policies, regulations, and laws and become involved at the local, state, and national levels to educate those in positions of power on needed changes to improve care for CYSHCN.

SUMMARY

Caring for CYSHCN and their families requires a holistic approach, including a plethora of resources from within and outside the provider's organization. Care providers in community agencies, clinics, hospitals, or educational systems must respect child and family autonomy through practice models of family-directed and family-centered care. Providers must communicate with each other and the families for joint problem solving and resource procurement. Providers must work with families in a culturally and linguistically respectful way to identify gaps in service delivery and advocate for system change at the microsystem, mesosystem, and macrosystem levels. Leadership, collaboration, and advocacy are essential if quality, cost-effective, community-based systems of care for families of CYSHCN are to be realized. Pediatric nurse practitioners are pivotal to making dramatic and effective changes for individuals and families and state and federal policy.

RESOURCES

Table 1.3   Resources for Pediatric Health Care Providers and Families

PROGRAM	WEBSITE	DESCRIPTION
2-1-1	211.org, then access by Zip code or city	Access to information on school lunch programs, summer food programs, and other government-sponsored programs (e.g., SNAP, WIC, soup kitchens, community gardens)
American Academy of Pediatrics Medical Home	https://www.aap.org/en/practice-management/medical-home	
Association of National & Child Health Programs	http://archived.amchp.org/modules/cyshcn-2019/story_html5.html	An overview of Title V CYSHCN programs. *This author highly recommends reviewing the history to better understand where we started and where we are today.*
Center for Parent Information & Resources	https://www.parentcenterhub.org/	Supporting the parent centers who serve families of children with disabilities
Disaster Preparedness for Children and Youth with Special Health Care Needs	https://www.aap.org/en/patient-care/disasters-and-children/professional-resources-for-disaster-preparedness/preparedness-for-children-and-youth-with-special-health-care-needs/	
Food Insecurity	https://frac.org/wp-content/uploads/FRAC_AAP_Toolkit_2021_032122.pdf	Screen and intervene toolkit for providers to address food insecurity
HealthFinder	www.healthfinder.gov	A service of the US Department of Health and Human Services

Continued

Table 1.3	Resources for Pediatric Health Care Providers and Families—cont'd	
PROGRAM	**WEBSITE**	**DESCRIPTION**
Healthy Food Bank Hub	Healthyfoodbankhub.feedingamerica.org	Includes a food bank locator and other tools and resources for food-insecure households
KidsHealth	https://kidshealth.org/	Site provides child-focused health information
My Plate	http://www.choosemyplate.gove/budget/downloads/MeetingYourMyPlateGoalsOnABudget.pdf	
Maternal & Child Health Timeline	https://mchb.hrsa.gov/about/timeline/index.asp	Excellent resource for providers to understand the history of maternal and child health in the United States
National Standard Online Toolkit	https://www.nashp.org/toolkit-national-standards-for-children-and-youth-with-special-health-care-needs/	
National Institute for Children's Health Quality	https://www.nichq.org/about	A mission-driven nonprofit committed to creating and promoting new approaches for lasting systems change to improve children's health

CYSHCN, Children and youth with special health care needs; *SNAP,* Supplemental Nutrition Assistance Program; *WIC,* Special Supplemental Nutrition Program for Women, Infants, and Children.

REFERENCES

Agrawal, R., Shah, P., Zebracki, K., Sanabria, K., Kohrman, C., & Kohrman, A. F. (2012). Barriers to care for children and youth with special health care needs: perceptions of Illinois pediatricians. *Clinical Pediatrics, 51*(1), 39–45. https://doi.org/10.1177/0009922811417288.

American Academy of Pediatric Dentistry. (2021). Overview. Retrieved September 29, 2022, from https://www.aapd.org/research/oral-health-policies–recommendations/management-of-dental-patients-with-special-health-care-needs/.

American Academy of Pediatrics. (8/27/2021). *The impact of the pandemic on households with CYSHCN.* Retrieved September 13, 2022. https://www.aap.org/en/patient-care/family-snapshot-during-the-covid-19-pandemic/the-impact-of-the-pandemic-on-households-with-cyshcn/.

American Academy of Pediatrics. (n.d.). What is medical home? Retrieved September 13, 2022, from https://www.aap.org/en/practice-management/medical-home/medical-home-overview/what-is-medical-home/.

American Academy of Pediatrics Committee on Child Health Financing. (n.d.). Scope of health care benefits for children from birth through age 26. Retrieved September 28, 2022, from https://publications.aap.org/pediatrics/article/129/1/185/31576/Scope-of-Health-Care-Benefits-for-Children-From.

Anderson, N. W., & Zimmerman, F. J. (2021). Trends in health equity among children in the United States, 1997–2018. *Maternal and Child Health Journal, 25,* 1939–1959. doi:10.1007/s10995-021-03253-w.

Association of Maternal & Child Health Programs (n.d.). Website. https://amchp.org/.

Barclay L. February 4). Limited time for pediatric visits compromises care: A newsmaker interview with Peter Holbrook, MD. *Medscape: Medical News* [online]. 2003. Available at www.medscape.com/viewarticle/448898. Retrieved March 4, 2003.

Berry, J. G., Perrin, J. M., Hoover, C., Rodean, J., Agrawal, R. K., & Kuhlthau, K. A. (2021). Health care insurance adequacy for children and youth with special health care needs. *Pediatrics, 148*(4). doi:10.1542/peds.2020-039891.

Bethell, C. D., Blumberg, S. J., Stein, R. E., Strickland, B., Robertson, J., & Newacheck, P. W. (2015). Taking stock of the CSHCN screener: a review of common questions and current reflections. *Academic pediatrics, 15*(2), 165–176. https://doi.org/10.1016/j.acap.2014.10.003.

Bethell, C. D., Read, D., Blumberg, S. J., & Newacheck, P. W. (2008). What is the prevalence of children with special health care needs? Toward an understanding of variations in findings and methods across three national surveys. *Maternal and Child Health Journal, 12*(1), 1–14. https://doi.org/10.1007/s10995-007-0220-5.

Bethell, C. D., Read, D., Stein, R. E. K., Blumberg, S. J., Wells, N., & Newacheck, P. W. (2002). Identifying children with special health care needs: Development and evaluation of a short screening instrument. *Ambulatory Pediatrics, 2*(1), 38–48. doi:10.1367/1539-4409(2002)002<0038:icwshc>2.0.co;2.

Bramlett, M. D., Blumberg, S. J., Ormson, A. E., George, J. M., Williams, K. L., Frasier, A. M., Skalland, B. J., Santos, K. B., Vsetecka, D. M., Morrison, H. M., Pedlow, S., & Wang, F. (2014). Design and operation of the National Survey of Children with Special Health Care Needs, 2009-2010. *Vital and Health Statistics.* Ser. 1, Programs and collection procedures, (57), 1–271.

Braveman, P., Arkin, E., Orleans, T., Proctor, D., Acker, J., & Plough, A. (2018). What is health equity? *Behavioral Science & Policy, 4*(1), 1–14. doi:10.1353/bsp.2018.0000.

Brown, T. W., McLellan, S. E., Scott, J. A., & Mann, M. Y. (2022). Introducing the blueprint for change: A national framework for a system of services for children and youth with special health care needs. *Pediatrics, 149*(Supplement 7). doi:10.1542/peds.2021-056150b.

Bunch L., Bandekar A. (2021). Changes in children's health coverage varied by poverty status from 2018–2020. Available at https://www.census.gov/library/stories/2021/09/uninsured-rates-for-children-in-poverty-increased-2018-2020.html. Retrieved September 13, 2022.

Burns, K. (2022). *Expansions to child tax credit contributed to 46% decline in child poverty since 2020.* Census.gov. https://www.census.gov/library/stories/2022/09/record-drop-in-child-poverty.html.

Centers for Disease Control and Prevention. (2021, June 16). *Health-related quality of life (HRQOL).* Retrieved September 28, 2022, from https://www.cdc.gov/hrqol/index.htm.

Centers for Disease Control and Prevention, National Center for Health Statistics. (2022, October 18). Index. Retrieved September 28, 2022, from https://www.cdc.gov/nchs/index.htm.

Child Stats. (n.d.). Welcome to America's children: Key national indicators of well-being. ChildStats.gov Forum on Child and Family Statistics. Retrieved July 2, 2022, from https://www.childstats.gov/.

Children's Defense Fund. (2020). Evaluating 2019 US census child poverty data in the wake of covid-19 fact sheet. Available at https://www.childrensdefense.org/wp-content/uploads/2020/09/Evaluating-2019-US-Census-Child-Poverty-Data-in-the-Wake-of-COVID-19.pdf. Retrieved August 26, 2020.

Children's Defense Fund. (2021). *The state of America's children, 2021*. Retrieved August 28, 2022, from https://www.childrensdefense.org/wp-content/uploads/2021/04/The-State-of-Americas-Children-2021.pdf.

Cohen, S. S., Toly, V. B., Lerret, S. M., & Sawin, K. J. (2022). The impact of covid-19 on systems of care for children and youth with special health care needs. *Journal of Pediatric Health Care.* doi:10.1016/j.pedhc.2022.09.009. Epub ahead of print. PMCID: PMC9492508.

Coleman, C. L., Morrison, M., Perkins, S. K., Brosco, J. P., & Schor, E. L. (2022). Quality of life and well-being for children and youth with special health care needs and their families: A vision for the future. *Pediatrics, 149*(Supplement 7). doi:10.1542/peds.2021-056150g.

Committee on Child Health Financing (2006). (2006). Scope of health care benefits from birth through age 21. *Pediatrics, 117*(3), 979–982.

Cross, T., Bazron, B., Dennis, K., & Issaces, M. (1989). *Towards a culturally competent system of care: A monograph on effective services for minority children who are severely emotionally disturbed. (Vol. I).* Washington, DC: Georgetown University Child Development Center.

Doherty, W., & Baird, M. A. (1987). *Family-centered medical care: A clinical casework.* Guilford Press.

Dunn, C. G., Kenney, E., Fleischhacker, S. E., & Bleich, S. N. (2020). Feeding low-income children during the covid-19 pandemic. *New England Journal of Medicine, 382*(18). doi:10.1056/nejmp2005638.

Federal Interagency Forum on Child and Family Statistics. (2021). *America's children: Key national indicators of well-being, 2021.* Washington, DC: US Government Printing Office.

Food and Nutrition Service, US Department of Agriculture. (n.d.). SNAP data tables. Retrieved August 2, 2022, from https://www.fns.usda.gov/pd/supplemental-nutrition-assistance-program-snap.

Ghandour, R. M., Hirai, A. H., & Kenney, M. K. (2022). Children and youth with special health care needs: A profile. *Pediatrics, 149*(s7), e2021056150D.

Gitterman, B., Chilton, L., Cotton, W., Duffee, J., Flanagan, P., Keane, V., Krugman, S., Kuo, A., Linton, J., McKelvey, C., Paz-Soldan, G., Daniels, S., Abrams, S., Corkins, M., de Ferranti, S., Golden, N., Magge, S., & Schwarzenberg, S. (2015). Promoting food security for all children. *Pediatric Clinical Practice Guidelines & Policies, 136*(5), 1431–1438. https://doi.org/10.1542/peds.2015-3301.

Guy-Evans, O. (2020). Bronfenbrenner's ecological systems theory. *Simply Psychology.* www.simplypsychology.org/Bronfenbrenner.html.

Hager, E. R., Quigg, A. M., Black, M. M., Coleman, S. M., Heeren, T., Rose-Jacobs, R., Cook, J. T., Ettinger de Cuba, S. A., Casey, P. H., Chilton, M., Cutts, D. B., Meyers, A. F., & Frank, D. A. (2010). Development and validity of a 2-item screen to identify families at risk for food insecurity. *Pediatrics, 126*(1), e26–e32. https://doi.org/10.1542/peds.2009-3146.

Hales, L., & Coleman-Jensen, A. (2022). *Food insecurity for households with children rose in 2020, disrupting decade-long decline.* US Department of Agriculture. Retrieved August 13, 2022, from https://www.ers.usda.gov/amber-waves/2022/february/food-insecurity-for-households-with-children-rose-in-2020-disrupting-decade-long-decline/.

Houtrow, A., Martin, A. J., Harris, D., Cejas, D., Hutson, R., Mazloomdoost, Y., & Agrawal, R. (2022). Health equity for children and youth with special health care needs: A vision for the future. *Pediatrics, 149*(Supplement 7), e2021056150F. doi:10.1542/peds.2021-056150F.

Kogan, M. (2022). *National survey of children's health (NSCH).* Maternal and Child Health Bureau. Retrieved September 29, 2022, from https://mchb.hrsa.gov/data-research/national-survey-childrens-health.

Kuo, D. Z., Rodgers, R. C., Beers, N. S., McLellan, S. E., & Nguyen, T. K. (2022). Access to services for children and youth with special health care needs and their families: Concepts and considerations for an integrated systems redesign. *Pediatrics, 149*(Supplement 7). doi:10.1542/peds.2021-056150h.

Lebrun-Harris, L. A., Canto, M. T., Vodicka, P., Mann, M. Y., & Kinsman, S. B. (2021). Oral health among children and youth with special health care needs. *Pediatrics, 148*(2). doi:10.1542/peds.2020-025700.

Lichstein, J. C., Ghandour, R. M., & Mann, M. Y. (2018). Access to the medical home among children with and without special health care needs. *Pediatrics, 142*(6). doi:10.1542/peds.2018-1795.

McLellan, S. E., Mann, M. Y., Scott, J. A., & Brown, T. W. (2022). A blueprint for change: Guiding principles for a system of services for children and youth with special health care needs and their families. *Pediatrics, 149*(Supplement 7). doi:10.1542/peds.2021-056150c.

Okoniewski, W., Sundaram, M., Chaves-Gnecco, D., McAnany, K., Cowden, J. D., & Ragavan, M. (2022). Culturally sensitive interventions in pediatric primary care settings: A systematic review. *Pediatrics, 149*(2). doi:10.1542/peds.2021-052162.

Perrin J. M., Bloom S. R., & Gortmaker S. L. (2007). The increase of childhood chronic conditions in the United States. *The Journal of the American Medical Association, 297*(24), 2755-2759.

Pilapil, M., Coletti, D. J., Rabey, C., & DeLaet, D. (2017). Caring for the caregiver: Supporting families of youth with special health care needs. *Current Problems in Pediatric and Adolescent Health Care, 47*(8), 190–199. doi:10.1016/j.cppeds.2017.07.003.

Price, J., Brandt, M. L., Hudak, M. L., Berman, S. K., Carlson, K. M., Giardino, A. P., Hammer, L., Heggen, K., Pearlman, S. A., & Sood, B. G. (2020). Principles of financing the medical home for children. *Pediatrics, 145*(1). doi:10.1542/peds.2019-3451.

Schickedanz, A., & Halfon, N. (2020). Evolving roles for health care in supporting healthy child development. *Future Child, 30*(2), 143–164. PMID: 33875912; PMCID: PMC8053141.

Schiff, J., Manning, L., VanLandeghem, K., Langer, C. S., Schutze, M., & Comeau, M. (2022). Financing care for CYSHCN in the next decade: Reducing burden, advancing equity, and transforming systems. *Pediatrics, 149*(Supplement 7). doi:10.1542/peds.2021-056150i.

Simpser, E., Hudak, M. L., Okun, A. L., Langley, J., Lin, E., Maynard, R., McNeal, D., Sajous, C., & Thornburg, J. B. (2017). Financing of pediatric home health care. *Pediatrics, 139*(3). doi:10.1542/peds.2016-4202.

Stefko, J. M., Stolfi, A., & Pascoe, J. M. (2022). Screening for children's chronic health conditions and their strengths and difficulties in primary care. *Journal of Developmental & Behavioral Pediatrics, 43*(1), e1–e8. doi:10.1097/DBP.0000000000000969.

Stein, R. E., & Silver, E. J. (1999). Operationalizing a conceptually based noncategorical definition: A first look at US children with chronic conditions. *Archives of Pediatric and Adolescent Medicine, 153*, 68–74.

Thorn, B., Kline, N., Tadler, C., Wilcox-Cook, E., Michaels, J., & Tran, V. (2018). *WIC participant and program characteristics 2016.* US Department of Agriculture, Food and Nutrition Service.

Ullmann, H., Madans, J., & Weeks, J. (2022). Children living in households that experienced food insecurity: United States, 2019-2020. *NCHS Data Brief, 432.* doi:10.15620/cdc:113966.

US Census Bureau (2021). About the foreign-born population. Retrieved August 5, 2022, from www.census.gov/topics/population/foreign-born/about.html.

US Census Bureau (2021). Uninsured rate of US children in 2021. Retrieved August 5, 2022, from https://www.census.gov/library/stories/2022/09/uninsured-rate-of-children-declines.html.

US Census Bureau. (2022). 2020 census results. Retrieved July 2, 2022, from https://www.census.gov/2020results.

US Census Bureau. (2022). Data. Retrieved September 13, 2022, from https://www.census.gov/data/.

US Department of Agriculture. (n.d.). Data. Retrieved August 23, 2022, from https://www.usda.gov/topics/data.

US Department of Agriculture. (n.d.). Definitions of food security. Retrieved August 23, 2022, from https://www.ers.usda.gov/topics/food-nutrition-assistance/food-security-in-the-u-s/definitions-of-food-security/#:~:text=Food%20insecurity%E2%80%94the%20condition%20assessed,may%20result%20from%20food%20insecurity.

US Department of Health and Human Services. (2022). Healthy people 2030 data-driven national objectives to improve health and well-being over the next decade. Retrieved September 13, 2022. https://health.gov/healthypeople.

van Dyck, P. C., McPherson, M., Strickland, B. B., Nesseler, K., Blumberg, S. J., Cynamon, M. L., & Newacheck, P. W. (2002). The national survey of children with special health care needs. *Ambulatory Pediatrics: The Official Journal of the Ambulatory Pediatric Association*, 2(1), 29–37. https://doi.org/10.1367/1539-4409(2002)002<0029:tnsocw>2.0.co;2.

Wagner, E. H. (1998). Chronic disease management: What will it take to improve care for chronic illness? *Effective Clinical Practice, 1*, 2–4.

Warren, M. D., McLellan, S. E., Mann, M. Y., Scott, J. A., & Brown, T. W. (2022). Progress, persistence, and hope: Building a system of services for CYSHCN and their families. *Pediatrics, 149*(Supplement 7). doi:10.1542/peds.2021-056150e.

Chronic Conditions and Child Development

Amee Moreno, Jessica Peck

Childhood development is influenced by internal and external factors, including physiologic state, psychological competence, social support systems, and external environment. Children with chronic medical conditions have developmental and behavioral risk factors that may impact the normal patterns of mastering developmental tasks (Lipkin & Macias, 2020). Children have more commonalities regarding their development than differences; therefore this chapter focuses on the common patterns of development of children with chronic conditions globally rather than disease-specific patterns (Villagomez et al., 2019).

Children with chronic conditions may experience delays in cognition, communication, motor, adaptive, and social skills compared with unaffected children. Differences range in severity from mild to global delays and intermittent to permanent. The presence of a chronic condition does not necessarily equate to the presence of a developmental delay or permanent disability. Many children with chronic conditions attain developmental milestones in a typical pattern without delays. Children with chronic conditions may experience developmental delays in a single domain (e.g., motor difficulty in a child with juvenile rheumatoid arthritis) or globally, affecting all developmental domains (e.g., those seen in a child with Down syndrome). Some children experience a normal sequence of milestones but in a delayed manner compared to their peers of the same chronologic age, such as children with a partially corrected congenital heart defect. Discrepancies in development across domains result from unevenly developed or damaged neurologic processes causing disruptions in selected developmental sequences (e.g., a child with autism). The greater the severity of a condition, the more likely the child will experience global delays, with some domains being more affected than others.

Development is continuous, and the maturation of structures and functions is interdependent. For example, an integrated nervous system is modeled through repeated use, such as the development of normal 20/20 vision or amblyopia in the absence of repeated use. Numerous physiologic and psychological variables can contribute to the occurrence and severity of maturational alterations associated with chronic conditions. For example, infants and mothers may have difficulty forming long-term emotional bonds if they are physically, cognitively (e.g., brain injury), or emotionally (e.g., postpartum depression) separated from each other. A child's culture also influences the attainment of developmental skills (Villagomez et al., 2019). For example, the language development of a school-age child is impacted by the amount of direct speech the child receives early in life, which is influenced by the cultural norms for parenting and childhood socialization (Villagomez et al., 2019).

Developmental deviations in a child with a chronic condition are not directly related to a specific diagnosis. Rather, the type, intensity, and duration of developmental changes evolve from the reciprocal interaction of condition-specific characteristics and child-specific attributes. These are more fully described in the next section. Because a child is still maturing, many potential and actual problems may be overcome if condition management programs proactively address these concerns. Specifically, clinical management requires capitalizing on the child's strengths to optimize development. Improved developmental and clinical outcomes are realized by the child when families and providers engage in active partnerships when designing and implementing treatment regimens.

CHARACTERISTICS OF THE CONDITION

The pathophysiology, severity, persistence, visibility, and prognosis of the condition and any iatrogenic insults that may have occurred influence a child's developmental outcome.

PATHOPHYSIOLOGY, SEVERITY, AND PERSISTENCE

The pathophysiologic mechanisms of a condition (e.g., chronic hypoxemia, aberrant serum glucose levels, malabsorption) and its related severity, persistence, and prognosis can affect development. The correlation between physiologic severity/persistence and developmental attainment is neither causal nor highly robust and moderated by a nexus of individual traits, available social support, and symptom management quality. Children in the least and most disabled groups are at greater risk than those at intermediate severity.

Conditions associated with multisystem involvement and neurologic impairment place children at greater global developmental risk because their condition physically, mentally, or psychologically interferes with their ability to complete age-appropriate developmental tasks. The interaction of pathophysiologic changes, availability for learning, and contact with the environment further compromise developmental attainment.

The pathophysiologic changes that children with mild conditions lack sufficient severity or are ameliorated by treatment, so they readily adapt to them, and thus the potential for developmental insult is minimized. When conditions are marked by occasional exacerbations, have limited visibility, or appear to cause only marginal problems, they may be ignored or denied by children and their families (Joachim & Acorn, 2000; Carroll et al., 2020). This denial is often motivated by an effort to normalize the child's condition; yet when mild conditions are not recognized by others but do affect a child's performance, the child may be held to unrealistic expectations, such as is frequently seen in children with attention-deficit/hyperactivity disorder. Unfortunately when denial interferes with symptom recognition, management regimens, and appropriate behavioral expectations, children may have poorer developmental outcomes.

Developmental limitations may be secondarily imposed by the condition's pathophysiology and management. Conditions that are painful, embarrassing, or energy depleting place a child at greater risk for developmental delay. Tremendous exertion may be necessary to cope with intensive treatment protocols or the time-consuming activities of daily life. For example, children with cystic fibrosis may spend more than 3 hours each day receiving pulmonary care. Additional energy is also required in adjusting to new or exacerbated symptoms (e.g., persistent pain, malaise, fatigue). The activities of children who depend on technology are limited by physical constraints and the time needed to care for equipment such as ventilators and infusion pumps. Large expenditures of time and energy may limit children's opportunities to engage in recreational activities or predispose them to significant fatigue because participation requires too much effort. Moreover, parent-child interactions and other social activities are restricted in families where caregiving needs become the primary focus of daily living.

VISIBILITY

The visibility of a chronic condition may place the child at risk for stigmatization and can trigger self-consciousness (Carroll et al., 2020; Immelt, 2006). Stigmatization is an act or process in which an individual is negatively labeled or characterized because of possessing certain attributes or behaviors. Visible conditions (e.g., Down syndrome, myelodysplasia) place a child at risk for immediate stigmatization, and individuals may discredit the child's capabilities. For invisible conditions, such as inflammatory bowel disease, children may try to hide their condition and pass as normal,

creating stress for fear of discovery. Passing may also require ignoring aspects of condition management, such as adolescents with diabetes or phenylketonuria who ignore dietary recommendations, thus impairing their health status. Disclosing one's condition may promote stigmatization, as it frequently occurs in children with epilepsy (Sengül & Kurudirek, 2022). Children with deteriorating conditions may fear accidental disclosure.

PROGNOSIS

The natural course of a chronic condition influences developmental progression. Children with conditions associated with ongoing pathophysiologic deterioration may initially achieve milestones but then lose them as the condition worsens.

This is commonly noted when there is a progressive degeneration of the neurologic system (e.g., muscular dystrophy), but this is also a problem with any seriously compromised physiologic state. Even in nonprogressive conditions, developmental lags become noticeable as children mature and developmental expectations are higher. The uncertainty associated with a condition's trajectory that parents and children face is a major stressor and may influence a child's developmental outcomes (Szulczewski et al., 2017). Children thought to have limited or unknown outcomes may be deprived of a past-present-future perspective of learning about one's cultural heritage or forming goals and personal aspirations, which plays an instrumental role in shaping cognitive processes. If individuals do not believe that the information should be transmitted to the child or would upset the child, this lack of information limits children's ability to learn. Children may also be held to differing behavioral expectations than their peers by well-intentioned adults; however, this can contribute to anxiety in the child and strained relationships with siblings and peers. Differing expectations can create anxiety in the child and resentment in siblings and peers.

Predicting prognoses for children with chronic illness is complex due to the rapid advances in medicine, contributing to a rise in the prevalence and increased survival of children with chronic illness (Yu et al., 2021). The life expectancies for children with cerebral palsy, cystic fibrosis, organ transplantation, cancer, human immunodeficiency virus, and numerous other conditions continue to increase dramatically. Delivering a poor medical prognosis to the family without a broader perspective of the child's future may result in poorer psychological outcomes.

IATROGENIC INSULTS

Selected treatment protocols impose their risks. Developmental iatrogeny refers to health care interventions that hinder children from progressing through their normal developmental milestones. Therapeutic interventions commonly associated with developmental iatrogeny are the associations between aminoglyco- sides and hearing loss, cancer therapies, transplantation and late effects, and oxygen/steroid administration and retinopathy of prematurity (Erdmann et al., 2021; Farzal et al., 2016; Smolkin et al., 2008; Yim et al., 2018). Numerous other interventions, however, either directly or indirectly influence development. Many classes of drugs (e.g., anticonvulsants, steroids) have been shown to alter cognition, perceptual abilities, or behavior and make children less available for learning (Moavero et al., 2017).

CHARACTERISTICS OF THE CHILD

The developmental tasks associated with each age group present new challenges for children with chronic conditions. The age at the onset of the chronic condition affects adaptation and progression from one developmental stage to the next. Achieving a developmental skill that has never been acquired differs from regaining a previously learned and lost skill. Children with congenital conditions tend to have greater developmental plasticity and adaptive mechanisms and more readily acclimate to limitations imposed by their underlying disorder. Children with chronic conditions have higher rates of behavioral difficulties, with younger children most at risk.

Developmental milestones were updated by the American Academy of Pediatrics (AAP) and the Centers for Disease Control and Prevention in 2022, adding milestones to the 15- and 30-month screenings and transferring one-third of the expected developmental tasks to different ages, with most transferred to older age groups (Zubler et al., 2022). These changes were made to improve the early identification of autism and developmental delays in children (Zubler et al., 2022).

INFANCY

The major developmental tasks of infancy center around establishing trust and learning about the environment through sensorimotor exploration (Berk, 2006). Infants with congenital chronic conditions may experience difficulty accomplishing these expected developmental tasks. Caregivers mourning the loss of their idea of a perfect child may have decreased energy levels to care for a medically complex and demanding infant. If parents find little gratification in trying to meet their child's basic needs despite their best efforts, they may begin to view their child as vulnerable because of the extensive care required, and this attitude can affect future development. A poor prognosis may lead some parents to emotionally detach from their infants to prevent further emotional hurt. Infants subjected to prolonged or frequent hospitalizations may encounter repeated separations, the unpredictability associated with numerous caregivers, unreliable or inadequate care, and painful experiences. The culmination of these factors can inhibit infant attachment and the subsequent development of a trusting relationship. For infants whose conditions are physically limiting or painful, exploration and interaction with their environment are limited, further curtailing development.

TODDLERHOOD

The major developmental tasks of toddlerhood include acquiring a sense of autonomy, developing self-control, and forming symbolic representation through language acquisition (Berk, 2006). Developmental tasks of independence such as toileting, feeding, and development of friend groups may be discouraged by caregivers if the child's chronic condition requires careful limit setting and control of activities of daily living. For example, toddlers who are immunosuppressed may need social contact and play environment limitations. Children with bleeding disorders may need modified play environments or restrictions on exploring their environment. Mandatory prolonged dependency can make separation difficult and contribute to a fragile self-image.

Previously mastered development tasks may be lost in toddlers experiencing acute exacerbations of disease—with or without hospitalization. This behavioral regression is a means of social and emotional adaptation whereby children revert to earlier stages when they do not have the necessary psychic energy to maintain functioning at developmental levels already achieved (Freud, 1966). Behavioral regression is exacerbated by psychic and physiologic stress associated with fear, separation, pain, and other symptomatology. Depending on the severity and duration of a condition's exacerbation and the child's resilience and support, behavioral regression may deteriorate into behavioral disorders. Although regression can happen at any point along the developmental continuum, it is most commonly noted in this age group.

PRESCHOOL CHILDREN

The primary developmental task for preschoolers is acquiring a sense of initiative to successfully meet the challenges of their ever-expanding world (Berk, 2006). Preschoolers with chronic conditions may not have the physical energy or motivation to design and perform activities necessary to accomplish this task; therefore opportunities for learning about the environment, developing social relationships, and cultivating self-confidence and a sense of purpose are diminished. They may have difficulty forming a healthy self-concept, body image, and sexual identity, particularly if most of their body awareness is associated with disability and discomfort. The egocentricity and naive reasoning processes of preschoolers influence their understanding and interpretation of their condition. Although their understanding of illness and its relationship to morality is less enmeshed than previously thought, preschoolers may think that their thoughts or behaviors cause their symptoms. Regardless, developing self-esteem and motivation to undertake new tasks may be compromised by their condition.

SCHOOL-AGE CHILDREN

The developmental tasks for school-age children are increasing independence and mastery over their environment (Berk, 2006). Such activities contribute to gaining social skills, developing a sense of accomplishment, learning to cope effectively with stress, and acquiring the skills that result in self-sufficiency. Functional limitations in self-care, communication, mobility, stamina, and learning hinder children with chronic conditions from successfully participating in school and extracurricular activities that help develop independence and mastery (National Center for Chronic Disease Prevention and Health Promotion, 2017) and result in a poorer overall quality of life (Bai et al., 2017).

Parental and child perceptions of the impact of their condition affect a child's developing sense of self-worth and psychological adjustment. The child's dependency on the caregivers resulting from a treatment regimen or overprotective caregivers may create social and emotional barriers between the child and their unaffected peers.

Children with a condition that is not highly visible may try to hide its existence until forced by circumstances to admit otherwise when they recognize that it distinguishes them from their peers, placing them at risk for stigmatization, ostracism, and bullying (Carroll et al., 2020; Pinquart, 2017). When taught self-advocacy and social competency skills, including communicating condition-specific information to their peers, these children will be confident and able to build and sustain friendships. Failure to learn these skills may cause withdrawal, anxiety, and depression.

ADOLESCENCE

Adolescence is the transitional period from childhood to adulthood, developing socially and emotionally with the important task of searching for identity (Betz, 2007; Betz et al., 2013). These developmental tasks require that adolescents develop some level of independence from their parents:

1. Develop personal moral and ethical codes for behavior
2. Assume greater responsibility for academic endeavors and career planning
3. Master social rules
4. Avoid high-risk behaviors that threaten the adolescent's well-being

Adolescents with chronic conditions often have chronic dependency related to their condition and may experience psychological difficulties. Personal goal setting and career planning typically occur during adolescence; however, adolescents with chronic illnesses need assistance and a social network that includes their caregivers, friends, interdisciplinary services, and professionals (Traino et al., 2019). Adolescents are prone

to two dangers in planning for the future: They may (1) overemphasize the potential barriers that accompany their condition and succumb to a sense of futility or despair, and (2) deny realistic limitations and set themselves up for failure by holding unrealistic expectations. Adolescence is the time for assuming responsibility for the care of their condition, but adolescents' relative inexperience and the complexity of care needs may preclude this from happening. For an adolescent who requires complex care or has a limited life expectancy, transitioning from parental care to self-care is more difficult to achieve and may go unmet.

Puberty is a time of rapid change and uncertainty for adolescents and may be more difficult for teens with chronic conditions. Delayed puberty accompanies many conditions, emphasizing the differences between affected and unaffected youths. Body image and self-concept may be impacted by limitations related to the adolescent's chronic illness and the sequelae. Because this is a particularly difficult time to be viewed as different by one's peers, some adolescents may withdraw from social activities and relationships that promote healthy psychosexual development. Others may choose to engage in risky behaviors (e.g., smoking, unprotected sex), with some literature supporting higher rates compared to youths without chronic illness (Alley et al., 2021; Horner-Johnson et al., 2021). Adolescents with chronic conditions, however, are particularly vulnerable to sexual exploitation as a way of seemingly being accepted by their peers. The exposure of youth with chronic conditions to sex education is generally consistent but often insufficient as it rarely addresses condition-specific issues. Although pubertal development may be slower and social isolation more common, youth with disabilities are as interested in pursuing intimate sexual relationships and are as sexually experienced as their counterparts (Alley et al., 2021; Horner-Johnson et al., 2021).

INDIVIDUAL CHARACTERISTICS

Despite great odds, many children have psychological and interpersonal resources that allow them to overcome the limitations of their disability and excel in life. A child's characteristics that underlie their behavior (i.e., temperament, motivation, resilience, locus of control, intellect, attitudinal qualities, interpersonal skills) influence developmental attainment and adaptation to the child's condition. Some behavioral traits, such as temperament, are inborn, and others, such as self-concept, develop over time. Social and environmental factors influence the refinement of modifiable traits. A child's self-esteem is linked to fully mastering a variety of physical, intellectual, social, and emotional tasks during the appropriate developmental period, and failure of such developmental tasks can impact physical and psychosocial health. Although children with chronic conditions are at a higher risk for developing behavioral problems, many are remarkably resilient

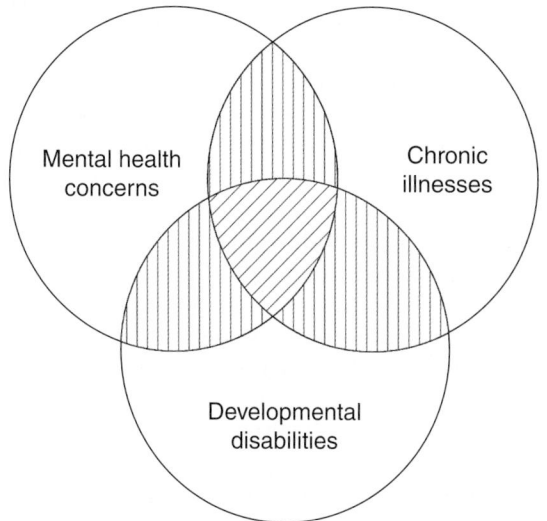

Fig. 2.1 **Cooccurring conditions.**

and confidently approach life's challenges. Many learn to rapidly identify threats to their integrity, respond confidently to those who are prejudiced against them, and reject insults from biased individuals. These children often work to simultaneously educate those around them, dispelling myths and inaccuracies that might interfere with their developmental competence.

Children often live with multiple chronic conditions. Two or more conditions can occur within the same domain—chronic illnesses, developmental disabilities, mental health problems, or across domains (Fig. 2.1) (Vessey, 1999). Children with multiple chronic conditions are at increased risk for psychosocial problems, although disease severity alone may not affect a child's psychological outcome. Risk factors known to place children at greater risk for coexisting psychiatric conditions include (1) poor self-esteem, (2) inappropriate or underdeveloped coping mechanisms, (3) family dysfunction, (4) familial or geographic isolation, (5) poverty, (6) school absenteeism, and (7) peer victimization (Brady et al., 2021; Iannucci & Nierenberg, 2022). Boys experiencing behavioral problems tend toward externalizing disorders (e.g., conduct or oppositional disorders) that are more readily detected than disorders of girls, who tend toward internalizing disorders (e.g., depression). Children with coexisting physical and psychiatric disorders may not have their psychiatric condition adequately treated due to prioritization of the needs of the physical disorder (Brown et al., 2022).

The interrelationships of a child's self-esteem, perceived autonomy, temperament, internal locus of control, perceptual and communication skills, cognitive appraisal of the condition, and coping skills in conjunction with family support, community mentoring, and peer relationships all contribute to the child's adaptive abilities (Chew et al., 2018; Meijer et al., 2002). When children are provided with the protective factors needed to balance out risk exposure, improved resilience and developmental attainment are more likely to occur.

ROLE OF FAMILY AND SOCIAL NETWORKS

Healthy childhood development is largely influenced by a variety of repeated positive interactions between the child and the environment.

A child's caregivers are important influences on a child's development and a strong predictor of emotional well-being during early childhood (Chew et al., 2018). Although maternal and paternal responses and roles differ, many parents are tremendously resilient despite the demands of the child's condition and effectively balance their role in normative parenting with meeting specific demands of the condition (Qiu et al., 2021). Conversely, parental guilt, despair, or unfinished grief over the loss of the fantasized child may negatively affect a child's development. Other factors include parental depression, anxiety, poor self-esteem, and a chronically stressful environment. Children with disabilities are at higher risk for child abuse and neglect (Maclean et al., 2017). Well-functioning families enhance their child's development, whereas dysfunctional family systems may curtail development (Coffey, 2006; Knafl & Gillis, 2002; Qiu et al., 2021). Other factors that influence development in children with the chronic illness include culture, language, religion, and socioeconomic status of the family. Access to resources, coping abilities, and social support largely impact successful adaptation for children with chronic illnesses and their families.

As children mature, their environmental and social networks expand to include extended family members, teachers, friends, and acquaintances as influences that impact developmental maturation. Individuals emerge as advocates for the child, offering practical and tangible support, providing intellectual stimulation, and taking pride in the child's accomplishments. For children whose conditions are associated with disfigurement, their development may be unwittingly at risk because of the reactions of others. Many uninformed individuals automatically assume that a physical handicap is associated with cognitive impairment. Children may be spoken of as if they are not present, or questions may be addressed to nearby family members or peers. The damage that can be done to a child's sense of self-worth is inestimable. The family can be helped to educate significant others about the child's strengths and limitations, mainstream their child into community activities, and use effective methods for working with insensitive individuals.

DEVELOPMENTAL PERSPECTIVES OF THE BODY, ILLNESS, MEDICAL PROCEDURES, AND DEATH

How children view their own body, illness, medical procedures, and death vary depending on their experiences, age, and cognitive abilities. Children with chronic conditions often have significant knowledge about specific topics related to their illnesses based on their experiences. Variability in their understanding ranges from a proficient understanding of their disease to an incomplete understanding of other related areas such as anatomy, physiology, illness, and specific medical management such as procedures, surgery, and pharmacotherapy. It is imperative to confirm a child's understanding of pertinent topics, as many children will utilize vocabulary that can be misleading and result in inaccurate perceptions. The child's beliefs impact their understanding of themselves, their abilities, and adherence to treatment and influence their school performance, functional status, and psychosocial competence.

UNDERSTANDING OF THE BODY

Understanding of the body occurs along a developmental spectrum. Toddlers can point to various body parts when asked, whereas preschoolers can conceptualize their external body parts and the relationships between them. Most preschoolers can name some of their internal body parts, including the heart, brain, and blood; however, they generally have a limited understanding of the internal workings of body parts based on their experiences, cognitive level, and perceptual abilities. Children may describe their internal body parts, functions, and relationships to each other abstractly, possibly influenced by their imagination. Physiologic processes of the body are viewed individually without regard to the relationships between body systems. It is not until later in childhood that children begin to understand the complex relationships between body systems and physiologic processes as their ability to reason and differentiate develops. Children may then begin to organize the levels of the body and understand how they integrate into one another. As the child moves into adolescence, they may attain knowledge from school science classes and develop an even more complex understanding of body functions. Children with chronic illnesses may have experiences that allow them different perspectives of the internal body without a greater understanding of the internal body compared to their unaffected peers. They may focus on the area of their body impacted by their chronic illness but do not necessarily have a more or less sophisticated understanding of the organ or body system involved.

UNDERSTANDING OF ILLNESS, MEDICAL PROCEDURES, AND TREATMENTS

Children's understanding of illness, medical procedures, and treatments are directly related to their level of understanding of their body. Children with chronic illness may develop negative perceptions of their condition because of the impact of their illness and treatment. Providers and other trusted support people may assist them in developing positive images of their illness as the child matures.

An infant's understanding of illness, medical procedures, and treatment extends so far as its intrusion on personal comfort. The developmental task of attachment may be curtailed because of illness-related hospitalization, subsequent familial separation, unpredictable routines, and pain leading to irritability and withdrawal.

Toddlers begin to understand the concept of illness. For children with chronic conditions, this is usually interpreted by how the condition interferes with desired activities. Many condition-specific treatments and procedures (e.g., injections of insulin, wearing a seizure helmet) are particularly onerous for this age group. As children develop, they begin to form ideas and articulate their feelings about illness. Because preschoolers are egocentric and engage in magical thinking, they often ascribe the causes of illness and associate treatments to their thoughts or behaviors, especially related to other temporally occurring events. The purpose of a procedure is viewed as independent of a child's health status, and little discrimination about its diagnostic or therapeutic purpose is made except by children who have undergone repetitive procedures. All procedures are designed to make them "better" or "sicker." Many associate treatments with punishment, and because preschoolers' understanding of body boundaries is not well developed, virtually all invasive procedures are perceived as threats to their body integrity.

School-age children develop views of illness and begin reflecting on their evolving causal reasoning. Illness is initially perceived as occurring from contamination of, or physical contact with, the causal agent. With the maturation of their understanding, children begin to believe that illnesses are caused by external events (e.g., germs that enter the body). School-age children are often intrigued with medical procedures and may be excited to engage in their care. Multistep procedures and their purposes can be understood by school-age children, who can classify and order variables. Medical information may be interpreted literally, resulting in a misunderstanding by the child, necessitating confirmation and clarification of the provided teaching. School-age children respect health care personnel and their role. Although they sometimes express affection for their caregivers, children are often ambivalent about their relationships with health care providers.

With the development of formal operations, adolescents acquire more knowledge about illness and pathophysiology. Illness causation is recognized as a complex, multifaceted process. Initial biologic and physiologic explanations that form the basis for illness later evolve into psycho-physiologic descriptions with an understanding of the relationship between behavior and emotion related to the illness. Adolescents can understand the efficacy of specific medical procedures and the relationships between procedures and their health status, although their sense of invincibility and desire for experimentation affect their decision making. Informed decisions about alternative treatments are possible. Adolescents view the health care provider's authority as extending only as far as their willingness to adhere to recommended therapeutic regimens. Although the need for therapeutic adherence is understood, treatments may not be automatically accepted and integrated into an adolescent's daily activities.

UNDERSTANDING OF DEATH

Some may view death as the ultimate experience of separation and loss for children and their families. Children's understanding of death is formed along a developmental progression and reflects their cognitive maturation and experience (Menendez et al., 2020). Infants do not comprehend death but may respond to the phenomena associated with death, such as pain or separation. By late toddlerhood and preschool age, children may describe death in terms of its occurrence and attributes with magical thinking and an egocentric viewpoint. They may perceive their impending death as punishment, yet do not view death as permanent but rather as sleep or separation from the family. The permanence of death is not realized until early childhood when the concepts of reversibility and irreversibility are learned. Children in this age group often personify death as a fictional creature or monster. For dying children, this newfound knowledge enhances their fears of the unknown. Adolescents, with their new metacognitive abilities, conceptualize death as a life cycle process, readily comprehending the emotional, social, and financial implications of the loss occurring from death for themselves and their families. Adolescents of all age groups may have the most difficulty dealing with death because of their level of understanding.

Children with chronic conditions are often subjected to many intrusive and painful experiences and may have experienced the death of friends in the hospital, even some with the same chronic illness. These experiences can exacerbate fear and anxiety about death. Depending on individual experience, a child's understanding of death may not follow the projected trajectory. Even preschool-age children may express fear of separation, even though death may not yet be conceptualized as irreversible.

Separation, mutilation, and loss of control impact the conceptualization of death for the dying child. Care must be taken to prevent unnecessary separation and help these children maintain their autonomy, sense of mastery, and other developmental skills whenever possible.

PRIMARY CARE PROVIDER'S ROLE IN PROMOTING DEVELOPMENT

Many chronic conditions are not curable; therefore provider management must focus on overall supportive care to minimize disease symptomatology and complications while optimizing physical, cognitive, and psychosocial function. Understanding the unique familial dynamics and adopting a patient and family-centered approach supports the overall goal of optimal function of the child with chronic illness. This model of care was previously called family-centered care but was replaced with patient and family-centered care (PFCC), referring to the approach that engages both the family and child and treats both as members of the health care team (Garzon Maaks et al., 2020). PFCC recognizes that the family is the constant in the child's life and, as such, is vital to children successfully meeting their greatest potential. The goal of PFCC is caregiver empowerment and child advocacy (Garzon Maaks et al., 2020). Elements of PFCC include the following: (1) acknowledgment of the unique needs of the family; (2) support of the family's needs to care for the child; (3) shared decision making between the family and providers, with caregivers considered to be equal members of the decision-making team to the extent they feel comfortable; and (4) acknowledgment and respect of cultural differences (Garzon Maaks et al., 2020).

The patient-centered health care home (PCHH) is a model of care for children with chronic illnesses that ideally provides access to coordinated, culturally competent PFCC. Elements of the PCHH include (1) a plan of care with input from the provider, child, and family; (2) a central record that is confidential and accessible to the family; (3) care coordination, including information sharing with the child, family, and other caregivers; (4) caregiver support, including mental health services; and (5) communication (Garzon Maaks et al., 2020).

The primary care provider is integral to the PCHH and should utilize a PFCC model to build a holistic management plan that incorporates specific disease management and mitigates functional limitations. Developmental considerations for each child can be made according to diagnosis and then individualized based on the unique needs of the child and family.

ASSESSMENT AND MANAGEMENT

Maturational alterations are rarely immutable and should not be thought of as such. Children with chronic conditions require comprehensive care, including developmental surveillance, to achieve their optimal level of functioning. Developmental lags or behavioral problems should be identified as soon as possible, and vigorous intervention should ensue, followed by careful observation for progress with modifications in the treatment plan as necessary. Many interventions, such as physical therapy, occupation therapy, and speech therapy, are most effective when initiated in the preclinical period when slight changes in development may be detected but gross manifestations are not yet evident. Early intervention may prevent or ameliorate many secondary problems resulting from neglect or mistreatment of the original condition; therefore a watch and wait approach to developmental delay is not recommended. For example, although a child may experience hearing loss from aminoglycosides, subsequent language and cognitive delays may be prevented with aggressive intervention.

Like all children, developmental surveillance should be incorporated into every primary care visit for children with chronic conditions, as the primary care provider serves as the child's medical home, providing continuous and comprehensive care. Developmental surveillance is a systematic approach to the early identification of developmental disorders in children (Lipkin & Macias, 2020). It incorporates the following components: (1) eliciting a parent's concerns; (2) obtaining a developmental history; (3) observing the child; (4) identifying risks, strengths, and protective factors; (5) maintaining a record; and (6) sharing opinions and findings (AAP, 2022). The AAP algorithm for the developmental surveillance of all children serves as a structured foundation for the developmental surveillance of children with chronic conditions. Developmental alterations detected in the surveillance process should prompt standardized developmental screening or referral to a specialist for evaluation (Lipkin & Macias, 2020).

For children with mild conditions, the standard surveillance schedule is probably sufficient. Providers must normalize developmental surveillance, and caregivers should be counseled that ongoing surveillance is the standard of care for all children, not because their child has a chronic condition. This will help allay fears that their child is unduly vulnerable and create self-fulfilling prophecies. Additional and ongoing assessment throughout a child's lifetime is warranted for those children at risk for specific delays. Any parental observations regarding developmental differences should be assessed as they correlate with their children's developmental differences.

Standardized developmental assessment instruments are useful and necessary adjuncts to a complete history and physical examination for a comprehensive developmental evaluation. When used at regular intervals, these instruments provide objective data so that small developmental changes can be detected. Considering the ever-growing number of children with special needs being cared for in the community, primary care practitioners need a compendium of readily administered standardized instruments from which to draw (Table 2.1). They should not rely only on broadband developmental screening instruments designed to identify global delay rather than provide in-depth information on the type and severity of developmental problems. Focused instruments provide specific information that is useful as part of an in-depth evaluation.

Instruments should be carefully chosen and results thoroughly interpreted because most of these are norm referenced instead of criterion referenced. Other instruments and results are invalid if they measure one developmental construct based on performance in a different area of development (e.g., a child's cognitive development with a tracheostomy should not be assessed by an instrument requiring verbal responses). Timed tests may also bias results particularly if a child has a motor or learning deficit. If a child tires easily it is best to perform developmental assessments in short intervals so as not to obscure the child's true capabilities. Last, screening instruments must be culturally relevant to be valid.

When developmental alterations are detected, the pediatric primary care provider can either provide treatment or, more likely, refer the child to subspecialists with expertise in the area of concern. Referrals should ideally be made to individuals who are part of the specialty team or within the child's school setting, but additional local referrals may be necessary if the specialty team is far away or school services are inadequate. Adding another layer of care providers requires coordination of services if the child is to receive appropriate care without overlaps, gaps, or too many demands to cause fatigue. The PCHH model provides the framework needed to support the necessary coordination of services, and the primary care provider helps ensure that care is seamless and integrated across disciplines.

Obtaining services may require that the child's condition and associated problems be diagnostically labeled, although federal legislation has made this less common. Providing a label may help validate the concerns of children and families and direct future interventions and activities, but it must be done judiciously. Labeling often sets children apart from their peers and may result in different treatment by family members, teachers, and significant others. Diagnostic labels assigned in childhood follow children into adulthood and might prevent them from pursuing selected careers, joining the military, or being eligible for insurance. Although it is usually feasible to label specific disease entities, labeling associated with developmental manifestations should be done carefully. The ultimate long-term goal of care is for a child to reach and sustain optimal levels of functioning. Developing precise, measurable, short-term goals helps ensure that optimal functioning is obtained.

The use of person-centered language is essential. A child should not be labeled as diabetic but as a child who has diabetes. Another example is children with Down syndrome rather than Down syndrome children. The "Spread the Word to End the Word" campaign in 2009 was initiated by two college students to raise awareness of the disrespect and harm caused by using the R-word (retarded) in a demeaning way. It encourages people to take an annual pledge to refrain from negative use and is supported by more than 200 organizations working to eliminate the word used in public and in health professions. In 2010 Rosa's law

Table 2.1   Instruments Used in Developmental Assessment

TEST/SCORE	AGE LEVEL	METHOD	COMMENTS	TIME; EXAMINER QUALIFICATIONS REQUIRED
General Development				
AAIDD Diagnostic Adaptive Behavior Scale Authors: M. Tasse, R. Schalock, D. Thissen, G. Balboni, S. Borthwick-Duffy, S. Spreat, K. Widaman, D. Zhang Source: American Association on Intellectual and Developmental Disabilities (AAIDD) Website: https://www.aaidd.org/dabs	4–21 yr	Observation Performance tasks	Provides precise diagnostic information regarding significant limitations in adaptive behavior Assesses adaptive behavior through conceptual, social, and practical skills Paper-and-pencil interview assessment followed by purchasing a scoring token for online scoring platform	15–30 min/domain, 1–2 hr in full
Ages and Stages Questionnaires (ASQ), 3rd ed. Authors: D. Bricker, J. Squires, J. Clifford, J. Dolata, J. Farrell, G. Fink, R. Hoselton, Y. Kim, K. Murphy, L. Potter, M. Davis, E. Twombly, S. Yockelson Source: Paul H. Brookes Publishing Co. Website: https://agesandstages.com/	1–66 mo	Parent-completed questionnaire with provider scoring	21 questionnaires and scoring sheets at age 2, 4, 6, 8, 9, 10, 12, 14, 16, 18, 20, 22, 24, 27, 3, 33, 36, 42, 48, 54, and 60 mo Series of age-specific questions for parents Screens communication, gross motor, fine motor, problem solving, and personal adaptive skills Pass/fail scoring for domains	10–15 min for parents to complete, 2–3 min for professionals to score
Alberta Infant Motor Scale (AIMS) Authors: M. Piper, J. Darrah Source: Elsevier (2021) Website: www.elsevier.com; www.apta.org	Birth–18 mo	Observation Performance-based, norm-referenced observational tool	58 items to measure gross motor developmental milestones Assesses postural control in four position-centric subscales: supine, prone, standing, and sitting positions Assesses delays or atypical motor performance and evaluates motor development over time Should not be used in infants with diagnosed altered movement patterns (spina bifida, muscle spasticity, etc.)	20–30 min Rehabilitation therapists; health care professionals with knowledge of motor development in infants
Battelle Developmental Inventory (BDI-3), 3rd ed. (2020) Author: J. Newborg Source: Riverside Publishing Co. Website: http://riversideinsights.com	Birth–7 yr 11 mo	Structured observation and/or interview format Scored in a web-based platform	Assesses developmental readiness for school, eligibility for special education services, including individualized family service plans and individualized education programs Full BDI spans five domains: communication, social, emotional, adaptive, motor, cognitive	Screening test takes 10 min for numeracy, 30 min for literacy Interviewer can choose one domain, or any combination as needed
Bayley Scales of Infant and Toddler Development, 4th ed. (2019) Authors: N. Bayley, G. Aylward Source: Pearson Assessments Website: https://pearsonassessments.com	16 days–42 mo	Observation Demonstration Caregiver responses support scoring Paper-and-pencil assessment with online scoring platform	Extensive formal assessment tool to diagnose developmental delays, including early identification of intellectual delay Items scored per domain: cognitive (81), language (42 in receptive, 37 in expressive), motor (46 in fine motor, 59 in gross motor) Also includes a socioemotional scale and adaptive behavior scale	30–70 min depending on age of child Qualified practitioner to examine and evaluate an infant; training provided for a fee

Continued

Table 2.1   Instruments Used in Developmental Assessment—cont'd

TEST/SCORE	AGE LEVEL	METHOD	COMMENTS	TIME; EXAMINER QUALIFICATIONS REQUIRED
Newborn Behavioral Observations (NBO) (1995) Author: T.B. Brazelton Source: Brazelton Touchpoints Center Website https://www.brazeltontouchpoints.org	Birth–3 mo	Interactive relationship-based tool that informs parents about their baby's communication strategies	Designed as a serial assessment weekly, biweekly, or monthly Evaluates 18 neurobehavioral observations items in the areas of habituation, orientation, motor maturity, variation, self-quieting, and social summarized by AMOR (autonomic, motor, organization of state, and responsiveness) Evidence is limited in effectiveness as an intervention to improve parent-infant interaction. Should be used primarily for research or as a supplemental tool	20–30 min Administer by trained examiner
Child Behavior Checklist (CBCL/6–18) (2001) Author: T.M. Achenbach Source: Achenbach System of Empirically Based Assessment (ASEBA) Website: www.aseba.org	Preschool version: 1.5–5 yr School-aged version: 6–18 yr	Observation/ interview Separate assessments for parents or caregivers, teachers or school staff, and youth	Helps identify problematic behavior Scored according to eight empirically based syndromic scales: aggressive behavior, anxious/depressed, attention problems, rule-breaking behavior, somatic complaints, social problems, thought problems, withdrawn/depressed	Problem items completed by most parents in 10 min with additional competence items 5–10 min Scoring: 3 min via computer, 20 min by hand Trained professional needed to interpret Available in >90 languages
Child Development Inventory (CDI) (1992) Author: H. Ireton Source: Child Development Review Website: https://www.childdevelopmentinventory.com	15 mo–6 yr	Parent-completed questionnaire	300-item inventory to identify parental concerns about health, growth, vision, hearing, development, and behavior Measures social, self-help, motor, expressive language, and general developmental quotients and age equivalents for different developmental domains Appropriate for more in-depth evaluation	30–50 min
Child Development Review–Parent Questionnaire (CDR-PQ) (2006) Author: H. Ireton Source: Child Development Review Website: www.childdevelopmentinventory.com	Infant: Birth–18 mo Child: 18 mo–kindergarten	Parent-completed questionnaire	Assess developmental skills across five domains: social, self-help, gross motor, fine motor, and language skills	10–20 min
The Early Screening Inventory, 3rd ed. (2019) Authors: S. Meisels, D. Marsden, L. Henderson, M. Wiske Source: Pearson Learning Group Website: www.pearsonassessments.com	3–5 yr 11 mo	Observation Parent questionnaire to assess perception of development	Helps identify children who may need special education services in school Assesses socioemotional development and adaptive behaviors (e.g., interactions with adults and peers, social communication and skills for self-help) Includes a parent checklist	15–20 min Must be a trained professional Available in English and Spanish

TEST/SCORE	AGE LEVEL	METHOD	COMMENTS	TIME; EXAMINER QUALIFICATIONS REQUIRED
Hawaii Early Learning Profile (HELP) (2014) Authors: S.F. Furuno, K.A. O'Reilly, C.M. Kosaka, T.T. Inatsuka, B. Zeisloft-Dalby Source: Vort Corporation Website: www.vort.com	Birth–36 mo 3–6 yr	Observation and parent interview	Comprehensive, family-centered curriculum-based assessment 685 developmental tasks used to assess six domains: cognition, language, gross motor, fine motor, socioemotional, and self-help Supports federal requirements for Part C of Individuals with Disabilities Education Act and Head Start	Each domain takes 15–30 min to administer Domains may be selected for individual use Administration manual required for proper use, 5-hour training course offered
Modified Checklist for Autism in Children Revised (MCHAT-R/F) (2009) Authors: D. Robins, D. Fein, M. Barton Source: M-Chat Screen Website: www.mchatscreen.com	16–30 min	Parent-report screening tool	20-item questionnaire Assesses for specific risk and early detection of autism spectrum disorder (ASD), allowing early interventions and promoting improved diagnosis High false positive rate, so red flags should be followed up with further assessment Screening for ASD is recommended by the American Academy of Pediatrics for all children ages 18–24 mo during well visits	10 min Must be used in its entirety, cannot be modified Follow-up tool should be used for children who screen positive
Parents' Evaluation of Developmental Status–Revised with Follow-Up (PEDS-R/f) (2022) Author: F.P. Glascoe Source: Ellsworth & Vandermeer Press, LLC Website: www.pedstest.com	Birth–8 yr	Parent interview form	10 items crossing developmental domains, including expressive/receptive language, gross/fine motor, behavior, social help, school and social skills, global/cognitive and psychosocial challenges Improves the ability for parents to raise concerns with cultural responsiveness Revised tool adds two questions to elicit parental concerns Should be used as a prompt to evaluate the need for further screening	2–10 min Available in English, Spanish, and Chinese
Pediatric Symptom Checklist (PSC-35) (1999) Youth PSC (Y-PSC) PSC-17 Y-PSC-17 Authors: M. Murphy, M. Jellinek Source: Bright Futures Website: https://brightfutures.org	6–18 yr (2–5 yr version also)	PSC-35: parent checklist Y-PSC: self-report for adolescents PSC-17: shortened version of PSC Y-PSC-17: shortened version of Y-PSC	35-item parent report questionnaire focused on daily behaviors and moods Psychosocial screen to recognize areas of recognition of cognitive, emotional, and behavioral problems to prompt early intervention Scores above the designated cutoff indicate the need for further evaluation	3–5 min

Continued

Table **2.1**   Instruments Used in Developmental Assessment—cont'd

TEST/SCORE	AGE LEVEL	METHOD	COMMENTS	TIME; EXAMINER QUALIFICATIONS REQUIRED
Vision				
Allen Picture Card Test of Visual Acuity Author: H.F. Allen Source: Western Ophthalmics Corporation Website: www.west-op.com	26 yr, able to cooperatively follow direction with intelligible expressive language	Observation Interview style "Name the picture"	Preschooler screening test for visual acuity No pretraining needed for preschool children	Time varies
HOTV (matching symbol test) Author: O. Lippmann Source: Veatch Instruments Website: www.veatchinstruments.com	≥3 yr, or able to identify shapes and cooperatively follow directions	Flashcards	Good for young children or those who do not like to verbalize Children name the four letters *H, O, T, V* on a chart for testing at 10–20 ft and match them to a demonstration card Avoids the problem with image reversal and eye-hand coordination that can occur with the letter *E*	Time varies
Snellen Tumbling E Test Author: H. Snellen Source: American Academy of Ophthalmology; American Association of Ophthalmology Website: www.paao.org	≥3 yr	Observation using two persons as a team in screening	Intended as a screening measure for central acuity of preschool-age children and other children who have not learned to read	Time varies
Language/Cognitive				
The Bzoch-League Receptive Expressive Emergent Language Scale (REEL), 3rd ed. (2006) Authors: K.R. Bzoch, R. League Source: Pearson Assessments Website: www.pearsonassessments.com	Birth–36 mo	Paper-and-pencil inventory Parent interview	To identify young children who have language impairments or other disabilities that interfere with language development	20 min
Kaufman Brief Intelligence Test (KBIT-2 Revised) (2022) Authors: A.S. Kaufman, N.L. Kaufman Source: Pearson Assessments Website: www.ags.pearsonassessments.com	4–90+ yr	Structured test format	Quick measure of verbal and nonverbal ability Identifies learners who may benefit from educational enrichment Evaluates cognitive ability of a child after intervention or a significant life event	15–30 min
McCarthur-Bates Communicative Development Inventory (CDI-2e), 2nd ed. Authors: L. Fenson, V. Marchman, D. Thal, P. Dale, J. Reznick, E. Bates Source: Brookes Publishing Website: www.brookespublishing.com	8–37 + mo developmentally delayed children	Parent or caregiver report measuring vocabulary development	Measures vocabulary development (words and sentences) in children with prognosis for language delay Includes an extensive vocabulary checklist containing words that children typically produce in the second and third years; parents are asked to review and check all words that their child can spontaneously produce	20–40 min to complete, 10–15 min to score Administered by a speech therapist or pathologist, primary care provider, or nurse

TEST/SCORE	AGE LEVEL	METHOD	COMMENTS	TIME; EXAMINER QUALIFICATIONS REQUIRED
Peabody Picture Vocabulary Test (PPVT-5), 5th ed. Author: D. Dunn Source: Pearson Assessments Website: http://ags.pearsonassessments.com	2–6 yr through 90+	Individual "point to" response test	Measures receptive vocabulary acquisition Assesses strengths and weaknesses in semantics and language development	10–15 min Administer by a qualified clinician
Hearing				
Biologic AuDX PRO FLEX Source: Natus Website: www.natus.com	Age depends on test selected	Diagnostic oto-acoustic emissions (OAE)	Flexible tabletop device offering screening or diagnostic acoustic immittance. Capabilities include screening tympanometry; diagnostic tympanometry; screening audiometry; diagnostic audiometry; screening OAE, diagnostic OAE, input-output OAE, threshold estimation OAE	A few minutes, depending on child cooperation
Psychosocial Development				
ASQ: Social-Emotional (ASQ: SE-2), 2nd ed. Authors: D. Bricker, J. Squires, J. Clifford, J. Dolata, J. Farrell, G. Fink, R. Hoselton, Y. Kim, K. Murphy, L. Potter, M. Davis, E. Twombly, S. Yockelson Source: Paul H. Brookes Publishing Co. Website: https://agesandstages.com/	1–72 mo	Parent-completed questionnaire with provider scoring	9 questionnaires and scoring sheets at age 2, 6, 12, 18, 24, 30, 26, 48, 60 mo Series of age-specific questions for parents Screens self-regulation, compliance, social-communication, adaptive functioning, autonomy, affect, and interaction with people Pass/fail scoring for domains	10–15 min for parents to complete, 1–3 minutes for professionals to score
CDI-2 (2010) Author: M. Kovacs Source: Pearson Assessments Website: www.pearsonassessments.com	7–17 yr	Paper-and-pencil self-report	Assesses cognitive, affective, and behavioral signs of depression Contains 28 items and is designed for schools, child guidance clinics, pediatric practices, and child psychiatric settings First-grade reading level Four subscales include negative mood/physical symptoms, negative self-esteem, interpersonal problems, ineffectiveness	5–10 min
Piers-Harris Children's Self-Concept Scale, 3rd ed. (2018) Authors: E.V. Piers, S. Shemmassian, D. Herzberg Source: Western Psychological Services Website: www.wspublish.com	6–22 yr	Self-report Descriptive statements used by groups or individuals	Assesses a raw self-concept score plus cluster scores for 58 items in six domains: behavior adjustment, freedom from anxiety, intellectual and school status, happiness and satisfaction, physical appearance and attributes, and social acceptance Version 3 includes popularity, bullying, social isolation, and body image Test title: "The Way I Feel about Myself"	10–15 min

Continued

Table **2.1**   Instruments Used in Developmental Assessment—cont'd

TEST/SCORE	AGE LEVEL	METHOD	COMMENTS	TIME; EXAMINER QUALIFICATIONS REQUIRED
Stress and Anxiety				
Generalized Anxiety Disorder-7 (GAD-7) (2006) Authors: R. Spitzer, K. Kroenke, J. Williams, B. Lowe Source: Pfizer Website: www.phqscreeners.com	≥12 yr	Self-report	Screening questionnaire measuring severity of various signs of anxiety. Documented sensitivity and specificity for generalized anxiety, panic, social anxiety, and posttraumatic stress disorder Cut-off points of 5, 10, and 15 suggest mild, moderate, and severe levels of anxiety	≤5 min Available in the public domain in several languages
KySS Worries Questionnaire (2022) Authors: B. Melnyk, P. Lusk Source: National Association of Pediatric Nurse Practitioners (NAPNAP) Website: www.napnap.org	10–21 yr	Self-report questionnaire	15-item Likert-scale questionnaire that identifies common pediatric worries Parent version has 13 items	
Revised Children's Manifest Anxiety Scale (RCMAS-2), 2nd ed. (2008) Authors: C.R. Reynolds, B.O. Richmond Source: Western Psychological Services Website: www.wpspublish.com	6–19 yr	Self-report	Designed to assess the level and nature of anxiety in children and adolescents. For children age >9 yr it can be administered in a group Based on 28 items and 9 items making up the "Lie Scale"	10–15 min
Screen for Child Anxiety Related Disorders (SCARED) Authors: B. Birmaher, D. Brent, L. Chiappetta, L. Bridge, J. Monga, M. Baugher Source: University of Pittsburgh Website: www.pediatricbipolar.pitt.edu	8–17 yr	Self-report for children, teens, and their parents	41-item self-report questionnaire that identifies anxiety-related disorders on a Likert scale of 0–3 Suggestive of panic disorder, generalized anxiety disorder, separation anxiety, social anxiety disorder, and significant school avoidance	
State-Trait Anxiety Inventory for Children (STAIC) (1997) Authors: C.D. Spielberg, C.D. Edwards, R.E. Lushene, J Montuori, D. Platzek Source: Mind Garden Website: www.mindgarden.com	Upper elementary and junior high school students Best for ages 9–12	Self-administered in groups or individually	Measures anxiety in elementary school children Test title: "How I Feel Questionnaire" Two 20-item Likert scales to differentiate between anxiety proneness to anxious behavior and transient state anxiety	20 min
Family Function				
Feetham Family Functioning Survey (FFFS) (1982) Authors: S. Feetham, S. Humenick Source: Springer Website: www.springerpub.com	Family	Self-reporting	25 questions evaluating six areas of functioning: household tasks, child care, sexual and moral relations, interaction with family and friends, community involvement, and sources of support Used for identifying specific areas of dysfunction in a stressed family	10 min

TEST/SCORE	AGE LEVEL	METHOD	COMMENTS	TIME; EXAMINER QUALIFICATIONS REQUIRED
Home Observation for Measurement of the Environment (HOME) (1984) Authors: R. Bradley, B. Caldwell Source: Home Inventory LLC, University of Arkansas–Little Rock Website: www.ualr.edu/crtldept/home4.htm	Birth–3 yr; 3–6 yr; middle childhood (6–10 yr); early adolescence (10–15 yr)	Interview Direct observation of the interaction between care-taker and child	Two instruments designed to assess the quantity and quality of social, emotional, and cognitive support available to a child within the home Inventory for birth–3 yr contains 45 items; 3–6 yr contains 55 items; 6–10 yr contains 59 items, and 10–15 yr contains 40 items	Each inventory takes approximately 1 hr
Stress and Anxiety				
RCMAS Authors: C.R. Reynolds, B.O. Richmond Source: Western Psychological Services Website: www.wpspublish.com	6–19 yr	Self-report	Designed to assess the level and nature of anxiety in children and adolescents For children age >9 yr it can be administered in a group Based on 28 items and 9 items making up the "Lie Scale"	10–15 min
STAIC (1997) Authors: C.D. Spielberg, C.D. Edwards, R.E. Lushene, J Montuori, D. Platzek Source: Mind Garden Website: www.mindgarden.com	Upper elementary and junior high school students	Self-administered in groups or individually	Measures anxiety in elementary school children Test title: "How I Feel Questionnaire"	20 min
STAIC (1984) Authors: C.D. Spielberger, C.D. Edwards, J. Montuori, R. Lushene Source: Mind Garden Website: www.mindgarden.com	Sixth-grade reading level	Group administration	Two 20-item scales Designed to assess anxiety as an emotional state (S-Anxiety) and individual differences in anxiety proneness as a personality trait (T-Anxiety).	10–20 min
Family Function				
FFFS (1982) Authors: S. Feetham, S. Humenick Source: Springer Website: www.springerpub.com	Family	Self-reporting	25 questions evaluating six areas of functioning: household tasks, child care, sexual and moral relations, interaction with family and friends, community involvement, and sources of support Used for identifying specific areas of dysfunction in a stressed family	10 min
HOME (1984) Authors: R. Bradley, B. Caldwell Source: Home Inventory LLC, University of Arkansas–Little Rock Website: www.ualr.edu/crtldept/home4.htm	Birth–3 yr; 3–6 yr; middle childhood (6–10 yr); early adolescence (10–15 yr)	Interview Direct observation of the interaction between care-taker and child	Two instruments designed to assess the quantity and quality of social, emotional, and cognitive support available to a child within the home Inventory for birth–3 yr contains 45 items; 3–6 yr contains 55 items; 6–10 yr contains 59 items, and 10–15 yr contains 40 items	Each inventory takes approximately 1 hr

was passed by the US Congress to remove the terms mental retardation and mentally retarded from all federal documentation and replace them with intellectual disabilities. This inspiring story began with a mother who did not want her child to be referred to as retarded at school. Some advocates use the general term differently abled rather than disabled. The most important element of family care planning within this domain is to empower the child and family with the agency to clearly articulate their preferred language. For example, the Deaf community has an oppositional stance to person-first language because of the debate over how Deaf persons identify (or not) with disability culture. All patients should have care that is respectful of and responsive to individual and/or family preferences (Crocker & Smith, 2019).

FOSTERING PSYCHOSOCIAL HEALTH

Effective therapeutic interventions can strengthen a child's resiliency and improve general well-being and quality of life while preventing or mitigating coexisting psychological problems. Effective coping strategies, including seeking social support, managing condition-related stressors, and developing good social skills, help children with chronic conditions reduce the likelihood of developing behavioral problems. Fostering a good parent-child relationship is the gateway to promoting childhood resilience (Hallas, 2019). Other strategies are listed in Box 2.1.

Children with and without chronic conditions enjoy participating in the same activities. The role of schools should not be undervalued because they provide a measure of independence and opportunities for self-mastery and self-esteem building that are not readily achieved at home. Specialty camps help youth cope with their conditions, improve self-care skills, and foster healthy self-esteem (McCarthy, 2015). Other extracurricular activities, including a wide range of sports that showcase children's skills and encourage peer interaction, are equally useful but must be selected considering condition-specific limitations (Box 2.2). Participation in sports is associated with higher levels of physical activity and general measures of fitness in youth with chronic diseases or physical disabilities (Lankhorst et al., 2021). Sports participation for all children is generally beneficial, including children with disabilities and chronic conditions, particularly cognitive and behavioral disabilities. Benefits for participation generally spanning domains of increased holistic wellness must be balanced with barriers to participation, generally spanning domains of safety and access. The Council on Children with Disabilities and the Council on Sports Medicine and Fitness within the AAP published the guidelines *Promoting the Participation of Children and Adolescents with Disabilities in Sports, Recreation, and Physical Activity*, which provides critical guidance for guiding families in individualized decision making (Carbone et al., 2021).

Box 2.1   Fostering Resilience

- Encourage the child's unique talents and interests, fostering conditions for expression.
  Identify the child's and family's assets; help them develop assertiveness and self-advocacy skills.
- Nurture positive self-esteem and self-efficacy in all family members.
- Help youth see that their chronic condition is not an insurmountable problem and find ways to express hope and intentional gratitude.
  Reassure and diminish their sense of guilt over having a chronic illness.
- Help all family members develop flexible coping skills.
  Provide clear and consistent expectations with clear rules.
- Teach needed communication and problem-solving skills.
  Label emotions with clear words while encouraging healthy expression.
  Foster stress management activities, including meditation, yoga, controlled breathing, and exercise.
  Normalize asking for help.
  Pay special attention to emotional needs of siblings, who may feel overlooked or resentful.
- Encourage academic attainment in youth.
- Encourage children to make social connections in school and through participation in extracurricular activities.
  Foster sustainable friendships.
- Promote volunteerism in the community and other contributions to others.
- Help families develop healthy habits and youth develop appropriate self-care skills.
- Support youth in developing values, beliefs, and goals for their life.
- Encourage parents to role model appropriate behavior.
- Assist parents to set realistic but high expectations.

Modified from Fostering Resilience. (n.d.). Website. https://www.fosteringresilience.org.

ANTICIPATORY GUIDANCE AND EDUCATION

Children with chronic conditions require the same anticipatory guidance as their unaffected peers, although this needs to be adapted to their developmental (rather than chronologic) age and condition-specific limitations (Hallas, 2019). Primary care providers need to help prepare children for self-care behaviors and the development of self-advocacy skills for dealing with the health care community. This is important for children and adolescents with chronic conditions because they are likely to use the health care system often throughout their lives. The transition between pediatric and adult care is a complex endeavor exacerbated by provider and system obstacles. Often adult providers are not equipped to care for transitioning youth with chronic conditions and the accompanying social complexity. Recommendations from the National Association of Pediatric Nurse Practitioners (NAPNAP, 2020a) on facilitating these transitions are

Box 2.2 Categorization of Sports by Physical Contact Potential

Box 2.2 Categorization of Sports by Physical Contact Potential

HIGH-CONTACT SPORTS
- Basketball
- Boxing
- Cheerleading
- Diving
- Dodge ball
- Football
- Gymnastics
- Hockey
- Judo
- Kick boxing
- Lacrosse
- Mountaineering
- Parachuting
- Rugby
- Skiing/snowboarding
- Soccer
- Trampolining
- Water polo
- Wrestling

RESTRICTED-CONTACT SPORTS
- Baseball
- Cycling
- Fencing
- Football, touch
- Horseback riding
- Racquetball
- Rafting/sea kayaking
- Skating
- Skiing, cross-country and water
- Softball
- Surfing
- Squash
- Tae Kwon Do
- Track-and-field events
- Volleyball

NONCONTACT SPORTS
- Archery
- Badminton
- Bowling
- Canoeing/kayaking
- Crew/rowing
- Dance
- Fishing
- Golf
- Hiking
- Pilates
- Rope jumping
- Running
- Sailing
- Scuba diving
- Snowshoeing
- Swimming
- Tennis
- Track
- Yoga

Note: Depending on intensity of activity and of participants, amount of contact can change.

Modified from Rice, S.G., & Council on Sports Medicine and Fitness. (2008). Medical conditions affecting sports participation. Pediatrics, 121, 841–848.

Box 2.3 Supporting Youth Transition to Adult Care

Each transition should be individualized and developmentally sensitive.

Transition planning should begin as early as 12 years of age to ensure adequate time for acquiring management skills and networks.

Transitions should be planned using best practices as outlined by the American Academy of Pediatrics.

Transition readiness should be formally assessed using validated scales.

Underserved and vulnerable populations need special attention to avoid gaps in care.

Pediatric-focused advanced practice registered nurses should lead care coordination and evidence-based practice standard development.

Modified from National Association of Pediatric Nurse Practitioners. (2020a). Supporting the transition from pediatric to adult-focused health care. https://www.napnap.org/position-statements-and-white-papers/.

found in Box 2.3. Educating children and adolescents about their condition helps empower them to negotiate with the health care system effectively.

To accomplish primary care objectives, children must acquire developmentally appropriate knowledge of anatomy, physiology, associated pathophysiology, and complexities of the health care system. Adequate comprehension of their condition should not be assumed simply because children use medical jargon, appear comfortable with the health care environment, or have been diagnosed for an extended period. Accurate, developmentally appropriate information needs to be incorporated into the primary care of all children with chronic conditions because learning is more likely to occur in a nonthreatening environment where children are in a comparatively good state of health rather than when they are sick or hospitalized. A comprehensive plan managed by the primary care provider in conjunction with parents, subspecialty providers, and school support services will help ensure that this learning occurs. Teaching methods must be altered to fit the child's developmental age. Children will learn best when the material presented to them remains within one level of their current cognitive functioning. Information also needs to be reiterated with greater complexity as the child matures. Incorporating a child's voice into care planning in an environment of complex intersections of ethical and legal parameters with parental authority in decision making is one of pediatric care professionals' biggest challenges in care planning.

A multisensory approach (i.e., one that brings all of the child's senses to bear on the learning task at hand) is more likely to be effective with preschool- and school-age children than more traditional lecture methods. Materials need to be selected according to their age appropriateness, cultural relevance, and accuracy of information. For example, anatomically correct rag dolls or models, doll hospitals, and play equipment are highly effective teaching aids to use with younger children. For older youth, an ever-expanding array of professionally developed audiovisual media (e.g., books, videos, interactive computer programs, websites, and health applications on smartphones) are available and useful adjuncts to individualized teaching plans. Practitioners should examine all materials in advance to determine if the information presented will correspond to the child's experiences and treatment plan.

THERAPEUTIC ADHERENCE

Promoting therapeutic adherence is a critical role of the primary care provider especially considering current health care trends that shift the onus of treatment responsibilities to the family. It should be noted the term compliance is outdated and should not be used because of its association with paternalism, lack of patient agency and autonomy, and expectations of obedience to an authoritarian provider figure. Condition management programs must be tailored to the child to maximize the likelihood of therapeutic adherence. A meta-analysis of interventions designed to promote adherence to pediatric treatment regimens for chronic conditions demonstrated that condition-specific education is necessary but insufficient in promoting adherence (Hommel et al., 2017). Interventions with greater efficacy include those that use behavioral, cognitive-behavioral, self-regulatory skill training, or combined approaches. Therapeutic adherence is further enhanced by effective self-management when youth actively participate in health care decisions; feel supported by parents, peers, and practitioners; have the energy, motivation, and willpower to manage their treatment regimen; and the interventions are culturally responsive (Catarino et al., 2021).

Revisiting adherence strategies needs to be an ongoing component of clinical management because adherence tends to diminish over time. Older children and adolescents should begin to take responsibility for more of the care regimens. Useful steps in this process include reeducating youth about their conditions, helping parents and teens negotiate care responsibilities, and assisting parents in shifting from close supervision so that by early adulthood youth assume responsibility for all or most of their care when possible (Catarino et al., 2021). Peers should be involved because they are an increasingly important part of a youth's social support system and, along with parental involvement, have a profound impact on their successful transition to self-care (Lewis et al., 2017).

Assistive aids may help promote independence and therapeutic adherence. For example, digital and technological devices such as smartphones, smartwatches, and other advances, including smart glucose monitoring, help youth remember to monitor vital signs, assess lab values, and take medications on time. Smartphone applications can be used in biometric monitoring and decision making on treatments. Youth are more likely

Box 2.4 Promoting Therapeutic Adherence

Teach children in a developmentally appropriate manner about the following:
- Anatomy and physiology
- Pathophysiology of their condition
- Medication and treatment use and effectiveness
- How to tell friends, teachers, and others about the condition

Explore the thoughts and feelings of children and parents about the treatment plan:
- Revisit as children mature
- Incorporate culturally relevant information

Adjust the treatment plan to fit within the child's and family's lifestyle.

Suggest the use of props to serve as reminders:
- Beepers or watch or cell phone alarms for medication reminders
- Coordinate medications with mealtimes
- Adjust medications to the minimal number of pills and doses necessary
- Incorporate a reward system; use sticker charts or tokens with younger children

to be receptive to gathering and interpreting information from a technological source than from traditional education methods. Technology has significantly impacted care delivery for children with chronic conditions such as asthma, cystic fibrosis, and diabetes (Low & Manias, 2019). For youth with physical or emotional disabilities, companion animals help create independence, improve socioemotional functioning, and enhance work/school function (Rodriguez et al., 2020). Therapeutic adherence can be encouraged through open discussion and the adoption of activities such as those listed in Box 2.4.

In evaluating therapeutic adherence, the clinician should seek information from both the child and parents and, when appropriate, other sources (e.g., schools). Besides inquiring about the prescribed treatment plan, information regarding complementary and alternative therapies needs to be discussed (Hallas, 2019) because families and youth frequently use these as adjuncts or replacement measures. Evidence indicates that neither parents nor children are necessarily accurate in their reports, particularly in the absence of skilled and specific questioning by the health care provider (Stubbe, 2018). Although nonadherence is an issue, determining the reason is critical before instituting any action. Nonadherence is usually not deliberate or consistent but due to misunderstanding the instructions, poor time management, forgetfulness, inability to afford a recommended or prescribed therapy, or other related behaviors. Some families with consistent but nondeliberate nonadherence may be too overwhelmed with the complexity and volume of care elements required in daily living to maintain a long-term, sustained management plan. Smaller groups of children (and their parents) might deliberately choose not to adhere to a treatment regimen because they believe it is ineffective, fear side effects, find it too costly, or have personal or religious objections. Other families choose certain treatments as priorities and adhere to them while not adhering to others they feel are of little value. Still, others remain in denial as to the severity or ramifications of the condition. Interventions must specifically address the reason for nonadherence, and a referral for mental health counseling and/or a support group may be appropriate. ·

ADVOCACY

Many professionals are called on to care for the complex needs of children with chronic conditions. Although all have the same goal—to help the child reach maximum potential—conflicts may arise over the best approach for realizing it. Primary care providers are uniquely positioned to advocate for a child by identifying treatment options and their implications, informing the child and family of available resources, and helping coordinate interdisciplinary services. Advocacy extends to helping families acquire and maintain health insurance, financial resources, and transportation needed for receiving necessary services. This is especially critical in light of the changing service delivery and reimbursement patterns for chronic conditions.

EMERGENCY CARE

Children with chronic conditions are at higher risk for severe acute illnesses, often potentially preventable and tangential to the condition. Children with multiple diagnoses or increased complexity are most at risk for emergency care utilization (Berry et al., 2017). They are also at higher risk for neglect or abuse from family members and others (Committee on Child Abuse and Neglect and Committee on Children with Disabilities, 2001). Clinicians can advocate for children's physiologic and psychological safety by helping ensure ongoing assessments and instituting appropriate interventions. Providers should also help families prepare for emergency care of their child should it be necessary. Because children with chronic conditions may require different and complex services not usually needed by the developmentally and physiologically normative child, encouraging the family to ensure that the child wears a medical alert bracelet and providing a completed emergency information form to day care, school, camp, and extracurricular activity personnel will help ensure that the child receives prompt care should this be necessary. For children on ventilators or who are differently abled, a care plan should be filed with the local fire department and utility services in case of fire, flood, or power outage. A general emergency information form (in both English and Spanish), selected condition-specific forms, and disaster preparedness information is available from the AAP at https://www.aap.org/en/patient-care/disasters-and-children/.

COUNSELING

Careful attention must be paid to the mental and emotional health of children with chronic conditions. Growing up is difficult, and the incidence of violence, substance abuse, depression, suicide, and other risks continues to climb among all children. Children with chronic conditions—especially those with diminished self-esteem—may be particularly vulnerable to mental health problems. Maladaptive health behaviors increase the frequency and incidence of mental health conditions. Beneficial interventions include health promotion, promotion of self-management, cognitive behavioral therapy, behavioral therapy, parent training, and motivational interviewing. Improved psychologic functioning is associated with improved outcomes in physical health parameters (Rohan & Verma, 2020).

Despite the prevalence of mental health concerns among children, many do not receive specialty mental health services; children from Black, Hispanic, and poor families are disproportionately underserved (Bartek et al., 2021). Primary care providers are responsible for identifying and appropriately managing psychosocial problems. The longitudinal relationship that such individuals have with children and families is critical in helping to recognize that mental health problems might develop or may already exist. Mental health presentations in children with chronic illnesses can be overshadowed by symptoms associated with their chronic condition and may go unrecognized and undiagnosed. Mental and behavioral health conditions are among the top five chronic conditions (affecting 13–20% of children in the United States) contributing to functional impairments. Integrating mental health services into primary care delivery is critical to increasing access and decreasing stigmatization associated with specialty care referral. NAPNAP (2020b) issued recommendations in their 2020 position statement that are summarized in Box 2.5.

The National Network of Child Psychiatry Access Programs I (2022) is a national collaborative that highlights and connects existing and emerging child psychiatry networks and consultations to increase the availability of expertise to facilitate delivery of mental health services in primary care environments. Advanced practice registered nurses can use the website database to explore resources available to them by state, which may include services such as an on-call child psychiatrist available free of charge (funded by state budget allocations), clinical algorithms, and educational resources. Integration of care is especially important for children with chronic illness who may already be managing complex care from multiple specialists and may see mental health appointments as a lower priority or a bridge too far in light of competing needs.

It is essential for pediatric providers to recognize and appreciate the potential for psychological impairment in children with chronic conditions. Mental

Box 2.5	Integration of Mental Health Services Into Primary Care

Use standardized screenings for all patients, not just those with assumed mental health needs or presentations.

Support integration of research into evidence-based practice recommendations for diagnosis and treatment of mental health.

Promote positive parenting practices to strengthen family connections and optimize social emotional health.

Deliver anticipatory guidance, health promotion, and recommended standardized screenings as recommended, to include mental health concerns.

Educate patients and their families about early signs of mental health presentations with tangible guidance how and when to access care for mental health presentations.

Treat commonly presenting and easily managed mental health conditions in primary care environments.

Encourage pediatric care providers to obtain additional specialty education and certification in mental health management.

Advocate for policies that support reimbursement for mental health services provided in primary care.

Develop a robust interprofessional network, including collaboration with mental health professionals and a strong referral network.

Enrich curricula in advanced practice registered nurse education to ensure adequate preparation for mental health services provision in primary care.

Modified from National Association of Pediatric Nurse Practitioners. (2020b). NAPNAP position statement on the integration of mental health care in pediatric primary care settings. https://www.jpedhc.org/article/S0891-5245(20)30128-0/pdf.

health presentations may initially manifest as global behavioral or achievement problems or aberrant behaviors (e.g., psychosomatic complaints, extreme apprehension, deliberate therapeutic nonadherence, or nontherapeutic communication) to family members and others. Adopting a mindset open to a clinical narrative inclusive of mental health, conducting a careful health history, and providing an atmosphere for collaborative, respectful discussion will help identify children at risk. Families should be interviewed together and separately with careful consideration of unique perspectives and honoring child voices in care planning. It is important to explore this possibility in discussions with all family members, stressing that information will be kept confidential unless the child is at risk. Because standardized behavioral screening instruments are not extensively validated with populations of children with chronic conditions, careful observation and in-depth interviewing with an individualized approach are important.

If no concerns are apparent, then the focus is on primary prevention, where holistic measures can be undertaken to promote optimal mental health. Therapeutic interventions include counseling, life and communication skills training, health education, support groups, or combinations of these to promote the development of resilience and coping skills. Referral to a mental health professional may be appropriate to help a child adapt to a new diagnosis or a deteriorating prognosis to manage complex diagnoses with comorbidities or conditions that do not respond to first-line interventions, including cognitive and pharmacologic interventions.

Secondary prevention seeks to treat emotional or mental distress symptoms early to prevent long-term sequelae of mental illness. When concerns are present, an accurate diagnosis in accordance with the *Diagnostic and Statistical Manual of Mental Disorders V-TR* (American Psychiatric Association, 2022) is important. After a diagnosis is established, appropriate interventions must be promptly initiated, including individual or group counseling or other behavioral interventions, judicious use of psychotropic medications, or referral to a mental health provider. Current insurance and health care delivery infrastructure, accompanied by family resistance to mental health intervention, can be a significant barrier to the referral process. Moreover, limited mobility may make seeking services while maintaining privacy difficult for children and families. Primary care providers can facilitate connection and care coordination.

HOSPITALIZATION

Hospitalization is not uncommon with this population of children, and care is usually transferred to the subspecialty team during this time. Pediatric primary care providers can assist in a smooth transition. In addition to giving information about the child's physical condition, parents must be encouraged to inform the subspecialty team about developmental enrichment programs, school services, or any other ancillary or programmatic support the child is receiving. If the hospitalization is planned, every effort should be made for hospital-based educators or tutors to confer with school officials before the child's admission to create a mutually agreed-upon plan to minimize school disruption. Pediatric care providers should be familiar with federally mandated, state-facilitated school-based services, including individualized education programs (IEPs) and 504s. Properly preparing the child and family—especially for new situations—also smooths the adjustment to hospitalization. Preparation must include procedural information about situations the child and family will encounter, definitions of medical jargon specific to the condition, and opportunities to process (i.e., through play, role-playing, or discussion) new situations they may experience. For families who are nonassertive or overly aggressive, primary care providers can help to appropriately empower the child and family members for self-advocacy by working through these tasks.

Monitoring the child's adjustment to hospitalization and how it affects their future development is also an important part of advocacy. A child's personality and the severity of the condition affect adaptation to hospitalization. Hospitalization is an intrusion into the lives of many children with chronic conditions, but other children have positive memories of previous hospitalizations and may see the hospital as a safe and familiar environment. Children may perceive the staff as friends and are often relieved to have a temporary respite from the stress of school, the harassment of other children, or the demands of daily activities. Primary care providers need to recognize that some children will occasionally seek hospitalization intentionally to remove themselves from home or particularly onerous school situations, although this is uncommon.

PALLIATIVE CARE

Palliative care is designed to relieve, rather than cure, symptoms caused by a child's condition. Palliative care helps children live more comfortably and improves their quality of life. It is not limited to dying children but is appropriate for all children with severe chronic conditions for which there is no cure. Palliative care services are vastly underused. Families often confuse palliative care with hospice care and fear a recommendation for palliative care means the health care team has given up hope for their child. Primary care providers must understand the differences between palliative and hospice care and communicate these clearly to the families.

Palliative care should be integrated into the care of children diagnosed with severe or profound disabilities or life-threatening or terminal conditions, regardless of the outcome. Even when restorative treatments are still being tried, palliative care measures can be instituted. Palliative care teams can assist with complex pain, symptom management, quality of life, prognostic appraisal, goal setting, and family support (Linebarger et al., 2022). The emphasis should be on symptom management, including pain, gastrointestinal complaints (e.g., nausea, vomiting, constipation, diarrhea), and psychosocial distress (e.g., anger, anxiety, depression, suicide ideation). Primary care providers need to be comfortable providing or referring for palliative care, whether directly or in tandem with a multidisciplinary palliative care team.

DYING AND HOSPICE CARE

The medical home and primary care providers are crucial for children who are dying and require hospice. For children with a downward clinical course, early discussions of hospice care before all curative options are exhausted are appropriate. End-of-life conversations should utilize a trauma-informed and culturally sensitive approach (Linebarger et al., 2022). End-of-life management can occur in many settings, including primary care provider clinic appointments, home-based settings, and intensive care units. Hospitalization and home care have advantages and disadvantages, and

the decision of which to pursue should be coordinated with the child's wishes and the family's capabilities, resources, and support network. Although some parents and children may feel more secure being in the hospital and surrounded by professionals they trust, increasingly families are choosing for children to die at home where they are in familiar surroundings, separation is minimized, care is individualized, and they are in greater control of their situation. Primary care providers can be instrumental in facilitating either option.

For families who choose for their child to die at home, primary care providers, as members of the larger interdisciplinary team, help plan for a seamless transition from hospital to home and provide hospice care during this difficult time. The need to identify child-appropriate services is critical when arranging hospice home care services for dying children and their families. Home hospice agencies that provide pediatric services need to provide not only appropriate end-of-life care for children of various ages but also bereavement counseling to other family members, including siblings.

Many hospice agencies are less comfortable managing the care of dying children, and pediatric hospice care is not always available. Therefore the primary care provider needs to remain closely involved in coordinating the child's care, regularly communicating with hospice staff and family members while supporting hospice caregivers in managing symptoms and prescribing medications. The primary care provider must be respectful of and responsive to the family's culture, spiritual belief system, and rituals.

Children should participate in decision making to the fullest extent possible. Primary care providers need to acknowledge that children frequently are aware of their impending death and help them communicate their wishes to their families and others. Some adolescents with chronic, life-threatening conditions may seek to discontinue treatment, and providers must balance the adolescents' and their parents' desires and help mediate these conversations with the help of a hospital's ethics committee or palliative care/hospice personnel, which can assist with shared decision making and advance care planning (Linebarger et al., 2022).

The psychosocial and emotional needs and fears of dying children need to be addressed from their cognitive level of development. Children often become anxious or depressed and should be reassured that they are not responsible for their illness and encouraged to talk about their feelings or express them. Pharmacologic interventions may be considered. Primary care providers can help family members with this by modeling ways to communicate these sensitive issues and offering insights into how children's developmental levels affect their ability to conceptualize death. Many children are deeply spiritual, and their faith should be acknowledged and respected. Helping family members and other significant individuals communicate effectively with the child and each other makes death easier to bear. The primary care provider continues to have a responsibility in the child's care after their death as the family may require support following the death of the child.

SUMMARY

Children with chronic conditions are at a higher risk for detrimental developmental sequelae than their nonaffected peers. The severity and persistence of the condition, the child's individual traits, family functioning, and the available network of social and structural supports all influence the child's developmental outcomes. Comprehensive prospective care can often eliminate or significantly ameliorate negative outcomes. Careful assessment using an interdisciplinary approach helps identify potential or emerging problems associated with the child's disease progression, functional status, social interactions, or global development. Individualized intervention strategies—including therapeutic management, education, counseling, and advocacy—can be designed and implemented to help children with chronic conditions reach their developmental potential. Partnering with families is essential to ensure optimal outcomes.

RESOURCES

BRIGHT FUTURES

A national health promotion and disease prevention initiative that addresses children's health needs in the context of family and community. Diverse resources are available to help improve and maintain the health of all children and adolescents.
    Website: www.brightfutures.aap.org

CHILDREN'S HOSPICE AND PALLIATIVE CARE COALITION

A social movement led by children's hospitals, hospices, home health, and grassroots agencies to improve care for children with life-threatening conditions and their families.
65 Nielson St. #108
Watsonville, CA 95076
(831) 763-3070
Website: www.childrenshospice.org

FAMILY VOICES

A national grassroots network that advocates for health care services and provides information for families with children and youth with special health care needs.
3411 Candelaria NE, Suite M
Albuquerque, NM 87107
(888) 835-5669
Website: www.familyvoices.org

STARLIGHT STARBRIGHT CHILDREN'S FOUNDATION

Improves the quality of life for children with serious medical conditions by providing entertainment, education, and family activities that help them cope with the pain, fear, and isolation of prolonged illness.
5757 Wilshire Blvd., Suite M100
Los Angeles, CA 90036
(310) 479-1212
Website: www.starlight.org

REFERENCES

Alley, J., Owen, R. Y., Wawrzynski, S. E., Lasrich, L., Ahmmad, Z., Utz, R., & Adkins, D. E. (2021). Illness, Social disadvantage, and sexual risk behavior in adolescence and the transition to adulthood. *Archives of Sexual Behavior, 50*(1), 205–217. doi:10.1007/s10508-020-01747-2.

American Academy of Pediatrics. 2022. *Developmental surveillance and screening.* https://www.aap.org/en/patient-care/developmental-surveillance-and-screening-patient-care/.

American Psychiatric Association. (2022). *Diagnostic and statistical manual of mental disorders* (5th ed, text revision). Author.

Bai, H., van Herten, M., Landgraf, J., Korfage, I., & Raat, H. (2017). Childhood chronic conditions and health related quality of life: Findings from a large population-based study. *PloS One, 12*(6), e0178539. doi:10.1371/journal.pone.0178539.

Bartek, N., Peck, J., Garzon, D., & VanCleve, S. (2021). Addressing the clinical impact of covid-19 on pediatric mental health. *Journal of Pediatric Health Care, 35*(4), 377–386.

Berk, L. E. (2006). *Development through the lifespan. Upper saddle river* (NJ). Allyn & Bacon.

Berk, L. E. (2017). *Development through the lifespan* (7th ed.). Allyn & Bacon.

Berry, J. G., Rodean, J., Hall, M., Alpern, E. R., Aronson, P. L., Freedman, S. B., Brousseau, D. C., Shah, S. S., Simon, H. K., Cohen, E., Marin, J. R., Morse, R. B., O'Neill, M., & Neuman, M. I. (2017). Impact of chronic conditions on emergency department visits of children using medicaid. *The Journal of Pediatrics, 182,* 267–274. https://doi.org/10.1016/j.jpeds.2016.11.054.

Betz, C. L. (2007). Facilitating the transition of adolescents with developmental disabilities: Nursing practice issues and care. *Journal of Pediatric Nursing, 22,* 103–115.

Betz, C. L., Lobo, M. L., Nehring, W. M., & Bui, K. (2013). Voices not heard: A systematic review of adolescents' and emerging adults' perspectives of health care transition. *Nursing Outlook, 61*(5), 311–336. doi:10.1016/j.outlook.2013.01.008.

Betz, C. L., & Redcay, G. (2002). Lessons learned from providing transition services to adolescents with special health care needs. *Issues in Comprehensive Pediatric Nursing, 25,* 129–149.

Brady, A., Deighton, J., & Stansfeld, S. (2021). Chronic illness in childhood and early adolescence: A longitudinal exploration of co-occurring mental illness. *Developmental Psychopathology, 33*(3), 885–898. doi:10.1017/S0954579420000206.

Brown, A., Noone, K., Rapee, R. M., Kangas, M., Anderson, V., & Bayer, J. K. (2022). Preventing internalizing problems in preschoolers with chronic physical health conditions. *Journal of Child Health Care, 26*(2), 228–241. doi:10.1177/13674935211013192.

Burke, S. O., Kauffmann, E., LaSalle, J., Harrison, M. B., & Wong, C. (2000). Parents' perceptions of chronic illness trajectories. *The Canadian Journal of Nursing Research = Revue Canadienne De Recherche En Sciences Infirmieres, 32*(3), 19–36.

Cantrell, M. A. (2007). Health-related quality of life in childhood cancer: State of the science. *Oncology Nursing Forum, 34,* 103–111.

Carbone, P., Smith, P. J., Lewis, C., & LeBlanc, C. (2021). Promoting the participation of children and adolescents with disabilities in sports, recreation, and physical activity. *Pediatrics (Evanston), 148*(6), 1–. https://doi.org/10.1542/peds.2021-054664.

Carroll, L., Graff, C., Wicks, M., & Diaz Thomas, A. (2020). Living with an invisible illness: a qualitative study exploring the lived experiences of female children with congenital adrenal hyperplasia. *Quality of Life Research, 29*(3), 673–681. doi:10.1007/s11136-019-02350-2.

Catarino, M., Charepe, Z., & Festas, C. (2021). Promotion of self-management of chronic disease in children and teenagers: A scoping review. *Healthcare (Basel), 9*(12), 1642.

Chew, J., Carpenter, J., & Haase, A. M. (2018). Young people's experiences of living with epilepsy: The significance of family resilience. *Social Work in Health Care, 57*(5), 332–354. doi:10.1080/00981389.2018.1443195.

Christia., B., D'Auria, J. P., & Fox, L. C. (1999). Gaining freedom: Self-responsibility in adolescents with diabetes. *Pediatrics, 25*, 255–260. , 266.

Coffey, J. S. (2006). Parenting a child with chronic illness: A metasynthesis. *Pediatric Nursing, 32*, 51–59.

Committee on Child Abuse and Neglect and Committee on Children with Disabilities. (2001). Assessment of maltreatment of children with disabilities. *Pediatrics, 108*, 508–512.

Council on Children with Disabilities; Council on Sports Medicine and Fitness. (2021). Promoting the participation of children and adolescents with disabilities in sports, recreation, and physical activity. American Academy of Pediatrics. *Pediatrics, 148*(6), e2021054664.

Crocker, A. G., & Smith, S. N. (2019). Person-first language: Are we practicing what we preach? *Journal of Multidisciplinary Healthcare, 12*, 125–129.

Erdmann, F., Frederiksen, L. E., Bonaventure, A., Mader, L., Hasle, H., Robison, L. L., & Winther, J. F. (2021). Childhood cancer: Survival, treatment modalities, late effects and improvements over time. *Cancer Epidemiology, 71*(Pt B), 101733. https://doi.org/10.1016/j.canep.2020.101733.

Farmer, J. E., Clark, M. J., Sherman, A., Marien, W. E., & Selva, T. J. (2005). Comprehensive primary care for children with special health care needs in rural areas. *Pediatrics, 116*(3), 649–656. https://doi.org/10.1542/peds.2004-0647.

Farzal, Z., Kou, Y.-F, St. John, R., Shah, G. B., & Mitchell, R. B. (2016). The role of routine hearing screening in children with cystic fibrosis on aminoglycosides: A systematic review. *Laryngoscope, 126*(1), 228–235. doi:10.1002/lary.25409.

Frank, R. G., Thayer, J. F., Hagglund, K. J., Vieth, A. Z., Schopp, L. H., Beck, N. C., Kashani, J. H., Goldstein, D. E., Cassidy, J. T., Clay, D. L., Chaney, J. M., Hewett, J. E., & Johnson, J. C. (1998). Trajectories of adaptation in pediatric chronic illness: the importance of the individual. *Journal of Consulting and Clinical Psychology, 66*(3), 521–532. https://doi.org/10.1037//0022-006x.66.3.521.

Freud, A. (1966). *The ego mechanism of defense.* International Universities Press.

Friedrichsdorf, S. J., & Kang, T. I. (2007). The management of pain in children with life-limiting illnesses. *Pediatric Clinics of North America, 54*, 645–672.

Garwick, A. W., Patterson, J. M., Meschke, L. L., Bennett, F., & Blum, R. (2002). The uncertainty of preadolescents' chronic health conditions and family distress. *Journal of Child and Family Nursing, 8*, 11–31.

Garzon Maaks, D., Barber Starr, N., Brady, M., Gaylord, N., Driessnack, M., & Duderstadt, K. (2020). *Burns' pediatric primary care.* Elsevier.

Glascoe, F. P. (1999). Using parents' concerns to detect and address developmental and behavioral problems. *Journal of Society of Pediatric Nurses, 4*, 24–35.

Graef, J. W., Wolfsdorf, J. I., & Greenes, D. S. (2008). *Manual of Pediatric Therapeutics.* Lippincott Williams & Wilkins.

Hallas, D. (Ed.). (2019). *Behavioral pediatric healthcare for nurse practitioners: A growth and developmental approach to intercepting abnormal behaviors.* Springer.

Hommel, K., Ramset, R., Rick, K., & Ryan, J. (2017). *Adherence to pediatric treatment regimes.* In *Handbook of pediatric psychology.* Guilford Press.

Horner-Johnson, W., Senders, A., Higgins Tejera, C., & McGee, M. G. (2021). Sexual health experiences among high school students with disabilities. *Journal of Adolescent Health, 69*(2), 255–262. doi:10.1016/j.jadohealth.2021.03.001.

Iannucci, J., & Nierenberg, B. (2022). Suicide and suicidality in children and adolescents with chronic illness: A systematic review. *Aggression and Violent Behavior, 64*, 101581. doi:10.1016/j.avb.2021.101581.

Immelt, S. (2006). Psychological adjustment in young children with chronic medical conditions. *Journal of Pediatric Nursing, 21*, 362–377.

Joachim, G., & Acorn, S. (2000). Stigma of visible and invisible chronic conditions. *Journal of Advanced Nursing, 32*, 243–248.

Knafl, K. A., & Gillis, C. L. (2002). Families and chronic illness: A synthesis of current research. *Journal of Family Nursing, 8*, 178–198.

Lankhorst, K., Takken, T., Zwinkels, M., van Gaalen, L., Te Velde, S., Backx, G. F., Verschuren, O., Wittink, H., & de Groot, J. (2021). Sports participation, physical activity, and health-related fitness in youth with chronic disease and physical disabilities: The health in adapted youth sports study. *Journal of Strength and Conditioning Research, 35*(8), 2327–2337.

Lewis, P., Klineberg, E., Towns, S., Moore, K., & Steinbeck, K. (2017). The effects of introducing peer support to young people with a chronic illness. *Journal of Child and Family Studies, 25*, 2541–2553.

Linebarger, J. S., Johnson, V., & Boss, R. D. (2022). Guidance for pediatric end-of-life care. *Pediatrics, 149*(5). https://doi.org/10.1542/peds.2022-057011.

Lipkin, P., & Macias, M. M. (2020). Promoting optimal development: Identifying infants and young children with developmental disorders through developmental surveillance and screening. *Pediatrics (Evanston), 145*(1), 1. doi:10.1542/peds.2019-3449.

Low, J., & Manias, E. (2019). Use of technology-based tools to support adolescents with chronic disease: Systematic review and meta-analysis. *Journal of Medical and Internet Research, 7*(7), e12042.

Maclean, M., Sims, S., Bower, C., Leonard, H., Stanley, F. J., & O'Donnell, M. (2017). Maltreatment risk among children with disabilities. *Pediatrics (Evanston), 139*(4), 1. doi:10.1542/peds.2016-1817.

McCarthy, A. (2015). Summer camp for children and adolescents with chronic conditions. *Pediatric Nursing, 41*(5), 245–250.

Meijer, S. A., Sinnema, G., Bijstra, J. O., Mellenbergh, G. J., & Wolters, W. H. G. (2002). Coping styles and locus of control as predictors for psychological adjustment of adolescents with a chronic illness. *Social Science & Medicine, 54*(9), 1453–1461. https://doi.org/10.1016/S0277-9536(01)00127-7.

Melnyk, B. M., Moldenhauer, Z., Veenema, T., Gullo, S., McMurtrie, M., O'Leary, E., Small, L., & Tuttle, J. (2001). The KySS (Keep your children/yourself Safe and Secure) campaign: a national effort to reduce psychosocial morbidities in children and adolescents. *Journal of Pediatric Health Care: Official Publication of National Association of Pediatric Nurse Associates & Practitioners, 15*(2), 31A–34A. https://doi.org/10.1067/mph.2001.113665.

Menendez, D., Hernandez, I. G., & Rosengren, K. S. (2020). Children's emerging understanding of death. *Child Development Perspectives, 14*(1), 55–60. doi:10.1111/cdep.12357.

Moavero, R., Santarone, M. E., Galasso, C., & Curatolo, P. (2017). Cognitive and behavioral effects of new antiepileptic drugs in pediatric epilepsy. *Brain & Development (Tokyo. 1979), 39*(6), 464–469. doi:10.1016/j.braindev.2017.01.006.

National Association of Pediatric Nurse Practitioners. 2020a. Supporting the transition from pediatric to adult-focused health care. https://www.napnap.org/position-statements-and-white-papers/.

National Association of Pediatric Nurse Practitioners. 2020b. NAPNAP position statement on the integration of mental health care in pediatric primary care settings. https://www.jpedhc.org/article/S0891-5245(20)30128-0/pdf.

National Center for Chronic Disease Prevention and Health Promotion. 2017. Chronic health conditions and academic achievement. https://www.cdc.gov/healthyschools/chronic_conditions/pdfs/2017_02_15-CHC-and-Academic-Achievement_Final_508.pdf.

National Network of Child Psychiatry Access Programs I (2022). Integrating physical and behavioral health for every child. https://www.nncpap.org/.

Pinquart, M. (2017). Systematic review: Bullying involvement of children with and without chronic physical illness and/or physical/sensory disability-a meta-analytic comparison with healthy/nondisabled peers. *Journal of Pediatric Psychology, 42*(3), 245–259. doi:10.1093/jpepsy/jsw081.

Qiu, Y., Xu, L., Pan, Y., He, C., Huang, Y., Xu, H., Lu, Z., & Dong, C. (2021). Family resilience, parenting styles and psychosocial adjustment of children with chronic illness: A cross-sectional study. *Frontiers in Psychiatry, 12*, 646421. doi:10.3389/fpsyt.2021.646421.

Rodriguez, K. E., Bibbo, J., & O'Haire, M. E. (2020). The effects of service dogs on psychosocial health and wellbeing for individuals with physical disabilities or chronic conditions. *Disability and rehabilitation, 42*(10), 1350–1358. https://doi.org/10.1080/09638288.2018.1524520

Rohan, J., & Verma, T. (2020). Psychological considerations in pediatric chronic illness: Case examples. *International Journal of Environmental Research and Public Health, 17*(5), 1644.

Santucci, G., & Mack, J. W. (2007). Common gastrointestinal symptoms in pediatric palliative care: Nausea, vomiting, constipation, anorexia, cachexia. *Pediatric Clinics of North America, 54*, 673–689.

Schmidt., C. K. (2001). Development of children's body knowledge, using knowledge of the lungs as an exemplar. *Issues in Comprehensive Pediatric Nursing, 24*, 177–191.

Schwartz, C. L., Hobbie, W., Constine, L. S., & Ruccione, K. (2015). *Survivors of Childhood and Adolescent Cancer: A multidisciplinary approach.* Springer.

Sengül, Y., & Kurudirek, F. (2022). Perceived stigma and self-esteem for children with epilepsy. *Epilepsy Research, 186*, 107017. doi:10.1016/j.eplepsyres.2022.107017.

Slaughter, V., & Griffiths, M. (2007). Death understanding and fear of death in young children. *Clinical Child Psychology and Psychiatry, 12*, 525–535.

Smolkin, T., Steinberg, M., Sujov, P., Mezer, E., Tamir, A., & Makhoul, I. R. (2008). Late postnatal systemic steroids predispose to retinopathy of prematurity in very-low-birth-weight infants: a comparative study. *Acta Paediatrica (Oslo, Norway: 1992), 97*(3), 322–326. https://doi.org/10.1111/j.1651-2227.2008.00629.x.

Spencer, N., Devereux, E., Wallace, A., Sundrum, R., Shenoy, M., Bacchus, C., & Logan, S. (2005). Disabling conditions and registration for child abuse and neglect: a population-based study. *Pediatrics, 116*(3), 609–613. https://doi.org/10.1542/peds.2004-1882.

Stewart., J. L. (2003). Children living with chronic illness: An examination of their stressors, coping responses, and health outcomes. *Annual Review of Nursing Research, 21*, 203–243.

Stewart, J. L., & Mishel, M. H. (2000). Uncertainty in childhood illness: A synthesis of the parent and child literature. *Scholarly Inquiry in Nursing Practice, 14*, 299–319.

Stubbe, D. (2018) Complementary and alternative medicine: If you don't ask, they won't tell 16 (pp. 60–62). *American Psychiatric Publishing* (pp. 60–62)

Szulczewski, L., Mullins, L. L., Bidwell, S. L., Eddington, A. R., & Pai, A. L. H. (2017). Meta-analysis: Caregiver and youth uncertainty in pediatric chronic illness. *Journal of Pediatric Psychology, 42*(4), 395–421. doi:10.1093/jpepsy/jsw097.

Traino, K. A., Bakula, D. M., Sharkey, C. M., Roberts, C. M., Ruppe, N. M., Chaney, J. M., & Mullins, L. L. (2019). The role of grit in health care management skills and health-related quality of life in college students with chronic medical conditions. *Journal of Pediatric Nursing, 46*, 72–77. doi:10.1016/j.pedn.2019.02.035.

Turnidge, J. (2003). Pharmacodynamics and dosing of aminoglycosides. *Infectious Disease Clinics of North America, 17*, 503–528.

Vessey, J. A. (1999). Psychologic comorbidity and chronic conditions. *Pediatric Nursing, 25*, 211–214.

Villagomez, A. N., Muñoz, F. M., Peterson, R. L., Colbert, A. M., Gladstone, M., MacDonald, B., Wilson, R., Fairlie, L., Gerne, G., Patterson, J., Boghossian, N., Burton, V., Cortes, M., Katikaneni, L., Larson, J., Angulo, A., Joshi, J., Nesin, M., Padula, M., Padula, S., et al. (2019). Neurodevelopmental delay: Case definition & guidelines for data collection, analysis, and presentation of immunization safety data. *Vaccine, 37*(52), 7623–7641. doi:10.1016/j.vaccine.2019.05.027.

Yim, C. L., Tam, M., Chan, H. L., Tang, S. M., Au, S. C. L., Yip, W. W. K., Ko, S. T. C., Rong, S. S., Chen, L. J., Ng, D. S., & Yam, J. C. S. (2018). Association of antenatal steroid and risk of retinopathy of prematurity: a systematic review and meta-analysis. *The British Journal of Ophthalmology, 102*(10), 1336–1341. https://doi.org/10.1136/bjophthalmol-2017-311576.

Yu, J., Perrin, J. M., Hagerman, T., & Houtrow, A. J. (2021). Underinsurance among children in the United States. *Pediatrics, 149*(1). https://doi.org/10.1542/peds.2021-050353.

Zubler, J. M., Wiggins, L. D., Macias, M. M., Whitaker, T. M., Shaw, J. S., Squires, J. K., Pajek, J. A., Wolf, R. B., Slaughter, K. S., Broughton, A. S., Gerndt, K. L., Mlodoch, B. J., & Lipkin, P. H. (2022). *Evidence-Informed Milestones for Developmental Surveillance Tools. Pediatrics, 149*(3), e2021052138. https://doi.org/10.1542/peds.2021-052138.

School and the Child With a Chronic Condition

3

Jennifer Hill, Wendy Lord Mackey, Neesha Ramchandani

In the United States, almost half of school-aged children ages 6 to 17 years have at least one chronic health condition (National Survey of Children's Health, 2020–2021). It is therefore important to understand these children's rights, provisions for, and care in the school setting.

ROLE OF SCHOOL IN A CHILD'S LIFE

School plays a vital role in children's lives. It is the second most influential environment for children after that of the family (Council on School Health [COSH], 2016). School plays an influential role in children's development of their sense of self and understanding of their place in relation to their peers. School participation is especially important for children with chronic conditions because it gives them a chance to interact with their peers and participate in, or at the very least be exposed to, normal childhood activities (Lum et al., 2017). Most children genuinely enjoy school despite any protestations. This may be particularly true for children with chronic conditions because they may have fewer opportunities to socialize outside the school setting. Additionally, including children with various chronic ailments in school and extracurricular activities can also benefit their peers in developing a sense of acceptance and respect for individuals with special needs.

In the United States, legislation has been in place since the 1970s to ensure all children, including those with chronic conditions, receive the education they are entitled to (Cornett & Knackstedt, 2020). This is discussed in more detail later. Recent data have found that approximately 90% of US children are in the primary and secondary public school system (Research.com, 2023), a number that has remained relatively stable over the past few decades (Riley-Lawless, 2006).

LAWS ON EDUCATION OF CHILDREN WITH CHRONIC CONDITIONS

"In these days, it is doubtful that any child may reasonably be expected to succeed in life if he is denied the opportunity of an education. Such an opportunity […] is a right which must be made available to all on equal terms."

Brown v. Board of Education, 1954, p. 875

The provision of free public elementary and secondary education is a right of all children regardless of race, ethnic background, religion, gender, or citizenship, as well as the presence or absence of disability as declared by the 14th Amendment to the US Constitution. This is an expansion of the Universal Declaration of Human Rights of 1948, article 26, stating everyone has the right to education.

Legislative and judicial rulings over the past half century have dramatically improved the role of public educational institutions in providing services to children with chronic conditions. The modern-day education rights of children with disabilities in the United States are the result of three landmark court decisions and governing laws enacted by Congress (Cornett & Knackstedt, 2020). This change in public policy began with the civil rights movement when the landmark decision of Brown v. Board of Education (1954) banned segregated schools and affirmed education as a right of all US citizens. The principle of "separate is not equal" was used almost 20 years later in Pennsylvania Association for Retarded Citizens v. Pennsylvania (1972) to challenge the state's right to exclude children with intellectual disabilities from public education (National Council on Disability, 2000). That same year, the Supreme Court ruled that a free and public education must be provided to all school-age children regardless of disability or degree of impairment (Mills v. Board of Education of the District of Columbia, 1972). This momentous Supreme Court decision paved the way for the federal government to enact legislation supporting public education for all children regardless of their health or ability.

Currently, the educational rights of children with disabilities attending schools are governed by four federal laws: Rehabilitation Act Section 504, Individuals with Disabilities Act (IDEA), Americans with Disabilities Act (ADA), and Every Student Succeeds Act (ESSA). Section 504 and IDEA civil laws are enforced by the US Department of Education Office for Civil Rights as their programs and activities receive federal funding (Lee, 2018). ADA is enforced by the US Department of Justice and the Office for Civil Rights; laws specific to education and health are under the jurisdiction of each state, obliging them to protect, respect, advocate, and provide education to all children within their borders,

49

| Table 3.1 | Comparison of Civil Rights Laws for Children With Disabilities | | | |

WHAT THESE LAWS PROVIDE	IDEA	SECTION 504	ADA
Legal rights for people with disabilities	x	x	x
An Individualized Education Plan (IEP) for eligible K–12 students	x		
Special education and related services to meet a student's unique needs	x		
A 504 plan for eligible K–12 students		x	
Accommodations (e.g., audiobooks, extra time to complete tasks) for K–12 students	x	x	
Accommodations for college students		x	
Reasonable accommodations in workplaces (with 15 or more employees)			x
A requirement that public schools find and evaluate (at no cost to families) children who may have a disability	x		
Education funding for schools	x		
A free appropriate public education (FAPE) in the least restrictive environment (LRE) for students	x	x	
Procedural safeguards that protect families' rights (e.g., access to school records)	x	x	
Due process (or an impartial hearing) for resolving disputes between families and schools	x	x	
Freedom from discrimination at private schools (including colleges and universities) that get federal funding		x	x
Freedom from discrimination in workplaces (with 15 or more employees)			x
Access to places that offer goods and services to the public (e.g., restaurants, websites)			x

Modified from Lee, A. IDEA, Section 504 and the ADA, which laws do what. https://www.understood.org/articles/at-a-glance-which-laws-do-what/. Accessed June 6, 2023.

including those with chronic conditions. Provisions of these laws vary greatly across the country and may vary even within a single school district. Table 3.1 provides a visual of provisions under each law.

Important statutory changes in language were formalized in 2010 with Rosa's law (PL 111-256), where any reference to mental retardation was changed to intellectual disability, and any reference to a mentally retarded individual was changed to an individual with intellectual disability in all US federal law (US Government Printing Office, 2010). This law was enacted in response to a parent of a child with Down syndrome who lobbied to eliminate the derogatory term and replace it with inclusive, people-first language that describes an individual's thinking ability (Special Olympics, 2010). This coincided with a revolution sweeping the nation to eliminate the R-word to show respect for a population stigmatized throughout history.

REHABILITATION ACT SECTION 504

The Rehabilitation Act of 1973 (PL 93-112) was the first civil rights law for individuals with disabilities. It was enacted to prohibit discrimination of qualified persons based on disability. Section 504 of the Rehabilitation Act of 1973 (PL 93-112), a subsection of the act, was originally aimed at providing job opportunities and training to adults with disabilities; however, it is now interpreted as conferring the same rights and expectations to schools and the education of children with disabilities. It has two primary goals: the removal of barriers to education for children with disabilities and the prevention of discrimination against those with disabilities. Thus there is an emphasis on the right to reasonable accommodations to allow equal access to learning and activities. Section 504 states:

"No otherwise qualified individual with a disability in the United States, as defined in section 706(8) of this title, shall, solely by reason of her or his handicap, be excluded from participation in, be denied the benefits of, or be subjected to discrimination under any program or activity receiving Federal financial assistance or under any program or activity conducted by any Executive agency or by the United States Postal Service."

29 U.S.C. §794(a) (1973)

The act defines a person with a disability as someone who has a mental or physical impairment that significantly limits one or more major life activities, has a record of such impairment, or is regarded as having such impairment. As referenced in 34 Code of Federal Regulations Part 104.3, physical or mental impairment includes:

"(A) any physiological disorder, cosmetic disfigurement or anatomical loss affecting one or more of the following systems: respiratory, including speech; cardiovascular;

reproductive; digestive; genitourinary; hematologic and lymphatic; skin; and endocrine or (B) any mental or psychological disorder such as mental retardation, organic brain syndrome, emotional or mental illness and specific learning disabilities."

Furthermore, "major life activities" refers to self-care, performing manual tasks, walking, seeing, hearing, speaking, breathing, learning, and working. This list is not all inclusive, with other functions being considered major life activities. A student who has a chronic condition that meets one of the defined criteria is eligible for services provided by Section 504. It requires that the educational needs of the child with a disability be met, and strategies for classroom adaptation be implemented so the student can be educated as adequately as children without disabilities in the least restrictive environment (LRE).

The school administration is responsible for student accommodation plans (i.e., 504 plans). However, the 504 plan does not need to be written, does not include special education services, and applies to all levels of education, including college and university education. The plan provides a blueprint for the school to allow students full participation in school programming with a focus on removing barriers to learning. The key words in implementing this law are "reasonable accommodations." An accommodation may include changes in the environment, such as preferential seating in the classroom, test taking in a quiet environment, or integration of assistive technologic devices. For example, an accommodation may be as simple as allowing a child with Crohn disease to use the bathroom facilities in the nurse's office and having a signal to the teacher when the student must quickly exit the classroom or allowing a student with diabetes to keep glucose testing supplies or a snack on hand in the classroom. Children with hematologic or respiratory conditions may need accommodation in physical education that allows them to rest more often or avoid contact sports. Children with a food or latex allergy may need extensive plans that include cafeteria personnel, art teachers, classroom material purchasing considerations, and notifying families of other children in the class. Other accommodations may include extended time for assessments, organizational assistance, using behavioral management techniques, having exceptions made in the school's uniform policy, having an additional set of books at home, or alternative testing or homework/class assignments to demonstrate knowledge. Accommodation does not change what students learn, just how they learn it by maximizing access to learning and removing barriers to learning.

A school accommodation evaluation can be requested by the student, the student's parent or guardian, or any individual working with the student. The school may appoint a team to determine student eligibility for necessary accommodation. The assessment may include a meeting with the parent/guardian; classroom observation of the student; input from involved teachers, school nurse, support faculty; review of the medical records; or input from medical providers. The Office of Civil Rights in the US Department of Education has jurisdiction over the implementation of Section 504, and conflicts between parents and school districts are mediated through this office.

According to the Advocacy Institute (2015), national trends of students served under Section 504 alone represent 1.5% of overall student enrollment. Gender distribution is predominantly male (62.3% vs 37.7%) and does not vary significantly across states. There is a predominant overrepresentation of students identifying as White receiving 504 accommodations and an underrepresentation of Hispanic or Latino students. This trend is consistent in 49 of 51 states. New Hampshire has the highest percentage (4.8%) of students with 504 plans, and New Mexico and Wisconsin have the lowest (0.4%).

INDIVIDUALS WITH DISABILITIES EDUCATION IMPROVEMENT ACT

From a historical perspective, an early attempt at special education for children with disabilities was initially made in 1965 with the enactment of the Elementary and Secondary Education Act (PL 89-10). After several amendments, Congress passed the Education for All Handicapped Children Act (PL 94-142) in 1975, as an educational bill of rights entitling children with disabilities between the ages of 5 and 18 years to a free and appropriate public education (FAPE), including the provision of related services to those who qualify (Education for All Handicapped Children Act, 1975). Prior to this law, Congress identified 1 million children with disabilities excluded from the public school systems and 4 million who were denied appropriate educational services for equal opportunity (IDEA, 2021; US Department of Education, 2008a).

In 1986, PL 99-457 was passed, which included the Handicapped Infants and Toddlers Program, Part H (Infant and Toddler Program, 1986). PL 99-457 extended services to children from birth to 21 years of age and required interagency and interdisciplinary collaboration, the development of a child identification system, a care manager designated for the family, and the implementation of an individualized family service plan for children from birth through 2 years, analogous to the individualized educational program (IEP) for older children. This amendment dramatically increased the school systems' role in providing early intervention services to infants and toddlers at elevated risk for developing hindering conditions and preschool programs for children 3 to 5 years with developmental delays. These laws were ultimately updated and renamed in 1990 as the Individuals with Disabilities Education Act (PL 101-476). IDEA was reauthorized in 2004 (PL 108-446) and most recently amended in December 2015 through the ESSA (PL 114-95).

Today, IDEA is a federal law that entitles the provision of FAPE for eligible children from infancy through 21 years of age through early intervention and special education and related services (PL 94-142). IDEA defines FAPE as "special education and related services provided at public expense, under public supervision and direction, without charge and in conformity with an Individualized Educational Program (IEP) even if those children are advancing from grade to grade" (34 CFR S300.101). Eligible children refer to those with a disability that would adversely impact academic performance and therefore require and benefit from early intervention or special education services (Lipkin et al., 2015). In this law, Congress states:

"Disability is a natural part of the human experience and in no way diminishes the right of individuals to participate in or contribute to society. Improving educational results for children with disabilities is an essential element of our national policy of ensuring equality of opportunity, full participation, independent living, and economic self-sufficiency for individuals with disabilities."

IDEA, 20 U.S.C. §1400 General Provisions

The IDEA statute is divided into four parts:
- Part A contains general provisions, including the purpose, goals, and definitions.
- Part B is focused on Assistance for Education of All Children with Disabilities and describes how the federal government aids states in the education of children with disabilities from ages 3 to 21 years. It further outlines how state agencies must supervise and monitor the statute and outline the basic rights and responsibilities of children with disabilities and their parents or guardians.
- Part C is Infants and Toddlers with Disabilities; it outlines the early intervention services provided to infants and toddlers with disabilities and their families, birth through 2 years of age.
- Part D, National Activities to Improve Education of Children with Disabilities, authorizes programs to improve teacher preparation and credentialing in the education of children with disabilities (US Department of Education, 2008a). The final regulations were published in 2006.

The purpose of IDEA is to ensure that children with disabilities receive assistance with the additional educational needs that result from their disability so that they can progress in the general curriculum in an educational setting. The following are the basic legal principles and mandated components of IDEA (20 U.S.C. §1400):
1. *Zero reject.* A student cannot be excluded from a local school district because of a disability. Therefore even children with the most severe disabilities and those with significant health and medical needs must be included in the educational process.
2. *Child find.* The school district is responsible for identifying and locating children with disabilities from birth to age 21 and then for informing the parents of the available special education services. The identified children are to be evaluated at no cost to the families, and then the school must provide appropriate educational programs to these students.
3. *Nondiscriminatory testing.* Materials used for testing must be racially and culturally appropriate, "comprehensive and validated for the purpose for which they are being used and be administered by trained personnel" in a nondiscriminatory manner, and in the native language of the child (Centers for Disease Control and Prevention [CDC], 2008, p. 81). Parents may seek one independent evaluation at public expense if they disagree with the district's evaluation.
4. *FAPE.* This applies to all children with disabilities in the state where the family resides. This includes the opportunity to participate in physical education, including specially designed activities, if physical education is provided to nondisabled students.
5. *LRE.* This speaks to the placement of the child, with the regular classroom being the preferred site. Children with disabilities should be educated with their nondisabled peers. "Special classes, separate schooling, or other removal of children with disabilities from the regular education environment occurs only when the nature of the severity of the disability is such that education in regular classes with the use of supplementary aids and services cannot be achieved satisfactorily" (National Council on Disability, 2008, p. 91). Getting children with disabilities into regular classrooms was referred to as mainstreaming and inclusion. The premise of this principle is that all students, no matter how severe their disability, have some aspects of their development that are typical. (See the options for special education listed later.)
6. *Development of an IEP.* This is described in the following section and includes the educational program development process and the specific IEP.
7. *Procedural due process.* Due process is to be explained to the families and followed for mediation and for resolving conflicts among parents, school personnel, and educational professionals. It includes the evaluation process, protection of parental participation rights, and prevention of expelling a student or changing a student's educational placement without following due process.
8. *Parental participation.* Parents are to be involved in developing an IEP. They must provide consent for the initial evaluation as well as for follow-up evaluations, and their participation in the decisions made about placement and accommodation should be supported. Parents should be encouraged and supported in speaking up for the needs of their children. They should have access to all.

Individualized Education Program
The key component of IDEA was the development of the IEP; it is mandated for every student who qualifies under IDEA. The IEP should outline the accommodations and

Members of the Individualized Educational Program Team, as Required Under the Individuals With Disabilities Education Act of 2004

- Parents/guardians of the child
- At least one regular teacher of the child
- At least one special education teacher or paraprofessional of the child—a school district representative who is qualified to provide/supervise the provision of special education, knowledgeable about the general curriculum, knowledgeable about the availability of district resources
- An individual who can interpret the instructional implications of the evaluation results
- At the discretion of the parent or the school district, other individuals who have knowledge or special expertise about the child, such as a health care provider
- When appropriate, the child with the disability

instructional approaches necessary to allow the child to participate in the learning environment and to progress in the same curriculum as the child's peers. The desired academic content standards should be those set by the state under ESSA (PL 114-95).

The team that determines eligibility and develops the IEP must include the parents/guardians of the child, at least one regular education teacher of the child, at least one special education teacher of the child, a representative of the public agency, and someone who can interpret the instructional implications of the evaluation (this could be the psychologist who administered the tests). Whenever it is appropriate, the child should also be included. Box 3.1 lists the people required by law to be part of the IEP team. This team is also responsible for evaluating the child's progress toward the goals, determining if the plan is effective, and making changes as needed. A complete reevaluation is required at least every 3 years; if it is done more frequently, by law, it does not have to be done more than once a year (Lipkin et al., 2015).

The law requires that testing evaluations be free and the child be evaluated in all areas related to the suspected disability: health, vision, hearing, social and emotional status, general intelligence, academic performance, communication ability, and motor abilities. Input from the parents/guardians, teachers, and other professionals with knowledge of the child's condition is included in the evaluation process. Evaluations done previously or external to the school setting can also be submitted for review during this preplacement phase. These preplacement evaluations are often helpful in documenting the child's abilities and disabilities. The preplacement must be comprehensive enough to determine eligibility and what related accommodations or services the child will need. The findings from this evaluation process serve as the foundation for the child's IEP. This is also where input from primary care and specialty health care providers would be most beneficial.

Informed parental consent must be obtained prior to conducting an initial evaluation or reevaluation. The parents/guardians must be given information about IDEA, special education services, related services, parental rights, and the appeal process. IDEA requires that procedural safeguards be established to protect the rights of the parents/guardians and the child. Once initiated, the school system has 60 workdays to complete the preplacement evaluation process.

The IEP must include the present level of the child's academic and functional performance, including how the disability or chronic condition affects the child's ability to learn or participate in the learning environment; outline measurable academic and functional goals annually and short-term objectives for children with significant cognitive disabilities; describe how and when the child's progress will be measured and reported; list the specific interventions that will be provided, including the amount of special education and related services that will be provided, the supplementary aids and accommodations that are needed, and the extent to which the child will not participate with nondisabled peers in a regular class or school activities; provide dates and places where services will be provided; and, by age 16, make transition plans for postsecondary goals (Rief, 2016). Box 3.2 provides a summary of content included in a student's IEP document.

Special education is defined by IDEA as specially designed instruction that meets the unique needs of a student with a disability through adaptation of the content, methodology, or delivery of instruction. Special education services can be provided in a regular classroom, special classroom or facility, home, private nonprofit preschool, private school, college, hospital, and even state prison. Placement falls under the principle of the LRE. Children eligible for services who attend private schools are still eligible through the public school system, but parents will need to bring them to public schools for placement evaluation services.

Of school-age students served under IDEA in Fall 2020, 95% were enrolled in public schools; 3% of students served under IDEA were enrolled in separate schools (public or private) for students with disabilities, 2% were placed in regular private schools, and less than 1% each were home schooled or in hospitals, in separate residential facilities (public or private), or in correctional facilities.

Inclusion is the term used when a child receiving special education services is in a regular day care, preschool, or school program. This environment is seen as the least restrictive, providing children with the fullest educational potential. They receive special education services (e.g., speech, physical therapy, occupational therapy) in the classroom or are removed briefly for services and then return to the classroom when the intervention is completed.

Box 3.2   Content Included in an Individualized Educational Program (IEP) Document

A statement of the child's present levels of academic achievement and functional performance, including how the identified disability affects the child's progress in the school's general curriculum.

A statement of measurable annual goals, including academic and functional goals that address the child's needs and allow progress in the general education curriculum.

Special educational and related services and accommodations to be provided, including assistive technology devices. All services required to meet the educational goals, including supplemental aids (e.g., communication devices), must be identified.

An explanation of the extent, if any, as to which the child is not included in regular education programs with nondisabled children in the general education setting as well as extracurricular and nonacademic settings.

A statement of any individual accommodations necessary for participation in state and districtwide assessments. If the child cannot participate in these standard tests, alternative assessments aligned to alternative achievement standards, including short-term objectives, must be described, including how and when the child's progress toward meeting annual goals will be measured.

Projected date for the initiation of services and modifications and the anticipated frequency, location, and duration of the accommodations.

Beginning no later than the child's 16th birthday, the IEP must list measurable postsecondary goals based on age-appropriate transition assessment related to training, education, employment, and (when appropriate) independent living skills and transition services needed to assist the child in reaching these goals.

Beginning no later than 1 year before the child reaches the age of majority under state law, the IEP must include a statement that the child has been informed of rights under Part B of the Individuals with Disabilities Education Act, if any, that will transfer to the child on reaching the age of majority.

Children with severe disabilities or who are medically fragile will require services in special classrooms often found within regular school settings; in special schools, institutions, or hospitals; or at home (if the individual is unable to attend other facilities). Even children who are profoundly handicapped are required by law to receive educational services for a designated period each week.

Related services are defined by IDEA (§300.24) as "transportation and such developmental, corrective, and other supportive services as may be required to assist a child with a disability to benefit from special education and includes the early identification and assessment of disabling conditions in children." These services may be used in evaluating students with disabilities to determine needed services or augment the education and include services such as audiology, counseling, speech therapy, social work, nutritional services, physical therapy, occupational therapy, transportation,

and interpretation services. In some situations, a child may not need special education but may qualify and benefit for a related service only (Morin, 2023). The term also includes school health services such as of the school nurse and supplemental aids and supports needed to enable children with disabilities to be educated with their peers to the most appropriate extent (§300.3).

Children with disabilities whose parents place them in nonpublic schools are referred to as parentally placed private school children (§300.13, §300.36, §§300.145–300.147). These children are also eligible to receive the benefits and services under the law. It is the responsibility of local education agencies and state education agencies to ensure that children with disabilities participate equitably in the state's implementation of IDEA: "Parentally placed children with disabilities do not have an individual entitlement to services they would receive if they were enrolled in a public school. Instead, the local education agencies are required to spend a proportionate amount of IDEA federal funds to provide equitable services to this group of children" (US Department of Education, 2008b, p. 1). Therefore the services provided, if any, may be different from those provided in a public school.

According to the National Center for Education Statistics (2022), 7.2 million children living in the United States receive special education under IDEA, accounting for 15% of all public school students. To be eligible for services, the child must be adversely affected by one or more disabilities within IDEA categories (Box 3.3). Fig. 3.1 offers representation of percentages of students (3–21 years) by disability type served by IDEA.

From a race and ethnicity lens, the percentages of students receiving services through IDEA were fairly uniform, with the highest percentage of students identifying as American Indian/Alaskan Native (19%) and the lowest percentage of students identifying as Asian (8%) (National Center for Education Statistics, 2022). With respect to gender, in school-age students, 18% of male students received services versus 10% of female students (National Center for Education Statistics, 2022).

When considering students served by IDEA (aged 14–21 years) who exited the system, differences were noted by ethnicity/race and type of disability. Students identifying as Black had the lowest percentage (65%) who graduated from a regular high school and the highest graduating with an alternative diploma (12%) when compared to other groups (US Department of Education, 2022). Students graduating with a regular high school diploma were highest in students with speech and language impairments (85%) and lowest in children with multiple disabilities (45%). The highest percentage of students who dropped out were those with emotional disturbance (33%) and the lowest in students with autism (7%) (US Department of Education, 2022).

According to data from the academic year 2021-2022, 95% of students receiving IDEA services were enrolled

Box 3.3 **Categories of Disabilities Entitled to Special Education per the Individuals With Disabilities Education Act**

Autism: A developmental disability significantly affecting verbal and nonverbal communication and social interaction.
Deaf blindness: Children with both deafness and blindness; communication with others is severely impaired.
Deafness: Children with a hearing deficiency that impairs processing of linguistic information through hearing with or without amplification.
Hearing impairment: Permanent or fluctuating hearing loss that adversely affects the child's educational process.
Mental retardation: Significant subaverage general intelligence existing with deficits in adaptive behavior.
Multiple disabilities: Concomitant impairments other than deaf/blindness resulting in severe educational problems that cannot be addressed in a special education program solely for one impairment.
Orthopedic impairments: Severe orthopedic impairments that adversely affect the child's educational performance.
Other health impairments: Limited strength, vitality, or alertness, including a heightened alertness to environmental stimuli, that results in limited alertness with respect to the educational environment, resulting from chronic or acute health problems, such as asthma, a heart condition, lead poisoning, tuberculosis, rheumatic fever, nephritis, sickle cell anemia, hemophilia, epilepsy, leukemia, diabetes, attention-deficit/hyperactivity disorder, or Tourette syndrome, and that adversely affects a child's educational performance.
Serious emotional disturbance: A child who exhibits over a prolonged period one or more of the following characteristics: an inability to learn that cannot be explained by intellectual, sensory, or health factors; an inability to build or maintain satisfactory interpersonal relationships; inappropriate behavior or feelings; depression or unhappiness; and a tendency to develop physical symptoms or fears associated with personal or school problems.
Specific learning disability: A disorder in one or more of the psychological processes involved in understanding or using spoken or written language; term does not apply to children who have learning problems primarily caused by other disabilities listed here or environmental, cultural, or economic disadvantages.
Speech or language impairment: A communication disorder caused by impaired articulation, problems with language development, or voice impairment that adversely affects a child's educational performance.
Traumatic brain injury: Acquired injury to the brain resulting in total or partial functional and/or psychosocial impairment.
Visual impairments (including blindness): Visual impairments, including ones that can be corrected, that adversely affect a child's educational performance.

DISABILITIES AS DEFINED FOR CHILDREN 3–9 YEARS OF AGE
Children experiencing developmental delays, as defined by the state, in one or more of the following developmental areas: physical, cognitive, communication, social, emotional, or adaptive development.
Children meeting these requirements are eligible for services from their school district at age 3 years.

DISABILITIES AS DEFINED FOR INFANTS AND TODDLERS
Infants and toddlers from birth to age 2 years who (1) experience delay in cognitive, physical, communicative, social/emotional, or adaptive development; (2) are diagnosed with a physical or mental condition that has a high probability of resulting in developmental delay; or (3) are at risk of having developmental delays if early intervention services are not provided.

Modified from US Department of Education, Office of Special Education Programs. (2007). Children with disabilities receiving special education under part B of the Individuals with Disabilities Education Act. Office of Management and Budget No. 18200-043. US Government Printing Office.

in the public school system, 3% in schools for students with disabilities, 2% in private schools, and less than 1% were homebound, in hospitals, or in correctional facilities (National Center for Education Statistics, 2022). Sixty-six percent of these children spent 80% of their day mainstreamed in the general education classroom with their peers (US Department of Education, 2022). Over 363,000 infants and toddlers with disabilities and their families are enrolled in IDEA Part C, early intervention services (US Department of Education, 2022). Federal enforcement of IDEA is through the Office of Special Education and Rehabilitation Services in the US Department of Education through each state's office.

AMERICANS WITH DISABILITIES ACT

The Americans with Disabilities Act of 1990 (PL 101-336) is an antidiscrimination law that further protects the civil rights of individuals with disabilities in everyday life. Initially passed by Congress in 1990 and amended in 2008, ADA is based on the 1964 Civil Rights Act, which prohibited employment and accommodation discrimination by the private sector against women and racial and ethnic minorities. Before the ADA, no federal law prohibited discrimination against people with disabilities in the private sector. The federal government has a crucial role in enforcing the standards and ensuring individuals with disabilities have the same opportunities as those without disabilities in all public institutions, services, programs, or activities, regardless of whether they receive any federal funding (Office of Civil Rights, 2005).

Educational institutions are addressed specifically in Title II of the ADA, ensuring reasonable accommodations so that students with disabilities can participate in school activities and access school services (CDC, 2008). Educational opportunities, extracurricular activities, and facilities must be accessible to all students, parents, and employees regardless of ability, including anyone with a physical, sensory, cognitive, or mental disability of any severity.

Although this law has minimal effect on school programs, it has been extremely helpful in facilitating the

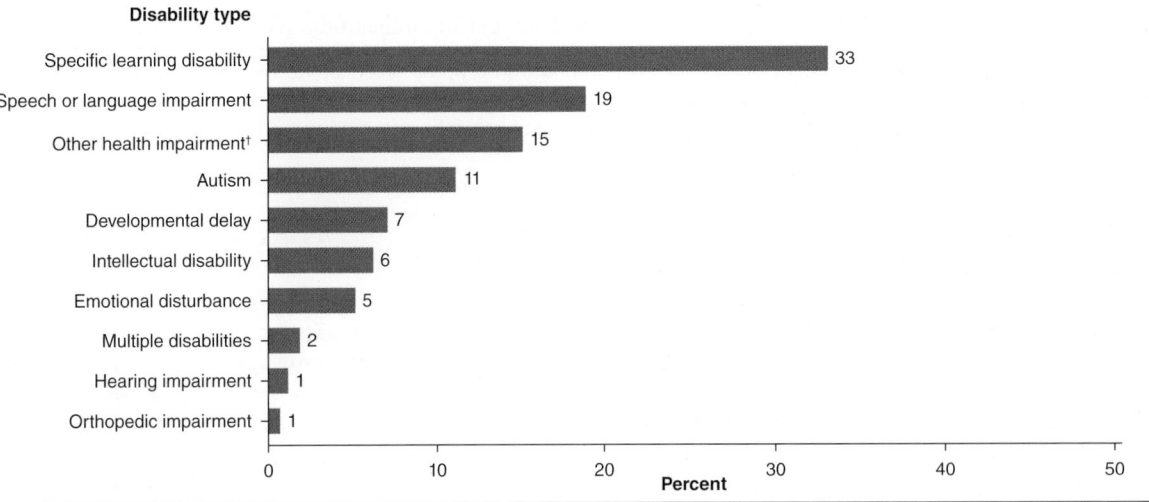

Disability type

† Other health impairments include having limited strength, vitality, or alertness due to chronic or acute health problems such as a heart condition, tuberculosis, rheumatic fever, nephritis, asthma, sickle cell anemia, hemophilia, epilepsy, lead poisoning, leukemia, or diabetes. Note: Data are for the 50 states and the District of Columbia only. Visual impairment, traumatic brain injury, and deaf-blindness are not shown because they each account for less than 0.5 percent of students served under IDEA. Due to categories not shown, detail does not sum to 100 percent. Although rounded numbers are displayed, the figures are based on unrounded data.

Fig. 3.1 Percentage of students (3–21years) by disability type served by the Individuals with Disabilities Education Act *(IDEA).* (From US Department of Education, Office of Special Education Programs. [2020]. IDEA section 618 data products: State level data files. https://www2.ed.gov/programs/osepidea/618-data/state-level-data-files/index.html#bcc.)

transition of students with disabilities into employment positions and independent housing, as well as ensuring accessibility for parents and staff with disabilities. ADA defines a person with a disability as one with a physical or mental impairment that limits one or more major life activities, has a history of such impairment, or is perceived by others as having an impairment. Supreme Court decisions have indicated that the disability must be present and limit the person's major life activities for them to be protected under the ADA. If a person's disability (i.e., severe myopia or severe hypertension) can be mitigated by corrective therapy, that individual is no longer protected under ADA (*Sutton v. United Airlines, Inc,* 119 S. Ct 2139, 1999; *Murphy v. United Parcel Service, Inc,* 119 S. Ct. 2133, 1999). ADA is enforced by the US Department of Justice and the Office for Civil Rights (Mayerson & Mayer, 2000).

EVERY STUDENT SUCCEEDS ACT

The No Child Left Behind Act (NCLB) (2001), built on the Elementary and Secondary Education Act of 1965, improved children's academic achievement and aimed to make schools more accountable for student outcomes. Although initially designed to assist children who were poor and disadvantaged, the intent of NCLB was to improve all students' achievement and ensure that all children have a fair, equal, and significant opportunity to receive a high-quality education and achieve at or above state standards. Prior to this act, students with disabilities were excluded from state reports on standard academic measures such as reading, science, and math standards, thus leading to lower expectations for those with disabilities (Lehr &

Thurlow, 2003; Thurlow, 2004). NCLB law provided a transparent report card of how children with disabilities performed in the school system by mandating that students with disabilities be held to the same standard and expectations as those without disabilities. Multiple studies documented the benefits of NCLB (e.g., the dropout rate of students with disabilities who left special education dropped from 33.6% in 2003 [pre-NCLB] to 18.5% by 2014) (US Department of Education, 2014, 2016). Unfortunately, this well-intentioned law created several loopholes that negatively impacted several aspects of the American public education system, including the sector with disabilities (National Council on Disability, 2018).

To address these concerns, NCLB was replaced with the Every Student Succeeds Act (PL 114-95) on December 10, 2015. The purpose is "to provide all children significant opportunity to receive a fair, equitable, and high-quality education, and to close educational achievement gaps." This law is based on the notion of standards-based reform, which calls for clear and measurable standards for all students, assessing each student against a concrete standard and ensuring curriculum, assessment, and professional development align with those standards. ESSA requires each state to define rigorous academic standards expected for students within their borders and measure competence in accordance with those standards. However, ESSA does make provisions for alternative assessments to address the needs of students with significant cognitive disabilities, although no more than 1% of a state's student population may be offered alternatives (Klein, 2018). Furthermore, this law allows for dedicated resources and support for vulnerable children, including those with disabilities (The White House, 2015). The National Council on Disability notes recommendations to ensure students with disabilities are supported by their school, district, and state with the implementation of ESSA (National Council on Disability, 2018). Oversight and guidance of state implementation of the law is the responsibility of the US Department of Education, with the financial backing of $21 billion in federal funds (Klein, 2018). Implementing IDEA and providing adequate special education services require collaborative efforts between federal, state, and local education agencies, parents, teachers, and school administrators.

The intent of IDEA is honorable, and it is an improvement over previous inequities and lack of services for children with disabilities. Problems exist, however, with funding, eligibility, responsibility for services, and the actual implementation of services to the targeted child. The lack of adequate funding to support public education and services for children with special needs is the basis for most controversies.

ROLE OF HEALTH PROFESSIONALS IN DETERMINING SPECIAL EDUCATION SERVICES

Children with chronic conditions live longer, and medical technology enables them to participate in school; concern has surfaced about the qualifications of school personnel to provide services to children with special needs. Many schools are without the services of a full-time school nurse and have aides, secretaries, and even teachers performing skills for which they are ill prepared and limited. National data indicate 39% of public schools have a school nurse all day, every day; another 35% of schools have a school nurse who works part time in one or more schools, leaving 26% of schools without any school nurse coverage (National Association of School Nurses [NASN], 2022). The "American Academy of Pediatrics' policy has previously supported ratios of 1 school nurse to 750 students in the healthy student population and 1:225 for student populations requiring daily professional nursing services. However, using a ratio for workload determination in school nursing is inadequate to fill students' increasingly complex health needs" (COSH, 2016).

Although we failed to meet the Healthy People 2010 objective to have one school nurse for every 750 students, a current objective of Healthy People 2030 is to increase the proportion of secondary schools with a full-time registered nurse. The NASN (2022) urges Congress to pass the One School, One Nurse Act that would work to enable every public school to have a full-time registered nurse on staff so that children are safe, healthy, and ready to learn. As more children enter schools with chronic conditions, the school nurse has the breadth of knowledge to provide optimum care in the school setting.

Many public schools have established school-based clinics (referred to as wellness centers or school-based health centers [SBHCs]) to care for the school's children enrolled in the services. The SBHC model encompasses an integrative health care model by an interdisciplinary team of health professionals, including primary care, mental health care, and dental care (Keeton et al., 2012). This may include these same services to children with chronic conditions. SBHCs improve student access to health care services by decreasing financial, geographic, age, and cultural barriers. SBHCs represent a collaborative commitment with the school community to support child and adolescent health and academic success (COSH, 2016).

School districts that identify therapeutic interventions for children with special needs in the IEP process are generally required to pay for these services, although Medicaid fee-for-service or other public funding can often be billed if the child is eligible. For children covered by Medicaid managed care or state children's insurance plans (SCHIP), coverage varies substantially among plans. Private insurance will not usually cover services provided in the school setting. School systems are also financially responsible for providing the necessary equipment to support the child's educational program but can attempt to obtain reimbursement or funding from other sources, such as Maternal and Child Health Bureau Title V services, Medicaid, SCHIP, or other private health insurance plans.

The primary care provider's role starts with early identification and assessment of children with disabilities, as well as children at risk for disabilities, as part of the mandated child find regulations of IDEA. If the primary care provider identifies a child at risk, the family should be referred to the school district's special education office to determine the appropriate public agency to evaluate the child.

To initiate the IEP process, the parents or caretakers must request a special education assessment in writing. The primary care provider can provide the parents with a sample letter to initiate this process and inform them of their rights and their child's rights under IDEA (Box 3.4). A written letter by the primary care provider describing the child's diagnosis, known limitations, available test results, and need for medical treatments is a critical component because it provides medical documentation to support the request and can guide the comprehensiveness of the evaluation. This initial request determines the IEP assessment plan, so it is important to identify all areas of delay or potential risk.

The primary care provider can be part of the comprehensive multidisciplinary assessment process by providing health records and physical findings, with parental consent, to the IEP team.

The primary care provider may participate in additional assessments or referrals to other specialists. Although the IEP team is responsible for explaining the assessment findings to the parents and child, the primary care provider may be able to offer additional insight or interpretation.

The primary care provider's role can be helpful in making recommendations for interventions and reviewing the plan with the family to determine its appropriateness

Box 3.4	Sample Letter to Begin Special Education Assessment Process

Today's Date (include month, day, and year)

Your Name
Street Address
City, State, Zip Code
Daytime telephone number

Name of Principal or Special Education Administrator
Name of School
Street Address
City, State, Zip Code

Dear (person's name),

I am writing to request that my son/daughter, (child's name), be evaluated for special education services.
I am worried that (child's name) is not doing well in school and believe he/she may need special services in order to learn. (Child's name) is in the____ grade at (name of school). (Teacher's name) is his/her teacher.

Specifically, I am worried that (child's name) does/does not (give a few direct examples of your child's problems at school).

I understand that I have to give written permission in order for (child's name) to be evaluated. Before the evaluation begins, I have some questions about the process that I need to have answered (list any questions you may have). I would be happy to talk with you about (child's name). You can send me information or call me during the day on (daytime telephone number). Thank you for your prompt attention to my request.

Sincerely,

Your name

cc: Your child's principal (if letter is addressed to an administrator)
Your child's teacher(s)

From Siegel, L.M. (2001). *The complete IEP guide: How to advocate for your special ed child.* Consolidated Printers, Inc.

Box 3.5	Questions to Ask When Evaluating the Appropriateness of an Individualized Education Plan

1. What does the child know about the condition? How much of the care is the child responsible for? What help will the child require?
2. Is the child's general health stable, improving, or worsening? Is the child terminally ill?
3. Are any classes or school activities contraindicated by the child's condition? Is the child placed in the least restrictive environment?
4. Is preferential seating in the classroom recommended? Are assistive devices required?
5. What modifications in diet exist? Does the child require any assistance in feeding?
6. What physical restrictions and exercise limitations exist? How are they best managed at school? Can the child access all school services? Is fatigue a problem?
7. What medications or treatments does the child receive during the school day? Can dosage times or treatments be modified around school hours?
8. Does the child require counseling, special therapies (e.g., occupational, physical, speech), adaptive equipment, protective devices, or transportation?
9. Does the child need assistance with any activities of daily living (i.e., toileting)?
10. What precautions, first aid interventions, and emergency procedures should school personnel be able to implement? Does the child wear a medical alert bracelet?

the school. The primary care provider can request specific accommodations to be included in the 504 plans. Although 504 plans are less comprehensive than IEPs, the process is also less formal, and often a simple letter from the primary care provider or even a note on a prescription pad with the diagnosis and recommended accommodations will provide sufficient documentation for the family and school.

Ongoing support and involvement of the primary care provider will facilitate a child's adjustment to school. Although the school district is the lead agency for services provided in the school setting, school personnel often welcome input from the child's primary care provider in coordinating health care information and services among specialty clinics, the school, and the child and family. If the school district has a nurse assigned to oversee health care services for children with chronic conditions, the primary care provider should establish a link with that individual.

School nurses work within an educational setting and practice across multiple health care domains, including public health, community agencies, hospitals, and insurance systems, to orchestrate and provide complex care for many of the nation's 50 million public school students (McClanahan & Weismuller, 2015). Interprofessional collaboration in the school setting requires collaboration between health and non-health professionals with expert skills and knowledge bases to deliver comprehensive care to students with chronic health conditions in the school setting. Core

for the child. If the provider and family think the plan is insufficient to meet the child's developmental and cognitive needs, it can be rejected and additional recommendations made to the IEP team. Recommendations supported by assessment findings or relevant literature are more likely to be accepted and incorporated into the plan. The primary care provider should act as an advocate for the parents and child. Box 3.5 lists multiple questions the primary care provider can ask to determine the appropriateness of the interventions identified on the IEP.

Although the aforementioned information speaks to the primary care provider's role in accessing and ensuring appropriate special education for children, the provider should also be an advocate for students who need Section 504 accommodation plans. Children and families should be assisted in identifying those accommodations that would facilitate learning in the school environment and then be supported in advocating for those rights in competencies for interprofessional collaborative practice were developed in 2011 and updated in 2016 by the Interprofessional Education Collaborative (IPEC) Expert Panel to promote patient-centered health care to improve safety, quality, accessibility, and efficiency for population health goals (Fleming & Willgerodt, 2017). The IPEC core competencies are as follows:

- Values/Ethics for Interprofessional Practice: open communication and maintenance of mutual respect and shared values
- Roles and Responsibilities: understanding one's own and one's partners' roles and responsibilities in supporting individual patient and population health care needs
- Interprofessional Communication: communication with partners in health and other fields and specialties that supports a team approach and ensures timely responses to health promotion and disease prevention
- Teams and Teamwork: apply relationship-building values and principles of team dynamics to plan, deliver, and evaluate patient/population-centered care, programs, and policies that are appropriate, safe, effective, and equitable

The role of the school medical consultant is based on the medical and social needs of the community, the school district's priorities, and state regulations. This role requires critical knowledge of multifaceted aspects of school, child, and public health to ensure the provision of cost-effective and legally sound quality health services within the school setting (Box 3.6) (COSH, 2016).

Before initiating any discussion with the school that could involve the release of medical information about the child, it is important for primary care providers to seek the permission of the child and the family and adhere to Health Insurance Portability and Accountability Act regulations.

The primary care provider should know that school district personnel, including nurses and advanced practice registered nurses (APRNs) who are school district employees, are bound by Family Educational Rights and Privacy Act (FERPA) guidelines. FERPA is a federal law designated to protect the privacy and appropriate access to student education records from primary school through graduate school (20 U.S.C. § 1232g; 34 CFR Part 99). Although this will not be a problem for most families, establishing open communication and the limits of confidentiality within the school district may need to be explored. Autonomy in disease management is gained gradually as parents, teachers, friends, and health care providers participate in supporting a child's learning.

FRAMEWORKS THAT GUIDE SCHOOL NURSING PRACTICE

In 2015, the NASN developed the Framework for 21st-Century School Nursing Practice to help guide

Box 3.6	Critical Knowledge Base for the School Medical Consultant

- Public health, including risk assessment, management, and resources
- Infectious diseases to reduce spread of communicable disease, outbreak control, pandemic liaison, and surveillance
- Immunizations and screenings
- Legal knowledge
  - State and district school and public health laws, regulations, and policies
  - IDEA, Section 504, and ADA
  - FERPA and HIPAA
- Developmental and adolescent health
- Physical education and sports medicine
  - Physical education programming
  - Injury prevention and conditioning
  - Concussion management
  - Adaptive physical education
- Emergency preparedness
- Environmental and occupational health considerations
- Counseling and social service resources
- Nutrition services
- Health education
- Staff health promotion and family/community involvement

Modified from Americans with Disabilities Act, Family Education Rights and Privacy Act, Health Insurance Portability and Accountability Act, Individuals with Disabilities Education Act.

school nurses to provide the best care possible for students while they are in school (Maughan et al., 2016; NASN, 2020). This student-centered framework provides a structure for nursing care of children while they are in school within the context of their family and school community while also focusing on the key principles of care coordination, leadership, quality improvement, and community/public health. These principles are surrounded by the standard of practice principle, which is the foundation for using evidence-based nursing practice and providing clinically competent and quality care (Maughan et al., 2016; NASN, 2020) (Fig. 3.2). The Framework for 21st-Century School Nursing Practice is aligned with the Whole School, Whole Community, Whole Child (WSCC) model, which outlines a collaborative approach between learning and health (Association for Supervision and Curriculum Development [ASCD] & CDC, 2014) (Fig. 3.3). The American Academy of Pediatrics (AAP) COSH has used NASN's framework, along with the medical home and medical neighborhood models, the dental home model, the chronic care model (Wagner, 1998; Fig. 3.4), care coordination frameworks, the principles of an effective system of care for children and youth with special health care needs, and the WSCC model, to develop a common framework that can guide an integrated, collective approach to chronic condition management in schools (AAP COSH, 2021).

Framework for 21st Century School Nursing Practice™

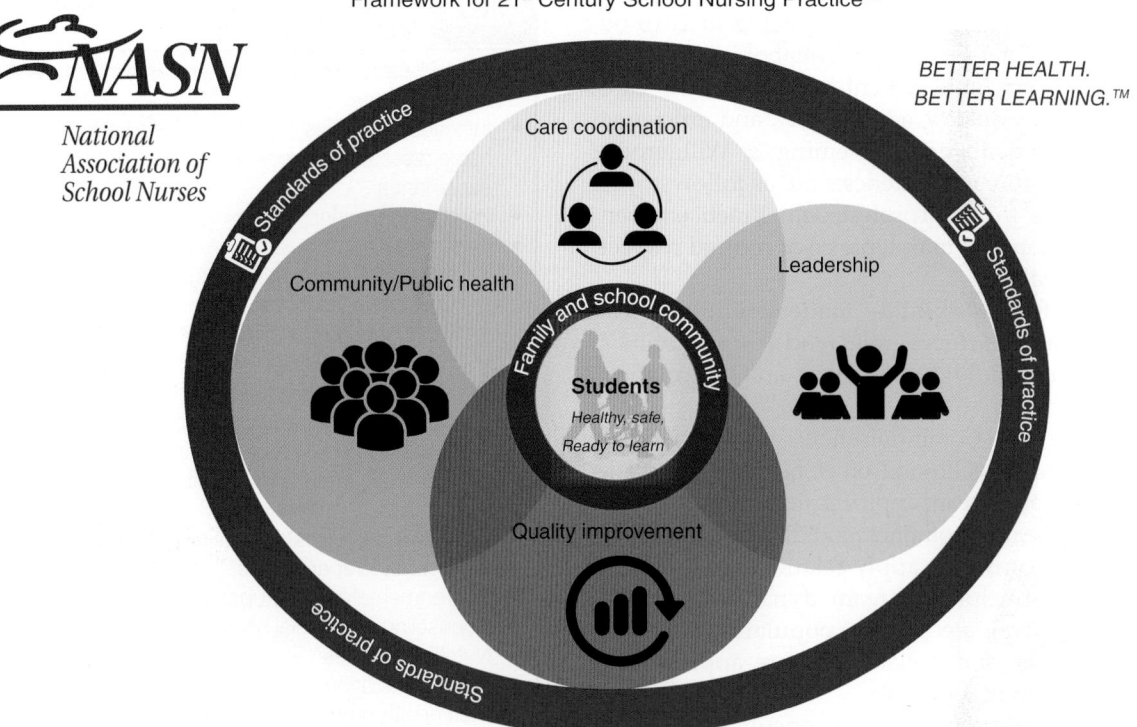

Fig. 3.2 **Framework for 21st-Century School Nursing Practice.** (From Maughan, E.D., Bobo, N., Butler, S., & Schantz, S. [2016]. Framework for 21st century school nursing practice. National Association of School Nurses. *NASN School Nurse, 31*(1), 45–53; National Association of School Nurses. [2020]. Framework for 21st century school nursing practice: Clarification and updated definitions. *NASN School Nurse, 35*(4), 225–233.)

ROLE OF THE SCHOOL NURSE

The school nurse wears many hats when caring for a child with a chronic condition. The school nurse holds an important leadership role in providing school health services for children with chronic conditions (COSH, 2016; Selekman, 2019). This person assesses the student's health, identifies health problems needing to be addressed at school to enable the student to participate fully in the educational process, and develops a plan in conjunction with the student's health care provider and family to address these issues. The nurse often functions as the coordinator/case manager of care for children with chronic conditions while they are in school and is responsible for ensuring continuity of care between school and home. The school nurse also provides or supervises the acute, chronic, episodic, and emergency health care of all students in the assigned school; encourages self-management where appropriate; acts as the liaison among the family, health care professionals, the school, and the community; is an advocate for the child and family; and coordinates the school health services team (CDC, 2017; COSH, 2016; Fleming & Willgerodt, 2017; McCabe, 2020; Maughan et al., 2018; NASN, 2017).

When children with chronic conditions require medical interventions in school, an individualized health plan (IHP), analogous to the IEP for educational services, is necessary (Gereige et al., 2022). As outlined earlier, this plan needs to be in writing and approved by the parents and school officials. The school nurse obtains information from the parents, from the student, and, with parent/student permission, from other health care providers responsible for the child's medical care and establishes goals and objectives for medical care and therapies in the school setting. The contents of the IHP are often included in the school 504 form/plan and incorporated directly into the IEP, which may bypass the need for a separate IHP document.

The school nurse is in an ideal position to coordinate care with the primary care provider, specialists, and local public health and social services agencies (COSH, 2016; Fleming & Willgerodt, 2017; Maughan et al., 2018). The nurse "is the constant in the student's school experience over the years. It is the nurse who can see the whole picture of what is happening with a student over time" (Selekman & Gamel-McCormick, 2006). The nurse can see the child daily and identify changes in health status, the effectiveness of newly prescribed interventions or medications, and the effectiveness of the IEP-related services and assistive technologic devices in meeting the educational goals for the child. Potential problems and strategies can be proactively identified and implemented, or changes in the child's condition can be easily communicated.

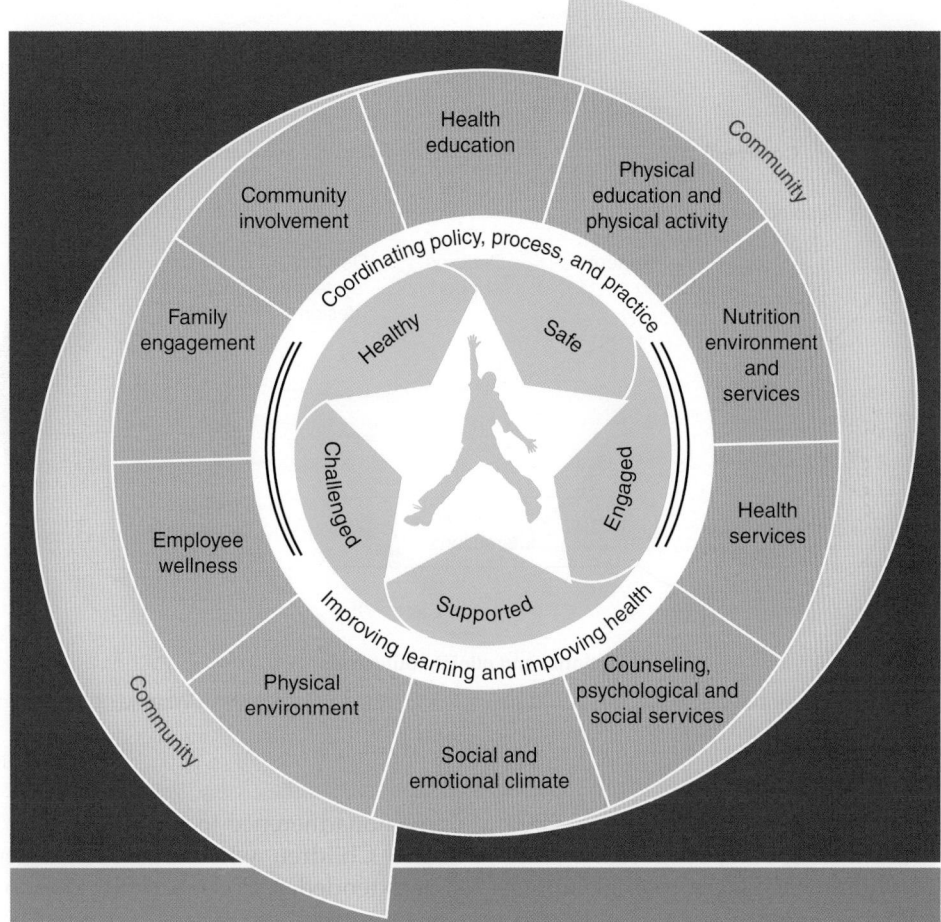

Fig. 3.3 Whole School, Whole Community, Whole Child model. (From Association for Supervision and Curriculum Development & Centers for Disease Control and Prevention. [2014]. Whole school whole community whole child: A collaborative approach to learning and health. https://www.cdc.gov/healthyschools/wscc/wsccmodel_update_508tagged.pdf.)

COLLABORATION WITH SCHOOL-BASED APRNs

An optimum potential for collaboration occurs when a school nurse and APRN are both in the same facility. Having a school-based health/wellness center in a school facilitates the coordination of care and continuity of care for a child with a chronic condition (COSH, 2016). If the APRN is an employee of the school, either the APRN or the school nurse could be the team leader for the IEP team for children with health-related conditions. In cases where the school nurse covers multiple schools in the district, it then becomes the school-based APRN's responsibility to take the lead in the care of children with chronic conditions or to communicate with the responsible person within the school about the child. It should be noted, however, that most SBHCs are free-standing entities that are not under the direction or employment of the school or school district.

FACILITATING THE SCHOOL EXPERIENCE

Children with chronic conditions face more challenges related to school attendance, achievement, and social relationships than their so-called healthy peers (Lum et al., 2017). For children with chronic conditions,

their condition severity and perceived limitations interfere with normal school activities for 6.5% of students; about 1.5% are unable to regularly attend school (Council on Children with Disabilities, 2005; Kaffenberger, 2006). Nevertheless, school is important for children with chronic conditions because it offers them a sense of normalcy and allows them to experience school-related developmental tasks such as regular attendance, academic achievement, and social competence alongside their peers. Therefore it is important to understand the challenges faced by children with chronic conditions both in the school setting and with their ability to attend school, and what can be done to help minimize the impact of a child's chronic condition on attendance, academic performance, and social interactions in school.

FACTORS THAT IMPACT THE SCHOOL EXPERIENCE

Several factors have been identified over the years that either hinder or enhance the school experience and academic success for children with chronic illness. Findings from a systematic meta-review that analyzed

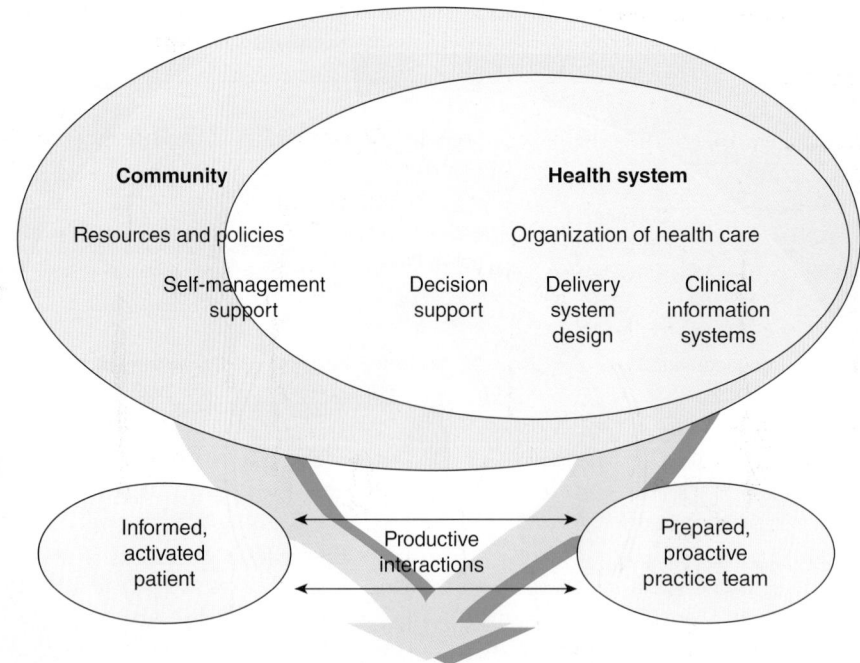

Fig. 3.4 Chronic care model. (From Wagner, E.H. [1998]. Chronic disease management: What will it take to improve care for chronic illness? *Effective Clinical Practice*, 1(1), 2–4.)

18 peer-reviewed papers published since the year 2000 are discussed later (Lum et al., 2017). Additionally, factors in the home environment play a role, including support for the school experience and ensuring adequate sleep, nutrition, and care (Madan-Swain et al., 2004; Shaw & McCabe, 2008; Wodrich & Cunningham, 2008).

Academic Performance

A child having a chronic illness may not impact academic performance, nor does it affect classroom behavior. However, greater disease severity, younger age at diagnosis, treatments with stronger side effects, and diseases and treatments that affect cognitive functioning all have a negative effect on academic performance. Additionally, a weak association was found between lower socioeconomic status and physical sequelae of treatment negatively impacting academic performance. Despite the challenges faced, the presence of academic and social support helped improve academic performance compared to children with chronic illnesses who did not receive these supports (Lum et al., 2017).

Absenteeism

Children who have a chronic illness are more likely than their unaffected peers to miss school, though illness alone is rarely a suitable excuse for academic difficulty and school failure. Other factors that result in increased absenteeism from school include greater disease severity, frequent hospitalization, low socioeconomic status, belonging to a minority ethnic group,

and nonadherence to the medication/treatment regimen. Children who have been absent from school for extended periods, whether due to hospitalization or other reasons, may additionally be anxious about returning to school and have concerns about participating and keeping up with schoolwork (Lum et al., 2017). School refusal is fivefold higher, and absenteeism averages 16 days per year among students with chronic conditions compared with 3 days per year for nonaffected youth (McDougall et al., 2004; Shiu, 2001).

Students who have chronic absenteeism, defined as missing 15 or more days of school in an academic year, are much less likely to reach early learning milestones, are more likely to drop out of school before completing 12th grade, and have poorer outcomes later in life (Allison et al., 2019; US Department of Education, 2019). Therefore it is important that information regarding a student's academic performance, social skills, support networks, capabilities in performing activities of daily living, health care needs, and stamina for handling the demands of the school day be assessed and acted upon to best help the child cope with the limitations that may be encountered in school because of the chronic condition while helping the child maintain independence. In fact, greater support from school staff is associated with fewer days of missed school for a child with a chronic condition (Lum et al., 2017).

The pattern of absences is more predictive of poor academic performance than the number of days missed, with frequent short-term interruptions more disruptive than a single, long absence. The primary reasons for absenteeism are exacerbations in the child's condition, treatment side effects, fatigue, health care appointments, and family dysfunction. Repeated absenteeism not only affects academic performance but can create a downward spiral in a child's self-concept, peer relations, and school connectedness (Allison et al., 2019; Kearney & Bensaheb, 2006; US Department of Education, 2019), especially in this era of high-stakes testing. Parental guilt and anxiety can further contribute to absenteeism by fostering school resistance or school phobia. These consequences are difficult to reverse.

Interpersonal School Experiences

Having a chronic illness may negatively impact the child's relationship with teachers and peers. Children with chronic conditions often endure teasing and bullying about their appearance, physical functioning, and/or academic performance. There is evidence that teachers and peers exhibit negative attitudes and behaviors toward children with chronic conditions, such as being unsupportive, dismissive, and inflexible. The affected child is also concerned about being different from their peers, being able to keep up with their peers, and being understood by their peers. In addition, greater disease severity is linked to poorer peer relationships and social isolation. However, all relationships with teachers and peers are not compromised by the presence of a chronic illness. Social support at school has been associated with better relationships at school between the child and their teachers and peers compared to the relationships of those without social support. Greater social support may also be associated with greater awareness of the illness by teachers and peers, which may make them more supportive and understanding of the affected child (Lum et al., 2017).

Engagement With School

Children with chronic illnesses are eager to attend school because it provides a sense of normalcy for them (Clay, 2004; Wilkie, 2012). However, many are also nervous or hesitant to attend school because they have a lower sense of confidence, body image issues secondary to the disease or treatments for it, they feel different than their peers, and educational goals and aspirations may have changed because of their illness, and they have a sense of being treated differently by their teachers. Despite this last point, experiences with teachers have mostly been described as positive. Poorer engagement with the school has been linked to poorer peer relationships, poor school-oriented support from within the hospital for those who may be hospitalized, and poorer academic functioning. Conversely, better school experiences have been linked to better school support both from within the school and/or hospital (such as a structured hospital-to-school liaison) and supportive adjustments to school or work requirements to accommodate for the challenges imposed on the child by their chronic illness (Lum et al., 2017).

Additional Factors That Impact School Experience

In addition to the abovementioned condition manifestations and management, a child's perceived sense of safety both in school and traveling to and from school, and components of the school's physical environment, can impact the child's ability to learn (Madan-Swain et al., 2004; Shaw & McCabe, 2008; Wodrich & Cunningham, 2008). Disease processes (e.g., poor oxygen diffusion, repeated hypoglycemia), side effects from various interventions (e.g., chemotherapies, long-term steroid use, cranial radiation), and associated fatigue may affect academic motivation and learning (e.g., concentration, memory, information processing) (Shaw & McCabe, 2008). The coexistence of psychosocial problems such as anxiety, depression, or family difficulties further exacerbates the student's potential for poor academic performance.

ACCOMMODATIONS TO FACILITATE THE SCHOOL EXPERIENCE

Primary and specialty care providers of children with chronic conditions need to work in conjunction with the child, family, school personnel (ideally the school nurse), and auxiliary personnel such as school bus drivers and coaches to ensure a successful school experience. Information about the child's condition is generally only disclosed on a need-to-know basis so that the child can be treated normally in school as much as possible while ensuring services are in place to provide an optimal learning environment and safe supervision (Clay, 2004; Wilkie, 2012). During follow-up visits, clinicians should include questions that can help identify and optimally manage symptomatology that impairs students' motivation and academic performance. For many children with chronic conditions, school nurses and counselors are critical partners for primary and specialty care providers because of their ability to provide regular observations about students' health, their ability to engage in self-care, and the effectiveness of treatment protocols, including the availability of needed medications and supplies (Bethell et al., 2012; Erickson et al., 2006).

Because schools vary widely in their resources and commitment to students with chronic conditions, student needs must be addressed on a case-by-case basis (Bethell et al., 2012). For underresourced schools, the primary care or specialty provider can assume a leadership role in helping staff access accurate condition-specific information and receive the necessary training. Students' school experiences are enriched when school personnel are educated about specific conditions, the implications of each condition, related treatments or interventions on academic success, and support services are in place (Johnson et al., 2022; Lum et al., 2017). This can help teachers and other school personnel understand whether a child's behavior or academic performance is related to the chronic condition or warrants further assessment or other intervention (Johnson et al., 2022). Support from family, school personnel, and peers is the biggest indicator of success for a child with a chronic condition in the school environment (Lum et al., 2017, 2019).

Absenteeism

School absenteeism can be reduced by families and health care professionals working together. First, parents must clearly communicate their expectations about school to their children and facilitate their attendance. With regard to follow-up visits and treatments, families should try to schedule health care visits around school hours or during school vacations when possible. Alternatively, if visits can be consolidated into one or fewer days, the child will not have to miss as many half days of class. However, insurance reimbursement constraints may preclude several appointments from being scheduled on the same day in the current health care environment.

If a prolonged absence is anticipated, primary care and specialty providers can help parents arrange for home instruction. School policies vary, and delays because of child ineligibility, poor coordination of services, or unavailable teachers may be encountered before homebound education is initiated. If schools are not approached before the requisite length of absenteeism (i.e., usually 2–4 weeks) is met, additional delays are likely to be encountered before services are arranged. Most schools are willing to work with families in maintaining their child's education by providing homework assignments, communicating with hospital-based teachers, helping parents become informal tutors, and arranging for tutorial services or even remote audio or video participation from home to the classroom via Zoom or another videoconferencing service to begin as soon as the child is eligible. If hospitalizations are frequent or prolonged absences are anticipated, a specific objective should be included in the child's IEP or IHP to ensure uninterrupted schooling. This is one example of how case management and care coordination can benefit the child and family. More information about the transition from hospital/home to school appears in "Transition Between Hospital and School."

Mobility Concerns

Several children with chronic conditions have either temporary or permanent mobility concerns at some point during their school experience. Mobility is affected by physical impairments, diminished strength, and fatigue. Regardless of the cause, limited mobility can affect students' ability to achieve and compete. Physical changes can limit some children from participating fully in physical education, recess, sports, and afternoon activities. In the worst-case scenario, limited mobility will hinder children from participating in critical learning activities.

If mobility is a problem, appropriate adaptations must be addressed in a student's IEP meetings. Two major approaches are used to facilitate a child's mobility: structuring the environment and improving mobility. School districts have eliminated many physical obstacles in compliance with the ADA, but individual schools may be more difficult to navigate than others. When choosing a school is an option, its physical layout (e.g., number of floors, width of hallways, presence of elevators, location of bathrooms) needs to be considered. Providing the child with two sets of books, one for the classroom and one for home, eliminates the problem of transporting them. Scheduling classes in rooms close to one another and scheduling a study hall or lunch after physical education class gives the student more time to change and prevent tardiness. Class buddies can be assigned to assist a student in getting from one class to the next.

For students with more permanent mobility issues, their ability to get around will be improved and normalization promoted if appropriate assistive devices are used. For example, an adolescent in a large high school may prefer to use a wheelchair when traveling long distances between classes rather than limiting the class schedule to classes that are near each other. Adaptive aids can help children write, reach books on library shelves, or respond to questions in the classroom. Backpacks on rollers may assist the student in dragging rather than lifting books and supplies. For students who drive, access to handicapped parking needs to be ensured.

Fatigue

Fatigue is an integral part of many chronic conditions that affect children's overall quality of life, including school success and participation in scholastic activities. Severe fatigue affects approximately 20% of children with chronic illnesses (Nap-van der Vlist et al., 2019). Fatigue may be a symptom of the disease (e.g., in heart disease or sickle cell disease), a physiologic side effect of treatment (e.g., chemotherapy, radiation), associated with time-consuming therapies (e.g., chest physiotherapy for cystic fibrosis), or a side effect of medications (e.g., those given for epilepsy, or secondary to low blood sugar in someone with diabetes).

Strategies for reducing fatigue focus on structuring a child's educational experience in a way that is not physically taxing while promoting academic success and peer acceptance. For example, the child could be encouraged to use an MP3 or other digital recorder for note taking, serve as a scorekeeper rather than participating in a vigorous activity during physical education, or be assigned easy classroom chores such as sharpening pencils with an electric sharpener. Choosing classes in close proximity is particularly important in large schools or those with several buildings. Scheduling a study hall period immediately after lunch allows the child to nap (ideally in a different setting) without missing instructional time. Another strategy is arranging the student's schedule so that the most important classes are either in the morning or in the afternoon; that way, if only half-day sessions are possible, the student can still learn the important content. The homework demands of various courses should also be considered when planning a child's schedule. It is better to defer one class than to have children take on a rigorous schedule that portends failure. Selected courses may be taken during summer school to lighten a child's academic load. Prospective academic planning is important, as schools have limited summer offerings. When fatigue is an issue, students and families must be helped in setting reasonable expectations around participation in school activities.

Medications and Treatments

If medications are required during the school day, the general guidelines and criteria of each state and school district must be followed:

1. A legal prescriber must authorize the medication.
2. Parents must give written permission for medication to be administered.
3. The medication should be properly labeled in its original container.
4. The medication must be stored properly (at room temperature, refrigerated, etc.) in a locked area.
5. The school must document that the medication was administered.

Schools are responsible for having written policies regarding student confidentiality and medication storage and, in the absence of a school nurse if the state nurse practice act allows, designate an individual trained in medication administration (NASN, 2017).

Orders for any over-the-counter medications must also be given to ensure smooth coordination among providers, the school, and the family. When it is desired that children carry their own medications, such as with an asthma inhaler, EpiPen, or glucagon, these must be cleared with the school district because policies vary across jurisdictions. If a student will likely need to take medications ordered as needed or on school field trips, clearly defined protocols should be made for their administration (Butler et al., 2020).

Medications that can interfere with learning need to be prescribed judiciously. Steroids, a mainstay with many chronic conditions, can lead to dysthymia, anxiety, sleep disturbances, weight gain, and other distressing symptoms that may interfere with academic performance and social acceptance (The Royal Children's Hospital, 2018). Other medications, including some analgesics, anticonvulsants, antidepressants, and antipsychotics, also affect academic performance. When monitoring a drug's efficacy in managing a specific condition, its side effects on learning must be assessed.

Clinicians should alter treatment protocols around school schedules for several pragmatic reasons when possible. A child with a chronic condition wants to be considered normal. Requiring the child to go to the nurse for medications may be met with resistance, which puts the child at risk of not receiving the necessary treatment. School nurses can adopt unobtrusive methods, such as instant messaging or vibrating beepers, to remind students about coming to take their medications. There are some cases, however, when the treatment provided by the school nurse is the best way of guaranteeing that the medication or treatment was given, usually because of an unstable home environment; therefore some primary care providers set up the schedule so that the child is guaranteed to have the treatment at least 5 days per week in the school setting.

Even in the best of circumstances, there may not be adequate time or qualified personnel within the school to administer medications or oversee treatments. As children enter adolescence, exploring ways to help them develop self-care behaviors (e.g., self-medication, intermittent clean catheterizations, and checking blood glucose levels) is often appropriate. Such activities will help children become more autonomous, which is an important developmental goal.

More Specific Condition-Related Accommodations

Accommodations for specific conditions and their treatments are beyond the scope of this chapter. However, providers should be aware that each chronic condition has specific issues that may need to be addressed in the school setting in addition to what has been discussed above. Seasoned clinicians and professional organizations related to those conditions can provide guidance regarding school accommodation for these issues.

SOCIAL AND EMOTIONAL NEEDS

Students with chronic conditions have an array of social and emotional needs that can impact motivation, learning, and school success. Common internal (e.g., anxiety, depression, suicide ideation) and external (e.g., impulsivity, anger) psychosocial problems are associated with school stress (Mattson et al., 2019; Shaw & McCabe, 2008). Associated peer rejection, increased high-risk behaviors (including substance abuse), increasing somatization, and deteriorating self-esteem peak in adolescence (Erickson et al., 2005; Mattson et al., 2019; Shiu, 2001). Effective coping strategies and a healthy self-concept are paramount if children with chronic conditions are to become resilient in handling the demands of their condition and school pressures (Lum et al., 2019). These can be established through normative school activities and by recognizing areas of academic and extracurricular achievement. Children who excel in a specific academic area or participate in sports and other extracurricular activities are more likely to be successful because these activities help build self-esteem and enhance other spheres of development (Dale et al., 2019; Dimitri et al., 2020).

Developing healthy self-esteem in students with chronic conditions is not without difficulty. These children face unique stressors associated with their conditions that are further exacerbated by insensitive policies or a lack of privacy when taking medications or performing management tasks. They are more likely to be teased; many may experience bullying or even ostracism (Faith et al., 2015).

Helping youth with chronic conditions develop a social support network will positively influence their psychosocial adjustment and self-esteem (Faith et al., 2015; Lum et al., 2017, 2019). Opportunities must be created for these youth to interact with nonaffected peers in nonacademic settings, including sports teams, clubs, and other extracurricular activities. They benefit from interventions to strengthen their coping abilities, helping them deal constructively with peer rejection, loneliness, or isolation. Incorporating social skills training into children's educational plan is one way to help them and their families become more confident in their interactions with others and their use of effective behaviors when dealing with discrimination. School personnel can assist by dealing with the inappropriate behavior of other students and developing an awareness of what it is like to have a chronic condition.

Students' self-concepts are enhanced when they can successfully communicate information about their condition and its management to their friends and school personnel, thus creating a supportive environment and enhancing their own safety and security. This is especially important for adolescents who are increasingly independent of their parents. The primary care or specialty provider can role-play situations with students, such as determining what friends they may trust and how to communicate selected information.

Parents, teachers, and school professionals often are challenged with how to best help foster emotional development and school connectedness in children with chronic conditions. Teachers and parents may be overprotective, be anxious that care needs will be addressed, have lowered academic expectations, or impose less discipline (Clay, 2004; Power et al., 2019). They may need help to acknowledge that children with chronic conditions experience the same developmental stressors as their peers and therefore need to be treated similarly and taught the same coping skills. Using a variety of techniques to help these children normalize their school experience will be beneficial to developing their self-concept.

For a variety of reasons, the process of ensuring appropriate educational placement and accommodations for children with special health care needs can be contentious and stressful for families: inadequate school funding for special education, lack of a funding stream for 504 accommodations, and differing perspectives and lack of trust between parents and educators. From the school's perspective, parents may deny the presence of a chronic condition, refuse to test, or dispute the IEP team's finding that their child has special needs. From the parents' perspective, schools may delay or deny educational assessments, deny recommended therapies or educational aides, fail to provide adequate education in separate classes, or fail to enforce plans that are in place. Primary care and specialty providers are sometimes put in the middle of this process and, at other times, may be unaware that encouraging the parent to ask for an IEP does not necessarily lead to a speedy and mutually satisfactory result. As a trustworthy third party, the primary care and/or specialty provider can effectively reinforce the benefits of adequate evaluation when communicating with the parents and the need for specific interventions when communicating with educational professionals.

ENSURING SAFETY

School systems are responsible for ensuring that students with chronic conditions are in a safe environment. Schools should have policies and procedures in place to handle emergency situations, including: "(1) developing campus-wide communication with local emergency medical services (EMSs); (2) establishing and practicing a medical emergency response plan (MERP) involving school nurses, primary care providers, athletic trainers, and EMS...; (3) identifying students at risk for life-threatening emergencies and ensuring each has an individualized emergency care plan; (4) training staff and students in first aid and CPR (cardiopulmonary resuscitation); (5) having emergency equipment in schools for life-threatening emergencies; and (6) implementing lay rescuer Automated External Defibrillator (AED) programs" (Ugalde et al., 2018, p. 399). Primary care and specialty providers can assist families in ensuring that these policies and procedures contain sufficient information to handle common emergencies associated with their child's condition.

Because many chronic conditions or their treatments place children at greater risk for infection, illness, or injury, each student's risks must be assessed individually. For example, students with asthma may have numerous classroom triggers (Akar-Ghibril & Phipatanakul, 2020). Impaired sensory function (e.g., cataracts, diminished vision) and lowered immunity may result from long-term use of steroids. The school's policy on notifying parents of possible exposure to communicable diseases must be clarified. Depending on the child's chronic condition, specific areas of concern may include strep throat, measles, varicella, meningitis, hepatitis A and B, salmonella, shigella, or SARS-CoV-2 infections. Latex allergy is another potential threat for students with chronic conditions. Although students with myelodysplasia are the most likely to be affected, any child with repeated exposure to latex is at greater risk.

For children on life-sustaining equipment such as ventilators, adaptive electrical equipment must be periodically inspected with a reserve generator made available. Provisions for transporting a student with a physical disability during emergencies such as fires and earthquakes need to be determined and disseminated to all school personnel. Faculty and staff need to rehearse plans to retrieve students with mobility or cognitive deficits from classrooms, especially those not on the first floor.

Many students with chronic conditions participate in intramural and varsity athletics. Athletic trainers and coaches need to be informed and prepared to handle condition-specific emergencies such as hypoglycemia, seizures, or asthma attacks (Gereige et al., 2022). Because such emergencies rarely occur, providing individualized procedure cards to be included in field emergency kits is useful, particularly if the team travels. Other students' conditions may prohibit them from participating in regular school teams. Special Olympics programs (www.specialolympics.org) may be an alternative. For younger children, adaptations to playground equipment may be necessary and should be individualized. Regardless of the level of play, appropriate safety equipment must be used under adult supervision. Strengthening exercises also help prevent injury.

Under IDEA (2004), school buses may transport children with chronic conditions as young as 3 years of age for related services. Children with disabilities need individualized evaluation to determine the appropriate restraint system for their age, size, and disability. School buses need to be equipped with appropriate safety devices (i.e., communication system, fire extinguisher, first aid kit) that meet federal motor vehicle safety standards (FMVSS). Buses need to be equipped with height- and weight-appropriate, forward-facing seats with dynamically tested three-point restraints and/or four-point tie-down devices for wheelchairs that allow the passenger to face forward that meet FMVSS if transporting disabled children. Certified transit wheelchairs should be used whenever possible; lapboards should be removed and stored separately. Strollers are not permitted. Students under 50 pounds should be restrained with safety vests. Oxygen, suctioning equipment, or other specialized equipment needs to be stored appropriately and labeled. An aide/health paraprofessional (aka health para) or nurse should accompany selected medically fragile children. The school nurse will develop emergency action plans that direct lay personnel in the emergency measures to take for a particular child's condition until medical assistance arrives. Written emergency evacuation plans should be in place, with drills held yearly (Committee on Injury, Violence, and Poison Prevention, 2007).

TRANSITION BETWEEN HOSPITAL AND SCHOOL

Primary care and specialty providers are an important part of the team establishing school reintegration programs for youth who have had prolonged absences or dropped out (Betz & Redcay, 2002; Hinton & Kirk, 2015; Shaw & McCabe, 2008). Students are excited to return to school and reestablish some normalcy but are also nervous about rejoining their peers and concerned whether they will be able to keep up academically (Lum et al., 2017). Those returning to school with developmental changes or new disfigurements are especially at risk of having trouble when they return to school (Xie et al., 2020). A positive experience of reentry can provide children with a sense of accomplishment and social acceptance, strengthen faltering self-esteem, and lessen maladaptive emotional responses to their condition (Hinton & Kirk, 2015; Lum et al., 2017).

Experiences with school reintegration for children with chronic illnesses have been strongly linked to the model of support available in the school and hospital. A good model for school reintegration includes the following components: "1) structured communication and collaboration pathways between the hospital, school, and family, such as that performed by school liaison personnel; 2) a clear understanding of the educational implications of the illness and the roles and responsibilities of teachers, school psychologists, nurses, and medical specialists in facilitating a successful return to school; and 3) flexible adjustments that allow the ill child to attend partial school days or reduce homework load" (Lum et al., 2017).

Primary care and specialty providers can help promote a smooth transition from the hospital/home back to school by proactively engaging the child, family members, and school personnel in determining strategies to facilitate school reentry. For children who are returning to school after a prolonged hospitalization, a three-phase approach is used. In phase 1, families are helped to identify school and community support. In phase 2, communication occurs between hospitals and health care providers, and school personnel (i.e., principal, school nurse, counselor) to help make the transition a positive experience for the child. An appropriate IEP or IHP (or both) should be initiated, addressing individualized educational strategies for the child and peer and teacher education. Last, in phase 3, the follow-up to ensure that the transition has been successful is undertaken (Kliebenstein & Broome, 2000; Madan-Swain et al., 2004; Gereige et al., 2022).

Since most children with chronic conditions no longer experience long hospitalizations but rather have shorter hospital stays followed by longer home recuperation with more outpatient services, transition planning may be more complex. Children who are out of school but not in the hospital have less access to hospital teachers, and parents may assume increasing health care and educational responsibilities. Given current circumstances, it is important that schools tailor a student's educational program to allow for flexible attendance, offer differentiated instruction, and provide mechanisms for social support (Lum et al., 2017; Shaw & McCabe, 2008).

As mentioned earlier, if a prolonged absence is anticipated, primary care and specialty providers can help parents arrange for home instruction. School policies vary, and delays because of child ineligibility, poor coordination of services, or unavailable teachers may be encountered before homebound education is initiated. If schools are not approached before the requisite length of absenteeism (i.e., usually 2–4 weeks) is met, additional delays are likely to be encountered before services are arranged. Most schools are willing to work with families in maintaining their child's education by providing homework assignments, communicating with hospital-based teachers, helping parents become informal tutors, and arranging for tutorial services or even remote audio or video participation from home to the classroom via Zoom or another videoconferencing service to begin as soon as the child is eligible. If hospitalizations are frequent or prolonged absences are anticipated, a specific objective should be included in the child's IEP or IHP to ensure uninterrupted schooling.

The two primary goals in the transition from hospital/home to school are to help the child and family anticipate situations they may encounter and to prepare teachers and classmates for the child's return. One helpful approach to preparing the child for reentry is role-playing, wherein the primary care provider plays the role of a classmate, and the child plays oneself. The purpose is to act out a variety of scenarios that may occur during the first day back at school so that the child can develop answers to potentially embarrassing questions or situations that may arise. Another useful strategy is to ask close friends to accompany the child and serve as a buffer on the return to school. Parents may also take the child for several drop-in visits or sponsor a welcome back class party designed to promote peer acceptance.

A variety of approaches can be used to help teachers and classmates adjust. Two-way videoconferencing while the child is still in the hospital or homebound using a videoconferencing platform such as Zoom is available and easy for teachers and students to use. A child may be encouraged to write a letter or record a video for classmates about the experience of being in the hospital or undergoing treatment, which is then shared with teachers or classmates several days before the child's return. Providing visual images of a child—either by video or in photographs—allows time for sanctioned staring or for classmates to ask questions or express their concerns without fear of recrimination. This is particularly important if the child has undergone major physical changes (e.g., alopecia secondary to chemotherapy, scarring from burns). Role-playing, science projects, literature assignments, and video presentations can be used by teachers to promote understanding and acceptance within the child's peer group. Careful advance planning will improve the likelihood of a successful return to school for the child.

The decision to repeat a grade must be made with great care. This setback can cause feelings of shame, inadequacy, and inferiority, but the decision to remain in the same grade may also enhance feelings of success because the work requirements may be easier. New classmates provide a second chance to form friendships.

SCHOOL AND THE STUDENT WITH A TERMINAL CONDITION

School is an appropriate activity for many children who are terminally ill because it provides a sense of normality, opportunities for socialization, and personal achievement. For children to have a successful school experience, the following must be considered:

1. A priori discussions on how and when information regarding the child's condition will be shared with the child, peers, school personnel, and other parents
2. Flexible academic programming tailored to the needs of the specific student so that school remains relevant as the child's condition declines (e.g., an adolescent enrolled in a college preparatory curriculum needs accommodation in place to develop achievable objectives rather than giving up all hope for the future)
3. Efforts and interventions in place to help the child maintain a positive self-concept and body image, which is especially important when a child begins to manifest physical and mental changes because of the illness (e.g., children who are dying often need to exhibit more control over their lives and environments; when possible, efforts must be made to help them reach the goals they have set for themselves)

"From 2000 to 2006, the percentage of schools in which health services staff were required to follow do-not-attempt-resuscitation (DNAR) orders increased from 29.7% to 46.2%, respectively. It is essential for childcare and school systems to be prepared to address requests from families and their doctors about DNAR orders" (AAP et al., 2010). Many students and school personnel have had little to no experience with educating or learning alongside terminally ill students. School administrators and health care providers need to be aware of legal policies related to DNAR orders in their individual states. School personnel need to partner with the school's nurse, social workers, and counselors, in consultation with palliative care or hospice programs, to provide education, support, and anticipatory guidance throughout this challenging time. After a child's death, developmentally appropriate bereavement counseling for students and staff is imperative.

DO NOT ATTEMPT RESUSCITATION ORDERS

The decision to withhold life-prolonging medical interventions at the end of life is a sensitive and emotionally challenging decision for families and terminally ill children. Every attempt to honor this decision should be made, as there may be legal consequences if it is not upheld (NASN, 2017). Comprehensive planning for

Box **3.7**	Components of a Do Not Attempt Resuscitation (DNAR) Order

The DNAR order within the individualized health care plan (IHCP) should outline the child's needs and provide specific directives for the staff to follow in the event of a cardiac or respiratory arrest. The elements of the plan should include:

- Identification of staff members who should be informed of and educated about the IHCP and the DNAR order.
- The location to which the child will be moved if serious distress or sudden death should occur at school or plans to remove onlookers from the area if the child cannot be moved.
- Which comfort measures should be offered to the child?
- Protocols for notification of the prearranged emergency medical services provider.
- Protocols for notification of the family and primary care provider.
- Protocols that define steps to take should the child die in school.
- Designation of the clinician who will pronounce the child's death (primary care provider, nurse practitioner, or physician assistant).
- A specific plan for removing the body from the school to a local health care facility or designated funeral home, including such details as the type of vehicle to be used, where it will park at the school, who will clear the corridors, and what kind of transport equipment will be required to move the body to the waiting vehicle.

Modified from Council on School Health & Council on Bioethics (2010). Honoring do-not-attempt-resuscitation requests in schools. *Pediatrics, 125*(5), 1073–1077.

end-of-life care for a child with a terminal condition may include disseminating the family's wishes that the child is not resuscitated if a cardiac arrest occurs. A comprehensive approach to responding to do not resuscitate (DNR) orders in the school requires school personnel to develop and implement a protocol to follow when a child with a DNR order attends school (Box 3.7). It should be noted that some facilities use the term *allow natural death* (AND) rather than DNR.

The National Education Association (NEA) has issued guidelines for DNR orders in schools if a school district and state honor DNR orders (NEA, 2000). The NEA has suggested the following minimum conditions if a school board is to honor DNR:

1. The request should be submitted in writing and be accompanied by a written order signed by the student's primary care provider.
2. The school should establish a team to consider the request and all available alternatives and, if no other alternative exists, develop a medical emergency plan.
3. Staff should receive training.
4. Staff and students should receive counseling.

In its statement, the NEA delineated the following elements of the medical emergency plan:

1. The student's teachers specify their actions if the student experiences a cardiac arrest or other life-threatening emergency.

2. Other school employees who supervise the student receive briefing sessions.
3. The student wears an identification bracelet indicating the DNR order.
4. The parents execute a contract with the local emergency medical service and send a copy to the superintendent.
5. The team reviews the plan annually.

In 2000, the Committee on School Health and Committee on Bioethics (2010) of the AAP released a joint policy statement on DNR orders in schools. This document is like that of the NEA but goes further in recommending that health care providers review the plan with the board of education and its legal counsel and update the plan every 6 months rather than yearly.

Individual states have highly varied DNR policies and laws that govern the actions of emergency medical personnel actions when treating students (Costante, 2001). Practitioners are encouraged to determine specific regulations for their state. Schools should develop protocols for responding to DNR orders in accordance with NEA guidelines, AAP policy, and state regulations and in a spirit of collaboration, respect, and sensitivity. Parents, educators, support personnel, and members of the health care team must be committed to a flexible process responsive to the child's changing needs. In some cases, it is appropriate for the child to be actively involved with the planning. Essential to this process is ongoing forums where parents and educators can discuss their concerns, share their values and preferences about how certain situations should be handled, and define or revise plans. Within these discussions, it is crucial to define the range of possible scenarios that are likely to occur for the child and to build contingency plans for how they should be handled. Hospice personnel may be helpful in guiding these discussions.

SUMMARY

It is beneficial for children with chronic conditions to be in school with their peers. There are several laws and policies in place to ensure these children receive the education they are entitled to while also getting the services they need to manage their condition. Taking an individual child's needs into consideration, making specific accommodations, and providing social and academic support can help ensure a successful school experience.

RESOURCES

Administration for Children and Families: https://www.childcare.gov.

American Academy of Pediatrics: https://www.healthychildren.org.

Centers for Disease Control and Prevention: www.cdc.gov/HealthyYouth/index.htm.

Council for Exceptional Children: https://exceptionachildren.org.

Disability Rights Education and Defense Fund: https://dredf.org.

Federation for Children with Special Needs: https://fcsn.org.

National Association of School Nurses: https://www.nasn.org.

National Association of State Boards of Education: https://www.nasbe.org.

Understand: https://www.understood.org.

U.S. Department of Education: https://sites.ed.gov; https://www.ed.gov.

REFERENCES

The Advocacy Institute. Analysis finds students with disabilities served under section 504 overwhelmingly white, disproportionately male. 2015. https://www.advocacyinstitute.org/resources/504analysisCRDC2012.shtml.

American Academy of Pediatrics. (2010). Policy statement: Honoring do-not-attempt resuscitation requests in schools. *Pediatrics, 125,* 1073–1077. doi:10.1542/peds.2010-0452.

American Academy of Pediatrics Council on School Health. (2016). Role of the school nurse in providing school health services. *Pediatrics, n137*(6), e20160852.

American Academy of Pediatrics Council on School Health. (2012). School-based health centers and pediatric practice. *Pediatrics, 129*(5).

Akar-Ghibril, N., & Phipatanakul, W. (2020). The indoor environment and childhood asthma. *Current Allergy and Asthma Reports, 20*(43). https://doi.org/10.1007/s11882-020-00941-5.

Allison, M. A., & Attisha, E. American Academy of Pediatrics Council on School Health. (2019). The link between school attendance and good health. *Pediatrics, 143*(2), e20183648.

American Academy of Pediatrics Council on School Health. Consensus statement on the core tenets of chronic condition management in schools. 2021. https://downloads.aap.org/AAP/PDF/Consensus%20Statement%20-%20Core%20Tenets%20of%20CCMS%20%202021-08%20.pdf?_ga=2.249230151.1973556024.1679068782-1823549654.1679068780.

Americans with Disabilities Act. (1990). *Public Law 101-336, 42 USC 12101 et seq.* Washington, DC: US Government Printing Office.

Association for Supervision and Curriculum Development & Centers for Disease Control and Prevention. Whole school whole community whole child: A collaborative approach to learning and health. 2014. https://files.ascd.org/staticfiles/ascd/pdf/siteASCD/publications/wholechild/wscc-a-collaborative-approach.pdf.

Bethell, C., Forrest, C. B., Stumbo, S., Gombojav, N., Carle, A., & Irwin, C. E. (2012). Factors promoting or potentially impeding school success: Disparities and state variations for children with special health care needs. *Maternal and Child Health Journal, 16*(Suppl 1), S35–S43. doi:10.1007/s10995-012-0993-z. PMID: 22488159.

Betz, C. L., & Redcay, G. (2002). Lessons learned from providing transition services to adolescents with special health care needs. *Issues in Comprehensive Pediatric Nursing, 25,* 129–149.

Brown v. Board of Education. U.S. Supreme Court 347, US, 483. 1954.

Butler, S. M., Boucher, E. A., Tobison, J., & Phan, H. (2020). Medication use in schools: Current trends, challenges, and best practices. *Journal of Pediatric Pharmacology Therapy, 25*(1), 7–24. https://doi.org/10.5863/1551-6776-25.1.7.

Centers for Disease Control and Prevention (2008). A CDC review of school laws and policies concerning child and adolescent health. *J School Health, 78*(2), 69–128.

Centers for Disease Control and Prevention (CDC). Managing chronic health conditions in schools: The role of the school nurse. 2017. Retrieved from https://www.cdc.gov/healthyschools/chronic_conditions/pdfs/2017_02_15-FactSheet. Role of School Nurses_FINAL_508.pdf

Clay, D. L. (2004). *Helping schoolchildren with chronic health conditions.* Guilford Press.

Committee on Injury, Violence, and Poison Prevention. (2007). School transportation safety. *Pediatrics, 120,* 213–220.

Cornett, J., & Knackstedt, K. M. (2020). Original sin(s): Lessons from the US model of special education and an opportunity for leaders. [Lessons from US model of special education]. *J Edu Admin, 58*(5), 507–520. https://doi.org/10.1108/JEA-10-2019-0175.

Costante, C. (2001). Do not resuscitate in the school setting: Determining the policy and procedures. In Schwab, N., & Gerlman, M. (Eds.), *Legal issues in school health services: A resource for school administrators, school attorneys, and school nurses.* Sunrise River Press.

Council on Children with Disabilities. (2005). Care coordination in the medical home: Integrating health and related systems of care for children with special health care needs. *Pediatrics, 116,* 1238–1244.

Council on School Health. (2016). Role of the school nurse in providing school health services. *Pediatrics, 137*(6), e20160852. doi:10.1542/peds.2016-0852. PMID: 27217476.

Council on School Health & Council on Bioethics. (2010). Honoring do-not-attempt-resuscitation requests in schools. *Pediatrics, 125*(5), 1073–1077. https://doi.org/10.1542/peds.2010-0452.

Dale, L. P., Vanderloo, L., Moore, S., & Faulkner, G. (2019). Physical activity and depression, anxiety, and self-esteem in children and youth: An umbrella systematic review. *Mental Health and Physical Activity, 16,* 66–79. https://doi.org/10.1016/j.mhpa.2018.12.001.

Dimitri, P., Joshi, K., & Jones, N. on behalf of the Moving Medicine for Children Working Group. (2020). Moving more: Physical activity and its positive effects on long-term conditions in children and young people. *Archives of Disease in Chilhoodd, 105*(11), 1035–1040.

Education for All Handicapped Children Act. Public Law 94-142. 1975.

Erickson, C. D., Splett, P. L., Mullet, S. S., et al. (2006). The healthy learner model for student chronic condition management—I. *Journal of School Nursing, 22,* 310–318.

Erickson, J. D., Patterson, J. M., Wall, M., & Neumark-Sztainer, D. (2005). Risk behaviors and emotional well-being in youth with chronic health conditions. *Children's Health Care, 34*(3), 181–192. https://doi.org/10.1207/s15326888chc3403_2.

Elementary and Secondary Education Act of 1965: H. R. 2362, 89th Cong., 1st Sess., Public Law 89-10. Reports, Bills, Debate and Act. Washington, DC: US Government Printing Office.

Every Student Succeeds Act, 20 U.S.C. 6301 § 1001, Statement of Purpose.

Every Student Succeeds Act. Public Law 114-95. 2015.

Faith, M. A., Reed, G., Heppner, C. E., Hamill, L. C., Tarkenton, T. R., & Donewar, C. W. (2015). Bullying in medically fragile youth: A review of risks, protective factors, and recommendations for medical providers. *Journal of Developmental and Behavioral Pediatrics, 36*(4), 285–301. doi:10.1097/DBP.0000000000000155.

Family Educational Rights and Privacy Act. 20 U.S.C. § 1232g; 34 CFR Part 99.

Fleming, R., & Willgerodt, M. A. (2017). Interprofessional collaborative practice and school nursing: A model for improved health outcomes. *OJIN, 22*(3) Manuscript 2.

Fletcher, J., Lyon, G. R., Fuchs, L., & Barnes, M. (2018). *Learning disabilities: From identification to intervention* (2nd ed.). Guilford Press.

Gereige, R. S., Gross, T., & Jastaniah, E. AAP Council on School Health, AAP Committee on Emergency Medicine.

(2022). Individual medical emergencies occurring at school. *Pediatrics, 150*(1), e2022057987.

Hinton, D., & Kirk, S. (2015). Teachers' perspectives of supporting pupils with long-term health conditions in mainstream schools: A narrative review of the literature. *Health Social Care Community, 23*(2), 107–120.

IDEA 2021 Fact Sheet — Section 2014 of the American Rescue Plan Act of 2021 and the Individuals with Disabilities Education Act (July 1, 2021) | OSEP Policy Support 21-02

Individuals with Disabilities Education Act. (1991). *20 U.S.C. 1400 et seq. Public Law 101-119*. Washington, DC: U.S. Government Printing Office.

Individuals with Disabilities Education Improvement Act. (2004). *Public Law 108-446*. Washington, DC: U.S. Government Printing Office.

Individuals with Disabilities Education Act Data. Data tables for OSEP state reported data. 2007. Available at https://www.ideadata.org. Retrieved November 4, 2008.

Infant and Toddler Program, Part H. (1986). *Public Law 99-457*. Washington, DC: U.S. Government Printing Office.

Johnson, E., Atkinson, P., Muggeridge, A., Cross, J. H., & Reilly, C. (2022). Impact of epilepsy on learning and behaviour and needed supports: Views of children, parents and school staff. *European Journal of Paediatric Neurology, 40*, 61–68. doi:10.1016/j.ejpn.2022.08.001. Epub 2022 Aug 20. PMID: 36031701.

Kaffenberger, C. (2006). School re-entry for students with chronic illness: A role for professional counselors. *Professional School Counseling, 9*, 223–230.

Kearney, C. A., & Bensaheb, A. (2006). School absenteeism and school refusal behavior: A review and suggestions for school-based health professionals. *Journal of School Health, 76*, 3–7.

Keeton, V., Soleimanpour, S., & Brindis, C. D. (2012). School-based health centers in an era of health care reform: Building on history. *Current Problems in Pediatric and Adolescent Health Care, 42*(6), 132–156.

Klein, A. (2018). *What's in store for states on federal ESSA oversight*. Education Week.

Kliebenstein, M. A., Broome M. E. School re-entry for the child with chronic illness: parent and school personnel perceptions. *Pediatr Nurs*. 2000 Nov-Dec;26(6):579–82. PMID: 12026357.

Lee A. IDEA, section 504 and the ADA, which laws do what. Understood. 2018. https://www.understood.org/articles/at-a-glance-which-laws-do-what.

Lehr, C., & Thurlow, M. (2003). *Putting it all together: Including students with disabilities in assessment and accountability systems*. NCEO Policy Directions 16. Accessed March 11, 2023. https://nceo.info/Resources/publications/onlinePubs/Policy16.htm.

Lipkin P. H., Okamoto J; Council on Children with Disabilities; Council on School Health. The Individuals With Disabilities Education Act (IDEA) for Children With Special Educational Needs. *Pediatrics*. 2015 Dec;136(6):e1650–62. doi: 10.1542/peds.2015-3409. PMID: 26620061.

Lum, A., Wakefield, C. E., Donnan, B., Burns, M. A., Fardell, J. E., & Marshall, G. M. (2017). Understanding the school experiences of children and adolescents with serious chronic illness: A systematic meta-review. *Child Care Health Development, 43*, 645–662. doi:10.1111/cch.12475.

Lum, A., Wakefield, C. E., Donnan, B., et al. (2019). Facilitating engagement with school in students with chronic illness through positive education: A mixed-methods comparison study. *School Psychology, 34*(6), 677–686. https://doi.org/10.1037/spq0000315.

Madan-Swain, A., Katz, E. R., & LaGory, J. (2004). School and social reintegration after a serious illness or injury. In Brown, R. T. (Ed.), *Handbook of pediatric psychology in school settings*. Erlbaum.

Mattson, G., & Kuo, D. Z. Committee on Psychosocial Aspects of Child and Family Health, Council on Children with Disabilities, , Yogman, M., et al. (2019). Psychosocial factors in children and youth with special health care needs and their families. *Pediatrics, 143*(1), e20183171. https://doi.org/10.1542/peds.2018-3171.

Maughan, E. D., Bobo, N., Butler, S., & Schantz, S. (2016). Framework for 21st century school nursing practice: National Association of School Nurses. *NASN School Nurse, 31*(1), 45–53. doi:10.1177/1942602x15618644.

Maughan, E. D., Cowell, J., Engelke, M. K., McCarthy, A. M., Bergren, M. D., & Vessey, J. A. (2018). The vital role of school nurses in ensuring the health of our nation's youth. *Nursing Outlook, 66*, 94–96. https://doi.org/10.1016/j.outlook.2017.11.002.

Mayerson, A. B., & Mayer, K. S. (2000). *Defining disability in the aftermath of Sutton: Where do we go from here?* Disability Rights Education and Defence Fund (DREDF). [online]Available at. http://64.143.22.161/articles/mayerson.html.

McCabe, E. M. (2020). School nurses' role in self-management, anticipatory guidance, and advocacy for students with chronic illness. *NASN School Nurse*, 339–343.

McClanahan, R., & Weismuller, P. C. (2015). School nurses and care coordination for children with complex needs: An integrative review. *Journal of School Nursing, 31*(1), 34–43. doi:10.1177/1059840514550484.

McDougall, J., King, G., de Wit, D. J., Miller, L. T., Hong, S., Offord, D. R., LaPorta, J., & Meyer, K. (2004). Chronic physical health conditions and disability among Canadian school-aged children: A national profile. *Disability and rehabilitation, 26*(1), 35–45. https://doi.org/10.1080/09638280410001645076.

Mills v. Board of Education of the District of Columbia. U.S. Court of Appeals 348F, Supp. 866. 1972.

Morin A. Related services for kids who learn and think differently. Understood. https://www.understood.org/en/articles/related-services-for-kids-with-learning-and-thinking-differences-what-you-need-to-know. Accessed 3/7/2023. 2023.

Nap-van der Vlist, M. M., Dalmeijer, G. W., Grootenhuis, M. A., & Nijhof, S. L. (2019). Fatigue in childhood chronic disease. *Archives of Disease in Childhood, 104*, 1090–1095. doi:10.1136/archdischild-2019-316782.

National Council on Disability (2008). Finding the Gaps: A Comparative Analysis of Disability Laws in the United States to the United Nations Convention on the Rights of Persons with Disabilities. Washington, DC: Author.

National Association of School Nurses. *Position statement: One school one nurse act*. 2022. Available at www.nasn.org. Retrieved March 7, 2023

National Association of School Nurses. (2020). Framework for 21st century school nursing practice: Clarification and updated definitions. *NASN School Nurse, 35*(4), 225–233. doi: 10.1177/1942602×20928372.

National Association of School Nurses. (2017). *Medication administration in schools (Position Statement)*. Author. From. https://files.eric.ed.gov/fulltext/ED581613.pdf.

National Association of School Nurses. The school health services team: Supporting student outcomes (Position Statement). 2017. https://www.nasn.org/nasn-resources/professional-practice-documents/position-statements/ps-team.

National Council on Disability. *Back to school on civil rights*. 2000. Available atwww.ncd.gov/newsroom/publications/backtoschool_1.html.

National Education Association. *Providing safe health care: The role of educational support personnel*. 2000. Available at www.nea.org/esphome/images/safecare.pdf.

National Survey of Children's Health. NSCH 2020-2021: Number of current or Lifelong health conditions, nationwide, age in 3 groups website. www.childhealthdata.org. Accessed March 17, 2023.

National Center for Education Statistics. (2022). *Students with disabilities. Condition of education*. US Department of

Education, Institute of Education Sciences. Retrieved [date], from. https://nces.ed.gov/programs/coe/indicator/cgg.

National Council on Disability. (IDEA Series) *Every Student Succeeds Act and students with disabilities.* Washington, DC. 2018.

No Child Left Behind Act. (2001). *Public Law 107-110.* Washington, DC: U.S. Government Printing Office.

Office of Civil Rights, US Department of Education. *Protecting students with disabilities.* 2005. Available at www.ed.gov/about/offices/list/ocr/504faq.html. Retrieved July 29, 2008.

Office of the Law Revision Counsel, (December 3, 2004). Individuals with Disabilities Education Act. U.S. Code, Title 20, Chapter 33, Subchapter I. Section 1400- Short title; findings; purposes. Subchapter 1- General Provisions, §1400. Short title; findings; purposes. 20 USC Chapter 33- Education of individuals with disabilities. https://uscode.house.gov/.

Pennsylvania Association for Retarded Citizens v. Pennsylvania. U.S. Court of Appeals, 343 F. 1972.

Pelentsov, L. J., Laws, T. A., & Esterman, A. J. (2015). The supportive care needs of parents caring for a child with a rare disease: A scoping review. *Disability Health Journal, 8,* 475–491. https://doi.org/10.1016/j.dhjo.2015.03.009.

Power, T. G., Dahlquist, L. M., & Pinder, W. (2019). Parenting children with a chronic health condition. In Bornstein, M. H. (Ed.), *Handbook of parenting: Children and parenting* (pp. 597–624). Routledge/Taylor & Francis Group https://doi.org/10.4324/9780429440847-18.

Rehabilitation Act of 1973, Public Law 93–112, 87 Stat. 355, enacted September 26, 1973, 29 U.S.C. § 701 et seq.

Research.com. 101 American school statistics: 2023 data, trends & predictions| Research.com. Accessed 3/17/23. 2023.

Riley-Lawless, K. (2006). The demographics of children and adolescents. In Selekman, J. (Ed.), *School nursing: A comprehensive text.* F.A. Davis.

Rief, S. (2016). *How to reach and teach children with ADD/ADHD: Practical technique, strategies, and interventions* (3rd ed.). National Professional Resources, Inc.

Selekman, J. (2019). *School nursing: A comprehensive text.* F.A. Davis.

Selekman, J., & Gamel-McCormick, M. (2006). Children with chronic conditions. In Selekman, J. (Ed.), *School nursing: A comprehensive text.* F.A. Davis.

Shaw, S. R., & McCabe, P. C. (2008). Hospital-to-school transition for children with chronic illness: Meeting the new challenges of an evolving health care system. *Psychology in Schools, 45,* 74–87.

Shiu, S. (2001). Issues in the education of students with chronic illness. *International Journal of Disability, Development, and Education, 48,* 269–281.

Siegel, L. M. (2001). *The complete IEP guide: How to advocate for your special ed child* (2nd ed.). Consolidated Printers.

Special Olympics. Rosa's law. Special Olympics: North America. 2010. http://www.specialolympics.org/Regions/north-america/News-and-Stories/Rosa-s-Law.aspx.

The Royal Children's Hospital. Kids health information: Corticosteroid use. 2018. https://www.rch.org.au/kidsinfo/fact_sheets/Corticosteroid_medicine/. Accessed 3/22/23.

Thurlow, Martha. (Fall 2004). NCLB and the inclusion of students with disabilities in the accountability and assessment systems, testimony before the House Education and Workforce Committee. *Beacon.* Accessed October 30, 2017. http://www.harborhouselaw.com/articles/highstakes.nclb.inclusion.thurow.htm.

Ugalde, M. R., Guffey, D., Minard, C. G., Giardino, A. P., & Johnson, G. A. (2018). A survey of school nurse emergency preparedness 2014-2015. *Journal of School Nursing, 34*(5), 398–408. doi:10.1177/1059840517704702.

US Bureau of the Census. 2020 state population estimates by age, sex, race, and Hispanic origin. Data accessed July 2021 from http://www.census.gov/popest.

US Constitution 14th Amendment U.S. Const. Amend.XIV

US Department of Education. (2006). 34 CFR, Parts 300 & 301: Assistance to states for the education of children with disabilities and preschool grants for children with disabilities. Final rules. *Federal Register, 71,* 46540–46845.

US Department of Education. *Office of Special Programs' IDEA* website. (2008a). Available at http://idea.ed.gov/explore/view/p/%2Croot%2Cstatute%2CI%2C. Retrieved July 29, 2008.

US Department of Education. (2008b). *The Individuals with Disabilities Education Act (IDEA): Provisions related to children with disabilities enrolled by their parents in private school.* Washington, DC: Author.

US Department of Education, ED*Facts* Metadata and Process System (*EMAPS*): IDEA part C child count and settings survey, 2020. Data obtained July 7, 2022.

US Department of Education. Chronic absenteeism in the nation's schools: A hidden educational crisis. 2019. https://www2.ed.gov/datastory/chronicabsenteeism.html.

US Department of Education. 43rd annual report to Congress on the implementation of the Individuals with Disabilities Education Act, 2021. 2022. http://www.ed.gov/about/reports/annual/osep

US Department of Education (2014). Office of Special Education and Rehabilitative Services, Office of Special Education Programs. In , *36th annual report to Congress on the implementation of the Individuals with Disabilities Education Act.* Author. Accessed October 30, 2017. http://www2.ed.gov/about/reports/annual/osep/2014/parts-b-c/36th-idea-arc.pdf. 24.

US Department of Education (2016). Office of Special Education and Rehabilitative Services, Office of Special Education Programs. In , *38th annual report to Congress on the implementation of the Individuals with Disabilities Education Act.* Author. Accessed October 30, 2017. http://www2.ed.gov/about/reports/annual/osep/2016/parts-b-c/38th-arc-for-idea.pdf.

US Department of Justice, Introduction to the Americans with Disabilities Act. https://www.ada.gov/topics/intro-to-ada/.

US Department of Education, Office for Civil Rights. (2022). *Case processing manual.* US Government Printing Office.

US Department of Education, ED*Facts* Data Warehouse (EDW): IDEA part B child count and educational environments collection, 2020-21. Data extracted as of July 7, 2021, from file specifications 002 and 089. Modified from U.S. Department of Education, Office of Special Programs' IDEA Website (2008).

US Government Printing Office. Public Law. 2010. Retrieved from: http://www.gpo.gov/fdsys/pkg/BILLS-111s2781enr/pdf/BILLS-111s2781enr.pdf.

Universal Declaration of Human Rights of 1948, article 26

Vocational Rehabilitation Act. (1973). *Public Law 93-112, 29 USC, Section 504, 45CFR.* Washington, DC: U.S. Government Printing Office.

Wagner, E. H. (1998). Chronic disease management: What will it take to improve care for chronic illness? *Effective Clinical Practice, 1*(1), 2–4.

White House. (2015). *Fact Sheet. Congress acts to fix no child left behind.* Office of the Press Secretary, Briefing Room.

Wilkie, K. J. (2012). Absence makes the heart grow fonder: Students with chronic illness seeking academic continuity through interaction with their teachers at school. *Australasian Journal of Special Education, 36*(1), 1–20. doi:10.1017/jse.2012.4.

Wodrich, D. L., & Cunningham, M. M. (2008). School-based tertiary and targeted interventions for students with chronic medical conditions: Examples from type 1 diabetes mellitus and epilepsy. *Psychology in Schools, 45,* 52–62.

Xie, Q. W., Chan, C. L., & Chan, C. H. (2020). The wounded self-lonely in a crowd: A qualitative study of the voices of children living with atopic dermatitis in Hong Kong. *Health and Social Care in the Community, 28,* 862–873.

Transitions to Adulthood

4

Rachel Whitfield, Gladesia Tolbert

ADOLESCENT TRANSITION TO ADULTHOOD

The transition to adult care is complicated for a child with a chronic illness. Most youth with special health care needs do not receive the necessary support to successfully transition from pediatric to adult care (White & Cooley, 2018). Youth with chronic health conditions and special health care needs face challenges in attaining self-management skills. In concurrence with a physical or developmental disability, complete independence may not always be attainable (Betz et al., 2021). During the transition period, obstacles noted have been linked to poor health outcomes, inadequate follow-up, and increased morbidity and mortality (Okumura et al., 2022). Often health systems and families are reactive and begin fast-tracking the continuation of care once the adolescent approaches adulthood (Pritchard & Rees, 2016). A proactive response is warranted to enhance preparedness and avoid potential adverse outcomes and trauma associated with a lapse in health care.

Young people with long-term conditions are living longer, with 90% of all youth with chronic health conditions surviving into adulthood (Betz et al., 2021). Despite this trajectory, the process of health care transition is often overlooked and unplanned (White et al., 2020). In 2018, Benson et al. reported less than half of youth receiving subspecialty care acquire the knowledge, attitudes, and skills necessary to transition to adult services effectively. Consequently, many young adults entering adulthood do not continue care with a primary care provider resulting in higher emergency department visits, medical complications, and treatment failure (Spencer et al., 2018; White & Cooley, 2018). Lack of transition planning significantly contributes to this gap in care and loss of follow-up. Pediatric and adult health care providers have reported increased difficulty transitioning youth with medical complexity (White & Cooley, 2018). Lebrun-Harris et al. (2018) reported that among youth with special health care needs, only 17% receive recommended transition planning. It is of special concern that adolescents with intensive daily management requirements may be overlooked, resulting in serious life-threatening consequences (Betz et al., 2021).

UNDERSTANDING TRANSITION

Health care transition (HCT) is the planned process of shifting from pediatric to adult health care systems (Okumura et al., 2022; Saulsberry et al., 2019). Successful HCT aims to prepare adolescents to manage their medical care with optimal health outcomes. HCT is comprised of three phases: transition preparation, transfer, and adult care integration (White & Cooley, 2018). HCT occurs during adolescence, which is a critical period to gain the necessary skills to develop independence. Self-management is a prerequisite for optimal transition from pediatric to independent adult care. Transitioning from adolescence to adulthood can be filled with uncertainties, and many youth may be unprepared to manage essential life skills. Attaining health management skills adds additional learning needs and independence (Okumura et al., 2022).

Transitioning youth with a chronic illness or disability to adult care services is an even more complex process requiring coordination and continuity of care (Zhou et al., 2016). The National Survey of Children's Health reported that nearly 31% of adolescents have one or more moderate to severe chronic illnesses (Alderman & Breuner, 2019). A quarter of chronically ill adolescents have at least one unmet health need, which may affect the adolescent's physical growth, development, and adult health trajectory (Alderman & Breuner, 2019). However, only 18% to 23% of adolescents receive transition management, with most pediatric providers beginning this process between 18 and 20 years of age (Lebrun-Harris et al., 2018). Findings revealed that most pediatric providers begin transition planning between 18 and 20 years of age (Lebrun-Harris et al., 2018). HCT should incorporate a planned, proactive approach from dependence to developmentally appropriate self-management (Okumura et al., 2022). This approach should be included in routine health care visits beginning at age 12 (Lebrun-Harris et al., 2018; White & Cooley, 2018).

Children who grow up with a pediatric-onset chronic condition are not only required to adjust to the uncertainties of multifaceted life transitions from childhood to adulthood but also must simultaneously cope with the daily challenges of their health condition (Sattoe & van Staa, 2021). Meeting these challenges is even more demanding for those with chronic health conditions, particularly those with a physical disability. Pritchard and Rees (2016) reported that adolescents with a physical disability are often inaccurately assumed to be lacking in mental capacity. This assumption has been an obstacle to these adolescents' engagement in active decisions surrounding their care (Pritchard & Rees, 2016).

Teamwork remains a vital component in coordinating care during the HCT process (White & Cooley, 2018). In 2006, Gall et al. (2006) introduced a shared management model. In this model, the authors outline the shift as youth gradually adapt from being receivers of their care to leaders of their care. When adolescents become leaders, the parents' role changes to consultants, and health care providers become resources.

Learning health management skills and engaging in self-management involve a wide range of specialized tasks and awareness to maintain stability and prevent complications that can interfere with daily functioning. To maximize positive outcomes and decrease barriers, adolescents must have time to ease into this transition with education reinforced in all settings (Betz et al., 2021). Structured transition interventions improve adherence, health literacy, and patient satisfaction and reduce emergency department visits and hospitalizations (Lebrun-Harris et al., 2018).

ADOLESCENCE AND EMERGING ADULTHOOD: A UNIVERSAL TIME OF CHANGE

Adolescence is the stage of life between childhood and adulthood, occurring between 10 and 24 years of age (Alderman & Breuner, 2019; Arain et al., 2013). The primary goal of adolescence is to achieve a sense of identity and become independent, responsible adults. To achieve this goal, healthy cognitive, psychosocial, physical, and sexual development is necessary for all adolescents. Adolescents have unique attributes that must be addressed to ensure quality health needs are met (Alderman & Breuner, 2019). Unique biologic and psychosocial changes occur rapidly during the period of adolescence.

Shaped by hormonal, physical, psychological, and social change, the adolescent period is marked by pubertal hormonal changes and physical maturation (Arain et al., 2013). The timing and physiology of puberty have been associated with differences between racial groups and adolescents with chronic conditions. Some chronic conditions, such as obesity and trauma, may result in early puberty. Delayed pubertal onset may also be associated with the development of chronic illnesses (Alderman & Breuner, 2019). Developmental delays can subsequently affect the progression of key psychosocial developmental milestones and self-care management. Providers need to gain familiarity with normal adolescent social and cognitive development and how these developmental changes shape the complex needs of an adolescent with chronic health conditions (Alderman & Breuner, 2019).

Cognitive and psychosocial development in adolescents is not congruent, although both rely on significant brain structure changes (Sanders, 2013; Vijayakumar,

2018). These necessary changes enable adolescents to achieve mental and emotional developmental progress. The establishment and nurturing of intimate relationships, the development of identity, future perspective, independence, self-confidence, self-control, and social skill development occur during this period (Vijayakumar, 2018).

FACTORS MODERATING INDIVIDUAL TRANSITION

Cognitive development, psychosocial development, problem solving, degree of autonomy, peer relationships, and sexuality are all factors that influence an adolescent's ease and success in the transition to adulthood.

COGNITIVE DEVELOPMENT

Jean Piaget proposed that adolescents are in the formal operational stage of his four stages of cognitive development. In this stage, adolescents begin to plan for the future, think hypothetically, and assume adult responsibilities. Further brain development must occur for the formal operational stage to commence (Sanders, 2013). Brain development remains under construction during adolescence and is ongoing through early adulthood. Complete brain development is not achieved until approximately 25 years of age. Researchers in brain development found that during adolescent development, changes in signaling regulate impulse control, placing adolescents at an increased propensity for high-risk behaviors. Adverse childhood experiences have been shown to impact brain development, impacting health choices (Alderman & Breuner, 2019; Vijayakumar, 2018).

While physical changes, including accelerated growth, development of secondary sexual characteristics, and pubertal maturation, occur rapidly during adolescence, social, emotional, and cognitive function skills are still in process (Arain et al., 2013). Brain development occurs from back to front, with the limbic structures of the midbrain maturing before the prefrontal cortex. The limbic and paralimbic structures of the brain guide the social-emotional system, while the prefrontal and parietal cortical structures control the cognitive system. The limbic system accounts for reactive, unconscious thought and rapid automatic processing leading to reward-seeking behavior and a heightened response to emotionally loaded situations. As the brain develops during adolescence, it becomes more efficient as so-called *pruning* of gray matter and synapses occurs (Alderman & Breuner, 2019; McNeely & Blanchard, 2009). The prefrontal cortex, the region of the brain responsible for abstract thinking, rational decision making, emotional regulation, and executive function, is the last to develop (Vijayakumar, 2018).

PSYCHOSOCIAL DEVELOPMENT

Psychosocial development occurring during the adolescent period is comprised of acquiring developmental skills leading to autonomy, identity, and future orientation (Sanders, 2013). Establishing autonomy includes the adolescent striving to become emotionally and financially independent of parents or guardians (Sanders, 2013). Most adolescents seek independence gradually. Anticipatory guidance for parents promoting the emerging need for independence is helpful for parents to adjust to this normal developmental stage (Sanders, 2013).

As adolescents transition into adulthood, they begin thinking about their future roles as adults. Erik Erikson defined eight stages of psychosocial development, with adolescents' primary goal to achieve identity. Erikson proposed that adolescents develop a sense of self and look toward their future. During this period, adolescents may begin experimentation with a range of behaviors and activities to figure out their identity (Sanders, 2013). Within this theory, adolescents who have an unhealthy dependence on their parents may experience more role confusion than adolescents who pursue their interests.

Adolescents with a chronic illness may have more difficulties developing positive self-image and identity due to their limited ability to reach independence and the impact of their illness on body image. Inadequate achievement of self-identity can lead to low self-esteem, underachievement, mental health problems, substance use, and increased risk-taking behaviors (Sanders, 2013). Acceptance and praise of the adolescent are important during this stage to help promote the establishment of a secure identity. Once identity is achieved, the ability for future orientation becomes more within reach. During this late adolescent stage, youth have gained increased cognitive maturity and are able to identify realistic goals. During this time, the expectation is for youth to have increased autonomy, have more responsibility, and be treated as adults (Sanders, 2013).

PROBLEM SOLVING AND AUTONOMY

Studies of youth with chronic conditions have identified that problem-solving and autonomy skills are related to positive health outcomes (Beacham & Deatrick, 2013; Holmbeck et al., 2002; Sawin et al., 2002). Knowledge about health care, specific chronic conditions, and experience in making decisions are prerequisites for making decisions about health. Practicing decision making in other areas (e.g., what clothes to purchase, hairstyle, what to do with friends, how to budget money) allows youth to gain confidence through experience. Health care choices are impossible for adolescents to make without strong decision-making skills to build upon. Experience is essential to solving potential health care dilemmas; giving simple choices (e.g., whether to take the medication with applesauce or gelatin) should be offered as early as developmentally possible so that there is a gradual movement to making all choices about health care management.

Health care autonomy is a developmental key that links caregiver management and self-care. Health care autonomy typically occurs during late adolescence, with many health care providers and caregivers expecting children with chronic conditions to master the skill of self-care earlier. Health care autonomy is the ability to evaluate options, make decisions, and define health-related goals with the confidence to stand by the decisions and develop strategies to meet health-related goals (Beacham & Deatrick, 2013).

The development of autonomy is integral to the development of self-care in children with chronic conditions providing the foundation for child health and well-being. Chronic health conditions can lead to decreased well-being for children in terms of missed school days, social interactions, and activities, as well as a loss of wages and increased medical expenses for the parents (Beacham & Deatrick, 2013). Families and caregivers face the challenges of managing all facets of the child's condition early in the child's life and then transitioning the management responsibilities to the child.

ATTITUDES, BELIEFS, PERCEPTIONS, AND PEER RELATIONSHIPS

An adolescent's attitudes, beliefs, and perceptions, such as hope, communication, self-efficacy, coping, and future expectations, can significantly impact outcomes. Problem solving and autonomy are critical skills necessary to develop self-management and independence; attitudes and beliefs have been found to be the strongest predictors of mental health measures, such as depression, behavior problems, and health-related quality of life.

Establishing meaningful friendships with others is the hallmark of successful social interaction. Friendships are the basis for the social, emotional, and practical support needed to become truly integrated into society and are one measure of success in community integration. The social skills necessary for successful peer relationships are reading verbal and nonverbal cues from others, making judgments about those cues, and responding appropriately. Mastering social skills can be hard for many individuals with learning disabilities, chronic health conditions, or neurodevelopmental deficits. Social immaturity, isolation, limited social life, and a lack of social skills may all be present in youth with chronic conditions (Murphy & Young, 2005; Zimmerman et al., 2022). The social expectation for displays of affection, caring, anger, and frustration must be learned in adolescence if not acquired during childhood. Transition plans must aggressively identify mechanisms for integrating youth with chronic conditions with their peers in educational, recreational, sports, and social activities. Adults who have successfully transitioned report that peer and inclusion activities are fundamental to independence.

SEXUALITY

Sexuality is a basic component of full adult life. Developing an identity as a sexual being is a universal developmental task of adolescents and young adults and should not be confused with sexual activity. Youth with chronic conditions are sexual beings with desires and interests similar to those of their unaffected peers, yet society often views and treats them as asexual. Adolescent women with chronic health conditions who experience pregnancy may be at increased risk of dropping out of school because of pregnancy or child-bearing issues.

Sex education should focus on the physical changes of puberty, along with integrated alterations caused by their condition, to have a successful transition (Engelen et al., 2019; Murphy & Young, 2005; Buran et al., 2006). Discussions over time should include abuse and pregnancy prevention, access to reproductive health care, and responsible sexual decision making. Body image and the development of sexual sense are especially impaired by chronic conditions, with these issues of sexuality not routinely addressed by school programs, caregivers, health care providers, or other transition team members (Engelen et al., 2019; Murphy & Young, 2005; Buran et al., 2006).

Condition-specific information is critical. For example, it is important for youth with spina bifida, who have a very high incidence of latex allergy, to avoid latex condoms. Likewise, women with spinal cord injuries may not be good candidates for oral contraceptives because of their high risk for deep vein thrombosis. Young women with epilepsy treated with select anticonvulsants have an increased risk of fetal anomalies if the type and dose of the medications are not altered before conception. It is also important to realize that seizure medication can interact with some oral contraceptives, decreasing their effectiveness (American Academy of Neurology, 1998).

DEVELOPMENTAL STAGES AND TRANSITION PLANNING

The early adolescent stage between 11 and 14 years is an opportune time to begin transitioning to adult care as it is a time of transforming and developing lasting health behaviors (Got Transition, 2022). During this period, the priority is to promote less dependence on caregivers and encourage increased involvement of adolescents in their health needs. Providers need to begin one-on-one time with adolescents during preventive care visits. One-on-one time promotes the development of trust and improves the adolescent's comfort level talking to a health care provider. During this stage it is ideal for the provider to begin discussing the need for decision-making guidance and guardianship with adolescents with intellectual and developmental disabilities (Got Transition, 2022).

During middle adolescence, between the age of 15 and 17, assessing for current self-care skills and promoting new self-care skills are priorities. Designated one-on-one time with the provider remains a key component of preventive visits, which sets the groundwork to prepare the adolescent for an adult model of care, including discussion of privacy and consent laws. Anticipatory guidance on self-care skills, readiness, and transferring to an adult clinician is provided. Motivational interviewing is recommended to assess readiness and confidence in self-care and transferring to an adult provider. In a patient with intellectual and developmental disabilities, a guardianship plan must be in place before age 18 (Got Transition, 2022).

The late adolescent period is between 18 and 21 years of age; although the cognitive function is still developing, age 18 is considered the legal adult age in most states. Without legal guardianship documentation, privacy and confidentiality should be protected at this stage, and young adults should begin receiving an adult model of care. At 18, young adults should begin receiving an adult model of care and should be seen individually for the complete visit duration (Got Transition, 2022). Many young adults leave home and gain adult responsibilities while pursuing education, employment, and independent living during this period. During preventive health visits, a final transition readiness assessment should be completed to identify any remaining skills necessary to complete their trajectory toward independent health care management (Got Transition, 2022).

Adolescents often face situations that place them at risk due to incomplete brain development and the gradual progression toward autonomy and executive functioning (Alderman & Breuner, 2019). They may engage in risk-taking behaviors, such as drug and alcohol use, electronic cigarette use, and unprotected sex. Most adolescent health visits are to seek treatment for preventable conditions, some of which may have long-term health consequences (Alderman & Breuner, 2019). Unintentional injuries, homicide, and suicide are the leading causes of morbidity and mortality in this age group. Young adults are vulnerable due to risky behaviors, low health care utilization, and increased susceptibility to worsening chronic conditions (White & Cooley, 2018). Health care can be low in priority compared with other transition tasks of adolescence, such as education, housing, relationships, and employment (White & Cooley, 2018). These developmental challenges are not isolated to healthy adolescents. Adolescents with chronic health conditions face similar developmental challenges, with the added concerns of adjustments related to their medical issues (Alderman & Breuner, 2019) (Table 4.1).

BARRIERS TO HEALTH CARE TRANSITION

For successful planning and HCT to occur, barriers must be recognized and addressed. Several factors have contributed to the lack of transition preparation and planning. HCT has progressed from a pediatric-only responsibility to a shared multidisciplinary responsibility with the inclusion of adult care clinicians

Table 4.1 Developmentally Based Skills Checklist

HEALTH PROMOTION AND CONDITION MANAGEMENT	MEDICATIONS, SUPPLIES, AND OTHER EQUIPMENT	HEALTH CARE SYSTEM
Early Adolescence (11–14 yr)		
Knows simple anatomy, physiology, and pathology Able to tell health care providers what is wrong Discusses diagnosis and management plans with parents and providers Knows name(s), dates, and significance of any chronic illness and significant injuries Can perform appropriate first aid Knows cardiopulmonary resuscitation Knows any allergies and can outline avoidance and emergency treatment actions Takes responsibility to monitor chronic condition and quickly notify parents of any new developments Manages aspects of chronic condition in predictable or common situations, accessing consultation for family or other resource people in unfamiliar situations If assistance with ADLs needed, can identify needs and preferences and knows the tasks to be carried out by others Has opportunity to develop decision making and has responsibilities at home Knows about basic money management (e.g., function of checking and saving accounts) and manages small personal resources	Knows names of medication taken, dose, reason, expected response Is aware of amount of regularly taken medication remaining in container and alerts parents or caregiver when low Understands the difference between illicit drugs and medications Takes medications for chronic condition correctly Knows use and care of equipment and supplies and can notify parents when problems occur	Knows the difference in kinds of health care providers (e.g., obstetrician vs. optometrist) Knows date of and reason for next health appointment Knows where primary care providers and specialists are located and how to contact them
Middle Adolescence (15–17 yr)		
Knows date of last menstrual period (girls) and keeps record on personal or family calendar (i.e., may be early task for females with early-onset menses) Knows the basics of own health history, including family history Knows year of last tetanus shot Knows about TSE and BSE; performs regularly Manages chronic conditions in less predictable situations; seeks consultation when needed; requires minimal day-to-day supervision Can plan ahead to anticipate problem areas and generate options If assistance with ADLs needed, knows care well enough to direct others in the steps Has increasing responsibility in family Has a savings or checking account and manages it with supervision from parents if needed	Calls pharmacy to reorder own medications or calls own provider about need for refill Knows the difference between generic and proprietary medication Selects own medications for minor illnesses (e.g., URI, headaches) Orders new supplies or equipment with supervision; can reorder these materials independently Arranges for transportation to get medication supplies or for appointments	Makes own health care appointments Knows basic facts of own health insurance; knows limitations and issues for insurance in ordering supplies or medications and other equipment
Late Adolescence and Emerging Adulthood (18–25 yr)		
Manages stable chronic condition independently; uses parents or professionals to get advice regarding complex situations but makes management decisions Participates in discussions regarding adult health care options Understands the connection among mind, body, and spirit in health and illness Engages in healthy lifestyle activities; chooses healthful foods; exercises regularly; avoids caffeine, tobacco, illicit substances; gets adequate amount of sleep If assistance for ADLs needed participates in the hiring, supervision, and termination of attendant caregiver	Independently manages medication, manages assessment and repair of any equipment, and pays for or arranges payment for medications and supplies	Understands the complexities of own health insurance plan Understands effect of change in employment or school status on insurance options Keeps updated file of own health records Takes responsibility to initiate contact with providers when transition to new living or educational environment occurs

ADLs, Activities of daily living; BSE, breast self-examination; TSE, testicular self-examination; URI, upper respiratory infection.

(White & Cooley, 2018). This necessary partnership between adult and pediatric clinicians and collaboration between health care delivery systems can be challenging. Transition training and education among health care providers are key. To reach optimal adult health, increased awareness is needed among youth, young adults, and their families of the importance of health maintenance and continuity of care (White & Cooley, 2018).

Significant barriers may influence adolescents' willingness to participate in health care management and subsequent transition planning. Some of these deterrents include fear of lack of confidentiality, judgment of health care providers, and stigma (Aeschbach et al., 2021). Inadequate preparedness, insufficient self-management skills, system-level barriers, lack of resources, care coordination, and poor communication between providers have been cited as barriers to transition (Okumura et al., 2022).

Barriers summarized by White and Cooley (2018) include adolescents' hesitation to leave their pediatric provider and institution and fear of a new health care system. It also may be difficult to gain control of their health care from parents' authority. These adolescents and families may have limited to no experience with one-on-one time with the pediatric provider (White & Cooley, 2018). Adolescents who are not allowed to be adequately involved in decisions surrounding their health can become frustrated, leading to detrimental effects on their self-esteem and fostering the development of mistrust of health care providers (Pritchard & Rees, 2016).

Other logistical barriers include inexperience with insurance issues and loss of coverage, health care records access, and prescription refill management (White & Cooley, 2018). Although many youth desire to manage their health care, some may be less interested due to anxiety about the unknown and limited knowledge or experience with the adult health care system, including where and how to access care. Inadequate support and lack of preparation have been recurring barriers. Adult care providers with specialized knowledge of pediatric-onset chronic conditions may be limited, posing an additional barrier to these youth (Boxes 4.1 and 4.2) (White & Cooley, 2018).

FACTORS MODERATING TRANSITION

Comorbidities can complicate this already delicate process. Adolescents with mental health conditions are more likely to be lost to follow-up care during the transitional period. This is particularly concerning as an increased rate of mental health conditions peak during young adulthood. Mental and behavioral challenges can limit a patient's ability to participate in self-care and health care decision making. A shortage of mental and behavioral health providers exacerbates these challenges. Partnerships with family members, mental health providers, and community agencies

Box 4.1 Youth, Young Adult, and Family Transition Barriers

FEAR OF A NEW HEALTH CARE SYSTEM AND/OR HOSPITAL
Not wanting to leave their pediatric clinician and pediatric institution
Anxiety about how to relinquish control around managing their youth condition
Anxiety of not knowing the adult clinicians, adult health care system, and logistical issues (i.e., finding parking, making appointments, finding a primary care provider who is taking new patients, transferring patient records, and insurance issues)
Changing and/or different therapies recommended in adult health care
Families' fear that adult clinicians will not listen to and value their expertise
Negative beliefs about adult health care

INADEQUATE PLANNING
Inadequate preparation and support from clinicians on the transition process and adult model of care
Not having seen clinician alone
Youth and young adults less interested in health compared with broader life circumstances
Adolescents' age, sex, and race and/or ethnicity and their parents' socioeconomic status can affect transition preparation

SYSTEM DIFFICULTIES
Lack of communication and coordination and transfer of medical records between adult and pediatric clinician or system
Limited availability of adult primary and specialty clinicians
Difficulty in locating adult clinicians who have specialized knowledge about and community resources for youth with pediatric-onset chronic diseases
Loss of insurance coverage among young adults and cost of care barriers

From White, P. H., & Cooley, W. C. (2018). Supporting the health care transition from adolescence to adulthood in the medical home. *Pediatrics, 142*(5), 1–20.

encouraging self-advocacy early on can help bridge this gap (White & Cooley, 2018).

Youth with medical complexities include those with several chronic health conditions affecting multiple organ systems. Transitioning to this special population poses a unique set of challenges requiring a high level of care, coordination, and frequent consultation. For this high level of coordination to care, individualized transition planning is fundamental. Collaboration must occur among inpatient and outpatient care teams in pediatric and adult institutions (White & Cooley, 2018).

Survival rates for chronic conditions have increased into adulthood; therefore ensuring continuity of care for patients with pediatric-onset chronic illnesses is of vital importance. Saulsberry et al. (2019) describes a subset of patients who develop increased disease severity during the transition of the health care transfer period. This time of transition is deemed a high-risk time, resulting in increased incidents of poor outcomes. For example, between the ages

Box **4.2**	Adult and Pediatric Clinician Transition Barriers

COMMUNICATION AND/OR CONSULTATION GAPS

Lack of communication, coordination, guidelines, and protocols between the pediatric and adult systems

Inadequate communication from pediatric clinicians, often with a lack of medical records and follow-up recommendations

Lack of long-term follow-up guidelines with care information for youth with special health care needs

Gap in consultation with pediatric clinicians

Adult clinicians' concerns about not enough adult subspecialty or mental health care clinicians to care for young adults

TRAINING LIMITATIONS

Lack of knowledge and/or training in pediatric-onset conditions and adolescent development and behavior

Difficulty meeting psychosocial needs of young adults with pediatric-onset conditions

Caring for adult patients reliant on caregivers

CARE DELIVERY, CARE COORDINATION, AND/OR STAFF SUPPORT GAPS

Lack of care coordination and follow-up

Lack of mental health and supportive services

Unfamiliarity with local and regional resources for young adults with chronic conditions

Lack of adequate infrastructure and training

Administrative constraints and lack of time and reimbursement

Lack of coverage for young adults

LACK OF PATIENT KNOWLEDGE AND ENGAGEMENT

Young adults' lack of knowledge about disease treatments, medications, and medical history

Lack of information about community resources and/or support groups

Dependency on parents or guardians

Lack of self-advocacy, decision-making skills, and self-care skills

Poor adherence to care

Unrealistic expectations of youth or young adult knowledge of adult medical system and lack of readiness for adult care

LACK OF COMFORT WITH ADULT CARE

Unrealistic youth, young adult, and family expectations of time and attention

Concerns regarding loss of strong relationships with previous clinicians (patient, parent, and/or staff)

Pediatric clinician's lack of confidence in adult clinician and in the stylistic differences between pediatric and adult care, particularly for some youth and young adults with intellectual or developmental disabilities or behavioral health conditions

Parents' reluctance to relinquish responsibility

Parents unaware of changes in privacy issues

From White, P. H., & Cooley, W. C. (2018). Supporting the health care transition from adolescence to adulthood in the medical home. *Pediatrics*, *142*(5), 1–20.

of 20 and 24 there is a rise in mortality for patients with sickle cell disease coinciding with the time frame they leave pediatric health care (Saulsberry et al., 2019).

Social determinants of health should be considered in all adolescents during each health care visit. Social complexities are the source of many disparities in receiving adequate health care access and utilization. These disparities may affect the care received among ethnic and minority groups, refugee populations, and those with language and cultural differences, as well as those who are lesbian, gay, bisexual, transgender, and queer. Youth affected by poverty, homelessness, and foster care need specific resources to enhance their transition process. Engaging with community health workers and the involvement of social workers, schools, and community centers can be advantageous for these patients (White & Cooley, 2018).

HEALTH CARE TRANSITION PLANNING

The process of adapting from a mentality of being a recipient of care to managing health care is a process requiring commitment and planning. Streamlining the process of transitioning adolescents to adult care has been ever evolving. The American Academy of Pediatrics (AAP), the American Academy of Family Physicians (AAFP), and the American College of Physicians (ACP) recommend that the HCT process be more interdisciplinary with the inclusion of nurses and social workers (White & Cooley, 2018). Li et al. (2022) recommend incorporating dedicated time for transition readiness into clinic visits. Health care providers should integrate separate transition visits, focusing on planning and advocacy.

A change in clinical practice is essential to support the education needed to assist these patients (Betz et al., 2021). Due to the rising need for adult providers to care for patients with childhood-onset illnesses, new initiatives and improvements to transition have arisen. Pediatric to adult-based HCT has become a priority nationwide. HCT planning models have been developed to ease this process (Betz et al., 2021; White & Cooley, 2018). The transition theory is an application framework for transitioning youth to adulthood. Meleis's transition theory recognizes transition as a complex process. Meleis addresses the need for readiness assessment, the influence of environment and community, and health care inequities (Lestishock et al., 2021). As outlined by White and Cooley (2018), there are nine overarching tenets/principles for successful HCT (Box 4.3).

THE SIX CORE ELEMENTS OF HEALTH CARE TRANSITION

In 2018, a clinical report on HCT, a collaborative effort by AAP, AAFP, and ACP, recommended establishing a widely adopted approach to transitioning (White & Cooley, 2018). Got Transition, a federally funded national resource center on HCT, developed a structured clinical approach to HCT. The Six Core Elements of Health Care Transition is a structured clinical approach created for health care providers to assist youth in their transition to adult care (Got Transition, 2022). The goal of this approach is to guide health care systems, professionals, and clinicians in improving

Box **4.3**	Nine Overarching Tenets/Principles for Successful Health Care Transfer

1. Importance of youth-centered and/or young adult–centered, strength-based focus
2. Emphasis on self-determination, self-management, and family and/or caregiver engagement
3. Acknowledgment of individual differences and complexities
4. Recognition of vulnerabilities and need for a distinct population health approach for youth and young adults
5. Need for early and ongoing preparation, including the integration into an adult model of care
6. Importance of shared accountability, effective communication, and care coordination between pediatric and adult clinicians and systems of care
7. Recognition of the influences of cultural beliefs and attitudes as well as socioeconomic status
8. Emphasis on achieving health equity and elimination of disparities
9. Need for parents and caregivers to support youth and young adults in building knowledge regarding their own health and skills in making health decisions and using health care

From White, P. H., & Cooley, W. C. (2018). Supporting the health care transition from adolescence to adulthood in the medical home. *Pediatrics*, *142*(5), 1–20.

how adolescents and young adults manage their health care safely and effectively as they transition from a pediatric to an adult model of care.

The six core elements include policy/guide, tracking and monitoring, readiness, planning, transfer of care, and transition completion (Got Transition, 2022):

Core Element 1: *Transition and Care Policy/Guide* is implemented in early adolescence, between 12 and 14. The second, third, and fourth stages all occur between 14 and 18. For Core Element 1, the clinician develops the transition and care policy/guide and shares it with the patient and family.

Core Element 2: *Tracking and Monitoring* involves the progress via an individual registry within the electronic medical record.

Core Element 3: *Transition Readiness* is where the readiness and self-care assessment occurs. In this stage, the clinician assesses self-care skills and offers customized education.

Core Element 4: *Transition Planning* is the individualized HCT plan developed within the medical summary. This phase is delivered in collaboration with adolescents and parents/caregivers. The transition planning will continue until the youth transfers out of pediatric care. Transition planning is an individual, customized approach encompassing building health literacy and independent self-care skills.

Core Element 5: *Transfer of Care* is a systematic process for transferring care to an adult clinician established during this phase. Coordination of care is necessary for youth with special health care needs requiring multiple clinicians and subspecialists. When transferring to multiple clinicians, Got Transition (2022)

suggests staggering transitions so that the transfers to primary and subspecialty clinicians do not occur simultaneously. It is ideal that all transfers to an adult care system occur while health insurance remains active to avoid any disruptions in coverage.

Core Element 6: *Transfer Completion* is the final stage of the approach, during which the pediatric provider confirms the youth has transferred successfully to an adult clinician and offers transition support and pediatric consultation as needed.

These elements outline the basic components of a structured transition process, with sample tools for each (Got Transition, 2022) (Table 4.2). They are intended to be customized for all practice settings and applied to different transition care models (White & Cooley, 2018). The HCT intervention can be molded to fit individual health complexities and social determinants of adolescent health and include a timeline and step-by-step approach with sample tools for transition planning. There are three versions of the Six Core Elements approach. One version is for pediatric practices, another is tailored to adult practices, and the last is for family medicine clinicians who care for patients throughout their lifespans. The sample tools included in the Six Core Elements for pediatric practices include a transition policy, tracking and monitoring (and forms), readiness assessment, transition planning, patient education, and transfer of care tools.

ACCESS TO HEALTH CARE AS AN ADULT

Successful HCT is linked with better health outcomes, such as improved long-term adherence to treatment plans, increased quality of life, and self-care skills. It has also been shown to increase attendance at adult visits and decrease the time between the last pediatric visit and the initial visit to an adult care provider (White & Cooley, 2018). Data from the 2021 National Healthcare Quality and Disparities Report (NHQDR) show that 16% of adults and 6% of children were not scheduled for their routine care within the time frame the appointment was needed. Having timely access to comprehensive and quality health care services improves overall health outcomes and reduces unnecessary disability and premature deaths, as well as the overall cost of health care for the consumer (Agency for Healthcare Research, 2021). A transition planning, tracking, and follow-through process is vital for the successful transition of youth into adult care (White et al., 2018). This process should begin early in adolescence and continue through young adulthood. Historically, HCT has been primarily the responsibility of pediatric care providers. A more recent paradigm shift includes a shared responsibility by the pediatric and adult care clinicians and the medical team, along with the utilization of technology such as electronic medical records and telemedicine for communication throughout the transition process (White & Cooley, 2018).

Table 4.2 Six Core Elements of Transition Approach Roles for Pediatric and Adult Practices[a]

PRACTICE/ PROVIDER	1. TRANSITION POLICY	2. TRACKING AND MONITORING	3. TRANSITION READINESS/ ORIENTATION TO ADULT PRACTICE	4. TRANSITION PLANNING/ INTEGRATION INTO ADULT CARE	5. TRANSFER OF CARE/INITIAL VISIT	6. TRANSITION COMPLETION/ ONGOING CARE
Pediatric	Create and discuss with youth/family	Track progress of youth/family readiness for transition	Transition RA	Develop transition plan including needed RA skills	Transfer of care with information and communication to adult clinician	Obtain feedback on the transition process
Adult	Create and discuss with YA/guardian, if needed	Track progress to increase YA's knowledge of health and adult health care system	Share/discuss welcome and FAQs letter with YA and caregiver, if needed	Obtain transfer package, communicate with pediatric PCP	Review transfer package, address YA concerns about new practice, clarify adult approach to care	Confirm completion of transfer with pediatric practice, obtain feedback, continue self-care skill building

[a]Providers caring for youth/young adults throughout the lifespan would complete both sets of core elements without the transfer process.
FAQ, Frequently asked questions; *PCP,* primary care provider; *RA,* readiness assessment; *YA,* young adult.
From Got Transition. (2022). The Six Core Elements of Health Care Transition. Available at: http://gottransition.org/six-core-elements/.

Without structured HCT interventions, the young adult has an increased likelihood of experiencing poor health outcomes due to delayed care, medication complications, decreased well-being, difficulty with treatment and medication adherence, and increased cost to the young adult and medical system due to increased emergency department utilization and hospitalizations (Quinn et al., 2020). Despite these findings, many young adults report a lack of preparation for HCT and regard health care as a low priority compared to education, employment, housing, relationships, and recreation while transitioning to adulthood. From 2020 to 2021 only 20% of children with special needs received the services necessary for a successful transition into adult care, and only 16% of children without special needs received the services necessary for a successful transition into adult care (Maternal and Child Health Bureau, 2021).

Many barriers exist to obtaining quality structured transition planning; as outlined previously, the clinician must also consider the many disparities of vulnerable populations in the US health care system. Social determinants of health consider one's environment and help clinicians anticipate health disparities and inequalities that youth may experience (Fig. 4.1). Social determinants of health include economic stability, access to quality education, access to quality health care, environment, and community (Healthy People, 2030). Adolescents and young adults with decreased access to education, fair wage employment, unsafe environments, and unstable living conditions are vulnerable to experiencing health disparities and inequalities and ultimately have decreased likelihood of a successful transition.

Vulnerable populations are those at higher risk for health disparities because of age, gender, disability,

Social determinants of health

Fig. 4.1 Social determinants of health. (From Healthy People 2030, US Department of Health and Human Services, Office of Disease Prevention and Health Promotion. [2022, October 21]. https://health.gov/healthypeople/objectives-and-data/social-determinants-health.)

geography, socioeconomic status, and risk status related to sex and gender (Centers for Disease Control and Prevention, 2022). There are specific traits that make youth particularly vulnerable; those who are aging out of foster care, those in the juvenile justice system, and those in racial, ethnic, and socioeconomic minorities are all included as vulnerable populations and should be accounted for when considering transition planning (Quinn et al., 2020).

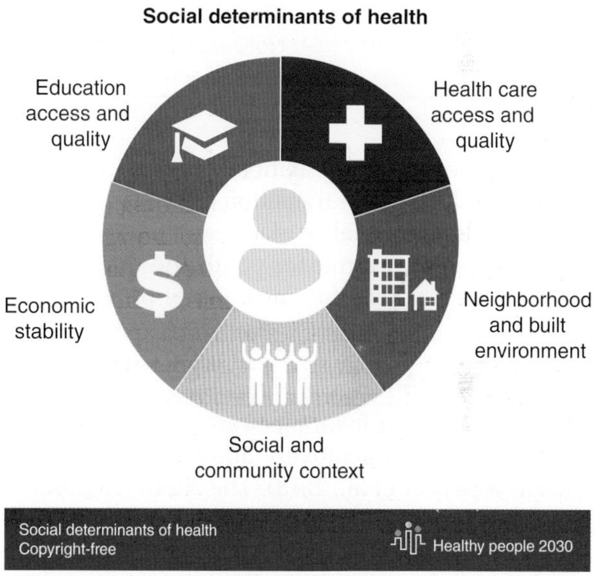

Clinicians must apply a comprehensive multidisciplinary approach when transitioning youth to adult care. Barriers that both clinicians and youth experience, social determinants of health, and vulnerabilities

Table 4.3   Types of Health Insurance Coverage Available to Youth

PLAN	DESCRIPTION
Public	
Medicaid	Provides free or low-cost health coverage based on income, age, or health status. Coverage and eligibility vary by state and funded through federal and state funds.
Medicare	A federal insurance program for people with certain disabilities, health conditions or over the age of 65.
Other: Children's Health Insurance Program	Provides low-cost health coverage for children in families that do not qualify for Medicaid due to income but would endure financial hardship to purchase private coverage. Coverage and eligibility vary by state and funded through federal and state funds.
Private	
Health Maintenance Organization	Covers contracted providers and institutions, focused on health. Typically lower out of pocket cost. Can only use in network care except in emergencies.
Preferred Provider Organization	Can see any provider within designated network. Can see providers outside of network for a higher cost.
Exclusive Provider Organization	A managed care plan that only covers contracted providers and institutions. Can only use in-network care except in emergencies.
Point of Service	Pay less when you use providers within the network but requires referrals.
Catastrophic	Low monthly premiums and high deductible. An affordable way to cover worst-case scenarios. Typically for people younger than 30.
Other	
Student Health Plan	Offered through postsecondary institutions.
Direct Primary Care	Not insurance coverage. A program where the consumer pays the practice directly for a defined set of services.

specific to adolescent populations must be considered throughout all stages of transition planning. A team of clinicians, nurses, social workers, and adult care providers must all play a role for youth and their families to experience a successful, meaningful transition into adulthood.

HEALTH INSURANCE

Ensuring linkage to insurance care during childhood has been shown to positively affect health outcomes in adults (Spencer et al., 2018). The 2021 NHQDR outlines that with expanded access to insurance coverage, low-income adults and those with chronic conditions have improved medication adherence, increased use of preventative care, and a positive outlook on their perceived health care status. Evidence also suggests that increasing access to insurance coverage decreases disparities in access to care and increases equity in the care provided. Adolescents and young adults are most likely to lack insurance coverage, which can cause delays in care, increased cost of care delivered, and potential tax consequences for lack of coverage due to the Affordable Care Act (ACA) requirements. Understanding the options for medical coverage and coordinating coverage can be difficult for youth to navigate independently; health care team members can play an integral role in ensuring youth have a smooth and coordinated transition into adult care and coverage.

Youth may have questions about the different types of health insurance and coverage available and how to enroll. Table 4.3 outlines the various types of coverage

available. Medicaid or the Children's Health Insurance Program (CHIP) covers most youth with chronic health conditions. Over 72 million Americans are enrolled in Medicaid and CHIP programs, with approximately 9.6 million children enrolled in CHIP (CHIP, n.d.). The coverage that Medicaid and CHIP provide is mandated by federal law, but details and eligibility criteria vary by state. Continuing Medicaid after age 18 varies by state regulations and depends on income, health conditions, and eligibility for Supplemental Security Income (SSI). Those who exit foster care at 18 and are on Medicaid while in foster care are not eligible for other Medicaid coverage and may continue coverage until age 26.

The ACA of 2010 provided many options for youth transitioning out of pediatric coverage to adult coverage. The ACA removed the ability for insurance companies to deny coverage for preexisting conditions; this is essential for chronically ill youth and young adults. Many states expanded Medicaid coverage with the ACA's enactment, making these programs more accessible for youth. In most states, youth who have job-based or Marketplace insurance coverage through their parent's plan are now eligible for coverage up to the age of 26 if they are claimed as tax dependents or live in their parent's home, regardless of school enrollment, marital status, or if they have adopted or are adopting a child. Additional benefits offered through the ACA include free preventative care, more options for young adults, removing lifetime and annual coverage limits, assured coverage for birth control methods, mental health, and substance abuse programs.

Those who do not meet the eligibility requirements for Medicaid and are not covered by a parent's plan are eligible to enroll in health insurance through the ACA Marketplace, which provides many options for insurance coverage for the young adult. Youth in college also have the option to enroll in a school-based student health plan.

The Consolidated Omnibus Budget Reconciliation Act (COBRA) of 1985 protects people from losing insurance by allowing them to pay the full premium for the insurance plan for a limited time. COBRA coverage is short term and typically very expensive to carry. The ACA provides options outside of this to ensure medical coverage into early adulthood.

Social Security Disability Insurance is available for those who qualify for SSI. To qualify for SSI, those over the age of 18 must be low income and age 65 years or older, blind, or have a severe physical or mental disability preventing them from working. SSI is also available for people under 18 with a physical or mental condition that causes severe functional limitations for an extended period or will result in death. If minors receive SSI, they must apply for redetermination to continue the benefit as an adult; this is a process that the health care team should begin with the youth and their guardian prior to their 18th birthday to ensure no gaps in coverage occur.

TRANSITION PLANNING IN THE SCHOOL SYSTEM

Transitioning of care includes consideration of transitioning their education, which is essential to well-being and important for the health care provider to consider when planning. The recommendation is that youth receiving special education services begin the transition planning process by age 16 (US Department of Education, 2017). Like HCT planning, when transition planning occurs in the school system, it should be individualized, multidisciplinary, and cross organizational lines; however, schools lack resources and the ability to successfully provide transition services from school to adult life (Snell-Rood et al., 2020). The Individuals with Disabilities Education Act (IDEA) requires public schools to provide transition services as part of the Individualized Education Program (IEP). The reauthorized 2004 IDEA defines transition services as:

> *A results-oriented process that is focused on improving the academic and functional achievement of the child with a disability to facilitate the child's movement from school to post-school activities, including postsecondary education, vocational education, integrated employment (including supported employment), continuing and adult education, adult services, independent living, or community participation. Based on the individual child's needs, taking into account the child's strengths, preferences, and interests; and includes instruction, related services, community experiences, the development of employment and other post-school adult living objectives, and, when appropriate, acquisition of daily living skills and functional vocational evaluation (pp. 34 CFR 300. 43[a]) (20 USC 1401 [34]).*

Studies have shown that participants of school-based transition programs were not individualized, lacked consideration for students' abilities and needs, and included unrealistic goals that were not relevant to the long-term goals of students and their families (Kuhn et al., 2022; Snell-Rood et al., 2020). School systems attempting to implement school-based, evidence-based transition programs report an inability to streamline communications between health care services, disability services, and educational services, making it difficult for families to navigate through the process and lacking resources to implement comprehensive transition programs (Kuhn et al., 2022). Adoption of effective school-based transition services is largely dependent on the socioeconomic status of the community where the school is located, and those in lower socioeconomic communities tend to receive lower-quality programming and are less likely to adopt the program creating an inequity of services provided throughout the country (Kuhn et al., 2022).

POSTSECONDARY EDUCATION

Postsecondary education is often the primary goal for most students with disabilities (US Department of Education, 2017); the National Center for Education Statistics showed that over 17% of students entering a postsecondary education institution registered for disability services. IDEA requires that the IEP include postsecondary education goals related to training, education, employment, and appropriate independent living skills. Regular review of the IEP will ensure that the goals remain appropriate as the student matures and their needs and abilities change. Educators should encourage students who receive disability services to take courses that challenge them academically in preparation for college-level courses. It is also important for students to participate in community service programs and school clubs and activities. Guidance counselors can also play a role in transition planning with additional discussion of career goals and college requirements to reach those goals (US Department of Education, 2017).

Parent or guardian input is also vital to implementing a meaningful postsecondary transition plan; a study of parent participation in school-based transition programs showed a low level of family participation at almost a quarter of the schools studied (Kuhn et al., 2022). The educator and health care team should encourage parents and guardians to discuss career plans, the college environment, and necessary support services for the youth to be successful in the postsecondary education environment.

Other considerations when transitioning youth to postsecondary education include the educator support staff, school guidance counselors, and parents/guardians discussing how to pay for postsecondary education and eligible scholarships and financial aid. It is important to also choose the correct college environment, such as local colleges, community colleges, and available resources and accessibility for students with disabilities. Throughout the preparation for postsecondary education, state-sponsored vocational rehabilitation teams can provide support before, during, and after whichever postsecondary education option the student chooses (US Department of Education, 2017).

VOCATIONAL TRAINING AND THE TRANSITION

The Rehabilitation Act and the Workforce Innovation and Opportunity Act provide state-sponsored vocational rehabilitation (VR) services and job training for youth with disabilities entering the workforce. The state-sponsored VR services are individualized to meet each person's needs. The VR services provided under the Rehabilitation Act have criteria for inclusion in the programs, and students are required to apply for participation in these programs. Frequent and ongoing communication between the school, the family, and the VR service program is vital to successfully coordinate services as youth transition out of the educational system and into a VR program.

In addition to vocational counseling and job skills development, which includes guidance on searching for jobs, gaining skills to obtain a job, and resume preparation, many state VR agencies provide more individualized services. Transition services include the VR team working with students and their special education staff to provide guidance and support when transitioning from high school to a working environment based on mutually agreed upon goals. The state VR agency also provides an Individual Plan for Employment (IPE), which is developed in collaboration with the youth and includes work goals and the necessary steps to achieve those goals, a time frame for achieving the established vocational goals, the costs of the services needed to achieve the goals, and youth responsibility (Whitney et al., 2012). The Job Accommodations Network allows individuals to search for their state-sponsored VR agency.

TRANSITION FROM HOME TO COMMUNITY LIVING

An important component of transitioning to adulthood is independent and community living. Ideally, education about the life skills required to successfully integrate into community living occurs throughout primary school; however, it is the responsibility of educators, guardians, and the health care team. Important skills for independent living include grooming, personal safety, making healthy choices, using public transportation, budgeting and money

management, and building community with others (PACER's National Parent Center on Transition and Employment, 2023).

There are many federally funded programs to protect those with disabilities from discrimination. Americans with Disabilities Act (ADA) ensures that housing is accessible and safe for disabled persons; section 504 of the Rehabilitation Act prevents discrimination in housing programs that receive government funds. The Fair Housing Act protects people from discrimination when attempting to rent or buy a home, seeking financing to purchase a home, or assistance to obtain housing. Medicaid beneficiaries can receive home placement services through the Home and Community-Based Services (HCBS, n.d.) program provided. The HCBS program provides services to those with intellectual, developmental, and physical disabilities and those with mental illness. The primary purpose of the HCBS program is to prevent the institutionalization of those with disabilities who can live independently with some assistance. This program is monitored by the Centers for Medicare and Medicaid for quality. The types of services provided through the HCBS program vary widely by state.

COORDINATION OF TRANSITION PLANNING

The ideal approach to transitioning youth to adulthood includes interdisciplinary coordination and communication between the pediatric and adult health care teams and communication with the school-based transition teams and community programs for vocational training and housing. However, health care providers report communication and coordination as significant barriers in the process. In one survey, over 50% of the adult care providers who participated reported that they are willing to accept a young adult with chronic or behavioral conditions despite lacking adequate resources for care coordination, community resources, specialist care, and ability to have access to pediatric providers for consultation when care is initiated (White et al., 2020). Continued involvement of the pediatric primary care providers is essential during the transfer of care and transfer completion phases to ensure a meaningful and successful transition.

The families of chronically ill youth report frustrations with the lack of coordination and resources available during the transition process. The health care team must provide families with psychological support, education, and medical care needed throughout a transition process. Transitioning to adult care should begin early and continue at least annually throughout adolescence. Implementing a comprehensive, evidence-based program such as Got Transition is one way for the health care team to equip adolescents to transition into adulthood. The Got Transition program provides comprehensive, evidence-based resources for clinicians, youth and young adults, and parents and caregivers of youth. Primary care providers should begin discussing transitioning to adult care between age 12 and 14. Over the ages of 14 to 18, the pediatric primary care provider should assess readiness for transition and the HCT planning. During the readiness assessment phase of the transition, health literacy discussions occur along with conversations about youth health history, current chronic conditions, medications and why they take them, and plans for insurance coverage in young adulthood. The pediatric primary care provider should also assess the youth and their family's knowledge of available resources in the community for occupational assistance, food, housing, mental health, and medications. Once they demonstrate sufficient health literacy, youth are ready to transfer care, ideally between age 18 and 23. The pediatric primary care provider is recommended to provide initial support to the adult care provider early in the transition and surveys youth and their caregivers' perception of the process.

The pediatric health care team is one piece of a successful transition puzzle. Youth and their parents or guardians must work synergistically with the pediatric and future adult health care teams, their educational team, and the appropriate supportive government agencies to ensure that these youth function to the full extent of their abilities and lead fulfilling adult lives.

RESOURCES

GENERAL INFORMATION AND EDUCATION

Got Transition: gottransition.org.
Pacer Center: Pacer.org.
Six Core Elements of Health Care Transition: Sample Plan of Care: gottransition.org/6ce/?leaving-plan-care.

ADULT CARE AND HEALTH INSURANCE

Social Security Administration: Supplemental Security Income: ssa.gov/ssi.
Centers for Medicaid & Medicare Services: medicaid.gov.

POSTSECONDARY EDUCATION AND VOCATIONAL TRAINING

National Technical Assistance Center on Transition: transitionta.org/.
Institute for Educational Leadership: iel.org.
Association of University Centers on Disabilities: aucd.org.

HOUSING RESOURCES

USA.gov: Housing Help: www.usa.gov/housing-help.
Child Welfare Information Gateway: childwelfare.gov.

HEALTH INSURANCE

Healthcare.gov.
Medicaid.gov.

REFERENCES

Aeschbach, C., Burrough, W., Olejniczak, A., & Koepsel, E. (2021). Teaching adolescents to manage their own health care. *Journal of School Nursing, 37*(5), 404–411. http://doi:10.1177/1059840519867363.

Agency for Healthcare Research. (2021). National healthcare quality and disparities report. Agency for Healthcare Research and Quality; Pub. No. 21(22)-0054-EF.

Alderman, E. M., & Breuner, C. C. (2019). Unique needs of the adolescent. *Adolescent Health,* 3–14. https://doi.org/10.1542/9781610024310-part01-ch01.

American Academy of Neurology. (1998). Practice parameter: Management issues for women with epilepsy. *Neurology, 51,* 944–948.

Arain, M., Haque, M., Johal, L., Mathur, P., Nel, W., Rais, A., Sandhu, R., & Sharma, S. (2013). Maturation of the adolescent brain. *Neuropsychiatric Disease and Treatment, 9,* 449–461. https://doi.org/10.2147/NDT.S39776.

Beacham, B. L., & Deatrick, J. A. (2013). Health care autonomy in children with chronic conditions. *Nursing Clinics of North America, 48*(2), 305–317. https://doi.org/10.1016/j.cnur.2013.01.010.

Benson, N., Cunningham, C., Braun, L., et al. (2018). Transitioning pediatric patients to adult health care: A quality improvement needs assessment. *Journal of Pediatric Health Care, 32*(3), 216–222. https://doi.org/10.1016/j.pedhc.2017.09.014.

Betz, C., Mannimo, J., & Disabato, A. (2021). Survey of US pediatric nurses' role in health care transition planning: Focus on assessment of self-management abilities of youth and young adults with long-term conditions. *Journal of Child Health Care, 25*(3), 468–480. https://doi.org/10.1177/1367493520953649.

Buran, C. F., Brei, T. J., Sawin, K. J., Stevens, S., & Neufeld, J. (2006). Further development of the adolescent self management and independence scale: AMIS II. *Cerebrospinal Fluid Research, 3*(Suppl 1), S37. https://doi.org/10.1186/1743-8454-3-S1-S37.

Centers for Disease Control and Prevention (CDC). (2022, February 22). *Populations and vulnerabilities.* Retrieved October 23, 2022, from https://www.cdc.gov/nceh/tracking/topics/PopulationsVulnerabilities.htm.

Children's Health Insurance Program (CHIP). (n.d.). *Medicaid.* Retrieved October 19, 2022, from https://www.medicaid.gov/chip/eligibility/index.html.

Cooley, W. C., & Sagerman, P. J. (2011). Supporting the health care transition from adolescence to adulthood in the medical home. *Pediatrics, 128*(1), 182–200. https://doi.org/10.1542/peds.2011-0969.

Engelen, M. M., Knoll, J. L., Rabsztyn, P. R., Maas-van Schaaijk, N., & van Gaal, B. (2019). Sexual health communication between healthcare professionals and adolescents with chronic conditions in western countries: An integrative review. *Sexuality and Disability, 38*(2), 191–216. https://doi.org/10.1007/s11195-019-09597-0.

Gall, C., Kingsnorth, S., & Healy, H. (2006). Growing up ready. *Physical & Occupational Therapy in Pediatrics, 26*(4), 47–62. https://doi.org/10.1080/j006v26n04_04.

Got Transition (2022). *Six core elements of health care transition.* https://www.gottransition.org/six-core-elements/.

Healthy People 2030, US Department of Health and Human Services, Office of Disease Prevention and Health Promotion. Social determinants of health. Retrieved October 21, 2022, from https://health.gov/healthypeople/objectives-and-data/social-determinants-health.

Holmbeck, G. N., Johnson, S. Z., Wills, K. E., McKernon, W., Rose, B., Erklin, S., & Kemper, T. (2002). Observed and perceived parental overprotection in relation to psychosocial adjustment in preadolescents with a physical disability: The mediational role of behavioral autonomy. *Journal of*

Consulting and Clinical Psychology, 70(1), 96–110. https://doi.org/10.1037/0022-006X.70.1.96.

Home & Community-Based Services. (n.d.). Medicaid. Retrieved October 25, 2022, from https://www.medicaid.gov/medicaid/home-community-based-services/index.html.

Kuhn, J., Szidon, K., Kraemer, B., Steinbrenner, J. R., Tomaszewski, B., Hume, K., & DaWalt, L. (2022). Implementation of a multi-family autism transition program in the high school setting. *Autism : The international Journal of research and practice, 26*(3), 615–627. https://doi.org/10.1177/13623613211065533.

Lebrun-Harris, L. A., McManus, M. A., Ilango, S. M., Cyr, M., McLellan, S. B., Mann, M. Y., & White, P. H. (2018). Transition planning among us youth with and without special health care needs. *Pediatrics, 142*(4), e20180194. https://doi.org/10.1542/peds.2018-0194.

Lestishock, L., Nova, S., & Disabota, J. (2021). Improving adolescent and young adult engagement in the process of transitioning to adult care. *Journal of Adolescent Health, 69*(3), 424–431. https://doi.org/10.1016/j.jadohealth.2021.01.026.

Li, L., Polanski, A., Lim, A., & Strachan, P. H. (2022). Transition to adult care for youth with medical complexity: Assessing needs and setting priorities for a health care improvement initiative. *Journal of Pediatric Nursing, 62*, 144–154. https://doi.org/10.1016/j.pedn.2021.08.006.

Maternal and Child Health Bureau, Child and Adolescent Health Measurement Initiative (2021). Child Resource Data Center for Child and Adolescent Health. Retrieved 2022, from https://www.childhealthdata.org/browse/survey/results?q=9604&r=1.

McNeely, C., & Blanchard, J. (2009). *The teen years explained: A guide to healthy adolescent development.* Baltimore: John Hopkins Bloomberg School of Public Health, Center for Adolescent Health. Retrieved October 1, 2022 from. https://www.jhsph.edu/research/centers-and-institutes/center-for-adolescent-health/_docs/TTYE-Guide.pdf.

Murphy, N., & Young, P. C. (2005). Sexuality in children and adolescents with disabilities. *Developmental Medicine & Child Neurology, 47*(9), 640–644.

Office of Special Education and Rehabilitative Services–What to know about youth transition services for students with disabilities. US.

Okumura, M. J., Kuo, D. Z., Ware, A. N., Cyr, M. H., & White, P. H. (2022). Improving health care transitions for children and youth with special health care needs. *Academic Pediatrics, 22*(2S), S7–S13. https://doi.org/10.1016/j.acap.2021.03.014.

PACER's National Parent Center on Transition and Employment. (2023). *Transition to adult health care.* https://www.pacer.org/transition/learning-center/health/transition-to-adult-health-care.asp.

Pritchard, A. W., & Rees, S. A. (2016). Challenges and "obstacles": Reframing our perspective on the transition into adulthood for young people with life-limiting and life-threatening conditions. *Journal of the Royal College of Physicians of Edinburgh, 46*(4), 223–227. https://doi.org/10.4997/jrcpe.2016.402.

Sanders, R. A. (2013). Adolescent psychosocial, social, and cognitive development. *Pediatrics in Review, 34*(8), 354–359. https://doi.org/10.1542/pir.34.8.354.

Sattoe, J. N., & van Staa, A. L. (2021). *The development of self-management in young people with chronic conditions: A transitional process.* In *Self-management of young people with chronic conditions: A strength-based approach for empowerment and support* (pp. 37–54). Springer.

Saulsberry, A. C., Porter, J. S., & Hankins, J. S. (2019). A program of transition to adult care for sickle cell disease. *Hematology, 2019*(1), 496–504. https://doi.org/10.1182/hematology.2019000054.

Sawin, K. J., Buran, C. F., Brei, T. J., & Fastenau, P. S. (2002). Sexuality issues in adolescents with a chronic neurological condition. *The Journal of perinatal education, 11*(1), 22–34. https://doi.org/10.1624/105812402X88579.

Snell-Rood, C., Ruble, L., Kleinert, H., McGrew, J. H., Adams, M., Rodgers, A., Odom, J., Wong, W. H., & Yu, Y. (2020). Stakeholder perspectives on transition planning, implementation, and outcomes for students with autism spectrum disorder. *Autism: The International Journal of Research and Practice, 24*(5), 1164–1176. https://doi.org/10.1177/1362361319894827.

Society for Adolescent Health and Medicine (2020). Transition to adulthood for youth with chronic conditions and special health care needs. *The Journal of Adolescent Health: Official Publication of the Society for Adolescent Medicine, 66*(5), 631–634. https://doi.org/10.1016/j.jadohealth.2020.02.006.

Spencer, D. L., McManus, M., Call, K. T., Turner, J., Harwood, C., White, P., & Alarcon, G. (2018). Health care coverage and access among children, adolescents, and young adults, 2010–2016: Implications for future health reforms. *The Journal of Adolescent Health: Official Publication of the Society for Adolescent Medicine, 62*(6), 667–673. https://doi.org/10.1016/j.jadohealth.2017.12.012.

US Department of Education (Department), Office of Special Education and Rehabilitative Services. A transition guide to postsecondary education and employment for students and youth with disabilities (2017). Retrieved October 26, 2022, from https://www2.ed.gov/about/offices/list/osers/transition/products/postsecondary-transition-guide-may-2017.pdf?utm_content=&utm_medium=email&utm_name=&utm_source=govdelivery&utm_term.

Vijayakumar, N. (2018). Puberty and the human brain: Insights into adolescent development. *Neuroscience and Biobehavioral Reviews, 92*, 417–436. http://doi.org/10.1016/j.neubiorev.2018.06.004.

White, P. H., & Cooley, W. C. (2018). Supporting the health care transition from adolescence to adulthood in the medical home. *Pediatrics, 142*(5). https://doi.org/10.1542/peds.2018-2587.

White, P. H., Ilango, S. M., Caskin, A. M., de la Guardia, M. G. A., & McManus, M. A. (2020). Health care transition in school-based health centers: A pilot study. *Journal of Schools Nursing.* https://doi.org/10.1177/1059840520975745.

Whitney, J., Smith, L. M., & Duperoy, T. (2012). Vocational rehabilitation (VR): A young adult's guide [English and Spanish versions]. *Psychiatry Information in Brief, 9*(5). https://doi.org/10.7191/pib.1070.

Zhou, H., Roberts, P., Dhaliwal, S., & Della, P. (2016). Transitioning adolescent and young adults with chronic disease and/or disabilities from pediatric to adult care services – an integrative review. *Journal of Clinical Nursing, 25*(21-22), 3113–3130. https://doi.org/10.1111/jocn.13326.

Zimmerman, C., Garland, B. H., Enzler, C. J., Hergenroeder, A. C., & Wiemann, C. M. (2022). The roles of quality of life and family and peer support in feelings about transition to adult care in adolescents with gastroenterology, renal, and rheumatology diseases. *Journal of Pediatric Nursing, 62*, 193–199. https://doi.org/10.1016/j.pedn.2021.04.032.

Ethics and the Child With a Chronic Condition

Elise M. Geithner

DECISION MAKING ALONG THE COURSE OF CHRONIC CONDITIONS

The course of a chronic condition is likely to include diagnosis and treatment; periods of recovery, exacerbations, stability, or instability; and in some cases deterioration and death. These phases are often punctuated by recurring ethical issues, including:

1. Defining what constitutes a life worth living
2. Recognizing the threshold for certainty in diagnosis and treatment
3. Choosing a decision maker to decide about treatment or nontreatment
4. Determining the role of minors in making treatment decisions
5. Deciding whether to pursue experimental or innovative therapies
6. Knowing how to resolve conflicts

The range of chronic conditions in childhood and adolescence is paralleled by the range of values held by people with chronic conditions or caregivers of those with chronic conditions. Competing ethical obligations can create a set of problematic situations for children, families, and health care providers.

THE ETHICAL DOMAIN

A moral or ethical course of action is based on guiding principles of doing what is right (i.e., ethics is concerned with "what ought to be" and how individuals think about and discuss this). Ethics is concerned with individual and group behaviors, choices, and character. Ethical questions arise alongside but differ from fundamental social, legal, political, professional, and scientific questions. For example, public policies and laws (e.g., the death penalty) set boundaries for human behavior but do not necessarily correspond to an individual's sense of "what ought to be." It is within this context that ethical discourse occurs.

There are many ways of discerning the ethical dimensions of an issue or quandary. The discernment process is complex and influenced by emotions, scientific facts, values, interpersonal relationships, culture, religion, the essence of who we are, and myriad situational factors—all of which shape the way ethical questions are framed.

Ethical questions arise because an individual is unsure of the right thing to do or the proper outcome to pursue. For example, primary care providers may be concerned about whether to offer an experimental treatment protocol to a family when the likelihood of altering the natural course of the child's condition is remote, and pursuing such treatment will require the family to pay out-of-pocket costs. Ethical questions may also arise because there are genuine value conflicts about the right thing to do or the proper outcomes to pursue. For example, primary care providers and families may disagree about whether it is justified to continue aggressive treatment for a child with end-stage cystic fibrosis. The providers may reason that continued treatment is burdensome and will prolong death; in contrast, the parents may believe that extending life is the appropriate goal to be pursued despite the burden endured by the child. In both instances, careful consideration of the judgments and the justifications used to defend one's position and behavior is warranted.

Ethical deliberation involves discerning, analyzing, and articulating ethically defensible positions and acting on them. Ethical thinking provides a reasoned account of an ethical position and helps one move beyond intuition or emotions. Ethical deliberation aims not to achieve absolute certainty about what is right but to achieve reliability and coherence in behavior, choices, character, process, and outcomes.

Ethical theories and principles provide a foundation for ethical analysis and deliberation (Table 5.1) and a guide for organizing and understanding ethically relevant information in a dilemma or conflict situation. These theories and principles suggest directions and avenues for resolving competing claims and supply reasons that justify moral action. Ethical principles are universal but not absolute. Each case involves particular principles and values integral to the decision-making process. One must balance the claims generated from competing principles relevant to a particular case. Moreover, factors such as family dynamics, the nature of relationships, contextual features, integrity, and faithfulness to commitments are also morally relevant to the decision-making process. Even when one chooses a morally justifiable course of action, there are always unmet obligations when resolving ethical dilemmas (i.e., a moral remainder).

Ethical theories and principles must be applied systematically within the decision-making process. Ethical

Table 5.1   Ethical Theories: Telological vs. Deontological

	TELEOLOGICAL THEORY	DEONTOLOGICAL THEORY (TYPICALLY CALLED KANTIAN THEORY)
Definition	Focuses on the rightness or wrongness of actions by examining the consequences and on accomplishing a certain goal or end.	Focuses on whether the actions are performed in accordance with duty. The intrinsic quality of the act itself or its conformity to a rule—not its consequences—determines whether an act is right or wrong.
Consequences	A consequential theory in which the moral right or moral wrong depends on the outcome of the action.	A nonconsequential theory in which the moral right or moral wrong does not depend on the outcome of the action.
Weakness	It is not always possible to predict the consequences of the action.	It is rigid and objective.

Box 5.1   Process to Facilitate Ethical Decision Making

1. Identify the ethical problem(s); distinguish them from clinical, administrative, or legal problems.
2. Identify key players (including family members and their roles); identify your role.
3. Identify the ethical issue(s); describe/define the issue(s) in terms of principles, values of key players, and potential conflicts.
4. Identify preferences of the key players regarding the decision to be made.
5. Identify the decision maker(s).
6. Identify options, the range of permissible actions for this situation, and the ethical ramifications of each action.
7. Make decision/facilitate decision/abide by decision.
8. Evaluate the decision-making process and your role in the process.
9. Consider what you would do differently in the future and why.

Box 5.2   A Moral Framework for Decision Making

- Beneficence
  - Balancing benefit and burden
- Respect for persons
  - Informed consent
- Justice
  - Macro- and microallocation of resources
  - Individual vs. societal needs
- Ethic of care

analysis is enhanced when a framework that provides a systematic process of decision making is used, and mistakes are avoided by using only logic and reason (Box 5.1). In addition, because some decisions (e.g., those to withhold or withdraw certain therapies) help determine the timing and consequences of death, other important social, ethical, and religious values come into play.

A MORAL FRAMEWORK FOR DECISION MAKING

A specific framework provides a mechanism for individuals, families, and providers dealing with the ethical dimensions of difficult situations. For adults, a morally defensible framework for decision making is relatively straightforward and widely accepted (President's Commission for the Study of Ethical Problems in Medicine and Biomedical and Behavioral Research [President's Commission], 1983) (Box 5.2). Consistent with the Western view of autonomy, treatment options should promote the individual's well-being according to that individual's understanding of it. When

individuals lack the capacity to make choices for themselves, someone else must represent their values and preferences. Ethical decision making is a process with multiple contributors; it is a combination of the health provider's expertise on the available choices and the individual's or surrogate's expertise on which choices best promote that individual's life goals and values. This decision-making process is also influenced by the family system, culture, religious and spiritual affiliations, and personal values and preferences (Blustein, 1998; Jonsen et al., 1998; Schwartz, 2016).

Ethical decision making is more complex for children because most lack the capacity to make independent decisions. Children have not formulated life goals and values to base such decisions. The capacity to be involved in decision making varies according to a child's level of maturity, and as a result it is generally assumed that children need surrogate decision makers (American Academy of Pediatrics [AAP] Committee on Bioethics, 2017). However, more recent findings suggest that child decision making is based on more factors than stages of cognitive development (Alderson et al., 2006; Jeremic et al., 2016). A growing body of research supports the involvement of children in their health care decisions (Beidler & Dickey, 2001; Martenson & Fagerskiold, 2007; Olszewski & Goldkind, 2018). Decisions made on behalf of children lack a key feature of the moral framework for adults: individuals' unique assessment of their own well-being. Despite this, minors can be involved in meaningful decisions about their health care (discussed later). The moral principles involved in adult decision making do, however, provide a valuable framework for making decisions on behalf of children (Diekema, 2019; Ross, 1997; Savage, 1997). It is often useful to use ethical principles as an organizational framework for addressing ethical issues in decision making for children.

BENEFICENCE

The primary principles involved in decision making are beneficence (i.e., doing good) and its corollary, nonmaleficence (i.e., avoiding or minimizing harm). Treatment options should include those that benefit the infant or child and outweigh the associated burdens and harms. This best-interest standard is often used as a hallmark when making decisions for children; it establishes a presumption in favor of life because existence is usually required for other interests to be advanced. Generally, life should be saved when possible. When life cannot be saved or the chance of survival is minimal, however, burdensome treatment should not be provided, and palliative care should be considered to manage the child's symptoms and promote comfort (Hynson & Sawyer, 2001; Moresco & Moore, 2021). Burdens for children with chronic conditions include repeated pain and suffering associated with invasive procedures, symptoms, or disability and emotional distress caused by fear, immobilization, prolonged hospitalization, or isolation from family and friends. Decisions about a child whose chances of dying are great might reasonably focus on the comfort of dying instead of on therapies to prolong life.

An additional standard, the relational potential standard, has also been suggested as an adjunct to the best-interest standard when balancing the benefits and burdens of various courses of action (McCormick, 1974; Wightman et al., 2019). This standard focuses on the child's cognitive and intellectual capacities, the degree of neurologic impairment, the prognosis of reversing the neurologic condition, and whether the outcome of the condition can be altered through treatment or therapy. For example, infants or children who are permanently unconscious have no capacity to feel either pleasure or pain, so their best interests are limited to prolonging biologic life. Because such children cannot be burdened in the usual sense, and most of the reasons for treatment (e.g., better function, fewer symptoms, the opportunity for human relationships, or greater opportunity to achieve life's goals) are gone, many would argue that treatment is not obligatory (Fost, 1999). The Baby Doe regulations in 1984 (PL 98-457), for example, regard permanent unconsciousness as a condition that does not require life-sustaining treatment; yet there are a wide range of views on the degree of neurologic impairment that justifies limiting or forgoing treatment.

The challenge for children, parents, and health care providers is understanding the unique meaning of health, sickness, disability, suffering, care, and death for a child in a particular situation. The meaning that these concepts give to an individual's life is influenced by that individual's values, interests, aims, rights, and duties. A holistic understanding of a child's life, a recognition of important values that give direction to treatment decisions, and the tenor of the professional-family-child relationship evolve and change over time; therefore discovering the threshold for balancing benefits and burdens in a certain case may change as the child's condition changes. For example, the initial goals for a newborn with multiple congenital anomalies resulting in neurologic impairment and severe physical disability may be to understand the extent of the child's condition and to preserve life. In this instance, parents and professionals may agree to tolerate a high degree of burden to the child to diminish the uncertainty surrounding diagnosis and prognosis. However, 2 years later, after the diagnosis and prognosis have been clarified, parents and professionals may have a different view of how much burden the child must tolerate sustaining life especially when continued treatment will not alter the prognosis and may impose significant burdens.

Beneficence is promoted by helping the child and family construct a meaningful life by balancing the burdens of the condition with the positive dimensions of living. Beneficence is expressed by identifying individualized care outcomes that enhance the child's well-being (e.g., adequately managing symptoms, accommodating to limitations imposed by the chronic condition, and maximizing functional capacities). Therefore treatment interventions must be designed to contribute to the individualized goals that enhance the quality of life and promote the child's sense of integrity despite the limitations related to the condition.

Parents and professionals must openly discuss the uncertainty in diagnosis and prognosis and explore the extent of certainty necessary for parental and professional decision making. At times, the need for greater certainty of either parents or professionals may result in burdensome diagnostic evaluations that do not contribute to the child's well-being or outcome. Alternatively, parents may accept uncertainty when professionals are compelled to seek further evidence to support their recommendations. The dynamic nature of the condition's course may create special challenges for caregivers and parents. Ideally, the supporting adults create a shared vision and a common understanding of the balance of benefits and burdens that is acceptable for a certain child.

NONMALEFICENCE

Health care providers have a duty to prevent or remove harm, yet the interventions they pursue to benefit a child sometimes cause harm. Certain medical interventions are painful and uncomfortable and can cause permanent injury or disability. These unintended harms may be justified if they are proportional to the overall benefit the child will derive from the treatment. Unintended harm can occur with or without negligence. For instance, interacting with the health care system puts children at risk of iatrogenic harm, failure to adequately assess and treat pain can lead to increased suffering, and certain complementary and alternative medical therapies intended to help may pose the risk of harm when their side effects are unknown. In extreme cases, children with chronic conditions may receive intentional injuries because of maltreatment. Each of these categories of potential harm will be discussed further.

Medical Harms

Health care providers strive to prevent harm. With technologic interventions that support and improve health, there are often trade-offs regarding comfort, side effects, mobility restrictions, and unfortunately iatrogenicity. In the decision to accept treatment, parents and children (when developmentally appropriate) weigh the potential benefits against the known or potential harms that can occur with treatment. Chemotherapy usually causes side effects of temporary immunosuppression, gastrointestinal disturbances, hair loss, fatigue, and more permanent complications of peripheral neuropathy or sensorineural hearing loss. Even with careful symptom management, some children cannot escape the side effects during treatment or late effects years later (Erdmann et al., 2021). However, for many families, the potential benefit of cure (beneficence) over the burdens of treatment justifies the harm.

Other harms can befall children with chronic conditions who interact with health care professionals. Infiltrations of intravenous fluids, nosocomial infections, and skin breakdown are among the complications that can occur in an inpatient setting. The most common harm in pediatrics is medication error (Kaushal et al., 2001, 2004; Gonzales, 2010). Children have less physiologic ability to sustain a medication error, yet there are often more opportunities for error. More calculations and steps are required in ordering, dispensing, and administering medication to children than adults, increasing the likelihood of error at each juncture. Progress has been made in computerizing orders and altering how medications are administered, but the safety of children depends on the vigilance of the care providers (D'Errico et al., 2022; Ferranti et al., 2008; Wang et al., 2007).

Pain Assessment and Management

It is unequivocally substantiated that children have pain associated with disease and treatments. In 2001 standards for assessing and managing pain were required by the Joint Commission on Accreditation of Healthcare Organizations (2001) under the category "Rights, Responsibilities, and Ethics." The standard requires systematic assessment and monitoring of the child's response to treatment. Unless the pain provides a therapeutic, necessary use (aid in diagnosis or progression of symptoms), it should be treated, and then it should be reduced to the lowest possible level. When a child's pain is not treated adequately, the child experiences unjustified harm. Concern about oversedation, difficulty with assessment, or the dismissal of the child's self-report contributes to the undertreating of pain in children. Nonverbal children, very young children, or children with significant disabilities are especially vulnerable, and the health care providers must depend on the parents' interpretation of the child's behavior to assess pain and pain relief (Carter et al., 2002; Jordan et al., 2021). Health care providers must stay abreast of assessment techniques, interventions, and professional guidelines for relieving pain in children (AAP & American Pain Society, 2001; O'Donnell & Rosen, 2014).

New Therapies

Introducing new therapies for children with chronic conditions often raises ethical concerns. There are two categories of current therapies: complementary and alternative and experimental. Complementary and alternative medicine (CAM) has become increasingly popular. Micozzi (2001) identifies three major areas: alternative medical therapies (e.g., homeopathy and naturopathy), complementary medicine (e.g., psychoneuroimmunology, mind-body interventions, humor, expressive and creative arts therapies), and traditional medical systems (e.g., yoga, Chinese medicine, curanderismo). Yeon and Nam (2016) cite that CAM is used by 24% to 78% of children with neurologic diseases, including seizure disorders and cerebral palsy, versus 12% of healthy children. Numerous ethical issues revolve around their use, with the safety of the therapies being paramount (McClafferty et al., 2017; Vohra & Cohen, 2007). For parents to make an informed decision about using CAM, they need information. Health care providers can assist the parents in finding reliable information on CAM, although there is limited research evidence. As with all parents' decisions, the health care providers strive to ensure that parents have as much available information as possible to make their decision. The parent's choice of CAM may reflect their values stemming from their culture. Unless providers believe that the use of CAM represents a real danger to the child's health, parents are given wide latitude in its use. The health care provider and the parents can evaluate the available data, analyze the possible risks and benefits, and decide in the child's best interests.

Experimental treatments or procedures are also used for children. In addition, the National Institutes of Health (NIH) mandates that children be included in all federally funded research unless it is inappropriate, but the investigator must justify excluding children (NIH, 1998). Although research on children can be extremely crucial in discovering efficacious treatments, the NIH mandate is controversial. The Food and Drug Administration issued a Pediatric Rule requiring pharmaceutical companies to conduct clinical trials in children, but a federal court overturned this rule in late 2002 (Albert, 2002). Researchers must be aware of the different approaches necessary when conducting research on children (Punch, 2002; Ramanan et al., 2022).

Before children are included in clinical research, investigators must get approval from their institutional review board (IRB) to conduct their study in a particular institution. The IRB follows federal regulations for children, which stipulate four conditions under which a child may be included in a study. Briefly, those conditions are when the research (1) poses minimal risk to the child; (2) poses greater than minimal risk, but there is the possibility of direct benefit to the child; (3) poses greater than minimal risk, there is no direct benefit, but the research should generate generalizable knowledge about the disorder or condition; and (4) would not otherwise be approved but "presents an opportunity to prevent, or alleviate a serious problem affecting the health or welfare of children" (US Department of Health and Human Services, 1991, 2005, 2016). Many if not all oncology treatments for children are through the enrollment of the child in a national clinical trial. Parents must understand the nature of the research, risks, benefits, and alternatives. Again, the ethical imperative is to foster a complete and thorough understanding of the information for parents to make an informed decision. For children developmentally capable of giving assent, obtaining the child's assent is required unless the study offers the prospect of a direct benefit.

It is important for health care providers to be aware of the therapeutic misconception that parents may have. Although they are told that the child will be randomized into the standard or experimental therapy, parents may believe that the inclusion of the child in a study is for the child's good. Although it is hoped that the child will benefit from inclusion, clinical equipoise exists; that is, it is not known which treatment, the standard therapy or the experimental therapy, is better. It is ethical therefore to randomize the child into one of the two groups. However, the purpose of the study is to determine the better treatment, thereby helping children in the future but not guaranteeing the children in the study will be helped.

Primary care providers, children, and families must consider the balance of benefits and burdens of both CAM and experimental therapies. Parents and caregivers should engage in ongoing, open discussions about poorly tested therapies or experimental treatments to address these challenging situations. For example, when an innovative surgical procedure is considered for a young child with an orthopedic deformity, the health care provider must disclose the uncertainty surrounding its effectiveness.

Maltreatment

Globally, children with disabilities are more likely to be victims of maltreatment than their nondisabled peers (Legano et al., 2021). Maltreatment is three times higher in children with disabilities (3%–10% of the population) than in typically developing children (Legano et al., 2021). Many of the same factors that contribute to the maltreatment of children without chronic conditions are also present in families of children with chronic conditions, such as familial dysfunction, high levels of stress in the parents, low socioeconomic status (SES), and lower educational level of parents (Goldson, 2001; Legano et al., 2021). However, maltreatment of children crosses all SES and educational levels. Poor, uneducated parents are likely reported for suspected or actual abuse and neglect more often than parents of higher SES and educational levels. It is also likely that fatalities caused by maltreatment are underrecognized (Crume et al., 2002; McCarroll et al., 2021). Primary care providers should be aware of the increased risk and assess families for parenting stress and coping abilities. Recognition and early intervention may reduce the incidence of maltreatment (Committee on Child Abuse and Neglect and Committee on Children with Disabilities, 2001; Fortson et al., 2016). Advocacy in the political arena for improved services for families of children with disabilities or chronic conditions may also aid in reducing the parental stresses contributing to maltreatment.

AUTONOMY

A child's autonomy (self-determination) develops as the child matures. Before the child becomes an independent decision maker, parents make decisions for their children. Underlying the principle of autonomy is respect for persons.

RESPECT FOR PERSONS

A fourth principle involved in decision making is respect for persons. Respect for persons means respecting another person as sharing a common human destiny. Adult decisions focus on the individual's unique life goals and values out of respect for that individual and the integrity of each life. The uniquely human freedom of each person to create a meaningful life is highly valued. Even though children are neither autonomous nor self-determining, respect is still required because their lives also have a unique meaning. Treating individuals with respect is to acknowledge and value who they are outside of a medical context rather than only treating them according to how professional goals and values are advanced. Most children live in families that provide nurturance and care. The relationships that arise within families are inherently valuable to the well-being of children. To respect a child is to acknowledge the importance of the child's world and the relationships that are central to it. Unilateral decision making by health care professionals based solely on medical indications denies a child fullness of life and relationships that also benefit and sustain.

A central problem associated with parental or other surrogate decisions is the inherent difficulty of judging the quality of a child's life and the benefits and burdens that are experienced. The child, family members, and health care providers may attach different meanings to the child's life. Although life is valuable, professionals and surrogate decision makers cannot consider the prolongation of life exclusively. Decisions need to benefit and respect the child as an individual but recognize that the child relies on the family for nurturance and physical care. The values the parents place on their parenting roles may make it difficult for them to separate the benefits and burdens of parenting a child with special needs from the benefits and burdens that the child experiences. These decisions are even more complex for primary care providers as they attempt to discern what is best for the child in the family context. The choice of interventions can positively or negatively affect the comfort or ease with which a child lives.

Respect for others is enhanced and evidenced by nonjudgmental attitudes and behaviors. It is important to stress that being nonjudgmental does not mean relinquishing values or being blind or indifferent to personal principles. Instead, the goal is openness to different ways of viewing and acting on personal commitments and life circumstances. An essential dimension of nonjudgmental behavior is not imposing personal judgments on others.

Informed Consent

The standard of informed consent is derived from the principle of respect for persons. Autonomy (self-determination) is the central moral value expressed through the process of informed consent. Legally, informed consent requires disclosure, comprehension, and voluntary agreement or consent by the competent individual or surrogate. To every possible extent, relevant information about diagnosis and treatment—including a description of the nature and purpose of the treatment or procedure, the benefits and risks, the problems related to recovery, the likelihood of success, and alternative treatments—must be discussed with the surrogate and the child (AAP Committee on Bioethics, 2016; Claassen, 2000; Savage, 1997). The person giving consent (i.e., usually a parent) must understand relevant information, reason, and deliberate according to his or her values and preferences and the child's perceived values and preferences, and communicate the choices to others. Finally, consent must be given voluntarily without coercion. The informed consent process must be evaluated as the child matures and altered as necessary to include the child's expressed decisions or concerns.

VERACITY AND FIDELITY

As part of respect for persons, the health care provider has a duty to be truthful and faithful. In caring for children, the health care provider may feel a conflict in loyalties; sometimes the provider feels a conflict between being truthful with the child and following the request of the parents. For example, a conflict may arise when total parenteral nutrition (TPN) is recommended for a 12-year-old girl with Crohn disease. Her parents have requested that she not be told about her diagnosis or the length of time she is expected to need TPN. The health care team expresses their desire to engage the child in decisions affecting her care, but the parents are steadfast in demanding she not be told. In another example, a child who has sustained a spinal cord injury is told by his parents that his paralysis is not permanent. Despite his direct questions, his parents tell him that his condition is temporary, and he will walk again "soon." Although the relationships between providers and parents can become tense, open, honest communication and transparency in decision making can facilitate decisions in the child's best interests. If a mutually acceptable approach to veracity cannot be reached, health care providers can negotiate a smooth transfer of care to another appropriate health care provider when they believe they cannot in good conscience participate in a child's care; however, the transfer is not always feasible or desirable.

JUSTICE

Justice pertains to fair and equal treatment of others. Therefore justice also refers to an individual's access to adequate health care and the distribution of available health care resources. Caregivers promote justice by being fair in providing care and attending to children and their families. For example, the *Code of Ethics for Nurses* focuses on the delivery of care with respect for human dignity, which is not to be defined in terms of personal attributes, SES, or the nature of an illness (American Nurses Association, 2015). This provision requires that a criterion (e.g., age, gender, wealth, religious beliefs, social prejudice) should not be a factor in deciding between individuals competing for the same treatment. This provision strives for genuine impartiality, equal respect for all persons, and refusal to create a hierarchy of individual worth. Prejudicial treatment based on personal or other attributes is a violation of a moral norm and ideal precious to the health care professions for generations.

Consistent with the ethical obligations of justice, children with chronic conditions are legally protected from discriminatory treatment by state and federal laws. Section 504 of the Rehabilitation Act of 1973 (PL 93-112) grants protection from discrimination based on disability, whereas the Individuals with Disabilities Education Act (IDEA) of 2004 (PL101-476) guarantees access for children with disabilities to education by establishing a federal grant program to help states provide free and appropriate public education to all children in need of special education. The 1990 Americans with Disabilities Act (ADA) gives civil rights protection to individuals with disabilities by guaranteeing equal opportunity to public accommodations, employment, transportation, state and local government services, and telecommunications. Such laws create important obligations for parents and health care providers and must be considered in the ethical analysis of troubling cases.

Macroallocations of Justice

Health policies for children with chronic conditions address some of the concerns encompassed in the principle of justice. These policies include strategies to avoid discrimination, stigmatization, and the exploitation of dependence. Strategies to support health insurance reform, delivery of family-centered service, access to employment, and educational opportunities, as well as the community's role in supporting children and their families, are consistent with a justice perspective.

Issues involving the just distribution of health care resources arise at two levels. The macroallocation level refers to the share of societal resources allocated to specific societal goods (e.g., health care). Resources allocated to support the health, development, and education of children with chronic conditions reflect society's values and willingness to recognize and address these children's unique circumstances and needs. Unfortunately, health care coverage for children rarely includes habilitation-rehabilitation services, and access to long-term care and other services (e.g., home nursing, some durable and nondurable equipment, or services for children without clear diagnoses) is usually limited. Eligibility is often restricted based on income or physical, mental, or emotional disabilities. In addition, by not establishing uniform eligibility requirements for Medicaid or the Children's Health Insurance Program from state to state, children who depend on either of these insurance plans for support services and care in one state may not be able to obtain the same services if they move to another state. These issues reflect some of the challenges of devising a national health policy that supports the interests of children with chronic conditions.

Within health care, macroallocation refers to the division of a resource (e.g., money) among various services (e.g., transplantation programs, critical care, outpatient services) (Beauchamp & Childress, 2019). This issue is particularly relevant at the institutional level, where costs and priorities for allocating scarce resources are determined. In an era of cost containment and downsizing, institutions and programs providing specialized services to children with chronic conditions are particularly vulnerable. For example, providers may reason that the expenditures for specialized services for children with organ transplants consume a disproportionate share of the overall budget for pediatric care. They may conclude that more children can be helped if money is spent on preventive services. Such reasoning focuses on the consequences of actions by evaluating their utility based on how they can maximize the benefits and outcomes for the greatest number of children. Focusing on a single criterion, such as utility, may not account for other important moral values (e.g., protection of vulnerable populations and existing obligations toward those in the greatest need of services).

Microallocation of Justice

The term *microallocation* is applied at the individual level; these decisions involve determining the distribution of a specific resource. In general, the professional's main concern is for the individual, but the needs of others may impinge on an individual's care especially during periods of shortages of human and material resources. Health care providers participate in microallocation decisions when determining which child needs the greatest amount of care, thereby limiting care to others perceived as less needy. Microallocation issues arise when resources are limited to the point there is not enough to provide for all in need.

Beneficence and Justice

The ethical principles of beneficence and justice are central to resource allocation and rationing issues. The principle of beneficence requires health care providers to help others and promote good. This principle is evident on two levels: the societal level and the individual level (Beauchamp & Childress, 2019). Each level includes different considerations about allocating limited resources. To realize beneficence at the societal level, resources are allocated based on the needs of society. From a utilitarian perspective, the greatest good for the entire community is considered. The focus shifts from crisis care and doing good for the individual to preventive care and actions that benefit society. This shift is particularly important for children with chronic conditions because the greater emphasis on prevention may diminish the specialized services designed to meet their needs. As resources become scarce, difficult decisions must be made to balance the needs of individuals—especially those with chronic conditions—with the needs of society.

On the individual level, health care providers fulfill the duty of beneficence by allocating resources based on individual needs. Scarce resources are distributed to those with immediate needs without regard for the needs of other potential clients or the community at large. For example, when an infant is born with spina bifida, a cadre of medical, developmental, educational, and social resources is mobilized regardless of SES, cultural or religious heritage, or ability to pay. This initial commitment to provide equitable and fair services for all families may not be sustained. Cost constraints, lack of available resources, and accessibility of resources may limit services for some children as they mature.

ETHICS OF CARE

Traditional ethical reasoning requires providers to ascertain the individual's rights and weigh the ethical principles to resolve conflicting obligations. Applying ethical principles alone cannot resolve the clinical quandaries that arise while caring for a child with a chronic condition. The language and method used to analyze a particular case can clarify or confound the situation. For example, when children's rights are opposed to their parents' rights, an adversarial tension that may polarize discussion can be established. In contrast, if it is recognized that most parents are motivated to promote their child's interests, such polarity may be avoided. Considering other aspects of the moral life (e.g., virtue, individual experience) may reduce adversarial tensions between the rights of children and their parents and allow for a more comprehensive appreciation of the attitudes, values, and moral commitments of decision makers within the context of family relationships. This perspective is often referred to as an ethic of care.

From the care perspective, the resolution of ethical quandaries is focused on the child's needs in the context of the family's and the provider's corresponding responsibilities within the provider-family-child relationship. Primary care providers can focus on the special circumstances and context of the specific situation in which moral action occurs instead of merely considering the individual's interests and preferences in isolation. Becker and Grunwald (2000) identified contextual dynamics of ethical decision making in the neonatal intensive care unit, but their sociologic observations resonate with other health care settings that care for children with chronic conditions. Such a model supports efforts to help children and their families find unique meaning or purpose in living or dying and realize goals that promote a meaningful life or death. Engaging in medical decision-making conversations with patients and families can be difficult for providers if they have not received specific training and opportunities to practice these skills. deSante-Bertkau and Herbst (2021) implemented an educational module for pediatric residents to develop skills in facilitating shared medical decision making for pediatric and young adult patients.

From this vantage point, the values and expectations involved in certain roles and relationships are primary. Therefore advocating for a child with a chronic condition involves appreciating the relationships significant to the child and understanding how those relationships affect care. Children with chronic conditions develop an intricate web of relationships that support and sustain them throughout their lives. In keeping with a family-centered philosophy of care, families are viewed as essential partners in the treatment and care of a child. Professionals must recognize and respect these interconnections as central to a child's well-being. A care perspective also emphasizes the interrelationships of the health care team members. Therefore it recognizes that nurses, primary care providers, and other caregivers work collaboratively to advance the interests and goals of children with chronic conditions.

Ethical principles (e.g., beneficence, nonmaleficence, autonomy, respect for persons, veracity, fidelity, justice) and an ethic of care provide a framework for approaching ethical questions in clinical practice. It must also be acknowledged that although these are the most common, they may not be the only principles relevant to a particular case. The challenge for primary care providers is to discern how these and other principles can help illuminate ethical issues and guide the resolution of competing obligations.

THE PROCESS OF DECISION MAKING

SHARED DECISION MAKING

Traditionally, a shared decision-making model assumes that decisions are shared among children (if capable), parents, and professionals (Box 5.3). Treatment decisions must represent a combination of the individuals' expertise to select choices that best promote the life goals and values of the child. Parents do not have the expertise to act as surrogate health care professionals, and health care professionals cannot replace the expertise of parents. Shared decision making means that parents and professionals should agree on general treatment goals, but professionals may provide more input into the treatment modalities necessary to advance the agreed-on goals (Lee et al., 2020).

Endorsement of a model of shared decision making ideally means that parents and children (if capable) engage fully in the process by understanding the range of treatment possibilities and the consequences of each and sharing their goals, values, and aspirations in a meaningful way. Such a model goes beyond the legal requirements for disclosure, comprehension, and voluntary consent (Bauchner, 2001). Although professionals theoretically embrace the ideal of shared decision making as the desired model of parent-professional decision making, accomplishing it remains difficult (Ladd & Mercurio, 2003; Lee et al., 2020; Perrin et al., 2000).

ROLE OF PARENTS IN TREATMENT DECISION MAKING

Based on the moral framework of shared decision making described here, someone must represent the

Box 5.3   Shared Decision Making
• Role of parents
• Limits of parental authority
• Role of minors
• Legal issues in role of minors
• Reality of shared decision making

interests of the child. There is a strong presumption that parents will make judgments that are in the best interest of the child (Aarthun et al., 2019; Perrin et al., 2000). Parents are appropriate surrogates because their strong bonds of affection and commitment are likely to yield the greatest concern for the well-being of their children. Parents are expected to protect their children from harm and to do as much good for them as possible.

There is a direct connection between the well-being of parents and children; the identities of each are inextricably linked. For example, a woman who defines herself as a mother regards her welfare partly in terms of the welfare of her child. Harm to the child constitutes personal harm to the mother. Parents are identified as primary decision makers because of the importance of the family institution. Families play an essential role in maintaining the integrity of society. Children learn values of cooperation and commitment within the family context that can be generalized to other members of society.

Parents must be involved in treatment decisions for their infants and children because these decisions have lifelong consequences. Parents will be responsible for the ongoing physical, emotional, medical, and financial care of the infant or child who survives with serious disabilities and will live with the consequences of those decisions. The family will remember and have incorporated such momentous decisions into their lives long after health care professionals have forgotten a case.

LIMITS OF PARENTAL AUTHORITY

In addition to being members of their immediate families, children are also members of a broader community. A moral community shares an interest in the life and well-being of each member. Certain community standards of best interest (e.g., preservation of life) may override a family's interpretation of a child's best interest. Although there are compelling reasons to support parents' decision-making authority, such authority is not absolute. The interests of the parents and the family must take a high priority but should not override the fundamental respect for the infant's or child's best interest. Ideally, the family and providers engage in a partnership to include the child in decision making as appropriate (Cavet & Sloper, 2004; Sabatello et al., 2018).

Even when parents and professionals presume shared responsibility to promote the well-being of a child, there are times when parents should be disqualified as primary decision makers. This disqualification may result from incapacity or choosing a course of action that is clearly against the child's best interest (President's Commission, 1983). If a parent has a known psychiatric condition and is behaving irrationally or has a documented history of child abuse or neglect, the primary care provider may question the parental capacity to advocate on behalf of the child. If there is a dispute about parental intentions or capacity to function as decision makers, it is incumbent that those who substitute another decision maker provide convincing evidence of why the parents should be disqualified. For example, even though respect for religious beliefs is an important community value, so is the value of life. Although adults who are Jehovah's Witnesses can choose to forgo a lifesaving blood transfusion for themselves, they are often not permitted to make a similar decision for their children. Moreover, children are entitled to grow up and independently assess their religious beliefs.

In such circumstances, health care providers must advocate for children and uphold the community standard of best interest. There will always be cases in which such assumptions are challenged, but these are likely to be few. Those who challenge parental motives and commitments must prove that parents should be disqualified as decision makers instead of having parents prove that their motives and commitments are authentic. Safeguards to protect the interests of children, families, and professionals will continue to be necessary and prudent. Assessing when community standards should outweigh a family determination is extremely difficult.

When parents are disqualified, a surrogate decision maker should know all relevant facts and be able to perceive and represent the feelings and interests of those involved. Surrogate decision makers should also be free of serious conflicts of interest that may bias a decision. A court-appointed guardian ad litem often serves as a surrogate decision maker. In special circumstances, such as obtaining permission for withholding resuscitation for a child with significant disabilities who is a ward of the state, it is difficult to identify a single surrogate. The personnel in the child welfare agency may not know the child well, the foster parents may not know the child well, and the natural parents may not have any contact with the child. In these instances, an ethics consultation may aid in identifying key people and designing a process for deciding the child's best interests (Johnson et al., 2015; Savage & Michalik, 2002).

ROLE OF MINORS IN TREATMENT DECISION MAKING

Professionals who care for children and adolescents with chronic conditions are increasingly concerned about minors' role in making decisions about their health care. Many adolescents experience catastrophic physical and mental health problems associated with severe disabilities, malignancies, or cardiac, pulmonary, and hepatic organ disease without having the legal right to decide about their treatments.

As client advocates, primary care providers must be concerned with promoting adolescents' interests in decisions regarding their health care. The concerns of adolescents escalate when parents and primary care providers seem to disregard the adolescent's previously expressed preferences or embark on a course of treatment that is inconsistent with the adolescent's life goals and values. Many health professionals are questioning the adequacy of current decision-making models and searching for creative solutions perhaps through the advent of advance directives for minors. Advanced directives available for children and teens include *Voicing My Choices* and *My Wishes*, as well as the adult form *Five Wishes*, all of which are available in English and Spanish. These documents can be filled out by children and teens and used in discussions with the family and medical team to increase communication about difficult topics and allow young people's preferences to be honored (Wiener et al., 2022).

From a moral viewpoint, minors with decision-making capacities have a legitimate claim to be involved in decisions about their health care. This claim is based on a respect for persons that recognizes that adolescents and young adults can be self-determining and therefore should have a voice in their care and the extent of medical interventions provided. Such respect for them as individuals and members of families and society compels primary care providers to take their preferences seriously when treatment decisions are made. Moreover, adolescents' interpretations of the benefits and burdens of treatment should be considered.

The standards for determining the decision-making capacity of minors are the same as those for adults (AAP Committee on Bioethics, 1994, 2017):

1. The ability to comprehend essential information about their diagnosis and prognosis
2. The ability to reason about their choices in accordance with their values and life goals
3. The ability to make a voluntary informed decision, which includes being able to recognize the consequences of various courses of action

Based on our knowledge of conceptual development, most children do not reach this level of maturity until age 11 or 12 years (White, 1994), although there is wide variation and controversy concerning theories and stages of cognitive development (Alderson et al., 2006). These standards are straightforward, but applying them in clinical practice requires clinicians to be skilled in systematically assessing and documenting the decision-making capacity of minors.

Despite the importance of self-determination and well-being in justifying the participation of minors in treatment decisions, there is another competing value at stake: the interests of parents in making decisions for their minor children. It has traditionally been assumed that minors require surrogates to decide for them. Parents are generally identified as the appropriate surrogates for their children and have been afforded considerable discretion in making treatment decisions.

Currently, treatment decisions for adolescents are made through a joint determination by the primary care provider or health care team and the parent or guardian for the child. Joint decisions to withhold or withdraw therapeutic interventions are difficult for parents and health care providers to formulate. Parents may seek any possible intervention to prolong their child's life regardless of the burden. Alternatively, they may wish to relieve their child's suffering by forgoing certain life-sustaining treatments. The primary care provider or health care team and the parent or guardian may have different agendas for either continuing or initiating certain therapeutic interventions or, instead, forgoing certain interventions, yet both groups may interpret their decisions as being in the best interest of the child. Despite their assessments, neither group may truly understand the adolescent's perspective. In many cases, the adolescent may already understand the pain and consequences of the treatment options, including the finality of death. Unfortunately, parents and health care providers may hesitate to consider adolescents as legitimate decision makers about medical treatment.

As the decision-making model enlarges to include a definitive role for minors with decision-making capacity, health care providers must recognize that such a departure will also challenge the traditional decision-making process and may create conflicts between minors and their parents. The potential for such moral and legal conflicts will necessitate the determination of a mechanism for resolving disputes. Researchers combined information from three studies on decision making in pediatric oncology, published literature, and professional associations' positions to posit evidence-based practice guidelines for end-of-life decision making by adolescents, their parents, and health care providers (deSante-Bertkau & Herbst, 2021; Hinds et al., 2001). These guidelines may be useful outside the oncology setting as well.

Legal Viewpoint on the Role of Minors in Decision Making

The legal system has determined that adolescents in certain circumstances have specific rights and responsibilities associated with their decision-making capabilities for health care. Emancipated minors are children under 18 years of age who are in the armed forces or are financially self-supporting and live away from home (Dickens & Cook, 2005). Most states have legislation recognizing the rights and responsibilities of emancipated minors. Emancipation is rarely determined by the courts and is generally implied through factors such as marital status, pregnancy or parenthood, and financial self-sufficiency. Emancipated minors do not need parental consent for medical treatment and have rights similar to adults in refusing medical treatment (Dickens & Cook, 2005; Traugott & Alpers, 1997).

The courts have also classified some adolescents as mature minors in relation to their decision-making capacity for seeking and accepting health care interventions. Mature minors are at least 15 years of age and are thought to have the capacity to understand the nature and risk of medical interventions. Adolescents classified as mature minors may consent to treatment that benefits them and does not involve any substantial risk. Derish and Vanden Heuvel (2000) present the pro and con arguments for the mature minor's right to refuse life-sustaining treatment.

State statutes generally support a minor's (i.e., a 14- to 17-year-old's) rights to consent to ordinary medical care. For example, some state statutes support the right of minors to consent to specific medical treatment (e.g., contraceptive therapies) without parental notification and consent; the right to consent to abortion, however, is complex and varied. The Omnibus Reconciliation Act of 1990, also called the Patient Self-Determination Act (PSDA) of 1990, supports the right of adults (i.e., at least 18 years old) admitted to health care facilities to accept or refuse medical treatment. This age limit is based on the belief that only adults have the capacity and the right to determine what should be done to their bodies—even if executing this right means implementing their right to die. It is crucial, however, that health care providers do not ignore the plight of thousands of adolescents (i.e., 12- to 17-year-olds) who face similar catastrophic and terminal conditions but are not given this legal right.

Although the PSDA was created for adults, the spirit of the PSDA provides an opportunity to examine the potential role of minors in their treatment decisions and ultimately their right to determine the circumstances of their death. Many young children and adolescents likely have the capacity to help make their own treatment decisions and determine what is in their best interest. There has been minimal guidance from the courts or legislation on a minor's right to refuse lifesaving medical care. In the few decisions rendered, the application of the mature minor status was used to support the minor's decision-making capacity to refuse treatment and understand the consequences of this decision. Unfortunately, because minimal and vague legal guidelines are available to support a minor's right to refuse treatment, health care providers are reluctant to intervene and support the minor's decision to withhold treatment—especially if this opposes the parents' wishes.

Involving minors in decision making about treatment requires families and professionals to create a system that supports the participation of minors. Such a system must include comprehensive guidelines for assessment, intervention, and ongoing revision (Hallström & Elander, 2005; McCabe et al., 1996).

MAKING SHARED DECISIONS A REALITY

Regardless of the child's age, the family's composition and dynamics, or professionals' involvement, ethical concerns are resolved by an authentic model of shared decision making that accommodates the diverse ways children and families participate. To resolve ethical concerns it is necessary to move beyond a procedural model of informed consent to an authentic partnership in which parents, the child, and professionals create an alliance that promotes the child's interests. The foundation for this alliance is a mutual understanding of each other's aspirations and goals, perspectives on what makes life meaningful for the child, and concepts of benefit and burden. In addition, parents need to share their goals, values, and definition of being good parents, and professionals must share their uncertainties and boundaries of their professional responsibility.

Shared decision making requires a vision that results from collaboration and open, effective communication using language without technical terminology and jargon. One reason achieving shared decision making fails is that professionals may focus primarily on the decision itself instead of on the process. Parents also may have difficulty separating emotions from facts. A revised model of shared decision making would focus more on the context of the situation—especially the relational dimensions, the parents' unique concept of good parenting, and the factors that mediate decision making—rather than on the decision itself.

Professionals must begin to appreciate the parents' perspective in decision making and not try to force them into a traditional, rational, stepwise model that is incongruent with their perspective. Therefore the goals of the parent-professional relationship, the outcomes of the process, and the process itself must be closely scrutinized. For example, if the goal of the relationship with families is to get them to see the world in the same way as the professional, dissenting views cannot be articulated or respected. Parents should be engaged early in a variety of choices about their child's care so that their involvement is not reserved for required consent for treatment or decisions about life-sustaining treatment. Parents need and want professionals to be partners in the care of their child—regardless of the outcome—and want professionals to help them be good parents in the process. Therefore sharing in decision making must begin early in the management of the condition.

Authentic shared decision making does not mean that differences will not exist or that everyone will come to the same conclusion about when and how to advance the child's interests (deSante-Bertkau & Herbst, 2021). Nor does it mean that all participants will have the same skills, abilities, or preferences. Shared decision making is a process in which differences are discussed, differing opinions are valued, and the quality of care ultimately provided to the child and family is enhanced.

TRANSITION TO ADULTHOOD

In most states, people 18 years of age and older are legally responsible for giving or refusing consent for medical treatment. People with chronic conditions often continue to be treated by pediatric subspecialists into their 20s and 30s because children with these disorders (e.g., spina bifida, congenital heart disease) in the past did not survive into adulthood. Unfortunately, some pediatric health care providers operate under a child-focused decision-making model and do not transition to an adult model when young adults are legally able and willing to serve as primary decision makers. Many transition programs are in place or being developed, but these are not without ethical problems. Ideally, the adolescent or young adult would have increasingly participated in decision making as developmentally appropriate; however, in some families children with chronic conditions are prevented from participating because their parents see them as too immature and unable to make rational decisions. The child's lack of experience makes the parents' impression a self-fulfilling prophecy. Lacking the experience, the child is unable to participate or fears participating in decision making. The health care team can educate parents to identify and foster the capabilities for decision making in their child: understanding information, manipulating information, appreciating the impact of the decision on one's situation, and making a choice (Grisso & Appelbaum, 1998).

Many older adolescents and young adults demonstrate a sophisticated level of understanding of their conditions and treatment. The health care team members can honor the autonomy of older adolescents and young adults by preparing them to participate in decisions and acting on their choices after the informed consent process (Dickens & Cook, 2005). There are other older adolescents or young adults who—because of cognitive comorbidity or immaturity—do not have the capacity to make decisions. Although they may be legally competent because they have not been declared incompetent by the courts, their ability to reason may be legitimately questioned. An assessment of their decision-making capacity, specific to the decision, should be undertaken and documented. Traditionally, parents or guardians have retained decision-making authority in such circumstances. Clinicians must work to foster decision making within the family context. To avoid confusion, parents should be counseled to seek legal guardianship for adult children who lack decision-making capacity. Unfortunately, the cost of doing so is prohibitive for some families. Persons who lack the capacity to make decisions independently (e.g., those with severe developmental disabilities) should be respectfully allowed to participate in the decision-making process. As with young children, every child should be allowed to be prepared for medical interventions, receive developmentally appropriate explanations, and express preferences. The more important the decision in the life of the person, the greater the care in assessing that person's decision-making capacity pertinent to what the specific decision should be. Health care providers must be familiar with their institution's policies on surrogate decision making for adults who lack decisional capacity.

The 1999 Olmstead decision (*Olmstead v. LC*, PL 98-536) bolstered the move toward independent and assisted living. Young adults who previously would have remained at home or were placed in residential facilities may choose the most integrated setting versus the most restrictive one. The public entity, such as a state-supported institution, must facilitate placement in the most integrated setting appropriate to the needs of qualified individuals with disabilities. In the transition program, the health care provider knowledgeable about the Olmstead decision can assist in removing barriers often faced by young adults with chronic disabling conditions.

STRATEGIES FOR ETHICAL DECISION MAKING

INCREASED KNOWLEDGE OF ETHICS, LAWS, AND POLICIES

Professionals can enhance their effectiveness in resolving ethical conflicts by seeking opportunities to enhance their knowledge of and skills in ethical analysis and by identifying resources to assist them in resolving dilemmas. Further, knowledge of legal, public, and professional policies is advantageous. In particular, primary care providers who care for children with chronic conditions should be aware of pertinent state statutes and case laws that may affect their health care. Primary care providers must be particularly aware of institutional policies on discontinuing life-sustaining treatment if such policies exist and participate in developing them if they do not. Institutional policies that permit information to be withheld from parents or effectively deny parental access to divergent medical opinions should also be examined and challenged.

PROACTIVE DIALOGUE, ASSESSMENT, AND PLANNING

Children with chronic conditions and their families often have a high level of personal interaction with primary care providers. Because many chronic conditions persist over a lifetime, there are many natural opportunities to examine, revise, or abandon various goals or dimensions of the treatment plan. This is referred to as *advance care planning*. With proactive planning it is also possible and desirable to anticipate the ethical conflicts that accompany the treatment plan. Ongoing dialogue about the treatment plan is essential for optimal planning and must not be reserved for crisis situations associated with acute episodes of illness, deteriorating conditions, or death.

Many children with chronic conditions and their families and providers will confront difficult decisions about treatment that will create significant moral tension. Questions about parental acceptance of psychoactive medications to treat children with attention-deficit/hyperactivity disorder or to try an experimental protocol for treating cancer may arise. Such morally difficult decisions are best made when there is adequate time for education, discussion, and reflection. Therefore ethical issues should be anticipated and discussions begun early.

GENETIC TESTING: PRIVACY AND CONFIDENTIALITY

Ethical questions regarding genetic testing and new or experimental techniques for treating genetic disorders are arising. Genetic testing has long been accepted in newborn testing for the purposes of early identification for treatment. Technology has advanced to be able to identify many genetic disorders. Parents may be offered the opportunity to have genetic testing for themselves and their child to diagnose their child's condition. When signs and symptoms indicate that a child may have a genetic disorder, even if a cure is not available, the family may benefit by knowing the diagnosis, planning for the child's future needs, and learning the probability of future children being affected. Although parents may have an intense desire to discover their child's diagnosis, they may fear that their child will be stigmatized and discriminated against by insurance companies, schools, and eventually employers. The Health Insurance Portability and Accountability Act of 1996 (HIPAA; 2002) contained no special provisions protecting genetic information; however, newer federal legislation passed in 2008, the Genetic Information Nondiscrimination Act, was designed to protect Americans against discrimination based on their genetic information when it comes to health insurance and employment. Additionally, there is extensive relevant state legislation (see www.genome.gov/PolicyEthics/LegDatabase/pubsearch.cfm for a list of all legislation).

Although obtaining a blood test, buccal smear, or performing a skin biopsy in the office may seem rather benign, the ramifications of the findings can have profound consequences on the child's and family's future. Primary care providers can guard the privacy and confidentiality of a child's medical information by developing and implementing institutional policies on informed consent for genetic testing, special disposition of test results, and special procedures for releasing medical records containing test results (i.e., to schools, insurers, and others) (National Task Force on Confidential Student Health Information, 2000). Many institutions currently have special procedures for tests (e.g., human immunodeficiency virus) that protect individuals from unwarranted disclosure of information.

Presymptomatic genetic testing for adult-onset conditions (e.g., Huntington disease, breast cancer) generally is not recommended for children (AAP, 2005; AAP Committee on Bioethics, 2001, 2013; Ross & Moon, 2000), but decisions should always be made in the best interest of the child (Twomey, 2006). Predictive testing may be done according to the rule of earliest onset for selected conditions (Kodish, 1999) and at the parents'

discretion for late childhood–onset disorders, with the child's input where appropriate. However, government-sponsored predictive screenings "do not fulfill public health screening criteria" (Ross, 2002, p. 225).

Testing one member of the family can yield information about other members. Families need to be aware of the ramifications of testing. Genetic counselors are skilled in assisting families in making decisions to share or withhold information about a tested relative. Sometimes it is necessary to test relatives. Again, genetic counselors assist families in understanding the extent to which other family members need to be involved to yield useful information (Hodge, 2004; Stein et al., 2018). Guidelines in protecting the privacy of family members for genetics research may also prove useful for protecting privacy for nonresearch testing. Doukas and Berg (2001) proposed a family covenant model in working with families who have genetic testing. The family covenant recognizes the family as a unit and its members in the context of the family. With genetic knowledge increasing exponentially, professionals working with children with chronic conditions and their families should stay abreast of genetic advances and applicable laws. Programs such as the Ethical, Legal, and Social Implications branch of the National Human Genome Research Institute provide leadership in this area and post emerging news and information in this dynamic field (www.genome.gov). Professional organizations may also provide information and advocacy on advances in genetics.

Enormous advances in gene therapy and stem cell research are being realized. Hundreds of gene transfer protocols are underway or will be underway for conditions such as cystic fibrosis, hemophilia, sickle cell disease, muscular dystrophy, Fanconi anemia, Gaucher disease, and Canavan disease. As with any clinical trial, parents need as much information as possible to make an informed decision, and the child, if capable, should be included in the discussions. Additional ethical issues surrounding genetic advances, such as their availability and limitations, will need to be addressed.

STRATEGIES FOR DEALING WITH CONFLICT

Even when communication among children, parents, and professionals is optimal, conflicts arise. Good communication may illuminate points of real ethical dispute. Participants often prioritize values differently and employ processes to reach morally defensible conclusions. Therefore activities that promote multidisciplinary sharing, analysis, and decision making in an atmosphere of openness, objectivity, and diversity can lead to more tolerance of others' views.

When moral disagreements occur, strategies for resolution include the following:
1. Obtaining the most current factual information on points of controversy
2. Reaching a consensus about the language used for concepts or definitions

3. Agreeing on a framework of moral principles to guide discussions
4. Engaging in a balanced discussion of the positive and negative aspects of a viewpoint

Institutions can review difficult or disputed cases through institutional ethics committees and other means of efficiently accessing legal, governmental, and consultative services. An internal review process can serve several purposes:

1. Verifying the facts of the case
2. Confirming the propriety of decisions
3. Resolving disputes
4. Making referrals to public agencies when appropriate

Institutional ethics committees are often consultants to staff and families experiencing ethical conflict. Multidisciplinary membership (i.e., including a parent) provides a broad representation of different viewpoints. In general, these committees are primarily consultative without any binding authority; however, the opportunity for uninvolved parties to assist in reviewing difficult cases can provide constructive recommendations for resolution. Ethics committees or ethics consultants are increasing in home health agencies, nursing homes, and community health facilities.

Mechanisms to resolve conflicts between minors and their parents must be developed as the process of involving minors in treatment decisions unfolds. Based on a model of family-centered care, mechanisms supporting individual self-determination within the family system context are necessary. Strategies will also be needed to support families as they allow their minor children to be more involved in decision making. Mechanisms for examining the decision-making patterns of families and the roles of children and parents in other types of decisions within the family are also necessary. Finally, strategies to prepare minors to participate in decisions about health care through community or school educational programs and as part of routine health care encounters are important prerequisites (Cavet & Sloper, 2004; deSante-Bertkau & Herbst, 2021).

SUMMARY

The resolution of ethical conflicts requires that health care professionals recognize there is a moral problem, use a systematic process of moral reasoning, and take action. As a prerequisite to such analysis, primary care providers who care for children with chronic conditions and their families must examine their own values about the content and structure of treatment decisions. Such clarification is necessary to ensure that the ideal of authentic shared decision making becomes a reality.

RESOURCES

Alliance of Genetic Support Groups, Inc.: www.geneticalliance.org

American Nurses Association: www.nursingworld.org
American Society for Bioethics and Humanities: www.asbh.org
Academic Bioethics Centers: bioethics.od.nih.gov/academic.html
Center for Bioethics, University of Pennsylvania Medical Center: www.bioethics.upenn.edu
Center for Clinical Ethics and Humanities in Health Care, University of Buffalo: www.wings.buffalo.edu/faculty/research/bioethics
Council for Responsible Genetics: www.gene-watch.org.
Eubios Ethics Institute: www.eubios.info
International Society of Nurses in Genetics (ISONG): www.isong.org
Kennedy Institute of Genetics, Georgetown University: bioethics.georgetown.edu
MacLean Center for Clinical Ethics at University of Chicago: medicine.uchicago.edu/centers/ccme/index.htm
National Bioethics Advisory Commission: www.bioethics.gov
National Human Genome Research Institute: www.genome.gov
National Library of Medicine: www.nlm.nih.gov
National Reference Center for Bioethics Literature: bioethics.georgetown.edu/nrc/visitNRCBL.htm

REFERENCES

Aarthun, A., Oymar, K. A., & Akerjordet, K. (2019). Parental involvement in decision-making about their child's health care at the hospital. *Nursing Open, 6*(1), 50–58.

Albert T. *Federal court overturns FDA pediatric drug testing rule.* 2002. Available at www.ama-assn.org/amednews/2002/11/18/gvsc1118.htm. Retrieved November 19, 2008.

Alderson, P., Sutcliffe, K., & Curtis, K. (2006). Children's competence to consent to medical treatment. *Hastings Center Report, 36*(6), 25–34.

American Academy of Pediatrics. (2005). AAP publications retired and reaffirmed. *Pediatrics, 115*, 1438.

American Academy of Pediatrics Committee on Bioethics. (1994). Guidelines on forgoing life sustaining medical treatment. *Pediatrics, 3*, 533–535.

American Academy of Pediatrics Committee on Bioethics. (2017). Guidelines on forgoing life sustaining medical treatment. *Pediatrics, 140*(3), 1–9.

American Academy of Pediatrics Committee on Bioethics. (2001). *Ethical issues with genetic testing in pediatrics. Pediatrics, 107*(6), 1451–1455.

American Academy of Pediatrics Committee on Bioethics. (2013). Ethical and policy issues with genetic testing and screening of children. *Pediatrics, 131*(3), 620–622.

American Academy of Pediatrics Committee on Bioethics. (2016). Informed consent in decision-making in pediatric practice. *Pediatrics, 138*(2).

American Academy of Pediatrics & American Pain Society. (2001). The assessment and management of acute pain in infants, children and adolescents. *Pediatrics, 108*(3), 793–797.

American Nurses Association. *Code of ethics for nurses with interpretive statements.* Washington, DC. 2015

Americans with Disabilities Act of 1990. (1990). Available at www.ada.gov/pubs/ada.htm. Retrieved November 12, 2008.

Bauchner, H. (2001). Shared decision-making in pediatrics. *Archives of Disease in Childhood, 84*, 246.

Beauchamp, T. L., & Childress, J. F. (2019). *Principles of biomedical ethics* (8th ed.). United Kingdom: Oxford University Press.

Becker, P. T., & Grunwald, P. C. (2000). Contextual dynamics of ethical decision making in the NICU. *Journal of Perinatal and Neonatal Nursing, 14*(2), 58–72.

Beidler, S. M., & Dickey, S. B. (2001). Children's competence to participate in healthcare decisions. *JONA's Healthcare, Law, Ethics, and Regulation, 3*, 80–87.

Blustein, J. (1998). The family in medical decision-making. In Monagle, J. F., & Thomasma, D. C. (Eds.), *Health care ethics: Critical issues for the 21st century.* Aspen Systems.

Carter, B., McArthur, E., & Cunliffe, M. (2002). Dealing with uncertainty: Parental assessment of pain in their children with profound special needs. *Journal of Advanced Nursing, 38*, 449–457.

Cavet, J., & Sloper, P. (2004). Participation of disabled children in individual decisions about their lives and in public decisions about service development. *Children & Society, 18*(4), 278–290.

Child Abuse Amendments of 1984. (1984). *42 US Code 10401 et seq: Interpretive guidelines.* (45 CFR Part 1 1340:15 et eq.) Washington, DC: US Government Printing Office.

Claassen, M. (2000). A handful of questions: Supporting parental decision making. *Clinical Nurse Specialist, 14*(4), 189–195.

Committee on Bioethics. (1994). Guidelines for forgoing life-sustaining medical treatment. *Pediatrics, 93*(3), 532–536.

Committee on Child Abuse and Neglect and Committee on Children with Disabilities. (2001). Assessment of maltreatment of children with disabilities. *Pediatrics, 108*, 508–512.

Crume, T. L., DiGuiseppi, C., Byers, T., Sirotnak, A. P., & Garrett, C. J. (2002). Underascertainment of child maltreatment fatalities by death certificates, 1990–1998. *Pediatrics, 110*(2 Pt 1), e18. https://doi.org/10.1542/peds.110.2.e18.

Derish, M. T., & Vanden Heuvel, K. (2000). Mature minors should have the right to refuse life-sustaining medical treatment. *Journal of Law, Medicine & Ethics, 28*, 109–124.

D'Errico, S., Zanon, M., Radaelli, D., Padovano, M., Santurro, A., Scopetti, M., Frati, P., & Fineschi, V. (2022). Medication errors in pediatrics: Proposals to improve the quality and safety of care through clinical risk management. *Frontiers in medicine, 8*, 814100. https://doi.org/10.3389/fmed.2021.814100.

deSante-Bertkau, J., & Herbst, L. A. (2021). Ethics of pediatric and young adult medical decision-making: Case-based discussions exploring consent, capacity, and surrogate decision-making. *MedEdPORTAL, 17*(1).

Dickens, B. M., & Cook, R. J. (2005). Adolescents and consent to treatment. *International Journal of Gynecology and Obstetrics, 89*(2), 179B–184B.

Diekema, D. S. (2019). Decision making on behalf of children: Understanding the role of the harm principle. *Journal of Clinical Ethics, 30*(3), 207–212.

Doukas, D. J., & Berg, J. W. (2001). The family covenant and genetic testing. *American Journal of Bioethics, 1*(3), 2–10.

Erdmann, A., Rehmann-Sutter, C., & Bozzaro, C. (2021). Patients' and professionals' views related to ethical issues in Precision Medicine: A mixed research synthesis. *BMC Medical Ethics, 22*(1). https://doi.org/10.1186/s12910-021-00682-8.

Erdmann, F., Frederiksen, L. E., Bonaventure, A., Mader, L., Hasle, H., Robison, L. L., & Winther, J. F. (2021). Childhood cancer: Survival, treatment modalities, late effects and improvements over time. *Cancer epidemiology, 71*(Pt B), 101733. https://doi.org/10.1016/j.canep.2020.101733.

Ferranti, J., Horvath, M. M., Cozart, H., Whitehurst, J., & Eckstrand, J. (2008). Reevaluating the safety profile of pediatrics: a comparison of computerized adverse drug event surveillance and voluntary reporting in the pediatric environment. *Pediatrics, 121*(5), e1201–e1207. https://doi.org/10.1542/peds.2007-2609.

Fortson, B. L., Klevens, J., Merrick, M. T., et al. (2016). *Preventing child abuse and neglect: A technical package for policy, norm, and programmatic activities.* Atlanta, GA: National Center for Injury Prevention and Control, Centers for Disease Control and Prevention.

Fost, N. (1999). Decisions regarding treatment of seriously ill newborns. *JAMA, 281*(21), 2041–2043.

Goldson, E. (2001). Maltreatment among children with disabilities. *Infants and Young Children, 13*(4), 44–54.

Gonzales, K. (2010). Medication administration errors and the pediatric population: A systematic search of the literature. *Journal of Pediatric Nursing, 25*(6), 555–565.

Grisso, T., & Appelbaum, P. S. (1998). *Assessing competence to consent to treatment.* Oxford University Press.

Hallström, I., Elander, G. (2005). Decision making in paediatric care: an overview with reference to nursing care. *Nursing Ethics. 12*(3), 223–238.

Health Information Portability and Accountability Act (HIPAA). (2002). Available at www.hhs.gov/ocr/hipaa. Retrieved May 25, 2008.

Hinds, P. S., Oakes, L., Furman, W., Quargnenti, A., Olson, M. S., Foppiano, P., & Srivastava, D. K. (2001). End-of-life decision making by adolescents, parents, and healthcare providers in pediatric oncology: research to evidence-based practice guidelines. *Cancer nursing, 24*(2), 122–136. https://doi.org/10.1097/00002820-200104000-00007.

Hodge, J. G. (2004). Ethical issues concerning genetic testing and screening in public health. *American Journal of Medical Genetics Part C, 125*(1), 66–70.

Hynson, J. L., & Sawyer, S. M. (2001). Paediatric palliative care: Distinctive needs and emerging issues. *Journal of Paediatric and Child Health, 37*(4), 323–325.

Individuals with Disabilities Education Amendments of 1997. (1997). *Public Law 105-17.* Washington, DC: US Government Printing Office.

Individuals with Disabilities Education Improvement Act of 2004. (2004). *Public Law 108-446.* Washington, DC: US Government Printing Office.

Jeremic, V., Sénécal, K., Borry, P., Chokoshvili, D., & Vears, D. F. (2016). Participation of children in medical decision-making: Challenges and potential solutions. *Journal of bioethical inquiry, 13*(4), 525–534. https://doi.org/10.1007/s11673-016-9747-8.

Johnson, L. M., Church, C. L., Metzger, M., & Baker, J. N. (2015). Ethics consultation in pediatrics: Long-term experiences from a pediatric oncology center. *American Journal of Bioethics, 15*(5), 3–17.

Joint Commission on Accreditation of Healthcare Organizations. *Comprehensive accreditation manual for hospitals: The official handbook.* Oakbrook Terrace, IL. 2001.

Jonsen, A. R., Siegler, M., & Winslade, W. J. (1998). *Clinical ethics* (4th ed.). McGraw-Hill.

Jordan, A., Carter, B., & Vasileiou, K. (2021). "Pain talk": A triadic collaboration in which nurses promote opportunities for engaging children and their parents about managing children's pain. *Paediatric and Neonatal Pain, 3*(3), 123–133.

Kaushal, R., Bates, D. W., Landrigan, C., McKenna, K. J., Clapp, M. D., Federico, F., & Goldmann, D. A. (2001). Medication errors and adverse drug events in pediatric inpatients. *JAMA, 285*(16), 2114–2120. https://doi.org/10.1001/jama.285.16.2114.

Kaushal, R., Jaggi, T., Walsh, K., Fortescue, E. B., & Bates, D. W. (2004). Pediatric medication errors: what do we know? What gaps remain? *Ambulatory pediatrics: the official journal of the Ambulatory Pediatric Association, 4*(1), 73–81. https://doi.org/10.1367/1539-4409(2004)004<0073:pmewdw>2.0.co;2.

Kodish, E. (1999). Testing children for cancer genes: The rule of earliest onset. *Journal of Pediatrics, 135*(3), 390–395.

Ladd, R. E., & Mercurio, M. R. (2003). Deciding for neonates: Whose authority, whose interests? *Seminars in Perinatology, 27*, 488–494.

Lee, K. J., Hill, D. L., & Feudtner, C. (2020). Decision-making for children with medical complexity: The role of the primary care pediatrician. *Pediatric Annals, 49*(11), e473–e477.

Legano, L. A., Desch, L. W., Messner, S. A., Idzerda, S., Flaherty, E. G., COUNCIL ON CHILD ABUSE AND NEGLECT, & COUNCIL ON CHILDREN WITH DISABILITIES (2021). Maltreatment of children with disabilities. *Pediatrics, 147*(5), e2021050920. https://doi.org/10.1542/peds.2021-050920.

Martenson, E. K., & Fagerskiold, A. M. (2007). A review of children's decision-making competence in health care. *Journal of Clinical Nursing, 19*(7), 40–43.

Mccabe, M. A., Rushton, C. H., Glover, J., Murray, M. G., & Leikin, S. (1996). Implications of the Patient Self-Determination Act: guidelines for involving adolescents in medical decision making. *The Journal of adolescent health: official publication of the Society for Adolescent Medicine, 19*(5), 319–324. https://doi.org/10.1016/S1054-139X(96)00160-7.

McCarroll, J. E., Fisher, J. E., Cozza, S. J., & Whalen, R. J. (2021). Child maltreatment fatality review: Purposes, processes, outcomes, and challenges. *Trauma, Violence, & Abuse, 22*(5), 1032–1041.

McClafferty, H., Vohra, S., Bailey, M., Brown, M., Esparham, A., Gerstbacher, D., Golianu, B., Niemi, A. K., Sibinga, E., Weydert, J., Yeh, A. M., & SECTION ON INTEGRATIVE MEDICINE (2017). Pediatric integrative medicine. *Pediatrics, 140*(3), e20171961. https://doi.org/10.1542/peds.2017-1961.

McCormick, R. (1974). To save or let die: The dilemma of modern medicine. *JAMA, 229*(2), 172–176.

Micozzi, M. S. (2001). *Fundamentals of complementary and alternative medicine* (2nd ed.). Churchill Livingstone.

Moresco, B., & Moore, D. (2021). Pediatric palliative care. *Hospital Practice*, 1–9.

National Institutes of Health. *Policy and guidelines on the inclusion of children as participants in research involving human subjects.*1998. Available at http://grants1.nih.gov/grants/guide/notice-files/not98-024.html. Retrieved November 12, 2008.

O'Donnell, F. T., Rosen, K. R. (2014). Pediatric pain management: a review. *Mo Med., 111*(3), 231–237. PMID: 25011346; PMCID: PMC6179554.

Olmstead v. *LC* (PL 98-536) US Supreme Court decidedJune 22, 1999. Available at http://supct.law.cornell.edu/supct/html/98-536.ZO.html. Retrieved November 19, 2008.

Olszewski, A. E., & Goldkind, S. F. (2018). The default position: Optimizing pediatric participation in medical decision making. *American Journal of Bioethics, 18*(3), 4–9.

Omnibus Reconciliation Act (Patient Self-Determination Act [PSDA]), Title IV. *Section* 4206, h12456-h12457, *Congressional Record*, October 26, 1990.

Perrin, E. C., Lewkowicz, C., & Young, M. H. (2000). Shared vision: Concordance among fathers, mothers, and pediatricians about unmet needs of children with chronic health conditions. *Pediatrics, 105*(Suppl 1), 277–285.

President's Commission for the Study of Ethical Problems in Medicine and Biomedical and Behavioral Research. (1983). *Deciding to forgo life-sustaining treatment.* Washington, DC: US Government Printing Office.

Punch, S. (2002). Research with children the same or different from research with adults? *Childhood, 9*(3), 321–341.

Ramanan, A. V., Modi, N., & deWildt, S. N. (2022). Improving clinical paediatric research and learning from COVID-19: Recommendations by the Connect4Children expert advice group. *Pediatric Research, 91*, 1069–1077.

Ross, L. F. (1997). Health care decision-making by children: Is it in their best interest? *Hastings Center Report, 27*(6), 41–45.

Ross, L. F. (2002). Predictive genetic testing for conditions that present in childhood. *Kennedy Institute of Ethics Journal, 12*(3), 225–244.

Ross, L. F., & Moon, M. R. (2000). Ethical issues in genetic testing of children. *Archives of Pediatric and Adolescent Medicine, 154*(9), 873–879.

Sabatello, M., Janvier, A., Verhagen, E., Morrison, W., & Lantos, J. (2018). Pediatric participation in medical decision making: Optimized or personalized? *The American Journal of Bioethics: AJOB, 18*(3), 1–3. https://doi.org/10.1080/15265161.2017.1418931.

Savage, T. A. (1997). Ethical decision-making for children. *Critical Care Nursing Clinics of North America, 9*(1), 97–105.

Savage, T. A., & Michalik, D. R. (2002). Finding agreement to limit life-sustaining treatment for children who are in state custody. *Current Practices in Pediatric Nursing, 27*, 594–597.

Schwartz, M. S. (2016). Ethical decision-making theory: An integrated approach. *Journal of Business Ethics, 139*, 755–776.

Section 504 of the Rehabilitation Act of 1973. (1973). *Public Law 93-112*. Washington DC: US Government Printing Office.

Stein, Q., Loman, R., & Zuck, T. (2018). Genetic counseling in pediatrics. *Pediatrics in Review, 39*(7), 323–331.

Traugott, I., & Alpers, A. (1997). In their own hands: Adolescents' refusals of medical treatment. *Archives of Pediatric and Adolescent Medicine, 151*(9), 922–927.

Twomey, J. G. (2006). Issues in genetic testing of children. *MCN American Journal of Maternal and Child Nursing, 31*, 156–163.

US Department of Health and Human Services. (1991). Office for Human Research Protections. *45 CFR 46 Subpart B.* 46, 404–407.

US Department of Health and Human Services. (2008, January 3). Office for Human Research Protections (OHRP). OHRP 45 CR part 46. *Frequently asked questions.*

US Department of Health and Human Services. (2016, March 18). Office for Human Research Protections (OHRP). Children: In formation on special protections for children as research subjects. https://www.hhs.gov/ohrp/regulations-and-policy/guidance/special-protections-for-children/index.html. Retrieved August 25, 2022.

US Department of Health and Human Services. (2005). *Administration on Children, Youth and Families. Child maltreatment 2003.* Washington, DC: US Government Printing Office.

Vohra, S., & Cohen, M. H. (2007). Ethics of complementary and alternative medicine use in children. *Pediatric Clinics of North America, 54*, 875–884.

Wang, J. K., Herzog, N. S., Kaushal, R., Park, C., Mochizuki, C., & Weingarten, S. R. (2007). Prevention of pediatric medication errors by hospital pharmacists and the potential benefit of computerized physician order entry. *Pediatrics, 119*(1), e77–e85. https://doi.org/10.1542/peds.2006-0034.

White, B. C. (1994). *Competence to consent.* Washington, DC: Georgetown University Press.

Wiener, L., Bedoya, S., Battles, H., Sender, L., Zabokrtsky, K., Donovan, K. A., Thompson, L. M. A., Lubrano di Ciccone, B. B., Babilonia, M. B., Fasciano, K., Malinowski, P., Lyon, M., Thompkins, J., Heath, C., Velazquez, D., Long-Traynor, K., Fry, A., & Pao, M. (2022). Voicing their choices: Advance care planning with adolescents and young adults with cancer and other serious conditions. *Palliative & supportive care, 20*(4), 462–470. https://doi.org/10.1017/S1478951521001462.

Wightman, A., Kett, J., Campelia, G., & Wilfond, B. S. (2019). The relational potential standard: Rethinking the ethical justification for life-sustaining treatment for children with profound cognitive disabilities. *Hastings Center Report, 49*(3), 18–25.

Yeon, G. M., & Nam, S. O. (2016). The use of complementary and alternative medicine in children with common neurologic diseases. *Korean Journal of Pediatrics, 59*(8), 313–318.

Zaiger, D. S. (2000). National task force on confidential student health information offers guidelines. *Nasnewsletter.* 15(2), 1, 11. PMID: 11051993.

Managing Chronic Conditions via Telehealth

6

Kelli Garber, Ragan DuBose-Morris

INTRODUCTION

Since the beginning of the telecommunications age, societies have utilized new technologies to connect patients and providers over time and distance constraints. With the expansion of access through audio and visual means, health care has moved from the initial use of technologies for emergent/urgent health needs to services for chronic care patients (Genes, 2017). Defined as the transmission of health information across distances to support clinical services and patient contacts, telemedicine utilizes information and communication technologies through innovative applications such as videoconferencing, text- and image-based apps, remote monitoring, and telerobotics (Gogia, 2020). Expanding the scope of these services to include education, research, and other administrative functions broadens telemedicine to the provision of telehealth services. Telehealth, due to its "inclusion of preventative and promotive components" (Gogia, 2020), is the term used in this chapter.

Telehealth interventions, which began as a follow-up to in-person care, now facilitate the evaluation of patients in their home environments. While these technologic advances have traditionally been supported through academic centers, they are built on a foundation of rural and underserved clinical service provisions (Bashshur et al., 2014; Gogia, 2020). Either through provider-to-provider or patient-to-provider connections, the origin of telehealth practice to support pediatric patients is built on adult and specialty care models to improve access and reduce the need for an in-person consultation.

While the COVID-19 pandemic accelerated the development of these types of technologic support systems, decades of care innovations have already been documented in support of pediatric patients (Meyer et al., 2012; Silva et al., 2022). From primary care to specialty care and combinations of other clinical models, the evolution of health care services is being driven by technologic expertise and human ingenuity. Examples abound in the use of telehealth to support patients from prenatal development through adulthood into elder care. Examples include prenatal and newborn monitoring, virtual urgent care consultations, hospital-to-hospital support for complex cases, and direct-to-consumer interventions in community settings (American Academy of Pediatrics [AAP], 2022c).

In addition to the need for urgent clinical assessment across a variety of care settings, there is also the need for increasing chronic care management for our youngest patients (Curfman, McSwain, Chuo, Yeager-McSwain, et al., 2021; Milne Wenderlich & Herendeen, 2021). These needs stem from systemic issues related to access, quality, and costs associated with the provision of pediatric health care. These cost and procedural considerations flow across health care institutions and individual patients and their caregivers (Curfman et al., 2022). Telehealth is a tool that when used appropriately can mitigate social and systemic challenges.

As demonstrated through an increasing prevalence of telehealth services, increased provider access to patients and support for patients across the continuum remain priorities to improve overall care and reduce provider burnout (AAP, 2022b). Innovations and consultative services are just the beginning of the opportunities that exist to connect patients with care. New community-based and population health models have risen to the collective consciousness of policymakers, administrators, and clinicians as ways to specifically support children with chronic conditions (Bansa et al., 2019; Lesher et al., 2020). These models integrate telehealth as a tool for improved care.

OVERVIEW OF TELEHEALTH

Telehealth services are facilitated through a combination of real-time, asynchronous, remote monitoring and e-health/digital health technologies (Gogia, 2020). Often these telehealth practice models are divided into ambulatory and hospital-to-hospital (facility-to-facility) modalities (Curfman, McSwain, Chuo, Yeager-McSwain, et al., 2021). While ambulatory is most likely described as direct-to-consumer services, a variety of community-based sites also fall under this heading, including schools, federally qualified health centers, private practices, libraries and community centers, and other evolving locations for meeting the needs of pediatric patients where they live and gather.

Technology and types of services provided are dictated by the needs of the patient, the discretion of the provider, and the availability of connectivity through technology applications and telecommunication

03

Table **6.1**   Pediatric Telehealth Application Examples by Category

CATEGORY	APPLICATION EXAMPLE	SUPPORTING TECHNOLOGIES
Ambulatory	Asthma management	Direct-to-patient video applications and telehealth carts
Inpatient	Infection control protocols	Telehealth carts and in-room video systems
Facility-to-facility	Neonatal and pediatric intensive care unit consultations	Telehealth carts with peripherals (i.e., cameras, stethoscopes)
Hospital-to-home	Complex medical children—home ventilation management	Smart monitoring devices and direct-to-patient video applications
Remote patient monitoring	Implanted cardiovascular device monitoring	Blood pressure cuffs, glucose monitor, O_2 sensors, cardiac devices, mobile applications

Modified from Aalam, A.A., Hood, C., Donelan, C., Rutenberg, A., Kane, E.M., & Sikka, N. [2021]. Remote patient monitoring for ED discharges in the COVID-19 pandemic. *Emergency Medicine Journal, 38*[3], 229–231; American Medical Association. [2020]. *Telehealth implementation playbook*. https://www.ama-assn.org/terms-use; Curfman, A.L., McSwain, S.D., Chuo, J., Yeager-McSwain, B., Schinasi, D., Marcin, J., Herendeen, N., Chung, S.L., Rheuban, K., & Olson, C.A. [2021]. Pediatric telehealth in the COVID-19 pandemic era and beyond. *Pediatrics, 148*[3]; Foster, C., Schinasi, D., Kan, K., et al. [2022]. Remote monitoring of patient- and family-generated health data in pediatrics. *Pediatrics, 149*[2], e2021054137; Gutierrez, J., Rewerts, K., CarlLee, S., et al. [2022]. A systematic review of telehealth applications in hospital medicine. *Journal of Hospital Medicine, 17*[4], 291–302; Rosen, J.M., Adams, L.V., Geiling, J., et al. [2021]. Telehealth's new horizon: Providing smart hospital-level care in the home. *Telemed E-Health, 27*[11], 1215–1224; Vinadé Chagas, M.E., Rodrigues Moleda Constant, H.M., Cristina Jacovas, V., et al. [2021]. The use of telemedicine in the PICU: A systematic review and meta-analysis. *PLOS ONE, 16*[5], e0252409.

processes. For hospital-to-hospital care, telehealth modalities generally focus on the consultative model and provide decision-making support to help manage care in the most local and appropriate locations. In addition, monitoring services for pediatric patients can occur within formal settings (neonatal and pediatric intensive care units) or as part of remote patient monitoring applications within a patient's home (i.e., newborn, chronic care, or wound management) (Aalam et al., 2021; Foster et al., 2022; Vinadé Chagas et al., 2021). Overall, applications and technologies are deployed across care settings in a significant number of pediatric specializations (Table 6.1).

Telehealth applications help to provide a continuum of services that can link patients and health care systems through medical informatics and telecommunications to support patients through life cycles and across disease states (Ford et al., 2020). These applications, especially in hospital settings, have been shown to support a wide range of consultation, diagnosis, care coordination, mentoring, and monitoring processes between and within urban and rural settings (Gutierrez et al., 2022). These uses help to fill gaps in patient care, reduce access issues regardless of geographic location and time, and expand the team concept to include additional providers as well as patients and their caregivers. Traditional telehealth applications and technology are not necessary for the provision of all communication as the transfer of images and text is often shared through more traditional mobile devices and health system portal access. For example, decision making about pre- and postoperative care conducted using a patient/caregiver's personal device can reduce the need for patients to travel for in-person care (Jin et al., 2021).

BENEFITS

Telehealth has a history of use in cases where video communications easily facilitate clinical care. This can be seen most prominently in behavioral health through a long record of innovation aimed at improving access to specialty services (Keder et al., 2022). For both patients and providers, the benefits of telehealth can lead to high satisfaction and usability based on factors such as convenience, extended reach of the medical home model, reduction in infectious disease exposure, flexibility and efficiency for scheduling, and improved well-being for patients, their caregivers, and providers (Preminger, 2022).

Data are vague on the specific economic returns offered by telehealth based on changes in service delivery and innovation within care models (Curfman, McSwain, Chuo, Olson, et al., 2021). Deriving value measurements for cost expenditure and returns related to telehealth has been shown to improve pediatric care through small pilot studies, but larger research initiatives are needed to fully demonstrate the true impact of these care delivery models. New pediatric research collaboratives, such as Supporting Pediatric Research on Outcomes and Utilization of Telehealth, aim at increasing the number of patients, services, and institutions participating in telehealth research to accelerate the development of high-quality, high-impact pediatric programs (AAP, 2023).

CHALLENGES

Telehealth policies and funding remain the leading factors affecting the reduction in the adoption and uptake of telehealth. This is due to the complexities of reimbursement and the regulatory environment surrounding the types of care that can be provided (Kruse et al., 2021). Implementing new telehealth services and expanding current offerings require stability in terms of financial viability. Further complications are seen when providers must navigate a myriad of regulations related to the service level of care, originating and delivery sites, and frequency of care to determine how to address the specific needs of each patient via telehealth. This is especially true when dealing with chronic care conditions that require cross-team and interprofessional collaboration. Telehealth applications are further dependent upon the types of payment programs supporting the patient and the accessibility of reimbursement for the provider team as dictated by the Centers for Medicare and Medicaid Services (CMS) or third-party payers (Ray et al., 2020; Zhao et al., 2020).

Additional complications remain in terms of equity and the disparate nature of health care systems in general. While telehealth is an important tool to ensure equitable access to care, external factors such as broadband connectivity, telehealth literacy, and socioeconomic support contribute to the ongoing issues of equity (AAP, 2022d; Katzow et al., 2020). Beyond the considerations related to connectivity at the home or local access locations (schools, community centers, private practices, libraries, etc.), patients may also have concerns about utilizing limited data plans or having access to a smartphone or device during a scheduled telehealth visit. Many of these social determinants of health (SDoH) indicators are not currently displayed on electronic health record dashboards or evident through traditional patient intake forms, although this is an area of current health informatics research and development (Hughes et al., 2021).

While technology has advanced significantly since the early days of television and the National Aeronautics and Space Administration's use of biometrics on space flights (Gogia, 2019), most pediatric consultations still face constraints in terms of the physical exam and the ability of the provider to have a sufficient level of clinical information by which to make an informed diagnosis and treatment plan. Understanding the roles of the telehealth application and the types of clinical visits being conducted is essential to overcoming challenges related to perceived inequity between in-person and telehealth visits (Ansary et al., 2021). There are workarounds for physical exams that involve utilizing the patient, their caregivers, or clinical telepresenters at ambulatory sites to document clinical information (Milne Wenderlich & Herendeen, 2021). The onus of utilizing that clinical information for decision making still rests upon the provider of record, and the provider's comfort with the process is paramount to accountability.

IMPORTANCE OF NETWORKS

Health care networks that support the general connectivity of our society and access to health care serve as key predictors of economic stability for a community (Chatterjee et al., 2022). Equitable access to care is still highly dependent on broadband and cellular networks that comprise the backbone of connectivity for telehealth programs (Fig. 6.1) (DeGuzman & Jain, 2020; Kruse et al., 2021). Closing the gap in connectivity is an essential strategy for mitigating population health disparities and maintaining the continuity of care for individual patients, especially in pediatrics (Cahan et al., 2022; Wosik et al., 2020).

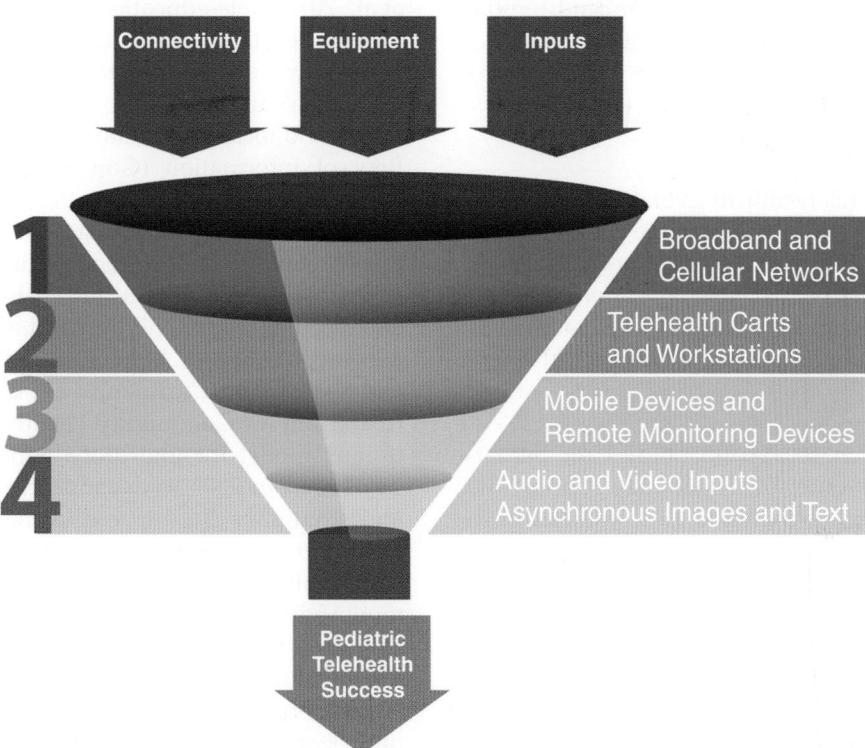

Fig. 6.1 Visualization of communication networks, equipment, and services supporting pediatric telehealth.

The US Federal Communications Commission has prioritized the development of broadband networks to connect rural and underserved communities across the country in support of education and health care initiatives (Whitacre & Biedny, 2022). In addition, targeted support for individual homes is being subsidized through evolving legislation that recognizes the need for telecommunication services in community settings such as homes, schools, and civic centers (Kang, 2021). By acknowledging the importance of internet connectivity, much like the initial rollout of telephone and electrical services across the country in the 20th century (Whitacre & Biedny, 2022), federal policymakers are recognizing the 21st-century value of connected homes to support health care and education as a way of reducing inequities and supporting future generations in their development as healthy citizens of a society.

PANDEMIC IMPLICATIONS: NEW AREAS OF CHRONIC CARE

The COVID-19 pandemic highlighted the need for innovative models of connectivity simply to maintain basic health services. Telehealth helped to serve as a tool of connectivity for millions of patients seeking care and avoiding exposure to infectious diseases during a time of a novel viral outbreak (Gilson et al., 2020). Telehealth adoption was accelerated by these two factors aligning with the reduction in federal, state, and payer restrictions during the public health emergency (PHE). Patterns of care underwent significant changes starting in 2020, and researchers continue to track the trends toward increased utilization of digital health applications to support ambulatory, urgent care, and remote patient monitoring services (Thronson et al., 2020).

TELEHEALTH APPLICATIONS IN PEDIATRIC CHRONIC CARE MANAGEMENT

The application of telehealth to pediatric care is not new, though the COVID-19 pandemic thrust virtual care to the forefront of health care delivery. Applications, including teleresearch, tele-education, teleconsultation, and telepractice, have been implemented to enhance pediatric care for years (Burke et al., 2015).

TELERESEARCH

Utilizing teleresearch to expand studies on pediatric patients with chronic conditions may support the development and dissemination of new knowledge to enhance patient care.

Teleresearch removes distance barriers for conducting research and recruiting patients, improves collaboration among researchers, and enhances the dissemination of translational research from academic medical centers to primary care clinicians (Burke et al., 2015; Chandler et al., 2020). Clinical trials may fail due to a lack of efficacy, safety concerns, or limited funding, as well as problems with patient recruitment, enrollment, and retention (Fogel & Raymond, 2020). Pediatric studies face these challenges as well as barriers such as less prevalent disease instances leading to smaller sample sizes, ethical concerns, and reluctance by caregivers and providers to enroll children (Joseph et al., 2015). Virtual or direct-to-family clinical trials can overcome some of these barriers by allowing for data collection remotely, even from the comfort of the participant's homes (Balevic et al., 2021; Khozin & Coravos, 2019). Often referred to as decentralized clinical trials, these models have been shown to be feasible and successful (Ali et al., 2020). They can expand the diversity of participants, improve recruitment and retention, improve efficiency, and reduce costs (Ali et al., 2020; Khozin & Coravos, 2019; Rosa et al., 2015; Sommer et al., 2018).

TELE-EDUCATION AND TELEMENTORING

Tele-education can be delivered through synchronous or asynchronous methods to a variety of audiences, including clinicians, patients, and families. Children with chronic conditions and their families often require support to enhance self-management to improve health outcomes (Lozano & Houtrow, 2018). The most common barriers to accessing self-management support resources are cost, transportation issues, physical symptoms, and insufficient knowledge (Jerant et al., 2005). Remote education can provide necessary support while overcoming many of these barriers. Virtual education for patients with chronic conditions has been shown to be as effective, if not more effective, than that delivered through traditional methods (Rush et al., 2018). Tele-education programs also enhance clinicians' ability to remain abreast of current recommendations, travel less often to obtain continuing medical education, and promote relationships between academic and local providers allowing for a bidirectional flow of information (González-Espada et al., 2009; Smith et al., 2009).

Telementoring has emerged as a valuable form of tele-education. In this model, telehealth technology is used to remotely educate health care providers to enhance the care of children and adolescents, improving the quality of care and reducing unnecessary and costly care (Curfman et al., 2022). Project ECHO (Extension for Community Healthcare Outcomes) is a unique model for interprofessional health education developed in 2003 to expand access to specialty care and strengthen the capacity of health care providers to deliver evidence-based specialized care in the local community (Arora et al., 2011). This hub-and-spoke model virtually connect specialists to geographically dispersed local clinicians to provide case-based learning, mentoring, and peer support on a regular basis for a predetermined period (Project ECHO, 2022b). In this model, specialized care can be provided in the medical home, reducing barriers such as transportation

Table 6.2	Telehealth Resources	
RESOURCE	**ADDRESS**	**DESCRIPTION**
Project ECHO	https://hsc.unm.edu/echo/	Main ECHO site with links to ECHO hubs across the country
Center for Connected Health Policy	https://www.cchpca.org/	Tracks federal and state legislation and regulation pertaining to telehealth
Telehealth Technology Resource Center	https://telehealthtechnology.org/	Provides free consultation and information on telehealth technology
National Consortium of Telehealth Resource Centers	https://telehealthresourcecenter.org/	Free consultation and resources on telehealth; divided into 12 regional resource centers and two national resource centers

and distance and enhancing communication and care coordination (Curfman et al., 2022). As of August 2022, there are over 3000 ECHO programs available around the world, including those focused on mental health, behavioral health, and specific medical conditions (Project ECHO, 2022a). Pediatric ECHO programs include those focused on sickle cell disease (Shook et al., 2016), anxiety and depression, Duchenne muscular dystrophy, the transition of care from pediatric to adult-focused care, addiction treatment, neurodevelopmental screening, obesity, asthma, and SDoH, among others (AAP, 2022a). While specific outcome studies on the ECHO model for all pediatric use cases have not been performed, a systematic review by Zhou et al. (2016) concluded that Project ECHO is an effective and potentially cost-saving model that enhances provider knowledge and increases access to health care. ECHO has also been shown to enhance networking opportunities and to provide access to quality continuing education leading to practice change for participant providers as well as second- and third-degree contacts (Agley et al., 2021). Successful outcomes have been demonstrated among interdisciplinary health care providers for improvement in perceived knowledge and self-efficacy in caring for children with medical complexity and palliative care (Lalloo et al., 2020, 2021), pediatric cardiology, respiratory and neonatology (Nhung et al., 2021), pediatric food (Leeds et al., 2022), and developmental and mental health disorders (Harrison et al., 2022). ECHO programs designed to facilitate early diagnosis and early intervention for patients with autism have been shown to be successful. Increasing provider self-efficacy and knowledge will lead to practice change, increasing utilization of autism-specific screening tools, enhancing patient-provider relationships, increasing access to care for families served by ECHO participants, and expediting patient access to autism services by 2 to 6 months (Mazurek et al., 2019). Interprofessional teams caring for pediatric patients with chronic conditions and special health care needs will benefit from participation in Project ECHOs related to the populations they serve. Researching available ECHOs in one's own state or region, as well as those available nationally, may facilitate participation. Table 6.2 includes resources for identifying available ECHOs.

TELECONSULTATION

Teleconsultation, also referred to as remote consultation, is generally defined as synchronous or asynchronous consultation across distances. It facilitates diagnostics or treatment between geographically separated health care providers or between health care providers and patients (Deldar et al., 2016). The most common type of teleconsultation connects patients with providers in underserved areas to pediatric subspecialists, increasing access to care, saving time and travel expenses for patients, and supporting local providers (Chandler et al., 2020). Common pediatric subspecialty telehealth applications include pediatric dermatology, emergency medicine, intensive care, neonatology, cardiology, surgery, and psychiatry.

Teleconsultation also includes connecting community hospitals or emergency departments to distant academic medical centers for triage, remote consultation, management, and facilitation of hospital transfers. The use of telehealth for pediatric critical care telemedicine consultation has been shown to enhance the assessment of patients, expedite treatment, support the transfer of patients to a lower level of care, and reduce costs (Harvey et al., 2017). Telehealth may be used to facilitate multidisciplinary care; enhance bidirectional communication between primary care providers, families, and specialists; and enhance communication while facilitating case management conferences (Curfman et al., 2022; Heard-Garris et al., 2017).

An emerging method of teleconsultation is e-consult. E-consults are asynchronous interactions between primary care providers and specialists to facilitate communication and care coordination (Porto et al., 2021). In this model, primary care providers submit patient-specific clinical inquiries to a specialist through electronic means such as secure email. Additional information, such as laboratory results and digital images, may also be shared. Once reviewed, the specialist may provide recommendations for care (avoiding the need for a face-to-face visit), request additional information, or recommend an in-person visit along with any necessary additional diagnostic tests (Keely et al., 2013). In addition to improved communication between primary care providers and specialists, e-consults have been shown to reduce the number of required face-to-face specialty consultations, leading to reduced wait times for patients required to be seen in person (Barnett et al., 2018; Keely et al., 2013). Patient and provider satisfaction with e-consults is generally positive (Liddy et al., 2016). Furthermore, an e-consult system is more convenient for patients as they can receive more specialized care in their medical homes (Porto et al., 2021). Primary care for children with chronic conditions may be enhanced by communication and collaboration with pediatric subspecialists and allied health team members. Utilizing teleconsultation, including e-consults, to improve interprofessional collaboration may benefit the patient, family, and care team.

TELEPRACTICE

Telepractice refers to the provision of care between a provider in one location and a patient in another (Burke et al., 2015). Ambulatory telehealth, presurgical assessments, follow-up appointments, posthospitalization or emergency department visits, and chronic condition management are all valuable telehealth applications (Curfman et al., 2022) that fall under the description of telepractice. Many different modalities can be utilized for telepractice, including synchronous audio-video communications with or without telemedicine peripheral devices, asynchronous platforms (e-visits), synchronous audio-only communications, and remote patient monitoring. The type of technology implemented depends on the care being provided as well as the originating site. Pediatric originating sites include schools, child care centers, group homes, camps, and juvenile detention facilities (Burke et al., 2015) as well as the child's home. Many types of pediatric care can be provided through telehealth, including medical care, behavioral and mental health services, and speech therapy (Burke et al., 2015; Kwok et al., 2022). It is important to note that no specific diagnosis, specialty, care setting, or population is fundamentally suitable or unsuitable for telehealth. The determination depends on individual patient factors, the necessary elements of the physical exam to support medical decision making, and the resources and technology available to support a remote examination (Curfman et al., 2022).

Using technology to extend clinical care beyond the provider's brick-and-mortar office has emerged as an important component of the health care continuum particularly since the onset of the COVID-19 pandemic. Prior to the pandemic, pediatric ambulatory telehealth use rose due to expanded direct-to-consumer and subspecialty care models, but use in primary care remained low (Barnett et al., 2017). The arrival of the COVID-19 pandemic propelled the adoption and implementation of telehealth across many use cases, as evidenced by the 154% increase in telehealth visits during the last week of March 2020 as compared to the same period in 2019 (Koonin et al., 2020a). Patients with chronic illness and their families experience stressors that may strain their resiliency, finances, and social capital (Lozano & Houtrow, 2018). Limited mobility, lack of transportation, and financial barriers may limit patients' access to essential primary care health services focused on the prevention and management of chronic illnesses, leading to poor continuity of care and less than ideal outcomes (Bates et al., 2020). These challenges may be exacerbated for those living in rural and underserved communities. Virtual office visits for new or established patients provide a way to improve access to personalized care by overcoming barriers such as transportation, cost, and time away from school or work for patients and parents (Burke et al., 2015).

SDoH are the conditions present where people live, learn, work, and play that affect health, functioning, and quality-of-life risks and outcomes (Centers for Disease Control and Prevention, 2021). SDoH contribute to health disparities and inequalities and have a major impact on people's health and well-being (Healthy People 2030, 2022). Direct-to-patient, in-home telehealth visits provide a unique opportunity to examine many of the patient's SDoH, leading to appropriate interventions to maximize the patient's health. These visits allow for evaluation of the patient's home environment, the risk for food insecurity, caregiver relationships, and interactions, and they allow family members who otherwise may not be able to participate in patient care visits to do so. These factors may be less easily observed in a traditional office visit.

Telehealth care has been shown to be effective in managing chronic conditions in pediatric patients in a variety of settings, with care comparable to or better than in-person services (Shah & Badawy, 2021). A systematic review conducted by Shah and Badawy (2021) evaluated the evidence for the use of telehealth for managing pediatric asthma, obesity, otitis media, mental health conditions, skin conditions, attention-deficit/hyperactivity disorder, type 1 diabetes, and cystic fibrosis–related pancreatic insufficiency. Most of the studies reviewed used synchronous videoconferencing, though additional interventions included smartphone-based apps, telephone counseling, and web-based screening visits. In addition to establishing consistency with care provided in person, patients and caregivers consistently reported higher levels of satisfaction with telehealth visits as compared to in-person visits. Recent literature has also shown that patients and families find telehealth easy to use and of comparable or superior quality to in-person care (Ray et al., 2020; Solomon et al., 2021; Weaver et al., 2020).

Children with developmental disabilities and complex health care also benefit from telehealth visits. Additional challenges for these patients may include psychological and behavioral barriers as well as logistical barriers, including the need for special transportation such as a vehicle with wheelchair capacity, special equipment, nursing support, or multiple caretakers to accompany them to an appointment. Furthermore, children with developmental disabilities may experience anxiety, fear, and disruptive behaviors when transitioning to unfamiliar environments such as a health care provider's office or clinic (Langkamp et al., 2015). Patients with intellectual disabilities and/or autism experience lower health care access rates than the general population resulting in unmet health needs (Doherty et al., 2020). Effective communication, reduced wait times, less stressful clinical environments, and greater interprofessional collaboration may help improve the health and well-being of these patients.

Telehealth promotes the implementation of these essential care elements by overcoming the need for specialized transport equipment and staff, allowing patients to remain in a familiar environment, maintaining a consistent routine, reducing stress for the patient and family, increasing the likelihood of a successful encounter, and possibly leading to a less stressful experience for the health care provider (Langkamp et al., 2015). Patients with medical complexity, including those requiring technology assistance at home, can also benefit from interprofessional collaboration between the primary care provider and home health staff. Physical exams and necessary diagnostic services may be conducted virtually in the home environment, leading to earlier intervention for potentially serious illnesses and reducing the need for hospitalization (Curfman et al., 2022). Furthermore, the use of remote patient monitoring to enhance the surveillance of chronic conditions may improve the quality of care and enhance outcomes (Noel & Ellison, 2020).

SCHOOL-BASED TELEHEALTH FOR PEDIATRIC CHRONIC CARE MANAGEMENT

With children spending most of their time in the school setting, extending the health care continuum to include the school site is an obvious solution to overcoming barriers to health care access, particularly for those with chronic conditions. School-based health centers (SBHCs) provide health services to students while they are at school as collaborations between local health care organizations and schools share the common goal of improving the health, well-being, and academic success of students (Goddard et al., 2021). Often, SBHCs deliver comprehensive care to students who otherwise may not receive it, thereby improving health equity (Knopf et al., 2016). SBHCs have been shown to improve educational and health-related outcomes (Community Preventive Services Task Force, 2016; Knopf et al., 2016). In recent years the number of SBHCs using telehealth has increased significantly. As of 2019, over 1 million students across 1800 public schools had access to some

form of school-based telehealth, representing 2% of students and nearly 2% of US public schools (Love et al., 2019). Telehealth may improve the efficiency and sustainability of SBHCs by allowing multiple schools to be served by the same provider on the same day (Garber et al., 2021). School-based telehealth (SBTH) programs have been shown to be successful in the provision of chronic care management for pediatric asthma (Chinnis & Stanley, 2022; Sanchez et al., 2019), diabetes, and children with speech impairments (Sanchez et al., 2019). Programs providing clinical evaluation and treatment for acute and chronic asthma, asthma education, and direct observation of daily preventative asthma medication administration have all shown promise in improving patient outcomes. SBTH programs have also been shown to reduce asthma symptoms and decrease missed school days, emergency room visits, and hospitalizations, as well as improve physical activity, lung function, and asthma knowledge (MacGeorge et al., 2021). Regarding type 1 diabetes management, SBTH programs have been shown to reduce hemoglobin A1c levels, reduce urgent diabetes-related calls from school nurses, reduce hospitalizations and emergency department visits, and improve scores on pediatric quality-of-life questionnaires (Izquierdo et al., 2009). The effectiveness of virtual speech-language services is also well documented. Studies following pediatric patients indicate that articulation, language, and fluency services can be delivered virtually as effectively as in-person therapy (McGill et al., 2019; Wales et al., 2017). Additionally, school-based language screenings are as effective as those completed in person (Raman et al., 2019). SBTH programs may also benefit children with complex medical needs by overcoming many of the challenges faced by this population when accessing health care. Cormack et al. (2016) found that the utilization of telehealth at a school for children with medical complexity was significantly higher than that of children enrolled in 12 regular schools within the same program.

The value of telehealth in the school setting extends beyond that of providing direct care to patients while at school. Allowing for more frequent follow-up visits and ongoing support of patients' families, as well as facilitating interprofessional communication with school personnel, enhances patient care. Furthermore, enabling participation by the health care team in meetings regarding individualized education plans and accommodations (i.e., 504 plans) and those related to individual health accommodations may enhance the student's overall education experience.

IMPLEMENTING A TELEHEALTH PROGRAM

Successful implementation and sustainability of a telehealth program require extensive planning and preparation (AlDossary et al., 2017). Many providers mistakenly focus primarily on the technology without attention to the many important components of a telehealth program. This poses a challenge to long-term sustainability. Essential to successful telehealth programs is a clear vision with attention to desired outcomes, identification of the population to be served, type of services to be provided, and necessary technology, as well as consideration of pertinent legal, regulatory, and reimbursement factors affecting telehealth care at the state and national levels (Rutledge et al., 2020). Various frameworks exist to promote successful programs. One such program is the telehealth service implementation model (TSIM). TSIM provides a framework for telehealth best practices, establishes common terminology for service development, and provides standardized processes to address specific telehealth issues (Ford et al., 2021). The framework is divided into six phases: pipeline, strategy, development, implementation, operations, and continuous quality improvement. Another helpful model is the four Ps of telehealth, which includes four key components: planning, preparing, providing, and performance evaluation (Rutledge, Gustin, et al., 2020). In this model, the planning phase includes identifying the population and health care issue to be addressed, selecting the technology, researching related legal and regulatory issues and reimbursement, and identifying the providers. The preparation phase includes protocol development, consenting processes, securing technology, and training for telehealth delivery. The providing phase refers to the actual delivery of telehealth, and the performance phase includes an evaluation of the impact of the telehealth program (Rutledge, Gustin, et al., 2020). Utilizing a framework to guide telehealth program development will enhance its efficiency and effectiveness by ensuring that all the important details are in place.

PRACTICES FOR TELEHEALTH ENCOUNTERS

Often cited but unfounded, limitations of telehealth include limited ability to perform a comprehensive physical exam, limited ability to build patient-provider relationships, fragmentation of care, and risk of overprescribing and overutilization of health care services (Barbosa et al., 2021). Ensuring telehealth care is provided through the medical home, when feasible, can mitigate many of these potential concerns. When coordinated through the medical home, telehealth care will promote continuity of care in a cost-efficient way and foster high-quality, high-value coordinated care (Curfman, Hackell, et al., 2021). Important to recognize is that telehealth does not change the standard of care. The same patient-centered, evidence-based care that is provided in person can be delivered across distances (Chike-Harris, 2020). Providers must consider the elements necessary to meet the standard of care for each telehealth encounter. If the standard of care cannot be met, the patient should be referred to in-person care with any necessary referrals or care coordination provided by the telehealth team (Garber

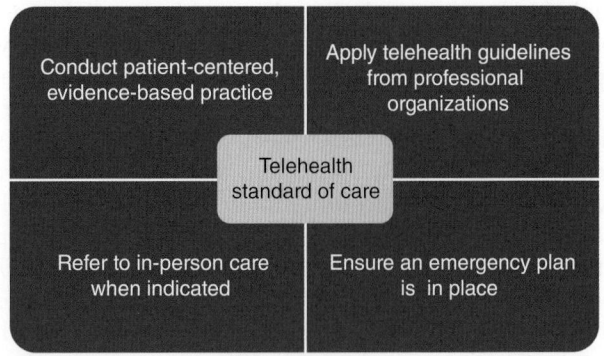

Fig. 6.2 Elements necessary to maintain the standard of care when practicing via telehealth.

et al., 2021). For example, if a specific element of the exam cannot be completed virtually but is necessary for medical decision making, the patient should not be diagnosed without that element. Knowledge of existing guidelines for telehealth related to the specific patient population or condition to be managed is also essential. Many professional organizations have established guidelines or recommendations for the application of telehealth. It is important for the provider to incorporate the guidelines specific to their discipline into their practice. Additionally, it is essential that telehealth providers ensure they have an emergency plan in place when providing virtual care. Having accurate and up-to-date contact information for the patient they are seeing and knowing the patient's physical location during the encounter is essential. Fig. 6.2 summarizes the essential elements to maintain the standard of care during telehealth encounters.

The providers who are conducting telehealth care benefit from patience, creativity, and flexibility. Utilizing available resources at patients' locations, employing the support of caregivers, and understanding the importance of meeting patients where they are rather than establishing arbitrary requirements benefit both the patient and provider while ensuring high-quality health care is provided virtually.

TELEHEALTH ETIQUETTE

The key to a successful telehealth encounter is the use of telehealth etiquette and "webside" manner. This is essential to optimizing the patient-provider relationship and leading to enhanced patient satisfaction and improved outcomes (Heath, 2016). A strong patient-provider relationship will result in patient-centered, team-based care that improves patient satisfaction and experience scores as well as positive outcomes (Heath, 2017). Telehealth etiquette refers to the soft skills or "screenside" etiquette demonstrated by a provider during a telehealth encounter (Gustin et al., 2020) and encompasses the webside manner. Bedside manner has long been recognized to mean the behaviors a provider uses during visits to make the patient feel comfortable, such as demonstrating a friendly, kind, understanding demeanor (Cambridge English Dictionary, 2022). Web-side manner refers to the provider's bedside manner applied across distances (Gonzalez, 2017). Essential to the patient-provider relationship is trust. This is especially important regarding pediatric care, as parents and caregivers often experience significant anxiety around their child's illness. An environment of trust is key to reducing this anxiety (McConnochie, 2019). Once trust is established and the patient and caregiver feel that their emotions are fully understood and respected, they will be more likely to understand and believe the diagnosis and treatment plan and to follow the guidance offered by the clinician.

The PEP Model for Telehealth Etiquette

Telehealth etiquette encompasses three aspects of the virtual visit: the provider's performance, environment, and privacy/security (PEP) considerations specific to a virtual encounter (Rutledge, Gustin, et al., 2020). The PEP model for telehealth etiquette has been developed to assist telehealth providers in prioritizing these key factors that are essential to a virtual patient encounter (Garber et al., n.d.). Performance includes professionalism, communication, and technology proficiency. Being punctual, establishing rapport, employing professional behavior such as avoiding eating and drinking during visits, and setting the agenda for each visit are all important aspects of professionalism. Another essential aspect of the provider's performance is relationship-centered communication. Creating a safe and supportive environment is necessary to establish a personal connection with the patient and family and to foster trust and collaboration (Windover et al., 2014). Communication during telehealth encounters may be limited by the inability to use touch or certain body language techniques to connect with the patient. As such, telehealth providers must modify their communication style to emphasize the use of voice, manner, and facial expression to overcome the absence of these important elements (McCormick, 2018). Communication considerations begin before the visit starts, continue during the visit, and end when the visit is closed (Chua et al., 2020). Specific elements to enhance communication during telehealth encounters are listed in Box 6.1.

The environment includes aspects of the provider's location and appearance (Garber et al., n.d.). Attention must be directed at reducing potential visual and auditory distractions. Lighting and framing are important aspects of the virtual visit (Sharma et al., 2019). To ensure the provider can be seen clearly and avoid casting a shadow, it is best to have the light shining from behind the camera rather than behind the provider. Furthermore, avoiding clutter and inappropriate items in the background, as well as the use of distracting virtual backgrounds, facilitates a more focused interaction. Ensuring there are no auditory distractions, such as music, television, email or cellphone alerts, or other

Box 6.1	**Essential Techniques for Effective Telehealth Communication**

- Ensure the camera is at eye level.
- Make eye contact by looking into the camera.
- Ensure a "passport view" of the provider in the screen.
- Use a friendly tone.
- Greet the patient.
- Be authentic and genuine.
- Convey respect to the patient.
- Set the agenda for the visit.
- Employ active listening.
- Express empathy both verbally and nonverbally.
- Employ verbal reflections rather than "mm-hmm," which can disrupt the conversational flow.
- Employ patient teach-back.
- Recognize and control bias.
- Overcome language barriers through interpreter use.
- Ensure shared decision making.
- Summarize the plan of care and necessary next steps.
- Ensure opportunity for the patient and caregiver to ask questions.
- Provide an appreciative closure statement ("I am glad you scheduled this visit. Thank you for allowing me to participate in your care.").

Modified from Chua, I.S., Jackson, V., & Kamdar, M. (2020). Webside manner during the COVID-19 pandemic: Maintaining human connection during virtual visits. *Journal of Palliative Medicine, 23*(11), 1507–1509; Garber, K.M., Gustin, T.S., Rutledge, C.M. (n.d.). Put PEP into telehealth: A framework for successful encounters. *Online Journal of Issues in Nursing*; Heath, S. (2017). 3 key traits of a positive patient-provider relationship. *Patient Engagement HIT*. https://patientengagementhit.com/news/3-key-traits-of-a-positive-patient-provider-relationship; Heath, 2017; McCormick, T.M. (2018). Three essential qualities that make a good telemedicine physician. *LinkedIn Corporation*. https://www.linkedin.com/pulse/three-essential-qualities-make-good-telemedicine-mccormick-md/.

background noises, is also important (Garber et al., n.d.). Technology placement is also a key element of the environment. The camera and computer should be placed on a stable platform with the camera at eye level (American Telemedicine Association, 2016). The provider must also ensure that the wifi in the environment is strong enough to ensure an uninterrupted virtual connection or should use a wired ethernet connection (Garber et al., n.d.).

Privacy and security are the third elements of the PEP model. It is always best practice to use a secure Health Insurance Portability and Accountability Act (HIPAA)–compliant platform when conducting telehealth encounters, in addition to utilizing vendors who agree to enter into a HIPAA business associate agreement in connection with the technology (US Department of Health and Human Services [HHS], 2020). It is important to note that the HIPAA privacy rule does extend to audio-only telephone services conducted over electronic phone lines, not traditional phone lines, in addition to video communications, necessitating providers to ensure they conduct visits from a private setting, avoid using a speakerphone, and confirm the patient identity at the start of the visit (Hennessy & Maguregui, 2022). Similarly, the HIPAA security rule applies to technologies, including smartphone applications, VoIP technologies, messaging services that store audio messages, and technologies that record or transcribe telehealth encounters (Hennessy & Maguregui, 2022). HHS does acknowledge that once the patient's information has been received by the patient's phone or other devices, the telehealth provider is no longer responsible for the privacy or security of the patient's information (HHS, 2022a).

Additional privacy and security considerations include the identification of anyone who is present for the visit at the patient or provider's location and whether they have permission to participate (Gustin et al., 2020). Securing the provider's location by closing the door and using a headset with a microphone rather than a speaker is also essential (Garber et al., n.d.).

HEALTH EQUITY AND TELEHEALTH

While telehealth has evolved to include a wide array of technology, applications, and use cases, it was originally conceived to extend access to care to those in rural and underserved communities (Barbosa et al., 2021). The expansion of telehealth during the COVID-19 pandemic highlighted several barriers faced by this population, including the digital divide, which refers to the gap between those with access to information and communications technology, such as telephone, television, computers, and the internet, and those without access (Hanna, 2021). As of 2022, only 50% of homes in the United States have access to broadband with speeds of 25 Mbps download or higher, which is required to sustain a telehealth connection, with 15% of homes having no internet access (The NPD Group, 2021). A Pew Research study conducted in 2021 also revealed that roughly 25% of adults with household incomes below $30,000 a year report not owning a smartphone, 41% do not own a desktop or laptop computer, and most of this population does not own a tablet (Vogels, 2021). Populations affected by the digital divide include those living in rural areas, older adults, people of color, and those with lower socioeconomic status, as well as those living with disabilities (Valdez et al., 2021). In fact, people with disabilities are 20% less likely to own a computer, smartphone, or tablet than people without disabilities (Anderson & Perrin, 2017). To optimize inclusivity, successful telehealth programs must consider the targeted population's digital literacy, health literacy, and literacy levels in addition to the digital divide. It is essential that telehealth programs be tailored to the end user's needs and understanding. Not all patients have the skills necessary to participate in a video visit or to understand the technologic terminology to follow instructions to do so. Education related to the telehealth encounter regarding what to expect and how to conduct the visit must be easy to understand and delivered in various formats, including audio, video, still images (such as screenshots), and writing. Empowering patients with detailed information enhances their experience with telehealth.

ACCESSIBILITY AND TELEHEALTH

The Americans with Disabilities Act (ADA) was signed into law on July 26, 1990. It prohibits discrimination and guarantees that those with disabilities have the same opportunities as those without disabilities. It is essentially an equal opportunity law for people who have disabilities (HHS, 2022b). While it has been updated since it was originally passed, the ADA initially focused on issues related to accessibility to physical structures and architecture (Noel & Ellison, 2020). The expansion of telehealth during the COVID-19 pandemic highlighted the need for inclusive telehealth platforms to ensure that all who need and wish to receive care via telehealth have access. Patients with disabilities, particularly those with chronic diseases, can benefit significantly from telehealth and must be assured access to the same virtual care as those without disabilities. Inclusive innovation will ensure accessible technologic designs for all (Noel & Ellison, 2020). Without it, health inequities for those with disabilities may be exacerbated.

The ADA (2005) requires that medical providers communicate effectively with consumers and their caregivers and further places the responsibility for providing effective communication on the covered entity (US Department of Justice, 2014). This includes providing sign language or spoken language interpreters and making written materials accessible to the blind through means such as braille, audio, or digital formats (Powers et al., 2017). Health care provided through telehealth is no different. Failure of a health care provider to implement measures to ensure that care provided through telehealth is accessible may result in unlawful discrimination (HHS, 2022b). Providers must ensure the availability of qualified sign language interpreters, translators, and readers, along with closed captioning, audio descriptions, and large text options (Valdez et al., 2021). This may require using telehealth technology that includes an option to add a third party. Additionally, adequate training for staff and for patients before, during, and after virtual visits may be necessary to ensure the avoidance of discrimination based on disability (HHS, 2022b).

TELEHEALTH LEGAL AND REGULATORY CONSIDERATIONS

Telehealth care is impacted by legislation and regulation at the federal and state levels. It is essential that primary care providers delivering care virtually be well informed about these important policy considerations. Fig. 6.3 depicts the key legal and regulatory considerations for telehealth providers. Telehealth is affected by many laws and regulations beyond those specifically aimed at telehealth. At the federal level, legislation pertaining to HIPAA requirements, Drug Enforcement Agency (DEA) requirements, and the Ryan Haight Online Prescribing and Consumer Protection Act must be considered along with CMS- and COVID-19-related

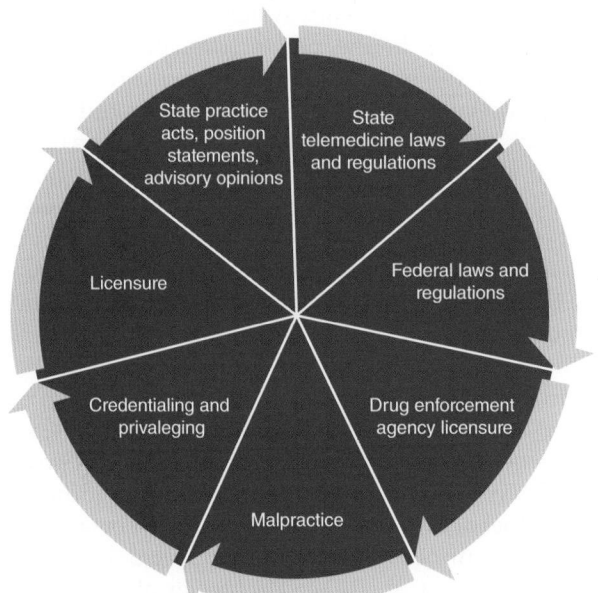

Fig. 6.3 **Key legal and regulatory considerations for telehealth providers.**

legislation and regulation (Center for Connected Health Policy, 2022a). Of specific interest to the primary care provider are laws surrounding the prescribing of controlled substances via telehealth. It is important to note that the DEA requires a separate DEA registration in each state where the provider prescribes controlled substances (DEA, 2020). While this requirement was lifted during the COVID-19 pandemic PHE, it remains to be seen at this time whether it will be reinstated following the PHE. The Ryan Haight Online Pharmacy Consumer Protection Act was enacted to prevent the illegal distribution and dispensing of controlled substances through the internet without a valid prescription (Implementation of the Ryan Haight Online Pharmacy Consumer Protection Act of 2008, 2020). This law requires that providers establish a patient-provider relationship in person before prescribing controlled medications via telehealth. It also requires a face-to-face physical examination every 24 months. Exceptions include if the patient is being treated by and is physically located in a DEA-registered facility or in the physical presence of a DEA-registered provider as long as the provider is acting in the usual course of practice, prescribing consistent with state laws, and is registered with the DEA in the state where the patient is physically located (DEA, 2020). Familiarizing one-self with the CMS legislation and regulation applicable to telehealth is also necessary, as this affects reimbursement for services provided via telehealth. Prior to the COVID-19 pandemic, many barriers to reimbursement existed, including those limitations related to geographic location, site type, provider type, eligible services, and modality. The introduction of the 1135 waiver during the PHE removed many of these barriers and improved provider telehealth reimbursement,

allowed for cross-state practice, expanded provider types, reduced cost sharing for patients, and allowed virtual visits to be conducted from the patient's home (Koonin et al., 2020b).

State laws and regulations must also be reviewed by telehealth providers before providing care. As with federal policy, state telehealth policy includes more than just telehealth legislation. Attention must be directed to state telehealth/telemedicine laws, practice acts, advisory opinions, and position statements put forth by licensing boards, Medicaid policy, and parity laws. State telehealth laws vary significantly, with no two states alike in how telehealth is defined, regulated, or reimbursed (Center for Connected Health Policy, 2022a). Though they vary significantly in content, state telehealth laws may include a definition of telemedicine or telehealth, prescribing guidance, guidelines regarding establishing a patient-provider relationship via telehealth, practice standards, consent requirements, and certification requirements (Center for Connected Health Policy, 2022a, 2022b). An excellent resource to review state and federal telehealth-related policy is the Center for Connected Health Policy (https://www.cchpca.org/).

The originating site (patient location) is the site of service, necessitating that the telehealth provider is familiar with and subject to the laws and regulations in the state where the patient is physically located (Center for Connected Health Policy, 2022a, 2022d). As such, the provider must be licensed in the originating site state. One exception exists for health care providers who work for the Veterans Administration (VA). In 2018, the Department of Veteran Affairs passed a final rule allowing telehealth practice regardless of the provider and patient's state locations (Federal Register, 2018).

For those working outside the VA, this may be accomplished through licensure in each state or, depending on the type of licensure, through interstate licensure compacts. As of 2022, 34 states have joined the Interstate Medical Licensure Compact, 33 states participate in the Physical Therapy Compact, 30 states have adopted the Psychology Interjurisdictional Compact (PSYPACT), 10 states participate in the Counseling Compact, 19 have joined the Audiology and Speech-Language Pathology Interstate Compact, 21 have passed the Emergency Medical Services Personnel Licensure Interstate Compact, 37 participate with the Nurse Licensure Compact, and only three have passed legislation to adopt the Advanced Practice Registered Nurse (APRN) Compact (Center for Connected Health Policy, 2022a, 2022c). The APRN Compact will not be enacted until at least seven states pass legislation (The National Council of State Boards of Nursing, 2020). Because APRN practice requirements vary significantly by state (American Association of Nurse Practitioners, 2022), it is particularly important that APRNs review and adhere to all originating state policies. For example, if the APRN is physically practicing in a state with full practice authority but is seeing a patient across state lines in a restricted practice state, that person must be licensed in that state but also meet all existing practice requirements, such as those pertaining to a practice agreement and supervision or collaboration. Moreover, some states issue special certificates or licenses or offer telehealth exceptions for out-of-state licensed providers wishing to practice in their state (Center for Connected Health Policy, 2022a, 2022d).

Additional provider considerations include credentialing and privileging, telehealth certification, and malpractice. Facilities accredited by The Joint Commission (TJC), such as hospitals or hospital-owned clinics, are required to ensure that all providers be credentialed and privileged (TJC, 2022). Credentialing refers to ensuring a provider is qualified to perform medical services; privileging refers to the provider's level of competence in a specific type of care (Jones, 2020). When conducting care between sites, the telehealth provider must be credentialed and privileged at both the originating and distant sites. This may be done through full credentialing at each location or through credentialing by proxy (Center for Connected Health Policy, 2022a, 2022c). While there are emerging telehealth certification programs across the United States, only one state (Washington) requires health professionals other than primary care providers to complete compliant telemedicine training that meets state guidelines (Washington State Hospital Association, 2018). Malpractice coverage for telehealth is another important consideration. It is essential that providers consult their malpractice carriers to ensure telehealth care is covered. Some carriers cover telehealth; others may require a separate rider or premium (Shah et al., 2020). When inquiring, it is important to ask whether the coverage extends across state lines.

FUTURE STATE

Advances in the technology supporting pediatric care will continue to expand the types of services that can be provided at a distance and across time/geographic constraints. Specifically, remote patient monitoring can support pediatric patients housed at home (instead of inpatient or skilled nursing settings) with their family members through device capture, measurement, transmission, and the display of biometric data (Foster et al., 2022). Automated messaging, patient portals, and asynchronous communication through apps and chatbots can be partnered with appropriate support buttressed by in-person diagnostic processes (Espinoza et al., 2020; Milne Wenderlich & Herendeen, 2021). These innovations continue to be honed to ensure a safety net of services for patients and their caregivers in settings conducive to long-term care.

Factor into the decision matrix the use of big data and artificial intelligence to advance the provision of

health care through health systems that further incorporate analytics in the patient care process (Zhang et al., 2021). The integration of more powerful analytic tools can result in better decision making, fuller relationships with customers, clearer determination of risk, and the alignment of strategic initiatives (Muruganantham et al., 2019). By integrating artificial intelligence into telehealth processes, clinician decision making may be enhanced when using video-based multimedia technologies and across synchronous and asynchronous platforms (Hah & Goldin, 2022). Examples of these technical innovations, along with the patient populations studied, are found in Fig. 6.4.

Guided by ethical frameworks that are used to ensure quality interactions and improve safety within the provision of digital health services, additional work is needed to safeguard patient privacy and confidentiality through processes supported by mutual trust (Keenan et al., 2022; Thomas et al., 2020). The increased use of telehealth creates opportunities for biomedical and ethical explorations focused on maintaining autonomy, reducing malfeasance, improving benefits for patients and providers, and securing the professional-patient relationship, all while leading from the concept of justice (i.e., fairness and equity). When telehealth is viewed as health care, the ethical underpinnings are indistinguishable from traditional and in-person care. Still, clinicians and administrators are required to define and adhere to revised standards of clinical care balanced upon health informatics industry standards for privacy, security, and fidelity (Keenan et al., 2022).

In addition to telehealth applications serving as a catalyst for changing models of health care as standalone tools, these applications are increasingly being integrated into existing health information technology systems (electronic health records, patient portals). These integrations have further influenced the need for system interoperability and data sharing (Thomas et al., 2020). During the same time, patient expectations have shifted to having real-time, 24/7 access to their private health information, access to their providers through asynchronous portals, and the ability to leverage their relationships within health care systems to access further specialized care. The expectation of privacy, while context dependent, is an area requiring refined practices and ongoing research through partnerships between health informatics professionals, frontline providers, and the patients they serve (Pool et al., 2022).

Educational opportunities based on established telehealth competencies are needed to support learners to meet the changing needs of clinical and research services in the 21st century (Dzioba et al., 2022). The modes of education delivery often require realignment to best facilitate simulated and real-world clinical experiences (Hah & Goldin, 2022). Undergraduate and graduate programs are inserting formal telehealth curriculum roadmaps into programs and developing

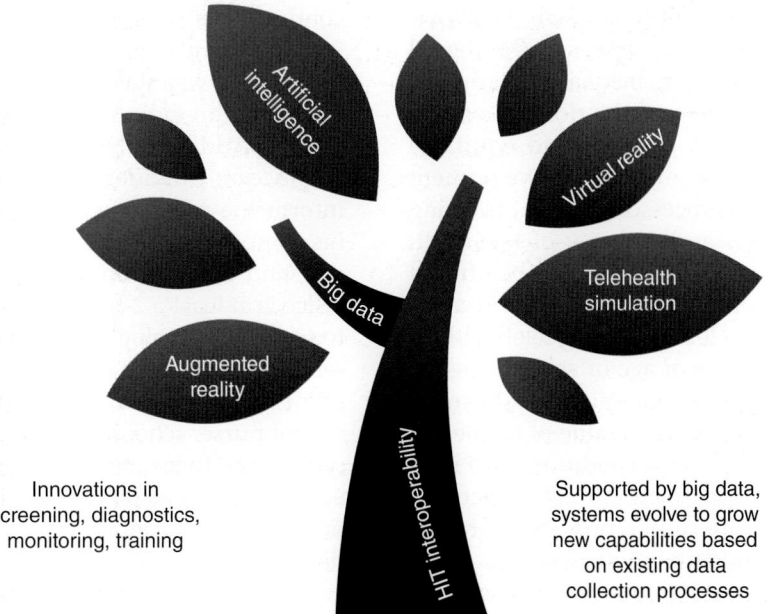

Fig. 6.4 **Examples of 21st-century pediatric telehealth support by artificial intelligence, virtual reality, augmented reality, and big data initiatives.** *HIT,* Health care information technology. (Modified from Bian, Y., Xiang, Y., Tong, B., Feng, B., & Weng, X. [2020]. Artificial intelligence-assisted system in postoperative follow-up of orthopedic patients: Exploratory quantitative and qualitative study. *Journal of Medical Internet Research, 22*[5], 1–8; Fierson, W.M. [2013]. Screening examination of premature infants for retinopathy of prematurity. *Pediatrics, 131*[1], 189–195; Jadczyk, T., Wojakowski, W., Tendera, M., Henry, T.D., Egnaczyk, G., & Shreenivas, S. [2021]. Artificial intelligence can improve patient management at the time of a pandemic: The role of voice technology. *Journal of Medical Internet Research, 23*[5], 1–11; Jung, S.Y., Lee, K., & Hwang, H. [2022]. Recent trends of healthcare information and communication technologies in pediatrics: A systematic review. *Clinical and experimental pediatrics*, [65(6), 291–299]; Lo, M., Gower, W., Byrnes, C., et al. [2021]. Real-world verification of artificial intelligence algorithm-assisted auscultation of breath sounds. *Frontiers in Pediatrics, 9,* 627337.)

new evaluation structures to ensure that learners move from beginner to competent and eventually to proficient skill levels (DuBose-Morris et al., 2021; Rutledge et al., 2021). Whether applied from an individual or team-based approach, digital health concepts and competencies are starting to be found within most health professions training programs. Significant expectations have been established through the release of the Association of American Medical Colleges Telehealth Competencies (2021) and the American Board of Pediatrics (2019) supplemental entrustable professional activities on telehealth. Practicing providers have an ethical obligation to maintain their knowledge base and continue to integrate new concepts grounded in evidence-based telehealth practice into their digital health toolbox.

The final component of telehealth service relates to the extensive research agenda necessary to validate clinical services, design effective population-based telehealth solutions, advance partnerships in support of equity, and promote clinical findings and operational activities through translational research dissemination for the sake of policymakers and health care funders (Fiks et al., 2022). Recognizing the substantial need for a national research agenda focused on children and youth with special health care needs, the Maternal and Child Health Bureau and the US Health Resources and Services Administration have gone so far as to establish a national research network specifically drawing on health system data to support innovation within this patient population (Stille et al., 2022). Telehealth is seen as a bridge between traditional health care systems and community settings, specifically in ways that address the needs of the most vulnerable and those with ongoing care needs. This can be seen in clinical operations and analyzed through integrated research protocols focusing on specific conditions and populations. The research agenda continues to focus on feasibility, appropriateness of interventions, the effect of rurality and medically underserved settings, and effective strategies for reducing disparities within pediatric populations (Van Cleave et al., 2022).

SUMMARY

Telehealth has been shown to be comparable to or better than in-person care, while patients and caregivers consistently report high levels of satisfaction with virtual visits. Cost savings, increased access to care, and improved outcomes with telehealth continue to be demonstrated. Exponential growth in telehealth utilization resulting from the COVID-19 pandemic has fueled the integration of telehealth into the future of health care. Telehealth has also helped to focus attention on the need to be intentional with the provision of services to reduce known issues in the digital divide and other metrics of health inequality (Ramsetty & Adams, 2020). Work remains to be done to ensure that telehealth is used in an effective and equitable way going forward through extensive development and quality improvement processes aimed at tracking not only the effectiveness and viability of telehealth but also the way in which care models can be offered to insert telehealth appropriately across the lifespan of populations (Calton et al., 2020). Moving telehealth as an integrated tool, regardless of age or stage, is essential for future clinical and research initiatives. Primary care providers should consider the value of telehealth in caring for patients with chronic conditions and integrate virtual care into their practice. Patient-focused, evidence-based quality care can be provided through telehealth. With careful planning, efficient and effective sustainable telehealth programs can be a successful part of the health care continuum.

CASE STUDY

Chase is a 15-year-old male student in 10th grade at a rural high school. He is cognitively delayed and cannot read. He has a history of severe asthma, for which he has been hospitalized several times. He lives with his mother, three siblings, and two younger cousins in a small house trailer that has no air conditioning. His mother is the sole provider for the family and works an hourly wage job 70 miles away. The family does not own a car, so she travels daily on "the beach bus" to work in a tourist area. The bus leaves at 7 a.m. and returns at 7 p.m. with no option for return during the day. Chase shares a room with his siblings but sometimes sleeps in a sleeping bag on the floor in the living room. He rides a bus for 2 hours to get to school each day. They live in a very rural area, and the closest pediatric office is over 30 miles away. He receives most of his health care from the local emergency department (ED) and rarely has a well visit. He gets his vaccinations from the local health department. Every time he is admitted to the hospital or seen in the ED, Chase is referred to a pediatric provider for follow-up, but the family is never able to get there due to transportation and scheduling issues. The literacy level of the family is low, and they are unable to fully understand the instructions sent home with them from the ED.

Thankfully, Chase's school has a SBTH program. He is evaluated and treated in the school nurse's office through real-time audio/videoconferencing with a nurse practitioner (NP). With the assistance of the school nurse, the NP can complete a thorough physical exam using telehealth peripheral devices, including a digital stethoscope, otoscope, and exam camera.

Chase was initially referred to the SBTH program by the school principal following two trips to the ED by ambulance in the first 2 weeks of school. The NP conducted a thorough asthma evaluation through telehealth and diagnosed him with severe persistent asthma. He was started on necessary medications consistent with evidence-based guidelines and followed closely. Additionally, the NP was able to consult a health care provider and pediatric pulmonologist to inform the patient's care plan due to the severity of his symptoms. Given the family's barriers to accessing care and the minimum distance to a pulmonologist's office is at least a 2-hour drive, he had never been able to see a pulmonologist, though he had been previously referred. Following his evaluation with the telehealth NP, asthma education was provided to the patient, school nurse, school staff, siblings attending the same school, and to his mother by phone. Additional asthma education was also provided via telehealth by a certified asthma educator who is a respiratory therapist. A detailed yet simplified (using photos and colors) asthma action plan was provided to the family and school nurse. The prescribed medications were arranged to be delivered to the school to overcome barriers to picking them up from the pharmacy. Additionally, with his mother's consent and completed medication administration school forms, the school nurse dosed the daily controller medicine at school. This allowed for consistency of administration and ensured compliance.

This case demonstrates how telehealth allowed for interprofessional collaboration with the clinical team, school nurse, school staff, and family, thereby enhancing the patient's care. Since receiving ongoing care for his asthma by seeing a pediatric provider on a regular basis, Chase's asthma has been well controlled. Once he began being followed by the SBTH program, he did not return to the ED for an asthma exacerbation. Furthermore, his academics improved; he learned to read and was able to graduate from high school!

KEY POINTS

- Telehealth is an efficient and effective method of care delivery.
- Telehealth improves access to care, reduces cost, and improves outcomes.
- Telehealth services are supported across multiple disciplines, community locations, modalities, and care models.
- Patients and caregivers report positive experiences and satisfaction with telehealth.
- Telehealth improves health equity but may also exacerbate inequities for certain populations.
- Care must be taken to ensure that telehealth is accessible to all, regardless of disabilities.
- Successful and sustainable telehealth programs necessitate detailed planning prior to implementation.
- Telehealth etiquette is important to a positive patient-provider experience and to the patient's perception of quality.

- Telehealth providers must review telehealth policy and ensure compliance with all laws and regulations in the originating site state (patient location).
- Telehealth research continues to identify opportunities to support adoption, health system integration, and improved health outcomes.

RESOURCES FOR TELEHEALTH

National Consortium of Telehealth Resource Centers: https://telehealthresourcecenter.org/.

Center for Connected Health Policy: https://www.cchpca.org/.

Center for Telehealth Innovation Education & Research (C-TIER): https://telehealtheducation-ctier.com/.

American Academy of Pediatrics Section on Telehealth Care (AAP SOTC): https://www.aap.org/en/community/aap-sections/telehealth-care/.

AAP SOTC Supporting Pediatric Research and Outcomes and Utilization of Telehealth (SPROUT): https://www.aap.org/en/community/aap-sections/telehealth-care/sprout/.

American Telemedicine Association: https://www.americantelemed.org/resource/.

REFERENCES

Aalam, A. A., Hood, C., Donelan, C., Rutenberg, A., Kane, E. M., & Sikka, N. (2021). Remote patient monitoring for ED discharges in the COVID-19 pandemic. *Emergency Medicine Journal, 38*(3), 229–231. https://doi.org/10.1136/emermed-2020-210022.

Agley, J., Delong, J., Janota, A., Carson, A., Roberts, J., & Maupome, G. (2021). Reflections on project ECHO: Qualitative findings from five different ECHO programs. *Medical Education Online, 26*(1). https://doi.org/10.1080/10872981.2021.1936435.

AlDossary, S., Martin-Khan, M. G., Bradford, N. K., Armfield, N. R., & Smith, A. C. (2017). The development of a telemedicine planning framework based on needs assessment. *Journal of Medical Systems, 41*(5), 74. https://doi.org/10.1007/s10916-017-0709-4.

Ali, Z., Zibert, J. R., & Thomsen, S. F. (2020). Virtual clinical trials: Perspectives in dermatology. *Dermatology, 236*(4), 375–382. https://doi.org/10.1159/000506418.

American Academy of Pediatrics. (2022). *Pediatric ECHOs.* Practice management. https://www.aap.org/en/practice-management/project-echo/pediatric-echos/.

American Academy of Pediatrics. *Telehealth: Indispensable care modality—a multistakeholder symposium to explore barriers and opportunities to improve equity and value of virtual care.* 2022b.

American Academy of Pediatrics. 2022c. Telehealth. https://www.aap.org/en/practice-management/care-delivery-approaches/telehealth/.

American Academy of Pediatrics; 2022d. *Ensuring equitable access to telehealth for diverse and underserved communities.* https://www.aap.org/en/practice-management/care-delivery-approaches/telehealth/ensuring-equitable-access-to-telehealth-for-diverse-and-underserved-communities/.

American Academy of Pediatrics. 2023. Supporting pediatric research on outcomes and utilizations of telehealth (SPROUT). https://services.aap.org/en/community/aap-sections/telehealth-care/sprout/

American Association of Nurse Practitioners. *State practice environment.* 2022. https://www.aanp.org/advocacy/state/state-practice-environment

American Board of Pediatrics. *Entrustable professional activities for general pediatrics.* 2019. https://www.abp.org/entrustable-professional-activities-epas

American Medical Association. *Telehealth implementation playbook.* 2020. https://www.ama-assn.org/terms-use

American Telemedicine Association. *A concise guide for telemedicine practitioners: Human factors quick guide - eye contact.* 2016

Americans with Disabilities Act. (2005). ADA business brief: Communicating with people who are deaf or hard of hearing in hospital settings. In *www.ada.gov* (p. 4). US Department of Justice Civil Rights Division. https://www.ada.gov/hospcombr.htm.

Anderson M, Perrin A. *Barriers to adoption and attitudes towards tech among older Americans.* 2017. https://www.pewresearch.org/internet/2017/05/17/barriers-to-adoption-and-attitudes-towards-technology/

Ansary, A. M., Martinez, J. N., & Scott, J. D. (2021). The virtual physical exam in the 21st century. *Journal of Telemedicine and Telecare, 27*(6), 382–392. https://doi.org/10.1177/1357633X19878330.

Arora, S., Thornton, K., Murata, G., Deming, P., Kalishman, S., Dion, D., Parish, B., Burke, T., Pak, W., Dunkelberg, J., Kristin, M., Brown, J., Jenkusky, S., Komaromy, M., Qualls, C. (2011). Outcomes of treatment for hepatitis C virus infection by primary care providers. *New England Journal of Medicine, 364*(23), 2199–2207. https://doi.org/10.1056/NEJMoa1009370.

Association of American Medical Colleges. *Telehealth competencies across the learning continuum* (Issue March). 2021. https://www.aamc.org/data-reports/report/telehealth-competencies

Balevic, S. J., Singler, L., Randell, R., Chung, R. J., Lemmon, M. E., & Hornik, C. P. (2021). Bringing research directly to families in the era of COVID-19. *Pediatric Research, 89*(3), 404–406. https://doi.org/10.1038/s41390-020-01260-1.

Bansa, M., Glassgow, A. E., Martin, M., Caskey, R., Paulson, A., Minier, M., Roper, P., Mitacek, R., Wilder, J., & Van Voorhees, B. (2019). Development of a community-based medical neighborhood for children with chronic conditions. *Progress in Community Health Partnerships: Research, Education and Action, 13*(1), 83–95. https://doi.org/10.1353/cpr.2019.0011.

Barbosa, W., Zhou, K., Waddell, E., Myers, T., & Dorsey, E. R. (2021). Improving access to care: Telemedicine across medical domains. *Annuls of Reviews in Public Health, 42*(1), 463–481. https://doi.org/10.1146/annurev-publhealth-090519-093711.

Barnett, M. L., Ray, K. N., Souza, J., & Mehrotra, A. (2018). Trends in telemedicine use in a large commercially insured population, 2005-2017. *JAMA, 320*(20), 2147–2149. https://doi.org/10.1001/jama.2018.12354.

Barnett, M. L., Yee, H. F., Mehrotra, A., & Giboney, P. (2017). Los Angeles safety-net program econsult system was rapidly adopted and decreased wait times to see specialists. *Health Affects, 36*(3), 492–499. https://doi.org/10.1377/hlthaff.2016.1283.

Bashshur, R., Shannon, G. W., Smith, B. R., Alverson, D. C., Antoniotti, N., Barsan, W. G., Bashshur, N., Brown, E. M., Coye, M. J., Doarn, C. R., Ferguson, S., Grigsby, J., Krupinski, E. A., Kvedar, J. C., Linkous, J., Merrell, R. C., Nexbitt, T., Poropatich, R., Rheuban, K. S., Sanders, J. H. (2014). The empirical foundations of telemedicine interventions for chronic disease management. *Telemedicine and E-Health, 20*(9), 769–800. https://doi.org/10.1089/tmj.2014.9981.

Bates, R. A., Henderson, K., & Rutledge, C. M. (2020). Telehealth basics. In: Schweickert, P. A., & Rutledge, C. M. (Eds.), *Telehealth essentials for advanced practice nursing* (pp. 23–44). SLACK Books. https://www.slackbooks.com/telehealth-essentials-for-advanced-practice-nursing/?utm_campaign=schweickerttelemedicine.

Bian, Y., Xiang, Y., Tong, B., Feng, B., & Weng, X. (2020). Artificial intelligence-assisted system in postoperative follow-up of orthopedic patients: Exploratory quantitative and qualitative study. *Journal of Medical Internet Research, 22*(5), 1–8. https://doi.org/10.2196/16896.

Burke, B. L. Jr., Hall, R. W., & Section on Telehealth Care. (2015). Telemedicine: Pediatric applications. *Pediatrics, 136*(1), e293–e308. https://doi.org/10.1542/peds.2015-1517.

Cahan, E. M., Matun, J., Bailey, P., Fernandes, S., Addala, A., Kibrom, S., Krissberg, J. R., Smith, S., Sha, S., Wang, E., Saynina, O., Wise, P., Chamberlain, L. J. (2022). The impact of telehealth adoption during COVID-19 pandemic on patterns of pediatric subspecialty care utilization. *Academic Pediatrics.* https://doi.org/10.1016/j.acap.2022.03.010.

Calton, B., Abedini, N., & Fratkin, M. (2020). Telemedicine in the time of coronavirus. *Journal of Pain Symptom Management, 60*(1), e12–e14. https://doi.org/10.1016/J.JPAINSYMMAN.2020.03.019.

Cambridge English Dictionary. *Bedside manner.* 2022. https://dictionary.cambridge.org/us/dictionary/english/bedside-manner

Center for Connected Health Policy. *State telehealth laws and reimbursement policies* (Issue February). 2022a. https://www.cchpca.org/2022/05/Spring2022_Infographicfinal.pdf

Center for Connected Health Policy. *State telehealth laws and reimbursement policies report, Spring 2022.* 2022b. https://www.cchpca.org/resources/state-telehealth-laws-and-reimbursement-policies-report-spring-2022/

Center for Connected Health Policy. *Telehealth policy 101: Credentialing and privileging.* 2022c. https://www.cchpca.org/policy-101/?category=credentialing-privileging

Center for Connected Health Policy. *Telehealth policy 101: Cross state licensing and compacts.* 2022d. https://www.cchpca.org/policy-101/?category=cross-state-licensing-compacts

Centers for Disease Control and Prevention. (2021). *Social determinants of health.* Centers for Disease Control and Prevention, Social Determinants of Health. https://www.cdc.gov/socialdeterminants/index.htm.

Chandler, A. L., Beavers, J. C., & Hall, R. W. (2020). Telemedicine in pediatrics: Possibilities and pitfalls. *Pediatrics in Review, 41*(7), 376–378. https://doi.org/10.1542/pir.2019-0171.

Chatterjee, P., Lin, Y., & Venkataramani, A. S. (2022). Changes in economic outcomes before and after rural hospital closures in the United States: A difference-in-differences study. *Health Services Research, 57*(5), 1020–1028. https://doi.org/10.1111/1475-6773.13988.

Chike-Harris, K. E. (2020). The role of the advanced practice registered nurse in implementing telehealth practice. In: Schweickert, P., & Rutledge, C. M. (Eds.), *Telehealth essentials for advanced practice nurses.* SLACK Books.

Chinnis, S., & Stanley, A. (2022). A new model of care: Pediatric asthma management. *Online Journal of Rural Nursing and Health Care, 22*(1), 42–56. https://doi.org/10.14574/ojrnhc.v22i1.685.

Chua, I. S., Jackson, V., & Kamdar, M. (2020). Webside manner during the COVID-19 pandemic: Maintaining human connection during virtual visits. *Journal of Palliative Medicine, 23*(11), 1507–1509. https://doi.org/10.1089/jpm.2020.0298.

Community Preventive Services Task Force. (2016). School-based health centers to promote health equity. *American Journal of Preventive Medicine, 51*(1), 127–128. https://doi.org/10.1016/j.amepre.2016.01.008.

Cormack, C. L., Garber, K., Cristaldi, K., Edlund, B., Dodds, C., & McElligott, L. (2016). Implementing school-based telehealth for children with medical complexity. *Journal of Pediatric Rehabilitative Medicine, 9*(3), 237–240. https://doi.org/10.3233/PRM-160385.

Curfman, A. L., Hackell, J. M., Herendeen, N. E., Alexander, J. J., Marcin, J. P., Moskowitz, W. B., Bodnar, C. E. F., Simon, H. K., McSwain, S. D., & Section on Telehealth Care, Committee on Practice and Ambulatory Medicine, Committee on Pediatric Workforce. (2021). Telehealth: Improving access to and quality of pediatric health care. *Pediatrics, 148*(3), e2021053129. https://doi.org/10.1542/peds.2021-053129.

Curfman, A. L., Hackell, J. M., Herendeen, N. E., Alexander, J., Marcin, J. P., Moskowitz, W. B., Bodnar, C. E. F., Simon, H. K., & McSwain, S. D. (2022). Telehealth: Opportunities to improve access, quality, and cost in pediatric care. *Pediatrics, 149*(3), e2021056035. https://doi.org/10.1542/peds.2021-056035.

Curfman, A. L., McSwain, S. D., Chuo, J., Olson, C. A., & Simpson, K. (2021). An economic framework to measure value of pediatric telehealth. *Telemedicine and E-Health, 27*(12), 1440–1442. https://doi.org/10.1089/tmj.2020.0520.

Curfman, A. L., McSwain, S. D., Chuo, J., Yeager-McSwain, B., Schinasi, D., Marcin, J., Herendeen, N., Chung, S. L., & Rheuban, K., Olson, C. A. (2021). Pediatric telehealth in the COVID-19 pandemic era and beyond. *Pediatrics, 148*(3). https://doi.org/10.1542/peds.2020-047795.

DeGuzman, P. B., & Jain, N. (2020). Can public libraries be leveraged to expand access to telehealth? Exploration of a strategy to mitigate rural health disparities. *MedRxiv, 6*(165), 1–13. https://doi.org/10.1101/2020.08.18.20177287.

Deldar, K., Bahaadinbeigy, K., & Tara, A. (2016). Teleconsultation and clinical decision making: A systematic review. *Acta Informatica Medica, 24*(4), 286. https://doi.org/10.5455/aim.2016.24.286-292.

Doherty, A. J., Atherton, H., Boland, P., Hastings, R., Hives, L., Hood, K., James-Jenkinson, L., Leavey, R., Randell, E., Reed, J., Taggart, L., Wilson, N., & Chauhan, U. (2020). Barriers and facilitators to primary health care for people with intellectual disabilities and/or autism: An integrative review. *BJGP open, 4*(3), bjgpopen20X101030. https://doi.org/10.3399/bjgpopen20X101030.

Drug Enforcement Administration. (2020). *DEA policy: Exception to separate registration requirements across state lines* (pp. 1–2). US Department of Justice. https://www.deadiversion.usdoj.gov/GDP/(DEA-DC-018)(DEA067). DEA state reciprocity (final)(Signed).pdf.

DuBose-Morris, R., McSwain, S. D., McElligott, J. T., King, K. L., Ziniel, S., & Harvey, J. (2021). Building telehealth teams of the future through interprofessional curriculum development: A five-year mixed methodology study. *Journal of Interprofessional Care,* 1–9. https://doi.org/10.1080/13561820.2021.2005556.

Dziob, C., LaManna, J., Perry, C. K., Toerber-Clark, J., Boehning, A., O'Rourke, J., & Rutledge, C. (2022). Telehealth competencies: Leveled for continuous advanced practice nurse development. *Nurse Educator, 47*(5), 293–297. https://doi.org/10.1097/NNE.0000000000001196.

Espinoza, J., Crown, K., & Kulkarni, O. (2020). A guide to chatbots for COVID-19 screening at pediatric health care facilities. *JMIR Public Health Surveillance 2020, 6*(2), E18808. *Https://Publichealth.Jmir.Org/2020/2/E18808,* 6(2), E18808. https://doi.org/10.2196/18808.

Federal Register. (2018). Authority of health care providers to practice telehealth. https://www.federalregister.gov/documents/2018/05/11/2018-10114/authority-of-health-care-providers-to-practice-telehealth

Fierson, W. M. (2013). Screening examination of premature infants for retinopathy of prematurity. *Pediatrics, 131*(1), 189–195. https://doi.org/10.1542/PEDS.2012-2996.

Fiks, A. G., Kelly, M. K., Nwokeji, U., Ramachandran, J., Ray, K. N., & Gozal, D. (2022). A pediatric telemedicine research agenda: Another important task for pediatric chairs. *Journal of Pediatrics.* https://doi.org/10.1016/j.jpeds.2022.07.048.

Fogel, J. L., & Raymond, J. K. (2020). Implementing telehealth in pediatric type 1 diabetes mellitus. *Pediatric Clinics of North America, 67*(4), 661–664. https://doi.org/10.1016/j.pcl.2020.04.009.

Ford, D., Harvey, J. B., McElligott, J., King, K., Simpson, K. N., Valenta, S., Warr, E. H., Walsh, T., Debenham, E., Teasdale,

C., Meystre, S., Obeid, J. S., Metts, C., & Lenert, L. A. (2020). Leveraging health system telehealth and informatics infrastructure to create a continuum of services for COVID-19 screening, testing, and treatment. *Journal of the American Medical Informatics Association: JAMIA, 27*(12), 1871–1877. https://doi.org/10.1093/jamia/ocaa157.

Ford, D., Harvey, J., Mcelligott, J., Valenta, S., & Warr, E. (2021). In Valenta, S., & Ford, D. (Eds.), *TSIM: The telehealth framework - a comprehensive guide to telehealth implementation.* Independent Publishers Group. https://www.tsimtelehealth.com/.

Foster, C., Schinasi, D., Kan, K., Macy, M., Wheeler, D., Curfman, A. (2022). Remote monitoring of patient- and family-generated health data in pediatrics. *Pediatrics, 149*(2), e2021054137. https://doi.org/10.1542/peds.2021-054137.

Garber KM, Gustin TS, Rutledge CM (n.d.). Put PEP into telehealth: A framework for successful encounters. Online Journal of Issues in Nursing.

Garber, K., Wells, E., Hale, K. C., & King, K. (2021). Connecting kids to care: Developing a school-based telehealth program. *Journal of Nurse Practice, 17*(3), 273–278. https://doi.org/10.1016/j.nurpra.2020.12.024.

Genes, N. (2017). Alexander Graham Bell and the birth of telemedicine. *Telemedicine.* http://www.telemedmag.com/article/alexander-graham-bell-and-the-birth-of-telemedicine/.

Gilson, S. F., Umscheid, C. A., Laiteerapong, N., Ossey, G., Nunes, K. J., & Shah, S. D. (2020). Growth of ambulatory virtual visits and differential use by patient sociodemographics at one urban academic medical center during the COVID-19 pandemic: Retrospective analysis. *JMIR Medical Information, 8*(12). https://doi.org/10.2196/24544.

Goddard, A., Sullivan, E., Fields, P., & Mackey, S. (2021). The future of telehealth in school-based health centers: Lessons from COVID-19. *Journal of Pediatric Health Care, 35*(3), 304–309. https://doi.org/10.1016/j.pedhc.2020.11.008.

Gogia, S. (2019). Rationale, history, and basics of telehealth. *Fundamentals of Telemedicine and Telehealth,* 11–34. https://doi.org/10.1016/B978-0-12-814309-4.00002-1.

Gogia, S. (2020). Fundamentals of telemedicine and telehealth. In *Fundamentals of telemedicine and telehealth.* Elsevier. https://doi.org/10.1016/C2017-0-01090-X.

González-Espada, W. J., Hall-Barrow, J., Hall, R. W., Burke, B. L., & Smith, C. E. (2009). Achieving success connecting academic and practicing clinicians through telemedicine. *Pediatrics, 123*(3), e476–e483. https://doi.org/10.1542/peds.2008-2193.

Gonzalez, R. (2017). Telemedicine is forcing doctors to learn "webside" manner. *Wired.* https://www.wired.com/story/telemedicine-is-forcing-doctors-to-learn-webside-manner/.

Gustin, T. S., Kott, K., & Rutledge, C. (2020). Telehealth etiquette training: A guideline for preparing interprofessional teams for successful encounters. *Nurse Educator, 45*(2), 88–92. https://doi.org/10.1097/NNE.0000000000000680.

Gutierrez, J., Rewerts, K., CarlLee, S., Kuperman, E., Anderson, M. L., & Kaboli, P. J. (2022). A systematic review of telehealth applications in hospital medicine. *Journal of Hospital Medicine, 17*(4), 291–302. https://doi.org/10.1002/jhm.12801.

Hah, H., & Goldin, D. (2022). Moving toward AI-assisted decision-making: Observation on clinicians' management of multimedia patient information in synchronous and asynchronous telehealth contexts. *Health Information Journal, 28*(1), 1–14. https://doi.org/10.1177/14604582221077049.

Hanna, K. T. (2021). *What is the digital divide and how is it being bridged?* TechTarget. https://www.techtarget.com/whatis/definition/digital-divide.

Harrison, J. N., Steinberg, J., Wilms Floet, A. M. L., Grace, N., Menon, D., German, R., Chen, B., Yenokyan, G., & Leppert, M. L. O. (2022). Addressing pediatric developmental and mental health in primary care using tele-education. *Clinical Pediatrics, 61*(1), 46–55. https://doi.org/10.1177/00099228211059644.

Harvey, J. B., Yeager, B. E., Cramer, C., Wheeler, D., & McSwain, S. D. (2017). The impact of telemedicine on pediatric critical care triage. *Pediatric Critical Care Medicine, 18*(11), e555–e560. https://doi.org/10.1097/PCC.0000000000001330.

Healthy People 2030. (2022). *Social determinants of health.* Health. Gov. https://health.gov/healthypeople/priority-areas/social-determinants-health.

Heard-Garris, N., Arora, S., & Lurie, N. (2017). Building physician networks as part of the Zika response. *Disaster Medicine and Public Health Preparedness, 11*(2), 259–261. https://doi.org/10.1017/dmp.2017.24.

Heath, S. (2016). 4 best practices for improving patient-provider communication. *Patient Engagement HIT.* https://patientengagementhit.com/news/4-best-practices-for-improving-patient-provider-communication.

Heath, S. (2017). 3 key traits of a positive patient-provider relationship. *Patient Engagement HIT.* https://patientengagementhit.com/news/3-key-traits-of-a-positive-patient-provider-relationship#:~:text=Empathy%2C strong communication%2C and shared, a positive patient-provider relationship.

Hennessy, J. J., & Maguregui, A. T. (2022). HIPAA & telehealth: FAQs from HHS guidance on audio-only telehealth. *Health Care Law Today.* June. https://www.foley.com/en/insights/publications/2022/06/hipaa-telehealth-faqs-hhs-audio-only-telehealth.

Hughes, H. K., Hasselfeld, B. W., Cooper, L. A., Thornton, R. L. J., & Commodore-Mensah, Y. (2021). A process for developing a telehealth equity dashboard at a large academic health system serving diverse populations. *Journal of Health Care for the Poor and Underserved, 32*(2), 198–210. https://doi.org/10.1353/hpu.2021.0058.

Implementation of the Ryan Haight Online Pharmacy Consumer Protection Act of 2008, Pub. L. No. 2020–21310. 2020. https://www.deadiversion.usdoj.gov/fed_regs/rules/2020/fr0930_2.htm#:~:text=110-425)(hereafter%2C by means of the internet

Izquierdo, R., Morin, P. C., Bratt, K., Moreau, Z., Meyer, S., Ploutz-Snyder, R., Wade, M., & Weinstock, R. S. (2009). School-centered telemedicine for children with type 1 diabetes mellitus. *The Journal of Pediatrics, 155*(3), 374–379. https://doi.org/10.1016/j.jpeds.2009.03.014.

Jadczyk, T., Wojakowski, W., Tendera, M., Henry, T. D., Egnaczyk, G., & Shreenivas, S. (2021). Artificial intelligence can improve patient management at the time of a pandemic: The role of voice technology. *Journal of Medical Internet Research, 23*(5), 1–11. https://doi.org/10.2196/22959.

Jerant, A. F., Friederichs-Fitzwater, M. M. von., & Moore, M. (2005). Patients' perceived barriers to active self-management of chronic conditions. *Patient Education Counseling, 57*(3), 300–307. https://doi.org/10.1016/j.pec.2004.08.004.

Jin, M. L., Brown, M. M., Dhir, P., Nirmalan, A., & Edwards, P. A. (2021). Telemedicine, telementoring, and telesurgery for surgical practices. *Current Problems in Surgery,* 100987. https://doi.org/10.1016/j.cpsurg.2021.100987.

Jones, J. (2020). *Introduction to privileges: Credentialing versus privileging and CMS requirements.* VerityStream. https://veritystream.com/resources/details/blog/2020/05/08/introduction-to-privileges-credentialing-versus-privileging-and-cms-requirements#:~:text=Credentialing is %22the process of,content of patient care services.%22.

Joseph, P. D., Craig, J. C., & Caldwell, P. H. Y. (2015). Clinical trials in children. *British Journal of Clinical Pharmacology, 79*(3), 357–369. https://doi.org/10.1111/bcp.12305.

Jung, S. Y., Lee, K., & Hwang, H. (2022). *Recent trends of healthcare information and communication technologies in pediatrics: A systematic review.* In Clinical and experimental pediatrics, 65(6), 291–299. https://doi.org/10.3345/cep.2020.01333.

Kang, C. F. C. C. (2021). Approves a $ 50 monthly high-speed internet subsidy. *New York Times.* https://www.nytimes.com/2021/02/25/technology/fcc-broadband-low-income-subsidy.html.

Katzow, M. W., Steinway, C., & Jan, S. (2020). Telemedicine and health disparities during COVID-19. *Pediatrics, 146*(2), e20201586. https://doi.org/10.1542/peds.2020-1586.

Keder, R. D., Mittal, S., Stringer, K., Wallis, K. E., Wallace, J. E., & Soares, N. S. (2022). Society for Developmental & Behavioral Pediatrics position statement on telehealth. *Journal of Developmental and Behavioral Pediatrics, 43*(1), 55–59. https://doi.org/10.1097/DBP.0000000000001046.

Keely, E., Liddy, C., & Afkham, A. (2013). Utilization, benefits, and impact of an e-consultation service across diverse specialties and primary care providers. *Telemedicine and E-Health, 19*(10), 733–738. https://doi.org/10.1089/tmj.2013.0007.

Keenan, A. J., Tsourtos, G., & Tieman, J. (2022). Promise and peril-defining ethical telehealth practice from the clinician and patient perspective: A qualitative study. *Digital Health, 8.* https://doi.org/10.1177/20552076211070394.

Khozin, S., & Coravos, A. (2019). Decentralized trials in the age of real-world evidence and inclusivity in clinical investigations. *Clinical Pharmacology and Therapeutics, 106*(1), 25–27. https://doi.org/10.1002/cpt.1441.

Knopf, J. A., Finnie, R. K., Peng, Y., Hahn, R. A., Truman, B. I., Vernon-Smiley, M., Johnson, V. C., Johnson, R. L., Fielding, J. E., Muntaner, C., Hunt, P. C., Phyllis Jones, C., Fullilove, M. T., & Community Preventive Services Task Force (2016). School-based health centers to advance health equity: A community guide systematic review. *American Journal of Preventive Medicine, 51*(1), 114–126. https://doi.org/10.1016/j.amepre.2016.01.009.

Koonin, L. M., Hoots, B., Tsang, C. A., Leroy, Z., Farris, K., Jolly, T., Antall, P., McCabe, B., Zelis, C. B. R., Tong, I., & Harris, A. M. (2020a). Trends in the use of telehealth during the emergence of the COVID-19 Pandemic—United States, January-March 2020. *MMWR. Morbidity and Mortality Weekly Report, 69*(43), 1595–1599. https://doi.org/10.15585/mmwr.mm6943a3.

Koonin, L. M., Hoots, B., Tsang, C. A., Leroy, Z., Farris, K., Jolly, T., Antall, P., McCabe, B., Zelis, C. B. R., Tong, I., & Harris, A. M. (2020b). Trends in the use of telehealth during the emergence of the COVID-19 Pandemic—United States, January-March 2020. *MMWR. Morbidity and Mortality Weekly Report, 69*(43), 1595–1599. https://doi.org/10.15585/mmwr.mm6943a3.

Kruse, C. S., Williams, K., Bohls, J., & Shamsi, W. (2021). Telemedicine and health policy: A systematic review. *Health Policy and Technology, 10*(1), 209–229. https://doi.org/10.1016/j.hlpt.2020.10.006.

Kwok, E. Y. L., Chiu, J., Rosenbaum, P., & Cunningham, B. J. (2022). The process of telepractice implementation during the COVID-19 pandemic: A narrative inquiry of preschool speech-language pathologists and assistants from one center in Canada. *BMC Health Services Research, 22*(1), 81. https://doi.org/10.1186/s12913-021-07454-5.

Lalloo, C., Diskin, C., Ho, M., Orkin, J., Cohen, E., Osei-Twum, J. A., Hundert, A., Jiwan, A., Sivarajah, S., Gumapac, A., & Stinson, J. N. (2020). Pediatric project ECHO: Implementation of a virtual medical education program to support community management of children with medical complexity. *Hospital Pediatrics, 10*(12), 1044–1052. https://doi.org/10.1542/hpeds.2020-0067.

Lalloo, C., Osei-Twum, J.-A., Rapoport, A., Vadeboncoeur, C., Weingarten, K., van Zanten, S. V., Widger, K., & Stinson, J. (2021). Pediatric project ECHO: A virtual community of practice to improve palliative care knowledge and self-efficacy among interprofessional health care providers. *Journal of Palliative Medicine, 24*(7), 1036–1044. https://doi.org/10.1089/jpm.2020.0496.

Langkamp, D. L., McManus, M. D., & Blakemore, S. D. (2015). Telemedicine for children with developmental disabilities: A more effective clinical process than office-based care. *Telemedicine and E-Health, 21*(2), 110–114. https://doi.org/10.1089/tmj.2013.0379.

Leeds, S., Auerbach, M., & Tiyyagura, G. (2022). Impact of project ECHO on community pediatricians' food allergy knowledge. *Journal of Allergy and Clinical Immunology, 149*(2), AB42. https://doi.org/10.1016/j.jaci.2021.12.169.

Lesher, A. P., Fakhry, S. M., DuBose-Morris, R., Harvey, J., Langston, L. B., Wheeler, D. M., Brack, J. T., & McElligott, J. T. (2020). Development and evolution of a statewide outpatient consultation service: Leveraging telemedicine to improve access to specialty care. *Population Health Management, 23*(1), 20–28. https://doi.org/10.1089/pop.2018.0212.

Liddy, C., Drosinis, P., & Keely, E. (2016). Electronic consultation systems: Worldwide prevalence and their impact on patient care—a systematic review. *Family Practice, 33*(3), 274–285. https://doi.org/10.1093/fampra/cmw024.

Love, H., Panchal, N., Schlitt, J., Behr, C., & Soleimanpour, S. (2019). The use of telehealth in school-based health centers. *Global Pediatric Health, 6.* https://doi.org/10.1177/2333794X19884194.

Lozano, P., & Houtrow, A. (2018). Supporting self-management in children and adolescents with complex chronic conditions. *Pediatrics, 141*(Supplement_3), S233–S241. https://doi.org/10.1542/peds.2017-1284H.

MacGeorge, C. A., Andrews, A. L., & King, K. L. (2021). Telehealth for pediatric asthma. In: Ford, D., & Valenta, S. (Eds.), *Telemedicine: Overview and application in pulmonary, critical care, and sleep medicine* (1st ed., pp. 129–141). Springer Nature. https://doi.org/10.1007/978-3-030-64050-7_8.

Mazurek, M. O., Curran, A., Burnette, C., & Sohl, K. (2019). ECHO autism STAT: Accelerating early access to autism diagnosis. *Journal of Autism and Developmental Disorders, 49,* 127–137. https://doi.org/10.1007/s10803-018-3696-5.

McConnochie, K. M. (2019). Webside manner: A key to high-quality primary care telemedicine for all. *Telemedicine and E-Health, 25*(11), 1007–1011. https://doi.org/10.1089/tmj.2018.0274.

McCormick, T. M. (2018). Three essential qualities that make a good telemedicine physician. *LinkedIn Corporation.* https://www.linkedin.com/pulse/three-essential-qualities-make-good-telemedicine-mccormick-md/.

McGill, M., Noureal, N., & Siegel, J. (2019). Telepractice treatment of stuttering: A systematic review. *Telemedicine and E-Health, 25*(5), 359–368. https://doi.org/10.1089/tmj.2017.0319.

Meyer, B. C., Clarke, C. A., Troke, T. M., & Friedman, L. S. (2012). Essential telemedicine elements (tele-ments) for connecting the academic health center and remote community providers to enhance patient care. *Academic Medicine, 87*(8), 1032–1040. https://doi.org/10.1097/ACM.0b013e31825cdd3a.

Milne Wenderlich, A., & Herendeen, N. (2021). Telehealth in pediatric primary care. *Current Problems in Pediatric and Adolescent Health Care, 51*(1), 1–5. https://doi.org/10.1016/j.cppeds.2021.100951.

Muruganantham, A., Nguyen, P. T., Lydia, E. L., Shankar, K., Hashim, W., & Maseleno, A. (2019). Big data analytics and intelligence: A perspective for health care. *International Journal of Engineering and Advanced Technology, 8*(6S), 861–864. https://doi.org/10.35940/ijeat.F1162.0886S19.

Nhung, L. H., Dien, T. M., Lan, N. P., Thanh, P. Q., & Cuong, P. V. (2021). Use of project ECHO telementoring model in continuing medical education for pediatricians in Vietnam: Preliminary results. *Health Servics Insights, 14,* 117863292110368. https://doi.org/10.1177/11786329211036855.

Noel, K., & Ellison, B. (2020). Inclusive innovation in telehealth. *Npj Digital Medicine, 3*(1), 89. https://doi.org/10.1038/s41746-020-0296-5.

Pool, J., Akhlaghpour, S., Fatehi, F., & Gray, L. C. (2022). Data privacy concerns and use of telehealth in the aged care context: An integrative review and research agenda.

International Journal of Medical Informatics, 160(August 2021), 104707. https://doi.org/10.1016/j.ijmedinf.2022.104707.

Porto, A., Rubin, K., Wagner, K., Chang, W., Macri, G., & Anderson, D. (2021). Impact of pediatric electronic consultations in a federally qualified health center. *Telemedicine and E-Health, 27*(12), 1379–1384. https://doi.org/10.1089/tmj.2020.0394.

Powers, G. M., Frieden, L., & Nguyen, V. (2017). Telemedicine: Access to health care for people with disabilities. *Houston Journal of Health Law and Policy, 17*, 7–20. http://www.law.uh.edu/hjhlp/volumes/Vol_17/V17-Frieden-FinalPDF.pdf.

Preminger, T. J. (2022). Telemedicine in pediatric cardiology: Pros and cons. *Current Opinions in Pediatrics*, 1–7. https://doi.org/10.1097/MOP.0000000000001159.

Project ECHO. (2022). *Our programs*. The University of New Mexico. https://hsc.unm.edu/echo/partner-portal/programs/.

Project ECHO. (2022). *The ECHO model is a learning framework that results in sustainable change*. The University of New Mexico. https://hsc.unm.edu/echo/what-we-do/about-the-echo-model.html.

Raman, N., Nagarajan, R., Venkatesh, L., Monica, D. S., Ramkumar, V., & Krumm, M. (2019). School-based language screening among primary school children using telepractice: A feasibility study from India. *International Journal of Speech-Language Pathology, 21*(4), 425–434. https://doi.org/10.1080/17549507.2018.1493142.

Ramsetty, A., & Adams, C. (2020). Impact of the digital divide in the age of COVID-19. *JAMIA, 0*(April), 1–3. https://doi.org/10.1093/jamia/ocaa078.

Ray, K. N., Mehrotra, A., Yabes, J. G., & Kahn, J. M. (2020). Telemedicine and outpatient subspecialty visits among pediatric Medicaid beneficiaries. *Academic Pediatrics, 20*(5), 642–651. https://doi.org/10.1016/j.acap.2020.03.014.

Rosa, C., Campbell, A. N. C., Miele, G. M., Brunner, M., & Winstanley, E. L. (2015). Using e-technologies in clinical trials. *Contemporary Clinical Trials, 45*, 41–54. https://doi.org/10.1016/j.cct.2015.07.007.

Rosen, J. M., Adams, L. V., Geiling, J., Curtis, K. M., Mosher, R. E., Ball, P. A., Grigg, E. B., Hebert, K. A., Grodan, J. R., Jurmain, J. C., Loucks, C., Macedonia, C. R., & Kun, L. (2021). Telehealth's new horizon: Providing smart hospital-level care in the home. *Telemedicine Journal and E-Health : The Official Journal of the American Telemedicine Association, 27*(11), 1215–1224. https://doi.org/10.1089/tmj.2020.0448.

Rush, K. L., Hatt, L., Janke, R., Burton, L., Ferrier, M., & Tetrault, M. (2018). The efficacy of telehealth delivered educational approaches for patients with chronic diseases: A systematic review. *Patient Education and Counseling, 101*(8), 1310–1321. https://doi.org/10.1016/j.pec.2018.02.006.

Rutledge, C. M., Gustin, T. S., & Schweickert, P. (2020). Telehealth competencies: Knowledge and skills. In: Rutledge, C. M., & Schweickert, P. (Eds.), *Telehealth essentials for advanced practice nurses*. SLACK Books.

Rutledge, C. M., Hawkins, E. J., Bordelon, M., & Gustin, T. S. (2020). Telehealth education: An interprofessional online immersion experience in response to COVID-19. *Journal of Nursing Education, 59*(10), 570–576. https://doi.org/10.3928/01484834-20200921-06.

Rutledge, C. M., O'Rourke, J., Mason, A. M., Chike-Harris, K., Behnke, L., Melhado, L., Downes, L., & Gustin, T. (2021). Telehealth competencies for nursing education and practice: The four P's of telehealth. *Nurse Educator, 46*(5), 300–305. https://doi.org/10.1097/NNE.0000000000000988.

Sanchez, D., Reiner, J. F., Sadlon, R., Price, O. A., & Long, M. W. (2019). Systematic review of school telehealth evaluations. *Journal of School Nursing, 35*(1), 61–76. https://doi.org/10.1177/1059840518817870.

Shah, A. C., & Badawy, S. M. (2021). Telemedicine in pediatrics: Systematic review of randomized controlled trials. *JMIR Pediatrics and Parenting, 4*(1), E22696. *Https://Pediatrics.Jmir.Org/2021/1/E22696, 4*(1), E22696. https://doi.org/10.2196/22696.

Shah, E. D., Amann, S. T., & Karlitz, J. J. (2020). The time is now: A guide to sustainable telemedicine during COVID-19 and beyond. *American Journal of Gastroenterology, 115*(9), 1371–1375. https://doi.org/10.14309/AJG.0000000000000767.

Sharma, R., Nachum, S., Davidson, K. W., & Nochomovitz, M. (2019). It's not just facetime: Core competencies for the medical virtualist. *International Journal of Emergency Medicine, 12*(1), 8. https://doi.org/10.1186/s12245-019-0226-y.

Shook, L. M., Farrell, C. B., Kalinyak, K. A., Nelson, S. C., Hardesty, B. M., Rampersad, A. G., Saving, K. L., Whitten-Shurney, W. J., Panepinto, J. A., Ware, R. E., & Crosby, L. E. (2016). Translating sickle cell guidelines into practice for primary care providers with Project ECHO. *Medical Education Online, 21*, 33616. https://doi.org/10.3402/meo.v21.33616.

Silva, C. R. D. V., Lopes, R. H. Jr., de Goes Bay, O., Martinano, C. S., Fuentealba-Torres, M., Arcencio, R., Lapao, L., Dias, S., da Costat Uchoa, S. (2022). Digital health opportunities to improve primary health care in the context of COVID-19: Scoping review. *JMIR Human Factors, 9*(2), e35380. *2022;9(2):E35380 Https://Humanfactors.Jmir.Org/2022/2/E35380*. https://doi.org/10.2196/35380.

Smith, C., Fontana-Chow, K., Boateng, B. A., Azzie, G., Pietrolungo, L., Cheng-Tsallis, A., Golding, F., Tallett, S. (2009). Tele-education: Linking educators with learners via distance technology. *Pediatric Annals, 38*(10), 550–556. https://doi.org/10.3928/00904481-20090918-10.

Solomon, G. M., Bailey, J., Lawlor, J., Scalia, P., Sawicki, G. S., Dowd, C., Sabadosa, K. A., & Van Citters, A. (2021). Patient and family experience of telehealth care delivery as part of the CF chronic care model early in the COVID-19 pandemic. *Journal of Cystic Fibrosis: Official Journal of the European Cystic Fibrosis Society, 20*(Suppl 3), 41–46. https://doi.org/10.1016/j.jcf.2021.09.005.

Sommer, C., Zuccolin, D., Arnera, V., Schmitz, N., Adolfsson, P., Colombo, N., Gilg, R., & McDowell, B. (2018). Building clinical trials around patients: Evaluation and comparison of decentralized and conventional site models in patients with low back pain. *Contemporary Clinical Trials Communications, 11*, 120–126. https://doi.org/10.1016/j.conctc.2018.06.008.

Stille, C. J., Coller, R. J., Shelton, C., Wells, N., Desmarais, A., & Berry, J. G. (2022). National research agenda on health systems for children and youth with special health care needs. *Academic Pediatrics, 22*(2), S1–S6. https://doi.org/10.1016/j.acap.2021.12.022.

The Joint Commission. (2022). Credentialing and privileging - requirements for physician assistants and advanced practice registered nurses. *Hospital and Hospital Clinics*. https://www.jointcommission.org/standards/standard-faqs/hospital-and-hospital-clinics/medical-staff-ms/000002124/.

The National Council of State Boards of Nursing. *APRN compact*. 2020. https://www.ncsbn.org/aprn-compact.htm

The NPD Group. *Only 50% of homes in the continental US receive true broadband internet access, new NPD report reveals*. 2021. https://www.npd.com/news/press-releases/2022/new-npd-report-only-50-of-homes-in-the-continental-us-receive-true-broadband-internet-access/

Thomas, E. E., Haydon, H. M., Mehrotra, A., Caffery, L. J., Snoswell, C. L., Banbury, A., & Smith, A. C. (2022). Building on the momentum: Sustaining telehealth beyond COVID-19. *Journal of Telemedicine and Telecare, 28*(4), 301–308. https://doi.org/10.1177/1357633X20960638.

Thronson, L. R., Jackson, S. L., & Chew, L. D. (2020). The pandemic of health care inequity. *JAMA Network Open, 3*(10), e2021767. https://doi.org/10.1001/jamanetworkopen.2020.21767.

US Department of Health and Human Services. *Notification of enforcement discretion for telehealth | HHS.gov*. 2020. https://www.hhs.gov/hipaa/for-professionals/special-topics/

emergency-preparedness/notification-enforcement-discretion-telehealth/index.html

US Department of Health and Human Services. *Guidance: How the HIPAA rules permit covered health care providers and health plans to use remote communication technologies for audio-only telehealth | HHS.gov.* 2022a. https://www.hhs.gov/hipaa/for-professionals/privacy/guidance/hipaa-audio-telehealth/index.html

US Department of Health and Human Services, Division CR. (2022). *Guidance on nondiscrimination in telehealth: Federal protections to ensure accessibility to people with disabilities and limited English proficient persons* (pp. 1–12). Department of Health and Human Services (HHS) Office for Civil Rights (OCR) and the Department of Justice's (DOJ) Civil Rights Division. https://www.hhs.gov/sites/default/files/guidance-on-nondiscrimination-in-telehealth.pdf?mkt_tok=NzEwLVpMTC02NTEAAAGF6wlqVSjvddEfqp-OS6e6oj2wKBwoGP2Ff0UCAobPLeAiLfrsWC3U67H6SOb2D8YZS2WvjzEOI9PF387jHOsrz_GfEUW72bFeZZbzT2lNLcJs.

US Department of Justice. *ADA requirements: Effective communication.* 2014. https://www.ada.gov/effective-comm.htm

Valdez, R., Rogers, C. C., Claypool, H., Trieshmann, L., Frye, O., Wellbeloved-Stone, C., Kushalnagar, P. (2021). Ensuring full participation of people with disabilities in an era of telehealth. *Journal of American Medical Informatics Association,* 28(2), 389–392. https://doi.org/10.1093/jamia/ocaa297.

Van Cleave, J., Stille, C., & Hall, D. E. (2022). Child health, vulnerability, and complexity: Use of telehealth to enhance care for children and youth with special health care needs. *Academic Pediatrics,* 22(2), S34–S40. https://doi.org/10.1016/j.acap.2021.10.010.

Vinadé Chagas, M. E., Rodrigues Moleda Constant, H. M., Cristina Jacovas, V., Castro da Rocha, J., Galves Crivella Steimetz, C., Cotta Matte, M. C., de Campos Moreira, T., & Cezar Cabral, F. (2021). The use of telemedicine in the PICU: A systematic review and meta-analysis. *PLOS ONE,* 16(5), e0252409. https://doi.org/10.1371/journal.pone.0252409.

Vogels EA. *Lower-income Americans still less likely to have home broadband, smartphone.* 2021. https://www.pewresearch.org/fact-tank/2021/06/22/digital-divide-persists-even-as-americans-with-lower-incomes-make-gains-in-tech-adoption/

Wales, D., Skinner, L., & Hayman, M. (2017). The efficacy of telehealth-delivered speech and language intervention for primary school-age children: A systematic review. *International Journal of Telerehabilitation,* 9(1), 55–70. https://doi.org/10.5195/ijt.2017.6219.

Washington State Hospital Association. *Washington state telehealth training information.* 2018. https://www.wsha.org/policy-advocacy/issues/telemedicine/washington-state-telemedicine-collaborative/telemedicine-training/

Weaver, M. S., Robinson, J. E., Shostrom, V. K., & Hinds, P. S. (2020). Telehealth acceptability for children, family, and adult hospice nurses when integrating the pediatric palliative inpatient provider during sequential rural home hospice visits. *Journal of Palliative Medicine,* 23(5), 641–649. https://doi.org/10.1089/jpm.2019.0450.

Whitacre, B., & Biedny, C. (2022). A preview of the broadband fabric: Opportunities and issues for researchers and policymakers. *Telecommunications Policy,* 46(3), 102281. https://doi.org/10.1016/j.telpol.2021.102281.

Windover, A. K., Boissy, A., Rice, T. W., Gilligan, T., Velez, V. J., & Merlino, J. (2014). Optimizing relationship as a therapeutic agent. *Journal of Patient Experience,* 1(1), 8–13. https://doi.org/10.1177/237437431400100103.

Wosik, J., Fudim, M., Cameron, B., Gellad, Z. F., Cho, A., Phinney, D., Curtis, S., Roman, M., Poon, E. G., Ferranti, J., Katz, J. N., & Tcheng, J. (2020). Telehealth transformation: COVID-19 and the rise of virtual care. *Journal of the American Medical Informatics Association: JAMIA,* 27(6), 957–962. https://doi.org/10.1093/jamia/ocaa067.

Zhang, J., Wang, H. S., Zhou, H. Y., Dong, B., Zhang, L., Zhang, F., Liu, S. J., Wu, Y. F., Yuan, S. H., Tang, M. Y., Dong, W. F., Lin, J., Chen, M., Tong, X., Zhao, L. B., & Yin, Y. (2021). Real-world verification of artificial intelligence algorithm-assisted auscultation of breath sounds in children. *Frontiers in Pediatrics,* 9, 627337. https://doi.org/10.3389/fped.2021.627337.

Zhao, M., Hamadi, H., Haley, D. R., Xu, J., White-Williams, C., & Park, S. (2020). Telehealth: Advances in alternative payment models. *Telemedicine and E-Health,* 26(12), 1492–1499. https://doi.org/10.1089/tmj.2019.0294.

Zhou, C., Crawford, A., Serhal, E., Kurdyak, P., & Sockalingam, S. (2016). The impact of project ECHO on participant and patient outcomes. *Academic Medicine,* 91(10), 1439–1461. https://doi.org/10.1097/ACM.0000000000001328.

Asthma and Allergies

Jodi Shroba, Brenda Snyder

ASTHMA

ETIOLOGY

Asthma is a chronic lung disease characterized by variable and recurring symptoms, including airflow obstruction, bronchial hyperresponsiveness, and underlying inflammation. The National Heart, Lung, and Blood Institute (NHLBI, 2007) Guidelines for the Diagnosis and Management of Asthma define asthma as:

a chronic inflammatory disorder of the airways in which many cells and cellular elements play a role: in particular mast cells, eosinophils, T lymphocytes, macrophages, neutrophils and epithelial cells. In susceptible individuals, inflammation causes recurrent episodes of wheezing, breathlessness, chest tightness, and cough particularly in the at night or early morning. These episodes are usually associated with widespread but variable airflow obstruction that is often reversible either spontaneously or with treatment, The inflammation also causes an associated increase in the existing bronchial hyperresponsiveness to a variety of stimuli. Reversibility of airflow limitation may be incomplete in some patients with asthma.

In 2019, the Global Initiative for Asthma (GINA, 2022) report defined asthma as:

a heterogeneous disease, usually characterized by chronic airway inflammation defined by the history of respiratory symptoms such as wheeze, shortness of breath, chest tightness, and cough that vary over time and in intensity, together with variable expiratory airflow limitations.

Understanding asthma phenotypes has led to a better understanding of disease pathogenesis and additional asthma treatment options.

- Allergic asthma is identified as the most common phenotype, particularly among children. Approximately 60% of asthma is considered allergic. Inflammation in allergic asthma is initiated by the activity of antigen-presenting cells that promote the production of type 2 T-helper (Th2) cells from naïve T lymphocytes. Th2 cells then mediate the allergic asthma pathway through proinflammatory cytokines (i.e., interleukin-4 [IL-4], IL-5, IL-9, IL-13) leading to the production of immunoglobulin E (IgE) early in the cascade and, later, eosinophils. Allergic asthma is typically identified based on sensitization of allergen IgE testing (Kim et al., 2017).

- Nonallergic asthma has one or more different pathways leading to airway inflammation. Cytokines in the epithelium (IL-25, IL-33, thymic stromal lymphopoietin) activate type 2 innate lymphoid cells, from which IL-5 and IL-13 produce elevated levels of eosinophils, mucous hypersecretion, and airway inflammation and hyperreactivity (Fig. 7.1). Nonallergic asthma tends to develop later in life and more predominantly in women than in the allergic variety. The prevalence of nonallergic asthma is considered to be 10% to 33%. It appears to be associated with more severe asthma and lower responsiveness to standard therapy. Nonallergic asthma is diagnosed when allergic sensitization cannot be demonstrated using skin prick or in vitro IgE testing (Kim et al., 2017).

The development of asthma appears to involve the interplay between host factors (particularly genetics) and environmental exposures that occur at a crucial time in developing the immune system.

- Innate immunity. Numerous factors may affect the balance between Th1- and Th2-type cytokine responses in early life and increase the likelihood that the immune response will downregulate the Th1 immune response that fights infection and instead will be dominated by Th2 cells, leading to the expression of allergic diseases and asthma. This is known as the hygiene hypothesis, which postulates that certain infections early in life, exposure to other children (e.g., presence of older siblings and early enrollment in child care both offer a greater likelihood of exposure to respiratory infection), less frequent use of antibiotics, and country living are associated with a Th1 response and lower incidence of asthma. In contrast, the absence of these factors is associated with a persistent Th2 response and higher rates of asthma.

- Genetics. Asthma has an inheritable component, but the genetics involved remain complex. As the

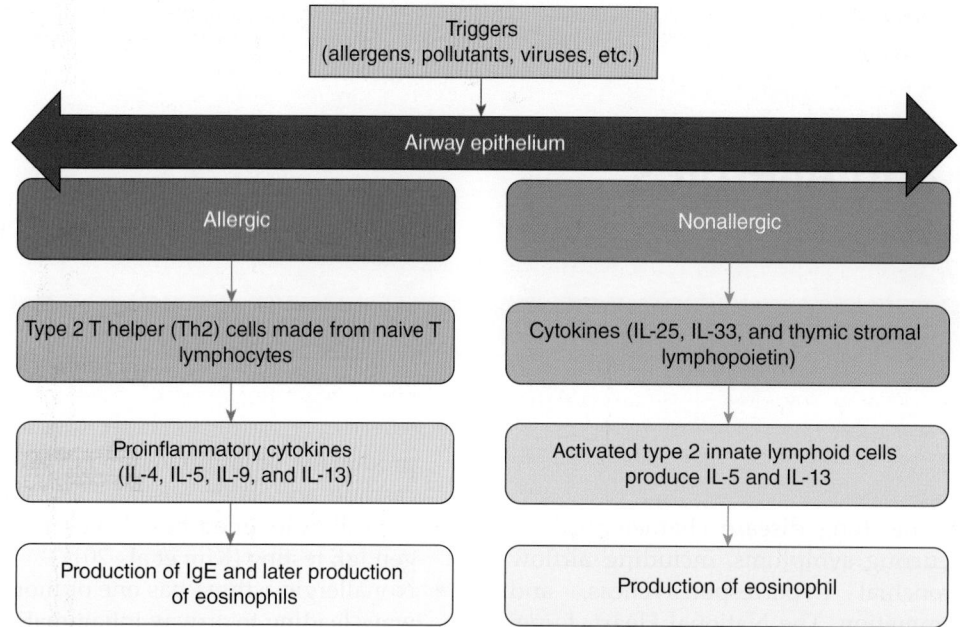

Fig. 7.1 **Asthma pathway.** This explains how exposure to an asthma trigger initiates the onset of symptoms by activation of an immune response. *IgE,* Immunoglobulin E; *IL,* interleukin. (Modified from Kim, H., Ellis, A., Fischer, D., et al. [2017]. Asthma biomarkers in the age of biologics. *Journal of Allergy and Clinical Immunology, 13,* 48.)

linkage of genetic factors to different asthma phenotypes becomes clearer, treatment approaches have become directed to specific patient phenotypes and genotypes.

- Environmental factors. Two factors are important in the development, persistence, and possibly the severity of asthma: airborne allergens (particularly sensitization and exposure to house-dust mites and Alternaria mold) and viral respiratory infections (including respiratory syncytial virus and rhinovirus). Other environmental factors include exposure to tobacco smoke, air pollution (ozone and particulate matter), and diet (NHLBI, 2007).

Asthma symptoms are the result of exposure to a trigger that leads to a cascade of physiologic changes creating the acute inflammatory episode that leads to symptoms of an asthma exacerbation: cough, wheeze, chest tightness, and shortness of breath. An acute asthma episode is initiated by at least one of two types of offending triggers: (1) inflammatory triggers (e.g., allergens, chemical sensitizers, viral infections) or (2) irritants (e.g., particulates in the air, smoke, cold air, exercise). Inflammatory triggers cause symptoms from an IgE-dependent release of mediators, increasing the frequency and severity of airway smooth muscle contraction and enhancing airway hyperresponsiveness through inflammatory mechanisms. Noninflammatory triggers and irritants cause a bronchospastic response that narrows the airways and may become more severe if there is already elevated responsiveness or chronic inflammation (Fig. 7.2).

An asthma trigger can cause an immediate, late, or mixed response. Initial exposure causes a reaction

ASTHMA

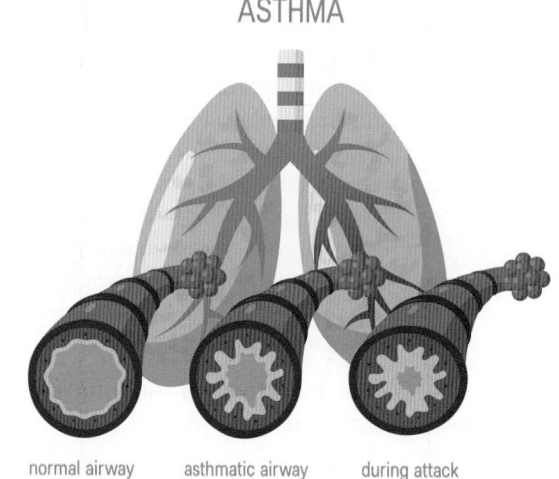

normal airway   asthmatic airway   during attack

Fig. 7.2 **Illustration of the normal airway, asthmatic airway, and an asthmatic airway during an attack.** (From OPHEA. [2023]. Creating asthma friendly environments. https://www.asthmafriendly.ca/home/about-asthma.)

within 10 to 20 minutes. The allergen/antigen binds to the allergen-specific IgE surface, causing activation of resident airway mast cells and macrophages. Proinflammatory mediators such as histamine and leukotrienes are released. These provoke contraction of the airway's smooth muscles, increased secretion of mucus, and vasodilation.

Consequently, microvascular leakage and exudation of plasma into the airway walls cause them to become thickened and edematous with subsequent airway lumen constriction. Additionally, plasma may pass through the epithelial layer to collect in the airway lumen itself, causing further problems in removing mucus and increasing airflow obstruction. This early response is therapeutically addressed through bronchodilation with short-acting beta-agonist (SABA) medications.

Subsequently, occurring up to a few hours later, the inflammatory response predominates. Recruitment, release into circulation, and activation of CD4+ T cells, eosinophils, neutrophils, basophils, prostaglandins, and other macrophages by the initial early-phase stimulation mediator release cause further airway wall inflammation and bronchospasm. Treatment for this process not only involves smooth muscle relaxation through SABA or long-acting beta$_2$-agonists (LABA) but also requires acute and long-term control with routine antiinflammatory medication. An ongoing cycle of proinflammatory mediator release leads to further cell activation, recruitment, and ultimately a cycle of persistently inflamed airways and bronchial hyperreactivity (Ratcliffe & Kieckhefer, 2010).

INCIDENCE AND PREVALENCE

Asthma is the most common noncommunicable childhood disease affecting approximately 14% of children globally and 8.6% of children in the United States. Furthermore, asthma accounts for more than 14 million missed school days per year and costs billions of dollars in health care utilization (Naja et al., 2018). It is one of the three leading causes of hospitalizations in children. In 2017, asthma resulted in an estimated 1.6 million emergency department (ED) visits and 183,000 hospitalizations in the United States (Pate et al., 2021).

The Centers for Disease Control and Prevention (CDC) analyzed asthma data from 2001 to 2016 collected through the National Health Interview Survey for children age 0 to 17 years to examine trends and demographic differences in health outcomes and health care use. The report found asthma was more prevalent among males (9.2%) than females (7.4%) and children age 5 years and older (~10%) than children less than 5 years of age (3.8%). Ethnic and racial differences were noted, with non-Hispanic Black children (15.7%) and children of Puerto Rican descent (12.9%) having a higher prevalence than among non-Hispanic White children (7.1%). Socioeconomic status also plays a factor with a higher prevalence in children living in low-income families (10.5%) than among those living in families with income at or above 250% of the federal poverty level (~7%). Asthma prevalence among children increased from 8.7% in 2001 to 9.4% in 2010 and then decreased to 8.3% in 2016 (Zahran, 2018).

Among children with asthma, the percentage who had an asthma attack in the past 12 months declined significantly from 2001 to 2016. Whereas asthma prevalence was lower among children age 0 to 4 years than among older children, the prevalence of asthma attacks (62.4%), ED/urgent care center (ED/UCC) visits (31.1%), and hospitalization (10.4%) was higher among children with asthma age 0 to 4 years than among those age 12 to 17 years (44.8%, 9.6%, and 2.8%, respectively) (Zahran, 2018). During 2016 to 2018, approximately 46% of the US population with current asthma reported having had one or more asthma attacks in the past 12 months, with 53% reported in children age 0 to 17 years (Pate et al., 2021). During the same 2-year period, approximately 11.9% (11.1–12.7%) of the US population with current asthma reported having one or more ED/UCC visits because of asthma within the past 12 months. Almost twice as many children with asthma reported ED/UCC visits (17.9%) than did adults (10.1%) (Pate et al., 2021). During 2016 to 2018, the asthma mortality rate was 10.8 per million among all ages, with a rate of 2.7 per million children reported (Pate et al., 2021).

DIAGNOSTIC CRITERIA

The diagnosis of asthma in children can be challenging as testing may be difficult to accurately perform in young children, and for some children testing may not show changes in lung function despite the clinical history.

Key points in the diagnosis of asthma are recommended by the NHLBI (2007) report:
- To establish a diagnosis of asthma, the clinician should determine the following:
  1. Episodic symptoms of airflow obstruction or airway hyperresponsiveness are present.
  2. Airflow obstruction is at least partially reversible.
  3. Alternative diagnoses are excluded.
- Recommended methods to establish the diagnosis are as follows:
  1. Detailed medical history
  2. Physical exam focusing on the upper respiratory tract, chest, and skin
  3. Spirometry to demonstrate obstruction and assess reversibility, including in children 5 years of age or older; reversibility (improvement) is determined either by an increase in forced expiratory volume in 1 second (FEV$_1$) of 12% or greater from baseline or by an increase of 10% or greater of predicted FEV$_1$ after inhalation of a short-acting bronchodilator
  4. Additional studies as necessary to exclude alternate diagnoses

When assessing the diagnosis of asthma, clinical history will be of utmost importance. Some important questions to ask during the history include:
- What are your child's symptoms (e.g., cough, wheeze, chest tightness, shortness of breath)?
- Do symptoms occur daily or in episodes due to a trigger? (This would include frequency and duration of symptoms and timing in the day [daytime, nighttime, or both].)
- What are your child's precipitating or aggravating factors (e.g., illness, exercise, emotions, strong smells, allergen exposure)?
- What medications were previously used to treat symptoms? What were the responses to those medications?

- Have there been hospitalizations or ED/UCC visits for treatment?
- Is there a family history of asthma?
- Is there a personal history of atopic disease?
- Does the child's home environment include pets, carpeting, and/or smoke exposure? What type of heating and cooling systems are in the home? What cleaning products are used and how often?

In infants and children younger than 4 years, asthma diagnosis is particularly difficult because of the lack of objective parameters. The need for chronic treatment is recommended in the following instances:

- Four or more episodes of wheezing in the past 12 months that lasted longer than 1 day and affected sleep
- Require SABA more than 2 days per week for 4 weeks
- Experienced two exacerbations that required oral corticosteroids within 6 months
- Elimination of other possible diagnoses and causes of similar (asthma-like) symptoms (NHLBI, 2007)

It is important to discern if dry skin patches with evidence of eczema are present or if there is a family history of asthma or atopy because these conditions heighten the suspicion of allergies and asthma in all children. Other conditions that prompt consideration of asthma include a history of recurrent pneumonia, recurrent croup with wheezing, frequent sinus infections, and posttussive emesis with chronic cough. In older children and teenagers, decreased ability to exercise with a complaint of shortness of breath, chest pain or pressure, and history of coughing or wheezing about 10 or 15 minutes after starting or completing exercise is indicative of exercise-induced bronchospasms (EIB) (Ratcliffe & Kieckhefer, 2010).

Diagnosis of EIB can be attempted with an exercise challenge resulting in a subsequent 15% decrease in FEV_1 before and after exercise at 5-minute intervals over 20 to 30 minutes of activity. Cold air challenge is also used to clarify this diagnosis and is generally conducted in a specialty center (NHLBI, 2007).

SYMPTOMS OF ASTHMA

Asthma symptoms can occur intermittently, episodically, or be persistent (chronic). Intermittent symptoms will occur when in the presence of a trigger and quickly resolve with SABA. Episodic symptoms will occur with illness or prolonged exposure to a trigger, such as staying in a home with a cat when a child is sensitized to cat dander. As directed by the asthma action plan, treatment will help resolve these symptoms, and removing inciting triggers or illness will also help resolve episodic symptoms. There can also be a seasonal pattern of symptoms when airborne allergens trigger exacerbations, such as during the spring when tree pollen is present and during fall when mold and ragweed can be prevalent. A return to school usually

| Box 7.1 | Asthma Symptoms |

ACUTE SYMPTOMS
- Cough
- Wheezing
- Chest tightness
- Prolonged expiratory phase
- Tachypnea
- Retractions, use of accessory muscles, and nasal flaring
- Agitation or altered mental state
- Hyperinflation, increased anterior-posterior diameter on x-ray (although radiography is not needed for the diagnosis of asthma or an acute exacerbation)

CHRONIC SYMPTOMS
- Chronic cough, especially at night
- Prolonged cough with colds and triggers
- Wheeze, although this may only be present with acute episodes or activity
- Shortness of breath with exercise
- Recurrent pneumonia, bronchitis, or sinusitis
- Seasonal pattern of symptoms
- Response to beta-agonist therapy

heralds further environmental exposures leading to exacerbations, especially since it coincides with the fall virus season.

Chronic or persistent symptoms occur 2 or more days/nights per week, indicating that asthma is not controlled. A visit with a primary care provider or asthma specialist is warranted to adjust the asthma action plan to gain control. It is also helpful to plan a return visit just before the child's problematic season to review the asthma action plan (Box 7.1).

TREATMENT

The current asthma treatment reflects the understanding that airway inflammation is predominant. The goals of asthma management are to optimize the control of asthma symptoms, decrease the risk of asthma exacerbations, and minimize the adverse effects of medications. Each therapy must be individualized to that patient. It is imperative to control underlying inflammation with long-term controllers. The goal of treatment is that each person should be able to participate in work, school, play, and sports without any limitations due to breathing. The hope of preventing airway remodeling and preserving the child's pulmonary function by treating airway hyperreactivity and inflammation through appropriate and timely anti-inflammatory treatment drives the current controller treatment regimens (NHLBI, 2007). Treat bronchoconstriction with short-acting rescue medication. Asthma is a chronic condition and can be successfully controlled with lifelong learning and family participation with the help of a health care provider. There are four essential components of asthma management: patient education, control of asthma triggers, monitoring for changes in symptoms or lung function, and pharmacologic therapy.

NHLBI Guidelines for Diagnosis and Management

The primary goal of treatment is to allow the child to live as normal a life as possible with as close to normal lung function as possible. The child should be able to participate in regular childhood activities, experience exercises of tolerance similar to peers, and attend school to grow intellectually and develop socially. The current Guidelines for the Diagnosis and Management of Asthma articulate best evidence-based practices and incorporate expert opinion to translate research findings into clinical practice (NHLBI, 2007; National Asthma Education and Prevention Program [NAEPP], 2020). This document provides a framework to guide clinical decision making by the primary care provider and serves as the basis for recommendations advocated in this chapter. Because knowledge is rapidly expanding, providers must regularly review updated online reports on best practices, evidence-based management strategies from the NHLBI Information Center (www.nhlbi.nih.gov), and other relevant professional

organizations such as the American Academy of Pediatrics (AAP; www.aap.org) and National Association of Pediatric Nurse Practitioners (www.napnap.org) (Ratcliffe & Kieckhefer, 2010).

Asthma severity is determined before initiating therapy. It is divided into intermittent, mild persistent, moderate persistent, and severe persistent levels with respect to frequency and timing of symptoms, interference with daily activities, objective parameters from pulmonary function testing, and the need for short-acting relief medications. Asthma severity is classified based on the most severe level of symptoms or impairment. If already on asthma therapy, severity is ascertained or inferred by the type of medications needed to maintain control (Fig. 7.3). Once treatment has started, asthma control is evaluated based on the level of impairment and risk when on a daily regimen. Risk and impairment influence the foundation of assessment of severity and management of asthma for subsequent ongoing treatment (Ratcliffe & Kieckhefer, 2010).

Since asthma is a chronic condition with episodic symptoms, asthma management entails treatment

Classifying asthma severity and initiating therapy in children

Key: FEV_1, forced expiratory volume in 1 second; FVC, forced vital capacity; ICS, inhaled corticosteroids; ICU, intensive care unit; N/A, not applicable

Notes:
- Level of severity is determined by both impairment and risk. Assess impairment domain by caregiver's recall of previous 2–4 weeks. Assign severity to the most severe category in which any feature occurs.
- Frequency and severity of exacerbations may fluctuate over time for patients in any severity category. At present, there are inadequate data to correspond frequencies of exacerbations with different levels of asthma severity. In general, more frequent and severe exacerbations (e.g., requiring urgent, unscheduled care, hospitalization, or ICU admission) indicate greater underlying disease severity. For treatment purposes, patients with ≥2 exacerbations described above may be considered the same as patients who have persistent asthma, even in the absence of impairment levels consistent with persistent asthma.

Components of severity		Intermittent		Persistent					
				Mild		Moderate		Severe	
		Ages 0–4	Ages 5–11	Ages 0–4	Ages 5–11	Ages 0–4	Ages 5–11	Ages 0–4	Ages 5–11
Impairment	Symptoms	≤2 days/week		>2 days/week but not daily		Daily		Throughout the day	
	Nighttime awakenings	0	≤2x/month	1–2x/month	3–4x/month	3–4x/month	>1x/week but not nightly	>1x/week	Often 7x/week
	Short-acting beta₂-agonist use for symptom control	≤2 days/week		>2 days/week but not daily		Daily		Several times per day	
	Interference with normal activity	None		Minor limitation		Some limitation		Extremely limited	
	Lung Function • FEV_1 (predicted) or peak flow (personal best) • FEV_1/FVC	N/A	Normal FEV_1 between exacerbations >80% >85%	N/A	>80% >80%	N/A	60–80% 75–80%	N/A	<60% <75%
Risk	Exacerbations requiring oral systemic corticosteroids (consider severity and interval since last exacerbation)	0–1/year (see notes)		≥2 exacerbations in 6 months requiring oral systemic corticosteroids, or ≥4 wheezing episodes/1 year lasting > 1 day AND risk factors for persistent asthma	≥2x/year (see notes) Relative annual risk may be related to FEV_1		→		→
Recommended step for Initiating Therapy (See "Stepwise Approach for Managing Asthma" for treatment steps.) The stepwise approach is meant to assist, not replace, the clinical decisionmaking required to meet individual patient needs.		Step 1 (for both age groups)		Step 2 (for both age groups)		Step 3 and consider short course of oral systemic corticosteroids	Step 3: medium-dose ICS option and consider short course of oral systemic corticosteroids	Step 3 and consider short course of oral systemic corticosteroids	Step 3: medium-dose ICS option OR step 4 and consider short course of oral systemic corticosteroids
		In 2–6 weeks, depending on severity, evaluate level of asthma control that is achieved. • Children 0–4 years old: If no clear benefit is observed in 4–6 weeks, stop treatment and consider alternative diagnoses or adjusting therapy. • Children 5–11 years old: Adjust therapy accordingly.							

Fig. 7.3 Classification of asthma and therapy to use in children and adults. (From National Heart, Lung, and Blood Institute [NHLBI]. [2007]. *Expert panel report 3: Guidelines for the diagnosis and management of asthma.* National Institutes of Health.)

Classifying asthma severity and initiating treatment in youths 12 years of age and adults

Assessing severity and initiating treatment for patients who are not currently taking long-term control medications

Components of severity		Classification of asthma severity ≥12 years of age			
		Intermittent	Persistent		
			Mild	Moderate	Severe
Impairment Normal FEV₁/FVC: 8-19 yr 85% 20-39 yr 80% 40-59 yr 75% 60-80 yr 70%	Symptoms	≤2 days/week	>2 days/week but not daily	Daily	Throughout the day
	Nighttime awakenings	≤2x/month	3–4x/month	>1x/week but not nightly	Often 7x/week
	Short-acting beta₂-agonist use for symptom control (not prevention of EIB)	≤2 days/week	>2 days/week but not daily, and not more than 1x on any day	Daily	Several times per day
	Interference with normal activity	None	Minor limitation	Some limitation	Extremely limited
	Lung function	• Normal FEV₁ between exacerbations • FEV₁ >80% predicted • FEV₁/FVC normal	• FEV₁ >80% predicted • FEV₁/FVC normal	• FEV₁ >60% but <80% predicted • FEV₁/FVC reduced 5%	• FEV₁ <60% predicted • FEV₁/FVC reduced >5%
Risk	Exacerbations requiring oral systemic corticosteroids	0–1/year (see note)	≥2/year (see note) → ← Consider severity and interval since last exacerbation. Frequency and severity may fluctuate over time for patients in any severity category. → Relative annual risk of exacerbations may be related to FEV₁.		
Recommended step for Initiating treatment (See "Stepwise approach for managing asthma" for treatment steps.)		Step 1	Step 2	Step 3	Step 4 or 5 and consider short course of oral systemic corticosteroids
		In 2–6 weeks, evaluate level of asthma control that is achieved and adjust therapy accordingly.			

Key: EIB, exercise-induced bronchospasm; FEV1, forced expiratory volume in 1 second; FVC, forced vital capacity; ICU, intensive care unit

Notes:
- The stepwise approach is meant to assist, not replace, the clinical decisionmaking required to meet invidual patient needs.
- Level of severity is determined by assessment of both impairment and risk. Assess impairment domain by patient's/caregiver's recall of previous 2–4 weeks and spirometry. Assign severity to the most severe category in which any feature occurs.
- At present, there are inadequate data to correspond frequencies of exacerbations with different levels of asthma severity. In general, more frequent and intense exacerbations (e.g., requiring urgent, unscheduled care, hospitalization. or ICU admission) indicate greater underlying disease severity. For treatment purposes. patients who had ≥2 exacerbations requiring oral systemic corticosteroids in the past year may be considered the same as patients who have persistent asthma. even in the absence of impairment levels consistent with persistent asthma.

Assessing asthma control and adjusting therapy in youths ≥12 years of age and adults

Components of control		Classification of asthma control (≥12 years of age)		
		Well controlled	Not well controlled	Very poorly controlled
Impairment	Symptoms	≤2 days/week	>2 days/week	Throughout the day
	Nighttime awakenings	≤2x/month	1–3x/week	≥4x/week
	Interference with normal activity	None	Some limitation	Extremely limited
	Short-acting beta₂-agonist use for symptom control (not prevention of EIB)	≤2 days/week	>2 days/week	Several times per day
	FEV₁ or peak flow	>80% predicted/personal best	60–80% predicted/personal best	<60% predicted/personal best
	Validated questionnaires ATAQ ACQ ACT	0 ≤0.75* ≥20	1–2 ≥1.5 16–19	3–4 N/A ≤15
Risk	Exacerbations requiring oral systemic corticosteroids	0–1/year	≥2/year (see note)	
		Consider severity and interval since last exacerbation		
	Progressive loss of lung function	Evaluation requires long-term followup care.		
	Treatment-related adverse effects	Medication side effects can vary in intensity from none to very troublesome and worrisome. The level of intensity does not correlate to specific levels of control but should be considered in the overall assessment of risk.		
Recommended action for treatment (See "Stepwise approach for managing asthma" for treatment steps.)		• Maintain current step. • Regular followup at every 1–6 months to maintain control. • Consider step down if well controlled for at least 3 months.	• Step up 1 step. • Reevaluate in 2–6 weeks. • For side effects, consider alternative treatment options.	• Consider short course of oral systemic corticosteroids. • Step up 1–2 steps. • Reevaluate in 2 weeks. • For side effects, consider alternative treatment options.

*ACQ values of 0.76–1.4 are indeterminate regarding well-controlled asthma.
Key: EIB, exercise-induced bronchospasm; ICU, intensive care unit

Notes:
- The stepwise approach is meant to assist, not replace, the clinical decisionmaking required to meet individual patient needs.
- The level of control is based on the most severe impairment of risk category. Assess impairment domain by patient's recall of previous 2–4 weeks and by spirometry/or peak flow measures. Symptom assessment for longer periods should reflect a global assessment, such as inquiring whether the patient's asthma is better or worse since the last visit.
- At present, there are inadequate data to correspond frequencies of exacerbations with different levels of asthma control. In general, more frequent and intense exacerbations (e.g., requiring urgent, unscheduled care, hospitalization, or ICU admission) indicate poorer disease control. For treatment purposes, patients who had ≥2 exacerbations requiring oral systemic corticosteroids in the past year may be considered the same as patients who have not-well-controlled asthma, even in the absence of impairment levels consistent with not-well-controlled asthma.
  ATAQ = Asthma Therapy Assessment Questionnaire°
  ACQ = Asthma Control Questionnaire°
  ACT = Asthma Control Test™
  Minimal Important Difference: 1.0 for the ATAQ; 0.5 for the ACQ; not determined for the ACT.

Before step up in therapy:

– Review adherence to medication, inhaler technique, environmental control, and comorbid conditions.

– If an alternative treatment option was used in a step, discontinue and use the preferred treatment for that step.

Fig. 7.3 Cont'd

based on the needs or severity of the child's underlying airway pathology, seasonal changes, and growth and development (Fig. 7.4). It requires the provider to either step up treatment if asthma symptoms emerge and remain uncontrolled or step down treatment after control has been achieved. Step-down therapy is advocated if the child's asthma has been under control for at least 3 months, reducing the inhaled corticosteroid (ICS) dose by 25% to 50% at a time to the lowest possible dose while maintaining control (NHLBI, 2007). Specific questions about day/nighttime symptoms versus global perceptions are needed to accurately assess asthma control, asking for both the parent's and child's perceptions (Ratcliffe & Kieckhefer, 2010).

Ages 0–4 years: Stepwise approach for management of asthma

Treatment	Intermittent asthma	Management of persistent asthma in individuals ages 0–4 years				
	Step 1	Step 2	Step 3	Step 4	Step 5	Step 6
Preferred	PRN SABA and At the start of RTI: Add short course daily ICS▲	Daily low-dose ICS and PRN SABA	Daily medium-dose ICS and PRN SABA	Daily medium-dose ICS-LABA and PRN SABA	Daily high-dose ICS-LABA and PRN SABA	Daily high-dose ICS-LABA + oral systemic corticosteroid and PRN SABA
Alternative		Daily montelukast* or Cromolyn,* and PRN SABA		Daily medium-dose ICS + montelukast* and PRN SABA	Daily high-dose ICS + montelukast* and PRN SABA	Daily high-dose ICS + montelukast*+ oral systemic corticosteroid and PRN SABA

For children age 4 years only. see Step 3 and Step 4 on Management of Persistent Asthma in Individuals Ages 5–11 Years diagram.

Assess control

- First check adherence, inhaler technique, environmental factors, ▲and comorbid conditions.
- **Step up** if needed; reassess in 4-6 weeks
- **Step down** if possible (if asthma is well controlled for at least 3 consecutive months)

Consult with asthma specialist if Step 3 or higher is required. Consider consultation at Step 2.

Control assessment is a key element of asthma care. This involves both impairment and risk. Use of objective measures, self-reported control, and health care utilization are complementary and should be employed on an ongoing basis, depending on the individual's clinical situation.

Abbreviations: ICS, inhaled corticosteroid; LABA, long-acting beta$_2$-agonist; SABA, inhaled short-acting beta$_2$-agonist; RTI, respiratory tract infection; PRN, as needed
▲Updated based on the 2020 guidelines.
* Cromolyn and montelukast were not considered for this update and/or have limited availability for use in the United States. The FDA issued a Boxed Warning for montelukast in March 2020.

Fig. 7.4 Stepwise approach to asthma management. (From Expert Panel Working Group of the National Heart, Lung, and Blood Institute (2020). 2020 focused updates to the asthma management guidelines: a report from the National Asthma Education and Prevention Program Coordinating Committee Expert Panel Working Group. *J Allergy Clin Immunol 146*(6), 1217–1270.

Asthma Action Plan

All children with asthma need a written action plan to be implemented in times of exacerbation and to describe the chronic management of their disease (Fig. 7.5). Children with even mild asthma may have a severe exacerbation that requires an emergency action plan in addition to a written daily management plan. The emergency action plan reduces the severity and length of the exacerbation and often prevents the need for emergent medical care (NHLBI, 2007).

The daily management plan provides a strategy to control underlying inflammation/daily symptoms and prevent exacerbations while allowing the child's caretakers or the child to plan for any contingency. For example, a written plan for everyday management may include morning and evening controller medications per metered-dose inhaler (MDI) with a spacer. An action plan to implement during exacerbation might additionally include the following:

- Begin or increase rescue SABA medication up to every 4 hours at home.

- Start oral steroid burst at the prescribed dose if symptoms are not improved or are getting worse after taking SABA.

Notify the primary care provider within 24 hours if starting oral steroids.

If symptoms do not respond to home management, the child needs further evaluation and treatment in a primary care provider's office if appropriate monitoring and treatment equipment are available there or in an ED or hospital setting. These settings offer the ability to monitor the child's breath sounds and air movement, work of breathing, oxygenation, and blood gases; administer oxygen as needed; perform spirometry; continuously monitor cardiac and respiratory status; and give medications frequently in a controlled environment (Ratcliffe & Kieckhefer, 2010).

Pharmacologic Therapy

Quick relief or rescue medications. The first medication for an acute exacerbation is a quick reliever (i.e., SABA). This inhaler will inhibit the early

Notes for individuals ages 0–4 years diagram

Quick-relief medications	• Use SABA as needed for symptoms. The intensity of treatment depends on severity of symptoms: up to 3 treatments at 20-minute intervals as needed. • **Caution:** Increasing use of SABA or use >2 days a week for symptom relief (not prevention of EIB) generally indicates inadequate control and may require a step up in treatment. • Consider short course of oral systemic corticosteroid if exacerbation is severe or individual has history of previous severe exacerbations.
Each step: Assess environmental factors, provide patient education, and manage comorbidities▲	• In individuals with sensitization (or symptoms) related to exposure to pests‡: conditionally recommend integrated pest management as a single or multicomponent allergen-specific mitigation intervention. ▲ • In individuals with sensitization (or symptoms) related to exposure to identified indoor allergens, conditionally recommend a multi-component allergen-specific mitigation strategy. ▲ • In individuals with sensitization (or symptoms) related to exposure to dust mites. conditionally recommend impermeable pillow/mattress covers only as part of a multicomponent allergen-specific mitigation intervention, but not as a single component intervention. ▲
Notes	• If clear benefit is not observed within 4-6 weeks and the medication technique and adherence are satisfactory. the clinician should consider adjusting therapy or alternative diagnoses.
Abbreviations	EIB, exercise-induced bronchoconstriction; SABA, inhaled short-acting beta$_2$-agonist. ▲Updated based on the 2020 guidelines. ‡ Refers to mice and cockroaches, which were specifically examined in the Agency for Healthcare Research and Quality systematic review.

Notes for individuals ages 5–11 years diagram

Quick-relief medications	• Use SABA as needed for symptoms. The intensity of treatment depends on severity of symptoms: up to 3 treatments at 20-minute intervals as needed. • In Steps 3 and 4, the preferred option includes the use of ICS-formoterol 1 to 2 puffs as needed up to a maximum total daily maintenance and rescue dose of 8 puffs (36 mcg). ▲ • **Caution:** Increasing use of SABA or use >2 days a week for symptom relief (not prevention of EIB) generally indicates inadequate control and may require a step up in treatment.
Each step: Assess environmental factors, provide patient education, and manage comorbidities▲	• In individuals with sensitization (or symptoms) related to exposure to pests‡ conditionally recommend integrated pest management as a single or multicomponent allergen-specific mitigation intervention. ▲ • In individuals with sensitization (or symptoms) related to exposure to identified indoor allergens, conditionally recommend a multi-component allergen-specific mitigation strategy.▲ • In individuals with sensitization (or symptoms) related to exposure to dust mites. conditionally recommend impermeable pillow/mattress covers only as part of a muticomponent allergen-specific mitigation intervention, but not as a single component intervention.▲
Notes	• The terms ICS-LABA and ICS-formoterol indicate combination therapy with both an ICS and a LABA. usually and preferably in a single inhaler. • Where formoterol is specified in the steps, it is because the evidence is based on studies specific to formoterol. • In individuals ages 5–11 years with persistent allergic asthma in which there is uncertainty in choosing, monitoring, or adjusting anti-inflammatory therapies based on history, clinical findings, and spirometry, FeNO measurement is conditionally recommended as part of an ongoing asthma monitoring and management strategy that includes frequent assessment.
Abbreviations	EIB (exercise-induced bronchoconstriction): FeNO (fractional exhaled nitric oxide): ICS (inhaled corticosteroid); LABA (long-acting beta$_2$-agonist); SABA (inhaled short-acting beta$_2$-agonist). ▲Updated based on the 2020 guidelines. ‡ Refers to mice and cockroaches, which were specifically examined in the Agency for Healthcare Research and Quality systematic review.

Fig. 7.4 Cont'd

Treatment	Intermittent asthma	Management of persistent asthma in individuals ages 12+ years				
	Step 1	Step 2	Step 3	Step 4	Step 5	Step 6
Preferred	PRN SABA	Daily low-dose ICS and PRN SABA or PRN concomitant ICS and SABA▲	Daily and PRN combination low-dose ICS-formoterol▲	Daily and PRN combination medium-dose ICS-formoterol ▲	Daily medium-high dose ICS-LABA + LAMA and PRN SABA▲	Daily high-dose ICS-LABA + oral systemic corticosteroids + PRN SABA
Alternative		Daily LTRA* and PRN SABA or Cromolyn,* or Nedocromil,* or Zileuton,* or Theophylline,* and PRN SABA	Daily medium-dose ICS and PRN SABA or Daily low-dose ICS-LABA, or daily low-dose ICS + LAMA,▲or daily low-dose ICS + LTRA,* and PRN SABA or Daily low-dose ICS + Theophylline* or Zileuton,* and PRN SABA	Daily medium-dose ICS-LABA or daily medium-dose ICS + LAMA, and PRN SABA▲ or Daily medium-dose ICS + LTRA,* or daily medium-dose ICS + Zileuton,* and PRN SABA	Daily medium-high dose ICS-LABA or daily high-dose ICS + LTRA,* and PRN SABA	
		Steps 2–4: Conditionally recommend the use of subcutaneous immunotherapy as an adjunct treatment to standard pharmacotherapy in individuals ≥ 5 years of age whose asthma is controlled at the initiation, build up, and maintenance phases of immunotherapy▲			Consider adding asthma biologics (e.g., anti-IgE, anti-IL5, anti-IL5R, anti-IL4/IL13)**	

Assess control

- First check adherence, inhaler technique, environmental factors, ▲ and comorbid conditions.
- **Step up** if needed: reassess in 2–6 weeks
- **Step down** if possible (if asthma is well controlled for at least 3 consecutive months)

Consult with asthma specialist if Step 4 or higher is required. Consider consultation at Step 3.

Control assessment is a key element of asthma care. This involves both impairment and risk. Use of objective measures. self-reported control, and health care utilization are complementary and should be employed on an ongoing basis, depending on the individual's clinical situation.

Abbreviations: ICS, inhaled corticosteriod; LABA, long-acting beta$_2$-agonist: LAMA, long-acting muscarinic antagonist; LTRA, leukotriene receptor antagonist; SABA, inhaled short-acting beta$_2$-agonist
▲Updated based on the 2020 guidelines
* Cromolyn, Nedocromil, LTRAs including Zileuton and montelukast, and Theophylline were not considered for this update, and/or have limited availability for use in the United States, and/or have an increased risk of adverse consequences and need for monitoring that make their use less desirable. The FDA issued a Boxed Warning for montelukast in March 2020.
** The AHRQ systematic reviews that informed this report did not include studies that examined the role of asthma biologics (e.g., anti-IgE, anti-IL5, anti-IL5R, anti-IL4/IL13). Thus, this report does not contain specific recommendations for the use of biologics in asthma in Steps 5 and 6.
■Data on the use of LAMA therapy in individuals with severe persistent asthma (Step 6) were not included in the AHRQ systematic review and thus no recommendation is made.

Fig. 7.4 Cont'd

Notes for individuals ages 12+ years diagram

Quick-relief medications	• Use SABA as needed for symptoms. The intensity of treatment depends on the severity of symptoms: up to 3 treatments at 20-minute intervals as needed. • In steps 3 and 4, the preferred option includes the use of ICS-formoterol 1 to 2 puffs as needed up to a maximum total daily maintenance and rescue dose of 12 puffs (54 mcg). ▲ • **Caution:** Increasing use of SABA or use >2 days a week for symptom relief (not prevention of EIB) generally indicates inadequate control and may require a step up in treatment.
Each step: Assess environmental factors, provide patient education, and manage comorbidities▲	• In individuals with sensitization (or symptoms) related to exposure to pests‡: conditionally recommend integrated pest management as a single or multicomponent allergen-specific mitigation intervention. ▲ • In individuals with sensitization (or symptoms) related to exposure to identified indoor allergens, conditionally recommend a multi-component allergen-specific mitigation strategy. ▲ • In individuals with sensitization (or symptoms) related to exposure to dust mites, conditionally recommend impermeable pillow/mattress covers only as part of a multicomponent allergen-specific mitigation intervention, but not as a single component intervention.▲
Notes	• The terms ICS-LABA and ICS-formoterol indicate combination therapy with both an ICS and a LABA, usually and preferably in a single inhaler. • Where formoterol is specified in the steps. it is because the evidence is based on studies specific to formoterol. • In individuals ages 12 years and older with persistent allergic asthma in which there is uncertainty in choosing, monitoring, or adjusting anti-inflammatory therapies based on history. clinical findings, and spirometry, FeNO measurement is conditionally recommended as part of an ongoing asthma monitoring and management strategy that includes frequent assessment. • Bronchial thermoplasty was evaluated in Step 6. The outcome was a conditional recommendation against the therapy.
Abbreviations	EIB, exercise-induced bronchoconstriction; FeNO, fractional exhaled nitric oxide; ICS, inhaled corticosteroid; LABA, long-acting beta$_2$-agonist; SABA, inhaled short-acting beta$_2$-agonist. ▲Updated based on the 2020 guidelines. ‡ Refers to mice and cockroaches, which were specifically examined in the Agency for Healthcare Research and Quality systematic review.

Fig. 7.4 Cont'd

bronchospastic response. These beta-agonists may cause tachycardia and tremor of the hands. Parents may also notice hyperactivity, irritability, and sleeplessness. There is an isomer of albuterol, levalbuterol (Xopenex), that may have fewer side effects and can be used in place of albuterol. At times it may be hard to get this medication approved by insurance (Ratcliffe & Kieckhefer, 2010).

Using an air compressor with an updraft nebulizer and aerosol mask to deliver a beta-adrenergic medication is available; however, children and even infants can be treated with MDI by using a spacer/mask with equally effective results. There are also spacers with mouthpieces for older children. The spacer is attached to the MDI and allows the medication to get into the lungs as opposed to getting left on the lips, tongue, or back of the throat when not using a spacer, which leads to a less therapeutic treatment (Fig. 7.6). Dry powder inhalers (DPI) involve inhaling a powder form of the medication. This medication will need the inspiratory effort of at least a 5- to 6-year-old child. The provider must know how to use the proper technique in delivering inhalers, and the office staff must also teach the patient to allow proper medication adherence and management of well-controlled asthma.

Fig. 7.6 compares delivery of medicine with and without an aerochamber.

Inhaled corticosteroids. ICS are called controller or maintenance medications and are the most effective drugs used in asthma to suppress airway inflammation. This occurs mainly by the downregulation of proinflammatory proteins. Corticosteroids seem to reverse components of asthma-induced structural changes (airway remodeling), including the bronchial wall's increased vascularity. ICS can reduce the number of inflammatory cells in the airways, including eosinophils, T lymphocytes, mast cells, and dendritic cells. Epithelial cells may be a major cellular target for ICS, which are the mainstay of modern asthma management (Hossney et al., 2016). The preferred treatment for those with more than intermittent asthma is

Ages 5–11 years: Stepwise approach for management of asthma

	Intermittent asthma	Management of persistent asthma in individuals ages 5–11 years				
Treatment	Step 1	Step 2	Step 3	Step 4	Step 5	Step 6
Preferred	PRN SABA	Daily low-dose ICS and PRN SABA	Daily and PRN combination low-dose ICS-formoterol▲	Daily and PRN combination medium-dose ICS-formoterol▲	Daily high-dose ICS-LABA and PRN SABA	Daily high-dose ICS-LABA + oral systemic corticosteroid and PRN SABA
Alternative		Daily LTRA,* or Cromolyn,* or Nedocromil,* or Theophylline,* and PRN SABA	Daily medium-dose ICS and PRN SABA or Daily low-dose ICS-LABA, or daily low-dose ICS + LTRA,* or daily low-dose ICS +Theophylline,* and PRN SABA	Daily medium-dose ICS-LABA and PRN SABA or Daily medium-dose ICS + LTRA* or daily medium-dose ICS + Theophylline,* and PRN SABA	Daily high-dose ICS + LTRA* or daily high-dose ICS + Theophylline,* and PRN SABA	Daily high-dose ICS + LTRA* + oral systemic corticosteroid or daily high-dose ICS + Theophylline* + oral systemic corticosteroid, and PRN SABA
		Steps 2–4: Conditionally recommend the use of subcutaneous immunotherapy as an adjunct treatment to standard pharmacotherapy in individuals ≥ 5 years of age whose asthma is controlled at the initiation, build up, and maintenance phases of immunotherapy▲			Consider Omalizumab**▲	

Assess control

- First check adherence, inhaler technique, environmental factors, ▲and comorbid conditions.
- **Step up** if needed; reassess in 2–6 weeks
- **Step down** if possible (if asthma is well controlled for at least 3 consecutive months)

Consult with asthma specialist if Step 4 or higher is required. Consider consultation at Step 3.

Control assessment is a key element of asthma care. This involves both impairment and risk. Use of objective measures, self-reported control, and health care utilization are complementary and should be employed on an ongoing basis, depending on the individual's clinical situation.

Abbreviations: ICS, inhaled corticosteroid; LABA, long-acting beta$_2$-agonist; LTRA, leukotriene receptor antagonist; SABA, inhaled short-acting beta$_2$-agonist
▲Updated based on the 2020 guidelines.
* Cromolyn, Nedocromil, LTRAs including montelukast, and Theophylline were not considered in this update and/or have limited availability for use in the United States, and/or have an increased risk of adverse consequences and need for monitoring that make their use less desirable. The FDA issued a Boxed Warning for montelukast in March 2020.
** Omalizumab is the only asthma biologic currently FDA-approved for this age range.

Fig. 7.4 Cont'd

ICS. There are a variety of brands available, such as a hydrofluoroalkane (HFA) inhaler, DPI, or nebulizer solution (Table 7.1).

Even young children can use ICS via MDI with a spacer/mask or nebulizer, thus reducing their need for systemic treatment. Children using a spacer with ICS should rinse their mouth and spit and then wipe the facial area that was covered by the mask after use to prevent the development of thrush. The nebulized medication should be administered via a mask, directing the mist away from the eyes to prevent a theoretical but potential complication of cataract formation (Ratcliffe & Kieckhefer, 2010).

Long-acting beta$_2$-agonists. For the child with moderate or severe persistent asthma whose symptoms remain uncontrolled with ICS, a LABA such as salmeterol (Serevent) or formoterol (Foradil) should be added to the regimen and its effects evaluated (Table 7.2). Currently, pediatric LABA use is only recommended when paired with ICS and is never used as an independent agent for EIB or maintenance asthma therapy. The typical duration is at least 12 hours after a single dose.

SMART therapy. Single maintenance and reliever (SMART) therapy is a treatment option for those 4 years and older with uncontrolled asthma. With this therapy, the patient will use a combination inhaler of ICS-formoterol as both a controller medication and a quick reliever. ICS-formoterol can be administered with 1 to 2 puffs once or twice daily as a maintenance medication, then additional puffs can be used as a quick reliever. The maximum number of puffs is 8 (36 µg formoterol)

Asthma action plan

For: _____ Doctor: _____ Date: _____

Doctor's phone number: _____ Hospital/Emergency department phone number: _____

	Doing well	Daily medications medicine	How much to take	When to take it

GREEN ZONE

Doing well
- No cough, wheeze, chest tightness, or shortness of breath during the day or night
- Can do usual activities

And, if a peak flow meter is used,
Peak flow: more than _____
(80 percent or more of my best peak flow)
My best peak flow is: _____

Daily medications medicine
_____
_____
_____
_____
_____

How much to take
_____
_____
_____
_____

When to take it
_____
_____
_____
_____

Before exercise	☐ _____	☐ 2 or ☐ 4 puffs	5 minutes before exercise

YELLOW ZONE

Asthma is getting worse
- Cough, wheeze, chest tightness, or shortness of breath, or
- Waking at night due to asthma, or
- Can do some, but not all, usual activities

–Or–

Peak flow: _____ to _____
(50 to 79 percent of my best peak flow)

1st ➤ **Add: quick-relief medicine—and keep taking your GREEN ZONE medicine.**

_____ _____ Number of puffs   Can repeat every _____ minutes
(quick-relief medicine)   or ☐ Nebulizer, once   up to maximum of _____ doses

2nd ➤ **If your symptoms (and peak flow, if used) return to GREEN ZONE after 1 hour of above treatment:**
☐ Continue monitoring to be sure you stay in the green zone.
   –Or–
If your symptoms (and peak flow, if used) do not return to GREEN ZONE after 1 hour of above treatment:
☐ Take: _____ _____ Number of puffs   or ☐ Nebulizer
   (quick-relief medicine)
☐ Add: _____ mg per day   For _____ (3–10) days
   (oral steroid)
☐ Call the doctor ☐ before/ ☐ within_____ hours after taking the oral steroid.

RED ZONE

Medical alert!
- Very short of breath, or
- Quick-relief medicines have not helped,
- Cannot do usual activities, or
- Symptoms are same or get worse after 24 hours in Yellow Zone

–Or–

Peak flow: less than _____
(50 percent of my best peak flow)

Take this medicine:
☐ _____ _____ Number of puffs   or ☐ Nebulizer
   (quick-relief medicine)
☐ _____ mg
   (oral steroid)

Then call your doctor NOW. Go to the hospital or call an ambulance if:
- You are still in the red zone after 15 minutes AND
- You have not reached your doctor.

Danger signs	• Trouble walking and talking due to shortness of breath	➤	• Take _____ puffs of _____ (quick relief medicine) AND
	• Lips or fingernails are blue		• Go to the hospital or call for an ambulance _____ NOW! (phone)

See the reverse side for things you can do to avoid your asthma triggers.

Fig. 7.5 Example of an asthma action plan (AAP). All patients should have an AAP at home to help with the daily management of asthma and steps to take when asthma is flared. (From: National Heart Lung and Blood Institute (NHLB). Retrieved May 11, 2022, from https://www.nhlbi.nih.gov/resources/asthma-action-plan-2020.)

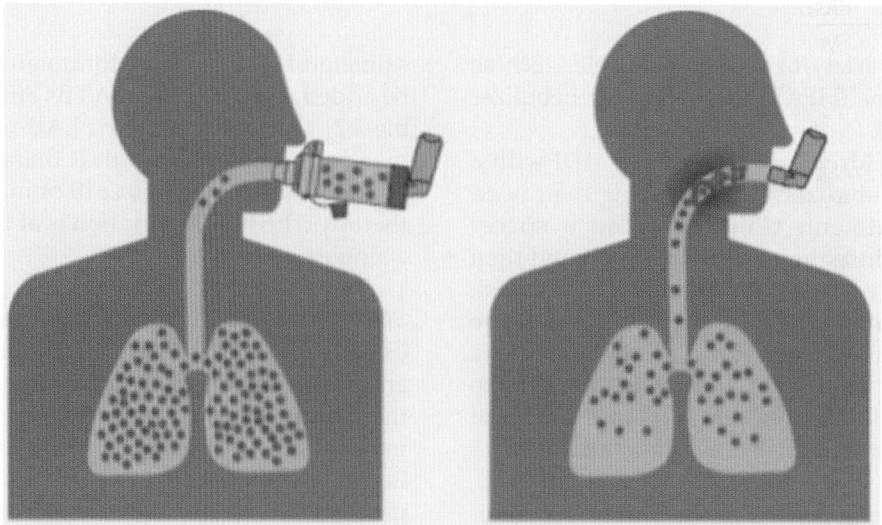

Fig. 7.6 Comparison between deposition of medicine with the use of an aerochamber for delivery *(left)* and inhalers without an aerochamber *(right).* (Copyright Trudell Medical International.)

Table 7.1 List of Inhaled Corticosteroid Inhalers

GENERIC NAME	BRAND NAME	STRENGTHS	RECOMMENDED AGES	DOSAGE
Beclomethasone dipropionate	Qvar RediHaler	40 µg 80 µg	4–11 yr ≥12 yr	1–2 puffs twice a day 1–2 puffs twice a day of 40 or 80 µg
Budesonide	Pulmicort Flexhaler	90 µg 180 µg	6–17 yr ≥18 yr	180 µg twice a day (360 µg max) 360 µg twice a day (720 µg twice a day max)
Budesonide	Pulmicort Respules	0.25 mg/2 mL 0.5 mg/2 mL 1 mg/2 mL	12 mo–8 yr	0.5–1 mg once a day or in divided doses
Ciclesonide	Alvesco	80 µg 160 µg	≥12 yr	80 or 160 µg 1 puff twice a day
Fluticasone furoate	Arnuity Ellipta inhalation powder	50 µg 100 µg 200 µg	5–11 yr ≥12 yr	50 µg once daily 100 or 200 µg once daily
Fluticasone propionate	Flovent Flovent Diskus	44 µg 110 µg 220 µg 50 µg 100 µg 250 µg	≥4 yr	Dosing will vary: 1–2 puffs twice a day 1 puff 1–2 times a day Dosing will be adjusted based on asthma control
Fluticasone propionate	ArmonAir RespiClick	55 µg 113 µg 232 µg ArmonAir Digihaler (connects with a companion mobile application)	≥12 yr	1 puff twice a day
Mometasone	Asmanex Twisthaler	110 µg 220 µg	4–11 yr ≥12 yr	1 puff daily 1–4 puffs daily
Mometasone furoate	Asmanex inhaler	100 µg 200 µg	≥12 yr	1–2 puffs twice daily

Modified from the American Academy of Allergy, Asthma & Immunology (AAAAI) (2020b). Visit https://www.aaaai.org/tools-for-the-public/drug-guide/inhaled-corticosteroids/ for additional information and updates.

Table 7.2 List of Combination Inhalers (ICS + LABA)

GENERIC NAME	BRAND NAME	STRENGTHS	RECOMMENDED AGES	DOSAGE
Budesonide-formoterol	Symbicort	80 µg/4.5 160 µg/4.5	≥12 yr	2 puffs twice a day
Fluticasone furoate–vilanterol	Breo Ellipta	100 µg/25 200 µg/25	≥18 yr	1 puff daily
Fluticasone-salmeterol	Advair Diskus Advair HFA	100/50 250/50 500/50	4–11yr ≥12 yr can use any strength	1 puff twice daily
Fluticasone propionate–salmeterol	AirDuo RespiClick AirDuo DigiHaler (connects with a companion mobile application)	55/14 113/14 232/14	≥12 yr	1 puff twice a day
Fluticasone propionate–salmeterol	Wixela Inhub inhalation powder	100/50 250/50 500/50	4–11 yr ≥12 yr can use any strength	1 inhalation twice a day
Mometasone-formoterol	Dulera	50/5 100/5 200/5	5–11 yr ≥12 yr use 100 or 200 µg strength	2 puffs twice a day

ICS, Inhaled corticosteroids; LABA, long-acting beta2-agonist. Modified from the American Academy of Allergy, Asthma & Immunology (AAAAI) (2020c). Visit https://www.aaaai.org/tools-for-the-public/drug-guide/long-acting-beta-agonists-(labas) for additional information and updates.

for children ages 4 to 11 years and 12 (54 µg formoterol) for those over age 12 years. This dose of formoterol is based on 4.5 µg/inhalation. SMART therapy is only recommended using formoterol as LABA and not recommended with inhalers containing salmeterol. The benefits of this therapy include a reduction of exacerbations, reduced use of oral steroids, and improved asthma control (NAEPP, 2020; Reddel et al., 2022). Children ages 4 to 11 years may have a lower risk of growth suppression than those on higher-dose ICS therapy alone (NAEPP, 2020). This is not a US Food and Drug Administration (FDA)–approved therapy, so patients may have challenges with this therapy due to the cost and insurance formularies. A 1-month supply may not last the entire month, and this should be discussed with patients when initiating SMART therapy (NAEPP, 2020).

Leukotriene receptor antagonists. Another class of asthma controller medications is leukotriene receptor antagonists (LTRAs). Medications that block leukotriene receptors are less effective than ICS for treating asthma in most patients; however, some patients have a good response to monotherapy with LTRAs. The FDA has added a black box warning of serious neuropsychiatric events to the package of montelukast (Sawicki & Haver, 2023).

Systemic corticosteroids. Children with frequent symptoms or exacerbations, even with combination therapy, may require systemic corticosteroid treatment in either a short burst (3–10 days) or a longer period (NHLBI, 2007). In children who require prolonged or repeated short treatments, reevaluation is needed every 2 to 3 months. Evaluation includes review and documentation of treatment, effects, appropriate use of medication and delivery devices, review of any comorbidities, environmental evaluation for new triggers/allergies, and family understanding of the treatment regimen. At each visit, a thorough interval history is necessary to determine any adverse effects of corticosteroid therapy. Oral/systemic corticosteroid use is prevalent in asthma management, and the risks of acute and chronic complications increase with the cumulative oral corticosteroid dosage (Ratcliffe & Kieckhefer, 2010).

To prevent problems with growth suppression or, more seriously, suppression of the hypothalamic-pituitary-adrenal (HPA) axis, the total dose of oral, inhaled, and topical corticosteroids should be adjusted to the cumulative lowest level necessary to maintain symptom control. Awareness of potential HPA suppressive effects may include severe chickenpox, the risk to bone density, insulin intolerance, systemic hypertension, cataract development, and ocular hypertension (Ratcliffe & Kieckhefer, 2010). Appropriate and timely assessment of adrenal function, depending on steroid exposure, is controversial; if concerned, consultation with an endocrinologist is advised. There can also be effects on bone metabolism. When appropriate doses of ICS are used, this outweighs growth concerns.

Anticholinergics. Anticholinergic agents block cholinergic reflex bronchoconstriction by antagonizing the effect of acetylcholine at muscarinic receptors and may be most useful in children with bronchitis symptoms of increased mucous secretion when used with beta-agonists or antiinflammatory agents. These agents, however, are not particularly helpful against allergic challenges and do not block late-phase response or inhibit mediators from mast cells. Ipratropium bromide (Atrovent) and tiotropium (Spiriva) are the only two anticholinergics approved for use in asthma. Ipratropium bromide can be used with SABA (DuoNeb or Combivent) for acute exacerbations. The combination product may benefit children who respond poorly or adversely to SABA. Side effects include dry mucous membranes, blurred vision, constipation, and urinary retention.

Biologics. Biologics are targeted therapies that can be added to reduce disease burden. The first biologic available was omalizumab, which is an anti-IgE monoclonal antibody. Additional biologic therapies targeting eosinophilic asthma have become available for use. Biologics have also been successful in therapy for other atopic diseases, such as atopic dermatitis (AD), nasal polyps, chronic idiopathic urticaria, and eosinophilic esophagitis (EoE). They are also under investigation as a therapy for food allergies. The therapies available for children are all subcutaneous injections given in various dosing schedules based on the medication (Table 7.3). Overall risks are low, and they are generally well tolerated; however, they do suppress parts of the immune system. The most common side effect is injection site reactions, although other symptoms may include sore throat, myalgia, headache, fatigue, weakness, and back pain. The risks and benefits of biologic therapy should be discussed with patients as part of the shared decision-making process to identify the best treatment.

Treatment of Exercise-Induced Bronchospasm

EIB is a phenotype of asthma. When a child experiences EIB, a SABA can be used to block the symptoms that inhibit the child's continued exercise. When taken to prevent EIB, these agents should be inhaled with a spacer if using MDI formulation approximately 15 to 30 minutes before participation in scheduled exercise. Protection against symptoms of EIB typically lasts 3 to 4 hours with SABA. Long-term control asthma medications are taken daily to prevent symptoms and attacks. They help relieve the narrowing and inflammation of the bronchial tubes. It may take 2 to 4 weeks for these drugs to reach their maximum effect. Prescription of SABA is still required for rescue from acute symptoms

Table 7.3   Biologic Therapy

	MEPOLIZUMAB (NUCALA)	BENRALIZUMAB (FASENRA)	OMALIZUMAB (XOLAIR)	DUPILUMAB (DUPIXENT)	TEZEPELUMAB (TEZSPIRE)
Targets	Anti-IL-5 antibody	Anti-IL-5 antibody	Anti-IgE antibody	Anti-IL-4 and IL-13 antibody	Antithymic stromal lymphopoietin antibody
Indications	Severe asthma with eosinophilic phenotype	Severe asthma with eosinophilic phenotype	Moderate-severe asthma Also used in chronic idiopathic urticaria and uncontrolled nasal polyps	Moderate-severe asthma Also used in atopic dermatitis and chronic rhinosinusitis with nasal polyps	Severe uncontrolled asthma with no phenotype or biomarker limitations
Age for asthma use	6+	12+	6+	6+	12+
Dosage	40 mg SQ (6–11 yr), 100 mg SQ (12+ yr) every 4 wk for asthma	30 mg every 4 wk x 3 doses, then every 8 wk	Asthma: 75–375 mg SQ every 2 or 4 wk; based on total IgE and weight (kg)	For dose information, SEE package insert at https://www.regeneron.com/downloads/dupixent_fpi.pdf	210 mg administered SQ once every 4 wk
Side effects	Injection site reactions	Injections site reactions	Injection site reactions Anaphylaxis (patients with history of anaphylaxis are at most risk)	Injections site reactions; hypersensitivity	Injection site reactions; hypersensitivity Most common adverse reactions: pharyngitis, arthralgia, back pain
Lab requirements/ suggestions	Eosinophils >150 within last 6 wk or 300 within past 12 mo	CBC: no specific range for eosinophil count, but evidence of efficacy exists for eosinophil counts >150/µL	IgE ≥30; positive blood or skin test to the perennial allergen	CBC: no specific range for eosinophil count, but evidence of efficacy exists for eosinophil counts >150/µL	None

CBC, Complete blood count; *IgE*, immunoglobulin E; *IL*, interleukin; *SQ*, subcutaneous.
Modified from American College of Allergy Asthma and Immunology. (2022). Biologic cheat sheet. https://college.acaai.org/wp-content/uploads/2022/08/ACAAI_BiologicsCheatSheet_082222.pdf; Brusselle, G., & Koppelman, G. (2022). Biologic therapies for severe asthma. *New England Journal of Medicine, 386,* 157–171.

(NHLBI, 2007). Wearing a mask or scarf over the mouth, if feasible, or an extended warmup session before activity (such as 10–15 minutes of fast walking, then slow jogging before running) may reduce EIB symptoms in conjunction with medication.

Immunotherapy and Environmental Remediation
Immunotherapy can be considered when a specific symptom-producing allergen is identified in the child's environment, one that cannot be eliminated and leads to increasing asthma therapy. This type of therapy needs to be done in a provider's office for observation and potential management of anaphylaxis. Additional environmental remediations in the home can also help reduce exposure to asthma triggers. Both topics will be discussed in the section on allergy treatment. A reduction in symptoms may improve along with the use of medications.

TESTING
Spirometry can be performed in children older than 5 years of age. The accuracy of spirometry is highly dependent on the user's ability to perform the test. Spirometry starts with the patient taking a full breath and then exhaling as long as possible. It is used to assess airway obstruction and reversibility. Spirometry parameters are adjusted according to sex, age,

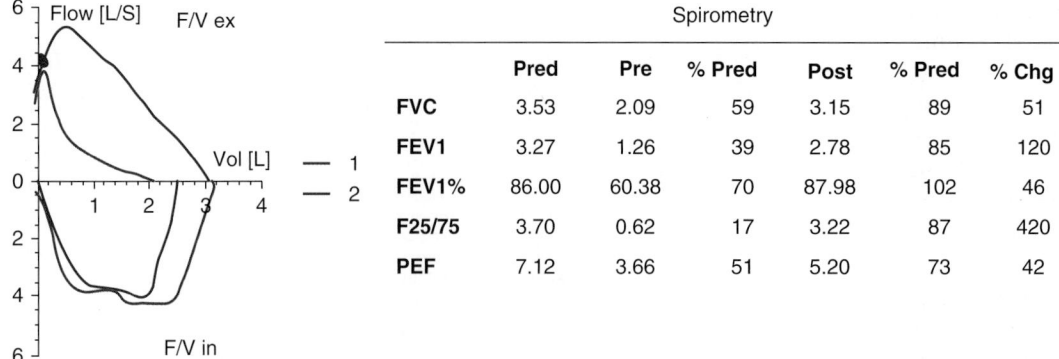

Fig. 7.7 Example of spirometry, including pre- and postbronchodilation. *Blue line* represents prebronchodilation with obstruction noted based scooped curve; *red line* represents postbronchodilation after albuterol was given with reversibility achieved due to change of >12% in FEV1. *%Chg,* Percentage of reversibility between pre- and posttesting; *F25/75,* middle half of FVC; *FEV1,* forced expiratory volume in 1 second; *FEV1%,* percentage expired in 1 second; *FVC,* forced vital capacity; *PEF,* peak expiratory flow; *Pre,* actual values; *Pred,* predicted values; *%Pred,* percentage based on predicted value; *Post,* actual values after albuterol given.

height, and ethnicity. American Thoracic Society recommendations define a significant bronchodilator response as an increase in FEV_1 of 12% or more and/or 200 mL in both adults and children (Gallucci et al., 2019) (Fig. 7.7). In patients able to perform spirometry, it should be performed at diagnosis or at the initiation of treatment, after 3 to 6 months of controller therapy, and then yearly or sooner if clinically warranted.

Common terminology of spirometry:
- FVC: total volume of air exhaled during maximal forced expiration effort
- FEV_1: the volume of air exhaled in the first second of testing
- FEV_1/FVC ratio (FEV_1%): the percentage of FVC expired in 1 second
- Forced expiratory flow: the middle half of the FVC from 25% to 75% of exhalation
- Peak expiratory flow (PEF): the maximal flow achieved with maximally forced expiration

Fig. 7.7 provides an example of spirometry that includes pre- and postbronchodilation.

PEF may be used as an additional functional test in the monitoring of asthma at home. It may be helpful for adults with poor perception of symptoms; however, it can be unreliable based on the user's technique. Therefore most guidelines do not routinely recommend its use in pediatric patients.

Fractional exhaled nitric oxide (FeNO) measures eosinophilic airway inflammation and the amount of exhaled nitric oxide. FeNO can be used in conjunction with history, clinical findings, and spirometry for asthma monitoring and as a diagnostic tool when the diagnosis of asthma remains elusive despite use of other tools. Caution with interpretations as comorbid conditions such as atopy can increase levels, and behaviors such as smoking can decrease levels. Eosinophilic inflammation is steroid responsive, which can

be used to assess asthma control and responsiveness to treatment. FeNO levels below 20 ppb in children are considered low limits and not indicative of eosinophilic inflammation. Levels greater than 50 ppb (>35 ppb in children 5–12 years of age) are consistent with elevated type 2 inflammation and support the diagnosis of asthma.

Bronchial provocation tests include the direct inhalation of different substances such as methacholine, histamine, mannitol, inhalation of allergens, or the use of stimuli such as exercise, inhalation of cold air, and hyperventilation with dry air. Within the pediatric population the exercise test may be a precious tool for evaluating indirect bronchial hyperresponsiveness. Compared to the baseline, a reduction in postexercise FEV_1 is considered a sign of bronchial obstruction induced by exercise. A positive exercise challenge for children is considered a fall in FEV_1 greater than 12% of predicted or PEF greater than 15% (Gallucci et al., 2019).

ASTHMA CONTROL SCORES

Asthma control scores can be used as part of clinical history to assess asthma control through simple questions answered by the child and parent. These questionnaires collect information regarding exacerbations, limitations to daily activities, use of reliever medication, and nocturnal awakenings. The Asthma Control Test (ACT) and Asthma Control Questionnaire (ACQ) are validated and recommended for use (Gallucci et al., 2019).
- ACT (>12 years of age) includes five questions: three related to symptoms, one related to medication use, and one about overall control during the past 4 weeks with separate sections for parent and child; a score of 19 or less indicates poor symptom control.
- C-ACT (4–11 years) includes seven items and is divided into two parts. The first part is addressed

to the child and consists of four questions on the perception of asthma control, limitation of activities, coughing, and awakenings at night. The second part is completed by parents and consists of three questions (daytime complaints, daytime wheezing, and awakenings at night) with six response options. The score ranges from 0 (poorest asthma control) to 27 (optimal asthma control).

- ACQ includes seven questions: five related to symptoms, one on rescue treatment use, and one on FEV_1 finding; the control is assessed over the preceding week. For children with normal FEV_1, a version of a five-point questionnaire is preferable.
- TRACK (a test for respiratory and asthma control in kids) is a validated questionnaire designed to assess asthma control exclusively in young children (<4 years). It includes five questions: three on symptoms and two on medication use. A score below 80 indicates asthma may not be controlled.

DIFFERENTIAL DIAGNOSIS

Symptoms of asthma can also be seen in other childhood diseases. It is important to obtain a good clinical history and perform any testing that is clinically indicated. Other conditions should be considered and eliminated during the evaluation of asthma. Common diseases in the differential include:

- Upper airway diseases: allergic rhinitis (AR), sinusitis, and gastroesophageal reflux
- Obstruction in airways: foreign body aspiration, vascular rings, laryngotracheomalacia, tracheal stenosis or bronchostenosis, tumors, bronchiolitis, cystic fibrosis, bronchopulmonary dysplasia, and vocal cord dysfunction (a paradoxic fold motion disorder causing the vocal cords to close when they should be open, causing difficulties on inhalation)

OTHER CONDITIONS CAUSING COUGH AND WHEEZE

Because children display a variety of common symptoms with asthma, other conditions must be considered and eliminated before initiating treatment.

A child with a history of premature birth and bronchopulmonary dysplasia resulting in relatively smaller, scarred airways may show subsequent asthma-like symptoms. Children with a history of cough, wheezing, recurrent pneumonia, or sinusitis and otitis, even with no evidence of malabsorption, may need a repeat sweat chloride test for cystic fibrosis. In young children, monophonic wheezing or stridor may indicate foreign body aspiration in the trachea or esophagus. Similar symptoms may also be due to tracheal airway compression from an aberrant vessel, tracheal stenosis, tracheomalacia or bronchomalacia, pertussis, and primary ciliary dyskinesia. Gastroesophageal reflux with ascending aspiration or dysphagia leading to descending aspiration may also cause chronic congestion, coughing, stridor with laryngomalacia, and wheezing. Environmental tobacco exposure can lead to increased coughing and secretions (Ratcliffe & Kieckhefer, 2010).

COMORBIDITIES AND ASSOCIATED PROBLEMS WITH ASTHMA

Allergies

All children who have allergies do not have asthma, but many children with asthma have allergies. Sensitization to aeroallergens can trigger airway inflammation and lead to asthma exacerbations. A strong history of allergic reactions associated with respiratory symptoms or unsuccessful escalation of therapy suggests consideration for skin-prick tests or ImmunoCAP allergy blood testing in conjunction with total IgE level to determine specific problematic allergens. It is vital to review possible allergens and triggers with the family, discussing avoidance or, at the minimum, modification of the child's environment to reduce exposures (see this chapter for additional material on AR) (Ratcliffe & Kieckhefer, 2010).

Gastroesophageal Reflux

Gastroesophageal reflux (GER) is found in many children with chronic lung disease. Reflux of gastric secretions into the esophagus can initiate a reflex vagal response with increased production of airway secretions and cough. The cough itself can induce reflux episodes. Management of GER includes upright positioning following thickened feedings for infants, smaller feedings, and the use of medications that reduce acidity or increase gastric motility.

Illness and Sinusitis

Chronic infections of the sinuses with fever, pain, and thick postnasal secretions can irritate lower airways and trigger asthma exacerbation. Treatment of the infection is necessary to reduce this trigger and may involve routine nasal washes with antibiotic/saline solutions, intermittent nasal or oral steroids, and antibiotics. Treatment may be needed over a prolonged period because chronic sinusitis is a notoriously difficult infection to eradicate.

Sensitivity to Aspirin and Nonsteroidal Antiinflammatory Drugs

Aspirin and nonsteroidal antiinflammatory drugs (NSAIDs) may precipitate an asthma episode in adults and children. Aspirin is rarely indicated in children, and parents should be taught to read over-the-counter (OTC) drug labels because aspirin can be combined with other substances, especially cold remedies. Ibuprofen is commonly used in children and may have cross sensitivity to aspirin and NSAIDs. If NSAID sensitivity is suspected, referral to a specialist for confirmatory diagnosis is warranted (Ratcliffe & Kieckhefer, 2010).

Box 7.2   List of Common Allergens

ENVIRONMENTAL ALLERGENS
- Indoor allergens
  - Dust mites
  - Animal dander
  - Cockroaches
- Outdoor allergens
  - Molds
  - Pollens (trees, grass, and weeds)

FOOD ALLERGENS
- Cow's milk
- Eggs
- Peanuts
- Tree nuts
- Soy
- Fish
- Shellfish
- Sesame

Swallowing Disorders

Some infants and young children have dysphagia or swallowing disorders that may cause episodes of microaspiration with or without obvious symptoms of cough. The aspiration of food or formula into the lungs will trigger a chronic inflammatory response that will exacerbate a child's asthma and require escalating therapy. If suspected, a video fluoroscopic swallowing study can document aspiration with resulting feeding adaptations required until the swallow is normally developed. Adaptations may include thickened feedings, positioning, or occupational therapy evaluation.

ALLERGIES

ETIOLOGY

Allergy is an adverse health effect of the body on what is perceived as a foreign substance or allergen. Allergens are not always harmful and can trigger a positive response. A positive or beneficial response results in the development of immunity, whereas a negative or unwanted response results in the development of atopy or an IgE-mediated condition. The term *atopy* is often used interchangeably with the term *allergy*. Atopy refers to the genetic tendency to develop allergic diseases such as AR, asthma, and AD (eczema). Atopy is typically associated with heightened immune responses to common allergens, especially inhaled and food allergens (Box 7.2) (American Academy of Allergy Asthma & Immunology [AAAAI], n.d.-b). Although allergy is a broad topic, this chapter will specifically cover the common chronic conditions of allergic rhinoconjunctivitis and food allergies (Table 7.4). Medication allergies, allergic reactions to insect bites and venom, and AD are briefly overviewed in this chapter (Fig. 7.8).

Allergy is the result of an immunologically based acquired change in the body of an individual child. In most cases, the response to a foreign substance can be classified as either a Th1 or a Th2 response, referring to the type of cytokine that is activated. A Th1 response is linked to the development of immunity that protects against many infections, and a Th2 response contributes to atopy and allergy symptoms. Allergic reactions involve the production of antigen-specific mediators and a complex cascade of reactions. Histamines or other mediators are released from a mast cell or basophil, which causes inflammation. The resulting respiratory, dermatologic, and eye symptoms vary with the individual's sensitivities and may include sneezing; itching of the nose, ears, and eyes; and rhinitis, wheezing, conjunctivitis, and rash. When the offending agent is a particular food, the child may experience abdominal pain, diarrhea, vomiting, and skin rashes, alone or in addition to respiratory symptoms within minutes to a few hours of ingestion. For the purpose of this chapter, food allergies will refer to IgE-mediated reactions; however, the term is also commonly used for less specific food reactions and intolerances that are a result of nonallergic causes, such as pharmacologic, toxic, or metabolic mechanisms, as well as gastrointestinal (GI) intolerances, such as lactose (Fig. 7.9) (Sloand et al., 2010).

The *allergic march* is a widely used term to define the progression of allergic disease from infancy through adulthood. The progression usually begins as AD in infancy, then progresses to food allergies, AR with sensitization to aeroallergens, and asthma.

INCIDENCE AND PREVALENCE

AR is one of the most common chronic diseases in the United States. Incidence reports are between 10% and 30% of children and adults in the United States and other developed nations (Brown, 2019; Schuler & Montejo, 2019). The incidence and prevalence of allergies are very low until the age of 2 years, but then extend upward throughout childhood. There is a steady increase in the prevalence of allergies to 15% by age 7 years. Allergies account for an average 2 million lost school days per year and indirect costs such as lost productivity for working parents. The annual direct and indirect costs of AR to society are estimated to be $25 billion (Brown, 2019). In contrast, food allergies affect 32 million Americans, with approximately 8% of children (1 in 13) carrying a diagnosis of food allergies (Food Allergy Research and Education [FARE], n.d.-b). Overall, food allergies cost $24.8 billion annually or $4184 per child. The total cost comprises significant direct medical costs for food allergies ($4.3 billion) and even larger costs borne by families ($20.5 billion) (Gupta et al., 2013). Each year about 200,000 people require treatment in the ED for allergic reactions to foods (FARE, n.d.-b). Over 170 different foods have been reported to induce an allergic reaction; however, the top 9 are the most common (FARE, n.d.-b):
- Shellfish: 8.2 million
- Milk: 6.1 million

Table 7.4 Medications Used in the Treatment of Allergic Rhinoconjunctivitis

	ROUTE	AGE	DOSING	ADVERSE EFFECTS
Systemic Antihistamines				
Allegra (fexofenadine HCl)	Oral	≥12 yr 2–11 yr	180 mg once daily or 60 mg twice daily 30 mg twice daily	Headache
Alavert OTC (loratadine)	Oral (quick dissolving tablets)	≥6 yr	10 mg once daily	Nervousness, wheezing, dry mouth
Claritin OTC (loratadine)	Oral	≥6 yr 2–5 yr	10 mg once daily 5 mg once daily	≥12 yr: headache, somnolence, fatigue, dry mouth <12 yr: nervousness, wheezing, fatigue
Clarinex (desloratadine)	Oral	≥12 yr 6–11 yr 12 mo–5 yr 6–11 mo	5 mg once daily 2.5 mg once daily 1.25 mg 1 mg	Sore throat, dry mouth
Zyrtec (cetirizine HCl)	Oral	≥6 yr 2–5 yr 6–23 mo	5–10 mg once daily 2.5–5 mg once daily or 2.5 twice daily 2.5 mg once daily	≥12 yr: somnolence, fatigue, dry mouth <12 yr: headache, somnolence
Benadryl OTC (diphenhydramine HCl)	Oral	2–6 yr 6–11 yr >12 yr 6–11 yr	6.25 mg three or four times daily 12.5–25 mg three or four times daily 25–50 mg three or four times daily 5 mg/kg/day in 3 or 4 divided doses	Drowsiness, excitability
Chlor-Trimeton OTC (chlorpheniramine maleate)	Oral	>12 yr 6–12 yr 4–6 yr	4 mg every 4–6 hr 2 mg every 4–6 hr 1 mg every 4–6 hr	Drowsiness, excitability
Topical Antihistamines				
Astelin (azelastine HCl)	Nose	≥12 yr 5–11 yr	2 sprays/nostril twice daily 1 spray/nostril twice daily	Bitter taste, headache, somnolence
Patanase (Olopatadine)	Nose	6–11yr >12 yr	1 spray/nostril twice daily 2 sprays twice daily	Transient burning, stinging, discomfort
Alaway (ketotifen fumarate) Zaditor (ketotifen fumarate) Olopatadine 0.1% Olopatadine 0.2%	Eyes	>3 yr >2 yr	1 drop to the affected eye Twice daily, every 12 hr 1 drop twice a day 1 drop once a day	
Topical Mast Cell Stabilizers				
Nasalcrom (cromolyn sodium)	Nose	≥2 yr	1 spray each nostril every 4–6 hr Prevention: Begin 1 wk before exposure to a known allergen	Transient stinging, sneezing
Opticrom (cromolyn sodium)	Eyes	≥4 yr	1–2 drops/affected eye four to six times daily	Transient stinging or burning on instillation
Topical Steroids				
Flonase (fluticasone propionate)	Nose	2–11 yr ≥12 yr	1 spray/nostril daily 2 sprays/nostril daily	Epistaxis, headache, pharyngitis
Nasacort (triamcinolone acetonide)	Nose	2–5 yr >6 yr	1 spray/nostril daily 1–2 sprays daily	Epistaxis, pharyngitis, increased cough
Nasonex (mometasone furoate)	Nose	2–11 yr ≥12 yr	1 spray daily 2 sprays/nostril daily	Epistaxis, pharyngitis, headache

Data from Crisalida, T., Kaline, M.A., & Turkeltaub, M. (2002). *Allergies and asthma pocket guide.* Adelphi Inc.; Boguniewicz, M. (2007). Allergic disorders. In W.W. Hay, M.J. Levin, J.M. Sondheimer, & R.R. Deterding (Eds.), *Current pediatric diagnosis and treatment* (18th ed.). Lange Medical Books/McGraw-Hill; Sloand, E., & Caschera, J. (2010). Allergies. In P.J. Allen, J. Vessey, & N.A. Schapiro (Eds.), *Primary care of the child with a chronic condition* (5th ed., pp. 145–167). Elsevier.

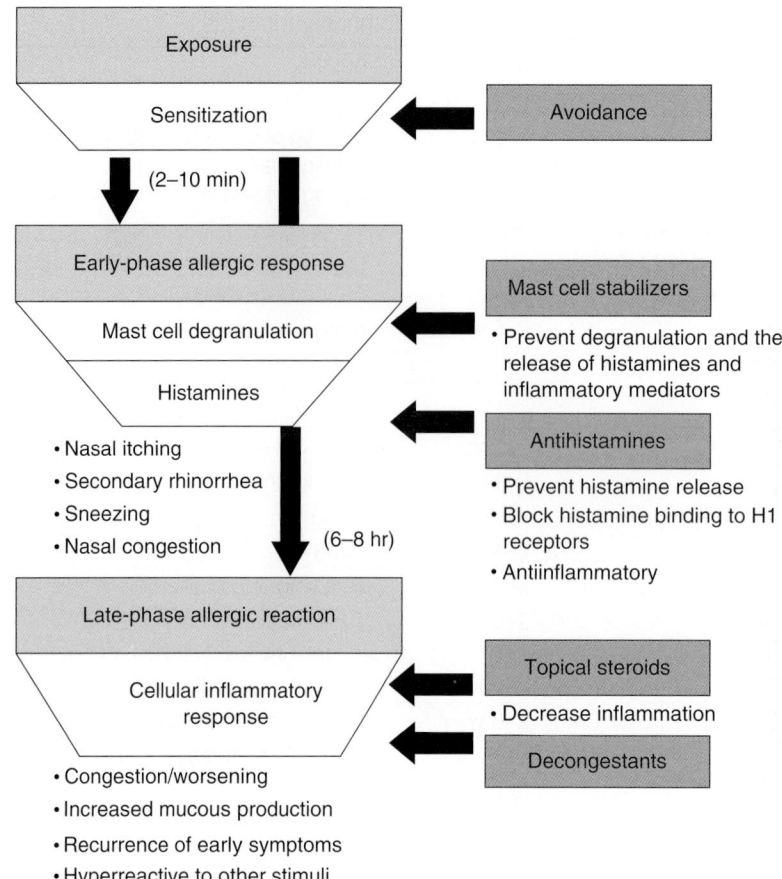

Fig. 7.8 **Etiology of allergic responses and the corresponding treatment.** *EGID*, Eosinophilic gastrointestinal disease.

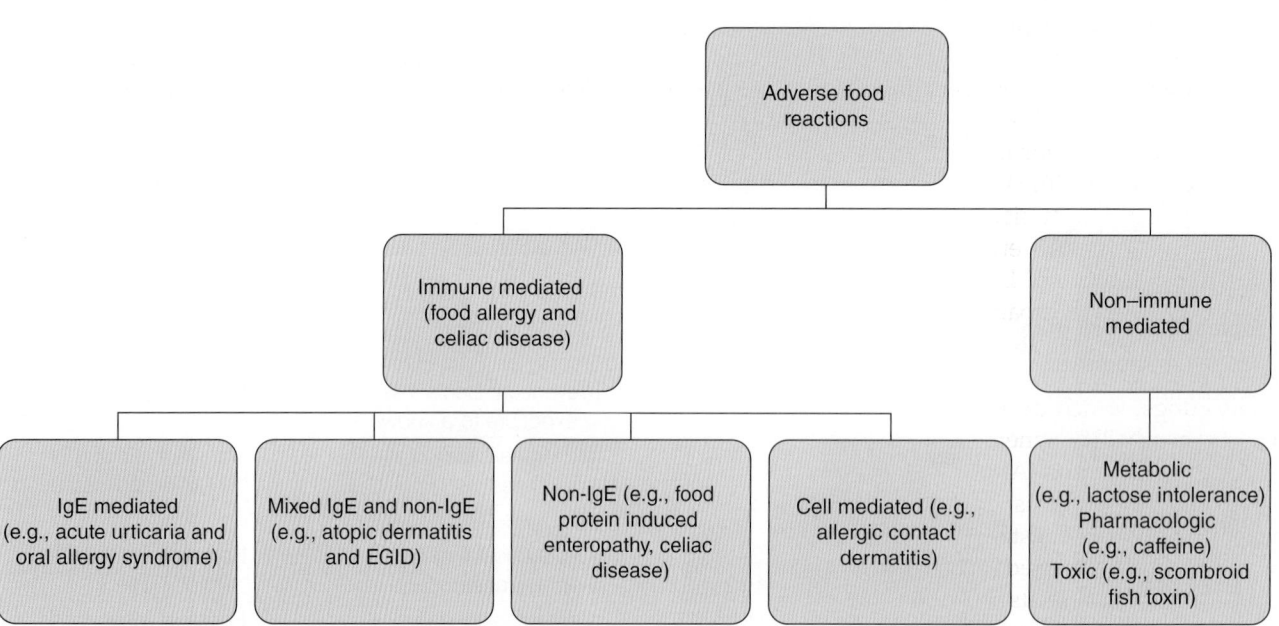

Fig. 7.9 **Classification of adverse food reactions.** *IgE*, Immunoglobulin E. (Modified from Sampson, H.A., Aceves, S., Bock, S., et al. [2014]. Food allergy: A practice parameter update—2014. *Journal of Allergy and Clinical Immunology, 134*[5], 1016–1025.)

- Peanut: 6.1 million
- Tree nuts: 3.9 million
- Egg: 2.6 million
- Fin fish: 2.6 million
- Wheat: 2.4 million
- Soy: 1.9 million
- Sesame: 0.7 million

Theories Behind the Increase in Allergies

There has been a significant worldwide increase in the development of allergies, with nearly 30% of the world's population affected (Rothenberg, 2022), with many theories hypothesized for this increase. The leading theory is the hygiene hypothesis, which was first formulated in 1989 by epidemiologist David P. Strachan, who found an inverse relationship between family size and the development of allergic disease. It was proposed that a lower incidence of infection in early childhood could be a cause of the rise in allergic diseases. Subsequently, the concept evolved into the broader notion that declining microbial exposure was a major causative factor for the increasing incidence of allergic diseases. The hygiene hypothesis suggests that loss of symbiotic relationships with evolutionary relevant microorganisms prevents the necessary stimulus to train the immune system to develop tolerogenic responses and is therefore proposed to be the underlying cause of the allergy epidemic. Indeed, less frequent bathing and showering appear to be protective against aeroallergen sensitization in children without current allergies (Zhang et al., 2021).

A wide range of lifestyle factors that contribute to an altered microbial exposure has been examined, such as clean food and water, sanitation, usage of antibiotics and vaccines, birth delivery modes (e.g., usage of cesarian section), and geographic migratory patterns (e.g., the move from farm to urban living) (Rothenberg 2022; Zhang et al., 2021). Several studies showed that farm and large family size distinctly reduce the prevalence of hay fever (Ahrens & Posa, 2017). The allergy-protective influence of living on a farm and being in contact with a very broad variety of animals has been reported by several studies (Ahrens & Posa, 2017). Birth cohort studies found a favorable effect of exposure to dogs, which decreased the risk of AD in children by nearly 25%, whereas no association was found with exposure to cats (Ahrens & Posa, 2017).

Another hypothesis behind allergic symptoms becoming more persistent includes climate change, which is the term used to describe human-induced global warming and its impact on weather patterns. Global warming and related changes in rainfall patterns, hurricanes, and winds have modified many aspects of pollination, including its seasonality, timing of the release, quantity, and geographic distribution (Rothenberg, 2022). These climate changes have increased the length of pollination and created new sources of pollen due to invasive species (Zhang et al., 2021). Furthermore, plants produce more pollen at high atmospheric levels of carbon dioxide. Pollens are not only allergen carriers but also release lipid mediators, which have proinflammatory and immunomodulatory effects on allergic responses. One of the consequences of climate change is the increased occurrence of extreme weather conditions, including thunderstorms (known to exacerbate asthma), flooding (known to contribute to mold growth), prolonged heat waves (causing several health issues and increased exposure to indoor allergens such as dust mites, cockroaches, and molds), and air pollution (from wildfires and dust storms) (Rothenberg, 2022).

Dietary changes may also play a role in the increasing prevalence of allergic diseases and asthma, and children with high levels of butyrate and propionate (≥95th percentile) in feces at the age of 1 year have been shown to have significantly less atopic sensitization between 3 and 6 years. Moreover, a recent meta-analysis of observational studies has indicated a direct association between obesity or overweight and the risk of AR in children (Zhang, 2021). It is reasonable to expect that a complex interplay of genetics and environmental conditions is responsible for allergy development.

Regarding the development of food allergies, there is a strong relation between filaggrin gene mutations and AD. This hypothesis states that skin barrier defects promote sensitization to allergens. Skin barrier defects, in general, have been established in the list of risk factors for food allergy development, along with heredity, route, and timing of exposure to food allergens (e.g., the introduction of solid foods), vitamin D sufficiency, dietary fat, antioxidants, obesity, and exposure to infections (Ahrens & Posa, 2017). The dual allergen exposure hypothesis postulates that allergic sensitization results from cutaneous exposure and tolerance as a result of oral exposure to foods (Ahrens & Posa, 2017; Du Toit et al., 2015).

One of the greatest breakthroughs in food allergy development is the Learning Early About Peanut (LEAP) trial, a randomized controlled trial in high-risk infants performed in the United Kingdom. This study hypothesized that infants at high risk for the development of peanut allergy would have a decreased incidence with the early introduction of peanuts. There were 640 infants between the ages of 4 and 11 months with severe eczema, egg allergy, or both assigned to introduce peanuts, and the others were avoided for a length of 60 months. Among the 530 infants in the intention-to-treat population who initially had negative results on the skin-prick test, the prevalence of peanut allergy at 60 months of age was 13.7% in the avoidance group and 1.9% in the consumption group (p <.001). Among the 98 participants in the intention-to-treat population who initially had positive test results, the prevalence of peanut allergy was 35.3% in

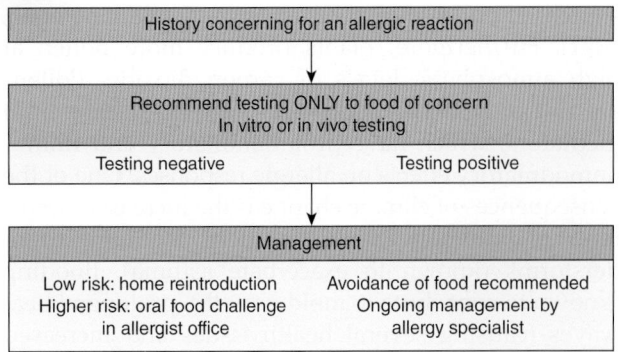

Fig. 7.10 **Algorithm for food allergy diagnosis.** (Modified from Anvari, S., Miller, J., Chih-Yen, Y., et al. [2019]. IgE mediated food allergy. *Clinical Review in Allergy and Immunology, 57*, 244–260.)

the avoidance group and 10.6% in the consumption group (*p* = .004) (Du Toit et al., 2015). The LEAP study showed that early oral introduction of peanuts could prevent allergy in high-risk, sensitized infants and in nonsensitized infants (Du Toit et al., 2015). Based on the results of this trial, the early introduction of peanuts is recommended. Subsequent trials have also shown the early introduction of eggs into the infant's diet also reduces the risk (Peters et al., 2021).

The role of early diet diversification is an important concept in the development of food allergies. Studies have shown that restricted food patterns, especially allergenic foods in the first year of life, might increase the risk of asthma and allergies in childhood, whereas an increased diversity of food within the first year of life seems to have a protective effect on asthma, food allergy, and food sensitization and is associated with increased expression of a marker for regulatory T cells (Ahrens & Posa, 2017).

DIAGNOSTIC CRITERIA

In primary care practices, allergies are most often diagnosed based on the clinical presentation and response to antihistamine therapy. Diagnostic tests, including in vivo skin testing and in vitro testing, may be indicated if the allergy symptoms are severe or persistent to assess for the child's triggers. Identifying allergens can encourage the family to avoid the offending agents (Fig. 7.10).

In Vivo Skin Testing

Skin testing is usually done in the allergist's office. This process involves a skin-prick test to expose the individual to a small amount of allergen. A positive test results in a reaction caused by IgE antibodies to the allergen, and the patient will develop a wheal and flare where pricked. Skin testing can be blocked if the patient is on antihistamines, therefore it is recommended to stop oral antihistamines 7 days prior to testing but remain on asthma medications. Skin testing has good sensitivity and specificity and can be completed in about 20 minutes in the office, which allows patients to leave with real-time results.

In Vitro Testing

Blood testing for specific IgE antibodies uses an enzyme-linked immunosorbent assay (ELISA). The most common form of ELISA testing is ImmunoCAP. Blood testing is more expensive and less specific than skin testing but can be useful if skin testing is not an option due to overwhelming AD, behavioral concerns, or the inability to stop antihistamines. The benefits of blood testing include there being no medication interference with results and no risk of allergic reaction to testing.

Elevated total serum IgE is consistent with atopy but is not a specific indicator for allergies. Blood eosinophilia may be used as a screening test, but it has a low sensitivity. A nasal smear with eosinophils clearly indicates allergies but does not implicate a specific allergen.

Blood testing for environmental allergies is typically only repeated if there is concern for additional allergen development. However, yearly blood testing is performed on food allergies to monitor for loss of sensitization (resolution of allergy to food previously considered an allergen). Allergen panels for foods should never be performed. Only testing for foods that have a history and/or suspicion of reaction should be tested.

In summary, no single screening test is recommended for identifying people with allergies. Positive testing identifies sensitization to allergens. Patient history of symptoms and medication response is the most valuable and practical diagnostic tool used in conjunction with diagnostic testing.

Other Tests

Component resolved diagnostics (CRD) refers to specific IgE testing that is directed toward specific antigens or epitopes. Testing for specific epitopes can increase specificity by distinguishing clinically relevant IgE from IgE directed at nonallergic components (Oriel & Wang, 2021). CRD testing is available for multiple foods and aeroallergens, such as animal dander.

There are many alternative tests for allergies available, such as IgG-specific testing, applied kinesiology, hair analysis, lymphocyte stimulation, and provocation neutralization; currently none of these are recommended as validated tools in the diagnostic workup for IgE-medicated allergies (Anvari et al., 2019).

Oral Challenge

Considered the gold standard of food allergy testing, these are performed in the allergist's office under medical supervision. During these procedures the child is given increasing amounts of the suspected food to reach a certain amount of protein (typically 5–8 g). These challenges can be done in many ways, including double blinded, single blinded, open, or placebo controlled. Double-blind challenges are usually performed as part of the research, whereas an open

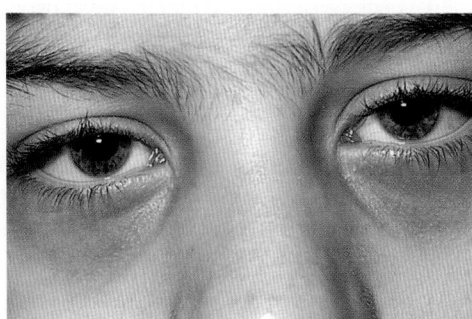
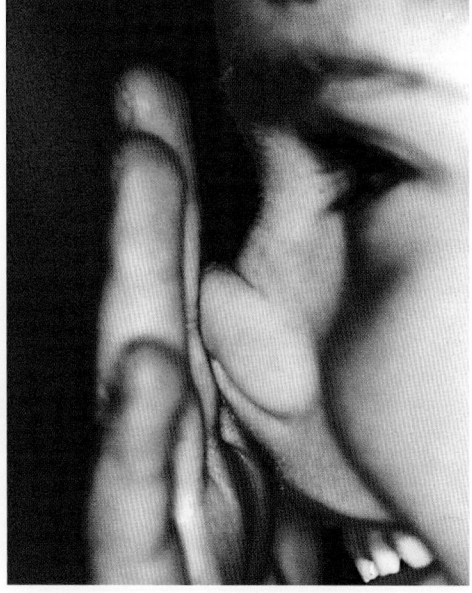

Fig. 7.11 **Clinical presentation of allergic rhinitis.** (From Chong, H., Green, T., Larkin, A. Allergy and immunology. In: Zitelli, B., McIntire, S., Nowalk, A. (2018). *Zitelli and Davis' Atlas of Pediatric Physical Diagnosis*. Phladelphia: Elsevier.).

challenge is the easiest to complete and is most often used in clinical practice. Oral challenges can be performed to confirm the diagnosis or to determine if the child has outgrown an allergy.

SYMPTOMS OF ALLERGIES

AR is a global concern. The incidence of this disease imposes a heavy burden on general well-being and has a significant financial impact from both direct and indirect costs for the management of the disease. Symptoms of AR include nasal itching, nasal congestion, rhinorrhea with clear nasal discharge, and bouts of sneezing. Clinical signs include pale, bluish boggy nasal mucosa and turbinated, clear nasal discharge as well as nasal obstruction. Specific signs of AR include a crease across the nose (allergic salute), allergic shiners (dark circles under the eyes), Dennie Morgan sign (lines under the lower lid margin), throat clicking or clucking, nose twitching, and facial grimacing (Fig. 7.11).

Allergic conjunctivitis or ocular allergy occurs when the conjunctiva becomes irritated. Like all allergies, allergic conjunctivitis starts when the immune system identifies an otherwise harmless substance as an allergen. This causes your immune system to overreact and produce antibodies called immunoglobulin (i.e., IgE). These antibodies travel to cells that release chemicals that cause an allergic reaction, such as painful, itchy, watery eyes that become red and swollen (AAAAI, n.d.-c). Allergic conjunctivitis may occur in combination with AR, or it may occur alone. The hallmark symptom is significant itching of the eyes.

There are other general symptoms that can be present with rhinitis or conjunctivitis. These may include postnasal drip, throat clearing, dry throat, itchy ears or

Box 7.3	Differential Diagnosis for Allergies

- Asthma
- Acute viral rhinitis
- Vasomotor rhinitis
- Acute infectious sinusitis, pharyngitis, and conjunctivitis
- Rhinitis medicamentosa
- Substance abuse
- Urticaria
- Gastroenteritis and other gastrointestinal problems

throat, dry cough, headache, fullness in the ear, or ear popping. Symptoms may be similar to a cold. They can be present for weeks or months (Box 7.3).

Children are typically afebrile with these symptoms. Some children may exhibit behavior manifestations due to allergies. At times children may misbehave at school or at home due to their symptoms. They can become irritable, have sleep deprivation, and decrease their ability to concentrate. Some of these symptoms could be due to lack of sleep or the use of OTC medications. Providers need to ensure that they do not confuse these symptoms for attention-deficit/hyperactivity disorders, which may be very similar.

Children with AR may display allergic shiners and adenoid facies, resulting from long-standing mouth breathing. The features of adenoid facies include a long and narrow face, narrow and upturned nose, short upper lip, exposed upper incisors, recessed lower jaw, and forward head posture.

Food allergies may manifest with a wide variety of symptoms, affecting the skin, oral area, GI system, respiratory system, and cardiovascular system. Mild symptoms can include skin rash, stomachache, nausea,

Table 7.5	Symptoms of an Allergic Reaction Due to Ingestion of Allergenic Food

SYSTEM	SYMPTOMS
Skin	Hives, itchy rash, swelling of the face and extremities
Mouth	Itching, tingling, or swelling of lips, tongue, and/or mouth
Nasal	Sneezing, nasal congestion, nasal drainage
Gastrointestinal	Nausea, abdominal cramps, vomiting, diarrhea
Throat	Tightening of the throat, hoarseness, hacking cough
Respiratory	Shortness of breath, repetitive coughing, and wheezing
Cardiovascular	Thready pulse, low blood pressure, fainting, pallor, blue skin
Other	Sense of impending doom

Box 7.4 Avoidance of Allergens at Home

- Do not use aerosol products.
- Use dehumidifiers in damp places, such as basements.
- Do not allow smoking in the family's home or car.
- Control dust with vacuuming, air filtration systems, wet mopping, and keeping dust catchers (e.g., stuffed toys, open shelving) out of bedrooms.
- Keep windows closed or use air conditioning.
- Enclose pillows and mattresses in hypoallergenic covers.

diarrhea, nasal congestion, and sneezing, but some children have much more severe symptoms, such as respiratory distress and anaphylaxis. Symptoms typically begin within minutes to 2 hours after ingestion (Table 7.5).

Anaphylactic Reactions

Anaphylaxis occurs when any of the following three criteria occurs:

1. Sudden onset of an illness, with involvement of the skin, mucosal tissue, or both and at least one of the following: respiratory compromise, reduced blood pressure, associated symptoms of end-organ dysfunction
2. Two or more of the following that occur rapidly after exposure to a likely allergen: skin/mucosal involvement, respiratory compromise, reduced blood pressure, GI symptoms
3. Reduced blood pressure after exposure to a known allergen (Yue et al., 2018)

Biphasic reactions are possible when patients experience a recurrence of symptoms within 72 hours of the initial anaphylactic event without reexposure to the trigger. The risk of a biphasic reaction was greater with hypotension on presentation and an unknown inciting trigger (Yue et al., 2018).

Up to 5% of the US population has suffered anaphylaxis, although fatal outcomes are rare and constitute less than 1% of total mortality risk (Turner et al., 2017). The majority of fatal food anaphylaxis is caused by peanut and tree nut hypersensitivity. Of note, these foods also tend to induce persistent sensitivity in the majority of children, in contrast to other foods (milk, soy, eggs, wheat) that are usually outgrown. As children get older and develop other atopic symptoms, such as asthma, it is not uncommon for them to experience more severe anaphylaxis symptoms. Therefore those children with

asthma who concurrently have food allergies should be identified as high risk for an anaphylactic reaction. Recognition of signs and symptoms of a reaction and prompt treatment are the most important aspects of the successful management of anaphylaxis.

TREATMENT

The first line of defense against seasonal allergies is avoidance (Box 7.4), which may be difficult for some children depending on their family lifestyle. It is important to consider medication, education for the child and family about the condition, and a management plan. A referral to an allergist for immunotherapy may be an option. Each treatment plan needs to be individualized, along with shared treatment between the parents and the affected child.

Pharmacologic Therapy

Rhinitis and conjunctivitis. Many OTC and prescription medications can be used to control allergy symptoms (see Table 7.5). Antihistamine usage helps decrease itching, sneezing, and rhinorrhea within 1 hour of its dosing.

Rhinitis. Intranasal steroids (INS) are very effective and the first-line treatment for persistent nasal symptoms. It can be used in children as young as 2 years of age. INS has a potent antiinflammatory property that directly modulates the pathophysiology of AR. The use of these agents in seasonal disease leads to a reduction in inflammatory cells and cytokines within the normal mucosa and secretions of patients with AR. Reducing nasal symptoms improves the quality of life and sleep of patients with AR. The continuous use of INS is recommended and more efficacious than intermittent use. The onset of action is 3 to 36 hours after the first dose. It is reasonable to assess that efficacy should be reached after 1 week of therapy, and if none is observed the treatment might be considered ineffective (Seidman et al., 2015).

As well as diminished nasal symptoms, INS has beneficial effects on allergic eye symptoms, including itchiness, tearing, redness, and puffiness. Some studies suggest that INS can also improve asthma symptoms. There are a few side effects of INS, including tearing, dryness, stinging, blood-tinged secretions, and epistaxis. With the proper technique of pointing away from the septum and toward the outer ear, this can minimize epistaxis.

Intranasal antihistamines that are H1 receptor antagonists are very efficient in treating AR. Two are FDA approved in the United States: azelastine and olopatadine. For the treatment of nasal symptoms, intranasal antihistamines have shown equality or superiority to oral antihistamines in numerous well-designed, controlled, and blinded studies (Seidman et al., 2015). The most common adverse events with intranasal antihistamines are bitter taste, epistaxis, headache, somnolence, and nasal burning. There is a rapid onset within 15 to 30 minutes.

Conjunctivitis. There are a wide variety of eye drops available to relieve symptoms of allergic conjunctivitis. The mast cell stabilizers are very effective and include ketotifen fumarate (Zaditor) and cromolyn sodium (Opticrom). They vary in frequency and administration, which can be particularly important with a younger child who is fearful of or combative with eye drops. Some of the mast cell stabilizers are approved for children as young as 2 years old. Olopatadine hydrochloride (Patanol) is a mast cell stabilizer that also has antihistamine properties. Eye drops containing steroids are not recommended for children. In addition to pharmacotherapy, the child may gain some relief from ocular itching with the application of cool compresses, especially during a period of acute discomfort. Storing the eye drops in the refrigerator will help improve symptoms due to the cooling sensation.

Immunotherapy

Immunotherapy is an effective treatment when used in carefully selected situations. Allergen immunotherapy, also known as allergy shots, is a form of long-term treatment that decreases symptoms for many people with AR, allergic asthma, conjunctivitis, or stinging insect allergy. Children who have severe allergies and for whom avoidance and medications are not effective in relieving nasal symptoms may benefit from immunotherapy. Allergy shots decrease sensitivity to allergens and often lead to lasting relief of allergy symptoms even after treatment is stopped. This makes it a cost-effective, beneficial treatment approach for many children (AAAAI, 2020a). Both the patient/family and the allergist should base the decision regarding allergy shots on the following:

- Length of allergy season and severity of symptoms
- How well medications and/or environmental controls are helping the allergy symptoms
- Patient's desire to avoid long-term medication use
- Time available for treatment (allergy shots require a 3–5-year commitment)
- Cost, which may vary depending on region and insurance coverage (AAAAI, 2020a)

Immunotherapy is not used for the treatment of ocular symptoms alone or for food allergies. A pediatric allergist should be consulted, who will test the child for specific allergies and will prepare the appropriate extract that is needed for that individualized child.

Allergy shots work like a vaccine. Your body responds to injected amounts of a particular allergen, given in gradually increasing doses, by developing immunity or tolerance to the allergen. The child becomes desensitized to the allergen. Immunotherapy should be given in a supervised facility with proper staff and equipment to identify and treat adverse reactions to allergy injections. This could be done with a provider who is an allergist or a provider who has been adequately trained to supervise the proper instructions for allergy shots. If there is no improvement after 1 year of maintenance therapy, other treatment options may be necessary.

Reactions may occur with immunotherapy. There can be redness or swelling at that site, which is a normal response that may happen immediately or several hours after the injection. There could be serious anaphylaxis with swelling in the throat, wheezing or tightness in the chest, nausea, and dizziness. Most serious reactions develop within 30 minutes of allergy injections, therefore it is recommended the patient wait in the doctor's office for at least 30 minutes after receiving allergy shots (AAAAI, 2020a).

Complementary and Alternative Therapies

Many Americans integrate complementary and alternative medicine (CAM) therapies into overall health strategies for themselves and their children. Pediatric clinicians should have some knowledge regarding CAM because they may be asked to advise patients regarding these therapies or provide a referral to CAM practitioners. Clinicians should discuss with their patients what CAM therapies are being used and answer questions that arise (Kemper, 2022).

There are several CAM therapies being used:

- Integrative medicine uses patient-centered care that focuses on the whole person.
- Complementary medicine (e.g., massage, biofeedback, hypnosis, acupuncture, herbs, support groups, guided imagery) does not replace conventional medicine but supports the patient and family.
- Alternative therapies are used in place of conventional care.
- Folk therapies are provided by family and cultural tradition.
- Holistic care involves the whole patient (body, mind, emotion, spirit, relationships).

CAM has been used as an alternative therapy for many years but is not routinely prescribed by allergists. Research is ongoing to evaluate the mechanisms and effectiveness of this type of treatment.

Food Allergies

The current treatment of food allergies is avoidance of the allergen and preparation for allergic reactions should they occur. A careful reading of food labels and knowledge of cross-contamination/cross-contact is essential for the successful management of food allergies. The second important aspect of treatment is the recognition of signs and symptoms of an allergic reaction and prompt treatment of symptoms. It is also important that those providing care for children with food allergies, such as teachers, day care providers, and other caregivers, be properly trained on how to manage food allergies.

When an allergic reaction occurs, there are two medications that can be used. For mild symptoms use of antihistamines such as cetirizine or diphenhydramine is recommended. When symptoms are consistent with anaphylaxis, the first-line treatment is the prompt use of epinephrine. The dosing of epinephrine is 0.01 to 0.3 mg. The most common and easiest way to give epinephrine is with an autoinjector. Epinephrine autoinjectors are manufactured by several companies but come in doses of 0.15 mg for those under 25 kg and 0.3 mg for those above 25 kg. There is also an infant dose of 0.1 mg for those under 15 kg (Auvi-Q). Epinephrine will vasoconstrict the blood vessels to maintain blood pressure and bronchodilate the airways to improve respirations and decrease edema that may be causing airway collapse (Anvari et al., 2019). Autoinjectors come in packs of two, and in some cases the second dose is required quickly; therefore it is important for children to have a two-pack supply in all locations where they spend time, such as home and school. Seeking medical care in the ED/UCC is recommended after epinephrine is used. The patient should be observed for at least 4 hours for complete resolution of symptoms. All children should also carry an emergency food allergy plan to follow in case of a reaction (Fig. 7.12).

Oral Immunotherapy

Oral immunotherapy (OIT) is a treatment where children are given small increasing doses of their allergen to desensitize them to it. This treatment is not a cure, but it can help lessen reactions upon accidental exposures. Dosing is typically increased every 2 weeks until a maintenance dose is reached. OIT requires the child to take the dose every day indefinitely. At the time of publication there is only one FDA-approved product for peanut OIT (Palforzia), which is indicated for those age 4 to 17 years. Patients can undergo OIT for other foods using commercial-grade products that are not FDA approved for OIT. This treatment should only be performed in an allergist's office.

In addition, epicutaneous immunotherapy (EPIT) is currently under evaluation. EPIT involves the allergen being absorbed through the skin. Sublingual immunotherapy (SLIT) is another form that is currently being evaluated. SLIT involves placing the allergen in droplet form under the tongue in increasing doses. Both options also reduce allergy reactions but are not a cure.

Early Introduction

Based on the LEAP trials, new guidelines regarding the early introduction of allergenic foods were created in 2017 by the National Institutes of Allergy and Infectious Disease (NIAID) (Table 7.6).

Fleischer et al. (2021) published consensus guidelines from North American allergy societies. These guidelines recommend the introduction of peanuts and eggs starting at 6 months of age but not before 4 months. Introductions should be done after tolerance of complementary foods. Screening can be done prior but is not required for peanut and egg (Fleischer et al., 2021). Current guidelines also recommend that the mother eat a diverse diet and not restrict any allergenic foods during pregnancy and the breastfeeding period. Hydrolyzed formulas do not prevent food allergies or sensitization and should only be used in those with a diagnosed milk allergy, milk protein intolerance, or other medical condition in which a specialized formula is required (Greer et al., 2019).

Education

Education regarding how to manage a child's food allergies is of utmost importance to keep the child safe. A few essential components of food allergy education are provided here.

Reading labels. The Food Allergen Labeling and Consumer Protection Act of 2004 required that companies clearly label foods containing milk, egg, soy, wheat, peanut, tree nut, fish, and crustacean shellfish on packaged goods (Oriel & Wang, 2021). It also required the allergen to be listed in unambiguous terms (i.e., milk for casein and whey) (Oriel & Wang, 2021). Sesame was required on all packaging in the United States in 2023. Precautionary advisory labeling (PAL), which is unregulated and not mandated by law, includes the terms "may contain" or "manufactured on shared equipment." PAL can be confusing as these labels do not reliably correspond with the absence of detectable allergenic proteins (Oriel & Wang, 2021). Children at a young age can be taught to avoid their known allergens as they grow more independent and spend more time away from home.

Eating in restaurants. Eating in restaurants can be anxiety provoking for children and families with food allergies. Looking at menus prior to arriving at the restaurant can identify safe foods. While at the restaurant, telling the server and manager about allergies can help alert the kitchen to take precautions when cooking the child's food. If allergen information is not readily available, the best option is to avoid the food item in question.

School safety. All children should have an emergency action plan and an epinephrine injector available at school. At the beginning of the year, the family can

FOOD ALLERGY & ANAPHYLAXIS EMERGENCY CARE PLAN

Name: _____ D.O.B.: _____

Allergic to: _____

Weight: _____ lbs. Asthma: ☐ Yes (higher risk for a severe reaction) ☐ No

NOTE: Do not depend on antihistamines or inhalers (bronchodilators) to treat a severe reaction. USE EPINEPHRINE.

☐ Special Situation/Circumstance - If this box is checked, the child has an extremely severe allergy to the following food(s) _____.

Even if the child has MILD symptoms after eating (ingesting) this food(s), Give Epinephrine immediately.

For ANY of the following SEVERE SYMPTOMS

LUNG Shortness of breath, wheezing, repetitive cough

HEART Pale or bluish skin, faintness, weak pulse, dizziness

THROAT Tight or hoarse throat, trouble breathing or swallowing

MOUTH Significant swelling of the tongue or lips

SKIN Many hives over body, widespread redness

GUT Repetitive vomiting, severe diarrhea

OTHER Feeling something bad is about to happen, anxiety, confusion

OR A COMBINATION of symptoms from different body areas

1. **INJECT EPINEPHRINE IMMEDIATELY.**
2. **Call 911.** Tell emergency dispatcher the person is having anaphylaxis and may need epinephrine when emergency responders arrive.
- Consider giving additional medications following epinephrine:
  » Antihistamine
  » Inhaler (bronchodilator) if wheezing
- Lay the person flat, raise legs and keep warm. If breathing is difficult or they are vomiting, let them sit up or lie on their side.
- If symptoms do not improve, or symptoms return, more doses of epinephrine can be given about 5 minutes or more after the last dose.
- Alert emergency contacts.
- Transport patient to ER, even if symptoms resolve. Patient should remain in ER for at least 4 hours because symptoms may return

MILD SYMPTOMS

NOSE Itchy or runny nose, sneezing

MOUTH Itchy mouth

SKIN A few hives, mild itch

GUT Mild nausea or discomfort

FOR MILD SYMPTOMS FROM MORE THAN ONE BODY SYSTEM, GIVE EPINEPHRINE.

FOR MILD SYMPTOMS FROM A SINGLE BODY SYSTEM (E.G. SKIN, GI, ETC.), FOLLOW THE DIRECTIONS BELOW:
1. Antihistamines may be given, if ordered by a healthcare provider.
2. Stay with the person; alert emergency contacts.
3. Watch closely for changes. If symptoms worsen, give epinephrine.

MEDICATIONS/DOSES

Epinephrine Brand or Generic: _____
Epinephrine Dose: ☐ 0.1 mg IM ☐ 0.15 mg IM ☐ 0.3 mg IM
Antihistamine Brand or Generic: _____
Antihistamine Dose: _____
Other (e.g., inhaler/bronchodilator if wheezing): _____

PATIENT OR PARENT/GUARDIAN AUTHORIZATION SIGNATURE   DATE   HEALTHCARE PROVIDER AUTHORIZATION SIGNATURE   DATE

© 2023, **Food Allergy Research & Education** (FARE - FoodAllergy.org). Used with Permission.

Fig. 7.12 Emergency food allergy plan to follow in case of a reaction. (From Food Allergy Research & Education [FARE]. Copyright 2023. Used with permission.)

meet with the school staff and nurse to discuss allergies and ways to keep the child safe at school. An individualized health plan or 504 can be created for the student. Careful planning with lunchroom staff can help identify foods that are safe for the child to eat. In addition, the child with allergies should never share or trade food with others. There is no need for an allergen-safe table unless the child is not able to safely sit around other children due to behavioral or developmental delays or young children who may have difficulties communicating.

DIFFERENTIAL DIAGNOSIS FOR COMMON ILLNESSES FOR ALLERGIES

Acute Viral Rhinitis

Acute viral rhinitis, or upper respiratory infection (URI), is the most frequent infection in all children and is easily confused with AR. Both may cause

Table 7.6	Summary of the Addendum Guidelines for Early Introduction of Peanut to Infants by NIAID		
ADDENDUM GUIDELINE	INFANT CRITERIA	RECOMMENDATIONS	EARLIEST AGE OF PEANUT INTRODUCTION
1	Severe eczema, egg allergy, or both	Strongly consider evaluation with peanut-specific IgE and/or skin-prick test and, if necessary, an oral food challenge. Based on test results, introduce peanut-containing foods.	4–6 mo
2	Mild-moderate eczema	Introduce peanut-containing foods.	~6 mo
3	No eczema or any food allergy	Introduce peanut-containing foods.	Age-appropriate and in accordance with family preferences and cultural practices

IgE, Immunoglobulin E; NIAID, National Institute of Allergy and Infectious Diseases.

cough, nasal congestion, and discharge. Usually the nasal discharge in URI is time limited (<2 weeks); however, this situation is more difficult to evaluate when the child has a history of recurrent bouts of URI, a common case in school-age children or children in day care.

The diagnosis of seasonal AR is usually straightforward. The clinician who is knowledgeable about local environmental pollens can correlate the clinical signs and symptoms with the seasonal time frame, recorded pollen counts, and personal and family health history and make the diagnosis. The clinician can also differentiate URI from allergies by evaluating for erythematous nasal mucosa, fever, and purulent nasal discharge, all of which are commonly seen in URI.

Vasomotor Rhinitis
Vasomotor rhinitis is a diagnosis made after ruling out AR. Symptoms can be similar to nasal congestion and rhinorrhea. A complaint of an itchy nose or eyes is usually absent. Symptoms occur with exposure to odors, irritants in the air, weather/seasonal change, or air pollution.

Acute Infectious Sinusitis, Pharyngitis, and Conjunctivitis
Acute sinusitis, pharyngitis, and conjunctivitis can be mistaken for allergies. The affected child may have nasal obstruction, sore throat, headache, red eyes, and fatigue. In these cases, the clinician must be alert for signs of infection, such as lymphadenopathy, fever, erythema, and purulent discharge. There is often a history of contagious contact in the family, school, or day care setting. Some of the hallmark signs of allergies, such as pruritus and clear discharge, are not present with infections. A rapid strep test or throat culture can help determine if antibiotics are needed. Infectious conjunctivitis can be differentiated from allergic causes of red eye, primarily with history and physical evidence of infection, such as purulent discharge, the presence of periauricular lymph nodes, and eye crusting. For a child who has recurrent pharyngitis, recurrent otitis media, or snoring, a referral to pediatric otolaryngology should be considered.

Rhinitis Medicamentosa
Rhinitis medicamentosa is severe rebound nasal congestion that occurs as a result of the frequent, prolonged use of OTC nasal decongestant sprays. When the child stops using the spray, the rebound congestion is acute and intensely uncomfortable.

Gastroenteritis and Other Gastrointestinal Problems
GI symptoms such as stomach upset, diarrhea, and vomiting are common symptoms in children, with a myriad of causes other than food allergies, including lactose intolerance, acute gastroenteritis, parasitic infestations, and colic. Intolerance to food is an inability of the body to digest the food, but it is not an allergy because it is not an IgE-mediated reaction driven by the immune system. Differentiating between actual allergies and intolerance is important. Typically, a child with allergies to food will have skin or respiratory symptoms in addition to GI symptoms.

Acute gastroenteritis has an onset of less than 1 week, may or may not be accompanied by a fever, and is always time limited. With a bacterial cause, critical aspects of the history include the presence of bloody diarrhea, fever, chills, and cramps. When caused by a virus, the diarrhea is typically watery. A wait-and-see approach is reasonable in the case of mild gastroenteritis, focusing more on adequate intake of fluids and maintaining hydration. Other helpful clues for discriminating between food allergies and gastroenteritis include the season at the time of presentation (viral, more likely in winter and summer) and contact with other sick individuals. The diagnosis of a parasitic infestation depends ultimately on stool cultures, but a history of recent travel or blood or mucus in the stool increases the likelihood of parasitic infection.

> **Box 7.5**   **Oral Allergy Syndrome Cross-Reacting Pollens and Foods**
>
> Ragweed → bananas, melons (watermelon, cantaloupe, honeydew), zucchini, cucumber
> Birch → apples, pears, peaches, apricots, cherries, plums, prunes, nectarines, kiwi, carrots, celery, potatoes, peppers
> Grass → peaches, celery, melons, tomatoes, oranges

OTHER ALLERGIC CONDITIONS

Oral Allergy Syndrome

Oral allergy syndrome (OAS) is also called pollen allergy food syndrome. This condition occurs in those with pollen allergies, and when they eat certain fruits and vegetables patients will develop symptoms such as itchiness or swelling of the mouth, face, lip, tongue, and throat. The protein found in certain pollens is common to the protein found in fruits and vegetables and confuses the immune system. This rarely causes systemic symptoms as the protein is neutralized in the GI tract.

Symptoms of OAS can be reduced by avoiding eating these raw foods especially during allergy season. Reducing symptoms can also occur by baking or microwaving the food as high temperatures break down the proteins. Also, canned foods may limit the reaction (Box 7.5). Pretreatment with an antihistamine is recommended when symptoms develop. Some studies have shown allergy shots can improve the symptoms of OAS (AAAAI, 2020c).

Eosinophilic Esophagitis

EoE is a chronic condition where there is an accumulation of eosinophils in the esophagus leading to inflammation. The symptoms of EoE can vary based on age. Infants and toddlers may refuse to eat, vomit their food, or not grow properly. School-age children often will have decreased appetite, recurring abdominal pain, and trouble swallowing or vomiting. Teenagers and adults will have the same symptoms, but in addition they often have difficulty swallowing solid foods, which could lead to food impaction (AAAAI, 2022). The treatment options for EoE are as follows:

- Proton pump inhibitors (PPIs) have been found to reduce esophageal inflammation in some patients with EoE. Thus PPIs are often used as the first treatment for EoE.
- Swallowed corticosteroids can also help reduce inflammation. It is important to be on the lowest dose to treat, to eliminate the side effects of corticosteroids.
- An empiric elimination diet can include a combination of dairy, egg, wheat, soy, peanut/tree nut, and fish/shellfish.
- Dupilumab (Dupixent) is the only FDA-approved drug to date for EoE (AAAAI, 2022).

Stinging Insects

Stinging insect bites for most individuals cause redness and swelling at the site; however, some may be allergic and develop systemic reactions or anaphylaxis. The most serious reactions are caused by five types of insects: yellow jackets, honeybees, paper wasps, hornets, and fire ants. For most patients, care of the site with ice, pain medication, and lotion is all that is required. If patients have systemic reactions, they should be treated promptly with epinephrine, be prescribed epinephrine autoinjectors for future emergencies, and be referred to an allergist for ongoing care. Allergy shots may be an option for those with stinging insect allergies.

Drug Allergy

We will not discuss all medications here, but it is important for primary care providers to understand penicillin (PCN) allergies because the label "PCN allergic" is commonly attached in childhood, where common childhood infections can be confused with an allergy. In addition, even in those with true allergies, over 90% will lose this tendency in a 10-year period. Consequently, although approximately 10% of the population is labeled as being allergic to penicillin, over 90% of these individuals are negative on allergy testing and can tolerate penicillin (AAAAI, 2020d). Typically, allergic reactions to PCN will occur in the first 24 to 48 hours of taking the medication. If a reaction is suspicious for allergic reaction, then referral to an allergist is recommended.

Urticaria

Urticarial lesions are described as circumscribed, raised, erythematous plaques, often with central pallor. They may be round, oval, or serpiginous in shape and vary in size. They will be intensely pruritic. Urticaria is defined in two ways: acute (occurrence being present <6 weeks) and chronic (occurs several times a week for >6 weeks). Acute urticaria can be caused by a multitude of reasons, including infection, allergic reaction to foods or drugs, and physical triggers (cold, heat, exercise, vibratory, aquagenic). Chronic urticaria is rarely caused by allergies, and therefore IgE testing is not warranted. Treatment of urticaria includes antihistamines but may require four times the dose (AAAAI, n.d.-d).

ASSOCIATED PROBLEMS OF ALLERGIES AND TREATMENT

Children with allergies often are brought to the clinician with one or more clinical manifestations because there is a strong association between sensitization and symptoms of allergy. Children with asthma, eczema, or rhinitis are more likely to be sensitized to one or more allergens than those without these conditions. Besides asthma and AD (eczema), other associated problems include URIs (sinusitis, pharyngitis, and acute otitis media), eustachian tube obstruction, sleep apnea, and dental malocclusion.

Asthma

One of the most prominent associated conditions is asthma. Studies show that 88% of children with asthma were sensitized to at least one inhalant allergen. When a child is affected by both conditions, both must be aggressively treated.

Atopic Dermatitis (Eczema)

AD is a chronic inflammatory rash characterized by severe pruritus, overall dryness of the skin, and a pattern of exacerbation and remission. Patients with AD have higher rates of allergic diseases than the general population. Up to 80% of children with AD develop asthma and/or AR later in childhood (Spergel, 2022). While allergies do not cause AD, they may be triggers to the flaring of the skin.

Sleep Apnea

Children with AR may be more prone to obstructive sleep apnea because of upper airway edema and lymphoid hypertrophy. Children with allergies who have habitual snoring or evidence of disturbed sleep should receive further workup for obstructive sleep apnea syndrome (OSAS). Once snoring is recognized in a child, a more focused history and examination are necessary to identify the child's potential for OSAS. Detailed information regarding the quality of the snoring and the subsequent pauses, snorts, or gasps are important in distinguishing OSAS from primary snoring. A trial of allergy medications and environmental measures may help alleviate the problem. Referral to a pediatric otolaryngologist or pediatric sleep specialist may be indicated when symptoms persist.

Upper Respiratory Infections

Sinusitis, pharyngitis, and acute otitis media sometimes complicate AR. Clinicians should be careful to follow the current treatment guidelines and avoid the overuse of antibiotics. Children who have recurrent bouts of these related infections should be referred to a pediatric otolaryngologist for consultation. In cases of a persistent cough or recurrent respiratory tract infections, a pediatric pulmonologist may be consulted.

Eustachian Tube Obstruction

Allergies often involve inflammation of the eustachian tubes, which may cause obstruction, accumulation of fluid in the inner ear, and infection. Hearing can be affected, and if the inflammation is chronic, speech problems can develop. This is of particular concern between the ages of 6 months and 3 years, a critical period for speech development.

Dental Malocclusion

AR causes mouth-breathing in many children. The result may be dental malocclusion, causing an overbite that could benefit from an orthodontic referral.

PRIMARY CARE MANAGEMENT FOR ASTHMA AND ALLERGY

HEALTH CARE MAINTENANCE

Summary of Primary Care Needs for the Child with Allergies.

GROWTH AND DEVELOPMENT

Asthma

The practitioner should measure height and weight, calculate body mass index, and record these measurements on the child's growth charts at each acute care and monitoring visit. Major deviations from population norms (i.e., <10th or >90th percentile) or departure (i.e., two or more zones) from the child's individualized curve should be noted and assessed in detail to determine if a lack of asthma control or treatment may be influencing growth. Genetic, social, and nutritional factors unassociated with asthma must be considered when evaluating patterns in growth. Alterations may need to be monitored over time for their significance to be appreciated. During a series of acute exacerbations, a plateau or small drop in weight may take place; however, with improved health status, catchup growth should occur. If it does not, the cause of the weight loss should be further explored.

The first year of ICS use may lead to a temporary decrease in growth velocity, but this should disappear in subsequent years (NHLBI, 2007). Primary care providers need to carefully monitor growth at least every 6 to 12 months after the age of 2 years to evaluate the cost-benefit ratios of treatment protocols. The use of ICS for more than 12 months in children with asthma has a limited impact on annual growth velocity. In ICS users there is a slight reduction of about 1 cm in the final adult height (Loke et al., 2015). Adjunctive long-term control therapy may reduce the need for high-dose inhaled or systemic steroids and thus minimize the dose-dependent undesirable effects of treatment (NHLBI, 2007).

Delays in development are rarely documented in asthma. Delays may be found due to the limitations placed on the child with asthma. These limitations may be in physical activities or social experiences. Physical activity in children with asthma is recommended, although they may have to adjust the sport they play or pretreat with albuterol prior to the activity to be successful. In addition, well-controlled asthma can limit absences from school and social activities.

Allergies

Allergies may result in inadequate food intake and consequently affect growth. Chronic congestion may cause a child to have a poor appetite or allergies to various common foods and may severely limit a child's intake. Mener et al. (2015) performed a meta-analysis that suggests short-term intranasal corticosteroids for the treatment of AR in children may decrease short-term growth velocity; however, the effect on longer-term growth velocity is not clear. Providers should carefully monitor the growth of children receiving long-term steroids.

First-generation antihistamines can cause sedation and may not be appropriate for daily use as they can interfere with the ability to concentrate and focus on school, which can affect the ability to learn. Second-generation antihistamines are less sedated and more appropriate for daytime use. Sedation can also alter the ability to operate machinery and drive automobiles. A child with severe seasonal allergies may need to avoid outdoor activities and sports, even when fully medicated. When this is the case, providers, parents, and children can work together to identify other age-appropriate activities that would be enjoyable for the child and enhance development.

DIET

Asthma
Obesity is a risk factor for asthma, which can lead to an increase in symptoms, frequency of symptoms, more severe exacerbations, and reduced response to asthma medications (Peters et al., 2018). Providers should discuss diet and ways to increase physical activity in the child's lifestyle. Reducing portion sizes, high-calorie/high-fat food intake, and substituting juice and sugary drinks should be discussed. Advocating changes by the entire family rather than focusing just on the child's habits is more effective in stabilizing the child's weight.

Allergy
The current feeding recommendations include the introduction of allergenic foods in infants. After the introduction of complementary foods, allergenic foods can be introduced one at a time, starting around 4 to 6 months of age. Those at high risk of developing food allergies may be referred to an allergist for additional evaluation (Fleischer et al., 2021). Discussion regarding the introduction of allergenic foods should occur at 2-, 4-, and 6-month well-child exams.

Managing the diet of a child with food allergies can be particularly challenging. Because avoidance is the mainstay of treatment, parents must become experts in deciphering food labels and be continually vigilant for hidden sources of the offending food. Several websites provide useful tips for identifying hidden foods on product labels (see Asthma and Allergy Resources, later). Equally challenging is making sure the child with food allergies is getting all nutrients in adequate amounts. For example, a child who has an allergy to milk must consume other sources of calcium and vitamin D or take a supplement. Helping parents find an alternative is an important aspect of the primary care provider's role in promoting good health. In situations of multiple food allergies, providers may refer the family to a nutritionist.

Children with poorly controlled AR may complain of a lack of taste and smell. This may affect their eating and appetite. Ensuring adequate intake of a well-balanced variety of foods may take extra effort for a child with allergies.

SAFETY

Asthma
Medications kept in the home must be safely stored in their original containers in a locked location that is inaccessible to infants and young children. Children will need age-appropriate responsibility for medication administration. Practitioners can help parents identify their child's developmental capabilities and limits for safely assisting with medication by providing age-normative suggestions. For example, when a child is an infant or a toddler, the parents must speak about the medications as such—not as candy. With maturation, toddlers can be taught how to hold facemasks or take slow breaths to assist in therapy. Preschool-age children typically have the manual dexterity to take part in medicinal therapy by helping parents assemble inhalers or count doses in the parent's presence. Young school-age children may be asked to get the medication and take it in the presence of a parent. When older school-age children can tell time, they can assume greater responsibility to prompt the parent when medication is needed, get the medication, take the medication in the parent's presence, and return it to its proper storage place. School-age children should also become increasingly responsible for taking needed medication while at school. Parents can monitor and encourage safe and knowledgeable use by discussing or having a child count and record on a calendar the number of times medication was taken. During adolescence, more autonomy should be given for independently taking, self-carrying, and replenishing both controller and rescue medication and ensuring that the medication is in all needed locations (e.g., home, school, sports bag). Parents need to be reminded that one consistent finding in successful adolescent adherence to prescribed regimens is the continued support and age-appropriate assistance of their parents. With age and increasing time spent away from parents, children must independently recognize when their treatment is not effective and seek assistance. An episode that does not respond to treatment as expected may herald a particularly severe exacerbation requiring the need for systemic corticosteroids (Ratcliffe & Kieckhefer, 2010).

Electrical burns are possible when equipment (e.g., nebulizers and dehumidifiers) is run in the child's presence. Infants and young children should never be left alone where they can reach equipment, cords, or open sockets. School-age children and adolescents should be properly instructed in the safe use of electrical equipment and demonstrate their use to parents or providers before being encouraged to use the equipment independently (Ratcliffe & Kieckhefer, 2010).

Allergies

Children with food allergies must always have injectable epinephrine available in case of an allergic reaction. It is important that all caregivers know how to use epinephrine injectors, and as children age they should be aware of symptoms and know how to use epinephrine devices. A medical alert bracelet to identify the child's allergy is recommended.

IMMUNIZATIONS

Children with asthma and allergies can receive childhood vaccinations, including COVID-19 vaccination, unless there is a history of previous allergic reaction or known allergen to a component of the vaccine. The number of reported possible allergic reactions to vaccines is high, but confirmed vaccine-triggered allergic reactions are rare, affecting less than 1 in 100,000 (Nilsson et al., 2017). Egg allergy is no longer considered a contraindication to influenza and measles, mumps, rubella (MMR) vaccines.

Steroid therapies that are short term (<2 weeks), alternate day scheduling, physiologic replacement, or topical (skin or eyes) and aerosol treatments are not considered contraindications to the use of live virus vaccines. The immunosuppressive effects of corticosteroid treatment vary, but many clinicians consider a dose equivalent to either 2 mg/kg of body weight or a total of 20 mg/day of prednisone for 2 or more weeks to be considered immunosuppressive and raise a concern about the safety of vaccination with live virus vaccines (e.g., MMR, varicella, live attenuated influenza vaccine, yellow fever). Providers should wait at least 1 month after discontinuation of therapy or reduction of dose before administering a live virus vaccine to patients who have received highly systemically absorbed doses of corticosteroids for 2 weeks or more. Inactivated vaccines and toxoids can be administered to all immunosuppressed patients in usual doses and schedules, although the response to these vaccines may be suboptimal (Immunize.org, n.d.).

Infants and children may have frequent signs of respiratory infection; these signs alone, in the absence of specifically published contraindication, should not be the basis for deferring immunizations (AAP, 2008b). Inadequate immunization with subsequent risk of infection is of greater concern. Only if the child is currently ill with moderate or severe illness with or without fever should a vaccine be delayed.

Children with asthma may experience complications with influenza (e.g., increased wheezing, bronchitis, pneumonia, increased school absences and medical care visits). Therefore, despite recent or current prednisone bursts, children with asthma should annually receive an influenza vaccine after the age of 6 months.

The flu vaccine is available as a shot or a nasal spray. The Asthma and Allergy Foundation of America (AAFA, 2022) recommends the following:

- Ages 6 months to 4 years: Get the flu shot.
- Ages 4 and older: If your asthma is under control with no symptoms, you can get the flu shot or the nasal spray vaccine.
- Ages 4 and older: If you have recent asthma episodes or wheezing, get the flu shot.

Routine pneumococcal immunization is recommended. Ongoing immunization of children after 24 months who are on high-dose oral corticosteroids with the 23-valent vaccine is warranted because of their presumed high-risk status for serious infection (CDC, 2022).

SCREENING

- Diet and exercise: Routine screening is recommended.
  - Children with asthma and allergies can still fully participate in physical activity. If the family reports trouble participating, then discussion regarding pretreating sport with a bronchodilator or finding an activity that would be suited for the child is recommended.
- Anemia: Routine screening is recommended.
  - Children on a restricted diet for food allergies may be iron deficient and may need supplementation.
- Cholesterol on 9- to 11-year-olds: Routine screening is recommended.
- Vision: Routine screening is recommended.
  - Daily high-dose corticosteroids may cause inflammatory changes, cataracts, and glaucoma in adults; refer to an eye doctor if abnormal findings are present during a routine exam.
  - Ocular symptoms or the use of ocular medications for the treatment of allergic conjunctivitis may require closer evaluation of a child's eyes on physical examination.
- Hearing: Routine screening is recommended. A child with allergies may require more frequent hearing screens to evaluate for a hearing deficit that may be secondary to recurrent otitis media or transient congestion.
- Dental: Routine screening is recommended.
  - Inhaled medication may lead to an increased risk of dental caries. Rinsing the mouth after inhaling all medications should be routinely taught.
  - Malocclusion may occur due to prolonged mouth breathing.
- Blood pressure: Routine screening is recommended. Since there is a link between obesity and asthma, obesity and hypertension, more frequent evaluation in an asthmatic child that is classified as obese is recommended (US Preventive Services Task Force, 2020).

Condition-Specific Screening

- Review of medication use. Routine monitoring of medication use is important to maintain good asthma and allergy control. Also, review the use of quick relieving medication as this may indicate that asthma is not well controlled. For children with seasonal allergies, review their seasons and when to make sure of medication.

- Lung function. Ongoing monitoring in the office setting can assess current function, airway obstruction, and the effects of treatment. Spirometry should be done at diagnosis, following any changes in treatment, and annually. Spirometry should always be evaluated in the context of clinical history because, when used alone, it can underestimate disease severity and control (Ratcliffe & Kieckhefer, 2010).
- Allergic triggers. A biannual review of possible environmental allergens and irritants is helpful. Repeat testing may be warranted if implicated in asthma exacerbations or if medication is not controlling symptoms, as immunotherapy may be a treatment option. A review of environmental remediations is also recommended. Allergy testing can be done at any age; however, pollen allergies are typically not seen until between 3 and 6 years of age. Indoor triggers such as animal dander and dust mite can be a trigger in infants and toddlers. Referral to an allergist is recommended for poor control of allergy and asthma symptoms due to environmental allergens.
- Food allergies. Have IgE testing every 1 to 2 years to identify if children are losing sensitization to food.

DEVELOPMENTAL ISSUES

Sleep Patterns

Asthma. Sleep patterns are common in healthy young children as well as in older children and adolescents with asthma. When young children have sleep disturbances, parental sleep is also typically disrupted. Those children with poorly controlled asthma, along with their parents, report significant sleep issues. When sleep is disrupted by nocturnal asthma symptoms, there is evidence that deficient sleep leads to increased daytime asthma symptoms (Meltzer & Pugliese, 2017). As providers, we need to determine if there are any night symptoms of asthma during our history and assessment with each clinic visit. Nocturnal symptoms represent an exaggeration of existing bronchial hyperresponsivity; optimizing daytime control and reducing environmental irritants in the child's room often reduce symptoms.

Most young children find a nighttime ritual soothing. Primary care providers can assist parents in establishing a bedtime ritual that is relaxing and easily implemented by the family.

Allergies. Nasal obstruction and itching can disrupt the sleep of children with allergies. It can result in restlessness, shortened naps, and waking during the night. For example, for patients with AR, circadian rhythms can lead to a peak in nasal congestion during the early morning hours, adversely affecting sleep quality. Furthermore, histamine, an inflammatory mediator released during an allergic reaction, might contribute to disturbed sleep because it is involved in

the regulation of the sleep-wake cycle and arousal but also can induce symptoms of rhinitis, directly leading to sleep disruption. Typical sleep-related problems seen in patients with AR include sleep-disordered breathing, sleep apnea, and snoring, all of which are associated with nasal congestion/obstruction (Koinis-Mitchell et al., 2021).

The resulting sleep deprivation can cause irritability and an inability to concentrate, disturbing home and school activities. When this happens, providers should be careful not to mislabel a child with attention-deficit/hyperactivity disorder or a learning disability. In turn, daytime sleepiness may be attributed to the sedative effects of some antihistamines rather than a lack of sleep. The clinician must be alert for these more subtle signs of allergies, be certain that the child's treatment plan is appropriately aggressive, and ensure the plan is well understood by the child and family to promote adherence. In addition, clinicians must encourage a reasonable bedtime and consistent bedtime ritual.

Carpets, stuffed toys, curtains, or anything that retains dust should be removed from the sleeping room, and the change in symptoms should be noted. Dust mite covers for the pillow and mattress can be tried at a low cost. Pets should remain out of the sleeping room, and windows should be kept closed, reducing pollen and grass allergens. Mold-producing agents such as houseplants should be removed. The regional American Lung Association may have a home environmentalist program that can provide a comprehensive in-home assessment if requested by the family.

Toileting

Toileting needs are typically not altered by a child's asthma. Bowel and bladder training is achieved at the expected ages.

Food allergies with accompanying symptoms of diarrhea can cause additional challenges in the toddler who is toilet training. When this occurs, it is best to caution the parent to wait until the diarrhea subsides before proceeding with toilet training.

Discipline

Asthma. Parents may report that they find it difficult to deal with discipline for fear of upsetting the child and initiating an asthma exacerbation. Because children with asthma may experience some degree of bronchospasm with intense crying, the parental concern is understandable. Crying cannot be entirely avoided, but parents should be reassured that most discipline can be implemented by rewarding desirable behaviors if this is done routinely and begins early in a child's life. The inconsistent limit setting for undesirable behavior only confuses children and makes it more difficult for them to learn and internalize the limits chosen by their parents. Another parental concern is that the child's irritability, refusals, or acting-out behavior is caused by illness or medications. Medications and illness may influence the child's behavior, but the consistency of parental expectations is of greater importance. Blaming illness or medication does not remove the necessity to help a child develop behaviors desired by the family and social networks (Ratcliffe & Kieckhefer, 2010).

Allergies. Caregivers must be reminded that behavioral manifestations may be due to inadequately treated allergies. Itchy eyes, nose, skin, and ears can be extremely uncomfortable. Children can feel totally miserable but be unable to fully verbalize the symptoms. This is especially true with young children but can also apply to older children or adolescents. Sometimes, children just feel bad, get irritable, and cry or act out in some other way. The whole family can be disrupted, and parents may feel compelled to employ stronger disciplining methods. However, if the true underlying cause of the misbehavior is allergies, caregivers should be encouraged to seek help in reevaluating the treatment plan with the provider and adapt as necessary to achieve better control of allergy symptoms.

Child Care

Asthma. Most families find it necessary to use child care services on either a regular or sporadic basis. Having a child with asthma should not prohibit this. Because URIs trigger exacerbations of asthma in many children less than 5 years of age, a smaller site with less chance of exposure to these infections may reduce the number of asthma exacerbations. Parents should evaluate the child care environment for any known triggers. Licensed child care centers prohibit exposure to secondhand smoke and are evaluated for dust mite catchers (e.g., carpets, stuffed toys, or furniture), molds or mildew, and animals. If unlicensed, private, or in-home child care arrangements do not need to meet state requirements, parents must take the initiative to evaluate these known triggers. With proper communication and explanation, child care can be safely accomplished with a responsible, interested caretaker. Whether child care is at a center or is home based, provided by a relative, neighbor, or professional, information must be shared by parents to ensure success in asthma management.

Parents are responsible for providing all relevant information to the caretaker; that is, what triggers the child's asthma, early warning signs of an impending asthma episode, what the caretaker should do first, what should be done next if the action is not fully effective, how the parent and other responsible parties (i.e., including health care provider) can be reached, and what information must be passed on to emergency personnel if they are called. The recommended way to provide this information is in written format, using an asthma action plan created by the health care provider. Examples of this asthma action plan can be found earlier in this chapter. Parents can be encouraged to share the action plan they receive, or the provider can obtain parental permission to mail a copy directly to the child care provider, whichever best ensures that the child care site obtains the needed paperwork.

If the child care provider is to give any treatments, the parent must demonstrate the procedures and observe the provider's repeat performance. In addition, center-based programs may require written prescriptions from the primary health care provider and written permission from the parent for the child care provider to perform the treatment. Parents must maintain close contact with the child care provider to learn about changing triggers or emerging early warning signs.

Anyone in repeated contact with the child who observes responses to treatments should also relay that information to the parent. This information can then be integrated into the overall routine reevaluation of the treatment plan. Treatment modifications should be immediately related to the child care provider so that a consistent approach is provided to the child regardless of the setting. Frequent and open communication is the key to successful child care arrangements. At times, direct communication between the child care site and the health care provider, with parental consent, may be beneficial (Ratcliffe & Kieckhefer, 2010).

Allergies. Child care providers are usually very vigilant about contagious conditions, and it is not unusual for a child with red teary eyes, a runny nose, cough, or sneezing to be sent home for fear that other children will be exposed to the illness. Parents of children with allergies can be quite frustrated when this happens repeatedly. If the red eyes or runny nose is exclusively allergy related, the clinician can work with the parents to reassure the day care center that the child poses no threat to the other children. Usually, a statement from the clinician verifying that this is not a contagious condition is sufficient. It may also be helpful to send additional written information to reinforce the facts. There are excellent resources for parents and caregivers that can be used (See Asthma and Allergy Resources, later).

One critical issue in day care concerns the child who has a severe food allergy. Day care providers must be informed of the allergy and whatever additional information they need to fully understand the problem and how it should be handled. Ideally, a food allergy action plan should be in place, as described in the earlier section on anaphylaxis. In cases of severe food allergies, an EpiPen of 0.3 mg, 0.15 mg, or 0.10 mg and oral antihistamine should be kept at the day care center with explicit instructions. When there are multiple food allergies, a list of offending foods can be posted in both the day care kitchen and classroom areas, especially if the day care center employs multiple caregivers. Clear distinctions should be made between food intolerances, mild food allergies, and severe food allergies. Information should be distributed to all parents who may also bring food into the school or day care setting to avoid accidental exposure to the offending food.

Schooling

Asthma. Poorly controlled asthma can lead to an increase in school absences. Parents report that communicating with school personnel is essential but often difficult. Many teachers do not recognize a cough as a sign of poorly controlled asthma but instead mistake it for an infectious disease that should be managed at home. Teachers and administrators may attempt to limit the child more than the parents or primary care provider believes necessary, especially regarding sports participation. With appropriate warmup, pacing, hydration, and preventive pharmacologic therapy, almost all children with asthma will be able to participate in active school activities on a regular basis. Field trips also do not need limitations, although a SABA and a copy of the asthma management plan should accompany the child on each field trip.

Fitting in with school peers and maintaining positive peer relationships are essential to the child's full development. Parents can actively arrange peer gatherings, encourage the child to join clubs or organizations, and allow the child age-appropriate independence in visiting friends to ensure social experiences. Friends may question why the child is taking medications, and simple explanations about the child's asthma should be given with the assurance that asthma is not contagious. This might also be done in school as a class presentation with the teacher's assistance because with asthma, one of the most common chronic conditions of childhood, several children in any classroom may have it. Parents are encouraged to discuss their child's asthma with the parents of their child's peers so that all may have an honest understanding of the child's condition and abilities as well as any temporary limitations or needs for treatment (Ratcliffe & Kieckhefer, 2010).

Allergies. Up to 25% of individuals with AR miss time from school or work. Those who do go to school or work are significantly less productive and less able to learn often due to poor sleep or sedating effects of medications.

The school setting can be a source of many allergens. Common sources of allergic triggers in school include chalk dust, classroom pets, plants, upholstered furniture or pillows, and carpeting. School-age children should be seated as far away from the blackboard as possible if it is a chalk-type board to minimize exposure to chalk dust. Other less obvious sources of allergens include mold and industrial cleaning agents. If a child's allergies are much worse during school days,

with improvement during the weekends or vacations, then a review of products used in the building is recommended. For children with specific environmental allergies, school personnel can be instructed to close the windows when the grass is being cut or leaves are being raked. Depending on school regulations, the school nurse or designated person may be able to administer medications as needed, such as antihistamines, to a child with acute symptoms.

Physical education, recess period activities, and after-school sports programs do not usually cause additional problems for the child with allergies unless such activities take place outside during the high-pollen season. School personnel may have to alter the child's schedule to avoid being outside on high-pollen days. The family and the school nurse can collaborate to be aware of those days and make appropriate adjustments.

School nurses and teachers should be informed about a child with AR or allergic conjunctivitis. Even with appropriate treatment, the child may sometimes have inflamed eyes or a runny nose. Like day care providers, school personnel will usually take any potential exposure to an infectious condition very seriously, so they must be reassured that the child is not contagious and is getting proper treatment. As in the day care situation, clinicians and parents must provide the necessary documentation to allay any fears of school personnel.

The school-age child who is treated with antihistamines may be drowsy during school, decreasing school performance. Children usually do better if treated with a second-generation antihistamine, which typically does not cause sedation. Conversely, the school-age child who is taking a decongestant may be overactive and therefore have trouble focusing on schoolwork. For both reasons, providers must be careful to recommend the minimum medication with the least adverse side effects while achieving optimum symptom control.

Food allergies are a common cause of anaphylactic reactions that occur outside the hospital. Discussions with school personnel, including the principal, teachers, nurses, cafeteria workers, and other school personnel, are imperative. School nurses can play a key role in the safety and care of children with allergies by ensuring that each child has current information about allergies and treatment on file and that appropriate personnel is fully aware of the plan for care. An emergency health care plan should include specifics regarding the child's allergies, typical reactions, and a plan to administer epinephrine. Emergency epinephrine should always be available in school and on field trips. The school emergency plan should be updated at least yearly, including emergency contact information. All school personnel who may be in a setting to respond to an anaphylactic emergency should have a copy of the plan. Attaching a photo of the child is useful for rapid identification.

Sexuality

Asthma. As noted earlier, pubertal development may be delayed if asthma has not been adequately controlled to allow regular growth. Systemic corticosteroids historically have been associated with delays in development because of their effect on the adrenal glands and corticosteroid production.

Allergies. Age-appropriate anticipatory guidance regarding sexuality should be provided for preadolescents and adolescents with allergies similar to that given to their peers. If there is a known allergy to latex, information about the avoidance of latex condoms and diaphragms should be discussed. In this case the child must also be aware of the risk for anaphylaxis along with a plan of action, including epinephrine.

Transition to Adulthood

Asthma. As youth with asthma enter adulthood, it is important that they continue to increase and periodically update their understanding of asthma and its management. Formal review and updating education might take place before a move to college or a switch in primary care providers. College students need to have access to their medications and an emergency care provider while away from home. If persons with a history of moderate to severe asthma are currently symptom free, they should be reminded to inform their adult provider of their asthma history because symptoms may return later in life. If the history is complex, a formal request for the transfer of records to the adult health care provider should be made. Maintaining a smoke-free work environment is essential. Some vocations that involve inhaled irritants or allergens and overexposure to known triggers (e.g., work with laboratory animals, cleaning fluids, or painting products) may be best avoided (Ratcliffe & Kieckhefer, 2010).

Allergies. Most children with allergies will progress to adulthood with some allergy symptoms. For this reason, children and adolescents must be encouraged to move gradually toward independence in their self-management care. As with most chronic conditions, such a transition must start early, with young children learning the basics of their condition and care. By adolescence, the parents can assume a supportive role while the teenager practices self-care. Young adults with food allergies may take additional risks by not always carrying epinephrine injectors, not reading food labels, or ingesting foods that may contain their allergen. It is important to discuss with adolescent patients to continue safe allergen practices as well as educate their peers about their food allergies and how to use epinephrine injectors.

FAMILY CONCERNS

Asthma. Family members may express guilt during the child's exacerbations because of the genetic nature of asthma. Parents should be reminded that there is little they could have done to prevent asthma in their children, but they can help prevent exacerbations. Given the familial nature of asthma, cultural and ethnic considerations are important. In the United States, minority ethnicity and poverty continue to be linked to potentially reduced access to care, lower quality of care, and reduced implementation of recommended care with subsequent higher risks of morbidity and mortality.

Providers must be child advocates for reducing environmental exposures that cause asthma and its exacerbation (e.g., prenatal tobacco smoke, preterm birth, housing with poor ventilation, mold and mildew, and early URI). Providers can support policies and legislation that ensure comprehensive systems with the ability to meet the needs of children with asthma and universal access to health care because both have been found to influence asthma outcomes. Exploring the values, beliefs, and health practices of diverse families can assist in optimizing the care of the child. Individualized plans help ensure the greatest acceptance and implementation of the recommended care by tailoring the management program to the cultural realities of the child and family.

Prenatal exposure to tobacco is linked to developing asthma, and smoking by a family member is also associated with increased asthma flareups. Changing the smoking habits of family members is difficult for health care providers and family members alike. When advising families to eliminate smoke from their child's environment, the practitioner should convey resources for smoking cessation or, at minimum, risk avoidance. If unable to stop smoking, parents must be reminded to only smoke outside (i.e., not in another room, near an open window, or in the car) and wear a smoking jacket (i.e., an outer layer to prevent smoke retention on clothes). In-home smoking can lead to a more frequent need for systemic steroids, can lead to hospitalizations with extended stays, and in some extreme situations may be considered child endangerment.

Many parents express ambivalence about long-term medication regimens, especially when the child has been taking medications for years. Although parents acknowledge the effectiveness of these regimens, many also hold the belief that long-term medication—especially steroids—can be harmful to their children. Helpful approaches for supporting parents include acknowledging and discussing these common feelings while presenting the belief that more detrimental effects of asthma come from poor control. It is also useful to reinforce that the long-term treatment program will continue to be tailored to their individual child, trying to decrease medication to the minimum amount needed for symptom control.

Asthma, like all chronic conditions, can disrupt the life of the child's family. Disruption comes not only from disease but also from management activities. It is important to recognize the effort families exert and point out successes for them to reflect on, as well as continue to implement the simplest, most effective treatment regimen (Ratcliffe & Kieckhefer, 2010).

Allergies. When managing a child's allergies, it is important to recognize the strong familial link and the likelihood that several other family members may also have allergies. The provider should inquire about allergies in other family members to ascertain how they are managing their condition and discourage the sharing of medications. Altering the home environment by installing air conditioning, removing carpeting, or even getting rid of the family pet may be essential to controlling allergen exposure. Following local pollen reports can be helpful in controlling outdoor allergies.

Food allergies require the vigilance of the whole family. Avoiding foods often necessitates change on the part of the entire family. Using nutritionists specializing in food allergies can help the family maintain a balanced diet while avoiding offending foods. Linking families to resources and support groups is a critical aspect of management. As with any chronic condition, dealing with food allergies is a disruption of normal daily life. The families of children with food allergies must live with constant uncertainties and fear for this reason, a careful and accurate diagnosis must be made, followed by education and emotional support. Treating allergies, whether others in the family share the condition, will always include treating the family as a unit.

RESOURCES

Primary care providers should become familiar with the local offices of national organizations (see the list that follows) to identify community-based services in the area that can complement their health care services. Many of these community-based services have programs that are useful to children and parents for the daily management of asthma and allergies. Consider adding a lending library or links to educational organizations on your office's website.

ASTHMA AND ALLERGY RESOURCES

Air Now: www.airnow.gov
Allergic-Child: www.allergicchild.com
Allergies and Asthma Network: allergyasthmanetwork.org
Allergy and Asthma Network: www.breatherville.org
American Academy of Allergies, Asthma, and Immunology: www.aaaai.org
American College of Allergy, Asthma, and Immunology: www.acaai.org
American Association for Respiratory Care: www.aarc.org
American Lung Association: www.lungusa.org
Association of Asthma Educators: www.asthmaeducators.org
Asthma and Allergy Foundation of America: www.aafa.org
Centers for Disease Control and Prevention: www.cdc.gov
Food Allergy Awareness Connection Team (FAACT): www.foodallergyawareness.org
Food Allergy Research and Education (FARE): www.foodallergy.org
Food Equality Initiative: www.foodequalityinitiative.org
Kids with Food Allergies: www.kidswithfoodallergie.com
Mission Allergy: www.missionallergy.com
National Allergy: www.natlallergy.com
National Heart, Lung, and Blood Institute: www.nhlbi.nih.gov; www.nhlbi.nih.gov/health-topics/asthma-management-guidelines-2020-updates
National Jewish Health: www.nationaljewish.org
Pollen Count: www.pollen.com
Snack Safely: www.snacksafely.com
US Environmental Protection Agency: www.epa.gov

Health Care Maintenance

GROWTH AND DEVELOPMENT
- It is important to monitor height, weight, and body mass index and evaluate anything outside of normal expectations.
- Prolonged steroid use may affect growth; monitor carefully.
- First-generation antihistamines and disordered sleep can impede a child's ability to learn.
- Delayed development is only noted when unnecessary limitations are placed on the child.

DIET AND EXERCISE
- Children who are overweight should be encouraged to increase exercise and eat a well-balanced diet without excess caloric intake.
- Introduction of food, including allergenic foods, should begin between 4 and 6 months and before 11 months of age after complementary foods have been tolerated.
  - If considered high risk for the development of food allergies, then referral to an allergist is recommended.
- Offer a wide variety of healthy foods.
- Children with food allergies may need guidance in selecting appropriate substitutions or supplementations to ensure a balanced diet. A referral to a nutritionist may be necessary.

Continued

Health Care Maintenance—cont'd

SAFETY
- Children with food allergies need injectable epinephrine for home and school.
  - This includes having an emergency action plan for reactions.
- Regular instruction regarding the use of epinephrine is needed. It is safer to give epinephrine than to withhold treatment.
- A medical alert bracelet identifying the allergy and treatment is recommended.
- Altering the home environment by installing air conditioning, removing carpeting, fixing water issues, remediation of insect and rodent infestations, and limiting exposure to animals is essential to controlling allergen exposure.
- Medication safety changes with developmental age and adjustments in mediation handling and storage are needed.
- Using quick relievers too often or lack of response should be monitored and may require prompt treatment in ED or a change in asthma management.

IMMUNIZATIONS
- Routine immunizations are recommended.
- There is no contraindication to the influenza vaccine in children who are allergic to egg.

SLEEP PATTERN
- A regular bedtime routine is recommended.
- Exacerbations in asthma or seasonal allergies may interfere with sleep.
- Reduce environmental triggers in the bedroom.
- Daytime use of first-generation antihistamines may cause daytime drowsiness.

TOILETING
- Toilet training is routine.

DISCIPLINE
- Rewarding positive behavior and creating behavioral expectations are recommended.
- Monitor for illness and medications causing changes in mood and behavior, and if noted then a change in medication is necessary.
- Discipline should not be avoided out of concern that upsetting the child will induce an asthma attack.

CHILD CARE
- A clear description of environmental allergies, food allergies, and asthma triggers, including an emergency plan and medications, should be at all locations that the child spends time.
  - Child care providers should be trained in how to:
    - Recognize signs and symptoms of an allergic reaction and an asthma attack
    - Use an epinephrine injector and quick reliever inhalers (albuterol)

SCHOOLING
- School personnel should have written documentation of known allergens and asthma triggers.
- A written emergency plan and medications should be in the school nurse's office.
  - Plans and medications should accompany children on all field trips.
- Triggers (e.g., chalk dust, classroom pets, plants, mold, carpeting) should be identified and measures taken to reduce exposure for the child.
- Encourage participation in physical activity. Alternative activities may be necessary on high pollen days or if a child's asthma is flared.
- Discuss medication use with school personnel as some medications may make the child drowsy.
- Children with asthma and allergies may need an individualized health plan or 504 plan on file.

SEXUALITY
- Latex allergy may be a concern for a sexually active adolescent; education should be provided.

TRANSITION TO ADULTHOOD
- As children mature into adolescents, they gradually increase their participation and responsibility for care.
- Begin discussing a transition plan from a pediatric provider to an adult care provider.
- Allergic and asthma symptoms may improve in adolescence and young adults, but discuss the importance of having medication available if symptoms return.
- Discuss vocational issues.

FAMILY CONCERNS
- Care of an allergic and asthmatic family requires assistance from the entire family as changes in the home environment and diet may be necessary to keep the child safe.
- Smoking is detrimental to a child's health, and encouragement of family members to quit smoking is recommended.
- Medication sharing among family members is discouraged.

REFERENCES

Ahrens, B., & Posa, D. (2017). Prevention of allergies in childhood – where are we now? *Allergologie Select, 1*(2), 200–213. https://doi.org/10.5414/ALX01807E.

American Academy of Allergy Asthma & Immunology n.d.-a American Academy of Allergy Asthma & Immunology. (n.d.-a).

American Academy of Allergy Asthma & Immunology. (n.d.-b). Atopy defined. *Childhood Asthma Control Test (C-ACT).* Retrieved May 11, 2022, from https://www.aaaai.org/Tools-for-the-Public/Allergy,-Asthma-Immunology-Glossary/Atopy-Defined#:~:text=Share%20this%20page%3A,inhaled%20allergens%20and%20food%20allergens.

American Academy of Allergy Asthma & Immunology. (n.d.-c) Eye (ocular) allergy. Retrieved May 30, 2022, from https://www.aaaai.org/Conditions-Treatments/Allergies/Eye-(Ocular)-Allergy.

American Academy of Allergy Asthma & Immunology. (n.d.-d) Hives (urticaria) and angioedema overview. Retrieved May 29, 2022, from https://www.aaaai.org/Tools-for-the-Public/Conditions-Library/Allergies/Hives-(Urticaria)-and-Angioedema-Overview.

American Academy of Allergy Asthma & Immunology. (2020a). Immunotherapy can provide lasting relief. Retrieved May 30, 2022, from https://www.aaaai.org/Tools-for-the-Public/Conditions-Library/Allergies/Immunotherapy-can-Provide-Lasting-Relief.

American Academy of Allergy Asthma & Immunology. (2020b). Inhaled corticosteroids. Retrieved May 15, 2022, from https://www.aaaai.org/Tools-for-the-Public/Drug-Guide/Inhaled-Corticosteroids.

American Academy of Allergy Asthma & Immunology. (2020c). Long acting beta agonists (LABAS) Retrieved May 30, 2022, from https://www.aaaai.org/tools-for-the-public/drug-guide/long-acting-beta-agonists-(labas).

American Academy of Allergy Asthma & Immunology. (2020d). Oral allergy syndrome (OAS). Retrieved May 30, 2022, from https://www.aaaai.org/Tools-for-the-Public/Conditions-Library/Allergies/Oral-allergy-syndrome-(OAS).

American Academy of Allergy Asthma & Immunology. (2020e). Penicillin allergy–what do you need to know? Retrieved May 15, 2022, from https://www.aaaai.org/tools-for-the-public/conditions-library/allergies/penicillin-allergy.

American Academy of Allergy Asthma & Immunology. (2022). Eosinophilic esophagitis (EOE). Retrieved June 15, 2022, from https://www.aaaai.org/tools-for-the-public/conditions-library/allergies/eosinophilic-esophagitis.

American College of Allergy Asthma and Immunology. (2022). Biologic cheat sheet. Retrieved May 4, 2022, from https://college.acaai.org/wp-content/uploads/2022/04/ACAAI-Biologics-Cheat-Sheet-040522.pdf.

Anvari, S., Miller, J., Chih-Yen, Y., Davis, C. (2019). IgE mediated food allergy. *Clinical Review in Allergy and Immunology, 57,* 244–260.

Asthma and Allergy Foundation of America, 2022, Flu (influenza). from https://www.aafa.org/asthma/asthma-triggers/other-health-conditions/respiratory-infections/flu-influenza.aspx#:~:text=AAFA%20recommends%20the%20following%3A,wheezing%2C%20get%20the%20flu%20shot.

Brown, T. (2019). Diagnosis and management of allergic rhinitis in children. *Pediatric Annals, 48*(12), 485–488.

Brusselle, G., & Koppelman, G. (2022). Biologic therapies for severe asthma. *New England Journal of Medicine, 386,* 157–171.

Centers for Disease Control and Prevention (2022, January 24). Pneumococcal vaccination: Who and when to vaccinate. Retrieved June 24, 2022, from https://www.cdc.gov/vaccines/vpd/pneumo/hcp/who-when-to-vaccinate.html UpToDate.

deShazo, R., & Kemp, S. (2022, April 26). *Allergic rhinitis: Clinical manifestations, epidemiology, and diagnosis.* UpToDate. https://www.uptodate.com/contents/allergic-rhinitis-clinical-manifestations-epidemiology-and-diagnosis.

Du Toit, G., Roberts, G., Sayre, P. H., Bahnson, H. T., Radulovic, S., Santos, A. F., Brough, H. A., Phippard, D., Basting, M., Feeney, M., Turcanu, V., Sever, M. L., Gomez Lorenzo, M., Plaut, M., Lack, G., & LEAP Study Team (2015). Randomized trial of peanut consumption in infants at risk for peanut allergy. *The New England Journal of Medicine, 372*(9), 803–813. https://doi.org/10.1056/NEJMoa1414850.

Fleischer, D. M., Chan, E. S., Venter, C., Spergel, J. M., Abrams, E. M., Stukus, D., Groetch, M., Shaker, M., & Greenhawt, M. (2021). A consensus approach to the primary prevention of food allergy through nutrition: Guidance from the American Academy of Allergy, Asthma, and Immunology; American College of Allergy, Asthma, and Immunology; and the Canadian Society for Allergy and Clinical Immunology. *The Journal of Allergy and Clinical Immunology. In practice, 9*(1), 22–43.e4. https://doi.org/10.1016/j.jaip.2020.11.002.

Food Allergy Research and Education. (n.d.-a) Food allergy and anaphylaxis emergency plan. Retrieved May 14, 2022, from https://www.foodallergy.org/living-food-allergies/food-allergy-essentials/food-allergy-101/food-allergy-action-plan-center.

Food Allergy Research and Education. (n.d.-b). Food allergy facts and statistics. Retrieved May 14, 2022, from https://www.foodallergy.org/resources/facts-and-statistics.

Gallucci, M., Carbonara, P., Pacilli, A. M. G., et al. (2019, Mar 5). Use of symptoms scores, spirometry, and other pulmonary function testing for asthma monitoring. *Frontiers in Pediatrics, 7,* 54.

Global Initiative for Asthma (GINA). (n.d.) Global strategy for asthma management and prevention 2022 report. Retrieved May 1, 2022, from https://ginasthma.org/wp-content/uploads/2022/07/GINA-Main-Report-2022-FINAL-22-07-01-WMS.pdf.

Greer, F., Sicherer, S., & Burks, W. (2019). The effects of early nutritional interventions on the development of atopic disease in infants and children: The role of maternal dietary restriction, breastfeeding, hydrolyzed formulas, and timing of introduction of allergenic complementary foods. *Pediatrics, 143*(4), e20190281.

Gupta, R., Holdford, D., Bilaver, L., Dyer, A., Holl, J., Meltzer, D. (2013). The economic impact of childhood food allergy in the United States. *JAMA Pediatrics, 167*(11), 1026–1031.

Hossney, E., Rosario, N., Lee, B. W., Singh, M., El-Ghoneimy, D., Yi Soh, J., Le Souef, P. (2016). The use of inhaled corticosteroids in pediatric asthma: Update. *The World Allergy Organization Journal, 9,* 26. https://doi.org/10.1186/s40413-016-0117-0.

Immunize.org. (n.d.). Ask the experts: Contraindications and precautions. Retrieved June 5, 2022, from https://www.immunize.org/askexperts/contraindications-precautions.asp.

Kim, H., Ellis, A., Fischer, D., Noseworthy, M., Olivenstein, R., Chapman, K., Lee, J. (2017). Asthma biomarkers in the age of biologics. *Journal of Allergy and Clinical Immunology, 13,* 48.

Kemper, K. J. (2022, May). Complementary and alternative medicine in pediatrics. *UpToDate.* Retrieved June 24, 2022, from https://www.uptodate.com/contents/complementary-and-alternative-medicine-in-pediatrics?topicRef=16359.

Koinis-Mitchell, D., Craig, T., Esteban, C. A., & Klein, R. B. (2012). Sleep and allergic disease: a summary of the literature and future directions for research. *The Journal of Allergy and Clinical Immunology, 130*(6), 1275–1281. https://doi.org/10.1016/j.jaci.2012.06.026.

Loke, Y. K., Blanco, P., Thavarajah, M., & Wilson, A. M. (2015). Impact of inhaled corticosteroids on growth in children with asthma: Systematic review and meta-analysis. *PloS One, 10*(7), e0133428. https://doi.org/10.1371/journal.pone.0133428.

Meltzer, L. J., & Pugliese, C. E. (2017). Sleep in young children with asthma and their parents. *Journal of Child Health Care, 21*(3), 301–311. https://doi.org/10.1177/1367493517712064.

Mener, D. J., Shargorodsky, J., Varadhan, R., & Lin, S. Y. (2015). Topical intranasal corticosteroids and growth velocity in children: a meta-analysis. *International Forum of Allergy & Rhinology, 5*(2), 95–103. https://doi.org/10.1002/alr.21430.

Murphy, K., & Solis, J. (2021). National Asthma Education and prevention program 2020 guidelines: What's important for primary care. *The Journal of Family Practice, 70*(6 Supplement), 19–28. https://doi.org/10.12788/jfp.0219.

Naja, A., Permaul, P., & Phipatanakul, W. (2018). Taming asthma in school-aged children: A comprehensive review. *Journal of Allergy and Clinical Immunology: In Practice, 6*(3), 726–735.

National Institute of Health: National Heart, Lung, and Blood Institute (NHLBI). 2007. Expert panel report 3: Guidelines for the diagnosis and management of asthma.

Nilsson, L., Brockow, K., Alm, J., Cardona, V., Caubet, J. C., Gomes, E., Jenmalm, M. C., Lau, S., Netterlid, E., Schwarze, J., Sheikh, A., Storsaeter, J., Skevaki, C., Terreehorst, I., & Zanoni, G. (2017). Vaccination and allergy: EAACI position paper, practical aspects. *Pediatric Allergy and Immunology: Official Publication of the European Society of Pediatric Allergy and Immunology, 28*(7), 628–640. https://doi.org/10.1111/pai.12762.

OPHEA Healthy Schools Healthy Communities (2023) Creating asthma friendly environment. https://www.asthmafriendly.ca/home/about-asthma.

Oriel, R., & Wang, J. (2021). Diagnosis and management of food allergy. *Immunology and Allergy Clinics of North America, 41*, 571–585.

Pate, C. A., Zahran, H. S., Qin, X., Johnson, C., Hummelman, E., Malilay, J. (2021). Asthma surveillance- United States, 2006-2018. *MMWR Surveillance Summary, 70*(No. SS-5), 1–32.

Peters, U., Dixon, A. E., & Forno, E. (2018). Obesity and asthma. *Journal of Allergy and Clinical Immunology, 141*(4), 1169–1179.

Peters, R., Krawiec, M., Koplin, J., Santos, J. (2021). Update on food allergy. *Pediatrics Allergy and Immunology, 32*, 647–657.

Ratcliffe, M., & Kieckhefer, G. (2010). Asthma. In Allen, P. J., Vessey, J., & Schapiro, N. A. (Eds.), *Primary care of the child with a chronic condition* (5th ed, pp. 168–196). Elsevier.

Reddel, H. K., Boteman, E. D., Schotz, M., Krishnan, J., Cloutier, M. (2022). A practical guide to implementing SMART in asthma management. *Journal of Allergy and Clinical Immunology: In Practice, 10*(1S), S31–S38.

Rothenberg, M. (2022). The climate change hypothesis for the allergy epidemic. *Journal of Allergy and Clinical Immunology, 149*(5), 1522–1524. 202.

Sampson, H. A., Aceves, S., Bock, S.a., James, J., Jones, S., Lang, D., Nadeau, K., Nowak-Wegrzyn, A., Oppenheimer, J., Perry, T., Randolph, C., Sicherer, C., Simon, R., Vickery, B., Wood, R., Bernstein, D., Blessing-Moore, J., Khan, D., Lang, D., Nicklas, R., et al. (2014). Food allergy: A practice parameter update-2014. *Journal of Allergy and Clinical Immunology, 134*(5), 1016–1025.

Sawicki, G., & Haver, K. (2023, February). Asthma in children younger than 12 years: Management of persistent asthma with controller therapies. *UpToDate*. Retrieved May 17, 2022, from https://www.uptodate.com/contents/asthma-in-children-younger-than-12-years-management-of-persistent-asthma-with-controller-therapies?search=leukotriene%C2%B1sawicki&source=search_result&selectedTitle=4~139&usage_type=default&display_rank=4.

Schuler, C., & Montejo, J. (2019). Allergic rhinitis in children and adolescents. *Pediatric Clinics of North America, 66*, 981–993.

Seidman, M. D., Gurgel, R. K., Lin, S. Y., Schwartz, S. R., Baroody, F. M., Bonner, J. R., Dawson, D. E., Dykewicz, M. S., Hackell, J. M., Han, J. K., Ishman, S. L., Krouse, H. J., Malekzadeh, S., Mims, J. W., Omole, F. S., Reddy, W. D., Wallace, D. V., Walsh, S. A., Warren, B. E., Wilson, M. N., … Guideline Otolaryngology Development Group. AAO-HNSF (2015). Clinical practice guideline: Allergic rhinitis. *Otolaryngology-Head and Neck Surgery: Official Journal of American Academy of Otolaryngology-Head and Neck Surgery, 152*(1 Suppl), S1–S43. https://doi.org/10.1177/0194599814561600.

Sloand, E., & Caschera, J. (2010). Allergies. In Allen, P. J., Vessey, J., & Schapiro, N. A. (Eds.), *Primary care of the child with a chronic condition* (5th ed., pp. 145–167). Elsevier.

Spergel J. (2022). Role of allergy in atopic dermatitis (eczema). *UpToDate*. Retrieved June 11, 2022, from https://www.uptodate.com/contents/role-of-allergy-in-atopic-dermatitis-eczema.

Trudell Medical International. (n.d.). Aerochamber use. Retrieved May 11, 2022, from https://aerochamber.com/patients-consumers.

Turner, P. J., Jerschow, E., Umasunthar, T., Lin, R., Campbell, D. E., & Boyle, R. J. (2017). Fatal anaphylaxis: Mortality rate and risk factors. *The Journal of Allergy and Clinical Immunology. In Practice, 5*(5), 1169–1178. https://doi.org/10.1016/j.jaip.2017.06.031.

US Department of Health and Human Services. (n.d.). *Asthma action plan*. National Heart Lung and Blood Institute. Retrieved May 11, 2022, from https://www.nhlbi.nih.gov/resources/asthma-action-plan-2020.

US Preventive Services Task Force. (2020). Screening for high blood pressure in children and adolescents: US Preventive Services Task Force recommendation statement. *JAMA, 324*(18), 1878–1883.

Yue, D., Ciccolini, A., Avilla, E., Waserman, S. (2018). Food allergy and anaphylaxis. *Journal of Asthma and Allergy, 11*, 111–120.

Zahran, H. S., Bailey, C. M., Damon, S. A., Garbe, P. L., Breysse P. N. (2018 Feb 9). Vital Signs: Asthma in Children - United States, 2001–2016. *MMWR Morb Mortal Wkly Rep. 67*(5):149–155. doi: 10.15585/mmwr.mm6705e1. PMID: 29420459; PMCID: PMC5812476.

Zhang, Y., Feng, L., & Zhang, L. (2021). Advances and highlights in allergic rhinitis. *Allergy, 76*(11), 3383–3389.

Anxiety Disorders and Obsessive-Compulsive Disorder

8

Girwan Khadka

INTRODUCTION

When parents describe symptoms of anxiety they see in their children, they can use a variety of words and phrases: worry, stress, tense, uneasy, fearful, nervous, apprehensive, and anxiety. Many things in a child's world can make the child feel these emotions, and often these feelings are appropriate for the situation. However, in a subset of children, these feelings of worry and anxiety persist even when the original trigger is no longer present. Anxiety can be considered disordered when their reaction to triggers for anxiety is excessive, developmentally inappropriate, and has significant adverse effects on their day-to-day functioning. Health care providers face this question regularly from parents: "Is what my child is experiencing normal or is this an anxiety disorder?" The health care provider utilizes assessment tools and appropriate rating scales, including a thorough diagnostic interview with children and their parents. These help distinguish between clinically significant anxieties requiring pharmacologic and psychological support and regular anxieties plentiful in life at any age.

Many anxieties are quite typical and common for certain ages in children. In their first year of life, generally 6–9 months of age, children can show anxiety related to strangers and unfamiliar people, which can be part of healthy development. Preschoolers may verbalize fear of unknown things such as monsters under the bed or the dark, which correspond with the cognitive development of their conception of the world around them and the beginning of learning what is real and what is not. School-aged children can have anxiety about things that have a real possibility of happening (e.g., injury to self or family members, natural disasters such as fire, thunderstorms, tornadoes). Older children and adolescents can have anxiety related to comparisons with their peers, such as their appearance, school performance, and social standing. As they venture out more and more into the outside world and their interactions with others increase, such comparisons are inevitable.

Anxieties that children and adolescents experience could simply be adaptive in nature or eustress (i.e., anxiety or stress about something that actually can propel them to take adaptive action to improve the situation). For example, consider a 17-year-old female who, instead of going out with her friends over the weekend, preps for her upcoming SAT exam because she is anxious to do well on it. In contrast, pathologic anxiety is characterized largely by attempts to avoid anxiety-provoking situations. For example, consider a 17-year-old male taking the SAT exam who binges on a Netflix show instead of studying because he is anxious about taking the exam. Thus for any anxiety to be considered a disorder (i.e., maladaptive, pathologic, or clinically significant), an individual has to experience anxiety that is persistent, excessive, age inappropriate, and that adversely affects daily functioning (American Psychiatric Association [APA], 2013).

INCIDENCE AND PREVALENCE OF ANXIETY IN CHILDREN AND ADOLESCENTS

Anxiety disorders are the most diagnosed mental health disorders among children and adolescents (Beesdo et al., 2009; Merikangas et al., 2010). A 2016 National Survey of Children's Health reported that among children aged 3 to 17 years, 7.1% had current anxiety problems (Ghandour et al., 2019). The lifetime prevalence of anxiety is between 6% and 20% (Augustyn et al., 2010; Beesdo et al., 2009; Kessler et al., 2005; Sakolsky & Birmaher, 2008). Anxiety is generally equal in ratio during early and late childhood, but it is seen more frequently in females, with a ratio of 2:1 to 3:1 by adolescence (APA, 2013; Augustyn et al., 2010). Of adults diagnosed with anxiety disorder, 70% report their symptoms started in childhood (Augustyn et al., 2010).

ANXIETY DISORDERS AND OBSESSIVE-COMPULSIVE DISORDER

The *Diagnostic and Statistical Manual of Mental Disorders*, Fifth Edition (DSM-5) takes a more developmental approach to understanding anxiety disorders than the revised DSM-IV-TR and is arranged in the DSM-5 according to the age of onset (APA, 2013). In the DSM-IV-TR, obsessive-compulsive disorder (OCD) and posttraumatic stress disorder (PTSD) were housed under anxiety disorders (APA, 2000). In a major departure from the DSM-IV-TR, OCD and trauma- and stress-related disorders now have their own diagnostic criteria categories separate from the anxiety disorders

Table 8.1	Anxiety, Obsessive-Compulsive, and Trauma and Stress-Related Disorders	
ANXIETY DISORDERS	**OBSESSIVE-COMPULSIVE AND RELATED DISORDERS**	**TRAUMA- AND STRESS-RELATED DISORDERS**
Separation anxiety disorder	Obsessive-compulsive disorder	Reactive attachment disorder
Selective mutism	Body dysmorphic disorder	Disinhibited social engagement disorder
Specific phobia	Hoarding disorder	Posttraumatic stress disorder
Social anxiety disorder (social phobia)	Trichotillomania (hair-pulling disorder)	Acute stress disorder
Panic disorder	Excoriation (skin-picking) disorder	Adjustment disorders
Agoraphobia	Substance/medication-induced obsessive-compulsive and related disorders	Other specified trauma- and stress-related disorders
Generalized anxiety disorder	Obsessive-compulsive and related disorders due to another medical condition	Unspecified trauma- and stress-related disorders
Substance/medication-induced anxiety disorder	Other specified obsessive-compulsive and related disorders	
Anxiety disorder due to another medical condition	Unspecified obsessive-compulsive and related disorders	
Other specified anxiety disorder		
Unspecified anxiety disorder		

Data from American Psychiatric Association. Diagnostic and Statistical Manual of Mental Disorders, Fifth Edition (DSM-5). American Psychiatric Association; 2013.

category. Though OCD and trauma- and stress-related disorders, which include PTSD, constitute separate categories in the DSM-5, anxiety remains an important attribute of the diagnostic criteria for these disorders. Table 8.1 shows these three criteria categories and the disorders under them as listed in the DSM-5.

For this chapter, the focus will be on the three anxiety disorders that have a high prevalence in the general pediatric population: separation anxiety disorder (SAD), social anxiety disorder or social phobia (SocAD), and generalized anxiety disorder (GAD). OCD, though in a separate diagnostic category from anxiety disorders in the DSM-5, will also be covered in this chapter.

SEPARATION ANXIETY DISORDER

SAD is characterized by developmentally inappropriate and excessive fear or anxiety concerning separation with whom the child/person is attached (APA, 2013). While SAD was presented as a childhood disorder until the DSM-IV-TR, the conceptualization of SAD has been augmented to include adults in the DSM-5. The lifetime prevalence of SAD in children is 4%, and the 12-month prevalence is between 1% and 4% (APA, 2013; Lavallee et al., 2011). The lifetime prevalence for adults is 6.6% (Shear et al., 2006), and the 12-month prevalence for adults is 0.9% to 1.9% (APA, 2013; Shear et al., 2006). In adolescents in the United States, the 12-month prevalence of SAD is 1.6% (APA, 2013). SAD has a median age of onset of 7 years (Kessler et al., 2005).

Diagnostic Criteria for SAD in the DSM-5

To qualify for a diagnosis of SAD, at least three of the following symptoms must cause significant impairment in social, academic, occupational, or other areas of functioning for at least 4 weeks for children/adolescents and more than 6 months for adults (APA, 2013):

- Recurrent excessive distress when anticipating or experiencing separation

- Persistent worry about losing attachment figures via illness, death, and disasters
- Worry about untoward event to self (kidnapping, having an accident) that would cause separation from major attachment figures
- Refusal to go from home to other places because of fear of separation
- Having nightmares related to separation
- Repeated somatic complaints when separation occurs or is about to occur

Clinical Manifestation of SAD at Time of Diagnosis

While the core presentation of SAD is the recurrent, persistent, and excessive distress of experiencing or anticipating separation from an attachment figure, younger children and older children can manifest SAD differently. Younger children can begin to manifest these symptoms with their reluctance to go to day care or school, which does not resolve despite being taken there for 4 weeks or more. Younger children can also try to avoid going to places where they would have to be separated from their attachment figures for any length of time by complaining about somatic symptoms such as stomachache or headache or needing to use the restroom frequently before departure from the home. Younger children may not express worries in concrete terms even when asked directly by their caregivers. On the other hand, older children can generally verbalize specific concerns or dangers, such as accidents, kidnapping, and death, even though there may not be a cause for concern. In older children, SAD can also be seen when they refuse to go for sleepovers with their friends even though they may otherwise be quite social.

In young adults and adults, SAD can be manifested in their limited ability to cope with major changes in their lives (e.g., moving away to college or moving for a job that puts them farther away from family and close friends). In adults, SAD can manifest in a variety of individuals, including family members, spouses, children, and close friends. Similar to children, adults who experience SAD are also excessively distressed about separation and worry about the safety and security of their close ones.

Understandably, children and adults with SAD demonstrate difficulty in daily adaptive functioning, including adults' ability to seek out and keep their jobs. Children with SAD demonstrate difficulty with academic achievement and social skills development—consequences manifesting from school refusal (APA, 2013). SAD can lead to social withdrawal, apathy, sadness, or difficulty concentrating in children (APA, 2013). For young adults leaving their homes for the first time for college, adjusting to this change can be very difficult, and they may choose to give up their educational pursuit to be back home with their families.

SOCIAL ANXIETY DISORDER (SOCIAL PHOBIA)

SocAD is characterized by intense fear or anxiety in a situation where a person could be scrutinized by others (APA, 2013). The DSM-5 augmented the diagnostic criteria for SocAD from that in the DSM-IV-TR to include fear or anxiety about doing something humiliating or embarrassing that could lead to rejection or offending others (Heimberg et al., 2014). Epidemiologic studies have identified a worldwide SocAD current prevalence of 5% to 10% and a lifetime prevalence of 8.4% to 15% (Koyuncu et al., 2019). The 12-month prevalence of SocAD in the United States is similar to the worldwide prevalence of 7% (APA, 2013) to 9% (Merikangas et al., 2010). SocAD has a median age of onset of 13 years (Kessler et al., 2005). SocAD appears more commonly in females than males, with a ratio of 1.5:1 to 2.2:1 (APA, 2013; Rose & Tadi, 2021).

Diagnostic Criteria for SocAD in the DSM-5
To qualify for the SocAD diagnosis, the following criteria must be met along with the symptoms causing significant impairment in social, academic, occupational, or other areas of functioning for at least 6 months for children as well as adults (APA, 2013):
- Fear or anxiety in social situations where an individual could face possible scrutiny by others. Social situations could include participating in social interactions such as having a conversation, meeting unfamiliar people; being observed while eating or drinking in the presence of others; and performing in front of others, such as giving a speech.
- Fear and anxiety about being negatively evaluated lead to feelings of humiliation, embarrassment, rejection, or that they may offend others.
- Social situations almost always provoke fear or anxiety.
- The social situations are either avoided or endured with intense fear or anxiety.

- The fear or anxiety is out of proportion to the actual threat posed by the social situation and the sociocultural context.

The DSM-5 notes two modifications for the diagnostic criteria specifically for children: (1) The anxiety must occur in peer settings and not only while interacting with adults, and (1) the fear/anxiety could be expressed by crying, tantrums, freezing, clinging to adults, shrinking, or failing to speak in social situations (APA, 2013).

Clinical Manifestations of SocAD at Time of Diagnosis
As noted previously, younger children can manifest SocAD more behaviorally by crying and throwing tantrums, while older children can manifest SocAD by demonstrating fear/anxiety or avoiding social situations. Examples of this would be rejecting the invitation to friends' birthday parties, being unwilling or anxious about walking the hallways at school between classes, eating in the cafeteria, going to the bathroom at school, or playing at recess. Children may also have difficulty reading or answering in class, ordering at restaurants, initiating conversations in the playground or other places with unfamiliar peers, and using public restrooms. Children with SocAD generally have the ability to develop age-appropriate friendships but manifest anxiety in bigger groups with unfamiliar people. Adolescents may experience SocAD in the context of dating. Adults with SocAD also try their best to avoid social situations; when they participate socially, they may endure it for short lengths of time while experiencing intense anxiety.

GENERALIZED ANXIETY DISORDER

GAD is characterized by excessive anxiety or worry about events and activities (APA, 2013) that may be happening in the home, school, work, or community setting. GAD affects about 1% of children and 1% to 3% of adolescents (APA, 2013; Beesdo et al., 2009; Gale & Millichamp, 2016). The female-to-male ratio for GAD is about 2:1 (APA, 2013; Bandelow & Michaelis, 2015).

Diagnostic Criteria for GAD in the DSM-5
To qualify for the GAD diagnosis, the following criteria must be met along with the symptoms causing significant impairment in social, academic, occupational, or other areas of functioning more days than not for at least 6 months for children as well as adults (APA, 2013):
- Excessive anxiety and worry (apprehensive expectation) about different events or activities at school or work
- The individual has difficulty controlling the worry.
- The anxiety/worry is associated with at least three of the six following symptoms for adults; for children, only one symptom is needed:
  - Feeling restless or on edge

Box **8.1**   Obsessions Versus Compulsions

Obsessions are characterized by (1) recurrent and persistent thoughts, urges, or images that are intrusive and unwanted that cause anxiety, which (2) the individual attempts to ignore or suppress or attempts to neutralize by engaging in another thought or action (i.e., by performing a compulsion).

Compulsions are characterized by (1) repetitive behaviors (e.g., handwashing, ordering things based on some arbitrary rule, repeatedly checking on things) or mental acts (e.g., praying, counting, repeating words silently) that are responses to the obsession, and the behaviors or aimed at preventing or reducing anxiety.

Modified from American Psychiatric Association. (2013). *Diagnostic and statistical manual of mental disorders* (5th ed.).

- Being easily fatigued
- Difficulty concentrating or mind going blank
- Irritability
- Muscle tension
- Sleep disturbance

Clinical Manifestation of GAD at Time of Diagnosis

For individuals with GAD, the issues they are anxious or worried about are generally relevant to their everyday lives. For example, children may worry about school and sports achievement, health and safety of self and close ones, and extreme weather. Adolescents can be additionally worried about social issues such as fitting in, dating, and appearance. Adults can worry about their family's well-being and physical health (APA, 2013). The issues that become sources of worry and anxiety for each age group (see earlier) are quite appropriate for their ages; however, what can make the worry and anxiety disordered is when the intensity, duration, or frequency of the anxiety and worry is out of proportion to the actual likelihood or impact of the anticipated event (APA, 2013).

OBSESSIVE-COMPULSIVE DISORDER

OCD is characterized by obsessions and/or compulsions (APA, 2013) (Box 8.1).

The lifetime and 12-month prevalence estimates of OCD in the United States are 2.3% and 1.2%, respectively (APA, 2013; Ruscio et al., 2010), while the prevalence is between 1.1% and 1.8% worldwide (APA, 2013). Females are affected by OCD slightly more in adulthood and males more in childhood (APA, 2013).

Diagnostic Criteria for OCD in the DSM-5

An individual is diagnosed with OCD when there is the presence of obsessions, compulsions, or both and when these obsessions and compulsions take at least 1 hour a day and are causing significant impairment in social, academic, occupational, or other areas of functioning. The DSM-5 has three specifiers for the diagnostic criteria of OCD: (1) with good or fair insight (when

the individual recognizes that the OCD beliefs are definitely or probably not true, (2) with poor insight (when the individual thinks the OCD beliefs are probably true), and (3) with absent insight/delusional beliefs (when the individual believes that the OCD beliefs are true) (APA, 2013).

Compulsive behaviors tend to relieve anxiety for a short time, which accounts for individuals engaging in them even though they may be progressively spending more and more time obsessing or engaging in compulsive behaviors (more than 1 hour a day), and this leads to significant impairment in social, occupational, academic, and other day-to-day functioning (APA, 2013). Young children may be unable to articulate why they engage in these behaviors or mental acts (APA, 2013).

The compulsions are not connected realistically to what they are supposed to neutralize or prevent (APA, 2013) For example, consider a child who may engage in the compulsion of always wearing the right sock only after wearing the left sock to prevent obsessive thoughts about getting into a car accident (i.e., the child wearing socks in a particular way has no bearing on having or not having a car accident).

Clinical Manifestation of OCD at Time of Diagnosis

Certain OCD themes are commonly seen in children and adolescents. Some OCD themes are related to fear of contamination, fear of harm or concern for safety, ordering/arranging, and scrupulosity (Sapyta et al., 2012) (Box 8.2).

ASSESSMENT OF ANXIETY DISORDERS AND OBSESSIVE-COMPULSIVE DISORDER IN A CLINICAL SETTING

Given that children and adolescents experience a variety of anxiety disorders, it is important to assess and determine the correct diagnosis before embarking on a treatment plan (pharmacologic and psychological) that would be most appropriate and evidence based for the diagnosis. The diagnosis of OCD also needs to be determined by using good differential skills because certain anxiety disorders can have features seen in OCD. For example, constant worrying is a feature of both GAD and OCD, but what leads to a differential between the two is that in GAD, children worry about real-life situations; in OCD, the worrying may not be rooted in reality and can be odd and irrational (APA, 2013). To achieve the goal of gathering relevant information needed for differential diagnosis, a clinician should use a combination of a thorough diagnostic interview with caregivers and children/adolescents, any additional information from other relevant informants (e.g., teachers, coaches, close adult figures other than parents or guardians), and appropriate assessment tools such as rating scales.

| Box 8.2 | Themes of Obsessive-Compulsive Disorder |

Contamination: Obsessions associated with contamination could be manifested as preoccupation with keeping oneself safe from getting sick or dying. Children who have this obsession can engage in the following compulsions: excessive handwashing or using hand sanitizers incessantly; repeatedly cleaning surfaces that do not require it; refusing to use the restroom at school or in public places. These children may present in the clinic first for medical attention due to eczematous changes as a result of excessive handwashing or for encopresis due to refusal to use school or public restrooms (Augustyn et al., 2010).

Harm or concern for safety: Obsessions are associated with fear of being harmed or dying, which can extend to safety concerns for family members as well. The compulsions that children engage in are seeking repeated reassurances of safety and well-being from caregivers and engaging in superstitious behaviors with the belief that engaging in them will reduce the likelihood of harm. These compulsions are not realistically associated with any way of reducing harm (e.g., circling the car three times before getting into it, believing that this compulsion will prevent an accident).

Ordering/arranging: Obsessions associated with ordering and arranging are manifested with being very fastidious about things needing to be in a particular order, pattern, or symmetry. The compulsions observed with this obsession are ordering things based on odd or even numbers; needing the food on the plates to not touch; arranging items by color, number, shape, or any other rule; or repeatedly counting things.

Scrupulosity: Obsessions of scrupulosity are associated with a preoccupation with right and wrong (morality) or feeling bad about having a "bad" thought. In adolescents, this obsession can manifest as thoughts about harming others physically or sexually, which understandably can be extremely distressing to the youth. The compulsions that individuals engage in are confessing their "bad" thoughts to their parents, engaging in prayer or counting, and seeking reassurance from others that they are a "good" person.

DIAGNOSTIC INTERVIEW

A solid diagnostic interview is the backbone of any good assessment and can help the health care provider make good differential diagnoses, including anxiety disorders. The diagnostic interview should include questions related to current concerns, history of concerning issues, developmental history, medical history, and any past psychological and academic evaluations. Family psychiatric history is essential to identify during a diagnostic interview because psychiatric conditions tend to overlap within families and share common gene and environmental risk factors (Sullivan et al., 2000). It is important in a diagnostic interview to ask about the child's or adolescent's social history because that can provide important information about where and with whom the child or adolescent expresses significant anxiety, which can be very helpful with the differential diagnosis. The social history should include questions about relationships with family members and extended family, school and neighborhood peers, teachers, coaches, work colleagues, and romantic partners when appropriate. Additionally, information about daily adaptive functioning should be gathered, including the child's or adolescent's functioning at home: Does the child demonstrate age-expected independence vs. age-inappropriate dependence? Does the adolescent demonstrate appropriate self-direction or need constant monitoring? How is the child or adolescent functioning within the school/academic setting and extracurricular interests?

When focusing on current symptoms, the health care provider needs to ask about the intensity, duration, frequency, and level of distress the symptoms are causing and how they interfere with daily functioning. This information can help identify disordered anxiety, which is out of proportion in intensity, duration, and frequency to the stressor and can be inappropriate for the age. This information will help develop the differential diagnosis. Another piece of information to gather during the assessment is the length of time that the specific anxiety has occurred (e.g., at least 4 weeks for children diagnosed with SAD and more than 6 months for a diagnosis of SocAD). For OCD it is important to ask about the kinds of obsessive thoughts, urges, and images an individual has and the compensatory compulsive thoughts or behaviors utilized to neutralize the obsession. Gathering information about the themes of obsession and compulsions can be very helpful in developing appropriate therapy protocols to address OCD.

The DSM-5 has two additional criteria to be met for diagnosing most anxiety disorders (i.e., SAD, SocAD, GAD, OCD): (1) The disturbance is not attributable to the physiologic effects of a substance (e.g., an abused drug or a medication) or another medical condition (e.g., hyperthyroidism), and (2) the disturbance is not better explained by another mental disorder (APA, 2013). Evaluating these two criteria is paramount in making a good differential diagnosis and is integral to a good diagnostic interview.

When possible, it is helpful to collect information from those adults who are an essential part of the child's life because they can provide pertinent information to help make an accurate differential diagnosis. This can be done with one-on-one interviewing or rating scales.

PSYCHOMETRIC ASSESSMENT TOOLS

Psychometric assessment tools such as rating scales can be integral for the differential diagnosis of anxiety disorders and OCD. They can also help measure symptom severity (Myers & Winters, 2002; Storch et al., 2015). Self-report and parent-report measures are typically utilized to assess anxiety disorders and OCD in children and adolescents. Common measures used in clinical practice are discussed next.

Revised Children's Manifest Anxiety Scale, Second Edition

The Revised Children's Manifest Anxiety Scale, Second Edition (RCMAS-2), is a self-report measure for children and adolescents composed of 49 items (Reynolds & Richmond, 2008). The instrument has been normed for ages 6 to 19 years. It is also normed for sex (male and female). Norms are presented separately for ages 6 to 8, 9 to 14, and 15 to 19 years. The instrument has three anxiety-related scales: physiologic anxiety (items such as "Tired a lot" and "Often I feel sick in the stomach"), worry (items such as "Worry about what other people think about me" and "Worry about what is going to happen"), and social anxiety (items such as "Fear other kids will laugh at me in class" and "Am afraid to speak up in a group"). The total of these three scales then yields a total anxiety scale score. There are two validity scales: the inconsistent responding index and the defensiveness scale. These two scales help the examiner recognize a pattern of random responses from individuals and whether they have presented themselves in an overtly positive fashion. In this second edition of the RCMAS, a new cluster of 10 items has been included to assess performance anxiety. The RCMAS-2 generally takes 10 to 15 minutes to complete. There is also a short form, which comprises the first 10 items of RCMAS-2 and requires less than 5 minutes to complete. The items are easy to read and understand, written at a second-grade reading level. Reliability estimates for the scale scores for the RCMAS-2 are between .75 and .86 (Reynolds & Richmond, 2008). The internal consistency of the full scale is good (α = .90) (Wu et al., 2016).

Multidimensional Anxiety Scale for Children, Second Edition

The Multidimensional Anxiety Scale for Children, Second Edition (MASC-2), is a multirater assessment tool (self- and parent-report versions available) for assessing anxiety symptoms and comprises 50 items (March, 2012). The instrument has been normed for ages 8 to 19 years. Norms are presented separately for ages 8 to 11, 12 to 15, and 16 to 19 years. It is also normed for sex (male and female). The MASC-2 comprises the following six scales: separation anxiety/phobias, social anxiety, obsessions and compulsions, physical symptoms, harm avoidance, and GAD index. It also consists of a validity scale (inconsistency index), which examines a pattern of random responses from the rater. The measure takes 10 to 15 minutes to complete. A possible advantage of using the MASC-2 is this measure has a scale dedicated

to obsessions and compulsions and scales for other anxiety disorders. The MASC-2 has excellent internal reliability and test-retest reliability for the parent measure (coefficient α = .89 and .93, respectively) and for the self-measure (coefficient α = .92 and .89, respectively) (March, 2012).

Screen for Child Anxiety-Related Disorders

The Screen for Anxiety-Related Disorders (SCARED) is a multirater measure that can be completed by the parent (parent version) and the child (child version). Each version comprises 41 items (Birmaher et al., 1999). The instrument has been studied with children aged 9 to 18 (Birmaher et al., 1999). Unlike the RCMAS-2 and the MASC-2, this measure is not normed for different age groups, and there are no norms available separately for males and females. The SCARED tool measures the following five factors: panic/somatic, generalized anxiety, separation anxiety, social phobia, and school phobia. These factors have good internal consistency (coefficient α = .78 to .87), and the measure has strong discriminative validity with depressive and disruptive disorders (Birmaher et al., 1999). The questionnaire can be completed in about 10 minutes. The SCARED is considered a good screener for anxiety disorders that can be used in primary care (Sakolsky & Birmaher, 2008); however, a formal diagnosis of an anxiety disorder will require a thorough diagnostic interview (Birmaher et al., 1999) and other normed anxiety scales. Unlike the RCMAS-2 and MASC-2, the SCARED, including the scoring instructions, is free. Table 8.2 shows the three assessment tools described previously that can be utilized for the assessment of SAD, SocAD, and GAD.

Children's Yale-Brown Obsessive-Compulsive Scale

The Children's Yale-Brown Obsessive-Compulsive Scale (CY-BOCS) is a clinician-administered measure designed to rate the severity of obsessive and compulsive symptoms in children and adolescents aged 6 to 17 (Scahill et al., 1997). The CY-BOCS is divided into two sections: obsessions checklist and compulsion checklist (Box 8.3). The measure is administered in an interview format where questions are asked to both the child and the parent. Based on these answers, clinicians use their judgment to determine a total score. The CY-BOCS shows a high level of internal consistency (coefficient α = .87). The interrater agreement has good to excellent reliability, with scores of .84, .91, and .68 for the CY-BOCS total, obsession, and compulsion scores, respectively (Scahill et al., 1997). The CY-BOCS is available to use clinically for free.

Two other sections in the CY-BOCS assess the severity of both obsessions and compulsions on a scale of 0 (no symptoms) to 4 (extreme symptoms) by asking five questions related to obsessions and five questions related to compulsions. These five questions are related

Table 8.2	Assessment Tools to Assess SAD, SocAD, and GAD		
ASSESSMENT TOOLS	**REVISED CHILDREN'S MANIFEST ANXIETY SCALE, SECOND EDITION (RCMAS-2)**	**MULTIDIMENSIONAL ANXIETY SCALE FOR CHILDREN, SECOND EDITION (MASC-2)**	**SELF-REPORT FOR CHILDHOOD ANXIETY-RELATED DISORDERS (SCARED)**
Number of items	49 items	50 items	41 items
Type	Self-report	Self-report and parent report	Self-report and parent report
Norms	Normed by age and sex	Normed by age and sex	Not normed
Anxiety screened or identified	General anxiety, social anxiety, performance anxiety, physical symptoms of anxiety	Separation anxiety/phobias, generalized anxiety, social anxiety, performance anxiety, obsessions/compulsions, panic, avoidance, physical symptoms of anxiety	General anxiety, separation anxiety, social anxiety, school phobia, physical symptoms of anxiety
Ages	6–19 yr	8–19 yr	9–18 yr
Length of time to complete	10–15 min; short version also available (5 min)	10–15 min	10 min
Free?	No	No	Yes

GAD, Generalized anxiety disorder; *SAD*, separation anxiety disorder; *SocAD*, SAD or social phobia.

Box 8.3	Obsessions and Compulsions Checklists of the CY-BOCS

OBSESSIONS CHECKLIST (ASKS ABOUT THE CHILD'S CURRENT AND PAST OBSESSIONS THAT FALL UNDER DIFFERENT CATEGORIES)	**COMPULSIONS CHECKLIST (ASKS ABOUT THE CHILD'S CURRENT AND PAST COMPULSIONS THAT FALL UNDER DIFFERENT CATEGORIES)**
Contamination	Washing/cleaning
Magical	Checking
Aggressive	Repeating
Sexual	Counting
Hoarding/saving	Ordering/arranging
Thoughts/superstitious	Hoarding/aaving
Somatic	Superstitious
Religious	Rituals involving other persons
Miscellaneous	Miscellaneous

CY-BOCS, Children's Yale-Brown Obsessive-Compulsive Scale.

to time spent (on obsession and compulsion), obsession-free/compulsion-free interval, interference (from obsession and compulsion), resistance against (obsession and compulsion), and control (over obsession and compulsion). The severity index score for obsession and compulsion has a maximum score of 20 each, which is then combined to yield a total score (with a maximum score of 40). A CY-BOCS score greater than or equal to 16 indicates clinically significant OCD (Piacentini & Bergman, 2000).

Rather than hard cutoffs, the scores shown in Box 8.4 can serve as a guideline in determining the severity of OCD symptoms in children and adolescents on the CY-BOCS (Storch et al., 2015).

TREATMENT OF ANXIETY DISORDERS AND OBSESSIVE-COMPULSIVE DISORDER

PSYCHOTHERAPEUTIC INTERVENTIONS FOR ANXIETY DISORDERS

Psychotherapeutic interventions for the pediatric population involve therapeutic conversations and interactions between a licensed therapist and a child or family. These therapies can help children and families understand and resolve problems, modify their behaviors, and make positive life changes. While various psychotherapeutic modalities are available for treating anxiety disorders, cognitive-behavioral therapy (CBT) is considered the most effective (Bandelow & Michaelis, 2015; Panganiban et al., 2019; Wehry et al., 2015) and evidence-based therapy for anxiety disorders. The American Academy of Child and Adolescent Psychiatry (AACAP) recommends that CBT be offered to patients 6 to 18 years old with SAD, GAD, SocAD, specific phobia, or panic disorder (Walter et al., 2020). A combination of CBT with pharmacotherapy is the superior choice in the treatment of children and adolescence for SAD, GAD, and SocAD (Mohatt et al., 2014).

There are different treatment protocols involving CBT that are available for the treatment of anxiety disorders in children and adolescents. One such CBT protocol with extensive research support for treating anxiety disorders in children is the Coping Cat program (Kendall, 1992), which consists of 14 to 18 sessions and takes 3 to 4 months. This protocol has shown efficacy in treating SAD, SocAD, and GAD (Kendall et al., 2010).

Coping Cat, as well as other CBT treatment protocols, have certain common components, which include psychoeducation, somatic symptoms management skills, cognitive restructuring, gradual exposure to

Box 8.4   Scores to Determine the Severity of OCD Symptoms in Children and Adolescents on the CY-BOCS

SCORES	LEVEL OF SEVERITY
0–13	Subclinical to mild symptoms
14–25	Moderate symptoms
26–34	Moderate-severe symptoms
35–40	Severe symptoms

CY-BOCS, Children's Yale-Brown Obsessive-Compulsive Scale; *OCD,* obsessive-compulsive disorder.

feared things/situations, and relapse prevention (Kennedy et al., 2017) (Box 8.5).

PSYCHOTHERAPEUTIC INTERVENTIONS FOR OBSESSIVE-COMPULSIVE DISORDER

For the treatment of OCD, exposure-based CBT is considered the first-line treatment for mild to moderate pediatric OCD (Peris & Schneider, 2017). The AACAP and the American Psychological Association Task Force on Promotion and Dissemination of Psychological Procedures have concluded that CBT with exposure/response prevention (E/RP) is the treatment of choice for children (American Psychological Association, 1995; Geller et al., 2012; Sapyta et al., 2012). The premise of exposure-based CBT or CBT with E/RP is to gradually expose a child to the triggers that set off the obsession while simultaneously avoiding engaging in the ritual or compulsion.

Similar to the CBT protocols for treating anxiety disorders, there are different iterations of exposure-based CBT. However, good CBT protocols for OCD will include these features: psychoeducation, cognitive restructuring, E/RP, and behavioral rewards (Peris & Schneider, 2017) (Box 8.6).

PHARMACOLOGIC INTERVENTIONS FOR ANXIETY DISORDERS

Selective serotonin reuptake inhibitors (SSRIs) and serotonin-norepinephrine reuptake inhibitors (SNRIs) have been most widely studied and viewed as more efficacious with fewer adverse reactions for the treatment of anxiety disorders than other classes of antidepressants (Panganiban et al., 2019). SSRIs and SNRIs work by increasing the effects of serotonin and norepinephrine, which are identified as neurotransmitters that regulate anxiety, mood, and social behavior. Several medications have been shown to be effective in treating childhood anxiety disorders, including duloxetine, sertraline, fluoxetine, fluvoxamine, paroxetine, and venlafaxine (AACAP et al., 2020). Of these medications, duloxetine is currently the only medication approved by the US Food and Drug Administration (FDA) for use in children and adolescents (Strawn et al., 2018). SSRI/SNRI medications can take 2 to 4 weeks to show their effects and can take an additional

Box 8.5   Cognitive-Behavioral Therapy Treatment Protocols

Psychoeducation: Receiving education about anxiety—how anxiety is an adaptive response to a stressful situation but can also become disordered when that anxiety remains persistent even after the removal of the stressful situation; how anxiety can affect daily functioning; how anxiety responses can be categorized in the flight, fight, or freeze model and how avoidance can become a maladaptive response to anxiety; learning about the intricate relationship of thoughts, feelings, and actions, and how they can exacerbate or alleviate anxiety.

Somatic symptoms management skills: Learning about the somatic responses to anxiety (e.g., muscle tension, rapid heartbeat, rapid breathing, sweating, dizziness); building skills to counteract the physiologic responses of anxiety by engaging in relaxing activities (e.g., deep and diaphragmatic breathing, progressive muscle relaxation, visualization).

Cognitive restructuring: Learning to identify and challenge negative and inaccurate thoughts/assumptions (e.g., black-and-white thinking), which contribute to anxiety symptoms; also learning to replace the problematic thoughts with more adaptive and balanced thoughts.

Gradual exposure to feared things/situations: Developing a hierarchy of things/situations that cause anxiety (e.g., getting inside a car) from least anxiety provoking to most anxiety provoking, and then gradually exposing themselves to more and more anxiety-provoking events (first, staring at the car from inside the home through a window; then, staring at the car from outside the home; then, getting closer to the car; then, touching the car; then, sitting in the car with the door open; and then, sitting in the car with the door closed) while simultaneously using cognitive and behavioral coping strategies and relaxation techniques in each step to manage anxiety.

Relapse prevention: Learning that even after treatment, anxiety may reappear but also assuring themselves that they have the tools necessary to address them; also, learning to continue to utilize the skills learned in therapy to prevent relapse of anxiety.

8 to 12 weeks for improvement (Strawn et al., 2018). It will be important to continue to track somatic symptoms, response to the medication, and side effects to evaluate the effectiveness of the medication and the dosage. This can be done through symptom checklist completion at regular intervals and providing updates to the prescribing health care provider.

A meta-analysis completed in 2022 (Stefánsdóttir et al., 2022) found that SSRIs and SNRIs effectively treat childhood anxiety disorders and are superior to pill placebo. Although the risk of serious adverse events (e.g., suicidal ideation with a plan, suicidal attempts, and self-injurious behaviors such as cutting) was low

| Box 8.6 | Exposure-Based Cognitive-Behavioral Therapy Protocols |

Psychoeducation: In addition to providing information about anxiety in general, parents and children should be educated about what obsessions and compulsions are, how they interact, and what role compulsions can play in sustaining obsessive-compulsive disorder (OCD). Presenting OCD as a neurobehavioral condition (Sapyta et al., 2012) can reduce the stigma and self-blame the individual may be engaging in. Because OCD can take overwhelming control of an individual's life, it is sometimes difficult for the person to separate the disorder from oneself; thus effective treatment for OCD generally begins with externalizing the OCD. This can be done by using terms such as "the worry monster/OCD troll makes you think that way" with children; with adolescents, it might work to use "the OCD brain vs. the rational brain."

Cognitive restructuring: Maladaptive thinking plays a key role in the development of obsessive thoughts, which then lead to maladaptive compulsions. Thus it is important in treatment to identify these maladaptive thoughts so that they can be challenged and then replaced with more adaptive and balanced thoughts. For example, maladaptive thinking is what leads a child to obsess about counting from 1 to 50 within 10 seconds, thinking that doing so will lead to having a good day at school. As a treatment, this notion will first need to be challenged (by having the child evaluate the validity of the thinking) and then replaced by finding more adaptive ways of increasing the chances of having a good day at school.

Exposure/response prevention (E/RP): In this stage, the parents, child, and clinician develop a hierarchy of fears that will then be addressed one at a time. The hierarchy will include triggers that cause the least anxiety moving up to triggers that cause the most anxiety. The child can be given a scale from 0 to 10 (where 0 is "no anxiety" to 10 is "extreme anxiety") to quantitatively label the severity of each trigger. It is also important in this stage to teach the child ways to "talk back to the worry monster/OCD troll" along with some cognitive restructuring techniques (e.g., when an obsession comes up, the child can engage in self-talk: "There is that worry monster telling me to do ____. But I know I don't need to do it!").

Behavioral rewards: Engaging in an E/RP protocol can understandably be quite stressful for a child. Thus using a rewards system that is salient to the child could help the child work against the urge to avoid the treatment plan and be a motivation to stay on the course of treatment despite the anxiety.

with SSRI/SNRI treatment, there was an increased risk of experiencing behavioral activation (e.g., aggressiveness, emotional lability, impulsivity, irritability, insomnia, hypomania/mania, paranoia) with SSRI/SNRI treatment (Stefánsdóttir et al., 2022).

The Child/Adolescent Anxiety Multimodal Study (CAMS)—a large-scale multimodal study that was completed in 2014 with 488 patients aged 7 to 17 years—compared the efficacy of CBT alone, sertraline therapy alone, and combination therapy of CBT plus sertraline against pill placebo in the treatment of anxiety disorders (Piacentini et al., 2014). The study focused on children who met the criteria for GAD, SAD, or SocAD and were studied over a 12-week acute treatment phase and a 6-month maintenance phase. The study found that 59.7% of the participants showed improvement with CBT alone, 54.9% showed improvement with sertraline alone, and 80.7% showed improvement with a combination of CBT and sertraline.

PHARMACOLOGIC INTERVENTIONS FOR OBSESSIVE-COMPULSIVE DISORDER

SSRIs (fluoxetine, fluvoxamine, paroxetine, citalopram, and sertraline) are effective treatments for pediatric OCD (Pediatric OCD Treatment Study [POTS] Team, 2004). SSRIs are considered the first-line treatment for OCD. Clomipramine (a tricyclic antidepressant) is considered the second-line medication; despite having more efficacy in reducing obsessive-compulsive symptoms in comparison with SSRIs, clomipramine results in a higher rate and severity of adverse effects in children (POTS Team, 2004; Sánchez-Meca et al., 2014). Only four medications have been approved by the FDA for children's treatment of pediatric OCD: clomipramine, fluoxetine, fluvoxamine, and sertraline.

POTS (POTS Team, 2004) is a seminal study that examined the impact of both manualized psychotherapy and medication on symptoms of OCD in children. The study had a sample of 112 patients aged 7 to 17 years; they were chosen based on their OCD diagnosis based on the DSM-5 and a score of 16 or higher on the CY-BOCS. The study looked at treating pediatric OCD for 12 weeks using sertraline alone, CBT alone, combined treatment (CBT and sertraline together), and placebo. CBT alone, sertraline alone, and combined treatment were all more efficacious than placebo. The clinical remission rate for combined treatment was 53.6%, for CBT alone 39.3%, for sertraline alone 21.4%, and for placebo 3.6%.

Additionally, combined treatment was more effective than either CBT or sertraline alone. The remission rate for combined treatment did not differ from that for CBT alone ($p = .42$) but differed from sertraline alone ($p = .03$) and from placebo ($p < .001$) (POTS Team, 2004). The main conclusion of the study was that children and adolescents with OCD should begin treatment with the combination of CBT plus a SSRI or CBT alone.

CONCLUSION

Anxiety disorders and OCD are very prevalent in the pediatric population. Given the variety of presentations of anxiety disorders and the overlap of certain symptoms from one disorder to another, a clinician needs to use excellent diagnostic skills to make a correct differential diagnosis. A good differential diagnosis is built upon certain clinical foundations, including receiving relevant current and historical information from the children, parents, and other relevant adults and utilizing valid rating scales to assist in the diagnostic process. It is only after health care providers and clinicians arrive at the diagnosis accurately that they can use corresponding evidence-based treatments (pharmacologic and psychological) that provide a higher likelihood of symptom amelioration. Once treatment begins it is important to continue receiving updated rating scales over time so that the health care providers and clinicians involved in the care of the child or adolescent can quantitatively receive real-time data to maintain or modify the course of treatment as needed. At the same time it is advisable to continue to get a child and caregiver report, particularly about changes in a child's day-to-day (adaptive) functioning, because the goal of any treatment is not just the improvement of symptoms but the qualitative improvement in functioning within the home, school, and community and with family, friends, and other important people in their lives.

PRIMARY CARE MANAGEMENT

HEALTH CARE MAINTENANCE

Growth and Development

Children with anxiety and OCD are generally thought to achieve normal growth and developmental milestones unless the child has additional conditions, such as pervasive developmental disorder or psychosis. There has been some concern raised about growth issues in children on long-term SSRIs, with more research needed on the topic. Some SSRIs have been associated with weight gain.

Parents and some providers may be concerned with distinguishing between developmentally normal rituals and obsessions of early childhood and the rituals and obsessions associated with OCD, particularly in families with a history of tics or OCD among first-degree relatives. Normal childhood rituals are similar to OCD-related rituals: needing things to be "just so," having lucky numbers, and having bedtime rituals. However, in children unaffected by OCD, the normal developmental rituals seem to aid in mastering anxiety and enhancing the child's socialization, whereas in OCD the rituals are distressing, isolating, and hinder activities of daily living.

Diet

Abrupt changes in dietary preferences may be a part of normal development or responses to contamination fears or other obsessions and anxiety. In addition, there is an association of OCD with eating disorders. A detailed discussion of food aversion and eating disorders is beyond the scope of this chapter; however,

the growth and body mass index charts of children with OCD should be carefully maintained. Any failure to make or maintain expected gains in height and weight, failure to progress through puberty, or secondary amenorrhea in the absence of pregnancy should prompt a more careful history, examination, and referral to the appropriate specialists. If the child is already seeing a psychotherapist, close communication between the primary care provider and the therapist is essential.

In looking for alternatives, parents sometimes try elimination diets or restrict the intake of foods thought to trigger obsessive-compulsive symptoms. Working with the family to ensure adequate caloric and nutritional intake is important.

Safety

Self-injurious behavior is associated with anxiety and OCD (APA, 2013). Suicidal ideation is increased in OCD and mood disorders (Bramante et al., 2023). Although parents may be unable to prevent all risky or self-injurious behaviors in older children and adolescents, they should be alert to the possibility of such behaviors and seek guidance from professionals with expertise in OCD.

Treating self-injurious behaviors can be difficult depending on whether the behavior is a complex tic or a compulsion (Jankovic, 1997). Adolescents with anxiety and OCD, like other adolescents with chronic conditions, may be more likely than their nonaffected peers to engage in risky behavior (Soleimani et al., 2017) (Box 8.7).

Immunizations

Children with anxiety and OCD should be vaccinated following the schedule recommended by the American Academy of Pediatrics (Centers for Disease Control and Prevention [CDC], 2022).

Box 8.7	Diagnosis

Sniffing, coughing, throat clearing
- Allergy
- Upper respiratory infection

Pharyngitis
- Streptococcal infection (observe for an increase in tics or OCD)

Headache
- Medication side effects (e.g., clonidine)
- Somatic preoccupation or obsession

Abdominal pain
- Constipation related to toileting issues (OCD)
- Constipation related to medication side effects
- Somatic preoccupation or obsession
- Self-injurious behavior
- Nail biting
- Trichotillomania

OCD, Obsessive-compulsive disorder.

Screenings

Vision. Routine screening is recommended.

Hearing. Routine screening is recommended.

Dental. Routine screening is recommended.

Blood pressure. Routine screening is recommended.

Hematocrit. Routine screening is recommended.

Urinalysis. Routine screening is recommended.

Tuberculosis. Routine screening is recommended.

Condition-Specific Screening
Additional monitoring is advised with selected medications.

Self-injurious behavior.

The primary care provider should be particularly vigilant in examining the skin, hair, nails, and scalp of children with OCD for signs of self-injurious behavior.

COMMON ILLNESS MANAGEMENT
Differential Diagnosis
OCD symptoms may begin or flare up explosively after a streptococcal infection. At this point, rigorously conducted research regarding diagnosis and treatments for pediatric autoimmune neuropsychiatric disorders associated with streptococcal infections (PANDAS) is scarce, and published studies have a high risk of bias (Sigra et al., 2018).

When a child with OCD complains of typical childhood symptoms, such as headaches and stomachaches, it is hard for parents and providers to discern the cause: Is the child obsessed with illness? Is there a serotonin imbalance implicated in headaches or stomachaches? Is the child constipated as a side effect of the medication? Or is there a serious health problem? After listening carefully to the child, parents may need to consult with the child's therapist and primary care provider. Changes in skin condition and musculoskeletal complaints may be due to bruising from tics, holding unusual positions as part of a tic, or self-injurious behavior.

Drug Interactions
Erythromycin and other macrolide antibiotics can interact with medications such as pimozide or aripiprazole (dopamine blockers) to prolong the QT interval (Taketomo, 2022). Dextromethorphan, a cough suppressant commonly found in over-the-counter medications and sometimes taken in high doses by adolescents for its psychoactive properties, may interact with fluoxetine to cause increased sedation, hallucinations, muscle dystonia, and hyperthermia, known as central serotonin syndrome. Ecstasy and related club or designer drugs may also cause central serotonin syndrome in interaction with SSRIs (Malcolm & Thomas, 2022). SSRIs, dopamine blockers, and other psychoactive medications are metabolized through cytochrome P (CYP) pathways and can each enhance or inhibit the metabolism on the same pathway of other medications the child might be taking. Fluoxetine and other CYP 2D6 pathway inhibitors can interact with codeine to prevent its breakdown into the active metabolite, thereby diminishing its analgesic properties (Taketomo, 2022). These examples should alert the provider to keep an accurate list of current medications and updated information about drug-drug interactions and ensure that parents and adolescents are aware of them.

Evidence shows that given the plethora of vitamins, supplements, and complementary and alternative medications available, many families of children with OCD use them, so it is imperative that the health care providers should open dialog with the child and family about possible drug interactions with any alternative treatment (e.g., St. John's wort, dimethylglycine, and trimethylglycine can interact with SSRIs) (Hoban et al., 2015).

DEVELOPMENTAL ISSUES
Sleep Patterns
Children with OCD can have difficulty falling asleep if the bedclothes do not feel right to them. Children with OCD, as noted previously, tend to have rituals they feel compelled to perform before bedtime, which can often delay sleep for several hours. If the child does not involve the parent in these rituals, the parent may not be aware of them. Like other rituals, bedtime rituals may be diminished with therapy and/or medication.

Toileting
Most children with anxiety and OCD are not diagnosed until school age, when toilet training is no longer an issue. Children who are diagnosed when they are older may have had difficulties with toilet training and had obsessions and rituals related to toileting. There may be increased encopresis and enuresis related to OCD symptoms (e.g., wetting or soiling connected to avoiding public bathrooms). As with other OCD symptoms, either CBT or medication or both combined may help.

Discipline
Increasing awareness and understanding by parents, health care providers, and educators of the significant impact of anxiety, OCD, and cooccurring mental, emotional, and behavioral conditions has become an important aspect of treatment (Robinson et al., 2013). When children with OCD begin treatment, there can be flare-ups of rituals. Parents will have to work with the child and therapist to decide which rituals to limit and which to ignore (Chansky, 2014; Rizzo & Gulisano, 2019).

Questions regarding the appropriateness of behavior, fairness to siblings, and consequences for behavior that is only partially under the child's control are complex, and families often benefit from support groups or other contacts (e.g., online support communities) with parents of children with anxiety or OCD (Dekel et al., 2020). Greene's seminal work in 2005 recommends the use of a basket system for prioritizing behaviors of explosive children, including children with anxiety or OCD; basket A contains the behaviors needed to maintain the safe child and family functioning, basket B contains the behaviors around which there is some room to teach the child negotiation skills, and basket C contains behaviors the parent is willing to ignore for the time being (such as maintaining a clean room). Even with essential behaviors, parents may have to modify how they customarily give commands and monitor adherence to break cycles of coercive parent-child interactions.

In addition to developing increased flexibility for acceptable behavior standards, parents may have to adjust their systems of consequences and rewards. Most children respond well to positive reinforcement, and children with anxiety and OCD, in particular, may need rewards because the acceptable behavior may provoke anxiety rather than being its own reward. According to Greene (2005), timeouts are not helpful for children who would like to behave well but lack the neurologic capability to work through frustrating situations without a meltdown. Greene recommends that parents help children avoid meltdowns by acting as their surrogate frontal lobe: modeling and teaching them flexibility, verbal skills, and the ability to shift gears. For children engaging in explosive behavior, a safe place to regroup is important (Dekel et al., 2020).

Child Care
The combination of structure and flexibility is important for children with anxiety and OCD. Although children may not be formally diagnosed during preschool, they may have increased problems with adaptability and peer relationships. Child care providers can give important information to parents concerned about their child's intellectual and social development.

Schooling
Children with anxiety and OCD are more likely to need additional educational support but are not often referred for such support. Children with anxiety, OCD, and attention-deficit/hyperactivity disorder may benefit from similar educational interventions (Carter et al., 1999).

Silent rituals associated with OCD, such as counting the number of times a letter occurs in reading or avoiding the number 3 in math problems, can slow the child considerably without being apparent to either teachers or parents (Carter et al., 1999). Conversely, the child's rituals may disrupt the class, sometimes leading to the inaccurate labeling of compulsions as symptoms of oppositional defiant disorder (Carter et al., 1999). Children may get stuck on one task, have rewriting compulsions, or have difficulty making choices. Individualizing a plan and creating alliances with teachers and school personnel when possible is key. Their observations may be invaluable in tracking responses to medication and behavioral treatment.

Two levels of educational support are available for children with anxiety and OCD attending public schools: written plans to provide access to educational programs/protection from discrimination (Section 504) and special education services (CDC, 2022). All children with OCD can qualify for Section 504 protection, which might include preferential seating, parent input into teacher selection, allowing a child to stop an activity if stuck, permission to leave the classroom to release tics, extra time on tests, and homework modification (Carter et al., 1999), with only a letter of diagnosis as documentation. Evaluations for services under the Individuals with Disabilities Education Improvement Act are more complex, but a parent can request an evaluation for an individualized education program (IEP) in writing.

Children with OCD frequently have difficulty initiating and maintaining friendships. Preoccupation with obsessions often leaves little time or energy for friends. In addition, the desire to hide their obsessions and rituals from peers may lead to social isolation, and bullying by peers is associated with more severe symptoms, depressive symptoms, isolation, and behavioral difficulties at home (Storch et al., 2006; Van Noppen et al., 2021). Children with OCD may benefit from socialization groups, in which social skills are explicitly taught, and from structured activities, such as religious or community youth groups or sports.

Sexuality
Children and adolescents with anxiety and OCD, unless affected by other conditions, typically have normal physical and sexual developmental. However, the psychosocial aspects of sexuality with the diagnosis of anxiety and OCD can be affected in several ways. Adolescents with OCD may avoid touch, including holding hands and kissing, because of contamination fears or have sexual obsessions (Fernández de la Cruz et al., 2013), including unwanted sexual thoughts, invasive thoughts that disrupt romantic or sexual activity, and obsessions or fears around being homosexual in teens who do not have same-sex attractions. In addition, the medications used for anxiety and OCD, most notably SSRIs, have some effect on libido and sexual functioning (Atmaca, 2020), which may be distressing for adolescents and affect medication adherence.

Adolescents with anxiety and OCD may feel uncomfortable discussing sexuality with their parents and may be reluctant to raise the issue with their health care providers, reinforcing the primary care provider's responsibility to discuss sexuality with all adolescents. Health care providers need to tailor their discussion to include how one feels about one's body, touch, and prevention of teen pregnancy along with sexually transmitted diseases.

Transition to Adulthood

Virtually all colleges receive some form of federal assistance and are required by law to provide services for students with disabilities. Although services vary from school to school, families who have struggled with public school systems for accommodations for their children with anxiety and OCD may find college disability services surprisingly easy to access. Parents should ensure that the adolescent will have an IEP or a 504 plan and is reevaluated within 3 years of entering college to facilitate the transition. Parents can help students contact college disability services and help their adolescents prepare and submit documentation of any past services, but the responsibility for using college disability services rests with the young adult.

Young adults with severe anxiety and OCD or other associated psychiatric conditions may have limited employment, education, housing, and health care options. Parents and adolescents may benefit from hiring a case manager or working with their school's vocational rehabilitation services team to address the transition to adulthood and independent living issues. Adults with OCD may not have received effective treatment as a child or adolescent. It may be, with early diagnosis and effective care, that future adult outcomes will be much improved.

FAMILY CONCERNS

Parents and siblings of children with anxiety or OCD experience stress in accommodating the child's rituals, and siblings may feel ashamed of the child's bizarre behavior at school. Health care providers are encouraged to have parents explain anxiety and OCD as medical conditions to the child's siblings and to validate the feelings of unfairness or embarrassment at their sibling's outbursts. Family meetings with the child's therapist to work out fair house rules may be helpful. Neuropsychiatric conditions have historically been associated with stigma and are difficult for family members to explain to friends, relatives, and school personnel. Parents may not be used to the role of advocate for their child and may not even be sure whether to disclose the diagnosis of anxiety or OCD. Families can benefit from sympathetic guidance from their primary providers as well as referral to the appropriate organizations and resources.

RESOURCES

American Academy of Child & Adolescent Psychiatry: https://www.aacap.org/AACAP

American Academy of Pediatrics: https://www.aap.org/en/patient-care/mental-health-minute/screening-tools

Child Mind Institute (anxiety): https://childmind.org/topics/anxiety

Child Mind Institute (complete guide to OCD): https://childmind.org/guide/parents-guide-to-ocd

International OCD Foundation: https://kids.iocdf.org

Nemours KidsHealth: https://kidshealth.org

OCD resources: https://www.ocdkidsmovie.com/ocdresources

 Summary

Primary Care Needs for the Child With Anxiety and Obsessive-Compulsive Disorder

HEALTH CARE MAINTENANCE

Growth and Development

- Growth is generally normal, although there are some concerns about the growth of children on long-term medication, such as SSRIs.
  - If growth slows or weight falls in older children/adolescents, consider an eating disorder.
  - Development is generally normal.
  - Rituals with OCD associated with isolation and distress increase when normal childhood rituals start to diminish.
  - Some parents report decreased flexibility and increased difficulties with regulation even before the emergence of specific symptoms.

Diet

- Abrupt changes in dietary preference may be due to obsessions/compulsions, especially around contamination.
  - Increased risk of eating disorders occurs in children with anxiety and OCD.

- Parents may restrict intake in an attempt to eliminate triggers from foods or food additives.

Safety

- Self-injurious behavior in OCD
- Adolescents may self-medicate with alcohol and/or recreational drugs for symptom relief.

Immunizations

- Children with anxiety and OCD should be vaccinated following the recommended schedule by the American Academy of Pediatrics (O'Leary et al., 2023).

Screening

- *Vision*. Routine screening is recommended.
- *Hearing.* Routine screening is recommended.
- *Dental.* Routine screening is recommended.
- *Blood pressure.* Routine screening is recommended. Children taking certain medications may need more frequent screening.
- *Hematocrit.* Routine screening is recommended.
- *Urinalysis.* Routine screening is recommended.

Continued

- *Tuberculosis.* Routine screening is recommended.

Condition-Specific Screening
- Careful observation for signs of self-injurious behavior

COMMON ILLNESS MANAGEMENT
Differential Diagnosis
- *Headache.* Medication side effects, somatic preoccupation, or obsession
- *Abdominal pain.* Constipation related to toileting issues (OCD), medication side effects, somatic preoccupation, or obsession

Drug Interactions
- SSRIs reduce the effectiveness of codeine for analgesia.
- St. John's wort and other supplements interact with SSRIs.

DEVELOPMENTAL ISSUES
Sleep Patterns
- Bedtime rituals can delay sleep for several hours; parents may not be aware of the extent of rituals.

Toileting
- Some obsessions and rituals are related to toileting.
- Some medications increase constipation.
- Avoidance of public toilets may lead to constipation and encopresis.

Discipline
- Children with OCD may need rewards for avoiding rituals.
- Timeouts may not be effective for children with rage attacks.
- Respect their feelings.
- Reassure the child.

Child Care
- A combination of structure and flexibility is needed.
- Day care providers can give valuable feedback about socialization skills.

Schooling
- Anxiety and OCD may not be apparent to teachers, or the child may disrupt the class.
- All children are eligible for Section 504 accommodations, some for IEPs.
- Peer relations may be impaired.

Sexuality
- Adolescents may avoid touch due to contamination fears.

REFERENCES

American Academy of Child and Adolescent Psychiatry, American Psychiatric Association, & Parents' Medication Guide Workgroup. (2020). *Anxiety disorders: Parents' medication guide* (p. 20). https://www.aacap.org/App_Themes/AACAP/docs/resource_centers/resources/med_guides/anxiety-parents-medication-guide.pdf.

American Academy of Pediatrics. (2022).

American Psychiatric Association. (2000). *Diagnostic and statistical manual of mental disorders* (4th ed.). Author.

American Psychiatric Association. (2013). *Diagnostic and statistical manual of mental disorders* (5th ed.). Author.

American Psychological Association. (1995). *Task force on psychological intervention guidelines. Template for developing guidelines: Interventions for mental disorders and psychosocial aspects of physical disorders.* Author.

Atmaca, M. (2020). Selective serotonin reuptake inhibitor-induced sexual dysfunction: Current management perspectives. *Neuropsychiatric Disease Treatment, 16,* 1043–1050. https://doi.org/10.2147/NDT.S185757.

Augustyn, M., Zuckerman, B. S., & Caronna, E. B. (2010). *The Zuckerman Parker handbook of developmental and behavioral pediatrics for primary care.* Lippincott Williams & Wilkins.

Bandelow, B., & Michaelis, S. (2015). Epidemiology of anxiety disorders in the 21st century. *Dialogue in Clinical Neuroscience, 17*(3), 327–335. https://doi.org/10.31887/DCNS.2015.17.3/bbandelow.

Beesdo, K., Knappe, S., & Pine, D. S. (2009). Anxiety and anxiety disorders in children and adolescents: Developmental issues and implications for DSM-V. *Psychiatric Clinics of North America, 32*(3), 483–524. https://doi.org/10.1016/j.psc.2009.06.002.

Birmaher, B., Brent, D. A., Chiappetta, L., Bridge, J., Monga, S., & Baugher, M. (1999). Psychometric properties of the screen for child anxiety related emotional disorders (SCARED): A replication study. *Journal of the American Academy of Child and Adolescent Psychiatry, 38*(10), 1230–1236. https://doi.org/10.1097/00004583-199910000-00011.

Bramante, S., Maina, G., Borgogno, R., Pellegrini, L., Rigardetto, S., & Albert, U. (2023). Assessing suicide risk in patients with obsessive-compulsive disorder: A dimensional approach. *Brazilian Journal of Psychiatry.* https://doi.org/10.47626/1516-4446-2022-2632.

Carter, A. S., Fredine, N. J., Findley, D., Scahill, L., Zimmerman, L., & Sparrow, S. S. (1999). *Recommendations for teachers.* Hoboken, NJ: John Wiley & Sons Inc.

Centers for Disease Control and Prevention. (2022, February 17). Birth–18 years immunization schedule. *Centers for Disease Control and Prevention.* Retrieved January 15, 2023, from https://www.cdc.gov/vaccines/schedules/hcp/imz/child-adolescent.html.

Chansky, T. (2014). *Freeing your child from anxiety, revised and updated edition: Practical strategies to overcome fears, worries, and phobias and be prepared for life—from toddlers to teens.* Harmony.

Committee On Infectious Diseases. (2022). Recommended childhood and adolescent immunization schedule: united states, 2022. *Pediatrics, 149*(3), e2021056056. https://doi.org/10.1542/peds.2021-056056.

Dekel, I., Dorman-Ilan, S., Lang, C., Bar-David, E., Zilka, H., Shilton, T., Lebowitz, E. R., & Gothelf, D. (2020). The feasibility of a parent group treatment for youth with anxiety disorders and obsessive-compulsive disorder. *Child Psychiatry Human Development, 52*(6), 1044–1049. https://doi.org/10.1007/s10578-020-01082-6.

Fernández de la Cruz, L., Barrow, F., Bolhuis, K., Krebs, G., Volz, C., Nakatani, E., Heyman, I., & Mataix-Cols, D. (2013). Sexual obsessions in pediatric obsessive-compulsive disorder: Clinical characteristics and treatment outcomes. *Depression and Anxiety, 30*(8), 732–740. https://doi.org/10.1002/da.22097.

Gale, C. K., & Millichamp, J. (2016). Generalized anxiety disorder in children and adolescents. *BMJ Clinical Evidence,* 1002.

Geller, D. A., & March, J. The AACAP Committee on Quality Issues (CQI). (2012). Practice parameter for the assessment and treatment of children and adolescents with obsessive-compulsive disorder. *Journal of the American Academy of Child and Adolescent Psychiatry, 51*(1), 98–113. https://doi.org/10.1016/j.jaac.2011.09.019.

Ghandour, R. M., Sherman, L. J., Vladutiu, C. J., Ali, M. M., Lynch, S. E., Bitsko, R. H., & Blumberg, S. J. (2019). Prevalence and treatment of depression, anxiety, and conduct problems in US children. *Journal of Pediatrics, 206,* 256–267.e3. https://doi.org/10.1016/j.jpeds.2018.09.021.

Greene, R. W. (2005). *The explosive child: a new approach for understanding and parenting easily frustrated, chronically inflexible children.* Rev. and updated. New York, Harper.

Heimberg, R. G., Hofmann, S. G., Liebowitz, M. R., Schneier, E. R., Smits, J. A., Stein, M. B., Hinton, D. E., & Craske, M. G. (2014). Social anxiety disorder in DSM-5. *Depression and Anxiety, 31*(6), 472–479. https://doi.org/10.1002/da.22231.

Hoban, C. L., Byard, R. W., & Musgrave, I. F. (2015). A comparison of patterns of spontaneous adverse drug reaction reporting with St. John's wort and fluoxetine during the period 2000-2013. *Clinical and Experimental Pharmacology and Physiology, 42*(7), 747–751. https://doi.org/10.1111/1440-1681.12424.

Jankovic J. (1997). Tourette syndrome. Phenomenology and classification of tics. *Neurol Clin. 15*(2), 267–275. doi: 10.1016/s0733-8619(05)70311-x. PMID: 9115460.

Kendall, P. C. (1992). *Coping cat workbook.* Workbook Pub Incorporated.

Kendall, P. C., Furr, J. M., & Podell, J. L. (2010). Child-focused treatment of anxiety. In: Weisz, J. R., & Kazdin, A. E. (Eds.), *Evidence-based psychotherapies for children and adolescents* (2nd ed., pp. 45–59). Guilford Press.

Kennedy, S., Mash, J., Tawfik, S., & Ehrenreich-May, J. (2017). Anxiety disorders. In: Flessner, C. A., & Piacentini, J. C. (Eds.), *Clinical handbook of psychological disorders in children and adolescents: A step-by-step treatment manual* (pp. 122–168). Guilford Publications.

Kessler, R. C., Berglund, P., Demler, O., Jin, R., Merikangas, K. R., & Walters, E. E. (2005). Lifetime prevalence and age-of-onset distributions of DSM-IV disorders in the National Comorbidity Survey Replication. *Archives of General Psychiatry, 62*(6), 593–602. https://doi.org/10.1001/archpsyc.62.6.593.

Koyuncu, A., İnce, E., Ertekin, E., & Tükel, R. (2019). Comorbidity in social anxiety disorder: Diagnostic and therapeutic challenges. *Drugs Context, 8,* 212573. https://doi.org/10.7573/dic.212573.

Lavallee, K., Herren, C., Blatter-Meunier, J., Adornetto, C., In-Albon, T., & Schneider, S. (2011). Early predictors of separation anxiety disorder: Early stranger anxiety, parental pathology and prenatal factors. *Psychopathology, 44*(6), 354–361. https://doi.org/10.1159/000326629.

Malcolm, B., & Thomas, K. (2022). Serotonin toxicity of serotonergic psychedelics. *Psychopharmacology, 239*(6), 1881–1891. https://doi.org/10.1007/s00213-021-05876-x.

March, J. S. (2012). *Multidimensional anxiety scale for children* (2nd ed). Multi-Health Systems.

Merikangas, K. R., He, J. P., Burstein, M., Swanson, S. A., Avenevoli, S., Cui, L., Benjet, C., Georgiades, K., & Swendsen, J. (2010). Lifetime prevalence of mental disorders in US adolescents: Results from the National Comorbidity Survey Replication–Adolescent Supplement (NCS-A). *Journal of the American Academy of Child and Adolescent Psychiatry, 49*(10), 980–989. https://doi.org/10.1016/j.jaac.2010.05.017.

Mohatt, J., Bennett, S. M., & Walkup, J. T. (2014). Treatment of separation, generalized, and social anxiety disorders in youths. *American Journal of Psychiatry, 171*(7), 741–748. https://doi.org/10.1176/appi.ajp.2014.13101337.

Myers, K., & Winters, N. C. (2002). Ten-year review of rating scales. II: Scales for internalizing disorders. *Journal of the American Academy of Child and Adolescent Psychiatry, 41*(6), 634–659. https://doi.org/10.1097/00004583-200206000-00004.

O'Leary, S. T., Campbell, J. D., Ardura, M. I., Banerjee, R., Bryant, K. A., Caserta, M. T., Frenck, R. W., Gerber, J. S., John, C. C., Kourtis, A. P., Myers, A., Pannaraj, P., Ratner, A. J., Shah, S. S., Kimberlin, D. W., Barnett, E. D., Lynfield, R., Sawyer, M. H., Bernstein, H. H., … Frantz, J. M. (2023). Recommended childhood and adolescent immunization schedule: United States, 2023. *Pediatrics, 151*(3). https://doi.org/10.1542/peds.2022-061029.

Panganiban, M., Yeow, M., Zugibe, K., & Geisler, S. L. (2019). Recognizing, diagnosing, and treating pediatric generalized anxiety disorder. *JAAPA, 32*(2), 17–21. https://doi.org/10.1097/01.JAA.0000552719.98489.75.

Pediatric OCD Treatment Study (POTS) Team. (2004). Cognitive-behavior therapy, sertraline, and their combination for children and adolescents with obsessive-compulsive disorder: The Pediatric OCD Treatment Study (POTS) randomized controlled trial. *JAMA, 292*(16), 1969–1976. https://doi.org/10.1001/jama.292.16.1969.

Peris, T., & Schneider, B. (2017). Obsessive-compulsive disorder. In: Flessner, C. A., & Piacentini, J. C. (Eds.), *Clinical handbook of psychological disorders in children and adolescents: A step-by-step treatment manual* (pp. 273–298). Guilford Publications.

Piacentini, J., Bennett, S., Compton, S. N., Kendall, P. C., Birmaher, B., Albano, A. M., March, J., Sherrill, J., Sakolsky, D., Ginsburg, G., Rynn, M., Bergman, R. L., Gosch, E., Waslick, B., Iyengar, S., McCracken, J., & Walkup, J. (2014). 24- and 36-week outcomes for the Child/Adolescent Anxiety Multimodal Study (CAMS). *Journal of the American Academy of Child and Adolescent Psychiatry, 53*(3), 297–310. https://doi.org/10.1016/j.jaac.2013.11.010.

Piacentini, J., & Bergman, R. L. (2000). Obsessive-compulsive disorder in children. *Psychiatric Clinics of North America, 23*(3), 519–533. https://doi.org/10.1016/S0193-953X(05)70178-7.

Reynolds, C. R., & Richmond, B. O. (2008). *Revised children's manifest anxiety scale* (2nd ed.). Pearson.

Rizzo, R., & Gulisano, M. (2019). Treatment options for TIC disorders. *Expert Reviews in Neurotherapy, 20*(1), 55–63. https://doi.org/10.1080/14737175.2020.1698950.

Robinson, L. R., Bitsko, R. H., Schieve, L. A., & Visser, S. N. (2013). Tourette syndrome, parenting aggravation, and the contribution of co-occurring conditions among a nationally representative sample. *Disability and health journal, 6*(1), 26–35. https://doi.org/10.1016/j.dhjo.2012.10.002.

Rose, G. M., & Tadi, P. (2021). *Social anxiety disorder.* StatPearls Publishing. http://www.ncbi.nlm.nih.gov/books/NBK555890/.

Ruscio, A. M., Stein, D. J., Chiu, W. T., & Kessler, R. C. (2010). The epidemiology of obsessive-compulsive disorder in the National Comorbidity Survey Replication. *Molecular Psychiatry, 15*(1), 53–63. https://doi.org/10.1038/mp.2008.94.

Sakolsky, D., & Birmaher, B. (2008). Pediatric anxiety disorders: Management in primary care. *Current Opinions in Pediatrics, 20*(5), 538–543. https://doi.org/10.1097/MOP.0b013e32830fe3fa.

Sánchez-Meca, J., Rosa-Alcázar, A. I., Iniesta-Sepúlveda, M., & Rosa-Alcázar, Á. (2014). Differential efficacy of cognitive-behavioral therapy and pharmacological treatments for pediatric obsessive–compulsive disorder: A meta-analysis. *Journal of Anxiety Disorders, 28*(1), 31–44. https://doi.org/10.1016/j.janxdis.2013.10.007.

Sapyta, J. J., Freeman, J., Franklin, M. E., & March, J. S. (2012). Obsessive-compulsive disorder. In: Szigethy, E., Weisz, J., & Findling, R. L. (Eds.), *Cognitive-behavior therapy for children and adolescents* (pp. 299–330). American Psychiatric Pub.

Scahill, L., Riddle, M. A., Mcswiggin-Hardin, M., Ort, S. I., King, R. A., Goodman, W. K., Cicchetti, D., & Leckman, J. F. (1997). Children's Yale-Brown obsessive compulsive scale: Reliability and validity. *Journal of the American Academy of Child and Adolescent Psychiatry, 36*(6), 844–852. https://doi.org/10.1097/00004583-199706000-00023.

Shear, K., Jin, R., Ruscio, A. M., Walters, E. E., & Kessler, R. C. (2006). Prevalence and correlates of estimated DSM-IV child and adult separation anxiety disorder in the National Comorbidity Survey Replication. *American Journal of Psychiatry, 163*(6), 1074–1083. https://doi.org/10.1176/ajp.2006.163.6.1074.

Sigra, S., Hesselmark, E., & Bejerot, S. (2018). Treatment of pandas and pans: A systematic review. *Neuroscience &*

Biobehavioral Reviews, 86, 51–65. https://doi.org/10.1016/j.neubiorev.2018.01.001.

Soleimani, M. A., Pahlevan Sharif, S., Bahrami, N., Yaghoobzadeh, A., Allen, K. A., & Mohammadi, S. (2017). The relationship between anxiety, depression and risk behaviors in adolescents. *International Journal of Adolescent Medicine and Health, 31*(2). https://doi.org/10.1515/ijamh-2016-0148.

Stefánsdóttir, Í. H., Ivarsson, T., & Skarphedinsson, G. (2022). Efficacy and safety of serotonin reuptake inhibitors (SSRI) and serotonin noradrenaline reuptake inhibitors (SNRI) for children and adolescents with anxiety disorders: A systematic review and meta-analysis. *Nordic Journal of Psychiatry, 0*(0), 1–10. https://doi.org/10.1080/08039488.2022.2075460.

Storch, E. A., De Nadai, A. S., Conceição do Rosário, M., Shavitt, R. G., Torres, A. R., Ferrão, Y. A., Miguel, E. C., Lewin, A. B., & Fontenelle, L. F. (2015). Defining clinical severity in adults with obsessive–compulsive disorder. *Comprehensive Psychiatry, 63,* 30–35. https://doi.org/10.1016/j.comppsych.2015.08.007.

Storch, E. A., Ledley, D. R., Lewin, A. B., Murphy, T. K., Johns, N. B., Goodman, W. K., & Geffken, G. R. (2006). Peer victimization in children with obsessive-compulsive disorder: relations with symptoms of psychopathology. *Journal of clinical child and adolescent psychology : the official journal for the Society of Clinical Child and Adolescent Psychology, American Psychological Association, Division 53, 35*(3), 446–455. https://doi.org/10.1207/s15374424jccp3503_10.

Strawn, J. R., Geracioti, L., Rajdev, N., Clemenza, K., & Levine, A. (2018). Pharmacotherapy for generalized anxiety disorder in adult and pediatric patients: An evidence-based treatment review. *Expert Opinions in Pharmacotherapy, 19*(10), 1057–1070. https://doi.org/10.1080/14656566.2018.1491966.

Sullivan, P. F., Neale, M. C., & Kendler, K. S. (2000). Genetic epidemiology of major depression: Review and meta-analysis. *American Journal of Psychiatry, 157*(10), 1552–1562. https://doi.org/10.1176/appi.ajp.157.10.1552.

Taketomo, C. K. (2022). *Pediatric & neonatal dosage handbook: An extensive resource for clinicians treating pediatric and neonatal patients.* Lexicomp/Wolters Kluwer.

Vaccination recommendations by the AAP. American Academy of Pediatrics. (2023, July 10). https://www.aap.org/en/patient-care/immunizations/vaccination-recommendations-by-the-aap/.

Van Noppen, B., Sassano-Higgins, S., Appasani, R., & Sapp, F. (2021). *Cognitive-behavioral therapy for obsessive-compulsive disorder: 2021 update.* Focus (American Psychiatric Publishing). *19*(4), 430–443. https://doi.org/10.1176/appi.focus.20210015.

Walter, H. J., Bukstein, O. G., Abright, A. R., Keable, H., Ramtekkar, U., Ripperger-Suhler, J., & Rockhill, C. (2020). Clinical practice guideline for the assessment and treatment of children and adolescents with anxiety disorders. *Journal of the American Academy of Child and Adolescent Psychiatry, 59*(10), 1107–1124. https://doi.org/10.1016/j.jaac.2020.05.005.

Wehry, A. M., Beesdo-Baum, K., Hennelly, M. M., Connolly, S. D., & Strawn, J. R. (2015). Assessment and treatment of anxiety disorders in children and adolescents. *Current Psychiatry Report, 17*(7), 52. https://doi.org/10.1007/s11920-015-0591-z.

Wu, L.-M., Liu, Y., Chen, H.-M., Tseng, H.-C., & Lin, W-T. (2016). Psychometric properties of the RCMAS-2 in pediatric cancer patients. *European Journal of Oncology Nursing, 20,* 36–41. https://doi.org/10.1016/j.ejon.2015.07.008.

Attention-Deficit/Hyperactivity Disorder

9

Jamie Neal Lewis, Megan Bolch, Simone Moody, Hanein Edrees

ETIOLOGY

Attention-deficit/hyperactivity disorder (ADHD) was first described in 1775 in a German medical textbook by Melchoir Adam Weikard. In it, he depicted children and adults who had problems with inattention, distractibility, overactivity, and impulsivity (Barkley, 2015a). In 1798, Scottish physician Alexander Crichton wrote a more detailed description of two types of attention disorders: distractibility, shifting, and diminished power of attention (Barkley, 2015a). The 1800s brought more descriptions of attention disorders, including poems by German pediatrician Heinrich Hoffman in 1865 about an impulsive and fidgety child called "Fidgety Phil" and a daydreamy child called "Johnny Head-in-Air" (Barkley, 2015a). ADHD has had different names, including organic driveness, restlessness syndrome, brain-injured child, minimal brain damage, minimal brain dysfunction, hyperkinetic impulse disorder, hyperactivity syndrome, and physiologic hyperactivity (Barkley, 2015a).

The core symptoms of ADHD are inattention, hyperactivity, and impulsivity. ADHD is defined by the *Diagnostic and Statistical Manual of Mental Disorders*, Fifth Edition Text Revision (DSM-5-TR) as "a persistent pattern of inattention and/or hyperactivity-impulsivity that interferes with functioning or development" that has "persisted for at least six months that is inconsistent with developmental level and that negatively impacts directly on social and academic/occupational activities" (American Psychiatric Association [APA], 2022).

ADHD is a neurodevelopmental disorder intrinsic to the individual with multiple etiologies, including genetic factors, neurologic factors such as structural and functional brain abnormalities, neurotransmitter deficiencies, pregnancy, birth complications, and environmental toxins. ADHD can also be acquired following traumatic brain injuries (TBI) and is not caused by poor parenting (Barkley, 2015a). ADHD is likely a central nervous system disorder (Zayats & Neale, 2020).

ADHD is highly heritable at about 80% and is now considered one of the most genetically influenced mental health disorders (Barkley, 2015a). Twin studies reveal heritability at less than 100%, suggesting an environmental role in the development of ADHD (Faraone & Larsson, 2019). Genome-wide association studies have revealed candidate genes that may account for symptoms of ADHD (Grimm et al., 2020). Genetic studies also indicate that symptoms of ADHD occur when there is a defect in the dopamine transporters (Drechsler et al., 2020).

There is an increased risk for symptoms of ADHD following neurologic insults to the brain, such as hypoxic-anoxic injury, premature birth, and low birth weight (Rajaprakash & Leppert, 2022). Complications from birth, such as intrapartum hemorrhage, toxemia, and prolonged delivery, are also associated with symptoms of ADHD. Complications during pregnancy, such as preeclampsia, are associated with ADHD (Dachew et al., 2019). ADHD symptoms are more likely to occur in children with seizure disorders and with focal stroke to the putamen (Barkley, 2015a). Most children with ADHD will not have a history of significant brain injury (Barkley, 2015a). Prenatal exposure to alcohol (Mattson et al., 2019), opioids (Conradt et al., 2019), and tobacco (Rajaprakash & Leppert, 2022) are all associated with attention deficits. Children with complex cardiac defects such as ventricular septal defect, transposition of the greater arteries, and tetralogy of Fallot that have been surgically corrected are at increased risk of developing ADHD (Holst et al., 2020). Environmental toxins, such as elevated lead levels, have consistently been associated with ADHD symptoms (Barkley, 2015a). The risks of ADHD are higher in children with epilepsy, intellectual disabilities, autism spectrum disorders, cerebral palsy, Tourette syndrome, and learning disabilities (Rajaprakash & Leppert, 2022).

There are associations between ADHD and specific genetic syndromes, as chromosomal differences have been discovered in children with ADHD and certain developmental disorders (Grimm et al., 2020). Fragile X syndrome is one of the most common genetic syndromes associated with ADHD, with reports revealing that 59% of males with fragile X syndrome meet the diagnostic criteria for ADHD. One-third of children with neurofibromatosis type 1 display symptoms of ADHD. Tuberous sclerosis is associated with a 30% to 60% prevalence of ADHD. Turner and Klinefelter syndromes are associated with ADHD. Two-thirds of children with Williams syndrome display symptoms of ADHD. Velocardiofacial/DiGeorge syndrome (22q.11 deletion syndrome) is associated with ADHD in 40% of children (Grimm et al., 2020).

Neuroanatomic research indicates ADHD is associated with delayed brain maturation especially in the prefrontal cortex (Barkley, 2015a). Additionally, evidence suggests that small cerebellar volume, specifically in the vermis, and decreased white matter integrity in children and adults are associated with ADHD (Barkley, 2015a). Executive functioning defects are hypothetically linked to poor processing in the dorsolateral prefrontal cortex (Stahl, 2013). Neurotransmitter dysfunction has been implicated in the pathophysiology of ADHD. There are imbalances in the dopamine and norepinephrine pathways in the prefrontal cortex, which cause deficient signaling and decreased neurotransmission of these two neurotransmitters (Stahl, 2013). This may explain why children with ADHD respond to stimulants such as methylphenidate and amphetamine, as they increase dopamine availability in the synapse. Nonstimulants may increase the norepinephrine in the synapse by blocking the norepinephrine transporter (Barkley, 2015a).

Barkley has expanded the overview of ADHD to include problems with emotional impulsivity and poor emotional self-regulation and extended the dimensions to include deficits in executive functioning (Barkley, 2015c). In 1997, Barkley surmised that behavioral inhibition is a key foundational executive function and, when deficient in ADHD, causes additional deficits in other executive functions, including working memory and emotional and motivational self-regulation (Barkley, 2015c).

INCIDENCE AND PREVALENCE

ADHD is one of childhood's most common neurobehavioral disorders (Mick & Faraone, 2008; Rajaprakash & Leppert, 2022; Wolraich et al., 2019). Prevalence estimates range from 7% to 15% and vary based on historical changes in clinical diagnostic criteria, sample (e.g., ages and geographic region), and research methods (Wolraich et al., 2019). A meta-analysis in 2015 indicated a worldwide estimate of 7.2% (Thomas et al., 2015). National data reported that 9.4% of children aged 2 to 17 years have a diagnosis of ADHD, including 2.4% of children from 2 to 5 years of age (Danielson et al., 2018). According to the Centers for Disease Control and Prevention (CDC), the estimated number of children aged 3 to 17 years diagnosed with ADHD is 6 million (9.8%) using parental survey data from 2016 to 2019 (Bitsko et al., 2022). Prevalence estimates from studies that use clinical interviews in addition to parent and teacher report measures are known to be more precise in applying diagnostic criteria from the DSM-5. They are likely more accurate in identifying ADHD because they assess for functional impairment (Barkley, 2015a).

Prevalence rates of ADHD in children vary based on age and generally increase throughout development (Rajaprakash & Leppert, 2022). Danielson et al. (2018) reported that 2.1% of preschool children ages 2 to 5, 8.9% of 6- to 11-year-olds, and 11.9% of 12- to 17-year-olds meet the criteria for a diagnosis of ADHD. The median age of diagnosis was approximately 7 years, with one-third of children diagnosed before age 6 (Visser et al., 2015). Symptoms often persist into adolescence and adulthood, although primary symptomatology may differ across stages of development. For example, hyperactive and impulsive symptoms tend to decrease, while inattentive symptoms often persist (Molina et al., 2009). Changes in symptoms also may impact diagnosis and subsequent access to treatment.

Males are more than twice as likely than females to receive a diagnosis of ADHD (Danielson et al., 2018). This may be because more males have noticeable signs of hyperactivity, and more females exhibit symptoms consistent with the inattentive type of ADHD, leading to a delayed or missed diagnosis. Additionally, males are more likely to be diagnosed with cooccurring externalizing conditions such as oppositional defiant disorder (ODD) (Elia et al., 2008). Females with ADHD are more likely to have cooccurring internalizing conditions such as anxiety and depression (Tung et al., 2016). Across age groups, Black (12%) and White (10%) non-Hispanic children are more often diagnosed with ADHD than Hispanic children (8%) or Asian non-Hispanic children (3%) (Bitsko et al., 2022).

DIAGNOSTIC CRITERIA

The diagnostic criteria for ADHD, as defined by the DSM-5-TR (2022), consist of individuals with significant ADHD symptoms that persist for at least 6 months. Several symptoms are present before the age of 12 years, and several symptoms occur in more than one setting, interfere with or reduce an individual's functioning, and another mental disorder does not better explain symptoms. The DSM-5-TR specifiers include three presentations of ADHD: predominately inattention presentation (ADHD-I), predominantly hyperactive-impulsive presentation (ADHD-H/I), and combined presentation (ADHD-C). For a diagnosis of ADHD-I, at least six of nine possible symptoms of inattention must be present and have persisted for at least 6 months for children and adolescents 16 years old and younger (Box 9.1). For a diagnosis of ADHD-H/I, at least six of nine possible symptoms of hyperactivity or impulsivity must be present and have persisted for at least 6 months for children and adolescents 16 years old and younger. For individuals 17 years old and older, five of nine symptoms of inattention or hyperactivity-impulsivity are required for diagnosing ADHD. ADHD-C is diagnosed when symptom criteria are met for the inattentive and hyperactive-impulsive categories.

The American Academic of Pediatrics (AAP) Clinical Practice Guideline for the Diagnosis, Evaluation, and Treatment of Attention-Deficit/Hyperactivity Disorder

| Box 9.1 | Diagnostic Criteria for Attention-Deficit/Hyperactivity Disorder From DSM-5-TR |

A persistent pattern of inattention and/or hyperactivity-impulsivity that interferes with functioning or development, as characterized by (1) and/or (2):

1. Inattention: Six (or more) of the following symptoms have persisted for at least 6 months to the degree that is inconsistent with developmental level and that negatively impacts social and academic/occupational activities:
   a. Often fails to give close attention to details or makes careless mistakes in schoolwork, at work, or during other activities (e.g., overlooks or misses details, work is inaccurate).
   b. Often has difficulty sustaining attention in tasks or play activities (e.g., has difficulty remaining focused during lectures, conversations, or lengthy reading).
   c. Often does not seem to listen when spoken to directly (e.g., mind seems elsewhere, even in the absence of any obvious distraction).
   d. Often does not follow instructions and fails to finish schoolwork, chores, or duties in the workplace (e.g., starts tasks but quickly loses focus and is easily sidetracked).
   e. Often has difficulty organizing tasks and activities (e.g., difficulty managing sequential tasks; difficulty keeping materials and belongings in order; messy; disorganized work; has poor time management; fails to meet deadlines).
   f. Often avoids, dislikes, or is reluctant to engage in tasks that require sustained mental effort (e.g., schoolwork or homework; for older adolescents and adults, preparing reports, completing forms, reviewing lengthy papers).
   g. Often loses things necessary for tasks or activities (e.g., school materials, pencils, books, tools, wallets, keys, paperwork, eyeglasses, mobile telephones).
   h. Is often easily distracted by extraneous stimuli (for older adolescents and adults, it may include unrelated thoughts).
   i. Is often forgetful in daily activities (e.g., doing chores, running errands; for older adolescents and adults, returning calls, paying bills, keeping appointments).
2. Hyperactivity and Impulsivity: Six (or more) of the following symptoms have persisted for at least 6 months to a degree that is inconsistent with developmental level, and that negatively impacts social and academic/occupational activities:
   a. Often fidgets with or taps hands or feet or squirms in the seat.
   b. Often leaves seat in situations in which remaining seated is expected (e.g., leaves place in the classroom, in the office, or other workplace, or in other situations that require remaining in place).
   c. Often runs about or climbs in situations in which it is inappropriate (in adolescents or adults, may be limited to feeling of restlessness).
   d. Often unable to play or engage in leisure activities quietly.
   e. Is often "on the go" or acting as if "driven by a motor" (e.g., is unable to be or uncomfortable being still for extended time, as in restaurants, meetings; may be experienced by others as being restless or difficult to keep up with).
   f. Often talks excessively.
   g. Often blurts out an answer before a question has been completed (e.g., completes people's sentences; cannot wait for turn in conversation).
   h. Often has difficulty waiting their turn (e.g., while waiting in line).
   i. Often interrupts or intrudes on others (e.g., butts into conversations, games, or activities; may start using other people's things without asking or receiving permission; for adolescents and adults, may intrude into or take over what others are doing).
A. Several inattentive or hyperactive-impulsive symptoms were present prior to age 12 years.
B. Several inattentive or hyperactive-impulsive are present in two or more settings (e.g., at home, school, or work; with friends or relatives, in other activities).
C. There is clear evidence that the symptoms interfere with, or reduce the quality of, social, academic, or occupational functioning.
D. The symptoms do not occur exclusively during schizophrenia or another psychotic disorder and are not better explained by another mental disorder (e.g., mood disorder, anxiety disorder, dissociative disorder, personality disorder, substance intoxication, or withdrawal).

From the *Diagnostic and Statistical Manual of Mental Disorders, Fifth Edition, Text Revision*. Copyright 2022 by the American Psychiatric Association. All Rights Reserved.

in Children and Adolescents (2019) recommends that primary care clinicians evaluate children and adolescents 4 to 17 years old for ADHD when symptoms of inattention, hyperactivity, or impulsivity are present, and the child displays behavioral or academic problems (Wolraich et al., 2019).

In 2020, the Society for Developmental and Behavioral Pediatrics defined complex ADHD "based on age (<4 years or presentation at age >12 years), presence of coexisting conditions (neurodevelopmental, mental health, medical or psychosocial factors adversely affecting health and development), moderate to severe functional impairment, diagnostic uncertainty, or inadequate response to treatment." Recommended evaluation includes verifying previous diagnoses and screening for coexisting conditions. Treatment includes psychoeducation about ADHD and coexisting conditions, using evidence-based approaches to focus on areas of functional impairment, not just symptom control. Because ADHD is a chronic health condition, treatment should be ongoing with regular monitoring of patients throughout their lifespan (Barbaresi et al., 2020).

Table 9.1   Changes from the DSM-IV-TR to the DSM-5 and DSM-5-TR

DSM-IV-TR	DSM-5 AND DSM-5-TR
Few examples of ADHD symptoms Six or more symptoms of inattention and/or hyperactivity-impulsivity required for all ages	Additional examples of ADHD symptoms Five or more symptoms of inattention and/or hyperactivity-impulsivity required for individuals age ≥17 years
Some symptoms present prior to 7 years old	Several symptoms present prior to 12 years old
Impairment is present in more than one setting	Several symptoms are present in more than one setting
Symptoms result in impairment in social, academic, or occupational functioning Specify ADHD predominantly inattentive type, predominantly hyperactive-impulsive type, or combined type No severity specifier	Symptoms interfere or reduce the quality of functioning socially, at school, or at work Specify ADHD predominantly inattentive presentation, predominately hyperactive-impulsive presentation, or combined presentation Specify mild, moderate, or severe
Partial remission specifier without criteria	Partial remission specifier used if symptom criteria have not been met for at least 6 months, but there is ongoing functional impairment
ADHD not otherwise specified	Other specified ADHD Unspecified ADHD

ADHD, Attention-deficit/hyperactivity disorder; *DSM-5*, Diagnostic and Statistical Manual of Mental Disorders, Fifth Edition; *DSM-IV-TR*, DSM Fourth Edition Text Revision; *DSM-5-TR*, DSM Fifth Edition Text Revision.

There were several notable changes in the ADHD diagnostic criteria from the DSM-IV-TR (2000) to the DSM-5 (2013). There were no changes in the ADHD diagnostic criteria from the DSM-5 to the DSM-5-TR (2022). Changes from the DSM-IV-TR to the DSM-5 and DSM-5-TR are summarized in Table 9.1. DSM diagnostic changes were intended to diagnose ADHD more accurately by providing more guidance on how symptoms present and more flexibility on the criteria based on updated research. These changes may contribute to the increasing prevalence rate of ADHD (Epstein & Loren, 2013). A limiting factor of the DSM-5 diagnostic criteria is that it does not capture developmental course differences in the presentation of ADHD or the proposed theory of ADHD as a dimensional disorder (Epstein & Loren, 2013).

DIAGNOSTIC MEASURES

According to the AAP ADHD Clinical Practice Guideline (Wolraich et al., 2019), a diagnosis of ADHD should include an evaluation to determine if DSM-5 criteria are met. This evaluation should include multiple informants to capture the child's symptoms and functioning in multiple settings. Typical informants include parent(s)/guardian(s) and the child's teacher(s). Information is obtained through standardized rating scales by caregivers (e.g., parent and teacher) and interviews with parent(s)/guardian(s) and the child (Barkley, 2015a; Wolraich et al., 2019). For middle and high school students with multiple teachers, consider obtaining ratings from two or more teachers or other adults who have regular interactions with the adolescent. For preschool-age children, reliable information from a second setting may be difficult to establish if the child does not attend day care or school. If a preschooler suspected to have ADHD does not meet the diagnostic criteria, behavioral intervention and ongoing monitoring are encouraged (Wolraich et al., 2019).

Standardized rating scales should include ADHD-specific symptom ratings from reporters in more than one setting (e.g., parent and teacher). Examples of ADHD rating scales for school-age children and adolescents include the Vanderbilt ADHD Diagnostic Parent and Teacher Rating Scales (Wolraich et al., 2003), ADHD Rating Scale 5 (DuPaul et al., 2016), Connors 3 (Conners, 2008), Swanson, Nolan, and Pelham Rating Scales (SNAP-IV; Swanson et al., 2012), and the Disruptive Behavior Disorder Rating Scale (DBDRS; Pelham et al., 1992) (Table 9.2). ADHD rating scales for preschoolers include the ADHD Rating Scale-IV Preschool Version (McGoey et al., 2007) and the Connors Early Childhood (Conners, 2009) (Table 9.3). Assessing child interference or reduction in functioning in the home, school, and social settings can be done through standardized rating scales such as the Vanderbilt, Connors, Impairment Rating Scale (Fabiano et al., 2006), and the Home Situations Questionnaire and School Situations Questionnaire (Barkley & Murphy, 2006) and a clinical interview.

Information from a clinical interview is obtained from the parent(s)/guardian(s) and the child or adolescent. Parent(s)/guardian(s) should serve as the primary source of information for ADHD symptoms and impairment, as child and adolescent reports tend to be less reliable (Barkley, 2015). An individual, private interview with adolescents is recommended to screen for conditions such as substance use, sleep problems, and internalizing disorders (e.g., anxiety and depression) (Pliszka & American Academy of Child and Adolescent Psychiatry [AACAP] Work Group on Quality Issues, 2007).

Most children and adolescents with ADHD have a cooccurring condition. Therefore the AAP ADHD Clinical Practice Guideline recommends that primary care clinicians screen for cooccurring disorders (Wolraich et al., 2019). Broad-band measures of child and

Table **9.2**	School-Age and Adolescent ADHD Rating Scales			
ADHD RATING SCALES	**AGE RANGE**	**RESPONDERS**	**DESCRIPTION**
Vanderbilt ADHD Diagnostic Rating Scales	6–12 yr	Parent Teacher	Presentations of ADHD, ODD, CD, anxiety/depression screening, academic and behavioral impairment
ADHD Rating Scale-5 (ADHD-5)	5–17 yr	Parent Teacher	Presentations of ADHD
Conners 3	6–18 yr	Parent Teacher Child	Presentations of ADHD, ODD, CD, aggression, executive functioning, anxiety and depression screening, learning and social problems, impairment
SNAP-IV Rating Scales	6–18 yr	Parent Teacher	Presentations of ADHD, ODD
Disruptive Behavior Disorder Rating Scales	5–18 yr	Parent Teacher	Presentations of ADHD, ODD, CD

ADHD, Attention-deficit/hyperactivity disorder; *CD,* conduct disorder; *ODD,* oppositional defiant disorder.

Table **9.3**	Preschool ADHD Rating Scales			
ADHD RATING SCALES	**AGE RANGE**	**RESPONDERS**	**DESCRIPTION**
ADHD Rating Scale–IV Preschool Version (ADHD-IV)	3–5 yr	Parent Teacher	Presentations of ADHD
Connors Early Childhood	2–6 yr	Parent Teacher	Behavior scales, including inattention/hyperactivity, anxiety and mood/affect, developmental milestones, impairment

ADHD, Attention-deficit/hyperactivity disorder.

adolescent emotional, behavioral, social, and adaptive functioning, such as the Achenbach System of Empirically Based Assessment (ASEBA) or the Behavior Assessment System for Children, Third Edition (BASC-3), may be used as a screener for ADHD and other conditions (Barkley, 2015a). These measures include parent, teacher, and self-report, tend to be used in mental health specialty care settings, and are available at a cost. The Pediatric Symptom Checklist is a free, brief parent report and youth report screening measure of child and adolescent attention, internalizing (anxiety and depression), and externalizing (conduct) symptoms available in multiple languages (Jellinek et al., 1988).

Similarly, the Preschool Pediatric Symptom Checklist is a brief, publicly available report of young children's social-emotional and behavioral functioning (Sheldrick et al., 2012). ADHD-specific measures include screenings for emotional, behavioral, and developmental disorders, such as the Vanderbilt ADHD Parent Diagnostic Rating Scale and the Disruptive Behavior Disorder Rating Scale, which assess for all ODD and conduct disorder (CD) symptoms. Anxiety and depression can be screened through broad-band assessment, some ADHD-specific rating scales, and other measures commonly used in pediatric practice. If applicable, trauma and posttraumatic stress can be screened through clinical interviews and assessments. Learning problems may be screened on rating scales, including academic impairment, such as the Vanderbilt or Connors, or through educational history. Other developmental/physical conditions can be screened through history and physical exams. Hearing

and vision testing are encouraged as part of the medical evaluation. For children with suspected learning or intellectual disorders, cognitive testing by specialists is indicated (Barbaresi et al., 2020). Neuropsychological testing is not indicated for a diagnosis of ADHD unless there are suspected central nervous system conditions such as a TBI or stroke (Barbaresi et al., 2020; Wolraich et al., 2019).

CLINICAL MANIFESTATIONS AT TIME OF DIAGNOSIS

The core symptoms of ADHD are impulsivity, inattention, and hyperactivity. ADHD is associated with impairments across multiple facets of a child's life. It is a chronic disorder; following the chronic care, a medical home model is recommended. Referral to subspeciality care (i.e., developmental-behavioral health care providers, nurse practitioners, and psychologists) may be needed for complex ADHD. According to the National Survey of Children's Health in 2011, the median age of onset was 6 years, although for severe ADHD the median age was 4 years. Symptoms of ADHD may be identified in early childhood; however, referral for evaluation is frequently made during school years when the demands for sustained attention and behavior are increased and potentially disrupting to the school environment. Even then, children (most often females) with the inattentive type often go undetected. Children with the inattentive form of ADHD are less likely to exhibit the level of behavior difficulty observed in those with the combined or hyperactive-impulsive type (APA, 2000). Children with predominantly inattentive presentation may have high levels of sluggish cognitive tempo, with symptoms such as daydreaming, drowsiness, slowness to respond, and hypoactivity (Barkley, 2015c). As mentioned, difficulties with emotional impulsivity, emotional dysregulation, and impairments with executive functioning are often seen.

◎ Clinical Manifestations at Time of Diagnosis

POSSIBLE BEHAVIORAL MANIFESTATIONS
- Suspensions from day care or preschool
- Hyperactivity: inability to sit still, fidgeting, toe-tapping
- Impulsivity: blurting out answers, difficulty taking turns, emotional impulsivity
- Difficulties with attention specifically related to persistent effort
- Sluggish cognitive tempo: increase in daydreaming
- Poor emotional self-regulation
- Disorganization at school, home, or work
- Executive function difficulties
- Difficulties with social interaction
- Older adolescents: possible criminal behavior, drug or alcohol use disorders

From Wolraich, M. L., et. al. (2019). Clinical practice guideline for the diagnosis, evaluation, and treatment of attention-deficit/hyperactivity disorder in children and adolescents. *Pediatrics*, 144(4), e20192528; Barkley, R. A. (Ed.). (2015). *Attention-deficit hyperactivity disorder: A handbook for diagnosis & treatment* (4th ed.). The Guilford Press.

ADHD IN PRESCHOOL CHILDREN

For preschool-age children, reliable information from a second setting may be difficult to establish if the child does not attend day care or school; however, informants from at least two settings are critical in making an accurate diagnosis (O'Neill et al., 2014). Early symptoms of ADHD are associated with an increased risk of negative outcomes across domains (i.e., behavior, social, emotional, and academic) (O'Neill et al., 2017). A diagnosis of ADHD for preschool-age children tends to remain stable over time (Riddle et al., 2013), but the presentation may change. In the preschool period, hyperactive-impulsive symptoms are more likely to be present and then decline over time, whereas inattentive symptoms starting in the preschool period have a more variable developmental trajectory (O'Neill et al., 2017). Evidence supports that the risk of accidental injury increases with age for preschoolers with ADHD. Therefore providers in acute care settings may assist with early identification and referral for services (Allan et al., 2021).

ADHD IN OLDER ADOLESCENTS AND ADULTS

Symptom presentation in older adolescents and adults often differs from that of younger children, with hyperactivity often declining in adolescents and impulsivity/inattentiveness persisting (Riddle et al., 2013). Outcomes of childhood ADHD may include externalizing symptoms such as CD or ODD, internalizing symptoms such as anxiety and depression, substance

use, driving problems, and broad academic, occupational, or social functioning difficulties (Owens et al., 2015). Symptoms presenting in adults may be considered subthreshold (less than six symptoms) according to DSM-5-TR criteria, but these symptoms often can include significant functional impairments.

In adolescence, teenagers face the challenges of managing complex educational, extracurricular, and personal activities, which can result in increased difficulties for adolescents who have symptoms of ADHD. Specific difficulties may include academic failure or related challenges, employment problems such as job turnover or decreased performance, substance use, driving problems, poor social interactions, and risk-taking behaviors (Owens et al., 2015). With the risk for such significant life impairments, in recent years it has become more widely accepted that older adolescents and adults with suspected signs or symptoms of ADHD should be further assessed to ensure that individuals undiagnosed or with late onset of symptoms are identified and adequately managed. Long-term follow-up studies indicate if this occurs, improved academic outcomes and decreased rates of mood symptoms, substance abuse, criminal behavior, motor vehicle accidents, and injuries can result (Boland et al., 2020; Rajaprakash & Leppert, 2022).

TREATMENT

ADHD is a chronic health condition that can cause significant functional impairment in multiple settings. Treatment of ADHD must encompass behavioral, educational, and general health care needs (Barkley, 2015a). The US Food and Drug Administration (FDA)–approved medications for ADHD have strong efficacy and safety data (Cortese et al., 2018). Accurate and early diagnosis and appropriate treatment can improve long-term outcomes in children with ADHD (Rajaprakash & Leppert, 2022). Screening and management for problems that may exacerbate symptoms of ADHD include sleep problems, other mental health disorders, pain symptoms, and safety of the children (Rajaprakash & Leppert, 2022). A multimodal approach is recommended with involvement from the family, primary care provider, teachers, psychologists, social workers, and school nurses. The efficacy of management can be ascertained with feedback from parents and teachers using validated questionnaires, clinical interviews, and input from the child.

BEHAVIORAL INTERVENTION

The AAP recommends behavior therapy as a first-line treatment for children with ADHD (Wolraich et al., 2019) (Box 9.2). Behavior therapy is recommended prior to medication management for preschool-age children with ADHD or at high risk for ADHD. There are limited exceptions in which medication management may be considered for preschool-age children

Box **9.2**   Behavior Management Strategies

STRATEGY: POSITIVE REINFORCEMENT
- *Description:* Immediate reward given for desired behavior; tangible reinforcers, such as small treats, stickers, or inexpensive toys, are the most effective. Other reinforcers include special privileges or activities.
- *Example:* Child performs targeted behavior and receives previously agreed-on reinforcer. Child completes task, receives praise and small treat.

STRATEGY: WITHDRAWAL OF PRIVILEGES (COST-RESPONSE INTERVENTION)
- *Description:* Undesirable behavior results in loss of desired privilege.
- *Example:* Access to computer time or favorite TV show is withdrawn if targeted misbehavior occurs. Alternatively, time-out removes child temporarily from setting where misbehavior occurred.

STRATEGY: TOKEN ECONOMIES
- *Description:* Tokens are awarded for each appropriate behavior, which can be accumulated and used to acquire a desired activity or object. Alternatively, the child starts with a given number of tokens, and each incidence of targeted misbehavior results in loss of a token. A certain number of tokens must be acquired or retained by child to access special privileges or items.
- *Example:* Desired behavior occurs; token is awarded. Alternatively, undesirable behavior occurs, token is withdrawn. Different numbers of tokens can be traded for small toys, games, or special privileges at the end of a specified time period.

From Barkley, 2015a; DuPaul, G.J., & Kern, L. (2011). *Young children with ADHD: Early identification and intervention.* American Psychological Association; Evans, S.W., Owens, J.S., Wymbs, B.T., et al. (2018). Evidence-based psychosocial treatments for children and adolescents with attention deficit/hyperactivity disorder. *Journal of Clinical Child and Adolescent Psychology, 47*(2), 157–198.

with ADHD (e.g., lack of access to behavior therapy and inadequate response to behavior therapy). Behavior therapy and medication management are recommended for school-age children with ADHD. For adolescents with ADHD, medication management is recommended, while behavior therapy or training interventions for organization and time management are encouraged if available. The APP recommends that educational interventions and supports are included in treatment for children of all ages (Wolraich et al., 2019). In a recent individual participant data meta-analysis, behavioral interventions were found to be equally effective for children with ADHD across demographic variables such as child age, sex, socioeconomic status, IQ, medication status, and common cooccurring conditions such as ODD, depression, and anxiety (Groenman et al., 2022). Behavioral intervention efficacy studies have become more ethnically and racially diverse over time; however, an overrepresentation of parents with a high level of education and an underrepresentation of other underserved populations remains (Evans et al., 2018).

Behavior therapy for children and adolescents with ADHD targets functional impairments in the home,

school, and social settings. Behavioral parent training (BPT), behavioral classroom management, and behavioral peer interventions are well-established treatments for children with ADHD (Evans et al., 2018). These treatments involve modifying behaviors at the point of performance at home, school, and in social settings for optimal improvement in functioning. Example behavioral goals include on-task behavior and timely completion of routines, emotion regulation, following classroom rules, assignment completion and accuracy, and appropriate peer interactions. Unsafe behaviors are prioritized and can be targeted through behavioral techniques such as caregiver education, stimulus control (e.g., safe storage of dangerous items), close monitoring of child behavior, and reinforced practice of safety skills (DuPaul & Kern, 2011). BPT has the strongest evidence base among psychosocial treatments for children with ADHD (Evans et al., 2018). Modifying antecedents (e.g., planning and preventing undesired behavior) and positive reinforcement (e.g., praise and rewards for desired behavior) have been found to be the most effective components. The effect sizes for BPT programs for children with ADHD are strongest when children are younger, and their behavior is more malleable (Dekkers et al., 2022). As children progress through adolescence, BPT is classified as a possibly efficacious treatment (Evans et al., 2018) as opposed to well established. Typical developmental differences in adolescence, such as increased independence and fewer opportunities for parents to modify the adolescent's environment, limit the effectiveness of BPT.

Behavioral classroom management is another well-established intervention for ADHD (Evans et al., 2018). Antecedent and consequence-based strategies (e.g., effective instruction, structure, praise, contingency management) are effective at managing impairments related to ADHD in the school setting (Staff et al., 2022). Daily report cards are an evidenced-based tool that utilizes antecedent and consequence-based strategies and has been shown to reduce ADHD-related symptoms and impairment in addition to other disruptive behaviors in the classroom (Fabiano et al., 2010; Iznardo et al., 2020). Parents and guardians are encouraged to advocate for the use of these evidence-based tools and partner with school personnel to decrease classroom impairments (Chacko et al., 2017).

Behavioral peer-based intervention is a well-established treatment for children with ADHD (Evans et al., 2014, 2018; Fabiano et al., 2006). This evidence base was established from the Summer Treatment Program, an intervention for ADHD that targets child impairment across various domains, including social functioning (Pelham & Fabiano, 2008). Behavioral peer intervention consists of reinforcement of social skills in real-world settings to reduce social impairments. Caregiver involvement is required to implement these programs, as teaching social skills alone is not an evidence-based treatment. These interventions are challenging to implement in social settings where parents and teachers are absent, as the point of performance feedback from a caregiver may be limited or impossible (Chacko et al., 2017).

Training Interventions

The AAP ADHD Clinical Practice Guideline recommends the use of training interventions for adolescents with ADHD (Wolraich et al., 2019). Training interventions are one of the latest evidence-based additions to the ADHD psychosocial treatment, and their efficacy varies based on skill type and the amount of training time (Evans et al., 2018). Training interventions with a well-established evidence base include repeated practice and performance feedback for real-world organization tasks such as managing school assignments (Evans et al., 2018).

Pharmacologic Therapy

The AAP ADHD Clinical Practice Guidelines recommend treatment based on the child's age. When starting pharmacotherapy in children, a common principle used is "start low, go slow"—that is, start with a low dose and titrate slowly over time. In children age 4 to exactly 6 years, treatment starts with evidence-based BPT or behavioral classroom interventions. Methylphenidate can be considered. Treatment for elementary and middle school children ages 6 to exactly 12 years begins with prescribing FDA-approved medications for ADHD along with parent training or behavioral classroom interventions. An individualized education program (IEP) may be helpful. Treatment for adolescents age 12 to exactly 18 years begins with prescribing FDA-approved medications for ADHD with the assent of the adolescent (Wolraich et al., 2019).

The goals of treatment are to minimize ADHD symptoms and decrease functional impairment in the child's life while minimizing the adverse effects of medications. Stimulants have been used in children since the 1930s and continue to be first-line medications in the treatment of ADHD (Posner et al., 2020). Nonstimulants such as selective norepinephrine reuptake inhibitors (SNRIs) and two alpha$_2$-agonists are considered second-line therapy for school-age children and adolescents due to lower efficacy compared to stimulants or if treatment with stimulants is not effective (Posner et al., 2020). No other interventions have been shown to be as effective in treating core symptoms of ADHD (Rajaprakash & Leppert, 2022). Stimulants include different formulations of methylphenidate and amphetamine but have similar mechanisms of action (Posner et al., 2020). Dopamine or norepinephrine are released into the synapse from the presynaptic neuron and then are reversibly attached to their receptors on the postsynaptic neuron. Methylphenidate works by increasing extrasynaptic dopamine and norepinephrine by blocking their reuptake (Stahl, 2013; Partain et al.,

2019). Amphetamine works by blocking the reuptake of dopamine and norepinephrine and facilities neurotransmitter release into the extraneuronal space (Partain et al., 2019). A meta-analysis of over 10,000 children and adolescents found that methylphenidate and amphetamine formulations had moderate to large effect sizes when assessed by clinicians and teachers (Cortese et al., 2018). Methylphenidate and amphetamine are both available in short- and long-acting preparations (Rajaprakash & Leppert, 2022). Response to stimulants is individualized, with about 40% of children responding to both the methylphenidate family and amphetamine family and 40% responding to only one family (Wolraich et al., 2019).

Stimulant medications

Prescribing principles. Stimulants are not usually dosed on weight and typically begin at the lowest dose with weekly titration to an effective dose while monitoring for adverse effects (Rajaprakash & Leppert, 2022). For children age 6 years and older, start with the lowest dose of the desired stimulant and titrate to effect. It is generally helpful to divide the day into thirds: morning, afternoon, and evening. Individuals may have parts of the day when they have the greatest need for symptom control. Mornings can be particularly troublesome for kids with ADHD. An individual who needs better symptom control in the morning may benefit from a long-acting (i.e., extended-release) stimulant with a higher short-acting/immediate-release component; an individual who needs better symptom control in the afternoon may benefit from a long-acting stimulant with a lower short-acting/immediate-release component (Partain et al., 2019).

The effectiveness of stimulants is determined by assessing behavioral changes in the child, such as improved attention and focus and decreased hyperactivity. It is reasonable for parents to start the medication on the weekend to observe the child for 2 days of use. Questionnaires such as the Vanderbilt Rating Scale can be given to parents and teachers for subjective measurements over time. The ADHD Medication Guide (www.adhdmedicationguide.com) can be found online and is a helpful tool for visualization and updated summarization of medications. However, choices may be limited by insurance coverage. It is important to ask the family practical questions to assist with stimulant titration, such as: (1) When does the child take the medication? (2) What time does it wear off? (3) Is the medication helpful? and (4) Is the child experiencing adverse effects? (Rajaprakash & Leppert, 2022).

Treatment with stimulants has shown to be effective in reducing ADHD symptoms in numerous short-term trials lasting approximately 3 months, and both methylphenidate and amphetamine had moderate to large effect sizes (Posner et al., 2020). All stimulants have shown a higher efficacy than placebo for the

Table 9.4   Methylphenidate Short-Acting/Immediate-Release Preparations

MEDICATION	DOSAGE FORM	STARTING DOSE	TITRATION	MAXIMUM DOSE	DURATION	NOTES
Methylphenidate (Ritalin)	5-, 10-, 20-mg tablet	2.5 mg twice daily	Up to 7.5 mg BID to TID per day over 2–4 wk	2 mg/kg or 60 mg daily	3–4 hr	Can be crushed
Methylin solution	5 mg/mL; 10 mg/5 mL liquid	Same	Up to 10 mg TID	Same	3–4 hr	Grape flavor
Methylphenidate chewable	2.5-, 5-, 10-mg chewable	Same	Up to 10 mg TID	Same	3–4 hr	Grape flavor
Dexmethylphenidate (Focalin)	2.5-, 5-, 10-mg tablet	2.5 mg twice daily	Up to 10 mg BID	Same	4–6 hr	

BID, Twice a day; *TID*, three times a day.
From Feder, J.D., Tien, E., & Puzantian, T. (2018). *The child medication fact book for psychiatric practice*. Carlat Publishing, LLC; Rajaprakash, M., & Leppert, M. L. (2022). Attention-deficit/hyperactivity disorder. *Pediatric Review, 43*(3), 135–147.

Table 9.5   Amphetamine Short-Acting/Immediate Release

MEDICATION	DOSAGE FORM	STARTING DOSE	TITRATION	MAXIMUM DOSE	DURATION	NOTES
Evekeo (amphetamine), Evekeo ODT	5, 10 mg 5, 10, 15, 20 mg	3–5 yr: 2.5 mg daily; >6 yr: 5 mg daily	Increase by 2.5 mg every week	20 mg BID	3–5 hr	
Procentra (dextroamphetamine oral solution)	5 mg/mL	3–5 yr: 2.5 mg daily; >6 yr: 5 mg daily	Increase by 2.5 mg every week; 5 mg every week for >6 yr	20 mg BID	3–5 hr	Bubble gum flavor
Zenzedi (dextroamphetamine)	2.5, 5, 7.5, 10, 15, 20, 30 mg	As above	As above	As above	3–5 hr	
Adderall (mixed amphetamine salts)	5, 7.5, 10, 15, 20, 30 mg	As above	As above	As above	4–6 hr	

BID, Twice a day.
From Feder, J.D., Tien, E., & Puzantian, T. (2018). *The child medication fact book for psychiatric practice*. Carlat Publishing, LLC; Rajaprakash, M., & Leppert, M. L. (2022). Attention-deficit/hyperactivity disorder. *Pediatric Review, 43*(3), 135–147.

short-term management of ADHD. Amphetamines may be less tolerated in children and adolescents but may be slightly more efficacious (Cortese et al., 2018).

Stimulants come in a variety of formulations and delivery systems, including tablets, capsules (many of which can be opened and sprinkled), solutions, chewables, orally disintegrating tablets, and skin patches. The technologies vary in the delivery systems and include a spheroidal oral drug absorption system used for Ritalin LA and Focalin XR, an osmotic release oral system used for Concerta, and Diffucaps used for Metadate CD (Partain et al., 2019). Methylphenidate has D- and L-isomers, with the D-isomer being more potent. Amphetamine also has D- and L-isomers, with the D-isomer identified as more potent for dopamine binding, but the D- and L-isomers are equally effective on norepinephrine binding (Stahl, 2013). Insufficient evidence supports stimulant pharmacogenetic testing (Wolraich et al., 2019).

Short-acting/immediate-release formulations. Most of the short-acting amphetamines (Evekeo, Adderall, Dexedrine, Zenzedi, Procentra) and their generics are FDA approved for children age 3 years and older, with the exception of the D- and L-amphetamine sulfate orally disintegrating tablet (Evekeo ODT) (Tables 9.4 and 9.5). However, methylphenidate has the most safety and efficacy data in preschool children (Wolraich et al., 2019). Shorting-acting methylphenidates include Ritalin, Methylin, and Focalin and their generics. Short-acting preparations of either class last 3 to 6 hours and can be given two times a day (after breakfast and lunch). They generally take effect in 30 minutes. Some children may benefit from a third dose in the later afternoon to help with evening activities. Some children may have increasing ADHD symptoms as the medication wears off.

Intermediate and long-acting (extended-release) formulations. There are a limited number of intermediate-acting methylphenidate preparations, which have a duration of 6 to 8 hours, including methylphenidate hydrochloride extended-release and Metadate ER. There are multiple preparations of long-acting methylphenidates and amphetamines, which have 8 to 12 hours of duration (Tables 9.6 and 9.7). Depending on the delivery system, they can take 30 to 90 minutes to take effect. The long-acting methylphenidates include

| Table 9.6 | Methylphenidate Extended Release | | | | | |

MEDICATION	DOSAGE FORM	STARTING DOSE	TITRATION	MAX DOSE	DURATION	NOTES
Aptensio XR	10, 15, 20, 30, 40, 50 60 mg	10 mg daily	Increase in 10-mg increments every week	60 mg	12+ hr (2nd peak at 7–8 hr)	Capsules can be opened and swallowed
Concerta	18, 27, 36, 54 mg	18 mg daily	Increase by 18 mg every week	6–12 yr: 54 mg; >13 yr: 72 mg	12 hr	Must be swallowed whole, OROS technology
Cotempla XR ODT	8.6, 17.3, 25.9 mg	8.6 mg daily	Increase in 8.6-mg increments every week	51.8 mg	12–13 hr	Dissolves in mouth, grape flavor
Daytrana transdermal patch	10, 15, 20, 30 mg	10 mg daily	Increase to the next incremental patch	30 mg	Up to 12 hr	Can cause skin irritation, takes 1–2 hr to take effect
Focalin XR (dexmethylphenidate)	5, 10, 15, 20, 25, 30, 35, 40 mg	5 mg daily	Increase in 5-mg increments every week	40 mg	8–12 hr	Can be opened and swallowed, SODAS technology
Jornay PM:-take between 6:30 and 9:30 pm	20, 40, 60, 80, 100 mg	20 mg at HS	20 mg every week	100 mg	12–14 hr	Delayed release and extended release, taken at night
Metadate CD Metadate ER	CD: 10, 20, 30, 40, 50, 60 mg ER: 10, 20 mg	CD: 10 mg daily ER: 10 mg daily	Increase by 10-mg increments every week	60 mg	8–10 hr 6–8 hr	Capsules can be opened and swallowed
QuilliChew ER	20, 30, 40 mg	10–20 mg daily	Increase by 10 mg every week	60 mg	12–13 hr	Scored tablets, cherry flavor
Quillivant XR oral suspension	25 mg/5mL	5–10 mg daily	Increase by 5 mg every week	60 mg	12–13 hr	Banana flavor
Ritalin LA	10, 20, 30, 40, 60 mg	10 mg daily	Increase by 10 mg every week	60 mg	8–12 hr	Capsules can be opened and swallowed, SODAS technology
Astarys: prodrug (dexmethylphenidate + serdexmethylphenidate)	26.1/5.2, 39.2/7.8, 52.3/10.4 mg	26.1/5.2 daily	Increase to next capsule size	52.3/10.4 mg		

OROS, Osmotic-controlled release oral delivery system; SODAS, spheroidal oral drug absorption system.
From Feder, J.D., Tien, E., & Puzantian, T. (2018). *The child medication fact book for psychiatric practice*. Carlat Publishing, LLC; Rajaprakash, M., & Leppert, M. L. (2022). Attention-deficit/hyperactivity disorder. *Pediatric Review, 43*(3), 135–147.

Aptensio XR, Metadate CD, Ritalin LA, Concerta, Focalin XR, Daytrana (a skin patch), and their generic equivalents. The long-acting methylphenidates without a generic version available include Adhansia XR, Cotempla XR-ODT, Quillivant XR, Azstarys, and Jornay PM (which is a long-acting release/delayed onset taken at night). There are no intermediate-acting formulations of amphetamines. The long-acting formulations of amphetamines include Adzenys ER, Dyanavel XR, Adderall XR, Mydayis XR, Dexedrine Spansules, and Vyvanse (which comes in a chewable as well). Long-acting formulations may need to be augmented with a short-acting formulation in the mid to late afternoon if symptoms are not well controlled in the evening.

Prodrugs. There are prodrugs in each class of stimulants. Prodrugs may be a good choice for patients with ADHD or their parents with cooccurring substance use disorder (SUD) due to their ability to be broken down into an active ingredient in gastric acid. FDA-approved prodrugs are Vyvanse (lisdexamfetamine) and Azstarys (dexmethylphenidate and serdexmethylphenidate).

Stimulants are used in preschool children if they do not exhibit improved symptom control or have at least moderate ongoing functional impairment despite behavioral interventions (Rajaprakash & Leppert, 2022; Wolraich et al., 2019). Preschool children are more likely to have mood lability and dysphoria with stimulants. Although most short-acting amphetamines

Table 9.7 **Amphetamine Extended Release**

MEDICATION	DOSAGE FORM	STARTING DOSE	TITRATION	MAX DOSE	DURATION	NOTES
Adderall XR (mixed amphetamine salts)	5, 10, 15, 20, 25, 30 mg	5–10 mg daily	Increase by 5–10 mg every week	6–12 yr: 30 mg 13–17 yr: 40 mg	10–12 hr	Can be opened and swallowed
Adzenys ER (oral suspension) Adzenys XR ODT	1.25 mg/mL 3.1, 6.3, 9.4, 12.5, 15.7, 18.8 mg	2.5 mg 6.3 mg	Increase by 2.5 mg every week Increase by 3.1 mg every week	18.8 mg	10–12 hr	Orange flavor; 3.1 mg is equivalent to 5 mg of mixed amphetamine salts
Dexedrine Spansules	5, 10, 15 mg	5 mg once daily	Increase by 5 mg every week	20 mg twice daily	5–10 hr	
Dyanavel XR oral suspension Dyanavel XR	2.5 mg/mL 2.5, 5, 7.5, 10, 12.5, 15, 17.5, 20 mg	2.5 mg 2.5 mg	Increase by 2.5 mg every week	20 mg	13 hr	Bubble gum flavor, 2.5 mg = 4 mg mixed amphetamine salts
Mydayis (mixed amphetamine salts)	12.5, 25, 37.5, 50 mg	12.5 mg	Increase by 12.5 mg every week	50 mg	14–16 hr	Can be opened and swallowed
Vyvanse–Prodrug (lisdexamfetamine) Vyvanse chewable	10, 20, 30, 40, 50, 60, 70 mg Same, stops at 60 mg	10 mg	Increase by 10 mg every week	70 mg	10–13 hr	Capsule can be opened and dissolved in water, chewable is strawberry flavor

From Feder, J.D., Tien, E., & Puzantian, T. (2018). *The child medication fact book for psychiatric practice*. Carlat Publishing, LLC; Rajaprakash, M., & Leppert, M. L. (2022). Attention-deficit/hyperactivity disorder. *Pediatric Review, 43*(3), 135–147.

are FDA approved for this age, methylphenidate is the recommended first-line stimulant (Wolraich et al., 2019). There is not sufficient evidence to recommend nonstimulants for this age group.

Adverse effect profiles of all stimulants are similar and include appetite suppression, insomnia, dry mouth, nausea, abdominal pain, headaches, and increased tics (Posner et al., 2020; Rajaprakash & Leppert, 2022) (Box 9.3). Adverse effects do not assume a need to change or stop stimulants unless they are persistent or functionally impairing (Rajaprakash & Leppert, 2022). Some mild adverse effects may improve over time and be managed with minimal intervention. If sleep onset or maintenance insomnia occurs, giving the stimulant earlier and reviewing good sleep hygiene may resolve the problem. A trial of melatonin may be beneficial if these changes do not suffice (Rajaprakash & Leppert, 2022). If appetite suppression is significant or ongoing, giving the medication after breakfast and recommending calorie-dense foods and snacks (i.e., peanut butter) may be beneficial. Other strategies include allowing extra snacks in the evenings after the medication has worn off, holding the medication on weekends, or taking drug holidays on nonschool days (Rajaprakash & Leppert, 2022). Hallucinations and other psychotic symptoms have rarely occurred (Wolraich et al., 2019).

Box 9.3 **Common Adverse Effects of Stimulants**

- Appetite suppression
- Insomnia
- Dry mouth
- Nausea
- Abdominal pain
- Headaches
- Increase in tics
- Decreased height trajectory
- Abuse/misuse potential
- Cardiovascular events

Additional areas of concern with stimulants include decreased height trajectory, abuse potential, and cardiovascular events. One result of the prospective Multimodal Treatment of Attention-Deficit/Hyperactivity Disorder (MTA) study showed long-term stimulant use for 16 years was associated with decreased height trajectory, reduced adult height (1–3 cm), and an increase in weight and body mass index (Greenhill et al., 2020; Posner et al., 2020). The benefits of stimulant use may outweigh this risk. Stimulants potentially have euphorigenic effects on mood, increasing the risk of SUD and dependence. However, long-term research has found that stimulant use has no effect on or may decrease the risk of SUD (Posner et al., 2020). Stimulant diversion is a concern and should be discussed with adolescents and adults during visits. On average, stimulant medications increase patient heart rate by one to two beats per minute and increase systolic and diastolic blood pressure by 1 to 4 mm Hg; however, 5% to 15% of patients may have a significantly higher increase in these parameters. Because stimulants have sympathomimetic properties there has been concern about increased cardiovascular risks. Early research suggested an association between stimulants and sudden cardiac death; however, subsequent large studies have found no relationship between significant cardiovascular events and stimulants (Posner et al., 2019). The most current policy statement from the AAP regarding cardiovascular monitoring for patients under consideration for stimulants recommends a careful cardiac assessment, physical exam, and targeted cardiac history assessment, including the patient's history of cardiac disease, palpitations, syncope, or seizures, as well as family history of sudden death in children or young adults, hypertrophic cardiomyopathy, long QT syndrome, or Wolff-Parkinson-White syndrome (Perrin et al., 2008; Wolraich et al., 2019). Routine electrocardiogram (ECG) or subspecialty cardiology evaluation before starting therapy with stimulants is not recommended unless one of the previously identified cardiac risks is noted (Perrin et al., 2008).

Nonstimulant medications. Four nonstimulants that are FDA approved for use in the treatment of ADHD in children and adolescents include the SNRIs Strattera (atomoxetine) and Qelbree (viloxazine), as well as the alpha$_2$-agonists Intuniv (extended-release guanfacine) and Kapvay (extended-release clonidine). They have been shown to reduce core symptoms of ADHD in school-aged children and adolescents but with smaller effect sizes compared to stimulants (Posner et al., 2020; Wolraich et al., 2019). SNRIs are known for their antidepressant effects and work on ADHD symptoms by inhibiting norepinephrine transports, which increase dopamine and norepinephrine in the prefrontal cortex (Stahl, 2013). The alpha$_2$-agonists work on ADHD symptoms by mediating norepinephrine effects in the prefrontal cortex (Stahl, 2013) and act on the brainstem by reducing peripheral vascular resistance; it therefore can lower blood pressure (Mechler et al., 2022).

Prescribing nonstimulants. Nonstimulants can be trialed in children older than 6 years when stimulants have shown to be ineffective or if adverse effects are impairing (Rajaprakash & Leppert, 2022) (Table 9.8). They can also be used in conjunction with stimulants to extend or enhance their effects. Intuniv and Kapvay have the additional benefits of inducing sleep onset and can be taken at night. Qelbree and the alpha$_2$-agonists are dosed using the lowest dose and titrating up. Atomoxetine is dosed using the patient's weight (Mechler et al., 2022).

The adverse effects of alpha$_2$-agonists include sedation, decreased heart rate, blood pressure, headaches, fatigue, dry mouth, dizziness, irritability, and abdominal pain (Rajaprakash & Leppert, 2022; Wolraich et al., 2019). Rebound hypertension can occur if Intuniv or Kapvay are discontinued suddenly; therefore a taper is recommended. Alpha-agonists have been used in children with ADHD, tics, mild anxiety, and ODD (Pringsheim et al., 2015; Rajaprakash & Leppert, 2022).

Adverse effects of the SNRIs include increased heart rate and blood pressure, sleepiness, abdominal pain, and decreased appetite. Atomoxetine and viloxazine

Table **9.8** Nonstimulants						
MEDICATION	**DOSAGE FORM**	**STARTING DOSE**	**TITRATION**	**MAX DOSE**	**DURATION**	**NOTES**
Intuniv (guanfacine ER)	1, 2, 3, 4 mg	1 mg	Do not increase faster than 1 mg per week	4 mg (up to 7 mg in adolescents has been reported)	24 hr	Do not stop suddenly (rebound hypertension)
Kapvay (clonidine XR)	0.1, 0.2 mg	0.05 mg at HS	Increase by 0.05–0.1 mg every week; give divided twice daily	0.4 mg daily	12–16 hr	Titrate up slowly (orthostatic hypotension); do not stop suddenly (rebound hypertension)
Strattera (atomoxetine)	10, 18, 25, 40, 60, 80, 100 mg	Based on weight: <70 kg, start 0.5 mg/kg, titrate to 1.2 mg/kg; >70 kg, start 40 mg		1.4 mg/kg	24 hr	Must be swallowed whole
Qelbree (viloxazine)	100, 150, 200 mg	100 mg	100 mg every week	400 mg	24 hr	

From Feder, J.D., Tien, E., & Puzzantian, T. (2018). *The child medication fact book for psychiatric practice.* Carlat Publishing, LLC; Rajaprakash, M., & Leppert, M. L. (2022). Attention-deficit/hyperactivity disorder. *Pediatric Review, 43*(3), 135–147.

have a black box warning of increased risk of suicidal thoughts due to the antidepressant effects, and all patients treated with these need to be monitored closely for this as well as changes in behavior during the first few months of treatment and following dose changes (Mechler et al., 2022). Atomoxetine has a rare association with hepatitis and has been linked to decreased height trajectory (Wolraich et al., 2019). Atomoxetine can be given once daily or twice daily if abdominal pain occurs. The benefits of this medication may not be noted until several weeks after initiation (Rajaprakash & Leppert, 2022).

Third-line medications. Bupropion is a norepinephrine-dopamine reuptake inhibitor that has been used but is not FDA approved for ADHD. Tricyclic antidepressants (TCAs) such as desipramine and nortriptyline have been used for treatment but have varying degrees of success and are also not FDA approved due to the paucity of safety and efficacy data in children (Stahl, 2013). The central nervous system stimulant modafinil is used to treat excessive sleepiness in adults but is not FDA approved for ADHD due to a lack of safety and efficacy data (Cortese et al., 2018).

Ongoing monitoring. It is reasonable to obtain symptom rating scales on a regular basis from teachers and parents to help guide treatment decisions. The patient should be monitored regularly with height, weight, heart rate, and blood pressure documented with each visit (see Health Care Maintenance, later) with additional screenings for the development of comorbidities such as sleep problems, anxiety, depression, or suicidal thoughts (Box 9.4).

Complementary and Alternative Therapies

The term *complementary and alternative medicine* refers to a range of interventions or treatments distinct from conventional medicine and standard care practices of

Box 9.4	Associated Problems of ADHD and Treatment

- Learning disabilities
- Conduct disorder (CD), oppositional defiant disorder, and other mental health disorders
- Coexisting psychiatric conditions
- Anxiety disorders
- Mood disorders
- Tourette syndrome and tic disorders
- Drug and alcohol abuse/tobacco use
- Psychosocial sequelae: low self-esteem, inadequate social skills, academic difficulties, multiple failures, family conflict, exercising of poor judgment, altered peer relationships, antisocial behavior (especially with ADHD and CD), psychosomatic complaints, failure to reach potential, and labeling with a mental health professional after a comprehensive physical examination by the primary care provider.

ADHD, Attention-deficit/hyperactivity disorder.

medical professionals (Bader & Adesman, 2015). Complementary medicine includes treatments that are used in combination with standard medical care, whereas alternative medicine includes treatments used in place of standard care (Lofthouse & Hurt, 2014). Although the word "medicine" is utilized in name and definition, it is important to note that most of these approaches do not involve pharmacologic interventions or medicines. Additionally, although some have been subject to research, these interventions are not routinely subject to scientific rigor or experimental evaluation to confirm their effectiveness, making them different from evidenced-based medicine or treatments. They will be referred to as complementary and alternative treatments (CATs) in this chapter.

The majority of caregivers who elect to explore or implement CATs with their children do so for a variety of reasons, such as finding evidenced-based treatments (i.e., stimulant medication or behavioral therapy) ineffective, intolerable due to factors such as side effects, or personally unacceptable (Lofthouse & Hurt, 2014). Previous surveys have suggested using CATs alone or in conjunction with other treatments to be commonplace, with reports up to 60% of patients diagnosed with ADHD (Wu et al., 2022). The frequency of use is associated with the chronicity of ADHD.

CATs vary significantly and include dietary changes, nutritional supplements, yoga or meditation, herbal products, biofeedback, attention training, and occupational therapy interventions. A host of dietary changes are considered CATs, including eliminating certain foods or drinks (e.g., dairy products or caffeine), restricting dietary substances such as food dyes, and limiting sugar intake. Only limited evidence suggests the negative effects of food additives on some subgroups of children, but these effects are not restricted to the ADHD population and extend to nonclinical samples (Searight et al., 2012). Although caregivers often believe that sugar ingestion can lead to behavioral changes such as hyperactivity, no scientific evidence supports this claim (Hurt & Arnold, 2015).

Nutritional supplements include macronutrients, micronutrients, and metabolites, and the assumption is that children with ADHD may have insufficient amounts of a particular substance, which contributes to their ADHD symptoms (Hurt & Arnold, 2015). Supplementation of minerals such as lead, iron, magnesium, and zinc has been most studied in response to the thought that these minerals are cofactors for neurotransmitter synthesis, uptake, and breakdown. Findings are inconsistent, and potential improvements appear to occur at times when added to traditional drug therapies (e.g., zinc and methylphenidate combined) (Searight et al., 2012). The efficacy of fish oil or omega-3 fatty acid supplementation has been explored through meta-analytic reviews involving randomized, placebo-controlled trials, including small but significant treatment effects for hyperactive and inattentive symptoms (Bloch & Qawasmi, 2011; Sonuga-Barke et al., 2013), yet other studies found no treatment effects (Hirayama et al., 2004; Voigt et al., 2001). Adjunctive supplementation of omega-3 fatty acids may benefit children whose response to evidenced-based treatments is unsatisfactory (Hurt & Arnold, 2015).

Cognitive training, such as a commercially available computerized training program called Cogmed, is designed to improve working memory and focus in individuals with ADHD. Cogmed includes visual-spatial and verbal tasks where the individual views the pattern on the screen and then applies it to later screens. In addition to practical factors such as time and cost, this intervention has been subject to scrutiny given that it does not appear to target working memory and that any initial improvements are not maintained posttreatment (Rapport et al., 2015; Searight et al., 2012). Various forms of occupational therapy, such as sensory integration training and the interactive metronome, have also been explored, with limited studies and inconclusive results. Mind-body therapies such as yoga, massage, meditation, and homeopathy have not been studied rigorously and thus lack evidence of effectiveness (Bader & Adesman, 2015).

More recently, in 2020 the FDA approved the first ever video game therapy (EndeavorRx) by prescription for children ages 8 to 12 with attentional disorders. This digital, mobile-based app is intended for use in combination with behavioral and medication treatment. Two randomized controlled trials have yielded some initial positive outcomes on measures of attention without adverse effects, particularly as an adjunct treatment to medication (Kollins et al., 2020, 2021). Skepticism remains among some in the ADHD field, and additional exploration of the efficacy of this novel intervention is needed.

The external trigeminal nerve stimulation (eTNS) Monarch eTNS System was also recently FDA approved for the treatment of pediatric ADHD as a monotherapy in 7- to 12-year-olds. A small double-blind, randomized controlled trial of eTNS showed efficacy in decreasing ADHD symptoms after 1 month of treatment in children with pediatric ADHD age 8 to 12 years. The stimulator device is available by prescription only and is worn across the forehead; it emits low-level electrical stimulation targeting the trigeminal nerve and areas of the brain thought to be implicated in ADHD. The most common side effects of eTNS were drowsiness, increased appetite, trouble sleeping, teeth clenching, headache, and fatigue. Of note, the study did not enroll children taking ADHD medications, so the safety and effectiveness of this device in children taking ADHD medication are unknown. Treatment response durability and long-term safety are unknown (McGough et al., 2019).

In summary, CATs are widely utilized for children with ADHD, and health care providers should be aware of their prevalent use to inform meaningful conversations with patients and caregivers (Wu et al., 2022).

ANTICIPATED ADVANCES IN DIAGNOSIS AND MANAGEMENT

Multimodal advances in genetic, imaging, and phenotypic data are emerging. As ADHD is viewed as a multifactorial disorder, it is suspected of being mediated by multiple genes (Faraone, 2019). A recent genome-wide association meta-analysis identified significant risk loci associated with ADHD in or near genes involved in neurodevelopmental processes, including *FOXP2* (Demontis et al., 2019). Other examinations exploring candidate genes in methylphenidate response show a small impact regarding variants in dopamine transporter and dopamine receptor D4, catechol-O-methyltransferase, and norepinephrine transporter, though results are inconsistent. Testing for this may be helpful for clinicians especially when the desired clinical response has not been achieved (Brown et al., 2019).

Research in the diagnostic utility of neuroimaging is still being explored. Neuroimaging studies have shown abnormalities in prefrontal structures, basal ganglia, and the corpus callosum in individuals with ADHD compared to controls. Other studies show neural activity and connectivity differences during task execution and at rest in the frontoparietal, ventral, or dorsal attention networks (Albajara Sáenz et al., 2019). Current pharmacologic treatments for ADHD target the dopaminergic and noradrenergic systems. New treatments and repurposing emerging medications, such as amantadine, may be promising, but further research is needed.

Overall, a number of areas are being investigated for diagnostic and therapeutic utility and are opening potential avenues of research.

ASSOCIATED PROBLEMS OF ADHD AND TREATMENT

Because ADHD is a chronic condition that causes symptoms and dysfunction over long periods, the AAP recommends that primary care providers manage the child with ADHD as they would children with special health care needs, using the standards of the chronic care model and the medical home. Longitudinal studies reveal that ADHD treatments are frequently not continued over time resulting in impairments into adulthood with increased risk for early death, suicide, and SUD. People with ADHD have lower educational achievement and increased rates of incarceration than people without ADHD. Without treatment for ADHD, people with ADHD are at higher risk of depression, interpersonal issues, accidents and injuries, motor vehicle accidents, criminality, and violent reoffending (Wolraich et al., 2019). Females with ADHD have deficits in social skills and relationships compared to peers with more parent-reported peer conflict; males have fewer close friends, trouble keeping friends, and more parent-reported social problems (Barkley, 2015).

Those with ADHD may be prone to internet and video game addiction or having problematic usage (Barkley, 2015c). Teens who game more than 1 hour per day had elevated symptoms of ADHD, especially inattention (Barkley, 2015c). According to Barkley (2015), "parents report that their children with ADHD are inattentive while engaging in risky activities and are more heedless or thoughtless of the consequences of their actions (impulsive), thus placing themselves in a situation or engaging in activities that are more likely than usual to result in physical harm." Children admitted to hospitals for injuries are three times more likely to have ADHD. Children with ADHD are more likely to have accidental poisonings as well. Driving problems are considerable in teens with ADHD, with outcomes revealing "more traffic citations, more license suspensions, more damage during crashes, less safe driving behavior, more impulsive errors and slow reaction times" (Barkley, 2015c).

LEARNING DISABILITIES

From a large-scale study on the national prevalence of developmental disabilities utilizing the National Health Interview Survey from 2009 to 2017, estimates of the prevalence of learning disabilities among children age 3 to 17 was 7.74% (Zablotsky et al., 2019). Learning disabilities and ADHD often intersect and cooccur in children, with prevalence rates ranging from 33% to 45% or above (DuPaul & Landberg, 2015). Despite some similar known genetic, environmental, and cognitive factors (Sexton et al., 2012) the treatment is often different with overlapping environmental modifications and behavioral interventions. For example, while psychopharmacologic treatment has strong evidence for treating ADHD in children (Sexton et al., 2012), no specific medications are designed to treat learning disabilities in isolation.

Evaluation of children with ADHD should include knowledge and careful attention to the possibility of an underlying learning deficit or disability. When concerns exist, referrals to the school for further evaluation or an outside specialist who is qualified and proficient in psychological assessment and can conduct a direct and comprehensive evaluation of learning are warranted. Using sound norm references and measures of academic achievement is necessary. In addition, direct observation and curriculum-based measurement of impacted areas such as math, reading, or writing are critical to accurate diagnosis and intervention (DuPaul & Landberg, 2015). Multimodal, ongoing learning assessment is also key to identifying goals and ensuring successful outcomes.

CONDUCT DISORDER, OPPOSITIONAL DEFIANT DISORDER, AND OTHER MENTAL HEALTH DISORDERS

Over half of the children with ADHD have additional behavioral or conduct problems (Bitsko et al., 2022).

Early intervention is important to prevent an escalation in these disruptive behaviors. Without intervention, children with ADHD and additional disruptive behavior problems are at higher risk for negative outcomes (Groenman et al., 2022). Fortunately, these cooccurring conditions can be treated together because behavioral interventions are well established for ADHD and disruptive behavior disorders (Chacko et al., 2015).

OTHER COEXISTING PSYCHIATRIC CONDITIONS

ADHD coexists with multiple mental health, developmental, and medical disorders. Preschoolers may present with underlying or associated symptoms of autism spectrum disorders, developmental delays, language disorders, hearing loss, and motor delays. School-age children may present with learning disabilities, speech and language impairments, anxiety, ODD, and CD. Adolescents may present with sleep disorders, substance use, learning disability, or new-onset mood and anxiety disorders (Rajaprakash & Leppert, 2022). Females with and without ADHD are at higher risk for adolescent mood and anxiety disorders (Barkley, 2015c). Males and females with ADHD are at increased risk for cigarette use. Evidence suggests no increased risk for the development of alcohol use disorders, but there is an increased risk for later illicit drug use and marijuana use (Barkley, 2015c).

DRUG AND ALCOHOL ABUSE/TOBACCO USE

Individuals with ADHD are at risk for developing SUD, with a two to three times higher likelihood of developing cigarette smoking/e-cigarette use, nicotine use, cannabis use, or SUD compared to peers (Wilens et al., 2011). Adolescents with ADHD show a higher risk of earlier initiation of nicotine and poorer results in cessation intervention programs (van Amsterdam et al., 2018). A possible explanation is the association of both ADHD and SUD with the dopamine system, the brain's reward system. For example, cocaine increases dopamine and has a similar effect to that provided by stimulant medications for ADHD (Szobot & Bukstein, 2008). Literature on the self-medication hypothesis, which theorizes that individuals with ADHD use drugs or alcohol to manage ADHD symptoms, is mixed (Taubin et al., 2022). There is also speculation that youth with ADHD may overestimate their competence, have difficulty evaluating the negative consequences of substance abuse, or have high impulsivity and difficulty with the decision-making process of how to refuse or avoid using these products (Szobot & Bukstein, 2008). Despite this, SUD and the risk for SUD in youth with ADHD are underidentified. Screening and identifying individuals at risk is key to preventing negative outcomes. Treatment includes both psychotherapy and pharmacotherapy.

The question remains regarding the effects of stimulants on the increasing risk of SUD, although there is no evidence that treatment with stimulants increases the risk for later SUD. Studies have shown that earlier-onset and longer duration of treatment of ADHD were associated with the largest risk reduction for future SUD (Taubin et al., 2022). Treatment of ADHD appears to have a protective effect on developing SUD in adolescence, but effects have not been found in adulthood (Biederman, 2008).

PSYCHOSOCIAL AND HEALTH-RELATED SEQUELAE

Psychosocial consequences of children with ADHD begin in childhood, tend to persist into adulthood, and impact a variety of domains (Cherkasova et al., 2022). In the school setting, children with ADHD are more likely to have trouble with work completion and accuracy and poorer academic achievement in core subjects. Poor executive functioning will likely worsen educational outcomes as children progress into middle and high school and are expected to become more independent (DuPaul & Landberg, 2015). In addition to educational impairments, children with ADHD display more disruptive behaviors in the classroom and are more likely to be suspended and expelled from school (Martin, 2014; Robb et al., 2011). Children with ADHD are also more likely to experience grade retention, have fewer years of education, and are less likely to graduate high school (Barbaresi et al., 2020; DuPaul & Landberg, 2015). Consequently, children with ADHD are more likely to have poorer occupational attainment and performance (Barkley, 2015b).

Family and social relationships are often impaired for children with ADHD. Children with ADHD are more likely to have impaired parent-child relationships and other family relationship stressors, such as sibling conflict and divorced parents (Johnston & Chronis-Tuscano, 2015). Adults with ADHD are at increased risk for interpersonal challenges and poorer marital and intimate relationship satisfaction (Barkley, 2015b). Children with ADHD are more likely to experience peer rejection and victimization, have fewer friendships, and display more disruptive peer interactions and bullying of their peers (McQuade & Hoza, 2015). As children with ADHD approach adolescence and adulthood, they are more likely to abuse substances and engage in risky driving and sexual behavior (Pollak et al., 2019).

Given the aforementioned psychosocial sequelae it is not surprising that ADHD negatively impacts self-esteem if left untreated (Harpin et al., 2016) and increases the likelihood of emotional problems (Stern et al., 2020) and suicidality (Balazs & Kereszteny, 2017). Furthermore, children with ADHD and conduct problems are more likely to engage in criminal behavior and become incarcerated (Erskine et al., 2016).

Beginning in early childhood, the risk of a variety of physical injuries increases for those with ADHD (Allan et al., 2021; Kang et al., 2013). One study of preschoolers presenting to urgent care or the emergency department found that children with ADHD were more likely to experience injuries such as poisoning, contusions, bike injuries, foreign body injury, abrasions, and sprains/strains (Allan et al., 2021). Overall, individuals with ADHD have poorer health-related outcomes (Nigg, 2013) and are at a higher risk of a shorter life expectancy compared to those without ADHD, especially for individuals with impaired behavioral inhibition (Barkley & Fischer, 2019; London & Landes, 2022).

PROGNOSIS

Although there once was a historical belief that individuals with ADHD may outgrow their symptoms, the persistence of ADHD into adolescence and adulthood has been well established through longitudinal research. The disorder's persistence rates vary based on survey methods (e.g., parental vs self-report), diagnostic measures or criteria, and symptom threshold utilized. From a variety of studies, estimates include 50% to 80% of adolescents and 35% to 65% of adults having persistent symptoms that continue from childhood into adulthood (Owens et al., 2015).

With treatment, many children with ADHD become successful adults in various domains. Depending on factors such as symptom severity, it also is expected that these individuals will likely have at least some continued impairments throughout their adult lives. Prospective follow-up studies have confirmed heterogeneity in outcomes, but the differences in why this occurs are largely unclear (Klein et al., 2012; Kuriyan et al., 2013). The MTA data from Hechtman et al. (2016) found that individuals with higher levels of persistent symptoms of ADHD fared worse than those individuals with less persistent symptoms in terms of a variety of outcomes, including functional (e.g., times fired/quit a job), sexual (e.g., risky sexual behavior), emotional (e.g., anxiety and mood disorders), and substance abuse outcomes. In addition to the personal costs for families of children with ADHD regarding treatment and related health care, there are significant economic costs associated with ADHD (Barkley, 2015b). According to a review of 44 studies, primarily in North America and Europe, estimates for the economic impact of ADHD nationally were significant, ranging from $356 million to $20.27 billion (Chhibber et al., 2021).

Treatment over the life course has been shown to improve prognosis with respect to some limited functional outcomes. For example, medication treatment of children with ADHD has been found in several studies to result in higher rates of adult employment, suggesting the long-term benefits of employment status (Barkley, 2015a). Although the known positive impact of a combination of behavioral and pharmacologic interventions is well documented for ADHD in the short term, continued study of the impact of these treatments on lifelong outcomes is needed.

PRIMARY CARE MANAGEMENT

HEALTH CARE MAINTENANCE

Growth and Development

Primary care providers must pay careful attention to the routine measurement of weight, physical growth parameters, and appetite (i.e., about every 6 months) in children taking stimulant medication (AAP, 2022; Cortese et al., 2018). There have been stimulant-related decreases in growth rates after the start of treatment, though this may be temporary and diminish over time. The potential effect on growth with stimulant medication may be due to their adverse effect on appetite or acute inhibition of growth hormone with increases in synaptic dopamine (Faraone, 2019). A 3-year follow-up of data from the prospective MTA study reported that growth in newly medicated children was 2 cm and 2.7 kg less than the control group (Swanson et al., 2007). The growth reduction was seen mostly in the first year of treatment, and the effects were not seen in the third year, though there was no evidence of growth rebound (Swanson et al., 2007). However, several studies in a systemic analysis indicated that within 2 years of discontinuing treatment, accelerated growth rate compensated for the initial height and weight decreases (Faraone, 2008). The growth rate may be slowed by approximately 1 cm/year for 1 to 3 years, but then it approaches normal with no long-term effects on health (Vitiello, 2008). Higher doses of stimulants may cause more growth reduction. A study found no difference in peak height velocity or final adult height between those treated with stimulants and those that were not (Harstad, 2014). If the height and weight plotted on growth charts decrease and cross two percentile lines, a drug holiday may be discussed using a risk-benefit balance (Pliszka & AACAP Work Group on Quality Issues, 2007). The possibility of drug holidays is discussed in this chapter under managing adverse medication side effects; if there is continued poor growth despite management strategies, referral to an endocrinologist or specialist is warranted.

Children with ADHD should demonstrate the normal progression of attaining developmental milestones, especially in the early years. Continuous developmental and behavioral surveillance and screening are important and recommended during preventive health care visits. As the child reaches the preschool years, some delay in the development of a longer attention span and increased activity level may signal a need for a referral for psychoeducational evaluation.

The Individuals with Disabilities Education Improvement Act (2004) requires that children at risk for developing ADHD be assessed in the first 3 years of life if signs and symptoms are evident. Health care providers have more responsibility to develop and use tools that can identify components of ADHD at an earlier age. Because children may learn to compensate for their disabilities, and in some cases the nature of their disabilities changes as they grow and develop, it is important to reevaluate their cognitive, motor, and psychosocial level of development at each well-child visit. Screening tools used in the initial assessment of ADHD can be used periodically to monitor their progress with treatment interventions.

Diet

There are no dietary restrictions, and no empiric evidence suggests that diets that restrict sugars, refined carbohydrates, food additives, or food colors result in any improvement in the symptomatology, nor do they cause ADHD (Barkley & Murphy, 2006). Recent data suggest small but clinically significant effects of artificial food colors on behavior in children with or without ADHD diagnosis (Hurt & Arnold, 2015).

Children taking stimulant medication may have a decreased appetite, and their increased activity level may warrant an increased caloric intake, late evening meals, and taking medication after meals if indicated. Meals and snacks that are high in protein and calories and easy to eat should be encouraged to enhance nutritional status; because of the timing of medications, it may be easier to promote a healthy breakfast intake, and bedtime before and after the action of the stimulants has peaked. Nutritional supplements may also be encouraged. Children may also experience a stomachache as a side effect of the medications; if this is the case, medication should be taken on a full stomach. Behaviorally, children with ADHD may be easily distracted from the meal and leave the table before they have finished eating; establishing a mealtime routine may be beneficial. Parents and caregivers should look for windows of opportunity to provide nutritious foods and well-balanced meals.

Safety

There are a number of safety issues for children and adolescents with ADHD. Children with ADHD have an increased risk for accidents and unintentional injuries and are much more likely than children without ADHD to be seen in emergency departments. One study showed that children with ADHD who had a visit for an injury by 3 years of age were six times as likely to have a subsequent visit by the age of 6 years (Allan et al., 2021). As children grow and independent activities increase, so does the opportunity to engage in activities with greater risk of physical harm. Close caregiver monitoring and anticipatory guidance are needed.

Some adolescents and adults are at increased risk for adverse driving outcomes, including traffic citations, vehicular crashes, and greater likelihood of license suspension/revocation, most notably in younger drivers. Driving is an activity that requires multiple tasks and decision making simultaneously. Many adolescents with ADHD have decreased judgment of speed, space, and distance and impairments in attention, which may lead to increased motor vehicle accidents in this population (Barkley & Murphy, 2006). Other symptoms that may be present in individuals with ADHD, such as aggression, excessive anger, and irritability, may have additional driving risks. Few reports have shown the impact of ADHD treatment on driving. Still, providing medication coverage and symptom control during driving should be considered.

Misuse or diversion of stimulants continues to be a significant problem among high school and college students. Among college students, rates of stimulant misuse have been reported to range between 8% and 34%, even up to 50% (Taubin et al., 2022). Students with ADHD are sometimes solicited to sell or give their stimulant medications to others. The primary motivator for misuse is performance enhancement, though data on the stimulant enhancement of cognitive performance is mixed (Taubin et al., 2022). Medication safety strategies are crucial when counseling patients. Standard precautions for keeping medications safely secured should be followed for the child with ADHD, siblings, classmates, and schools because many of the medications can be stolen and sold. Safe storage and use of weekly pill boxes or organizers may be helpful for children who are self-administering their medications. Clinicians should monitor symptoms, prescription refills, and requests. Many states require participation in prescription drug monitoring programs to help curb misuse. The use of extended-release and longer-acting stimulant medications and the use of the methylphenidate patch has lowered the potential for abuse. Clinicians may also consider using nonstimulant medications to reduce abuse potential.

Immunizations

No changes in the routine schedule of immunizations are needed.

Screenings

Vision. Comprehensive vision testing should be performed during the diagnostic period. Vision problems, such as refractive errors and strabismus, may present with ADHD symptoms, especially inattention and difficulty reading and remembering what was read. The AAP and the American Association for Pediatric Ophthalmology and Strabismus have developed screening guidelines for vision problems at different ages,

Hearing. Comprehensive audiometric testing should also be performed during the diagnostic period. Some indicators of hearing loss may be misinterpreted as ADHD symptoms, such as inattentiveness or not responding when spoken to. Routine screening at recommended intervals should then occur.

Dental. Routine screening is recommended.

Blood pressure. Blood pressure alterations may occur as a result of receiving stimulants, tricyclics, clonidine, or guanfacine. Thus blood pressure should be monitored every 3 to 6 months (Barkley & Murphy, 2006). Children not taking medication for ADHD should have routine blood pressure screening.

Hematocrit. Routine screening is recommended.

Lead. Routine screening is recommended for up to 72 months if not previously completed. Lead-associated cognitive deficits and behavioral problems can occur.

Tuberculosis. Routine screening is recommended.

It is also recommended that practitioners screen for comorbid conditions, including emotional or behavioral conditions (e.g., anxiety, depression, ODD, CD, substance use), developmental conditions (e.g., learning and language disorders, autism spectrum disorders), and physical conditions (e.g., tics, sleep apnea).

Condition-Specific Screenings

As mentioned, if considering medication for the treatment of ADHD, a thorough cardiac and physical exam should be completed, as well as an assessment of individual cardiac disease or family history of hypertrophic cardiomyopathy, long QT syndrome, Wolff-Parkinson-White syndrome, or sudden death especially in children or young adults (Wolraich et al., 2019).

Learning Issues

Due to the increased risk for academic and school-related problems in children with ADHD and that learning disabilities often cooccur with attention issues, monitoring this area closely and conducting a thorough screening for learning concerns are essential. Follow-up with school resources or referrals to specialists qualified in assessment may be necessary.

Psychological Screening

Due to the high incidence of comorbidity of ADHD with other psychological and psychiatric conditions, the child's general mental health and potential related mood concerns, such as anxiety and depression, should be evaluated at each medical visit. As part of the 2022 Bright Futures, the AAP recommends assessment of behavioral, social, and emotional functioning as part of all well visits and depression and suicide risk screening annually for ages 12 to 21 years.

COMMON ILLNESS MANAGEMENT

Differential Diagnosis

The symptoms of ADHD overlap with several conditions, including neurologic or developmental conditions, emotional and behavioral disorders, psychosocial or environmental factors, and certain medical conditions. It is important to differentiate ADHD from these conditions or if they are comorbid.

Comprehensive vision and audiology evaluations are essential for ADHD evaluations and as part of the differential diagnosis.

Neurodevelopmental or developmental conditions such as learning disabilities, communication disorders, or autism spectrum disorder may mimic or coexist with ADHD. Children with learning disabilities may display inattention due to a lack of understanding, interest, or limited ability. Comprehensive psychological testing and speech and language evaluations may be needed. Emotional and behavioral disorders include anxiety disorders, mood disorders, ODD, CD, obsessive-compulsive disorder, adjustment to stressors, and posttraumatic stress disorder. Inattention and restlessness may be seen in anxiety disorders, though these symptoms are due to worry and rumination rather than inattention in ADHD. Poor concentration and distractibility are also seen in depressive disorders, yet additional features define these disorders (depressed mood, loss of interest, weight changes). It is also important to assess for SUD due to the overlap between symptoms of both disorders and cooccurrence. A period of abstinence from substances is recommended during the evaluation process.

A number of medical conditions may mimic ADHD. Endocrine disorders, such as thyroid disease and medications for thyroid disease, may cause fatigue, difficulty concentrating, hyperactivity, and restlessness. Lead toxicity and iron deficiency anemia may be associated with cognitive, motor, and behavioral problems (Konofal et al., 2004). Iron deficiency may also contribute to ADHD; many children may benefit from iron supplementation (Konofal et al., 2004). As mentioned, symptoms of inattention and hyperactivity may be symptoms of a sleep disorder. History and screening with a potential referral for a sleep study will help differentiate. Seizure disorders and antiseizure medications can mimic symptoms of ADHD; however, ADHD is a comorbidity seen in epilepsy, with the prevalence of ADHD two to three times higher in individuals with seizure disorders compared to control groups (Williams et al., 2016). Epilepsy and antiseizure medications are associated with cognitive deficits, including attention (Williams et al., 2016).

Additionally, childhood absence seizures may be misdiagnosed as ADHD due to frequent episodes of inattention and staring or daydreaming. Clinical features of absence seizures include automatisms (mouth chewing movements, eye fluttering) and sudden return to activity after the seizure ends (lasting 3–30 seconds) (Albuja & Qutubuddin Khan, 2022). An EEG, referral to neurology, and neuropsychological testing for comorbid conditions may be necessary for a definitive diagnosis.

Psychosocial and environmental factors may affect behavior and social-emotional functioning. Childhood traumatic stress or adverse childhood experiences may be misdiagnosed as ADHD due to the significant overlap of symptoms. A comprehensive assessment that includes history from multiple respondents, caregiver stress, caregiver mental health conditions, socioeconomic status, and other social determinants of health may help clarify the diagnosis and potential comorbidities.

The symptoms or treatments for ADHD may sometimes compromise diagnostic or recovery phases of some medical illnesses. Side effects of stimulant medications or the characteristics of the conditions themselves (e.g., anorexia, weight loss, stomachache, headache, insomnia) may mask the symptoms of other physical and psychological illnesses. The lack of appetite, insomnia, and difficulty with rest may interfere with recovery and the intake of fluids and nutrients needed. Children with ADHD require no modification in diagnosing or treating common childhood illnesses, keeping in mind the potential medication interaction (Box 9.5).

Drug Interactions

Amphetamines are metabolized via the cytochrome P450 CYP2D6 pathway; therefore concomitant use of medications that are CYP2D6 inhibitors (i.e., bupropion, duloxetine, fluoxetine, paroxetine) may increase the amphetamine concentration. Consider using a lower dose of Vyvanse in patients taking CYP2D6 inhibitors due to the increased risk of serotonin syndrome (hyperreflexia, clonus, hyperthermia, diaphoresis, tremor, autonomic instability, mental status changes). Methylphenidates are mostly metabolized via the carboxylesterase-1 pathway, and the P-glycoprotein transporter protein may be involved in distribution and transport. Carbamazepine may induce methylphenidate and lower its concentration. Other identified medications, including phenobarbital, phenytoin, and rifampin, can also affect the concentration of methylphenidate. Methylphenidate may increase imipramine, amitriptyline, and clomipramine concentrations. Atomoxetine is metabolized by CYP2C19, and patients who are poor CYP2D6 metabolizers may have higher concentration levels and better response but an increased risk of adverse effects. Guanfacine is metabolized by CYP3A4, and concomitant use of CYP3A4 inducers and inhibitors should be avoided if possible. Carbamazepine, phenobarbital, phenytoin, rifampin, modafinil, armodafinil, oxcarbazepine greater than 1200 mg/day, topiramate greater than 400 mg/day, and St. John's wort can reduce guanfacine concentrations. Strong and moderate CYP3A4 inhibitors (clarithromycin, diltiazem, erythromycin, grapefruit juice, ketoconazole, fluoxetine, and fluvoxamine) can increase the guanfacine concentration (Kim & Heo, 2020). There are not enough data on clonidine and viloxazine to make recommendations.

In general, alcohol may increase the adverse effects of methylphenidate. Stimulants can lower the seizure threshold. Monoamine oxidase inhibitors (MAOIs) can

Box 9.5   Differential Diagnosis

MEDICAL CONDITIONS
- Vision or hearing impairments
- Seizure disorders
- Iron deficiency/iron deficiency anemia
- Lead poisoning or other toxins
- Endocrine disorders, such as thyroid diseases
- Sleep disorders
- Neurologic disorders, such as central nervous system infections or tumors

NEURODEVELOPMENTAL DISORDERS
- Learning disability
- Communication disorders
- Autism spectrum disorders
- Fetal alcohol spectrum disorders

EMOTIONAL AND BEHAVIORAL DISORDERS
- Anxiety disorders
- Mood disorders
- Oppositional defiant disorder/conduct disorder
- Adjustment disorder
- Posttraumatic stress disorder
- Obsessive-compulsive disorder
- Substance use disorder

PSYCHOSOCIAL FACTORS
- Caregiver stress
- Caregiver mental health conditions
- Childhood adverse experiences, such as neglect or abuse

From American Psychiatric Association. (2022). *Diagnostic and statistical manual of mental disorders* (5th ed., text rev.).

enhance the hypertensive effects of stimulants. Bupropion can lower the seizure threshold. Guanfacine and clonidine have multiple interactions that can increase the risk of lowering blood pressure and causing central nervous system depression.

DEVELOPMENTAL ISSUES

Sleep Patterns

Sleep problems are reported in 25% to 55% of children with ADHD and are thought to be due to increased activity levels throughout the day and evening, distractions from tasks, and difficulty shutting down their brains. These children are more likely to have an increased prevalence of sleep disorders, poor sleep hygiene, and restless leg syndrome (Stein et al., 2022). Families report difficulty falling asleep (initial insomnia), bedtime resistance, daytime sleepiness, nightmares, enuresis, and sleep talking (Ricketts et al., 2018). Stimulants, especially extended-release formulations, can delay sleep onset (considered >30 minutes) in children (Stein et al., 2022). A systematic approach to screening for sleep problems is necessary for ADHD evaluations and ongoing management. Screening tools, such as the BEARS screening questions and the Children's Sleep Habits Questionnaire, may be used in clinical settings (see Table 9.9). Positive screenings should be followed by a focused history and

intervention, with potential referral to a subspecialist. Recommendations may include adjusting the timing of medications, improving sleep hygiene, establishing a bedtime routine, avoiding electronics and caffeine, and maintaining a sleep-promoting bedroom environment. There are currently no approved medications for sleep-related problems in ADHD. In addition to behavioral interventions, melatonin (1–6 mg) may be given 30 to 60 minutes before desired sleep time (Stein et al., 2022). There are theoretical risks of long-term use of melatonin, including the impact on other hormones. Adults in the United States report a significant increase in the use of exogenous melatonin at doses of 5 mg or more. This raises safety concerns given that some melatonin content may be 478% higher than the labeled melatonin (Li et al., 2022). Melatonin is available by prescription only in many countries.

Toileting

Children with ADHD are 3.4 times more likely to have nocturnal enuresis (Barkley, 2015a). One study found that 15% of children with ADHD have enuresis or encopresis. Additionally, children with ADHD will likely have difficulty with bowel training and constipation (Barkley, 2015a). These children are at increased risk for severe nocturnal enuresis, dysfunctional voiding, and constipation (Kovacevic et al., 2018).

Discipline

A variety of strategies are used to reduce the need for discipline in children with ADHD. Providing education about ADHD and related impairments may help families set realistic expectations regarding their child's behavior. Furthermore, antecedent-based strategies and positive reinforcement reduce the need for discipline and are more effective at reducing disruptive behavior compared to punishment (van der Oord & Tripp, 2020). Minor misbehavior that is attention maintained (e.g., complaining, interrupting) can be extinguished through consistent removal of attention (i.e., ignoring). However, it is important to emphasize to families that initial attempts at planned ignoring are likely to escalate disruptive behavior before it extinguishes, and that planned ignoring works best when paired with reinforcement of desired behavior (Chacko et al., 2015). In the context of behavioral interventions, mild discipline is reserved for highly impairing and dangerous disruptive behavior, such as aggression, destruction of property, elopement, stealing, and repeated noncompliance, and is used in combination with positive parenting techniques. Evidence-based behavioral interventions include punishment techniques such as time-out and response costs (Chacko et al., 2015). The use of physical punishment, such as spanking, is discouraged. Spanking is associated with a host of negative child outcomes, including increased aggressive behavior, poorer parent-child relationships, the development of mental health conditions, and

| Table 9.9 | Sleep-Related Screening Tools |

SCREENING TOOL	AGE RANGE	RESPONDERS	DESCRIPTION
BEARS Sleep Screening Tool	2–18 yr	Parent Self	Examines 5 major sleep domains: B = Bedtime Issues E = Excessive Daytime Sleepiness A = Night Awakenings R = Regularity and Duration of Sleep S = Snoring
Children's Sleep Habits Questionnaire	3–12 yr	Parent	Assesses behavioral and medically based sleep problems, including bedtime resistance, sleep onset and duration, anxiety, sleep-disordered breathing, parasomnias, daytime sleepiness
Sleep Habits Questionnaire	Adolescent to Adult	Parent Self	Assesses behavioral and medically based sleep problems for adolescents
Pediatric Sleep Questionnaire-Sleep Related Breathing Disorder Scale (PSQ-SRBD Scale)	3–18 yr	Parent	Screens for obstructive sleep apnea features, including snoring, observed apneas, difficulty breathing during sleep, daytime sleepiness, inattentive or hyperactive behavior
Epworth Sleepiness Scale for Children and Adolescents (ESS-CHAD)	12–18 yr	Parent Self	Assess daytime sleepiness, propensity to fall asleep in 8 situations

From Mindell, J.A., & Owens, J.A. (2015). A clinical guide to pediatric sleep, diagnosis and management of sleep problems (3rd ed.). Lippincott Williams & Wilkins; Owens, J. A., Spirito, A., & McGuinn, M. (2000). The children's sleep habits questionnaire (CSHQ): Psychometric properties of a survey instrument for school-aged children. Sleep, 23(8), 1043–1051; Chervin, R.D., Hedger, K., Dillon, J.E., & Pituch, K.J. (2000). Pediatric sleep questionnaire (PSQ): Validity and reliability of scales for sleep-disordered breathing, snoring, sleepiness, and behavioral problems. Sleep Medicine, 1(1), 21–32; Johns, M.W. (1991). A new method for measuring daytime sleepiness: The Epworth sleepiness scale. Sleep, 14(6), 540–545.

a higher risk of physical abuse (Gershoff & Grogan-Kaylor, 2016).

Child Care

Child care settings that include a structured and consistent environment with routines and procedures are ideal for children with ADHD. Toddlers and preschoolers with ADHD need careful and close monitoring and supervision, with a low caregiver-to-child ratio being the ideal situation. They also need increased opportunities for physical outlets such as active play due to symptoms of hyperactivity. It is recommended that families speak directly with child care directors and staff regarding their experience and skills in working with children with ADHD. Ensuring a positive child care environment with developmentally appropriate and evidenced-based behavioral management strategies is critical to combat potential negative consequences and establish a strong working partnership. For instance, an epidemiologic review of preschool children with ADHD found that more than 40% had been suspended, and about 16% had been expelled from their school or day care (Egger et al., 2006). Given these rates, parents should know the specific evidence-based behavioral management procedures utilized in child care programs.

Caregivers of children with severe ADHD may want to consider resources such as respite care as a means of temporary relief if the ADHD and related behaviors are creating considerable strain on the family. Formal resources for respite care, such as ARCH National Respite Network and Resource Center or the local state developmental disability agency, may

provide direction. Medicaid waiver funding for respite care varies from state to state but also may be available.

Schooling

ADHD and its related symptoms have a major effect on the education of children and adolescents; problems in both the academic and behavioral arenas are common in the school setting. Of promising note, support for school-based behavioral interventions is well established as first-line treatments, with effect sizes for interventions such as contingency management relatively similar to pharmacotherapy and those for academic interventions superior to pharmacotherapy (Pfiffner & DuPaul, 2015). This underscores the need for focused efforts on the early identification of children with ADHD to help implement school-based interventions and improve educational outcomes.

A comprehensive evaluation by a qualified professional to determine if the child has ADHD often leads to recommendations, including two categories of school-based services, interventions, and accommodations. The first category includes interventions to help the child meet age-appropriate academic or behavioral goals (e.g., point systems, training interventions, and daily report cards). The second category includes changes to the student's program to improve the negative impact of the ADHD on school-related outcomes (e.g., accommodations such as extended time to complete tests or assignments and reduced class or homework demands) (Wolraich et al., 2019).

Further evaluation by the school district may occur to determine if the child is eligible for an educational plan, which provides accommodations and support for a child with a defined disability such as ADHD. Two federal laws (Section 504 of the Rehabilitation Act of 1973 [Section 504] and the Individuals with Disabilities Education Act [IDEA]) protect individuals with disabilities and guarantee a free and appropriate public education. These educational plans provide appropriate accommodations and modifications in the school environment to support a child with a disability such as ADHD. Both federal statutes also advocate for the least restrictive environment, which allows a child with a disability to be educated with peers without disabilities to the maximum extent appropriate (US Department of Education, 2019). Depending on their needs, these children may be eligible for supports or accommodations under IDEA, Section 504, or both provisions. It is helpful for clinicians to be aware of the eligibility criteria in the state where they practice (Wolraich et al., 2019). Most importantly, the school district is legally required to uphold this plan and be accountable for providing appropriate accommodations and modifications to the school environment.

Teacher education regarding ADHD is one of the primary necessary steps in helping foster a positive teacher-student relationship and setting the stage for interventions to improve academic and social functioning. Teachers need to have a solid understanding of the biologic basis of ADHD. Education should also center on the premise that ADHD is not a lack of skill or knowledge but a "problem of sustaining attention, effort, and motivation and inhibiting behavior in a consistent manner over time, especially when consequences are delayed, absent, or weak" (Pfiffner & DuPaul, 2015, p. 597). As such, it is much more difficult for children with ADHD to complete similar academic work and social behavior of their peers.

Flexibility and willingness to be creative in using tools to help the child with ADHD succeed in the classroom are qualities to look for in teachers. A combination of positive (praise and tangible rewards) and negative consequences has been shown to be ideal, and these strategies should be implemented immediately, consistently, and frequently (Pfiffner & DuPaul, 2015). Practical strategies such as allowing frequent breaks and opportunities to engage in active play for younger children, breaking content into smaller chunks, and providing additional prompts through visually based systems are equally important.

A collaborative approach between the school and home is important for successful schooling. Active and engaged teachers and staff, as well as supportive administrators, are critical, but a reciprocal relationship focused on mutual motivation toward helping the child succeed will provide the best outcomes. Strong family and school partnerships and coordination will aid the management of ADHD, which should include understanding the social determinants of health (Wolraich et al., 2019). Fostering effective communication between the home and school has been at the crux of various efforts to design and implement school-based interventions. One example is the school-home daily report card, which involves the provision of contingencies in the home based on the teacher's report of the child's behavioral performance at school (Barkley, 2013; Kelley, 1990).

As children progress in school, they should be involved in goal setting and evaluation of interventions because multicomponent treatments that involve parents, teachers, and youth are known to produce the most favorable results in various areas of difficulty (Pfiffner & DuPaul, 2015). Other strategies that have research support in the schooling of children with ADHD include self-regulation strategies where students monitor and evaluate their academic and social behaviors and reward themselves based on these evaluations. In two meta-analytic reviews of the impact of self-regulation interventions for students with ADHD in the school setting, effect sizes for behavioral and academic outcomes were large (DuPaul et al., 2012; Reid et al., 2005). Additionally, organizational training aimed at instructing the child or adolescent in managing materials, time, and homework is another training that shows some promising benefits (Pfiffner & DuPaul, 2015) (Box 9.6).

Sexuality

Primary care providers play a significant role in addressing sexual and reproductive health in pediatric patients with ADHD. National guidelines and recommendations provide guidance on sexual and reproductive health information, services, and counseling. Education should be developmentally appropriate and individualized. Role-playing can be helpful because problem solving may be difficult. Using a calendar for females to predict oncoming menses may be helpful. The risk of unsafe sexual behaviors generally increases during adolescence. ADHD is associated with risky sexual behavior, including earlier sexual activity and early pregnancy (Schoenfelder & Kollins, 2016). There are little data on reducing health risks for youth with ADHD. Guidelines include early screening, intervention, and treatment to strengthen environmental and family/social supports. Opportunities for open dialogue regarding puberty and sexuality must be made available by parents, counselors, or clinicians. Adolescents need to be made aware of community resources that offer information and services related to their developing sexuality.

Transition To Adulthood

The transition of older adolescents into adulthood is a critical point for families of children with ADHD. One-half to two-thirds of children with ADHD will continue to have symptoms as adults with some degree of continued impairments (Agnew-Blais et al., 2016). Executive functioning and problem-solving skills are

Box 9.6   **Behavioral, Educational, and Environmental Strategies for the Child With ADHD**

- Identify the child's strengths and build on them.
- Provide immediate and specific positive reinforcement for effort and achievement; reinforce positive behaviors (catch the child "being good").
- Make a hierarchy of rules; implement rules and consequences consistently and immediately.
- Provide parent coaching and child coaching.
- Provide learning activities when medication is at its peak.
- Get the child's attention first; put the child's head or shoulders gently in your hands or ensure eye contact; ask the child to repeat instructions (speak in a neutral tone).
- Give verbal *and* written instructions; list the steps on a 3 × 5 card, whiteboard, or other visual.
- Remind the child of expected behavior before an activity.
- Use hands-on activities (e.g., role-playing) for instruction.
- Use a notebook or planner for daily homework assignments.
- Help the child to develop a relationship with an older student or adult mentor to promote positive social interaction.
- Decrease the length of tasks, plan frequent breaks, divide large projects into smaller components.
- Post a daily schedule and make to-do lists (use pictures or visual schedules if necessary).
- Pace the child; do not let the child get overloaded.
- Provide assistance and coaching with organizational skills and tools.
- Use a timer to help structure tasks.
- Anticipate change and provide warnings for transitions.
- Build the child's self-esteem and self-confidence at every opportunity.
- Use calm reminders or prompts (e.g., "What should you be doing now?").
- Model positive behaviors (e.g., respectful language and calm tone of voice).
- Assist the child to feel "connected" with the school and their peers.

LEARNING ENVIRONMENT
- Allow structured "brain" breaks or opportunities for movement (e.g., stretching, passing out papers, nondistracting fidget tools).
- Decrease clutter (desks, worksheets, classroom).
- Seat the child in the front of the room, away from doors, windows, and distractions.
- Seat the child near a peer who is a positive role model (e.g., on-task).
- Provide a structured environment with clear guidelines.
- Provide consistency; maintain daily routines.
- Use calendars, organizational tools, structured schedule, untimed, oral testing if needed or testing in separate quiet room.
- Give additional time to process and respond to questions.
- Use technologic devices or apps for assistance with specific skills such as handwriting or organizational challenges (e.g., computer, iPad, speech to text programs).

From Children and Adults with Attention-Deficit/Hyperactivity Disorder, 2006. https://chadd.org.

needed in independent adult life and may be more difficult in individuals with ADHD. Other barriers to transition include limited adult mental health services and access and availability of services in adulthood (Price et al., 2019).

Planning for the transition and working on the developmental tasks of separation from parents and family are important. Establishing a sense of identity and independent living and formulating personal and occupational goals often require professional help. It is important to introduce steps of self-care skills around 14 years of age or earlier. As children enter adolescence, working on self-management skills in daily living and health care decisions, including being responsible for taking their medication, is important. However, parents must maintain control of the medications because many are controlled substances.

Fostering a smooth transition includes empowering youth with ADHD to understand their condition, recognize symptoms in adulthood and possible future challenges with ADHD, continue monitoring

and self-managing these symptoms, and the need for longer-term treatment (Price et al., 2019). Strategies to discourage the misuse of prescription medications should be discussed. The health care provider is responsible for assisting these young people in transitioning to adult health care services to a provider familiar with ADHD treatment and management in adulthood.

It is also important to identify potential support services and accommodations they may need as they enter postsecondary education or obtain a job. Reassessment for learning disabilities, executive functioning problems, and other coexisting conditions may be needed 1 to 2 years prior to high school graduation. Some students with ADHD need a formal transition plan through the school IEP or an individualized written rehabilitation plan for vocational rehabilitation programs. If the disability is disclosed, Section 504 and the ADA requires colleges to provide accommodations and service when necessary. Counselors, therapists, and coaches may be sought out for further support. Empowering individuals with ADHD with knowledge and skills while nurturing their self-esteem will help them lead successful and happy lives.

Family Concerns

With the knowledge that ADHD is a chronic and pervasive condition impacting various aspects of the child's functioning, it is important to consider the impact it has on families. Bidirectional family influences (parent-child and child-parent processes) are key to understanding the course of this disorder. Although parenting or family dynamics have not been identified as a cause of this disorder (Chacko et al., 2015; Muñoz-Silva et al., 2017), children who have ADHD often exhibit challenging behaviors that affect the family, which is particularly true for children with comorbid conditions such as ODD or CD. Barriers such as the associated costs and time invested in the long-term management of children with ADHD can be overwhelming for families. Evidenced-based care of ADHD calls for a multimodal treatment plan, which may be difficult for families to access with few resources or limited social support.

Research has consistently shown that parents of children with ADHD experience increased levels of stress and parent-child conflict and are more likely to exhibit ineffective parenting practices (e.g., inconsistent, overly directive or punitive, lax) (Chacko et al., 2015; Theule et al., 2013). This can lead to patterns of maladaptive coping by parents and negativity toward their child, a coercive cycle in which the overall adjustment and behaviors of the child are negatively impacted, and parenting practices worsen (Chacko et al., 2015). Parents of children with ADHD are commonly affected by this disorder. A recent meta-analysis indicated that 20% of parents of children with ADHD have ADHD themselves (Cheung & Theule, 2016), but other sources have suggested estimates closer to 50%. Parents of children with ADHD also have elevated rates of psychopathology, such as depression, anxiety, substance abuse, interparental conflict, and divorce (Cheung & Theule, 2016; Johnston & Chronis-Tuscano, 2015), which need to be considered in the context of treatment. Additionally, although not well researched, sibling relationships may be affected in various ways (e.g., parents having to provide increased attention to the needs of a sibling with ADHD).

On a positive note, reductions in negative outcomes such as parenting stress have been linked to parenting improvements with evidence-based interventions such as BPT. These interventions also may help prevent more significant disruptive behavior in children with ADHD (Chacko et al., 2015). Core components of BPT, such as increasing praise and positive attention and quality time, using effective commands, and implementing incentive systems within a framework of consistent structure, discipline, and routines, are vital to the family (Chacko et al., 2015). Parents may benefit from resources and social support focused on advocating for their child with ADHD. Resources offered through national organizations such as the AAP and Children and Adults with Attention-Deficit/Hyperactivity Disorder (CHADD, 2018) are beneficial, in addition to working with ADHD specialists in their area. The CDC has numerous videos on positive parenting skills. Supports to reduce barriers to treatment and help families access and navigate educational, behavioral, and medical interventions for ADHD are critical (Paidipati et al., 2021).

RESOURCES

BOOKS ON ADHD FOR PARENTS AND TEACHERS

Barkley, R.A. (2016). Managing ADHD in the school: The best evidence-based methods for teachers. PESI Publishing & Media.

Barkley, R.A. (2020). *Taking charge of ADHD: The complete authoritative guide for parents* (4th ed.). The Guilford Press.

Children and Adults with Attention-Deficit/Hyperactivity Disorder (CHADD). (2006). *CHADD educator's manual.* Author.

Gallagher, R., Spira, E.G., & Rosenblatt, J.L. (2018). *The organized child: An effective program to maximize your kid's potential in school and in life.* The Guilford Press.

Guare, R., Dawson, P., & Guare, C. (2013). *Smart but scattered teens: The "executive skills" program for helping teens reach their potential.* Guilford Press.

Hinshaw, S.P. (2022). *Straight talk about ADHD and girls: How to help your daughter thrive.* The Guilford Press.

Wolraich, M.L., & Hagan, J.F. (2019). *ADHD: What every parent needs to know.* American Academy of Pediatrics.

BOOKS ON ADHD FOR CHILDREN

Hutton, J.S. (2016). *ADH-me!* Blue Manatee Press.

Quinn, P.O., & Stern, J.M. (2012). *Putting on the brakes: Understanding & taking control of your ADD or ADHD* (3rd ed.). Magination Press.

Spodak, R., & Stefano, K. (2011). *Take control of ADHD: The ultimate guide for teens with ADHD.* Prufrock Press, Inc.

Stumpf, T. (2014). *Journal of an ADHD kid: The good, the bad, and the useful.* Woodbine House.

Taylor, J.F. (2006). *The survival guide for kids with ADD or ADHD.* Free Spirit Publishing.

PARENTING RESOURCES

The Incredible Years (evidence-based programs for parents, children, and teachers): https://incredible-years.com

Triple P–Positive Parenting Program (evidence-based parenting program): https://www.triplep.net/glo-en/home

Parent-Child Interaction Therapy (evidence-based treatment for young children with behavioral problems): http://www.pcit.org

Centers for Disease Control and Prevention (essentials for parenting; resources for parents and caregivers): https://www.cdc.gov/parents/essentials/index.html

Centers for Disease Control and Prevention (positive parenting tips): https://www.cdc.gov/ncbddd/childdevelopment/positiveparenting/index.html

HealthyChildren.org (from the American Academy of Pediatrics): https://www.healthychildren.org

Organizations

ADD Warehouse: www.addwarehouse.com

American Academy of Child and Adolescent Psychiatry: www.aacap.org

American Academy of Pediatrics: www.aap.org

AAP ADHD toolkit: https://publications.aap.org/toolkits/pages/ADHD-Toolkit

Attention Deficit Disorder Association: www.add.org

Children and Adults with Attention-Deficit/Hyperactivity Disorder: www.chadd.org

Health Resource Center (National Clearinghouse for Postsecondary Education for People with Disabilities): www.acenet.edu

Learning Disabilities Association of America: https://ldaamerica.org

National Center for Learning Disabilities: www.ncld.org

National Information Center for Children and Youth with Disabilities: www.nichcy.org

National Initiative for Children's Healthcare Quality: www.nichq.org

National Institute of Mental Health, Office of Communications and Public Liaison, Information Resources and Inquiries Branch: www.nimh.nih.gov

Understood for All Inc.: www.understood.org

 Summary

Primary Care Needs for the Child With Attention-Deficit/Hyperactivity Disorder

HEALTH CARE MAINTENANCE

Growth and Development

- Medications for ADHD can cause appetite suppression; assess height and weight every 3 to 6 months.
- Early identification of developmental delays and problem behaviors that do not fall within normal ranges will promote early interventions and decrease morbidity.

Diet

- A nutritious diet with adequate protein and calories for growth is important. Decreased appetite may occur in children taking stimulant medication.
- Assess weight and height every 3 to 6 months.
- Additional snacks, the timing of medications, or nutritional supplementation may be considered in children with poor appetite. Further referral may also be warranted.
- Stomachache may be a side effect of stimulants and nonstimulants. Give medication on a full stomach.

Safety

- There is a risk of injury because of impulsive behaviors and altered judgment. Adolescents of driving age may need closer monitoring and support.
- Children with ADHD have an increased incidence of injuries and may have more injury visits at age 6 years.
- Use of long-acting stimulants, patches, and nonstimulant medication options have decreased the risk of stimulant misuse.
- Medication should be kept safely out of reach of young children. Refills and requests may be monitored through state drug monitoring programs.

Immunizations

- Routine schedule is recommended.

Screening

- *Vision.* Comprehensive visual testing is done initially as part of differential diagnosis.
- *Hearing.* Comprehensive audiometric testing is done initially as part of differential diagnosis. Children may have difficulty with audiometric testing because of attention needed.
- *Dental.* Routine screening is recommended.

- *Blood pressure.* Routine screening is recommended. In children taking medications for ADHD, blood pressure should be monitored every 3 to 6 months.
- *Hematocrit.* Routine screening is recommended.
- *Lead.* Routine screening is recommended up to 72 months if not previously completed.
- *Urinalysis.* Routine screening is not recommended.
- *Tuberculosis.* Routine screening is recommended.

Condition-Specific Screening

- *Learning issues.* Testing may be needed in the diagnostic process or to assess for cooccurring learning concerns, including cognitive and academic assessments, speech and language assessments.
- *Psychological.* Comprehensive assessment of the child's general mental health and potential related mood concerns should be evaluated at each visit. Screening for suicidal ideation, mood and anxiety, and social-emotional functioning should be included annually.
- *Cardiac function.* A thorough cardiac and physical exam is required. ECG is not necessary for most children taking stimulants or nonstimulants. Indications for ECG are listed earlier.

COMMON ILLNESS MANAGEMENT

Differential Diagnosis

- ADHD symptoms overlap with several conditions, including neurologic or developmental conditions, emotional and behavioral disorders, psychosocial or environmental factors, and certain medical conditions.
- Irritability, anorexia, weight loss, and insomnia are common side effects of stimulants.
- Increased inattention or somnolence may indicate that medication dosage needs to be decreased.

Drug Interactions

- Stimulants should not be given with MAOIs.
- There may be some negative interaction when combining dextroamphetamine with beta-adrenergic blockers, phenothiazines, and guanethidine.
- TCAs and warfarin are affected by methylphenidate.

Continued

- TCAs decrease the effect of clonidine.

DEVELOPMENTAL ISSUES

Sleep Patterns

- Children with ADHD are at increased risk of sleeping problems. These can be exacerbated when taking stimulant medication if given late in the day or in large doses.
- It is important to screen for sleep disorders during evaluation for ADHD and ongoing follow-up.

Toileting

- Nocturnal enuresis is common. Children with ADHD may be at increased risk for dysfunctional voiding and constipation.

Discipline

- Children may have difficulty responding to directions and may not understand discipline or learn from past experiences. Consistency in expectations is important.
- Behavior modification may be effective. A bad behavior must be differentiated from a bad child.
- Antecedent-based strategies and positive reinforcement are more effective compared to punishment.

Child Care

- Children perform better in a small, structured, consistent, and safe environment with constant adult supervision.

Schooling

- Education strategies to decrease distraction in a regular classroom, in addition to creative teaching modalities appropriate to the specific learning needs of the child, should be implemented. Building a child's self-esteem and confidence is essential. Children should be helped to learn to compensate for their disability.
- Development of the IEP or accommodation plan is a team effort.

Sexuality

- ADHD is associated with risky sexual behavior. Education should be individualized and developmentally appropriate when discussing reproductive health and sexuality.
- Open dialogue regarding puberty and sexuality must be made available by parents, counselors, or clinicians.

Transition to Adulthood

- Professional help may be necessary to facilitate the transition to more autonomous living and work situations; peer coaching may be helpful.
- The child needs to be empowered to understand the condition, how it manifests, what accommodations are needed, and what treatments are used.
- Career development counseling may be helpful in identifying postsecondary education and/or vocation based on a child's strengths and weaknesses.

Family Concerns

- The child and the family need to readjust to this disability at every new developmental stage. Family counseling can provide information and emotional support.

REFERENCES

Adesman, A. (2022). Cohen Children's Medical Center of New York. *The ADHD medication guide*. http://www.adhdmedicationguide.com/.

Agnew-Blais, J. C., Polanczyk, G. V., Danese, A., Wertz, J., Moffitt, T. E., Arseneault, L. (2016). Evaluation of the persistence, remission, and emergence of attention-deficit/hyperactivity disorder in young adulthood. *JAMA Psychiatry, 73*(7), 713–720. doi: 10.1001/jamapsychiatry.2016.0465.

Albajara Sáenz, A., Villemonteix, T., & Massat, I. (2019). Structural and functional neuroimaging in attention-deficit/hyperactivity disorder. *Developmental Medicine and Child Neurology, 61*(4), 399–405. https://doi.org/10.1111/dmcn.14050.

Albuja, A. C., & Qutubuddin Khan, G. (2022). Absence seizure. *Springer Reference*. https://doi.org/10.1007/springerreference_183783.

Allan, C. C., DeShazer, M., Staggs, V. S., Nadler, C., Crawford, T. P., Moody, S., Chacko, A. (2021). Accidental injuries in preschoolers: Are we missing an opportunity for early assessment and intervention? *J Pediatr Psychol, 46*(7), 835–843. doi: 10.1093/jpepsy/jsab044.

American Psychiatric Association. (2022). *Diagnostic and statistical manual of mental disorders* (5th ed., text revision). American Psychiatric Association Publishing.

Bader, A., & Adesman, A. (2015). Complementary and alternative medicine for ADHD. In Barkley, R. A. (Ed.), *Attention-deficit hyperactivity disorder, fourth edition: A handbook for diagnosis & treatment* (pp. 728–738). The Guilford Press.

Balazs, J., & Kereszteny, A. (2017). Attention-deficit/hyperactivity disorder and suicide: A systematic review. *World Psychiatry, 7*(1), 44–59. https://doi.org/10.5498/wjp.v7.i1.44.

Barbaresi, W. J., Campbell, L., Diekroger, E. A., Froehlich, T. E., Liu, Y. H., O'Malley, E., Pelham, W. E., Jr., Power, T. J., Zinner, S. H., Chan, E. (2020). Society for developmental and behavioral pediatrics clinical practice guideline for the assessment and treatment of children and adolescents with complex attention-deficit/hyperactivity disorder. *J Dev Behav Pediatr, 41*(Suppl 2S), S35–S57. doi: 10.1097/DBP.0000000000000770.

Barkley, R. A. (2013). *Defiant children: A clinician's manual for parent training* (3rd ed.). Guilford Press.

Barkley, R. A. (Ed.). (2015a). *Attention-deficit hyperactivity disorder: A handbook for diagnosis & treatment* (4th ed.). The Guilford Press.

Barkley, R. A. (2015b). Educational, occupational, dating, and marital, and financial impairments in adults with ADHD. In Barkley, R. A. (Ed.), *Attention-deficit hyperactivity disorder, fourth edition: A handbook for diagnosis & treatment* (pp. 314–342). The Guilford Press.

Barkley, R. A. (2015c). Psychological assessment of children with ADHD. In Barkley, R. A. (Ed.), *Attention-deficit hyperactivity disorder, fourth edition: A handbook for diagnosis & treatment* (pp. 455–474). The Guilford Press.

Barkley, R. A., & Fischer, M. (2019). Hyperactive child syndrome and estimated life expectancy at young adult follow-up: The role of ADHD persistence and other potential predictors. *Journal of Attention Disorders, 23*(9), 907–923. https://doi.org/10.1177/1087054718816164.

Barkley, R. A., & Murphy, K. R. (2006). *Attention-deficit hyperactivity disorder: A clinical workbook* (3rd ed.). Guilford Press.

Barnes, P. M., Powell-Griner, E., McFann, K., & Nahin, R. L. (2005). Complementary and alternative medicine use among adults: United States, 2002. *Advance Data*, (343), 1–19.

Biederman, J., & Spencer, T. (2008). Psychopharmacological interventions. *Child and Adolescent Psychiatric Clinics of North America, 17*(2), 439–458.

Bitsko, R. H., Claussen, A. H., Lichstein, J., Black, L. I., Jones, S. E., Danielson, M. L., Hoenig, J. M., Davis Jack, S. P., Brody, D. J., Gyawali, S., Maenner, M. J., Warner, M., Holland, K. M., Perou, R., Crosby, A. E., Blumberg, S. J., Avenevoli, S., Kaminski, J. W., Ghandour, R. M. (2022). Contributor. Mental Health Surveillance Among Children – United States, 2013–2019. *MMWR Suppl., 71*(2), 1–42. doi: 10.15585/mmwr.su7102a1.

Bloch, M. H., & Qawasmi, A. (2011). Omega-3 fatty acid supplementation for the treatment of children with attention-deficit/hyperactivity disorder symptomatology: Systematic review and meta-analysis. *Journal of American Child and Adolescent Psychiatry, 50*(10), 991–1000. https://doi.org/10.1016/j.jaac.2011.06.008.

Boland, H., DiSalvo, M., Fried, R., Woodworth, K. Y., Wilens, T., Faraone, S. V., Biederman, J. (2020). A literature review and meta-analysis on the effects of ADHD medications on functional outcomes. *J Psychiatr Res, 123*, 21–30. doi: 10.1016/j.jpsychires.2020.01.006.

Brown, J. T., Bishop, J. R., Sangkuhl, K., Nurmi, E. L., Mueller, D. J., Dinh, J. C., Gaedigk, A., Klein, T. E., Caudle, K. E., McCracken, J. T., de Leon, J., Leeder, J. S. (2019). Clinical pharmacogenetics implementation consortium guideline for cytochrome P450 (CYP)2D6 genotype and atomoxetine therapy. *Clin Pharmacol Ther, 106*(1), 94–102. doi: 10.1002/cpt.1409.

Chacko, A., Allan, C. C., Uderman, J., Cornwell, M., Anderson, L., & Chimiklis, A. (2015). Training parents of youth with ADHD. In Barkley, R. A. (Ed.), *Attention-deficit hyperactivity disorder: A handbook for diagnosis and treatment* (pp. 513–536). The Guilford Press.

Chacko, A., Allan, C. C., Moody, S. S., Crawford, T. P., Nadler, C., & Chimiklis, A. (2017). Behavioral interventions. In Goldstein, S., & DeVries, M. (Eds.), *Handbook of DSM-5 disorders in children and adolescents* (pp. 617–636). Springer International Publishing/Springer Nature. https://doi.org/10.1007/978-3-319-57196-6_32.

Children and Adults with Attention-Deficit/Hyperactivity Disorder (CHADD). (2018). *Classroom accommodations*. Retrieved February 14, 2023, from https://chadd.org/for-educators/classroom-accommodations/.

Cherkasova, M. V., Roy, A., & Molina, B. (2022). Review: Adult outcome as seen through controlled prospective follow-up studies of children with attention-deficit/hyperactivity disorder followed into adulthood. *Journal of American Child and Adolescent Psychiatry, 61*(3), 378–391. https://doi.org/10.1016/j.jaac.2021.05.019.

Cheung, K., & Theule, J. (2016). Parental psychopathology in families of children with ADHD: A meta-analysis. *Journal of Child and Family Studies, 25*(12), 34513461. https://doi.org/10.1007/s10826-016-0499-1.

Chhibber, A., Watanabe, A. H., & Chaisai, C. (2021). Global economic burden of attention-deficit/hyperactivity disorder: A systematic review. *PharmacoEconomics, 39*(4), 399–420. https://doi.org/10.1007/s40273-020-00998-0.

Conners, C. K. (2009). *Connors early childhood*. Multi-Health Systems (MHS).

Conners, C. K. (2008). *Connors 3*. Multi-Health Systems (MHS).

Conradt, E., Flannery, T., Aschner, J. L., Annett, R. D., Croen, L. A., Duarte, C. S., Friedman, A. M., Guille, C., Hedderson, M. M., Hofheimer, J. A., Jones, M. R., Ladd-Acosta, C., McGrath, M., Moreland, A., Neiderhiser, J. M., Nguyen, R. H. N., Posner, J., Ross, J. L., Savitz, D. A., Ondersma, S. J., Lester, B. M. (2019). Prenatal opioid exposure: Neurodevelopmental consequences and future research priorities. *Pediatrics, 144*(3), e20190128. doi: 10.1542/peds.2019-0128.

Cortese, S., Adamo, N., & Del Giovane, C. (2018). Comparative efficacy and tolerability of medications for attention-deficit hyperactivity disorder in children, adolescents, and adults: A systematic review and network meta-analysis. *Lancet Psychiatry, 5*(9), 727–738. https://doi.org/10.1016/s2215-0366(18)30269-4.

Dachew, B. A., Scott, J. G., Mamun, A., & Alati, R. (2019). Pre-eclampsia and the risk of attention-deficit/hyperactivity disorder in offspring: Findings from the ALSPAC birth cohort study. *Psychiatry Research, 272*, 392–397. https://doi.org/10.1016/j.psychres.2018.12.123.

Danielson, M. L., Bitsko, R. H., Ghandour, R. M., Holbrook, J. R., Kogan, M. D., Blumberg, S. J. (2018). Prevalence of parent-reported ADHD diagnosis and associated treatment among US children and adolescents, 2016. *J Clin Child Adolesc Psychol., 47*(2), 199–212. doi: 10.1080/15374416.2017.1417860.

Dekkers, T. J., Hornstra, R., van der Oord, S., Luman, M., Hoekstra, P. J., Groenman, A. P., van den Hoofdakker, B. J. (2022). Meta-analysis: Which components of parent training work for children with attention-deficit/hyperactivity disorder? *J Am Acad Child Adolesc Psychiatry, 61*(4), 478–494. doi: 10.1016/j.jaac.2021.06.015.

Demontis, D., Walters, R. K., & Martin, J. (2019). Discovery of the first genome-wide significant risk loci for attention deficit/hyperactivity disorder. *Nature Genetics, 51*(1), 63–75. https://doi.org/10.1038/s41588-018-0269-7.

Drechsler, R., Brem, S., Brandeis, D., Grünblatt, E., Berger, G., Walitza, S. (2020). ADHD: Current concepts and treatments in children and adolescents. *Neuropediatrics, 51*(5), 315–335. doi: 10.1055/s-0040-1701658.

DuPaul, G. J., & Eckert, T. L. (1997). The effects of school-based interventions for attention deficit hyperactivity disorder: A meta-analysis. *School Psychology Review, 26*(1), 5–27.

DuPaul, G. J., Eckert, T. L., & Vilardo, B. (2012). The effects of school-based interventions for attention deficit hyperactivity disorder: A meta-analysis 1996–2010. *School Psychology Review, 41*(4), 387–412.

DuPaul, G. J., & Kern, L. (2011). *Young children with ADHD: Early identification and intervention.* American Psychological Association. https://doi.org/10.1037/12311-000.

DuPaul, G. J., & Landberg, J. M. (2015). Educational impairments in children with ADHD. In Barkley, R. A. (Ed.), *Attention-deficit hyperactivity disorder, fourth edition: A handbook for diagnosis & treatment* (pp. 169–190). The Guilford Press.

DuPaul, G. J., Power, T. J., Anastopoulos, A. D., & Reid, R. (2016). *ADHD rating scale-5: Checklists, norms, and clinical interpretation.* Guilford Press.

DuPaul, G. J., & Stoner, G. (2014). *ADHD in the schools: Assessment and intervention strategies* (3rd ed.). Guilford Press.

DuPaul, G. J., Reid, R., Anastopoulos, A. D., Lambert, M. C., Watkins, M. W., Power, T. J. (2016). Parent and teacher ratings of attention-deficit/hyperactivity disorder symptoms: Factor structure and normative data. *Psychol Assess., 28*(2), 214–225. doi:10.1037/pas0000166.

Egger, H. L., Kondo, D., & Angold, A. (2006). The epidemiology and diagnostic issues in preschool attention-deficit/hyperactivity disorder: A review. *Infants Young Child, 19*(2), 109122. https://doi.org/10.1097/00001163-200604000-00004.

Elia, J., Ambrosini, P., & Berrettini, W. (2008). ADHD characteristics: I. Concurrent co-morbidity patterns in children & adolescents. *Child and Adolescent Psychiatry and Mental Health, 2*(1), 15. https://doi.org/10.1186/1753-2000-2-15.

Epstein, J. N., & Loren, R. E. (2013). Changes in the definition of ADHD in DSM-5: Subtle but important. *Neuropsychiatry, 3*(5), 455–458. https://doi.org/10.2217/npy.13.59.

Erskine, H. E., Norman, R. E., Ferrari, A. J., Chan, G. C., Copeland, W. E., Whiteford, H. A., Scott, J. G. (2016). Long-term outcomes of attention-deficit/hyperactivity disorder and conduct disorder: A systematic review and meta-analysis. *J Am Acad Child Adolesc Psychiatry, 55*(10), 841–850. doi: 10.1016/j.jaac.2016.06.016.

Evans, S. W., Owens, J. S., & Bunford, N. (2014). Evidence-based psychosocial treatments for children and adolescents with attention-deficit/hyperactivity disorder. *Journal of Clinical Child and Adolescent Psychology, 43*, 527–551. https://doi.org/10.1080/15374416.2013.850700.

Evans, S. W., Owens, J. S., Wymbs, B. T., Ray, A. R. (2018). Evidence-based psychosocial treatments for children and adolescents with attention deficit/hyperactivity disorder. *J Clin Child Adolesc Psychol., 47*(2), 157–198. doi: 10.1080/15374416.2017.1390757.

Fabiano, G. A., Pelham, W. E., Jr., Waschbusch, D. A., Gnagy, E. M., Lahey, B. B., Chronis, A. M., Onyango, A. N., Kipp, H., Lopez-Williams, A., Burrows-Maclean, L. (2006). A practical measure of impairment: Psychometric properties of the impairment rating scale in samples of children with attention deficit hyperactivity disorder and two school-based samples. *J Clin Child Adolesc Psychol., 35*(3), 369–385. doi: 10.1207/s15374424jccp3503_3.

Fabiano, G. A., Vujnovic, R. K., Pelham, W. E., Waschbusch, D. A., Massetti, G. M., Pariseau, M. E., Naylor, J., Yu, J., Robins, M., Carnefix, T., Greiner, A. R., & Volker, M. (2010). Enhancing the effectiveness of special education programming for children with attention deficit hyperactivity disorder using a daily report card. *School Psychology Review, 39*(2), 219–239. https://doi.org/10.1080/02796015.2010.12087775.

Faraone, S. V., & Larsson, H. (2019). Genetics of attention deficit hyperactivity disorder. *Molecular Psychiatry, 24*(4), 562–575. https://doi.org/10.1038/s41380-018-0070-0.

Feder, J. D., Tien, E., & Puzantian, T. (2018). *The child medication fact book for psychiatric practice.* Carlat Publishing, LLC.

Findling, R. L., Candler, S. A., Nasser, A. F., Schwabe, S., Yu, C., Garcia-Olivares, J., O'Neal, W., Newcorn, J. H. (2021). Viloxazine in the management of CNS disorders: A historical overview and current status. *CNS Drugs, 35*(6), 643–653. doi: 10.1007/s40263-021-00825-w.

Gershoff, E. T., & Grogan-Kaylor, A. (2016). Spanking and child outcomes: Old controversies and new meta-analyses. *Journal of Family Psychology, 30*(4), 453–469. https://doi.org/10.1037/fam0000191.

Greenhill, L. L., Swanson, J. M., Hechtman, L., Waxmonsky, J., Arnold, L. E., Molina, B. S. G., Hinshaw, S. P., Jensen, P. S., Abikoff, H. B., Wigal, T., Stehli, A., Howard, A., Hermanussen, M., Hanć, T. (2020). MTA Cooperative Group. Trajectories of growth associated with long-term stimulant medication in the multimodal treatment study of attention-deficit/hyperactivity disorder. *J Am Acad Child Adolesc Psychiatry, 59*(8), 978–989. doi:10.1016/j.jaac.2019.06.019.

Grimm, O., Kranz, T. M., & Reif, A. (2020). Genetics of ADHD: What should the clinician know? *Current Psychiatry Reports, 22*(4). https://doi.org/10.1007/s11920-020-1141-x.

Groenman, A. P., Hornstra, R., & Hoekstra, P. J. (2022). An individual participant data meta-analysis: Behavioral treatments for children and adolescents with attention-deficit/hyperactivity disorder. *Journal of the American Academy of Child and Adolescent Psychiatry, 61*(2), 144–158. https://doi.org/10.1016/j.jaac.2021.02.024.

Harstad, E. B., Weaver, A.L., Katusic, S. K., Colligan, R. C., Kumar, S., Chan, E., Voigt, R. G., Barbaresi, W. J. (2014). ADHD, stimulant treatment, and growth: a longitudinal study. *Pediatrics, 134*(4):e935–44. doi:10.1542/peds.2014-0428.

Harpin, V., Mazzone, L., Raynaud, J. P., Kahle, J., Hodgkins, P. (2016). Long-term outcomes of ADHD: A systematic review of self-esteem and social function. *Journal of Attention Disorders, 20*(4), 295–305. doi: 10.1177/1087054713486516. Epub 2013 May 22. PMID: 23698916.

Hechtman, L., Swanson, J. M., Sibley, M. H., Stehli, A., Owens, E. B., Mitchell, J. T., Arnold, L. E., Molina, B. S., Hinshaw, S. P., Jensen, P. S., Abikoff, H. B., Perez Algorta, G., Howard, A. L., Hoza, B., Etcovitch, J., Houssais, S., Lakes, K. D., Nichols, J. Q. (2016). MTA Cooperative Group. Functional adult outcomes 16 years after childhood diagnosis of attention-deficit/hyperactivity disorder: MTA results. *Journal of the American Academy of Child and Adolescent Psychiatry, 55*(11), 945–952.e2. doi:10.1016/j.jaac.2016.07.774. Epub 2016 Sep 2. Erratum in: *J Am Acad Child Adolesc Psychiatry.* 2017 Jul;56(7):628. Erratum in: *J Am Acad Child Adolesc Psychiatry.* 2018 Mar;57(3):225.

Hirayama, S., Hamazaki, T., & Terasawa, K. (2004). Effect of docosahexaenoic acid-containing food administration on symptoms of attention-deficit/hyperactivity disorder - a placebo-controlled double-blind study. *European Journal of Clinical Nutrition, 58*(3), 467–473. https://doi.org/10.1038/sj.ejcn.1601830.

Holst, L. M., Kronborg, J. B., Jepsen, J. R. M., Christensen, J. Ø., Vejlstrup, N. G., Juul, K., Bjerre, J. V., Bilenberg, N., Ravn, H. B. (2020). Attention-deficit/hyperactivity disorder symptoms in children with surgically corrected ventricular septal defect, transposition of the great arteries, and tetralogy of Fallot. *Cardiology in the Young, 30*(2), 180–187. doi:10.1017/s1047951119003184.

Hurt, E., & Arnold, L. E. (2015). Dietary management of ADHD. In Barkley, R. A. (Ed.), *Attention-deficit hyperactivity disorder, fourth edition: A handbook for diagnosis & treatment* (pp. 630–640). The Guilford Press.

Iznardo, M., Rogers, M. A., Volpe, R. J., Labelle, P. R., Robaey, P. (2020). The effectiveness of daily behavior report cards for children with ADHD: A meta-analysis. *Journal of Attention Disorders, 24*(12), 1623–1636. doi:10.1177/1087054717734646.

Jellinek, M. S., Murphy, J. M., Robinson, J., Feins, A., Lamb, S., Fenton, T. (1988). Pediatric symptom checklist: Screening school-age children for psychosocial dysfunction. *Journal of Pediatrics, 112*(2), 201–209. doi:10.1016/s0022-3476(88)80056-8.

Johnston, C., & Chronis-Tuscano, A. (2015). Families and ADHD. In Barkley, R. A. (Ed.), *Attention-deficit hyperactivity disorder, fourth edition: A handbook for diagnosis & treatment* (pp. 191–209). The Guilford Press.

Kang, J. H., Lin, H. C., & Chung, S. D. (2013). Attention-deficit/hyperactivity disorder increased the risk of injury: A population-based follow-up study. *Acta Paediatrica, 102*(6), 640–643. https://doi.org/10.1111/apa.12213.

Kelley, M. L. (1990). *School-home notes: Promoting children's classroom success.* The Guilford Press.

Kim, E., & Heo, Y. A. (2020). Consider clinically relevant pharmacokinetic drug interactions when co-prescribing drugs in attention-deficit/hyperactivity disorder. *Drugs and Therapy Perspectives, 36*(9), 386–388. https://doi.org/10.1007/s40267-020-00749-3.

Klein, R. G., Mannuzza, S., Olazagasti, M. A., Roizen, E., Hutchison, J. A., Lashua, E. C., Castellanos, F. X. (2012). Clinical and functional outcome of childhood attention-deficit/hyperactivity disorder 33 years later. *Archives in General Psychiatry, 69*(12), 1295–1303. doi:10.1001/archgenpsychiatry.2012.271.

Kollins, S. H., Childress, A., Heusser, A. C., Lutz, J. (2021). Effectiveness of a digital therapeutic as adjunct to treatment with medication in pediatric ADHD. *NPJ Digital Medicine, 4*(1), 58. doi:10.1038/s41746-021-00429-0.

Kollins, S. H., DeLoss, D. J., Cañadas, E., Lutz, J., Findling, R. L., Keefe, R. S. E., Epstein, J. N., Cutler, A. J., Faraone, S. V. (2020). A novel digital intervention for actively reducing severity of paediatric ADHD (STARS-ADHD): A randomised controlled trial. *Lancet Digital Health, 2*(4), e168–e178. doi:10.1016/S2589-7500(20)30017-0.

Konofal, E., Lecendreux, M., Arnulf, I., Mouren, M. (2004). Iron deficiency in children with attention-deficit/hyperactivity disorder. *Archives in Pediatric and Adolescent Medicine, 158*(12), 1113–1115. doi:10.1001/archpedi.158.12.1113.

Kovacevic, L., Wolfe-Christensen, C., Rizwan, A., Lu, H., Lakshmanan, Y. (2018). Children with nocturnal enuresis and attention deficit hyperactivity disorder: A separate entity? *Journal of Pediatric Urology, 14*(1), 47.e1–47.e6. doi:10.1016/j.jpurol.2017.07.002.

Kuriyan, A. B., Pelham, W. E., Jr., Molina, B. S., Waschbusch, D. A., Gnagy, E. M., Sibley, M. H., Babinski, D. E., Walther, C., Cheong, J., Yu, J., Kent, K. M. (2013). Young adult educational and vocational outcomes of children diagnosed with ADHD. *Journal of Abnormal Child Psychology, 41*(1), 27–41. doi:10.1007/s10802-012-9658-z.

Li, J., Somers, V. K., Xu, H., Lopez-Jimenez, F., Covassin, N. (2022). Trends in use of melatonin supplements among US adults, 1999–2018. *JAMA, 327*(5), 483–485. doi:10.1001/jama.2021.23652. PMID: 35103775; PMCID: PMC8808329.

Lofthouse, N., & Hurt, E. (2014). Complementary and alternative treatments for preschool children with ADHD. In Ghuman, J. K., & Ghuman, H. S. (Eds.), *ADHD in preschool children: Assessment and treatment* (pp. 180–209). Oxford University Press.

London, A. S., & Landes, S. D. (2022). Attention deficit hyperactivity disorder and the age pattern of adult mortality. *Biodemography and Social Biology, 67*(1), 28–39. https://doi.org/10.1080/19485565.2021.2020618.

Martin, A. J. (2014). The role of ADHD in academic adversity: Disentangling ADHD effects from other personal and contextual factors. *School Psychology Quarterly, 29*(4), 395–408. https://doi.org/10.1037/spq0000069.

Mattson, S. N., Bernes, G. A., & Doyle, L. R. (2019). Fetal alcohol spectrum disorders: A review of the neurobehavioral deficits associated with prenatal alcohol exposure. *Alcoholism: Clinical and Experimental Research, 43*(6), 1046–1062. https://doi.org/10.1111/acer.14040.

McGough, J. J., Sturm, A., Cowen, J., Tung, K., Salgari, G. C., Leuchter, A. F., Cook, I. A., Sugar, C. A., Loo, S. K. (2019). Double-blind, sham-controlled, pilot study of trigeminal nerve stimulation for attention-deficit/hyperactivity disorder. *Journal of American Child and Adolescent Psychiatry, 58*(4), 403–411.e3. doi:10.1016/j.jaac.2018.11.013. Epub 2019 Jan 28.

McQuade, J. D., & Hoza, B. (2015). Peer relationships of children with ADHD. In Barkley, R. A. (Ed.), *Attention-deficit hyperactivity disorder, fourth edition: A handbook for diagnosis & treatment* (pp. 210–222). The Guilford Press.

Mechler, K., Banaschewski, T., Hohmann, S., Häge, A. (2022). Evidence-based pharmacological treatment options for ADHD in children and adolescents. *Pharmacology and Therapeutics, 230*, 107940. doi:10.1016/j.pharmthera.2021.107940.

Mick, E., & Faraone, S. (2008). Genetics of attention deficit hyperactivity disorder. *Child Adolesc Psychiatr Clin North Am, 17*(2), 261–284.

Molina, B. S. G., Hinshaw, S. P., Swanson, J. M., Arnold, L. E., Vitiello, B., Jensen, P. S., Epstein, J. N., Hoza, B., Hechtman, L., Abikoff, H. B., Elliott, G. R., Greenhill, L. L., Newcorn, J. H., Wells, K. C., Wigal, T., Gibbons, R. D., Hur, K., Houck, P. R. (2009). MTA Cooperative Group. The MTA at 8 years: prospective follow-up of children treated for combined-type ADHD in a multisite study. *Journal of American Child and Adolescent Psychiatry, 48*(5), 484–500. doi:10.1097/CHI.0b013e31819c23d0.

Morgan, P. L., Staff, J., Hillemeier, M. M., Farkas, G., Maczuga, S. (2013). Racial and ethnic disparities in ADHD diagnosis from kindergarten to eighth grade. *Pediatrics, 132*(1), 85–93. doi:10.1542/peds.2012-2390.

Muñoz-Silva, A., Lago-Urbano, R., & Sánchez-García, M. (2017). Family impact and parenting styles in families of children with ADHD. *Journal of Child and Family Studies, 26*, 2810–2823.

Nigg, J. T. (2013). Attention-deficit/hyperactivity disorder and adverse health outcomes. *Clinical Psychology Reviews, 33*(2), 215–228. https://doi.org/10.1016/j.cpr.2012.11.005.

O'Neill, S., Schneiderman, R. L., Rajendran, K., Marks, D. J., Halperin, J. M. (2014). Reliable ratings or reading tea leaves: Can parent, teacher, and clinician behavioral ratings of preschoolers predict ADHD at age six? *Journal of Abnormal Child Psychology, 42*(4), 623–634. doi: 10.1007/s10802-013-9802-4.

O'Neill, S., Rajendran, K., Mahbubani, S. M., Halperin, J. M. (2017). Preschool predictors of ADHD symptoms and impairment

during childhood and adolescence. *Current Psychiatry Reports, 19*(12), 95. doi: 10.1007/s11920-017-0853-z.

Owens, E. B., Cardoos, S. L., & Hinshaw, S. P. (2015). Developmental progression and gender differences among individuals with ADHD. In Barkley, R. A. (Ed.), *Attention-deficit hyperactivity disorder, fourth edition: A handbook for diagnosis & treatment* (pp. 223–255). The Guilford Press.

Paidipati, C. P., Deatrick, J. A., Eiraldi, R. B., Ulrich, C. M., Lane, J. M., Brawner, B. M. (2022). Caregivers' perspectives on the contextual influences within family management for ethnically diverse children with ADHD. *J Spec Pediatr Nurs., 27*(2), e12365. doi: 10.1111/jspn.12365.

Partain, P., White, J., & Hammerness, P. (2019). New stimulant formulations for pediatric attention-deficit/hyperactivity disorder: A case-based approach for the primary care provider. *Current Opinions in Pediatrics, 31*(1), 166–174. doi:10.1097/MOP.0000000000000718.

Pelham, W. E. Jr., Gnagy, E. M., Greenslade, K. E., Milich, R. (1992). Teacher ratings of DSM-III-R symptoms for the disruptive behavior disorders. *Journal of the American Academy of Child and Adolescent Psychiatry, 31*(2), 210–218. doi: 10.1097/00004583-199203000-00006. Erratum in: *J Am Acad Child Adolesc Psychiatry* 1992 Nov;31(6):1177.

Perrin, J. M., Friedman, R. A., Knilans, T. K. (2008). Black box working group; section on cardiology and cardiac surgery. Cardiovascular monitoring and stimulant drugs for attention-deficit/hyperactivity disorder. *Pediatrics, 122*(2), 451–453. doi: 10.1542/peds.2008-1573.

Pfiffner, L. J., & DuPaul, G. J. (2015). Treatment of ADHD in school settings. In Barkley, R. A. (Ed.), *Attention-deficit hyperactivity disorder, fourth edition: A handbook for diagnosis & treatment* (pp. 596–629). The Guilford Press.

Pliszka, S. (2007). AACAP Work Group on Quality Issues. Practice parameter for the assessment and treatment of children and adolescents with attention-deficit/hyperactivity disorder. *Journal of American Child and Adolescent Psychiatry, 46*(7), 894–921. https://doi.org/10.1097/chi.0b013e318054e724.

Price, A., Mitchell, S., Janssens, A., Eke, H., Ford, T., Newlove-Delgado, T. (2022). In transition with attention deficit hyperactivity disorder (ADHD): Children's services clinicians' perspectives on the role of information in healthcare transitions for young people with ADHD. *BMC Psychiatry, 22*(1), 251. doi: 10.1186/s12888-022-03813-6.

Pollak, Y., Dekkers, T. J., Shoham, R., & Huizenga, H. M. (2019). Risk-taking behavior in attention deficit/hyperactivity disorder (ADHD): A review of potential underlying mechanisms and of interventions. *Current Psychiatry Reports, 21*(5), 1–11. https://doi.org/10.1007/s11920-019-1019-y.

Posner, J., Polanczyk, G. V., & Sonuga-Barke, E. (2020). Attention-deficit hyperactivity disorder. *The Lancet, 395*(10222), 450–462. https://doi.org/10.1016/s0140-6736(19)33004-1.

Pringsheim, T., Hirsch, L., Gardner, D., Gorman, D. A. The pharmacological management of oppositional behaviour, conduct problems, and aggression in children and adolescents with attention-deficit hyperactivity disorder, oppositional defiant disorder, and conduct disorder: a systematic review and meta-analysis. Part 1: psychostimulants, alpha-2 agonists, and atomoxetine. *Can J Psychia* PMID: 25886655; PMCID: PMC4344946.

Rajaprakash, M., & Leppert, M. L. (2022). Attention-deficit/hyperactivity disorder. *Pediatric Review, 43*(3), 135–147. https://doi.org/10.1542/pir.2020-000612.

Reid, R., Trout, A. L., & Schartz, M. (2005). Self-regulation interventions for children with attention deficit/hyperactivity disorder. *Exceptional Child, 71*(4), 361–377.

Ricketts, E. J., Sturm, A., McMakin, D. L., McGuire, J. F., Tan, P. Z., Smalberg, F. B., McCracken, J. T., Colwell, C. S., Piacentini, J. (2018). Changes in sleep problems across attention-deficit/

hyperactivity disorder treatment: Findings from the multimodal treatment of attention-deficit/hyperactivity disorder study. *Journal of Child and Adolescent Psychopharmacology, 28*(10), 690–698. doi: 10.1089/cap.2018.0038.

Riddle, M. A., Yershova, K., Lazzaretto, D., Paykina, N., Yenokyan, G., Greenhill, L., Abikoff, H., Vitiello, B., Wigal, T., McCracken, J. T., Kollins, S. H., Murray, D. W., Wigal, S., Kastelic, E., McGough, J. J., dosReis, S., Bauzó-Rosario, A., Stehli, A., Posner, K. (2013). The preschool attention-deficit/ hyperactivity disorder treatment study (PATS) 6-year follow-up. *J Am Acad Child Adolesc Psychiatry. 52*(3), 264–278.e2. doi:10.1016/j.jaac.2012.12.007.

Robb, J. A., Sibley, M. H., Pelham, W. E. Jr., Foster, E. M., Molina, B. S., Gnagy, E. M., Kuriyan, A. B. (2011). The estimated annual cost of ADHD to the US education system. *School Mental Health, 3*(3), 169–177. doi: 10.1007/s12310-011-9057-6.

Roy, A., Garner, A. A., Epstein, J. N., Hoza, B., Nichols, J. Q., Molina, B. S. G., Swanson, J. M., Arnold, L. E., Hechtman, L. (2020). Effects of childhood and adult persistent attention-deficit/hyperactivity disorder on risk of motor vehicle crashes: Results from the multimodal treatment study of children with attention-deficit/hyperactivity disorder. *Journal of American Child and Adolescent Psychiatry, 59*(8), 952–963. doi:10.1016/j.jaac.2019.08.007.

Schoenfelder, E. N., & Kollins, S. H. (2016). Topical review: ADHD and health-risk behaviors: Toward prevention and health promotion. *Journal of Pediatric Psychology, 41*(7), 735–740. https://doi.org/10.1093/jpepsy/jsv162.

Shuai, L., Daley, D., Wang, Y. F., Zhang, J. S., Kong, Y. T., Tan, X., Ji, N. (2017). Executive function training for children with attention deficit hyperactivity disorder. *Chin Med J (Engl). 130*(5), 549–558. doi:10.4103/0366-6999.200541.

Searight, H. R., Robertson, K., Smith, T., Perkins, S., Searight, B. K. (2012). Complementary and alternative therapies for pediatric attention deficit hyperactivity disorder: A descriptive review. *ISRN Psychiatry, 2012,* 804127. doi: 10.5402/2012/804127.

Sexton, C. C., Gelhorn, H. L., Bell, J. A., Classi, P. M. (2012). The co-occurrence of reading disorder and ADHD: Epidemiology, treatment, psychosocial impact, and economic burden. *Journal of Learning Disabilities, 45*(6), 538–564. doi: 10.1177/0022219411407772.

Sheldrick, R. C., Henson, B. S., Merchant, S., Neger, E. N., Murphy, J. M., Perrin, E. C. (2012). The preschool pediatric symptom checklist (PPSC): Development and initial validation of a new social/emotional screening instrument. *Academic Pediatrics, 12*(5), 456–467. doi:10.1016/j.acap.2012.06.008.

Sonuga-Barke, E. J., Brandeis, D., Cortese, S., Daley, D., Ferrin, M., Holtmann, M., Stevenson, J., Danckaerts, M., van der Oord, S., Döpfner, M., Dittmann, R. W., Simonoff, E., Zuddas, A., Banaschewski, T., Buitelaar, J., Coghill, D., Hollis, C., Konofal, E., Lecendreux, M., Wong, I. C., Sergeant, J. (2013). European ADHD guidelines group. Nonpharmacological interventions for ADHD: Systematic review and meta-analyses of randomized controlled trials of dietary and psychological treatments. *American Journal of Psychiatry, 170*(3), 275–289. doi:10.1176/appi.ajp.2012.12070991.

Staff, A. I., van der Oord, S., Oosterlaan, J., Hornstra, R., Hoekstra, P. J., van den Hoofdakker, B. J., Luman, M. (2022). Effectiveness of specific techniques in behavioral teacher training for childhood ADHD behaviors: Secondary analyses of a randomized controlled microtrial. *Research on Child and Adolescent Psychopathology, 50*(7), 867–880. doi:10.1007/s10802-021-00892-z.

Stahl, S. M. (Ed.). (2013). *Stahl's essential psychopharmacology: Neuroscientific basis and practical applications* (4th ed.). Cambridge University Press.

Stein, M. A., Zulauf-McCurdy, C., & DelRosso, L. M. (2022). Attention deficit hyperactivity disorder medications and sleep. *Child and Adolescent Psychiatric Clinics of North America, 31*(3), 499–514. https://doi.org/10.1016/j.chc.2022.03.006.

Stern, A., Agnew-Blais, J. C., & Danese, A. (2020). Associations between ADHD and emotional problems from childhood to young adulthood: A longitudinal genetically sensitive study. *Journal of Child Psychology and Psychiatry, 61*(11), 1234–1242. https://doi.org/10.1111/jcpp.13217.

Swanson, J. M., Elliott, G. R., Greenhill, L. L., Wigal, T., Arnold, L. E., Vitiello, B., Hechtman, L., Epstein, J. N., Pelham, W. E., Abikoff, H. B., Newcorn, J. H., Molina, B. S. G., Hinshaw, S. P., Wells, K. C., Hoza, B., Jensen, P. S., Gibbons, R. D., Hur, K., Stehli, A., Davies, M., March, J. S., Conners, C. K., Caron, M., Volkow, N. D. (2007). Effects of stimulant medication on growth rates across 3 years in the MTA follow-up. *Journal of American Child and Adolescent Psychiatry, 46*(8), 1015–1027. doi:10.1097/chi.0b013e3180686d7e.

Swanson, J. M., Schuck, S., Porter, M. M., Carlson, C., Hartman, C. A., Sergeant, J. A., Clevenger, W., Wasdell, M., McCleary, R., Lakes, K., Wigal, T. (2012). Categorical and dimensional definitions and evaluations of symptoms of ADHD: History of the SNAP and the SWAN rating scales. *International Journal of Psychoeducational Assessments, 10*(1), 51–70.

Szobot, C., & Bukstein, O. (2008). Attention deficit hyperactivity disorder and substance use disorders. *Child adolesc Psychiatr Clin North Am, 17*(2), 309–323.

Taubin, D., Wilson, J. C., & Wilens, T. E. (2022). ADHD and substance use disorders in young people: Considerations for evaluation, diagnosis, and pharmacotherapy. *Child and Adolescent Psychiatric Clinics of North America, 31*(3), 515–530. https://doi.org/10.1016/j.chc.2022.01.005.

Theule, J., Wiener, J., Tannock, R., & Jenkins, J. M. (2013). Parenting stress in families of children with ADHD. *Journal of Emotional and Behavioral Disorders, 21*(1), 3–17. https://doi.org/10.1177/1063426610387433.

Thomas, R., Sanders, S., Doust, J., Beller, E., Glasziou, P. (2015). Prevalence of attention-deficit/hyperactivity disorder: A systematic review and meta-analysis. *Pediatrics, 135*(4), e994–e1001. doi:10.1542/peds.2014-3482. Epub 2015 Mar 2. PMID: 25733754.

Tung, I., Li, J. J., Meza, J. I., Jezior, K. L., Kianmahd, J. S. V., Hentschel, P. G., O'Neil, P. M., & Lee, S. S. (2016). Patterns of comorbidity among girls with ADHD: A meta-analysis. *Pediatrics, 138*(4). https://doi.org/10.1542/peds.2016-0430.

US Department of Education (2019). https://sites.ed.gov/idea.

van Amsterdam, J., van der Velde, B., Schulte, M., & van den Brink, W. (2018). Causal factors of increased smoking in ADHD: A systematic review. *Substance Use & Misuse, 53*(3), 432–445. https://doi.org/10.1080/10826084.2017.1334066.

Van der Oord, S., & Tripp, G. (2020). How to improve behavioral parent and teacher training for children with ADHD: Integrating empirical research on learning and motivation into treatment. *Clinical Child and Family Psychology Review, 23*(4), 577–604. https://doi.org/10.1007/s10567-020-00327-z.

Visser, S. N., Zablotsky, B., Holbrook, J. R., Danielson, M. L., Bitsko, R. H. (2015). Diagnostic experiences of children with attention-deficit/hyperactivity disorder. *National Health Statistics Reports*, (81), 1–7.

Vitiello, B. (2008). Understanding the risk of using medications for attention deficit hyperactivity disorder with respect to physical growth and cardiovascular function. *Child Adolesc Clin North Am, 17*(2), 459–474.

Voigt, R. G., Llorente, A. M., Jensen, C. L., Fraley, J. K., Berretta, M. C., Heird, W. C. (2001). A randomized, double-blind, placebo-controlled trial of docosahexaenoic acid supplementation in children with attention-deficit/hyperactivity disorder. *Journal of Pediatrics, 139*(2), 189–196. doi:10.1067/mpd.2001.116050.

Wilens, T. E., Martelon, M., Joshi, G., Bateman, C., Fried, R., Petty, C., Biederman, J. (2011). Does ADHD predict substance-use disorders? A 10-year follow-up study of young adults with

ADHD. *Journal of American Child and Adolescent Psychiatry, 50*(6), 543–553. doi:10.1016/j.jaac.2011.01.021.

Wilens, T. E., Woodward, D. W., Ko, J. D., Berger, A. F., Burke, C., Yule, A. M. (2022). The impact of pharmacotherapy of childhood-onset psychiatric disorders on the development of substance use disorders. *Journal of Child and Adolescent Psychopharmacology, 32*(4), 200–214. doi:10.1089/cap.2022.0016.

Williams, A. E., Giust, J. M., Kronenberger, W. G., & Dunn, D. W. (2016). Epilepsy and attention-deficit hyperactivity disorder: Links, risks, and challenges. *Neuropsychiatric Disease Treatment, 12,* 287–296. https://doi.org/10.2147/NDT.S81549.

Wolraich, M. L., Hagan, J. F., & Allan, C. (2019). Clinical practice guideline for the diagnosis, evaluation, and treatment of attention-deficit/hyperactivity disorder in children and adolescents. *Pediatrics, 144*(4), e20192528. https://doi.org/10.1542/peds.2019-2528.

Wolraich, M. L., Lambert, W., Doffing, M. A., Bickman, L., Simmons, T., Worley, K. (2003). Psychometric properties of the Vanderbilt ADHD diagnostic parent rating scale in a referred population. *Journal of Pediatric Psychology, 28*(8), 559–567. doi:10.1093/jpepsy/jsg046.

Wu, J., Li, P., Luo, H., & Lu, Y. (2022). Complementary and alternative medicine use by ADHD patients: A systematic review. *Journal of Attention Disorders,* 10870547221111557. Advanced online publication. https://doi.org/10.1177/10870547221111557.

Zablotsky, B., Black, L. I., Maenner, M. J., Schieve, L. A., Danielson, M. L., Bitsko, R. H., Blumberg, S. J., Kogan, M. D., Boyle, C. A. (2019). Prevalence and trends of developmental disabilities among children in the United States: 2009–2017. *Pediatrics, 144*(4), e20190811. doi:10.1542/peds.2019-0811.

Zayats, T., & Neale, B. M. (2020). Recent advances in understanding of attention deficit hyperactivity disorder (ADHD): How genetics are shaping our conceptualization of this disorder. *F1000Research, 8,* 2060. https://doi.org/10.12688/f1000research.18959.2.

10 Autism Spectrum Disorder

Cy Nadler, Melissa Campbell, July Jean Cuevas, Elizabeth Hastings, Jamie Neal Lewis, Jo Ann Youngblood

INTRODUCTION

Autism was not always a familiar term for pediatric primary care providers. However, escalating prevalence rates, expanded scientific investigation, public advocacy, and even reality TV has vaulted autism into professional and public awareness. Increased awareness and research advances have brought other changes, including how the medical profession defines autism, the implications of a diagnosis, and multifaceted perspectives from within the autism community. Even the terms used are experiencing evolution. Person-first language (i.e., "a person with autism") is still the default in medical contexts, putting the person first before the disability. However, it is important to acknowledge that most adult self-advocates prefer identity-first language (i.e., "autistic person") because autism is a core part of who they are. Other commonly applied medical and behavioral terms may also carry stigma (Dwyer et al., 2022). Respect for the preferences of individuals and families is paramount, with immense variability in how youth on the spectrum present their associated health and behavioral challenges, and vital for supporting their transitions to adulthood. The role of a pediatric primary care provider is not to be an autism expert—instead, it is to help patients and their families navigate their journeys by building foundational knowledge and awareness of the resources available. By continuing to seek out new knowledge, health care providers can learn from the patients and families and be well positioned to meet the clinical needs of youth on the autism spectrum.

ETIOLOGY

GENETIC FACTORS

The etiology of autism spectrum disorder (ASD) is complex and not completely understood in large part because there appear to be many causal and contributing factors (and their interactions) that can increase the likelihood of a person receiving an ASD diagnosis. Genetics plays a leading role, but there is no single autism gene. Numerous rare genetic variations (inherited, de novo mutations, and copy number variations) related to autism have been identified, but these variations account for only approximately 20% of ASD cases (Savatt & Myers, 2021).

Evidence is also beginning to suggest that the cumulative effect of multiple genetic variants (polygenetic risk) plays an important role in risk for ASD as well as other neurodevelopmental disorders and psychiatric disorders; in fact, some of the same genetic pathways appear to increase the risk for a range of conditions, including ASD (Jansen et al., 2020). There is also significant heritability in ASD, with estimates in the range of 64% to 91% (Tick et al., 2016). When one child in a family is diagnosed with ASD, rates of diagnosis for subsequent siblings are between 8% and 17% higher than for youth without this family history (Hansen et al., 2019).

There is significant variation in the phenotype and genetic variations found in ASD, which suggests a multifactorial etiology in most cases. Disruptions of common biologic pathways have also been associated with ASD, including chromatin remodeling, synaptic cell adhesion, scaffolding, neuronal signaling, and development (Jiang et al., 2022). Evidence for gene-environment interactions is also emerging, including interactions between specific gene variants and prenatal exposure to air pollution, ASD-associated copy number variants, and maternal prenatal infection (Lyall et al., 2017). Epigenetic mechanisms (related to the molecular information that regulates cell processes such as imprinting and gene expression) are also under investigation. These may help explain gene-environmental interactions or associations with environmental exposures (Srancikova et al., 2021). Three genetic syndromes (Rett syndrome, fragile X, and Angelman syndrome) are caused by epigenetic dysregulation and are associated with ASD.

ENVIRONMENTAL FACTORS

Environmental risks are also thought to play a role in the etiology of ASD. Advanced parental age is associated with slight increases in the likelihood of ASD (Janecka et al., 2019) as well as a shortened interpregnancy interval (e.g., <12 months between children) (Lyall et al., 2017). Prenatal nutrition has been evaluated as a possible factor, and periconceptional folic acid supplementation has been associated with a decreased likelihood of ASD (Friel et al., 2021). Prenatal exposure to maternal medications is also an area of ongoing research. While there is conflicting evidence regarding selective serotonin reuptake inhibitor (SSRI) use, prenatal exposure to antiepileptic medications and beta$_2$-adrenergic receptor antagonists has been associated with an increased likelihood of ASD (Janecka et al., 2018). Moreover, premature birth is associated with an increased likelihood of subsequent ASD diagnosis (as well as other developmental concerns), which may reflect a range of interacting contributory factors (McGowan & Sheinkopf, 2021). Importantly, all these findings are primarily drawn from large observational datasets that are not always able to control for other factors that may explain associations with ASD (e.g., maternal depression itself may increase the likelihood of ASD diagnosis, potentially explaining why SSRI use also has a small association) (Hagberg et al., 2018).

Immune factors are an environmental factor of interest, although this pathway is not completely understood. Children born to mothers hospitalized with an infection (bacterial or viral) during their pregnancy were more likely to have ASD (Zerbo et al., 2015). Maternal autoimmune disorders may also play a role, but this is not well understood at this time. Endocrine-disrupting chemicals (EDCs), which interfere in the activity of hormones critical to neurodevelopment, have also been evaluated as a risk factor for ASD, but what if any role EDCs play in the development of ASD is still unclear (Moosa et al., 2018). EDC exposure is ubiquitous, but there has been conflicting evidence for prenatal pesticide exposures and polychlorinated biphenyls (industrial products and chemicals). Exposure to bisphenol A has not been associated with an increased risk of ASD.

This review of etiologic considerations cannot conclude without mention of vaccines (specifically the measles-mumps-rubella [MMR] vaccine). Concerns emerged in the late 1990s based on a small case study that was eventually retracted because (per the journal's editor) "it was utterly clear, without any ambiguity at all, that the statements in the paper were utterly false" (Qian et al., 2020). In lieu of other clear-cut explanations for autism at that time, fears proliferated leading to persistent vaccine hesitancy. Decades of rigorous research since then have not identified any positive associations between MMR vaccination and later ASD diagnosis; in fact, some studies show a slightly reduced likelihood for vaccinated children (DeStefano & Shimabukuro, 2019). Pediatric primary care providers need to be prepared to receive concerns and questions from families about this controversial area with confidence, calm, and concrete information about vaccine safety, as well as the unfortunately increasing health risks associated with delaying or forgoing critical vaccinations (Olson et al., 2020).

INCIDENCE AND PREVALENCE

CURRENT ESTIMATES

Many pediatric primary care providers (as well as parents and families) will be aware of the increasing rates of ASD diagnosis over the past several decades.

Of note, the incidence of ASD is rarely a focus given the challenges in following large cohorts to determine new-onset ASD within a given timeframe; as described later, variations in ASD presentation (as well as social determinants impacting access to diagnostic evaluation) lead to vastly different ages of initial identification of developmental differences that have their origins long before a formal diagnosis.

The Autism and Developmental Disabilities Monitoring (ADDM) Network is a Centers for Disease Control and Prevention (CDC)–funded program created to collect epidemiologic data on youth with ASD and other developmental disabilities from representative sites within the United States. Using an evolving chart review methodology that considers medical and school records, ADDM has produced estimates about every 2 years regarding the prevalence of ASD for 8-year-olds during a given surveillance year, beginning in 2000 (1 in 150 children); as of this chapter's publication, the most recent average estimate for ADDM sites was a prevalence of 23 per 1000 (1 in 44) for the 2018 surveillance year (Maenner et al., 2021). Notably, that composite estimate reflects significant variability among the reporting sites, from 16.5 per 1000 (Missouri) to 38.9 per 1000 (California). There is little reason to believe that such substantial regional differences are due to environmental factors; instead, it appears that differences in service delivery (including access to diagnostic evaluation centers) are a major driver in regional prevalence differences.

CONTRIBUTING FACTORS

Why has the observed prevalence tripled in the last 20 years? Methodologic changes are important to consider. First, revisions to the diagnostic criteria for ASD have shifted and broadened the study population. Specifically, the fifth edition of the *Diagnostic and Statistical Manual of Mental Disorders* (DSM-5; American Psychiatric Association [APA], 2013) combined multiple previous categories (including autistic disorder, Asperger syndrome, and pervasive developmental disorder not otherwise specified) into a single ASD code. This change is caused by a lack of consistency in differentiating the separate categories.

The updated DSM allowed for criteria that can be met currently or by history and were tailored in part to capture younger children and individuals with mild symptoms that would not have been captured in previous editions (Table 10.1). Youth with ASD who do not have cooccurring intellectual disability account for some of the largest prevalence increases over the last 20 years. Among other methodologic considerations, approaches for counting children in prevalence studies are also evolving, and the proliferation of clinical and community identification of ASD and related developmental conditions, directly and indirectly, influences the observed prevalence rates in large cohort studies (Fombonne, 2018). Recommendations for universal

Table 10.1 Severity Levels for Autism Spectrum Disorder (Examples of Level Of Support Needs)

SEVERITY LEVEL	SOCIAL COMMUNICATION	RESTRICTED, REPETITIVE BEHAVIORS
Level 3 "Requiring very substantial support"	Severe deficits in verbal and nonverbal social communication skills cause severe impairments in functioning, very limited initiation of social interactions, and minimal response to social overtures from others. For example, a person with few words of intelligible speech who rarely initiates interaction and, when he or she does, makes unusual approaches to meet needs only and responds to only very direct social approaches.	Inflexibility of behavior, extreme difficulty coping with change, or other restricted/repetitive behaviors markedly interfere with functioning in all spheres. Great distress/difficulty changing focus or action.
Level 2 "Requiring substantial support"	Marked deficits in verbal and nonverbal social communication skills; social impairments apparent even with supports in place; limited initiation of social interactions; and reduced or abnormal responses to social overtures from others. For example, a person who speaks simple sentences, whose interaction is limited to narrow special interests, and who has markedly odd nonverbal communication.	Inflexibility of behavior, difficulty coping with change, or other restricted/repetitive behaviors appear frequently enough to be obvious to the casual observer and interfere with functioning in a variety of contexts. Distress and/or difficulty changing focus or action.
Level 1 "Requiring support"	Without supports in place, deficits in social communication cause noticeable impairments. Difficulty initiating social interactions, and clear examples of atypical or unsuccessful responses to social overtures of others. May appear to have decreased interest in social interactions. For example, a person who is able to speak in full sentences and engages in communication but whose to-and-fro conversation with others fails, and whose attempts to make friends are odd and typically unsuccessful.	Inflexibility of behavior causes significant interference with functioning in one or more contexts. Difficulty switching between activities. Problems of organization and planning hamper independence.

From the *Diagnostic and Statistical Manual of Mental Disorders* (DSM-5-TR). (2022). American Psychological Association.

screening for ASD in primary care by the American Academy of Pediatrics (AAP; described later) have also contributed substantially to increased awareness and identification (Hyman et al., 2020).

ASD has historically been identified in males compared to females, with estimates typically close to 4:1 (Maenner et al., 2021). Compelling evidence suggests that females who might otherwise meet the criteria for a diagnosis tend to be diagnosed later and that the accurate male-to-female sex ratio may be closer to 3:1 (Loomes et al., 2017). Studies have shown that females on the spectrum with no intellectual impairment or language delays demonstrate subtle characteristics of social and communication difficulties that may be less likely to prompt referral or diagnosis (Rubenstein et al., 2015). Recent data suggest that commonly used diagnostic tools may systematically exclude females from ASD research (D'Mello et al., 2022).

IDENTIFICATION AND DIAGNOSTIC ASSESSMENT

SCREENING IN PRIMARY CARE

The AAP recommends that pediatric primary care providers engage in continuous developmental surveillance at well-child visits, which includes reviewing the child's developmental history, eliciting concerns from the family, and observing the child. Many developmental resources are available for use in primary care, including the AAP's Bright Futures and CDC Milestones Tracker smartphone application. Developmental surveillance for ASD includes asking about social-emotional milestones, such as responding to name by 12 months, pointing to show interest in an object, making eye contact, preferring to be alone, delayed language, or making repetitive movements such as flapping hands, rocking, or spinning in circles. Providers should always ask families about any regression in developmental skills; if a parent reports regression in skills, this should be fully evaluated (Hyman et al., 2020).

Some misconceptions about language development in children may influence how health care providers manage concerns about developmental delays (Feldman, 2019). Children raised in a bilingual household can learn both languages, even children with delays such as trisomy 21. These children may have a smaller vocabulary in each language at a given time, but their vocabularies in both languages are comparable to children exposed only to one language. Another common myth is that males learn language slower than females and will catch up if given enough time; males experience higher rates of both speech and language disorders and ASD, so any concerns about delayed language in males and females should be evaluated and treated. Another cultural belief is that later-born children may appear to have delayed language because their older siblings talk for them. Children who are not firstborn may experience less adult-generated language directed toward them but have the benefit of experiencing conversations between adults and their older siblings (as well as their older siblings as role models); later-born children acquire language at the same age as firstborn children and should be referred for evaluation if language delays are a concern (Feldman, 2019).

Surveillance alone is not enough to identify children who need further evaluation, and the AAP recommends using standardized screening tools to identify these children. The AAP recommends universal developmental screening during well-child visits at 9, 18, and 30 months and specific autism screening at ages 18, 24, and 30 months (Hyman et al., 2020) (Fig. 10.1). For autism screening, the Modified Checklist for Autism in Toddlers (Robins et al., 2014) is one of the most used tools for meeting the AAP screening guideline. The Parent's Observation of Social Interaction (POSI) tool is widely used (Smith et al., 2013). The POSI can also be embedded within a general developmental screening tool called the Survey of Well-being in Young Children (Sheldrick & Perrin, 2013), which covers cognitive, language, and motor milestones. Other commonly used general developmental screening tools that are well suited for primary care include the Ages and Stages Questionnaires (Squires et al., 2009) and Parents' Evaluation of Developmental Status (PEDS) (Glascoe, 2000).

The screening tools focus primarily on early core social communication deficits. Screening tests are not diagnostic but help identify which children require further evaluation for their symptoms. When a screen yields a concern, the pediatric primary care provider should refer the child for further evaluation and intervention. A specific diagnosis is not required for children to receive services through early intervention (birth up to 3 years) or local public school districts (≥3 years). Simultaneous referral for evaluation and services is highly recommended, as this will help the child begin receiving services as quickly as possible. Note that early screening does not always identify children with more subtle presentations of ASD or those who do not have early cognitive delays. Children with milder symptoms may not be identified until elementary school age when their social skills, communication abilities, and behavioral rigidities interfere with their daily functioning. While validated screening tools exist

Commonly used ASD screening tests

Autism screening tests	Description	Age range	Average No. items	Administration time	Forms available EHR compatible	Psychometric properties	Scoring method	Cultural considerations	Source	Key references
M-CHAT-R/F	Parent-completed questionnaire designed to identify children at risk for autism from the general Population; follow-up clinician administered questions and repeat questionnaire required for specificity	16–30 mo	20	5–10 min	Yes	Standardization sample included 16071 children screened; 115 had positive screen results, 348 needed evaluation, 221 were evaluated, and 105 diagnosed with an ASD; validated by using the ADI-R, ADOS-G, CARS, and DSM-IV-TR; sensitivity: 0.91; specificity: 0.95 for low-risk 18- and 24-mo-old children with follow-up questionnaire and interview; 45% of children with a score ≥3 on the initial screen and ≥2 on follow-up had ASD; 95% had clinically significant developmental delay	Risk categorization for questionnaire (pass/need interview/ fail); after interview (pass/fail)	Available in multiple languages; see test information for details	http://mchat screen.com/	Ref 51
SCQ	Parent-completed questionnaire; designed to identify children at risk for ASD from the general population; based on items in the ADI-R	4 + y	40	5–10 min	No	Validated by using the ADI-R and DSM-IV on 200 subjects (160 with pervasive developmental disorder, 40 without pervasive developmental disorder); for use in children with mental age of at	Risk categorization (pass/fail)	Available in multiple languages; see test information for details.	Western Psychological Corporation: www. wpspublish.com	Refs 77 and 572

Fig. 10.1 **Commonly used autism spectrum disorder screening tests.** (From Hyman, S.L., Levy, S.E., Myers, S.M., et al. [2020]. Identification, evaluation, and management of children with autism spectrum disorder. *Pediatrics*, 145[1]. Copyright 2022, American Psychiatric Association. All rights reserved.)

Continued

Autism screening tests	Description	Age range	Average No. items	Administration time	Forms available EHR compatible	Psychometric properties	Scoring method	Cultural considerations	Source	Key references
						least 2 y and chronologic age 4+ y; available in 2 forms: lifetime and current. overall test: sensitivity: 0.85 (moderate), specificity: 0.75 (moderate); sensitivity can be improved with lowering cutoff for children younger than 5 y and 5–7 y, specificity poor for younger children				
STAT	Clinician-directed, interactive, and observation measure; requires training of clinician for standardized administration; not for population screening	24–35 mo; <24 mo (exploratory)	12	20–30 min	No	Validated by comparison with ADOS-G results in 52 children 24–35 mo (26 with autism, 26 with developmental delay); sensitivity: 0.83, specificity: 0.86, PPV: 0.77, NPV: 0.90, for <24 mo: sensitivity: 0.95, specificity: 0.73, PPV: 0.56, NPV: 0.97; screening properties improved for children > 14 mo	12 activities to observe early social-communicative behaviour; risk categorization (high risk/low risk)	English	http://stat.vueinnovations.com/	Refs 573 and 574
Promising autism screening tests the infant/toddler checklist (Communication and symbolic behavior scales developmental profile)	Parent questionnaire: screens for language delay	6–24 mo	24	15 min	No	PPV DD: 0.43 (6–8 mo); PPV DD: 0.79 (21–24 mo)	Identifies language delays (alone/ with ASD); risk for ASD; risk status for social speech, symbolic composites, and total score	Available in multiple languages; see test information for details	Paul H. Brookes Publishing CO Inc: 800-638-3775 or www.brookespublishing.com	Ref 59
Early screening for autism and communication disorders	Parent questionnaire; research edition 47 items	12–36 mo	47	10-15 min	No	Sensitivity: 0.85–0.91; specificity: 0.82–0.84; PPV: 0.55–0.81;NPV: 0.88–0.98	Investigation ongoing of subset (24 items)	English	https://firstwordsproject.com.screen-my-child/	Not in peer-reviewed literature
First-year inventory	Parent questionnaire; promising in high risk population to identify risk in 12-mo-old infants	12 mo	63	10 min	No	Sensitivity, specificity, PPV not reported	Scores at risk; promising in high-risk (infant sibling) cohort (Rowberry et al 575)	English	https://www.med.unc.edu/ahs/pearls/research/first-year-inventory-fyi-development/	Ref 575
Parent's observation of social interactions	Parent questionnaire used to assess autism risk; ASD screening included on 18–24, and 30-mo The Survey of Well-Being of Young Children forms	16–35 mo	7	~5 min	Available through patient tools, epic, and CHADIS; available for free download as pdfs from www.theswyc.org	Sensitivity: 83%–93% average 88.5% specificity: 42%–75% average 56.9%	3 of 7 symptoms in at-risk range	Available in multiple languages; see test information for details	Free download from www.theswyc.org	Publications and User's Manual available at www.theswyc.org; Refs 576 and 577
Rapid interactive screening test for autism in toddlers 13	Clinician observation: administered by trained examiner	12–36 mo	9 interactive items	20–30 min	No	Cutoff >15; sensitivity: 1; specificity: 0.84; PPV: 0.88; NPV: 0.94; needs further study in larger samples	9 interactive activities; total score summed, cutoff score of 15 (for that sample)	English	https://umassmed.edu/AutismRITA-T/about-the-test/	Ref 578

The AAP does not approve/endorse any specific tool for screening purposes. This table is not exhaustive, and other tests may be avilable ADOS-G, Autism Diagnostic Observation Schedule – Generic; CARS, Childhood Autism Rating Scale; CHADIS, Comprehensive Health and Decision Information System; EHR, electronic health record; ICD-10, *Internatoinal Classification of Diseases, 10th revision:* IMFAR, International Meeting fot Autism Research; NPV, negative predictive value; PPV, positive predictive value.

Fig. 10.1 cont'd

for children older than 30 months, they are not typically used in primary care settings (Hyman et al., 2020).

Any child with a concern elicited by either surveillance or screening should be referred for intervention and evaluation. Wait-and-see approaches have consistently resulted in delayed identification and access to care, so prolonged monitoring for developmental progress rather than referral is not recommended. It is critical for pediatric primary care providers to explicitly engage families in conversation about concerns as they are identified (via screening, surveillance, or other means). By engaging in direct communication about possible developmental differences, providing education about what supports families can access, and demystifying the possible outcomes of further assessment, caregivers can be empowered to advocate and support their children. Demonstrating comfort with the possibility that a child needs evaluation and support will model for families that such diagnostic possibilities do not fundamentally change who their child is; these categories help ensure that children receive the proper care and have all the support they need to remain happy and healthy.

HEALTH DISPARITIES

Like other areas of health care, research on the early identification of autism and timely delivery of quality support has revealed historical and ongoing health disparities. Children from minoritized families, families with lower incomes, families who speak languages other than English, and families in rural areas often experience delayed access to ASD diagnosis (Aylward et al., 2021). Among other factors, inconsistent adherence to primary care screening and referral guidelines may contribute to delayed identification (Wallis et al., 2020). Unfortunately, these disparities likely contribute to and exacerbate a range of later inequalities in access to treatment and supportive services for children of Black, Hispanic, and Asian descent and children from low-income families (Aylward et al., 2021; Carbone et al., 2020). Stigma regarding the diagnosis of ASD also remains, as does the uncertainty of how the diagnostic process works in some communities. Unfortunately, later identification and reduced access to care (including due to language and logistic barriers such as child care and transportation) contribute to poor health and developmental outcomes (Aylward et al., 2021). Pediatric primary care providers help ensure that families of children with identified ASD concerns receive diagnostic support in a timely fashion and that proactive support and community partnerships can be critical for mitigating these disparities (Feinberg et al., 2021; Kuhn et al., 2021).

DIAGNOSTIC CRITERIA

Diagnostic evaluation for possible ASD is purely clinical; there are no biologic or imaging tests used to confirm the diagnosis (Hyman et al., 2020). The diagnosis is confirmed or ruled out through a comprehensive developmental evaluation that includes direct observations, a thorough diagnostic interview to obtain information about the developmental history and current functioning, and standardized testing to evaluate the language, adaptive, and cognitive/developmental abilities (Hyman et al., 2020). Information gathered through the evaluation process is then used to determine whether the child (or adult) meets the diagnostic criteria for ASD in the DSM (Box 10.1). The ASD-specific features within social communication (SC) and restricted/repetitive behavior (RRB) might be ascertainable for some children using a more streamlined evaluation. Addressing all the developmental areas noted increases confidence in the diagnosis and the appropriate specifiers, including a descriptive rating of the child's current level of support needed within the SC and RRB domains.

In most cases, individuals who meet the criteria for an ASD diagnosis will continue to do so across their lifespan (although their presentation and support needs will undoubtedly change over time). Similarly, in cases where children have been rigorously evaluated and found not to meet the criteria for ASD, their diagnostic status may remain unchanged, and reevaluations might be appropriate and recommended if the initial evaluation occurred when the child was very young. As noted, females and Black, Hispanic, and other minoritized youth may be at higher risk for delayed identification. In some cases, a child who did not initially meet the criteria may not have made the same social, communication, or behavioral gains observed in same-age peers over several years following an initial evaluation, which may signal a need to reconsider ASD.

After a child has received an ASD diagnosis, repeated diagnostic assessments related to ASD are rarely warranted. In most cases the true areas of interest are related to the child's cognitive, achievement, or mental health needs, and these assessments may or may not be available from the source of a child's original ASD diagnosis.

DIAGNOSTIC TOOLS

Because of the nuances of presentation in ASD, using standardized tools to identify and document an individual's clinical phenotype is considered the best practice. That could include using a structured interview that relies on research-derived scoring algorithms, such as the Autism Diagnostic Interview-Revised (Rutter et al., 2003). It could include using a questionnaire (completed by a parent, teacher, or other informant) that rates the target child's difficulties in SC and RRB areas, such as the Social Responsiveness Scale (Constantino & Gruber, 2012). Some health care providers will use a standardized rating tool such as the

Box 10.1 Autism Spectrum Disorder

DIAGNOSTIC CRITERIA

A. Persistent deficits in social communication and social interaction across multiple contexts, as manifested by all of the following, currently or by history (examples are illustrative, not exhaustive; see text):

1. Deficits in social-emotional reciprocity, ranging, for example, from abnormal social approach and failure of normal back-and-forth conversation; to reduced sharing of interests, emotions, or affect; to failure to initiate or respond to social interactions.
2. Deficits in nonverbal communicative behaviors used for social interaction, ranging, for example, from poorly integrated verbal and nonverbal communication; to abnormalities in eye contact and body language or deficits in understanding and use of gestures; to a total lack of facial expressions and nonverbal communication.
3. Deficits in developing, maintaining, and understanding relationships, ranging, for example, from difficulties adjusting behavior to suit various social contexts; to difficulties in sharing imaginative play or in making friends; to absence of interest in peers.

B. Restricted, repetitive patterns of behavior, interests, or activities, as manifested by at least two of the following, currently or by history (examples are illustrative, not exhaustive; see text):

1. Stereotyped or repetitive motor movements, use of objects, or speech (e.g., simple motor stereotypies, lining up toys or flipping objects, echolalia, idiosyncratic phrases).
2. Insistence on sameness, inflexible adherence to routines, or ritualized patterns of verbal or nonverbal behavior (e.g., extreme distress at small changes, difficulties with transitions, rigid thinking patterns, greeting rituals, need to take same route or eat same food every day).
3. Highly restricted, fixated interests that are abnormal in intensity or focus (e.g., strong attachment to or preoccupation with unusual objects, excessively circumscribed or perseverative interests).
4. Hyper- or hyporeactivity to sensory input or unusual interest in sensory aspects of the environment (e.g., apparent indifference to pain/temperature, adverse response to specific sounds or textures, excessive smelling or touching of objects, visual fascination with lights or movement).

C. Symptoms must be present in the early developmental period (but may not become fully manifest until social demands exceed limited capacities, or may be masked by learned strategies in later life).

D. Symptoms cause clinically significant impairment in social, occupational, or other important areas of current functioning.

E. These disturbances are not better explained by intellectual development disorder (intellectual disability) or global developmental delay. Intellectual developmental disorder and autism spectrum disorder frequently co-occur; to make comorbid diagnoses of autism spectrum disorder and intellectual developmental disorder, social communication should be below that expected for general developmental level.

Note: Individuals with a well-established DSM-IV diagnosis of autistic disorder, Asperger's disorder, or pervasive developmental disorder not otherwise specified should be given the diagnosis of autism spectrum disorder. Individuals who have marked deficits in social communication, but whose symptoms do not otherwise meet criteria for autism spectrum disorder, should be evaluated for social (pragmatic) communication disorder.

- *Specify* current severity based on social communication impairments and restricted, repetitive patterns of behavior:
  - Requiring very substantial support
  - Requiring substantial support
  - Requiring support
- *Specify* if:
  - With or without accompanying intellectual impairment
  - With or without accompanying language impairment
- *Specify* if:
  - Associated with a known genetic or other medical condition or environmental factor (Coding note: Use additional code to identify the associated genetic or other medical condition.)
  - Associated with a neurodevelopmental, mental, or behavioral problem
- *Specify* if:
  - With catatonia (refer to the criteria for catatonia associated with another mental disorder, p. 135, for definition) (Coding note: Use additional code F06.1 catatonia associated with autism spectrum disorder to indicate the presence of the comorbid catatonia.)

DSM-5, Diagnostic and Statistical Manual of Mental Disorders, Fifth Edition.
From American Psychiatric Association. (2022). *Diagnostic and statistical manual of mental disorders* (5th ed., text rev.).

Childhood Autism Rating Scale (Schopler et al., 2010) to help them integrate their direct behavioral observations with the gathered history, other test scores, and collateral information.

Frequently, health care providers will use a tool that standardizes the observational context and helps them elicit and categorize their direct observations of a child. The gold standard measure is the Autism Diagnostic Observation Schedule (ADOS-2) (Lord et al., 2012). The ADOS involves presenting a series of social activities, play, and leisure items, as well as varying levels of communication presses that provide opportunities to observe an individual's social response patterns, verbal and nonverbal communication style, behavioral flexibility, interests, and repetitive or sensory-related behaviors. Trained administrators select a module or version of the ADOS based on the child's (or adult's) language level so that the test experience is comfortable for the participant and does not overly tax the participant's verbal communication abilities (which are not part of the DSM diagnostic criteria for ASD). The module for toddlers and individuals with no more than single-word speech involves commonly encountered play items, eating a snack, looking at a book, and other familiar routines. The module for individuals with phrase-level speech starts to integrate more conversational presses and creative activities. Finally, the modules for youth and adults with fluent (full-sentence) verbal communication add opportunities to sample the person's understanding of social relationships and emotional experiences. Administration of the ADOS typically lasts about 45 minutes, at which time the examiner will code detailed observations using a research-supported algorithm.

Pediatric primary care providers should keep in mind that no single test is sufficient for confirming a diagnosis of ASD. Multidisciplinary diagnostic teams are commonly employed to ensure a thorough evaluation considering all development and behavior aspects (Hyman et al., 2020). Given the significant demand for evaluation services, workforce shortages (especially in rural areas), and emerging science around efficient diagnostic practices (Zwaigenbaum & Warren, 2021), multidisciplinary teams are also not required unless regional or insurance requirements dictate otherwise. The team typically begins with the primary care provider and referrals to include developmental-behavioral pediatricians, neurologists, psychologists, and other providers with training related to ASD. Regional differences exist regarding what professional credentials are required to diagnose ASD via state or insurance regulations. Pediatric and primary care nurse practitioners who care for pediatric patients are among the professions approved in many regions and are well positioned to participate as part of the team.

While no specific test is necessary or sufficient from a clinical perspective, insurance providers increasingly require specific tests to verify an ASD diagnosis before authorizing certain treatment or other supportive services, including applied behavioral analysis (ABA). However, identified developmental delays (even without a specific diagnosis) will qualify children for state-administered early intervention programs (<3 years of age). Most allied health interventions (speech therapy, occupational therapy, etc.) will not require an ASD diagnosis.

DIFFERENTIAL DIAGNOSIS AND COOCCURRING PSYCHIATRIC/DEVELOPMENTAL CONDITIONS

One factor that makes ASD diagnostic evaluations complex is the need to ensure that other developmental and mental health conditions do not better account for the presenting features. Diagnosticians must also ensure that these very same conditions are not overshadowed due to the clear presence of ASD. Providers should be wary about assuming that a newly emerging problem is just the autism rather than something else that requires the attention and trust of the families and youth they serve when they report concerns.

About 46% of preschool-aged youth with ASD meet the criteria for global developmental delay (i.e., delays in multiple areas of development, such as fine/gross motor, receptive/expressive language) (Christensen et al., 2016). By age 8, about 35% of youth with ASD will continue to have substantial delays that merit a diagnosis of intellectual disability (Maenner et al., 2021). Language delays (expressive, receptive, articulation, etc.) commonly lead to positive ASD screens but also frequently cooccur with ASD; prevalence estimates vary in part because of overlapping diagnostic criteria.

Up to 94% of individuals with ASD have at least one cooccurring psychiatric condition, and almost 40% have at least two cooccurring conditions (Hossain et al., 2020). Thus when a patient presenting in primary care has been diagnosed or suspected of ASD, health care providers should continuously monitor for comorbidities that may emerge. Table 10.2 shows estimated ranges of cooccurrence for the most common psychiatric conditions associated with ASD, including attention-deficit/hyperactivity disorder (ADHD), disruptive behavior disorders, and anxiety disorders. Depending on a child's age, it may not be appropriate yet to definitively diagnose certain conditions (e.g., an extremely hyperactive 18-month-old may be at risk for

Table 10.2 Prevalence Estimates of Cooccurring Psychiatric and Developmental Conditions Among People With Autism Spectrum Disorder[a]

PSYCHIATRIC COMORBIDITY	ESTIMATED PREVALENCE RANGE
Anxiety disorders	1.47–54%
Attention-deficit/hyperactivity disorder	25.7–65%
Bipolar and mood disorders	5–33%
Depressive disorders	2.5–47.1%
Disruptive, impulse-control and conduct disorders	12–48%
Eating disorders	1.4–7.9%
Obsessive-compulsive and related disorders	9–22%
Schizophrenia spectrum/other psychotic disorders	4–67%
Substance use disorders	0.7–36%
Tourette syndrome/tic disorders	2.6–36%

[a]Data sources include youth and adults.
From Hossain, M.M., Khan, N., Sultana, A., Ma, P., McKyer, E.L.J., Ahmed, H.U., & Purohit. N. (2020). Prevalence of comorbid psychiatric disorders among people with autism spectrum disorder: An umbrella review of systematic reviews and meta-analyses. *Psychiatry Research*, 287, 112922.

a diagnosis of ADHD in the future but is too young at present to be diagnosed).

Keep in mind that cooccurring psychiatric conditions impose their own distinct (and likely interacting) risk factors for patients: for instance, up to 11% of youth with ASD experience a psychiatric hospitalization before adulthood that is typically driven by intense and dangerous behaviors directed toward themselves, others, and property (Siegel & Gabriels, 2013). Self-injurious behavior (SIB) is unfortunately common in people with ASD with and without intellectual disability (up to 50% and 12%, respectively) (Laverty et al., 2020). SIB refers to nonsuicidal, self-inflicted physical injury (e.g., hair pulling, head banging, skin picking). Distinct from nonsuicidal SIB, youth with ASD are also at heightened risk for suicidal ideation and behaviors. Estimates for suicide risk in youth with ASD range from 10.9% to 50%, and the risk extends into adulthood (Segers & Rawana, 2014). This increased risk is present for youth with and without cognitive delays. Health professionals should regularly screen for suicide and other safety risks using standardized screening tools when possible. When the risk is determined to be present, engage the patient and family/caregivers in safety planning. An essential part of safety planning is means restriction (i.e., temporarily limiting the individual's access to objects that could be used as lethal methods of suicide [knives, rope, firearms, medications] as well as objects or settings that may increase risk during SIB [sharps]). Multiple studies have shown that means restriction of a person at risk of suicide is effective in preventing suicide completion and reducing the lethality of attempts (Yip et al., 2012).

MEDICAL AND GENETIC EVALUATION

A complete etiologic evaluation after an ASD diagnosis is recommended, including a thorough physical exam, perinatal history, perinatal exposure to teratogens, and detailed family history, including three generations. Findings in physical exams and history obtained by parents can guide the next steps in the etiologic evaluation to avoid unnecessary tests. The medical evaluation to determine the etiology of an ASD diagnosis in children should include genetic testing. Identifying a genetic diagnosis provides clinicians and families with information about prognosis and recurrence risk that could help identify and, in some cases, prevent comorbid medical conditions (Hyman et al., 2020). A number of genetic conditions have been associated with a higher likelihood of ASD, including those discussed in this section.

Angelman syndrome is a neurodevelopmental disorder characterized by intellectual disability, motor dysfunction, speech impairment, hyperactivity, and seizures. The most common cause of Angelman syndrome is the loss of the maternally inherited *UBE3A* gene by deletion of the 15Q11-q13 region. Individuals with Angelman syndrome frequently have a cooccurring ASD diagnosis (Margolis et al., 2015).

Down syndrome is characterized by developmental delays and intellectual disability without a regression in skills. The most common cognitive deficits in children with Down syndrome are in the communication, language, and memory domains. Sociability is typically a strength in children with Down syndrome, with an increased prevalence of ASD (some estimates as high as 16%). A recent study showed that in children with Down syndrome and ASD, their social impairments were less than those with ASD alone, but their cognitive impairments were more significant than those with children with Down syndrome or ASD alone (Hamner et al., 2020).

Fragile X syndrome is the most common cause of inherited intellectual disability (causing 1–2% of intellectual disability) and is associated with ASD. Fragile X is characterized by a long face, prominent forehead and jaw, large ears, joint laxity, and macroorchidism in males (after puberty) and is caused by a trinucleotide expansion of the *FMR1* gene. Of those with fragile X, 60% to 74% meet the criteria for ASD (Hyman et al., 2020; Mila et al., 2018).

Rett syndrome is a degenerative neurodevelopmental disorder caused by a mutation in the *MECP2* gene (Hyman et al., 2020; Neul, 2022). Rett syndrome is characterized by typical development until approximately 6 to 18 months, when children enter stage 1 (stagnation), fail to make developmental progression at the expected rate, and begin to show developmental delays. During stage 2, regression starts between age 1 and 4 years, and these children lose purposeful hand use, develop hand stereotypies (repetitive movements), and lose expressive language skills. Some children also become more socially withdrawn at this stage. Following this is stage 3, the plateau where developmental regression ceases, and some developmental skills are regained, but language and purposeful hand movements are not often regained.

Tuberous sclerosis is a genetic disorder caused by a mutation in the *TSC1* or *TSC2* gene with a clinical presentation of hypopigmented macules, angiofibromas, shagreen patches (connective tissue nevi), brain tubers, ungual fibromas, cardiac rhabdomyomas, and retinal hamartomas and is associated with ASD. There is an increased prevalence of ASD in patients with tuberous sclerosis (26–45%). There is a higher risk of ASD in children with the *TSC2* mutation, with early-onset or refractory seizures, and location, type, and size of brain lesions (Hyman et al., 2020; Specchio et al., 2020).

INCREASING DIAGNOSTIC ACCESS

Because of persistently long waiting lists for diagnostic evaluations at specialty centers (as well as distance and economic barriers limiting family access), streamlined diagnostic models have emerged as a significant area of interest for researchers and practitioners alike. One approach seeks to enable primary care providers to move beyond surveillance and screening to actual ASD diagnosis in primary care. Models to support this involve providing an initial workshop or training period, followed by recurring case-based consultation (Mazurek et al., 2019). While the need for increased access to diagnostic support is universally recognized, and primary care settings are among the earliest points of contact where youth with emerging developmental delays can be identified, more research is needed to both scale primary care diagnostic models and ensure they do not create new problems in the diagnosis-to-services pipeline (Wieckowski et al., 2022). Note that as payers increasingly demand specific procedures in diagnostic evaluations before subsequently authorizing services, diagnoses confirmed in primary care that relies solely on abbreviated tests may not be accepted. Finally, models that rely on regular consultation and continuing education assume that the pediatric primary care provider will be able to engage in long-term participation, remain aware of evolutions in best practices, and clearly understand the limits of their competencies. All providers interested in ASD and related disability supports are encouraged to engage with opportunities for education (whether they seek to become diagnosticians or not), especially as the models discussed here continue to mature over time.

Even before the COVID-19 pandemic, telehealth-based models for autism diagnostic assessment were pursued as potential avenues for increasing access to care, especially for families living great distances from traditional centers. Even as pandemic conditions waned, these models have continued to grow in popularity because of their efficiency and growing research support. Most telehealth evaluation paradigms focus on young children and include a parent-mediated observation, where the health care providers coach the parent to perform specific tasks with the child on camera (often based on ADOS-2 tasks). Several protocols have been developed for administering and coding these structured observations virtually, with the TELE-ASD-PEDS protocol emerging as a leader for community adoption and empiric support (Jang et al., 2022; Wagner et al., 2021). Available data show that telehealth diagnostic approaches (primarily for young children) have a strong concordance with in-person evaluations, although more research is needed.

BIOMARKER-BASED ASSESSMENT

Pediatric primary care providers should be aware of the emerging science around biomarker-based (or informed) diagnostic assessment. As noted earlier, ASD is defined and diagnosed behaviorally; however, approaches that rely on technology and algorithm-based interpretations of various biomarkers are under investigation. Some have started to be marketed commercially (although acceptance and adoption are limited, at least as of this chapter's publication). Visual attention and eye-tracking paradigms have existed for decades, but the integration of machine learning and less expensive hardware (including tablets and smartphones) has led to some promising possible approaches. Similarly, researchers and health care providers have long relied on video recordings of youth in their natural environments to help ascertain behavioral characteristics of ASD, but automated and algorithm-based scoring of smartphone video clips is also of interest as diagnostic support (Washington et al., 2020). One such approach recently approved by the Food and Drug Administration (FDA) as a diagnostic aid (although not as an actual stand-alone diagnostic test) integrates information reported by parents and health care providers along with a machine learning–based analysis of video clips (Kanne et al., 2018; Megerian et al., 2022). Other researchers are pursuing blood and saliva assays that target algorithm-identified correlates (but not causal markers) of ASD diagnosis (Vargason et al., 2020). Many of these approaches are intended for eventual integration into primary care settings to improve access to diagnosis (and leverage a massive commercial market). More research is needed on virtually all these biomarker-based models before they can confidently be recommended. Further research on how to create novel diagnostic service settings must address how to support families as they navigate complex service systems, seek insurance authorizations for care (as mentioned earlier), and understand the holistic needs of each child (in a culturally sensitive way).

PROGNOSIS

The long-term outcomes for children with ASD vary substantially in the same way as clinical presentation varies (Hyman et al., 2020). There is a small minority of children whose symptoms worsen with age. Early diagnosis and intervention, as well as family support for individuals with ASD, is important. While significant advances have been made in the field, clearly more provider education is needed, together with timely, empathetic, and ongoing support to families of children with ASD. ASD is a lifelong condition, and families must learn to shift their focus on therapies as their child grows into adulthood. Effective communication between providers and families is essential to building supportive relationships that can positively affect not only the individual with ASD but also the family over a lifetime. Keep in mind that professionally defined optimal outcomes for individuals with ASD have evolved significantly along with an understanding of the condition; pediatric primary care providers can help families and individual patients maintain a focus on the quality of life and an emphasis on strengths, self-determination, and self-identified goals (Leadbitter et al., 2021).

PRIMARY CARE MANAGEMENT

The AAP's medical home model envisions the primary care provider serving as the coordinator of services for children and youth, including those with special needs. The medical home should be accessible, continuous, comprehensive, family centered, coordinated, compassionate, and culturally sensitive for all (Hyman et al., 2020; Kuo & Torrest, 2022). Concrete steps to create an inclusive care environment are outlined in Table 10.3 (Brasher et al., 2022).

GROWTH AND DEVELOPMENT

Children with ASD are at a higher risk for developing obesity than typically developing peers. Multiple factors may contribute to this; among them, 50% to 90% of children with ASD have feeding problems, which include selective eating patterns, rituals, and food refusal, and these problems persist past early childhood (Curtin et al., 2020). Children with ASD also engage in less physical activity compared with their typically developing peers due, for some, to low muscle tone and delay in meeting motor milestones. Children with ASD also engage in more sedentary activities, primarily screen time, than their typical peers. Therefore pediatric primary care providers must monitor the growth (height, weight, body mass index [BMI]) of their patients with ASD.

The AAP recommends pediatric primary care providers screen, assess, and manage weight in a child with ASD. The AAP and the US Preventive Services Task Force recommend screening for obesity and overweight in children 6 years and older and offer comprehensive, intensive behavioral intervention or refer for intensive behavioral intervention to improve weight. The provider should discuss their concerns with the caregivers and the child (if the child has an appropriate developmental level). In these discussions, providers must be positive role models, use nonjudgmental language, and provide a safe, nonstigmatizing

Table **10.3** Techniques to Support Care Interactions for Patients With Autism Spectrum Disorder

ADJUSTMENT	TECHNIQUE	RATIONALE
Sensory modifications	• Reduce/dim lights • Reduce noise exposure/ensure patient is located away from excessive noise/high-traffic areas (eg, nurse's station, elevator, extremely vocal patients or those in pain, front desk)	In addition to the core symptoms of ASD (eg, social interaction deficits, communication difficulties, repetitive behaviors), individuals with ASD often have strong sensory reactions to light, sound, tactile, smell and taste. These heightened sensory reactions can lead to mounting anxiety and inability to cope.
Communication modifications	• Identify every individual's preferred communication method (eg, verbal, sign language, written, technology assistance, writing board, picture exchange card system) • Use clear, concise communication • Use visual supports as needed • Explain what you are doing in advance • Speak in a quieter tone	Individuals with ASD have varying degrees of communication abilities and preferences in which they would like to communicate. Individuals with ASD tend to be literal and concrete. Therefore, direct and clear communication should be used, without jargon or innuendos. Individuals with ASD may prefer/rely on visual supports to communicate. In addition, individuals with ASD have an insistence of sameness and thus prefer to be communicated in advance before procedures or assessments are performed. Communicating in a quieter tone can also prevent sensory overload.
Personnel modifications	• Use the minimum amount of personnel for any visit, encounter, or procedure • Schedule visits during less busy times of the day • Allow extra time during procedures, assessments, and visits	Having too many personnel during a visit, encounter, or procedure may increase anxiety and sensory overload for individuals with ASD. Individuals with ASD will be able to cope better during visits with less stimuli, which typically occurs at certain times of the day (eg, before/after lunch, etc.). Moving quickly through procedures, assessment, or visits will likely increase anxiety in individuals with ASD.
Preference modification	• Document every individual's likes, dislikes, and triggers	Care of individuals with ASD should be highly customizable. Individuals with ASD have varying likes, dislikes, and triggers. Documentation of these preferences should be kept and communicated between nurses and other health care providers.

From Brasher, S., Stapel-Wax, J. L., & Muirhead, L. (2022). Racial and Ethnic Disparities in Autism Spectrum Disorder: Implications for Care. *Nursing Clinics*, 57(3), 489-499.

environment (Curtin et al., 2020). The pediatric primary care provider should comprehensively assess obesity in children with ASD with an elevated BMI (≥85th percentile) the same as they would for a typically developing child. The history should include information about diet, such as food selectivity, gastrointestinal (GI) or neurologic symptoms, and constitutional symptoms that may indicate depression or hypothyroid disorder. History should also focus on environmental factors, such as physical activity opportunities, mealtimes, and food available to the child (Curtin et al., 2020). Physical and laboratory examinations are also the same for children with ASD as they are for their typically developing peers. Physical exam should include height, weight, pulse, blood pressure measurement, and BMI calculation and evaluation of the thyroid, respiratory, cardiovascular, GI systems, skin, and neurologic findings (particularly those that might limit physical activity).

If there is a concern for hypothyroidism, a thyroid level should be drawn, and blood glucose, lipids, and liver enzymes should be checked in all children with obesity (Curtin et al., 2020). For an in-depth overview of health support recommendations for youth and ASD-specific modifications, see Table 10.4 (Curtin et al., 2020).

REVIEW OF SYSTEMS AND IMMUNIZATIONS

Youth with ASD benefit from the same rigorous schedule of health care monitoring recommended for their neurotypical peers. Health care providers should guard against diagnostic overshadowing for physical health conditions (e.g., attributing physical illness symptoms to the presence of ASD rather than investigating and treating potentially underlying physical illness). Of note, individuals with ASD are at heightened risk for health problems in virtually every body system (Croen et al., 2015). All routine screening recommendations (e.g., vision, dental, blood pressure, hematocrit, urinalysis, tuberculosis, liver function) should be completed. Similarly, the AAP recommends a full immunization schedule for all children starting at birth unless there are contraindications. Follow AAP's newest guidelines on the immunization schedule. Children and adolescents with ASD should also be protected against more novel and rapidly mutating viruses, including influenza and coronavirus. Follow AAP's guidelines for influenza and COVID immunization.

COMMON PSYCHOSOCIAL CONDITION MANAGEMENT

There is no one-size-fits-all approach to accommodating and supporting individuals with ASD. Intervention should always be tailored to individuals, considering their strengths, needs, and risk factors to maximize outcomes. In many cases, support plans should be developed irrespective of an individual's diagnostic profile (e.g., whether they meet criteria for ADHD, supports that address extreme hyperactivity may be warranted).

BEHAVIORAL INTERVENTION

Many of the evidence-based approaches commonly used for youth with ASD are based on ABA principles. ABA is the science of learning and behavior change, applying the principles of behavioral learning theory (such as reinforcement, modeling, shaping) to address skill deficits, build independence, and improve safety and adaptive functioning. Research suggests that children with ASD who receive early intensive behavioral interventions demonstrate significant improvements in cognitive abilities and social interaction (Leaf et al., 2021). ABA-based interventions may be highly structured or more naturalistic/developmental, depending on the needs of the individual. They may take place as part of a comprehensive program or a focused intervention targeting a specific skill or behavior. ABA-based approaches (whether explicitly described as such or not) are embedded into most general and special education programs (e.g., the practice of skills with feedback from teachers, offering praise and other forms of reinforcement to encourage success).

ABA therapy is the term often used to refer to intensive early intervention in young children. A large body of research indicates that youth with ASD between the ages of 2 and 5 years benefit from structured programs (often 20+ hours/week) that target fundamental learning to learn skills (i.e., imitation, eye contact, joint attention, instructional control, functional communication) (Klinger et al., 2021). Note that it is never too late for a person to receive evidence-based ABA supports. ABA therapy can come under different packages or approaches, which a family may choose based on availability, personal preference, or individual fit to the person's needs. Typically, traditional ABA therapy is implemented by board-certified behavior analysts (BCBAs) or behavioral technicians under the supervision of a BCBA. Still, other professionals (speech-language pathologists, psychologists, occupational therapists, etc.) may also use ABA-based techniques in their intervention and support contexts.

As noted, targeting delays or difficulties in communication is one of the highest priorities for both early intervention and ongoing support, especially for youth with ASD who engage in behaviors that are dangerous or disruptive. Functional communication training (FCT) encompasses a range of effective behaviorally based approaches for systematically teaching individuals to use specific, safe, and effective means to express their wants and needs rather than unsafe or ineffective alternatives (Gerow et al., 2018). One common FCT strategy is the Picture Exchange Communication System (PECS) (Bondy & Frost, 2011). Typically implemented by a speech-language pathologist or behavioral professional, children are taught to hand over a picture or icon printed on a PECS card in exchange for a highly preferred item. A gradual, stepwise approach is used (with highly motivating rewards) to build children's understanding of communication with another

| Table 10.4 | American Academy of Pediatrics (AAP) Healthy Lifestyle Recommendations and Autism Spectrum Disorder (ASD)–Specific Modifications | |

AAP RECOMMENDATIONS FOR GENERAL PEDIATRIC POPULATION[a]	ASD-SPECIFIC RECOMMENDATIONS
Assessment	
Primary care providers should assess all children's weight status on at least a yearly basis to include calculation of height, weight, and BMI for age and plot on standard growth charts. Assessing dietary patterns qualitatively should occur at each well-child visit. For children and youth with concerns about weight status, assessments should also include readiness to change and identify specific dietary practices that may be appropriate targets for change: • Frequency of eating fast food or at restaurants • Excessive consumption of sugar-sweetened beverages • Excessive portion sizes for age Additional dietary assessment elements can include: • Excessive consumption of 100% fruit juice • Frequency and/or quality of breakfast • High intake of energy-dense foods • Low consumption of fruits and vegetables	Measuring and/or weighing some children with ASD may be challenging. Be flexible with measurement, such as leaving shoes on or holding a favorite object to obtain the best possible height or weight. Parents can hold or stand on the scale with the child and then be weighed separately. If child is uncooperative on a stadiometer, have them stand against a wall and use a straight edge to mark the wall and measure height. Alternatively, allow the parent to obtain height or weight. Using spinning toys, which entertain or distract the child, may be useful for encouraging children to stand on scales and stadiometers. Segmental heights may be required for children who use a wheelchair or cannot stand long enough to obtain a height. Arm span or knee height can also be used to determine height.[b] Complete vital signs (especially blood pressure) at the end of the visit after the child has calmed down or acclimated to the visit. Assess for food selectivity; simple screening questions • Does your child eat from all food groups on a daily basis? • Is your child specific about brands or food presentation (e.g., only eats a certain type of chip, flavor of yogurt, or type of fast food)? • What are your and your child's favorite foods? Patterns of concern to look for include: • Low or no consumption of entire food groups (fruits, vegetables, meat, dairy, or grains) • High consumption of sugar-sweetened beverages • High consumption of high-fat or high-sugar food items (e.g., baked goods and candy) • Child sneaks food, binges on food, or has vomited from overeating
Treatment Recommendations	
Primary care providers should address weight management and/or lifestyle issues with all patients on at least a yearly basis irrespective of weight status. All children ages 2–18 yr with BMI values between the 5th and 84th percentile should follow preventive recommendations (see below). A staged approach should be taken to treat children ages 2–19 yr whose BMI is >85th percentile on the basis of child age, BMI, related comorbidities, parental weight status, and progress in treatment. The child's primary caregivers and family should be involved in the process.	Do not assume that parents of children with ASD are unconcerned about their children's weight status. The staged approach per AAP guidance for prevention and intervention is also appropriate for children with ASD. Include school and other treatment personnel (e.g., behavior specialists) to support behavior change. Consider including eating and/or physical activity goals in IEPs.
Stage 1: Prevention Plus	
May be implemented by the primary care providers with some training in pediatric weight management or behavioral counseling. Goal: weight maintenance with growth resulting in decreasing BMI with increasing age.	May be implemented by the primary care providers with some training in pediatric weight management or behavioral counseling. Goal: weight maintenance with growth resulting in decreasing BMI with increasing age.

| Table 10.4 | American Academy of Pediatrics (AAP) Healthy Lifestyle Recommendations and Autism Spectrum Disorder (ASD)–Specific Modifications—cont'd |

AAP RECOMMENDATIONS FOR GENERAL PEDIATRIC POPULATION[a]	ASD-SPECIFIC RECOMMENDATIONS
Monthly follow-up assessment recommended; after 3–6 mo, if no improvement in BMI and/or weight status is noted, stage 2 is indicated, which is a structured weight management protocol (see below). Stage 1 recommendations include: • Consume >5 servings of fruits and vegetables per day • Minimize and/or eliminate sugar-sweetened beverages • Limit screen time to ≤2 hr/day • No television in the room where the child sleeps • Engage in >1 hr daily physical activity The child and family should be counseled to adopt the following eating behaviors: • Eating breakfast on a daily basis • Limiting meals eaten outside the home • Eating family meals at least 5–6 times/wk • Allowing the child to self-regulate meals and avoiding overly restrictive behaviors Providers should acknowledge cultural differences and assist families in making appropriate adaptations to the recommendations.	Monthly follow-up assessments; after 6 mo, if no improvement in BMI and/or weight status has been noted, advance to stage 2, a structured weight management protocol (see below). Involving the parent(s) is essential; providers should work with the family and recommend: • Targeting gradual reduction (ideally elimination) of sugared drinks and juices, including 100% fruit juices • Developing viable strategies to manage portions and/or access to energy-dense foods (e.g., removing temptation by eliminating certain energy-dense foods from the home or storing them out of sight) • Serving fruits and/or vegetables that the child likes at each meal • See additional suggestions for working with families and schools around healthy eating and physical activity. Providers and family members should work together to set only 1–2 realistic and obtainable goals to work on each month.

Stage 2: Structured weight Management Protocol

May be implemented by primary care providers highly trained in weight management. Goal: weight maintenance that results in decreasing BMI as age and/or height increase. Weight loss should not exceed 1 lb/mo for children 2–11 yr of age or an average of 2 lb/wk for older overweight or obese children and adolescents. If there is no improvement in BMI and/or weight status after 3–6 mo, then stage 3 is recommended (see below). Stage 2 recommendations include: • Consumption of a balanced macronutrient diet with small amounts of energy-dense foods • Provision of structured daily meals and snacks (breakfast, lunch, dinner, and 1–2 snacks/day) • Supervised active play of >60 min/day • No more than 1 hr/day of screen time • Increased monitoring of target behaviors (e.g., screen time, physical activity, dietary intake, and restaurant logs) by provider, patient, and/or family • Reinforcement for achieving targeted behavior goals (not weight goals)	May be implemented by primary care providers highly trained in weight management. Goal: weight maintenance that results in decreasing BMI as age and/or height increase. Weight loss should not exceed 1 lb/mo for children 2–11 yr of age or an average of 2 lb/wk for older children and adolescents with overweight or obesity If there is no improvement in BMI or weight status after 6 mo, stage 3 is recommended (see below). Stage 2 recommendations include: • All of stage 1 for children with ASD recommendations and stage 2 recommendations from the AAP are also appropriate • Add the services of professionals who can work as a team • Occupational or speech therapist to address sensory issues associated with extreme food selectivity if applicable • Behavioral specialist for resistance to making behavioral changes • Dietitian for dietary counseling and/or support with limited food repertoire • Use a posted meal and snack schedule (e.g., pictorial schedule if appropriate for the child's age and ability level) • Use a snack box with preselected and/or preportioned snacks to manage and/or limit snacking • Implement a reward chart for completing physical activity, trying new fruits and vegetables, and drinking water

Continued

Table 10.4	American Academy of Pediatrics (AAP) Healthy Lifestyle Recommendations and Autism Spectrum Disorder (ASD)–Specific Modifications—cont'd

AAP RECOMMENDATIONS FOR GENERAL PEDIATRIC POPULATION[a]	ASD-SPECIFIC RECOMMENDATIONS
Stage 3: Comprehensive Multidisciplinary Intervention	
Patients whose BMI or weight status has not improved after 3–6 mo should be referred to a multidisciplinary team that specializes in obesity treatment. Goal: weight maintenance or gradual weight loss until BMI is <85th percentile; as above, weight loss should not exceed 1 lb/mo for children 2–5 yr of age or 2 lb/wk for older children and adolescents with obesity. Eating and activity goals are the same as in stage 2 and should include: • Planned negative energy balance achieved through structured diet and physical activity • A structured behavior modification program, including monitoring and development of short-term diet and physical activity goals • Involve primary caregivers and/or family members for behavioral modification for children <12 yr of age • Training families to improve the home environment • Frequent office visits, weekly visits for a minimum of 8–12 wk, and subsequent monthly visits on a monthly basis to aid in maintaining new behaviors • Systematic evaluation of body measurements, dietary intake, and physical activity should be conducted at baseline and specific intervals throughout the program	Patients whose BMI or weight status has not improved after 3–6 mo should be referred to a multidisciplinary team that specializes in obesity treatment. Goal: weight maintenance or gradual weight loss until BMI is <85th percentile; as above, weight loss should not exceed 1 lb/mo for children 2–5 yr of age or 2 lb/wk for older children and adolescents with obesity. Recommendations are the same as in stage 2 and the AAP's stage 3 but may also include 1 or more of the following strategies, tailored to the individual child: • Use food lists and/or guides such as the Stoplight Approach with support from a dietitian to help select snacks and/or guide meals • Remove trigger foods such as sugared beverages, chips, sweets, and other high-energy–dense foods from the house • Plan for a favorite food to be consumed 1 time/wk to prevent deprivation but do not use as a reward • Consider having family track calorie intake using a web-based application with assistance from the dietary team • Identify locations for accessible physical activity
Stage 4: Tertiary-Care Protocol	
Recommended for children >11 yr of age with BMI >95th percentile who also have significant comorbidities and have not been successful in stages 1–3 or for children with BMI of >99th percentile who have shown no improvement in stage 3. Treatment should include continued diet and activity counseling and consideration of additions such as meal replacements, low-calorie diets, medication, and possibly surgery.	Recommended for children >11 yr of age with BMI >95th percentile who also have significant comorbidities and have not been successful in stages 1–3 or for children with BMI of >99th percentile who have shown no improvement in stage 3. Treatment should include continued diet and activity counseling and consideration of the following strategies overseen by a team specializing in weight management of children with experience in working with children and youth with ASD and their families: • Family tracking of calorie intake by using a paper- or web-based application • Use of meal replacements if the child does not have strong food aversions • Medications to counteract the effects of second general antipsychotics (SGAs) if medically appropriate Consultation to evaluate candidacy for surgical intervention; guidance from the American Society for Metabolic and Bariatric Surgery indicates that ASD should not be a contraindication for bariatric surgery. Intervention should be considered on a case-by-case basis for the patient's needs and ability to engage in the dietary and/or lifestyle changes required before and after surgery.[c]

BMI, Body mass index; *IEP,* individualized education plan.

[a]Barlow, S.E., & Expert Committee. (2007). Expert Committee recommendations regarding the prevention, assessment, and treatment of child and adolescent overweight and obesity: Summary report. *Pediatrics, 120*(4), S164–S192.

[b]Bittner, M., Goudy, L., Dillon, S.R., Mcnamara, S., & Adams, D. (2018). Exercise identified as an evidence-based practice for students with autism spectrum disorder. *Palaestra Journal, 32*(1), 15–20.

[c]Pratt, J.S.A., Browne, A., Browne, N.T., et al. (2018). ASMBS pediatric metabolic and bariatric surgery guidelines, 2018. *Surgery for Obesity and Related Diseases, 14*(7), 882–901.

From Curtin, C., Hyman, S.L., Boas, D.D., et al. (2020). Weight management in primary care for children with autism: Expert recommendations. *Pediatrics, 145*(1), S126–S139.

person to obtain their wants, needs, and ability to engage in these exchanges independently. Many children graduate to building full sentences using icons of words and pictures (i.e., a sentence strip). Using visual supports to develop a communication repertoire can also serve as a stepping stone for improving verbal communication by pairing words with pictures (and lots of practice and encouragement). Many other communication modalities can be taught in similar ways, ideally guided by children's preferences and strengths; these include the use of sign language, technology-based solutions (e.g., the use of a keyboard or communication application with icons on a tablet), and single- or multibutton switches that speak for them. Speech-language pathologists are an essential part of the treatment team when a child has functional communication impairments, and identifying an appropriate alternative/augmentative communication system that can be accessible to the child in all settings (not just at school) is critical for improving independence, safety, and emotional well-being at any age.

Other applications of ABA principles occur within the child's daily routines and activities, including play (Hyman et al., 2020). Naturalistic developmental behavioral interventions (NDBIs) use the fundamentals of ABA and developmental principles to target developmental skills (Schreibman et al., 2015). In contrast to traditional ABA approaches that may engage a child up to 40 hours per week in intensive, therapist-delivered intervention, NDBIs are far less time intensive and capitalize on naturally occurring learning opportunities. NDBIs also typically enlist parents and caregivers to learn engagement and teaching strategies (e.g., following the child's interests, modeling, reinforcing attempts using a child's preferred activities and items) to maximize a child's exposure to enriched supports without the need for strict structure. Indeed, parent involvement and parent-mediated intervention are known factors that increase the likelihood of intervention effectiveness (Klinger et al., 2021). Intervention may occur virtually anywhere, but teaching frequently occurs in a classroom, home, or therapy setting. The Early Start Denver Model is the most well-researched NDBI (Waddington et al., 2016). Other examples of NDBIs include Pivotal Response Training and Reciprocal Imitation Training (Schreibman et al., 2015).

Youth with ASD frequently benefit from mental/behavioral health support, with modifications based on their language and learning needs. Parent management training (sometimes called behavioral parent training) teaches parents and caregivers to use behavioral principles to improve the quality of parent-child interactions and increase a child's success with following parental instructions (Nadler & Blum, 2022). These approaches enjoy a substantial evidence base for treating disruptive behavior disorders in typically developing children and have been successfully adapted for use with children with ASD and other disabilities. One such parent training

package, the Research Units in Behavioral Intervention parent training program, is an evidence-based combination of traditional parent management training and ABA-based strategies tailored for use with children with ASD (e.g., using visual supports, teaching functional communication and other skills) (Bearss et al., 2015).

Notably, behaviorally based approaches can also successfully be applied to intense aggression, SIB, and other high-intensity behavioral symptoms in both youth and adults. This may occur in school settings as well as in specialized behavioral units of hospitals or residential facilities where careful control over environmental contingencies (e.g., access to privileges) can be modified to help individuals achieve lower rates of severe behaviors while increasing functional communication and other adaptive behavior (Kurtz et al., 2020). Note that access to specialized treatment centers is extremely limited.

On an outpatient basis, intervention approaches investigated for typically developing youth have growing evidence bases for youth with ASD as well. For instance, programs based on cognitive-behavioral therapy to reduce anxiety and depression symptoms show success (with some adaptations) for youth on the spectrum (White et al., 2018). Related interventions focused on enhancing social skills are also commonly recommended, which can yield benefits for mood challenges and improve social communication and independence (see Sexuality, later).

PHARMACOLOGIC SUPPORTS

Behavioral, psychosocial, and allied health/educational supports represent first-line approaches for addressing mental/behavioral health challenges in youth with ASD. Specific medication types are commonly used in ASD to target cooccurring ADHD, anxiety, sleep disturbances, and other behavioral/medical conditions (Hollocks et al., 2019; Simonoff et al., 2020) (Table 10.5). Only second-generation atypical antipsychotics are FDA approved in children age 5 years and older to treat autism-associated irritability, including aggression, temper, tantrums, SIB, and quickly changing moods. SSRIs and other mood stabilizers are often used to treat anxiety, depression, and mood instability in individuals with ASD. The most used SSRIs are fluoxetine, sertraline, escitalopram, and citalopram. Stimulants (methylphenidate and amphetamines) and nonstimulants (alpha-agonists and atomoxetine) are used to treat ADHD symptoms. Despite being more likely to be prescribed psychiatric medications, youth on the spectrum appear to show lower rates of favorable response and higher rates of adverse effects (Patel et al., 2020).

ADVERSE EXPERIENCES

Pediatric primary care providers should be aware of this population's higher rates of adverse experiences (Hoover & Kaufman, 2018). Individuals with any intellectual or developmental disability appear four

Table 10.5	Common Pharmacologic Symptom Targets in Youth With Autism Spectrum Disorder (ASD)	
SYMPTOMS	MEDICATION	ADDITIONAL INFORMATION
Agitation, irritability, aggressive behaviors, quickly changing moods	Atypical antipsychotics	Risperidone is FDA approved for children with ASD age 5–16 yr; aripiprazole is FDA approved for children with ASD age 6–17 yr
Anxiety/depression	SSRIs, SNRIs	Black box warning
Attention-deficit/hyperactivity disorder	Stimulants, nonstimulants	Often used in combination

FDA, US Food and Drug Administration; SNRI, serotonin and norepinephrine reuptake inhibitor; SSRI, selective serotonin reuptake inhibitor.

times more likely to experience adverse childhood experiences than neurotypical peers, dramatically increasing their risk for other adverse health outcomes (McNally et al., 2021). Most notably, physical/sexual abuse and neglect have long been observed at higher rates for youth and adults with disabilities. This finding extends directly to youth with ASD, and pediatric primary care providers should routinely screen for this as they would for neurotypical youth. Unfortunately, youth with ASD experience maltreatment at about twice the rate of neurotypical peers (McDonnell et al., 2019).

Bullying is also among the adverse experiences more frequently encountered by youth with ASD. Bullying can include physical, verbal, social, and online acts of victimization. In their review of the literature, Humphrey and Hebron (2015) describe youth with ASD as having a "double disadvantage" when it comes to bullying because they are at higher risk and have worse outcomes compared to neurotypical peers. Protective factors for bullying include positive relationships and social skills (Humphrey & Hebron, 2015). They recommend important components to bullying prevention based on a review of research: social skills training, peer education (to improve understanding of autism), teacher/staff training, and developing a zero-tolerance school culture. Note that children with individualized education plans (IEPs) or a 504 have protections against bullying under the Individuals with Disabilities Education Act (IDEA). See Resources (later) for antibullying information.

Social camouflaging refers to the suppression, compensation, or masking of certain autistic traits in social settings by adolescents and adults with ASD. Social camouflaging might be more commonly used or reported by females than males. A small number of studies have been done using qualitative interviews with autistic adolescents and adults. People on the spectrum report being motivated to camouflage by their desire for friendship, social pressure, and avoiding discrimination or negative feedback from others (Hull et al., 2017). A major takeaway from the self-reports of autistic individuals is that social camouflaging often causes stress, feelings of exhaustion, and challenges to a person's self-concept/self-esteem (Hull et al., 2017). Many individuals with ASD report needing time alone to recover after camouflaging in the social environment.

Unintentional injury is another form of adverse experience. In particular, elopement and wandering are major safety concerns for children on the spectrum. Children with ASD are eight times more likely to elope or wander off from safety between the ages of 7 and 10 than their typically developing siblings, and nearly half of the children with ASD ages 4 to 10 tend to wander or bolt from safe settings (Anderson et al., 2012). More than one-third of children with ASD who wander/elope are never or rarely able to communicate their name, address, or phone number (Anderson et al., 2012). Accidental drowning is another risk factor that providers and families should consider. Youth with ASD are almost three times as likely to drown than their neurotypical peers, and historical estimates have suggested that accidental drowning has accounted for up to 91% of US deaths reported in children with ASD under age 15 (Peden & Willcox-Pidgeon, 2020). According to a study by the National Autism Association, accidental drowning accounts for 71% of lethal outcomes, followed by traffic injuries at 18% (McIlwain & Fournier, 2011). Other dangers include dehydration, heat stroke, hypothermia, falls, physical restraint, and encounters with strangers. Increased risks are associated with autism severity.

Law enforcement interaction can lead to adverse experiences, and about 20% of youth with ASD have been stopped/questioned by law enforcement personnel despite being less likely to commit crimes (Rava et al., 2017). The higher rates of mental and behavioral health conditions, elopement, and communication deficits likely contribute to this increased risk (see Resources [later] for safety planning guidance). Be sure to check in regularly with patients and families regarding safety concerns. Proactive planning and identification of likely high-risk situations can reduce negative outcomes.

Extremism and criminal conduct have emerged as concerns in recent years in large part due to media attention on the possible connection between ASD and violent or extremist behaviors. A small collection of studies suggests that individuals with ASD are more likely to be the victim rather than the perpetrator of a violent crime (Allely & Faccini, 2017). Clinically, immediate action to preserve safety should be taken when any child (especially one with cooccurring psychiatric challenges) appears at risk for harming oneself or others.

COMMON MEDICAL ILLNESS MANAGEMENT

SLEEP DISORDERS

Youth with ASD are at least twice as likely to have sleep problems compared to neurotypical youth, with some studies estimating that up to 80% of youth on the spectrum have sleep difficulties (Malow et al., 2012; Reynolds et al., 2019). Poor sleep has a negative impact on daytime behaviors, and fatigue may even exacerbate difficulties with social communication and restricted and repetitive behaviors. Poor sleep can also contribute to aggression and SIB.

Medical causes for sleep disturbances should always be ruled out. Acute illnesses such as viral respiratory and GI infections can affect sleep due to the intensity of symptoms, including fever, cough, diarrhea, and vomiting. Possible chronic conditions must also be considered. Obstructive sleep apnea can present as a child having difficulty falling asleep, waking at night, snoring, or loud and heavy mouth breathing. A referral should be made for evaluation in a sleep clinic that may include a sleep study. Restless leg syndrome may occur when a child has difficulty settling down to sleep at night, has a restless sleep, feels the need to move the legs to get comfortable (although not all patients with ASD will be able to verbalize this), and wakes in the night. Restless leg syndrome can be due to iron deficiency or low ferritin levels and is often responsive to iron supplementation. Melatonin is often recommended to assist with sleep onset difficulties. Other agents used for sleep difficulties include alpha-agonists (clonidine, guanfacine) as well as trazodone and gabapentin, which are helpful with both sleep onset and sleep maintenance.

Using a tool such as the Children's Sleep Habits Questionnaire (Owens et al., 2000) or the BEARS Sleep Screening Tool (Owens & Dalzell, 2005) can help elicit information about sleep habits and concerns. If a medical condition is identified, it should be treated prior to significant behavioral intervention, allowing for greater success with behavioral treatments. In many cases, sleep challenges are appropriately characterized as behavioral insomnia of childhood, reflecting that children have firmly established sleep-onset associations (e.g., insisting that a parent be present with them while they fall asleep) and/or difficulties with limit setting (e.g., children sneaking food or screen time during the night). Pediatric primary care providers can coach families on simple environmental adjustments to ensure a sleep-conducive environment (e.g., low light, cooler temperature, quiet/constant sound via white noise machine). Providers can also provide guidance on establishing consistent evening routines, limiting screen time in the hour leading up to bedtime, and increasing physical activity and light exposure during the day. The provider should work with the family to identify the goals and meet with them regularly to reassess, adjust, and determine if more advanced behavioral approaches are needed (Kirkpatrick et al., 2019).

GASTROINTESTINAL AND TOILETING PROBLEMS

Many children with ASD take longer than is typical to learn how to use the toilet. This delay can stem from a variety of reasons. First, many children with ASD have a general developmental delay; they learn new skills, including toileting, more slowly than other children. When approaching toilet training with children on the spectrum, their developmental level must be considered to determine if they are ready or where to start. Look for signs of readiness, such as longer periods of staying dry between diaper changes and any attempts to communicate when they are wet/soiled. Second, many children who have ASD have great difficulty breaking long-established routines (such as transitioning from voiding in a diaper to a toilet). It is common for children with ASD to develop anxiety around toileting. Anxiety may manifest as behavior problems such as tantrums or refusals or avoidance behaviors, such as hiding or withholding stool. In these cases, the fear must be addressed first before toileting skills. A gradual exposure model is usually effective in helping children overcome their fear of the toilet. ABA principles, such as positive reinforcement and repeated, stepwise practice, are practical. Finally, communication challenges add to the problem for many children on the autism spectrum. Some children must be taught how to ask to use the toilet using their most effective form of communication (e.g., words, signs, pictures). Many children with communication delays benefit from a visual schedule or prompt to help them learn a new skill or routine.

GI symptoms, including constipation, diarrhea, and reflux, are more common in children with ASD than those with delays or typically developing children. Not surprisingly, they are also more likely to have feeding challenges, which may contribute to GI symptoms. It is important to rule out medical problems contributing to toileting, such as constipation.

FEEDING AND EATING PROBLEMS

Up to 90% of children with ASD have some type of problem related to food intake (Curtin et al., 2015), which may contribute to GI symptoms such as constipation. Food selectivity may be based on texture, color, temperature, or presentation and extends well beyond picky eating observed in typically developing children. In some cases, food selectivity may be related to certain rituals or compulsions, sensory differences, or other core features of ASD. Despite issues with food selectivity, youth on the spectrum also face at least a 50% increased risk for obesity compared to peers (Sammels et al., 2022). This may be related to several factors, including restricted (but unhealthy) diets and weight gain related to pharmacologic management (e.g., atypical antipsychotics). Providers should identify feeding concerns as early as possible to support families with anticipatory behavioral strategies (Curtin et al., 2015).

Pica is another type of feeding concern that occurs at a higher rate among children with ASD, characterized as the persistent eating of nonnutritive, nonfood substances (APA, 2013). Prevalence rates are higher in children with ASD, both with and without intellectual impairment. A recent study found pica occurred in children with ASD with and without intellectual disability (28.1% and 14%, respectively)—both higher than occurrence in the population control group (3.5%) (Fields et al., 2021). Behavioral management strategies for pica include prevention (eliminating access to objects/substances that could cause harm if ingested), immediate interruption of the behavior, and redirection to a more appropriate behavior based on the determined function (sensory input, attention, etc.).

Up to 23% of youth with a diagnosed eating disorder (anorexia nervosa, bulimia nervosa, or binge eating disorder) also meet diagnostic criteria for ASD, perhaps explained by overlapping cognitive rigidity related to food and/or body image (Numata et al., 2021). Traditional eating disorder treatments can be adapted for youth on the spectrum, but outcomes data remain limited at this time.

EPILEPSY AND SEIZURE DISORDERS

Seizure disorders have long been associated with ASD. In some cases this may be the result of shared or overlapping genetic etiologies. Epilepsy is especially common in children with cooccurring ASD and intellectual disability, with approximately 20% of this group affected (Besag, 2018). For youth with ASD without intellectual disability, epilepsy prevalence is approximately 8% (Besag, 2018). Management of seizures does not necessarily change in the presence of an ASD diagnosis, but higher rates of other cooccurring mental health and medical conditions may complicate medication management.

ALLIED HEALTH AND EDUCATIONAL SUPPORTS

Children with ASD vary widely in their speech and language abilities, motor skills, sensory processing, and cognitive and academic abilities (Hyman et al., 2020). Individuals must be assessed in all these areas to determine what specialized services they need. The school district will usually evaluate these areas of functioning as part of an IEP evaluation. Many children will need to be referred for an outpatient assessment and therapy (i.e., speech-language, occupational, physical, and feeding therapy) to address specific challenges or deficits.

Coach the family to request an evaluation for an IEP or 504 plan in writing to ensure the school/district responds, and remind them that a medical diagnosis of ASD does not necessarily mean a child will qualify for special education services under the educational eligibility of autism. Refer the family to local advocacy groups for assistance with these if needed. Request that parents bring copies of educational plans to keep on file in the medical record and provide coaching and feedback to families if the plans do not seem to be meeting a child's academic, social-emotional, adaptive, or behavioral needs. Keep in mind that IEPs can and should address any areas that will limit a child's ability to benefit from the educational environment, including self-care tasks (e.g., toileting) and safety. Note that children who are home schooled or attend private school are still eligible to seek IEP-based services through the local public district (e.g., speech therapy). Encourage open and honest communication between the family and teachers to maintain good relationships and work together to navigate any conflicts that arise (Larcombe et al., 2019). When necessary, refer families to the regional Parent Training and Information Center to help them navigate situations where a school may not be fulfilling their mandated educational obligations (see Resources at the end of this chapter).

COMPLEMENTARY AND ALTERNATIVE APPROACHES

Autism has been described as a "21st-century fad magnet" (Metz et al., 2015), likely driven by the significant heterogeneity in presentation (as well as etiology). Estimates vary, but up to 95% of families have utilized at least one complementary and alternative medicine (CAM) approach (Höfer et al., 2017), including a wide variety of natural and interventional approaches (Box 10.2) (Lindly et al., 2018). Pediatric primary care providers must inquire about CAMs, recognize that new trends will continuously emerge, and be prepared to provide nonjudgmental but sound advice. Gluten-free diets (and variations) remain among the most popular CAMs, despite the sparse evidence of consistent effects on behavior, health, and developmental outcomes (Batarseh et al., 2022). Practically speaking, youth on the spectrum who already have challenges consuming a variety of nutritious foods may face even more challenges if food intake is further restricted; families who are interested in experimenting with diets and other benign vitamins/supplements should be encouraged to do so under the guidance of a nutritionist or dietician. Some common supplements can even be dangerous if consumed in large quantities, such as vitamin B_6.

Products and supplements that include cannabidiol (CBD) have become increasingly accessible and occasionally encouraged by nonprofessional sources as a more natural solution to behavioral challenges than traditional pharmacology. Providers have limited evidence to guide such recommendations and must consider legal factors, polypharmacy, and other health concerns (Duvall et al., 2019). One nonpharmacologic approach gaining in availability and popularity is the application of neurofeedback methodologies to improve core autism traits and associated behavioral

Box 10.2   Complementary and Alternative Treatments

NATURAL PRODUCTS OVERALL	94%
Herbal or nonvitamin supplements	61%
Specific vitamins and/or minerals	58%
Multivitamins/minerals	55%
Essential oils	23%
Herbal teas	10%
Cannabis	3%
Mind and body practices overall	81%
Massage therapy	35%
Yoga	26%
Qigong	26%
Meditation	19%
Biofeedback	16%
Music therapy	10%
Equestrian therapy	10%
Movement therapy	6%
Progressive relaxation	6%
Chiropractic/osteopathic manipulation	5%
Skin brushing	6%
Acupuncture	3%
Hydrotherapy	3%
Deep breathing exercises	3%
Other modalities overall	81%
Special diets	74%
Naturopathy	26%
Homeopathy	16%
Nebulizer or vaporizer	10%
Chelation	6%
Hyperbaric oxygen therapy	6%
Books	3%

Data reflect parent self-reports from a multisite sample (n = 352).
From Lindly et al. (2018).

or mental health concerns; this approach involves the use of noninvasive brain scanning (i.e., electroencephalography) and often a combination of audio and visual feedback (sometimes in the form of video games, etc.) to influence brain electrical activity. There is some evidence that this methodology can improve attention and executive functioning deficits associated with ADHD, but the effects are small and require much more research to determine whether these or other positive effects might be achieved for youth on the autism spectrum (Riesco-Matías et al., 2021). Of note, these programs are not always covered by insurance, and counseling on pursuing them should explicitly address the time and financial costs versus benefits (especially when evidence-based alternatives are available).

LIFESPAN CONSIDERATIONS

HOLISTIC FAMILY SUPPORT

Pediatric primary care providers can begin to provide both practical and social support to families even before a formal ASD diagnosis (Schiller et al., 2021). Some families may have difficulty understanding ASD, fear seeking an evaluation, or struggle to accept the outcome of the assessment. Other caregivers may feel relieved because their concerns have been validated, and they now have an opportunity to better understand and support their child. Caregivers commonly report growing awareness that their child may not experience what they had dreamed for them, or they may develop concerns about who will be available to support their child across the lifespan and in their absence. Note that caregivers of children with ASD tend to have higher rates of anxiety, depression, and stress compared to those of typically developing children; medical disorders; and other developmental disorders. Families may not have help from extended family or friends because they lack knowledge about ASD (Lindsey & Barry, 2018). Even if a child with ASD is an identified patient, encouraging adult caregivers to take care of their own physical and mental health needs may be an important component of helping them be the best supporters they can be for their child. Similarly, siblings may have a complicated relationship with a child with ASD; some sibling relationships are described as warm and close, while others reflect increased behavioral conflicts (Rixon et al., 2021). Consider recommending support for individual family members as needed and family-based therapies that bring everyone together.

SEXUALITY

Individuals on the autism spectrum are interested in sexuality and relationships, and this is a normal and healthy part of their development. Unfortunately, people with neurodevelopmental disorders often lack developmentally appropriate sexual education. For some people with developmental disabilities, sexual education is ignored completely. Individuals with ASD are at increased risk of sexual victimization and inappropriate sexual behaviors, including unintentional sexual offending (Pecora et al., 2016). Several studies have shown higher rates of sexual abuse and coercive sexual victimization in youth with ASD, and higher rates of sexual coercion, unwanted sexual contact, and rape in adults with ASD, compared to the general population. Some of this increased vulnerability may be related to differences in social perspective-taking, misunderstanding of nonverbal cues in others, and executive functioning deficits (Pecora et al., 2016).

It is important for health care professionals to encourage and assist families in providing developmentally appropriate sexual education to youth and to help adults with ASD access sexual health information. Pecora et al. (2016) recommend a combination of social skills training, relationship education, and sexual education to support youth on the spectrum. Some specific evidence-based programs include PEERS for young adults, Sexuality Education for Youth on the Autism

Spectrum, and Tackling Teenage programs (Pecora et al., 2016). Social stories and video modeling are effective strategies for teaching social skills and reducing inappropriate behaviors (Pecora et al., 2016). Sexual education is ongoing throughout childhood, adolescence, and adulthood and is not a one-time event.

Health care professionals need to be aware of issues surrounding sexual orientation and gender diversity when caring for people on the spectrum. Although prevalence rates vary, most studies agree that people with ASD are more likely than neurotypical peers to identify as LGBTQ+. Pecora et al. (2016) report that 15% to 35% of people with ASD identified as LGBTQ+ across several studies (compared to about 5% in the general population). George and Stokes (2018) found that people with ASD were two to three times more likely to be transgender than people in the general population. The reasons for the connection between ASD and gender/sexual identity diversity are not fully understood, and it is probably multiple reasons (Pecora et al., 2016). Providers need to recognize the intersection of disability and gender/sexuality to talk about this with clients. Sexual and gender minorities face a significantly increased risk of victimization and discrimination. Patients with ASD will benefit from community referrals for gender-affirming medical and mental health care and support groups.

COMMUNITY RESOURCES

Pediatric primary care providers are well positioned to support families as they navigate their children's and their families' evolving needs. At every visit the primary care provider needs to ask if families have questions about their child's health and what assistance they may need. Parents frequently need help finding specific interventions for problems, such as toilet training and sleep issues (Nordahl-Hansen et al., 2018). Always review the child's current services (such as an IEP at school, community ABA therapy), and check on safety concerns and current sources of stress. Accessing therapies and other supports can be difficult for families, especially in rural and other low-resource settings. The wait time for a diagnostic evaluation may exceed a year for some families, and access to ABA is surprisingly limited despite being one of the most sought services. Pediatric primary care providers can familiarize themselves with local and regional resources and connect with advocacy groups that can provide navigation on issues such as child care, guardianship and legal concerns, social skills opportunities, and more. The primary care provider should ensure that the patient becomes registered with the state- and county-based developmental disability support systems. These agencies often help families fund or link to respite care, supplemental therapies, vocational support, crisis support, and a host of other resources. See Resources at the end of this chapter for key links to help develop a toolkit for local and regional connections.

TRANSITION PLANNING

Children eligible for special education support can continue to attend public school up to age 21, but educational and other planning for the transition to adulthood should begin by age 14. In addition to considering educational and vocational goals, some families may consider legal guardianship when their child becomes an adult. This process should begin as early as possible so that families are ready to file by the child's 18th birthday. It is useful to complete an assessment as part of the transition process (e.g., Harris et al., 2021); this is an expansion of the HEEADSSS screening process (Home Environment, Education/Employment, Eating, Activities, Drugs, Sexuality, Suicide/Depression, Safety), including ASD (Autism-Specific Safety Risks, Social Skills, and Daily Life and Independence). Identify an adult provider and confirm the first appointment. Consider a discussion with the new adult provider. Review health insurance status for adulthood, as many may qualify for Medicaid in their state. Assess patient/family benefits such as Social Security Income (SSI), Division of Developmental Disabilities (DDD), and Special Needs Trust (Harris et al., 2021).

NEURODIVERSITY

Finally, the language, approaches, and conceptualizations surrounding ASD presented in this chapter will continue to evolve (Wright Stein et al., 2022). Beyond the active ASD research community, changes we anticipate in the future will also be informed (and driven) by the neurodiversity movement. Including and honoring self-advocates' perspectives in developing health care models and approaches, listening and responding to concerns raised by the community, and acknowledging areas of disagreement (with parents, caregivers, health care providers, and researchers) are critical for building understanding. Pediatric primary care providers are encouraged to learn from their patients and the communities they serve, prioritize shared decision making, and remain committed to their professional growth as the best clinical practices for health care for youth with ASD continue to evolve (Brown et al., 2021; Donaldson et al., 2017; Nicolaidis, 2012).

RESOURCES

SCREENING AND IDENTIFICATION

American Academy of Pediatrics: https://www.aap.org/en/patient-care/screening-technical-assistance-and-resource-center/screening-tool-finder
Centers for Disease Control and Prevention: https://www.cdc.gov/ncbddd/actearly/index.html

PSYCHOSOCIAL AND BEHAVIORAL SUPPORTS

Autism Society: https://autismsociety.org
Autism Speaks: https://Autismspeaks.org

Help Is in Your Hands: https://helpisinyourhands. org

Interacting with Autism: http://www. interactingwithautism.com

Vanderbilt University Medical Center: https://vkc. vumc.org/vkc/resources/autism

HEALTH CARE RESOURCES

Got Transition: https://gottransition.org

Society for Developmental & Behavioral Pediatrics: https://sdbp.org/adhd-guideline/ cag-guidelines

AASPIRE Toolkit: https://autismandhealth.org

SAFETY RESOURCES

Autism Society's Take Me Home program. https:// www.firstresponderautismtraining.com/ take-me-home

Autism Speaks' Autism Safety Project. https://www. autismspeaks.org/autism-safety

Autism Speaks' Wandering Prevention. https:// www.autismspeaks.org/wandering-prevention

AWAARE Collaboration (working to prevent wandering incidents and deaths in the autism community) https://www.inclusivechildcare.org/ resource-library/website/awaare-collaboration

Interacting with Law Enforcement | Autism Speaks. https://www.autismspeaks.org/interacting-law-enforcement

PACER National Bullying Prevention Center: www. pacer.org/bullying

Project Lifesaver (provides in-depth training regarding wandering behavior and tracking technologies to law enforcement agencies). https://projectlife-saver.org/resources/wandering-prevention

The Big Red Safety Box (a set of elopement/wandering-related resources from the National Autism Association). https://nationalautismassociation. org/big-red-safety-box

Tracking services available to help locate loved ones via devices: EmFinders, LoJack SafetyNet, Care Trak.

IDENTIFYING STATE/REGIONAL RESOURCE AGENCIES

Center for Parent Information and Resources: https:// www.parentcenterhub.org/find-your-center

National Association of State Directors of Developmental Disabilities Services: https://www.nasddds.org/ state-agencies

NURSING AND HEALTH CARE PROFESSIONALS

American Academy of Developmental Medicine & Dentistry: https://www.aadmd.org

American Academy of Pediatrics: https://www.aap. org/en/patient-care/autism

Centers for Disease Control and Prevention: https:// www.cdc.gov/ncbddd/developmentaldisabilities/ links.html

Echo Autism: https://echoautism.com

SAFE Initiative: https://safedbp.org

Society for Developmental and Behavioral Pediatrics: https://sdbp.org

---

Summary

Primary Care Needs for Children With Autism Spectrum Disorder

GROWTH AND DEVELOPMENT

- Children with ASD are at higher risk for obesity than typically developing peers.
- Pediatric primary care providers should screen, assess, and manage weight in children with ASD.
- Physical exam should include height, weight, pulse, and blood pressure measurement, as well as BMI calculation and evaluation of the thyroid, respiratory, cardiovascular, GI systems, skin, and neurologic findings

REVIEW OF SYSTEMS AND IMMUNIZATIONS

- Individuals with ASD are at heightened risk for health problems in every body system.
- Health care providers should guard against diagnostic overshadowing for physical health concerns (e.g., attributing physical illness symptoms to the presence of ASD rather than investigating and treating potentially underlying physical illness).
- Follow AAP's newest guidelines on the immunization schedule.

BEHAVIORAL AND MENTAL HEALTH
Behavioral and Psychosocial Supports

- Young children with ASD and substantial impairments benefit from 20+ hours per week of structured programs based on principles of ABA between the ages of 2 and 5 years.
- ABA-based interventions are also effective for youth with ASD of any age.
- FCT is one of the highest priorities for early intervention and ongoing support.
- Youth with ASD often benefit from mental and behavioral health support, such as behavioral parent training and cognitive-behavioral intervention.

Mental Health Comorbidities

- Cooccurring conditions are essentially the rule rather than the exception for ASD. Up to 94% of individuals with ASD have at least one cooccurring psychiatric condition.
- Pediatric health care providers should always consider cooccurring psychiatric and medical conditions when caring for a child with diagnosed (or suspected) ASD.

Challenging Behaviors and Self-Injury, Behavioral Management

- Children and adolescents with ASD are more likely to have inpatient psychiatric stays than typically developing peers; however, they also face increased barriers to accessing appropriate psychiatric facilities.

Continued

- SIB is common in people with ASD across the lifespan, and behavioral intervention based on ABA is the most effective intervention. Behavioral intervention can be provided at different levels of intensity (in-home, outpatient, residential).
- Youth with ASD are at increased risk for suicidal ideation and behaviors. It is important to screen regularly for suicide risk using standardized screening tools.
- When suicidal risk is determined to be present, engage the family in safety planning, including means restriction (temporarily limiting access to lethal methods).

Sexuality Considerations
- Developmentally appropriate sex education is extremely important for children and adolescents with ASD and should include a combination of social skills training, relationship education, and sexual education.
- Health care professionals need to be aware of and sensitive to issues surrounding sexual orientation and gender identity, as 15% to 35% of individuals with ASD identify as LGBTQ+.

Unintentional Injury and Safety
- Elopement and accidental drowning are among the most common safety concerns for children and youth with ASD. Proactive safety planning and education with families is necessary.

Law Enforcement Interaction
- Proactive safety planning and identification of high-risk situations with families is necessary because individuals with ASD (and frequent cooccurring conditions) are at increased risk for interacting with law enforcement.

Adverse Experiences
- Health care providers need to be aware of the higher rates of adverse experiences (i.e., bullying) experienced by youth with any intellectual or developmental disability (including ASD).
- Important components of bullying prevention include social skills training, peer education, teacher/staff training, and zero-tolerance school culture.
- Children with IEPs/504s have legal protections against bullying under IDEA (see Resources).
- Children and adults with disabilities (including ASD) have higher rates of physical/sexual abuse and neglect. Regular screening is necessary.

Extremism and Criminal Conduct
- Studies suggest that individuals with ASD are more likely to be the victim of a violent crime rather than the perpetrator. Immediate action to preserve safety should be taken when any child appears at risk of harming themselves or others.

COMMON ILLNESS MANAGEMENT
Gastrointestinal
- GI symptoms such as constipation, diarrhea, and reflux are more common in children with ASD.
- Feeding challenges may contribute to GI symptoms.

Toileting Problems
- Delays in toileting are common for children with ASD.
- Consider the role of developmental readiness, anxiety, and communication deficits.
- Many children benefit from ABA-based behavioral teaching, including gradual exposure, positive reinforcement, and repeated stepwise practice, as well as use of visuals.
- Rule out medical problems contributing to toileting, such as constipation.

Feeding and Diet
- Approximately 75% of children with ASD have problems related to eating, including selective eating.

Pica
- Pica is more common in children with ASD and other developmental disabilities compared to the general population. Behavioral intervention is recommended, including prevention, immediate interruption, and redirection.

Sleep
- Children with ASD are more likely to have behavioral and medical sleep disorders.
- Pediatric primary care providers should screen, evaluate, treat, or refer for medical and behavioral sleep disorders.
- Behavioral treatments for sleep disorders are effective in children with autism.
- If a medical sleep condition is identified, it should be treated first, prior to significant behavioral treatments, to increase the chance of success.

ALLIED HEALTH AND EDUCATIONAL
- Children with ASD need to be assessed in multiple areas of functioning, including language abilities, motor skills, sensory processing, cognitive abilities, and academic achievement.
- This can often be done through the school district as part of an IEP, although many children will benefit from referrals to outpatient therapies (speech-language, occupation, physical, feeding therapy).

COMPLEMENTARY AND ALTERNATIVE APPROACHES
- Up to 95% of families have utilized some complementary or alternative approach for their child on the spectrum.
- Gluten-free diets are commonly tried, although there is sparse evidence of consistent effects on behavior, health, and developmental outcomes.
- Products containing CBD have become increasingly popular. There is limited evidence to guide these recommendations.
- Neurofeedback is gaining in popularity and has shown some evidence for improving ADHD symptoms but little evidence for affecting core autism symptoms.
- Health care providers should provide nonjudgmental advice and aim to support families with the most robust research evidence and safety considerations.

LIFESPAN CONSIDERATIONS
- Families face numerous stressors before and after receiving a diagnosis of ASD.
- Encourage social support and assistance to families following a diagnosis.
- Ask at every visit if families have questions about their child's health and what assistance they may need. Review current services the child has in place (such as an IEP for school, ABA therapy, and safety concerns) and identify those specific areas of need.
- Encourage the family to request in writing an evaluation for an IEP or 504 plan. Refer the family to local advocacy groups for assistance with these if needed.
- Begin discussing transition plans early (by age 14), including considerations of guardianship for some patients.

REFERENCES

Allely, C. S., & Faccini, L. (2017). A conceptual analysis of individuals with an autism spectrum disorder engaging in mass violence. *Journal of Forensic and Crime Studies, 1*(1), 1–5.

American Psychiatric Association (APA). (2013). *Diagnostic and statistical manual of mental disorders* (5th ed.). Washington, DC: Author.

Anderson, C., Law, J. K., Daniels, A., Rice, C., Mandell, D. S., Hagopian, L., & Law, P. A. (2012). Occurrence and family impact of elopement in children with autism spectrum disorders. *Pediatrics, 130*(5), 870–877. doi:10.1542/peds.2012-0762.

Aylward, B. S., Gal-Szabo, D. E., & Taraman, S. (2021). Racial, ethnic, and sociodemographic disparities in diagnosis of children with autism spectrum disorder. *Journal of Developmental and Behavioral Pediatrics, 42*(8), 682.

Batarseh, H., AbuMweis, S., Almakanin, H. A., & Anderson, C. (2022). Gluten-free and casein-free diet for children with autism spectrum disorder: A systematic review. *Advances in Neurodevelopmental Disorders*, 1–10.

Bearss, K., Johnson, C., Smith, T., Lecavalier, L., Swiezy, N., Aman, M., McAdam, D. B., Butter, E., Stillitano, C., Minshawi, N., Sukhodolsky, D. G., Mruzek, D. W., Turner, K., Neal, T., Hallett, V., Mulick, J. A., Green, B., Handen, B., Deng, Y., Dziura, J., Scahill, L. (2015). Effect of parent training vs parent education on behavioral problems in children with autism spectrum disorder: A randomized clinical trial. *JAMA, 313*(15), 1524–1533. doi:10.1001/jama.2015.3150.

Besag, F. M. (2018). Epilepsy in patients with autism: Links, risks and treatment challenges. *Neuropsychiatric Disease and Treatment, 14*, 1.

Bondy, A., & Frost, L. (2011). *A picture's worth: PECS and other visual communication strategies in autism*. Woodbine House.

Brasher, S., Stapel-Wax, J. L., & Muirhead, L. (2022). Racial and ethnic disparities in autism spectrum disorder: Implications for care. *Nurse Clinic, 57*(3), 489–499.

Brown, H. M., Stahmer, A. C., Dwyer, P., & Rivera, S. (2021). Changing the story: How diagnosticians can support a neurodiversity perspective from the start. *Autism, 25*(5), 1171–1174.

Campbell, K., Carbone, P. S., Liu, D., & Stipelman, C. H. (2021). Improving autism screening and referrals with electronic support and evaluations in primary care. *Pediatrics, 147*(3).

Carbone, P. S., Campbell, K., Wilkes, J., Stoddard, G. J., Huynh, K., Young, P. C., & Gabrielsen, T. P. (2020). Primary care autism screening and later autism diagnosis. *Pediatrics, 146*(2), e20192314. doi:10.1542/peds.2019-2314.

Christensen, D. L., Bilder, D. A., Zahorodny, W., Pettygrove, S., Durkin, M. S., Fitzgerald, R. T., Rice, C., Kurzius-Spencer, M., Baio, J., & Yeargin-Allsopp, M. (2016). Prevalence and characteristics of autism spectrum disorder among 4-year-old children in the autism and developmental disabilities monitoring network. *Journal of Developmental and Behavioral Pediatrics: JDBP, 37*(1), 1–8. https://doi.org/10.1097/DBP.0000000000000235.

Constantino, J. N., & Gruber, C. P. (2012). *The social responsiveness scale* (2nd ed.). Western Psychological Services.

Constantino, J. N., Abbacchi, A. M., Saulnier, C., Klaiman, C., Mandell, D. S., Zhang, Y., Hawks, Z., Bates, J., Klin, A., Shattuck, P., Molholm, S., Fitzgerald, R., Roux, A., Lowe, J. K., & Geschwind, D. H. (2020). Timing of the diagnosis of autism in african american children. *Pediatrics, 146*(3), e20193629. https://doi.org/10.1542/peds.2019-3629.

Croen, L. A., Zerbo, O., Qian, Y., Massolo, M. L., Rich, S., Sidney, S., & Kripke, C. (2015). The health status of adults on the autism spectrum. *Autism: The International Journal of Research And Practice, 19*(7), 814–823. https://doi.org/10.1177/1362361315577517.

Curtin, C., Hubbard, K., Anderson, S. E., Mick, E., Must, A., & Bandini, L. G. (2015). Food selectivity, mealtime behavior problems, spousal stress, and family food choices in children with and without autism spectrum disorder. *Journal of Autism and Developmental Disorders, 45*, 3308–3315.

Curtin, C., Hyman, S. L., Boas, D. D., Hassink, S., Broder-Fingert, S., Ptomey, L. T., Gillette, M. D., Fleming, R. K., Must, A., & Bandini, L. G. (2020). Weight management in primary care for children with autism: Expert recommendations. *Pediatrics, 145*(Suppl 1), S126–S139. https://doi.org/10.1542/peds.2019-1895P.

DeStefano, F., & Shimabukuro, T. T. (2019). The MMR vaccine and autism. *Annual Review of Virology, 6*(1), 585.

D'Mello, A. M., Frosch, I. R., Li, C. E., Cardinaux, A. L., & Gabrieli, J. D. (2022). Exclusion of females in autism research: Empirical evidence for a "leaky" recruitment-to-research pipeline. *Autism Research, 15*(10), 1929–1940.

Donaldson, A. L., Krejcha, K., & McMillin, A. (2017). A strengths-based approach to autism: Neurodiversity and partnering with the autism community. *Perspectives in ASHA Special Interest Groups, 2*(1), 56–68.

Duvall, S. W., Lindly, O., Zuckerman, K., Msall, M. E., & Weddle, M. (2019). Ethical implications for providers regarding cannabis use in children with autism spectrum disorders. *Pediatrics, 143*(2).

Dwyer, P., Ryan, J. G., Williams, Z. J., & Gassner, D. L. (2022). First do no harm: Suggestions regarding respectful autism language. *Pediatrics. 149*(Suppl 4):e2020049437N. doi: 10.1542/peds.2020-049437N. PMID: 35363298; PMCID: PMC9066426.

Feinberg, E., Augustyn, M., Broder-Fingert, S., Bennett, A., Weitzman, C., Kuhn, J., Hickey, E., Chu, A., Levinson, J., Sandler Eilenberg, J., Silverstein, M., Cabral, H. J., Patts, G., Diaz-Linhart, Y., Fernandez-Pastrana, I., Rosenberg, J., Miller, J. S., Guevara, J. P., Fenick, A. M., & Blum, N. J. (2021). Effect of family navigation on diagnostic ascertainment among children at risk for autism: A randomized clinical trial from DBPNet. *JAMA Pediatr. 175*(3), 243–250. doi:10.1001/jamapediatrics.2020.5218.

Feldman, H. (2019). How young children learn language and speech: Implications of theory and evidence for clinical Practice. *Pediatric Reviews, 40*(8), 398–411. doi:10.1542/pir.2017-0325.

Fields, V. L., Soke, G. N., Reynolds, A., Tian, L. H., Wiggins, L., Maenner, M., DiGuiseppi, C., Kral, T. V. E., Hightshoe, K., & Schieve, L. A. (2021). Pica, autism, and other disabilities. *Pediatrics, 147*(2), e20200462. https://doi.org/10.2196/33391.

Fombonne, E. (2018). The rising prevalence of autism. *Journal of Child Psychology and Psychiatry, 59*(7), 717–720.

Friel, C., Leyland, A. H., Anderson, J. J., Havdahl, A., Borge, T., Shimonovich, M., & Dundas, R. (2021). Prenatal vitamins and the risk of offspring autism spectrum disorder: Systematic review and meta-analysis. *Nutrients, 13*(8), 2558. doi:10.3390/nu13082558.

George, R., & Stokes, M. A. (2018). Gender identity and sexual orientation in autism spectrum disorder. *Autism, 22*(8), 970–982.

Gerow, S., Davis, T., Radhakrishnan, S., Gregori, E., & Rivera, G. (2018). Functional communication training: The strength of evidence across disabilities. *Exceptional Children, 85*(1), 86–103.

Glascoe, F. P. (2000). Early detection of developmental and behavioral problems. *Pediatric Reviews, 21*(8), 272–280.

Hagberg, K. W., Robijn, A. L., & Jick, S. (2018). Maternal depression and antidepressant use during pregnancy and the risk of autism spectrum disorder in offspring. *Clinical Epidemiology, 10*, 1599.

Hamner, T., Hepburn, S., Zhang, F., Fidler, D., Robinson Rosenberg, C., Robins, D. L., & Lee, N. R. (2020). Cognitive profiles and autism symptoms in comorbid Down syndrome and autism spectrum disorder. *Journal of Developmental and Behavioral Pediatrics, 41*(3), 172–179. doi:10.1097/DBP.0000000000000745.

Hansen, S. N., Schendel, D. E., Francis, R. W., Windham, G. C., Bresnahan, M., Levine, S. Z., Reichenberg, A., Gissler, M., Kodesh, A., Bai, D., Yip, B. H. K., Leonard, H., Sandin, S., Buxbaum, J. D., Hultman, C., Sourander, A., Glasson, E. J., Wong, K., Öberg, R., & Parner, E. T. (2019). Recurrence risk of autism in siblings and cousins: A multinational, population-based study. *Journal of the American Academy of Child and Adolescent Psychiatry, 58*(9), 866–875. doi:10.1016/j.jaac.2018.11.017.

Harris, J. F., Gorman, L. P., Doshi, A., Swope, S., & Page, S. D. (2021). Development and implementation of health care transition resources for youth with autism spectrum disorders within a primary care medical home. *Autism, 25*(3), 753–766.

Hine, J. F., Wagner, L., Goode, R., Rodrigues, V., Taylor, J. L., Weitlauf, A., & Warren, Z. E. (2021). Enhancing developmental–behavioral pediatric rotations by teaching residents how to evaluate autism in primary care. *Autism, 25*(5), 1492–1496. doi:10.1177/1362361320984313. Epub 2021 Jan 5. PMID: 33401941; PMCID: PMC8255322.

Höfer, J., Hoffmann, F., & Bachmann, C. (2017). Use of complementary and alternative medicine in children and adolescents with autism spectrum disorder: A systematic review. *Autism, 21*(4), 387–402.

Hollocks, M. J., Lerh, J. W., Magiati, I., Meiser-Stedman, R., & Brugha, T. S. (2019). Anxiety and depression in adults with autism spectrum disorder: A systematic review and meta-analysis. *Psychological Medicine, 49*(4), 559–572.

Hoover, D. W., & Kaufman, J. (2018). Adverse childhood experiences in children with autism spectrum disorder. *Current Opinion in Psychiatry, 31*(2), 128.

Hossain, M. M., Khan, N., Sultana, A., Ma, P., McKyer, E. L. J., Ahmed, H. U., & Purohit, N. (2020). Prevalence of comorbid psychiatric disorders among people with autism spectrum disorder: An umbrella review of systematic reviews and meta-analyses. *Psychiatry Research, 287*, 112922.

Hull, L., Petrides, K. V., Allison, C., Smith, P., Baron-Cohen, S., Lai, M. C., & Mandy, W. (2017). Putting on my best normal": Social camouflaging in adults with autism spectrum conditions. *Journal of Autism and Developmental Disorders, 47*(8), 2519–2534. doi:10.1007/s10803-017-3166-5.

Humphrey, N., & Hebron, J. (2015). Bullying of children and adolescents with autism spectrum conditions: A 'state of the field' review. *International Journal of Inclusive Education, 19*(8), 845–862.

Hyman, S. L., Levy, S. E., & Myers, S. M.; Council on Children with Disabilities, Section on Developmental and Behavioral Pediatrics (2020). Identification, evaluation, and management of children with autism spectrum disorder. *Pediatrics, 145*(1), e20193447. https://doi.org/10.1542/peds.2019-3447.

Imm, P., White, T., & Durkin, M. S. (2019). Assessment of racial and ethnic bias in autism spectrum disorder prevalence estimates from a US surveillance system. *Autism, 23*(8), 1927–1935.

Janecka, M., Hansen, S. N., Modabbernia, A., Browne, H. A., Buxbaum, J. D., Schendel, D. E., Reichenberg, A., Parner, E. T., & Grice, D. E. (2019). Parental age and differential estimates of risk for neuropsychiatric disorders: Findings from the Danish birth cohort. *Journal of the American Academy of Child and Adolescent Psychiatry, 58*(6), 618–627. doi:10.1016/j.jaac.2018.09.447.

Janecka, M., Kodesh, A., Levine, S. Z., Lusskin, S. I., Viktorin, A., Rahman, R., Buxbaum, J. D., Schlessinger, A., Sandin, S., & Reichenberg, A. (2018). Association of autism spectrum disorder with prenatal exposure to medication affecting neurotransmitter systems. *JAMA Psychiatry, 75*(12), 1217–1224. doi:10.1001/jamapsychiatry.2018.2728.

Jang, J., White, S. P., Esler, A. N., Kim, S. H., Klaiman, C., Megerian, J. T., Morse, A., Nadler, C., & Kanne, S. M. (2022). Diagnostic evaluations of autism spectrum disorder during the COVID-19 pandemic. *Journal of Autism and Developmental Disorders, 52*(2), 962–973. doi:10.1007/s10803-021-04960-7.

Jansen, A. G., Dieleman, G. C., Jansen, P. R., Verhulst, F. C., Posthuma, D., & Polderman, T. J. (2020). Psychiatric polygenic risk scores as predictor for attention deficit/hyperactivity disorder and autism spectrum disorder in a clinical child and adolescent sample. *Behavior Genetics, 50*(4), 203–212.

Jiang, C. C., Lin, L. S., Long, S., Ke, X. Y., Fukunaga, K., Lu, Y. M., & Han, F. (2022). Signalling pathways in autism spectrum disorder: Mechanisms and therapeutic implications. *Signal Transduction and Targeted Therapy, 7*(1), 229. doi:10.1038/s41392-022-01081-0.

Kanne, S. M., Carpenter, L. A., & Warren, Z. (2018). Screening in toddlers and preschoolers at risk for autism spectrum disorder: Evaluating a novel mobile-health screening tool. *Autism Research, 11*(7), 1038–1049.

Kirkpatrick, B., Louw, J. S., & Leader, G. (2019). Efficacy of parent training incorporated in behavioral sleep interventions for children with autism spectrum disorder and/or intellectual disabilities: A systematic review. *Sleep Medicine, 53*, 141–152.

Klinger, L. G., Cook, M. L., & Dudley, K. M. (2021). Predictors and moderators of treatment efficacy in children and adolescents with autism spectrum disorder. *Journal of Clinical Child and Adolescent Psychology, 50*(4), 517–524.

Kuhn, J., Levinson, J., Udhnani, M. D., Wallis, K., Hickey, E., Bennett, A., Fenick, A. M., Feinberg, E., & Broder-Fingert, S. (2021). What happens after a positive primary care autism screen among historically underserved families? Predictors of evaluation and autism diagnosis. *Journal of Developmental and Behavioral Pediatrics, 42*(7), 515–523. doi:10.1097/DBP.0000000000000928.

Kuo, A. A., & Torrest, A. (2022). Meeting the primary care needs of autistic individuals. *Pediatrics, 149*(Supplement 4).

Kurtz, P. F., Leoni, M., & Hagopian, L. P. (2020). Behavioral approaches to assessment and early intervention for severe problem behavior in intellectual and developmental disabilities. *Pediatric Clinics, 67*(3), 499–511.

Larcombe, T. J., Joosten, A. V., Cordier, R., & Vaz, S. (2019). Preparing children with autism for transition to mainstream school and perspectives on supporting positive school experiences. *Journal of Autism and Developmental Disorders, 49*(8), 3073–3088. doi:10.1007/s10803-019-04022-z.

Laverty, C., Oliver, C., Moss, J., Nelson, L., & Richards, C. (2020). Persistence and predictors of self-injurious behaviour in autism: A ten-year prospective cohort study. *Molecular Autism, 11*(1), 1–17.

Leadbitter, K., Buckle, K. L., Ellis, C., & Dekker, M. (2021). Autistic self-advocacy and the neurodiversity movement: Implications for autism early intervention research and practice. *Frontiers in Psychology, 12*(Article 635690), 1–7.

Leaf, J. B., Cihon, J. H., Ferguson, J. L., Milne, C. M., Leaf, R., & McEachin, J. (2021). Advances in our understanding of behavioral intervention: 1980 to 2020 for individuals diagnosed with autism spectrum disorder. *Journal of Autism and Developmental Disorders, 51*(12), 4395–4410.

Lindly, O. J., Thorburn, S., Heisler, K., Reyes, N. M., & Zuckerman, K. E. (2018). Parents' use of complementary health approaches for young children with autism spectrum disorder. *Journal of Autism and Developmental Disorders, 48*, 1803–1818.

Lindsey, R. A., & Barry, T. D. (2018). Protective factors against distress for caregivers of a child with autism spectrum disorder. *Journal of Autism and Developmental Disorders, 48*(4), 1092–1107.

Loomes, R., Hull, L., & Mandy, W. P. L. (2017). What is the male-to-female ratio in autism spectrum disorder? A systematic review and meta-analysis. *Journal of the American Academy of Child and Adolescent Psychiatry, 56*(6), 466–474.

Lord, C., Rutter, M., DiLavore, P., Risi, S., Gotham, K., & Bishop, S. (2012). *Autism diagnostic observation schedule: ADOS-2.* Western Psychological Services.

Lyall, K., Croen, L., Daniels, J., Fallin, M. D., Ladd-Acosta, C., Lee, B. K., Park, B. Y., Snyder, N. W., Schendel, D., Volk, H., Windham, G. C., & Newschaffer, C. (2017). The changing epidemiology of autism spectrum disorders. *Annual Review* of Public Health, 38, 81–102. doi:10.1146/annurev-publhealth-031816-044318.

Maenner, M. J., Shaw, K. A., Bakian, A. V., Bilder, D. A., Durkin, M. S., Esler, A., Furnier, S. M., Hallas, L., Hall-Lande, J., Hudson, A., Hughes, M. M., Patrick, M., Pierce, K., Poynter, J. N., Salinas, A., Shenouda, J., Vehorn, A., Warren, Z., Constantino, J. N., … Cogswell, M. E. (2021). Prevalence and characteristics of autism spectrum disorder among children aged 8 years—autism and developmental disabilities monitoring network, 11 Sites, United States, 2018. Morbidity and mortality weekly report. Surveillance Summaries (Washington, D.C.: 2002), 70(11), 1–16. https://doi.org/10.15585/mmwr.ss7011a1.

Malow, B. A., Byars, K., Johnson, K., Weiss, S., Bernal, P., Goldman, S. E., Panzer, R., Coury, D. L., & Glaze, D. G. (2012). Sleep committee of the autism treatment network. A practice pathway for the identification, evaluation, and management of insomnia in children and adolescents with autism spectrum disorders. Pediatrics, 130(Suppl 2), S106–S124. doi:10.1542/peds.2012-0900I. PMID: 23118242; PMCID: PMC9923883.

Margolis, S. S., Sell, G. L., Zbinden, M. A., & Bird, L. M. (2015). Angelman syndrome. Neurotherapy, 12(3), 641–650.

Maye, M., Sanchez, V. E., Stone-MacDonald, A., & Carter, A. S. (2020). Early interventionists' appraisals of intervention strategies for toddlers with autism spectrum disorder and their peers in inclusive childcare classrooms. Journal of Autism and Developmental Disorders, 50(11), 4199–4208.

Mazurek, M. O., Kuhlthau, K., Parker, R. A., Chan, J., & Sohl, K. (2021). Autism and general developmental screening practices among primary care providers. Journal of Developmental and Behavioral Pediatrics, 42(5), 355–362.

Mazurek, M. O., Curran, A., Burnette, C., & Sohl, K. (2019). ECHO autism STAT: Accelerating early access to autism diagnosis. Journal of Autism and Developmental Disorders, 49(1), 127–137.

McDonnell, C. G., Boan, A. D., Bradley, C. C., Seay, K. D., Charles, J. M., & Carpenter, L. A. (2019). Child maltreatment in autism spectrum disorder and intellectual disability: Results from a population-based sample. Journal of Child Psychology and Psychiatry, 60(5), 576–584.

McGowan, E. C., & Sheinkopf, S. J. (2021). Autism and preterm birth: Clarifying risk and exploring mechanisms. Pediatrics, 148(3).

McIlwain, L., & Fournier, W. Lethal outcomes in autism spectrum disorders (ASD) wandering/elopement. 2011. Retrieved from National Autism Association: http://nationalautismassociation.org/wpcontent/uploads/2012/01/Lethal-Outcomes-In-Autism-SpectrumDisorders_2012.pdf.

McNally, P., Taggart, L., & Shevlin, M. (2021). Trauma experiences of people with an intellectual disability and their implications: A scoping review. Journal of Applied Research in Intellectual Disabilities, 34(4), 927–949.

Megerian, J. T., Dey, S., Melmed, R. D., Coury, D. L., Lerner, M., Nicholls, C. J., Sohl, K., Rouhbakhsh, R., Narasimhan, A., Romain, J., Golla, S., Shareef, S., Ostrovsky, A., Shannon, J., Kraft, C., Liu-Mayo, S., Abbas, H., Gal-Szabo, D. E., Wall, D. P., & Taraman, S. (2022). Evaluation of an artificial intelligence-based medical device for diagnosis of autism spectrum disorder. NPJ Digit Med., 5(1), 57. doi:10.1038/s41746-022-00598-6. PMID: 35513550; PMCID: PMC9072329.

Metz, B., Mulick, J. A., & Butter, E. M. (2015). Autism: A twenty-first century fad magnet. In Controversial therapies for autism and intellectual disabilities (pp. 189–215). Routledge.

Mila, M., Alvarez-Mora, M. I., Madrigal, I., & Rodriguez-Revenga, L. (2018). Fragile X syndrome: An overview and update of the FMR1 gene. Clinical Genetics, 93(2), 197–205.

Monz, B. U., Houghton, R., Law, K., & Loss, G. (2019). Treatment patterns in children with autism in the United States. Autism Research, 12(3), 517–526.

Moosa, A., Shu, H., Sarachana, T., & Hu, V. W. (2018). Are endocrine disrupting compounds environmental risk factors for autism spectrum disorder? Hormones and Behavior, 101, 13–21.

Nadler, C., & Blum, N. J. (2022). Behavioral parent training and consultation. In Feldman, H., Elias, E., Stancin, T., Blum, N., & Jimenez, M. (Eds.), Developmental-behavioral pediatrics (5th ed.). Elsevier.

Neul, J. L. (2022). The relationship of Rett syndrome and MECP2 disorders to autism. Dialogues in Clinical Neuroscience, 14, 253–262.

Nicolaidis, C. (2012). What can physicians learn from the neurodiversity movement? American Journal of Ethics, 14(6), 503–510.

Nordahl-Hansen, A., Hart, L., & Øien, R. A. (2018). The scientific study of parents and caregivers of children with ASD: A flourishing field but still work to be done. Journal of Autism and Developmental Disorders, 48(4), 976–979.

Numata, N., Nakagawa, A., Yoshioka, K., Isomura, K., Matsuzawa, D., Setsu, R., Nakazato, M., & Shimizu, E. (2021). Associations between autism spectrum disorder and eating disorders with and without self-induced vomiting: An empirical study. Journal of Eating Disorders, 9(1), 5. https://doi.org/10.1186/s40337-020-00359-4.

Olson, O., Berry, C., & Kumar, N. (2020). Addressing parental vaccine hesitancy towards childhood vaccines in the United States: A systematic literature review of communication interventions and strategies. Vaccines, 8(4), 590.

Owens, J. A., & Dalzell, V. (2005). Use of the 'BEARS' sleep screening tool in a pediatric residents' continuity clinic: a pilot study. Sleep Med., 6(1), 63–69. doi: 10.1016/j.sleep.2004.07.015. Epub 2005 Jan 12. PMID: 15680298.

Owens, J. A., Spirito, A., & McGuinn, M. (2000). The children's sleep habits questionnaire (CSHQ): Psychometric properties of a survey instrument for school-aged children. Sleep, 23(8), 1043–1052.

Patel, J. N., Mueller, M. K., Guffey, W. J., & Stegman, J. (2020). Drug prescribing and outcomes after pharmacogenomic testing in a developmental and behavioral health pediatric clinic. Journal of Developmental and Behavioral Pediatrics, 41(1), 65–70.

Pecora, L. A., Mesibov, G. B., & Stokes, M. A. (2016). Sexuality in high-functioning autism: A systematic review and meta-analysis. Journal of Autism and Developmental Disorders, 46(11), 3519–3556.

Peden, A. E., & Willcox-Pidgeon, S. (2020). Autism spectrum disorder and unintentional fatal drowning of children and adolescents in Australia: An epidemiological analysis. Archives of Disease in Childhood, 105(9), 869–874.

Qian, M., Chou, S. Y., & Lai, E. K. (2020). Confirmatory bias in health decisions: Evidence from the MMR-autism controversy. Journal of Health Economics, 70, 102284.

Rava, J., Shattuck, P., Rast, J., & Roux, A. (2017). The prevalence and correlates of involvement in the criminal justice system among youth on the autism spectrum. Journal of Autism and Developmental Disorders, 47(2), 340–346.

Reynolds, A. M., Soke, G. N., Sabourin, K. R., Hepburn, S., Katz, T., Wiggins, L. D., Schieve, L. A., & Levy, S. E. (2019). Sleep problems in 2- to 5-year-olds with autism spectrum disorder and other developmental delays. Pediatrics, 143(3), e20180492. doi:10.1542/peds.2018-0492.

Riesco-Matías, P., Yela-Bernabé, J. R., Crego, A., & Sánchez-Zaballos, E. (2021). What do meta-analyses have to say about the efficacy of neurofeedback applied to children with ADHD? Review of previous meta-analyses and a new meta-analysis. Journal of Attention Disorders, 25(4), 473–485.

Rixon, L., Hastings, R. P., Kovshoff, H., & Bailey, T. (2021). Sibling adjustment and sibling relationships associated with clusters of needs in children with autism: A novel methodological approach. Journal of Autism and Developmental Disorders, 51(11), 4067–4076.

Robins, D. L., Casagrande, K., Barton, M., Chen, C. M. A., Dumont-Mathieu, T., & Fein, D. (2014). Validation of the modified checklist for autism in toddlers, revised with follow-up (M-CHAT-R/F). *Pediatrics, 133*(1), 37–45.

Rubenstein, E., Wiggins, L. D., & Lee, L. C. (2015). A review of the differences in developmental, psychiatric, and medical endophenotypes between males and females with autism spectrum disorder. *Journal of Developmental and Physical Disabilities, 27*(1), 119–139.

Rutter, M., Le Couteur, A., & Lord, C. (2003). *Autism diagnostic interview revised.* Los Angeles, CA: Western Psychological Services; 29, 30.

Sammels, O., Karjalainen, L., Dahlgren, J., & Wentz, E. (2022). Autism spectrum disorder and obesity in children: A systematic review and meta-analysis. *Obesity Facts, 15*(3), 305–320.

Savatt, J. M., & Myers, S. M. (2021). Genetic testing in neurodevelopmental disorders. *Frontiers in Pediatrics, 9*, 526779.

Schiller, V. F., Dorstyn, D. S., & Taylor, A. M. (2021). The protective role of social support sources and types against depression in caregivers: A meta-analysis. *Journal of Autism and Developmental Disorders, 51*(4), 1304–1315.

Schopler, E., Van Bourgondien, M. E., Wellman, G. J., & Love, S. R. (2010). *Childhood autism rating scale, second edition* (CARS-2). Torrance, CA: Western Psychological Services.

Schreibman, L., Dawson, G., Stahmer, A. C., Landa, R., Rogers, S. J., McGee, G. G., Kasari, C., Ingersoll, B., Kaiser, A. P., Bruinsma, Y., McNerney, E., Wetherby, A., & Halladay, A. (2015). Naturalistic developmental behavioral interventions: Empirically validated treatments for autism spectrum disorder. *Journal of Autism and Developmental Disorders, 45*(8), 2411–2428. doi:10.1007/s10803-015-2407-8.

Segers, M., & Rawana, J. (2014). What do we know about suicidality in autism spectrum disorders? A systematic review. *Autism Research, 7*(4), 507–521.

Sheldrick, R. C., & Perrin, E. C. (2013). Evidence-based milestones for surveillance of cognitive, language, and motor development. *Academic Pediatrics, 13*(6), 577–586.

Siegel, M., & Gabriels, R. L. (2013). Psychiatric hospital treatment of children with autism and serious behavioral disturbance. *Child and Adolescent Psychiatric Clinics, 23*(1), 125–142.

Simonoff, E., Kent, R., Stringer, D., Lord, C., Briskman, J., Lukito, S., Pickles, A., Charman, T., & Baird, G. (2020). Trajectories in symptoms of autism and cognitive ability in autism from childhood to adult life: Findings from a longitudinal epidemiological cohort. *Journal of the American Academy of Child and Adolescent Psychiatry, 59*(12), 1342–1352. doi:10.1016/j.jaac.2019.11.020.

Smith, N. J., Sheldrick, R. C., & Perrin, E. C. (2013). An abbreviated screening instrument for autism spectrum disorders. *Infant Mental Health Journal, 34*(2), 149–155.

Specchio, N., Pietrafusa, N., Trivisano, M., Moavero, R., De Palma, L., Ferretti, A., Vigevano, F., & Curatolo, P. (2020). Autism and epilepsy in patients with tuberous sclerosis complex. *Frontiers in Neurology, 11*, 639. doi:10.3389/fneur.2020.00639.

Squires, J., Bricker, D. D., & Twombly, E. (2009). *Ages & stages questionnaires* (pp. 257–282). Baltimore, MD: Paul H. Brookes.

Srancikova, A., Bacova, Z., & Bakos, J. (2021). The epigenetic regulation of synaptic genes contributes to the etiology of autism. *Reviews in Neuroscience.*

Tick, B., Bolton, P., Happé, F., Rutter, M., & Rijsdijk, F. (2016). Heritability of autism spectrum disorders: A meta-analysis of twin studies. *Journal of Child Psychology and Psychiatry, 57*(5), 585–595.

Vargason, T., Roth, E., Grivas, G., Ferina, J., Frye, R. E., & Hahn, J. (2020). Classification of autism spectrum disorder from blood metabolites: Robustness to the presence of co-occurring conditions. *Research in Autism Spectrum Disorder, 77*, 101644.

Waddington, H., van der Meer, L., & Sigafoos, J. (2016). Effectiveness of the early start Denver model: A systematic review. *Review Journal of Autism and Developmental Disorders, 3*(2), 93–106.

Wagner, L., Corona, L. L., Weitlauf, A. S., Marsh, K. L., Berman, A. F., Broderick, N. A., Francis, S., Hine, J., Nicholson, A., Stone, C., & Warren, Z. (2021). Use of the TELE-ASD-PEDS for autism evaluations in response to COVID-19: Preliminary outcomes and clinician acceptability. *Journal of Autism and Developmental Disorders, 51*(9), 3063–3072. doi:10.1007/s10803-020-04767-y.

Wallis, K. E., Guthrie, W., Bennett, A. E., Gerdes, M., Levy, S. E., Mandell, D. S., & Miller, J. S. (2020). Adherence to screening and referral guidelines for autism spectrum disorder in toddlers in pediatric primary care. *PloS One, 15*(5), e0232335. doi:10.1371/journal.pone.0232335.

Washington, P., Park, N., Srivastava, P., Voss, C., Kline, A., Varma, M., Tariq, Q., Kalantarian, H., Schwartz, J., Patnaik, R., Chrisman, B., Stockham, N., Paskov, K., Haber, N., & Wall, D. P. (2020). Data-driven diagnostics and the potential of mobile artificial intelligence for digital therapeutic phenotyping in computational psychiatry. *Biological Psychiatry: Cognitive Neuroscience and Neuroimaging, 5*(8), 759–769. doi:10.1016/j.bpsc.2019.11.015.

White, S. W., Simmons, G. L., Gotham, K. O., Conner, C. M., Smith, I. C., Beck, K. B., & Mazefsky, C. A. (2018). Psychosocial treatments targeting anxiety and depression in adolescents and adults on the autism spectrum: Review of the latest research and recommended future directions. *Current Psychiatry Reports, 20*(10), 1–10. doi:10.1007/s11920-018-0949-0.

Wieckowski, A. T., Zuckerman, K. E., Broder-Fingert, S., & Robins, D. L. (2022). Addressing current barriers to autism diagnoses through a tiered diagnostic approach involving pediatric primary care providers. *Autism Research.*

Wright Stein, S., Alexander, R., Mann, J., Schneider, C., Zhang, S., Gibson, B. E., Gabison, S., Jachyra, P., & Mosleh, D. (2022). Understanding disability in healthcare: Exploring the perceptions of parents of young people with autism spectrum disorder. *Disability and Rehabilitation, 44*(19), 5623–5630. doi:10.1080/09638288.2021.1948114.

Yip, P. S., Caine, E., Yousuf, S., Chang, S. S., Wu, K. C. C., & Chen, Y. Y. (2012). Means restriction for suicide prevention. *Lancet, 379*(9834), 2393–2399.

Zerbo, O., Qian, Y., Yoshida, C., Grether, J. K., Van de Water, J., & Croen, L. A. (2015). Maternal infection during pregnancy and autism spectrum disorders. *Journal of Autism and Developmental Disorders, 45*(12), 4015–4025.

Zwaigenbaum, L., & Warren, Z. (2021). Commentary: Embracing innovation is necessary to improve assessment and care for individuals with ASD: A reflection on Kanne and Bishop (2020). *Journal of Child Psychology and Psychiatry, 62*(2), 143–145.

11

Bleeding Disorders

Lucy Delaney Carter Reardon, Mindy Eldridge

PATHOPHYSIOLOGY

Hemostasis is the blood clot formation process at the vessel injury site. When a blood vessel wall is disrupted, the hemostatic response must be quick, localized, and carefully regulated. The multistep process of clot formation is called coagulation. The coagulation cascade is a complex chemical process that uses up to 10 different proteins (or coagulation factors) to form a hemostatic plug at the site of vascular injury. When a blood vessel is injured, blood starts to flow. Vasoconstriction is the first thing that will occur to control bleeding. Platelets will then rush to the injury site and bunch together around the wound, helping form a plug. Tissue factors also come into this process when a blood vessel is injured to help stop bleeding. Tissue factors will stimulate clotting factors to produce fibrin, a strandlike substance that surrounds the platelet plug. The fibrin clot becomes meshlike, which keeps the plug firm and stable. Over the next days to weeks, the clot strengthens and then dissolves as the wound heals. Those with a bleeding disorder have abnormalities with key proteins in the coagulation cascade. This chapter focuses on common hereditary bleeding disorders: hemophilia A (factor VIII deficiency), hemophilia B (factor IX deficiency), and von Willebrand disease (vWD) (UpToDate, n.d) (James, 2022a) (Fig. 11.1).

HEMOPHILIA

People with hemophilia have low levels of clotting factor proteins, specifically factors VIII and IX. Both are necessary components for hemostasis. Hemophilia A (classic hemophilia or factor VIII deficiency) involves factor VIII protein; hemophilia B (Christmas disease or factor IX deficiency) involves factor IX protein. The severity of hemophilia is determined by the amount of factor in the blood (Table 11.1). The lower the amount of factor, the more likely the affected person will bleed (Centers for Disease Control and Prevention [CDC], 2020).

The exact number of people living with hemophilia in the United States is not completely known. In a study conducted by the CDC and US Hemophilia Treatment Center Network, the current number of males with hemophilia living in the United States is estimated between 30,000 and 33,000. The prevalence of hemophilia in the United States is 12 cases per 100,000 US males for hemophilia A and 3.7 cases per 100,000 US males for hemophilia B. The estimated incidence of hemophilia among US births is 1 per 5617 male births for hemophilia A and 1 per 19,283 male births for hemophilia B. Among all males with hemophilia, 4 in 10 are in the severe category. Looking at the distribution of race and ethnicity in the US population, the White race is more commonly affected. Hispanic ethnicity is equally common, whereas Black race and Asian descent are less common among persons with hemophilia (Soucie et al., 2020). Globally, it is estimated that 43% of the world's hemophilia population lives in Bangladesh, Indonesia, and China, although only 12% have a hemophilia diagnosis (Shetty, 2014).

ACQUIRED/INHERITANCE

In people with hemophilia there is a mutation in the gene for either factor VIII or IX. This mutation impacts the ability to produce factor VIII or IX proteins. The genes for factors VIII and IX are located on the X chromosome. There are no genes for clotting factors on the Y chromosome. Therefore hemophilia is inherited in an X-linked recessive pattern. For males, this means they only have one allele for factor VIII and one allele for factor IX. If males have a hemophilia allele on their only X chromosome, they will have the disorder.

Females inherit two copies of factor VIII or IX gene—one from their mother and one from their father. A female with a hemophilia allele on one X chromosome usually has a normal allele on the other X chromosome that can produce a normal clotting factor. A female with this phenotype is called heterozygous or a carrier. Typically, female carriers have normal factor VIII or IX levels; however, even with normal levels, carriers can still have bleeding symptoms with traumatic events, surgeries, or experience menorrhagia. Carriers can also have low factor VIII or IX levels and be diagnosed with mild, moderate, or severe forms of hemophilia based on their factor levels. Females can also have hemophilia if they inherit hemophilia alleles from both of their parents or if they inherit one hemophilia allele and their other X chromosome has a spontaneous mutation.

For a mother that is a carrier (heterozygous) of hemophilia, and the father does not have hemophilia, each male offspring has a 1 in 2 (50%) chance of having hemophilia. Each female offspring has a 1 in 2 (50%) chance of being a carrier (heterozygous). Overall, for a carrier, there is a 1 in 4 (25%) chance for each pregnancy

What happens when a person has *a bleeding* disorder

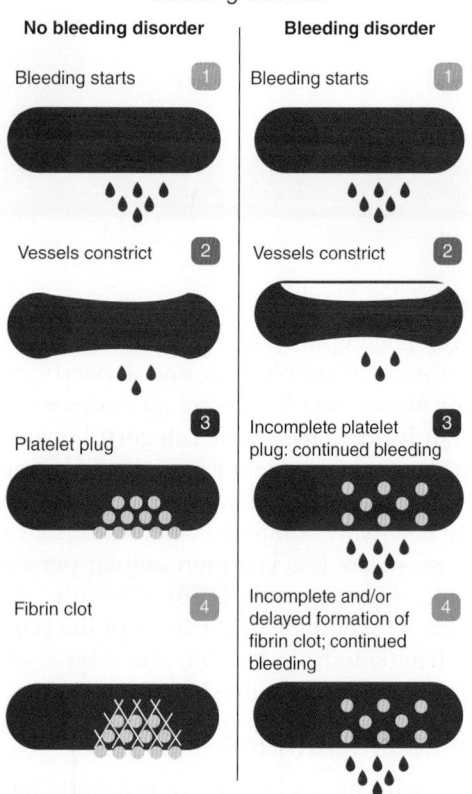

No bleeding disorder	Bleeding disorder
Bleeding starts **1**	Bleeding starts **1**
Vessels constrict **2**	Vessels constrict **2**
Platelet plug **3**	Incomplete platelet plug: continued bleeding **3**
Fibrin clot **4**	Incomplete and/or delayed formation of fibrin clot; continued bleeding **4**

Fig. 11.1 **Blood clot formation process.** (From Steps for Living. [2011]. What happens when a person bleeds. National Bleeding Disorders Foundation. https://stepsforliving.hemophilia.org/basics-of-bleeding-disorders/what-happens-when-a-person-bleeds/.)

Table 11.1 **Severity of Hemophilia**

SEVERITY	BLOOD CLOTTING FACTOR LEVEL
Normal	50–150%[a]
Mild	>5–<40%
Moderate	1–5%
Severe	<1%

[a]The classification of individuals with factor VIII levels between 40% and 50% remains unresolved. Some patients can bleed more than normal with factor VIII levels >40%.
From Makris, M., Oldenburg, J., Mauser-Bunschoten, E.P., et al. (2018). The definition, diagnosis and management of mild hemophilia A: Communication from the SSC of the ISTH. *Journal of Thrombosis and Haemostasis, 16*, 2530–2533; and Blanchette, V.S., Key, N.S., Ljung, L.R., et al. (2014). Definitions in hemophilia: Communication from the SSC of the ISTH. *Journal of Thrombosis and Haemostasis, 12*, 1935–1939.

that the baby will be a male offspring with hemophilia and a 1 and 4 (25%) chance the baby will be a heterozygous female offspring. There is a 1 in 2 (50%) chance that the baby (male or female offspring) will not get the hemophilia allele (CDC, 2021a).

For a father with hemophilia, he can only pass the X chromosome to his female offspring, so they will get the father's hemophilia allele and be heterozygous (carriers). A father cannot pass down a hemophilia allele to his male offspring as the hemophilia allele is on the X chromosome, and the father passes his Y chromosome to his male offspring. Overall, there is a 1 in 2 (50%) chance that the child will be a male offspring

who will not have hemophilia and a 1 and 2 (50%) chance the child will be a female offspring who is heterozygous (carrier) (CDC, 2021a) (Fig. 11.2).

Rarely, a person can develop acquired hemophilia (AH), an autoimmune disorder characterized by bleeding that occurs in a patient who has no personal or family history of hemophilia. In AH, the body produces inhibitors that attack clotting factors (most commonly factor VIII). AH is predominantly a disease of the elderly (between ages 60 and 80) and is rarely seen in children. In approximately 50% of the patients, no underlying disorder or triggering event can be identified (idiopathic form). The remaining 50% have coexisting disorders or conditions, including autoimmune disorders such as lupus, rheumatoid arthritis, multiple sclerosis, Sjögren syndrome, irritable bowel syndrome (IBS) or ulcerative colitis, infections, diabetes, hepatitis, blood (hematologic) cancer, or certain solid tumors. AH has also been associated with drugs such as penicillin or interferon, and an association with pregnancy has been reported mainly in the postpartum period (National Organization for Rare Disorders, 2022).

CLINICAL MANIFESTATIONS AT TIME OF DIAGNOSIS

The majority of children with hemophilia are diagnosed at birth because of known family history. It is recommended that male newborns of known carriers not diagnosed prenatally be tested for hemophilia by cord blood sampling of factor VIII or IV antigen levels, especially prior to circumcision (Kulkarni & Lusher, 2001; Kulkarni et al., 2006; Street et al., 2008). Circumcision is among the first surgical procedures performed on an infant or young male, with approximately 35% of male infants with hemophilia having prolonged bleeding following a circumcision (Liu et al., 2019). For patients without a family history, prolonged bleeding at circumcision should prompt additional laboratory investigation.

In addition, neonates with no family history of hemophilia and unexplained subgaleal or intracranial hemorrhage postdelivery should be screened for a hereditary bleeding disorder. It is estimated that 3.5% to 4% of neonates with hemophilia may experience an intracranial hemorrhage compared to full-term healthy neonates at 0.4%; this risk increases with the use of delivery instruments or traumatic measures during delivery (Shibahara et al., 2021a). Intracranial hemorrhage may be life threatening, and one-half of newborns with an intracranial hemorrhage develop neurologic deficits. Clinical manifestations of hemophilia and other bleeding disorders in infancy outside of bleeding with circumcision and intracranial hemorrhage include excessive bruising and hematomas, cephalohematoma, or bleeding following venipuncture, heel sticks, or immunizations (Kulkarni & Lusher, 2001; Kulkarni et al., 2006; Maclean et al., 2004; Street et al., 2008).

As stated, in approximately one-third of children the occurrence of hemophilia represents a new

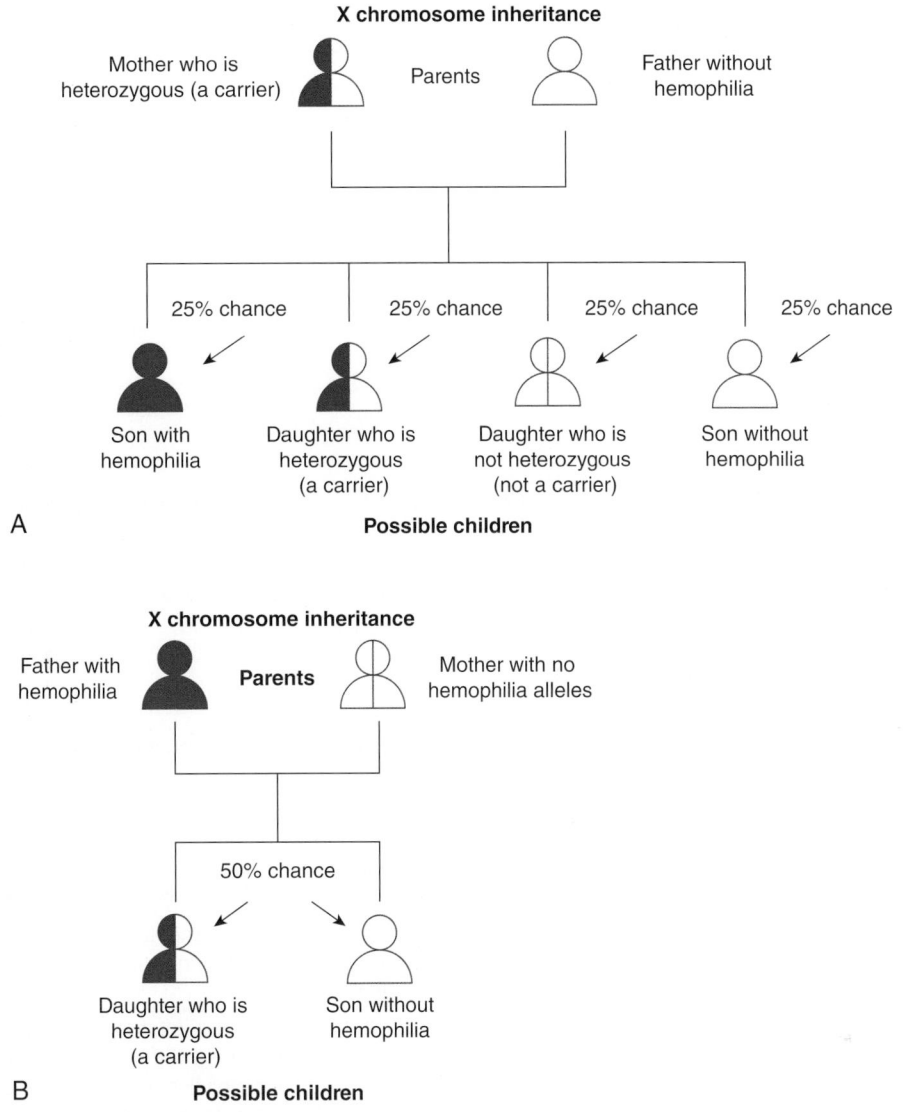

Fig. 11.2 **Hemophilia inheritance.** (From Centers for Disease Control and Prevention. [2021]. How hemophilia is inherited. https://www.cdc.gov/ncbddd/hemophilia/inheritance-pattern.html#:~:text=It%20almost%20always%20is%20inherited/.)

(spontaneous) mutation. Diagnosis is often made when these children begin to crawl and walk. Common symptoms include easy bruising, oral bleeding especially from a torn frenulum, hemarthroses (bleeding into joints), and intramuscular hemorrhages (bleeding into muscles) (Montgomery et al., 2008).

By 12 to 18 months of age, most children with severe hemophilia are diagnosed because of positive family history or unusual bleeding (Jones, 2002). Before diagnosis, parents may be questioned about child abuse because of excessive bruising. Children who first show signs of bleeding later in childhood or in adolescence more often have mild to moderate hemophilia.

A frequent misconception is that children with hemophilia can bleed to death from a typical childhood cut or scratch, but this does not occur. They may, however, demonstrate joint bleeding (i.e., hemarthrosis), muscle hematomas, excessive postoperative bleeding, or excessive or prolonged oral bleeding following frenulum tears, lost deciduous teeth, tooth eruption, and

dental extractions (Jones, 2002). If there is a suspicious bleeding pattern for the patient, utilization of the International Society of Thrombosis and Haemostatis ISTH-SSC Bleeding Assessment Tool gives insight into what would be considered a normal bleeding pattern versus an abnormal bleeding pattern (Elbatarny et al., 2014) (Table 11.2).

TESTING/DIAGNOSTIC CRITERIA

Testing for hemophilia includes a veinous blood sampling that measures the amount of circulating factor VIII or IX protein antigen or activity levels within the body. These screening tests are called clotting factor assays. When testing factors VIII and IX antigen levels in plasma, there are three most common assays available, including clot-based assay, chromogenic activity assay, and immunoassay. Appropriate diagnosis for all bleeding disorders requires access to laboratory facilities that are equipped with the appropriate resources and expertise to accurately perform factor assays (CDC, 2011).

Table **11.2**   ISTH-SSC Bleeding Assessment Tool

SYMPTOMS (UP TO THE TIME OF DIAGNOSIS)	0[§]	1[§]	2	3	4
Epistaxis	No/trivial	>5/yr or >10 min	Consultation only	Packing or cauterization or antifibrinolytic	Blood transfusion or replacement therapy (use of hemostatic blood components and rFVIIa) or desmopressin
Cutaneous	No/trivial	For bruises ≥5 (>1 cm) in exposed areas	Consultation only	Extensive	Spontaneous hematoma requiring blood transfusion
Bleeding from minor wounds	No/trivial	>5/yr or >10 min	Consultation only	Surgical hemostasis	Blood transfusion, replacement therapy or desmopressin
Oral cavity	No/trivial	Present	Consultation only	Surgical hemostasis, iron therapy	Blood transfusion, replacement therapy or desmopressin
GI bleeding	No/trivial	Present (not associated with ulcer, portal hypertension, hemorrhoids, angiodysplasia)	Consultation only	Surgical hemostasis, iron therapy	Blood transfusion, replacement therapy or desmopressin
Hematuria	No/trivial	Present (macroscopic)	Consultation only	Surgical hemostasis, iron therapy	Blood transfusion, replacement therapy or desmopressin
Tooth extraction	No/trivial or none done	Reported in ≤25% of all procedures, no intervention[b]	Reported in ≥25% of all procedures, no intervention[b]	Resuturing or packing	Blood transfusion, replacement therapy or desmopressin
Surgery	No/trivial or none done	Reported in ≤25% of all procedures, no intervention[b]	Reported in ≥25% of all procedures, no intervention[b]	Surgical hemostasis or antifibrinolytic	Blood transfusion, replacement therapy or desmopressin
Menorrhagia	No/trivial	Consultation only[a] or Changing pads more frequently than every 2 hr or Clot and flooding or PBAC score >100[c]	Time off work/school >2/yr or Requiring antifibrinolytics or hormonal or iron therapy	Requiring combined treatment with antifibrinolytics and hormonal therapy or Present since menarche and >12 mo	Acute menorrhagia requiring hospital admission and emergency treatment or Requiring blood transfusion, replacement therapy, desmopressin or Requiring dilatation and curettage or endometrial ablation or hysterectomy
Postpartum hemorrhage	No/trivial or no deliveries	Consultation only[a] or Use of syntocinon or Lochia >6 wk	Iron therapy or Antifibrinolytics	Requiring blood transfusion, replacement therapy, desmopressin or Requiring examination under anesthesia and/or the use of uterine balloon/package to tamponade the uterus	Any procedure requiring critical care or surgical intervention (e.g., hysterectomy, internal iliac artery legation, uterine artery embolization, uterine brace sutures)
Muscle hematomas	Never	Posttrauma, no therapy	Spontaneous, no therapy	Spontaneous or traumatic, requiring desmopressin or replacement therapy	Spontaneous or traumatic, requiring surgical intervention or blood transfusion

Table 11.2   ISTH-SSC Bleeding Assessment Tool—cont'd

SYMPTOMS (UP TO THE TIME OF DIAGNOSIS)	0§	1§	2	3	4
Hemarthrosis	Never	Posttrauma, no therapy	Spontaneous, no therapy	Spontaneous or traumatic, requiring desmopressin or replacement therapy	Spontaneous or traumatic, requiring surgical intervention or blood transfusion
CNS bleeding	Never			Subdural, any intervention	Intracerebral, any intervention
Other bleedings^	No/trivial	Present	Consultation only[a]	Surgical hemostasis, antifibrinolytics	Blood transfusion or replacement therapy or desmopressin

In addition to the guidance offered by the table, it is mandatory to refer to the text for more detailed instructions.

§Distinction between 0 and 1 is of critical importance. Score 1 means that the symptom is judged as present in the patient's history by the interviewer but does not qualify for a score 2 or more.

[a]Consultation only: The patient sought medical evaluation and was either referred to a specialist or offered detailed laboratory investigation.

[b]Example: One extraction/surgery resulting in bleeding (100%): the score to be assigned is 2; two extractions/surgeries, one resulting in bleeding (50%): the score to be assigned is 2; three extractions/surgeries, one resulting in bleeding (33%): the score to be assigned is 2; four extractions/surgeries, one resulting in bleeding (25%): the score to be assigned is 1.

[c]If already available at the time of collection.

^Include: umbilical stump bleeding, cephalohematoma, cheek hematoma caused by sucking during breast/bottle feeding, conjunctival hemorrhage or excessive bleeding following circumcision or venipuncture. Their presence in infancy requires detailed investigation independently from the overall score.

Normal range is <4 in adult males, <6 in adult females, and <3 in children.

From Rodeghiero, F., Tosetto, A., Abshire, T., Arnold, D.M., Coller, B., James, P., Neunert, C., Lillicrap, D., ISTH/SSC Joint VWF and Perinatal/Pediatric Hemostasis Subcommittees Working Group. (2011). ISTH/SSC bleeding assessment tool: A standardized questionnaire and a proposal for a new bleeding score for inherited bleeding disorders. Journal of Thrombosis and Haemostasis, 8(9), 2063–2065; Elbatarny, M., Mollah, S., Grabell, J., Bae, S., Deforest, M., Tuttle, A., Hopman, W., Clark, D.S., Mauer, A.C., Bowman, M., Riddel, J., Christopherson, P.A., Montgomery, R.R.; Zimmerman Program Investigators, Rand, M.L., Coller, B., James, P.D. (2014). Normal range of bleeding scores for the ISTH-BAT: Adult and pediatric data from the merging project. Haemophilia, 20(6), 831–835; and Kuiper, P. (n.d.). ISTH-SSC bleeding assessment tool. Bleeding Score. https://bleedingscore.certe.nl/

If there is a suspected diagnosis of hemophilia or another bleeding disorder, it can be helpful to run the following laboratory tests: complete blood count (CBC), activated partial thromboplastin time (aPTT) test, prothrombin time (PT) test, and appropriate factor assays. A CBC result can be normal in people with a bleeding disorder; however, if heavy bleeding has taken place, the hemoglobin and red blood cell count can be lower than normal. An aPPT test measures how long it takes for blood to clot, specifically measuring if clotting factors VII, IX, XI, and XII are low, which indicates it takes longer than normal for blood to clot, therefore causing a prolonged/higher result. A PT test also measures how long it takes blood to clot, specifically measuring if clotting factors I, II, V, VII, and X are low, which if it takes longer than normal for blood to clot then this causes a prolonged/higher result. Those with hemophilia A and B will likely have normal PT levels (CDC, 2011). While a prolonged aPTT is consistent with hemophilia, a normal aPTT does not exclude the possibility of a mild form of hemophilia, especially hemophilia B (factor IX deficiency). Thus regardless of the aPTT result, mixing studies are done to determine whether the patient has a factor deficiency or an inhibitor (Hoots & Shapiro, 2023).

A diagnosis of hemophilia A includes a factor VIII level less than 50%; a diagnosis of hemophilia B includes a factor IX level less than 50%. The severity of one's hemophilia diagnosis is categorized as severe, moderate, or mild; severe hemophilia is a factor level result less than 1%, moderate hemophilia is a factor level result of 1% to 5%, mild hemophilia is 6% to 40%. Normal factor VIII and IX coagulant levels are generally 50% to 150% (0.50–1.5 U/dL) (Srivastava et al., 2020). When a patient is under the stress of illness or trauma there may be a transient elevation in the factor VIII level. For this reason it is recommended that a patient be tested or, at times, retested when the stressor is resolved to give a more accurate factor VIII level (Hoots & Shapiro, 2023).

TREATMENT

Comprehensive Care at a Hemophilia Treatment Center

The standard of care for hemophilia, vWD, and other bleeding disorders is lifelong management with a collaborative interdisciplinary approach facilitated by local hemophilia treatment centers (HTCs). These centers, funded in part by the US government but also found internationally, provide comprehensive management of inherited coagulation disorders.

The core team consists of a hematologist, specialized hemophilia nurse coordinator, physical therapist, and social worker. Extended team members can include a genetic counselor, dental hygienist, or dentist; women's health providers, orthopedic providers, nutritionists, gastroenterologists, psychologists, and infectious disease specialists are other team members that are often either part of the team or able to provide consultative services (National Bleeding Disorders Foundation [NBDF], 2022j).

With the advent of patients' exposure to human immunodeficiency virus (HIV) and hepatitis C in the

1980s through blood product transfusions, HTCs have also been mandated by the government to either provide or procure comprehensive management for individuals exposed to HIV, while individuals exposed to hepatitis C are often seen by a liver specialist as an adjunct to the HTC team. Some of the many services provided by HTCs include interdisciplinary comprehensive evaluations, counseling and support services, child and family education, carrier detection, access to new technology treatment products through clinical trials, surgical treatment coordination, and instruction on home infusion (Sharathkumar & Pipe, 2008; Soucie et al., 2000).

All children, adolescents, and adults with hemophilia, vWD, and other bleeding disorder diagnoses should receive regular comprehensive evaluations at the nearest HTC. The frequency of these evaluations can range from every 3 months to every other year, depending on the severity of the patient's bleeding disorder, use of prophylaxis treatment, and other issues the child or family may be having.

At these visits, patients and their families are seen by the members of the core interdisciplinary team. The family and primary care provider receive updated information on the status of a child's health and development, treatment options, and new treatment products, and readiness for home therapy is evaluated. HTCs work closely in collaboration with primary care practitioners, other specialties, hospital staff, residential facilities, personal care assistants, schools, child care facilities, and justice systems to provide comprehensive, coordinated, and accessible care for the day-to-day management of a patient's bleeding disorder care and advocacy (NBDF, 2022j). A federally funded study found that individuals receiving care at HTCs were 30% less likely to die than those who did not receive comprehensive hemophilia care (Hoots, 2003; Soucie et al., 2000).

General Guidelines to Control Bleeding for all Bleeding Disorder Diagnoses

The primary goal of treatment for any patient who has hemophilia, vWD, or other bleeding disorder diagnosis is the prevention of bleeding episodes. The second goal is the early and aggressive treatment of bleeding episodes using a multidisciplinary team approach. Each bleeding episode should be treated on a case-by-case basis. When a bleeding episode is identified or suspected, therapy must be instituted promptly (NBDF, 2022j).

Pharmacologic Therapy for Hemophilia

When looking at pharmacologic therapies utilized in the treatment of hemophilia, they include factors VIII and IX product replacements (plasma derived and recombinant derived), bypassing agents, desmopressin acetate (DDAVP), emicizumab-kxwh (Hemlibra), and antifibrinolytic agents. When treating someone with a bleeding disorder, goals include prevention of bleeding and treatment of a bleed or injury.

One of the top ways to treat those with hemophilia is to replace their missing blood clotting factor. Factors VIII and IX clotting factor products are injected intravenously into patients to help achieve coagulation (CDC, 2019a). Plasma-derived factor products are generated from plasma collected from many people and separated into components such as clotting factor proteins that are then freeze-dried into the product. These products go through a strenuous testing process to ensure all potential viruses are killed before they are made available for use. In 1992, recombinant factor products were introduced into treatment options for hemophilia patients. Recombinant factor products are generated using genetically engineered DNA technology, with no human plasma or albumin. This means that recombinant products are preserved with the removal of bloodborne viruses (CDC, 2019a). There have been advances in the half-life of these products in which some products are categorized as standard half-life, while others are categorized as extended half-life products. The treatment product of choice should be determined by consulting with the patient's hematologist. This information should be updated at least yearly to incorporate changes in manufacturing technologies and dosing corrections as factor concentrate dosing is based on a patient's weight (NBDF, 2022h). For a list of products, see Tables 11.3 to 11.5.

The development of factor replacement concentrates is a wonderful advancement in the treatment of patients with bleeding disorders; however, these products are remain expensive. The price of factor products alone for a severe hemophilia patient who is receiving prophylactic therapy can cost $200,000 to $500,000 per year. The out-of-pocket costs for the patient vary based on insurance coverage, access to copay assistance programs, and state-funded assistance programs (Washington et al., 2019).

Vials of factor concentrate come in various sizes with varying numbers of factor units per vial. When a child is prescribed a specific dose of factor (i.e., expressed in factor VIII or IX units), this is considered a minimum dose, and the child should be given the full number of vials that provide the desired dose without discarding any of the factor from an individual vial. This minimum dosing rule is due to the high cost of the medication and the lack of adverse sequelae from a dose slightly higher than that originally prescribed.

Bypassing agents are used to treat hemophilia patients with inhibitors as well as other bleeding disorders (see Inhibitors, later).

DDAVP. DDAVP is a medication available in intravenous, intranasal, and subcutaneous forms that can be utilized for patients with mild hemophilia A and vWD. Desmopressin acts similarly to an antidiuretic hormone naturally occurring within the body. Once DDAVP is given, Weibel-Palade bodies (WPBs) in endothelial cells are released and increase two to five times the plasma levels of both von Willebrand factor (vWF) and factor VIII within 30 to 60 minutes (Xu et al., 2004). This can

Table **11.3**   Products Available to Treat Patients With Hemophilia A

| PRODUCT | PROPHYLAXIS | DOSING | | HALF-LIFE (HOURS)[a] | COMMENTS |
		MINOR BLEEDING/ SURGERY	MAJOR BLEEDING/ SURGERY		
Recombinant Factor VIII Products, Standard Half-Life					
Advate	**Adult and peds:** 20–40 units/kg IV TIW or every other day *or* 50–75 units/kg IV BIW or every 3 days	25 units/kg	50 units/kg	9–12	
Kovaltry	**Adults (age ≥12 yr):** 20–40 units/kg IV 2–3 times per week **Peds (age <12 yr):** 25–50 units/kg IV 2–3 times per week	25 units/kg	50 units/kg	12–14	
Novoeight	**Adult (age ≥12 yr):** 20–50 units/kg IV TIW *or* 20–40 units/kg every other day **Peds (age <12 yr):** 25–60 units/kg IV TIW *or* 25–50 units/kg IV every other day	25 units/kg	50 units/kg	8–12	
Nuwiq	**Adults (age ≥12 yr):** 30–40 units/kg IV every other day **Peds (age <12 yr):** 30–50 units/kg IV every other day or TIW	25 units/kg	50 units/kg	12–17	
Recombinate	**Adult and peds:** 20–40 units/kg IV TIW or IV every other day *or* 50–75 units/kg IV BIW or IV every 3 days	25 units/kg	50 units/kg	15	
Xyntha	**Adults (age ≥12 yr):** 30 units/kg IV TIW **Peds (age <12 yr):** 25 units/kg IV every other day	25 units/kg	50 units/kg	8–11	
Plasma Containing Factor 8 Products, Standard Half-Life					
Alphanate	**Adult and peds:** 20–40 units/kg IV TIW or every other day *or* 50–75 units/kg BIW or every 3 days	15–25 units/kg	40–50 units/kg	18	
Hemofil M	**Adult and peds:** 20–40 units/kg IV TIW or every other day *or* 50–75 units/kg BIW or every 3 days	25 units/kg	50 units/kg	15	
Koate	**Adult and peds:** 20–40 units/kg IV TIW or every other day *or* 50–75 units/kg BIW or every 3 days	25 units/kg	50 units/kg	16	
Monoclate	**Adult and peds:** 20–40 units/kg IV TIW or every other day *or* 50–75 units/kg BIW or every 3 days	15–25 units/kg	40–50 units/kg	17.5	
Wilate	**Adults[b] (age ≥12 yr):** 20–40 units/kg IV every 2–3 days	30–40 units/kg	35–50 units/kg	11	

Continued

Table 11.3 Products Available to Treat Patients With Hemophilia A—cont'd

PRODUCT	DOSING				
	PROPHYLAXIS	MINOR BLEEDING/ SURGERY	MAJOR BLEEDING/ SURGERY	HALF-LIFE (HOURS)[a]	COMMENTS
Extended Half-Life Recombinant Factor 8 Products					
Adynovate	**Adults (age ≥12 yr):** 40–50 units/kg IV BIW **Peds (age <12 yr):** 55 units/kg IV BIW (max: 70 unit/kg)	10–30 units/kg	30–50 units/kg	13–16	
Afstyla	**Adults (age ≥12 yr):** 20–50 units/kg IV 2–3 times weekly **Peds (age <12 yr):** 30–50 units/kg IV 2–3 times weekly	25 units/kg	50 units/kg	10–14	
Eloctate	**Age ≥6 yr:** 50 units/kg IV every 4 days. Regimen can be adjusted to dosing range of 25–65 units/kg IV every 3–5 days. **Age ≤6 yr:** 50 units/kg IV BIW. Regimen can be adjusted to dosing range of 25–65 units/kg IV every 3–5 days.	20–30 units/kg	40–50 units/kg	13–20	
Esperoct	**Adults (age ≥12 yr):** 50 units/kg IV every 4 days **Peds (age <12 yr):** 65 units/kg IV BIW	**Adults (age ≥12 yr):** 40 units/kg **Peds (age <12 yr):** 65 units/kg	**Adults (age ≥12 yr):** 50 units/kg **Peds (age <12 yr):** 65 units/kg	17–22	
Jivi	**Adults[c] (age ≥12 yr):** 30–40 units/kg IV BIW. Can be adjusted 45–60 units/kg every 5 days.	10–30 units/kg	30–50 units/kg	17–21	
Factor ixa- and Factor X-directed Antibody					
Hemlibra (Emicizumab)	**Adult and peds:** **Loading dose:** 3 mg/kg weekly SQ for 4 wk, then start maintenance dosing **Maintenance dose:** 1.5 mg/kg SQ weekly or 3 mg/kg SQ every 2 wk, or 6 mg/kg SQ every month			646 (~4 wk)	**Black box warning:** Thrombotic microangiopathy and thromboembolism Cases of thrombotic microangiopathy and thrombotic events were reported when on average a cumulative amount of >100 U/kg/24 hr of activated prothrombin complex concentrate (aPCC) was administered for 24 hr or more to patients receiving Hemlibra prophylaxis. Monitor for the development of thrombotic microangiopathy and thrombotic events if aPCC is administered. Discontinue aPCC and suspend dosing of Hemlibra if symptoms occur.

BIW, Twice weekly; *IV,* intravenously; *SQ,* subctutaneously; *TIW,* three times weekly.
[a]Half-lives are approximate. For children, half-lives are generally shorter than adults when assessed in pharmacokinetic studies. The half-life should be determined for the individual patient. Refer to product information and institutional guidelines for additional dosing and monitoring information.
[b]No FDA indications for use in children with hemophilia A.
[c]Not indicated in children age <12 yr.

Table 11.4   Products Available to Treat Patients With Hemophilia B

PRODUCT	PROPHYLAXIS	DOSING MINOR BLEEDING/ SURGERY	MAJOR BLEEDING/ SURGERY	HALF-LIFE[a] (HOURS)	COMMENTS
Recombinant Factor IX Products, Standard Half-Life[b]					
BeneFIX	**Adults and peds:** 100 units/kg weekly IV *or* 40–70 units/kg IV 2–3 times weekly	70 units/kg	120 units/kg	16–19	
Ixinity	**Adults (age ≥12 yr):** 40–70 units/kg IV BIW	60 units/kg	110 units/kg	24	
Rixubis	**Adults (age ≥12 yr):** 40–60 units/kg IV BIW **Peds (age <12 yr):** 60–80 units/kg IV BIW	60 units/kg	110 units/kg	23–26	
Plasma Containing Factor IX products, standard half-life[b]					
AlphaNine SD	40–60 units/kg IV 2–3 times per week	20–50 units/kg 2 times daily	50–100 units/kg 2 times daily	18	
Mononine	40–60 units/kg IV 2–3 times per week	20–30 units/kg	Up to 75 units/kg	23	
Extended Half-life Recombinant Factor IX Products[b]					
Alprolix	**Adult (age ≥12 yr):** 50 units/kg IV every 7 days *or* 100 units/kg every 10 days **Peds (age <12 yr):** 60 units/kg every 7 days	30–60 units/kg	80–100 units/kg	54–90	
Idelvion	**Adults (age ≥12 yr):** 25–40 units/kg every 7 days IV *or* 50–75 units/kg every 14 days **Peds (age <12 yr):** 40–55 units/kg every 7 days	30–60 units/kg	60–100 units/kg	104	
Rebinyn	**Adults and peds:** 40 units/kg IV every 7 days	40 units/kg	80 units/kg	103–115	
Bypassing Agents[c]					
NovoSeven (recombinant factor VIIa)	**Adult and peds:** 90 μg/kg IV every 2 hr adjustable based on severity of bleeding			3	**Black box warning:** • Serious arterial and venous thrombotic events following administration of NovoSeven RT have been reported. • Discuss the risks and explain the signs and symptoms of thrombotic and thromboembolic events to patients who will receive NovoSeven RT. • Monitor patients for signs or symptoms of activation of the coagulation system and for thrombosis

Continued

Table 11.4   Products Available to Treat Patients With Hemophilia B—cont'd

| PRODUCT | DOSING | | | HALF-LIFE[a] (HOURS) | COMMENTS |
	PROPHYLAXIS	MINOR BLEEDING/ SURGERY	MAJOR BLEEDING/ SURGERY		
FEIBA (antiinhibitor coagulant complex)	**Adult and peds:** Prophylaxis: 85 units/kg IV every other day Mild bleeding: 50–100 units/kg IV Major bleeding: 100 units/kg IV *Do not exceed a single dose of 100 units/kg body weight and a daily dose of 200 units/kg body			The safety and efficacy of FEIBA has not been evaluated in neonates. Dosing for >7 years of age.	**Black box warning:** • FEIBA can cause thromboembolic events following doses >200 units/kg per day and in patients with thrombotic risk factors. • Monitor patients receiving FEIBA for signs and symptoms of thromboembolic events. • Use of antifibrinolytics (tranexamic acid and aminocaproic acid) within approximately 6–12 hr after administration of FEIBA is not recommended.
SEVENFACT	**Adults (age ≥12 yr):** Mild to moderate bleeding: 75 µg/kg repeated every 3 hr until hemostasis is achieved *or* Initial dose of 225 µg/kg. If hemostasis is not achieved within 9 hr, additional 75 µg/kg doses may be administered every 3 hr until hemostatis is achieved. Severe bleeding: 225 µg/kg, followed if necessary 6 hr later with 75 µg/kg every 2 hr			1.6	**Black box warning:** • Serious arterial and venous thrombotic events may occur following administration of SEVENFACT. • Discuss the risks and explain the signs and symptoms of thrombotic and thromboembolic events to patients who will receive SEVENFACT. • Monitor patients for signs or symptoms of activation of the coagulation system and for thrombosis.

BIW, Twice weekly; *IV,* intravenously; *TIW,* three times weekly.
[a]Half-lives are approximate. For children, half-lives are generally shorter than adults when assessed in pharmacokinetic studies. The half-life should be determined for the individual patient. Refer to product information and institutional guidelines for additional dosing and monitoring information.
[b]First 10 to 20 treatments with factor IX product should be given in monitored setting.
[c]Available to treat patients with hemophilia A or hemophilia B with inhibitors.

Table 11.5   Other Hemostatic Agents Used for Mild Hemophilia A and von Willebrand Disease

PRODUCT	DOSING	COMMENTS

DDAVP	0.3 µg/kg (SQ or IV) daily, no more than 3 days in a row
	IV: give in 50 mL of NS over 30 min
		• For mild to moderate bleeding
		• Must fluid restrict while on medication (3/4 maintenance) to prevent hyponatremia
		• Prior to prescribing, patients should undergo DDAVP challenge to test for adequate response to medication
		• Nasal spray (Stimate) option is currently off market
		• Caution should be taken with patients who have history of seizure disorder due to risk of hyponatremia.
		• Contraindicated in following:
		  1. Children age <2 yr
		  2. Type 3 vWD, will not respond
		  3. Type 2B vWD, will cause or worsen thrombocytopenia
		  4. History of cardiovascular disease, increase risk of thrombosis
		  5. Adults age >65 yr

Tranexamic acid (Lysteda)	25 mg/kg PO every 8–12 hr or 10 mg/kg IV every 8–12 hr	• For mucous membrane bleeding and menorrhagia • Do not give if patient has hematuria • Continue to take 2–3 days after bleeding has stopped • Only oral agent comes in 650-mg tablets
Aminocaproic acid (Amicar)	100 mg/kg every 6 hr PO or IV Max dose: 6 g	• For mucous membrane bleeding and menorrhagia • Do not give if patient has hematuria • Continue to take 2–3 days after bleeding has stopped

work to increase the patient's own vWF and factor VIII levels so that they do not have to use clotting factors to stop bleeding episodes (CDC, 2019a).

DDAVP has been successfully used for patients to prevent bleeding complications in connection with dental or surgical procedures and for acute bleeding such as joint, muscle, or mucosal (oral, nasal, gastrointestinal [GI], menstrual) bleeding. Not all patients with mild hemophilia A or vWD respond adequately to DDAVP; a test of treatment or DDAVP challenge needs to be performed on these patients before DDAVP can be utilized for their bleeding plan of care. DDAVP should not be utilized for patients under 2 years of age, those with cardiovascular disease, diagnosis of seizure disorder, or pregnant women with preeclampsia. After DDAVP is given, free fluid intake restrictions are frequently recommended because of the effect of hyponatremia. Other side effects associated with DDAVP are headache, flushing, hypotension, and hypertension (UpToDate, n.d.) (James, 2022c).

Hemlibra. Hemlibra is a recombinant, humanized, bispecific immunoglobulin G4 (IgG4) monoclonal antibody that bridges activated factor IXa and factor X, thus substituting the need for activated factor VIIIa. Hemlibra is currently US Food and Drug Administration (FDA) approved for use in patients with a diagnosis of moderate to severe hemophilia A with and without inhibitors, and it is being explored in treatment for patients with vWD type 3 diagnoses and other bleeding disorder diagnoses. Hemlibra is administered via a subcutaneous injection initially weekly for a 4-week loading dose, then maintenance doses can be adjusted to weekly, every 2 weeks, or every 4 weeks depending on the patient and health care provider's preferences. All doses of Hemlibra are weight based. Once Hemlibra loading doses are completed and maintenance doses continued, Hemlibra sustains factor VIII levels that allow for adequate hemostasis (NBDF, 2022i).

Due to the low binding affinity of Hemlibra, factor VIII products and nonactivated prothrombin complex concentrate (non-aPCC) bypassing agents can be utilized in conjunction with Hemlibra for acute bleeding, injury, or invasive procedure. Hemlibra has a black box warning in place for its use in conjunction with aPCC bypassing agents such as factor VIII (FEIBA) due to a thrombotic event. Hemlibra has a half-life of 4 weeks, therefore once taken it can take up to 6 months for it to be excreted from a patient's body (NBDF, 2022i). Risks associated with Hemlibra include patients who use Hemlibra prophylactically and use replacement factor VIII products for breakthrough bleeding can still develop an inhibitor, bruising at the injection site, and burning with injections. The use of Hemlibra can give false results in laboratory tests, including aPTT, aPTT-based factor VIII activity, factor VIII inhibitor titers (unless chromogenic Bethesda assay is used), aPTT-based activated protein C, and activated clotting time (CDC, 2019a).

Antifibrinolytic agents. Antifibrinolytic agents are medications with antifibrin properties that are used to help prevent or slow the breakdown of clots. During the hemostasis process, a clot is formed and stays together with the use of a protein called fibrin. Once appropriate healing has taken place, clots go through a process called fibrinolysis, in which the fibrin breaks down. Fibrinolysis also ensures that an excess of clots is not formed (Subramaniam, n.d.). For patients with hemophilia, vWD, and other bleeding disorders, the process of hemostasis is not guaranteed. Antifibrinolytic agents are used singularly and in conjunction with other treatment products to protect a clot from breaking down. Antifibrinolytic agents are frequently given for a few days after bleeding has stopped to ensure hemostasis of a clot is completed. These medications are commonly used in the treatment of mucous membrane–related bleeding (epistaxis, menstrual bleeding, oral bleeding, GI bleeding); however, they are also used for other bleeding-related injuries and procedures. The dosing of antifibrinolytic medications is weight based (Indiana Hemophilia & Thrombosis Center, n.d.).

When envisioning a clot made by a patient with a bleeding disorder, the clot does not like to stay together. Clots must stay together to allow complete hemostasis to occur and healing to take place. Antifibrinolytic agents act like a net surrounding the clot and protecting it from breaking apart too early in the hemostasis process.

Aminocaproic acid. Aminocaproic acid (Amicar) is an antifibrinolytic agent that inhibits plasminogen activation in the clotting process by competing with protein plasminogen activators and preventing the degradation of fibrin clots. Amicar is available intravenously or orally (liquid and pill). Amicar has a half-life of approximately 80 minutes, and redosing must occur within a strict 6-hour time frame (CDC, 2019a).

Tranexamic acid. Tranexamic acid (Lysteda) is an antifibrinolytic agent that binds to plasminogen in the hemostasis process and prevents it from interacting with fibrin, thereby stabilizing the clot and preventing blood loss. Lysteda is available intravenously and orally (tablet). Lysteda has a longer-acting half-life of 3 hours compared to Amicar (Indiana Hemophilia & Thrombosis Center, n.d.).

Hormonal Therapy

For females with a diagnosis of hemophilia, hemophilia symptomatic carrier, vWD, or other bleeding disorders where they experience heavy bleeding symptoms, particularly heavy menstrual bleeding, hormonal therapy is an available treatment option. The hormones estrogen and progesterone have many effects on the female body, including sexual function and pregnancy. High levels of estrogen have been shown to slightly increase blood clotting factor levels for females and thus have shown to be effective in decreasing menorrhagia through their effect on the lining of the uterus. At the same time, progestin in combination with estrogen has been shown to be effective in decreasing bleeding from ovarian cysts. Heavy menstrual bleeding takes a physical and mental toll on patients with a bleeding disorder, and having the option of hormonal control can drastically impact their lives (Steps for Living, 2013c).

Prophylaxis

Prophylaxis is the regularly scheduled venous infusion of clotting factor concentrate with the goal of preventing most bleeding episodes. The use of home therapy and prophylactic therapy has revolutionized the care of children with hemophilia. The Medical and Scientific Advisory Council (MASAC) of the National Bleeding Disorders Foundation has recommended that prophylaxis be considered the standard of care for patients with severe (<1%) hemophilia A or B, including those with inhibitors. Prophylaxis therapy should also be considered for patients with mild and moderate hemophilia who have a severe genetic phenotype. The World Federation of Hemophilia (WFH) has provided these detailed recommendations for prophylaxis:

- Prophylaxis should be initiated at an early age, ideally before age 3 years and prior to the second joint bleed; prophylaxis may be considered within the first 6 months of life to reduce the occurrence of intracranial hemorrhage.
- Prophylaxis should be individualized by dose and frequency and sufficient to prevent all bleeds at all times.
- Options for prophylaxis include plasma-derived or recombinant standard half-life factor, extended half-life factor, and/or Hemlibra. For patients with inhibitors, the use of bypassing agents is needed (see Table 11.4) (NBDF, 2022h).

Furthermore, the WFH (Srivastava et al., 2020) broke down the term *prophylaxis* in its guidelines to clarify whether prophylaxis is continuous (including primary/secondary/tertiary) or intermittent. Following are the definitions:

- Continuous (regular) prophylaxis: replacement factor given to prevent bleeding for at least 45 weeks (85%) of a year
  - Primary prophylaxis: continuous prophylaxis started in individuals before age 3 who have not had a bleeding episode but are at high risk of bleeding. With severe factor deficiency (e.g., factor VIII or IX activity level <1%) it is recommended to receive primary prophylaxis due to the high risk of spontaneous bleeding and efficacy of prophylaxis in preventing bleeding and its complications.
  - Secondary prophylaxis: continuous prophylaxis for individuals who have had more than one bleeding episode (e.g., two or more bleeds into a target joint, evidence of joint disease by physical examination or radiography), but before the onset of chronic arthropathy.
  - Tertiary prophylaxis: continuous prophylaxis started after the onset of arthropathy to prevent further damage.
- Intermittent (short-term) prophylaxis: administered for several weeks to months and then discontinued; may be used in specific circumstances such as high-impact physical activities, joint bleeding, or surgical procedures. The individual bleeding phenotype must be considered in decision making.

Venous access is necessary for the delivery of standard half-life factor, extended half-life factor, and bypassing agents. Peripheral venipuncture is the first choice for venous access, but this can be difficult and traumatic for patients, especially young patients with hemophilia or patients with poor venous access due to anatomy and/or scarring. Central venous access devices (i.e., implanted port-a-cath) may be utilized to improve venous access. However, these devices are not without complications, the most common being infection. Each child needs to be evaluated individually with a thorough discussion with the family and caregivers in making a choice to use an implanted device (Valentino & Kapoor, 2005).

Prophylaxis has been shown to improve life expectancy for hemophilia patients. During the 1960s, the average life expectancy for a patient with hemophilia was about 12 years; now people diagnosed with hemophilia can anticipate a near-normal life expectancy (Ahle, 2020).

Acute Bleeding Episodes

In patients with hemophilia with acute bleeding, the immediate goal is to raise the factor activity to a level sufficient to achieve hemostasis. The location and severity of the bleeding, the half-life of the product administered, and presence of an associated injury or occurrence in a target joint are all things that need to be considered when determining the targeted factor activity for the treatment of acute bleeding.

The first rule when a patient with hemophilia is experiencing a serious or life-threatening bleed or sustained head trauma is to treat first, evaluate second, then plan further therapy. MASAC guidelines recommend that factor replacement should be given before any diagnostic studies (x-rays, computed tomography scans, etc.) are performed to evaluate a suspected bleeding problem, especially in the case of head trauma or suspected intracranial hemorrhage. Also, for routine joint bleeding, no radiographic studies are indicated (NBDF, 2022c).

Serious or life-threatening bleeding includes:
- Potential/suspected bleeding in the central nervous system (CNS)
- Ocular bleeding
- Bleeding in the hip
- Deep muscle bleeding with neurovascular compromise or the potential for neurovascular complications
- Intraabdominal and GI bleeding

- Bleeding that could affect the airway (e.g., into the throat or neck)
- Bleeding severe enough to result in anemia and potentially require red blood cell transfusion(s)
- Prolonged bleeding that is not adequately responding to home-based therapy
- Iliopsoas bleeding
- Significant injuries such as motor vehicle accidents or falls from distances of several feet or more (UpToDate, n.d.) (James, 2022b).

Hemarthroses.   Bleeding into a joint (hemarthrosis) is one of the most common manifestations of hemophilia. Joint bleeds are characterized by a reduced range of motion associated with pain or other unusual sensation (tingling), palpable swelling, or warmth to the joint. Bleeding into hip joints is concerning due to the greater risk of increased intraarticular pressure and osteonecrosis of the femoral head.

Target joints can develop in some patients due to repeated bleeding episodes, and chronic inflammation may occur with repeat bleeding in the joint.

The major aspects of the assessment and management of joint bleeding include the following:

- Factor should be infused promptly at the first sign of joint bleeding (i.e., at the onset of tingling, pain, or typical symptoms of joint bleeding rather than waiting for reduced range of motion or swelling).
- Additional interventions to reduce bleeding, pain, and inflammation include RICE (rest, ice, compression, and elevation) interventions to affected joints and analgesics as needed (generally avoiding agents with antiplatelet activity such as nonsteroidal anti-inflammatory drugs [NSAIDs]). Selective cyclooxygenase-2 inhibitors may be used.
- Clinical evaluation is used to distinguish an acute bleed from other conditions, such as pain due to chronic arthropathy, acute fracture or sprain, or infection. In many cases this assessment is based on the history and physical examination rather than radiography or ultrasound examinations. (UpToDate, n.d.) (James, 2022b)

Muscle/soft tissue bleeding.   Muscle bleeding may present with aching, stiffness, pain, or swelling. In muscle groups such as the upper arm, forearm, wrist, volar hand, and anterior or posterior tibial compartment, soft tissue hemorrhage may result in the development of a compartment syndrome with impingement on the neurovascular bundle. This may be associated with tingling, numbness, and in severe situations loss of distal arterial pulses. Therapy should be initiated as soon as possible (at the first sign of symptoms or immediately after injury or trauma). Severe muscle bleeds usually require more than one-factor infusion. Surgical decompression is undertaken only if medical therapy fails to forestall progression and in consultation with a comprehensive HTC.

Minor bleeding.   Minor bleeding such as small bruises, small cuts and scrapes, epistaxis, and mouth bleeds may be treated with local measures, including ice, pressure, or elevation. Bruising is common in children with hemophilia. Small cuts and scrapes usually do not require factor replacement; however, if a cut or laceration needs sutures, factor replacement may be necessary. Topical therapies, including antifibrinolytic agents or other adjunctive local therapies, may also be helpful. Epistaxis (nose bleeding) is a common manifestation in children with bleeding disorders; local measures such as pressure, tilting the head forward (this prevents blood from pooling in the posterior pharynx, thereby avoiding nausea and airway obstruction), and applying ice to the bridge of the nose is usually sufficient (Hemophilia of Georgia, n.d.). At times, episodes of epistaxis may be prolonged or may result in a larger volume of blood loss that will necessitate replacement therapy.

Inhibitors

Patients with hemophilia (and vWD type 3) have a risk of developing inhibitors due to the use of clotting factor concentrates (CFCs) for prophylactic and/or on-demand treatment for bleeding. In other words, inhibitors are IgG alloantibodies that the body produces in response to exogenous clotting factor VIII or IX. Inhibitors will neutralize (or inhibit) the function of the infused CFCs, thus the CFCs will be ineffective in stopping or preventing bleeding (Srivastava et al., 2020). The development of inhibitors occurs in approximately 1 in 5 people with hemophilia A and 3 in 100 people with hemophilia B (Guh et al., 2011). Inhibitor development is uncommon in vWD but has been reported in individuals with type 3 vWD (reported prevalence in inhibitor development with type 3 vWD is 6–10%) (UpToDate, n.d.) (James, 2022a). Inhibitor development is one of the most serious medical complications for people with bleeding disorders because it is difficult to treat bleeds and it is costly. Bleeding disorder patients with inhibitors are twice as likely to be hospitalized for a bleeding complication and are at increased risk of death (CDC, 2019b).

It is still unknown what exactly causes inhibitor development, but multiple research studies have identified potential risk factors (Box 11.1). It should be noted that for hemophilia B patients with inhibitors, inhibitor development is almost exclusively seen in patients with severe hemophilia B and occurs commonly in patients with null variants in which no endogenous clotting factor is produced due to large deletion, frameshift, and nonsense variants. Inhibitor development in hemophilia B is overall associated with a similar disease burden as hemophilia A, but anaphylaxis occurs in 50% of hemophilia B patients with inhibitors and, as stated, more frequently in those with null mutations. Anaphylaxis may be the first symptom of factor IX inhibitor development. Therefore newly diagnosed hemophilia B patients should be treated in a clinic or hospital setting capable of managing severe allergic reactions for the initial 10 to 20 exposures to factor IX CFCs (Srivastava et al., 2020).

Box 11.1	Potential Risk Factors for Inhibitor Development

- Race (Black African or Hispanic ancestry)
- Family history of inhibitors
- Genotype, immune regulatory genes
- Immunocompromised or body under stress
- Severity of hemophilia (more frequent in severe vs mild/moderate)
- Increase frequency and dosing of clotting factor concentrate (CFC):
  o In hemophilia A, 79% of inhibitor development occurs within the first 20 exposures and the remainder (21%) within the first 75 exposures of CFC.
  o In hemophilia B, most inhibitors occur after a median exposure of 9–11 exposures, and before 20 exposures, typically before 2 years of age.

Modified from Srivastava, A., Santagostino, E., Dougall, A., et al. (2020). WFH guidelines for the management of hemophilia, 3rd edition. *Haemophilia*.

Inhibitors are diagnosed with a blood test that measures if an inhibitor is present and the amount of inhibitor (inhibitor titer) in the blood. These titers are measured by the assay Bethesda unit (BU) or Nijmegen-modified Bethesda unit (NBU). Per WFH guidelines, the definition of a positive inhibitor is a Bethesda titer of greater than 0.6 BU for hemophilia A and 0.3 BU or greater for hemophilia B. There are two types of inhibitors, low responding and high responding. The low-responding inhibitor is an inhibitor below 5 BU and typically tends to be transient, meaning that the level will drop below the definition threshold within 6 months of initial detection without any change in the treatment regimen. A high-responding inhibitor is an inhibitor of 5 BU or more and tends to be persistent and may fall or become undetectable after a long period without central venous catheter (CVC) exposure. However, the inhibitor level will increase 3 to 5 days after receiving CFCs. It is important to perform routine inhibitor screening during the time of greatest risk for inhibitor development, at least every 6 to 12 months after CFC prophylaxis therapy is initiated and annually thereafter. Other indications for inhibitor testing include:

- After initial factor exposure

- After intensive factor exposure (e.g., daily exposure >5 days)
- Recurrent bleeds or target joint bleeds despite adequate CFC replacement therapy
- Suboptimal clinical or laboratory response to CFC replacement therapy
- Before surgery
- Suboptimal postoperative response to CFC replacement therapy (Srivastava et al., 2020)

Inhibitor testing is not routinely monitored in patients with vWD but should be considered when there is refractory bleeding and/or poor response to infusions of vWF concentrates.

Treatment for people with inhibitors is one of the biggest challenges in the care of people with bleeding disorders (Fig. 11.3). A person with an inhibitor should consider seeking care at a HTC that can provide a team of health care providers who are experienced with bleeding disorders and have specialized medical expertise for inhibitor treatment.

Treatment options for people with inhibitors include:
- High-dose CFCs: This is a good option for those with low-responding inhibitors. CFC is given at higher amounts or increased frequency to overcome the inhibitor and yet have enough CFC left to form a clot.
- Bypassing agents: This is a good option for high-responding inhibitors. Instead of replacing the missing factor with factor VIII or IX CFCs, a bypassing agent is used to go around (bypass) the factors that are blocked by the inhibitor to form a normal clot. Close monitoring is needed when taking a bypassing agent to make sure that blood is not clotting too much or clotting in the wrong places in the body. It should be noted for hemophilia B patients with inhibitors who had an allergic reaction/anaphylaxis to factor IX CFC therapy, the WFH recommends recombinant factor VIIa (i.e., NovoSeven) to treat acute bleeds and does not advise the use of aPCC (i.e., FIEBA) as it contains factor IX and may cause or worsen an allergic reaction (Srivastava et al., 2020).
- Products that mimic factor VIII (i.e., emicizumab [Hemlibra]): As discussed earlier, this is an option for hemophilia A patients with inhibitors because

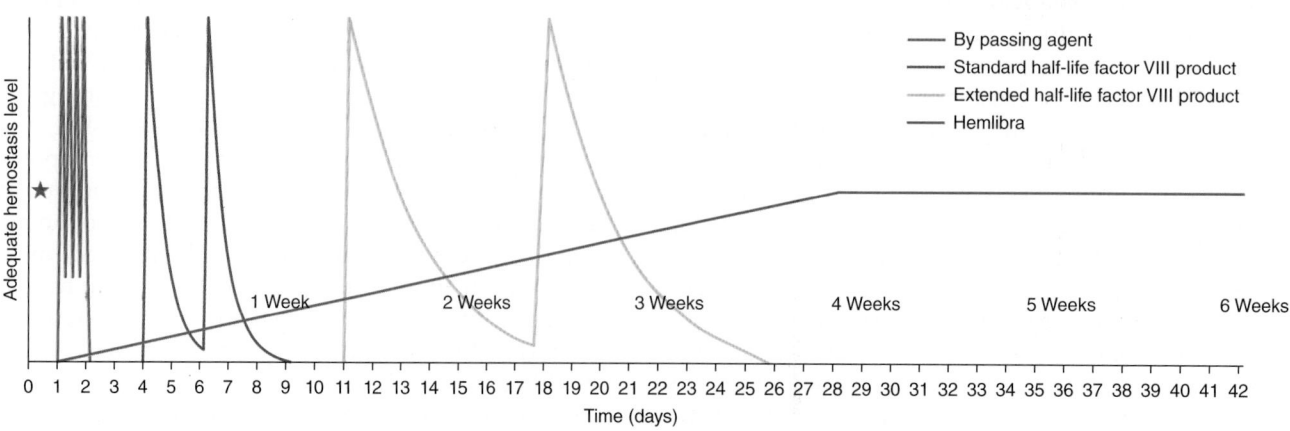

Fig. 11.3 Comparison of hemophilia A treatments. Graph is for demonstration purposes only; every patient is different.

it replaces the function of factor VIII without being affected by inhibitors.

- Immune tolerance induction (ITI) therapy: The goal of this therapy is to stop the inhibitor from blocking the factor in the blood and to teach the body to accept the factor as a normal part of blood. ITI therapy requires the patient to receive large amounts of factor every day for many weeks or months. It should be noted that since inhibitor prevalence is low in hemophilia B, experience with ITI is limited. Also, the success rate is lower, especially in a patient with an allergic reaction to factor IX CFCs (Srivastava et al., 2020).

Physical Therapy

Physical therapy is a vital adjunct therapy in the treatment of patients with hemophilia and other bleeding disorders and is one of the reasons physical therapists are core members of the HTC teams. Some adverse effects related to joint bleeds and injuries for hemophilia patients and other bleeding disorders include acute injury, muscle bleeding, hemarthroses, chronic synovitis, and hemophilic arthritis. The introduction of physical therapy to these patients has allowed for the rehabilitation and strengthening of muscles and joints as well as prophylactic techniques to be taught to protect a patient from injury and extend the time before surgical interventions are required. Physical therapy is also a crucial part of the treatment of hemophilia patients' pre- and postsurgical procedures. It may be that a patient would require a treatment plan of care, including factor infusion, before physical therapy in an attempt to prevent any damage. The options of physical therapy interventions and involvement with hemophilia patients are ever expanding in their quality of life (NBDF, 2022b).

OB-GYN Delivery

Although factor VIII levels in females generally rise above 50% during pregnancy, carriers whose baseline levels are below 50% may be at particular risk for postpartum hemorrhage. Factor VIII and IX levels should be checked at the start of the third trimester before anticipated delivery to assess the possible need for hematologic interventions, including factor products and antifibrinolytics at delivery. Treatment for epidural placement is a typical consideration in hematologic treatment plans.

Factor IX levels do not rise in pregnancy, and carriers with low levels of factor IX are more likely to need hematologic support with delivery (Kadir & Aledort, 2000; Kulkarni & Lusher, 2001; Peyvandi, 2005; Street et al., 2008). For a pregnant patient with hemophilia or who is a hemophilia carrier, it is important that the delivering provider be aware of the diagnosis and can coordinate with the patient's hematology providers to develop a treatment plan of care to ensure a safe delivery for mom and baby (CDC, 2011).

Some safety measures include not using forceps or a vacuum extractor to assist in delivery. If the baby has a risk of a hemophilia A or B diagnosis, then special cord blood collection for lab testing will need to be done to avoid veinous punctures. It is important to know a baby's diagnosis as soon as possible so steps can be taken to prevent bleeding. If there is a risk of bleeding disorder diagnosis in a male, it is recommended that circumcision not be completed until the diagnosis is known. Babies that should be tested for hemophilia include those born to families with a history of hemophilia, those who have mothers with a diagnosis or are carriers of hemophilia, and those that experience bleeding symptoms with birth, including head bleeds (CDC, 2011).

After delivery of the baby, a mother with a bleeding disorder will experience a fall in factor levels that were previously increased due to hormones; thus an increased amount of bleeding can occur. This mother is at increased risk for postpartum hemorrhage and bleeding after cesarean surgery, which may require treatment to help stop the bleeding (CDC, 2011).

Surgical Intervention

Surgery is a complicated and, at times, scary situation for those with a bleeding disorder diagnosis due to the increased risk of bleeding and healing complications. Luckily with the use of factor replacement products, antifibrinolytics, and other therapies, surgical procedures can be executed in a safe environment. Whether the procedure is a dental filling, spinal injection, circumcision, or joint replacement, communication and coordination of a patient's treatment plan of care with the performing provider and the hemophilia provider or team should always occur within a timely manner preoperatively (Mistry et al., 2017). For many procedures, factor products are given, and then factor levels are checked after the factor product infusion is completed to ensure a patient's factor levels are within a safe range for the procedure. This safe range can be altered depending on the procedure type, the patient's baseline levels, and the provider. Factor levels may also be checked postoperatively to ensure they are high enough for healing to take place and there is no risk of postoperative hemorrhage. If there is no treatment plan in place for an elective procedure, then surgical interventions should be postponed until a plan is determined by the appropriate provider. It is important that those with a family history of a bleeding disorder have had all testing completed and a diagnosis confirmed or denied before a surgical procedure takes place (Geraghty, n.d.).

Pain Management

Patients with a bleeding disorder diagnosis can experience acute and chronic pain due to bleeding. Of patients with hemophilia, 40% to 70% experience chronic pain, which impacts their quality of life (NBDF, 2022d). Prevention of bleeding and early treatment with the appropriate therapies are the best methods of preventing and treating pain in these patients. The restrictions associated with these patients' use of NSAIDs further complicate the treatment of their pain. NSAIDs have an antiplatelet effect in which it inhibits platelet aggregation or platelet plug from properly forming, which results in bleeding. Acet-aminophen is an appropriate medication to be given for pain; however, it must be understood by the patient and provider that acetaminophen has a limit on the dose per 24 hours, and frequently acetaminophen is found in cold medications and some opioid prescriptions (Lennie, 2020). The use of opioids is sometimes appropriate in the treatment of patients with bleeding disorder who experience acute and chronic pain, with the requirement of frequent evaluation by the provider. For many of these patients with chronic pain, a multidisciplinary approach and/or nonpharmacologic management is needed and appropriate. Patients with a bleeding disorder diagnosis and pain should have a treatment individualized to their personal needs and goals. Taking time to develop this treatment plan with patients' involvement is a critical component in pain control (NBDF, 2022d).

VON WILLEBRAND DISEASE

vWD is a bleeding disorder in which blood does not clot properly due to deficiency or abnormality of the blood protein, vWF. vWF performs two major roles in hemostasis: It first mediates the adhesion of platelets to sites of vascular injury, making it essential for platelet plug formation (clot formation); it then functions as a carrier protein that stabilizes coagulation factor VIII. In a person with vWD, because the vWF levels are low and/or do not work the way they should, forming a clot may take longer or form incorrectly, and bleeding might take longer to stop. The current classifications include types 1 and 3, which are characterized by quantitative deficiencies. Types 2A, 2B, 2M, and 2N are qualitative variants. Table 11.6 provides further details on each diagnosis.

Table 11.6 von Willebrand Disease Types

TYPE	CLINICAL FEATURES	LABORATORY FINDINGS
Type 1 (partial quantitative deficiency)	• Approximately 75% of individuals with vWD have this type • Variable bleeding severity from mild to severe • Autosomal dominance inheritance	• vWF activity and antigen both decreased. • Factor VIII activity normal or reduced • Ristocetin-induced platelet aggregation (RIPA) decreased (or can be normal) • Multimer electrophoresis: all multimers present and decreased • In type 1C, the vWF level at 4 hr post-DDAVP trial shows rapid reduction in vWF
Type 2 (Qualitative Variant)		
Type 2A (selective deficiency of high-molecular-weight multimers, reduced binding to platelet GPIB)	• Approximately 10–20% of individuals with vWD have this type • Moderate to severe bleeding • Mostly autosomal dominance; occasional autosomal recessive inheritance	• vWF activity decreased out of proportion to vWF antigen • Factor VIII activity normal or reduced • RIPA decreased • Multimer electrophoresis: large multimers decreased
Type 2B (enhanced binding to high-molecular-weight multimers to platelet GPIb; may have decrease in circulating high-molecular-weight multimers)	• Approximately 5% of individuals with vWD have this type • Moderate to severe bleeding • Thrombocytopenia • Autosomal dominance inheritance	• vWF activity decreased out of proportion to vWF antigen • Factor VIII activity normal or reduced • Thrombocytopenia • RIPA increased • Multimer electrophoresis: usually decreased large multimers
Type 2M (reduced binding of vWF to platelet GPIb)	• Not common • Moderate to severe bleeding • Autosomal dominance or recessive inheritance	• vWF activity decreased out of proportion to vWF antigen • Factor VIII activity normal or reduced • RIPA decreased • Multimer electrophoresis: all multimers present and decreased
Type 2N (reduced binding of vWF to factor VIII)	• Not common • Similar to hemophilia A with joint, soft tissue, and GU bleeding • Autosomal recessive inheritance	• vWF activity and antigen normal • Factor VIII levels low (5–15%) • RIPA normal • Multimer electrophoresis: normal
Type 3 (severe quantitative deficiency/absence of vWF)	• Rare • Similar to hemophilia A • Autosomal recessive inheritance	• vWF activity and antigen absent or markedly decreased • Factor VIII levels low (1–10%) • RIPA absent or very low • Multimer electrophoresis: undetectable or too faint to visualize

From Connell, N.T., Flood, V.H., Brignardello-Petersen, R., Abdul-Kadir, R., Arapshian, A., Couper, S., Grow, J.M., Kouides, P., Laffan, M., Lavin, M., Leebeek, F.W.G., O'Brien, S.H., Ozelo, M.C., Tosetto, A., Weyand, A.C., James, P.D., Kalot, M.A., Husainat, N., & Mustafa, R.A. (2021). Clinical presentation and diagnosis of von Willebrand disease and guidelines on the management of von Willebrand disease. *Blood Advances, 5*(1), 301–325.

vWD is the most common inherited bleeding disorder, found in up to 1% of the US population. In other words, 3.2 million (or 1 in every 100) people in the United States have vWD. vWD occurs equally among males and females, but females are more likely to notice symptoms due to heavy or abnormal menses and after childbirth. vWD occurs equally across all races and ethnicities (CDC, 2019b).

The diagnosis of vWD and determining the accurate type of vWD can be challenging. The American Society of Hematology (ASH), the International Society of Thrombosis and Haemostasis (ISTH), the NBDF (formerly the National Hemophilia Foundation), and the WFH created evidence-based guidelines to help support clinicians in decisions on vWD diagnosis (James et al., 2021). Fig. 11.4 provides the algorithm that summarizes these guidelines.

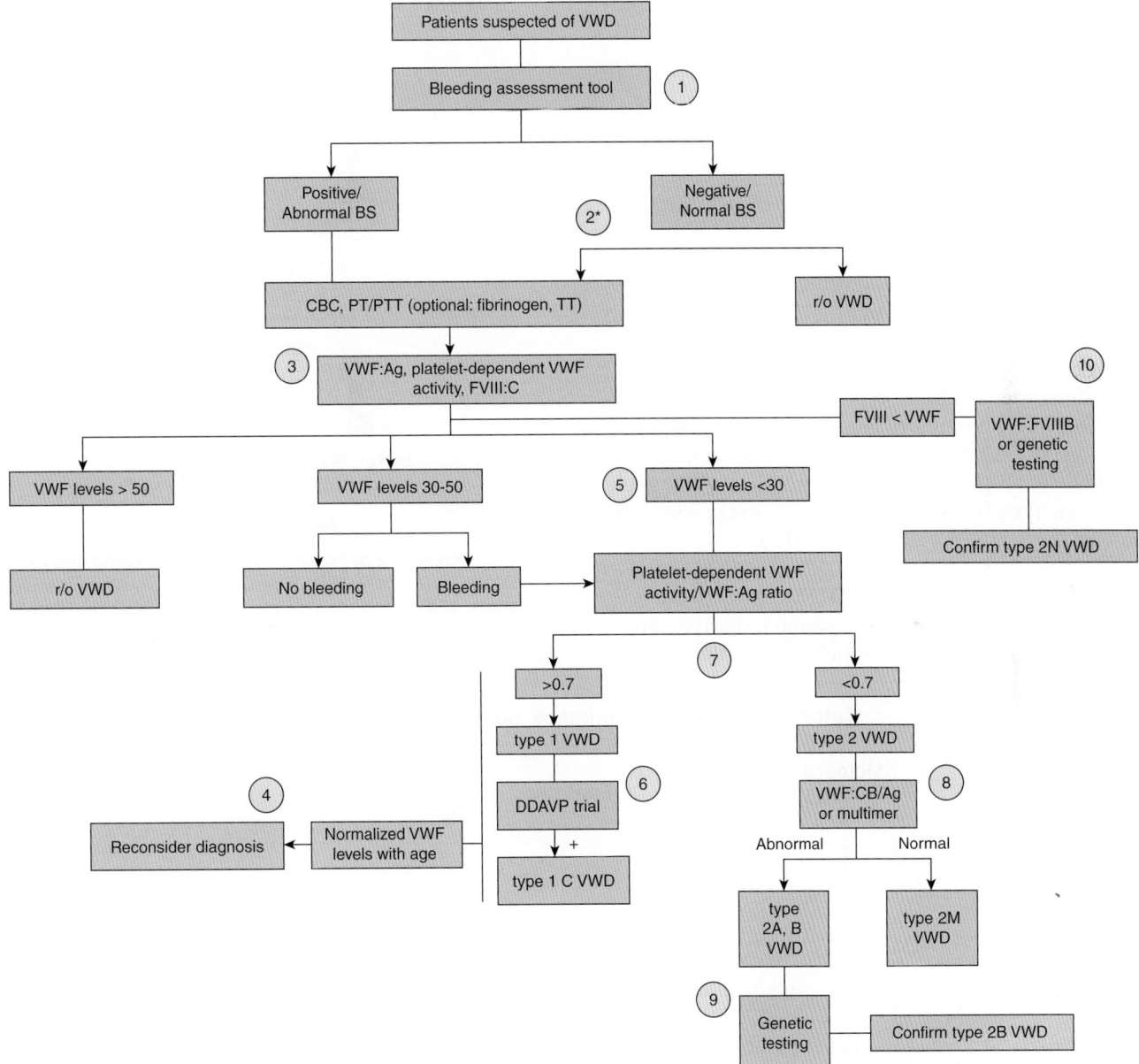

Fig. 11.4 An overall algorithm addressing the diagnosis of von Willebrand disease (VWD). The numbers in the yellow circles correspond to guideline questions. von Willebrand factor *(VWF)* levels refer to vWF antigen *(VWF:Ag)* and/or platelet-dependent vWF activity. The algorithm says vWF level 30–50 for simplicity; this refers to vWF levels of 0.30–0.50 IU/mL, with the caveat that the lower limit of the normal range as determined by the local laboratory should be used if it is <0.50 IU/mL. *Men and children, referred to a hematologist and/or first-degree relative affected with vWD. *BS,* Bleeding score; *CBC,* complete blood count; *DDAVP,* desmopressin; *FVIII,* factor VIII; *FVIII:C,* FVIII coagulant activity; *PT,* prothrombin time; *PTT,* partial thromboplastin time; *r/o,* rule out; *TT,* thrombin time; *VWF:CB/Ag,* ratio of vWF collagen binding to antigen; *VWF:FVIIIB,* vWF FVIII binding. (From James, P.D., Connell, N.T., Ameer, B., Di Paola, J., Eikenboom, J., Giraud, N., Haberichter, S., Jacobs-Pratt, V., Konkle, B., McLintock, C., McRae, S.R., Montgomery, R., O'Donnell, J.S., Scappe, N., Sidonio, R., Flood, V.H., Husainat, N., Kalot, M.A., & Mustafa, R.A. [2021]. ASH, ISTH, NHF, WFH 2021 guidelines on the diagnosis of von Willebrand disease. *Blood Advances,* 5[1], 280–300.)

ACQUIRED/INHERITANCE

Most people with vWD are born with it. In people with vWD there is a change in the gene for making the vWF protein, called a vWD allele. vWD allele can be passed down from either the mother or father or sometimes from both parents (CDC, 2021b).

Type 1 Vwd and Most Type 2 Vwd

The inheritance pattern for type 1 vWD and most type 2 vWD is autosomal dominant, meaning a child will inherit vWD if the child gets a vWD allele from one parent who has the disorder. There is a 1 in 2 (50%) chance of getting a vWD allele and having vWD (Fig. 11.5).

In rare situations, both parents may have vWD. When this happens, the child could either inherit one vWD allele and one normal allele and have vWD like the parents (1 in 2 chance [50%]) or get two vWD alleles and have a more severe form of the disease than the parents (1 in 4 chance [25%]). There is a 1 in 4 (25%) chance the child will not inherit a vWD allele from either parent. If that is the case, the child will not have vWD and cannot pass it down to offspring (Fig. 11.6).

If one parent as severe type 1 vWD that was inherited from both parents (meaning the parent has two vWD alleles), and the other parent does not have a vWD allele, all children will get only one vWD allele and have type 1 vWD that is less severe than the affected parent (CDC, 2021b) (Fig. 11.7).

Type 3 vWD and Type 2N vWD

Types 3 and 2N vWD have autosomal recessive inheritance patterns. This type of inheritance pattern occurs

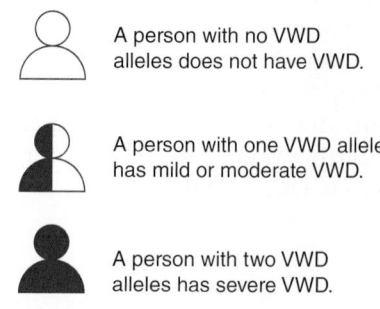

In autosomal dominant inheritance:

A person with no VWD alleles does not have VWD.

A person with one VWD allele has mild or moderate VWD.

A person with two VWD alleles has severe VWD.

A

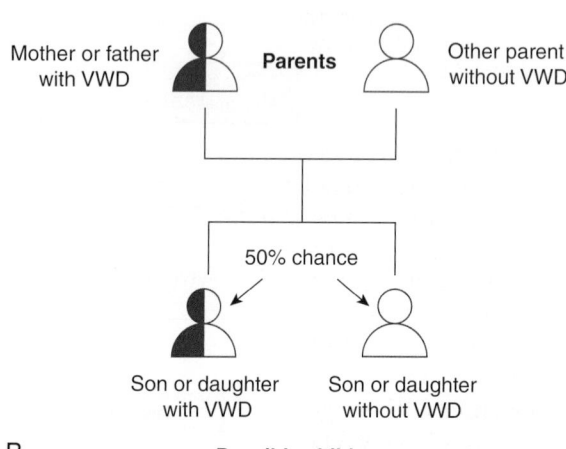

Autosomal dominant inheritance one parent with vWD

Mother or father with VWD   Parents   Other parent without VWD

50% chance

Son or daughter with VWD   Son or daughter without VWD

B   Possible children

Fig. 11.5 Inheritance pattern for type 1 von Willebrand disease *(VWD)* **and most type 2 vWD.** (From Centers for Disease Control and Prevention. [2021]. How von Willebrand disease is inherited. https://www.cdc.gov/ncbddd/vwd/inherited.html#:~:text=VWD%20can%20be%20passed%20down/.)

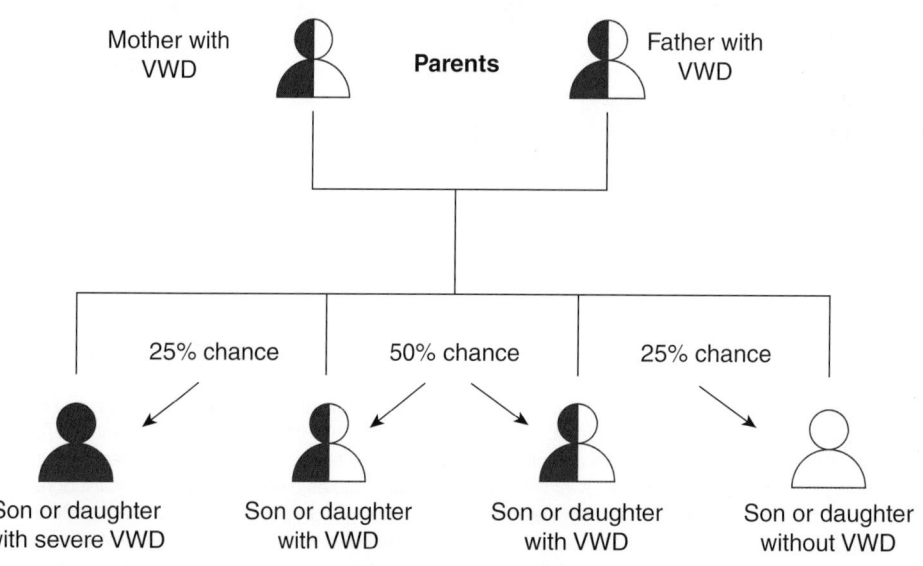

Autosomal dominant inheritance both parents with vWD

Mother with VWD   Parents   Father with VWD

25% chance   50% chance   25% chance

Son or daughter with severe VWD   Son or daughter with VWD   Son or daughter with VWD   Son or daughter without VWD

Possible children

Fig. 11.6 **Autosomal dominant inheritance when both parents have von Willebrand disease (VWD).** (From Centers for Disease Control and Prevention. [2021]. How von Willebrand disease is inherited. https://www.cdc.gov/ncbddd/vwd/inherited.html#:~:text=VWD%20can%20be%20passed%20down/.)

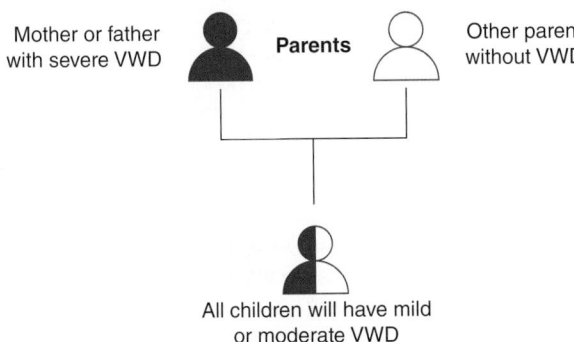

Autosomal dominant inheritance one parent with severe type 1 vWD

Mother or father with severe VWD

Parents

Other parent without VWD

All children will have mild or moderate VWD

Fig. 11.7 **Autosomal dominant inheritance when one parent has severe type 1 von Willebrand disease** *(VWD).* (From Centers for Disease Control and Prevention. [2021]. How von Willebrand disease is inherited. https://www.cdc.gov/ncbddd/vwd/inherited. html#:~:text=VWD%20can%20be%20passed%20down/.)

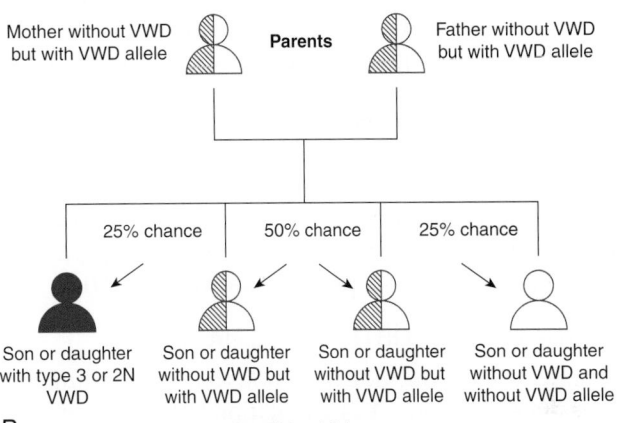

In autosomal recessive inheritance:

A person with no VWD alleles does not have VWD.

A person with one VWD allele does not have VWD.

A person with two VWD alleles has severe VWD.

A

Autosomal recessive inheritance

Mother without VWD but with VWD allele

Parents

Father without VWD but with VWD allele

25% chance | 50% chance | 25% chance

Son or daughter with type 3 or 2N VWD

Son or daughter without VWD but with VWD allele

Son or daughter without VWD but with VWD allele

Son or daughter without VWD and without VWD allele

B   **Possible children**

Fig. 11.8 **Type 3 and type 2N von Willebrand disease** *(VWD)* **autosomal recessive inheritance pattern.** (From Centers for Disease Control and Prevention. [2021]. How von Willebrand disease is inherited. https://www.cdc.gov/ncbddd/vwd/inherited. html#:~:text=VWD%20can%20be%20passed%20down/.)

when both parents have one vWD allele and one normal allele, but they do not have vWD. When two vWD alleles are present, the person will have vWD. To have vWD, the child must get the vWD allele from both parents (1 in 4 chance). A child may also get the vWD allele from one parent (1 in 2 chance). If this happens, the child will not have vWD but can pass down the vWD allele to offspring. There is also a 1 in 4 chance that the child will not get a vWD allele; therefore the child will not have vWD and will not pass it down to offspring (Fig. 11.8).

A type 3 or 2N vWD parent will give a vWD allele to the child, but the child will not have vWD if the other parent does not have a vWD allele. However, all children can pass down the vWD allele to their children (CDC, 2021b) (Fig. 11.9).

Acquired von Willebrand Syndrome

Acquired von Willebrand syndrome (AVWS) is a disorder characterized by low levels of vWF due to reduced production or enhanced removal of vWF from circulation. It is distinguished from inherited vWD by a lack of prior personal bleeding, a negative family history of vWD, and a nongenetic cause. The true prevalence of AVWS is unknown because many cases may be clinically silent or mild and remain undiagnosed. Also underreporting is likely because testing is not routinely performed on individuals who are not bleeding.

Certain diagnoses have been associated with a higher prevalence of developing AVWS, including:

- Lymphoproliferative disorders
- Myeloproliferative neoplasms
- Autoimmune disorders
- Congenital cardiac anomalies/aortic stenosis
- Left ventricular assist device or extracorporeal membrane oxygenation
- Wilms tumor (UpToDate, n.d.) (James, 2022a)

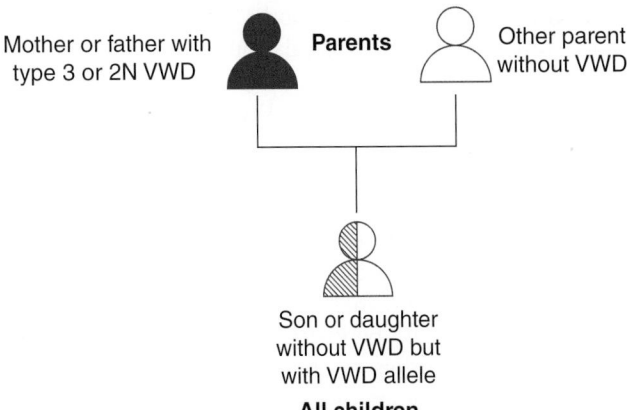

Autosomal recessive inheritance one parent with vWD

Mother or father with type 3 or 2N VWD

Parents

Other parent without VWD

Son or daughter without VWD but with VWD allele

All children

Fig. 11.9 **Autosomal recessive inheritance when one parent has von Willebrand disease** *(VWD).* (From Centers for Disease Control and Prevention. [2021]. How von Willebrand disease is inherited. https://www.cdc.gov/ncbddd/vwd/inherited.html#:~:text=VWD%20 can%20be%20passed%20down/.)

CLINICAL MANIFESTATIONS AT TIME OF DIAGNOSIS

vWD is commonly revealed by frequent and prolonged bleeding of mucous membranes and frequent bruising. The main forms of mucous membrane bleeding associated with vWD include epistaxis, oral bleeding, GI bleeding, and menstrual bleeding (James & Lillicrap, 2006; Kessler, 2007; Lillicrap, 2007).

Diagnostic testing is often requested when these symptoms are found, when there is a positive family history of the disorder, or when an increased PTT is obtained during routine preoperative screening (James, 2023). vWD is also frequently detected after bleeding occurs during or after a surgical procedure and at times with heavy postpartum bleeding or a family history of frequent miscarriages. In some types of vWD diagnoses, patients can experience bleeding in joints and other areas of the body (e.g., hemophilia patients) (CDC, 2019b).

Despite the relatively high incidence of this disorder, it is often not diagnosed because the common symptoms of epistaxis and heavy menstrual bleeding are often not brought to medical attention. If there is a suspicious bleeding pattern for the patient, utilization of the ISTH-SSC Bleeding Assessment Tool (see Table 11.2) gives insight into what would be considered a normal bleeding pattern versus an abnormal bleeding pattern. Box 11.2 also can be helpful (Elbatarny et al., 2014).

TESTING/DIAGNOSTIC CRITERIA

Testing for vWD includes a veinous blood sampling that measures the amount of circulating vWF protein antigen and activity levels within the body. These screening tests are called clotting factor assays. Appropriate diagnosis for all bleeding disorders requires access to laboratory facilities that are equipped with the resources and expertise to accurately perform factor assays. Because the levels of vWF antigen and activity are acute phase reactants and may vary over time and be influenced by a person's stress level, recent exercise, recent illness, amount of estrogen in the body, inflammatory states, and some medications, coagulation testing may need to be repeated to establish a diagnosis (CDC, 2019b).

If a suspected diagnosis of vWD or another bleeding disorder occurs, it can be helpful to run the following laboratory tests: CBC, aPTT, PT, and appropriate factor assays. A CBC result can be normal in people with a bleeding disorder; however, if heavy bleeding has taken place, the hemoglobin and red blood cell count can be lower than normal. Individuals with low hemoglobin levels should be further evaluated with ferritin levels or iron studies to ensure they are not exhibiting iron deficiency anemia secondary to loss of blood (James, 2022). An aPPT test measures how long it takes for blood to clot, specifically measuring if clotting factors VII, IX, XI, or XII are low, which indicates it takes longer than normal for blood to clot, therefore causing a prolonged/higher result. Some with vWD will have longer aPPT results; however, those with mild vWD diagnosis can have normal aPPT results. A PT test also measures how long it takes blood to clot, specifically measuring if clotting factors I, II, V, VII, and X are low, which if it takes longer than normal for blood to clot then this causes a prolonged/higher result. Those with vWD will likely have normal PT levels.

Box 11.2	What Is Abnormal Bleeding?
Epistaxis	Occurs ≥5 times/year
	Bleeds for >10 min
	Occurs with no injury
	Requires frequent cautery
Bruising	Occurs with no injury
	Occurs ≥4 times/month
	Takes longer to heal
Menstrual bleeding	Cycling more than every 3–4 wk
	Cycles lasting >6–7 days
	Changing a pad or tampon more than every 2 hr on heavy days, and bleeding through clothing
	Pictoral Blood Assessment Chart (PBAC) score >100
	Diagnosis of anemia
Oral bleeding	Gum bleeding daily with brushing teeth/oral hygiene
	Continued bleeding >1 day after dental cleaning
Gastrointestinal bleeding	Black tarlike stool
Postpartum bleeding	Requirement of blood transfusion after delivery
	Heavy bleeding continues after 2–3 mo postpartum
Surgery	Requirement of blood transfusion with surgery
	Surgery site oozing >3 hr after surgery

From Centers for Disease Control and Prevention. (2019a). Treatment of hemophilia. https://www.cdc.gov/ncbddd/hemophilia/treatment.html; and National Bleeding Disorders Foundation. (2022e). MASAC document 264—Recommendations regarding diagnosis and management of inherited bleeding disorders in girls and women with personal and family history of bleeding. https://www.hemophilia.org/healthcare-professionals/guidelines-on-care/masac-documents/masac-document-264-masac-recommendations-regarding-diagnosis-and-management-of-inherited-bleeding-disorders-in-girls-and-women-with-personal-and-family-history-of-bleeding/.

The specific clotting assays used to diagnosis vWD include factor VIII clotting activity, von Willebrand antigen, von Willebrand activity or ristocetin cofactor, vWF multimer, and platelet aggregation and secretion testing. There are some types of vWD in which factor VIII levels are low; therefore measuring the amount of factor VIII in the blood is helpful in diagnosis. von Willebrand antigen measures the amount of circulating vWF in the blood. von Willebrand activity or ristocetin cofactor measures the effectiveness or how well the vWF works in the blood. von Willebrand multimers are used to measure the makeup and structure of the vWF protein and are used in designating the type of vWD diagnosis. Lastly, platelet aggregation and secretion tests are used to measure how well platelets work in the clotting cascade; this can be impactful in distinguishing the type of vWD diagnosis (CDC, 2019b). For example, patients with type 2B vWD can experience thrombocytopenia when their vWD levels increase with stress, inflammation, or pregnancy (James, 2022). Similarly to factor VIII patients, when they are under the stress of illness or trauma, there may be a transient elevation of their von Willebrand levels. For this reason, it is recommended that a patient be tested or, at times, retested when the stressor is resolved to give a more accurate von Willebrand level (Hoots & Shapiro, 2023).

The diagnostic criteria of vWD and determining the accurate type of vWD can be challenging. The ASH, ISTH, NBDF, and WFH created evidence-based guidelines to help support clinicians in decisions on vWD diagnosis (see Fig. 11.4).

TREATMENT

Pharmacologic Therapy for von Willebrand Disease

When looking at pharmacologic therapies utilized in the treatment of vWD, frequently the treatment is dependent upon the subtype of the diagnosis. Management remains challenging because of the wide variability in each vWD patient's bleeding symptoms; there is wide variability in clinical practice and a gap of high-certainty evidence to guide clinical decision making (Connell et al., 2021). Primary care providers are urged to consult the patient's hematologist, the local HTC, or the NBDF for the most current treatment recommendations (NBDF, 2022g).

DDAVP. Desmopressin acetate, a synthetic analog of vasopressin, is the treatment of choice for persons with types 1, 2A, 2M, and 2N vWD but not subtype 2B if these patients have shown to be responsive to DDAVP in a DDAVP trial or challenge (NBDF, 2022g). Once DDAVP is given, WPBs in endothelial cells are released and increase two to five times the plasma levels of both vWF and factor VIII within 30 to 60 minutes (Xu et al., 2004). This can work to increase the patient's own vWF and factor VIII levels so they do not have to use clotting factors to stop bleeding episodes (CDC, 2019b).

DDAVP has been successfully used for patients to prevent bleeding complications in connection with dental or surgical procedures and for acute bleeding such as joint, muscle, or mucosal (oral, nasal, GI, menstrual) bleeding. Not all patients with vWD, including types 1, 2A, 2M, and 2N, respond adequately to DDAVP; a test of treatment or DDAVP challenge needs to be performed on these patients before DDAVP can be utilized for their bleeding plan of care. Unlike a DDAVP challenge for patients with hemophilia, a DDAVP challenge for those with vWF mutations brings concern associated with rapid clearance of vWF. For this reason it is recommended in a DDAVP challenge on a patient with vWD diagnosis that von Willebrand antigen, von Willebrand activity, and factor VII level be checked before DDAVP is given, 30 to 60 minutes after DDAVP is given and 4 to 6 hours after DDAVP is given (Lavin & O'Donnell, 2016). All DDAVP challenges should take place in a clinical-based setting. A successful response to a DDAVP challenge requires an increase of over two times the baseline vWF activity level, and that level must be sustained along with factor VIII greater than 0.5 IU/mL at 4 hours after DDAVP being given (NBDF, 2022g).

DDAVP should not be utilized for patients under 2 years of age, those with cardiovascular disease, diagnosis of seizure disorder, or pregnant women with preeclampsia. After DDAVP is given, free fluid intake restrictions are frequently recommended because of the effect of hyponatremia, and it should not be given more often than once every 24 hours. Other side effects associated with DDAVP are headache, flushing, hypotension, and hypertension (UpToDate, n.d.) (James, 2022c).

von Willebrand factor replacement products. One of the top ways to treat those with vWD types 2B, 3, and types 1, 2A, 2M, and 2N that do not respond to DDAVP is to replace their missing blood clotting factor. Factor VIII/vWF concentrate products are injected intravenously, and their higher-molecular-weight multimers of vWF help the patient achieve coagulation. There are human plasma-derived products and recombinant products available and FDA approved (NBDF, 2022g). vWF replacement products can be used in conjunction with antifibrinolytics and hormonal therapy. Like those with hemophilia, the use of factor replacement concentrates in a patient's treatment can cause financial strain due to the price of these products (see Tables 11.5 and 11.7 for a full list).

Oral antifibrinolytic agents, hormonal therapy. Antifibrinolytic agents (tranexamic acid and aminocaproic acid) and hormonal therapy are both utilized in the treatment of vWD and hemophilia. See previous sections for further information.

Prophylaxis. Typically, patients with vWD will have less frequent and clinically severe bleeding, so bleeding treatment is usually episodic at the time of bleeding (either from injury/trauma, anticipated invasive surgery, menstruation, or labor). More clinically severe forms of vWD (in any type of vWD) may need long-term prophylactic therapy, especially if there is a history of repeat bleeding in joints, nose, and GI tract (Franchini et al., 2021). ASH, ISTH, NBDF, and WFH guidelines define vWD prophylaxis as a period of 3 months of treatment with a vWF product given at a minimum of once a week or, for females with heavy menstrual bleeding using vWF product, at least once per menstrual cycle (NBDF, 2022g). Per the 2021 vWD guidelines (Connell et al., 2021), long-term prophylaxis rather than no prophylaxis is suggested for patients with vWD with a history of severe and frequent bleeds; however, this is a conditional recommendation based on low certainty/lack of research on the long-term effects of prophylaxis on other outcomes.

Bleeding Management for Acute Minor Bleeding and Minor Surgery

Minor bleeding is defined as bleeding that:
- Causes less than 2 g/dL decrease in hemoglobin
- Leads to transfusion of less than 2 units of whole or red blood cells

Table 11.7 Products Available to Treat Patients With von Willebrand Disease

PRODUCT	PROPHYLAXIS	DOSING MINOR BLEEDING/ SURGERY	DOSING MAJOR BLEEDING/ SURGERY	HALF-LIFE[a] (HOURS)	COMMENTS
Plasma VWF (All Contain VWF Multimers)					
Humate P	**Adults and peds:** 40–80 RCoF units/kg IV every 8–12 hr. Adjust the dosage based on the extent and location of bleeding.			11	Labeled in factor VIII and risto-cetin cofactor units
Wilate	**Adults and peds:** 20–60 RCoF units/kg IV every 12–24 hr. Adjust the dose and frequency based on the extent and location of bleeding.			16	Labeled in factor VIII and risto-cetin cofactor units
Recombinate VWF					
vonVendi	**For type 3 von Willebrand adults (age ≥18 yr):** 40–60 RCoF units/kg IV 2 times weekly	40–50 RCoF units/kg every 8–24 hr	Initial dose: 50–80 RCoF units/kg, then 50–60 RCoF every 8–24 hr	19–23	

RCoF, Ristocetin cofactor; *VWF*, von Willebrand factor.

[a]Half-lives are approximate. For children, half-lives are generally shorter than adults when assessed in pharmacokinetic studies. The half-life should be determined for the individual patient. Refer to product information and institutional guidelines for additional dosing and monitoring information.

- Is not life threatening
- Is located in noncritical areas or organs (UpToDate, n.d.) (James, 2022c)

The treatment goal for minor bleeding/surgeries is still similar to that in major bleeding surgeries: vWF activity levels should be increased to 50% or more with a combination of tranexamic acid with either desmopressin or factor concentrate (Connell et al., 2021). In settings of minor bleeding or minor surgical interventions, DDAVP can provide adequate coverage. This applies to the majority of type 1 vWD patients who have demonstrated adequate response to DDAVP. For patients who do not have an adequate response to DDAVP (or type 3 or severe type 1 and 2 vWD), vWF concentrate should be given.

Antifibrinolytic agents may be appropriate, either alone or in conjunction with DDAVP, for certain scenarios of epistaxis, mucosal bleeding, and surgeries involving the oropharynx or urogenital tract. In current guidelines (2021) for vWD management, tranexamic acid should be used in patients with type 1 vWD with baseline vWF activity levels greater than 30% and mild bleeding symptoms undergoing minor mucosal procedures (e.g., colonoscopy) (Connell et al., 2021).

Bleeding Management for Acute Major Bleeding and Major Surgery

The management of major bleeding due to injury or surgery in vWD mirrors the management of acute bleeding in hemophilia. The immediate goal is to increase the level of vWF in circulation and stabilize the clot that is formed at the site of injury. Things that need to be taken into consideration when formulating a treatment plan for acute bleeding include the patient's type of vWD, baseline vWF activity level, location and severity of bleeding, half-life of the product administered, and presence of associated injury. Examples of major bleeding in patients with vWD include:

- Bleeding that causes a decrease in hemoglobin of 2 g/dL or more
- Bleeding that leads to transfusions of 2 units or more of whole or red blood cells
- Bleeding into a closed space or compartments such as intracranial, spinal, or joint bleeding
- Uncontrolled surgical or traumatic bleeding
- Pregnant women with baseline vWF activity of less than 50 IU/dL during or after delivery and/or invasive procedures
- Any bleeding requiring treatment in a person with type 3 or severe type 1 or 2 vWD

In any of these situations, vWF should be administered without delay. DDAVP can also be considered for management; however, the rise in vWF levels may not be sufficient or last long enough for major bleeds or surgeries. Also DDAVP can be given for only 3 days because of the risk of tachyphylaxis and hyponatremia. If prolonged treatment is needed, vWF concentrate should be given. Antifibrinolytic agents are a useful adjunct for the management of major bleeds/surgeries but are not sufficient to treat bleeding by itself.

In addition, as discussed in Acute Bleeding Episodes, the definitions of serious/life-threatening bleeding and minor bleeding also apply to patients with vWD. Note too that patients with vWD and severe bleeding phenotypes can also experience hemarthroses and soft tissue/

muscle bleeds. Refer to this earlier section for further details on definitions of serious bleeding, hemarthroses, soft tissue/muscle bleeds, and minor bleeding.

For surgery management, the patient should receive an initial dose of vWF concentrate prior to surgery at a dose that will target vWF activity to approximately 100 IU/dL. Postoperatively per the 2021 guidelines on vWD management (Connell et al., 2021), the goal of treatment is to keep both factor VIII and vWF levels above 50 IU/dL for at least 3 days. The length of therapy is individualized and can range from 3 to 7 or more days.

There are a variety of vWF concentrates available (see Table 11.7). The decision on whether to use plasma-derived or recombinant vWF concentrate is usually based on cost and availability.

OB-GYN Delivery
Treatment for pregnant female patients with vWD needs to be a team-based approach between the obstetrician, primary clinician, and hematologist (or HTC) with expertise in the management of vWD. Ideally, baseline vWF activity and factor VIII activity are obtained prior to pregnancy. Like hemophilia carriers and pregnancy, the high levels of estrogen that occur during pregnancy will increase vWF and factor VIII levels in pregnant patients with vWD, causing higher levels during pregnancy. Consequently, after delivery, vWF and factor VIII levels will rapidly decline.

vWF and factor VIII activity should be monitored throughout pregnancy and after delivery (for type 2B vWD patients, the platelet count should be monitored). Typically, levels should be checked during the first and third trimesters to determine a delivery plan. vWF concentrate and antifibrinolytic agents can be used in pregnancy along with DDAVP. DDAVP should only be given as a single dose close to the time of delivery (after the cord is clamped), and fluids should be restricted to maintenance levels for 24 hours after delivery of the dose to avoid hyponatremia (NBDF, 2022f). Regional anesthesia can be considered. Per 2021 vWD guidelines (Connell et al., 2021), pregnant patients with vWD who wish to receive spinal, epidural, or combined spinal-epidural pain management during labor must have a vWF activity level between 50% and 150% prior to delivery of neuraxial anesthesia. vWF activity levels should be maintained at 50 IU/dL while the epidural is in place and for at least 6 hours after removal (NBDF, 2022f). For delivery (vaginal or cesarean), vWF and factor VIII should be maintained at 50 IU/dL or more for at least 3 to 5 days after delivery (UpToDate, n.d.) (James, P., James A., 2022). Even if the pregnant patient with vWD did not require treatment during pregnancy, she is still at risk for serious bleeding after delivery and during the first 3 weeks postpartum. The 2021 vWD guidelines recommend that tranexamic acid be given after the delivery of the baby in all patients with type 1 vWD or low VWF levels in any other type of vWD (Connell et al., 2021).

Newborns at risk for mild vWD should receive normal newborn care. If there is a family history of more severe types of vWD, a pediatric hematologist should be consulted. Neonatal vWF and factor VIII activity levels tend to be higher for approximately 6 months of life, so testing for mild vWD should be done (or repeated) at 6 months of age. Circumcisions and other elective surgical procedures should be delayed until the infant's vWF and factor VIII activity levels have been determined (UpToDate, n.d.) (James, P., James A., 2022).

THE FUTURE: ANTICIPATED ADVANCES IN DIAGNOSIS AND MANAGEMENT OF BLEEDING DISORDERS
The future treatment options for bleeding disorder diagnoses are vast, and innovative approaches are frequently being explored. Current clotting factor concentrates have never been safer, and pharmaceutic companies continue to develop products with higher purity (Great Lakes Hemophilia Foundation, n.d.). In the aftermath of the HIV and hepatitis C epidemics, the NBDF has adopted a zero-tolerance policy when faced with the potential of pathogen transmission. This strategy is intended to ensure that persons with hemophilia do not become infected with a recognized or emerging pathogen as a result of treatment with a factor concentrate (Matthew et al., 2005).

In addition to the focus on developing newer, more efficient factor products, some therapies are focused on other methods to stop bleeding. Some of these innovative treatments are still in the clinical trial phases of research and have not been approved by the FDA. Antitissue factor pathway inhibitor (anti-TFPI) and RNA interference (RNAi) are two therapies that are focused on restoring hemostatic balance by blocking components of the clotting cascade that decrease clotting and thus result in more clot formation. Anti-TFPI works to block the anticoagulant TFPI, whereas RNAi therapy works to block the anticoagulant antithrombin. Both therapies are novel in that they do not rely on replacing a specific clotting protein, such as factor VIII, factor IX, or vWF, and can be used in the prevention of bleeding for all bleeding disorders no matter the diagnosis (Great Lakes Hemophilia Foundation, n.d.).

Hemophilia has certain characteristics that make it attractive as a model for gene therapy approaches. Gene therapy works to deliver genes without genetic mutation to the liver, where factors VIII and IX are developed in the body, and the regeneration of the nonmutated genes will correct the disorder. The many approaches of gene therapy, including gene transfer, cell therapy, and gene editing (i.e., CRISPR), are still being explored in human clinical trials (Great Lakes Hemophilia Foundation, n.d.).

PRIMARY CARE MANAGEMENT

IMMUNIZATIONS

For those with a bleeding disorder diagnosis, it is recommended that patients follow the American Academy of Pediatrics and the CDC vaccine recommendations based on the patient's age. Some precautions that can be made for those with a bleeding disorder include using a small gauge needle (≤23 g), applying pressure to the injection site for 2 to 5 minutes after injection is completed, applying a cool pack or ice to the injection site before and after injection, giving certain vaccines subcutaneous versus intramuscular, giving one vaccine per limb, spreading out vaccines between 1 and 2 weeks, and infusing prophylactic factor treatment (if applicable) before vaccines are given (NBDF, 2022a).

For all vaccines, patients and families should be warned of the risks of hematoma, warmth, redness, mild swelling, bruising at the site, and fever. Patients should not use NSAIDs in the treatment of fever or pain; acetaminophen is a safe alternative if given appropriately (NBDF, 2022a).

Differential Diagnoses

- *Headaches and head injury*. Rule out intracranial bleeding, especially with concurrent vomiting and absence of GI symptoms.
- *Anemia*. Rule our frequent epistaxis, GI bleeding, heavy menstrual bleeding symptoms.
- *Visual disturbance*. Rule out intraocular, cranial bleeding, or retinal hemorrhage.
- *Fever*. If an indwelling venous access device is present, blood cultures must be drawn and intravenous antibiotics started.
- *Sore throat*. Throat cultures present a risk for posterior pharyngeal bleeding.
- *Mouth bleeding*. This often requires factor replacement in addition to topical measures and antifibrinolytic agents.
- *Abdominal pain*. Rule out GI bleeding. Rule out iliopsoas muscle bleeding with groin pain and decreased hip extension. Rule out heavy menstrual bleeding.
- *Gait disturbance/decrease in joint range of motion*. Rule out bleeding in and around the ankle, knee, hip, and iliopsoas muscle. Rule out scoliosis. Rule out hemarthrosis and osteoarthritis.
- *Dysuria and hematuria*. Rule out testicular bleeding, renal or ureteral bleeding, and infection.
- *Heavy menstrual bleeding*. May occur in women with bleeding disorder diagnoses.
- *Numbness, tingling, and pain*. Rule out nerve compression caused by bleeding.
- *Drug interactions*. Products that contain aspirin are contraindicated. Prolonged use of other substances that can affect platelet aggregation (e.g., NSAIDs) should be avoided.
- *HIV/hepatitis C*. Rule out exposure to blood products or factor products before 1986

In the newborn period, when there is a family history of a bleeding disorder or other high level of suspicion, circumcision, heel sticks, and intramuscular immunizations and injections should ideally be delayed until a definitive diagnosis is made. Vitamin K may be given subcutaneously instead of intramuscularly to reduce the risk of hematoma development. It is best if phlebotomy is performed by a skilled technician in pediatrics to avoid significant tissue hematomas (CDC, 2011).

GROWTH AND DEVELOPMENT

Monitoring the weight and height of a child with a bleeding disorder is especially important because obesity places added stress on joints and muscles, and limb length might be increased by bony overgrowth of the epiphysis on one side from chronic arthropathy. Repeated bleeding into a joint may result in a permanent contracture of that joint, with leg length discrepancy. Gait disturbances caused by scoliosis may predispose individuals with hemophilia to joint or muscle bleeding.

A thorough baseline and ongoing assessment of developmental parameters and neurologic status are useful in follow-up for head trauma and screening of potentially undiagnosed or unreported intracranial bleeding. Normal development is anticipated unless there is a history of intracranial bleeding.

DIET

It is especially important for children with bleeding disorders to meet the recommended requirements for protein and calcium intake because of their role in bone and muscle formation. A nonconstipating diet may prevent rectal bleeding that can occur when hard stools are passed. When a child has mouth bleeding, a soft diet and avoidance of foods that are hot or have sharp edges (e.g., chips) and straws (because the sucking action can disturb the clot) are recommended. As mentioned, weight management to prevent obesity is important to decrease stress on weight-bearing joints.

PHYSICAL ACTIVITY

Remaining physically active for those with a bleeding disorder diagnosis is very important for their overall health. Regular physical activity has been shown to decrease joint bleeding, decrease anxiety and depression, and provide healthy weight management. Involvement in sports can also assist in maintaining strong muscles, promoting joint stability, and building good social interactions. Some physical activities are riskier for those with a bleeding disorder. Some contact sports (e.g., tackle football, hockey, boxing, rugby, and some forms of martial arts) in which there is an increased risk of head trauma or other injuries to joints are not recommended for those with a bleeding disorder (Steps for Living, 2017c). Participation in physical activity must be taken with appropriate precautions, including wearing helmets and other protective equipment when advised. It is always recommended to discuss with the provider managing the patient's bleeding disorder when a new physical activity is started.

SAFETY

Prevention of bleeding is the first step in safety for a patient with a bleeding disorder. For many with a bleeding disorder, this means protective measures are highly encouraged, including wearing protective gear for a sport or physical activity.

Protection against head injury is of primary importance. Some patients with a bleeding disorder use a soft helmet when learning to move and walk to reduce the risk of head injury. All protective measures can be specific to that individual's needs and will change depending upon the patient's stage of life. Some safety precautions that can be considered are:
- Wearing appropriate and good-fitting shoes
- Decreasing causes of injury (sharp objects)
- Wearing a helmet when appropriate
- Wearing sports-appropriate equipment (knee pads, shin guards, mouth guards)
- Ensuring car seat, highchair, and swings have secure straps and are installed correctly

It is often difficult for parents and families to cope with their inability to prevent bleeding episodes despite diligent efforts to prevent injury. Fear of injury to the patient may even interfere with guardian-patient bonding.

Use of a medical identification/medical alert band or emblem that includes diagnosis and treatment recommendations is required for safety and recommended for all those with a bleeding disorder diagnosis. These can be worn around a patient's neck, wrist, or ankle. Medical information should be checked yearly and updated as necessary.

Families participating in a home infusion should follow accepted guidelines for infection control, including the use of gloves to mix and administer factor concentrates and the disposal of infectious wastes and sharp objects in approved containers that are disposed of appropriately.

All products that contain aspirin are contraindicated for patients with a bleeding disorder. For their safety, extreme caution should also be exercised with prolonged use of other medications that can affect platelet aggregation (e.g., NSAIDs). It is important to educate patients and their families on how to read medication labels (e.g., choosing those with acetaminophen over those with acetylsalicylic acid) and to enlist the help of the pharmacist when in doubt about the use of a particular product.

DISCIPLINE

Some families tend to overprotect children with a bleeding disorder and may be stricter with unaffected siblings. Positive disciplinary techniques that are age appropriate, developmentally appropriate, and do not include physical punishment should be recommended for all patients. Primary care providers should evaluate the disciplinary style of the patient's family and offer to counsel them on alternative discipline measures if potentially injurious methods are used.

ABUSE CONCERNS

If a child with a bleeding disorder has excessive bruising before and after diagnosis, parents and caregivers often encounter questions about suspected child abuse from health care providers or stare from friends, relatives, teachers, and strangers. Compounding the parents' distress may be guilt regarding the inheritance of the bleeding disorder.

CHILD CARE

Contact with the proposed source of child care can help allay fears and clarify the caretaker's responsibilities with regard to the prevention and management of bleeding episodes. HTC personnel or the primary care provider may provide this service. It is helpful to emphasize that early recognition of bleeding (e.g., mild swelling or a slight change in range of motion) and rapid access to medical evaluation and treatment are of primary importance for patients with bleeding disorders.

Child care providers should be discouraged from trying to make treatment decisions without the input of the parents/guardian, which is especially important when seemingly mild head injuries occur. To find the safest environment possible, parents may be encouraged to seek out sources of child care that have smaller numbers of children per provider, protective ground cover under outside activity spaces, and a staff willing to learn about the special needs and activity requirements of a child with a bleeding disorder. Some facilities may be fearful of admitting children with bleeding disorders because of their fear of liability. HTC teams can provide education and help allay concerns.

FINANCIAL CONCERNS

Reimbursement for high-priced factor replacement products and other medications has become an area of real concern as families reach the maximum lifetime amount of insurance reimbursement. Families who may face this problem need early intervention and counseling about insurance options. This is generally provided by the social worker at HTC.

HEALTH DISPARITIES AND CULTURAL INFLUENCES

Different racial and ethnic groups may have varying feelings about and experiences with disability and chronic conditions. As a result, individuals with a bleeding disorder diagnosis may receive little understanding from their own ethnic community and may even encounter racial bias in the delayed diagnosis of a hemarthrosis (e.g., a Black man with a swollen joint may be assumed to be having a sickle cell episode instead of being treated with a prompt infusion of factor concentrate). In many Asian cultures it is a sign of weakness to tell others about an illness or disease. Many Hispanics are hesitant to join organized support networks for their disorder because they fear stigmatization. Women are a medically underserved group in whom the effects of bleeding disorders or carrier diagnoses have been overlooked.

SCHOOLING

Teachers, school nurses, and athletic coaches should be informed of a child's bleeding disorder. Families and children may be reticent to disclose the diagnosis to others for fear of discrimination because of the past connection between hemophilia and HIV. School personnel are more often concerned with the prevention of bleeding (which may not be possible) and emergency management. Many HTCs offer school education visits by the program's nurse coordinator and social worker. These educational visits are most helpful upon the entrance to a new school and should be done with the permission and—ideally—participation of the patient and family. It is not uncommon for children and adolescents with a bleeding disorder to encounter peer disbelief about the disability and the need for crutches or a sling created by a bleeding episode. For many patients, the development of a 504 plan or individualized health plan may be needed to advocate for the patient's specific needs at school (Steps for Living, 2013e).

It is very important to consider the emotional impact and effect on mental health from having a bleeding disorder diagnosis for a young patient. Alterations in body image and self-esteem may be precipitated by chronic joint arthropathy, limitations on physical activity, or stress of heavy menstrual bleeding caused by the bleeding disorder. From the time of diagnosis, the family may be assisted in guiding the patient toward skills, careers, and sports that place less stress on joints and are not associated with high rates of injury. It is critical that children have activities and skills at which they can excel. The advent of prophylaxis has enabled more normal active play without the fear of increased injury and bleeding.

Participation in sports should be encouraged. Advances in prophylaxis have made it easier and safer for people with bleeding disorders to take part in a variety of activities; however, bleeding caused by injury is still a possibility. Anecdotal reports have demonstrated that fewer bleeding episodes are reported among children who are regularly active than among sedentary children. However, different activities carry different risks. Whenever a child is interested in participating in a sport, it should be discussed with HTC (Steps for Living, 2017c).

The development of a support network for these patients is vital to overall health. Many regional hemophilia organizations and HTCs host summer camps for young patients with bleeding disorders. These camps are opportunities for patients to meet peers with a bleeding disorder diagnosis, and many camps teach basic life skills and self-infusion and enhance a patient's community support (Steps for Living, 2013a).

SCREENING RECOMMENDATIONS

Vision

Routine screening is recommended. Following an eye injury, referral to an ophthalmologist is recommended, with follow-up until a resolution is obtained.

Hearing

Routine screening is recommended. Attempts at removing earwax with a curette may result in bleeding. Flushing the ear with warm water to remove cerumen is safer.

Dental

Invasive dental procedures can often be prevented through careful oral hygiene, fluoride treatments, and regular dental evaluations. An initial dental evaluation is recommended at 2 to 3 years of age in part to help the child establish a positive relationship with the dentist and to impress on parents the importance of preventive care. Hygiene should include flossing under parental supervision. Pediatric dentists with expertise in the management of persons with bleeding disorders are often associated with the local HTC. If necessary, local dentists can manage most procedures with consultation from the HTC. The HTC should be consulted about whether prophylactic treatment with factor concentrate, desmopressin, and/or antifibrinolytics is necessary for anesthetic infiltrates below the gum line and dental extractions. Treat for infections before any procedures.

Blood Pressure

Routine screening is recommended.

Hematocrit

Annual screening for anemia is recommended.

Hemoglobin

Annual screening for anemia is recommended.

Ferritin

Annual screening for anemia is recommended, particularly for menstruating females.

Urinalysis

Routine screening is recommended. More frequent screening is recommended if hematuria is present.

CONDITION-SPECIFIC SCREENING RECOMMENDATIONS

Liver Function Studies

Patients who have received any blood bank products (excluding factor concentrates) in the past year should have liver function studies performed.

HIV Antibody Testing

Pretest and posttest counseling is recommended for individuals exposed to blood products before 1986 who have not previously been tested.

Factor VIII Level

Those with hemophilia A who have received factor replacement product in the past year but are not on Hemlibra should be tested.

Factor VIII Inhibitor Level

Those with hemophilia A who have received factor replacement products in the past year should be tested.

Factor IV Level

Those with hemophilia B who have received factor replacement products in the past year should be tested.

Factor IV Inhibitor Level

Those with hemophilia B who have received factor replacement products in the past year should be tested.

DRUG INTERACTIONS/MEDICATION MANAGEMENT

All products that contain aspirin are contraindicated. Caution should also be exercised with prolonged use of other medications that can affect platelet aggregation (e.g., NSAIDs). It is important to educate parents on how to read medication labels (e.g., choosing those with acetaminophen over those with acetylsalicylic acid) and enlist the help of the pharmacist when in doubt about the use of a particular product.

SEXUALITY

As patients get older, it is natural to think about how their bleeding disorder can affect their sexuality and sexual interactions. Safe-sex counseling (e.g., including decision-making skills; values clarification; and instruction in the use of protection to prevent transmission of HIV, hepatitis B and C, and other sexually transmitted infections) should be offered to all adolescent patients. The risks associated with unplanned pregnancies and genetics associated with bleeding disorders should be discussed with the patient. When discussing a patient's sexual history it is important to discuss these things in private with the patient alone without a parent/guardian present so that the patient understands provider-patient confidentiality.

Sexual intercourse, like most physical activities, has its risks of bleeding and injury. Some common bleeding symptoms after intercourse are bruises, hematomas, muscle bleeds, joint bleeds, pain, limited motions, and swelling.

Patients with a penis should look out for any injury to the penis, which may be shown by external bleeding, swelling, pain, and discoloration of the urine. Sex may also increase the risk of internal bleeding to deep pelvic muscles in patients with and without a penis, which can be harder to recognize. Bleeding in these deep pelvic muscles can cause pain in the low back, abdomen, pelvic region, groin, and upper thigh as well as numbness and tingling. Bleeding in this area can affect more than the muscle, called a psoas bleed. Psoas bleeds and penis bleeds can be quite serious, and it is important to seek medical treatment immediately.

For patients without a penis, vaginal bleeding can occur before, during, and after sexual intercourse. It can also be a painful experience. If it is a painful experience, or bleeding occurs for longer than a couple of days, or patients need to change a pad more than twice a day, then they should be seen by their HTC provider. There are always options for treatment and safety measures that can make sexual activities safe for patients and their partners.

The subject of sexuality is sensitive in nature, and patients with a bleeding disorder may be exceptionally more reluctant to discuss the topic due to their bleeding. Many HTCs have designated interdisciplinary clinics for adolescents and young patients without a penis with gynecology teams for this reason (Steps for Living, 2013b).

TRANSITION TO ADULTHOOD

Arranging efficient transfer for adolescents from pediatric to adult care can be one of the greatest challenges. The transition from adolescence to adulthood can be particularly stressful for some individuals with bleeding disorders. When they approach adulthood, such individuals have their comprehensive HTC medical care transferred from the pediatric hematology service to the adult hematology service.

This is usually the time when the responsibility for medical care is transferred from the guardian to the young adult. It is helpful if this expected transition is discussed with the child and family when the child is still young. The open and ongoing discussion about this expected transition of care may help allay some of the stress, sadness, and anger the patient and family feel when they must transfer care to new providers.

The choice of college may also be influenced by the availability of specialized medical care in the area, and the patient's choice of career may be influenced by physical limitations. As adolescents make the transition to adulthood they may no longer be eligible for medical coverage under their parent's insurance policy and may have difficulty finding coverage that will accommodate the medications needed in the management of their diagnosis. In many states there are special programs that cover individuals with a bleeding disorder, or individuals may be eligible for a federal government program (e.g., Medicare, Medicaid, Supplemental Security Income) due to disability (Bolton-Maggs, 2007; Steps for Living, 2013d; Valentino et al., 2006).

RESOURCES

Foundation for Women & Girls with Blood Disorders (https://www.fwgbd.org/resources/patient-resources)

Healthychildren.org (https://www.healthychildren.org/English/health-issues/conditions/chronic/Pages/bleeding-disorders-in-children-von-willebrand-disease-and-hemophilia.aspx)

National Bleeding Disorders Foundation (https://www.hemophilia.org/who-we-are)

Summary

Primary Care Needs for the Child With Bleeding Disorders

GROWTH AND DEVELOPMENT
- Monitoring and preventing obesity is important because of added stress on joints.
- Developmental screening should be done annually, and specific screenings outlined as follow-up for head trauma or screening for undiagnosed or unreported intracranial bleeding.

DIET
- Adequate protein and calcium intake are of particular importance because of the role of both in bone and muscle formation.
- Nonconstipating diet will help prevent rectal bleeding.
- A soft diet and avoiding foods with sharp edges are necessary when a child has mouth bleeding.
- Obesity should be avoided because it places extra stress on joints.

SAFETY
- Recommended protective safety equipment
  Wearing appropriate and good-fitting shoes
  Decreasing causes of injury (sharp objects)
  Wearing a helmet when appropriate
  Wearing sports-appropriate equipment (knee pads, shin guards, mouth guards)
  Ensuring car seat, highchair, and swings have secure straps and are installed correctly
- It is generally recommended that some contact sports are considered dangerous and should be avoided (e.g., rugby, hockey, football, wrestling, some forms of martial arts). Participation in other contact sports is acceptable.
- The child should wear a medical identification emblem that includes information regarding diagnosis, treatment products, and contact with a health care provider. The information should be updated annually.
- Activities that increase the chance of testicular bleeding in males should be discouraged.
- Families participating in a home infusion program should follow accepted guidelines for universal precautions and disposal of infectious wastes.

IMMUNIZATIONS
- Routine immunizations are recommended.
- Parenteral immunizations are often given subcutaneously.
- Some children may require factor replacements before immunization injections if given intramuscularly.
- Injectable vaccines should be given with a 25-gauge needle.
- Firm pressure should be applied over the immunization site for 5 minutes. Ice may be applied before and after with pressure.

SCREENING
- *Vision.* Routine screening is recommended. Following an eye injury, referral to an ophthalmologist is recommended, with follow-up until a resolution is obtained.
- *Hearing.* Routine screening is recommended. Attempts at removing earwax with a curette may result in bleeding; flushing the ear with warm water to remove cerumen is safer.

- *Dental.* Invasive dental procedures can often be prevented through careful oral hygiene, fluoride treatments, and regular dental evaluations. An initial dental evaluation is recommended at 2 to 3 years of age, in part to help the child establish a positive relationship with the dentist and to impress on parents the importance of preventive care. Hygiene should include flossing under parental supervision. Pediatric dentists can manage most procedures with consultation from the HTC. The HTC should be consulted about whether prophylactic treatment with factor concentrate, desmopressin, and/or antifibrinolytics is necessary for anesthetic infiltrates below the gum line and dental extractions. Treat for infections before any procedures.
- *Blood Pressure.* Routine screening is recommended.
- *Hematocrit.* Annual screening for anemia is recommended.
- *Hemoglobin.* Annual screening for anemia is recommended. More frequent screening is recommended if a history of low ferritin or frequent bleeding occurs.
- *Ferritin.* Annual screening for anemia is recommended, particularly for menstruating females. More frequent screening is recommended if a history of low ferritin or frequent bleeding occurs.
- *Urinalysis.* Routine screening is recommended. More frequent screening is needed if hematuria is present.
- If blood product has been received in the past year, a factor VIII or IX inhibitor screen (i.e., specifically for persons with hemophilia) and liver function studies are indicated.

COMMON ILLNESS MANAGEMENT
Differential Diagnosis
- *Headaches and head injury.* Rule out intracranial bleeding, especially with concurrent vomiting and absence of GI symptoms.
- *Visual disturbance.* Rule out intraocular bleeding or retinal hemorrhage.
- *Fever.* If an indwelling venous access device is present, blood cultures must be drawn and intravenous antibiotics started.
- *Sore throat.* Throat cultures present a risk for posterior pharyngeal bleeding. Cultures should not be taken from an uncooperative child.
- *Mouth bleeding.* Mouth bleeding often requires factor replacement in addition to topical measures and antifibrinolytic agents.
- *Abdominal pain.* Rule out GI bleeding. Rule out iliopsoas muscle bleeding with groin pain and decreased hip extension.
- *Gait disturbance.* Rule out bleeding in and around the ankle, knee, hip, and iliopsoas muscle. Rule out scoliosis.
- *Dysuria and hematuria.* Rule out testicular bleeding, renal or ureteral bleeding, and infection. Antifibrinolytics should never be given when hematuria is present.
- *Heavy menstrual bleeding.* May occur in hemophilia carriers or females with vWD. DDAVP or estrogen therapy may be helpful. Checking ferritin levels is recommended.

- *Numbness, tingling, and pain*. Rule out nerve compression caused by bleeding.
- *Drug interactions*. Use of other substances that can affect platelet aggregation (e.g., NSAIDs) should be avoided.

DEVELOPMENTAL ISSUES
Sleep Patterns
- Standard developmental counseling is advised.

Toileting
- Counseling on the prevention and management of constipation is advised to prevent possible rectal bleeding caused by straining.

Discipline
- Recognize the potential for overprotection of the affected child and the use of deferential disciplinary methods when compared with unaffected siblings.
- Pulling a child by the arm may result in shoulder or elbow joint bleeding or soft tissue bleeding.
- Physical punishment may result in internal bleeding.
- Parents should be counseled about the use of time-outs, distractions, and other nonphysical methods of limit-setting.

Child Care
- Contact with the child care provider by the primary health care provider or HTC staff to discuss prevention and management of bleeding episodes and trauma is advised.
- The importance of early recognition and treatment of bleeding should be stressed.
- Child care centers with smaller numbers of children, protective ground cover, and a low child-to-provider ratio are suggested.
- Recognize that the child care providers may have fears regarding liability for injuries.

Schooling
- School visits are most helpful upon enrollment in a new school and ideally include the child and parent(s).
- Because of the difficulty in understanding the acute onset and resolution of bleeding episodes, peer acceptance may be poor.
- Acknowledge potential fear of HIV infection among school personnel; educate regarding transmission and current safety of treatment.
- Recognize potential alterations in body image and self-esteem because of chronic joint arthropathy or limitations on physical activity.

- Intracranial bleeding may result in learning problems.
- It is generally recommended that competitive contact sports are considered dangerous and should be avoided. Patients should consult their health care provider for questions.

Sexuality
- Delay circumcision until the child with a positive family history is screened for a bleeding disorder.
- Safe-sex counseling is recommended to prevent sexually transmitted diseases.
- Genetic counseling is recommended to discuss reproductive risks and the risk of offspring diagnosis.

Transition to Adulthood
- The transfer of medical care from a pediatric center to an adult hemophilia center can be difficult.
- Educational and career opportunities may be restricted because of physical limitations and the need to be near a treatment center.
- Obtaining health care coverage for a bleeding disorder may be difficult and may limit employment opportunities. Individuals may be eligible for Supplemental Security Income if their disabilities are significant.

FAMILY CONCERNS
- Child abuse may be suspected.
- Parents may experience guilt regarding the hereditary nature of a bleeding disorder.
- The fear of injury to an infant may decrease parent-infant bonding.
- Parents may fear the inability to prevent bleeding episodes despite attempts to prevent injury.
- The potential for undiscovered infectious diseases may be a concern.
- The family may experience uncertainty regarding the viral safety of blood products and all medications.
- Insurance problems may occur as children and adults reach lifetime maximum amounts of reimbursement.
- A lack of insurance coverage risks patients' inability to access medications needed for the management of their diagnosis.

Health Disparities and Cultural Influences
- Minorities, including women, are at increased risk of delayed bleeding disorder diagnosis.
- Increased hesitancy to seek care is due to patients' culture, racial bias, history of being overlooked, and fear of stigmatization.

REFERENCES

Ahle S. (2020). The high price of hemophilia. ASH Clinical News. https://www.ashclinicalnews.org/spotlight/feature-articles/high-price-hemophilia/.

Bolton-Maggs, P. H. (2007). Transition of care from paediatric to adult services in haematology. *Archives of Diseases in Childhood, 92*, 797–801.

Centers for Disease Control and Prevention. (2011). Diagnosis of hemophilia. https://www.cdc.gov/ncbddd/hemophilia/diagnosis.html#:~:text=Screening%20tests%20are%20blood%20tests.

Centers for Disease Control and Prevention. (2011). Information on hemophilia for women. https://www.cdc.gov/ncbddd/hemophilia/women.html.

Centers for Disease Control and Prevention. (2019a). Treatment of hemophilia. https://www.cdc.gov/ncbddd/hemophilia/treatment.html.

Centers for Disease Control and Prevention. (2019b). What is von Willebrand disease? https://www.cdc.gov/ncbddd/vwd/facts.html.

Centers for Disease Control and Prevention. (2020). What is hemophilia. https://www.cdc.gov/ncbddd/hemophilia/facts.html.

Centers for Disease Control and Prevention. (2021a). How hemophilia is inherited. https://www.cdc.gov/ncbddd/hemophilia/inheritance-pattern.html#:~:text=It%20almost%20always%20is%20inherited.

Centers for Disease Control and Prevention. (2021b). How von Willebrand disease is inherited. https://www.cdc.gov/ncbddd/vwd/inherited.html#:~:text=VWD%20can%20be%20passed%20down.

Connell, N. T., Flood, V. H., Brignardello-Petersen, R., et al. (2021). ASH, ISTH, NHF, WFH 2021 guidelines on the management of von Willebrand disease. *Blood Advances, 5*(1), 301–325. https://doi.org/10.1182/bloodadvances.2020003264.

Elbatarny, M., Mollah, S., Grabell, J., et al. (2014). Normal range of bleeding scores for the ISTH-BAT: Adult and pediatric data from the merging project. *Haemophilia, 20*(6), 831–835. https://doi.org/10.1111/hae.12503.

Franchini, M., Seidizadeh, O., Mannucci, P.M. Prophylactic management of patients with von Willebrand disease. *Therapeutic Advances in Hematology.* 2021;12. https://doi.org/10.1177/20406207211064064.

Great Lakes Hemophilia Foundation. (n.d). Future therapies. (n.d.). Retrieved October 12, 2022, from https://glhf.org/resources/facts-about-bleeding-disorders/future-therapies/.

Geraghty, S. (n.d.). Hemophilia and hospitalization a self learning program. *Hemophilia.org.* Retrieved October 12, 2022, from. https://www.hemophilia.org/sites/default/files/document/files/Hemophilia-and-Hospitalization-A-Self-Learning-Program.pdf.

Guh, S., Grosse, S. D., McAlister, S., Kessler, C. M., & Soucie, J. M. (2011). Healthcare expenditures for males with haemophilia and employer-sponsored insurance in the United States, 2008. *Haemophilia, 18*(2), 268–275. https://doi.org/10.1111/j.1365-2516.2011.02692.x.

Hemophilia of Georgia. (n.d.). Nosebleeds. *HoG handbook.* Retrieved September 9th, 2022, from https://www.hog.org/handbook/article/3/33/nosebleeds.

Hoots W. K., Shapiro A. D. Clinical manifestations and diagnosis of hemophilia. UpToDate. 2022. Retrieved March 8, 2023, from https://www-uptodate-com.proxy.hsl.ucdenver.edu/contents/clinical-manifestations-and-diagnosis-of-hemophilia?search=Hemophilia&source=search_result&selectedTitle=1~150&usage_type=default&display_rank=1#H1.

Hoots, W. K. (2003). Comprehensive care for hemophilia and related inherited bleeding disorders: Why it matters. *Current Hematology Reports, 2*(5), 395–401.

Hoots, W. K., & Shapiro, A. D. (2023). *Treatment of bleeding and perioperative management in hemophilia A and B.* UpToDate. https://www.uptodate.com/contents/treatment-of-bleeding-and-perioperative-management-in-hemophilia-a-and-b.

Indiana Hemophilia & Thrombosis Center. (n.d.). What are antifibrinolytic agents? https://www.ihtc.org/antifibrinolytic-agents.

James, P. Clinical presentation and diagnosis of von Willebrand diseases. *UpToDate.* (2022). Retrieved March 8, 2023, from https://www-uptodate-com.proxy.hsl.ucdenver.edu/contents/clinical-presentation-and-diagnosis-of-von-willebrand-disease?search=von%20willebrand&source=search_result&selectedTitle=1~150&usage_type=default&display_rank=1#H3771951064.

James, P. (2022a). Clinical presentation and diagnosis of von Willebrand disease. *UpToDate.* Retrieved August 11, 2022 from https://www.uptodate.com/contents/clinical-presentation-and-diagnosis-of-von-willebrand-disease/print.

James, P. (2022b). von Willebrand disease (VWD): Treatment of major bleeding and major surgery. *UpToDate.* Retrieved October 12, 2022 from https://www.uptodate.com/contents/von-willebrand-disease-vwd-treatment-of-major-bleeding-and-major-surgery.

James, P. (2022c). von Willebrand disease (VWD): Treatment of minor bleeding, use of DDAVP, and routine preventive care. *UpToDate.* Retrieved August 11, 2022 from https://www.uptodate.com/contents/von-willebrand-disease-vwd-treatment-of-minor-bleeding-use-of-ddavp-and-routine-preventive-care?topicRef=1372&source=related_link.

James, P., James A., (2022). von Willebrand disease (VWD): Gynecologic and obstetric considerations. *UpToDate.* Retrieved August 11, 2022 from https://www.uptodate.com/contents/von-willebrand-disease-vwd-gynecologic-and-obstetric-considerations?topicRef=1372&source=see_link.

James, P., & Lillicrap, D. (2006). Genetic testing for von Willebrand disease: The Canadian experience. *Seminars in Thrombosis and Hemostasis, 32,* 546–552.

James, P. D., Connell, N. T., Ameer, B., et al. (2021). ASH, ISTH, NHF, WFH 2021 guidelines on the diagnosis of von Willebrand disease. *Blood Advvances, 5*(1), 280–300. https://doi.org/10.1182/bloodadvances.2020003265.

James, P. (2023). Clinical presentation and diagnosis of von Willebrand disease. *UpToDate.* https://www.uptodate.com/contents/clinical-presentation-and-diagnosis-of-von-willebrand-disease/print.

James, P. (2023). *von Willebrand disease: Treatment of major bleeding and major surgery.* UpToDate. https://www.uptodate.com/contents/von-willebrand-disease-vwd-treatment-of-major-bleeding-and-major-surgery.

James, P. (2023). *von Willebrand disease: Treatment of minor bleeding, use of DDAVP, and routine preventive care.* UpToDate. https://www.uptodate.com/contents/von-willebrand-disease-vwd-treatment-of-minor-bleeding-use-of-ddavp-and-routine-preventive-care?topicRef=1372&source=related_link.

Jones, P. (2002). *Living with haemophilia* (5th ed.). Oxford University Press.

Kadir, R. A., & Aledort, L. M. (2000). Obstetrical and gynaecological bleeding: A common presenting symptom. *Clinical & Laboratory Haematology, 22*(Suppl 1), 12–16.

Kessler, C. M. (2007). Diagnosis and treatment of von Willebrand disease: New perspectives and nuances. *Haemophilia, 13*(Suppl 5), 3–14.

Kuiper, P. (n.d.). ISTH-SSC bleeding assessment tool. Bleeding Score. https://bleedingscore.certe.nl/.

Kulkarni, R., & Lusher, J. M. (2001). Review: Perinatal management of newborns with haemophilia. *British Journal of Haematology, 112,* 264–274.

Kulkarni, R., Ponder, K. P., James, A. H., et al. (2006). Unresolved issues in diagnosis and management of inherited bleeding disorders in the perinatal period: A white paper of the Perinatal Task Force of the Medical and Scientific Advisory Council of the National Hemophilia Foundation, USA. *Haemophilia, 12,* 205–211.

Lavin, M., O'Donnell, J. S. (2016). New treatment approaches to von Willebrand disease. *Hematology Am Soc Hematol Educ Program. 2016*(1), 683–689. doi: 10.1182/asheducation-2016.1.683.

Lennie, D. Managing pain. Great Lakes Hemophilia Foundation. 2020. https://glhf.org/managing-pain/.

Leung, L. K. (2022). Overview of hemostasis. *UpToDate.* Retrieved from https://www.uptodate.com/contents/overview-of-hemostasis.

Leung, L. K. (2023). Overview of hemostasis. *UpToDate.* https://uptodate.com/contents/overview-of-hemostasis.

Lillicrap, D. (2007). Von Willebrand disease—phenotype versus genotype: Deficiency versus disease. *Thrombosis Research, 120*(Suppl 1), S11–S16.

Liu, J. L., Michaud, J. E., Ludwig, W. W., & Gearhart, J. P. (2019). Diagnosis of hemophilia in newborn circumcision: A case presentation. *Urology Case Reports, 23,* 101–102. https://doi.org/10.1016/j.eucr.2019.01.017.

MacLean, P. E., Fijnvandraat, K., Beijlevelt, M., Peters, M. (2004). The impact of unaware carriership on the clinical presentation of haemophilia. *Haemophilia. 10*(5): 560–564. doi: 10.1111/j.1365-2516.2004.00955.x.

Makris, M., Oldenburg, J., Mauser-Bunschoten, E. P., Peerlinck, K., Castaman, G., Fijnvandraat, K; subcommittee on Factor VIII, Factor IX and Rare Bleeding Disorders. (2018). The definition, diagnosis and management of mild hemophilia A: communication from the SSC of the ISTH. *J Thromb Haemost.* 16(12), 2530–2533. doi: 10.1111/jth.14315.

Matthew, P., Manno, C. S., & Aledort, L. M. (2005). Therapeutic choices in the current millennium: Hemophilia workshop highlights. *Pediatric Blood Cancer,* 14, 611–615.

Mistry, T., Dogra, N., Chauhan, K., & Shahani, J. (2017). Perioperative considerations in a patient with hemophilia A: A case report and review of literature. *Anesthesia: Essays and Research,* 11(1), 243. https://doi.org/10.4103/0259-1162.181432.

Montgomery, R. R., Cox-Gill, J., & DiPaola, J. (2008). Hemophilia and von Willebrand disease. In Nathan, D. G., Orkin, S. H., & Ginsburg, D. et al (Eds.), *Hematology of infancy and childhood* (7th ed.). Elsevier.

National Bleeding Disorders Foundation. (2022a). MASAC document 221—Recommendations on administration of vaccines to individuals with bleeding disorders. Retrieved October 13, 2022, from https://www.hemophilia.org/healthcare-professionals/guidelines-on-care/masac-documents/masac-document-221-recommendations-on-administration-of-vaccines-to-individuals-with-bleeding-disorders.

National Bleeding Disorders Foundation. (2022b). MASAC document 238—Recommendations regarding physical therapy guidelines in patients with bleeding disorders. Retrieved October 12, 2022, from https://www.hemophilia.org/healthcare-professionals/guidelines-on-care/masac-documents/masac-document-238-recommendations-regarding-physical-therapy-guidelines-in-patients-with-bleeding-disorders.

National Bleeding Disorders Foundation. (2022c). MASAC document 257—Guidelines for emergency department management of individuals with hemophilia and other bleeding disorders. https://www.hemophilia.org/healthcare-professionals/guidelines-on-care/masac-documents/masac-document-257-guidelines-for-emergency-department-management-of-individuals-with-hemophilia-and-other-bleeding-disorders.

National Bleeding Disorders Foundation. (2022d). MASAC document 260—Management of chronic pain in persons with bleeding disorders: Guidance for practical application of the Centers for Disease Control's opioid prescribing guidelines. Retrieved October 12, 2022, from https://www.hemophilia.org/healthcare-professionals/guidelines-on-care/masac-documents/masac-document-260-management-of-chronic-pain-in-persons-with-bleeding-disorders-guidance-for-practical-application-of-the-centers-for-disease-controls-opioid-prescribing-guidelines.

National Bleeding Disorders Foundation. (2022e). MASAC document 264—Recommendations regarding diagnosis and management of inherited bleeding disorders in girls and women with personal and family history of bleeding. Retrieved October 12, 2022, from https://www.hemophilia.org/healthcare-professionals/guidelines-on-care/masac-documents/masac-document-264-masac-recommendations-regarding-diagnosis-and-management-of-inherited-bleeding-disorders-in-girls-and-women-with-personal-and-family-history-of-bleeding.

National Bleeding Disorders Foundation. (2022f). MASAC document 265—Guidelines for pregnancy and perinatal management of women with inherited bleeding disorders and carriers of hemophilia A or B. Retrieved October 12, 2022, from https://www.hemophilia.org/healthcare-professionals/guidelines-on-care/masac-documents/masac-document-265-masac-guidelines-for-pregnancy-and-perinatal-management-of-women-with-inherited-bleeding-disorders-and-carriers-of-hemophilia-a-or-b.

National Bleeding Disorders Foundation. (2022g). MASAC document 266—Recommendations regarding the treatment of von Willebrand disease. Retrieved October 12, 2022, from https://www.hemophilia.org/healthcare-professionals/guidelines-on-care/masac-documents/masac-document-266-masac-recommendations-regarding-the-treatment-of-von-willebrand-disease.

National Bleeding Disorders Foundation. (2022h). MASAC document 267—Recommendation concerning prophylaxis for hemophilia A and B with and without inhibitors. https://www.hemophilia.org/healthcare-professionals/guidelines-on-care/masac-documents/masac-document-267-masac-recommendation-concerning-prophylaxis-for-hemophilia-a-and-b-with-and-without-inhibitors.

National Bleeding Disorders Foundation. (2022i). MASAC document 268—Recommendation on the use and management of emicizumab-kxwh (Hemlibra) for hemophilia A with and without inhibitors. https://www.hemophilia.org/healthcare-professionals/guidelines-on-care/masac-documents/masac-document-268-recommendation-on-the-use-and-management-of-emicizumab-kxwh-hemlibrar-for-hemophilia-a-with-and-without-inhibitors.

National Bleeding Disorders Foundation. (2022j). MASAC document 269—Standards and criteria for the care of persons with congenital bleeding disorders. Retrieved October 12, 2022, from https://www.hemophilia.org/healthcare-professionals/guidelines-on-care/masac-documents/masac-document-269-standards-and-criteria-for-the-care-of-persons-with-congenital-bleeding-disorders.

National Organization for Rare Disorders. (2022). Acquired hemophilia. https://rarediseases.org/rare-diseases/acquired-hemophilia/#:~:text=Acquired%20hemophilia%20(AH)%20is%20.

Peyvandi, F. (2005). Carrier detection and prenatal diagnosis of hemophilia in developing countries. *Semin Thromb Hemost.* 31(5), 544–554. doi: 10.1055/s-2005-922226.

Steps for Living. (2013a). All about camps. https://stepsforliving.hemophilia.org/first-step/family-life/all-about-camps.

Steps for Living. (2013b). Dating and sex. https://stepsforliving.hemophilia.org/step-up/dating-and-sex.

Steps for Living. (2013c). Hormonal therapy. https://stepsforliving.hemophilia.org/step-out/non-factor-treatment/hormonal-therapy.

Steps for Living. (2013d). Health insurance. https://stepsforliving.hemophilia.org/step-out/financial-health/health-insurance.

Steps for Living. (2013e). Working with your school. https://stepsforliving.hemophilia.org/first-step/child-care-and-school/working-with-your-school.

Steps for Living. (2017). Physical activity. https://stepsforliving.hemophilia.org/resources/physical-activity.

Sharathkumar, A., & Pipe, S. W. (2008). Bleeding disorders. *Pediatric Reviews,* 29(4), 121–130.

Shetty, S. (2014). Haemophilia – diagnosis and management challenges. *Mol Cytogenet.* 7(Suppl 1 Proceedings of the International Conference on Human), I44. doi: 10.1186/1755-8166-7-S1-I44.

Shibahara, M., Shibata, E., Kinjo, Y., et al. (2021). Impact of the induction of labor on hemophilia carriers and their newborn infants. *Journal of Medical Cases,* 12(1), 5–8. https://doi.org/10.14740/jmc3597.

Soucie, J. M., Miller, C. H., Dupervil, B., Le, B., & Buckner, T. W. (2020). Occurrence rates of haemophilia among males in the United States based on surveillance conducted in specialized haemophilia treatment centres. *Haemophilia,* 26(3), 487–493. https://doi.org/10.1111/hae.13998.

Soucie, M. J., Nuss, R., Evatt, B., et al. (2000). Mortality among males with hemophilia: Relations with source of medical care. *Blood,* 96(2), 437–442.

Srivastava, A., Santagostino, E., Dougall, A., Kitchen, S., Sutherland, M., Pipe, S. W., Carcao, M., Mahlangu, J., Ragni,

M. V., Windyga, J., Llinás, A., Goddard, N. J., Mohan, R., Poonnoose, P. M., Feldman, B. M., Lewis, S. Z., van den Berg, H. M., Pierce, G. F; WFH Guidelines for the Management of Hemophilia panelists and co-authors. (2020). WFH Guidelines for the Management of Hemophilia, 3rd edition. *Haemophilia.* 26(Suppl 6), 1–158. doi:10.1111/hae.14046. Epub 2020 Aug 3. Erratum in: Haemophilia. 2021 Jul;27(4):699.

Street, A. M., Ljung, R., Lavery, S. A. (2008). Management of carriers and babies with haemophilia. *Haemophilia.* 14(Suppl 3), 181–187 . doi: 10.1111/j.1365-2516.2008.01721.x.

Subramaniam V. (n.d.). Antifibrinolytics. *Hemophilia News Today.* https://hemophilianewstoday.com/antifibrinolytics/.

TBH Creative. (2019). Severity of hemophilia. Indiana Hemophilia & Thrombosis Center. https://www.ihtc.org/severity-of-hemophilia.

UpToDate. (n.d.). Www.uptodate.com. https://www.uptodate.com/contents/overview-of-hemostasis.

UpToDate. (n.d.). Www.uptodate.com. Retrieved August 11, 2022, from https://www.uptodate.com/contents/clinical-presentation-and-diagnosis-of-von-willebrand-disease/print.

UpToDate. (n.d.). Www.uptodate.com. Retrieved August 11, 2022, from https://www.uptodate.com/contents/von-willebrand-disease-vwd-gynecologic-and-obstetric-considerations?topicRef=1372&source=see_link.

UpToDate. (n.d.). Www.uptodate.com. Retrieved August 11, 2022, from https://www.uptodate.com/contents/von-willebrand-disease-vwd-treatment-of-minor-bleeding-use-of-ddavp-and-routine-preventive-care?topicRef=1372&source=related_link.

UpToDate. (n.d.). Www.uptodate.com. Retrieved August 12, 2022, from https://www.uptodate.com/contents/treatment-of-bleeding-and-perioperative-management-in-hemophilia-a-and-b.

UpToDate. (n.d.). Www.uptodate.com. Retrieved October 12, 2022, from https://www.uptodate.com/contents/von-willebrand-disease-vwd-treatment-of-major-bleeding-and-major-surgery.

UpToDate. (n.d.). Www.uptodate.com. Retrieved October 12, 2022, from https://www.uptodate.com/contents/image?imageKey=HEME%2F110532.

Valentino, L., & Kapoor, M. (2005). Central venous access devices in patients with hemophilia. *Expert Review of Precision Medicine and Drug Development,* 2(6), 699–711.

Valentino, L., Santagostino, E., Blanchette, V., et al. (2006). Managing the pediatric patient and the adolescent/adult transition. *Seminars in Thrombosis and Hemostasis,* 32(2), 28–31.

Washington, D., Anderson-Cook, A., Maeda, J. et al. Working Paper Series Congressional Budget Office prices for and spending on specialty drugs in Medicare part D and Medicaid: An in-depth analysis. 2019. https://www.cbo.gov/system/files/2019-03/55011-Specialty_Drugs_WP.pdf.

Xu, L., Nichols, T. C., McCorquodale, S., Dillow, A., Merricks, E., & Ponder, K. P. (2004). DDAVP-induced increase of factor VIII activity in blood is likely due to release of factor VIII that is synthesized by endothelial cells. *Blood,* 104(11), 692. https://doi.org/10.1182/blood.v104.11.692.692.

12

Bone Marrow Transplantation

Nancy Shreve

ETIOLOGY

Bone marrow transplantation or hematopoietic stem cell transplantation (HSCT) continues to evolve as a treatment option for various acquired and congenital disorders. Over the past 50 years, HSCT has evolved from fundamental laboratory experiments and rudimentary procedures to a now highly sophisticated therapy that is a standard of care and potentially curative treatment for many diseases in adults and children. HSCT involves a nonfunctioning, damaged, or diseased bone marrow replaced with healthy blood stem cells from one's own body or a donor. Malignant and nonmalignant hematologic diseases, congenital and acquired immune system diseases, solid tumors, and inherited metabolism disorders are cured or controlled with HSCT (D'Souza et al., 2020). Recently the field of HSCT has expanded to additional cellular therapies, specifically chimeric antigen receptor T-cell (CAR-T) therapy, that use genetically engineered immune system cells to eliminate cancer cells (Goldsmith et al., 2022). The HSCT specialty integrates many medical disciplines, including hematology/oncology, immunology, organ transplantation, and transfusion therapy. As more and more children become recipients of successful HSCT or cellular therapy, primary care providers will play key roles in survivors' long-term care (Jesudas et al., 2013).

In the infancy of HSCT development, laboratory experiments were inspired by studying the radiation effects of nuclear weapons used in World War II. These early studies led to a better understanding of hematopoiesis, the dose-dependent toxicity of radiation, and the discovery that intravenous (IV) infusion of bone marrow cells could restore hematopoiesis after the bone marrow was ablated with lethal doses of radiation (Singh & McGuirk, 2016). Early clinical applications of infusion of bone marrow in patients with diseases proved unsuccessful primarily as there were few long-term survivors. Very little was known about hematopoiesis, immune responses, and antigen typing. Edward Donnall Thomas, who would later receive the 1990 Nobel Prize in Medicine for advances related to bone marrow transplant, is credited with pioneering work in the field and performing one of the first bone marrow transplants in 1956 when a child with leukemia received bone marrow from her identical twin.

Fundamental discoveries began to move the field of allogeneic transplants forward. The development of human leukocyte antigen (HLA) typing allowed for more suitable immunologic matching of donors to recipients and gave way to the first successful HLA-matched sibling transplant in 1968 for a male with severe combined immunodeficiency (SCID). Recognition of immunologic reactions, including graft rejection and graft versus host disease (GvHD), established the need for a conditioning therapy prior to transplant and immunosuppression following the transplant. Understanding the role of donor-derived T cells in the establishment of GvHD led to specific therapies targeted to remove or limit T-cell response. One important breakthrough in the field was the understanding that donor-derived immune cells could eradicate existing leukemia cells, known as the graft versus leukemia (GvL) effect, which improved the chance of cure (Singh & McGuirk, 2016).

Initially, allogeneic HSCT was limited in availability as only about 30% of patients have matched siblings. Improved HLA typing and successful prevention and treatment of GvHD led to the widespread use of unrelated matched donors. In 1979, the first successful unrelated donor transplant for a patient with leukemia was performed. Matched unrelated donor searches led to the creation of donor registries around the world. The National Marrow Donor Registry, established in 1987 in the United States, has facilitated over 100,00 matched unrelated stem cell transplants (Be the Match; see Resources, later).

In the 1990s, alternative stem cell sources other than bone marrow, including peripheral blood stem cells (PBSC) and umbilical cord blood (UCB), further changed the landscape of HSCT. The use of PBSC mobilized from the bone marrow into the peripheral blood by colony-stimulating factors (CSF) could be used as an alternative to bone marrow resulting in faster hematologic recovery and avoiding the anesthetic used in a bone marrow harvest. UCB stem cells also grew in popularity as a stem cell source with the advantage of being readily available as a frozen, off-the-shelf product that resulted in less GvHD.

Autologous transplants were utilized for cancers responsive to high doses of ablative chemoradiotherapy regimens that required a rescue of stem cells to overcome the severe myelosuppression. Improved techniques for stem cell cryopreservation aided in the feasibility of autologous stem cell collection.

Most recently, HSCT has expanded to previously excluded populations, namely the elderly and those with significant comorbidities due to the toxic effects of high chemotherapy and/or radiation doses. The reduced intensity and nonmyeloablative allogeneic transplants have proven successful in disease response and decreased organ toxicity. Haploidentical transplants, which use a half-matched family member (usually a sibling, child, or parent), have expanded donor options even further. This allows transplants to be more available to ethnic and minority groups that traditionally had a limited unrelated donor pool.

There are two basic types of HSCT, autologous and allogeneic. Autologous HSCT involves the use of the patient's stem cells, which are collected and stored before cytotoxic chemotherapy and/or radiation and then infused following this myeloablative therapy (Box 12.1). This is sometimes referred to as a stem cell rescue because the stem cells are used to ensure recovery of hematopoiesis resulting in the production of red blood cells (RBC), white blood cells (WBC), and platelets. In the pediatric population, this type of transplant is primarily utilized for the treatment of solid tumors, including high-risk neuroblastoma, recurrent Wilms tumor, brain tumors, recurrent lymphomas, and sarcomas. The preferred source of stem cells is the peripheral blood rather than the bone marrow because of the ease of collection, faster engraftment time, and therefore a shorter period of neutropenia during the posttransplant period. Autologous transplants are associated with lower transplant-related mortality as compared to allogeneic transplants; however, the potential for relapse or recurrent primary disease continues to be challenging.

An allogeneic HSCT involves using healthy blood stem cells from a suitably matched healthy donor when the patient's hematopoietic system is diseased or dysfunctional (Box 12.2). The patient receives high doses of chemotherapy and/or radiation followed by an infusion of donor cells. The donor cells replace the recipient's hematologic and immune systems. Donor options include an identical twin (syngeneic transplant); a related (family member) matched, mismatched, or haploidentical donor; or an unrelated matched or mismatched donor. Traditionally, HLA-identical family members, most often siblings, are the preferred source of allogeneic stem cells because they pose the lowest risk of GvHD and transplant-related mortality. However, there are more and more options for donor sources, including matched unrelated donors and haploidentical donors, that are proving to be successful alternatives.

Donor compatibility/matching is determined using a genetically transmitted set of cell surface proteins (HLA) that form humans' major histocompatibility complex. The best possible donors are ones that have HLA types that most closely match the recipient's HLA type. There are two main classes of HLAs: class I antigens (HLA-A, HLA-B, and HLA-C) and class II antigens (HLA-Dr, HLA-DQ, and HLA-DP), both of which are key in determining histocompatibility in transplantation. There are many specific HLA proteins within each class of antigen. The genes that encode these antigens are on the short arm of chromosome 6. These genes are linked and inherited within families as clustered groups or haplotypes. Each person has two haplotypes; one set is inherited from each parent. The most closely matched donor for an allogeneic HSCT is an HLA-identical sibling who shares two sets of identical haplotypes with the recipient. Siblings receiving the same HLA haplotype from each parent would be HLA identical (fully matched) and express the same HLAs on the surface of their cells. There is only a 25% chance that a child's sibling will be an identical match. In cases without a matched sibling, the next step is starting a search for an alternative donor source, including a partially matched family member, a well-matched unrelated volunteer donor via worldwide donor registries, or banked UCB.

HLA typing of the child and the child's siblings and parents requires either a simple blood draw or a buccal mucosal swab. This is often obtained as soon as it is determined that a stem cell transplant is a potential treatment for the patient.

Indications for an allogeneic transplant include hematologic malignancies and nonmalignant disorders, including primary immunodeficiencies, inherited bone marrow failure syndromes, and inherited disorders of inborn errors of metabolism (Kanate et al., 2020). The transplant-related mortality rate is higher than autologous transplants due to immune differences between the donor and recipient and to the immunosuppression needed to achieve donor engraftment and to prevent GvHD. In allogeneic transplant for malignant disease, the antitumor effect comes from both the cytotoxic effects of the conditioning therapy and the potential immune effect mediated by donor

---

Box **12.1**   **Autologous Transplant**

Administer high doses of chemotherapy and/or radiation to eliminate malignant disease. Recipient needs autologous stem cell rescue to reestablish hematopoiesis.

Box **12.2**   **Allogeneic Transplant**

Administer high doses of chemotherapy and/or radiation and immunosuppressant therapies to destroy malignant or defective bone marrow, make space for new donor stem cells to grow, and suppress the recipient's immune response to prevent rejection of stem cells.

In malignant diseases, the goal is to have a graft-versus-disease effect in which the new donor cells eliminate the cancer cells.

lymphocytes that target malignant cells, which is referred to the graft versus tumor or GvL effect. This immune response has also made it possible to reduce the intensity of the conditioning regimens.

Chemotherapy or radiation therapy is used in autologous and allogeneic transplants and is often referred to as conditioning therapy or preparative regimen. It is given in the days immediately prior to the transplantation of stem cells. This conditioning therapy serves to (1) destroy malignant cells or defective bone marrow, (2) make space in the bone marrow for the transplanted stem cells to grow, and (3) suppress the recipient's immune response to prevent rejection of the infused stem cells.

The type of transplant (autologous vs allogeneic), conditioning therapy, and stem cell source are determined by the child's diagnosis, clinical condition, and type of donor selected or available.

The most common concerns following HSCT include the following:

1. Preventing graft rejection mediated by recipient T lymphocytes that survived the conditioning regimen
2. Preventing donor cells from activating an immunologic response against the recipient causing tissue injury (i.e., GvHD)
3. Preventing and treating opportunistic infections and viral reactivation during the early months after HSCT
4. Allowing for immunologic reconstitution so that the donor-derived cells recognize and control pathogens in the host body
5. Organ toxicities related to conditioning therapy
6. Long-term effects of the conditioning therapy and transplant-related complications
7. Disease relapse

Overall transplant-related mortality has decreased over time partly due to improvements in donor selection, improved conditioning therapy, prevention/treatment of infections, and GvHD.

Although HSCT is a type of organ transplant, there are important fundamental differences between allogeneic HSCT and solid organ transplantation. In solid organ transplantation, a limited number of donor cells with immunologic activity are transferred into the host with the transplanted organ. Without adequate immune suppression, the recipient's immune system will recognize the organ as foreign and possibly reject the organ. To prevent organ rejection, lifelong administration of immunosuppressive medications is given (Hoegy et al., 2019). In HSCT, however, the conditioning therapy the recipient receives before transplantation eliminates most of the host's immune system. The transplant of donor stem cells contains all the necessary cellular elements for the complete reconstitution of the hematopoietic and immunologic systems in the recipient. Thus the immune system following transplantation comes from the donor, is generated by graft, and eventually replaces the HSCT recipient's immune system (Martin et al., 2012). Immune tolerance between the donor and recipient can usually be achieved within 6 to 12 months, thus allowing for a taper and eventually the discontinuation of immunosuppressive medications following allogeneic HSCT in the majority of children (Hansen et al., 2008).

INCIDENCE AND PREVALENCE

In 2020, 11,557 autologous transplants and 8326 allogeneic transplants were performed by US transplant centers registered with the Center for International Blood and Marrow Transplant Research (CIBMTR). Of the allogeneic transplants, nearly 1000 were in children less than age 18 years. Bone marrow remains the most used stem cell source for matched-related and matched-unrelated transplants in recipients under age 18 years. The number of UCB transplants has been decreasing overall. The number of haploidentical transplants in pediatric patients is rising significantly, with less than 100 per year from 2000 to 2013 to nearly 300 in 2020. The stem cell source for these haploidentical transplants was closely divided between peripheral blood and bone marrow (Auletta et al., 2019).

The number of transplants throughout the world continues to grow. It is estimated that 50,000 allogeneic HSCT take place each year worldwide. The CIBMTR database receives information from over 550 centers in 56 countries worldwide; they report more than 254,663 autologous, 251,053 allogeneic related and unrelated donors, and 15,057 cord blood transplants in 2018 (D'Souza et al., 2020). However, access to transplants varies significantly by country, with less developed countries having limited access to transplants partly due to a lack of local donor registries (Aljurf et al., 2019).

DIAGNOSTIC CRITERIA

CRITERIA FOR TRANSPLANT ELIGIBILITY

Referral and Consultation

Children being considered for transplantation are referred by their pediatric hematologist/oncologist, immunologist, or geneticist to the HSCT team for evaluation. Children and their families require comprehensive evaluation and counseling by an experienced multidisciplinary team. Frequent and effective communication between the transplant team and referring primary care providers is crucial. It is essential for potential HSCT recipients to be referred and evaluated promptly. In certain diseases, such as Hurler syndrome, outcomes can be improved if a transplant occurs early in the disease process or at a very young age. Research has shown that early HLA typing (at the time of diagnosis), rapid donor identification, and early referral to the HSCT team improve treatment outcomes (Pagel et al., 2020). Furthermore, patients who receive transplants earlier in their disease stage show better outcomes than those transplanted with advanced disease (Pidala et al., 2014). For many malignant diseases, transplanting patients while in remission dramatically improves disease outcomes. To assist practitioners in knowing when to appropriately refer patients, the National Marrow Donor Program (NMDP), Be the Match, and American Society for Transplantation and Cellular Therapy (ASTCT) jointly developed HSCT consultation timing guidelines based on clinical practice, medical literature, evidence-based reviews, and the National Comprehensive Cancer Network (NCCN) guidelines for the treatment of cancer.

Factors that impact a child's eligibility for transplant include type and stage of disease, remission status, underlying patient characteristics, comorbid conditions, and availability of a suitable donor. Identifying comorbidities prior to transplant can help better predict outcomes, result in adjustments of conditioning regimens, assist in appropriate donor selection, and guide and facilitate informed decision making. An established HSCT-specific comorbidity index can be used to predict transplant-related mortality and overall survival (Forlanini et al., 2022).

Pretransplant Workup

A pretransplant evaluation occurs 4 to 6 weeks prior to transplant and often takes place at the transplant center, but the primary care provider and local facilities may be requested to assist. Although testing is somewhat individualized, common evaluations include the following:

- Echocardiogram and electrocardiogram
- Pulmonary function testing (if patient is old enough to comply)
- Creatinine clearance or glomerular filtration rate
- Chest x-ray
- Computed tomography (CT) scans (evaluating for infectious disease)
- Hearing testing
- Complete eye exam
- Viral serologies and infectious disease markers
- Dental evaluation and treatment as necessary
- Complete ophthalmologic exam
- Nutritional assessment
- Ferriscan (evaluation of iron overload in certain patients)
- Review of allergies, medication history
- Bone marrow aspirate/biopsy and lumbar puncture for specific malignant diseases
- Performance status scale determination (Lansky or Karnofsky scale)
- Psychological/developmental evaluation
- A dental assessment to evaluate for any dental-related infection is completed.
- A baseline ophthalmology exam

The transplant workup is often a time of anxiety and uncertainty for the child and family; these feelings are further intensified by any transplant delays or unexpected problems, such as an infection or a relapse of the disease.

Human Leukocyte Antigen Typing

Tissue or HLA typing is used to identify genetically compatible hematopoietic system cell donors and recipients. HLAs are proteins found on the surface of almost all nucleated cells in the body. These antigens are responsible for the body's ability to recognize self from nonself on a cellular level. If an allogeneic transplant is required, a donor search is initiated. Generally, HLA typing is completed initially on siblings and immediate family members. Unrelated donor searches are initiated through national and international registries if the situation warrants an unrelated donor. These searches are initiated through coordinators at the transplanting institution. Be the Match in the United States is the world's largest and most diverse registry, with more than 19 million potential donors and more than 249,000 cord blood units. They partner with other international registries to assist in searching for the best potential matches for patients. The NMDP reports that they can now find potential matches for 76% to 97% of patients, depending on their ethnic background.

The NMDP, in collaboration with the CIBMTR, developed and published matching guidelines that are utilized when determining potential donors (Dehn et al., 2019). Ultimately, the transplant center provider is responsible for determining the best match for the patient. At times there may be more than one potential match, and priority may be given to one potential match over the other based on specific donor or recipient characteristics. Donor characteristics (e.g., age, size, sex, number of pregnancies [parity], and viral status [particularly the donor's cytomegalovirus (CMV) status]) are considered when selecting the most appropriate donor.

Donor Workup

All donors have standard evaluations, including a complete history and physical, laboratory testing, and evaluation for infectious diseases. There are specific findings that could make a potential donor ineligible for donation. For example, if a person has human immunodeficiency virus (HIV), hepatitis, or an autoimmune disease, then donation is not possible. A full list of these criteria can be found in the donor registry. Donors will donate either bone marrow or PBSC. Bone marrow donors have cells harvested in the operating room while asleep, and PBSC donors receive a colony-stimulating medication subcutaneously for approximately 5 days prior to donation. The PBSC are collected via an apheresis machine from a peripheral IV or specially placed apheresis catheter.

Donor workup can be completed at the transplant center performing the transplant, which is usually the case for many sibling donors. However, for sibling donors living in other cities or for an unrelated donor, the donor may be asked to travel to a facility that can perform the harvesting of the bone marrow or stem cells.

Being a donor is voluntary and requires informed consent. For older children, assent is obtained. Identified risks for donors may include complications related to anesthesia, pain related to colony-stimulating agents, placement and removal of IV lines, possible blood transfusion, infection, and fatigue. For sibling donors, there can be psychological benefits but also negative psychological effects of donation, including anger, guilt, blame, isolation, anxiety, and depression. Ethical considerations come to the forefront when a parent has a child with a potentially life-threatening disease and another child who is a potential donor or lifesaver, which may lead to pressure on the child to donate to save the sibling's life. Furthermore, siblings of donors have unique experiences and stressors in the posttransplant period. In recognition of the need to protect and promote the interests and well-being of the donor, the Bioethics Committee of the American Academy of Pediatrics (AAP) published recommendations regarding minor sibling donation. One recommendation is the appointment of a donor advocate to help protect the interests of the donor (Committee on Bioethics, 2010). Some transplant programs have developed programs in which donor advocates promote independent decision making, provide support and education to the donor prior to and during donation, and offer support following the procedure (even during stressful times when a recipient dies) (Hoag et al., 2018). The complex dynamics within families of recipient and sibling donors should be recognized when providing primary care follow-up for these families. Referral to psychologists may be considered for those with adjustment difficulties, anxiety, or depression.

For unrelated donors, anonymity is maintained, meaning the donor and recipient identification is not revealed to either person. Generally, contact information can be shared 1 year after the transplant if both parties consent. Donors and recipients sometimes correspond, and in some situations they meet each other and go on to develop meaningful and long-lasting bonds.

CONDITIONS COMMONLY TREATED WITH HSCT

There is a wide variety of conditions, including malignant and nonmalignant disorders, that HSCT commonly treats in children. Common malignant disorders include lymphomas, leukemias, and solid tumors such as brain tumors. The indications for nonmalignant disorders have greatly expanded in the last decade. Most of these conditions can be grouped into four general categories: inherited hemoglobinopathies, primary immune deficiency diseases, severe aplastic anemia/bone marrow failures, and inherited metabolic storage disorders (inborn errors of metabolism). Some of the more commonly treated disorders are listed in Table 12.1. However, there are many additional rare diseases in pediatrics that have been successfully treated with HSCT.

CLINICAL MANIFESTATIONS AT TIME OF DIAGNOSIS

HSCT is a treatment option for a wide and expanding variety of conditions, and clinical manifestations will vary accordingly. Children with malignant conditions are often in remission or have minimal residual disease when referred for HSCT and therefore exhibit no manifestations of their underlying condition. They may, however, exhibit treatment-related side effects, including anorexia, weight loss, specific organ dysfunction, or alopecia. Children with hemoglobinopathies, such as sickle cell disease (SCD) or beta-thalassemia, may exhibit symptoms of anemia and be transfusion dependent. Children with severe aplastic anemia will be pancytopenic and may have petechiae and bruising from thrombocytopenia. Primary immunodeficiencies may present with frequent infections. Hurler syndrome may not be easily apparent at birth but has specific clinical manifestations, including coarse facies with frontal bossing, flat nasal bridge, contractures, short stature, organomegaly, and kyphoscoliosis.

TREATMENT

STEM CELL COLLECTION

Stem cells can be harvested from bone marrow, peripheral blood, or umbilical cord blood, all of which are utilized within the field of a bone marrow transplant.

Bone Marrow Harvest

Hematopoietic stem cells from bone marrow were used as the traditional source of stem cells for many years. They continue to be utilized more frequently than PBSC in pediatric allogeneic transplant patients. Bone marrow harvest procedures take place under general or spinal anesthesia, usually in the operative. Bone marrow is harvested from the posterior iliac crests via multiple needle aspirations. The amount of bone marrow harvested is based on donor age, weight, patient weight, and the desired CD34+. Once the bone marrow is removed, it is filtered and processed in a specialized lab. In the case of a major ABO incompatibility between the donor and recipient, the bone marrow will be red cell or plasma depleted. The stem cell product is often given on the same day as the collection; however, it may be frozen if the plan is to transplant at a later date. Potential donor complications include difficulties related to anesthesia, pain, bleeding, hematoma, hypovolemia, and hypotension. Donors are most commonly discharged on the same day.

Table 12.1 Commonly Treated Disorders

INDICATION	DISORDER DETAILS	TRANSPLANT TYPE	RATIONALE	COMMENTS
Malignant Conditions				
Leukemias • Acute lymphoblastic leukemia (ALL) • Acute myeloid leukemia (AML)	ALL: production of abnormal lymphocytes; most common cancer in children, rapid progression AML: production of abnormal myeloid cells, various subtypes; linked to prognostic factors and treatment recommended	Allogeneic	High-dose chemotherapy and radiation kill malignant cells, and the new donor stem cells produce healthy blood cells. The new donor cells are also capable of recognizing and destroying the leukemia cells (graft-vs-leukemia effect)	HSCT used in high-risk disease (based on genetic or chromosomal abnormalities and/or response to initial chemotherapy treatment). Remission at the time of transplant results in best outcome
Myelodysplastic syndrome (MDS)	Hematologic malignancy associated with dysplastic changes resulting in decrease production of RBC, platelets, WBC. Distinction between MDS AML is based on blast percentages. MDS (30%) has tendency to develop into AML. Therapy-related MDS can develop years after treatment for another cancer	Allogeneic	As above	HSCT only curative option
Lymphomas	Cancers involving the lymphatic system, including lymph nodes, spleen, thymus gland, bone marrow	Allogeneic or autologous (depending on stage and type)		
Solid tumors • Brain tumor, neuroblastoma • Germ cell tumor		Autologous	High doses of chemotherapy and/or radiation therapy kills cancer cells responsible for these tumors. High doses of chemotherapy destroy normal stem cells, which need to be replaced by previously harvested stem cells to recover sufficiently	Eligibility for transplant depends on stage of disease. Tandem transplants (multiple autologous transplants) are done in a row to destroy the tumor most effectively. HSCT is often part of a clinical trial
Nonmalignant Conditions				
Inherited hemoglobinopathies		Allogeneic	Corrects abnormal hemoglobin production by replacing donor-derived healthy bone marrow	
Transfusion-dependent thalassemias	Inherited autosomal recessive disorder caused by a mutation in the *HBB* gene. This results in low levels of functional hemoglobin requiring chronic transfusions and subsequent iron overload			Ideally, HSCT is done prior to onset of hepatomegaly, portal fibrosis, or iron overload. Gene therapy is available as a clinical trial

Table 12.1   Commonly Treated Disorders—cont'd

INDICATION	DISORDER DETAILS	TRANSPLANT TYPE	RATIONALE	COMMENTS
Sickle cell disease	An autosomal recessive disorder caused by a mutation in the beta-globin chain leading to hemoglobin S—causes deformation of RBCs (sickle shape) accompanied with ischemia leading to multiple organ damage		HSCT restores normal hemato-poiesis with normal RBCs and potentially reverses or halts organ damage induced by the disease	Newborn screening used most widely for those who have had significant complications such as stroke, recurrent acute chest syndrome, or recurrent venooc-clusive pain crises
Primary immune deficiencies		Allogeneic	The specific defect in the im-mune system is corrected by replacing the immune/hemato-logic cells of a healthy donor	
Severe combined immu-nodeficiency (SCID)	Genetic disorders characterized by deficiencies in T and B cells and function and in some types, deficiencies in NK cells and function		An allogeneic transplant re-places the immune system of the recipient with healthy donor cells	All states screen for SCID
Chronic granulomatous disease	Inherited disorder in which phagocytes do not work properly leading to frequent serious bacterial and fungal infections and dysregu-lated inflammatory responses resulting in granuloma formation and other inflammatory disorders		Replace defective immune cells with normal donor-derived cells	
Wiskott-Aldrich syndrome	X-linked disease caused by mutations in the WAS gene leading to thrombocytopenia eczema, recurrent infections, autoimmune disease, and malignancy		HSCT corrects the underly-ing immunodeficiency and thrombocytopenia	
Severe aplastic anemia and bone marrow failures		Allogeneic		
Severe aplastic anemia	The body does not make enough RBC, WBC, or platelets			
Fanconi anemia	Inherited chromosome breakage syndrome characterized by physical abnormalities, pro-gressive bone marrow failure, and susceptibil-ity to cancers, including AML and squamous cell carcinoma			HSCT used when major bone mar-row failure occurs. Continue to be prone to developing malignan-cies post-HSCT; endocrinopa-thies common (thyroid, infertil-ity, growth hormone deficiency, hypogonadism)
Dyskeratosis congenita	Inherited bone marrow failure syndrome char-acterized by abnormal nails, reticular skin pigmentation, and oral leukoplakia and as-sociated with risk of development of aplastic anemia, MDS, leukemia, solid tumors		HSCT is the definitive cure to restore hematopoiesis, but it does not correct organ dysfunction	Monitor for pulmonary and liver fibrosis, increased cancer risk, including skin, head, neck, anorectal, esophagus, stomach, and lung

Continued

Table 12.1   Commonly Treated Disordersc—cont'd

INDICATION	DISORDER DETAILS	TRANSPLANT TYPE	RATIONALE	COMMENTS
Shwachman-Diamond syndrome	Autosomal recessive disorder resulting in bone marrow dysfunction, skeletal abnormalities, and pancreatic dysfunction with predisposition to MDS or AML			
Inherited metabolic storage disorders (inborn errors of metabolism)		Allogeneic		
Hurler syndrome (mucopolysaccharidosis type IH, MPS I)	Lacking an enzyme needed to break down long chains of sugar molecules called glycosaminoglycans, which build up and damage organs. It is characterized by skeletal abnormalities, cognitive impairment, heart disease, respiratory problems		Replaces enzyme-deficient stem cells with donor-derived enzyme-competent cells	HSCT stops the disease from causing more damage but does not reverse damage that already occurred. Transplant at an early age, usually before age 2 yr
Cerebral adrenoleukodystrophy (cALD)	A recessive condition in which a mutation in the ABCD1 gene on the X chromosome results in a buildup of very long chain fatty acids, which destroys the protective myelin sheath around brain nerve cells resulting in irreversible brain damage		HSCT provides healthy stem cells that produce the protein lacking in males with cALD. HSCT stops the progression of neurologic disease but does not improve the adrenal insufficiency that occurs with cALD	Newborn screening is available in some states. New gene therapy may be available for some not yet experiencing symptoms. Early treatment is necessary to avoid progressive neurologic disease

HSCT, Hematopoietic stem cell transplantation; NK, natural killer; RBC, red blood cell; WBC, white blood cell.

Peripheral Blood Stem Cell Collection

Hematopoietic stem cells normally reside in the bone marrow and are rarely detected in the peripheral blood. The PBSC must be mobilized to the peripheral blood to yield an adequate collection. PBSC collection is performed on most children receiving autologous HSCT. PBSC is the most common graft source for adult autologous and allogeneic transplants.

The process of apheresis is used to obtain PBSC. It involves using a commercially available automated blood separator that centrifuges the blood, transfers the stem cell layer into a collection bag, and returns the remaining blood components to the patient/donor via an IV line. In pediatric donors, it is common to place a temporary central venous catheter under anesthesia, which can be used for the removal of cells. The central venous catheter is removed following the procedure. The PBSC collection often occurs weeks or months before the planned transplant.

In autologous HSCT, apheresis is usually accomplished during the recovery phase of myelosuppressive chemotherapy and is enhanced by the administration of recombinant hematopoietic growth factors. Granulocyte CSF (G-CSF [filgrastim]) is commonly used and is administered daily by subcutaneous or IV infusion leading to the collection date. For healthy donors, chemotherapy is not utilized for mobilization, but they do receive G-CSF. Side effects of G-CSF include bone pain, headache, myalgia, and fatigue (Schmit-Pokomy, 2020). Some children who have been heavily treated with chemotherapy or radiation may experience poor mobilization of stem cells. In these cases, the chemokine antagonist plerixafor can be added to stimulate mobilization. This medication is given as a subcutaneous injection approximately 11 hours before the apheresis procedure. Side effects include gastrointestinal (GI) symptoms, injection-site reactions, headache, fatigue, arthralgias, and dizziness (Schmit-Pokomy, 2020). For allogeneic transplants, stem cell mobilization of healthy donor cells is accomplished by administering daily G-CSF starting approximately 5 days prior to the apheresis procedure. Assessing the number of peripheral blood CD34$^+$ cell counts by flow cytometry is used to determine when enough stem cells are present to begin apheresis, which will result in a successful stem cell yield.

Specific processes involved in apheresis vary among institutions. To provide more standardization based on current evidence, in 2014 the American Society of Blood and Marrow Transplantation established guidelines for peripheral blood progenitor cell mobilization based on current evidence (Duong et al., 2014). These guidelines specify preferred growth factors, dosing and timing of these growth factors, chemotherapy type and dose used for mobilization and when to initiate leukapheresis, and the target number of CD34 cell doses for collection and infusion (Duong et al., 2014). Specific pediatric recommendations include using a central apheresis catheter for young children, priming the apheresis machine with RBC or albumin for children less than 20 kg, and a target CD34+ cell dose of 2×10^6/kg for collection (Duong et al., 2014).

The primary advantage of PBSC over bone marrow is more rapid hematopoietic recovery, including neutrophil and platelet recovery and faster immune reconstitution. Additionally, no general anesthesia is needed compared to a bone marrow harvest procedure. Some studies have shown PBSC to be associated with a higher risk of GvHD than other stem cell sources, however.

Stem cell manipulation. Stem cells for autologous and allogeneic transplantation may be manipulated before infusion in an effort to reduce the risk of complications of disease recurrence. A blood cell separator is generally used for this purpose. For example, bone marrow products from related or unrelated donors are RBC depleted if the donor and the recipient are ABO incompatible. In autologous PBSC collection, particular stem cells may be selected for inclusion in the infusion, allowing the remainder of the pheresis product to be discarded and thereby facilitating the removal of potential tumor cell contamination. Likewise, a technique used at some transplant centers for allogeneic transplants involves the removal of T lymphocytes from unrelated donor marrow to decrease the risk of GvHD. Although T-lymphocyte depletion of donor marrow is an effective method of GvHD prevention, children who receive T-cell–depleted grafts are at an increased risk for graft rejection, disease recurrence, and delayed immunologic recovery after HSCT.

Apheresis procedures are normally well tolerated by the donor. The most common complications include (1) hypocalcemia related to the sodium citrate used to prevent the blood from clotting in the apheresis machine, (2) hypovolemia related to volume, and (3) thrombocytopenia from the collection of platelets into the product. Ionized calcium levels are carefully monitored before, during, and after the procedure, and calcium supplements and infusions are given during the procedure to maintain normal calcium levels. Fluid status is monitored closely through frequent vital sign monitoring and assessing for hypotension, tachycardia, lightheadedness, dysrhythmias, and diaphoresis. Platelet numbers are monitored carefully, and platelet transfusions may be necessary to keep them at a target range of above 50,000 mm^3.

Umbilical Cord Blood Collection

Cord and placental blood contain a large number of stem cells and have been used regularly as a stem cell source since the 1990s. The blood stem cells are collected from the umbilical cord and placenta after a baby is born and are frozen and stored at a cord blood bank for later use. These cells can be used in pediatric and adult populations but are used more commonly in pediatrics because a limited stem cell dose usually presents UCB units. When a higher stem cell dose is needed, two UCB units from different donors can be used for one transplant. This is referred to as a double cord transplant. UCB is an especially useful stem cell source if there is not an appropriately matched related or unrelated donor and for transplants that need to take place quickly because of a poor prognosis as the cells are readily available. UCB is easily harvested without additional risk to the mother or newborn. Advantages for UCB use include a lower incidence of GvHD, more tolerance of mismatched HLA, and lower risk of viral contamination than other stem cell sources. Some disadvantages include slower engraftment times resulting in longer periods of myelosuppression, increased potential for graft failure, possible transmission of infectious disease or undiagnosed genetic diseases, and the inability to gain more cells in the event of graft rejection or if there is a need for donor lymphocyte infusions (Dholaria et al., 2019).

PERITRANSPLANT PHASE

Conditioning Regimens

A child commonly begins the conditioning or preparative regimen 5 to 10 days before stem cell infusion. Admission to the transplant unit occurs when the preparative regimen begins or on the day of transplantation, depending on the institution. Preparative regimens consist of high-dose chemotherapy with or without total body irradiation (TBI) or total lymphoid irradiation and immunotherapeutic agents. Preparative regimen selection is determined by the underlying condition, HLA match and donor type, stem cell source, and goal of therapy.

The main purposes of the conditioning therapy include tumor cytoreduction and (ideally) disease eradication in the case of malignancy, marrow ablation to create space in the bone marrow for new stem cells, and sufficient immunosuppression to overcome host-mediated rejection of the donor cells.

Conditioning regimens can vary in intensity from myeloablative (most toxic) to nonmyeloablative to reduced intensity (least toxic) depending on recipient and disease factors. The chemotherapeutic agents listed in Table 12.2 are commonly used in pediatric HSCT. The selection of chemotherapy is based on several factors, including intensity of the transplant, mechanism of action of the chemotherapy agent, recipient comorbidities, and expected cumulative and noncumulative toxicities of each agent. A list of the more commonly used agents is provided later.

Total Body Irradiation

TBI is an effective cytotoxic modality that treats the entire body; it results in profound immunosuppression and is included in myeloablative conditioning regimens for malignancies that are sensitive to its effects, such as leukemias and lymphomas. To reduce toxicities, it is delivered in fractionated doses over several days. Shielding to protect vulnerable areas such as the lungs and boost doses can be given to areas that may harbor tumor cells, such as the central nervous system (CNS) and ovaries. Acute and late toxicities are listed in Table 12.3.

TBI is often avoided in children under the age of 3 to 4 years because of potential long-term toxicities, including negative effects on growth, neurocognition, and endocrine and metabolic functioning (Hoeben et al., 2022).

Conditioning Regimens for Autologous Stem Cell Transplants

Most pediatric autologous HSCT use myeloablative conditioning regimens to eradicate the existing disease. Regimens combine several drugs with nonoverlapping dose-limiting toxicities other than hematologic toxicity. The transplanted autologous donor cells are used to rescue the patient from the severe myelosuppression caused by the conditioning therapy. Unlike allogeneic transplants, there is no graft versus disease effect and no immunosuppressants needed to suppress donor T lymphocytes.

Tandem transplants are two or more sequential autologous transplants, usually about 6 to 10 weeks apart. The recipient gets a first course of myeloablative chemotherapy followed by infusion of autologous stem cells, then after a short recovery the recipient gets a second and sometimes third autologous transplant. Typically, each consecutive transplant uses a different high-dose regimen to maximize the antitumor effect. Improvements in supportive care and the use of PBSC and hematopoietic growth factors have enabled these to be possible in recent years. In the pediatric population, autologous tandem transplants are commonly used to treat neuroblastoma, primitive neuroectodermal tumors, atypical teratoid rhabdoid tumors, and medulloblastoma. Research has shown a survival advantage with tandem transplants compared to single transplants for select diseases (Guerra et al., 2017; Park et al., 2019).

Immunosuppressive Management

Immunosuppressive regimens vary according to the child's underlying diagnosis, cell source, preparative regimen, and institutional protocols. In addition to chemotherapy, allogeneic regimens contain immunosuppressants to prevent graft rejection and/or GvHD. Table 12.4 summarizes common immunosuppressants used in pediatric HSCT. Immunosuppressants are used to prevent rejection of the new graft and to prevent and treat GvHD in allogeneic HSCT.

The most successful immunosuppression agents to prevent GvHD include a calcineurin inhibitor (tacrolimus or cyclosporin) and methotrexate, cyclophosphamide, or antilymphocyte antibodies in the first week after transplant. Calcineurin inhibitors are initially

Table 12.2   **Commonly Used Chemotherapy Agents in Pediatric HSCT and Selected Toxicities**

CHEMOTHERAPEUTIC AGENT	EARLY SIDE EFFECTS AND MONITORING	LONG-TERM TOXICITIES AND CONSIDERATIONS
Busulfan	Venoocclusive disease Seizures Neurotoxicity Cardiotoxicity Hyperpigmentation of skin Requires therapeutic drug monitoring Pneumonitis	Pulmonary fibrosis Cataracts Infertility Secondary malignancy
Cyclophosphamide	Hemorrhagic cystitis (requires mesna and hydration) Nephrotoxicity Conjunctivitis Nasal congestion Headache/altered mental status Cardiac toxicity Pneumonitis	SIADH Cardiac toxicity Secondary nalignancy Infertility Pulmonary fibrosis
Melphalan	Severe mucositis Hypersensitivity Hyperpigmentation Pneumonitis (rare)	Secondary malignancy Infertility Peripheral neuropathy Pulmonary fibrosis
Thiotepa	Skin burns/rash, especially in intertriginous areas (excreted in sweat) Hyperpigmentation Nephrotoxicity Hepatotoxicity, late SOS	Central nervous system changes Pulmonary toxicity Secondary malignancy Infertility
Etoposide	Anaphylaxis Fevers chills Hypotension (w/ infusion) Metabolic acidosis Electrolyte imbalances Hyperpigmentation/erythema Peripheral neuropathy Pneumonitis	Pulmonary fibrosis Secondary acute leukemia
Fludarabine	Flulike symptoms Hyperpigmentation/erythema Rare severe neurologic toxicity Rare hemolytic anemia Nephrotoxicity	Peripheral neuropathy
Clofarabine	Skin rash, erythema, pruritis Hand-foot syndrome Hypotension, tachycardia Liver toxicity/VOD Acute kidney injury Systemic inflammatory response syndrome and capillary leak syndrome Anxiety	
Carboplatin	Ototoxicity Electrolyte imbalance Nephrotoxicity Hypersensitivity	Ototoxicity (hearing evaluations with dose adjustment) Peripheral neuropathy Secondary malignancy
Cytarabine	Fever, chills Hypersensitivity Dermatitis, erythema Conjunctivitis Headache, altered mental status	

HSCT, Hematopoietic stem cell transplantation; *SIADH,* syndrome of inappropriate antidiuretic hormone; *SOS,* sinusoidal obstructive syndrome; *VOD,* venoocclusive disease.

| Table 12.3 | Acute and Late Toxicities of Total Body Irradiation |

EARLY EFFECTS	LONG-TERM EFFECTS
Nausea/vomiting/diarrhea	Radiation fibrosis
Xerostomia/mucositis/ esophagitis	Cataracts
	Bronchiolitis obliterans
Skin erythema	Cardiotoxicity
Parotitis	Hypopituitarism
Fatigue	Bone growth disorders
Myelosuppression	Hypothyroidism
Radiation pneumonitis (inter-stitial pneumonitis)	Infertility
	Neurotoxicity
Idiopathic pneumonia syndrome	
Hepatic sinusoidal obstruc-tion syndrome	

From Oertel, M., Martel, J., Mikesch, J.-H., et al. (2021). The burden of survivorship on hematological patients—long-term analysis of toxicities after total body irradiation and allogeneic stem cell transplantation. *Cancers, 13(22)*, 5640.

administered as IV infusions but are eventually changed to oral administration. Therapeutic monitoring by obtaining routine blood trough levels is required and helps ensure adequate levels and avoid toxic ones. Both tacrolimus and cyclosporin are associated with drug-drug interactions; medications that inhibit or induce cytochrome P450 should be evaluated when using these medications. Close monitoring for nephrotoxicity and modifying doses or target levels for renal or hepatic dysfunction patients should be considered. Antifungals commonly used during HSCT, including fluconazole, voriconazole, and posaconazole, are PCP3A inhibitors and can markedly increase blood concentration levels of calcineurin inhibitors. Electrolyte abnormalities, most commonly hypomagnesemia, require monitoring and supplementation. Strict adherence to the administration schedule and timing of levels should be emphasized. Tapering immunosuppression may be institution or protocol specific. A person's risk for developing GvHD, conditioning therapy, and the underlying diagnosis are factors to consider when planning a taper schedule. Patients with high-risk malignancies may begin a taper early, such as day 60+, to potentially benefit from a GvL effect. Those with the nonmalignant disease may begin tapering later, such as day 180+ after transplant, as they do not benefit from a GvL effect.

Many strategies for immunosuppression continue to be investigated. One recent and successful strategy

| Table 12.4 | Commonly Used Immunosuppressive Agents, Uses, and Commonly Seen Toxicities in Pediatric HSCT |

CYCLOSPORINE	TACROLIMUS	METHOTREXATE	MYCOPHENOLATE MOFETIL	ALEMTUZUMAB (CAMPATH)	ANTITHYMOCYTE GLOBULIN	CORTICOSTEROIDS
Nephrotoxicity	Nephrotoxicity	Mucositis	GI effects	Infusion-related toxicities (fever, chills, hypotension, pulmonary edema)	Infusion-related toxicities	Hypertension
Hypertension	Hypertension	Hepatotoxicity	Myelosuppression	Serum sickness	Anaphylaxis	Hyperglycemia
Low magnesium	Low magnesium	Myelosuppression	Headache	Viral infections	Serum sickness	Muscle wasting
Tremors	Tremors	Nephrotoxicity		EBV-PTLD (post-transplant lymphoproliferative disease)		Sleep disturbance
Neurotoxicity	Neurotoxicity	Photosensitivity		Impaired immune reconstitution post-HSCT		Mood swings
Hyperkalemia	Hyperkalemia					Increased appetite
Hirsutism	Thrombotic microangiopathy					Weight gain
Thrombotic microangiopathy						Osteoporosis
						Delayed growth

EBV-PTLD, Epstein-Barr virus posttransplant lymphoproliferative disease; *GI*, gastrointestinal; *HSCT*, hematopoietic stem cell transplantation.

Table **12.5**	Transplant Timeline						
PRETRANSPLANT EVALUATION	CONDITIONING (CHEMO AND/OR RADIATION)	CELL INFUSION	INPATIENT RECOVERY	OUTPATIENT RECOVERY	HOME RECOVERY	RETURNING TO NORMAL
Days to weeks process	Day -7, -6, -5, etc.	Day 0	0–30 days	30–100 days	Day ±100–365	Day ±365 and annually
Extensive workup of donors and recipients	Number of days depends on exact treatment regimen	Monitoring for adverse reactions	• Early toxicities • Transfusion-dependence immunosuppressive therapy	• Early postengraftment • Continued symptom monitoring • Acute GvHD	• Late complications • Tapering immunosuppression • Chronic GvHD • Collaborate with primary care provider	• Long-term follow-up care with HSCT center • Evaluations by selected specialists (endocrine, cardiology, pulmonology) • Transition routine care to primary care provider

GvHD, Graft-versus-host disease; *HSCT*, hematopoietic stem cell transplantation.

uses posttransplant cyclophosphamide (PTCy) to eliminate alloreactive T lymphocytes and spare regulatory T cells, in combination with other immunosuppressive agents such as tacrolimus and mycophenolate mofetil. This regimen has been used successfully in haploidentical transplants and has greatly contributed to the significant increase in transplants for persons without a suitable HLA-matched related or unrelated donor (Carnevale-Schianca, 2021; Yao et al., 2021). PTCy use is beginning to broaden to other populations, including use in pediatric malignant and nonmalignant disorders (Even-Or et al., 2020).

Transplant Timeline

The days of the preparative regimen are referred to as negative days (day −5, −4, −3), all leading up to the day of the transplant. In certain cases, there may be a rest day when no chemotherapy is given immediately before the day of stem cell infusion (Table 12.5).

Transplant day (i.e., day 0) is the day the stem cells are infused into the recipient via a central venous catheter at the patient's bedside. If the stem cells are from the marrow of a related donor, the bone marrow harvest usually takes place the same day as the HSCT and is infused into the recipient shortly after collection. When using an unrelated donor, the freshly harvested marrow or stem cell product is escorted from the donor center, often requiring air transportation to the transplant center. In an autologous transplant, and sometimes with selected allogeneic donors, the stem cells have been cryopreserved and are thawed immediately prior to infusion into the recipient. Prior to the infusion of cells, the recipients are often premedicated, and there is frequent monitoring of vital signs and assessment for adverse reactions.

Once the cells are infused intravenously, they migrate to the bone marrow, and generally within 10 to 21 days production of bone marrow–derived cells begins. This is called hematopoietic engraftment. In many transplant centers, the children stay in the hospital while waiting for engraftment. Other institutional practices may allow for outpatient transplants with the waiting for engraftment taking place in the recipient's home with frequent outpatient follow-up visits.

Infection Prevention

Special precautions are taken to reduce the risk of infections in children who have undergone HSCT. Transplant centers use high-efficiency particulate air filter systems or laminar airflow rooms to decrease potential environmental pathogens during the acute phase of transplant. Neutropenia, immunosuppressants, alterations in mucosal integrity from treatment-related mucositis, and the presence of indwelling central venous catheters are significant risk factors contributing to infection during the early transplant period. Prophylactic antiinfective agents are prescribed to prevent *Pneumocystis jirovecii* pneumonia (PJP), fungal disease, and viral reactivations, including herpes simplex virus (HSV) and CMV. Additionally, most allogeneic and some autologous HSCT recipients receive passive antibody prophylaxis with IV immunoglobulin (IVIG). In an effort to further reduce infection risk, extensive counseling is provided for these children and their families regarding the prevention of infections through effective hand washing, appropriate food choices and preparation, and adherence to isolation policies that vary between institutions. Children are typically asked to stay in their room or a specialized unit while hospitalized. Visitors may be carefully screened for any symptoms of infection. The child uses a mask when outside the room or coming to clinic visits, and the child should avoid crowds, public spaces, and ill contacts. Children do not attend in-person school for the first months following the transplant and sometimes up to the first year posttransplant. They often utilize hospital-based schools, virtual schools, or homebound programs available through their home school.

Chimerism

Routine surveillance of the percentage of donor-derived versus residual recipient-derived hematopoietic cells is obtained in all allogeneic transplant recipients. This is referred to as chimerism testing and can be completed on either peripheral blood or bone marrow. Testing with single tandem repeats, which are highly repetitive DNA sequences with high variability between individuals, is commonly used to evaluate donor/recipient percentages. Serial chimerism testing allows the transplant team to assess for graft rejection and potential relapse. Institutional standards, treatment protocols, and the clinical course of each transplant recipient determine the frequency and timing of obtaining these samples. A full donor chimerism (percent of donor cells is ≥95%) is desired and usually necessary for disease cure in hematologic malignancy. Mixed donor chimerism is the coexistence of donor and recipient cells. In malignant disease it is associated with an increase in graft loss and recurrence of the original disease. In nonmalignant diseases, a mixed donor chimerism is often acceptable because disease control can still be maintained with the presence of some donor cells.

Consolidative Radiation Therapy and Chemotherapy

Some children require further antineoplastic treatment after HSCT. For example, in children with high-risk neuroblastoma, remission rates improved after HSCT with the addition of consolidative radiation therapy (XRT) to the primary tumor bed region. Following XRT, these children also receive a 6-month treatment course of 12-*cis*-retinoic acid (isotretinoin [Accutane]), an oral retinoid that is a differentiating agent for neuroblastoma and is thought to help control minimal residual disease (Park et al., 2019). Several US pediatric oncology centers offer posttransplant immunotherapy protocols in addition to retinoic acid for this high-risk population. Children with Hodgkin disease may receive post-HSCT XRT to the areas of previous disease after sufficient hematopoietic recovery. The transplant or oncology team closely monitors all children receiving XRT for treatment-related side effects and symptom management.

Donor lymphocyte infusions (DLI) are utilized to eradicate minimal residual disease, treat or prevent relapse, and promote donor engraftment in recipients with mixed donor chimerism (Dholaria et al., 2019). DLI works as an immunotherapy by promoting a GvL effect. The main complications associated with DLI are GvHD, which is observed in 40% to 60% of patients and bone marrow aplasia. Donor lymphocytes can be collected by lymphopoiesis or derived from cryopreserved stem cells originally collected for transplant purposes. DLI may be administered as a fresh product or a previously cryopreserved product.

Adoptive Immunotherapy/Chimeric Antigen Receptor T-Cell Therapy

CAR-T therapy is a type of cellular immunotherapy that has revolutionized the care of patients with specific malignancies (Feins et al., 2019). Since 2017 there have been six CAR-T products approved by the US Food and Drug Administration (FDA), with many more in the pipeline. Kymriah (tisagenlecleucel) is the only product approved for use in children and young adults. It is indicated for children and young adults with refractory or relapsed B-cell acute lymphoblastic leukemia. The therapy involves taking T cells from the patient using leukapheresis and sending them to an approved lab to be genetically modified. The cells are genetically modified to produce a protein receptor that will be able to recognize a specific antigen on the surface of cancer cells and then is able to destroy the cell. These modified T cells are multiplied in the millions and infused back into the patient. They are designed to continue multiplying while in the patient's body and eliminate cancer cells with the target antigen on their surface. They are sometimes referred to as a living drug (National Cancer Institute, 2022). Several days before CAR-T therapy is administered, the patient will receive lymphodepleting chemotherapy to prepare the body to accept these cells.

The two main toxicities post–CAR-T therapy include cytokine release syndrome (CRS) and neurotoxicity. CRS is an inflammatory response caused by the proliferation and activation of CAR-T cells (Neelapu et al., 2018). Common signs and symptoms include fever, hypotension, tachycardia, and hypoxia. This reaction often occurs in the first 24 hours after CAR-T therapy and can last 1 week or more. The second major complication, although less frequently seen, is neurotoxicity, referred to as immune effector cell-associated neurologic syndrome (ICANS). Symptoms related to ICANS include headache, confusion, tremors, aphasia, loss of consciousness, and seizures. Problems with attention, language, handwriting, disorientation, agitation, and somnolence are also observed (Neelapu et al., 2018). The ASTCT has developed a consensus grading of CRS, which helps guide the treatment and management strategies (Lee et al., 2019).

Complementary and Alternative Treatments

Complementary and alternative medicine (CAM) approaches encompass a wide variety of interventions, including nutritional-based specialized diets and supplements, aromatherapy, mind-body interventions such as yoga and tai chi, meditation and mindfulness, and physical interventions (e.g., massage, essential oils, healing touch, acupuncture, acupressure, heat, ice, electrostimulation).

Children may use a variety of CAM treatments during the conditioning phase and while recovering from HSCT to control or alleviate symptoms of their condition or treatment, including pain, nausea, fatigue, depression, and anxiety. These measures are used as adjuncts to conventional medical therapy, as opposed to those that replace standard care, and are often recommended by the HSCT or oncology team managing the medical interventions. Additionally, many programs offer child-life services, art and music therapy, and pet programs; these have been found helpful to children who are coping with the transplant experience. Some specific techniques include journaling, play therapy, distraction, mancala coloring, distraction, mindfulness, and diaphragmatic breathing. Virtual technology programs, including video games, have recently been utilized to improve the health of children with cancer (Cheng et al., 2021; Christopherson et al., 2021).

Biologically based therapies, including specific diets and nutritional and herbal supplements, are commonly utilized worldwide by pediatric cancer patients and their families (Kranjcec et al., 2022). These may include probiotics, antioxidants, cannabinoids, turmeric, vitamins, and mistletoe. These may be used as supportive care to help with the distressing symptoms related to cancer-related treatments, but there is some evidence that these types of therapies are used with curative intent by families (Diorio et al., 2020). There are limited controlled studies to establish the efficacy of these treatments; furthermore, they can cause harmful side effects and/or interact with other medications. Patients undergoing cancer care often do not reveal to their care team that they are using CAM therapies. It is therefore essential that providers openly discuss patients' thoughts regarding the use of CAM therapies to avoid any misunderstandings and unwarranted adverse effects.

Palliative Care

Palliative care focuses on symptom management, pain control, and psychological well-being before, during, and after recovery from HSCT. It has been demonstrated that pediatric oncology and HSCT patients and families have improved quality of life and decreased symptom burden when providing palliative care services (Uber et al., 2022). End-of-life care, including advance care planning discussions, hospice enrollment, comfort-focused therapies, and grief and bereavement counseling at the end of life, are facilitated with these services. The palliative care team can be utilized for pediatric patients and their families undergoing complex medical situations regardless of their prognosis. Reduction of parental distress and long-term grief has been seen with the use of palliative care teams in the pediatric oncology setting.

Due to the high risks related to transplant, the potential for dying during the first weeks and months following the transplant is a reality for many children and families. When patients face life-threatening complications during the transplant process, the need for escalation of intensive care can happen quickly. While the transplant team is focused on complex treatment management and lifesaving measures, a palliative care team can manage symptoms and facilitate difficult conversations around treatment choices (Mekelenkamp et al., 2021). Additionally, children with high-risk malignancies who experience a relapse after transplant may have few treatment options and little chance for cure. They are then faced with decision making around therapy goals and dealing with associated symptoms and psychological stress. Effective communication involves the consideration of the patient's developmental age, psychological state, maturational age, and ethnicity (Uber et al., 2022). Studies have demonstrated that parents prefer thorough prognostic information about their child's course to help in decision making, and children, most notably adolescents, and young adults, want to have an active role in conversations regarding their illness, prognosis, and treatment options. The palliative care team members are trained and skilled at these conversations and utilize specific communication strategies to address these complex discussions.

Research has demonstrated that families receiving palliative care reported improved communication, shorter hospitalizations, and fewer emergency department visits (Uber et al., 2022). The integration of palliative care services into the care of pediatric HSCT patients is variable at transplant centers, although it is recognized to be underutilized. Misconceptions that palliative care is only for the end of life or that it hastens death or diminishes hope for patients and families still exist, even though research does not support these ideas. Barriers to utilization include the availability of services, inadequate funding and reimbursement of palliative care services, and acceptance by HSCT team members (Uber et al., 2022). However, there continues to be advocacy for early and standardized integration of palliative care services in the complex care of pediatric transplant patients with the hope of improving quality of life, reducing symptom burden, facilitating communication (with patients, families, and among care team members), and providing ongoing psychosocial and spiritual support.

Anticipated Advances in Diagnosis and Management

Research and clinical advances continue to improve the survival of adults and children receiving HSCT. Data from CIBMTR show that day 100+ and 3-year survival rates for children undergoing allogeneic for all indications have improved significantly over time. From 2000 to 2009, the overall survival rate at day 100+ was 86%, and at 3 years was 60% compared to reports from 2010 to 2019, with survival rates of 93% and 74%, respectively (Phelan et al., 2022). Despite these advances, suitable donor availability, disease relapse, and transplant-related mortality due to complications and toxicities from HSCT, including GvHD, are continued challenges in the transplant field. Some of the areas under research include the following:

- Gene therapy. An emerging treatment modality for children with select genetic disorders, including primary immunodeficiencies, beta-thalassemia, and SCD, is gene therapy. For primary immunodeficiencies, including SCID, gene therapy uses autologous HSCT to deliver stem cells with added or edited versions of the missing malfunctioning gene that causes the underlying disorder. This therapy avoids the problems associated with using an allogeneic donor, including graft rejection and/or GvHD. Recent studies have demonstrated that gene therapy has equal or better outcomes as compared with allogeneic HSCT (Kohn & Kohn, 2021). In 2022 the FDA approved using Zynteglo, a gene therapy, for beta-thalassemia. In this therapy the patient's stem cells are genetically modified to produce functional beta-globin (Langer & Esrick, 2021).
- Consolidative therapies following HSCT. Even though disease relapse is the most common cause of death at day 100+ in children following autologous transplant and allogeneic transplant (CIBMTR), very few therapies are offered to patients to sustain remission after HSCT. Brentuximab vedotin, an anti-CD30 monoclonal antibody conjugate with monomethyl auristatin E, is undergoing investigation as consolidation therapy following autologous transplant in patients with Hodgkin lymphoma at high risk of relapse or disease progression (Moskowitz et al., 2015).
- Continued CAR-T development for other indications, developing off-the-shelf immunotherapies (Morgan et al., 2020).
- Continued expansion of donor cells. Methods are underway to expand the number of stem cells, in particular UCB sources, so these would be readily available for use with both pediatric and adult patients.
- Reduction of toxicities related to conditioning therapies. Toxicities related to conditioning regimens have immediate and long-term consequences for children. Additions of more effective antiemetics, successful use of less intensive chemotherapy doses, and medications that prevent mucositis have decreased these toxicities. The field continues to search for solutions to reduce toxicities related to primary treatment strategies and supportive care therapies without negatively affecting long-term survival. TBI contributes significantly to these toxicities.

POSTTRANSPLANT PHASE

Associated Problems of Hematopoietic Stem Cell Transplant and Treatment

Early complications posttransplantation. Acute or early complications refer to those that occur in the first 100 days after receiving conditioning therapy (Box 12.3). The severity and duration of these complications depend on the type of transplant, medications, and doses used in the conditioning therapy, receiving TBI, patient age, preexisting comorbidities, and performance status.

Myelosuppression. The decreased ability of the bone marrow to produce WBCs, neutrophils, platelets, and RBCs occurs due to chemotherapy and/or radiation therapy, which destroys the rapidly dividing stem cells in the bone marrow.

Neutropenia. Neutropenia is an absolute neutrophil count (ANC) of less than 500 cells/mm^3 and profound neutropenia (ANC <100 cells/mm^3). Neutrophils function to prevent infection by capturing and destroying bacteria and microorganisms. Persons with profound neutropenia are more susceptible to developing life-threatening bacterial infections. Rapid, profound, and prolonged neutropenia generally puts persons at the greatest risk of developing infections. Autologous HSCT recipients are at intermediate risk for infections with neutropenia expected for 7 to 10 days, while those undergoing allogeneic transplant with an anticipated duration of neutropenia lasting longer than 10 days and those with GvHD are considered at high risk (NCCN, 2021). Neutrophil engraftment depends on the type of transplant, stem cell source, stem cell dose, and if a CSF is used to facilitate recovery.

Thrombocytopenia. Profound thrombocytopenia, defined as a platelet count of less than 20,000 platelets per microliter, is also expected during the first weeks after receiving conditioning therapy. Platelets are needed to prevent bleeding and maintain vascular integrity. Many HSCT recipients receiving myeloablative transplants will require platelet transfusions for weeks following the transplant, and it may take 1 to 3 months for the platelet count to normalize. Patients are monitored closely for signs and symptoms of bleeding, including excessive bruising or petechiae, bloody or tarry stools, hematemesis, nosebleeds, or gingival bleeding. Although possible,

---

Box 12.3 **Early Complications: The First 100 Days**

- Mucositis
- Nausea/vomiting/diarrhea
- Anorexia (requiring enteral or parenteral feeding)
- Pancytopenia (anemia, neutropenia, thrombocytopenia)
- Infections
- Venoocclusive disease
- Engraftment syndrome
- Acute graft-versus-host disease
- Graft failure/graft rejection

serious spontaneous bleeding of the brain or lungs is uncommon; it generally occurs in persons with platelets less than 10,000 platelets per microliter. Prophylactic transfusion of random donor platelets for platelet counts of less than 10,000 platelets per microliter in pediatric patients undergoing an allogeneic transplant is a standard of care. A higher platelet transfusion threshold will be in place in some cases due to increased bleeding risk. These exceptions may include patients on anticoagulant therapy, patients undergoing invasive procedures such as a lumbar puncture, or patients with brain tumors. Measures to prevent bleeding are also implemented during the period of thrombocytopenia. These practices include the following:

- Using soft-bristle toothbrushes or sponges
- Avoiding rectal thermometers
- Use of stool softeners to prevent constipation
- Initiating hormonal therapy to prevent menstruation
- Taking fall-prevention measures
- Avoiding contact sports and rough activities
- Avoiding trauma during sexual relations

Anemia. Suppression of the bone marrow following chemotherapy and radiation also results in anemia requiring packed RBC transfusions until the donor's adequate hematopoietic function is restored by engrafting megakaryocytes and RBC precursors. In addition to conditioning therapy, there can be other causes of anemia in the transplant setting. These can include hemolysis, nutritional deficiency, hemolytic uremic syndrome, hemorrhage, transplant-associated thrombotic microangiopathy (TA-TMA), or kidney failure. Signs and symptoms of anemia include fatigue, pallor, headache, irritability, tachycardia, hypotension, and dyspnea. Institutional standards may guide transfusion thresholds, but often PRBCs are transfused for hemoglobin less than 7 g/dL or symptomatic anemia.

Transfusions. Blood products are irradiated to prevent transfusion-related GvHD. They may contain a small number of T lymphocytes, which if viable could cause a life-threatening reaction in the transfused child. Irradiation prevents these T lymphocytes from replicating and attacking host cells without altering the normal function of the transfused RBCs or platelets. CMV-negative or leukoreduced blood products are used for transfusions to avoid CMV transmission to an immunocompromised patient, most importantly if the recipient and donor are CMV negative on pretransplant serology studies. RBC transfusions are carefully typed as they must be compatible with the donor's and recipient's ABO antibodies and the donor's RhD status (Maziarz & Slater, 2021). The ABO and HLA genes are not inherited together; therefore a child may be HLA-A, -B, or -DR identical to the donor but have a minor or major incompatibility with the donor's RBCs. The isohemagglutinins may be present for weeks or more after HSCT and thus may react against donor RBCs (Maziarz & Slater, 2021).

Mucositis. Oral and oropharyngeal mucositis is an expected and early complication in 80% of pediatric patients undergoing HSCT. The degree of mucositis can be affected by the type of chemotherapy in the conditioning regimen and the presence of TBI. Chemotherapeutic agents that tend to cause the most severe mucositis include busulfan, melphalan, etoposide, and methotrexate.

Oral mucositis manifestations include erythema, ulceration, bleeding, and atrophy. It can result in pain, difficulty swallowing and talking, nutritional deficits, infections, and a decrease in quality of life. Patients report that mucositis is one of the most distressing symptoms associated with chemotherapy. Mucositis begins 4 to 10 days following chemotherapy initiation and can last as many as 2 to 3 weeks and heals with neutrophil engraftment. The breakdown of the oral mucosa becomes a portal of entry for infectious organisms. Mucosal barrier damage in the upper part of the digestive tract predisposes patients to infection with oral viridans streptococci and with gram-negative organisms with mucosal damage to the lower GI tract (Treleaven, 2009).

Dental evaluation and correction of caries, endodontic infections, or abscesses should take place as part of the pretransplant workup, and time for healing should be given prior to transplant (Tomblyn et al., 2009). Daily oral cavity observations allow for early identification of oral changes, and the use of standardized assessment tools assists in accurate and consistent evaluation, which can be communicated to all team members. Daily oral hygiene includes brushing with a soft toothbrush and doing frequent rinses. Although there is no definitive recommendation for the type of rinsing agent, normal saline is often used. Consistency of oral hygiene, regardless of oral care agent, is key to effective prevention and management. One evidence-based preventative practice found to reduce the severity of mucositis in older pediatric patients is cryotherapy (application of ice chips to oral mucosa) during short infusions of melphalan or 5-fluorouracil. The use of oral photobiomodulation (spectrum 620–750 mm) for pediatric patients undergoing allogeneic or autologous transplant is also a preventative strategy to reduce mucositis. Palifermin is an IV agent that effectively reduces mucositis when given in doses before the conditioning regimen. However, routine use is not indicated because of short-term adverse effects, high cost, limited availability, and potential negative effects on cancer outcomes (Patel et al., 2023). It has been used at some institutions on a case-by-case basis when there is a high risk of severe mucositis. Dietary changes such as avoiding spicy or citrus-containing foods or those with sharp edges that can further mucosal damage are avoided during this time. Oral and topical anesthetics include viscous lidocaine or magic mouthwash (Mawardi et al., 2021). When pain becomes moderate-severe, systemic analgesics are utilized. IV continuous or patient-controlled opioid analgesia is often needed to control mucositis-related pain.

Nutrition deficit. Nutritional support is a high priority during the bone marrow transplant experience. Prior to transplant, patients require a complete nutritional assessment, including weight, body mass index, anthropometric measurements, skinfold measurements, serum albumin, and dietary history. Patients who have received previous treatments, including chemotherapy, may have nutritional deficits at the time of transplant referral. Optimally, patients who have lost 10% to 20% of their body weight should receive nutritional intervention before transplant to improve their nutritional status.

Patients undergoing transplants are at high risk for developing nutritional deficits and malnutrition without close monitoring and active interventions. Common and expected early transplant complications, including nausea, vomiting, diarrhea, anorexia, taste changes, and mucositis, greatly affect the ability of children to maintain sufficient calories and hydration without intervention. Some difficulties, such as taste changes and anorexia, can persist for months posttransplant. It is common for pediatric patients to be supported with enteral or parenteral nutrition during the transplant process. There are no agreed-on standards for when enteral or parenteral nutrition should begin. Practices vary throughout institutions regarding enteral or parenteral nutrition preferences, and randomized clinical trials have been limited. A recent systematic review of randomized and nonrandomized studies evaluating enteral and parenteral nutrition in pediatric transplants concluded that enteral and parenteral nutrition have similar nutritional outcomes (Evans et al., 2019). However, there is evidence that enteral nutrition may be associated with a decrease in acute GvHD and may be preferred over total parenteral nutrition (TPN) (Evans et al., 2019; Zama et al., 2021).

Graft-versus-host disease. Acute and chronic GvHD are commonly occurring posttransplant complications. The primary care provider should be able to recognize common signs and symptoms. The transplant center providers will guide the treatment regimens.

Acute graft-versus-host disease. Acute GvHD is a common complication associated with significant morbidity and mortality following allogeneic HSCT. It occurs when activated donor-derived T cells (the graft) mount an immunologic attack on the donor-recipient cells (the host) after recognizing recipient antigens and cells as being foreign. It is theorized that for GvHD to occur, the following three requirements must be present: The graft must have immunocompetent T cells, the host (recipient) must be incapable of rejecting the donor cells (immunocompromised), and the recipient must express tissue antigens that are not present in the donor. HLA proteins expressed on the cell surfaces are essential to the activation of the allogeneic T cells (Zeiser & Blazar, 2017).

Pathogenesis involves a complex cascade of events described in three phases (Zeiser & Blazar, 2017):

1. The conditioning regimen causes damage to the skin, intestinal mucosa, and liver tissues resulting in bacterial translocation, secretion of inflammatory cytokines (including tumor necrosis factor-alpha and interleukins), and molecules that stimulate the immune response and enhance the presentation of antigens on the host tissues, thus making it easier for the mature donor T cells to recognize them and mount an inflammatory response.

2. T-lymphocyte activation, stimulation, and proliferation in host and donor T lymphocytes occur. Specifically, T lymphocytes CD4 and CD8 recognize alloantigens in HLA class 1 and 2, then activate, expand, and differentiate into effector T cells.

3. Activated effector T lymphocytes and phagocytes (monocytes and macrophages) also secrete cytokines, contributing to apoptosis and tissue damage within the target organs.

Acute GvHD involves complex immune pathways involving an extensive network of immune-mediated cells. Understanding these pathways and specific cells gives way to the current therapies for preventing and treating acute GvHD.

The three target host tissues in acute GvHD include the skin, GI tract (gut), and liver. Clinical signs include the following: an erythematous maculopapular skin rash, diffuse watery diarrhea, and elevated bilirubin.

- Skin is the most common organ affected by acute GvHD, with symptoms varying in intensity from a mild erythematous maculopapular rash that can be pruritic to generalized erythroderma with bullous lesions and epidermal necrolysis.

- GI symptoms are characterized by diarrhea and abdominal cramping and may include intestinal bleeding. This can be the most difficult to treat in children. Staging of GI GvHD is usually done by quantifying daily diarrhea output, which can be quite voluminous. Providing adequate fluid and electrolyte balance can be challenging. Infection must also be considered a cause of diarrhea, and stool cultures are sent for analysis.

- Although a common site for acute GvHD, the liver is rarely the site of single-organ involvement. The earliest and most common sign of liver involvement is a rise in the conjugated bilirubin and alkaline phosphatase; however, there are many other causes of liver abnormalities in these children, including venoocclusive disease (VOD), hepatic infections, and drug toxicity.

Acute GvHD involves a clinical diagnosis, and staging is based on defined criteria (Harris et al., 2016) (Table 12.6). However, other etiologies, including infection and drug toxicities, should be ruled out. Although tissue biopsies are not required to diagnose acute GvHD, they are often utilized to add to the understanding of the diagnosis and can help rule out

| Table **12.6** | Graft-Versus-Host Disease (GvHD) Target Organ Staging | | | |

STAGE	SKIN (ACTIVE ERYTHEMA ONLY)	LIVER (BILIRUBIN)	UPPER GI	LOWER GI (STOOL OUTPUT/DAY)
0	No active (erythematous) GvHD rash	<2 mg/dL	No or intermittent nausea, vomiting, anorexia	Adult: <500 mL/day or <3 episodes/day Child: <10 mL/kg/day or <4 episodes/day
1	Maculopapular rash <25% body surface area (BSA)	2–3 mg/dL	Persistent nausea, vomiting, anorexia	Adult: 500–999 mL/day or 3–4 episodes/day Child: 10–19.9 mL/kg/day or 4–6 episodes/day
2	Maculopapular rash 25–50% BSA	3.1–6 mg/dL	—	Adult: 1000–1500 mL/day or 5–7 episodes/day Child: 20–30 mL/kg/day or 7–10 episodes/day
3	Maculopapular rash >50% BSA	6.1–15 mg/dL	—	Adult: 1500 mL/day or >7 episodes/day Child: >30 mL/kg/day or >10 episodes/day
4	Generalized erythroderma (>50% BSA) plus bullous formation and desquamation >5% BSA	>15 mg/dL	—	Severe abdominal pain with or without ileus, or grossly bloody stool (regardless of stool volume)

Overall clinical grade (based on most severe target organ involvement):
Grade 0: No stage 1–4 or any organ.
Grade I: Stage 1 skin without liver, upper gastrointestinal (GI), or lower GI involvement.
Grade II: Stage 3 rash and/or stage 1 liver and/or stage 1 upper GI and/or stage 1 lower GI.
Grade III: Stage 2–3 liver and/or stage 2–3 lower GI, with stage 0–3 skin and/or stage 0–1 upper GI.
Grade IV: Stage 4 skin, liver, or lower GI involvement, with stage 0–1 upper GI.

other processes. Histologic grading data do not always correlate with clinical grading, but the evidence shows that clinical and histologic grades may be predictors of nonrelapse mortality (Narkhede et al., 2017).

Generally, acute GvHD occurs within the first 100 days posttransplant, classified as classic acute GvHD by the National Institutes of Health (NIH). Persistent, recurrent, or late acute GvHD occurs beyond the first 100 days posttransplant and is associated with immunosuppression tapering and donor lymphocyte infusions (Jagasia et al., 2015).

Chronic graft-versus-host disease. Chronic GvHD is considered a distinct clinical and pathophysiologic entity from acute GvHD. Compared to acute GvHD, less is known about the pathogenesis of chronic GvHD. In addition to inflammation caused by tissue injury and activation of donor T cells, it is also characterized by thymic injury, deficiency of regulatory T cells, and prolonged, uncontrolled B-cell activation leading to the production of autoantibodies. These mechanisms can result in tissue injury, repair, and fibrosis. It is often associated with higher morbidity and mortality and can significantly affect long-term quality of life. Classic chronic GvHD generally occurs 100+ days after HSCT, and the manifestations are numerous and diverse, often resembling other chronic immune disorders such as systemic lupus erythematosus, Sjögren syndrome, and rheumatoid arthritis. Common target organs include the skin, eyes, oral cavity, lungs, liver, GI system, musculoskeletal, genital, and hematopoietic systems. Because there are potentially so many organ systems involved and a variety of presentations, diagnosis can be challenging. In 2014 the NIH revised consensus criteria, including diagnostic guidelines describing each target organ's diagnostic and distinctive manifestations (Table 12.7) (Jagasia et al., 2015).

More recently it has been recognized that atypical manifestations may not be part of the traditional diagnostic or scoring criteria; these include immune-mediated cytopenias, myositis, pericardial or pleural effusions, myasthenia gravis, and nephrotic syndrome (Cuvelier et al., 2022).

Severe forms of chronic GvHD are predictive of prognosis and can be debilitating for patients as they can suffer from sclerotic skin impairing movement and altering function or can experience restrictive breathing from bronchiolitis obliterans syndrome (BOS), a pulmonary form of chronic GvHD. Quality of life can be severely impacted for those who experience severe forms of chronic GvHD.

Chronic GvHD can occur without having had acute GvHD (de novo), follow the resolution of acute GvHD, or be an extension of acute GvHD. In cases beyond 100 days where both acute and chronic manifestations occur simultaneously, it is referred to as chronic GvHD overlap syndrome. The degree of HLA compatibility is a known risk factor for developing acute GvHD. Other pediatric risk factors include malignancy versus nonmalignant disease, donors older than 8 years of age, use of TBI, high CD34+ cell dose, and female multiparous donor to the male recipient (Choi et al., 2017; Gatza et al., 2020).

Table 12.7	National Institutes of Health Defined Chronic Graft-Versus-Host Disease Target Organs and Manifestations

ORGAN	MANIFESTATIONS
Eyes	Dry eyes, keratoconjunctivitis sicca, punctate keratopathy
Mouth	Lichen planuslike features, ulcers, xerostomia
Lungs	Bronchiolitis obliterans or bronchiolitis obliterans syndrome
Gastrointestinal	Esophageal web, stricture of stenosis
Genitourinary	Lichen planus or lichen sclerosis-like features Females: vaginal scarring or clitoral/labial agglutination Males: phimosis or urethral/meatus scarring or stenosis
Skin	Poikiloderma, sclerotic features, lichen-planus, morphea, or lichen-sclerosus–like features Depigmentation, papulosquamous lesions
Musculoskeletal	Fasciitis, joint stiffness/contractures due to fasciitis or sclerosis

From Jagasia, M. H., Greinix, H. T., Arora, M., Williams, K. M., Wolff, D., Cowen, E. W., Palmer, J., Weisdorf, D., Treister, N. S., Cheng, G. S., Kerr, H., Stratton, P., Duarte, R. F., McDonald, G. B., Inamoto, Y., Vigorito, A., Arai, S., Datiles, M. B., Jacobsohn, D., ... Flowers, M. E. (2015). National institutes of health consensus development project on criteria for clinical trials in chronic graft-versus-host disease: I. The 2014 diagnosis and staging working group report. *Biol Blood Marrow Transplant, 21*(3), 389–401.e1.

Commonly cited risk factors for GvHD include:

- HLA antigen/allele mismatch
- Unrelated donor
- Older recipient age
- Higher conditioning intensity
- Multiparous female donor to a male host
- TBI
- Mobilized PBSC compared to bone marrow
- Higher CD34 cell dose in PBSC product
- Higher T-cell dose
- Occurrence of acute GvHD (a significant risk factor for chronic GvHD)
- ABO mismatch
- CMV seropositivity

Prevention of GvHD consists of multiple approaches. Initially, donor selection and stem cell sources may be selected based on the clinical concern related to the development of GvHD. For example, using cord blood or bone marrow is associated with less GvHD than PBSC (Ponce et al., 2021).

The mainstay in the prevention and treatment of GvHD includes immunosuppressive therapies. For acute GvHD prophylaxis, most commonly patients receive a calcineurin inhibitor such as cyclosporine A, tacrolimus, or sirolimus, all of which interfere with the proliferation of T lymphocytes. These may be combined with additional agents such as methotrexate or mycophenolate mofetil. A common GvHD

Box 12.4	Side Effects of Calcineurin Inhibitors

- Headache
- Diarrhea
- Nausea
- Vomiting
- Stinging/burning/soreness/itching of the affected skin
- Stomach upset
- Acne
- Muscle or back pain

prophylactic regimen is PTCy and calcineurin inhibitors in haploidentical transplants. More information is available under immunosuppressant therapy earlier in the chapter.

Calcineurin inhibitors, although instrumental as a prophylactic medication, require specific guidelines for administration and close monitoring for adverse reactions. The transplant centers most often guide the management of these medications, but monitoring for side effects is sometimes a shared responsibility. They are initiated approximately 48 hours prior to stem cell infusion and are tapered based on protocols, institutional guidelines, disease, risk of GvHD, desire for GvL effect, and type of transplant. For example, a patient at high risk for relapse and who will benefit from GvL may start tapering at day 60+, while a patient with the nonmalignant disease who will not benefit from a graft-versus-disease effect may not start tapering until day 180+. Generally, tapering lasts 4 to 12 weeks. The side effect profile of common calcineurin inhibitors (Box 12.4) is important to consider in the management of patients. Therapeutic drug monitoring of trough drug levels is required, and dose adjustments are based on established therapeutic goals. Cyclosporine, tacrolimus, and sirolimus are metabolized mainly by the CYP3A enzyme systems, and medications known to induce or inhibit these enzyme systems may result in increased or decreased metabolism of the calcineurin inhibitor. Antifungals commonly used during HSCT, including fluconazole, voriconazole, and posaconazole, are PCP3A inhibitors and can markedly increase blood concentration levels of calcineurin inhibitors. Calcineurin inhibitors are associated with the following adverse effects:

- Hypertension
- Electrolyte abnormalities (magnesium wasting, hyperkalemia)
- Renal insufficiency
- Neurotoxicity (tremors, headache, paresthesia, insomnia, agitation, seizures)
- Posterior reversible encephalopathy syndrome
- TA-TMA
- Cyclosporine A (additional side effects include hirsutism, glucose intolerance, gingival hyperplasia, hyperlipidemia)

Additional prophylactic approaches for GvHD include T-cell depletion. This can be done in vivo through the use of a polyclonal antibody (antithymocyte globulin [ATG]) or a monoclonal antibody (alemtuzumab [Campath-1]) as part of the conditioning regimen.

Ex vivo T-cell depletion by removing T lymphocytes from the stem cell graft prior to the infusion is another strategy to prevent GvHD. This can be done through physical separation techniques with either negative or positive selection techniques. Negative selection removes the unwanted components from the graft, while positive selection selects only the desired components from the graft, eliminating the undesired component. CD34+ lymphocyte selection is an example of positive selection.

Treatment of graft-versus-host disease. Despite the many options for prevention, developing GvHD is not uncommon. Although it occurs less in children than adults, it has been reported that 40% to 85% of pediatric patients experience grade II to IV acute GvHD. In pediatric patients, grade II to IV acute GvHD ranges from 40% to 85% depending on the degree of HLA mismatch and 27% in a transplant using an HLA fully matched sibling.

For stage I acute GvHD or mild chronic GvHD, targeted topical therapies may be used, such as steroid creams for skin GvHD, artificial tears associated with chronic ocular GvHD, or budesonide for GvHD of the GI tract. Frequent GvHD-focused reviews of systems and exams to evaluate for worsening of GvHD are essential in identifying the need to change or advance treatment.

Systemic steroids (methylprednisolone/prednisone) are the standard-of-care treatment for acute GvHD stages II to IV and newly diagnosed extensive chronic GvHD. A calcineurin inhibitor is often continued or added to the regimen. Due to the risk of developing fatal opportunistic infections and multiple complications associated with steroids, the goal is to taper the steroids as soon as clinically possible. For steroid-refractory GvHD, additional immunosuppressants are typically introduced by the specialist. However, there is not one definitive therapy used for steroid-refractory acute or chronic GvHD. Therapeutic options include methotrexate, mycophenolate mofetil, rituximab, etanercept, ATG, basiliximab, pentostatin, daclizumab, etanercept, infliximab, and alemtuzumab (Martin et al., 2012). Since 2017 there have been three new FDA-approved targeted agents for the treatment of refractory GvHD. These include ibrutinib (Bruton tyrosine kinase inhibitor), ruxolitinib (JAK-1/2 inhibitor), and belumosudil (ROCK2 inhibitor) for chronic GvHD and ruxolitinib for acute GvHD (Martini et al., 2022).

A nonpharmacologic approach to treat steroid-refractory GvHD includes extracorporeal photopheresis (ECP), which involves removing mononuclear cells collected by apheresis, treating the cells with methoxypsoralen, then exposing the solution to ultraviolet light and reinfusing them back into the patient. Randomized clinical trials using ECP for the treatment of GvHD are limited, but several smaller studies demonstrate partial response or better in a number of organ sites (Nygaard et al., 2020). The procedure is well tolerated, but not all centers have the availability or resources to perform ECP.

Graft failure and graft rejection. A successful transplant is dependent on the engraftment of donor hematopoietic stem cells and the subsequent population of the cells in the recipient. Failure to engraft or maintain engraftment is a rare but serious potential complication of allogeneic stem cell transplant. Hematopoietic recovery and donor engraftment are dependent on many factors, including primary disease, donor type, stem cell source and dose, cell manipulation, presence of GvHD, and presence of infection.

The ASTCT came to a consensus on standard definitions related to engraftment and graft failure. Primary graft failure is a lack of achievement of ANC at or above 500/μL by day 30+ associated with pancytopenia for PBSC and unstimulated bone marrow transplants and by day 42+ for cord blood transplant. Secondary graft failure is a decline in hematopoietic function (may involve hemoglobin and/or platelets and/or neutrophils) necessitating blood products or growth factor support after having met the standard definition of hematopoietic (neutrophils and platelets) recovery. When assessing for graft failure, measuring donor chimerism is standard practice, indicating the percentage of donor and recipient cells at any given time. Full donor chimerism is a finding of more than 95% donor cells in myeloid and lymphoid cell lineages. Mixed donor chimerism is 5% to 95% donor cells in the myeloid and lymphoid cell lineages. It is recommended to check donor chimerism at days 30+, 90+, 180+, and 365+ posttransplantation.

Evaluation of mixed donor chimerism is done with an understanding that mixed chimerism can be acceptable in certain situations. For many nonmalignant diseases, a full donor chimerism is not necessary to achieve long-term disease control. In contrast, for patients with oncologic disease, full donor chimerism is the goal to avoid relapse of the disease.

Graft failure is a rare but serious consequence of an allogeneic transplant. Studies have found the incidence of graft failure to be rare, with reports of 3.5%, 3.8%, and 7.7% (Wobma et al., 2020). Graft failure is associated with decreased survival due to relapse disease and development of serious and sometimes fatal infections, the longer length of stay, and subsequent higher health care costs (Wobma et al., 2020).

Management approaches are varied based on diagnosis, type of transplant, and presence of GvHD. Some general approaches include tapering immunosuppression for further engraftment of donor cells, stem cell boost, and second transplant.

In contrast to graft failure, poor graft function occurs when there is acceptable donor chimerism but frequent dependence on blood and/or platelet transfusions and/or growth factor support in the absence of other explanations, including disease relapse, drugs, infection, or immune-mediated event.

Sinusoidal obstructive syndrome/venoocclusive disease.
Sinusoidal obstructive syndrome (SOS; or VOD), is a potentially life-threatening early complication following HSCT. In the initial development of SOS, chemotherapy damages the sinusoidal endothelium of the liver, triggering the release of cytokines and adhesion molecules, which activate additional antiinflammatory pathways. A loss of endothelial cell structure leads to gaps in the endothelial barrier, allowing RBCs, WBCs, and cellular debris to pass through gaps and accumulate in the Disse space. There is sinusoid narrowing and detachment of endothelial cells with downstream embolization. There is blockage of blood flow and subsequent postsinusoidal obstruction. In severe cases, liver dysfunction can progress to multiorgan dysfunction syndrome and death (Mahadeo et al., 2020). Children are at higher risk of developing SOS, with a 20% to 60% prevalence compared to 10% for adults (Mahadeo et al., 2020).

The clinical presentation of SOS includes weight gain, ascites, painful hepatomegaly, and hyperbilirubinemia. Transfusion refractory thrombocytopenia is also commonly seen in these patients. Early identification resulting in earlier treatment is correlated with improved outcomes, while multiorgan dysfunction is associated with increased mortality.

Diagnosis of VOD/SOS remains a clinical diagnosis. Ultrasound is commonly used as a nondiagnostic assessment tool. A Doppler ultrasound can detect ascites, hepatomegaly, splenomegaly, portal vein dilation, and portal venous flow reversal, which may be considered a late finding of SOS/VOD. The use of ultrasound shear wave elastography, which measures the stiffness of the liver, is under investigation as another noninvasive radiologic tool to evaluate VOD/SOS (Reddivalla et al., 2018).

Prophylaxis and treatment strategies.
An initial strategy for preventing VOD/SOS is the evaluation of risk factors when planning for HSCT (e.g., avoiding agents highly associated with VOD/SOS in a person with existing hepatic dysfunction). Ursodiol is a common prophylactic agent because there is mixed evidence of a reduction in the incidence of SOS, and the product safety profile is satisfactory. Defibrotide is the pharmacologic treatment approved for SOS/VOD with renal or pulmonary dysfunction. Although not fully understood, defibrotide promotes endothelial stabilization through fibrogenetic and angiogenetic effects, reduces platelet adhesion and activation through its antithrombotic and profibrinolytic properties without systemic anticoagulant effects, and decreases vascular permeability and apoptosis due to calcineurin inhibitors and chemotherapy without interfering with the antitumor effects of cytotoxic rugs (Bonifazi et al., 2020). Supportive care measures are used throughout a patient's course with SOS/VOD. Patients with moderate-severe SOS/VOD can develop massive ascites, severe pain, hypoxia, pleural effusions, and renal dysfunction. A multidisciplinary team, including nurses, is integral to providing related interventions, including strict intake and output, weight and abdominal girth measures, fluid management, diuresis, analgesia, oxygen therapy, thoracentesis, paracentesis, and hemodialysis or hemofiltration. These complicated therapies may necessitate patient transfer to the intensive care unit for specialized care.

Engraftment syndrome.
Engraftment syndrome is an early inflammatory complication after autologous and allogeneic transplant near the time of neutrophil engraftment. It has been characterized by a group of symptoms that have been described in the literature as some of the following: noninfectious fevers, rash, weight gain, diarrhea, hypoxia, pulmonary edema not related to other reasons, capillary leak, renal and hepatic dysfunction, and rarely transient encephalopathy (Schmid et al., 2008). There have been some attempts to standardize diagnostic criteria, but there is no one standard in the pediatric HSCT field. It is often difficult to distinguish engraftment syndrome from acute GvHD because they have several overlapping clinical features (Spitzer, 2015). The pathophysiology of engraftment syndrome is unclear but hypothesized to be related to endothelial injury in the presence of activated granulocytes and increased cytokine production (Spitzer, 2015). One pediatric study documented a rise in proinflammatory cytokines followed by a rise in antiinflammatory cytokines in patients identified with engraftment syndrome (Khandelwal et al., 2016). The timing of the symptoms and clinical findings have been reported to occur within 3 days before to 7 days after engraftment (Cornell et al., 2015). Treatment approaches for engraftment syndrome consist of supportive care measures for mild symptoms and the use of systemic steroids for persistent moderate-severe symptoms.

Infection.
Despite advances in prophylaxis, early identification, and improved treatments, infections continue to pose a significant threat to the health and survival of children who receive HSCT. Risk factors for infection are well described and include the underlying disease, neutropenia and lymphopenia, mucosal barrier damage, central venous access devices, immunosuppressant therapies for GvHD, abnormal B- and T-cell function, and hypogammaglobulinemia. The complex interplay of these risk factors makes it hard to predict a person's exact risk.

Assessment for infections begins in the pretransplant workup phase. Dental screenings, radiologic evaluations of the chest, and screening for viral infections of both the recipient and donor can detect potential infectious threats prior to receiving a preparative regimen. Infections found in the pretransplant period are generally treated prior to starting the conditioning therapy and at times may delay the transplant. Providers need to consider the urgency of the transplant versus the risk of moving forward with a possible infection.

A recent study evaluating respiratory viral infections prior to HSCT found that moving ahead with transplant when patients had a positive viral nasal pharyngeal aspirate resulted in decreased survival and higher transplant-related mortality than those whose transplant was delayed (Ottaviano et al., 2019). Additionally, transplants that are nonurgent may be delayed to avoid the seasonality of viral infections. Outcomes of patients who developed a seasonal-related respiratory infection during the first 100 days posttransplant had higher mortality than those who did not develop infections (Hutspardol et al., 2015).

Specific bacterial, viral, and fungal infections occur at predictable times after transplant. The timeline is related to the timing of specific risks and the immune system recovery. The three phases include the preengraftment, postengraftment, and late phases (Fig. 12.1).

Bacterial infections. In the preengraftment phase, prolonged neutropenia and breaks in the mucosal and cutaneous barriers increase infection risks. Because the body is unable to fight infectious organisms and balance its natural flora, bacteria and fungi normally present in the GI tract may become potential pathogens. Translocated oral and bowel flora and indwelling central venous catheters are the primary source of gram-positive and enteric, gram-negative bacterial infections.

The focus on preventing infections during this period includes early identification of infections, use of prophylactic medications, and environmental controls. The evidence regarding the efficacy of infection control strategies continues to evolve. For example, for pediatric autologous transplant patients, there is substantial variability in center practices of providing infectious prophylaxis (Falcon et al., 2020). Antibacterial prophylaxis with levofloxacin during the neutropenic period is commonly practiced in many transplant centers (Gardner et al., 2022). Still, it is unclear if the efficacy outweighs the risks of multidrug-resistant organisms, the potential for an increased rate of *Clostridioides difficile (C. diff)*, and the increased rate of acute GvHD by disrupting the gut microbiome. However, recent recommendations from the Infectious Diseases Society of America and Children's Oncology Group (COG) emphasize that routine systemic antibacterial prophylaxis in children undergoing allogeneic HSCT is weak when examining benefits balanced with the potential impact on resistance (Lehrnbecher et al., 2020). Understanding patient risk and local resistance epidemiology is important in decision making regarding bacterial prophylaxis.

The development of fever with neutropenia is considered an emergency and requires a comprehensive

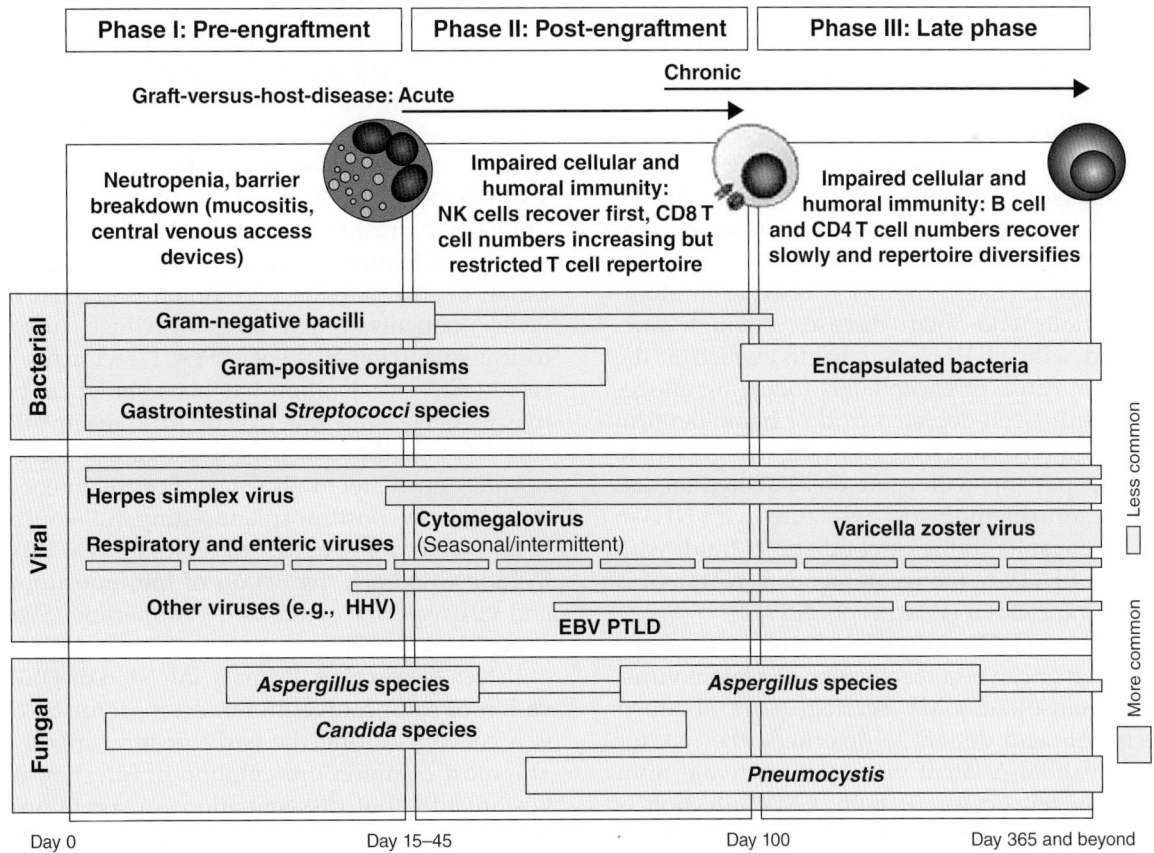

Fig. 12.1 Phases of opportunistic infections among allogeneic hematopoietic stem cell transplantation recipients. *EBV-PTLD*, Epstein-Barr virus posttransplant lymphoproliferative disease; *HHV*, human herpesvirus; *NK*, natural killer (Murray et al., 2017).

fever workup, including blood cultures, chest x-ray, and urine culture. Broad-spectrum antibiotics covering *Pseudomonas aeruginosa*, Enterobacteriaceae, and oral streptococci are started within 1 hour of fever onset. Most of this includes cefepime, piperacillin/tazobactam (Zosyn), or antipseudomonal carbapenem (e.g., Meropenem). For patients who are hemodynamically unstable, gram-positive coverage with vancomycin is added.

Postengraftment. During the first 100 days after HSCT, recipients of both autologous and allogeneic grafts have impaired cellular and humoral immunity. GvHD and immunosuppressive therapy, including Campath, increase the risk of infections in allogeneic transplant recipients. These children lack T-lymphocyte function and are at increased risk of viral infections that can result from primary infection or a reactivation of a latent infection. Fortunately, viral surveillance and improved viral prophylaxis and treatment options have expanded.

Viral surveillance with DNA polymerase chain reaction (PCR) testing is a sensitive and quantitative method of monitoring patients for viral reactivation. It has resulted in the early detection of viruses, preemptive antivirals, and improved outcomes related to serious viral infections. Early detection of a virus allows for an asymptomatic viremia or infection to be treated so it does not progress to viral infection or disease.

Routine surveillance for CMV, Epstein-Barr virus (EBV), adenovirus, and human herpesvirus 6 (HHV-6) is commonly utilized during the first 100 days posttransplant or until systemic immunosuppression has been discontinued. HHV-6 is related to the reactivation of a latent virus and occurs within the first month of transplant. Persons are normally infected early in life with HHV-6, passed from person to person through saliva, and are present in over 90% of the population over the age of 2 years. Viremia is often asymptomatic, but serious end-organ disease, although rare, is associated with HHV-6 encephalitis, which is the most frequent cause of encephalitis following allogeneic transplant. T-cell depleted cord or haploidentical recipients who have received ATG are at higher risk. Symptomatic patients with acute-onset altered mental status, short-term memory loss or seizures with HHV-6 PCR-positive results in the cerebral spinal fluid, with a diagnosis of HHV-6, the recommended treatment is foscarnet or ganciclovir (Ward et al., 2019).

Cytomegalovirus. CMV infection can occur as a primary infection or can be a reactivation of a latent virus. Before the transplant, CMV serologies are obtained from recipients and donors to determine the risk for CMV reactivation. A latent virus can reactivate from host or donor leucocytes, or both. CMV infection is often asymptomatic in the setting of frequent surveillance. CMV disease can affect any organ, including the lungs, GI tract, liver, CNS, and eyes. CMV infection is often asymptomatic in the setting of frequent surveillance. Preventative strategies for CMV infection include the selection of a lower-risk donor based on CMV risk status and the use of leukocyte-reduced blood products. Additionally, prophylactic therapy with letermovir, a recently approved agent for CMV prophylaxis, is recommended for allogeneic seropositive adult recipients and is administered from days 28 through 100 (Hakki et al., 2021). Studies have also demonstrated the safety and efficacy of CMV prophylaxis with letermovir use in children (Richert-Przygonska et al., 2022).

Preemptive CMV treatment with oral valganciclovir or IV ganciclovir is initiated when institutional viral thresholds have been met. Ganciclovir, valganciclovir, foscarnet, and cidofovir have been approved for the treatment of CMV disease. Cytopenias are commonly seen with ganciclovir and valganciclovir, while nephrotoxicity is often observed with foscarnet and cidofovir (Hakki et al., 2021).

Epstein-Barr virus. A primary EBV infection in young children presents as a self-limiting viral illness of the oropharynx and results in mononucleosis in older children and adults. The virus is latent in B cells for previously infected patients but can be reactivated during severe immunosuppression. Patients can develop asymptomatic EBV viremia but are also at risk of developing EBV posttransplant lymphoproliferative disease (EBV-PTLD), which is a rare but life-threatening disease caused by the opportunistic expansion of EBV-transformed donor B cells in a host with suppressed T-cell function (Pegorario & Favre, 2021). Clinical manifestations of PTLD include fever, malaise, sweats, weight loss, and enlargement of lymphoid tissue. The risk of developing PTLD is associated with T-cell depletion of the donor marrow, use of ATG, and unrelated or mismatched grafts (Landgren et al., 2009).

EBV PCR monitoring allowing for early identification of EBV viremia is commonly utilized for allogeneic patients. Single-dose rituximab given prior to transplant for allogeneic HSCT recipients at high risk of EBV reactivation has been shown to be effective in decreasing the risk of EBV reactivation and EBV-PTLD without increasing the risk of acute GvHD or infection (Patel et al., 2023). For treatment of EBV viremia in the posttransplant setting, full-course rituximab is commonly used. Strategies to treat EBV-PTLD include rituximab, reduction of immunosuppression, and virus-specific cytotoxic T-cell therapy (Styczynski et al., 2016).

Herpes simplex virus. Primary infection or HSV reactivation of seropositive immunocompromised children is a concern during the early posttransplant period. The most common presentation of infection is gingivostomatitis, but dissemination can occur in the GI tract, lungs, and liver. Routine surveillance testing is not typically done. A low yield and viremia can be easily detected when patients present with symptoms, including vesicular lesions, oral or genital mucosal ulceration, unexplained fevers, neurologic symptoms, or elevated liver enzymes not explained by something else (Patrick et al., 2015). Prophylaxis with acyclovir or valacyclovir in seropositive children before transplant is highly effective. Length of prophylaxis is determined based on the time from transplant, risk (including seropositivity prior to transplant), and institutional-specific guidelines. Treatment of HSV infection also utilizes acyclovir or valacyclovir in the treatment plan. Occasionally, acyclovir-resistant cases may require treatment with an alternative antiviral such as ganciclovir.

Varicella zoster virus. The varicella zoster virus (VZV) can be a serious infectious risk to children undergoing HSCT. Reactivating the latent virus, herpes zoster, and primary VZV infections can cause severe complications from dissemination. Prompt initiation of antiviral treatment is necessary to prevent dissemination. Varicella vaccination, which contains live virus, is recommended at 2 years posttransplant if the patient is no longer immunocompromised.

BK virus. A large majority of healthy people are infected with the BK virus sometime during their childhood. The virus lies latent in the uroepithelial cells of the bladder and reactivates during periods of significant immunosuppression. Urinary shedding can lead to hematuria, which may be asymptomatic in some, but it may also result in urinary urgency, frequency, dysuria, and pain in others. BK virus can be detected by PCR testing in the urine and the blood. Treatment is focused on supportive care, such as hyperhydration with diuresis, analgesics (including phenazopyridine), and antispasmodics. Therapeutic approaches can include decreasing immunosuppression and using the antiviral cidofovir, which has some activity against the BK virus.

Community-acquired respiratory virus infections. Community-acquired respiratory viral infections commonly occur in the pediatric population but can pose a substantial risk to children undergoing HSCT and contribute to morbidity and mortality (Lo et al., 2012). These infections include influenza A and B, respiratory syncytial virus (RSV), parainfluenza, rhinovirus, human coronavirus, metapneumovirus, adenovirus, coronaviruses, and most recently SARS-CoV-2. These viruses lead to lower tract respiratory infections or exacerbate existing HSCT pulmonary complications such as BOSns syndrome. A multicenter study documented that more than 16% of pediatric patients developed at least one respiratory viral infection in the first year posttransplant, with 48% requiring respiratory support and 14% with significant pulmonary sequelae. There are limited guidelines for the prevention, surveillance, and treatment of these infections in pediatric HSCT patients.

Patients with an active viral infection should be monitored closely for lower respiratory tract involvement. Chest x-rays or CT scans may be warranted. For patients with severe illness, consideration is given to decreasing immunosuppression if possible. Isolation procedures are put in place, which will include droplet and contact precautions. Supportive care alone is the treatment for parainfluenza, rhinovirus, human coronavirus, and metapneumovirus (Maziarz & Slater, 2021). Effective viral therapy is utilized for influenza A and B and chemoprophylaxis for immunocompromised transplant patients in close contact with an infected case (Centers for Disease Control and Prevention [CDC], 2022).

RSV can potentially result in serious consequences for young patients with HSCT. Despite potentially serious consequences, established guidelines based on controlled studies for treating RSV in pediatric patients with HSCT are limited. Individual patient risk is considered when defining a treatment approach. Consideration is given to the type of infections (upper vs lower tract respiratory infection), degree of immunosuppression, and severity of respiratory compromise. Aerosolized ribavirin with or without IVIG or palivizumab, an RSV-specific humanized monoclonal antibody, may be considered in patients at high risk for serious pulmonary complications.

COVID-19 virus emerged as a new threat to pediatric transplant patients. Data regarding the epidemiology, timeline, risk factors, and treatment approaches are limited. ASTCT published guidelines for managing COVID-19, but it must be recognized that evidence-based information is evolving (Waghmare et al., 2020). These guidelines recognize the need for screening patients for COVID-19 prior to admission and recommend delaying transplants in positive cases. Furthermore, COVID-19 vaccination and viral therapies are safely utilized in patients with HSCT. Because of rapidly changing information, the CDC should be utilized as the most reliable information source regarding vaccination and treatment for at-risk patients, including those who are immunocompromised (CDC, 2022).

Traditional pharmacologic approaches to the treatment of viruses have limitations in terms of toxicities, long-term efficacy, and resistance to treatment. One of the newest approaches is the use of viral-specific cytotoxic T lymphocytes to prevent and treat specific viral infections in patients with HSCT. In initial studies, donor-derived T cells were used, but the most recent research involves the use of third-party, partially HLA-matched T cells designed to target a number of specific viruses, including CMV, EBV, HHV-6, and BK virus. Optimally, these products would be considered off-shelf products, which could be readily available in a bank for patients to use either prophylactically or for treatment. Studies evaluating the viral-specific T cells have been promising, showing efficacy with few toxicities, including GvHD (Barrett et al., 2018).

Fungal disease. Children at the highest risk for fungal infection are those who have been neutropenic for a prolonged time or those with chronic GvHD. Significant morbidity and mortality are associated with fungal disease in the immunocompromised HSCT recipient. Fortunately, fungal disease has improved with the routine use of prophylactic antifungal therapy in high-risk patients (Styczynski et al., 2016).

Evidence-based recommendations for fungal prophylaxis in pediatric HSCT patients include systemic antifungal prophylaxis with an antifungal mold active agent with an echinocandin or mold-active azole during preengraftment or to those receiving systemic immunosuppression for GvHD treatment (Lehrnbecher et al., 2020).

Candida infections and aspergillosis are the most common infections in the posttransplant period. Candida is most often found in the oral cavity, whereas aspergillus is more commonly found in the lungs but can also affect the sinuses, CNS, or other organs. Mucormycosis is a serious and often devastating fungal infection with an overall mortality rate of 30% to 50% (Otto et al., 2019). In a review of pediatric cases, rhinosinusitis was the most frequent presentation, followed by disseminated disease and gastrointestinal, cutaneous, and pulmonary sites (Otto et al., 2019). Most frequently, infections develop in the lungs or the rhino-orbito-cerebral areas. Diagnosis requires tissue biopsy or culture from bronchoalveolar lavage (BAL) when a pulmonary site is involved. Treatment requires an amphotericin B product as first-line therapy. It should be noted that the commonly used voriconazole is not effective against mucormycosis. Surgical resection of fungal disease is an additional treatment approach used with antifungal therapy. This may include debridement of areas such as the sinuses or a single resection of the lungs or other organs.

Pneumocystis jirovecii pneumonia. PJP is an opportunistic, atypical fungus that causes pneumonia in immunocompromised persons. With adherence to prophylactic, PJP is rare, occurring in 0.63% of allogeneic and 0.28% of autologous transplant patients but is associated with high mortality (Williams et al., 2016). However, there are breakthrough infections when using second-line therapy or if prophylactic therapy is not used consistently. Effective prophylaxis combines trimethoprim-sulfamethoxazole, dramatically reducing infection incidence in patients following bone marrow transplant. It is recommended for 6 months posttransplant or up to 1 year or more if on immunosuppression. Intolerance to Bactrim is not uncommon due to allergic reactions such as rash, bone marrow suppression, or allergy. Alternatives to this medication include pentamidine, atovaquone, or dapsone. Pentamidine can be given either by IV or inhalation. Diagnosis is typically by microscopic visualization of the organisms in respiratory specimens from sputum or fluid from BAL. First-line treatment is 3 to 4 daily doses of Bactrim for 21 days with alternative medications of atovaquone or clindamycin when there is a significant sulfa allergy or intolerance.

Clostridioides difficile. C. diff is the leading cause of infectious diarrhea in HSCT recipients due to risk factors, including broad-spectrum antimicrobial exposure, immunosuppression, and disruption of bacterial microbiota and mucosa related to chemotherapy. New-onset diarrhea (three or more episodes) or loose stools, sometimes accompanied by abdominal cramping, nausea, vomiting, and fever, is the usual clinical picture of a person with C. diff infection. Serious secondary complications have been described, leading to dehydration, acute kidney injury, toxic megacolon, bowel perforation, and death (Alonso et al., 2022). C. diff infection is a clinical diagnosis determined when there is significant diarrhea and evidence of toxigenic C. diff or its toxins in the stool. Testing stool in asymptomatic persons is not recommended as they may be colonized with C. diff and test positive, leading to unnecessary treatment. Colonization occurs more commonly in children than adults.

The first-line treatment option is oral fidaxomicin, although oral vancomycin has also been used for the first episodes (Alonso et al., 2022). Oral metronidazole is used as an adjunctive agent in fulminant infection. Metronidazole is generally considered less efficacious than vancomycin or fidaxomicin. When possible, discontinuing antibiotic therapy contributing to the C. diff infection should be considered. Recurrence of infection in pediatric patients undergoing HSCT is common (Barbar et al., 2021; Spruit et al., 2020). New symptoms with a positive test after successful treatment within days to up to 12 weeks after cessation of treatment are considered a recurrence. Treatment regimens for recurrences contain fidaxomicin or vancomycin with different dosing regimens and longer duration than for the initial disease (Alonso et al., 2022). Consultation with an infectious disease expert can be helpful in recurrent cases.

Late effects. Improvements in the science of transplantation have allowed more children the opportunity for potentially curative therapy. However, this aggressive treatment has resulted in late effects for the increasing number of children who survive the transplant, resulting in the need for long-term follow-up care (Foord et al., 2020). The delayed or late sequelae that may develop can result from a combination of the following factors: (1) complications related to the condition for which transplantation was performed: (2) effects of previous treatment for the underlying disorder; (3) toxicities associated with the cytotoxic preparative regimen (usually high-dose chemotherapy with or without TBI); (4) toxic effects from treatment of posttransplant acute complications, most notably from use of immunosuppressive agents, including steroids for GvHD; and (5) physical effects of chronic GvHD. Most late effects of HSCT are a combination of these factors. Close attention must be paid to all previous therapies a child has received. Late effects can occur as early as 6 months posttransplant or many years later. Some of the most common late effects found in children who have undergone HSCT involve the endocrine system, which is particularly vulnerable to damage caused by radiation and some chemotherapeutic drugs. Impaired growth and pubertal development, infertility, and hypothyroidism are commonly seen.

Furthermore, patients who have been on long-term steroid therapy for chronic GvHD may result in decreased growth velocity, osteopenia and increased fractures, avascular necrosis (AVN), growth hormone deficiency, and adrenal insufficiency. Organ dysfunction resulting in specific cardiac, pulmonary, liver, eyes, and skin can be affected. Secondary cancers and relapse of their original disease are ongoing threats to survivors of HSCT.

Yearly evaluation in a dedicated long-term follow-up clinic at their transplanting institution is highly recommended. Multidisciplinary evaluations are necessary to fully assess sequelae related to HSCT. However, many children and families who reside far from the long-term follow-up clinic may require coordination of care locally with specialists such as oncologists or willing primary care providers. A recent randomized study found that a shared-care model in which local providers assisted early in the posttransplant care allowing the patient to be home sooner, resulted in similar nonrelapse mortality complications and improved quality of life compared with the usual model in which the transplant center provided all the care. In this study, interventions included a formal online care coordination plan, patient and physician engagement and education, and a shared patient-physician-transplanter portal (Abel et al., 2022).

Generally, the transplant and referring institutions coordinate the follow-up and surveillance testing schedule. It should include the evaluation and recognition of late effects, treatment options for late organ dysfunction, and evaluation for the detection of early relapse. To ensure optimum health care for general and specialty issues, good communication is critical among the various subspecialties and the primary care practitioner involved in caring for the child. The goal of treatment for every child who undergoes HSCT is not only to cure the underlying disorder but to minimize both the acute and long-term complications from the therapy. Some institutions have written electronic care summaries and care plans individualized for each patient. These can be useful for the patient and nontransplant providers involved in a patient's follow-up care.

PROGNOSIS

In children who have received autologous or allogeneic HSC transplants, relapse of their primary disorder is the most frequent cause of treatment failure. In malignant disorders, the vast majority of relapses occur within the first 2 years after HSCT. Since transplantation is usually the child's best option for a cure, additional treatment holds only a small likelihood of restoring the child to disease-free health; however, in recent years, immunotherapy has achieved some success, which uses the immune system to assist with disease eradication. Most recently, CAR-T therapy (specifically Kymriah) in children who relapse after HSCT has shown promising results in achieving a durable remission (Boettcher et al., 2022).

If the child is more than 1 year after HSCT when relapse occurs, a second transplant may be another option for cure if a hematologic remission can be achieved, although the toxicities to the child are often significant. Alternatively, there are several clinical trials at various centers nationwide for children with resistant or relapsed disease after HSCT. The primary transplant physician or oncologist will help review the availability of appropriate trials and discuss options with the child and parent. Families should clearly understand the trial's goals and weigh the benefits and risks. Some of these trials will require travel and transfer to other medical centers. If the child is not a candidate for further treatment or chooses not to pursue additional treatment options, the child's care may return to the referring center or primary oncologist for palliative therapy or end-of-life care.

The success of HSCT has a broad range and is greatly dependent on the child's original diagnosis, status of the disease at the time of transplant, organ function, type of transplant, and donor source. For example, from 2001 to 2019 the 5-year survival rate for children under age 18 years with severe aplastic anemia post-HSCT was approximately 90%, whereas survival rates from 2009 to 2019 in children under age 18 years with acute myeloid leukemia (AML) following allogeneic transplant ranged from approximately 50% to 65% depending on race (Auletta et al., 2019). Prognosis information therefore is individualized and should be discussed for adequate informed decision making.

PRIMARY CARE MANAGEMENT

The primary care provider plays a pivotal role in ongoing and long-term care of pediatric patients with HSCT. The timeline for transition of care varies for each patient depending on patient complications, availability of services at their home setting, and distance from the transplant center. Clear and open communication between the transplant center and the primary care team can help facilitate this transition and ease the patient's and family's anxiety related to returning home. Optimally, a detailed description of the transplant course, including complications and care plan, is conveyed to the primary care provider before the first visit. The primary care provider will assist the transplant team in identifying transplant-related complications and long-term effects of the transplant conditioning regimen and assist with routine health maintenance of the pediatric patient with HSCT. Fortunately there are useful resources outlining the surveillance of pediatric HSCT survivors for both the HSCT specialist and the primary care provider. COG created long-term follow-up guidelines for survivors of childhood, adolescent, and young adult cancer, including those treated with HSCT, which are readily available online (www.survivorshipguidelines.org). NMDP also has long-term follow-up guidelines for posttransplant patients (BeTheMatch.org, n.d.). Guidelines have also been developed for patients with specific transplanted diseases, including SCID, SCD and thalassemia, immune deficiencies, inherited marrow failure syndromes, and hemoglobinopathies (Dietz et al., 2017; Heimall et al., 2017; Shenoy et al., 2018).

HEALTH CARE MAINTENANCE

Growth and Development

Endocrine. Endocrine complications resulting from chemotherapy, radiation therapy, and steroids are common late effects seen in the pediatric transplant population. These include growth disturbances, hypothyroidism, and gonadal dysfunction.

Growth impairment has been reported to be as high as 50% to 85% in children undergoing transplant. This may be multifactorial but is associated with chronic GvHD, prolonged corticosteroid use, malnutrition, hypothyroidism, growth hormone deficiency, gonadal failure, and XRT (Wei & Albanese, 2014). More specifically, patients who have received TBI (10 Gy single fraction or 12 Gy fractionated TBI), and additional cranial radiation (≥18 Gy) are at particular risk (Chow et al., 2016).

Careful monitoring of growth by plotting height, weight, and body mass index on standardized growth charts and Tanner staging is recommended every 6 months in survivors of HSCT who have achieved skeletal maturity (Chow et al., 2016). Short stature is defined as 2 standard deviations below the mean for age. Children showing poor growth velocity should have a thyroid and bone age evaluation with a referral to an endocrinologist. Some survivors will be candidates for growth hormone replacement therapy, which has been shown to increase growth velocity and height, although some may not reach their genetic target height (Wei & Albanese, 2014).

Gonadal dysfunction and infertility. Pediatric survivors of HSCT are at risk for gonadal dysfunction resulting in delayed or arrested puberty, gonadal insufficiency, or impaired fertility. Conditioning therapies most closely associated with these effects include TBI, alkylating agents, and platinum-based agents; the dose used is important in calculating the risk for these complications. Counseling regarding fertility optimally occurs prior to treatment with chemotherapy or radiation, and should be given with the initial disease and then again prior to HSCT.

Fertility consultation services in teams have most recently been created in oncology programs to discuss the risks of infertility and preservation options. Specific options for adult female/pubertal include in vitro fertilization and embryo cryopreservation, oocyte cryopreservation, and ovarian tissue banking. Sperm banking has been the preferred method for adult men/pubertal males (Joshi et al., 2014). In recent years, fertility preservation is becoming available to children with the new surgical option of harvesting ovarian and testicular tissue, which is then cryopreserved for later use (Brodigan et al., 2021). Barriers to fertility preservation include lack of time due to urgency to begin treatment, costs, lack of insurance coverage, lack of knowledge and discussion around the issue, and difficulty in accessing reproductive specialists (Joshi et al., 2014).

Ovarian failure. Female recipients and their parents are informed of the potential risks of infertility and/or premature menopause prior to transplant. Exposure to high-dose cyclophosphamide, busulfan, and TBI is associated with ovarian failure (Joshi et al., 2014). Older age (>25 years) and pubertal status at the time of exposure increase the risk of ovarian dysfunction. Prepubescent females have a better chance of spontaneous menarche, but premature menopause is common (Wei & Albanese, 2014).

Clinical indicators of ovarian failure include failure to go through puberty, absent menstruation, and menopausal symptoms. Monitoring for elevated follicle-stimulating hormone, elevated luteinizing hormone, and low estradiol levels can be suggestive of ovarian failure and is usually started by age 13 years (Chow et al., 2016). Females with premature ovarian failure are referred to a gynecologist or endocrinologist to manage hormonal replacement therapy.

Testicular failure. Gonadal failure in males is related to high-dose conditioning therapy with TBI and age greater than 25 to 30 years, most often associated with infertility. The risk of Leydig (testosterone-producing) cell dysfunction after radiotherapy is correlated with the dose of radiation to the testes. Specifically, radiation doses below 12 Gy usually do not result in the need for testosterone replacement, but doses above 20 Gy in prepubertal males and above 30 Gy in pubertal and young adult males result in Leydig cell damage (Joshi et al., 2014). Males are monitored for Tanner stage, testicular volume, testosterone levels by age 14 years, and semen analysis to assess for fertility (Chow et al., 2016). Males at risk for gonadal failure are referred to an endocrinologist or urologist.

Thyroid dysfunction. Thyroid dysfunction, including hypothyroidism, Hashimoto thyroiditis, and thyroid nodules, have been reported as complications following pediatric HSCT. TBI and XRT to the thyroid are known risk factors (Chow et al., 2016). However, studies have documented thyroid dysfunction with non-radiation-based conditioning regimens (Cima et al., 2018). The incidence of hypothyroidism after TBI is 15%, and after busulfan and cyclophosphamide is 11% (Cima et al., 2018). COG recommends (1) annual monitoring of thyroid-stimulating hormone, free T_4, and assessment of thyroid-related symptoms in those with a history of neck radiation exposure, including TBI; and (2) an annual physical, including palpation of the thyroid for nodules (Chow et al., 2016). Patients receiving thyroid replacement therapy should have a thyroid evaluation once every 6 months.

Diet and Nutrition

Nutrition plays a key role during and after HSCT. Optimal nutrition is required to heal and maximize long-term growth and development potential. Nutrition is often compromised during the initial transplant process due to mucositis, nausea and vomiting, taste changes, diarrhea, and anorexia related to the conditioning therapy. As a result, the majority of patients with HSCT are supported on TPN or enteral nutrition for several weeks. Some patients, however, do not tolerate enteral nutrition due to nausea, vomiting, or diarrhea, or they may object to having a nasal gastric tube in place. Patients who fail or refuse enteral nutrition are often transitioned to TPN. In circumstances where the ability to eat normally is suspected to be long term, patients may have a gastrostomy tube (G-tube) inserted and nutritional supplements given via the G-tube. It is not uncommon for patients to be discharged from their transplant admission on parenteral or enteral nutrition. Parents are taught to administer this nutrition support at home, and providers follow weight and required lab work such as basic metabolic panel and electrolytes (including magnesium) as an outpatient. Nasogastric tube replacement is also needed periodically, which can be done at the hospital or in the physician's office when warranted.

Patients are encouraged to eat as tolerated during the transplant period. Transplant centers often have their own specific dietary guidelines for patients undergoing HSCT. Patients are encouraged to follow a food safety–based diet during neutropenia or immunosuppression. This is an alternative to the previously used neutropenic diet, which has not been found to reduce infections in transplant recipients and is restrictive and may be difficult to follow (Ma et al., 2022; Taggart et al., 2019). The US Department of Agriculture provides specific recommendations for transplant patients, which includes safe food choices, food preparation, and food storage information. A summary of these guidelines is outlined by BeTheMatch.org (Table 12.8). Nutritionists

---

Table 12.8   When Choosing Something to Eat

THESE FOODS ARE LOW RISK AND GENERALLY SAFE TO EAT:	THESE FOODS ARE HIGH RISK AND GENERALLY NOT SAFE TO EAT:
Dairy and Eggs	
• Pasteurized foods such as milk, eggs, yogurt, cottage cheese, tofu, and refrigerated juice; look for "pasteurized" on the label • Commercially packaged hard and semisoft cheeses, including cheddar, mozzarella, parmesan, Swiss and Monterey Jack	• Unpasteurized (raw) milk • Soft cheeses made from unpasteurized (raw) milk, such as feta, brie, or queso fresco • Foods that contain raw or undercooked eggs, such as homemade raw cookie dough, homemade eggnog, or homemade Caesar salad dressing
Fruits and Vegetables	
• Washed fresh fruits and vegetables • Cooked vegetables, including sprouts	• Unwashed fresh fruits and vegetables • Fruits and vegetables with bruises or bad spots • Raw sprouts, such as alfalfa or bean sprouts
Meat and Seafood	
• Meat or poultry cooked to a safe internal (inside) temperature • Seafood, when handled properly and cooked to a safe internal temperature	• Raw or undercooked fish or shellfish, including sashimi • Refrigerated smoked fish • Partially cooked seafood • Hot dogs, deli meats, and luncheon meats that have not been reheated
Packaged Foods	
• Prepared, packaged foods in boxes, cans or frozen, such as fruits and vegetables • Roasted and shelled nuts; look for "roasted" on the label • Commercially packaged peanut, almond, and soybean butter • Commercially packaged breads and cereals • Prepackaged snack foods such as pretzels, popcorn, and tortilla chips • Honey	• Frozen foods that are not frozen solid • Foods in damaged packaging (packages with dents or cracks) • Expired foods (check the expiration date on the packaging) • Bulk foods or items from self-service bins • Unroasted nuts or nujs in the shell

Courtesy National Marrow Donor Program.

are essential team members who meet with patients and families routinely during the transplant inpatient stay and often during outpatient follow-up. It is important to note that the ability to eat and drink does not always recover rapidly. Even though mucositis and nausea/vomiting may resolve, maintaining adequate nutrition and hydration in the months posttransplant can be challenging (BeTheMatch.org, n.d.).

Patients and parents may be asked to keep daily food/fluid records after returning home. Taste changes are common during the initial posttransplant period (Loves et al., 2018). However, until taste changes resolve, it is often difficult to find foods palatable to the child undergoing a transplant. Nutritional oral supplements or high-calorie, nutritious snacks are often utilized to gain or maintain weight. Poor appetite is treated with appetite stimulants, including cyproheptadine, megestrol, or dronabinol in certain situations. These have been found to be safe and efficacious in oncology patients and have been used in the posttransplant setting. Children experiencing specific problems, taking certain medications, or with specific underlying disease states may require additional dietary considerations. For example, patients with acute GvHD of the GI tract or patients on steroids with hypertension and hyperglycemia may be asked to alter their diet. Calcium and vitamin D supplements may be added for those who are deficient and at risk for osteopenia.

Tips for safe food storage (BeTheMatch, n.d.):

- Bring your groceries home and put them away right after leaving the store.
- Make sure refrigerated foods stay cold and frozen foods stay frozen until use.
- Throw away expired food and pay close attention to freshness.
- Make and store foods in small portions so they are used up quickly.
- Do not eat leftover foods that have been in the refrigerator for more than 2 days. Put a date on containers to monitor storage time.
- Do not eat foods that have been left out of the refrigerator for 2 or more hours.
  Tips for safe food preparation (BeTheMatch, n.d.):
- Wash hands with warm, soapy water before and after handling food.
- Use hot, soapy water with disposable sponges and paper towels or disinfectant kitchen wipes to clean areas where food is prepared and for washing dishes.
- Thaw frozen foods (including meat) in the refrigerator, not on the counter or in the sink.
- Wash all fruits and vegetables well before cutting them, even those that you peel before eating.
- The best way to wash fruits and vegetables is with running water. You can also scrub them with a produce brush. Do not use produce washes, soap, bleach, peroxide, or vinegar. Do not soak fruits or vegetables.
- Wash the top of cans and can opener with hot, soapy water before use.
- Use a side-opening can opener (to keep lids from falling inside).
- Avoid touching raw meat, poultry, and fish. Or, wear disposable gloves and wash hands well before and after touching raw meat, poultry, and fish.
- Use separate cutting boards, plates, and utensils for raw and cooked foods. Be especially careful to avoid contact between cooked meat and raw meat juices.
- Clean cutting boards with a solution of 1 tablespoon of bleach to 1 gallon of water, or wash them in the dishwasher.
- Cook meat and poultry to a safe internal (inside) temperature.
- Cook hot dogs and lunch meat until they are steaming.

Safety

Child safety should be reviewed with parents at primary care visits. First-time parents whose children become ill during infancy and who are now adjusting to the liberation of protective isolation often need additional anticipatory guidance. Infant and toddler safety guidelines that would normally have been reviewed are often ignored during the acute and often life-threatening treatment involved in transplant. For example, while under the care of the transplant team, children typically are not seeing their primary care team, so information such as safe sleeping practices and choking hazard information that the primary health care provider normally reviews on well-child visits may have been missed. Returning to their primary care provider can be delayed for over a year posttransplant depending on their transplant course and when they return to their home setting. Children returning home after transplant require multiple oral medications, supplies related to central venous catheter care, and at times IV medications. Parents should be reminded to store these supplies away from all their children. A sharps container should be in the home to properly dispose of needles and syringes.

Infection control practices are important to stay healthy when the patient returns home. Hand washing is the single most effective practice in preventing infections. Parents should teach and supervise the hand washing of small children. No ill contacts should be allowed in the home. Eating utensils, cups, glasses, and dishes should not be shared and should be washed with hot, soapy water or in the hot cycle of a dishwasher. The child's home should be cleaned often and free of mold, with any home or surrounding property construction delayed until immune reconstitution is established. If there are pets in the house, children should not have any direct contact with animal feces. Certain reptiles, such as snakes, lizards, turtles, and iguanas, should be avoided to reduce the risk of acquiring salmonellosis.

Their transplant provider should provide guidance on when to return to normal activities, such as attending school or large public events. This depends on the child's immune reconstitution and whether they remain on immunosuppression. Similarly, domestic and international travel should be discussed with the transplant provider and is dependent on the patient's immunocompetence, distance from the health care setting, and availability of health care in the place of desired travel.

In the early weeks of posttransplant, patients are often deconditioned. Loss of muscle mass and endurance are common after a lengthy hospitalization. Physical and occupational health can be helpful for those who have been severely affected. In general, physical activity is highly encouraged as tolerated. Patients with moderate-severe thrombocytopenia may have limitations on certain physical activities, such as climbing, cycling, and contact sports or when the risk of trauma is possible.

Immunizations

Following HSCT, most children partially or completely lose their immunity to vaccine-preventable diseases. Ablation of the bone marrow gradually removes immune memory from previous vaccination, and antibody titers to vaccine-preventable diseases decrease 1 to 4 years after transplant if not vaccinated. Vaccination is essential to reduce the patient's risks for vaccine-preventable illness (Majeed et al., 2020).

Reimmunization following transplant is recommended for both autologous and allogeneic transplant recipients. The reimmunization timing is based on several factors related to a person's ability to respond adequately to vaccines. These factors include time from transplant, time off immunosuppressive therapy, IVIG replacement, presence of GvHD, immune reconstitution (including absolute CD4), and absolute lymphocyte counts and immunoglobulin G (IgG) levels (Haynes et al., 2021). Many transplant centers develop reimmunization guidelines and update them frequently to capture the latest research. Table 12.9 shows an example of a post-HSCT vaccination schedule.

In general, patients without GvHD and after discontinuing immunosuppression begin killed virus vaccines 6 to 12 months posttransplant. Live virus vaccines are not given until at least 2 years posttransplant. Annual inactivated influenza vaccines should be administered to all household contacts of children undergoing transplantation. Siblings, family contacts, and health professionals should all be fully immunized to decrease the potential exposure of children undergoing or recovering from HSCT.

Primary care providers often assist in the completion of vaccinations during the posttransplant process. The transplant center provides a specific posttransplant immunization schedule for primary care providers to follow.

Screenings

The following recommendations include the COG report, "Late Effects Surveillance Recommendations among Survivors of Childhood Hematopoietic Cell Transplantation" (Chow et al., 2016).

Vision. Visual acuity and a fundoscopic evaluation should be completed annually on survivors of HSCT

Table 12.9 Sample Post-HSCT Vaccination Schedule

VACCINE	FIRST DOSE (MONTHS) AFTER HSCT	TIME POINTS FOR ADMINISTRATION	COMMENTS
Influenza	4–6	Yearly during flu season	Two doses for those under age 9 who have not received influenza vaccine post BMT
Pneumococcal conjugate	3–6	3 doses, 1–2-mo intervals, fourth dose	
Pneumococcal polysaccharide	12	1 dose if no chronic GvHD	
Hemophilus influenza B conjugate	6	3 doses, timing between intervals 0, 2, 4 mo	
Hepatitis B	6–12	3 doses, timing between intervals 0, 2, 6 mo	
Hepatitis A	6–12	2 doses, timing between intervals 0, 6 mo	
Meningococcal	6–12	2 doses	
Polio (IPV)	6–12		
Diptheria, acellular pertussis, and tetanus toxoids	6–12	3 doses	
Human papillomavirus (age 9–26 yr)	12	3 doses	
Measles, mumps, rubella (live virus)	24	2 doses, 2-mo interval	
Varicella virus (live virus)	24	2 doses, 2-mo interval	

GvHD, Graft-versus-host disease; *HSCT*, hematopoietic stem cell transplantation.

exposed to TBI or cranial radiation, busulfan, corticosteroids, and a history of chronic GvHD. Providers should assess patients for impaired vision, diplopia, halos, dry eyes, and irritation. Common posttransplant problems include posterior subcapsular cataracts and keratoconjunctivitis. Completing a Schirmer test or tear breakup time is utilized in patients suspected of having chronic GvHD of the eye. CMV retinitis is also a problem that has been identified in children after transplant. It is recommended that those with radiation exposure and a history of chronic GvHD have these screening exams conducted by an ophthalmologist at least every 1 to 3 years (Chow et al., 2016).

Additionally, children are at risk for CMV retinitis, which has been described as a condition that often has no early symptoms and may not be reported in young children. A delay in diagnosis can result in permanent vision loss, with late detection in children due to no symptoms (Al-Farsi & Al Jabri, 2022). Patients with CMV viremia and those at high risk should be considered for an ophthalmologic screening exam (Hiwarkar et al., 2014).

Hearing. Ototoxicity has not been well studied in pediatric patients with HSCT. However, data from childhood cancer literature describe hearing loss in patients who have received carboplatin, which is included in some HSCT conditioning regimens. Additionally, receiving aminoglycoside antibiotics and loop diuretics can increase the risk of ototoxicity. COG makes the following recommendations for screening for ototoxicity: All survivors should be screened annually for hearing difficulties, tinnitus, and vertigo, along with an otoscopic exam. Those at high risk (those exposed to cisplatin or carboplatin, cumulative pre- and HSCT cranial radiation ≥30 Gy) should have a complete audiology evaluation 1 year posttransplant; if any hearing loss is detected, they should continue to have a yearly performed.

Dental. Children receiving HSCT are particularly at risk for dental complications as they may receive these therapies during the formation and eruption of primary and permanent dentition. Risk factors associated with childhood cancer survivors include the following: younger age at treatment, higher radiation dose, and treatment with radiotherapy, chemotherapy, and HSCT. These were associated with an increased risk for dental agenesis, dental hypoplasia, root stunting, and enamel hypoplasia. The risk of dental caries in this population seems to be decreasing due to improved dental care (Gawade et al., 2014). Xerostomia is associated with TBI or radiation to the salivary glands and chronic GvHD of the oral mucosa. Xerostomia is known to increase the risk of dental caries and oral infections. Chronic GvHD of the oral mucosa is associated with unique symptomatology and can result in increased oral infections, decreased oral intake, nutritional deficiency, and increased health service (Fall-Dickson et al., 2019). In addition to recommended

pretransplant evaluation for caries and infection, patients should have routine dental follow-ups once they have adequate immune reconstitution. COG recommends that all childhood survivors of HSCT have dental exams and cleaning every 6 months and annual oral exams. Baseline panorex should be considered to evaluate root development. Special attention should be given to those with a history of XRT, chronic GvHD, and a review for secondary cancer (Chow et al., 2016).

Cardiovascular. When surviving long term, survivors of HSCT have a higher risk of cardiac dysfunction than the general population (Diesch-Furlanetto et al., 2021). Survivors of childhood HSCT have been found to have a significantly higher risk of cardiovascular complications when compared to their well siblings (Armenian et al., 2011). Similarly, a long-term outcome study showed adolescents and young adult cancer survivors to be at higher risk of developing long-term cardiac complications as compared to same-age siblings, although they had less risk than those survivors in younger age groups (Suh et al., 2020). Cardiac abnormalities, including cardiomyopathy, congestive heart failure, premature coronary artery disease, stroke, and valvular or conduction abnormalities, have the potential to occur years after HSCT, so vigilance in monitoring for these potential complications is necessary. Patients receiving chemotherapy and radiation therapy before HSCT may be at the highest risk for these complications because of cardiac toxicity and iron overload (Majhail et al., 2012).

Recommendations for cardiovascular monitoring include the following:

- Annual history and exam to screen for cardiac-related symptoms for those survivors treated with anthracyclines and/or chest radiation, including TBI
- Echocardiogram to assess cardiac function at intervals based on previous exposures and age (annually to every 5 years)
- Those exposed to cranial radiation, including TBI, screen for neurologic signs and symptoms of cerebrovascular disease
- Screen for modifiable cardiovascular risk factors, including diabetes and dyslipidemia, and tobacco use

Pulmonary. Late and long-term pulmonary complications in HSCT survivors can occur months to years following the completion of therapy. Risks may be related to prior therapy combined with additive risks from therapies related to transplant. Pulmonary fibrosis is known to develop following bleomycin, busulfan, carmustine, and lomustine. Risk increases with radiation exposure to the lung, including TBI.

Childhood transplant survivors specifically are at risk for idiopathic pneumonia syndrome and BOS.

Idiopathic pneumonia syndrome (or interstitial pneumonitis) generally occurs within the first several months post-HSCT but can occur later in the transplant course. Although not clearly defined, it is thought to be related to lung tissue injury from conditioning therapy and immunologic cell-mediated injury (Haider et al., 2020). Diagnosis requires evidence of widespread alveolar injury in the absence of a concurrent infection, iatrogenic fluid overload, or cardiac or renal dysfunction. Risk factors include myeloablative conditioning, TBI, age older than 40 years, and diagnosis of AML or myelodysplastic syndrome (MDS).

BOS is a nonspecific inflammatory injury of the small airways characterized by an obstructive pattern that can progress to fibrosis. The incidence is considered low in children, but if it occurs can result in significant morbidity and mortality (Walther et al., 2020). Patients may be asymptomatic in the early disease stages making early detection challenging. However, it can progress to cough and/or wheezing and dyspnea on exertion (Haider et al., 2020). Diagnosis is made through pulmonary function testing and high-resolution CT.

Other pulmonary complications in the transplant population include pleural effusions, pulmonary hypertension, cryptogenic organizing pneumonia, venous thromboembolic disease, interstitial lung disease, and diffuse alveolar hemorrhage (Haider et al., 2020).

COG recommendations for screening include:

- Survivors of HSCT who are at higher risk of developing pulmonary complications (those exposed to bleomycin, busulfan, nitrosoureas, chest radiation [including TBI]) or who have a history of chronic GvHD should be assessed annually for signs and symptoms of pulmonary dysfunction.
- Survivors should undergo pulmonary function testing at 1 year posttransplant or once age appropriate. Reevaluation of pulmonary function is per clinician discretion and guided by initial findings.
- Counseling regarding tobacco avoidance and smoking cessation is recommended.

Renal disease. Chronic kidney disease (CKD) following HSCT is estimated to occur in 50% of survivors. A recent pediatric single-center study showed 17% of pediatric patients with HSCT showed evidence of CKD 10 years after transplant (Lugthart et al., 2021). Risk factors include renal toxic conditioning agents, TBI, nephrotoxic antimicrobial use, and calcineurin inhibitors. COG guidelines recommend screening for hypertension annually and annual urinalysis to monitor for potential renal disease and begin nephroprotective interventions early. Electrolytes, including calcium, magnesium, and phosphate, should be checked at 1 year posttransplant and then as clinically indicated. Those with hypertension, proteinuria, and progressive renal insufficiency should be referred to a nephrologist (Chow et al., 2016).

Gastrointestinal. Liver disease is an area to monitor for long-term survivors of HSCT. This may be the result of previous SOS, GvHD, chronic infections, or iron overload related to chronic transfusions. COG recommends checking alanine aminotransferase and aspartate aminotransferase, bilirubin, and serum ferritin at 1 year posttransplant; for those with increased ferritin and who have received frequent transfusions, further workup for iron overload with a Ferriscan or liver biopsy may be indicated. Treatment of iron overload is completed with phlebotomy and/or chelation therapy.

Survivors with chronic GvHD of the gut and/or those who received TBI are at risk for developing esophageal or lower GI tract strictures. Those persons should be screened for GI-related symptoms, including dysphagia, heartburn, or lower GI tract symptoms (Chow et al., 2016).

Bone health. Childhood survivors of HSCT are at risk for reduced bone mineral density (BMD) and AVN. Risk factors for low BMD include younger age at diagnosis and transplant, White ethnicity, and GvHD therapy, including corticosteroids, methotrexate, and calcineurin inhibitors. TBI and craniospinal radiation are also risk factors. Growth hormone deficiency, hyperthyroidism, and hypogonadism can negatively affect bone density. AVN, which commonly affects the hips and knee joints, has been associated with age 5 years or older at transplant, female, malignancy diagnosis, myeloablative conditioning, and corticosteroid exposure.

COG recommends a BMD evaluation with either dual energy x-ray absorptiometry or quantitative CT scanning at 1 year posttransplant if patients meet the age requirement and then if clinically indicated after that time. Endocrine evaluation is indicated for children with a BMD z score 2+ standard deviations below the mean for age or if they have multiple fractures (Chow et al., 2016).

Skin. Patients who have received XRT and those having experience chronic GvHD of the skin are at higher risk of developing skin cancer, including melanoma. The skin is the most common organ affected in chronic GvHD. As described, skin manifestations can be numerous, including sclerosis of the skin. Associated changes (e.g., alopecia, nail dystrophy, vitiligo) may develop, which may be quite visible and have the potential to impact patients' quality of life.

COG recommends those patients with a history of TBI and chronic GvHD have annual full skin exams. Examination of the hair, nails, and external genitalia should be included for those with a history of chronic GvHD. Protecting skin from the sun and avoidance of tanning booths is recommended (Chow et al., 2016).

Immunologic. A number of patients continue to be at risk for infectious complications for a long period of time posttransplant. This is especially true for patients with chronic GvHD who are functionally asplenic and may have T- and/or B-cell dysfunction. This may result in hypogammaglobulinemia and secretory IgA deficiency. Patients who receive rituximab used for a number of transplant complications, including chronic GvHD and immune-related thrombocytopenia, may have B-cell aplasia. Similarly, CAR-T therapy (Kymriah), used for relapsed ALL posttransplantation, results in B-cell aplasia. These patients may require IVIG therapy to keep IgG levels above 400 mg/dL.

COG recommendations include the following:
- Use antibiotic prophylaxis against encapsulated organisms for those with active chronic GVHD.
- Those with a history of chronic GvHD should have annual history and physicals that assess for chronic conjunctivitis, sinopulmonary infections, and recurrent unusual severe infections.
- Screen for HIV and hepatitis C if exposed to blood products before universal virus testing of blood products.
- Survivors should receive vaccination according to standardized guidelines.

Secondary malignancies. Childhood survivors are at risk for the devasting complication of secondary malignancy. For those surviving 10 years or more after an allogeneic transplant, the risk of death from a subsequent neoplasm ranges from 5% to 12% (Wingard et al., 2011). Data show that posttransplant allogeneic patients' risk for developing cancer is higher than the general population (Tichelli et al., 2009). CIBMTR data show that in 2018–2019 the cause of death in autologous and allogeneic transplants under age 18 years at greater than 100 days posttransplant was 1% and 3%, respectively (Auletta et al., 2019).

Malignancies fall into three categories: lymphoma or lymphoproliferative disorder (PTLD), hematologic malignancies (MDS/AML), and solid tumors.

PTLD is a rare complication that most often occurs early (within 6 months of transplant) but has been reported to occur as many as 8 years post-HSCT (Majhail et al., 2012). It is highly associated with EBV infection. Prompt treatment of EBV viremia with rituximab (anti-CD20 monoclonal antibody therapy) is given to prevent the development of PTLD.

Development of secondary leukemia is reported to occur more commonly after an autologous transplant, while solid tumors appear to be more common after an allogeneic transplant (Chow et al., 2016). The transplant-related risk factors in the development of MDS include older age, TBI, use of PBSC, and large cumulative doses of alkylating agents (Pedersen-Bjergaard et al., 2000). Numerous types of solid tumors (oral, brain, thyroid, bone, soft tissue, skin cancers) are reported after transplant, and the risk increases with time from transplantation (Majhail et al., 2012). Risk factors include TBI and chronic

GvHD. Specific transplantable diseases or underlying conditions may be at greater risk of developing specific types of cancers. One example is patients with Fanconi anemia, who tend to have a higher incidence of squamous cell carcinomas. Patients and parents should be advised regarding the risk of developing secondary malignancies; routine screening and monitoring be performed in addition to avoidance of behaviors that could contribute to cancer development, such as tobacco use or unprotected sun exposure. For patients who received radiation to the chest or TBI, it is recommended that breast cancer screening starts at an earlier age (25 years or 8 years after radiation, whichever occurs later) but no later than age 40 years.

Neurocognitive. Research on neurocognitive effects in children who have completed HSCT is limited and often conflicting (Buchbinder et al., 2018). There are few prospective longitudinal studies to fully understand the long-term effects and how they evolve (Kelly et al., 2018). Potential transplant-specific risk factors cited include TBI and cranial radiation, calcineurin inhibitors, GvHD, infections (e.g., HHV-6, CMV, EBV), and primary disease that may already affect neurocognitive functions (e.g., adrenoleukodystrophy, SCD).

Previous therapies, underlying conditions, age at the time of transplant, parental support, and socioeconomic status all have the potential to influence neurocognitive functioning (Parris et al., 2020).

Based on limited available data, COG has the following recommendations:
- Screen all pediatric transplant patients yearly for educational and/or vocational progress.
- Formal neuropsychological evaluations should be considered at 1 year posttransplant for those with concerns.
- Survivors with neurocognitive deficits should be referred to a school liaison or a medical center that can assist in acquiring educational resources and/or social skills training.

Condition-Specific Screening/Monitoring
Physical examinations, laboratory studies, and procedures such as bone marrow biopsies or lumbar punctures are usually obtained at the transplant center or medical center of the referring subspecialist during the first year after HSCT. After the first year, the HSCT recipient may return to the transplant center only every few months or less often. Generally, each HSCT recipient will have an annual evaluation to assess for transplant-related complications and late effects. This may be done at the transplant center; they may also utilize local providers to assist in the evaluations and will include subspecialists, including an endocrinologist and ophthalmologist, as well as periodic echocardiograms and pulmonary function tests. Additional specialists may be required according to the child's

underlying disease. For example, children with Hurler syndrome require orthopedic evaluations, and patients with dyskeratosis congenita will have regular dermatology and pulmonary follow-ups.

Screening for Late Complications

The primary care provider plays a key role in screening for possible complications and late effects of treatment. Once the child returns to the community, it is the primary care provider's familiarity with late complications of HSCT (Table 12.10) and clinical manifestations of chronic GVHD (Table 12.11) that can aid in early recognition of potential problems and result in prompt consultation with the transplant team or referring subspecialist.

COMMON ILLNESS MANAGEMENT

Differential Diagnosis

Infection. Children who are immunocompromised may not be able to mount a typical response to infection (e.g., fever, erythema, edema) and therefore may not manifest signs and symptoms despite the presence of a true infection. A child who is still immunocompromised or taking immunosuppressants following HSCT is susceptible to complications from the common community-acquired respiratory viruses, including RSV,

adenovirus, influenza, parainfluenza, rhinovirus, and COVID-19, which can result in lower respiratory tract pneumonia or pneumonitis. In the early transplant period, when patients continue to be immunocompromised, it is important to limit exposures to ill persons by restricting contact with large groups of people. This may include schools, churches, theaters, concerts, airplane travel, or waiting rooms at medical offices. It is common for patients with HSCT to wear masks when out in public.

Guidelines for fever management may differ according to the transplanting institution. The arrangement and directions of what to do in the case of a fever should be communicated to the patient and/or parent and primary care office before the patient returns home from the transplant center. This will expedite the plans and avoid confusion and miscommunication if a fever develops. Patients and parents should be taught when and who to call when a fever or other concerning symptoms develop. Children within the first year of transplant or those still taking immunosuppressive medication should consult with the transplant team for any fevers. This may involve seeing the primary care provider, going to the emergency room, or seeing the transplant team. The primary care provider may be asked to provide the initial evaluation if the child lives more than 1 hour from

Table **12.10**	Late Complications of HSCT			
SYSTEM	**COMPLICATION**	**RISK FACTORS**	**PREVENTION/MONITORING**	**TREATMENT**

Immune	Infections	Immunosuppressants
		GvHD
		Inadequate immune
		   reconstitution
		Donor source
		Presence of central lines
			Prophylaxis with antibiotics,
			   antifungals, and antivirals
			PJP prophylaxis
			Consider functional asplenia
			Optimization of matching
			Donor selection
			Immunizations
				Targeted antimicrobials for
				   specific infections
				IVIG infusions for low IgG
				   levels

	Autoimmune
	   disorders
	(i.e., immune-
	   mediated
	   thrombocytopenia,
	   Evans syndrome)
		GvHD	Optimization of matching	IVIG, Promacta, rituximab,
				   steroids

Endocrine	Hypothyroidism	TBI, radiotherapy to
		   head/neck/mantle,
		   select chemotherapy
			Fractionation of TBI
			Annual thyroid screening
				Thyroid replacement

	Hypoadrenalism	Prolonged corticosteroid
		   use
		cALD diagnosis
			Use of steroid-sparing agents
			Stress dosing of steroids for
			   illness, procedures, fevers
				ACTH stimulation test-
				   ing—monitor status

	Gonadal failure	TBI, intensive
		   chemotherapy
			Sperm banking
			Ovarian and testicular tissue
			   preservation
				Hormone replacement
				   therapy

	Short stature	Prolonged corticosteroid use Specific diseases (Hurler syndrome)	Use of steroid-sparing agents	Growth hormone

Continued

| Table 12.10 | Late Complications of HSCT—cont'd |

SYSTEM	COMPLICATION	RISK FACTORS	PREVENTION/MONITORING	TREATMENT
Skeletal	Osteopenia/ osteoporosis	Prolonged corticosteroid use	Minimize steroid use Screening bone density scan, exercise, bisphosphonates, ovarian hormone replacement	Bisphosphonates Adequate calcium and vitamin D levels
	Avascular necrosis	Corticosteroid usage, male	Minimization of steroids	Joint replacement
Liver	GvHD	HLA disparity	Immunosuppressants	Immunosuppressants
	Hepatitis B or C		Hepatitis vaccines	Antiviral therapies
	Iron overload	Frequent red cell transfusions	Limit transfusions Monitor ferritin MRI of the liver (Ferriscan) Liver biopsy	Chelation therapy Therapeutic phlebotomy
Cardiac	Low ejection fraction cardiomyopathy, CHF	Anthracyclines TBI Chest radiation Iron overload	Monitor BP, cardiac rhythm with annual check Echocardiogram frequency based on exposures Reduce modifiable cardiovascular risk factors (smoking, diabetes, dyslipidemia), weight loss	Cardiology referral Pacemaker, surgical intervention
Renal	Acute or chronic renal failure	Medication induced (calcineurin inhibitors)	Suspend or adjust dosing of nephrotoxic drugs Adapt dosage of calcineurin inhibitors or change agent	Dialysis Renal transplant
Respiratory tract	Bronchiolitis obliterans infection	GvHD Immunosuppressants TBI	Pulmonary function testing High-resolution CT scan Follow vaccination schedule Avoid risk of exposures Avoid smoking	Steroids, GvHD treatment of lungs (fluticasone, azithromycin, montelukast) Treatment of infections
Eyes	Cataract formation	TBI, prolonged steroids Specific diseases (Hurler syndrome)	Slit lamp exam	Surgical repair
	Keratoconjunctivitis	GvHD Irradiation Infection	Ophthalmologic assessment (Schirmer testing, tear breakup time)	Artificial tears, cyclosporine ophthalmic solution, punctual plugs, lens implants, systemic treatment of GvHD
Musculature	Myopathy	Corticosteroid therapy	Decrease use of steroids Exercise, physical therapy	Decrease use of steroids Exercise, physical therapy
	Myositis	Chronic GvHD	GvHD: assess range of motion, exercise, physical therapy	Systemic treatment of chronic GvHD
Dentition and oral cavity	Cavities Sicca syndrome, oral GvHD	Chronic GvHD TBI	Dental hygiene, routine dental exams	Topical oral treatments Systemic treatment of GvHD
Malignancy	Secondary cancers	Chemotherapy, TBI Disease predisposition to cancer	Cancer screenings, mammography in females, self-exams (breast, skin, oral mucosa) Regular clinical assessments	Early detection Treatment of malignancy
	Relapse	High-risk disease	Disease surveillance exams Donor chimerism Blood counts and peripheral smears	Treatment of underlying malignancy Second transplant alternative treatment (i.e., CAR-T) Palliative care if appropriate

ACTH, Adrenocorticotropic hormone; *BP,* blood pressure; *cALD,* cerebral adrenoleukodystrophy; *CAR-T,* chimeric antigen receptor T cell; *CHF,* congestive heart failure; *CT,* computed tomography; *GvHD,* graft-versus-host disease; *HLA,* human leukocyte antigen; *HSCT,* hematopoietic stem cell transplantation; *IgG,* immunoglobulin G; *IVIG,* intravenous immunoglobulin; *MRI,* magnetic resonance imaging; *PJP, Pneumocystis jirovecii* pneumonia; *TBI,* total body irradiation.
From Tichelli et al., 2009.

Table 12.11   Clinical Manifestations of Chronic Graft-Versus-Host Disease (GvHD)

ORGAN	CLINICAL MANIFESTATION	EVALUATION	INTERVENTION
Skin	Erythematous papular rash (lichenoid) or thickened, tight, fragile skin (sclerodermatous)	Clinical and biopsy to confirm diagnosis of GvHD	Moisturize (petroleum jelly), treat local infections, protect from further trauma; topical steroid ointment may be used if it gives symptomatic relief to localized areas
Nails	Vertical ridging, fragile	Clinical	Nail polish may help decrease further damage
Sweat glands	Destruction leading to risk of hyperthermia		Avoid excessive heat
Hair	Scalp and body hair thin and fragile, can be partially or completely lost	Clinical	
Eyes	Dryness, photophobia, and burning	Regular ophthalmologic evaluation, including Schirmer test	Preservative-free tears during the day and preservative-free ointment at night
Mouth	Dry; sensitivity to mint, spicy food, tomato; whitish lacelike plaques in the cheeks and tongue identical to lichen planus; erythema and painful ulcerations, mucosal scleroderma with decreased sensitivity to temperature possible	Regular dental evaluation (with appropriate endocarditis prophylaxis); viral and fungal cultures at diagnosis and at any worsening	Avoid foods that are not tolerated; regular dental care preceded by appropriate endocarditis prophylaxis; topical steroid rinses followed by an antifungal agent for symptomatic relief
Respiratory tract	Bronchiolitis obliterans can manifest as dyspnea, wheezing, cough with normal computed tomography (CT) scan and marked obstruction at pulmonary function tests; chronic sinopulmonary symptoms and/or infections also common; with abnormal chest CT, must rule out infections; lung biopsy if clinically indicated	Pulmonary function tests, including FEV_1, FVC, DLCO, helium lung volumes; CT scan in symptomatic patients	Investigational therapy
Gastrointestinal	Abnormal motility and strictures; weight loss	Swallowing studies, endoscopy if clinically indicated; nutritional evaluation	No specific therapy is proven superior; FK-506 may concentrate in liver
Liver	Cholestasis (increased bilirubin, alkaline phosphatase); isolated liver involvement needs histologic confirmation	Liver function tests; liver biopsy if clinically indicated	No specific therapy is proven superior; FK-506 may concentrate in liver
Musculoskeletal	Fasciitis; myositis is rare; osteoporosis possible secondary to hormonal deficits, use of steroids, decreased activity	Periodical physical therapy evaluation to range of motion; bone density evaluation especially in patients using steroids	Aggressive physical therapy program
Immune system	Profound immunodeficiency; functional asplenia; high risk of pneumococcal sepsis, PCP, and invasive fungal infections; variable IgG levels	Assume all patients are severely immunocompromised and asplenic to 6 mo after GvHD has resolved	PCP prophylaxis (until 6 mo after no GvHD) and pneumococcal prophylaxis (lifetime); delay vaccinations
Hematopoietic system	Cytopenias; occasional eosinophilia	Counts; bone marrow aspirate and biopsy, antineutrophil and antiplatelet antibodies when indicated	Systemic treatment of GvHD
Others	Virtually all autoimmune diseases have been described in association with chronic GvHD	As clinically indicated	

DLCO, Diffusion capacity of lungs for carbon monoxide; *FEV$_1$,* forced expiratory volume in 1 sec; *FVC,* forced vital capacity; *IgG,* immunoglobulin G; *PCP, Pneumocystis jirovecii* (formerly *carinii*) pneumonia.

the transplant center. Children who are immunocompromised and receiving immunosuppressive medications or having a central venous catheter should be evaluated immediately to rule out an infection. A physical exam and laboratory analysis (including aerobic and anaerobic blood cultures peripherally and from each lumen of the central venous catheter) are performed, and a complete blood count is obtained. A urinalysis, urine culture, chest radiograph, throat culture, and nasal swab for rapid viral path testing are completed based on a patient's symptoms. Administration of antipyretics should be delayed until after the child is examined. Ibuprofen is avoided if thrombocytopenia or platelet function abnormality is suspected. Broad-spectrum IV antibiotics are generally initiated for a minimum of 48 hours if bacteremia is present or suspected. The antibiotic regimen is modified based on the organism identified and antimicrobial sensitivities. In these situations, admission to a hospital or transfer to the transplant center is often required. Decision making regarding management is usually completed collaboratively with the local physician and the HSCT specialist.

Children who are more than 1 year after HSCT, have demonstrated adequate immune recovery, are not on immunosuppressive medications, no longer have a central line, and have no evidence of GvHD may have less stringent fever management guidelines, and these should be communicated with those involved in the patient's care team.

Gastrointestinal symptoms. In the child who is immunocompromised, vomiting or diarrhea can be a sign of an opportunistic infection or GvHD, and therefore the transplant team should be consulted. Initially, a detailed history is provided regarding the volume of diarrhea within 24 hours, frequency, consistency, the appearance of the stool, odor, and any accompanying symptoms such as abdominal cramping, nausea, or pain. For a child with diarrhea, stool cultures, including bacterial, viral, and *C. diff*, should be obtained if the child is not able to keep down oral medications or immunosuppressive therapy because of vomiting. The transplant team should be contacted to discuss alternative forms of medication administration. Antiemetics are often prescribed on an as-needed basis and can be helpful in these situations. IV hydration should be considered for children with large fluid losses, symptoms of dehydration, and the inability to tolerate oral fluids.

Headache. Headache, although a common symptom in childhood and adolescence, can indicate a serious complication in the child who is immunocompromised following HSCT. The list of differential diagnoses is lengthy and includes infection, hypertension, dehydration, medication-induced toxicities, intracranial bleeding in those patients with severe thrombocytopenia, spinal fluid leak due to a recent lumbar puncture, and strain from impaired visual acuity. A detailed description of the headache is essential. If headaches are persistent or unusually severe, they should be evaluated, and consultation with the transplant provider is necessary.

Pain. A thorough history of the location, onset, precipitating factors, and qualities of the pain will help identify the cause in most children after HSCT. Because of the immunocompromised status of these children, the differential diagnosis primarily focuses on infectious etiology. Assessments should involve examination of the skin and oral pharynx for lesions. Herpes zoster can cause neuropathy and pain in a dermatomal distribution before visible vesicle formation and should be considered when children describe pain on the skin in a single dermatome. Mild myalgias are common as the child's activity level improves posttransplant.

Additionally, neuropathic pain secondary to chemotherapy may be present for some time following the transplant. Parents may have been advised to limit the acetaminophen and/or ibuprofen until they consult with the medical team. This is due to the concern about masking a fever in an immunocompromised patient. Pain that is persistent or severe requires a complete history and physical exam.

Rashes. Rashes and/or skin changes are commonly seen in patients following transplant. The differential diagnoses are many, but common reasons following transplant can be medication side effects, new environmental exposures, infections, eczema, extreme dryness, and GvHD of the skin. Assessment of the skin by a transplant provider is generally necessary for allogeneic transplant recipients. Digital photos or telemedicine appointments can be helpful for patients who are at a distance from the transplant center until the patient can be seen in person.

Medication Administration/Adherence/Drug Interactions

Children are administered multiple medications following HSCT. The regimens can be complex, and timeliness and accuracy of administration can be challenging for both older children and parents. Small studies have indicated poor adherence to the complex schedules following pediatric HSCT (McGrady et al., 2014; Pai et al., 2018). The addition of any medications, prescriptive or over the counter, increases the risk of drug interactions. Children who have received an allogeneic transplant usually receive cyclosporine or tacrolimus to prevent GvHD for months. The addition or discontinuation of other medications can greatly affect the absorption or clearance of these medications, causing a change in serum drug levels that can lead to organ toxicity or the development of GvHD. Primary care providers should consult the transplant team before prescribing or advising additional medications for these children. Families are also asked to disclose the use of any over-the-counter medications or CAM therapies. Reinforcing information that starting and stopping medication should be discussed with the transplant provider is also helpful. Most transplant teams include a pharmacist, who is a valuable resource when discussing medication changes and drug interactions.

Parents and families can utilize written medication schedules or electronic medication organizers to ensure medications are taken on time. Alarms can be set for medication reminders. In the early days of posttransplant there may be frequent medications that can be difficult to track. Reviewing a complete list of medications at each medical visit can help avoid medication errors or compliance concerns.

DEVELOPMENTAL ISSUES
Sleep Patterns
It is not uncommon for children recovering from HSCT to have disturbances in their sleep. Transitioning to sleeping at home versus a hospital setting is difficult. Both child and parent may have trouble adjusting if they are not in the same room as is typical in the hospital. Young children become accustomed to a parent with them at all times, and parents want to make sure they are available if they are needed quickly during the night. Children who are discharged on IV therapies or enteral feeds have their sleep interrupted by the noise and alarms of the pumps. Trouble getting to or staying asleep related to anxiety and altered sleep hours is a common complaint. Initiating and/or restoring good sleep routines and hygiene can be helpful. Steroids, which are commonly used to treat GvHD, can contribute to insomnia. Healthy sleep routines should be initiated when returning home, such as keeping a predictable bedtime routine, planning quiet activities in the evening, and avoiding overstimulating screen time, including video games and movies. For older children or teenagers, keeping phones or other devices off or outside the bedroom can be considered.

Toileting
In very young children it is common to see regression in toileting skills during and after hospitalization. Most often when the child's health improves and routines are reestablished, this regression resolves. Diarrhea, commonly seen posttransplant, can make toileting challenging for all patients. Older children and adolescents are often concerned with privacy and show embarrassment around issues related to urinating or stooling. This can make it challenging for the provider to fully understand the extent of issues such

as diarrhea or constipation. Taking extra care to allow for privacy and respectfully explaining the importance of understanding this aspect of care is a strategy to use with this population.

Discipline
Discipline can be challenging during the time of HSCT. In many cases, families have dealt with the child's condition and prognosis for months or years prior to transplantation. Patterns of discipline and behavior are often well established prior to hospitalization for HSCT. Because of the severity of the illness and the difficulty of treatment, parents may be more indulgent and less strict during this time as compared to their other children. It is sometimes hard to distinguish normal developmental behaviors, such as crying or tantrums, from medication-induced behavioral changes (e.g., behavioral changes associated with corticosteroids). Fear and anxiety related to painful procedures, prognosis, and isolation may contribute to unusual reactions or difficult behaviors. This can occur in both young and older adolescent children. Relationships between siblings, the transplant recipient, and parents are also affected by the change in routine. The primary care provider can be instrumental in helping facilitate normalcy within the family by reviewing with parents age-appropriate behavior, development, limit setting, and discipline. Parents should strive to achieve consistency in limit setting and discipline for all children in the household.

Child Care
Children who have received HSCT and are immunocompromised should avoid child care settings because of the risk of developing common community-acquired respiratory viruses or other communicable infections. If child care is required, in-home care is preferred.

Schooling
School plays a very important role in the development of a child. The transplant team, referring center, and parents should work together to ensure alternative forms of education during the child's hospitalization and the period of protective isolation after the transplant. This period may last between 6 and 12 months and may be longer for children with significant post-HSCT complications. Arrangements should be made for home study or hospital-based schooling until adequate immune function has been achieved. Virtual learning often allows for flexibility in timing and can allow patients to move at their own pace. The extended period of absence from school may result in school reentry difficulties. Factors found to influence the experience of reintegration to school include the following: structural support (continuity of education, supportive facilities, social, legal advice, and family-oriented rehabilitation program), health status (risk of infection, limited physical energy, and long-term

consequences), intrapersonal aspects (attitude of parents, character of the child), and social network (peer contact during treatment, supportive peers, supportive staff [teachers]). Another qualitative study examining adolescents and young adults returning to school and work after HSCT cite motivators to return, including feeling left behind, danger in dwelling on the medical experience, salvaging "my old life," a number of barriers to reentry (e.g., fatigue, cognitive difficulties, susceptibility to illness), and impact of breaks in school experiences (Brauer et al., 2017).

It should be recognized that not only do children and parents require assistance with the reentry process, but teachers and school staff also need to be considered when survivors of HSCT return to school (Inhestern et al., 2020). Teachers report that close contact with family and students, providing personalized attention, and receiving knowledge about the disease and ways to facilitate reentry would be helpful as they work with childhood cancer survivors (Galán et al., 2021).

Based on these findings, appropriate strategies that support successful reintegration should be employed. Consideration should be given to preparing patients and families prior to the transition, enabling continuous education in some form during the transplant process, finding ways to stay in touch with peers, and keeping open communication with peers and school staff to mobilize social support (Brauer et al., 2017). It should be recognized that children may return to school looking different than before (alopecia, wearing a mask, weight loss or gain). They may be more fatigued and need to take extra breaks. Preparing teachers and other students ahead of time is sometimes done through school visits from members of the transplant team. Children generally are encouraged to return to in-person school when protective isolation is no longer required. To the best of their abilities, they are encouraged to participate fully in all activities and classes, including physical education. Easily fatigued children may initially reenter school for a partial half-day and then transition to full-time hours. Parents are encouraged to meet with school counselors and teachers prior to resuming classes, and an individualized education program, including cognitive and behavioral evaluations, should be considered.

Sexuality

Many physical changes occur in children and young adults during and after transplantation secondary to surgery, medication side effects, transplant-related complications, and late effects. These changes can have negative effects on self-image. Fortunately, many of these changes are temporary, lasting only months, but others may be permanent. Physical changes may include alopecia, cushingoid features, scarring, striae, significant weight gain or loss, skin dyspigmentation, short stature, and hirsutism. The physical signs and symptoms of chronic GvHD may take years to improve or may never completely resolve.

Children who receive TBI during their preparative regimen are likely to be infertile because of the damaging effects of radiation on follicular development in ovaries and germinal epithelium in the testes. Small testicular volume and low to normal testosterone levels are seen in males after TBI, and some males will require testosterone therapy for pubertal progression and to maintain normal sexual function as young adults.

Delayed pubertal development may also affect self-esteem and peer acceptance. Adolescents who have received HSCT should have access to counseling. Sexually active young adults should be counseled on methods to reduce the risk of sexually transmitted infections and encouraged to practice cleanliness and safe sex with their partners. Barrier methods, particularly the use of condoms, should be encouraged. Intimate oral contact should be avoided until the mouth is completely healed.

Endocrine and fertility specialists play an important role before and after therapy for these children and young adults with a high rate of treatment-related infertility. Some children are often rendered infertile before referral for transplantation because of previous chemotherapy and irradiation. Optimally, children have been offered fertility preservation options when appropriate and in a timely manner before the start of treatment. This may include cryopreservation of unfertilized oocytes, sperm banking, ovarian tissue, and testicular tissue preservation. It must be recognized and communicated that the success of these preservation techniques is variable. Although many children and young adults are infertile after HSCT, successful pregnancies have occurred, and the likelihood of infertility should not be considered adequate birth control. Accordingly, appropriate birth control measures should be taken by sexually active young adults.

Genetic counseling should be offered for young adults who underwent HSCT for inherited conditions. Most transplant centers will have genetic counselors on staff. Initial genetic counseling may have been completed with parents at the time of diagnosis, but genetic counseling may be reintroduced as children reach an age where they can more fully understand their disease.

Transition to Adulthood

The struggle for independence for the adolescent is in sharp contrast to both the protective isolation before adequate immune recovery and the parent's need for close observation of their medically fragile adolescent. Transitioning responsibilities such as medication administration and scheduling appointments can be challenging for adolescents and their parents. Helping the adolescent prepare for that transition can be initiated at clinic visits. For example, questions about medical history, current health status, and medication reconciliation should be directed to the adolescent.

Normal adolescent issues still occur in young adults who have received HSCT. Practitioners caring for long-term survivors of HSCT should emphasize the importance of the routine use of sunscreen and abstinence from tobacco because of increased vulnerability to ultraviolet rays and carcinogens. Body piercing is not advised while the risk of developing GvHD or the immune system is still incompetent. Education focusing on a healthy lifestyle is important for these young adults. Maintaining a healthy weight, staying active with routine exercise, eating a varied diet, and limiting alcohol consumption may reduce the risk of further disease and complications as they age.

Focusing on education and future employment will be part of survivorship and moving into adulthood. In certain situations, community and national organizations may offer college scholarships to those who have undergone treatment for certain diseases. Social workers may have access to job training and career development services. Information about medical and life insurance is addressed during this time. Some childhood cancer survivor programs will apply to the HSCT population. For example, the Americans with Disabilities Act of 1990 protects any person diagnosed with cancer from discrimination in employment or housing and applies to many survivors of HSCT.

Family Concerns

HSCT is an intense and complicated form of treatment. Parents and children are often balancing the choice of potential long-term survival with the upfront risk of significant morbidity and mortality. The child and family face a series of intense stressors: the decision to accept the treatment, the search for a donor, the workup to determine the child's eligibility for transplant, enduring the cytotoxic preparative regimen followed by the anticlimactic infusion of the stem cells, the wait for blood count recovery, the potential for death from therapy-related complications, and discharge from the hospital and the eventual return home. Although transplant hospitalization is very stressful, parents often experience even more anxiety after discharge. Whereas nurses and doctors have been available to assess and treat their children, they now become responsible for administering daily medications and deciding what problems necessitate calling the transplant team. When children finally are allowed to return home, they may be at a significant distance from the security of the transplant team and medical center, and although they are home, their physical and social isolation has not ended.

Additionally, parents must now juggle their child's complex care with managing a household and meeting the needs of the other children and family members. Employment, child care, and financial constraints are also areas of stress during this time. Last, the threat of relapse or severe complications is ever present and looming. Providers often treat the entire family as they deal with the complexity of caring for someone who has undergone HSCT.

RESOURCES

Alex's Lemonade Stand Foundation for Childhood Cancer: www.alexslemonade.org
American Cancer Society: www.cancer.org
American Society for Transplantation and Cellular Therapy (for providers): www.astct.org
American Society of Clinical Oncology (for providers): www.asco.org
American Society of Hematology (for providers): www.hematology.org
Aplastic Anemia & MDS International Foundation: www.aamds.org
Association of Pediatric Hematology Oncology Nurses (for providers): www.aphon.org
Be The Match (for providers): https://bethematch.org
Blood and Marrow Transplant Information Network: www.BMTinfonet.org
Cancer.net (for parents): https://www.cancer.net
Children's Oncology Group: www.childrensoncologygroup.org
Cooley's Anemia Foundation: www.thalssemia.org
Dream Factory: https://www.dreamfactoryinc.org
Elephants and Tea (for parents): www.Elephantsandtea.com
Fanconi Anemia Research Fund: www.fanconi.org
Foundation for the Accreditation of Cellular Therapy (for providers): www.factglobal.org
Leukemia and Lymphoma Society: www.lls.org
Make-A-Wish: www.makeawish.org
National Clinical Trials Network: www.cancer.gov/research/infrastructure/clinical-trials/nctn
National Coalition for Cancer Survivorship: www.canceradvocacy.org
National Comprehensive Cancer Network (for providers): www.nccn.org
National Marrow Donor Program: www.Bethematch.org
National MPS Society: https://mpssociety.org/learn/diseases/mps-i
National Organization for Rare Disorders: http://rarediseases.org
Oncology Nursing Society (for providers): https://www.ons.org/
Sickle Cell Disease Association of America: https://www.sicklecelldisease.org
Stupid Cancer (for parents): https://stupidcancer.org

Summary

Primary Care Needs for the Child With Bone Marrow Transplant

HEALTH CARE MAINTENANCE
Growth and Development
- Height and weight should be measured at each visit and plotted on standard growth curve forms. Hypothyroidism and hormone deficiencies are common side effects of chemotherapy and radiation therapy.
- Children who receive transplants before puberty will often experience a delay in the onset and progression of puberty. Tanner staging should be done at each visit. Hormone replacement therapy may be needed for both males and females.
- Cognitive development has had limited studies in children with bone marrow transplants. Risks of cognitive impairment are similar to those of children with cancer receiving similar chemotherapy and radiation, especially cranial radiation and intrathecal chemotherapy.

Diet
- Optimal nutrition is required for healing and to maximize growth.
- A post-HSCT diet is instituted to reduce the risk of infection by avoiding foods with potential vectors for infection, such as unpasteurized products and undercooked meats.
- Nutritional support via enteral therapy or TPN is often needed for a few weeks after discharge. Occasionally children will have G-tube placement.
- Children receiving steroids may be placed on a low-sodium diet to reduce hypertension and calcium supplements to reduce the risk of osteopenia.

Safety
- Anticipatory guidance is important, especially for parents who had only parented when their child was sick and now must care for a more active and mobile child.
- Hand washing to prevent the spread of infections is critical. Eating utensils, cups, and glasses should not be shared.
- Avoid ill contacts and large groups of people while the child's immune system is suppressed.
- All medicines should be stored safely away from children, and needles and syringes should be deposited in a sharps container.

- The child should avoid pet care involving feces or litter boxes. Contact with certain pets, such as turtles and reptiles, is not recommended during immunosuppression.
- Physical activity may be restricted in children with thrombocytopenia.
- Travel to developing countries is not advised. Travel away from the transplant center should be arranged with the knowledge of the transplant team.

Immunizations
- Most children lose their immunity to previously administered vaccines following HSCT. Reimmunization often begins 1 year after transplant if there is no evidence of GvHD, and the child is not receiving steroids.
- Live virus vaccines pose the risk of active disease and are not administered until at least 2 years posttransplant.
- Influenza vaccine should be given annually to the child, all household or close contacts, and clinic and hospital personnel.

Screening
- *Vision.* An ophthalmologist familiar with the sequelae of high-dose chemotherapy and radiation should be involved in care.
  - Corticosteroid use can cause cataracts, chronic GvHD can result in keratoconjunctivitis, and CMV can cause retinitis.
  - Vision should be screened at each primary care visit, and a referral should be made for visual changes or abnormalities.
- *Hearing.* Routine screening is advised. Hearing loss may occur as a result of ototoxic drug therapy.
- *Dental.* Dental screening and restorative care should be done before the transplant to reduce potential sources of infection. Routine dental care should be resumed once the child's immune system is restored.
- *Blood pressure.* Take and record at each visit. Parents may be instructed to record blood pressure at home.
  - Steroids, calcineurin inhibitors, and nephrotoxic agents, which are commonly administered for post-HSCT, contribute to hypertension and the need for antihypertensive medications.

REFERENCES

Abel, G. A., Kim, H. T., Zackon, I., Alyea, E. P., Bailey, A., Winters, J. P., Meehan, K. R., Reagan, J. L., Walsh, J., Faggen, M., Sinclair, S., Joyce, A., Close, S., Emmert, A., Kallassy, I., Koreth, J., Antin, J. H., Cutler, C., Ho, V. T., & Soiffer, R. J. (2022). Non-relapse mortality and quality of life with shared care after allogeneic hematopoietic cell transplantation: A randomized control trial. *Blood, 140*(Supplement 1), 2135–2136. https://doi.org/10.1182/blood-2022-166996.

Al-Farsi, N., & Al Jabri, S. (2022). Cytomegalovirus retinitis in children post hematopoietic stem cell transplantation: Can we develop a screening protocol? *Oman Journal of Ophthalmology, 15,* 1–2.

Aljurf, M., Weisdorf, D., Alfraih, F., Szer, J., Müller, C., Confer, D., Hashmi, S., Kröger, N., Shaw, B. E., Greinix, H., Kharfan-Dabaja, M. A., Foeken, L., Seber, A., Ahmed, S., El-Jawahri, A., Al-Awwami, M., Atsuta, Y., Pasquini, M., Hanbali, A., … El Fakih, R. (2019). Worldwide Network for Blood &

Marrow Transplantation (WBMT) special article, challenges facing emerging alternate donor registries. *Bone Marrow Transplantation, 54*(8), 1179–1188. doi:10.1038/s41409-019-0476-6. Epub 2019 Feb 18. PMID: 30778127; PMCID: PMC6760540.

Alonso, C. D., Maron, G., Kamboj, M., Carpenter, P. A., Gurunathan, A., Mullane, K. M., & Dubberke, E. R. (2022). American Society for Transplantation and Cellular Therapy series: #5-Management of Clostridioides difficile infection in hematopoietic cell transplant recipients. *Transplantation and Cellular Therapy, 28*(5), 225–232. doi:10.1016/j.jtct.2022.02.013. Epub 2022 Feb 22. PMID: 35202891.

Armenian, S. H., Sun, C. L., Kawashima, T., Arora, M., Leisenring, W., Sklar, C. A., Baker, K. S., Francisco, L., Teh, J. B., Mills, G., Wong, F. L., Rosenthal, J., Diller, L. R., Hudson, M. M., Oeffinger, K. C., Forman, S. J., Robison, L. L., & Bhatia, S. (2011). Long-term health-related outcomes in survivors of childhood cancer treated with HSCT versus conventional therapy: A report from the Bone Marrow Transplant Survivor Study (BMTSS) and Childhood Cancer Survivor Study (CCSS). *Blood*, 118(5), 1413–1420. doi:10.1182/blood-2011-01-331835. Epub 2011 Jun 7. PMID: 21652685; PMCID: PMC3152502.

Auletta J. J., Kou J., Chen M., & Shaw B. E. (2019, September 19). Summary slides & reports. Retrieved March 29, 2023, from https://cibmtr.org/CIBMTR/Resources/Summary-Slides-Reports.

Barbar, R., Hayden, R., Sun, Y., Tang, L., & Hakim, H. (2021). Epidemiologic and clinical characteristics of Clostridioides difficile infections in hospitalized and outpatient pediatric oncology and hematopoietic stem cell transplant patients. *Pediatric Infectious Disease Journal*, 40(7), 655–662. https://doi.org/10.1097/inf.0000000000003126.

Barrett, A. J., Prockop, S., & Bollard, C. M. (2018). Virus-specific T cells: Broadening applicability. *Biology of Blood and Marrow Transplantation*, 24(1), 13–18. https://doi.org/10.1016/j.bbmt.2017.10.004.

BeTheMatch.org. (n.d.). Food safety. Donate marrow or blood stem cells. Retrieved March 29, 2023, from https://bethematch.org/patients-and-families/life-after-transplant/physical-health-and-recovery/food-safety/.

Boettcher, M., Joechner, A., Li, Z., Yang, S. F., & Schlegel, P. (2022). Development of CAR T Cell therapy in children-A comprehensive overview. *Journal of Clinical Medicine*, 11(8), 2158. doi:10.3390/jcm11082158.

Bonifazi, F., Barbato, F., Ravaioli, F., Sessa, M., Defrancesco, I., Arpinati, M., Cavo, M., & Colecchia, A. (2020). Diagnosis and treatment of VOD/SOS after allogeneic hematopoietic stem cell transplantation. *Frontiers in Immunology*, 11, 489. https://doi.org/10.3389/fimmu.2020.00489.

Brauer, E. R., Pieters, H. C., Ganz, P. A., Landier, W., Pavlish, C., & Heilemann, M. S. V. (2017). Snail mode to rocket ship mode: Adolescents and young adults' experiences of returning to work and school after hematopoietic cell transplantation. *Journal of Adolescent and Young Adult Oncology*, 6(4), 551–559. https://doi.org/10.1089/jayao.2017.0025.

Brodigan, K., Kapadia, M., Frazier, A. L., Laufer, M. R., Yu, R., Weil, B. R., Ginsburg, E. S., Duncan, C., & Lehmann, L. (2021). Safety of surgical fertility preservation procedures in children prior to hematopoietic stem cell transplant. *Transplantation and Cellular Therapy*, 27(8), 696.e1–696.e4. https://doi.org/10.1016/j.jtct.2021.04.001.

Buchbinder, D., Kelly, D. L., Duarte, R. F., Auletta, J. J., Bhatt, N., Byrne, M., DeFilipp, Z., Gabriel, M., Mahindra, A., Norkin, M., Schoemans, H., Shah, A. J., Ahmed, I., Atsuta, Y., Basak, G. W., Beattie, S., Bhella, S., Bredeson, C., Bunin, N., ... & Shaw B. E. (2018). Neurocognitive dysfunction in hematopoietic cell transplant recipients: Expert review from the late effects and Quality of Life Working Committee of the CIBMTR and complications and Quality of Life Working Party of the EBMT. *Bone Marrow Transplant*, 53(5), 535–555. doi:10.1038/s41409-017-0055-7. Epub 2018 Jan 17. PMID: 29343837; PMCID: PMC5985976.

Carnevale-Schianca, F., Caravelli, D., Gallo, S., Becco, P., Paruzzo, L., Poletto, S., Polo, A., Mangioni, M., Salierno, M., Berger, M., Pessolano, R., Saglio, F., Gottardi, D., Rota-Scalabrini, D., Grignani, G., Fizzotti, M., Ferrero, I., Frascione, P. M. M., D'Ambrosio, L., Gaidano, V., ... Fagioli, F. (2021). Post-transplant cyclophosphamide and tacrolimus—mycophenolate mofetil combination governs GVHD and immunosuppression need, reducing late toxicities in allogeneic peripheral blood hematopoietic cell transplantation from HLA-matched donors. *Journal of Clinical Medicine*, 10(6), 1173. https://doi.org/10.3390/jcm10061173.

Centers for Disease Control and Prevention. (2022, October 13). Current guideline. Retrieved March 29, 2023, from https://www.cdc.gov/transplantsafety/hc-providers/guidelines.html.

Cheng, L., Duan, M., Mao, X., Ge, Y., Wang, Y., & Huang, H. (2021). The effect of digital health technologies on managing symptoms across pediatric cancer continuum: A systematic review. *International Journal of Nursing Sciences*, 8(1), 22–29. https://doi.org/10.1016/j.ijnss.2020.10.002.

Choi, Y. B., Yi, E. S., Lee, J. W., Sung, K. W., Koo, H. H., & Yoo, K. H. (2017). Immunosuppressive therapy versus alternative donor hematopoietic stem cell transplantation for children with severe aplastic anemia who lack an HLA-matched familial donor. *Bone Marrow Transplantation*, 52(1), 47–52. https://doi.org/10.1038/bmt.2016.223.

Chow, E. J., Anderson, L., Baker, K. S, Bhatia, S., Guilcher, G. M., Huang, J. T., Pelletier, W., Perkins, J. L., Rivard, L. S., Schechter, T., Shah, A. J., Wilson, K. D., Wong, K., Grewal, S. S., Armenian, S. H., Meacham, L. R., Mulrooney, D. A., & Castellino, S. M. (2016). Late effects surveillance recommendations among survivors of childhood hematopoietic cell transplantation: A children's oncology group report. *Biology of Blood and Marrow Transplantation*, 22(5), 782–95. doi:10.1016/j.bbmt.2016.01.023.

Christopherson, U., Wells, S. J., Parker, N., Lyons, E. J., Swartz, M. D., Blozinski, A., Basen-Engquist, K., Peterson, S., & Swartz, M. C. (2021). Use of active video games with or without videoconferencing on health outcomes in adolescent and young adult cancer survivors: a systematic review. *Journal of cancer survivorship: Research and Practice*, 16(4), 714–727. https://doi.org/10.1007/s11764-021-01065-z.

Cima, L. N., Martin, S. C., Lambrescu, I. M., Stejereanu, L., Zaharia, C., Colita, A., & Fica, S. (2018). Long-term thyroid disorders in pediatric survivors of hematopoietic stem cell transplantation after chemotherapy-only conditioning. *Journal of Pediatric Endocrinology and Metabolism*, 31(8), 869–878. https://doi.org/10.1515/jpem-2018-0020.

Committee on Bioethics. (2010). Children as hematopoietic stem cell donors. *Pediatrics*, 125(2), 392–404. https://doi.org/10.1542/peds.2009-3078.

Cornell, R. F., Hari, P., & Drobyski, W. R. (2015). Engraftment syndrome after autologous stem cell transplantation: An update unifying the definition and management approach. *Biology of Blood and Marrow Transplantation*, 21(12), 2061–2068. https://doi.org/10.1016/j.bbmt.2015.08.030.

Cuvelier, G. D. E., Schoettler, M., Buxbaum, N. P., Pinal-Fernandez, I., Schmalzing, M., Distler, J. H. W., Penack, O., Santomasso, B. D., Zeiser, R., Angstwurm, K., MacDonald, K. P. A., Kimberly, W. T., Taylor, N., Bilic, E., Banas, B., Buettner-Herold, M., Sinha, N., Greinix, H. T., Pidala, J., Schultz, K. R., ... Wolff, D. (2022). Toward a Better Understanding of the Atypical Features of Chronic Graft-Versus-Host Disease: A report from the 2020 National Institutes of Health Consensus Project Task Force. *Transplantation and Cellular Therapy*, 28(8), 426–445. https://doi.org/10.1016/j.jtct.2022.05.038.

Dehn, J., Spellman, S., Hurley, C. K., Shaw, B. E., Barker, J. N., Burns, L. J., Confer, D. L., Eapen, M., Fernandez-Vina, M., Hartzman, R., Maiers, M., Marino, S. R., Mueller, C., Perales, M. A., Rajalingam, R., & Pidala, J. (2019). Selection of unrelated donors and cord blood units for hematopoietic cell transplantation: guidelines from the NMDP/CIBMTR. *Blood*, 134(12), 924–934. https://doi.org/10.1182/blood.2019001212.

Dholaria, B., Savani, B. N., Labopin, M., Luznik, L., Ruggeri, A., Mielke, S., Al Malki, M. M., Kongtim, P., Fuchs, E., Huang, X. J., Locatelli, F., Aversa, F., Castagna, L., Bacigalupo, A., Martelli, M., Blaise, D., Ben Soussan, P., Arnault, Y., Handgretinger, R., Roy, D. C., ... Mohty, M. (2020). Clinical applications of donor lymphocyte infusion from an HLA-haploidentical donor: consensus recommendations from the Acute Leukemia Working Party of the EBMT. *Haematologica*, 105(1), 47–58. https://doi.org/10.3324/haematol.2019.219790.

Diesch-Furlanetto, T., Gabriel, M., Zajac-Spychala, O., Cattoni, A., Hoeben, B. A., & Balduzzi, A. (2021). Late effects after haematopoietic stem cell transplantation in all, long-term follow-up and transition: A step into adult life. *Frontiers in Pediatrics, 9.* https://doi.org/10.3389/fped.2021.773895.

Dietz, A. C., Savage, S. A., Vlachos, A., Mehta, P. A., Bresters, D., Tolar, J., Bonfim, C., Dalle, J. H., de la Fuente, J., Skinner, R., Boulad, F., Duncan, C. N., Baker, K. S., Pulsipher, M. A., Lipton, J. M., Wagner, J. E., & Alter, B. P. (2017). Late effects screening guidelines after hematopoietic cell transplantation for inherited bone marrow failure syndromes: Consensus statement from the Second Pediatric Blood and Marrow Transplant Consortium International Conference on Late Effects after Pediatric HCT. *Biology of Blood and Marrow Transplantation: Journal of the American Society for Blood and Marrow Transplantation, 23*(9), 1422–1428. https://doi.org/10.1016/j.bbmt.2017.05.022.

Diorio, C., Kelly, K. M., Afungchwi, G. M., Ladas, E. J., & Marjerrison, S. (2020). Nutritional traditional and complementary medicine strategies in pediatric cancer: A narrative review. *Pediatric Blood Cancer, 67*(S3). https://doi.org/10.1002/pbc.28324.

D'Souza, A., Fretham, C., Lee, S. J., Arora, M., Brunner, J., Chhabra, S., Devine, S., Eapen, M., Hamadani, M., Hari, P., Pasquini, M. C., Perez, W., Phelan, R. A., Riches, M. L., Rizzo, J. D., Saber, W., Shaw, B. E., Spellman, S. R., Steinert, P., Weisdorf, D. J., … Horowitz, M. M. (2020). Current use of and trends in hematopoietic cell transplantation in the United States. *Biology of Blood and Marrow Transplantation: Journal of the American Society for Blood and Marrow Transplantation, 26*(8), e177–e182. https://doi.org/10.1016/j.bbmt.2020.04.013.

Duong, H. K., Savani, B. N., Copelan, E., Devine, S., Costa, L. J., Wingard, J. R., Shaughnessy, P., Majhail, N., Perales, M. A., Cutler, C. S., Bensinger, W., Litzow, M. R., Mohty, M., Champlin, R. E., Leather, H., Giralt, S., & Carpenter, P. A. (2014). Peripheral blood progenitor cell mobilization for autologous and allogeneic hematopoietic cell transplantation: Guidelines from the American Society for Blood and Marrow Transplantation. *Biology of Blood and Marrow Transplantation, 20*(9), 1262–1273. https://doi.org/10.1016/j.bbmt.2014.05.003.

Evans, J. C., Hirani, S. P., & Needle, J. J. (2019). Nutritional and post-transplantation outcomes of enteral versus parenteral nutrition in pediatric hematopoietic stem cell transplantation: A systematic review of randomized and nonrandomized studies. *Biology of Blood and Marrow Transplantation, 25*(8). https://doi.org/10.1016/j.bbmt.2019.02.023.

Even-Or, E., NaserEddin, A., Dinur Schejter, Y., Shadur, B., Zaidman, I., & Stepensky, P. (2020). Haploidentical stem cell transplantation with post-transplant cyclophosphamide for osteopetrosis and other nonmalignant diseases. *Bone Marrow Transplantation, 56*(2), 434–441. https://doi.org/10.1038/s41409-020-01040-9.

Falcon, C. P., Broglie, L., Phelan, R., Choi, S. W., Auletta, J. J., & Chewning, J. H. (2020). Infection prophylaxis patterns following pediatric autologous hematopoietic stem cell transplantation: A survey of pediatric transplant and cell therapy consortium centers. *Pediatric Transplantation, 24*(8), e13821. doi:10.1111/petr.13821.

Fall-Dickson, J. M., Pavletic, S. Z., Mays, J. W., & Schubert, M. M. (2019). Oral complications of chronic graft-versus-host disease. *JNCI Monographs, 2019*(53). https://doi.org/10.1093/jncimonographs/lgz007.

Feins, S., Kong, W., Williams, E. F., Milone, M. C., & Fraietta, J. A. (2019). An introduction to chimeric antigen receptor (CAR) T-cell immunotherapy for human cancer. *American Journal of Hematology, 94*(S1). https://doi.org/10.1002/ajh.25418.

Foord, A. M., Cushing-Haugen, K. L., Boeckh, M. J., Carpenter, P. A., Flowers, M. E. D., Lee, S. J., Leisenring, W. M., Mueller, B. A., Hill, J. A., & Chow, E. J. (2020). Late infectious complications in hematopoietic cell transplantation survivors: A population-based study. *Blood Advances, 4*(7), 1232–1241. https://doi.org/10.1182/bloodadvances.2020001470.

Forlanini, F., Zinter, M. S., Dvorak, C. C., Bailey-Olson, M., Winestone, L. E., Shimano, K. A., Higham, C. S., Melton, A., Chu, J., & Kharbanda, S. (2022). Hematopoietic cell transplantation-comorbidity index score is correlated with treatment-related mortality and overall survival following second allogeneic hematopoietic cell transplantation in children. *Transplantation and Cellular Therapy, 28*(3), 155.e1–155.e8. https://doi.org/10.1016/j.jtct.2021.11.015.

Galán, S., Tomé-Pires, C., Roy, R., Castarlenas, E., Racine, M., Jensen, M. P., & Miró, J. (2021). Improving the quality of life of cancer survivors in school: Consensus recommendations using a Delphi study. *Children (Basel, Switzerland), 8*(11), 1021. https://doi.org/10.3390/children8111021.

Gardner, J., Courter, J., Dandoy, C. E., Davies, S. M., & Teusink-Cross A. (2022). Safety and efficacy of prophylactic levofloxacin in pediatric and adult hematopoietic stem cell transplant patients. *Transplantation and Cellular Therapy, 28*(3). https://doi.org/10.1016/s2666-6367(22)00294-9.

Gatza, E., Reddy, P., & Choi, S. W. (2020). Prevention and treatment of acute graft-versus-host disease in children, adolescents, and young adults. *Biology of Blood and Marrow Transplantation, 26*(5). https://doi.org/10.1016/j.bbmt.2020.01.004.

Gawade, P. L., Hudson, M. M., Kaste, S. C., Neglia, J. P., Constine, L. S., Robison, L. L., & Ness, K. K. (2014). A systematic review of dental late effects in survivors of childhood cancer. *Pediatric Blood & Cancer, 61*(3), 407–416. https://doi.org/10.1002/pbc.24842.

Goldsmith, S. R., Ghobadi, A., Dipersio, J. F., Hill, B., Shadman, M., & Jain, T. (2022). Chimeric antigen receptor T cell therapy versus hematopoietic stem cell transplantation: An evolving perspective. *Transplantation and Cellular Therapy, 28*(11), 727–736. https://doi.org/10.1016/j.jtct.2022.07.015.

Guerra, J. A., Dhall, G., Marachelian, A., Castillo, E., Malvar, J., Wong, K., Sposto, R., & Finlay, J. L. (2017). Marrow-ablative chemotherapy followed by tandem autologous hematopoietic cell transplantation in pediatric patients with malignant brain tumors. *Bone Marrow Transplantation, 52*(11), 1543–1548. https://doi.org/10.1038/bmt.2017.166.

Haider, S., Durairajan, N., & Soubani, A. O. (2020). Noninfectious pulmonary complications of haematopoietic stem cell transplantation. *European Respiratory Reviews, 29*(156), 190119. https://doi.org/10.1183/16000617.0119-2019.

Hakki, M., Aitken, S. L., Danziger-Isakov, L., Michaels, M. G., Carpenter, P. A., Chemaly, R. F., Papanicolaou, G. A., Boeckh, M., & Marty, F. M. (2021). American Society for Transplantation and Cellular Therapy Series: #3-Prevention of cytomegalovirus infection and disease after hematopoietic cell transplantation. *Transplantation and Cellular Therapy, 27*(9), 707–719. https://doi.org/10.1016/j.jtct.2021.05.001.

Hansen, M. D., Filipovich, A. H., Davies, S. M., Mehta, P., Bleesing, J., Jodele, S., Hayashi, R., Barnes, Y., & Shenoy, S. (2008). Allogeneic hematopoietic cell transplantation (HCT) in Hurler's syndrome using a reduced intensity preparative regimen. *Bone Marrow Transplant, 41*(4), 349–353. doi:10.1038/sj.bmt.1705926. Epub 2007 Nov 19. PMID: 18026148.

Harris, A. C., Young, R., Devine, S., Hogan, W. J., Ayuk, F., Bunworasate, U., Chanswangphuwana, C., Efebera, Y. A., Holler, E., Litzow, M., Ordemann, R., Qayed, M., Renteria, A. S., Reshef, R., Wölfl, M., Chen, Y. B., Goldstein, S., Jagasia, M., Locatelli, F., … Levine, J. E. (2016). International, multicenter standardization of acute graft-versus-host disease clinical data collection: A report from the mount sinai acute GVHD international consortium. *Biology of Blood and Marrow Transplantation, 22*(1), 4–10. doi:10.1016/j. bbmt.2015.09.001. Epub 2015 Sep 16. PMID: 26386318; PMCID: PMC4706482.

Haynes, A. S., Curtis, D. J., Campbell, K., Giller, R. H., Quinones, R. R., Verneris, M. R., & Abzug, M. J. (2021). An immune recovery-based revaccination protocol for pediatric hematopoietic stem cell transplant recipients: Revaccination outcomes following pediatric HSCT. *Transplantation and Cellular Therapy, 27*(4), 317–326. https://doi.org/10.1016/j. jtct.2021.01.017.

Heimall, J., Buckley, R. H., Puck, J., Fleisher, T. A., Gennery, A. R., Haddad, E., Neven, B., Slatter, M., Roderick, S., Baker, K. S., Dietz, A. C., Duncan, C., Griffith, L. M., Notarangelo, L., Pulsipher, M. A., & Cowan, M. J. (2017). Recommendations for screening and management of late effects in patients with severe combined immunodeficiency after allogenic hematopoietic cell transplantation: A consensus statement from the Second Pediatric Blood and Marrow Transplant Consortium International Conference on Late Effects after Pediatric HCT. *Biology of Blood and Marrow Transplantation: Journal of the American Society for Blood and Marrow Transplantation, 23*(8), 1229–1240. https://doi.org/10.1016/j. bbmt.2017.04.026.

Hiwarkar, P., Gajdosova, E., Qasim, W., Worth, A., Breuer, J., Chiesa, R., Ridout, D., Edelsten, C., Moore, A., Amrolia, P., Veys, P., & Rao, K. (2014). Frequent occurrence of cytomegalovirus retinitis during immune reconstitution warrants regular ophthalmic screening in high-risk pediatric allogeneic hematopoietic stem cell transplant recipients. *Clinical Infectious Diseases : An official publication of the Infectious Diseases Society of America, 58*(12), 1700–1706. https://doi. org/10.1093/cid/ciu201.

Hoag, J., Igler, E., Karst, J., Bingen, K., & Kupst, M. J. (2018). Decision-making, knowledge, and psychosocial outcomes in pediatric siblings identified to donate hematopoietic stem cells. *Journal of Psychosocial Oncology, 37*(3), 367–382. https:// doi.org/10.1080/07347332.2018.1489443.

Hoeben, B. A. W., Pazos, M., Seravalli, E., Bosman, M. E., Losert, C., Albert, M. H., Boterberg, T., Ospovat, I., Mico Milla, S., Demiroz Abakay, C., Engellau, J., Jóhannesson, V., Kos, G., Supiot, S., Llagostera, C., Bierings, M., Scarzello, G., Seiersen, K., Smith, E., Ocanto, A., … Janssens, G. O. (2022). ESTRO ACROP and SIOPE recommendations for myeloablative Total Body Irradiation in children. *Radiotherapy & Oncology: Journal of the European Society for Therapeutic Radiology and Oncology, 173*, 119–133. https://doi.org/10.1016/j.radonc.2022.05.027.

Hoegy, D., Bleyzac, N., Rochet, C., De Freminville, H., Rénard, C., Kébaili, K., Bertrand, Y., Dussart, C., & Janoly-Dumenil, A. (2019). Medication adherence after pediatric allogeneic stem cell transplantation: Barriers and facilitators. *European Journal of Oncology Nursing : The official journal of European Oncology Nursing Society, 38*, 1–7. https://doi.org/10.1016/j. ejon.2018.11.006.

Hutspardol, S., Essa, M., Richardson, S., Schechter, T., Ali, M., Krueger, J., Fujii, H., Egeler, R. M., & Gassas, A. (2015). Significant transplantation-related mortality from respiratory virus infections within the first one hundred days in children after hematopoietic stem cell transplantation. *Biology of Blood and Marrow Transplantation: Journal of the American Society for Blood and Marrow Transplantation, 21*(10), 1802–1807. https://doi. org/10.1016/j.bbmt.2015.06.015.

Inhestern, L., Peikert, M. L., Krauth, K. A., Escherich, G., Rutkowski, S., Kandels, D., & Bergelt, C. (2020). Parents' perception of their children's process of reintegration after childhood cancer treatment. *PLOS One, 15*(10), e0239967. https://doi.org/10.1371/journal.pone.0239967.

Jagasia, M. H., Greinix, H. T., Arora, M., Williams, K. M., Wolff, D., Cowen, E. W., Palmer, J., Weisdorf, D., Treister, N. S.,

Cheng, G. S., Kerr, H., Stratton, P., Duarte, R. F., McDonald, G. B., Inamoto, Y., Vigorito, A., Arai, S., Datiles, M. B., Jacobsohn, D., … Flowers, M. E. (2015). National institutes of health consensus development project on criteria for clinical trials in chronic graft-versus-host disease: I. The 2014 diagnosis and staging working group report. *Biology of Blood and Marrow Transplantation, 21*(3), 389–401.e1. doi:10.1016/j. bbmt.2014.12.001.

Jesudas, R., Malesky, A., Chu, R., Fischer, H., & Kamat, D. (2013). Reviewing the follow-up care of pediatric patients' status post–hematopoietic stem cell transplantation for the primary care pediatrician. *Clinical Pediatrics, 52*(6), 487–495. https:// doi.org/10.1177/0009922813483361.

Joshi, S., Savani, B. N., Chow, E. J., Gilleece, M. H., Halter, J., Jacobsohn, D. A., Pidala, J., Quinn, G. P., Cahn, J. Y., Jakubowski, A. A., Kamani, N. R., Lazarus, H. M., Rizzo, J. D., Schouten, H. C., Socie, G., Stratton, P., Sorror, M. L., Warwick, A. B., Wingard, J. R., Loren, A. W., … Majhail, N. S. (2014). Clinical guide to fertility preservation in hematopoietic cell transplant recipients. *Bone Marrow Transplantation, 49*(4), 477–484. https://doi.org/10.1038/bmt.2013.211.

Kanate, A. S., Majhail, N. S., Savani, B. N., Bredeson, C., Champlin, R. E., Crawford, S., Giralt, S. A., LeMaistre, C. F., Marks, D. I., Omel, J. L., Orchard, P. J., Palmer, J., Saber, W., Veys, P. A., Carpenter, P. A., & Hamadani, M. (2020). Indications for hematopoietic cell transplantation and immune effector cell therapy: Guidelines from the American Society for Transplantation and Cellular Therapy. *Biology of Blood and Marrow Transplantation: Journal of the American Society for Blood and Marrow Transplantation, 26*(7), 1247–1256. https://doi.org/10.1016/j.bbmt.2020.03.002.

Kelly, D. L., Buchbinder, D., Duarte, R. F., Auletta, J. J., Bhatt, N., Byrne, M., DeFilipp, Z., Gabriel, M., Mahindra, A., Norkin, M., Schoemans, H., Shah, A. J., Ahmed, I., Atsuta, Y., Basak, G. W., Beattie, S., Bhella, S., Bredeson, C., Bunin, N., Dalal, J., … Shaw, B. E. (2018). Neurocognitive dysfunction in hematopoietic cell transplant recipients: Expert review from the late effects and quality of life working committee of the center for international blood and marrow transplant research and complications and quality of life working party of the european society for blood and marrow transplantation. *Biology of Blood and Marrow Transplantation, 24*(2), 228–241. https://doi.org/10.1016/j.bbmt.2017.09.004.

Khandelwal, P., Mellor-Heineke, S., Rehman, N., Lane, A., Smiley, K., Villanueva, J., Marsh, R. A., Grimley, M. S., Davies, S. M., & Filipovich, A. H. (2016). Cytokine profile of engraftment syndrome in pediatric hematopoietic stem cell transplant recipients. *Biology of Blood and Marrow Transplantation: Journal of the American Society for Blood and Marrow Transplantation, 22*(4), 690–697. https://doi. org/10.1016/j.bbmt.2015.12.016.

Kohn, L. A., & Kohn, D. B. (2021). Gene therapies for primary immune deficiencies. *Frontiers in Immunology, 12*. https:// doi.org/10.3389/fimmu.2021.648951.

Kranjcec, I., Abdovic, S., Buljan, D., Matijasic, N., Slukan, M., & Stepan, J. (2022). Complementary medicine practice and use of dietary supplements in pediatric cancer patients in Croatia. *Cureus.* https://doi.org/10.7759/cureus.30246.

Landgren, O., Gilbert, E. S., Rizzo, J. D., Socié, G., Banks, P. M., Sobocinski, K. A., Horowitz, M. M., Jaffe, E. S., Kingma, D. W., Travis, L. B., Flowers, M. E., Martin, P. J., Deeg, H. J., & Curtis, R. E. (2009). Risk factors for lymphoproliferative disorders after allogeneic hematopoietic cell transplantation. *Blood, 113*(20), 4992–5001. https://doi.org/10.1182/blood-2008-09-178046.

Langer, A. L., & Esrick, E. B. (2021). B-thalassemia: Evolving treatment options beyond transfusion and iron chelation. *Hematology, 2021*(1);600–606. https://doi.org/10.1182/hematology.2021000313.

Lee, D. W., Santomasso, B. D., Locke, F. L., Ghobadi, A., Turtle, C. J., Brudno, J. N., Maus, M. V., Park, J. H., Mead, E., Pavletic, S., Go, W. Y., Eldjerou, L., Gardner, R. A., Frey, N., Curran, K. J., Peggs, K., Pasquini, M., DiPersio, J. F., van den Brink, M. R. M., Komanduri, K. V., … Neelapu, S. S. (2019). ASTCT consensus grading for cytokine release syndrome and neurologic toxicity associated with immune effector cells. *Biology of Blood and Marrow Transplantation: Journal of the American Society for Blood and Marrow Transplantation, 25*(4), 625–638. https://doi.org/10.1016/j.bbmt.2018.12.758.

Lehrnbecher, T., Fisher, B. T., Phillips, B., Alexander, S., Ammann, R. A., Beauchemin, M., Carlesse, F., Castagnola, E., Davis, B. L., Dupuis, L. L., Egan, G., Groll, A. H., Haeusler, G. M., Santolaya, M., Steinbach, W. J., van de Wetering, M., Wolf, J., Cabral, S., Robinson, P. D., & Sung, L. (2020). Guideline for antibacterial prophylaxis administration in pediatric cancer and hematopoietic stem cell transplantation. *Clinical Infectious Diseases, 71*(1), 226–236. doi:10.1093/cid/ciz1082.

Lo, M. S., Lee, G. M., Gunawardane, N., Burchett, S. K., Lachenauer, C. S., & Lehmann, L. E. (2012). The impact of RSV, adenovirus, influenza, and parainfluenza infection in pediatric patients receiving stem cell transplant, solid organ transplant, or cancer chemotherapy. *Pediatric Transplantation, 17*(2), 133–143. https://doi.org/10.1111/petr.12022.

Loves, R., Tomlinson, D., Baggott, C., Dix, D., Gibson, P., Hyslop, S., Johnston, D. L., Orsey, A. D., Portwine, C., Price, V., Schechter, T., Vanan, M., Kuczynski, S., Spiegler, B., Tomlinson, G. A., Dupuis, L. L., & Sung, L. (2019). Taste changes in children with cancer and hematopoietic stem cell transplant recipients. *Supportive Care in Cancer: Official Journal of the Multinational Association of Supportive Care in Cancer, 27*(6), 2247–2254. https://doi.org/10.1007/s00520-018-4509-2.

Lugthart, G., Jordans, C. C. E., de Pagter, A. P. J., Bresters, D., Jol-van der Zijde, C. M., Bense, J. E., van Rooij-Kouwenhoven, R. W. G., Sukhai, R. N., Louwerens, M., Dorresteijn, E. M., & Lankester, A. C. (2021). Chronic kidney disease ten years after pediatric allogeneic hematopoietic stem cell transplantation. *Kidney International, 100*(4), 906–914. https://doi.org/10.1016/j.kint.2021.05.030.

Ma, Y., Lu, X., & Liu, H. (2022). Neutropenic diet cannot reduce the risk of infection and mortality in oncology patients with neutropenia. *Frontiers in Oncology, 12*. https://doi.org/10.3389/fonc.2022.836371.

Mahadeo, K. M., Bajwa, R., Abdel-Azim, H., Lehmann, L. E., Duncan, C., Zantek, N., Vittorio, J., Angelo, J., McArthur, J., Schadler, K., Chan, S., Tewari, P., Khazal, S., Auletta, J. J., Choi, S. W., Shoberu, B., Kalwak, K., Harden, A., Kebriaei, P., Abe, J. I., … Pediatric Acute Lung Injury and Sepsis Investigators (PALISI) Network and the Pediatric Diseases Working Party of the European Society for Blood and Marrow Transplantation (2020). Diagnosis, grading, and treatment recommendations for children, adolescents, and young adults with sinusoidal obstructive syndrome: An international expert position statement. *The Lancet Haematology, 7*(1), e61–e72. https://doi.org/10.1016/S2352-3026(19)30201-7.

Majeed, A., Harris, Z., Brucks, E., Hinchman, A., Farooqui, A. A., Tariq, M. J., Tamizhmani, K., Riaz, I. B., McBride, A., Latif, A., Kapoor, V., Iftikhar, R., Mossad, S., & Anwer, F. (2020). Revisiting role of vaccinations in donors, transplant recipients, immunocompromised hosts, travelers, and household contacts of stem cell transplant recipients. *Biology of Blood and Marrow Transplantation, 26*(2), e38–e50. doi:10.1016/j.bbmt.2019.10.030.

Majhail, N. S., Rizzo, J. D., Lee, S. J., Aljurf, M., Atsuta, Y., Bonfim, C., Burns, L. J., Chaudhri, N., Davies, S., Okamoto, S., Seber, A., Socie, G., Szer, J., Van Lint, M. T., Wingard, J. R., Tichelli, A., Center for International Blood and Marrow Transplant Research, American Society for Blood and Marrow Transplantation, European Group for Blood and Marrow Transplantation, Asia-Pacific Blood and Marrow Transplantation Group, … Sociedade Brasileira de Transplante de Medula Ossea (2012). Recommended screening and preventive practices for long-term survivors after hematopoietic cell transplantation. *Bone Marrow Transplantation, 47*(3), 337–341. https://doi.org/10.1038/bmt.2012.5.

Martin, P. J., Rizzo, J. D., Wingard, J. R., Ballen, K., Curtin, P. T., Cutler, C., Litzow, M. R., Nieto, Y., Savani, B. N., Schriber, J. R., Shaughnessy, P. J., Wall, D. A., & Carpenter, P. A. (2012). First- and second-line systemic treatment of acute graft-versus-host disease: Recommendations of the American Society of Blood and Marrow Transplantation. *Biology of Blood and Marrow Transplantation: Journal of the American Society for Blood and Marrow Transplantation, 18*(8), 1150–1163. https://doi.org/10.1016/j.bbmt.2012.04.005.

Martini, D. J., Chen, Y.-B., & DeFilipp, Z. (2022). Recent FDA approvals in the treatment of graft-versus-host disease. *Oncologist, 27*(8), 685–693. https://doi.org/10.1093/oncolo/oyac076.

Mawardi, H., Treister, N., Felemban, O., Alamoudi, W., Algohary, G., Alsultan, A., Alshehri, N., Tazi, I., Shaheen, M., Alsharani, M., Alshemmari, S., Arat, M., Bekadja, M. A., Al-Khabori, M., Okaily, S., Ali, N., Abujazar, H., Jastaniah, W., Hamidieh, A. A., Hashmi, S., … Aljurf, M. (2023). Current practice of oral care for hematopoietic stem cell transplant patients: A Survey of the Eastern Mediterranean Blood and Marrow Transplantation Group. *Hematology/Oncology and Stem Cell Therapy, 16*(1), 42–51. https://doi.org/10.1016/j.hemonc.2021.01.006.

Maziarz, R. T., & Slater, S. (2021). *Blood and Marrow Transplant Handbook: Comprehensive Guide for Patient Care.* Springer.

McGrady, M. E., Williams, S. N., Davies, S. M., & Pai, A. L. H. (2014). Adherence to outpatient oral medication regimens in adolescent hematopoietic stem cell transplant recipients. *European Journal of Oncology Nursing, 18*(2), 140–144. https://doi.org/10.1016/j.ejon.2013.11.007.

Mekelenkamp, H., Schröder, T., Trigoso, E., Hutt, D., Galimard, J. E., Kozijn, A., Dalissier, A., Gjergji, M., Liptrott, S., Kenyon, M., Murray, J., Corbacioglu, S., Bader, P., On Behalf Of The Ebmt-Nurses Group, & Paediatric Diseases Working Party (2021). Specialized pediatric palliative care services in pediatric hematopoietic stem cell transplant centers. *Children (Basel, Switzerland), 8*(8), 615. https://doi.org/10.3390/children8080615.

Morgan, M. A., Büning, H., Sauer, M., & Schambach, A. (2020). Use of cell and genome modification technologies to generate improved "off-the-shelf" CAR T and car NK cells. *Frontiers in Immunology, 11*. https://doi.org/10.3389/fimmu.2020.01965.

Moskowitz, C. H., Nademanee, A., Masszi, T., Agura, E., Holowiecki, J., Abidi, M. H., Chen, A. I., Stiff, P., Gianni, A. M., Carella, A., Osmanov, D., Bachanova, V., Sweetenham, J., Sureda, A., Huebner, D., Sievers, E. L., Chi, A., Larsen, E. K., Hunder, N. N., Walewski, J., … AETHERA Study Group (2015). Brentuximab vedotin as consolidation therapy after autologous stem-cell transplantation in patients with Hodgkin's lymphoma at risk of relapse or progression (AETHERA): A randomised, double-blind, placebo-controlled, phase 3 trial. *Lancet (London, England), 385*(9980), 1853–1862. https://doi.org/10.1016/S0140-6736(15)60165-9.

Murray, J., Agreiter, I., Orlando, L., & Hutt, D. BMT Settings, Infection and Infection Control. (2017). In: Kenyon, M., Babic, A., editors. The European Blood and Marrow Transplantation Textbook for Nurses: Under the Auspices of EBMT [Internet].

Cham (CH): Springer; 2018. Fig. 7.1, [Phases of opportunistic infections among...]. Available from: https://www.ncbi.nlm.nih.gov/books/NBK543675/figure/ch7.Fig1/. doi:10.1007/978-3-319-50026-3_7.

National Cancer Institute. (2022). Car T cells: Engineering immune cells to treat cancer. https://www.cancer.gov/about-cancer/treatment/research/car-t-cells.

Narkhede, M., Rybicki, L., Abounader, D., Bolwell, B., Dean, R., Gerds, A. T., Hanna, R., Hill, B., Jagadeesh, D., Kalaycio, M., Liu, H. D., Pohlman, B., Sobecks, R., Majhail, N. S., & Ky Hamilton, B. (2017). The association of histologic grade with acute graft-versus-host disease response and outcomes. *American Journal of Hematology, 92*(7), 683–688. https://doi.org/10.1002/ajh.24749.

Neelapu, S. S., Tummala, S., Kebriaei, P., Wierda, W., Gutierrez, C., Locke, F. L., Komanduri, K. V., Lin, Y., Jain, N., Daver, N., Westin, J., Gulbis, A. M., Loghin, M. E., de Groot, J. F., Adkins, S., Davis, S. E., Rezvani, K., Hwu, P., & Shpall, E. J. (2018). Chimeric antigen receptor T-cell therapy—assessment and management of toxicities. *Nature Reviews Clinical Oncology, 15*(1), 47–62. https://doi.org/10.1038/nrclinonc.2017.148.

Nygaard, M., Wichert, S., Berlin, G., & Toss, F. (2020). Extracorporeal photopheresis for graft-vs-host disease: A literature review and treatment guidelines proposed by the Nordic ECP Quality Group. *European Journal of Haematology, 104*(5), 361–375. https://doi.org/10.1111/ejh.13381.

Oertel, M., Martel, J., Mikesch, J. H., Scobioala, S., Reicherts, C., Kröger, K., Lenz, G., Stelljes, M., & Eich, H. T. (2021). The burden of survivorship on hematological patients—long-term analysis of toxicities after total body irradiation and allogeneic stem cell transplantation. *Cancers (Basel), 13*(22), 5640. doi:10.3390/cancers13225640.

Ottaviano, G., Lucchini, G., Breuer, J., Furtado-Silva, J. M., Lazareva, A., Ciocarlie, O., Elfeky, R., Rao, K., Amrolia, P. J., Veys, P., & Chiesa, R. (2020). Delaying haematopoietic stem cell transplantation in children with viral respiratory infections reduces transplant-related mortality. *British journal of haematology, 188*(4), 560–569. https://doi.org/10.1111/bjh.16216.

Otto, W. R., Pahud, B. A., & Yin, D. E. (2019). Pediatric mucormycosis: A 10-year systematic review of reported cases and review of the literature. *Journal of Pediatric Infectious Disease Society, 8*(4), 342–350. https://doi.org/10.1093/jpids/piz007.

Pagel, J. M., Othus, M., Garcia-Manero, G., Fang, M., Radich, J. P., Rizzieri, D. A., Marcucci, G., Strickland, S. A., Litzow, M. R., Savoie, M. L., Spellman, S. R., Confer, D. L., Chell, J. W., Brown, M., Medeiros, B. C., Sekeres, M. A., Lin, T. L., Uy, G. L., Powell, B. L., Bayer, R. L., ... Appelbaum, F. R. (2020). Rapid donor identification improves survival in high-risk first-remission patients with acute myeloid leukemia. *JCO Oncology Practice, 16*(6), e464–e475. https://doi.org/10.1200/JOP.19.00133.

Pai, A. L. H., Rausch, J., Drake, S., Morrison, C. F., Lee, J. L., Nelson, A., Tackett, A., Berger, S., Szulczewski, L., Mara, C., & Davies, S. (2018). Poor adherence is associated with more infections after pediatric hematopoietic stem cell transplant. *Biology of Blood and Marrow Transplantation: Journal of the American Society for Blood and Marrow Transplantation, 24*(2), 381–385. https://doi.org/10.1016/j.bbmt.2017.10.033.

Park, J. R., Kreissman, S. G., London, W. B., Naranjo, A., Cohn, S. L., Hogarty, M. D., Tenney, S. C., Haas-Kogan, D., Shaw, P. J., Kraveka, J. M., Roberts, S. S., Geiger, J. D., Doski, J. J., Voss, S. D., Maris, J. M., Grupp, S. A., & Diller, L. (2019). Effect of tandem autologous stem cell transplant vs single transplant on event-free survival in patients with high-risk neuroblastoma: A randomized clinical trial. *JAMA, 322*(8), 746–755. https://doi.org/10.1001/jama.2019.11642.

Parris, K. R., Russell, K. M., Triplett, B. M., & Phipps, S. (2020). Neurocognitive functioning in long-term survivors of pediatric hematopoietic cell transplantation. *Bone Marrow Transplantation, 56*(4), 873–882. https://doi.org/10.1038/s41409-020-01125-5.

Patel, C., Pasciolla, M., Abramova, R., Salerno, D., Gomez-Arteaga, A., Shore, T. B., Orfali, N., Mayer, S., Hsu, J., Phillips, A. A., Chaekal, O. K., Satlin, M. J., Soave, R., Kodiyanplakkal, R. P. L., Drelick, A., Plate, M., & Besien, K. V. (2023). Pre-hematopoietic stem cell transplantation rituximab for epstein-barr virus and post-lymphoproliferative disorder prophylaxis in alemtuzumab recipients. *Transplantation and Cellular Therapy, 29*(2), 132.e1–132.e5. https://doi.org/10.1016/j.jtct.2022.10.023.

Patrick, K., Ali, M., Richardson, S. E., Gassas, A., Egeler, M., Krueger, J., Lowry, J., Allen, U., & Schechter, T. (2015). The yield of monitoring for HSV and VZV viremia in pediatric hematopoietic stem cell transplant patients. *Pediatric Transplantation, 19*(6), 640–644. https://doi.org/10.1111/petr.12551.

Pedersen-Bjergaard, J., Andersen, M. K., & Christiansen, D. H. (2000). Therapy-related acute myeloid leukemia and myelodysplasia after high-dose chemotherapy and autologous stem cell transplantation. *Blood, 95*(11), 3273–3279. Erratum in: Blood 2000 Sep 1;96(5), 1680.

Pegoraro, F., & Favre, C. (2021). Post-transplantation lymphoproliferative disorder after haematopoietic stem cell transplantation. *Annals of Hematology, 100*(4), 865–878. https://doi.org/10.1007/s00277-021-04433-y.

Phelan, R., Chen, M., Bupp, C., Bolon, Y. T., Broglie, L., Brunner-Grady, J., Burns, L. J., Chhabra, S., Christianson, D., Cusatis, R., Devine, S. M., D'Souza, A., Eapen, M., Hamadani, M., Hengen, M., Lee, S. J., Moskop, A., Page, K. M., Pasquini, M., Pérez, W. S., ... Arora, M. (2022). Updated trends in hematopoietic cell transplantation in the United States with an additional focus on adolescent and young adult transplantation activity and outcomes. *Transplantation and Cellular Therapy, 28*(7), 409.e1–409.e10. https://doi.org/10.1016/j.jtct.2022.04.012.

Pidala, J., Lee, S. J., Ahn, K. W., Spellman, S., Wang, H. L., Aljurf, M., Askar, M., Dehn, J., Fernandez Viña, M., Gratwohl, A., Gupta, V., Hanna, R., Horowitz, M. M., Hurley, C. K., Inamoto, Y., Kassim, A. A., Nishihori, T., Mueller, C., Oudshoorn, M., Petersdorf, E. W., ... Anasetti, C. (2014). Nonpermissive HLA-DPB1 mismatch increases mortality after myeloablative unrelated allogeneic hematopoietic cell transplantation. *Blood, 124*(16), 2596–2606. https://doi.org/10.1182/blood-2014-05-576041.

Ponce, D. M., Politikos, I., Alousi, A., Carpenter, P. A., Milano, F., MacMillan, M. L., Barker, J. N., Horwitz, M. E., & American Society for Transplantation and Cellular Therapy Cord Blood Special Interest Group (2021). Guidelines for the prevention and management of graft-versus-host disease after cord blood transplantation. *Transplantation and Cellular Therapy, 27*(7), 540–544. https://doi.org/10.1016/j.jtct.2021.03.012.

Reddivalla, N., Robinson, A. L., Reid, K. J., Radhi, M. A., Dalal, J., Opfer, E. K., & Chan, S. S. (2020). Using liver elastography to diagnose sinusoidal obstruction syndrome in pediatric patients undergoing hematopoetic stem cell transplant. *Bone Marrow Transplantation, 55*(3), 523–530. https://doi.org/10.1038/s41409-017-0064-6.

Richert-Przygonska, M., Jaremek, K., Debski, R., Konieczek, J., Lecka, M., Dziedzic, M., Bogiel, T., Styczynski, J., & Czyzewski, K. (2022). Letermovir prophylaxis for cytomegalovirus infection in children after hematopoietic cell transplantation. *Anticancer Research, 42*(7), 3607–3612. https://doi.org/10.21873/anticanres.15848.

Schmid, I., Stachel, D., Pagel, P., & Albert, M. H. (2008). Incidence, predisposing factors, and outcome of engraftment syndrome in pediatric allogeneic stem cell transplant recipients. *Biology of Blood and Marrow Transplantation, 14*(4), 438–444. https://doi.org/10.1016/j.bbmt.2008.02.002.

Schmit-Pokorny, K., & Eisenberg, S. (2020). *Hematopoietic Stem Cell Transplantation: A Manual for Nursing Practice.* Oncology Nursing Society.

Shenoy, S., Gaziev, J., Angelucci, E., King, A., Bhatia, M., Smith, A., Bresters, D., Haight, A. E., Duncan, C. N., de la Fuente, J., Dietz, A. C., Baker, K. S., Pulsipher, M. A., & Walters, M. C. (2018). Late effects screening guidelines after hematopoietic cell transplantation (HCT) for hemoglobinopathy: Consensus Statement from the Second Pediatric Blood and Marrow Transplant Consortium International Conference on Late Effects after Pediatric HCT. *Biology of Blood and Marrow Transplantation: Journal of the American Society for Blood and Marrow Transplantation, 24*(7), 1313–1321. https://doi.org/10.1016/j.bbmt.2018.04.002.

Singh, A. K., & McGuirk, J. P. (2016). Allogeneic stem cell transplantation: A historical and scientific overview. *Cancer Research, 76*(22), 6445–6451. https://doi.org/10.1158/0008-5472.can-16-1311.

Spitzer, T. R. (2015). Engraftment syndrome: Double-edged sword of hematopoietic cell transplants. *Bone Marrow Transplantation, 50*(4), 469–475. https://doi.org/10.1038/bmt.2014.296.

Spruit, J. L., Knight, T., Sweeney, C., Salimnia, H., & Savaşan, S. (2020). Clostridium difficile infection in a children's hospital with specific patterns among pediatric oncology and hematopoietic stem cell transplantation populations. *Pediatric Hematology and Oncology, 37*(3), 211–222. https://doi.org/10.1080/08880018.2019.1711473.

Styczynski, J., van der Velden, W., Fox, C. P., Engelhard, D., de la Camara, R., Cordonnier, C., Ljungman, P., & Sixth European Conference on Infections in Leukemia, a joint venture of the Infectious Diseases Working Party of the European Society of Blood and Marrow Transplantation (EBMT-IDWP), the Infectious Diseases Group of the European Organization for Research and Treatment of Cancer (EORTC-IDG), the International Immunocompromised Host Society (ICHS) and the European Leukemia Net (ELN). (2016). Management of Epstein-Barr Virus infections and post-transplant lymphoproliferative disorders in patients after allogeneic hematopoietic stem cell transplantation: Sixth European Conference on Infections in Leukemia (ECIL-6) guidelines. *Haematologica, 101*(7), 803–811. https://doi.org/10.3324/haematol.2016.144428.

Suh, E., Stratton, K. L., Leisenring, W. M., Nathan, P. C., Ford, J. S., Freyer, D. R., McNeer, J. L., Stock, W., Stovall, M., Krull, K. R., Sklar, C. A., Neglia, J. P., Armstrong, G. T., Oeffinger, K. C., Robison, L. L., & Henderson, T. O. (2020). Late mortality and chronic health conditions in long-term survivors of early-adolescent and young adult cancers: A retrospective cohort analysis from the childhood cancer survivor study. *The Lancet Oncology, 21*(3), 421–435. https://doi.org/10.1016/S1470-2045(19)30800-9.

Taggart, C., Neumann, N., Alonso, P. B., Lane, A., Pate, A., Stegman, A., Stendahl, A., Davies, S. M., Dandoy, C. E., & Grimley, M. (2019). Comparing a neutropenic diet to a food safety-based diet in pediatric patients undergoing hematopoietic stem cell transplantation. *Biology of Blood and Marrow Transplantation: Journal of the American Society for Blood and Marrow Transplantation, 25*(7), 1382–1386. https://doi.org/10.1016/j.bbmt.2019.03.017.

Tichelli, A., Rovó, A., Passweg, J., Schwarze, C. P., Van Lint, M. T., Arat, M., & Socié, G. Late effects working party of the european group for blood and marrow Transplantation. (2009). Late complications after hematopoietic stem cell transplantation. *Expert Reviews in Hematology, 2*(5), 583–601. doi:10.1586/ehm.09.48.

Tomblyn, M., Chiller, T., Einsele, H., Gress, R., Sepkowitz, K., Storek, J., Wingard, J. R., Young, J. A., Boeckh, M. J., Center for International Blood and Marrow Research, National Marrow Donor program, European Blood and Marrow Transplant Group, American Society of Blood and Marrow Transplantation, Canadian Blood and Marrow Transplant Group, Infectious Diseases Society of America, Society for Healthcare Epidemiology of America, Association of Medical Microbiology and Infectious Disease Canada, & Centers for Disease Control and Prevention (2009). Guidelines for preventing infectious complications among hematopoietic cell transplantation recipients: A global perspective. *Biology of Blood and Marrow Transplantation: Journal of the American Society for Blood and Marrow Transplantation, 15*(10), 1143–1238. https://doi.org/10.1016/j.bbmt.2009.06.019.

Treleaven, J. (2009). Bacterial infections. *Hematopoietic Stem Cell Transplantation,* 453–455. https://doi.org/10.1016/b978-0-443-10147-2.50048-5.

Uber, A., Ebelhar, J. S., Lanzel, A. F., Roche, A., Vidal-Anaya, V., & Brock, K. E. (2022). Palliative care in pediatric oncology and hematopoietic stem cell transplantation. *Current Oncology Reports, 24*(2), 161–174. https://doi.org/10.1007/s11912-021-01174-z.

Waghmare, A., Abidi, M. Z., Boeckh, M., Chemaly, R. F., Dadwal, S., El Boghdadly, Z., Kamboj, M., Papanicolaou, G. A., Pergam, S. A., & Shahid, Z. (2020). Guidelines for COVID-19 management in hematopoietic cell transplantation and cellular therapy recipients. *Biology of Blood and Marrow Transplantation: Journal of the American Society for Blood and Marrow Transplantation, 26*(11), 1983–1994. https://doi.org/10.1016/j.bbmt.2020.07.027.

Walther, S., Rettinger, E., Maurer, H. M., Pommerening, H., Jarisch, A., Sörensen, J., Schubert, R., Berres, M., Bader, P., Zielen, S., & Jerkic, S. P. (2020). Long-term pulmonary function testing in pediatric bronchiolitis obliterans syndrome after hematopoietic stem cell transplantation. *Pediatric Pulmonology, 55*(7), 1725–1735. https://doi.org/10.1002/ppul.24801.

Ward, K. N., Hill, J. A., Hubacek, P., de la Camara, R., Crocchiolo, R., Einsele, H., Navarro, D., Robin, C., Cordonnier, C., & Ljungman, P; 2017 European Conference on Infections in Leukaemia (ECIL). (2019). Guidelines from the 2017 European Conference on Infections in Leukaemia for management of HHV-6 infection in patients with hematologic malignancies and after hematopoietic stem cell transplantation. *Haematologica, 104*(11), 2155–2163. doi:10.3324/haematol.2019.223073. Epub 2019 Aug 29.

Wei, C., & Albanese, A. (2014). Endocrine disorders in childhood cancer survivors treated with haemopoietic stem cell transplantation. *Children, 1*(1), 48–62. https://doi.org/10.3390/children1010048.

Williams, K. M., Ahn, K. W., Chen, M., Aljurf, M. D., Agwu, A. L., Chen, A. R., Walsh, T. J., Szabolcs, P., Boeckh, M. J., Auletta, J. J., Lindemans, C. A., Zanis-Neto, J., Malvezzi, M., Lister, J., de Toledo Codina, J. S., Sackey, K., Chakrabarty, J. L., Ljungman, P., Wingard, J. R., Seftel, M. D., … Riches, M. R. (2016). The incidence, mortality and timing of Pneumocystis jiroveci pneumonia after hematopoietic cell transplantation: A CIBMTR analysis. *Bone Marrow Transplantation, 51*(4), 573–580. https://doi.org/10.1038/bmt.2015.316.

Wingard, J. R., Majhail, N. S., Brazauskas, R., Wang, Z., Sobocinski, K. A., Jacobsohn, D., Sorror, M. L., Horowitz, M. M., Bolwell, B., Rizzo, J. D., & Socié, G. (2011). Long-term survival and late deaths after allogeneic hematopoietic cell transplantation. *Journal of Clinical Oncology, 29*(16), 2230–2239. https://doi.org/10.1200/jco.2010.33.7212.

Wobma, H., Jin, Z., Moscoso, S., Bhatia, M., Broglie, L., George, D., Garvin, J., & Satwani, P. (2020). Risk factors, clinical outcomes, and cost-of-care related to graft failure in pediatric allogeneic hematopoietic cell transplant recipients. *Biology of Blood and Marrow Transplantation, 26*(7), 1318–1325. https://doi.org/10.1016/j.bbmt.2020.03.009.

Yao, J. M., Yang, D., Clark, M. C., Otoukesh, S., Cao, T., Ali, H., Arslan, S., Aldoss, I., Artz, A., Amanam, I., Salhotra, A., Pullarkat, V., Sandhu, K., Stein, A., Marcucci, G., Forman, S. J., Nakamura, R., & Al Malki, M. M. (2022). Tacrolimus initial steady state level in post-transplant cyclophosphamide-based GvHD prophylaxis regimens. Bone marrow transplantation, *57*(2), 232–242. https://doi.org/10.1038/s41409-021-01528-y.

Zama, D., Gori, D., Muratore, E., Leardini, D., Rallo, F., Turroni, S., Prete, A., Brigidi, P., Pession, A., & Masetti, R. (2021). Enteral versus parenteral nutrition as nutritional support after allogeneic hematopoietic stem cell transplantation: A systematic review and meta-analysis. *Transplantation and Cellular Therapy, 27*(2), 180.e1–180.e8. https://doi.org/10.1016/j.jtct.2020.11.006.

Zeiser, R., & Blazar, B. R. (2017). Pathophysiology of chronic graft-versus-host disease and therapeutic targets. *New England Journal of Medicine, 377*(26), 2565–2579. https://doi.org/10.1056/nejmra1703472.

13

Cancer

Paige Johnson

ETIOLOGY

The definition of cancer is a disease in which cells grow uncontrollably and can spread to other parts of the body (National Cancer Institute [NCI], n.d.). Cancer is a result of the body failing to regulate cell production. A proliferation and spread of abnormal cells occur and, when left unchecked, may lead to the death of the host. Cancer can occur in any structure of the body, but common sites in childhood cancer are blood and bone marrow, brain and central nervous system (CNS), lymphatics, kidneys and adrenals, soft tissues, and bones (Table 13.1).

Although genetic factors or environmental exposures are known to place children at risk of developing cancer (see Table 13.1), the specific etiology of childhood cancer is yet to be identified. There are familial genetic predispositions that can place children at risk for developing cancer, in addition to genetic mutations/amplifications/deletions and gene rearrangement that can contribute to malignant transformations.

INCIDENCE AND PREVALENCE

An estimated 10,400 children and adolescents under the age of 15 years are diagnosed with cancer annually in the United States (American Cancer Society [ACS], 2022). It is the second leading cause of death of children under 14 years, after accidents. In 2019, the overall incidence of malignancy in children under 20 years was approximately 19.1 per 100,000/year (NCI, 2021a). A comparison of the incidence of the various childhood malignancies in the United States (see Table 13.1) illustrates a wide variation depending on site, with leukemia/lymphomas and brain/CNS tumors playing a large part in diagnoses (Yan et al., 2020). Childhood cancer incidence also varies by race, with White children comprising most cases and non-Hispanic Black children the lowest. Childhood cancers can be different based on age. Leukemias and brain/CNS tumors are the highest among children under 5 years, whereas lymphomas and epithelial cancers (skin, thyroid) are highest among those over 16 years of age (NCI, 2021a). Because of the recent treatment advances in oncology, 85% of children with cancer now survive 5 years or more (ACS, 2022). However, survival rates depend on the specific type of childhood cancer and other factors, including age, presence of metastases, and response to treatment.

DIAGNOSIS AND TREATMENT OPPORTUNITIES

Prompt referral to a pediatric cancer treatment center is a priority to ensure that a child has all the diagnostic requirements available to them and the opportunity to participate in a clinical trial. After a thorough history, physical examination, and laboratory tests, the workup may include radiologic examinations, tissue biopsies, bone marrow aspirate, bone marrow biopsy, and lumbar puncture, depending on the type of tumor suspected and the most frequent sites of metastases. If a biopsy is being considered outside of the comprehensive cancer institution, the primary care provider should consult the oncologist before proceeding. This ensures that the biopsy can be appropriately taken and that important molecular genetics and immunohistochemistry can be ordered and received in a timely manner.

The opportunity for children to participate in a clinical trial with a new cancer diagnosis enables them to get the most current treatment regimen possible that could include newer modalities available to improve outcomes and side effects/late effects. Of children diagnosed with cancer, 60% participate in clinical trials; the rate with adults is much lower (Children's Oncology Group [COG], 2018). Pediatric oncology clinical trials have given children opportunities to access new research areas in oncology, such as immunotherapy and targeted therapies, that can be more specific to cancer's genetic makeup and thus more effective in treatment.

CLINICAL MANIFESTATIONS AT TIME OF DIAGNOSIS

Pediatric cancer generally presents with vague symptoms, all determined by the type of cancer the child has developed (Box 13.1). Leukemia and lymphomas can present with fevers, repeated infections, bleeding, pallor, or the presence of lymphadenopathy. In comparison, children with solid tumors may present with symptoms of where the tumor is located, such as bone pain, fracture of a bone, abdominal distension, vomiting, and difficulty urinating and passing stool. Brain and CNS tumors can present as headaches, vision changes, early-morning vomiting, numbness/tingling/loss of function of extremities, and seizures (NCI, NIH, 2020). Retinal tumors can present with

Table 13.1   Common Pediatric Cancers

TYPE	SITE	INCIDENCE (AGES 0–14 YR)	ETIOLOGY	SIGNS/SYMPTOMS	TREATMENT
Leukemia					
	Bone marrow	4.7 per 100,000 children per year (Leukemia and Lymphoma Society [LLS])	*For ALL and AML:* Genetic factors Chromosomal abnormalities (trisomy 21, Bloom syndrome, Fanconi anemia, AT)	*For ALL and AML:* Pallor, fatigue, headache Fever, infection Purpura, bruising Lymphadenopathy Organomegaly Bone pain	
B-cell acute lymphoblastic leukemia (ALL)			Familial predisposition (ALL: infant identical twins) Environmental factors Ionizing radiation Chronic chemical exposure Use of alkylating agents for treatment of malignant disease (AML) Possible viral infection		Combination chemotherapy CNS prophylaxis Intrathecal chemotherapy Monoclonal antibodies
T-cell acute lymphoblastic leukemia (ALL)					Combination chemotherapy CNS prophylaxis
ALL with Philadelphia chromosome (Ph+ or Ph like)					Combination chemotherapy CNS prophylaxis Tyrosine kinase inhibitors (TKIs)
Acute myelogenous leukemia (AML)					Combination chemotherapy CNS prophylaxis Monoclonal antibodies
Central Nervous System (CNS)					
Infratentorial					
Medulloblastoma	Cerebellum/brainstem	3.2 per 100,000 children per year (National Institutes of Health [NIH])	*For all CNS cancers:* Genetic factors Heritable disease (NF, VHL, LFS) Familial Environmental factors Chronic chemical exposure Ionizing radiation Other primary malignancies Exogenous immunosuppression	*Early:* Decreased academic performance Fatigue Personality changes Intermittent headache *Late:* Morning headache Vomiting Diplopia/visual changes Brainstem/cerebellar Deficits of balance/positioning	Anticonvulsants, if symptoms present Treatment of hydrocephalus Corticosteroids Shunting Surgical resection (if operable) Radiation therapy Chemotherapy for some tumors HSCT in rare cases
Ependymoma	Midline cerebellar Ependymal lining of ventricular system or central canal of spinal cord				
Brainstem glioma	Brainstem				
Supratentorial					
Astrocytoma	Ventricles, midline diencephalon, cerebrum			*Supratentorial:* Nonspecific headache Seizures Hemiparesis	
Craniopharyngioma	Sella turcica				
Glioma	Visual pathway				
Pineoblastoma or germ cell tumor	Pineal region				

Table 13.1 Common Pediatric Cancers—cont'd

TYPE	SITE	INCIDENCE (AGES 0–14 YR)	ETIOLOGY	SIGNS/SYMPTOMS	TREATMENT
Lymphoma					
Non-Hodgkin lymphoma Lymphoblastic lymphoma	Generalized lymphade-nopathy Mediastinal mass Bone marrow	2.6 per 100,000 children per year (LLS)	*For all non-Hodgkin lymphomas:* Immunodeficiency (HIV) Exogenous immunosuppression Viral: associated with Epstein-Barr virus (EBV)	Generally rapid progression Dysphagia, dyspnea Swelling of neck, face, upper extremities Supradiaphragmatic lymphadenopathy Respiratory distress	Treatment of emergent symptoms Combination chemotherapy +/– CNS prophylaxis Monoclonal antibodies
Small nonclea/ed lymphoma, Burkitt lymphoma, non-Burkitt lymphoma	Abdomen Bone marrow Lymph nodes			Abdominal pain or swelling Change in bowel habits Nausea/vomiting GI bleeding Intestinal perforation (rarely) Inguinal/iliac adenopathy Intussusception	Treatment of emergent symptoms and tumor lysis syndrome Combination chemotherapy CNS prophylaxis Monoclonal antibodies
Large cell lymphoma	Lymph nodes Cutaneous lesions Mediastinum Abdomen Head, neck			As cited earlier, depending on site	
Hodgkin lymphoma	Single lymph nodes or lymphatic chains Mediastinal mass Spleen		Genetic factors Familial predisposition Environmental influence Iatrogenic or acquired immuno-deficiency (HIV, AT) Infectious etiology (EBV)	Lymphadenopathy Organomegaly Fatigue Anorexia/weight loss/fever	Combination chemotherapy Monoclonal antibodies Radiation therapy
Neuroendocrine					
Neuroblastoma	Anywhere along the sympathetic nervous system chain Most commonly abdomen, adre-nal gland, para-spinal ganglion, thorax, neck	0.85 per 100,000 children per year (Medical Science Monitor)	Genetic factors Autosomal dominant inherited predisposition in some children Familial predisposition Associated with fetal alcohol syndrome and fetal hydantoin syndrome	Dependent on primary site, site of metastases Metastases present in 70% of cases at diag-nosis (especially in bone marrow) Presence of a mass (abdomen, thoracic, cervical, pelvic, liver) Symptoms from compression of mass (Horner syndrome, edema of upper and lower extremities secondary to vascular compres-sion, hypertension caused by compression of renal vasculature, cord compression symptoms [paresis, paralysis, bowel/bladder dysfunction]) Diarrhea from vasoactive intestinal peptides produced by tumor cells Skin or subcutaneous nodules (infants only) Nonspecific symptoms (fever, weight loss, failure to thrive, generalized pain) Rarely syndrome of opsoclonus-myoclonus	Treatment of emergent symptoms Surgery (staging excision of tumor, evaluation of treatment) Radiation therapy Combination chemotherapy HSCT in some cases Monoclonal antibodies

Continued

Table 13.1 Common Pediatric Cancers—cont'd

TYPE	SITE	INCIDENCE (AGES 0–14 YR)	ETIOLOGY	SIGNS/SYMPTOMS	TREATMENT
Soft Tissue Sarcoma					
Rhabdomyosarcoma	Head and neck (most common)	1.1 per 100,000 children per year (NIH)	*For both sarcomas:* Genetic factors Associated with NF, LFS, Beckwith-Wiedemann syndrome Environmental factors Parental use of recreational drugs Possible viral etiology	*For both sarcomas:* Dependent on location and size of tumor	Surgical removal (if feasible) Radiation therapy for residual tumor Combination chemotherapy TKIs
Undifferentiated sarcoma	Abdomen Anywhere in body				
Renal Tumor					
Wilms tumor (nephroblastoma, renal embryoma)	Unilateral, bilateral	0.7 per 100,000 children per year (NIH)	Genetic factors Associated with aniridia, NF, Beckwith-Wiedemann syndrome, hemihypertrophy, Denys-Drash syndrome Familial predisposition Environmental factors Long-term chemical exposure (hydrocarbons/lead)	Asymptomatic mass Malaise, pain Microscopic or gross hematuria Hypertension	Complete surgical excision (if bilateral, nephrectomy of more involved site, excisional biopsy/partial nephrectomy of smaller lesion in remaining kidney) Combination chemotherapy Radiation therapy for high-risk tumors
Bone Tumors					
Osteosarcoma	Long bones of extremities	1 per 100,000 children per year (NIH)	Genetic factors Familial predisposition (hereditary retinoblastoma) Environmental factors Ionizing radiation Use of alkylating agents Possible genetic factors No strong or consistent association with constitution of chromosomal abnormalities or congenital diseases	Pain over involved area with or without swelling (often ≥3–5 mo) In the presence of metastatic disease nonspecific symptoms (fatigue, anorexia, weight loss, intermittent fever, malaise)	Combination chemotherapy Surgical excision of the tumor with limb salvage or amputation if the extent of disease or location does not allow complete excision Localized radiation therapy or surgical excision Combination chemotherapy
Ewing sarcoma	Bones of the extremities and central axis				
Retinoblastoma					
	Eye	1.2 per 100,000 per year (Fernandes, 2018)	Genetic factors Gene mutation (nonhereditary) Autosomal dominant (all bilateral retinoblastomas and 15% of unilateral)	Leukocoria (cat's-eye reflex) Squint Strabismus Orbital inflammation	Surgery (resection, enucleation with extensive disease; salvage of one eye attempted in bilateral disease) Radiation therapy Chemotherapy HSCT transplant

AT, Ataxia telangiectasia; *GI*, gastrointestinal; *HIV*, human immunodeficiency virus; *HSCT*, hematopoietic stem cell transplantation; *LFS*, Li-Fraumeni syndrome; *NF*, neurofibromatosis; *VHL*, von Hippel-Lindau syndrome.

Box 13.1 Child Cancer Symptoms

Continued, unexplained weight loss
Headaches with early-morning vomiting
Increased swelling or pain in bones, joints, back, or legs
Lump or mass (such as in the abdomen, neck, pelvis, or axilla)
Development of excessive bruising, bleeding, or rash
Constant/recurrent infections
A whitish color behind the pupil
Nausea that persists or vomiting with or without seizures
Constant tiredness or paleness
Eye or vision changes that occur suddenly or persists
Recurrent or persistent fevers of unknown origin

a white spot in the pupil (leukocoria). Nonspecific symptoms can include weight loss, diarrhea, low-grade fevers, malaise, or failure to thrive.

TREATMENT

Cancer treatment involves the concurrent or sequential use of surgery, chemotherapy, radiation therapy, hematopoietic stem cell transplantation (HSCT), and immunotherapy. Multi-institutional cooperative study groups and some specialty cancer treatment centers provide state-of-the-art treatment. These centers generally use a multidisciplinary approach combining the expertise of nurses, primary care providers, advanced practice nurses, nutritionists, social workers, art and child life therapists, and other specialists. In 2000, the COG was formed by merging four pediatric clinical trial cooperative groups (the Children's Cancer Group, the Pediatric Oncology Group, the National Wilms Tumor Study Group, and the Intergroup Rhabdomyosarcoma Study Group). The COG is now comprised of institutions in North America, Australia, New Zealand, and Europe and is the world's largest organization devoted exclusively to childhood cancer research (COG, 2022). Other institutions involved in childhood cancer treatment research include the NCI, St. Jude's Children's Research Hospital, and Dana Farber Cancer Institute.

Approximately 50% of children younger than 15 years with cancer in the United States are treated on a clinical trial; however, less than 20% of adolescents age 15 to 19 are enrolled in a clinical trial (Schapira et al., 2020). A remedy to this exclusion in a clinical trial would be to update protocols increasing the age of participation to include more adolescents and young adults; however, it has been seen that the lack of participation by adolescents on national clinical trials affects their survival and quality of life (Schapira et al., 2020). Adolescents and young adults with pediatric cancers treated in pediatric clinical trials have shown improved survival over those treated with adult treatment regimens.

A child's treatment protocol, determined by the type of cancer and the extent of the disease, consists of a schedule and combination of therapies shown to be effective in treating the condition. A particular disease protocol may have several treatment regimens based on an accepted treatment standard with slight variations based on specific disease factors, including genetic markers. Clinical trials look at improving the outcome of cancer by either introducing a new drug or schedule or modifying the way the standard of care chemotherapy is given. Before a child is assigned to a particular protocol, informed consent is obtained from the parents and, if appropriate, the child. If a child is treated on a research protocol, the family may elect to withdraw the child from the study at any time and have the child treated according to standard therapy.

Surgery

Surgical intervention is used to (1) obtain a biopsy specimen, (2) determine the extent of disease, (3) remove primary or metastatic lesions, (4) evaluate previously unresectable tumors, (5) provide a second look to evaluate the effects of chemotherapy and radiation on partially or nonresected tumors, and (6) relieve symptoms. Surgical procedures are also used to place indwelling venous access devices and to displace organs outside the radiation field (e.g., ovaries during pelvic irradiation).

Chemotherapy

Chemotherapy aims to interrupt the cell cycle of proliferating malignant cells while minimizing damage to normal cells. In combination with chemotherapy, different drugs are used to disrupt the cell cycle at different phases, increasing the exposure of the malignant cells to cytotoxic agents. The routes of chemotherapy administration include oral, intramuscular, intravenous, intrathecal, and intraventricular. Although most intravenous infusions have traditionally been administered in the hospital setting, some agents lend themselves to safe administration in the home. Eligibility for home infusion often depends on stable utilities in the home, parental reliability, and few side effects during an in-hospital trial of the agent.

Chemotherapeutic agents may be either phase-specific or nonspecific. Cell cycle–specific drugs kill cells only in a certain stage of the cell's development and are most effective on rapidly growing cells. Along with malignant cells, the cells of the bone marrow, hair follicles, and mucous membranes are susceptible to damage from these drugs. Cell cycle–nonspecific drugs kill cells regardless of their stage of development. They act on both dormant and dividing cells. Chemotherapeutic agents are further classified by their mechanism of action. The major classifications include alkylating agents, antimetabolites, vinca alkaloids, antibiotics, and corticosteroids.

Radiation Therapy

Radiation therapy is often used in conjunction with surgery and chemotherapy. Radiation causes the breakage of DNA strands, thus inhibiting cell division. Radiation therapy aims to destroy cancer cells while minimizing complications and long-term sequelae. The amount of radiation required depends on the type of cancer, the timing of the radiation, and any prior radiation treatment. Radiation can be used as a single method of treatment or part of a multimodal plan, including chemotherapy, surgery, or palliative. Palliative radiotherapy is used to relieve symptoms of an incurable disease after more conservative methods have proved ineffective.

There are many different types of radiation used with pediatric cancers. External beam radiotherapy is the most common delivery method for radiation treatments. Photons (a type of x-ray particle) are aimed by a machine into the tumor (ACS, 2022). It requires careful delivery to maximize the radiation reaching the tumor but limit its side effects to the healthy tissues surrounding the cancer. Proton therapy delivers radiation in a more confined matter to the tumor, minimizing side effects. Protons are particles that carry a charge and, when released into the body, deliver their radiation within the tumor region with fewer scatter effects to surrounding tissues. It is an important method of treating pediatric cancers to help reduce the radiation effects on growing tissues. Stereotactic and Gamma Knife radiation are very precise methods of delivering radiation, usually to brain tumors and under anesthesia. Total body irradiation is used with allogeneic bone marrow transplant patients to prepare the body to accept new bone marrow. Meta-iodobenzylguanidine (MIBG) therapy is a specialized type of radiation therapy targeting neuroblastomas, using an intravenous infusion of irradiated iodine (I-131) attached to a particle called MIBG to target this type of tumor.

The tumor's response to radiation depends on the type of tumor, the type and dose of radiation delivered, and the size of the area irradiated. These factors also influence the type and severity of side effects and long-term sequelae. Many side effects are similar to those of chemotherapy, but rather than a systemic response the side effects are generally related to the irradiated area. They include nausea and vomiting, diarrhea, mucositis, cataracts, skin changes, neurocognitive deficits, and growth and endocrine abnormalities.

Biotherapy

Biotherapy is a fast-developing area for the treatment of cancers that uses the knowledge of how the immune system works, how cells communicate with each other, and how cancer cells interact with each other and the immune system (Herring, 2019). It works differently than chemotherapy in that it targets a specific cell or cell marker and prevents growth or is cytostatic. (Chemotherapy is cytocidal and kills rapidly dividing cells without the ability to distinguish between cancer and healthy cells.) Biotherapy includes immunotherapy and targeted therapy as methods for treating cancer. Immunotherapy uses the body's ability to control cancer cells, and targeted therapy acts directly on a specific function or process that the cancer cell depends on for growth, division, or spread. It encompasses the use of T cells, B cells, natural killer (NK) cells, dendritic cells, and cytokines to identify and kill abnormal cells. The side effects of biotherapy are related to the stimulation of the immune system versus chemotherapy, where side effects are related to the suppression and destruction of rapidly dividing normal cells (Herring, 2019).

Immunotherapy can be passive or active. The most well-known passive or adoptive type of immunotherapy is chimeric antigen receptor T-cell (CAR-T) therapy. CAR-T therapy uses T cells in the body to target markers on the cancer cells and kill them. These T cells are taken from the patient's body and changed in the lab to add the CAR to the T cells, and then this infusion is given back to the patient. Currently, CAR-T therapy is used for leukemia and lymphomas and is a very promising area of treatment for other cancers.

Immunotherapy includes immunomodulators, checkpoint inhibitors, vaccines, and oncolytic viruses. These use the patient's immune system to do the cell-killing work (Herring, 2019). Immunomodulators include cytokines (interleukins and interferons) and growth factors (filgrastim, erythropoietin, and thrombopoietin). Cytokines are messengers between cells in the immune system to cause an inflammatory response when a foreign cell is detected. Checkpoint inhibitors are monoclonal antibodies. The immune system uses checkpoints to regulate immune responses. Many types of cancer cells can affect checkpoints or turn down their effect to allow the cancer cells to get through and proliferate. Checkpoint inhibitors prevent this inhibitory response of the T cells to allow them to attack the cancer cells. Vaccines can prevent cancer, such as the human papillomavirus vaccine (cervical/anal/penile cancers) and the hepatitis B vaccine (liver cancer). They also can be therapeutic to slow tumor growth or prevent a recurrence. Multiple vaccines in studies are now working toward preventing the recurrence of different pediatric cancers, such as neuroblastomas and some solid tumors (Herring, 2019; Olsen et al., 2021).

Targeted therapies also include monoclonal antibodies and small molecule inhibitors. They have fewer side effects because they target specific cells, there is less chance of drug resistance, and there are fewer cumulative dose-limiting side effects. They act on their own specific targets on the cell, not the whole cells, thus limiting the above-mentioned issues. Monoclonal antibodies are immunoglobins that bind with a specific receptor on the outside of the cell to start the immune response. They are easy to recognize in the name because they end with *-mab*. They are currently used in the treatment of multiple types of pediatric cancers and among other studies (Butler et al., 2021). Small molecule inhibitors are proteins that are small enough to cross the cell membrane of cancer cells to get inside and interact with proteins to interfere with pathways for cell proliferation (Herring, 2019). Tyrosine kinase inhibitors are the most recognized type of small molecule inhibitors; they end in -*nib*. They block receptor tyrosine kinase to stop the growth of many types of cancers that use this pathway, such as acute lymphoblastic leukemia (ALL) that is Philadelphia chromosome positive, chronic myeloid leukemia, myelodysplastic disorders, neurofibromatosis, and some solid tumors. Other types of biotherapies used in pediatric oncology include vascular endothelial growth factor inhibitors that induce angiogenesis (loss of blood flow to the tumor), differentiating agents (retinoids and arsenic) that make the cancer cells develop into normal cells or die, and gene therapy that injects genetic material to modify cells or alter the patient's cells (Herring, 2019).

Hematopoietic Stem Cell Transplantation

HSCT involves the infusion of hematopoietic stem cells to reconstitute a patient's hematopoietic system (NCI, 2022). It is designed to create a marrow space, suppress the immune system to prevent rejection, and kill malignant cells. HSCT is currently used in treating some cases of relapsed ALL, acute myelogenous leukemia, neuroblastoma, lymphoma, and brain tumors. It can also replace or modulate an absent or malfunctioning hematopoietic or immune system or treat some genetic disorders, such as severe combined immunodeficiency, Wiskott-Aldrich syndrome, or chronic granulomatous disease (NCI, 2022). Hematopoietic stem cells for transplantation come from bone marrow, peripheral blood, or umbilical cord blood. Donors of bone marrow or blood stem cells come from three sources: the affected person (autologous), an identical twin (syngeneic), or another histocompatible or incompatible donor (allogeneic) (NCI, 2022). This procedure allows for potentially lethal doses of chemotherapy with or without radiation to be given to rid the body of all malignant cells. The donor's marrow or blood stem cells replace the child's destroyed marrow and, after engraftment, should produce the donor's nonmalignant functioning cells.

There are many considerations when thinking of using HSCT as a mode of treatment for a child with cancer. Patients should be in remission of their disease after receiving chemotherapy because it has been found that children with residual disease do very poorly with transplants (NCI, 2022). There are significant risks and side effects that accompany HSCT, such as rejection of the bone marrow, graft-versus-host disease, infections, and venoocclusive disorder. Children who have lower risks of side effects and relapse should be chosen because those who have received multiple cycles of chemotherapy/radiation and those with multiple comorbid are at much higher risk of significant complications, including graft-versus-host disease, organ failure, sepsis, and death (NCI, 2022).

SUPPORTIVE CARE

Supportive care, an essential part of cancer care, is used to help mitigate the side effects of the therapies the child is receiving. Antiemetics are an essential part of supportive care. Nausea and vomiting can have profound physiologic and psychological effects on the child receiving therapy. Chemotherapies have varying degrees that are taken into consideration when designing a treatment plan. The mechanisms involved in nausea and vomiting are complex; no single drug will consistently control these side effects. The situation is further complicated by the wide variation in response of the individual child to both the chemotherapeutic agent and the antiemetic. The antiemetic should be given before nausea and vomiting occur and should be continued until the symptoms have resolved. Nausea and vomiting related to chemotherapy generally will not last longer than 48 hours after chemotherapy administration. However, some children experience delayed nausea and vomiting, particularly if cisplatin is used in the chemotherapeutic regimen. Radiation-induced nausea is generally limited to the first few hours following treatments directed toward the head or abdomen. There are many categories of antiemetics used with chemotherapies, such as H2 blockers (diphenhydramine), steroids (dexamethasone), selective 5-HT3 (ondansetron, palonosetron, granisetron), and NK1 receptor antagonists (fosaprepitant, aprepitant). Proper selection and timing of these medications can reduce nausea and vomiting significantly and minimize the potential for dehydration, nutritional deficiencies, and electrolyte imbalances in children receiving chemotherapy.

Anorexia and Weight Loss

During therapy, anorexia and weight loss are common and can be attributed to both the disease and its treatment. The psychological impact of cancer and the tumor's metabolic influence can contribute to weight loss. Nutrition is essential for the healing, growth, and development of the child, but treatment-induced nausea and vomiting, as well as changes in taste, may lead to food aversion. Therefore the child's weight must be closely monitored throughout treatment. Oral supplements, appetite stimulants, and in some cases nasogastric or gastrostomy feedings or hyperalimentation may be necessary to maintain the child's weight and nutrition.

Bone Marrow Suppression

Bone marrow suppression is another side effect of chemotherapy and radiation. Pancytopenia usually begins within 7 to 10 days after drug administration, with the nadir (i.e., the point at which the blood cell counts are the lowest) occurring at approximately 14 days. The marrow then recovers in 21 to 28 days. The exact time of the nadir varies depending on the specific chemotherapeutic agent. Close monitoring is necessary to determine the extent of marrow suppression. Leukopenia refers to the presence of a low number of all-white blood cells (WBCs), whereas neutropenia refers specifically to a low neutrophil cell count. Neutrophils are the body's main defense against bacterial infection. Infections are a major life-threatening complication of cancer and its treatment. Granulocyte colony-stimulating factor (G-CSF) is an essential part of many chemotherapy treatment plans to reduce the risk of prolonged neutropenia and infections. It promotes an increase in WBCs following chemotherapy. These injections are incorporated with many high-dose chemotherapy plans for solid tumors; they are not used with leukemia plans. Filgrastim is given daily as a subcutaneous injection starting at least 24 hours after the completion of chemotherapy. At the same time, peg-filgrastim is given as one injection.

Several precautions can be taken to reduce the risk of infection. Good hand-washing techniques by the child, the parents, all family members, and caregivers are paramount to reducing the spread of pathogens. Good personal hygiene by the child, including thorough dental care, is also important. A child with neutropenia should avoid individuals who are ill, crowded situations, and anyone with a communicable disease. Attending school and wearing masks should be discussed with the primary team. Rectal temperatures and suppositories should also be avoided because abrading the rectal mucosa increases the risk of introducing bacteria from the rectum into the bloodstream.

Anemia/Thrombocytopenia

Guidelines for transfusion are based on laboratory parameters and clinical symptoms. The thrombocytopenic child may require platelet transfusions because of the risk of serious hemorrhage. Transfusion is recommended if the platelet count is less than 10,000 to 20,000/mm³ and/or in the presence of bleeding. A transfusion is indicated in a child whose hemoglobin level is less than 7 to 8 g/dL and/or who is symptomatic (e.g., shortness of breath, headache, dizziness, fatigue). However, variations in transfusion practice guidelines exist between facilities. Epoetin alfa can be used to help with anemia in patients who do not have myeloid leukemia and are receiving myelosuppressive chemotherapy.

Alopecia

A distinguishing therapy-related complication is alopecia. It is generally a temporary condition that results from damage to the hair follicles by chemotherapy and radiation. Although the hair usually regrows after therapy, the texture and color may be slightly different. It is a traumatic experience sometimes for both the child and parents. Reassurance should be given, and options for head coverings should be discussed to bring comfort and confidence to the child/adolescent.

Fatigue

Fatigue is also a major and distressing consequence of childhood cancer and its therapy. It can be from many facets of therapy: anemia, poor nutrition, stress/worry, poor sleep, fever, and trying to do too much (COG, 2018). Fatigue can be managed through nutritional supplementation, transfusions, treatment of infections, some daily physical activity, and daily rest.

Toxicity From Chemotherapy

Chemoprotective agents are used to mitigate the toxic effects of chemotherapy on certain organs, such as the heart, kidneys, and CNS. Dexrazoxane is used to minimize the cardiotoxic effects of anthracyclines. Mesna is used to reduce the risk of hemorrhagic cystitis seen with cyclophosphamide and ifosfamide. Leucovorin is a folic acid derivative used as a rescue drug or antidote for high-dose intravenous methotrexate and for intrathecal methotrexate for children with Down syndrome or CNS methotrexate toxicity.

COMPLEMENTARY THERAPIES

Complementary therapies encompass a variety of interventions (e.g., the use of herbs, dietary supplements, cannabis, ice caps, essential oils) in hopes of treating the cancer or control of symptoms such as pain or nausea. Any supplement or major dietary change should be viewed in terms of its potential to interact with chemotherapeutic agents. Choices by families to use complementary therapy, in addition to chemotherapy/radiation/surgery, should be respected but also discussed for the potential of interaction with treatment. There are many items that can be used in conjunction with medical therapy that can be helpful to the comfort of the child.

 Associated Problems

Cancer and Treatment

- Vascular access: Most children require the use of an indwelling central venous access device (VAD).
- All lumens must be cultured if any fever is present.
Therapy-related complications
- Nausea and vomiting: Use antiemetics before and after chemotherapeutic administration, not on an as-needed (prn) basis.
- Anorexia and weight loss: Monitor weight regularly; early intervention is essential.
- Bone marrow suppression:
  - Hemoglobin <7–8 g/dL, consider transfusion
  - Platelets <10,000–20,000/mm³, consider transfusion
  - Absolute neutrophil count <500, high risk for infection; possible use of erythropoietin for treatment of anemia and granulocyte colony-stimulating factor for neutropenia unless having leukemia
- Infection: Blood cultures for all fevers
  - Intravenous antibiotics for fever and neutropenia or for any child with a central VAD; administer antibiotics within 1 hr of fever to reduce the risk of sepsis
- Alopecia
- Fatigue
- Late effects: see Table 13.2
- Relapse
- Death

ASSOCIATED PROBLEMS OF CANCER AND TREATMENT

Vascular Access

Children receiving intensive treatment require a central venous access device (VAD) to reduce frequent venipunctures for laboratory tests and the administration of chemotherapy, blood products, antibiotic therapy, and nutritional support. Access devices include tunneled catheters, peripherally inserted central catheters (PICCs), and implanted catheters. Many factors must be considered in the choice of VAD. Such factors include the child's frequency, duration, and type of therapy; the presence of a weakened immune system or other potential contraindications for surgery; the child's age; and the child's home environment. The patency of all long-term VADs is maintained through periodic flushing with heparin and/or saline. Complications of indwelling VADs include infection, occlusion of the catheter from thrombus and fibrin formation, damage to the external portion of the catheter, dislodgement, and (rarely) cardiac tamponade. Because this is the main source to administer all forms of therapy for the patient, the risk of infection is possible. With any fever, the central line should be on the top of the differential as a source of the infection.

Tunneled catheters include Hickman, Broviac, Cook, and Groshong catheters. These have internal and external portions. The catheter is inserted into the subclavian vein and advanced until the tip is at the right atrium. The external portion is the lumen(s) used to gain access to the line. They can be single, double, or triple lumen. The insertion site needs to be covered with a sterile dressing that is changed weekly or when the dressing becomes compromised. These lines must be flushed daily to prevent clotting.

Implanted ports include the mediport, port-a-cath, and infuse-a-port. These are implanted below the skin with the catheter tip at the junction of the superior vena cava and the right atrium. They can be single or double lumen. Venous access is achieved by puncturing the skin above the reservoir and passing a specially designed needle through the silicone membrane into the port receptacle. Topical anesthetics may be applied to port sites before accessing to reduce discomfort and fear.

PICCs are less invasive than the tunneled or implanted central line; however, these are meant to be used for short rather than long timeframes, as normally planned with chemotherapy. At times when central access is required and the child is not stable enough for anesthesia (e.g., mediastinal mass, critically ill), a PICC is warranted. PICCs are inserted in a large vein in the arm and threaded into the superior vena cava with the tip of the catheter at the top of the right atrium. Because they also have external lumens, a sterile dressing is applied to the insertion site and must be changed weekly or when compromised. These lines also must be flushed daily.

Peripheral intravenous lines are infrequently used for chemotherapy because of the risk of infiltration, and many drugs are irritants (causing inflammation) or vesicants (causing tissue death) that could damage surrounding tissue in the case of a leak. They are still used for procedures when an intravenous line is needed but a central line is not available or must be replaced.

Late Effects

As survival rates continually improve, the long-term effects of therapy are becoming evident. The goal of therapy is not merely improving survival but reducing physiologic and developmental morbidity. The development of second malignancies, impaired growth, diminished cognitive functioning, and organ damage are the areas of greatest concern. Factors that appear to influence the development of late effects include the child's age and stage of development at the time of diagnosis, the primary tumor, socioeconomic factors, and the therapy used. The American Academy of Pediatrics (AAP), working with COG, recommends that all primary care providers in pediatrics work with an oncologist to screen survivors of pediatric cancers for long-term side effects (AAP, 2021). They also recommend using the Long-Term Follow-up Guidelines for Survivors of Childhood, Adolescent, and Young Adult Cancers (COG, 2018) as a tool for screening survivors for long-term effects/complications (Table 13.2).

Relapse

Despite the advances in childhood cancer treatment, some children will experience a relapse of their disease. Relapse, like diagnosis, is a crisis period for the family. It poses a challenge for the oncology team because the best methods of treatment were used at diagnosis. Relapse often requires more experimental modes of treatment. The primary care provider, in cooperation with the oncology team, can support the family—and especially the child—through this difficult time.

Death

There may come a time when all possible viable treatment options have been exhausted. The care of the child moves from focusing on a cure to providing comfort and giving as much quality time as possible. The collaboration between the primary care provider and the oncology team can be invaluable during this time. Families often seek guidance and support in making decisions that they can live with long after the child's death. Knowledge of the community- and hospital-based hospice programs in their area can be beneficial in meeting many of the home care and support needs of families. All families need reassurance that they will not be abandoned at this time and that multidisciplinary resources will be made available to them as required.

Table 13.2 Late Effects of Antineoplastic Therapy on Body Systems

ADVERSE EFFECTS	CAUSATIVE AGENT	TIME INTERVAL	SIGNS AND SYMPTOMS	PREDISPOSING FACTORS	PREVENTIVE/DIAGNOSTIC MEASURES
Cardiovascular System					
Cardiomyopathy	Anthracycline chemotherapy	Weeks to years after therapy	Shortness of breath, dyspnea on exertion, orthopnea, chest pain, palpitation; if age <25 yr, possible abdominal symptoms (nausea/vomiting)	Comorbid with obesity, congenital heart disease, hypertension, diabetes mellitus, dyslipidemia, smoking, drug use Anthracycline therapy, especially if lifetime cumulative dose of ≥250 mg/m^2	Use of cardioprotectant drug-dexrazoxane with anthracyclines Yearly blood pressure and cardiac exam Echocardiogram (ECG) screening guidelines based on mg/m^2 given ECG first year of long-term follow-up to rule out prolonged QTC interval, then screen as clinically indicated Referral to cardiologist with subclinical abnormalities, left ventricular dysfunction, dysrhythmia or prolonged QTc interval
	Irradiation of chest, abdomen, spine (thoracic, total) or total body irradiation (TBI)				ECG guidelines based on total anthracyclines given with radiation For females considering pregnancy or who are pregnant ≥35 Gy chest radiation OR ≥15 Gy if combined with any dose of anthracycline
Pericarditis, pericardial fibrosis, valvular	Mediastinal irradiation	Few months to years	Chest pain, dyspnea, fever, paradoxic pulse, venous distention, friction rub, Kussmaul sign	Most common with doses of 40–60 Gy	Partial shielding of mediastinum Referral to cardiologist
Pulmonary System					
Pneumonitis followed by pulmonary fibrosis	Pulmonary irradiation	Months to years after treatment	Dyspnea, decreased exercise tolerance, pulmonary insufficiency	Increased risk with the following: Large lung volume in the radiation field Therapy during periods of pulmonary infection Use of radiation sensitizing chemotherapy TBI Doses >40 Gy	Careful monitoring of status with physical examination, chest radiograph, pulmonary function tests
	Bleomycin, carmustine, high-dose cyclophosphamide, busulfan			Higher doses of bleomycin (≥400 units/m^2 combined) Radiation to lungs or TBI	Yearly influenza vaccine Yearly pneumococcal vaccine Avoid smoking Encourage frequent rest periods High-dose steroids for severe cases Avoid high concentrations of oxygen

Continued

Table 13.2 Late Effects of Antineoplastic Therapy on Body Systems—cont'd

ADVERSE EFFECTS	CAUSATIVE AGENT	TIME INTERVAL	SIGNS AND SYMPTOMS	PREDISPOSING FACTORS	PREVENTIVE/DIAGNOSTIC MEASURES
Hematopoietic System					
Long-term suppression of marrow function	Extensive irradiation of marrow-containing bones Chemotherapy	Months to years following therapy	Fall in WBC and platelet counts; hypoplastic/aplastic bone marrow aspirates; diminished uptake of radioisotopes	Radiation doses: 30–50 Gy in older individuals Concomitant use of chemotherapy	Limitation of areas of marrow irradiated Monitoring of child's status with periodic bone marrow aspirates and peripheral blood cell counts
Alterations in immune system	Nodal irradiation affects cellular immunity Splenectomy or splenic irradiation affects humoral immunity	Weeks to years following therapy	Predisposition to infection	Adolescents more at risk than younger children	Pneumococcal vaccine and penicillin if splenectomy done Monitoring of child's status with periodic blood counts and tests of immune response
Gastrointestinal System					
Hepatic fibrosis-cirrhosis	Chemotherapy	Months to years following therapy	Persistent elevation of liver function tests after cessation of therapy; hepatomegaly, cirrhosis, jaundice, spider nevi	Daily low doses of methotrexate by mouth for long periods Long-term use of mercaptopurine	Monitor the child's status with liver function tests Perform liver biopsy if liver function test results remain persistently abnormal
Chronic enteritis	Radiation therapy	Months to years following therapy	Pain, recurrent vomiting, diarrhea, malabsorption syndrome, weight loss	Radiation doses >50 Gy Children with previous abdominal surgery Chemotherapy as radiation sensitizers (actinomycin, doxorubicin)	Avoid concomitant use of radiation sensitizers Careful monitoring of height and weight Supportive therapy when symptoms develop, including low-residue, low-fat, gluten- and milk-free diet
Hepatitis C infection	Blood transfusion before 1993	Months to years	Most patients asymptomatic	Other risk factors: IV drug use, high-risk sexual activity, use of clotting factors prior to 1987, organ transplants, long-term dialysis, sharing needles/razors/toothbrushes with those who have hepatitis C	Screen all recipients of transfusion before 1993 with AST/ALT and hepatitis C antibody; if positive (or negative with elevated ALT), monitor PCR-based RNA screen for hepatitis C and refer to gastroenterologist

Table 13.2 Late Effects of Antineoplastic Therapy on Body Systems—cont'd

ADVERSE EFFECTS	CAUSATIVE AGENT	TIME INTERVAL	SIGNS AND SYMPTOMS	PREDISPOSING FACTORS	PREVENTIVE/DIAGNOSTIC MEASURES
Kidney and Urinary Tract					
Nephritis–glomerular and/or tubular dysfunction	Radiation to renal structures (20–30 Gy)—may be enhanced by chemotherapy	Weeks to years after therapy	Decrease in renal function with elevated BUN and creatinine, proteinuria, anemia, hypertension, may have urinary wasting of magnesium, potassium, and calcium with cisplatin	Other nephrotoxic drugs (aminoglycosides, vancomycin, amphotericin, cyclosporine)	Periodically monitor renal status during and after therapy with blood pressure readings, urinalysis, CBC, BUN, and creatinine
	Cisplatin, ifosfamide, lomustine, carmustine, methotrexate (high doses)			Inadequate alkalinization of urine before methotrexate Urinary tract infections	Once progressive renal failure develops, treatment is supportive Electrolyte supplementation as needed Child should avoid rough contact sports after nephrectomy to protect remaining kidney
Renal Fanconi syndrome	Ifosfamide	Weeks to years after therapy	Urinary wasting of phosphorus, glucose, proteins, and inability to acidify urine; can lead to renal rickets with inhibition of growth and bone deformity	Age <3 yr at time of treatment, prior renal dysfunction, nephrectomy	Periodically monitor renal status during and after therapy with urinalysis and electrolytes and phosphorus Electrolyte supplementation as needed
Chronic hemorrhagic cystitis	Cyclophosphamide, ifosfamide Radiation therapy	Months to years after treatment	Sterile, painful hematuria; urinary frequency	Inadequate hydration during cyclophosphamide or ifosfamide therapy	Techniques to reduce bladder exposure during radiation therapy Frequent emptying of bladder during and 24 hr after therapy Adequate hydration before, during, and after therapy Concomitant use of mesna with chemotherapy Treatment of bladder hemorrhage with formalin instillation or cauterization of bleeding sites
Musculoskeletal System					
Impaired skeletal growth	Irradiation of skeletal structures and abdomen	Months to years following treatment	Growth retardation, reduction in sitting height, scoliosis, altered growth of facial skeleton	Effect of spinal irradiation to vertebral bodies in doses 10–20 Gy dependent on the age of the child; known damage >20 Gy Unilateral radiation results in asymmetric deformities Symmetric growth delay during periods of chemotherapy	Careful monitoring of the child's status with growth charts, radiographic studies, sitting and standing height Dose radiation reduction during periods of rapid growth
Delayed or arrested tooth development	Irradiation of maxilla or mandible Chemotherapy	Months to years	Teeth are small with pale enamel, malocclusion	Radiation during the period of dental growth and development	Dental examinations every 6 mo Good oral hygiene, including flossing Fluoride prophylaxis

Continued

Table **13.2** Late Effects of Antineoplastic Therapy on Body Systems—cont'd

ADVERSE EFFECTS	CAUSATIVE AGENT	TIME INTERVAL	SIGNS AND SYMPTOMS	PREDISPOSING FACTORS	PREVENTIVE/DIAGNOSTIC MEASURES
Avascular necrosis (AVN) and osteoporosis	Radiation	Months to years	AVN—joint pain often accompanied by slipped capital epiphysis of the femoral head	Poor calcium intake Increased body weight	Encourage calcium intake and low-impact exercise as preventive measures
	Steroids (particularly dexamethasone)		Osteoporosis—bone fractures		DEXA scan for osteoporosis
	Methotrexate (usually resolves at the end of therapy)				Referral to orthopedics
Endocrine System					
Thyroid gland dysfunction	Irradiation of thyroid gland, brain, and total body irradiation	Months to years	Hypothyroidism; may be asymptomatic and have abnormal thyroid function; nodular abnormalities, thyroid cancer	Cancer reported with varying radiation doses: 10–30 Gy Thyroid directly in the radiation field	Monitor thyroid function with T_3, free T_4, and TSH Hormonal replacement therapy for all children with abnormal thyroid tests since elevated TSH is associated with thyroid cancer Ultrasound
Injuries to gonads	Irradiation of gonads Chemotherapy (alkylating agents)	Months to years	Infertility, sterility, hormonal dysfunction, azoospermia, teratogenic during the first trimester of pregnancy	Testicular radiation (>6 Gy, azoospermia may be permanent) Ovarian radiation (≥5 Gy if pubertal, ≥10 Gy is prepubertal) Chemotherapy damage dependent on drug used, dose, duration of therapy, child's sex and age Radiation used in combination with HSCT	Tanner staging yearly Protection of testes/ovaries from the radiation field Gonadal dysfunction from chemotherapy may be reversible *Males (14 yr old):* check LH, FSH, testosterone levels *Females (12 yr old):* check LH, FSH, estradiol levels
Decreased growth rate	Irradiation of cranium and/or spine TBI Chemotherapy	Months to years	Reduction in height percentile or growth rate	Radiation therapy at younger age Higher cumulative radiation doses (≥20 Gy)	After completion of therapy, check standing and sitting heights 1–2 times each year Thyroid function tests, bone age, and growth hormone testing to be considered if rate declines

Table **13.2** Late Effects of Antineoplastic Therapy on Body Systems—cont'd

ADVERSE EFFECTS	CAUSATIVE AGENT	TIME INTERVAL	SIGNS AND SYMPTOMS	PREDISPOSING FACTORS	PREVENTIVE/DIAGNOSTIC MEASURES
Nervous System					
Peripheral sensory or motor neuropathies	Chemotherapy (vincristine, etoposide, cisplatin)	Months to years	Deficit in function Pain Decreased tendon reflexes	Chemotherapy with vinca alkaloids and heavy metals	Careful monitoring of child's status during and after therapy Physical and occupational therapy to help regain function or reduce the deficit
Central neuroendocrine dysfunction of hypothalamic-pituitary axis	Cranial irradiation; chemotherapy	Months to years	Growth hormone deficiency Panhypopituitarism with short stature; hypothyroidism; Addison disease	Dependent on the dose of radiation, age of the child, and concomitant use of chemotherapy Younger children who receive >18 Gy at greatest risk TBI ≥10 Gy in single fraction, ≥12 Gy fractionated	Careful monitoring of child's status with growth charts, Tanner staging, bone age at 9 yr then yearly to puberty Thyroid, hormone, insulin, and cortisol measurement may be necessary Treatment with replacement of deficient hormones
Encephalopathy	Cranial irradiation; chemotherapy, particularly IV methotrexate (high dose) and IT methotrexate	Months to years	May be asymptomatic but demonstrate abnormalities on head CT scans May have overt symptoms ranging from lethargy to somnolence, dementia, seizures, paralysis, and coma	Cranial radiation alone or with concomitant chemotherapy CNS leukemias/lymphomas Cranial radiation ≤24 Gy Younger children are more vulnerable	Monitor the child's status with careful physical examination, head MRI/CT scans, psychometric testing Reduce chemotherapy dose when preclinical radiographic findings appear
Neurocognitive deficits	Radiation therapy, chemotherapy	Months to years	Abnormal psychological tests with deficits in perceptual behavior, language development, and learning abilities Behavioral changes Diminished IQ	Younger children CNS tumors CNS leukemias/lymphomas Receiving higher doses of radiation or have larger fields	Careful monitoring with periodic neurocognitive/psychological evaluations Early intervention with multidisciplinary approach and specialized education programs

Continued

Table 13.2 Late Effects of Antineoplastic Therapy on Body Systems—cont'd

ADVERSE EFFECTS	CAUSATIVE AGENT	TIME INTERVAL	SIGNS AND SYMPTOMS	PREDISPOSING FACTORS	PREVENTIVE/DIAGNOSTIC MEASURES
Secondary (Malignancy Multiple Symptoms)					
Leukemia, especially AML	Alkylating agents Doxorubicin Etoposide	Years	Leukopenia Anemia Thrombocytopenia Fever Bone pain	Any malignancy receiving these chemotherapies, such as Ewing sarcoma (etoposide)	Monitor CBC Report persistent fever
Thyroid cancer	Irradiation of mediastinum, spine, head, or neck		Palpable mass/nodule Anterior cervical adenopathy	Younger age at the time of radiation therapy	If a thyroid nodule is present, obtain a thyroid ultrasound, thyroid function tests Biopsy or bone needle aspiration of nodule or node
Breast cancer	Irradiation of mediastinum, spine, or chest wall		Palpable mass	More common with those who received >20 Gy mantle area (prior to 1990)	Teach adolescents to do breast self-examination
Bone and soft tissue tumors	Irradiation of bone or soft tissue with primary tumor		Mass Pain	Those who received high-radiation doses (≥30 Gy; bone malignancies) NF1 mutation Bilateral or familiar retinoblastoma Gorlin syndrome	Dermatology skin checks Educate to seek assistance for any bone mass/pain.

ALT, Alanine transaminase; *AML,* acute myelocytic leukemia; *AST,* aspartate transaminase; *AVN,* avascular necrosis; *BUN,* blood urea nitrogen; *CBC,* complete blood count; *CNS,* central nervous system; *CT,* computed tomography; *DEXA,* dual energy x-ray absorptiometry; *FSH,* follicle-stimulating hormone; *HSCT,* hematopoietic stem cell transplantation; *IT,* intrathecal; *IQ,* intelligent quotient; *IV,* intravenous; *LH,* luteinizing hormone; *MRI,* magnetic resonance imaging; *PCR,* polymerase chain reaction; *RNA,* ribonucleic acid; *T₃,* triiodothyronine; *T₄,* thyroxine; *TSH,* thyroid-stimulating hormone; *WBC,* white blood cell.
From Children's Oncology Group. (2018). Long-term follow-up guidelines for survivors of childhood, adolescent, and young adult cancers. http://www.survivorshipguidelines.org/.

PRIMARY CARE MANAGEMENT

HEALTH CARE MAINTENANCE

Growth and Development

Although growth retardation secondary to chemotherapy often resolves when therapy is complete, it may persist for some children depending on the type of cancer they have and treatment. The effect of cranial/spinal radiation, or radiation targeting an immature skeletal bone, however, can be permanent. Radiation affects growth by damaging the epiphyseal plates of the long bones and the glands that are responsible for growth-related hormone production. A child's growth should be observed on a standardized growth curve, with growth patterns examined over time rather than as isolated measurements. Growth rates should be checked with each visit during therapy and then every 1 to 3 months for the first year after therapy; then, measurements should be taken every 6 months until linear growth is completed. Because of the risk of significant weight loss, weight should also be monitored at each visit.

Intellectual development can be affected by intrathecal chemotherapy and cranial/spinal radiation for those with leukemia involving the CNS. Avoidance of CNS radiation until children are 5 years old is essential to preserve brain development; however, sometimes it cannot be avoided because of the cancer. Therefore ongoing developmental assessment should be performed during and after therapy. Early identification and intervention are important in assisting the child in maintaining age-appropriate development. Neuropsychological testing is incorporated with many treatment plans as part of clinical trials and with neurooncology plans. These may be repeated after therapy has been completed if there are school concerns.

Diet

Maintaining adequate nutrition while a child is receiving treatment is challenging because of loss of appetite, taste changes, and weight loss. Well-balanced, nutritious meals should be offered. Small, frequent meals may be more appealing than the standard three meals daily. Working with a dietician can be very helpful in offering options for flavoring foods, smoothie recipes, or other recipes that could be more appetizing to children during therapy. Appetite stimulants can be used to maintain the needed calories during treatment and can be stopped when the child's appetite resumes during less intensive therapy or at the end of treatment.

Children receiving corticosteroids may experience an increased appetite and weight gain, but because corticosteroids usually are administered for limited periods of time, such symptoms generally are of short duration. However, some children develop long-term weight issues and have been on steroids as part of their treatment regimens.

Safety

Safety issues for a child with a malignant disease involve balancing normal participation in daily activities with taking appropriate precautions imposed by the treatment of a malignant disease. For the safety of all children, chemotherapeutic agents must be stored securely out of reach. Thorough hand washing should follow the handling of any chemotherapeutic agent, and parents should wear gloves when handling the medication. Pregnant women should avoid contact with the chemotherapeutic agents and the urine of children receiving chemotherapy. If circumstances make this impossible, gloves should be worn. Unused portions of chemotherapeutic drugs should be returned to the dispensing pharmacy for disposal with other potent chemicals.

External tunneled VADs must have a clean dressing applied to the exit site and the line secured to the chest to minimize any excessive tension on the catheter. Syringes and other supplies used to maintain the line should be stored properly out of reach of children. Children with external tunneled VADs should avoid lake or ocean swimming and hot tubs to reduce the risk of infection. They should also have extra clamps available in case of damage to the catheter lumen.

Exposure to ill contacts should be minimized for all immunosuppressed children. Frequent hand washing and wearing a mask around crowds are other interventions that can prevent infections. Contact sports should be avoided while the patient has low platelets and is at risk for bleeding or if the patient has a single organ (kidney). Many chemotherapeutic agents will alter the skin's tolerance for sun exposure. It is important that children should always wear sunscreen when outside. If the child has alopecia, a hat and sunblock should be worn to protect the scalp.

Immunizations

All vaccines should be avoided during chemotherapy treatment. It is not because there is a risk of getting the infection the vaccine is meant to prevent, but vaccines need a strong immune system available to work and produce antibodies with the vaccine. Children may not get an adequate response to the vaccines. Once therapy has been completed, vaccines can be resumed or caught up on based on recommendations from the Centers for Disease Control and Prevention (CDC) vaccine schedule and the child's oncology team. Annual influenza and COVID vaccinations are recommended during therapy to prevent these infections. Vaccinations are not repeated after chemotherapy unless the patient has undergone an allogenic bone marrow transplant. Vaccines will all be repeated after the child recovers immunity from the transplant, and then titers will be drawn to check for a response. There are further recommendations through the Advisory Committee on Immunization Practice for those with altered immunocompetence (CDC, 2022).

Screenings

It should be emphasized that Bright Futures screening recommendations should be used with all children, including those diagnosed with cancer. Additional screenings for these children can be found in the long-term follow-up guidelines by the COG.

Vision. Routine vision screening is advised. Brain tumors may manifest with impaired visual acuity caused by ocular nerve compression, increased intracranial pressure, or blurred vision caused by papilledema. A classic sign of retinoblastoma is the white eye reflex in place of the normal red reflex. Infant neuroblastoma can present with signs of Horner syndrome (miosis, ptosis, enophthalmos, anhidrosis). The development of cataracts is a late effect of alkylating agents and radiation to the eye.

Hearing. Routine screenings of a patient's hearing are advised. Unilateral hearing loss may indicate the presence of a mass. Children receiving radiation to the area, including the ear, or receiving cisplatin are at increased risk for hearing loss. Baseline audiogram evaluation by an audiologist prior to therapy is important and yearly for patients age 5 and under, every 2 years for those aged 6 to 12, then every 5 years at age 13 is recommended (COG, 2018).

Dental. Routine dental care is advised to occur prior to treatment if possible. However, if any procedures are needed, they must be done, and the patient must be healed prior to beginning myelosuppressive chemotherapy. If that is not possible because of the urgency to start treatment, however, working with the patient's dentist is important in case the child has problems. Dental cleanings should be delayed until the child is not neutropenic or thrombocytopenic. Both radiation therapy and chemotherapy place a child at risk for stomatitis, dental caries, and periodontal disease. Ideally, dental work requiring the manipulation of the oral tissues should be performed only if the absolute neutrophil count (ANC) is greater than 1000/mm³ and the platelet count is greater than 75,000/mm³ (Ritwik, 2018). The promotion of good oral hygiene by an interdisciplinary team is important in preventing stomatitis, infection, and caries.

Blood pressure. Blood pressure should be measured at every visit because of possible hypertension from corticosteroids, any renal involvement by cancer, potential renal toxicity of many chemotherapeutic agents, and cardiac toxicities from anthracyclines.

Hemoglobin/Hematocrit. Because of frequent hematologic analyses, routine screening is unnecessary while a child receives therapy. After therapy, the primary oncology team will perform the routine screening.

COMMON ILLNESS MANAGEMENT

Differential Diagnoses

Fever. The presence of fever (i.e., 101°F [38.3°C]) adds a critical dimension to diagnosis and treatment in the face of neutropenia. If adequate therapy is not initiated promptly, the result could be life-threatening sepsis. The first step in evaluating a fever is obtaining a complete blood count (CBC) with differential, aerobic, and anaerobic blood cultures from all central VAD lumens and cultures from other potential sites of infection as indicated by the history and physical examination. Obtaining a chest radiograph is not indicated in the absence of respiratory symptoms. A complete physical examination should be performed, including perineal/perianal areas. Respiratory panels may be needed if the patient is experiencing any respiratory symptoms. Expected signs of infection, such as erythema and edema, may be absent or diminished. A history of chills or rigors occurring with flushing a central VAD may indicate the presence of bacteremia.

Differential Diagnoses

FEVER
- Bacterial, viral, fungal, or protozoal infection
- Site: blood, venous access device, nasopharynx, skin, joints, perineal, perirectal areas

GASTROINTESTINAL SYMPTOMS
- Diarrhea: infectious causes or chemotherapy induced
- Constipation: vinca alkaloids (paralytic ileus)
- Vomiting: chemotherapy induced, anticipatory

HEADACHE
- Increased intracranial pressure caused by a mass lesion or shunt malfunction
- Cerebrospinal fluid leak with a recent history of lumbar puncture

PAIN
- Tumor related: caused by compression of nerves or invasion of bone
- Treatment related: mucositis, dermatitis, neurotoxicity, phantom limb pain, infection
- Procedure related: bone marrow, lumbar puncture, venipuncture

Admission to the hospital for treatment is generally required for the child who is febrile and neutropenic (i.e., ANC <500/mm³). In selected cases of moderate neutropenia (i.e., ANC 200–500/mm³) and with lower risk for sepsis (type of cancer, social factors), the child may be treated as an outpatient (Manji et al., 2012). While viruses are the most common cause of fever in pediatric cancer patients, bacterial causes are ruled out by blood culture. If the patient is bacteremic, then parenteral broad-spectrum antibiotics should be started immediately under the direction of the oncology team. Antibiotic choice is based on the suspected organism and (later) sensitivity reports. The length and manner of administration of antibiotics depend on the type of bacteria and resistance patterns. Because the

VAD communicates between the inside and outside of the body, it is possible it can be the source of infection and may need to be removed based on response to antibiotics.

Gastrointestinal symptoms. Fungal infections, such as candidiasis and aspergillosis, should be suspected with prolonged fevers despite antibiotic treatment. Aspergillosis should be a concern if the child lives on a farm or an old home with mold or any home with water damage and mold growth.

The child who is immunocompromised and at risk for *Pneumocystis jirovecii* (formerly *P. carinii*) may take trimethoprim/sulfamethoxazole, dapsone, or pentamidine prophylactically. The type of prophylaxis is determined by the presence of patient allergies to one of the medications and tolerance issues of the choice of drug. Prophylaxis is usually continued for approximately 6 months after the completion of therapy. Symptoms of *P. jirovecii* include dry cough, fever, dyspnea, and possibly respiratory distress.

Nausea, vomiting, and diarrhea, which are common side effects of cancer treatment, may be difficult to distinguish from infections caused by bacteria, protozoa, viruses, or *Clostridium difficile* toxins. The primary care provider may also need to establish the relationship between the symptoms and chemotherapy or radiation administration. During these symptoms it is important to monitor fluid intake and avoid dehydration, especially in children who are currently receiving chemotherapy. In some cases intravenous fluid replacement and antiemetics may be necessary. Stool cultures may help identify an infectious source of diarrhea. Blood chemistry values, especially blood urea nitrogen, creatinine, aspartate transaminase, and alanine transaminase, must be monitored closely to avoid damaging vital organs from concentrated levels of the chemotherapeutics and from delayed excretion because of dehydration. Many families are taught how to administer intravenous hydration at home.

Vinca alkaloids, such as vincristine and vinblastine, predispose children to the development of constipation. If dietary intervention is not successful, supplementation with a stool softener or laxative will be needed to prevent paralytic ileus. Suppositories and enemas should not be used without consultation with the oncology team because of the potential risk of infection related to reduced WBC counts.

Headache. Headache pain, which is usually benign late in childhood and adolescence, could indicate serious underlying difficulties in young children. Morning headaches associated with vomiting and minimal nausea should always arouse suspicion of increased intracranial pressure caused by a mass lesion or shunt malfunction in a child with a brain tumor. Headache following a lumbar puncture that resolves with lying down may be caused by a slow cerebrospinal fluid leak. This type of headache is best treated by bed rest, adequate hydration, and caffeine. While taking a thorough history, the primary care provider should note onset, any precipitating factors or symptoms, location, severity, and what if any medication gives relief. A thorough neurologic examination is imperative. Many headaches may be treated at home with acetaminophen and rest; however, if the headache symptoms are unrelieved by medication or there is any change in vision or neurologic function, then immediate evaluation is necessary.

Pain. Pain in children is often difficult to assess and requires understanding normal child development and age-appropriate verbal and behavioral cues. Most importantly, keep in mind that children rarely fabricate the presence of pain. The child with cancer poses additional challenges because of the multiple etiologies of pain, which may result from the malignancy, treatments, or procedures (e.g., bone marrow and spinal tap).

Tumor-related pain occurs with direct tumor invasion of the bone, impingement of the tumor on nervous tissue, or metastatic lesions. Compression of the spinal cord by a tumor may result in severe back pain, and immediate evaluation is imperative, because an untreated cord compression can rapidly progress to irreversible neurologic damage. Treatment-related pain can occur from mucositis, infection, radiation-induced dermatitis, neurotoxicity from chemotherapy (vincristine), abdominal pain, or phantom limb pain following the amputation of a limb. Management of disease-related pain relies on pharmacologic and behavioral approaches. A systematic assessment of the child's pain is needed to design an optimal plan. Specialized pain team involvement may be needed to help patients who have complex pain.

Pain resulting from procedures is greatly reduced with the use of conscious sedation (e.g., using a combination of a sedative [midazolam, diazepam] and an opioid [fentanyl, morphine]). Topical anesthetics are also used in combination with sedation to reduce procedural pain. The two primary methods of achieving topical anesthesia subcutaneous infiltration are with lidocaine and topical lidocaine/prilocaine creams. Topical anesthesia for procedures is achieved in 7 to 15 minutes. Nonpharmacologic therapies to reduce pain and distress include distraction, guided imagery, and hypnosis. Child life therapy can also assist children and adolescents in coping with the loss of control and pain associated with invasive procedures.

Drug Interactions

Children receiving therapy need to avoid aspirin-containing products because they impair platelet function. Acetaminophen is generally recommended;

however, its use during periods of neutropenia is discouraged because it may mask a fever. Multivitamins that are high in folic acid should be avoided because of the interference of folate with methotrexate. Vitamins low in folic acid are acceptable. Because of the number of drugs a child may be taking for therapy and the possibility of interaction, it is advisable that the primary care provider contact the pediatric oncology team before prescribing additional medications.

DEVELOPMENTAL ISSUES

Sleep Patterns

Disturbances in sleep patterns are common. The extent to which the child is affected will depend on the age at diagnosis, medication schedules, the frequency of hospitalizations, and general coping patterns of the child. Maintaining a consistent bedtime ritual when possible provides security during a time when many routines are disrupted. Parents should also be encouraged to bring transitional objects (e.g., a teddy bear, favorite blanket) to the hospital because these may help the child sleep during hospitalization.

Toileting

Diarrhea and constipation may occur with certain chemotherapy agents. Toilet training may be delayed, or regression may occur if treatment occurs during the toddler or preschool period. Severe constipation can contribute to encopresis.

Discipline

Discipline for a child with cancer should be the same as for all children. A consistent approach to establishing expectations and setting limits is important to the child's sense of security. Parents should be supported in maintaining normal patterns of discipline, although they may initially be ambivalent about disciplining their child who is ill. Cancer treatment imposes considerable role strain on parents. Those who maintain normal patterns of discipline may be judged for treating their children harshly, whereas parents who are more lenient may be seen as spoiling their children (Ernst et al., 2019). Consistency in discipline between parents and siblings is also important.

Child Care

The intensity of certain phases of therapy may make regular day care both impractical and potentially harmful to the child with cancer because of the increased risk of acquiring some infectious diseases in these settings. When a child has begun less intensive therapy, evaluating child care is possible. The caretaker must be educated about (1) the child's disease and notify the family immediately of any fever, signs and symptoms of infection, or increased bruising or bleeding; (2) reporting any communicable illness—especially chickenpox—in the other children; and (3) any medication or oral chemotherapeutic agent that must be administered during child care hours. In addition, the importance of good hand washing should be emphasized, especially before and after toileting, food preparation, and meals.

Schooling

The child who is too ill to participate in the regular classroom should be enrolled in a home study program. The role of health care providers, parents, and educators is to work as a team to assist the child in returning to school as soon after diagnosis as is medically possible. Returning to school provides a sense of normalcy and contributes to the child's hopefulness.

The child's school reentry must be carefully planned. When augmenting the child's participation in school activities, anticipatory guidance should include attention to the special precautions that need to be taken for the child's safety and learning needs. This can be achieved by mutual respect between parents and school personnel, a willingness to provide needed resources such as homebound education, and advocacy on the part of parents and the oncology team to educate school personnel about the special needs created by hospitalizations, chemotherapy-induced side effects, and long-term sequelae of surgery, radiation, and chemotherapy on learning abilities (CureSearch, 2017). In addition, establishing an individualized education program (IEP) can help define and anticipate the child's special needs. The teachers, school nurse, and school staff must be informed of the child's illness and implications that will influence attendance, social interaction, educational capacity, and the restrictions or special needs dictated by medical care. Early recognition of learning disabilities enhances prompt assessment and intervention. Finally, working with teachers and the oncology team, the child's classmates can be taught about the child's illness at an appropriate developmental level. The child also needs to be prepared to answer classmates' questions. The primary care provider can provide the family with support and resources to help ease the transition into school.

Sexuality

The child with cancer often struggles with an alteration in body image because of hair loss, weight loss or gain, or disfiguring surgery. A major task of these children is learning to deal with this change, be it temporary or permanent. This is especially true in adolescents, who, in addition to treatment, may be experiencing normal pubertal changes. Risks to future fertility will be assessed depending on the chemotherapy regimen, particularly with anthracyclines and brain or pelvic radiation, and then fertility salvage options can be discussed. In prepubescent females, ovarian salvage and freezing of the ovary can be done until patients decide they want to have children. Pubertal females can pursue ovarian salvage or egg harvesting to have available for when they desire children. Menstrual suppression can also help with fertility preservation. Pubertal males can use sperm banking for their future (Klipstein et al., 2020).

Young females receiving chemotherapy may experience delayed development of secondary sexual characteristics and amenorrhea, depending on where they are in their pubertal development. However, females should be counseled to use appropriate methods of birth control, because the effects of chemotherapy and radiation on fertility vary. Prevention of sexually transmitted infections (STIs) is critical, particularly in immunocompromised adolescents. After the cessation of therapy, development often occurs, and generally the menses will begin. A referral to an endocrinologist for hormonal supplementation should be done for those who are delayed. Males should also be evaluated for any delay in development related to chemotherapies or the possible loss of fertility as with testicular cancer. Tanner staging should be conducted at visits to record any delay in development.

Transition to Adulthood

In 2019, nearly 500,000 adult survivors of pediatric cancer were believed to be alive in the United States (NCI, 2021a). All these patients have the potential for comorbidities and complications related to their cancer and the treatments they were exposed to as pediatric patients. Because of this, most comprehensive pediatric oncology centers have created survivorship clinics that meet the needs of young adults after therapy and transition them to adult oncologists. Educating these patients about the possible long-term issues that can occur because of cancer and its treatments and providing them with treatment summaries and survivorship plans are essential to providing survivors with the tools necessary to care for themselves as adults and seek care as recommended (NCI, 2021b).

Family Concerns

Advances in medicine that have led to improved survival rates of children with cancer have also brought problems of chronic uncertainty. The uncertainty that families face centers around the basic issue of the child's survival. Family concerns often reflect the phase of treatment the child is experiencing. In the beginning, uncertainty is focused on whether remission will be obtained. If remission is achieved, will it be long term or will relapse occur? If relapse occurs, will the child enter remission again or die? At the end of treatment, families struggle with ambivalent feelings; they are grateful for the end of therapy yet fearful of the loss of their safety net of frequent contact with providers and the end of drugs that have maintained remission.

In addition to providing illness-related information, the health care team should help families cope with this uncertainty. Learning to cope with uncertainty is important to the health and well-being of all family members. Support for the child and family must be ongoing, not only at diagnosis but also long after the completion of therapy or the death of the child.

At diagnosis, parents often feel extreme guilt for not having brought the child to medical care sooner or for not being a more vocal advocate if providers did not realize the significance of the symptoms. The pediatric oncology team tries to support families through this difficult time by allowing individual and family counseling opportunities. Siblings of a child with cancer benefit from understanding what happens during clinic and hospital visits and from interventions directly addressing their need for communication and support.

The financial burden of a catastrophic illness is of monumental concern to the family. It affects the family's current financial status and has far-reaching implications for the child's future insurability. Insurance companies vary in reimbursement of medications and procedures they deem experimental. All these factors place a tremendous amount of stress on an already taxed family unit.

There are numerous local, regional, and national organizations available to provide information and educational resources about childhood malignant diseases. Local hospitals and cancer centers often provide support groups for family members. Informal parent-to-parent interactions based on the sense of having a common understanding of parenting a child with cancer can be a powerful source of support. Identifying local resources will provide a much welcomed service to these families.

RESOURCES

American Cancer Society (a volunteer organization offering educational programs, family services, rehabilitation support, and referral to local and regional resources): www.cancer.org

Association of Pediatric Hematology/Oncology Nurses (a professional organization for pediatric hematology/oncology nurses and other pediatric hematology/oncology health care professionals): www.aphon.org

Cancer Information Service, National Cancer Institute (a network of regional information centers that provide personalized answers to cancer-related questions from individuals, families, the general public, and health care professionals; also provides referral to local and regional resources): www.cancernet.nci.nih.gov

Candlelighters Childhood Cancer Foundation, Inc. (an international organization of parents whose children have had cancer; provides guidance and emotional support through local chapters, information, and referral to local and regional resources): www. candlelighters.org

Children's Oncology Group (a professional organization that conducts research for treatments of pediatric cancers and provides guidance to clinicians, patients, and families): https://www.childrensoncologygroup.org/patients-and-families-section

CureSearch (an organization that raises funds for childhood cancer research and provides family educational materials in conjunction with the Children's Oncology Group research trials): www.curesearch.org

Leukemia and Lymphoma Society (a volunteer organization offering educational programs, information, financial assistance, and referral to local and regional resources): www.leukemia.org

Pediatric Brain Tumor Foundation (an organization that provides leadership and funding to accelerate targeted therapies for pediatric brain tumors and support families with education, financial assistance, and emotional support): http://www.curethekids.org

---

 Summary

Primary Care Needs for the Child With Cancer

HEALTH CARE MAINTENANCE
Growth and Development
- Growth slows because of chemotherapy and radiation.
- Closely monitor weight; a child is at risk for significant weight loss because of disease and treatment and is also at risk for weight gain because of steroids.
- Periodic developmental screening is done to assess for age-appropriate behaviors.
- Neuropsychological testing is done for children who received cranial radiation.

Diet
- Maintain an adequate diet. Offer small, frequent meals if the child is experiencing anorexia. Work with a dietician on ways to improve the taste and consistency of foods to improve their palatability to patients. Increase fluid intake and high-fiber foods for constipation. Monitor diarrhea closely. Offer appetite stimulants.

Safety
- Ensure proper handling of chemotherapeutic agents at home and proper maintenance and protection of indwelling VADs.
- Avoid contact sports during chemotherapy and plan future participation with the oncology team.
- Because of photosensitivity related to medications and chemotherapy, children should wear sunscreen and hats to protect.

Immunizations
- Vaccines, except for influenza and COVID, should be avoided while receiving chemotherapy.
- Vaccines can be resumed at 6 months off therapy; primary care providers should follow the catchup schedule as needed.
- Children recovering from an allogeneic HSCT require special consideration with the readministration of vaccines and the follow-up schedule.

Screening
- *Vision.* Routine screening is recommended. A thorough assessment is warranted if visual abnormalities are detected. Visual changes may occur secondary to tumor growth, radiation, or chemotherapy.
- *Hearing.* Routine screening is recommended. Children receiving ototoxic drugs should have regular evaluations by an audiologist.
- *Dental.* Routine screening is recommended. A CBC may be done before an appointment to verify adequate ANC

and platelet count if needed for instrumentation. Meticulous oral hygiene is necessary to prevent infections.
- *Blood pressure.* Should be taken at each visit to evaluate for hypertension as a result of drug toxicity.
- *Blood counts.* Performed on a routine basis by the primary oncology team.
- *Urinalysis.* Screening is routine. Protein may be observed after radiation therapy, or hematuria may be seen after cyclophosphamide/ifosfamide therapy. Special urinary tract infection caution should be taken when only one kidney is present.

Condition-Specific Screening
- Close assessment is required for signs and symptoms of late effects of therapy or recurrence of malignancy (see Table 13.2).

COMMON ILLNESS MANAGEMENT
Differential Diagnosis
- *Fever.* Rule out neutropenia and infection. Do a septic workup as warranted. Prompt intervention is required with neutropenia or the presence of central VAD.
- *Pneumocystis jirovecii* prophylaxis is determined by patient allergies and tolerance.
- *Gastrointestinal symptoms.* For chemotherapy-induced constipation, ensure adequate hydration and begin stool softeners or laxatives as needed. Avoid suppositories and enemas.
- *Nausea and vomiting.* Determine the relationship between chemotherapy and radiation; rule out viral and bacterial infection. Give hydration fluid and antiemetics as needed.
- *Headache.* Perform a thorough neurologic examination. Consider the possibility of a brain tumor, CNS involvement, and lumbar puncture cerebrospinal fluid leak.
- *Pain.* Determine the source of pain; rule out tumor growth or cord compression. Do not treat with aspirin. Premedicate for painful procedures.

Drug Interactions
- No aspirin-containing products should be given. Acetaminophen is recommended except in times of neutropenia to avoid masking a fever.
- Low-folic-acid multivitamins may be taken. Consult with the oncology team before prescribing additional medication because of the risk of a drug interaction.

DEVELOPMENTAL ISSUES

Sleep Patterns

- Disturbances are common. Maintain a consistent bedtime schedule and routine when possible. A transitional object may increase security during hospitalization.

Toileting

- Standard developmental counseling is advised. Regression may occur.
- Constipation may occur with some therapies.

Discipline

- Use normal patterns of discipline; it is important to maintain consistency for all siblings.

Child Care

- Group child care should be avoided if possible because of the risk of communicable illnesses. Child care establishments should provide COVID precautions and cleaning requirements.
- Communicable diseases must be reported.
- Frequent hand washing for infection control is recommended.

Schooling

- The child should return to school as soon as possible.
- Ongoing communication between primary care providers and teachers is necessary. The education of school staff and classmates is crucial.

- Assist the family in developing an IEP. Periodically assess for school problems and learning disabilities.
- If the child is unable to participate in a regular school program, arrange for home tutoring.

Sexuality

- Give support for altered body image.
- Assess for appropriate Tanner staging. Any significant delay should be evaluated.
- Provide information about fertility preservation as appropriate. Egg harvest or ovarian preservation for females and sperm banking for adolescent males, as options before they begin chemotherapy or radiation.
- Provide contraception if appropriate and counsel regarding STI prevention.

Transition to Adulthood

- Transitioning pediatric cancer survivors to a survivorship program for monitoring long-term complications/effects of chemotherapy or radiation and adult care is essential.

Family Concerns

- The family must deal with chronic uncertainty.
- Insurance and catastrophic financial effects are also concerns.
- Address the needs of siblings.

REFERENCES

American Academy of Pediatrics. (2020). *American Academy of Pediatrics offers guidance for caring and treatment of long-term cancer survivors.* Retrieved April 24, 2023, from https://www.aap.org/en/news-room/news-releases/aap/2021/american-academy-of-pediatrics-offers-guidance-for-caring-and-treatment-of-long-term-cancer-survivors.

American Cancer Society. (2022). *Key statistics for childhood cancers.* Retrieved March 24, 2023, from https://www.cancer.org/cancer/cancer-in-children/key-statistics.html.

Butler, E., Ludwig, K., Pacenta, H. L., Klesse, L. J., Watt, T. C., & Laetsch, T. W. (2021). Recent progress in the treatment of cancer in children. *CA: A Cancer Journal for Clinicians, 71*(4), 315–332. https://doi.org/10.3322/caac.21665.

Centers for Disease Control and Prevention. (2023). *ACIP altered immunocompetence guidelines for immunizations.* Retrieved March 24, 2023, from https://www.cdc.gov/vaccines/hcp/acip-recs/general-recs/immunocompetence.html.

Children's Oncology Group. (2018). *Long-term follow-up guidelines for survivors of childhood, adolescent, and young adult cancers.* Retrieved March 24, 2023, from http://www.survivorshipguidelines.org/.

Children's Oncology Group. (2022). About us. Retrieved March 24, 2023, from https://childrensoncologygroup.org/about.

Children's Oncology Group. (n.d.). What is a clinical trial? Retrieved March 14, 2023, from https://childrensoncologygroup.org/index.php/what-is-a-clinical-trial.

CureSearch for Children's Cancer. (2017). *Preparing school staff for your child's return to school: Curesearch.* Retrieved February 24, 2023, from https://curesearch.org/Preparing-School-Staff-for-Your-Childs-Return-to-School.

Ernst, M., Brähler, E., Klein, E. M., Jüngar, C., Wild, P. S., Faber, J., Schneider, A., & Beutel, M. E. (2019). Parenting in the face of serious illness: Childhood cancer survivors remember different rearing behavior than the general population. *Psycho-Oncology, 28*(8), 1663–1670. https://doi.org/10.1002/pon.5138.

Fernandes, A. G., Pollock, B. D., & Rabito, F. A. (2018). Retinoblastoma in the United States: A 40-year incidence and survival analysis.

Journal of Pediatric Ophthalmology and Strabismus, 55(3), 182–188. https://doi.org/10.3928/01913913-20171116-03.

Herring, R. A. (2019). Chemotherapy/biotherapy. In *The pediatric chemotherapy and biotherapy curriculum.* Association of Pediatric Hematology/Oncology Nurses.

Klipstein, S., Fallat, M. E., Savelli, S.; COMMITTEE ON BIOETHICS; SECTION ON HEMATOLOGY/ONCOLOGY; SECTION ON SURGERY. (2020). Fertility preservation for pediatric and adolescent patients with cancer: Medical and ethical considerations. *Pediatrics, 145*(3), e20193994. doi: 10.1542/peds.2019-3994. Epub 2020 Feb 18. PMID: 32071259.

Manji, A., Beyene, J., Dupuis, L. L., Phillips, R., Lehrnbecher, T., & Sung, L. (2012). Outpatient and oral antibiotic management of low-risk febrile neutropenia are effective in children—a systematic review of prospective trials. *Supportive Care in Cancer, 20*(6), 1135–1145. https://doi.org/10.1007/s00520-012-1425-8.

National Cancer Institute, Surveillance, Epidemiology, and End Results Program. (n.d.). *Seer*Explorer overview.* Retrieved March 24, 2023, from https://seer.cancer.gov/statistics-network/explorer/overview.html.

National Cancer Institute. (n.d.). *What is cancer?* Retrieved March 13, 2023, from https://www.cancer.gov/about-cancer/understanding/what-is-cancer.

National Cancer Institute. (2021a). *Childhood cancer survivor study: An overview.* Retrieved February 24, 2023, from https://www.cancer.gov/types/childhood-cancers/ccss.

National Cancer Institute. (2021b). *Coping—care for childhood cancer survivors.* Retrieved January 24, 2023, from https://www.cancer.gov/about-cancer/coping/survivorship/child-care.

National Cancer Institute. (2022). *Pediatric hematopoietic stem cell transplantation and cellular therapy for Cancer (PDQ)–health professional version.* Retrieved February 24, 2023, from https://www.cancer.gov/types/childhood-cancers/hp-stem-cell-transplant.

National Cancer Institute, National Institutes of Health. (2020). *Childhood cancer of the brain and other nervous system—cancer stat facts.* Retrieved February 24, 2023, from https://seer.cancer.gov/statfacts/html/childbrain.html.

Olsen, H. E., Lynn, G. M., Valdes, P. A., Cerecedo Lopez, C. D., Ishizuka, A. S., Arnaout, O., Bi, W. L., Peruzzi, P. P., Chiocca, E. A., Friedman, G. K., & Bernstock, J. D. (2021). Therapeutic cancer vaccines for pediatric malignancies: Advances, challenges, and emerging technologies. *Neuro-Oncology Advances, 3*(1), vdab027. https://doi.org/10.1093/noajnl/vdab027.

Ritwik, P. (2018). Dental care for patients with childhood cancers. *Ochsner Journal, 18*(4), 351–357. https://doi.org/10.31486/toj.18.0061.

Schapira, M. M., Stevens, E. M., Sharpe, J. E., Hochman, L., Reiter, J. G., Calhoun, S. R., Shah, S. A., Bailey, L. C., Bagatell, R., Silber, J. H., Tai, E., & Barakat, L. P. (2020). Outcomes among pediatric patients with cancer who are treated on trial versus off trial: A matched cohort study. *Cancer, 126*(15), 3471–3482. https://doi.org/10.1002/cncr.32947.

Yan, P., Qi, F., Bian, L., Xu, Y., Zhou, J., Hu, J., Ren, L., Li, M., Tang, W. (2020). Comparison of incidence and outcomes of neuroblastoma in children, adolescents, and adults in the United States: A surveillance, epidemiology, and end results (SEER) program population study. *Med Sci Monit.* 26:e927218. doi: 10.12659/MSM.927218.

Celiac Disease

14

Patricia A. Bierly, Amy K. Williams

Celiac disease (CD) is an autoimmune-mediated enteropathy occurring in genetically predisposed individuals triggered by the ingestion of gluten. The prevalence of CD is estimated to be 1% of the world's population. CD can present with symptoms that are gastrointestinal or extraintestinal. The only treatment for CD is a lifelong gluten-free diet (GFD) (Melini, 2019). Removal of gluten often leads to the complete resolution of symptoms. Gluten is the broad term used to describe the proteins in grass-related grains, mainly wheat, rye, and barley. Gluten adds texture, flavor, and proteins to food.

ETIOLOGY

Aretaeus of Cappadocia, who lived in second-century Greece, is credited with writing the first description of a malabsorptive syndrome characterized by chronic diarrhea. Celiac is derived from the Greek word κοιλιακος (koiliakos), meaning "abdominal." CD was first reported in modern times as a disease entity by British pediatrician Samuel Gee. In 1888, Gee published a paper that described his clinical experience with a malabsorption syndrome in children. Gee noted that the cure for this affliction was likely related to diet. A substantial breakthrough in CD research came from Willem Karel Dicke in 1950 with his discovery of the harmful link between wheat and CD. Later, with the advent of improved intestinal biopsy techniques, gluten was found to cause small intestinal villous atrophy and crypt hyperplasia. The finding of the association of human leukocyte antigen (HLA) with the disease has helped expand knowledge of its genetic relevance. The discovery of gluten-dependent antibodies, particularly tissue transglutaminase (TTG), was instrumental in improving screening techniques (Rubin & Crowe, 2020). These advances in screening, genetics, and diagnostics have raised CD awareness.

CD is the most common autoimmune disorder, with a prevalence of 0.5% to 1% in the general population. CD occurs less often in areas (sub-Saharan Africa, Japan) that show low CD genes (predisposing genes and low gluten consumption) (Sahin, 2021). CD has increased in prevalence in Western countries between 1985 and 2000 and increased fivefold in the United States (Rubin & Crowe, 2020). Celiac is highest in first-degree relatives and high-risk groups such as type 1 diabetes mellitus, Williams syndrome, and immunoglobulin A (IgA) deficiency (Meijer et al., 2022). CD can occur at any age throughout the life span. It has two peaks: (1) after the intake of gluten in the first 2 years of life, and (2) in the second or third decade of life (Sahin, 2021).

CD is a unique autoimmune disease due to known elements: genetic HLA, DQ2, DQ8, autoantigen TTG, and an environmental trigger (gluten). There has been an increase in CD, questioning if gluten is the only trigger in genetically at-risk patients. Some theories include improved hygiene and lack of exposure to various microorganisms (Caio et al., 2019). The environmental trigger is the ingestion of gluten-containing products. These toxic proteins trigger a complex inflammatory cascade of T-cell–mediated immune events and include the proliferative production of inflammatory cytokines. Mucosal damage caused by chronic inflammation is cumulative and, in conjunction with increased intestinal permeability, distorts the absorptive capability of the small intestine (Caio et al., 2019).

In CD there is a genetic predisposition with an increased prevalence among first-degree relatives (10%–20%) depending on HLA and sex. Monozygotic twins have a concordance rate of approximately 75% to 80% (Meijer et al., 2022). The HLA complex is the major human histocompatibility complex. This group of genes is located on chromosome 6 and encodes cell surface antigen–presenting proteins on white blood cells and tissue cells. These genes have an essential function in the immune process. The *HLA-DQ2* allele combination is found in 90% to 95% of CD patients, and *HLA-DQ8* is present in the remaining 5% to 10%. However, about 30% of people without CD also have the *HLA-DQ2* gene (Sciurti et al., 2018). Thus carrying either *DQ2* or *DQ8* is necessary for the disease expression but not sufficient. In fact, in those of Western European ancestry, 30% to 40% carry *DQ2* or *DQ8*, but fewer than 3% are thought to eventually develop CD.

DIAGNOSTIC CRITERIA

The diagnostic criteria for CD include positive serologic markers, characteristic intestinal biopsies, and response to a GFD (Taraghikhah et al., 2020). Serologic tests aid in identifying patients for whom intestinal biopsy is indicated to confirm the diagnosis of CD. The currently

341

available tests include anti-TTG IgA and IgG antibodies, antiendomysial (anti-EMA) IgA, and deamidated gliadin antibodies (IgA and IgG). The North American Society of Pediatric Gastroenterology, Hepatology, and Nutrition (NASPGHAN) recommends the measurement of TTG IgA in the initial screening for CD (c).

The first marker used was the antigliadin in 1980. Due to low specificity, antigliadin is no longer used except for possible gluten intolerance/wheat sensitivity. The serologic studies that have higher predictive value include TTG, endomysial, and deamidated gliadin peptide (DGP). All have IgA and IgG markers. IgA class is highly sensitive and specific. There are many false-positive IgG antibodies except in IgA deficiency (Rubin & Crowe, 2020).

TTG is a normal gut enzyme released during cell injury. In those with CD, it modifies gliadin peptides (toxic protein factor of gluten) in the intestinal mucosa leading to an inflammatory cascade. TTG sensitivity ranges from 0.92 to 1.00 and specificity from 0.91 to 1.00. EMA IgA is as accurate as TTG (sensitivity 0.88–1.00, specificity 0.91–1.00) but is not recommended for initial screening because it is more expensive, time consuming, and prone to operator error in interpretation (Hill et al., 2016).

Antigliadin IgG and IgA are no longer recommended because of their variability and inferior specificity and sensitivity. Nevertheless, these serologic markers continue to be drawn as part of a panel and often are found to be elevated. Elevation of antigliadin IgA or IgG antibodies in the absence of TTG or EMA antibody positivity is considered a negative celiac screen.

DGP IgG should also be included in detecting CD in children 2 years of age and younger. Otherwise, DGP IgA is not as useful and is not recommended (Rubin & Crowe, 2020). Strict GFD compliance leads to normalization in serology between 12 and 24 months based on titer level and intestinal damage (Meijer et al., 2022).

In addition to antibody markers, genetic typing can aid diagnosis in that the absence of *HLA-DQ2* and *HLA-DQ8* essentially rules out CD. At this time, HLA typing is not recommended as part of routine screening, and many insurance companies may not cover it. Further supportive evidence of diagnosis is the reduction or resolution of antibodies after a period of a GFD (Hill et al., 2016).

All children with positive serologic markers should be referred to a gastroenterologist for esophagogastroduodenoscopy to obtain confirmatory biopsies, which remains the gold standard for diagnosis of CD (Hill et al., 2016). The guidelines for biopsy retrieval are to obtain four to six biopsies in the duodenum, given the patchy distribution of the disease. The histologic features include mucosal inflammation, villous atrophy, crypt hyperplasia, and lymphocyte infiltration of the epithelium (Fig. 14.1). Villous atrophy of the duodenum is characteristic but not specific to CD. Other causes include giardiasis, collagenous sprue, common variable immunodeficiency, autoimmune enteropathy, radiation enteritis, Whipple disease, tuberculosis, tropical sprue, eosinophilic gastroenteritis, human immunodeficiency virus enteropathy, intestinal lymphoma, Zollinger-Ellison syndrome, Crohn disease, and food allergies or intolerances other than to gluten (Villanacci et al., 2020). The diagnosis of CD should be based not only on intestinal biopsy but on serologic testing and clinical response to a GFD. A skilled endoscopist and pathologist familiar with CD morphology are essential in confirming the diagnosis (Fig. 14.2).

The European guidelines to forgo a small intestine biopsy are as follows: TTG IgA is 10 times the upper limit of normal and positive endomysial antibody

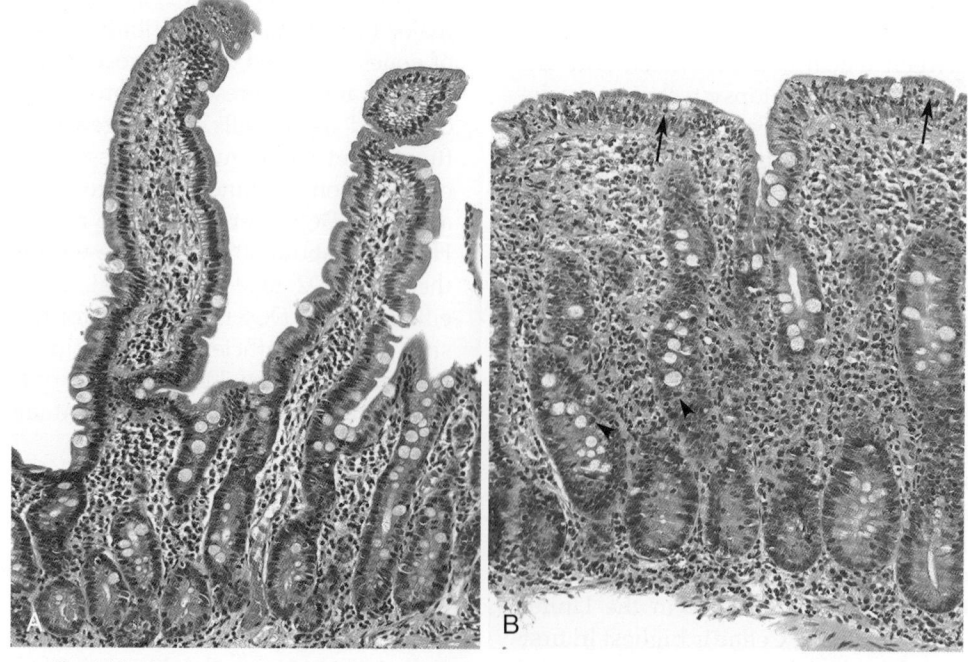

Fig. 14.1 **Biopsy of the duodenum.** (A) Normal. (B) Celiac disease. (Courtesy Teri Longacre, MD.)

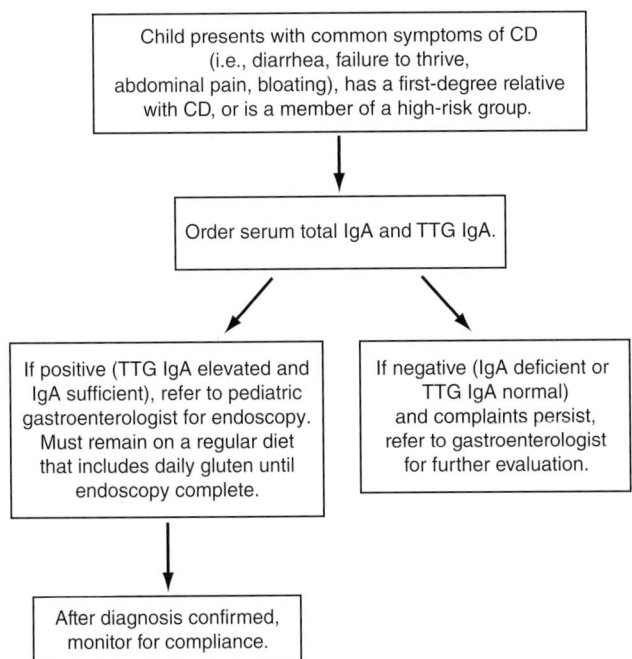

Fig. 14.2 **Diagnostic algorithm for celiac disease** *(CD)*. *IgA*, Immunoglobulin A; *TTG*, tissue transglutaminase.

Box flow diagram text:

Child presents with common symptoms of CD (i.e., diarrhea, failure to thrive, abdominal pain, bloating), has a first-degree relative with CD, or is a member of a high-risk group.

↓

Order serum total IgA and TTG IgA.

If positive (TTG IgA elevated and IgA sufficient), refer to pediatric gastroenterologist for endoscopy. Must remain on a regular diet that includes daily gluten until endoscopy complete.

If negative (IgA deficient or TTG IgA normal) and complaints persist, refer to gastroenterologist for further evaluation.

↓

After diagnosis confirmed, monitor for compliance.

Box 14.1 Clinical Manifestations at Time of Diagnosis

- Failure to thrive
- Diarrhea
- Abdominal distention/bloating/pain
- Nausea/vomiting
- Constipation
- Dermatitis herpetiformis
- Dental enamel defects
- Short stature
- Delayed puberty
- Osteoporosis
- Iron deficiency anemia

Data from Rubin, J. E., Crowe, S. E. (2020). Celiac disease. *Ann Intern Med*, 172(1), ITC1–ITC16.

IgA, celiac HLA positive for DQ2/DQ8, and clinical signs and symptoms. The diagnosis is confirmed with improvement in celiac serology and clinical response to the GFD (Al-Toma et al., 2019). This criterion has been accepted worldwide due to the lack of reproducibility of serologies (Caio et al., 2019). Other criteria proposed include the 4/5 rule, which indicates that four of five criteria are enough to establish the celiac diagnosis: (1) typical signs and symptoms of celiac, (2) antibody positive (TTG and EMA), (3) HLA DQ2 +/− DQ8 positive, (4) intestinal damage (i.e., minor lesions or villous atrophy), and (5) a clinical response to a GFD. In addition, the 4/5 rule helps health care providers identify the various subtypes of CD: seronegative (absence of criterion 2), potential CD (absence of criterion 4), non-classical symptoms (absence of criterion 1), and nonresponsive CD (absence of criterion 5).

CLINICAL MANIFESTATIONS AT TIME OF DIAGNOSIS

CD is thought to be one of the most common genetic disorders in the world and a frequent cause of malabsorption in children. Primary care providers must be aware of gastrointestinal and extraintestinal symptoms that may indicate CD because they vary widely among affected individuals (Box 14.1).

Infants and young children presenting symptoms of CD may have poor growth, chronic diarrhea, abdominal distention, muscle wasting, poor appetite, and irritability. These signs and symptoms generally manifest between 6 and 24 months of age, depending on when adequate amounts of gluten are introduced into the diet. The longer the diagnosis is delayed, the more malnourished a child may be. However, some children, such as those in high-risk groups, may have positive markers on screening and be clinically asymptomatic. Older children may present with gastrointestinal complaints such as recurrent abdominal pain, nausea, vomiting, bloating, and constipation. Extraintestinal manifestations of CD include short stature, pubertal delay, dental enamel defects, osteopenia, osteoporosis, and anemia secondary to iron, folate, or vitamin B$_{12}$ deficiency. A cutaneous manifestation of gluten enteropathy, dermatitis herpetiformis occurs in 13% of patients with CD. This is a severe erythematous pruritic skin rash that is rare in children (Salmi, 2019).

Other, less common manifestations may include neurologic and psychiatric syndromes such as peripheral neuropathy, cerebellar ataxia, migraines, and epilepsy (Therrien et al., 2020). In adults it has been found that elevations in liver transaminases and liver biopsies revealing nonspecific reactive hepatitis improve on a GFD (Therrien et al., 2020). Long-standing data demonstrate an increased risk of infertility, miscarriage, delayed menarche, and amenorrhea in females with delayed diagnosis or untreated CD (Therrien et al., 2020).

Providers should be aware of the classic symptoms of CD—diarrhea, abdominal distention, and failure to thrive—as well as the atypical symptoms mentioned previously.

Other forms of CD have been identified:
- Potential CD: abnormal celiac serology, positive genetics with normal histology, or minimal signs such as intraepithelial lymphocytes, with or without symptoms; scientific community has not universally agreed to start a GFD
- Refractory CD: persistent symptoms and atrophy after 12 months of a GFD, which may lead to ulcerative jejunitis, collagenous sprue, and intestinal lymphoma
- Seronegative CD: negative celiac serologies, clinical symptoms, and atrophy of small intestines
- Nonresponsive CD: symptoms, despite a GFD, do not differentiate active CD and associated conditions (Caio et at., 2019)

Primary care providers should also be cognizant of the rare phenomenon of celiac crisis, which can easily be mistaken for viral gastroenteritis. Signs and symptoms of a celiac crisis include severe acute diarrhea, marked abdominal distention, edema, dehydration, and electrolyte imbalances (Waheed et al., 2016).

 Treatment

GLUTEN-FREE GRAINS AND FLOURS AND FOODS DERIVED FROM GRAINS

The following are allowed on a gluten-free diet (GFD:
- Amaranth
- Arrowroot
- Beans
- Buckwheat
- Corn (maize)
- Distilled alcoholic beverages (e.g., wines, hard liquor)
- Distilled vinegars
- Flax
- Garfava
- Millet
- Montina
- Nut flours
- Oats (gluten-free oats)
- Potatoes
- Quinoa
- Rice
- Sorghum
- Soy
- Tapioca
- Teff

The following are not allowed on a GFD:
- Barley
- Beers, ales, lagers
- Malt, malt flavoring, malt vinegar
- Nondistilled alcoholic beverages
- Rye
- Triticale
- Wheat (durum, einkorn, faro, graham, kamut, semolina, and spelt)

From Celiac Disease Foundation. (n.d.). Gluten-free living. www.celiac.org.

The only known treatment for CD at this time is life-long adherence to a GFD. Gluten is a combination of the proteins gliadin and glutenin, which exist along with starch in grass-related grains, mainly wheat. Gliadin is the alcohol-soluble portion of gluten that is toxic in persons with CD. Rye and barley contain proteins very similar to gliadin: hordeins and secalins. Therefore a GFD excludes mainly wheat, rye, and barley. Malt, including malt syrups, extracts, and flavorings, should also be avoided because it is a partial hydrolysate of barley proteins. Triticale (combination of wheat and rye), kamut, spelt (faro), semolina (durum wheat), farina, einkorn, bulgar, and couscous are other grains that contain gluten and should be excluded (Aljada et al., 2021).

Oats were thought to cause mucosal damage in individuals with CD in the past, and a GFD with the inclusion of oats was not found to prevent mucosal healing or normalization of serologic markers (Comino et al., 2015). The concern over oat safety is its contamination with gluten in the harvesting, milling, and transport process. It is therefore very important that individuals confirm the product's purity before including it in their GFD.

In 2013, the US Food and Drug Administration (FDA) issued a final rule to define the term "gluten free" for voluntary use in labeling foods. This rule helps the consumer and those living with CD be confident that any items labeled "gluten free" meet a defined standard for gluten content. The final rule was issued under the Food Allergen Labeling and Consumer Protection Act of 2004 (FDA, 2013).

Clinical improvement on a GFD can usually be noticed within several days to several weeks, but it is unclear precisely how long it takes for the intestinal mucosa to recover completely. For now, the only known treatment is a GFD for life, though a small number of patients do not show clinical or histologic improvement with a GFD. In these cases the child needs to be followed closely by a gastroenterologist for further evaluation, including checking for compliance with the GFD, consideration of other diagnoses (e.g., lactose intolerance, small bowel bacterial overgrowth, food allergies, gastroparesis), and screening for complications of CD such as intestinal carcinoma, enteropathy-associated T-cell lymphoma, or refractory sprue (Rubin & Crowe, 2020).

The most common pitfall to a GFD is foods with hidden gluten. Assume all processed products contain gluten unless otherwise labeled or confirmed by the manufacturer. For example, it is possible that products such as cosmetics and toothpaste contain gluten (Box 14.2). Because beer is made from fermented grains, it should be avoided on a GFD. Gluten-free beers are available at specialty stores. Distilled forms

Box **14.2**	**Potential Gluten Pitfalls**[a]

- Breading and coating mixes
- Brown rice syrup
- Communion wafers
- Croutons
- Drugs and over-the-counter medications
- Energy bars
- Flour or cereal products
- Herbal supplements
- Imitation bacon
- Imitation seafood
- Marinades
- Nutritional supplements
- Panko (Japanese breadcrumbs)
- Pastas
- Play-Doh (This is a potential problem if hands are put on or in the mouth while playing with Play-Doh. Hands should be washed immediately after use.)
- Processed luncheon meats
- Sauces, gravies
- Self-basting poultry
- Soup bases
- Soy sauce or soy sauce solids
- Stuffings, dressing
- Thickeners (roux)
- Vitamins and mineral supplements

[a]Not a comprehensive list.
From Celiac Disease Foundation. (n.d.). Gluten-free living. www.celiac.org.

of alcohol are safe to drink if they are without gluten-containing additives. Closely examine liquors and premixed drinks for unsafe ingredients.

COMPLEMENTARY AND ALTERNATIVE THERAPIES

At this point, the only known treatment for CD is life-long adherence to a GFD.

ANTICIPATED ADVANCES IN DIAGNOSIS AND MANAGEMENT

Screening techniques that may eliminate the need for intestinal biopsy include the European guidelines of a TTG IgA of 10 times the upper limit of normal, a positive endomysial antibody IgA, and clinical symptoms with positive genetics. Not all countries adopted this due to the lack of reproducibility of TTG, as there is no universal standardization (Rubin & Crowe, 2020). Capsule endoscopy is currently being explored to monitor adherence and mucosal healing. Many ideas for nondietary treatments have been proposed, including techniques to genetically detoxify grains and modify gluten during manufacturing. Other proposals include immune cell–targeted therapy vaccinations to induce gluten tolerance, inhibition of intestinal permeability, and oral peptidase supplementation or other recombinant enzymes that digest gliadin in the gastrointestinal tract. There are several clinical studies in various phases of clinical research (Rubin & Crowe, 2020; Zhu, 2019).

ASSOCIATED PROBLEMS OF CELIAC DISEASE AND TREATMENT

The conditions most strongly associated with CD in children are first-degree relatives of individuals with proven CD (10–20% prevalence), autoimmune thyroiditis, type 1 diabetes mellitus, Down syndrome, Turner syndrome, Williams syndrome, selective IgA deficiency, and other autoimmune disorders, including dermatitis herpetiformis, systemic lupus erythematosus, liver disease, collagen vascular disease, rheumatoid arthritis, and Sjögren syndrome (Box 14.3) (Sahin, 2021). Current guidelines recommend routine periodic screening of asymptomatic children belonging to these groups beginning at age 3, after at least 1 year of adequate ingestion of gluten (Sahin, 2021). CD has an overlap in several endocrine disorders, including insulin-dependent diabetes, autoimmune thyroid conditions, adrenal insufficiency, hypoparathyroidism, infertility, and pituitary involvement (Sahin, 2021; Sange et al., 2020).

The clinical manifestations of CD vary widely as do the differential diagnoses. Depending on the symptoms, providers should consider inflammatory bowel disease (IBD), especially Crohn disease; small bowel bacterial overgrowth; giardiasis and other parasitic, bacterial, or viral gastroenteritis; food allergies;

Box **14.3**	High-Risk Groups

- Autoimmune thyroiditis
- Autoimmune liver disease
- First-degree relatives of celiac patients
- Juvenile chronic arthritis
- Selective immunoglobulin A deficiency
- Trisomy 21
- Turner syndrome
- Type 1 diabetes
- Williams syndrome

From Hill, I.D., Fasano, A., Guandalini, S., et al. (2015). NASPGHAN clinical report on the diagnosis and treatment of gluten-related disorders. *Journal of Pediatric Gastroenterology and Nutrition, 63*(1), 156–165; and Rubin, J.E., & Crowe, S.E. (2020). Celiac disease. *Annals of Internal Medicine, 172*(1), ITC1–ITC16.

eosinophilic enteropathy; malabsorptive syndromes; hypothyroidism; IgA deficiency; and protein-losing enteropathy. These may exist concurrently with CD (Sahin, 2021).

Because of the autoimmune nature of these conditions, there is a high crossover of CD with IBD. The prevalence of CD in IBD was reported to be between 0.5% and 3% (Bramuzzo et al., 2021). Thus the possibility of dual diagnosis should be considered especially if a child continues to be symptomatic on a GFD.

PROGNOSIS

The prognosis of children diagnosed and treated in a timely manner is excellent. Clinical improvement is usually apparent within the first few weeks on a GFD, but the complete restoration of the intestinal mucosa may take up to 2 years (Gidrewicz et al., 2017). Complications of untreated CD include short stature, dermatitis herpetiformis, dental enamel hypoplasia, recurrent stomatitis, fertility problems, osteoporosis, gluten ataxia, other neurologic disturbances, hyposplenism, refractory CD, and intestinal lymphoma. The risk of reduced bone mineral density in children with untreated CD is well documented, but a strict GFD improves bone mineralization in as quickly as 1 year (Shalin, 2021). Hyposplenism is a known complication in adults with untreated CD but is less commonly found in children. Individuals with untreated CD have an overall risk of intestinal cancer (adenocarcinoma and enteropathy-associated T-cell lymphoma) that is almost twice that of the general population (Shalin, 2021) Of patients with CD, 7% to 30% (5–19% in children) may have nonresponsive CD, which involves persistent symptoms and laboratory abnormalities in spite of a strict GFD for more than 12 months. Treatment is with the gluten contamination elimination diet and may prevent treatment with immunosuppression (Leonard et al., 2017). Persistent symptoms and intestinal villous atrophy characterize refractory CD despite strict adherence to the GFD for 12 months. There are two categories of refractory CD: type I and type II. Type I is characterized by the absence of aberrant T cells and type II by their presence. Al-toma et al. (2019) suggest that in these cases the diagnosis of CD should first be reexamined, along with assessing dietary compliance and excluding other causes of diarrhea, villous atrophy, and malignant complications of CD. Gluten immunosuppression beginning with corticosteroid induction is the treatment for type I refractory disease. Type II refractory CD is nonresponsive to medical treatment and has a poor prognosis, with a dismal 5-year survival rate of less than 50%. The most frequent cause of death in this group is the occurrence of T-cell lymphoma and recurrent infection (Al-toma et al., 2019). A potential promising therapy is autologous stem cell transplantation.

PRIMARY CARE MANAGEMENT

HEALTH CARE MAINTENANCE

In 2004, the National Institutes of Health Consensus Development Conference on Celiac Disease identified six key elements in managing individuals affected by CD, which remain relevant today. These elements include consultation with a skilled dietitian, education about the disease, lifelong adherence to a GFD, identification and treatment of nutritional deficiencies, access to an advocacy group, and continuous long-term follow-up by a multidisciplinary team (i.e., primary care providers, gastroenterologists, nurses, dietitians, social workers) (Box 14.4) (James, 2005). In this section we discuss important aspects of pediatric primary care in relation to a CD diagnosis.

Growth and Development

Growth and development can be significantly affected by undiagnosed or untreated CD. Children may experience growth delays as well as vitamin deficiencies. The assessment of anthropometric parameters is important in all children but particularly important in children with CD, who often have a suboptimal nutritional status at the time of diagnosis. Monitoring response in growth on the GFD is essential to ensure normal growth and development (Snyder et al., 2016).

Children with CD should have, at minimum, an annual visit with a primary care provider. At each visit the primary care provider should perform a thorough physical exam assessing for signs and symptoms of rickets, bone pain, tetany, acrodermatitis, coagulopathy,

Box 14.4 CELIAC: Six Key Elements in Management of Children With Celiac Disease

Consultation with a skilled dietitian
Education about the disease
Lifelong adherence to a gluten-free diet
Identification and treatment of nutritional deficiencies
Access to an advocacy group
Continuous long-term follow-up by a multidisciplinary team

Data from Rubin, J. E., Crowe, S. E. (2020). Celiac disease. *Ann Intern Med*, 172(1), ITC1–ITC16.

night blindness, dental enamel defects, muscle wasting, scant adipose tissue, protuberant abdomen, skin rash, nail abnormalities, or poor hair growth. These signs and symptoms may be indicative of refractory CD or noncompliance with the GFD (Valitutti et al., 2017).

Diet

The only treatment for CD is a strict GFD. A sudden change in diet can be overwhelming for a patient or family newly diagnosed with CD. The primary care provider needs to understand the basics of a GFD and provide resources (i.e., nutrition or dietary counseling) for patients and their families. The most fundamental tenet of the GFD is to avoid wheat, barley, and rye. Safe foods for those with CD include fresh fruits and vegetables, fresh meats and seafood, eggs, beans, seeds, and nuts. Obvious foods such as bread, pasta, cakes, pastries, and crackers should be avoided. Some foods may contain potentially risky ingredients that need further consideration before consumption by a person with CD. These include foods with caramel coloring, dressing or condiments with malt vinegar, processed meats, medications including over-the-counter vitamins, and any food from restaurants that should be assessed for cross-contamination (Robinson et al., 2015). The FDA identifies 20 parts per million (ppm) as the lowest level of detectable gluten in foods. All packaged products in the United States that carry a gluten-free label must have less than 20 ppm of gluten. Today many websites and smartphone applications can aid patients in making decisions about purchasing and consuming gluten-free foods. iPhone and Android applications can help users scan barcodes and ingredient lists to find potential gluten-containing ingredients. Other apps rely on user reviews and can help identify restaurants with safe kitchen environments for those with CD.

Safety

Children with CD have no special restrictions related to physical activity. The main safety risk for children with CD is the ingestion of gluten. Reactions to gluten vary considerably among individuals; some may not have an immediate or discernible reaction, whereas others may have severe reactions with varying symptoms a short time after consumption. Children and their caretakers, including parents, teachers, day care providers, coaches, and babysitters, should be informed about the child's condition and safe gluten-free foods. Families should be especially careful when eating out at restaurants where gluten contamination in the cooking process can easily occur. Social situations, including school parties, birthdays, and holidays, can be very challenging, as children with CD often feel left out. It will be important for parents and caregivers to prepare ahead of time to bring safe foods for the child to eat with friends and family. Common household items such as lipstick, toothpaste, and playdough may contain gluten. As individuals with CD approach adolescence, they are faced with temptations that involve risks such as alcohol consumption. Grain alcohols contain high amounts of gluten and should be avoided on a GFD. Adolescents should be counseled about this risk factor.

When patients with CD consume gluten, they will often have side effects, including severe abdominal pain and bloating, diarrhea, weight loss, dehydration, headache, joint pain, fatigue, or rash. When children experience these symptoms, supportive and symptomatic care is the only way to treat them. Individuals with celiac experience gluten exposure differently, so their treatment should be unique to their needs.

Immunizations

Children with CD should follow the current CDC childhood immunization schedule. There are no contraindications for vaccinating children with CD. However, it has been noted in multiple studies that there is a substantially higher frequency of nonprotective hepatitis B surface antibody concentrations in patients with CD fully immunized to hepatitis B as infants. Heshin-Bekenstein et al. (2015) determined that a single booster of either the standard hepatitis B vaccine or the newer pre-S vaccine is sufficient to raise hepatitis B surface antibody concentrations to protective levels in the vast majority of seronegative patients with CD.

Screenings

The following best practice recommendations attempt to provide a clear approach to the optimal management of CD in the pediatric population (Snyder et al., 2016).

Bone health. CD can affect a child's bone health in many ways, including pain, rickets, tetany, osteomalacia, osteopenia, osteoporosis, fractures associated with minimal trauma, or growth failure with or without symptoms of malabsorption. Bone mass and bone mineral density are restored rapidly upon initiation of a GFD. Guidance on age-appropriate calcium, vitamin D intake, and routine exercise should be provided during nutritional counseling at the time of diagnosis to promote bone health over time. Additionally, imaging studies should be used to evaluate bone health routinely for patients who do not adhere to a GFD (Snyder et al., 2016).

Hematology. Multiple hematologic disorders have been associated with CD, but anemia is by far the most common. Sometimes anemia can be the only clinical abnormality in patients with undiagnosed CD and may be the presenting feature in older children or young adults. Iron deficiency is the most common type of anemia in children with CD. Snyder et al. (2016) support the use of a combination of tests, including a complete blood count, ferritin, iron, and total iron binding capacity be obtained routinely for all children being evaluated for CD at the time of diagnosis.

Endocrine-associated disorders. Endocrine disorders frequently occur with CD primarily due to their shared HLA predisposition. Autoimmune thyroid disease and type 1 diabetes are the most common autoimmune diseases that occur with CD (Goodwin, 2019). Other diseases that can occur, but are much less common, include Addison disease, parathyroid disorders, and growth hormone deficiency. There are currently no recommendations to regularly screen patients with CD for type 1 diabetes; however, patients should be counseled on the signs and symptoms of type 1 diabetes so they can quickly communicate with the primary care provider if symptoms occur. At the time of diagnosis in children with CD, the primary care provider should screen for thyroid disease using a serum thyrotropin assay, which is accurate and widely available to screen for all common forms of hypothyroidism and hyperthyroidism (Snyder et al., 2016).

The liver and celiac disease. The liver is a common site for extraintestinal manifestations of undiagnosed and untreated CD. Therefore at the time of diagnosis, primary care providers should test for abnormalities in aspartate transaminase and alanine transaminase, which may indicate celiac hepatitis. As previously discussed in the vaccination section, providers should screen for hepatitis B immunization status and provide a booster dose to patients who have decreased surface antibodies (Snyder et al., 2016).

Nutritional Problems and Celiac Disease

Undiagnosed CD can cause intestinal inflammation leading to nutritional deficiencies (Husby et al., 2020). The GFD can pose many challenges to patients and their families, which may lead to deficiencies in both micronutrients and macronutrients. Nutrition is a dynamic issue for patients with CD and should be assessed regularly for compliance with the GFD. Additionally, multivitamin supplementation can be offered routinely to patients with CD at the time of diagnosis (Snyder et al., 2016).

Testing and Monitoring

There are several methods for diagnosing and monitoring CD, including serologic tests, genetic tests, and histology. Current guidelines by NASPGHAN state that positive serologic testing should be followed by a confirmatory small intestinal biopsy, which is the gold standard for diagnosis (Hill et al., 2016). However, the European Society of Paediatric Gastroenterology, Hepatology and Nutrition allows for a diagnosis based on serology alone (Husby et al., 2019). Additionally, routine testing with IgA anti-TTG antibodies at periodic intervals can help monitor compliance with a GFD (Snyder et al., 2016). HLA typing can be considered for at-risk children who test negative for TTG IgA antibodies and may determine whether continued monitoring for the development of CD is necessary (Snyder et al., 2016).

COMMON ILLNESS MANAGEMENT

Differential Diagnosis

Many of the classic symptoms of untreated CD can be difficult to differentiate from common childhood conditions. It is important to remember that the presentation of CD can vary widely and include gastrointestinal symptoms, extraintestinal manifestations, or be completely asymptomatic (Hill et al., 2016). Once patients with CD begin and remain compliant with a GFD, they typically remain healthy. Exacerbations of symptoms are usually only related to ingestions of gluten. However, it is important to complete a thorough evaluation of any complaints that may be related to CD or its associated symptoms before and after implementing a GFD.

Diarrhea. Chronic diarrhea is a hallmark complaint for patients with CD who have not yet been diagnosed. However, diarrhea may not occur chronically and may appear only intermittently, lessening parents' concerns and decreasing the likelihood of them mentioning diarrhea to the primary care provider. In children previously diagnosed with CD and on a GFD, acute diarrhea could indicate dietary noncompliance, intercurrent gastroenteritis, food intolerance or allergy, a side effect of antibiotics, or a concurrent diagnosis of IBD. The practitioner should consider CD if the course of diarrhea extends beyond a normal timeframe or if laboratory data reveal anemia. Severe, acute diarrhea accompanied by electrolyte imbalances should prompt consideration of celiac crisis and hospitalization. Persons with CD generally do not experience bloody diarrhea, so IBD or infectious colitis should be considered if a child has bloody stools. Persistent diarrhea despite a GFD should prompt further evaluation for the accuracy of the diagnosis as well as concurrent conditions such as lactose intolerance, small bowel bacterial overgrowth, underlying IBD, and food allergy.

Failure to thrive. Failure to thrive accompanies diarrhea in the classic description of CD (Khatib et al., 2016). Failure to thrive is a broad diagnosis that includes poor weight gain, short stature, and decreased weight for height. The physiologic basis of failure to thrive is inadequate nutrition, the cause of which is often multifactorial and includes both organic and nonorganic reasons. It is well accepted that children with delayed diagnosis of CD suffer growth delays caused by malabsorption. Proper adherence to a GFD will usually result in catching up and eventual normalization of growth. If catchup weight gain does not occur after the initiation of treatment, a careful diet history should be performed to ensure that all foods are completely gluten free and that the child is consuming enough calories for growth. If weight gain is not achieved despite adequate caloric intake and proper adherence to a GFD, other causes of malabsorption, such as pancreatic insufficiency, IBD, chronic parasitic infections, or food allergies, should be considered. Additionally, children with CD who do not achieve vertical catchup gain after a reasonable time on a GFD should be referred to an endocrinologist for evaluation of growth hormone deficiency.

Abdominal pain. Children with CD who have abdominal pain should elicit the same broad-based evaluation as all other children because this is a common complaint that could be related to anything from stress to constipation or more serious conditions such as IBD. Constipation can be a chronic and perplexing symptom, both in children with undiagnosed CD and in children who are compliant with a GFD after diagnosis. Dietary nonadherence as a cause of pain is another consideration and should prompt a thorough dietary review. Recurrent abdominal pain in children with CD who adhere to a strict GFD should prompt reconsideration of the diagnosis and evaluation of recurrent abdominal separation from CD. Irritable bowel syndrome (IBS) has also been linked to patients with CD. There are many overlapping symptoms of CD and IBS, including abdominal pain, diarrhea, bloating, and constipation. Therefore screening for CD in children with IBS and considering IBS in children with CD who are still experiencing abdominal pain should occur (Irvine et al., 2017).

DEVELOPMENTAL ISSUES

Sleep Patterns

Chronic fatigue may be a symptom of untreated CD. Nighttime bowel movements may also hinder the ability to get adequate sleep. After diagnosis and treatment with a GFD, sleep patterns of children with CD should be normal unless a coexisting condition exists.

Toileting

Chronic diarrhea, increased flatulence, and abdominal distention that may accompany undiagnosed CD may increase the difficulty of toilet training. It would be preferable to delay rigorous toilet training until symptom resolution is achieved on a GFD. Poor adherence to a GFD may induce a spectrum of symptoms, including abdominal pain, bloating, and diarrhea, that may affect the toileting regimen or evoke embarrassment in older children. Conversely, a minority of children with CD may have intractable constipation of unclear etiology.

Discipline

Behavioral expectations for children with CD should be the same as their peers. As children get older, they have more responsibility and power over their dietary choices, and strict adherence to a GFD may be difficult, especially when they are feeling well or have no immediate symptoms. Compliance numbers may be underestimated because children may be reluctant to admit they are not following medical advice. Knowledge of reported barriers to compliance may be useful in promoting adherence. These include the ability to manage emotions (depression and anxiety), the ability to resist temptation and exercise restraint, feelings of deprivation, the fear generated by inaccurate time pressures (planning and preparation of meals may take longer), competing priorities (work, job, school), assessing gluten-free content in foods (label reading), eating out (avoidance, fear, difficulty ensuring food safety), social events (not wanting to look or be different), and support of family and friends. One strategy to help with compliance may be a gluten-free household, where the entire family is gluten free for ease in grocery shopping and cooking (Itzlinger, 2018). Children should be encouraged by positive reinforcement for healthy food choices.

Child Care
Educating child care providers on a safe GFD is essential in providing a safe environment for children with CD.

Schooling
Children with CD should be held to the same academic expectations as their peers. Special gluten-free school lunches that are nutritionally balanced should be provided for these children. There should be no significant difference in the school performance of children with a well-controlled disease and their peers. Children with CD may face social stigma because of food choices that set them apart from their peers.

Sexuality
Delayed menarche is more prevalent in adolescent females with untreated CD. Issues surrounding poor self-esteem and body image may also affect the development of sexuality. At some point in adolescence, those with CD should be counseled on the complications of miscarriage and infertility in poorly treated celiac. There are no contraindications to contraceptive alternatives.

Transition to Adulthood
The pediatric primary care provider should begin preparing patients for transition to adult care during late adolescence. In children with CD, it will be important to provide guidance on finding an adult primary care provider and an adult gastroenterologist who can provide more specialized care throughout their adult life.

Family Concerns
Families with children who have CD are challenged to keep their children safe with gluten-free foods but also to provide nonaffected family members opportunities to enjoy their favorite foods that may contain gluten. Offering a consultation with a dietitian who is knowledgeable about a GFD at the time of diagnosis is very important. Follow-up with the dietician after several weeks or months on the GFD may be helpful because families often have additional questions after having experience with the gluten-free lifestyle. Other considerations include the higher cost of gluten-free products, which might present a financial burden for some families. These families may need additional assistance with creating affordable but well-balanced meals and snacks. National supermarkets (e.g., Whole Foods, Trader Joe's, Sprouts) are well stocked with gluten-free products, as are local health food and specialty stores. Large stores (e.g., Target, Walmart) often have designated gluten-free sections where many options for gluten-free substitutes are offered. Rural markets and food deserts may not carry many gluten-free options, so the availability of gluten-free foods for those who live in these areas may be a barrier.

The decision to impose the GFD on nonaffected family members while in the home is a very individual one and should be based on the common good (e.g., How many family members have the disease?), the family's lifestyle (e.g., Does everyone eat dinner together? Does the family eat out often?), and the personal preferences of the main food preparer and the individuals in question, as well as the ability to afford gluten-free foods in bulk.

RESOURCES
Many websites offer information on CD and the GFD. Health care providers should be aware of reputable sites. Many of these websites offer online or local support groups to provide families with additional information, practical advice, and a source of emotional and psychological support.
Beyond Celiac: www.beyondceliac.org
Canadian Celiac Association: www.celiac.ca
Celiac Disease Foundation: www.celiac.org
Gluten Intolerance Group: www.gluten.org
National Celiac Association: www.nationalceliac.org
North American Society for Pediatric Gastroenterology, Hepatology & Nutrition: www.naspghan.org

---

 Summary

Primary Care Needs for the Child With Celiac Disease

HEALTH CARE MAINTENANCE
Growth and Development
- Physical growth can be impaired as a result of malnutrition if diagnosis and treatment are not prompt.
- Routine visits to health care providers to monitor growth, monitor nutritional deficiencies, and review GFD.
- No deficits in cognition and development are specifically associated with celiac disease.

Diet
- Lifelong adherence to a GFD is the only known treatment.
- Increased risk of calcium, vitamin B12, and folate deficiency caused by limitations in diet.
- Recommend American Pediatric Association (APA) guidelines on food introduction.

Safety
- All caretakers should be educated about gluten-free foods.

Continued

- Reactions to gluten vary widely among individuals, from none to anaphylactic-type reactions; care must be taken to avoid the consumption of hidden gluten in foods.
- No special restrictions related to physical activity.

Immunizations
- Routine vaccines are recommended per CDC guidelines.

Screening
- *Vision.* Routine screening at regular well-child visits.
- *Hearing.* Routine screening at well-child visits.
- *Dental.* Increased risk of dental enamel defects in untreated celiac disease. Routine screening is recommended for those on GFD.
- *Blood pressure.* Routine screening at well-child visits.
- *Hematocrit.* Anemia is a common symptom in untreated celiac disease; it generally resolves on proper GFD. Currently, no set guidelines on the frequency of screening exist; it depends on clinical presentation and increased risk related to dietary restrictions (e.g., vegetarian GFD).
- Recommend full complete blood count (CBC) to screen for macrocytic anemia and iron deficiency.
- *Urinalysis.* Routine screening is recommended.
- *Tuberculosis.* The risk of tuberculosis is higher in persons with celiac disease for unknown reasons. No guidelines exist for more frequent screening; thus, routine screening is recommended at a minimum.

Condition-Specific Screening
- Recheck TTG IgA after 6 months on GFD to indirectly measure dietary compliance, then once yearly or as needed to monitor long-term compliance.
- No surveillance endoscopies are recommended after initial diagnosis.
- No consensus exists on whether or not to routinely screen asymptomatic family members, though some clinicians advise this given increased risk.

COMMON ILLNESS MANAGEMENT
Differential Diagnosis
- *Diarrhea and abdominal pain.* Rule out gluten ingestion (noncompliance versus accidental). Re-educate on GFD if necessary. If symptoms persist on GFD, consider lactose intolerance, small bowel bacterial overgrowth (SBBO), inflammatory bowel disease (IBD), concurrent infection, food allergy, etc.
- *Failure to thrive.* Malabsorption can lead to growth retardation. Generally, it normalizes on GFD, but the potential for short stature persists, especially with late diagnosis. If there is no catch-up gain on GFD, consider dietary noncompliance or other causes of malabsorption, such as pancreatic insufficiency, IBS, chronic parasitic infection, or food allergies.

DEVELOPMENTAL ISSUES
Sleep Patterns
- Normal unless there is a coexisting condition. Chronic fatigue is possible in untreated celiac disease.

Toileting
- No special needs if well on GFD. Symptoms of diarrhea, increased flatulence, bloating, and abdominal pain can make toilet training difficult in untreated celiac disease. Delay toilet training until symptoms resolve.

Discipline
- Same as peers. It may be difficult to adhere to GFD, especially in their teen years when able to make their own food purchases and choices. Offer positive reinforcement for making healthy food choices.

Child Care
- Essential to educate all care providers and schools about celiac disease and GFD.

Schooling
- Same academic standards as peers. Food choices that set children on GFD apart from peers may lead to social stigma.

Sexuality
- No contraindications to contraceptive measures. Delayed menarche and sexual development in untreated celiac disease can alter body image.

Transition to Adulthood
- Adolescent females should be counseled on the higher risk of infertility and miscarriages in untreated celiac disease.
- Lifelong dietary adherence should be emphasized because most adults with celiac disease do not receive routine dietary screening after transfer to adult care.

Family Concerns
- A strict GFD is a lifelong commitment. The decision about whether or not to impose this diet on members without celiac disease should be considered based on family circumstances. The higher cost of gluten-free foods may be a burden on family resources. Reputable websites (see Resources) offer food ideas and support groups locally or online.

REFERENCES

Aljada, B., Zohni, A., & El-Matary, W. (2021). The gluten-free diet for celiac disease and beyond. *Nutrients, 13*(11), 3993. doi:10.3390/nu13113993.

Al-Toma, A., Volta, U., Auricchio, R., Castillejo, G., Sanders, D. S., Cellier, C., Mulder, C. J., & Lundin, K. E. A. (2019). European Society for the Study of Coeliac Disease (ESsCD) guideline for coeliac disease and other gluten-related disorders. *United European Gastroenterology J, 7*(5), 583–613. doi:10.1177/2050640619844125. Epub 2019 Apr 13.

Bramuzzo, M., Lionetti, P., Miele, E., Romano, C., Arrigo, S., Cardile, S., Di Nardo, G., Illiceto, M. T., Pastore, M., Felici, E., Fuoti, M., Banzato, C., Citrano, M., Congia, M., Norsa, L., Pozzi, E., Zuin, G., Agrusti, A., Bianconi, M., Grieco, C., Giudici, F., Aloi, M., & Alvisi, P. (2021). Phenotype and natural history of children with coexistent inflammatory bowel disease and celiac disease. *Inflamm Bowel Dis, 27*(12), 1881–1888. doi:10.1093/ibd/izaa360.

Caio, G., Volta, U., Sapone, A., Leffler, D. A., De Giorgio, R., Catassi, C., & Fasano, A. (2019). Celiac disease: A comprehensive current review. *BMC Med, 17*(1), 142. doi:10.1186/s12916-019-1380-z.

Comino, I., Moreno, M. L., & Sousa, C. (2015). Role of oats in celiac disease. *World Journal of Gastroenterology and Nutrition, 61*(4), 400–403. https://doi.org/10.1097/MPG.0000000000000856.

Food and Drug Administration. (2013). *The Federal Register.* Federal Register Food Labeling; Gluten-Free Labeling of Foods. https://www.federalregister.gov/documents/2013/08/05/2013-18813/food-labeling-gluten-free-labeling-of-foods.

Gastroenterology. (2015). *21*(41), 11825–11831. Available from: http://www.wjgnet.com/1007-9327/full/v2.

Gidrewicz, D., Trevenen, C. L., Lyon, M., & Butzner, J. D. (2017). Normalization time of celiac serology in children on a gluten-free diet. *Journal of Pediatric Gastroenterology and Nutrition, 64*(3), 362–367. doi:10.1097/MPG.0000000000001270.

Goodwin, G. (2019). Type 1 diabetes mellitus and celiac disease: Distinct autoimmune disorders that share common pathogenic mechanisms. *Hormone Research in Paediatrics, 92*(5), 285–292. doi:10.1159/000503142.

Heshin-Bekenstein, M., Turner, D., Shamir, R., Bar-Meir, M., Dagan, R., Zevit, N., & Silbermintz, A. (2015). Hepatitis B virus revaccination with standard versus pre-S vaccine in previously immunized patients with celiac disease. *J Pediatr Gastroenterol Nutr, 61*(4), 400–403. doi:10.1097/MPG.0000000000000856. Erratum in: *J Pediatr Gastroenterol Nutr.* 2016 Mar;62(3):515.

Hill, I. D., Fasano, A., Guandalini, S., Hoffenberg, E., Levy, J., Reilly, N., & Verma, R. (2016). NASPGHAN clinical report on the diagnosis and treatment of gluten-related disorders. *J Pediatr Gastroenterol Nutr, 63*(1), 156–165. doi:10.1097/MPG.0000000000001216.

Husby, S., Koletzko, S., Korponay-Szabó, I., Kurppa, K., Mearin, M. L., Ribes-Koninckx, C., Shamir, R., Troncone, R., Auricchio, R., Castillejo, G., Christensen, R., Dolinsek, J., Gillett, P., Hróbjartsson, A., Koltai, T., Maki, M., Nielsen, S. M., Popp, A., Størdal, K., Werkstetter, K., & Wessels, M. (2020). European society paediatric gastroenterology, hepatology, and nutrition guidelines for diagnosing coeliac disease 2020. *J Pediatr Gastroenterol Nutr, 70*(1), 141–156. doi:10.1097/mpg.0000000000002497.

Husby, S., Murray, J. A., & Katzka, D. A. (2019). AGA clinical practice update on diagnosis and monitoring of celiac disease-changing utility of serology and histologic measures: Expert review. *Gastroenterology, 156*(4), 885–889. doi:10.1053/j.gastro.2018.12.010.

Irvine, A. J., Chey, W. D., & Ford, A. C. (2017). Screening for celiac disease in irritable bowel syndrome: An updated systematic review and meta-analysis. *American Journal of Gastroenterology, 112*(1), 65–76. https://doi.org/10.1038/ajg.2016.466.

Itzlinger, A., Branchi, F., Elli, L., & Schumann, M. (2018). Gluten-free diet in celiac disease—forever and for all? *Nutrients, 10*(11), 1796. doi:10.3390/nu10111796.

James, S. P. (2005). National institutes of health consensus development conference statement on celiac disease, June 28–30, 2004. *Gastroenterology, 128*(4), S1–S9. https://doi.org/10.1053/j.gastro.2005.02.007.

Khatib, M., Baker, R., Ly, E., Kozielski, R., & Baker, S. (2016). Presenting pattern of pediatric celiac disease. *Journal of Pediatric Gastroenterology and Nutrition, 62*(1), 60–63. https://doi.org/10.1097/MPG.0000000000000887.

Leonard, M. M., Cureton, P., & Fasano, A. (2017). Indications and use of the gluten contamination elimination diet for patients with nonresponsive celiac disease. *Nutrients, 9*(10), 1129. doi:10.3390/nu9101129.

Meijer, C. R., Auricchio, R., Putter, H., Castillejo, G., Crespo, P., Gyimesi, J., Hartman, C., Kolacek, S., Koletzko, S., Korponay-Szabo, I., Ojinaga, E. M., Polanco, I., Ribes-Koninckx, C., Shamir, R., Szajewska, H., Troncone, R., Villanacci, V., Werkstetter, K., & Mearin, M. L. (2022). Prediction models for celiac disease development in children from high-risk families: Data from the PreventCD cohort. *Gastroenterology, 163*(2), 426–436. doi:10.1053/j.gastro.2022.04.030.

Melini, V., & Melini, F. (2019). Gluten-free diet: Gaps and needs for a healthier diet. *Nutrients, 11*(1), 170. doi:10.3390/nu11010170.

Pinto-Sanchez, M. I., Silvester, J. A., Lebwohl, B., Leffler, D. A., Anderson, R. P., Therrien, A., Kelly, C. P., & Verdu, E. F. (2021). Society for the study of celiac disease position statement on gaps and opportunities in coeliac disease. *Nat Rev Gastroenterol Hepatol, 18*(12), 875–884. doi:10.1038/s41575-021-00511-8.

Robinson, B. L., Davis, S. C., Vess, J., & Lebel, J. (2015). Primary care management of celiac disease. *Journal for Nurse Practitioners, 40*(2), 28–34. https://doi.org/10.1097/01.NPR.0000459728.54533.ac.

Rubin, J. E., & Crowe, S. E. (2020). Celiac disease. *Ann Intern Med, 172*(1), ITC1–ITC16. doi:10.7326/AITC202001070.

Sahin, Y. (2021). Celiac disease in children: A review of the literature. *World Journal of Clinical Pediatrics, 10*(4), 53–71. doi:10.5409/wjcp.v10.i4.53.

Salmi, T. T. (2019). Dermatitis herpetiformis. *Clin Exp Dermatol, 44*(7), 728–731. doi:10.1111/ced.13992. Epub 2019 May 15.

Sange, I., Mohamed, M. W. F., Aung, S., Mereddy, N., & Hamid, P. (2020). Celiac disease and the autoimmune web of endocrinopathies. *Cureus, 12*(12), e12383. doi:10.7759/cureus.12383.

Sciurti, M., Fornaroli, F., Gaiani, F., Bonaguri, C., Leandro, G., Di Mario, F., & De' Angelis, G. L. (2018). Genetic susceptibility and celiac disease: What role do HLA haplotypes play? *Acta Biomed, 89*(9-S), 17–21. doi:10.23750/abm.v89i9-S.7953.

Snyder, J., Butzner, J. D., DeFelice, A. R., Fasano, A., Guandalini, S., Liu, E., & Newton, K. P. (2016). Evidence-informed expert recommendations for the management of celiac disease in children. *Pediatrics, 138*(3), e20153147. doi:10.1542/peds.2015-3147.

Taraghikhah, N., Ashtari, S., Asri, N., Shahbazkhani, B., Al-Dulaimi, D., Rostami-Nejad, M., Rezaei-Tavirani, M., Razzaghi, M. R., & Zali, M. R. (2020). An updated overview of spectrum of gluten-related disorders: Clinical and diagnostic aspects. *BMC Gastroenterol, 20*(1), 258. doi:10.1186/s12876-020-01390-0.

Therrien, A., Kelly, C. P., & Silvester, J. A. (2020). Celiac disease: Extraintestinal manifestations and associated conditions. *Journal of Clinical Gastroenterology, 54*(1), 8–21. doi:10.1097/MCG.0000000000001267.

Valitutti, F., Trovato, C. M., Montuori, M., & Cucchiara, S. (2017). Pediatric celiac disease: Follow-up in the spotlight. *Advances in Nutrition, 8*(2), 356–361. https://doi.org/10.3945/an.116.013292.

Villanacci, V., Vanoli, A., Leoncini, G., Arpa, G., Salviato, T., Bonetti, L. R., Baronchelli, C., Saragoni, L., & Parente, P. (2020). Celiac disease: Histology-differential diagnosis-complications. A practical approach. *Pathologica, 112*(3), 186–196. doi:10.32074/1591-951X-157.

Waheed, N., Cheema, H. A., Suleman, H., Fayyaz, Z., Mushtaq, I., Muhammad, & Hashmi, A. (2016). Celiac crisis: A rare or rarely recognized disease. *J Ayub Med Coll Abbottabad, 28*(4), 672–675.

Wei, G., Helmerhorst, E. J., Darwish, G., Blumenkranz, G., & Schuppan, D. (2020). Gluten degrading enzymes for treatment of celiac disease. *Nutrients, 12*(7), 2095. doi:10.3390/nu12072095.

Zhu, J., Mulder, C. J. J., & Dieleman, L. A. (2019). Celiac disease: Against the grain in gastroenterology. *J Can Assoc Gastroenterol, 2*(4), 161–169. doi:10.1093/jcag/gwy042.

15 Cerebral Palsy

Cheri Barber

Cerebral palsy (CP) was first described by Dr. William John Little in 1861. The definition of CP has evolved and was defined by an international consortium of experts in 2005 as "a group of permanent disorders of the development of movement and posture, causing activity limitation, that are attributed to non-progressive disturbances that occur in the developing fetal or infant brain. The motor disorders of CP are often accompanied by disturbances of sensation, cognition, communication, perception, or behavior and may be accompanied by a seizure disorder" (Rosenbaum et al., 2007; Sheu et al., 2022).

This revised definition was necessary because of increased knowledge of developmental neurobiology, the array of conditions that result in motor impairments that affect activities of daily living, and the antecedents and consequences of CP. In addition, advances in neuroimaging technology and the management of care for motor impairments have resulted in the need to reexamine the definition of CP. This condition should be described by the dominant movement or tone abnormality, brain morphology, and neurologic findings. However, despite the evolution in the clinical consensus of CP, the definition of CP continues to focus on the brain without acknowledging developmental spinal cord dysfunction (Brandenburg et al., 2019).

CLASSIFICATION OF CEREBRAL PALSY

Classifications are intended to improve communication among clinicians, researchers, patients, and caregivers. The topographic classification is used to describe the body parts that are affected by the condition, with health care providers using this terminology to explain where the motor difficulties take place in the body (Box 15.1). However, not all children have classic presentations of anatomic distribution (e.g., three affected limbs with one uninvolved limb or all extremities affected but not equally).

Recognizing the importance of accurately describing children's current clinical problems and their severity, evaluating their physical and quality-of-life status across time, and listing short- and long-term support needs have led to revisions in the classification systems over the past decade. There are four main types of CP: spastic, dyskinetic, ataxia, and mixed.

SPASTIC CEREBRAL PALSY

Spastic CP affects about 80% of people with CP (Centers for Disease Control and Prevention [CDC], 2022a). Spasticity describes the presence of increased muscle tone, which is noted through the passive range of motion of a joint. Characteristics of spastic CP include persistent primitive reflexes, exaggerated stretch reflexes, positive Babinski reflex, ankle clonus, and later development of contractures. This form of CP is most distinctly divided by the extremities involved and affects the majority of people with CP.

DYSKINETIC CEREBRAL PALSY (INCLUDES ATHETOID, CHOREOATHETOSIS, AND DYSTONIC)

Children with dyskinetic CP have problems with controlling the movement of their hands, arms, feet, and legs, making it difficult to sit and walk. Movements are uncontrollable and can be slow and writhing or rapid and jerky. A child with dyskinetic CP may have the face and tongue affected, causing difficulty with sucking, swallowing, and talking. Dyskinetic CP may cause muscle tone that can vary from too tight to too loose (CDC, 2022b). Children with this form of CP often display rigid muscle tone when awake and normal or decreased muscle tone when asleep.

ATAXIA

Ataxia occurs when neurologic damage is present in the cerebellum. Ataxia includes a range of conditions marked by the degree of muscle tone and coordination of movements and balance (CDC, 2022b). These conditions can range from ataxic to hypotonic to atonic. Children with ataxic CP walk with an unstable, wide-based gait and have problems with balance and coordination. They may have difficulty controlling their hands or arms when they reach for something or with quick movements or movements that need great control, such as handwriting.

MIXED

This motor dysfunction group of CP is characterized by more than one type of motor pattern, resulting from many defects in various areas of the brain. The first is mixed, which is also used when no one motor pattern is dominant. The most common type of mixed CP is spastic-dyskinetic CP (CDC, 2022b).

Box 15.1	Topographic Classifications

PREFIX AND SUFFIX

Key prefixes:
- *mono-* (one)
- *di-* (two)
- *tri-* (three)
- *quadri-* (four)
- *penta-* (five)
- *hemi-* (half)

Key suffixes:
- *-plegia* (paralyzed)
- *-paresis* (weakened)

TOPOGRAPHIC CLASSIFICATIONS

Monoplegia/monoparesis: one limb is affected.

Diplegia/diparesis: two limbs are affected; more often affects the legs than the arms

Triplegia/triparesis: some combination of three limbs is affected (e.g., one arm, one leg, the face are affected)

Hemiplegia/hemiparesis: arm and leg on one side of the body are affected

Double hemiplegia/double hemiparesis: all four limbs are affected, with one side of the body affected more than the other

Tetraplegia/tetraparesis: all four limbs are affected, but three limbs are affected more severely than the fourth

Paraplegia/paraparesis: lower half of the body as a whole is affected

Quadriplegia/quadriparesis: all four limbs are affected

Pentaplegia/pentaparesis: all four limbs and the head and neck region are affected

Table 15.1	Gross Motor Function Classification System (GMFCS)

GMFCS LEVEL	DESCRIPTION
Level I	Walks without limitations indoors or outdoors and climbs stairs without limitations. Speed, balance, and coordination are reduced.
Level II	Walks with limitations indoors or outdoors, climbs stairs holding on to a rail. Experiences limitations walking on uneven surfaces and inclines, in crowds or confined spaces.
Level III	Walks indoors or outdoors using a handheld mobility device and climbs stairs holding on to a railing. May require a self-propelled wheelchair when traveling longer distances, outdoors, or on uneven terrain.
Level IV	Self-mobility with great limitations and may use powered mobility.
Level V	Physical impairments restrict voluntary control of movement and have no means of independent mobility. Transported in a manual wheelchair.

Box 15.2	Communication Function Classification System (CFCS) Levels

CFCS LEVEL I

A person independently and effectively alternates between being a sender and receiver of information with most people in most environments.

CFCS LEVEL II

A person independently alternates between being a sender and receiver with most people in most environments, but the conversation may be slower.

CFCS LEVEL III

A person usually communicates effectively with familiar communication partners, but not unfamiliar partners, in most environments.

CFCS LEVEL IV

The person is not always consistent at communicating with familiar communication partners.

CFCS LEVEL V

A person is seldom able to communicate effectively even with familiar people.

SEVERITY

Reliable tools have been developed to assess the severity of multiple areas of function in those with CP. As CP is multidimensional, evaluation tools provide valuable information on a child's gross motor/mobility, fine motor, speech/communication, nutritional and functional status, and limitations. The Gross Motor Function Classification System (GMFCS) currently evaluates gross motor and mobility. This rating scale has five levels of severity, with GMFCS-I the least severe and GMFCS-V the most severe (Table 15.1) (Palisano et al., 1997, 2007; Paulson & Vargus-Adams, 2017).

Similarly, the Manual Abilities Classification System (MACS) (Fig. 15.1) is a simple, five-point ordinal classification system that provides information on the manual (hand use) function of a child (age 4–18 years) (Paulson & Vargus-Adams, 2017). The Communication Function Classification System (CFCS) (Box 15.2) assesses a child's communication abilities, with 31% to 88% of individuals with CP having a concomitant communication disorder (Hidecker et al., 2011; Paulson & Vargus-Adams, 2017).

INCIDENCE AND PREVALENCE

Based on international population-based studies, the CDC currently cites the prevalence of CP to be between 1 and nearly 4 per 1000 (CDC, 2022a). According to the latest data from 2010 compiled by the Autism and Developmental Disabilities Monitoring Network, the incidence of CP in the United States is about 2.9 in 1000 (about 1 in 345) (Durkin et al., 2016).

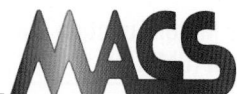

What do you need to know to use MACS?

The child's ability to handle objects in important daily activities, for example during play and leisure, eating and dressing.

In which situation is the child independent and to what extent do they need support and adaptation?

I. Handles objects easily and successfully.
At most, limitations in the ease of performing manual tasks requiring speed and accuracy. However, any limitations in manual abilities do not restrict independence in daily activities.

II. Handles most objects but with somewhat reduced quality and/or speed of achievement.
Certain activities may be avoided or be achieved with some difficulty; alternative ways of performance might be used but manual abilities do not usually restrict independence in daily activities.

III. Handles objects with difficulty: needs help to prepare and/or modify activities.
The performance is slow and achieved with limited success regarding quality and quantity. Activities are performed independently if they have been set up or adapted.

IV. Handles a limited selection of easily managed objects in adapted situations.
Performs parts of activities with effort and with limited success. Requires continuous support and assistance and/or adapted equipment, for even partial achievement of the activity.

V. Does not handle objects and has severely limited ability to perform even simple actions.
Requires total assistance.

Distinctions between Levels I and II
Children in Level I may have limitations in handing very small, heavy or fragile objects which demand detailed fine motor control, or efficient coordination between hands. Limitations may also involve performance in new and unfamiliar situations. Children in Level II perform almost the same activities as children in Level I but the quality of performance is decreased, or the performance is slower. Functional differences between hands can limit effectiveness of performance. Children in Level II commonly try to simplify handling of objects, for example by using a surface for support instead of handling objects with with both hands.

Distinctions between Levels II and III
Children in Level II handle most objects, although slowly or with reduced quality of performance. Children in Level III commonly need help to prepare the activity and/or require adjustments to be made to the environment since their ability to reach or handle objects is limited. They cannot perform certain activities and their degree of independence is related to the supportiveness of the environmental context.

Distinctions between Levels III and IV
Children in Level III can perform selected activities if the situation is prearranged and if they get supervision and plenty of time. Children in Level IV need continuous help during the activity and can at best participate meaningfully in only parts of an activity.

Distinctions between Levels IV and V
Children in Level IV perform part of an activity, however, they need help continuously. Children in Level V might at best participate with a simple movement in special situations, e.g. by pushing a button or occasionally hold undemanding objects.

Fig. 15.1 **Manual Abilities Classification System** *(MACS)*. (From National Center for Biotechnology Information, National Library of Medicine. [n.d.]. What do you need to know to use MACS? https://www.ncbi.nlm.nih.gov/core/lw/2.0/html/tileshop_pmc/tileshop_pmc_inline.html?title=Click%20on%20image%20to%20zoom&p=PMC3&id=5406689_children-04-00030-g002.jpg)

The reported incidence of CP has remained steady over the past several decades, with data from the CDC showing the prevalence of CP significantly more common in Black children than in White children and equal in White and Hispanic children (CDC, 2022a). However, prematurity and low birth weight are important risk factors; infants born at term account for about half of all children who develop CP with no identified risk factors. The birth prevalence was higher in twins, with 6.5 per 1000 live births (Sellier et al., 2021), with approximately half of the infants born with CP born prematurely. The birth and survival rates of premature babies with extremely low birth weight have continued to increase owing to considerable advances in perinatology, including modern methods of prenatal diagnostics, in utero transport, and intensive neonatal care (Sadowska et al., 2020). Most children with CP have been identified with spastic CP (82.9%) (CDC, 2022a).

ETIOLOGY AND RISK FACTORS

The etiology of CP is associated with a number of risk factors. There are numerous causes of CP, and sometimes a cause for the diagnosis is never clearly identified. The possible causes are delineated by the period in which the insult to the child's brain may have occurred (Sudip et al., 2022). Table 15.2 lists the risk factors for CP according to the following periods: preconception, prenatal, labor and delivery, and postnatal. During the prenatal period, both maternal and gestational risk factors are given. The most important etiologic risk factors for CP are premature birth, anoxia, and low birth weight. CP is thought to be increased in premature infants because the blood vessels are not fully developed in parts of the brain, allowing for damage and injury. More recent studies have shown that socioeconomic status also determines risk factors in CP etiology as well as smoking during pregnancy and education level of the mother (Başaran et al., 2023).

According to Moreno-De-Luca (2023), a growing body of evidence shows that a significant proportion of CP is caused by rare genomic variants; therefore it is important to understand genetic contributions to CP as new insights offer a unique window into the neurobiology of CP. By understanding the genetic basis of CP, the potential for new therapies and earlier diagnosis and interventions will increase (Moreno-De-Luca, 2023). A number of biochemical disorders and cerebral malformations may result in motor abnormalities and may be misdiagnosed as CP, such as hypotonia,

Table 15.2   Risk Factors for Cerebral Palsy According to the Period of Insult to the Child's Brain

PRECONCEPTION	PRENATAL	DURING BIRTH	AFTER BIRTH
Systemic illness of mother	Premature birth	Premature birth	Hypoxic ischemic encephalopathy
Use of drug and stimulants	Low birth weight	Cesarean section	Infection
Immune system disorders preceding pregnancy	Central nervous system (CNS) malformation	Vacuum-assisted delivery	Hyperbilirubinemia
Spontaneous abortions	Maternal diabetes mellitus	Delivery after the due date	Cerebrovascular accidents
Socioeconomic factors	Prolonged rupture of membranes	Prolonged labor	Intracranial hemorrhage
Poisoning	Maternal hemorrhage	Asphyxia	CNS infection
Infections	Multiple gestations	Meconium aspiration	Respiratory distress syndrome
Impaired fertility	Genetic factors	Breech vaginal delivery	Artificial respiratory support
Treatment of fertility	Encephalopathy of prematurity Congenital malformation Hypoxic ischemic encephalopathy In utero stroke	High fever during delivery	Hypoglycemia neonatal convulsions Traumatic brain injury Near drowning Meningitis
Genetic factors	In vitro fertilization Kernicterus Maternal disorder of clotting Meconium aspiration Fetal growth restriction Preeclampsia	Perinatal stroke	Sepsis Neonatal encephalopathy

From Paul, S., Nahar, A., Bhagawati, M., & Kunwar, A.J. (2022). A review on recent advances of cerebral palsy. *Oxidative Medicine and Cellular Longevity*, 1–20.

Duchenne muscular dystrophy, arginase deficiency, metachromatic leukodystrophy, adrenoleukodystrophy, hereditary progressive spastic paraplegia, dopa-responsive dystonia, Lesch-Nyhan disease, Rett syndrome, ataxia telangiectasia, Niemann-Pick disease type C, and mitochondrial cytopathies (Krigger, 2006; Pearson et al., 2019).

DIAGNOSIS

CP is a clinical diagnosis based on an assessment of the child's developmental, functional, and physical abilities. The detailed health history should include the family's medical history, the mother's and fetus's health during pregnancy, the infant's health at birth and up to the present, and the infant's development since birth. Additional testing, such as parental and infant genetic screening and testing, prenatal ultrasound or amniocentesis, cranial sonography or magnetic resonance imaging, and other designated developmental testing and evaluations of specific impairments should be included as warranted. When parents have related concerns, it is important for primary care providers to rule out other neurologic problems in conjunction with specialty consultations.

While there have been multiple calls for early diagnosis throughout the generations of CP research and care, historically there has been a general consensus that the signs of CP are not identifiable in the early postnatal stages (<12 months of age) and that it is not possible to diagnose a child with CP until 3 to 5 years of age (te Velde et al., 2019). However, in 2020, the 2017 international guidelines for early detection of CP were implemented in a study that aimed to reduce the age at which CP is diagnosed through a network of five diverse US high-risk infant programs (Maitre et al., 2020). The implementation phase was completed in 2018, only 15 months after the publication of the guidelines, yielding positive results for the early detection of CP by using quality improvement and science tools as being effective and feasible (Maitre et al., 2020). This was the first successful implementation of the international guidelines for the early diagnosis of CP across several clinical institutions in the United States. History or clinical findings that may be present in a child with CP are outlined in Box 15.3.

The importance of early intervention has been championed over the past several decades, and it is now universally accepted that diagnosis and treatment should be established at the earliest stage possible to ensure prevention or reduction of the complications of the condition, to support the child in maintaining functional potentials, and to maximize benefits of therapeutic interventions (Alberman & Goldstein, 1970; te Velde et al., 2019). Clinical signs that should warrant further evaluation are noted in Box 15.3.

| Box 15.3 | History or Clinical Findings That May be Present in a Child With Cerebral Palsy (CP) |

PERINATAL HISTORY
- Prematurity
- Low birth weight
- Neonatal encephalopathy
- Neonatal seizures
- Neonatal stroke or other known brain abnormality
- Congenital infection
- Chorioamnionitis
- Neonatal meningitis
- Known hypoxic event

DEVELOPMENTAL HISTORY
- Does not roll in either direction (age >6 mo)
- Unable to bring hands together (age >6 mo)
- Thumb in fist after 7 mo
- Inability to sit by 9 mo
- Milestones attained out of order (able to pull to stand before able to sit)
- Asymmetric creeping or crawling
- Inability to walk by 18 mo
- Persistent toe walking

EXAMINATION FINDINGS[a]
- Increased or decreased muscle tone
- Scissoring of the legs
- Asymmetric strength or reflexes
- Opisthotonus (rigid arching of the back)
- Persistent primitive reflexes
- Combination of ankle clonus, brisk deep tendon reflexes, and persistent Babinski after 18 mo

CLINICAL FEATURES THAT SHOULD PROMPT FURTHER EVALUATION
- Absent history of perinatal risk factor for brain injury
- Family history of sibling with similar neurologic symptoms
- Motor symptom onset after an initial period of normal development
- Developmental regression
- Progressive neurologic symptoms
- Paroxysmal motor symptoms or marked fluctuation of motor symptoms
- Clinical exacerbation in the setting of a catabolic state (e.g., febrile illness)
- Isolated generalized hypotonia
- Prominent ataxia
- Signs of peripheral neuromuscular disease (reduced or absent reflexes, sensory loss)
- Eye movement abnormalities (e.g., oculogyric, oculomotor apraxia, or paroxysmal saccadic eye-head movements)

[a]The presence of these elements does not mean that CP is present, and their absence does not mean that CP can be excluded.
Modified from Noritz, G.H., Davidson, L., Steingass, K., et al. (2022). Providing a primary care medical home for children's and youth with cerebral palsy. *Pediatrics*, 150(6), e2022060055; and Pearson, T.S., Pons, R., Ghaoui, R., & Sue, C.M. (2019). Genetic mimics of cerebral palsy. *Movement Disorders*, 34(5), 625–636.

Several clinical assessment diagnostic tools have been developed over the past decades to accurately identify CP in infants. Identification of persistent primitive reflexes has been utilized to identify signs of CP in infants since the 1970s (Capute, 1979; Molnar, 1979). In the 1990s, the Gross Motor Assessment (GMA) and the Hammersmith Infant Neurological Examination (HINE) assessment tools were introduced. The GMA assesses the spontaneous movement of infants. HINE is a scorable evaluation tool for assessing infants between the ages of 2 and 24 months. These more recent advances in infant assessment have proven accurate in identifying CP diagnoses in earlier infancy (Bosanquet et al., 2013; Novak et al., 2017) and "are highly sensitive and specific when performed by specially trained clinicians" (Noritz et al., 2022).

TREATMENT

There is no cure for CP, so the treatments used are largely symptomatic, with a focus on the quality of life and participation in society. CP is a multidimensional condition—it requires multidisciplinary care and cohesive collaboration among interdisciplinary providers (Box 15.4). The risks and benefits of any intervention should be carefully considered on a case-by-case basis. It is the role of the primary care provider to coordinate that collaboration. Box 15.5 outlines treatment modalities that are used in caring for the child with CP. The goals of treatment for children with CP are designed to maintain mobility and maximize the joint range of motion, as well as optimize muscle control and balance, communication, and performance of activities of daily living following the International Classification of Functioning, Disability, and Health (ICFDH) (van der Veen et al., 2022). Using ICFDH helps foster holistic, patient-centered care. Multiple studies have shown that therapies are more effective for improving motor function and self-care when the therapies are focused on goals that are set by the child and family. A continuum of comprehensive, interdisciplinary care should prevail across the lifespan. Box 15.6 outlines the assessment of tone in

| Box 15.4 | Multidisciplinary Team Members Involved in Care for Children With Cerebral Palsy |

- Audiologist
- Medical social worker
- Nursing
- Nutritionist
- Occupational therapist
- Pediatric gastroenterologist
- Pediatric neurologist
- Pediatric orthopedic surgeon
- Pediatric pulmonologist
- Pediatric surgeon
- Primary care nurse practitioner/provider
- Psychologist
- Speech-language therapist

| Box 15.5 | Treatment Modalities in the Care of Cerebral Palsy |

THERAPIES
- Physical therapy
- Gait analysis
- Neuromuscular electrical stimulation
- Occupational therapy
- Speech therapy
- Feeding therapy
- Behavioral therapy

ORTHOTIC DEVICES AND ADAPTIVE EQUIPMENT
- Braces
- Casting
- Splints
- Molded ankle-foot orthosis
- Adaptive equipment
- Boards
- Computers
- For functional use (e.g., eating utensils)
- Scooters and tricycles
- Switches
- Wheelchairs and standing devices

PHARMACOLOGIC THERAPY
- Botulinum toxin A
- Intrathecal baclofen
- Medications for:
  - Pain
  - Constipation
  - Urinary tract infections
  - Upper respiratory tract infections
  - Decubitus ulcers
  - Other secondary complications and conditions

SURGERY
- Orthopedic corrective (e.g., tendon transfers, muscle lengthening)
- Neurologic (e.g., neurectomies)
- Selective dorsal rhizotomy
- Feeding (e.g., gastrostomy)
- Dental

| Box 15.6 | Assessment of Tone in Infants |

NORMAL TONE
- Infant moves well against gravity and lacks high- or low-tone characteristics.

LOW TONE
- Infant lacks tone to move against gravity and resistance to passive movement; has low-tone postures (e.g., supine lying with arm abducted and/or legs abducted in a frog-legged position) or decreased movement.

HIGH TONE
- Infant becomes stiff when moving against gravity; the neck or extremities resist passive movement; infant has hypertonic head reactions (e.g., hyperextension of the neck when rolling over and/or head pushing when supine or when pulled to sitting position); infant has high tone posturing (e.g., increased extension of the head when supine lying, retracted shoulder girdle, lordosis of the back of extended lower extremities).

| Box 15.7 | Evaluations/Instruments Used for Management Decisions |

- Three-Dimensional Gait Analysis
- Nine-Hole Peg Test
- Activities Scale for Kids
- Assisting Hand Assessment
- Barry-Albright Dystonia Scale
- Bimanual Fine Motor Function
- Canadian Occupational Performance Measure
- Edinburgh Visual Gait Analysis Interval Testing Scale
- Energy Expenditure Measures
- Gillette Functional Assessment Questionnaire
- Goal Attainment Scale
- Gross Motor Function Measure
- Lifestyle Assessment Questionnaire for Cerebral Palsy
- Manual Ability Classification System
- Melbourne Assessment of Upper Limb Function
- Modified Ashworth Scale
- Pediatric Evaluation of Disability Inventory
- Pediatric Quality of Life Inventory
- Physician Rating Scale, Observational Gait Scale
- Pediatric Outcomes Data Collection Instrument
- Range of Motion
- Quality of Upper Extremity Skills Test
- Spinal Alignment and Range of Motion Measure
- Tardieu Scale
- Video Documentation
- WeeFIM (Functional Independence Measure for Children)
- Wong-Baker FACES Pain Rating Scale

Modified from Heinen, F., Molenaers, G., Fairhurst, C., et al. (2006). European consensus table 2006 on botulinum toxin for children with cerebral palsy. *European Journal of Paediatric Neurology, 10*, 215–225; Chaleat-Valayer, E., Bernard, J.-C., Morel, E., et al. (2006). Use of videographic examination for analysis of efficacy of botulinum toxin in the lower limbs in children with cerebral palsy. *Journal of Pediatric Orthopedics B, 15*, 339–347; and Krigger, K.W. (2006). Cerebral palsy: An overview. *American Family Physician, 73*, 91–100.

infants, Box 15.7 lists different evaluations that health care professionals can use for management decisions, and Box 15.8 lists the different interventions to treat spasticity.

PHYSICAL AND OCCUPATIONAL THERAPY

During infancy and toddlerhood, when most presumptive diagnoses take place, the first line of treatment involves physical and occupational therapy. These therapies aim to enhance motor development, minimize the development of contractures, and prevent deterioration or weakening of the muscles. For sitting and moving, gross motor skills, muscle control, balance, and coordination are needed. Fine motor skills, muscle control, and coordination are needed for writing and holding materials. Motor, cognitive, and language skills are also needed for self-care activities.

| Box 15.8 | Interventions to Treat Spasticity |

PHARMACOLOGIC

Baclofen: oral and intrathecal pump

Phenol intramuscular injection

Botulinum toxin intramuscular injection

Valium and clonazepam oral

Tizanidine and clonidine oral

Dantrolene oral

NONPHARMACOLOGIC

Physiotherapy

Occupational therapy

Use of adaptive equipment and orthoses

Orthopedic surgical procedures

Selective dorsal rhizotomy

Bowel and bladder control and prevention of pressure ulcers are important to learn.

Physical Therapy

Physical therapy started in the first few years of life has proven to be a cornerstone in CP treatment. Specific exercises used during therapy, such as stretching, resistance, and strength training, along with activities to maintain or improve muscle strength, balance, and motor skills, can help prevent contractures. Orthotic devices may also be used to improve mobility and stretch spastic muscles.

Occupational Therapy

Occupational therapy focuses on optimizing upper body function, improving posture, and making the most of the child's mobility by helping address new ways to meet everyday activities and routines at home, school, and within the community. Occupational therapy is an integral part of the interdisciplinary treatment of individuals with CP, promoting improvement in fine motor functioning and activities of daily living (Patel et al., 2020).

OTHER THERAPIES

Behavioral Therapy or Counseling

This may be needed at any point in a child's life and can be useful for the family in helping to live with a child with a chronic condition.

Physiotherapy

Physiotherapy has been shown to improve muscle strength, endurance, and joint range of movement for children with CP. By using passive, gentle range of motion exercises, physiotherapy exercises prevent or reduce joint contractures, increasing muscle strength with regular involvement of all major muscle groups (Patel et al., 2020). Specific physiotherapy exercises are

designed for each patient to improve balance, postural control, and gait and to assist with mobility and transfers (i.e., from bed to wheelchair).

Recreational Therapy

Recreational therapy is used to encourage participation in art and cultural programs, including sports and other events that help an individual expand their physical and cognitive skills and abilities. Parents will typically notice an improvement in their child's speech, self-esteem, and emotional well-being.

Speech Therapy

Speech therapy is typically recommended if an oromotor deficit is present. It can improve not only swallowing disorders but helps teach others varied ways of communication, such as sign language or the use of special communication devices such as a voice synthesizer for the computer.

ORTHOTIC DEVICES

Orthotic devices, which include braces and splints, usually accompany therapy when it alone no longer helps the child. Orthotic devices are used to provide stability to the joints, maintain optimal range of motion of the joints, prevent the occurrence or progression of contractures, and control involuntary movements. The most common types of orthoses are the short arm or leg cast or splint, the hand splint, and the molded ankle-foot orthosis, which is worn inside the shoe. Other types of adaptive equipment include devices for functional use (e.g., eating utensils), switches, computers, boards for positioning a child (e.g., on the side or in the prone or supine position), scooters, tricycles, and wheelchairs. Independent ambulation may be decreased in adolescents using orthotic devices because of contractures, a lack of motivation, or weight gain, and they may choose to use a wheelchair to maximize their energy. In each case, the orthosis is designed for a child and altered as the child grows or the condition changes.

PHARMACOLOGIC THERAPY

Decision making in pharmacologic treatment approaches includes age, adherence, degree of spasticity, dosage, comorbidity, costs, known adverse effects, and prior health and medication history. The most researched medications for the treatment of spasticity in CP include botulinum toxin A and intrathecal baclofen (ITB). Botulinum toxin A injections are used to treat focal spasticity with optimal effectiveness found between 1 and 6 years of age for lower extremity spasticity and between 5 and 15 years of age for spastic hemiplegia. Oral baclofen (although not approved by the US Food and Drug Administration and despite the efficacy data for children) remains a common treatment and first-line choice for spasticity (Reilly et al., 2020). Baclofen exhibits a high degree of pharmacokinetic and dosing variability within the pediatric population. Additional research continues to evolve as this becomes more widely used in pediatric CP. Common complications encountered during treatment with ITB include infection, cerebrospinal fluid leakage, and postdural spinal headache, with the most common complication related to pump and catheter complications (Imerci et al., 2019). Spasticity management with botulinum toxin A or ITB must be guided by a provider with expertise and experience in the use of these interventions. It is important to discuss all pharmacologic treatment decisions with parents, specifically addressing the possible outcomes so that the child and the parents have realistic expectations of the effect of the medication(s).

PAIN

Pain management in CP is discussed less frequently, although pain is common, especially in spastic CP. In a recent study, pain was one of the most frequent secondary conditions reported in CP, with females reporting pain more often than males (Eriksson et al., 2020). Pain is experienced most frequently in the joints of the lower extremities and reduces health-related quality of life, increasing stress in the parents and families (Eriksson et al., 2020). Treatment is generally focused on relieving the symptoms, maintaining the function, and increasing their participation in activities while preventing secondary conditions. Medications are prescribed for secondary conditions as they occur, which may include constipation, urinary tract infections (UTIs), upper respiratory infections, decubitus ulcers, among others.

SURGERY

Surgery is not an early choice of intervention for CP. Orthopedic and neurologic forms of surgery are the most common, but surgeries to enhance feeding, such as gastrostomy, gastroscopy, esophagoscopy, and correction of gastroesophageal reflux, as well as dental surgeries, are frequently done. Orthopedic surgery is not usually performed until after a child turns 6 years old. A child attains independent ambulation by this age if independence is at all possible. Orthopedic surgery is often recommended and performed when spasticity and stiffness are so severe that walking and moving about is difficult or painful to achieve. Surgeons can lengthen muscles and tendons, allowing greater leg movement and gait control, as well as correcting any extremity deformities. Orthopedic surgeries can be staggered at times appropriate to the child's age and level of motor development (Cerebral Palsy Research Network, 2022). The child's degree of spasticity, the child's size, and the effect of the spasticity on the child's life need to be considered when determining surgical interventions.

Selective dorsal rhizotomy is a widely utilized neurosurgical procedure performed on children with CP, which reduces spasticity primarily in the legs by interrupting the sensory component of the deep tendon reflex. Transient short-term side effects may include sensory or bowel/bladder symptoms, with long-term complications being rare. Potential anesthesia complications can occur in children with CP due to physiologic and motor impairments (Chin et al., 2020). The primary care provider, surgeon, parents, and child should discuss the risks and benefits carefully.

COMPLEMENTARY AND ALTERNATIVE THERAPIES

Complementary and alternative medicine (CAM) or therapies are used for children with CP and may include acupuncture, aquatic therapy, hippotherapy, massage therapy, music therapy, and stem cell therapy. These therapies lack scientific evidence and are not generally accepted by all professionals when compared to traditional therapies (Cerebral Palsy Research Network, 2022). CAMs may work with or to help support a traditional therapy or plan.

ASSOCIATED PROBLEMS OF CEREBRAL PALSY AND TREATMENT

Secondary conditions may be acute, chronic, or transitory and usually coexist with CP.

Plans for treatment, education, and habilitation must consider a child's individual symptoms and complaints.

Cognitive Impairments

Cognitive ability is one's intellectual capacity to reason, learn, or accurately perceive and informs many aspects of an individual's life (Boxes 15.9 and 15.10).

Box 15.9 Brain Functions That Fall Under Cognition
• Attention span • Comprehension • Decision making • Difficulty processing emotions and feelings • Language skills • Learning • Memory • Problem solving • Recognition • Speech proficiency

Box 15.10 Cognitive Impairment–Associated Conditions
• Anxiety • Attention-deficit/hyperactivity disorder • Behavioral challenges • Depression or moodiness • Fatigue • Inability to connect emotionally • Psychological disorders • Sleep disturbances

It is estimated that 30% to 50% of children with CP have some type of cognitive impairment. Examining cognitive impairment in pediatric patients with CP is important because cognitive deficits can affect their performance of functional activities and integration with the community and school (Song, 2013). In addition, 1 in 9 individuals with CP have autistic tendencies. Intellectual and developmental disabilities are usually most profound in children with abnormal motor behavior in all extremities, wherein more than 60% of the children have a normal intelligence quotient (IQ). Even if a child's IQ is normal, perceptual impairments and learning disabilities may exist.

Children with hemiplegia also have perceptual and attentional problems, with left hemiplegia experiencing more perceptual problems and inattention than children with right hemiplegia (Katz et al., 1998). Screening for cognitive impairments should occur regularly; if identified, interventions should begin immediately (Noritz et al., 2022).

Epilepsy

Approximately 35% to 62% of children with CP will be diagnosed with epilepsy (Noritz et al., 2022). Risk factors include the presence of neonatal seizures and structural brain abnormalities; despite the high numbers, there is little research to find the relationship between the two disorders of the brain. Primary care providers need to be aware of signs and symptoms that may present with seizures in CP patients, including apnea, staring, posturing, developmental regression, or sleepiness. Seizures are most seen in children with spastic quadriplegia and hemiplegia and are less common in children with dyskinesias and ataxia. Generalized tonic-clonic and minor motor types of seizures are the most common. Parents who have children with CP have identified the number-one stressor in caring for this chronic condition is seizures, which contribute to a lower quality of life.

As part of the interdisciplinary care team, the neurologist will prescribe and monitor the antiseizure medications. Some antiseizure medications, such as clobazam, is a benzodiazepine that is often used for epilepsy and has the added benefit of reducing tone in children with spasticity (Noritz et al., 2022). Other common benzodiazepines, such as diazepam, are used for spasticity in children and can improve seizure control.

Speech Impairments

The incidence of speech impairments in CP is common, with 60% to 80% of children with CP having some type of difficulty with communication (Noritz et al., 2022). A full evaluation with referral to a speech pathologist may be warranted as it is important to determine the etiology of the communication problem and the appropriate therapies. The CFCS is commonly used with this population to focus on expressive and receptive communication abilities (Paulson & Vargus-Adams, 2017). The same muscle tone problems that make it difficult for children with CP to move also create oromotor problems. Limitations in trunk movements and positioning may limit lung capacity, which is needed for strength in speaking both clearly and loudly. Problems in articulation (dysarthria) are caused by muscle tone deficiencies and are a muscle speech disorder that can affect 50% of children with CP (Noritz et al., 2022). Another common motor speech disorder that affects children with CP is apraxia, where the brain is unable to plan and coordinate the muscle movements needed to speak. Alternative communication systems may assist children with these conditions by using a communication board, book, or electronic device.

Sensory Deficits

Vision. Children with CP (50–90%) may have visual impairments or other ophthalmologic conditions, including refractive error, strabismus, amblyopia, cataracts, retinopathy of prematurity, and cortical blindness. In addition to the usual visual screenings recommended by the American Academy of Pediatrics (AAP) Bright Futures, ophthalmologic evaluations are recommended early in childhood and are most effective when initiated early. Those with more significant motor impairments tend to have more significant visual and oculomotor deficits making it more difficult to evaluate and may be underdiagnosed (Noritz et al., 2022).

Hearing. Children with CP experience hearing impairment at a greater frequency (4%–13%) than in the general population. The hearing loss is either sensorineural (i.e., damage to the auditory nerve or the inner ear) or more commonly conductive (i.e., because of anatomic abnormalities or frequent otitis media). Hearing impairments may further add to speech and communication delays with the recommendation for children with speech-language delays or a history of risk factors for delayed onset to be further evaluated with a formal audiology assessment by age 24 to 30 months (Noritz et al., 2022).

Other sensory deficits. As a result of damage to the parietal lobe of the brain, children with CP have deficits in other sensory functions. These include tactile hypersensitivity or hyposensitivity, dyspraxia (i.e., difficulty in using one's senses to plan movements), balance difficulties, and problems with proprioception, stereognosis, and movement.

Motor Impairments

Successful attainment of motor milestones is always delayed in children with CP. Some children's primitive reflexes persist, and protective reflexes never develop, thus permanently blocking their ability to ambulate. Poor muscle tone and control often lead to secondary physical problems (e.g., hip dislocation, scoliosis, contractures, fractures), which create further motor impairment and other medical problems related to basic physiologic functioning.

Subluxation and dislocation of the hip are common in children with CP, especially in spastic CP and in immobile children with spastic quadriplegia. Normal development of the hip structures is dependent on normal weight bearing and muscle tone, which is often lacking in the child with CP (Noritz et al., 2022). It is important for the primary care provider to do active surveillance of the hips with children who have CP to reduce the rate of hip subluxation and dislocation. This will allow for early detection of hip dysplasia and a referral to an orthopedic for treatment.

Abnormal muscle forces and asymmetric stresses on the spine can cause scoliosis in children with CP. Scoliosis can result from unequal muscle tension resulting from CP or from poor posture or positioning in seating and recumbent positions. Scoliosis is much more likely to occur in children with less ambulation capacity (Noritz et al., 2022). Stopping the progression of the curve and improving posture and seating are often achieved with spinal surgery, primarily spinal fusion. The decision to proceed with this type of intervention is individualized and depends heavily on the patient's factors and family goals. Spinal fusion is preferred after the completion of thoracic growth, which is typically around 10 years of age. Prior to that, growing rods can be placed and adjusted as the child grows.

Feeding and Eating Problems

Feeding and eating difficulties are common in children with CP primarily because of orofacial muscle impairments. Feeding difficulties among children with CP also play a role in the pathogenesis of malnutrition and add to the increased risk of growth failure (Sadowska et al., 2020). The consequence of malnutrition includes decreased cerebral function, impaired immune function, and diminished respiratory muscle strength, which can be life altering for any patient, especially a child with CP. Compromised cardiopulmonary functioning, as well as poor muscle tone (i.e., either hypertonic or hypotonic) in the neck, shoulders, and trunk, can impede the process of eating. Specifically, muscle tone and function deficits create problems with sucking, chewing, swallowing, and aspiration. Increased drooling and gastroesophageal reflux may also occur. Feeding and eating disabilities are most often seen in children with the athetoid type of CP. Early and severe feeding problems are a predictor for later growth, nutritional, and developmental outcomes.

Bowel Problems

Constipation is a common and often chronic condition in children with CP occurring in up to 75% (Noritz et al., 2022).

Low muscle tone or spastic abdominal muscles can prevent contractility and pressure to adequately advance and empty the bowel contents. Further reasons for constipation include limited mobility or ambulation; lack of exercise; inability to sense the signals of a bowel movement; painful defecations; inadequate fluid intake; a diet lacking in fruits, vegetables, and fiber; medications; a fear of toileting; poor positioning on the toilet; and behavior problems. Bowel incontinence, or encopresis, can also occur in CP. Good dietary and bowel management and education for patients and caregivers are imperative.

Urinary Problems

Problems with bladder control and urinary retention that occur in CP are often the result of neurologic insults with urinary incontinence affecting 25% to 40% of children with CP (Noritz et al., 2022). Intellectual and developmental disabilities may reduce a child's ability to sense bladder fullness and signals to urinate. A combination of incomplete bladder emptying, infrequent voiding, severe fluid restriction, and urinary reflux increases the likelihood of frequent UTIs, chronic constipation, improper perineal hygiene, and motor impairments. Prompt treatment of UTIs is imperative by the primary care provider or specialist.

Dental Problems

Children with CP are at an increased risk for oral health concerns such as dental caries, periodontal disease, tooth wear, and poor oral health related to their quality of life (Lansdown et al., 2021). Malocclusions commonly occur in children with CP because of orofacial muscle tone deficiencies. An overbite or underbite can affect chewing and speech. Tooth enamel defects also occur frequently and, if untreated, may lead to dental caries. Children who have seizures and take phenytoin (Dilantin) often experience hyperplasia (i.e., excessive growth of the gums). The primary care provider must be equipped to appropriately support and refer patients with CP. Through the promotion of good oral health and interdisciplinary collaboration, preventative strategies are essential to improving the health care outcomes for children and youth with CP (Fig. 15.2).

Pulmonary Effects

The pulmonary assessment in children with CP is often challenging due to alterations in positioning caused by abnormal muscle tone and spasticity, immobility, scoliosis, and contractures (Noritz et al., 2022). All of these can affect pulmonary function and place children with CP at a higher risk for respiratory infections (e.g., pneumonia). A baseline chest radiography for comparison is helpful when assessing acute illness. Respiratory infections often linger beyond the usual period because many children have difficulty coughing and blowing their nose. Aspiration and gastroesophageal reflux can also cause pneumonia. Health care providers and

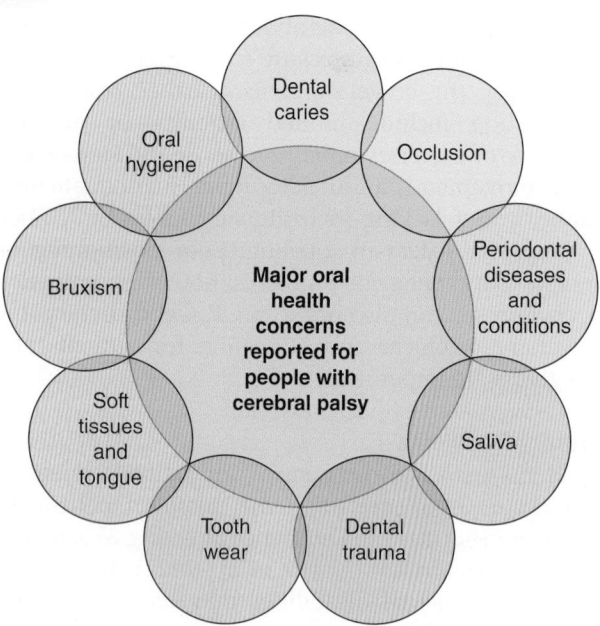

Fig. 15.2 Major oral health concerns reported for people with cerebral palsy.

families/caregivers need to be aware of the warning signs of respiratory infection and pneumonia because pneumonia is a leading cause of death in children with CP. Children with severe dysphagia who show abnormal respiratory rates and fatigue during feeding are likely hypoxemic, and having the ability to perform pulse oximetry can help augment the assessment and presentation when doing in-person and telehealth visits.

Skin Problems
Skin breakdown leading to raw and excoriated skin and decubitus ulcers is a common problem in children and adolescents with CP—especially when mobility is compromised. Thorough skin assessment and protection of bony prominences while a child is seated or recumbent are necessary. Prompt and aggressive treatment of any evidence of skin breakdown is necessary. During infancy, when children are in diapers, and later in adolescence, when females are menstruating, are times when vigilance is needed. Prevention strategies include frequent repositioning (every 2–3 hours), padding, wheelchair cushions, and special mattresses to protect the bony and dependent areas of the body.

Latex Allergy
Health care professionals who care for children with CP should be aware of the association between CP and latex allergy due to repeated exposures. Primary care providers should be mindful of the risk of anaphylaxis if a child has had repeated surgeries and ventriculoperitoneal shunts (Noritz et al., 2022).

Behavioral and Mental Health
Behavioral and mental health disorders are prevalent among children with CP and often affect their participation in social and community activities as well as their quality of life. Factors that contribute to this increased prevalence include the underlying brain disturbance, pain, physical difficulties, and the additional stress brought on by their chronic condition. The most common among this population include inattention, hyperactivity and impulsivity, disruptive behavior, anxiety, and depression (Noritz et al., 2022). In children with CP, the prevalence of autism spectrum disorder is 6% to 9% higher than in the general population. As a result of the exaggerated and prolonged existence of primitive reflexes, especially the startle reflex, infants and children with CP overreact to the mildest amounts of stimulation, causing frustration and fatigue.

PROGNOSIS

The prognosis, similar to treatment, depends on the type and severity of CP. In general, if the prognostic question refers to life expectancy, the current data show the most important factors associated with life expectancy depend on the degree of independent mobility and whether the child can self-feed (Noritz et al., 2022). Caution is necessary when discussing the prognosis with parents and should be done by health care providers who are well educated and versed in CP. There are a variety of disease trajectories for children with CP, and engagement with a palliative medicine specialist is recommended as part of this discussion.

PRIMARY CARE MANAGEMENT

Management of CP is best done by the primary care provider and medical home, along with a multidisciplinary team, due to the multiple associated conditions and complexities of support needed.

HEALTH MAINTENANCE
Growth and Development
Obtaining accurate measurements for height and weight can be challenging if a child experiences motor difficulty and has contractures. When height cannot be measured in either a standing or recumbent position, the upper arm length and lower leg length measurements are adequate. Accurate measuring also monitors spasticity, tone, contracture, and scoliosis changes. Triceps and subscapular skinfold thicknesses should also be obtained. Weight charts for males and females with CP, ages 2 to 20 years, are found at https://www.lifeexpectancy.org/articles/NewGrowthCharts.shtml (Brooks et al., 2011). Weight may be recorded from a standing position on a standardized scale or while the child is sitting or supine on a chair or hammock scale. Primary care providers may easily obtain an accurate weight by having a parent hold the child, step on the scale, and then subtract the parent's weight.

Management of CP is best done by a multidisciplinary team because of the multiple associated conditions and complexities of support needed. The team is needed to longitudinally observe the development of a child with CP. Periodic assessments of the child's mental, motor, language, self-care, and emotional development are warranted. Many general and specific screening instruments can be used by primary care providers and should be an important part of a child's care. Assessment of a child's cognitive status is important because of the presence of intellectual disabilities in many children with CP, as well as physical limitations and speech-language problems that may make determining a child's true cognitive abilities difficult. Standardized intelligence tests for infants and children are appropriate, but someone experienced in examining children with motor and language delays should conduct this assessment.

Motor assessment is most often completed by the physical or occupational therapist. Videotaping a child's movements, in combination with computer gait analysis, has greatly enhanced the abilities of the physical therapist and physiatrist to plan and treat motor deficits and complications.

However, primary care providers must accurately assess parental reports of language skills because parents often overestimate the number of spoken words by counting grunts and partial words. A speech therapist is the best person to assess language skills. Because of the many feeding and eating problems in infancy, a language assessment should be done in conjunction with a nutritional assessment when solid foods are introduced at about 6 months of age.

Self-care skills should be assessed throughout childhood and adolescence during history-taking at each primary health care visit. This assessment can be done through an interview, a questionnaire, or a standardized test (e.g., Functional Independence Measure for Children [WeeFIM] or Pediatric Evaluation of Disability Inventory). Emotional development is another important area for periodic assessment. Although there are a number of available instruments that measure self-concept and self-esteem, a good discussion with a trusted health professional is usually adequate for obtaining an understanding of how a child is coping at home, at school, and in other environments.

Nutrition

Undernutrition is most often seen during infancy in children with CP. Medical reasons must be ruled out before others can be addressed. Exercises to improve facial muscle tone can be initiated. External assistance or support can be applied if a child has trouble controlling the jaw or keeping the mouth closed. Children may also have oral tactile defensiveness and require a program of desensitization to different textures and a food plan developed around the foods they will eat. Other children do not feel the food or drink in their mouths, so most of the food or liquid falls out of the mouth, creating skin problems. These children may also drool excessively and are at risk for aspiration. General overall health status and better nutritional intake improve over time because of an increase in oromotor, gross motor, and fine motor skills.

As a result of hypersensitivity, parents may need to try different nipples until one is found that the infant prefers. The size of the nipple hole may also need to be increased if the thickened formula is prescribed with caution to observe, making sure flow is not too fast. Motor problems may inhibit a child from being an independent feeder. Adaptive equipment can be designed for a growing child at each developmental stage. A referral to a dietician and an occupational therapist can help support by suggesting ways to help a child with oromotor difficulties and supplement the diet to ensure that a child receives adequate calories. Determining optimal caloric intake depends on several factors, including mobility, type of CP, and the child's nutritional status (Noritz et al., 2022).

The diet and method of feeding are individually determined by a variety of factors: the shared decision making between the medical team, the patient, and the parent or guardian, with oral feeding being the goal for most patients and their families. Novak et al. (2020) in their systemic review of therapies for CP have recommended combined electrical stimulation with oral sensorimotor treatments as an emerging therapy. Depending on the clinical situation, some children with CP may need nonoral feeding with or without oral (i.e., oral feedings during the day with supplemental nonoral feedings during the night).

Children with CP (approximately 1 in 15) may benefit from a feeding tube to help improve nutritional status, weight gain, decrease the length of feedings, along with improving the experience of feeding for the child and family. Temporary nonoral feedings include nasogastric tube feeds or a gastrostomy tube (G-tube) or gastrojejunostomy tube (GJ-tube) for long-term feedings. G-tubes are placed percutaneously, endoscopically, or surgically; GJ-tubes are typically placed using fluoroscopy through an existing gastrostomy. Typically a decision is made to place a GJ-tube when there is ongoing severe vomiting, aspiration, or symptomatic gastroesophageal reflux disease.

Safety

Children with motor impairments and seizure disorders are at increased risk for injury. Special concern should be taken when physical activities, car seats, and environmental surroundings are chosen for children with CP. Children with CP may not be restricted in the type of physical activity (e.g., canoeing), but adult supervision is needed. Seizure precautions and helmets may be necessary for children with seizure disorders. Car seats should be appropriately padded and positioned to protect a child's head—especially if head control is an issue. These precautions apply to any seating arrangement. A child's environment should be free of sharp edges in case of unexpected falls and roomy enough for the child to maneuver. If the child is in a wheelchair, the home environment should be wheelchair accessible. Some engineers are specially trained to suggest adaptations to homes, day care settings, or schools to make them more wheelchair accessible. Home emergency plans should account for a child in a wheelchair, and local police and fire departments should be alerted.

Screenings

Vision. A pediatric ophthalmologist should assess the eyes of children with CP annually because of the many types of visual impairments that may occur (Jones et al., 2007; Noritz et al., 2022). Vision can also be screened each time the child comes for a primary care visit, and a referral made to an ophthalmologist by the preschool years. When performing a visual acuity test, children with motor problems may have difficulty showing which way an E points, and those with speech problems may have difficulty naming the letters.

Glasses often are prescribed for refractive errors. Contact lenses are contraindicated in children with CP because their motor impairments inhibit the placement and removal of the lenses. Glasses should be placed correctly on a child's face, and adaptive equipment (e.g., Velcro straps) may be recommended for comfortable and correct placement. Patching and surgery may be recommended for other vision complications associated with CP (e.g., strabismus, amblyopia).

Hearing. A pediatric audiologist should regularly check the hearing of a child with CP. An audiologist will use a tympanometer and evoked response audiometry for specific diagnostic information. The primary care provider should check the tympanic membranes at each visit (Jones et al., 2007; Noritz et al., 2022). Children with sensorineural hearing loss may be fitted with a hearing aid. Proper maintenance and use of hearing aids by children and families will help a child interact optimally with the environment.

Dental. Children with CP need a dentist who has experience with children with movement and motor disorders. The environment of the dentist's office must be accessible, with a chair that allows for easy transfer from a wheelchair if the child uses one. The chair must also protect fragile skin and support spastic extremities. Children with CP should visit the dentist at least every 6 months and more often if recommended (US Department of Health and Human Services [HHS], 2020). Sedation may be necessary for children with severe spasticity.

Malocclusions can be prevented through oromotor exercises to improve muscle tone around the oral cavity. An interdisciplinary team consisting of the nutritionist, occupational therapist, and speech-language pathologist can plan exercises to reduce the oral reflexes that can lead to the development of overbites or underbites. This team can also address drooling problems and help a child swallow saliva and keep the tongue in the mouth. If drooling persists, surgery may be warranted. Adaptive equipment (e.g., an altered toothbrush or a washcloth for washing teeth) may be appropriate (HHS, 2020).

Blood pressure. Routine screening is recommended.

Hemoglobin, hematocrit, and lead. Routine screening is recommended.

Urinalysis. Routine screening is recommended. A referral to a pediatric urologist may be needed if the child has chronic UTIs.

Motor and Movement Problems

A motor assessment should be done at each primary care visit. Body alignment and positioning; passive and active range of motion; and signs of hip dislocation, spinal deformities, contractures, and movement patterns (e.g., gait disturbances) should be assessed and measured when appropriate. Goniometric measurements of the joint mobility and motion of the knee and ankle can assist in screening for abnormalities in tone.

COMMON ILLNESS MANAGEMENT

Differential Diagnoses

Fever. Children experience many febrile episodes in their lives because of the many viruses and bacteria that are present in their environment. Children with CP are prone to respiratory infections and UTIs and may also get gastrointestinal infections. In each of these infections, fever is usually an accompanying symptom. A primary care provider must see children with CP if they are under 6 months of age, have had a fever over 38.6°C for 3 or more days without symptoms, appear acutely ill with undefined symptoms, or have had a seizure with a fever. The primary care provider needs a physical assessment and laboratory work for an accurate diagnosis and treatment.

Respiratory tract infections. Children with CP are susceptible to upper and lower respiratory tract infections (otitis media, sore throats, rhinorrhea, sinusitis, influenza). Asthma is more prevalent in premature infants with CP. Routine management of these problems is warranted with careful monitoring of the resolution of the infection. Sometimes these infections are not resolved with one round of antibiotics, and complications can occur (e.g., additional hearing loss from a case of otitis media). Referral to a specialist may be recommended.

Pain with or without infection is difficult to assess in children with severe CP. For example, the typical sign of pulling on the ear for an ear infection may not be present. Parents are often able to discern subtle signs in their child (e.g., increased irritability, decreased energy, fewer vocalizations, increased drooling) or to think that the child is not acting as usual. Children can also be asked yes-no questions to identify the source of pain. If a child uses a communication system, signs or symbols can be used to describe the pain. Children's pain scales (e.g., Wong FACES Scale) can be used by the primary care provider to further assess a child's pain.

It is important to stress the high probability of pneumonia occurring after an initial upper respiratory infection or bout of influenza in children with severe CP. Pneumonia can also be caused by aspiration and gastroesophageal reflux. Careful monitoring must be done to prevent a life-threatening situation. Children with CP are unable to expectorate well and handle increased secretions. Dehydration can easily occur. Hospitalization may be suggested as a preventive measure to ensure close observation of any changes in a child's health status. If a child is being cared for at home, parents must understand the importance of the treatment plan and contact their clinician if the condition worsens.

Dermatology issues. Skin problems arise from positioning in chairs and beds when bony prominences rub against hard surfaces. Decubitus ulcers can occur quickly, and vigilant skin management is warranted especially in nonmobile children. Protection of the bony prominences with soft protective coverings is usually enough, but medical attention should be obtained for persistent areas of redness. Assess for latex allergy.

Urinary tract problems. Common problems are incontinence, urgency, frequency, and retention. UTIs also occur more frequently in children with CP. The age of the child and any communication problems may impede obtaining detailed information on pain or other symptoms experienced by the child. A urinalysis and urine cultures must be ordered if there is any suspicion of a UTI or if the cause of the fever or other symptoms cannot be identified. After one or two UTIs have been diagnosed and treated in a child with CP, the parents and primary care provider may be better able to identify the signs and symptoms associated with this condition in the child. This information is especially important in a nonverbal child and should be recorded in the child's chart for further reference.

Antibiotic therapy and additional comfort measures (e.g., increased fluid intake, perineal hygiene after voiding, increased rest, and taking acetaminophen based on body weight) are recommended for UTIs. Follow-up is imperative after a UTI and should include a urine culture 2 to 3 days after initiation and at the conclusion of antibiotic therapy to assess its effect. If recurrent UTIs occur, referral to a pediatric urologist is recommended.

Gastrointestinal problems. Parents may note that a child has abdominal pain, straining with hard stools, rectal bleeding, soiled underwear, and a distended, hard abdomen when constipated. Documenting the signs and symptoms of this problem in infants or nonverbal children is especially important. Increased fluids, exercise, and a healthy diet with additional fiber are recommended. A bowel management program designed by an interdisciplinary team may be needed if constipation is an ongoing problem. A program of stool softeners, laxatives, suppositories, and enemas can be prescribed, as well as suggestions for proper positioning and seating on the toilet. The effectiveness of the program should be closely monitored and recorded.

A pattern for bowel elimination should be initiated and maintained. UTIs and impactions are complications of chronic constipation. Constipation is a very difficult long-term problem to deal with when a child is immobile and has a poor appetite. Bowel management programs must be individualized and evaluated periodically.

Drug Interactions

Medications may be prescribed to reduce spasticity. These medications should be used with caution if an adolescent with CP is pregnant. Diazepam (Valium) and baclofen should be monitored closely if used in a child with a seizure disorder because seizure control could be altered. Dantrolene (Dantrium) and baclofen are also affected by the concurrent use of alcohol, so drinking should be strongly discouraged in adolescents. Dantrolene should also be discouraged if a degree of spasticity is needed for daily functioning. Adverse respiratory symptoms and bowel function should also be monitored when using dantrolene. No other specific drug interactions have been noted with medications used to treat spasticity. The occurrence of constipation must be examined for its cause—whether because of diet or as a side effect of medications such as anticonvulsants or iron. Drug interactions must be assessed when a child with CP receives multiple medications.

DEVELOPMENTAL CONSIDERATIONS
Sleep Patterns
A clinical manifestation of CP in infancy is prolonged sleeping patterns interfering with nutritional intake and developmental stimulation. A variety of sleep problems (affecting 20%–40%) may exist with CP, such as insomnia, severe hypoxemia during sleep (which may require a sleep apnea monitor), difficulty in

falling asleep and staying asleep, and difficulties during the sleep-to-wake transition (Noritz et al., 2022). Sleep problems are important for the primary care provider to recognize and address because they may affect daytime functioning. Pain is significantly associated with sleep problems. During sleep, a neutral body position (i.e., with the neck and head slightly flexed) is encouraged. Bolsters or wedges can be used to facilitate appropriate positions and improve sleep quality. A side-lying position should be used for children who drool so that excessive fluid can drain out of the mouth instead of down the throat, which may cause choking. Behavioral strategies, such as bedtime fading and bedtime passes, can be implemented if sleep problems persist (Table 15.3).

Toileting

If children with CP are able to be toilet trained, then—like any other children—they will give their parents clues of their physical and neurologic readiness. The potty chair or toilet must adequately support the child's body and minimize the risk of skin breakdown from extended sitting. The child's feet must be able to touch the floor to assist the abdominal muscles in pushing. Special potty chairs can be made, or current chairs can be adapted with input from a physical or occupational therapist.

Discipline

Parents often discipline children who have special health and developmental needs differently from their siblings. As a result of their special needs and possible past health care emergencies, parents are often reluctant to discipline a child with CP. Parents must be consistent when disciplining all their children; both parents should agree with the type of discipline, and the discipline should be developmentally appropriate for a child's mental age.

Child Care

Many child care programs today include children both with and without chronic conditions. Depending on the child's degree of functional and cognitive severity, parents may choose an early intervention or an inclusive child care program. Children enrolled in an early intervention program will have an individualized family service plan developed for the child's development and family support. In an inclusive child care program, the providers will need instruction from the parents or a member of the child's interdisciplinary health care team on the best approaches for care and development. Parents of a child with CP must be aware that the risk for infection is greater in settings where children are together (e.g., in day care) and that issues of safety and accessibility are also important to consider.

Schooling

Children with CP may need to use different augmentative communication systems (e.g., communication boards, computers, keyboard voice synthesizers). Adaptive equipment for communicating, seating,

Table 15.3 Behavioral Sleep Interventions

BEHAVIORAL SLEEP INTERVENTIONS	DESCRIPTION
Extinction (crying it out)	Parents put the child to bed and ignore until morning (but monitor for concerns for safety or illness).
Graduated extinction (sleep training)	Parents put the child to bed and ignore crying and tantrums for a predetermined period before briefly checking on and reassuring the child. The time between checks is gradually increased. The time between checks should be determined based on the child's temperament and the parents' tolerance for crying.
Fading of parental presence	Parents put the child to bed and gradually fade their proximity to and interactions with the child during sleep-onset every few nights. For example, the parent can transition from lying next to the child to sitting in a chair next to the bed and progressively move the chair further from the bed every few nights until they are no longer in the room.
Scheduled awakenings	After establishing the baseline timing and number of night awakenings, parents wake the child up 15–30 min before the typical awakening and follow their typical response to spontaneous awakenings. The scheduled awakenings are then gradually faded out by increasing the time between them.
Positive routines	Parents develop a consistent bedtime routine of calm activities to establish a behavioral chain leading up to sleep onset and promote appropriate sleep associations. Use of a transitional object, such as a blanket or stuffed animal, can help promote appropriate sleep associations.
Bedtime pass	Parents provide the child with 1–2 tokens (the bedtime pass) that can be turned in for one request or contact with a parent after bedtime. If the child does not use the bedtime pass, then it can be turned in for a positive reinforcer in the morning.
Bedtime fading	The designated bedtime is temporarily delayed until it coincides with the child's usual onset of sleep. The bedtime is then gradually moved earlier. If the child fails to fall asleep as expected, the child is taken out of bed briefly before being put to bed again.

From Noritz, G. H., Davidson, L., Steingass, K., et al. (2022). Providing a primary care medical home for children's and youth with cerebral palsy. *Pediatrics, 150*(6), e2022060055.

writing, and reading may be needed and should be obtained. Occupational, physical, and speech therapy, as well as adaptive physical education, is often needed and individually planned for either group or individual sessions. An aide may be required to help a child with CP with personal needs. Transportation to and from school, transfer needs between classrooms, and emergency health and safety plans must also be arranged with school personnel.

The primary care provider plays an important role in assisting the parents and families of children with CP with the various therapies and school services available to them. The primary care provider can assess the school situation, including safety, performance, ambulation, and fatigue issues, during well- and sick-child visits.

Along with an interdisciplinary health plan, which is mandatory for children with CP, an accommodation plan or individualized education plan (IEP) is also necessary, which may include physical, occupational, speech, and behavioral therapy and other formal and informal support services. Today most children with CP participate in inclusive education. Special attention must be paid to a child's cognitive ability and social integration into the regular classroom by assisting the child with peer relationships and self-esteem.

During the middle and high school years, children with CP can be enrolled in vocational or college preparation programs, depending on career interests and the presence and degree of mental challenges. Adolescents with CP may also experience renewed social problems during these years as they cope with adolescent self-esteem issues and contemplate life after school. Work and social opportunities are not as prevalent in the adult years as they are during childhood for individuals with special health and developmental needs. Adolescents often experience depression when faced with the stigma of their condition and rejection in social situations. School performance also may decrease. Parents and professionals should look for signs that might alert them to these psychosocial issues during adolescence and offer support and professional counseling where needed.

Sexuality

Social isolation, long-term low self-esteem, and a poor body image can affect the development of intimate relationships. Sexuality education can help adolescents develop positive self-esteem and body image. Role modeling and exposure to social situations can be planned and executed. During their adolescent years, children do not often discuss sexuality and their feelings with their parents. Therefore peers, other adults, and support groups should be available to help adolescents with CP with these issues. In some cases, a referral to a sexuality counselor may be needed.

Female adolescents should begin to receive gynecologic care if they are sexually active. Because of spasticity, contractures, or poor muscle control, a female's position for such an examination should be adapted; the Sims position is often better than the lithotomy position. The female may also require assistance in positioning menstrual pads or tampons. Pregnancy is possible for females with CP.

Transition to Adulthood

The transition to adulthood in children with CP must address medical care, equipment needs, communication, activities of daily life, mobility, nutrition, vocational decisions, transportation, housing, and social needs. Proper preparation and handoff need to occur when the late adolescent or early adult with CP is leaving the care of the pediatric primary care provider and moving to adult care. It is important for the pediatric primary care provider to help the family find an adult provider who is familiar with CP and understands the medical changes that are common in the adult with CP and the challenges this person faces with transitioning of care (Noritz et al., 2022). Throughout life, optimal independence should be encouraged and learned helplessness avoided. Independence and self-advocacy should be stressed during the transitional period between adolescence and adulthood. Adolescents with CP need to actively choose a primary care provider and health care interdisciplinary team. Their participation in decision making about dietary choices, medications, surgical interventions if needed, and adaptive equipment is important.

Vocational decisions should be discussed and plans for successful employment determined. When deciding on a site for college or work, the physical layout, wheelchair accessibility, availability of personal aides, housing, and repair shop for wheelchairs and any other adaptive equipment must be considered, and resources identified. Independence in the use of public transportation should be planned. Individuals with mild CP may be able to drive. Independent living or assisted living arrangements must be discussed, and individuals should be placed on waiting lists early if living outside the home is desired because these lists are often years long. Social needs, including activities consistent with an individual's abilities, planned social programs, and opportunities to develop successful relationships, should be met. Guidance is available from the AAP (White & Cooley, 2018) (Fig. 15.3).

Family Considerations

It is important for the primary care provider to regularly assess the family's functioning to help guide the interventions and support services. The assessment should include evaluations of family stress, social abilities, as well as restrictions, resources, and adjustment of parents, caregivers, and siblings. By listening

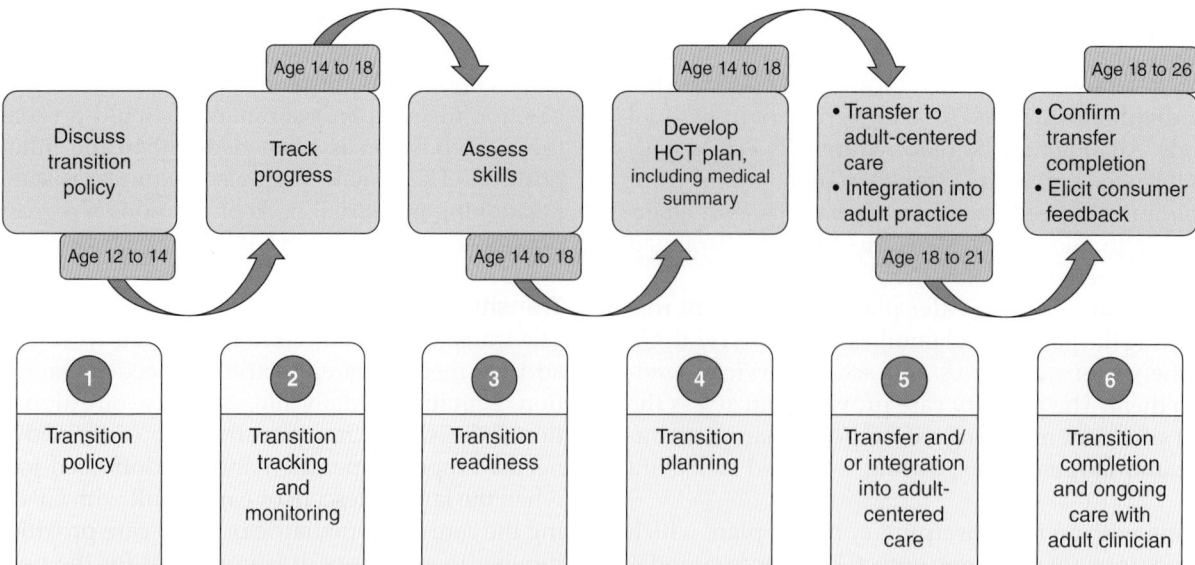

Fig. 15.3 **Six core elements of transition.** *HCT*, Health care transition. (From White, P.H., Cooley, W.C., Transitions Clinical Report Authoring Group, American Academy of Pediatrics, American Academy of Family Physicians, & American College of Physicians. [2018]. Supporting the health care transition from adolescence to adulthood in the medical home. *Pediatrics, 142*[5], e20182587.)

carefully, the primary care provider can better address the family's concerns and the child's needs. The health of the parents or caregivers is vital; if their health is compromised, outcomes for the children with and without CP will also suffer (Noritz et al., 2022). Respite care is highly recommended to give families time away from the constant responsibilities of caring for a child with CP. Social support, identification of and intervention with stressors, parenting skills for caring for a child with special needs, and early intervention programs are all very important for family well-being (Noritz et al., 2022; Pellegrino, 2007).

There are no specific cross-cultural or religious concerns for children with CP, although a stigma based on the diagnosis is attached to all families. The visibility of this condition may create more of a stigma in some cultures than in others, and in some cultures the child may be hidden from the outside world.

RESOURCES

PROVIDER RESOURCES

Gross Motor Function Classification System (well-established resources for providers): https://canchild.ca/en/resources/42-gross-motor-function-classification-system-expanded-revised-gmfcs-e-r

Gross Motor Function Measure (well-established resources for providers): https://canchild.ca/en/resources/44-gross-motor-function-measure-gmfm

ORGANIZATIONS

American Academy for Cerebral Palsy and Developmental Medicine: www.aacpdm.org

Cerebral Palsy Alliance: https://cerebralpalsy.org

Cerebral Palsy Foundation: https://www.yourcpf.org/people-and-partners

CP Channel (videos for parents about CP): https://www.yourcpf.org/cpproduct/cp-channel

CP Family Network: https://cpfamilynetwork.org/

CP Research Network: https://cprn.org

CP Toolkit for Families: https://cpnowfoundation.org/wp/wp-content/uploads/2015/11/CP-Tool-Kit.pdf

Disability Information and Resources (provides information on products, services, computer accessibility, home automation, environmental control, governmental and legislative disability information, legal advice and advocacy, sports, travel, recreation, and assistive technology): www.makoa.org

F-Words in Childhood Disability: https://www.canchild.ca/en/research-in-practice/f-words-inchildhood-disability/f-words-tools

Family Voices and Family-to-Family Health Information Centers: www.familyvoices.org

Healthy Bodies (puberty resources for children with disabilities; in English, Spanish, and Turkish): https://vkc.vumc.org/healthybodies

National Disability Sports Alliance: https://cpfamilynetwork.org/resources/resources-guide/national-disability-sports-alliance-ndsa

United Cerebral Palsy: http://www.ucp.org

US Department of Health and Human Services. Cerebral palsy: https://www.ninds.nih.gov/health-information/disorders/cerebral-palsy?search-term=cerebral+palsy

Summary

Primary Care Needs for the Child With Cerebral Palsy

HEALTH CARE MAINTENANCE
Growth and Development
- Different techniques should be used to obtain height, arm and leg lengths, and skinfold measurements.
- Weights may be attained via standing or sitting scales or recumbent lifts.
- Delayed development in motor and communication skills is common.
- Development strengths and weaknesses must be assessed and recorded.
- Intellectual and developmental disabilities and seizure disorders inhibit intellectual development.
- An exercise program may be individually developed.

Diet
- Undernutrition in infancy often leads to growth delay or impediment.
- Different nipples may be tried if hypersensitivity is an issue.
- Infants can have difficulty with sucking, swallowing, and chewing.
- Overweight conditions may occur in adolescence if mobility decreases.
- Drooling and aspiration can also be problems; caution needs to be taken with feedings and fluids.
- Assessment should be done early and repeatedly; referral to a nutritionist is commonly needed.
- Adaptive equipment is useful.
- Nutritional concerns may be lifelong, and placement of a gastrostomy tube may be warranted in severe cases.

Safety
- Children are at risk for injury because of spasticity, muscle control problems, delayed protective reflexes, and potential seizures.
- Positioning, modified car seats, and other adaptive equipment are often required.

Immunizations
- If the etiology for seizure activity is unknown, the pertussis vaccine may be deferred or an acellular vaccine used when age appropriate.
- The measles and varicella vaccines should be given as scheduled.
- Children with CP are at risk for complications of varicella and should be immunized.
- *Haemophilus influenzae* type B (Hib) vaccine and other immunizations should be given as scheduled.
- Children with CP are at risk for complications of influenza and should be immunized.
- Pneumococcal, meningococcal, rotavirus, hepatitis B, human papillomavirus vaccines should be given as recommended.
- Fever management is necessary to decrease the possibility of febrile seizures.

Screening
- *Vision*. A pediatric ophthalmologist should be seen during infancy because of the likelihood of vision problems. Vision should be checked for acuity, refractive errors, strabismus, retinopathy of prematurity, and cataracts.
- *Hearing*. Referral to a pediatric audiologist may be necessary during infancy to check for hearing problems and loss. Both sensorineural and conductive hearing loss is possible. Routine screening for conductive hearing problems and loss should be done.
- *Dental*. Children should be evaluated by a dentist experienced with children with motor problems every 6 months. Proper dental hygiene is needed. Administration of phenytoin may cause hyperplasia of the gums; proper preventive care and early treatment of this condition are important. Malocclusions can be prevented through oromotor exercises.
- *Blood pressure*. Routine screening is recommended.
- *Hematocrit*. Routine screening is recommended.
- *Urinalysis*. Routine screening is recommended. A referral to a pediatric urologist may be needed if the child has chronic UTIs.
- *Tuberculosis*. Routine screening is recommended.

Condition-Specific Screening
- A motor assessment, including assessment for scoliosis, hip dislocation, and contractures, should be done at every well-child visit.

COMMON ILLNESS MANAGEMENT
Differential Diagnosis
- *Fever*. Management of fever is routine except when the child is less than 6 months of age, has had a fever over 38.6°C for 3 or more days without symptoms, appears acutely ill with undefined symptoms, or has had a seizure with a fever, in which case the child needs to see the primary care provider for an accurate diagnosis and treatment.
- *Respiratory tract infections*. Respiratory infections should be promptly treated. Pneumonia may be life threatening to children with severe CP. Follow-up is important.
- *Dermatology issues*. Vigilant skin management is warranted because of high risk for decubiti, especially those children using wheelchairs. Assess for latex allergies.
- *Urinary tract problems*. Treatment for UTIs should be prompt, and follow-up is essential. Urinary tract abnormalities may also be present.
- *Gastrointestinal problems*. Constipation is a long-term problem for many children. A bowel management program may be needed.

Drug Interactions
- Diazepam (Valium) and baclofen may alter seizure control.
- Dantrolene (Dantrium) and baclofen are affected by the concurrent use of alcohol, so drinking should be strongly discouraged in the adolescent.
- Adverse respiratory symptoms and bowel function should also be monitored when using dantrolene.

DEVELOPMENTAL ISSUES
Sleep Patterns
- Correct positioning is needed during sleep because sleep apnea can occur.

Toileting
- Adaptive equipment is often needed for correct positioning on the toilet. Bladder and bowel training may be delayed.

Discipline
- It is important that consistent and age-appropriate discipline measures be taken.

Continued

Child Care
- Careful planning must be undertaken in choosing the best child care arrangements, especially regarding issues of safety, accessibility, health care needs, and increased rates of infection.

Schooling
- Use IEPs and inclusive classrooms. Specialized services and therapies for each child must be procured. Adaptive equipment and computers enhance a child's ability to learn. Behavioral and school problems can occur in adolescence because of poor self-esteem and body image.

Sexuality
- Opportunities for social activities should be arranged. Transportation needs are important to consider. Opportunities for same-sex and opposite-sex relationships are needed. Classes in social interaction and sexuality may be needed. Gynecologic examinations should begin for females with adaptations to the normal positioning. Reproductive issues should be discussed.

Transition to Adulthood
- A child's independence and self-advocacy should be promoted. Future residential and vocational plans need to be addressed.

FAMILY CONCERNS
- Respite care meets a family's needs.
- Effects on individual family members must be assessed and addressed. Special support groups are available for fathers and siblings.
- Family stigmas may be perceived.

REFERENCES

Alberman, E., & Goldstein, H. (1970). The "at risk" register: A statistical evaluation. *British Journal of Preventive & Social Medicine, 24*, 129–135.

Başaran, A., Kilinç, Z., Sari, H., & Gündüz, E. (2023). Etiological risk factors in children with cerebral palsy. *Medicine, 102*(15). https://doi.org/10.1097/md.0000000000033479.

Bosanquet, M., Copeland, L., Ware, R., & Boyd, R. (2013). A systematic review of tests to predict cerebral palsy in young children. *Developmental Medicine and Child Neurology, 55*, 418–426.

Brandenburg, J. E., Fogarty, M. J., & Sieck, G. C. (2019). A critical evaluation of current concepts in cerebral palsy. *Physiology, 34*(3), 216–229. https://doi.org/10.1152/physiol.00054.2018.

Brooks, J., Day, S. M., Shavelle, R. M., & Strauss, D. J. (2011). Low weight, morbidity, and mortality in children with cerebral palsy: New clinical growth charts. *Pediatrics, 128*, e299; originally published online July 18, 2011 (doi:10.1542/peds.2010-2801).

Capute, A. J. (1979). Identifying cerebral palsy in infancy through study of primitive-reflex profiles. *Pediatric Annals, 8*, 589–595.

Centers for Disease Control and Prevention. Data and statistics for cerebral palsy. (2022a). https://www.cdc.gov/ncbddd/cp/data.html.

Centers for Disease Control and Prevention. What is cerebral palsy? (2022b). Retrieved February 28, 2023, from https://www.cdc.gov/ncbddd/cp/facts.html.

Cerebral Palsy Research Network. Cerebral palsy alternative therapies. (2022). Retrieved March 13, 2023, from https://cprn.org/cerebral-palsy-alternative-therapies/.

Chaleat-Valayer, E., Bernard, J.C., Morel, E., Loustalet, E., Schneider, M., & Bagnol, M. (2006). Use of videographic examination for analysis of efficacy of botulinum toxin in the lower limbs in children with cerebral palsy. *Journal of Pediatric Orthopaedics B, 15*(5), 339–347. doi: 10.1097/01202412-200609000-00007.

Chin, E. M., Gwynn, H. E., Robinson, S., & Hoon, A. H. (2020). Principles of medical and surgical treatment of cerebral palsy. *Neurology Clinics, 38*(2), 397–416. https://doi.org/10.1016/j.ncl.2020.01.009.

Durkin, M. S, Benedict, R. E., Christensen, D., Dubois, L. A., Fitzgerald, R. T., Kirby, R. S., Maenner, M. J., Van Naarden Braun, K., Wingate, M. S., & Yeargin-Allsopp, M. (2016). Prevalence of Cerebral Palsy among 8-Year-Old Children in 2010 and Preliminary Evidence of Trends in Its Relationship to Low Birthweight. *Paediatr Perinat Epidemiol, 30*(5), 496–510. doi: 10.1111/ppe.12299.

Eriksson, E., Hägglund, G., & Alriksson-Schmidt, A. I. (2020). Pain in children and adolescents with cerebral palsy—a cross-sectional register study of 3545 individuals. *BMC Neurology, 20*(1). https://doi.org/10.1186/s12883-019-1597-7.

Hidecker, M. J., Paneth, N., Rosenbaum, P. L., Kent, R. D., Lillie, J., Eulenberg, J. B., Chester, K. Jr, Johnson, B., Michalsen, L., Evatt, M., & Taylor, K. (2011). Developing and validating the Communication Function Classification System for individuals with cerebral palsy. *Developmental Medicine & Child Neurology, 53*(8), 704–710. doi: 10.1111/j.1469-8749.2011.03996.x. Epub 2011 Jun 27. PMID: 21707596; PMCID: PMC3130799.

Imerci, A., Rogers, K. J., Pargas, C., Sees, J. P., & Miller, F. (2019). Identification of complications in paediatric cerebral palsy treated with intrathecal baclofen pump: A descriptive analysis of 15 years at one institution. *Journal of Child Orthopedics, 13*(5), 529–535. https://doi.org/10.1302/1863-2548.13.190112.

Jones, M. W., Morgan, E., & Shelton, J. E. (2007). Primary care of the child with cerebral palsy: A review of systems (part II). *Journal of Pediatric Health Care, 21*, 226–237.

Katz, N., Cermak, S., & Shamir, Y. (1998). Unilateral neglect in children with hemiplegic cerebral palsy. *Perceptual and Motor Skills, 86*, 539–550.

Krigger, K. W. (2006). Cerebral palsy: An overview. *American Family Physician, 73*, 91–100.

Lansdown, K., Irving, M., Mathieu Coulton, K., & Smithers-Sheedy, H. (2021). A scoping review of oral health outcomes for people with cerebral palsy. *Special Care Dental, 42*(3), 232–243. https://doi.org/10.1111/scd.12671.

Maitre, N. L., Burton, V. J., Duncan, A. F., Iyer, S., Ostrander, B., Winter, S., Ayala, L., Burkhardt, S., Gerner, G., Getachew, R., Jiang, K., Lesher, L., Perez, C. M., Moore-Clingenpeel, M., Lam, R., Lewandowski, D. J., & Byrne, R. (2020). Network implementation of guideline for early detection decreases age at cerebral palsy diagnosis. *Pediatrics, 145*(5), e20192126. doi: 10.1542/peds.2019-2126.

Molnar, G. E. (1979). Cerebral palsy: Prognosis and how to judge it. *Pediatric Annals, 8*, 596–605.

Moreno-De-Luca, A. (2023). It's time to offer genetic testing to all individuals diagnosed with cerebral palsy. *Parkinsonism and Related Disorders*, 105449. https://doi.org/10.1016/j.parkreldis.2023.105449.

Noritz, G. H., Davidson, L., & Steingass, K. (2022). Providing a primary care medical home for children's and youth with cerebral palsy. *Pediatrics, 150*(6), e2022060055. https://doi.org/10.1542/peds.2022-060055.

Novak, I., Morgan, C., Adde, L., Blackman, J., Boyd, R. N., Brunstrom-Hernandez, J., Cioni, G., Damiano, D., Darrah, J., Eliasson, A.C., de Vries, L. S., Einspieler, C., Fahey, M., Fehlings, D., Ferriero, D. M., Fetters, L., Fiori, S., Forssberg, H., Gordon, A. M., ... Badawi, N. (2017). Early, accurate diagnosis and early intervention in cerebral palsy: Advances in diagnosis and treatment. *JAMA Pediatrics, 171*(9), 897–907. doi: 10.1001/

jamapediatrics.2017.1689. Erratum in: JAMA Pediatr. 2017 Sep 1;171(9):919. PMID: 28715518; PMCID: PMC9641643.

Novak, I., Morgan, C., Fahey, M., Finch-Edmondson, M., Galea, C., Hines, A., Langdon, K., Namara, M. M., Paton, M. C., Popat, H., Shore, B., Khamis, A., Stanton, E., Finemore, O.P., Tricks, A., Te Velde, A., Dark, L., Morton, N., & Badawi, N. (2020). State of the evidence traffic lights 2019: Systematic review of interventions for preventing and treating children with cerebral palsy. *Current Neurology and Neuroscience Reports, 20*(2), 3. doi: 10.1007/s11910-020-1022-z.

Palisano, R., Rosenbaum, P., Walter, S., Russell, D., Wood, E., & Galuppi, B. (1997). Gross motor function classification system. *PsycTESTS Dataset.* https://doi.org/10.1037/t14000-000.

Patel, D. R., Neelakantan, M., Pandher, K., & Merrick, J. (2020). Cerebral palsy in children: A clinical overview. *Translations in Pediatrics, 9*(S1). https://doi.org/10.21037/tp.2020.01.01.

Paulson, A., & Vargus-Adams, J. (2017). Overview of four functional classification systems commonly used in cerebral palsy. *Children, 4*(4), 30. https://doi.org/10.3390/children4040030.

Pearson, T. S., Pons, R., Ghaoui, R., & Sue, C. M. (2019). Genetic mimics of cerebral palsy. *Movement Disorders, 34*(5), 625–636. https://doi.org/10.1002/mds.27655.

Pellegrino, L. (2007). Cerebral palsy. In Batshaw, M. L., Pellegrino, L., & Roizen, N. J. (Eds.), *Children with disabilities* (6th ed.). Baltimore: Brookes Publishing.

Reilly, M., Liuzzo, K., & Blackmer, A. B. (2020). Pharmacological management of spasticity in children with cerebral palsy. *Journal of Pediatric Health Care, 34*(5), 495–509. https://doi.org/10.1016/j.pedhc.2020.04.010.

Rosenbaum, P., Paneth, N., Leviton, A., Goldstein, M., Bax, M., Damiano, D., Dan, B., & Jacobsson, B. (2007). A report: the definition and classification of cerebral palsy April 2006. *Developmental Medicine & Child Neurology Suppl, 109*, 8–14. Erratum in: Dev Med Child Neurol. 2007 Jun;49(6):480.

Sadowska, M., Sarecka-Hujar, B., & Kopyta, I. (2020). Cerebral palsy: Current opinions on definition, epidemiology, risk factors, classification and treatment options. *Neuropsychiatric Disease and Treatment, 16*, 1505–1518. https://doi.org/10.2147/ndt.s235165.

Sellier, E., Goldsmith, S., McIntyre, S., Perra, O., Rackauskaite, G., Badawi, N., Fares, A., & Smithers-Sheedy, H; Surveillance of Cerebral Palsy Europe Group And The Australian Cerebral Palsy Register Group. (2021). Cerebral palsy in twins and higher multiple births: a Europe-Australia population-based study. *Developmental Medicine & Child Neurology, 63*(6), 712–720. doi: 10.1111/dmcn.14827.

Sheu, J., Cohen, D., Sousa, T., & Pham, K. L. (2022). Cerebral palsy: Current concepts and practices in musculoskeletal care. *Pediatrics in Review, 43*(10), 572–581. https://doi.org/10.1542/pir.2022-005657.

Song, C. S. (2013). Relationships between physical and cognitive functioning and activities of daily living in children with cerebral palsy. *Journal of Physical Therapy Science, 25*(5), 619–622. https://doi.org/10.1589/jpts.25.619.

Sudip, P., Nahar, A., Bhagawati, M., & Kunwar, A. J. (2022). A review on recent advances of cerebral palsy. *Oxidative Medicine and Cellular Longevity*, 1–20. https://doi.org/10.1155/2022/2622310.

te Velde, A., Morgan, C., Novak, I., Tantsis, E., & Badawi, N. (2019). Early diagnosis and classification of cerebral palsy: An historical perspective and barriers to an early diagnosis. *Journal of Clinical Medicine, 8*(10), 1599. doi: 10.3390/jcm8101599.

US Department of Health and Human Services. (2020). *Developmental disabilities & oral health.* National Institute of Dental and Craniofacial Research. Retrieved March 13, 2023, from. https://www.nidcr.nih.gov/health-info/developmental-disabilities.

van der Veen, S., Evans, N., Huisman, M., Welch Saleeby, P., & Widdershoven, G. (2022). Toward a paradigm shift in healthcare: Using the International Classification of Functioning, Disability and Health (ICF) and the capability approach (CA) jointly in theory and practice. *Disability and Rehabilitation*, 1–8. https://doi.org/10.1080/09638288.2022.2089737.

White, P., & Cooley, W. (2018). Supporting the health care transition from adolescence to adulthood in the medical home. *Pediatric Clinical Practice Guide Policies*, 1305. https://doi.org/10.1542/9781610021494-part05-supporting_the_healt.

16

Cleft Lip and Palate*

Jamie Nicole Tabb, Kelsey Reilly

ETIOLOGY

The embryology of cleft lip with or without cleft palate is distinctly different from cleft palate alone. The cleft lip occurs when the median nasal and premaxillary prominences fail to fuse with the lateral maxillary prominences. The lip and alveolar ridge or primary palate are fully formed between 6 and 7 weeks of gestation. The presence of a cleft lip can hinder the closure of the palate. A cleft palate results from a failure of the palatine shelves to fuse between 6 and 12 weeks of gestation (Mulliken, 2004; Stanier & Moore, 2004) (Box 16.1).

Although the specific cause is usually unknown, clefts can be divided into two categories: nonsyndromic and syndromic. The majority of clefts are nonsyndromic, meaning the cleft is not part of a pattern of malformation affecting other organs and systems. It is estimated that more than 70% of cleft lip and palate cases and cleft palate cases are nonsyndromic, isolated phenotypes with unclear etiology (Wilkins-Haug, 2022). The term *multifactorial* (multiple genetic and environmental influences) is used to describe the etiology of nonsyndromic clefts. Environmental factors that may increase the risk of a cleft are maternal folic acid deficiency and teratogens such as maternal alcohol and tobacco use (Romitti et al., 2007; Vieira, 2008). A positive family history of oral facial clefts increases the incidence of nonsyndromic clefts.

A syndrome is a collection of two or more major anomalies that occur together. There are more than 350 syndromes that include oral facial clefts. A cleft palate alone is far more often associated with a syndrome than a cleft lip or cleft lip and palate (Gorlin et al., 2001).

Syndromic clefts can be grouped into categories based on the underlying etiology or defect. (1) The first category would be single-gene disorders, such as Van der Woude syndrome. This condition is recognizable by the lower lip pits and has an autosomal dominant pattern of inheritance. Van der Woude syndrome is associated with a mutation in the interferon regulatory factor 6 (IRF6) gene. Stickler syndrome is another syndrome arising from a mutation of the COL2A1 gene and is most frequently autosomal dominant. Stickler syndrome can cause characteristic ophthalmologic anomalies such as myopia, hearing loss, spondyloepiphyseal dysplasia, and orofacial anomalies such as a flat midface, depressed nasal bridge, short nose, cleft palate, and micrognathia. (2) Another category is chromosomal syndromes, such as velocardiofacial syndrome, which is a microdeletion of chromosome 22, also known as DiGeorge syndrome or 22q11.2 deletion syndrome (Wilkins-Haug, 2022). This syndrome with velopharyngeal insufficiency or cleft palate is associated with cardiac malformation and developmental delay. (3) Teratogenic syndromes are also caused by any agent that can adversely affect embryonic development. Examples of teratogenic syndromes include fetal alcohol syndrome and fetal hydantoin syndrome. A few different drug classes have been recognized as potentially having a higher relative risk for the development of a cleft. The impact may be related to a genetically predisposed fetus or specific timing during organ development. These medications include but are not limited to antiseizure medications (phenytoin, sodium valproate, topiramate, methotrexate) and antiemetics (ondansetron [Zofran]) often when used in the first trimester. Cigarette smoking, maternal obesity, diabetes, and folate deficiency can also increase the risk for clefting, though they are variable in presentation (Wilkins-Haug, 2022). (4) The fourth category of syndromic clefts is called a sequence, such as a holoprosencephaly (underdevelopment of the premaxilla and nasal septum, brain abnormalities) and Pierre Robin sequence (U-shaped cleft palate, micrognathia [small lower jaw], glossoptosis [posteriorly rotated tongue]). Researchers postulate that in fetal development, micrognathia is the primary problem, and the cleft palate results from the

---

Box 16.1	Etiology of Cleft Lip and Palate

NONSYNDROMIC—MULTIFACTORIAL
- Environmental
- Genetic

SYNDROMIC
- Single-gene disorders
- Chromosomal abnormalities
- Teratogens
- Sequences

---

*A special thank you to our friend and colleague, Dr. David W. Low, for his contributions to this chapter. His medical illustrations and photos effectively highlight the complex evaluation and treatment required for comprehensive cleft lip and palate care. His teachings and dedication to cleft care are unparalleled.

tongue being placed superiorly, obstructing the movement of the maxillary shelves in the midline. Suboptimal mandibular growth has been thought to be caused by a variety of factors. The factors vary from positional malformation in utero, intrinsic causes from chromosomal or teratogenic influences, neurologic or neuromuscular abnormalities inhibiting the tongue from normal movement into the floor of the mouth in utero, or connective tissue disorders (St. Hilaire & Buchbinder, 2000). Both holoprosencephaly and Pierre Robin sequence can have devastating consequences in the newborn period by interfering with the airway and normal swallowing.

KNOWN GENETIC ETIOLOGY

The knowledge of genetic etiology for syndromic clefts that include single-gene mutations and chromosomal abnormalities is more advanced than understanding the genetic causes of nonsyndromic clefts. Genetic influences are thought to play a major role, and recently there has been considerable effort to map and identify genes that constitute risk factors for nonsyndromic clefts (Vieira, 2008). As noted, *IRF6* is an important contributor to cleft lip and palate, but the functional variant leading to the defect has not yet been defined. Inactivation of *MSX1* and genes in the fibroblast growth factor (FGF) family has also been shown to lead to cleft lip and palate (Vieira, 2008). Genes in the FGF/FGF receptor family have been shown to increase the risk for nonsyndromic cleft lip +/− palate through biologic pathways (Wang et al., 2013). A study by Lin-Shiao et al. (2019) demonstrated the role of transcription factor p63 in craniofacial development and mutations that may be involved in nonsyndromic cleft lip and palate cases. As more is understood about the genetic influences on nonsyndromic clefts, the question becomes more complex.

INCIDENCE AND PREVALENCE

Cleft lip and palate rank among the most commonly occurring birth defects (Centers for Disease Control and Prevention [CDC], 2020). According to the CDC, about 1 in every 1600 babies is born with a cleft lip and palate in the United States. That rate is 1 in every 2800 babies with cleft lip alone, and cleft palate alone accounts for about 1 in every 1700 babies in the United States (CDC, 2020). The generally accepted incidence rate of clefts worldwide is 1 in 700 births, although some ethnic differences exist (Murray, 2002). Indigenous Americans have an incidence of 14.3 per 10,000 births, Blacks have the lowest incidence rate at 5.8 per 10,000 births, and Asian/Pacific Islander and Hispanic Americans have higher rates of cleft lip and palate as compared to Whites (MyFace, n.d.) Incidence rates are based on varied reporting mechanisms, and problems occur with mixed studies of live births, stillbirths, and spontaneous abortions. No registry or national database exists documenting cleft birth defects. Clefts may or may not be recorded when they are components of a known syndrome.

Cleft lip and palate account for 50% of facial clefts, and a unilateral cleft lip occurs more often (75%) than a bilateral cleft lip (25%). A left-sided cleft lip occurs more often than a right-sided cleft lip. Cleft lip alone makes up 25% of clefts and occurs more frequently in males with or without cleft palate. Females are affected more often with cleft palate alone (American Cleft Palate-Craniofacial Association [ACPA], 2014; Fetal Medicine Foundation, 2022).

DIAGNOSTIC CRITERIA

A cleft lip is an obvious birth defect noted in the delivery room. It is described as unilateral or bilateral and incomplete or complete depending on whether the cleft extends into the nasal cavity (Fig. 16.1). A microform (forme fruste) cleft lip is characterized by minor notching or the appearance of a well-healed surgical scar or seam; however, microform cleft lip is usually only described by a craniofacial team or plastic and reconstructive surgeon.

The cleft palate may involve the primary palate (lip and alveolus anterior to the incisive foramen) and the secondary palate (hard and soft palates) (Fig. 16.2). A submucous cleft palate (SMCP) is characterized by a notch at the posterior spine of the hard palate and translucence at the midline (bifid uvula). The wide spectrum of variations in cleft lip and cleft palate types has made standardized and inclusive classification difficult (Koul, 2007). As a result, clinicians routinely draw a diagram or use physical descriptors to define tissue deficiencies. One proposed system to classify cleft lip and palate is the acronym L (Right Lip); A (Right Alveolus); H (Right Hard Palate); S (Soft Palate); H (Hard Palate Sn); A (SN Alveolus); L (Sn Lip) Lip, alveolus, hard palate, soft palate, hard palate, alveolus, lip; (LAHSHAL); the letters demonstrate clefting of the lip, alveolus, hard palate, and soft palate (Houkes, et al., 2023). Capital letters indicate a complete cleft and small letters indicate

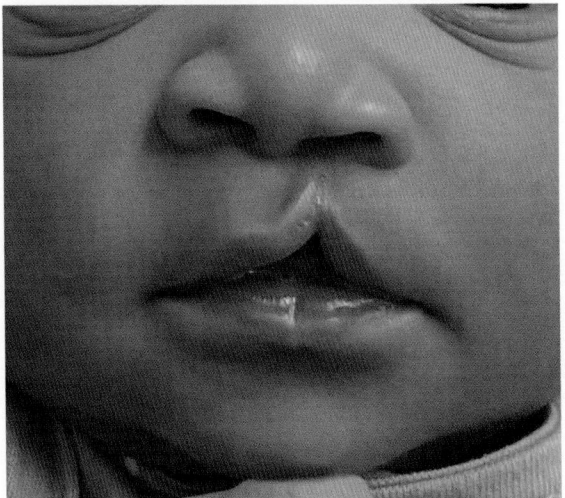

Fig. 16.1 A patient with a unilateral incomplete left cleft lip and left cleft nasal deformity, which includes left alar base widening and flatness of the nare on the affected side. (Courtesy David W. Low, MD.)

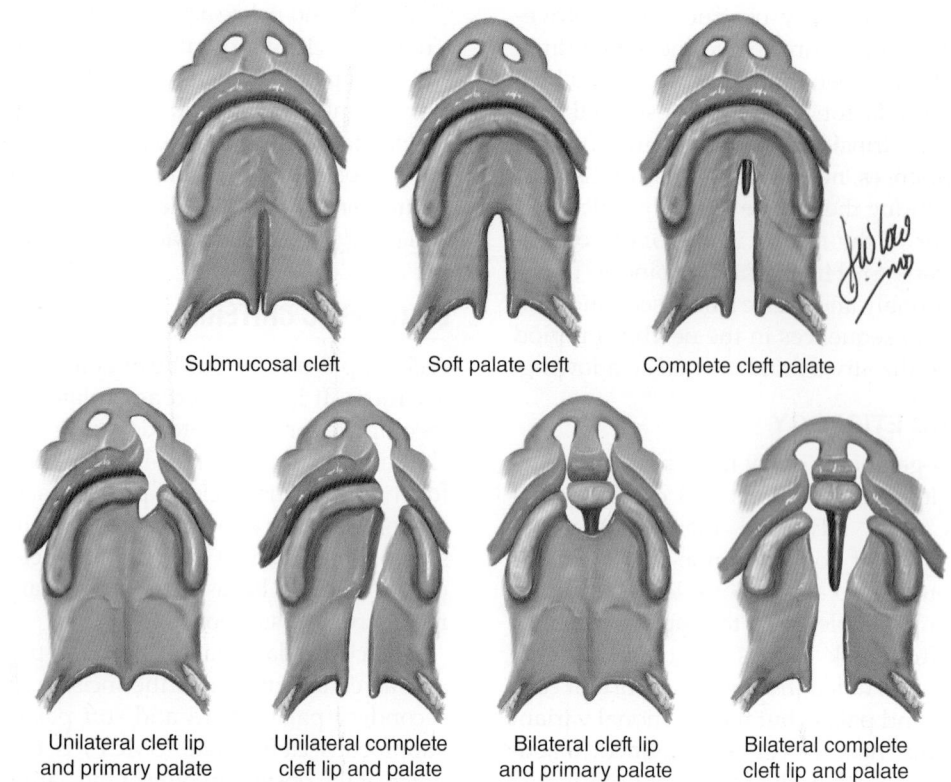

Fig. 16.2 **Illustration demonstrating a range of cleft lip and cleft palate anatomy from a submucous cleft palate through to a complete bilateral cleft lip and palate.** (Courtesy David W. Low, MD.)

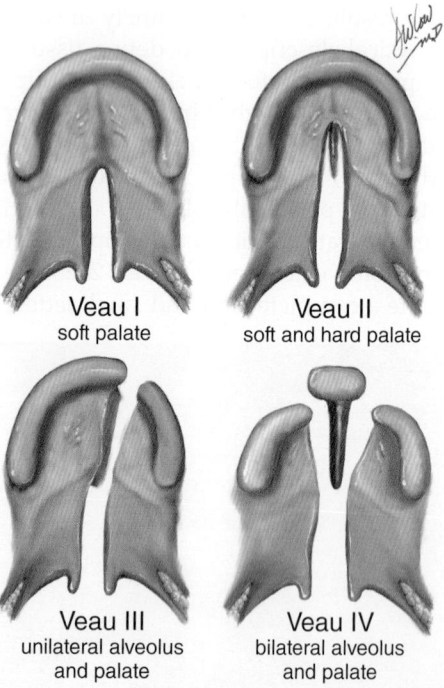

Fig. 16.3 **Veau classification of cleft palates.** Veau I involves only the soft palate. Veau II includes the soft and hard palates. Veau III is a cleft of the unilateral alveolus and palate. Veau IV involves clefting of the bilateral alveolus and palate. (Courtesy David W. Low, MD.)

an incomplete cleft. LAHSHAL would represent a complete bilateral cleft lip, bilateral cleft alveolus, and cleft palate (Tse, 2012). Cleft palates are often classified by the Veau system (Fig. 16.3). A Veau I cleft palate involves only the soft palate. A Veau II cleft involves the hard and soft palates. Veau III is a unilateral cleft that extends through the hard and soft palates to the alveolus. A Veau IV is a bilateral cleft extending through the hard and soft palates to the bilateral alveolar processes (Isaac & Chong, 2020; Wilkins-Haug, 2022).

A cleft lip can be diagnosed prenatally on ultrasound after about 13 to 14 weeks of gestation but is commonly noted on routine fetal anatomic surveys. Cleft palate, however, is not commonly perceived on prenatal ultrasound and requires more sophisticated imaging such as fetal magnetic resonance imaging (MRI). Fetal MRI has a sensitivity of 97% and specificity of 94% for the detection of cleft palate. It is worth noting that fetuses with orofacial clefting should undergo full body evaluation to assess for additional structural anomalies. A cleft lip in an atypical position may be related to amniotic band syndrome. Genetic testing should be offered or considered especially in the setting of presumed syndromic or multisystem involvement (Wilkins-Haug, 2022).

CLINICAL MANIFESTATIONS AT TIME OF DIAGNOSIS

The majority of babies born with cleft lip only or with cleft lip and palate do not have associated syndromes; however, all infants with clefts need a physical examination by a geneticist (Willner, 2000).

Infants with cleft palate only should be examined carefully for other anomalies. Some clefts of the palate are not detected by the staff in the delivery room. Infants who are unable to successfully breastfeed, are unable to latch on, or exhibit difficulties with bottle feedings with prolonged (>30–45 minutes) feeding times should be reexamined carefully for the presence of a cleft. Even a small cleft of the soft palate usually produces ineffective sucking as a result of the infant's inability to create a vacuum to draw the breastmilk or formula out of the nipple (Curtin, 1990). The mother may initially report that the baby will nurse for 45 minutes yet does not seem satisfied. The mother's breasts may still feel engorged at the end of a feeding, and there is never a feeling that the breast is empty of breastmilk. Frequent snacking can result in inadequate urine output and a fussy baby. After approximately 4 to 5 days of this feeding behavior, the infant becomes sleepier, lethargic, and exhibits signs of dehydration, including weight loss (Krishnamurthy et al., 2011). For some bottle-fed infants, the parents report that it may take more than 1 hour for the infant to consume 1 oz of formula. It is at this time that a palatal cleft may be noted. Somnolent, dehydrated 4-day-old infants may be hard to examine because they are resistant to opening their mouth. Insertion of a water-moistened gloved finger may be useful in examining palatal integrity (ACPA, 2004).

◉ Clinical Manifestations at Time of Diagnosis

- Cleft lip and palate: physical findings
- Cleft palate: difficulty feeding because of infant's inability to create suction
- Pierre Robin sequence: signs and symptoms of upper airway obstruction as a result of posterior position of tongue in the airway, micrognathia
- Submucous cleft palate: nasal-sounding speech

Pierre Robin sequence often presents with the findings of cleft palate, glossoptosis, and micrognathia (Box 16.2). Airway obstruction may not become evident until the infant is 2 weeks of age or until the first upper respiratory tract infection. Therefore it is prudent to observe these infants closely during the first months of life and consider a baseline pediatric pulmonary evaluation within the first weeks of life. These infants are able to maintain adequate oxygen and carbon dioxide saturation initially after birth but can tire over time with increased work of breathing. As infants grow, the size of the airway cannot accommodate their body's demand for more oxygen. There is increased respiratory effort demonstrated by retractions, nasal flaring, and stridor. With increased effort, the muscles of the tongue and nasopharynx or larynx collapse, especially during sleep, when the upper airway muscles are relaxed. The tongue is retropositioned in the mandible, and the infant has difficulty expiring carbon dioxide particularly when supine and during sleep when the ventilatory effort is diminished (Fig. 16.4). When this occurs, there is complete or partial obstruction of the airway, and although it appears that the

---

Box 16.2 Findings Apparent in Infants With Pierre Robin Sequence

- Increasing levels of carbon dioxide when measured serially as a result of carbon dioxide retention from intermittent upper airway obstruction with retropositioning of the tongue.
- Transient oxygen desaturations measured by pulse oximetry accompanied by increased work of breathing with chest wall retractions and gasping sounds as the tongue blocks the upper airway. These episodes usually self-correct within a short time as the infant repositions the tongue forward; however, the frequency may increase as the infant tires.
- Difficulty during feedings, especially when the nipple is removed from the mouth, and the infant is still swallowing residual breastmilk or formula. The tongue becomes retropositioned easily without the stimulus of the nipple to move it forward. Gagging sounds may be heard and become worse with supine positioning.
- Deceleration on the growth curve despite adequate intake of formula or expressed breastmilk. This should signal a possible worsening respiratory status.

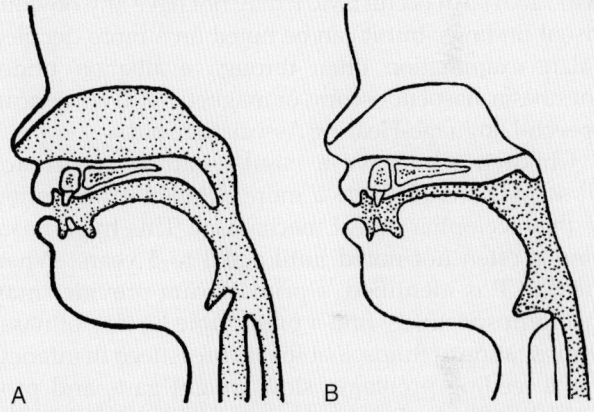

Anatomy of the roof of the mouth. The hard and soft palates separate the nasal cavity from the mouth. (A) Soft palate open. Muscles relax for breathing and making certain speech sounds. (B) Soft palate closed. Muscles in the soft palate and throat seal off the nasal cavity for swallowing foods and liquids and making certain speech sounds. (Modified from Mead Johnson & Co. (1997). *Looking forward: A guide for parents of the child with cleft lip and palate.* Author.)

Modified from Monasterio, F.O., Drucker, M., Molina, F., et al. (2002). Distraction osteogenesis in Pierre Robin sequence and related respiratory problems in children. *Journal of Craniofacial Surgery, 13,* 79–83; and Sidman, J.D., Sampson, D., & Templeton, B. (2001). Distraction osteogenesis of the mandible for airway obstruction in children. *Laryngoscope, 111,* 1137–1146.

---

child is breathing there are only intermittent breath sounds to auscultation. Oxygen saturation can drop, and carbon dioxide levels rise, thus necessitating treatment (Anderson et al., 2007; Smith & Senders, 2006).

The presentation of a child with SMCP is more elusive. The palpation of a posterior notch in the nasal spine at the juncture of the hard and soft palates, along with observation of translucence or blue discoloration of the soft palate (zona pellucida), is unusual unless there are clinical symptoms to warrant closer physical examination of the soft palate. There may or may not be a bifid uvula, which can also be a normal variant and a short soft palate with levator veli palatini muscle diastasis in

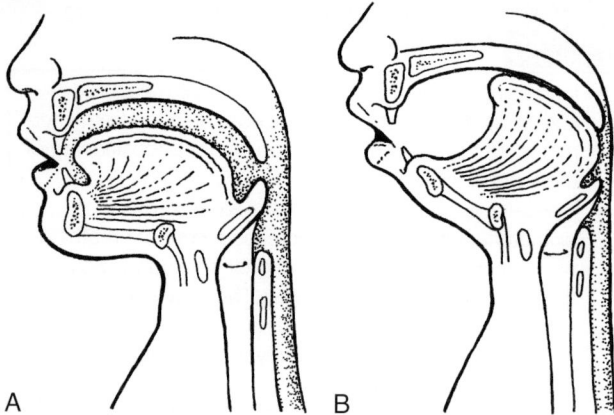

Fig. 16.4 Pierre Robin sequence. Anatomic features of the larynx. (A) Normal. (B) Mandibular hypoplasia. Note that posterior placement of the tongue makes the larynx appear more anteriorly situated than normal.

the midline. The SMCP is frequently undetected until preschool when the speech is unintelligible secondary to hypernasality or velopharyngeal insufficiency (Gorlin et al., 2001). An occult SMCP may not have any obvious visual findings, but it can be noted on a more detailed palate examination often through evaluation under anesthesia, nasoendoscopy, or magnetic MRI (American Speech-Language-Hearing Association, n.d.).

Children who have a nasal-sounding speech for all sounds should have a more detailed examination of their velopharyngeal mechanism. This hypernasal tone is often not noted until age 3 to 5 years. When the SMCP is identified, a primary care provider may then retrospectively find a predictable history of nasal regurgitation of fluids, inability to breastfeed in infancy, initial feeding problems, slow weight gain, and prolonged bottle-feeding times. In addition, a child may have a history of frequent episodes of serous and acute otitis media as a result of eustachian tube dysfunction associated with the cleft palate (Aniansson et al., 2002). Only SMCPs that are symptomatic require intervention (Ysunza et al., 2001).

TREATMENT

GOALS OF TREATMENT AND TEAM CARE

The goals of treatment are (1) to achieve optimum growth and function in speech, hearing, dental, and psychosocial development and (2) to achieve the optimal aesthetic repair. The ACPA believes that every individual with a cleft lip or cleft palate is best served by the multidisciplinary, coordinated approach offered by a cleft palate or craniofacial team (see Resources at the end of this chapter for listings). Parents may contact the team independently, or contact can be facilitated by their primary health care provider. Approved cleft and craniofacial teams have met the standards set forth by ACPA to provide experienced and qualified patient care that is interdisciplinary, coordinated, timely, and consistent (ACPA, 2019).

Treatment

- Establishment of adequate feeding
- Airway management for infants with Pierre Robin sequence
- Surgical reconstructive management
- Otolaryngology treatment
- Audiology and speech pathology management
- Dental care and orthodontic treatment

Newborns should be referred to a team before discharge from the birthing hospital. Older children can and should also be referred for team consultation because management occurs throughout the first 18 years of life. The team must include a qualified speech pathologist, an orthodontist, and a plastic surgeon. Other specialties on a cleft palate team often include audiology, otolaryngology, dental specialties (e.g., pediatric dentistry, prosthodontics, oral-maxillofacial surgery), genetics/dysmorphology, genetic counseling, nursing, social work, psychology, and pediatrics. Teams that care for children with more complex craniofacial deformities may also include members from anesthesia, neurosurgery, ophthalmology, radiology, and psychiatry.

Initial management of a newborn with a cleft involves diagnosis clarification (i.e., ruling out associated syndromes), psychosocial support for the grieving family of the child with a congenital birth defect, feeding support, and airway management for infants with Pierre Robin sequence and micrognathia.

Establishment of Adequate Feeding

Newborns with cleft lip and cleft palate have similar nutritional requirements as newborns born without cleft lip and cleft palate. In the early months of life it is important to maintain an appropriate diet for all newborns.

The goal of feeding is to maintain optimum nutrition using a technique that is as normal as possible. Infants with an isolated cleft lip or a cleft lip and alveolus (gum) do not generally experience any feeding difficulties. Infants with cleft palate, on the other hand, require some minor adaptations to establish effective feeding. Generating intraoral negative pressure is necessary to draw breastmilk or formula out of a nipple, and an infant with a cleft palate is unable to accomplish this because of the air leak through the nose. There is generally no problem with the infant's ability to swallow. Despite noisy feeding sounds, there is no increased risk of aspiration pneumonia in infants with cleft palate. Therefore the feeding technique must deliver the breastmilk or formula into the oral cavity so the baby can swallow it normally. Maintaining a sufficient diet is challenging in infants with cleft due to common feeding issues such as nasal regurgitation, ineffective sucking, frequent air intake, burping, and consequent longer feeding times (Singhal, 2022).

Although infants with a cleft lip or cleft lip and alveolus may be able to breastfeed with minor positioning modifications, infants with a cleft palate cannot breastfeed due to the inability to create a vacuum (Reilly et al., 2007). Babies with clefts are typically bottle fed with a one-way flow valve to increase the volume of breastmilk or formula that flows into the baby's mouth.

One of the more common feeding devices used is the Mead Johnson Cleft Lip and Palate Nurser (Fig. 16.5), which has a soft plastic compressible bottle and a cross-cut nipple that is slightly longer and narrower than regular nipples. The nipple, however, is not the crucial element of this device, as evidenced by some infants' preference for an orthodontic type of nipple that is also effective. The orthodontic nipple is useful in large clefts because it can span the distance between the edges of the cleft. This large nipple can provide some tongue stabilization during the sucking process, and its single hole provides a faster flow of breastmilk or formula. The soft plastic bottle allows the parent to control the rate of breastmilk or formula delivered, with rhythmic squeezing of the bottle timed to the infant's cues of swallowing. The nipple should be aimed at intact parts of the palate to take advantage of any possible nipple compression between the tongue and the palate.

Alternatives to the Mead Johnson nurser are available. The Medela Company distributes the Special-Needs Feeder (formerly the Haberman Feeder), which provides the flow of breastmilk or formula when the nipple is manually compressed by the caregiver or when the infant's gums apply pressure to the silicone nipple. There are varying flow rates to adjust to suit the baby's feeding ability and a one-way valve between the nipple and bottle to decrease the chances of air ingestion during natural pauses of feeding.

The Pigeon nipple, with its simple one-way valve system, is less expensive than the SpecialNeeds Feeder. It is commercially available (see Resources) with instructions for use in English and Japanese. The nipple is made of soft, easily compressible, nonlatex isoprene and has a one-way valve that fits into the nipple assembly. Therefore the breastmilk or formula flows only into the mouth, not back into the bottle, when the baby compresses the nipple.

Dr. Brown's Specialty Bottle system is also commercially available for babies with cleft palates. This bottle involves a one-directional flow valve within the nipple collar. Babies use their own tongue and jaw movements during sucking to express the breastmilk or formula into the mouth. The bottle is vented, which creates a positive-pressure flow that does not require a vacuum for feeding. This also helps eliminate air ingestion, thus reducing symptoms of gas, colic, or spit-up.

The Ross cleft palate nipple is intended for postoperative feeding and is not appropriate for newborns because the flow rate is too fast. Likewise, the Lamb nipple is an outdated, bulky device that causes gagging.

Whatever feeding method is chosen, there are principles or guidelines most effective in achieving appropriate weight gain. The family needs personalized teaching within the first week of life regarding assessment, feeding methodology, and evaluation of response to feeding by a practitioner experienced in the management of infants with clefts (ACPA, 2004). Ideally this practitioner should be a cleft palate or craniofacial team member. Consistency with a chosen technique for a minimum of 24 hours is important to allow both parent and infant to adapt. Continuous switching of nipples is confusing. Feedings should last no longer than 30 minutes, and the frequency should

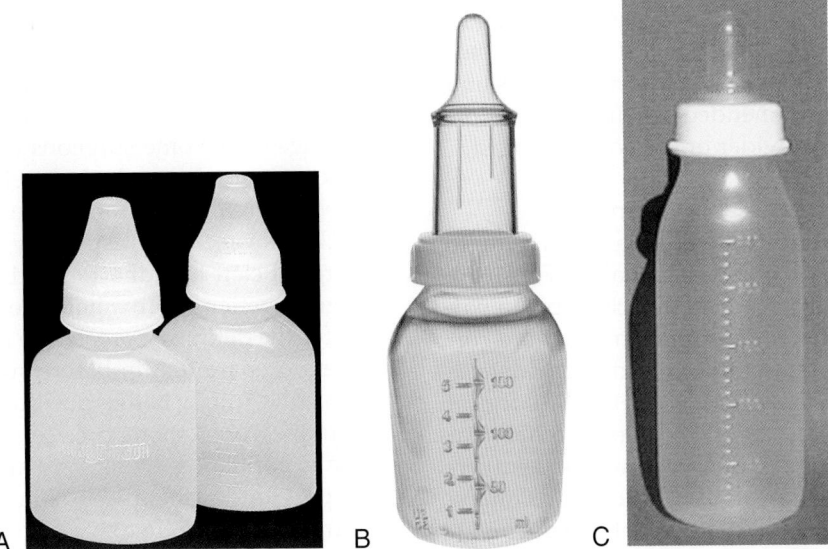

Fig. 16.5 (A) Mead Johnson Cleft Palate Nurser. (B) Haberman Special Needs Feeder. (C) Pigeon nipple and bottle. (A, Courtesy Mead Johnson & Co.; B, courtesy Medela, Inc.; C, courtesy Children's Medical Ventures.)

not be less than every 2.5 to 3 hours. These guidelines promote the conservation of energy and decrease caloric expenditure during the feeding process. It is helpful for parents to know how many ounces their child needs each day to grow normally. A quick, easy guide is a minimum of 2 oz breastmilk or formula per 1 lb of baby's weight every 24 hours. Therefore a 7-lb baby will need 14 oz each day.

The use of feeding appliances or presurgical orthopedic devices, such as an obturator, varies across the United States. The purpose of the obturator is to form negative pressure to allow proper breastmilk or formula removal during sucking from the breast or nipple. This can also help reduce nasal regurgitation. These devices assist the infant with a cleft by creating a barrier over the palatal cleft, enabling the baby to compress a nipple against a hard surface. Some groups anecdotally report improved feeding efficiency for both bottle feeding and breastfeeding using these plates. However, Masarei et al. (2007) found the use of presurgical orthopedics does not significantly improve feeding efficiency or general body growth.

Airway Management

Infants who have Pierre Robin sequence require a careful airway assessment, and effective airway management strategies must be in place before addressing feeding issues. These strategies may include placing a temporary nasopharyngeal airway or tracheostomy for severe upper airway obstruction, lip-tongue placation, or prone positioning. A surgical treatment that involves mandibular lengthening in the neonate is discussed in Surgical Reconstruction: Jaw Surgery, later. A feeding specialist, in conjunction with a craniofacial team, may develop the feeding plan for oral feeding with or without a nasogastric tube or gastrostomy tube. Infants with airway distress caused by obstructive etiology are postulated to have a higher incidence of gastroesophageal reflux; however, the association between Pierre Robin sequence and gastroesophageal reflux has not been proven. If an infant has symptoms of this condition, appropriate diagnostic studies and management are recommended as directed by the pediatric health care provider or gastroenterologist.

Surgical Reconstructive Management

It is important to know the normal anatomy in order to understand the repair of cleft lip and palate (Fig. 16.6). There is a frequent misconception that cleft lip and palate or both are merely surgical problems that are corrected in early childhood once the lip and palatal defects are closed. Parents who are very eager for the surgical repairs soon learn of the multidisciplinary rehabilitative services that must be coordinated with the surgeries. The specific timing of surgery also depends on the child's health, growth, and development. See the previous discussion of team-based cleft care for more information on this multidisciplinary approach.

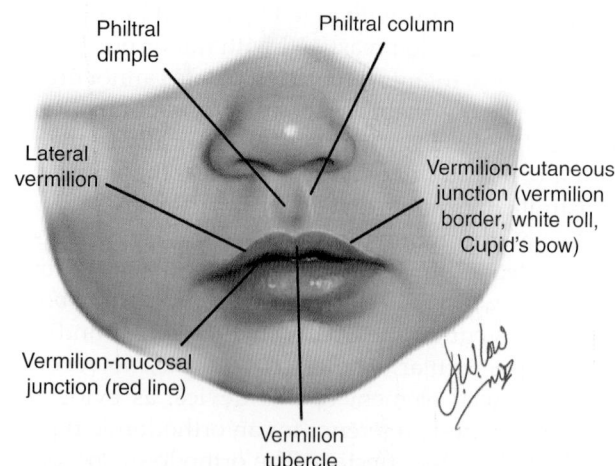

Fig. 16.6 Normal lip surface anatomy with external lip landmarks. Special attention is needed during cleft lip repair to align important structures, such as the vermilion-cutaneous junction, to yield a symmetric surgical result. (Courtesy David W. Low, MD.)

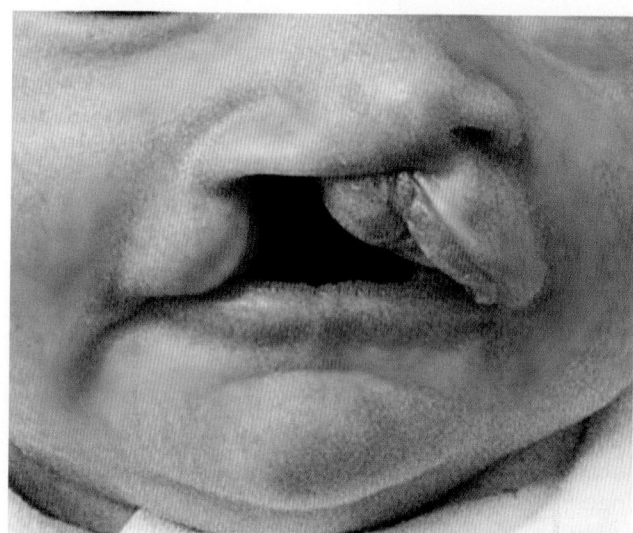

Fig. 16.7 A wide unilateral right cleft lip and cleft nasal deformity. Note the severe nasal deformity as a result of the wide cleft. (Courtesy David W. Low, MD.)

Surgical reconstruction of a cleft lip. Surgical repair of cleft lip is generally done between 3 and 6 months of age (Fig. 16.7). Some surgeons use the rule of 10s—10 weeks of age, a hemoglobin level of 10 g/dL, and 10 lb in body weight—in planning the repair. Occasionally if the cleft is very wide, especially in a unilateral defect, a surgical cleft lip adhesion is done at about 1 month of age to better approximate the lip tissue in preparation for the definitive procedure at the usual age. Some centers prepare the lip before surgery by moving the premaxilla into a better position with simple taping techniques or a more precise movement with orthodontic appliances (Peterson-Falzone et al., 2001). Box 16.3 provides further discussion of nasoalveolar molding treatment (Fig. 16.8).

At the time of the cleft lip repair, some surgeons may opt to repair the cleft nasal deformity with a

Box 16.3 Nasoalveolar Molding

Nasoalveolar molding (NAM) is a craniofacial orthodontic technique for infants with cleft lip and palate used to non-surgically narrow the cleft of the lip and gums, align the alveolar segments, and help improve the shape of the nose. The timing of this treatment is such to take advantage of pliable soft tissue and cartilage during infancy. Once the infant learns successful feeding skills and has established a pattern of weight gain, therapy can then be initiated within the first few weeks of life and continues through the cleft lip repair surgery. With this device there is a custom-fabricated intraoral acrylic mouthpiece that covers the roof of the mouth, which is similar to an orthodontic retainer, and this functions as a barrier to protect the nasal structures. As treatment progresses, the orthodontist adjusts this mouthpiece to gradually narrow and realign the cleft. Once the alveolar and lip clefts have narrowed, a nasal stent is added to help reshape the nose. Although time consuming and somewhat labor intensive, NAM effectively narrows the cleft and promotes better surgical outcomes during all stages of cleft surgery, including cleft lip repair, cleft palate repair, and alveolar bone grafting.

From Kurnik, N., Calis, M., Sobol, D. et al. (2021). A comparative assessment of nasal appearance following nasoalveolar molding and primary surgical repair for treatment of unilateral cleft lip and palate. *Plastic and Reconstructive Surgery, 148*(5), 1075–1084.

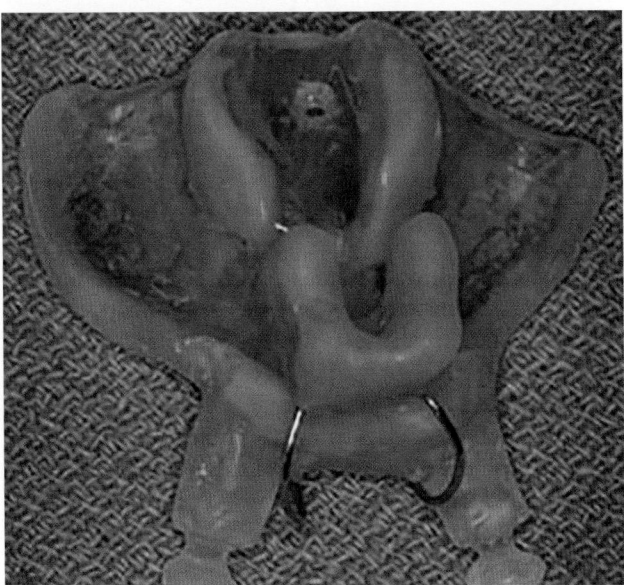

Fig. 16.8 Nasoalveolar molding device for bilateral cleft lip and palate. Acrylic mouthpiece with nasal stents that help reshape the nose.

simultaneous tip rhinoplasty to straighten the deviated nasal tip and improve projection. Primary gingivoperiosteoplasty is another surgical intervention that can close the alveolar cleft at the time of lip repair to limit the need for alveolar bone grafting in adolescence, but evidence remains inconclusive (El-Ashmawi et al., 2019). An anterior vomer flap can be utilized to close the anterior portion of the hard palate at the time of the lip repair to decrease the overall size of the palatal

defect and improve outcomes in formal palate repair (Agrawal & Panda, 2006).

Postoperative management for an infant with a cleft lip has changed dramatically over the years. Unrestricted breastfeeding or bottle feeding immediately after surgery has been shown to decrease the length of hospital stay, increase oral intake, and improve parental satisfaction without negatively affecting suture line integrity (Gailey, 2016). Surgery can be performed on an outpatient basis, with the infant discharged with elbow restraints. The lip area can be cleaned with soap, water, and often antibiotic ointment, per the surgeon's preference. Pain management is usually adequate with oral acetaminophen.

Surgical reconstruction of a cleft palate. Surgical repair of the cleft palate is usually done between 9 and 18 months of age. This is timed to provide the reconstructed palate needed for speech development. The repair is most commonly done all at one time in one stage. The postoperative management usually warrants a 1- or 2-night hospital stay for airway monitoring, pain management, and establishing adequate oral hydration. The use of elbow restraints, avoidance of pacifiers, and unrestricted use of straws and utensils for feeding for 2 weeks are routine. The patient can promptly resume use of the same preoperative bottle or cup after palatal surgery, but the exact timing may be variable depending on the center. Postoperative diet progresses from liquids to blenderized or soft food. The soft diet continues for several weeks after surgery. Good pain management usually requires the initial use of a narcotic medication (oxycodone) in conjunction with acetaminophen and ibuprofen. Regularly scheduled analgesia around the clock after surgery optimizes the success of oral feeding. Infants may require pain management at home with acetaminophen and ibuprofen around the clock for several days after surgery. Of note, an anesthetic nerve block at the time of the palate repair can effectively improve postoperative pain, limit opioid use, and enhance recovery (Moggi et al., 2020).

Secondary palatal surgery may be recommended by the speech pathologist to address persistent nasal speech after a period of speech therapy. The procedures may lengthen the palate (i.e., conversion to a Furlow palatoplasty [palatal lengthening with bilateral buccal myomucosal flaps]), create a smaller space in all dimensions (i.e., sphincter pharyngoplasty), or create a flap of tissue in the middle (i.e., pharyngeal flap) with two side ports to produce velopharyngeal sufficiency or closure during speech. This secondary palatal surgery is done for children of preschool age to achieve clear speech before school entry (Sie et al., 2001). This procedure is also used in school-age children who develop nasal speech after the adenoid pad involutes or is surgically removed.

Secondary lip revisions may be necessary before beginning school or during the school-age years and can occur separately or in combination with another planned surgical procedure. As previously noted, this may or may not include a tip rhinoplasty.

Surgical reconstruction of alveolar cleft. Repair of the bony defect along the gum or alveolar ridge appears to be optimal between maxillary growth completion and maxillary canine eruption, usually between 8 and 10 years of age (Craven et al., 2007), though the timing is variable across different institutions. Many centers elect to proceed with alveolar bone grafting at the stage of mixed dentition, between ages 6 and 8 years, after evaluation by an orthodontist for dental imaging, effective palatal expansion, and orthodontic treatment (Box 16.4). Roots of the teeth need to be anchored on bone, and generally iliac crest cancellous bone is harvested and packed into the alveolar cleft defect (Fig. 16.9). Dietary restrictions and the use of blenderized or soft food for 4 weeks are indicated. Once the bone has healed, implants can be used to replace missing teeth in the alveolar cleft (Kramer et al., 2005). A three-dimensional cone beam computed tomography (CT) helps to evaluate the take or solidification of the bone graft prior to the movement of the existing teeth. It is worth noting that some patients require a secondary bone graft if the imaging reveals an incomplete or insufficient bone graft taken to support the teeth or dental implant. Alveolar bone grafting can be combined with a cleft lip revision or tip rhinoplasty depending on patient needs and surgeon preference (Children's Hospital of Philadelphia [CHOP], n.d.).

Nasal reconstructive surgery (i.e., cleft rhinoplasty) is done when full growth or skeletal maturity has been attained (i.e., after menstruation in females and the growth spurt in males). A subset of teens with cleft lip and palate repaired in infancy also require midface oral-maxillofacial surgery to address facial imbalances that cannot be completely corrected by orthodontics (Good et al., 2007). Factors predisposing teenagers to jaw surgery include multiple missing teeth, secondary palate surgery for speech, and inconsistent team care (Oberoi et al., 2008). Further discussion of jaw surgery

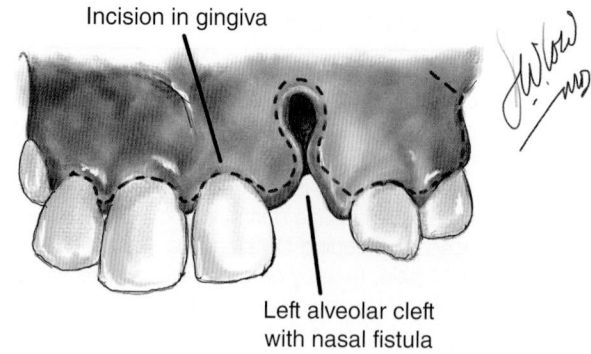

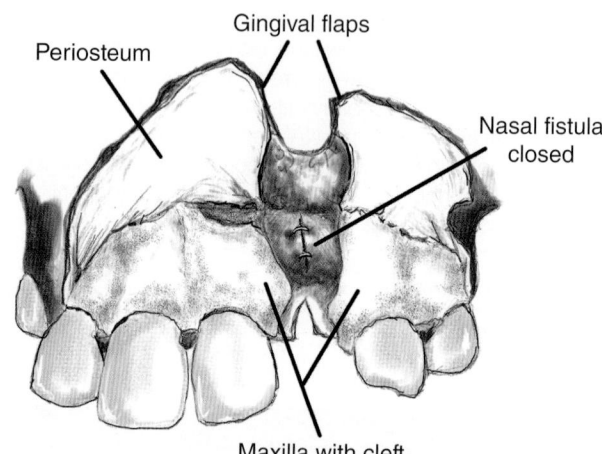

Fig. 16.9 Illustration demonstrating a left alveolar cleft with nasal fistula. The dotted lines represent the incisions made during alveolar bone grafting in the gingiva. The alveolar cleft is packed with iliac bone graft and closed with dissolvable sutures. (Courtesy David W. Low, MD.)

is presented next. Secondary speech, palatal, or lip revisional procedures may be elected to address aesthetic and functional concerns before the patient transitions to adult care. In ideal circumstances cleft care is completed by the age of 18 years.

Surgical reconstruction: jaw surgery. In the case of severe tongue-based obstruction in infancy, mandibular distraction may be needed. Mandibular distraction osteogenesis (MDO) is utilized when the mandible is hypoplastic or micrognathic and interferes with a baby's feeding and respiratory status, which can be seen in several different syndromes such as Pierre Robin sequence, hemifacial microsomia, or Treacher Collins syndrome. MDO helps to relieve airway obstruction by gradually lengthening the lower jaw and slowly depositing new bone while the soft tissues stretch to accommodate. Distraction osteogenesis involves surgically cutting the bone (osteotomy) and securing the distractor on both sides of the bone with screws. An external piece of the hardware protrudes from the skin that the health care provider or caregiver turns at a prescribed rate and interval for typically 2 to 3 weeks, averaging about 1 to 2 mm

---

Box 16.4   Cleft Orthodontic Treatment

Phases I and II orthodontic treatments are important adjuncts to cleft care. Phase I takes place at mixed dentition as the patient is beginning to lose baby teeth, typically 6 to 9 years of age. Phase II begins in early adolescence or older (14–18 years of age), and the teeth are both leveled and aligned. This treatment addresses and realigns teeth that are in an abnormal, missing, or displaced position. Prolonged or long-term orthodontic treatment may be needed but is patient specific. Bridges or dental implants can address missing teeth or notable gaps.

of lengthening per day. Weekly radiographs are used to monitor the hardware and progress. After consolidation to allow for bone strengthening and healing, these devices are removed with a separate surgery usually about 12 weeks later. Continued monitoring is needed to assess for relapse and ensure adequate jaw growth over time (CHOP, n.d.).

Orthognathic surgery may be needed to address jaw malocclusion and maxillary retrusion as a result of the underlying cleft palate defect. A LeFort I osteotomy is used to cut and advance the upper jaw for severe maxillary retrusion. Bilateral sagittal split osteotomy is a maneuver to cut and reposition the lower jaw to correct the malocclusion. A genioplasty can reposition the chin point to provide facial profile balance with this jaw advancement. Orthognathic surgery typically takes place at skeletal maturity (age 14–18 years) and is combined with comprehensive orthodontic treatment before and after surgery. Virtual surgical planning using an updated CT scan 4 to 6 weeks prior to surgery has improved the safety and effectiveness of this procedure by limiting operative time with advanced planning for surgical maneuvers and hardware placement (Fig. 16.10). Severe maxillary retrusion could be treated earlier as an intermediate phase with maxillary distraction osteogenesis when the discrepancy is beyond that which can be addressed in a single-stage operation (CHOP, n.d.).

Of note, many institutions have adopted measures to promote improved surgical outcomes, cost efficiency, and patient satisfaction after various major surgeries. Enhanced recovery after surgery (ERAS) is a comprehensive perioperative initiative that evaluates current practices and replaces them with evidence-based measures where applicable. Parenteral analgesia, intravenous fluids, and bedrest are just a few of these elements that can be tailored to improve perioperative care and recovery (ERAS Society, n.d.).

Otolaryngology Treatment

Otolaryngology management involves monitoring persistent serous otitis media and frequently placement of ventilation tubes in the tympanic membranes (Valtonen et al., 2005). Ventilation tubes should be considered if there is fluid in the middle ear space at the time of any other surgical procedures (i.e., cleft lip or palate repair). Because of the high incidence of middle ear problems, some centers favor the placement of ventilation tubes at the time of surgical palate repair for all children (Fig. 16.11) (Carbonell & Ruiz-Garcia, 2002; Goldstein et al., 2005).

A small percentage of children have chronic eustachian tube dysfunction after 5 years of age and may require multiple replacements of ventilating tubes to maintain normal hearing through the school-age years. The indication for tubes may be recurrent or persistent serous otitis media or severe retraction of the tympanic membrane in which there is little

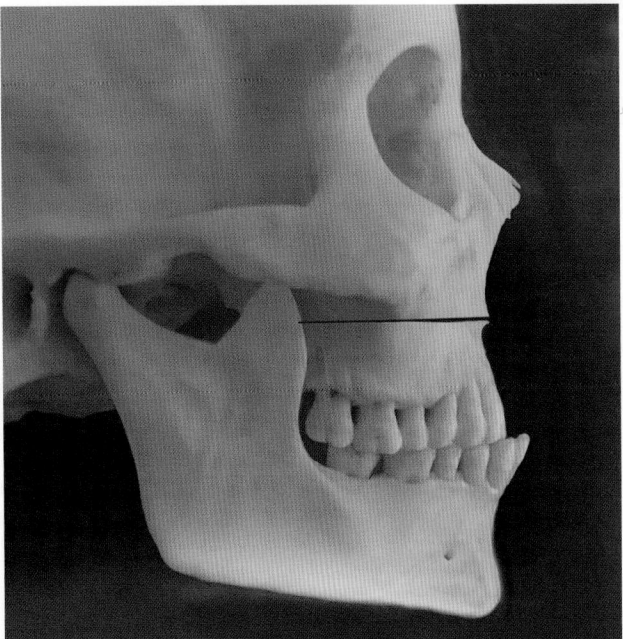
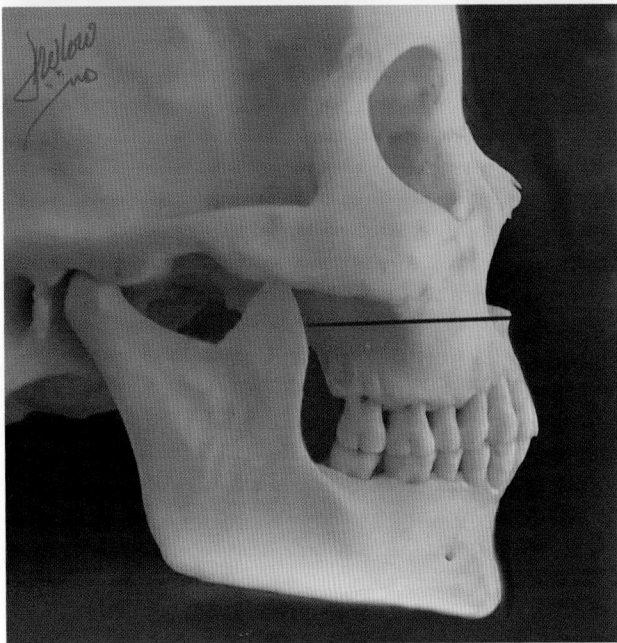

Fig. 16.10 Skull models representing jaw advancement during orthognathic surgery. Note in the top image that the upper jaw is set back behind the lower jaw (evident in the molar relationship). This demonstrates an Angle class III malocclusion. In the second model, the upper jaw has been advanced forward and normal occlusion achieved (Angle class I). (Courtesy David W. Low, MD.)

air present in the middle ear space, resulting in an increased risk for cholesteatoma. The tympanic membranes may be very scarred or weak and thin, which may result in persistent perforation of the tympanic membrane after extrusion of the ventilating tube. This membrane does not need to be patched surgically on an urgent basis if the hearing is not negatively affected because the perforation is functioning like a patent ventilating tube. When the child is a teenager, it may be patched when the eustachian tube

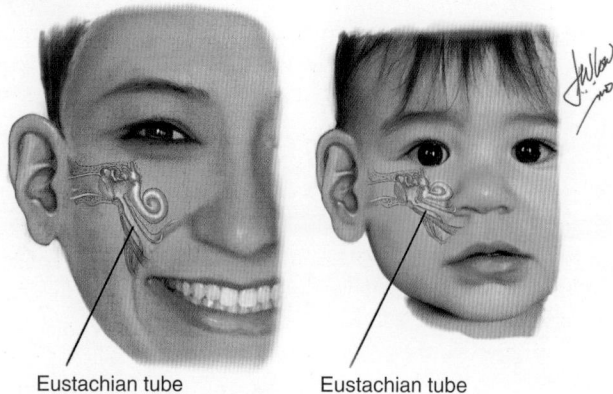

Eustachian tube   Eustachian tube

Fig. 16.11 Illustration demonstrating *anatomic* placement of the eustachian tubes relative to the palate. As discussed, eustachian tube dysfunction is common with cleft palate. Note the difference in size and angle of the eustachian tube, which is more horizontal in an infant and young child, as seen in the second photo. (Courtesy David W. Low, MD.)

functioning improves, and there are no recurrent infections (Muntz, 1993).

It is common practice to perform an adenoidectomy on the second set of middle ear ventilation tubes in the quest to avoid subsequent ear tube surgery; however, this practice is not common for children with cleft palate. Adenoidectomy is advocated for children without a cleft to prevent fluid accumulation in the middle ear and eustachian tube caused by blockage from an obstructing adenoid (Lous et al., 2005). For children with clefts, the adenoid tissue is often a factor in establishing velopharyngeal closure during a speech when the soft palate abuts the posterior pharyngeal wall at the level of the adenoid. As a result, an adenoidectomy is not usually recommended given the risk of developing velopharyngeal insufficiency or dysfunction.

When children with cleft lip and palate experience obstructive sleep apnea because of tonsil and adenoid hypertrophy, a modified surgical treatment plan is advocated. A tonsillectomy and superior (partial) adenoidectomy is generally done to preserve the inferior adenoid for velopharyngeal closure. Children with cleft lip and palate are not at a greater risk for this problem; however, the intervention is modified based on their underlying anatomic concerns for speech outcome.

Audiology and Speech Pathology Management

Diagnostic audiology evaluation and management are integral to the treatment plan for infants and children with cleft palate. Speech and language development are similarly monitored, and therapy is provided as appropriate (see Associated Problems, later).

Dental Care and Orthodontic Treatment

Dental care should begin early (1–2 years of age) with regular dental examinations every 6 months and fluoride supplements provided in nonfluoridated areas (Cheng et al., 2007) to preserve the health of the primary dentition. Children with bilateral or unilateral clefts of the alveolar ridge require considerable orthodontic management.

A child with a cleft palate alone requires regular pediatric dental care and orthodontic services. The anterior and lateral palatal growth may be restricted, especially if the cleft extends into the hard palate. Cleft palate repair results in scarring along areas that normally experience significant growth during childhood. As a result, a palatal expansion appliance may be necessary to achieve adequate dental occlusion.

Children with Pierre Robin sequence who have a significantly smaller mandible as compared with children with isolated cleft palate have been studied for catchup growth, and the results showed that the difference does not change after age 5 years (Daskalogiannakis et al., 2001). Some children, however, may need orthodontic management to deal with dental crowding, which may be a result of the small mandible.

Complementary and Alternative Therapies

Parents frequently ask the plastic surgeon if there are complementary or alternative therapies to reduce the visibility of the scar on the lip following cleft lip surgery. Some surgeons routinely cover the incision with paper tape or Steri-Strips until the wound is completely healed. This stabilizes the adjoining tissue and decreases the stress on the incision with movement from crying or smiling. Another therapy that has been used is a silicone patch or tape over the cleft lip scar. There are also over-the-counter scar creams with silicone that can help to improve scar appearance. In addition to topical silicone, scar massage is a helpful adjunct that can break down some of the scar-forming fibrinogen and soften the area; however, it is difficult to get an infant to hold still for a lip massage.

ADVANCES IN DIAGNOSIS AND MANAGEMENT

There continues to be a focus on fetal surgery for cleft lip and palate repair as it evolves with the advancement in imaging modalities, making it possible to diagnose cleft lip and palate antenatally. Proposed advantages of such surgical intervention include decreased scar formation in fetal wound healing, decreased potential costs as a result of less need for extensive postoperative care, orthodontia, and speech therapy, and minimized psychological trauma associated with a facial deformity.

Ongoing clinical research has focused on outcomes in cleft palate surgery, understanding the genetics of congenital cleft and craniofacial conditions, imaging considerations, and more. Currently there is a large multicenter study, the Cleft Outcomes Registry/Research Network (CORNET), funded by the National Institutes of Health, to compare surgical cleft palate repair techniques and their impact on speech, quality of life, and other outcomes. This prospective, observational study directly compares the surgical palatoplasty technique, either in the form of a straight-line repair (intravelar veloplasty) or zig-zag Furlow (double opposing Z-plasty). Sitzman et al., (2022) highlighted the differences in postoperative care after cleft palate repair. The majority of surgeons surveyed impose diet restrictions, typically pureed or soft foods, and upper extremity immobilizers for surgical site protection but lacked consensus on the duration of such measures, types of restrictions, postoperative use of bottles or sippy cups, pacifiers, and antibiotic therapy. This lack of agreement highlights the individual variation in each surgeon's practice. However, general agreement on the need for diet restrictions and immobilizers after surgery is consistent with prior studies on this topic. As mentioned, ERAS may help further standardize hospital postoperative care (Sitzman et al., 2022).

In a monumental study, three genes have been identified (*COBLL1*, *RIC1*, and *ARHGEF38*) that, when deleted, cause cleft lip or palate. This group of researchers analyzed DNA from patients with clefting in the United States and in the Philippines (Lansdon et al., 2023). Using a comparative genomic hybridization technique to seek out deleted sections of the DNA in patients with the disorder was compared with a control group that did not have clefting (Lansdon et al., 2023). Genetic research will continue to advance in this area of cleft lip and palate.

ASSOCIATED PROBLEMS OF CLEFT LIP AND PALATE AND TREATMENT

Audiology and Otolaryngology
Infants and children with an isolated cleft lip or cleft lip and alveolus generally do not have increased abnormal hearing as compared to the general population. However, infants and children with cleft palate have significant hearing and middle ear problems. Audiology testing is appropriate in children with cleft palate to monitor the degree of conductive hearing loss to guide the clinician in providing appropriate interventions and documenting the effectiveness of management. Hearing can be tested in newborns in the nursery by a screening known as automated auditory brainstem response screening or otoacoustic emissions (ACPA, 2004). If an infant does not pass the hearing screen, it is appropriate to proceed with more complex testing known as auditory brainstem response testing, which monitors the sensorineural auditory system.

Associated Problems

Cleft Lip and Palate and Treatment
- Audiology/otolaryngology
- Speech pathology
- Dental/orthodontic problems
- Psychosocial adjustment to a physical deformity

Children who are at least 6 to 9 months of age may be tested by behavioral audiology. This type of testing requires some degree of cooperation and is done when an infant can sit and respond to sounds. These findings should ideally correlate with the physical examination by the otolaryngologist so that a combined approach to management can then be devised.

The dynamic functioning of the eustachian tube, which serves as the communication link between the middle ear space and the back of the throat, is controlled by the palatal musculature. The child with a cleft palate has abnormal placement and underdevelopment of palatal musculature. As a result, the eustachian tube functions poorly. When a child develops an upper respiratory tract infection, fluid can accumulate in the middle ear space. This fluid usually drains into the oral cavity when the infection and swelling of the eustachian tube subside (see Fig. 16.11). In a child with cleft palate, however, the eustachian tube may only rarely open, and as a result the fluid remains behind the tympanic membrane on a long-term basis. Infants and children with cleft palate have a higher risk of developing chronic serous otitis media associated with eustachian tube dysfunction.

Monitoring children with ear tubes in place is usually done every 6 months and more frequently as necessary for blocked, infected, or prematurely extruded tubes. It is especially important to monitor for the presence of middle ear fluid and resultant conductive hearing loss in children who are rapidly acquiring speech-language skills and are already challenged by the cleft palate, which makes this acquisition more difficult.

Many parents query the primary care provider as to why the eustachian tube dysfunction continues after the surgical repair of the cleft palate. Even though palatal tissue is restored closer to normal, the dynamic mechanisms that control the influence of the palatal musculature on eustachian tube function are not normalized (Bluestone, 2004).

Speech Pathology
Children with a cleft lip only usually do not have significant speech articulation problems. These children may only require short-term therapy that focuses on bilabial sounds found in *m*, *b*, and *p*, which require competent lip closure. Children with clefts of the alveolus have additional challenges with anterior sounds as well as with managing air leakage from the front of the gums into the anterior nasal cavity before the alveolar bone graft surgery (Peterson-Falzone et al., 2001).

Children with cleft palate have problems with speech articulation as they try to correct the nasal air escape (Henningsson et al., 2008). The goal of palate surgery is to create a normally functioning palate before the emergence of compensatory mechanisms. The speech pathologist should meet the parents before surgery to explain normal speech-language development. Families must be taught that babies need to receive speech input directed at them and reciprocate in a turn-taking fashion with the use of body language and prespeech babbling behavior. Anticipatory guidance is standard practice for such families.

Following surgical closure of the cleft palate, the speech pathologist evaluates the success of the surgery. If formal speech therapy is needed, it can begin with children as young as 2 years. Without this intervention, these children can become frustrated in their inability to expand in expressive speech-language skills and may develop behavioral responses such as temper tantrums to communicate. In addition, the child is unable to communicate even simple desires to strangers who are unfamiliar with the child's speech repertoire.

Ongoing monitoring and parental guidance on a 6-month basis with the speech pathologist are appropriate during the toddler and preschool years. At some point during this time, the speech pathologist may determine that the child could benefit from regular speech therapy services. For children younger than 3 years, therapy may be provided by an infant development program (e.g., early intervention) that has specific speech therapy services or a speech pathologist who is community or hospital based. An intermediate unit can provide services after the age of 3 years, similar to early intervention programs. An individualized education program (IEP) is necessary for this isolated service because it is a component of special education services. The speech pathologist at the craniofacial or cleft palate center should continue to monitor progress every 6 to 12 months and provide feedback and suggestions to the speech pathologist providing the therapy.

The desired outcome following cleft palate surgery and speech therapy is clear articulation by 4 years of age. Although many variables have been studied, including the type of cleft, age of surgical repair, type of surgical technique used, initiation time, and length of speech therapy services, no one factor has been determined to provide the desired outcome (Peterson-Falzone et al., 2001). Rather it is a combination of factors that produces the optimal outcome.

Children who do not have clear speech development by 4 years of age may require secondary surgical palatal treatment—ideally before school entry. This surgery is particularly helpful if the articulation of sounds is good, but there is persistent nasal air emission as a result of a deficiency of palatal tissue or a palate that has inadequate motion, often demonstrated by nasoendoscopy or lateral videofluoroscopy. If secondary surgical or prosthetic management is done, follow-up speech therapy is usually needed to obtain maximum benefit from the intervention. It is not unusual for school-age children to receive speech therapy during school especially because they receive active orthodontic services that may further challenge speech articulation.

Dental and Orthodontic Problems

Children with a cleft lip and/or palate generally display poorer oral hygiene and higher susceptibility to caries associated with dental anomalies and defects of the repaired lip and palate (Cheng et al., 2007). Care should be taken not to remove teeth in the cleft area because they maintain alveolar bone mass in a dental arch that is deficient in the bone at the area of the cleft. Children often develop a crossbite from surgical closure of the palate, causing a collapse of the arches. The crossbite does not always need to be corrected in primary dentition, but some pediatric dentists offer early interceptive orthodontic treatment (see Box 16.3).

At 5 to 7 years of age, it is appropriate for a child with an alveolar cleft to have an orthodontic consultation, baseline records (e.g., photographs, dental study models, radiographs, examination), and a treatment plan. Initial management focuses on the expansion of the maxillary arch with a fixed active appliance in preparation for surgical grafting with iliac crest donor bone. The orthodontist usually indicates the appropriate time to perform the bone graft procedure. Following the grafting procedure, the expectation is that adjacent teeth will erupt into the arch. Dental implants combined with bone grafting can offer a reliable alternative to prosthetics for missing teeth (Kramer et al., 2005).

Orthodontic management is usually done in phases and may have periods of rest when the teeth are held in place by a passive retention type of appliance. The timing and phase of intervention depend on the maxillary and mandibular growth that occurs into the teen years. It is not uncommon for orthodontic management to span a period of 10 years. Compliance with the recommended regimen is crucial because the active movement of teeth depends on keeping frequent appointments, maintaining appliances, and practicing good oral hygiene. Maintaining regular pediatric dental care services during orthodontic treatment is also important.

Psychosocial Adjustment to a Physical Deformity

Parents of infants with a cleft are the first clients for the long-term psychosocial management of the child. According to observations, families who positively accommodate their child's chronic condition have children who appear to cope at a higher level than parents who exhibit negative adaptive behaviors (Klein et al., 2006). The degree of clefting is not predictive of the level of psychosocial functioning (Endriga & Kapp-Simon, 1999).

The first questions parents ask the primary care provider after the birth of a child with cleft lip or palate are "How did this happen?" and "Did I do something wrong?" (Bender, 2000). The parents should be reassured that clefts can occur in the healthiest of pregnancies and therefore should not blame themselves. The birth of an infant with facial malformation is a constant reminder of the physical condition. Bonding and attachment activities are related to the infant's face, and it takes some time to adjust and positively regard an abnormal face (Endriga & Kapp-Simon, 1999). Up to 25% of pregnant and postpartum women can experience some depressive symptoms (Bennett & Indman, 2006). With the added stress of the birth of a child with a difference, the mother's health should be assessed by the craniofacial team social worker, psychologist, or primary care provider. Most families learn over time to appreciate their infant's own personality and special way of expressing a wide smile. Some families have a secondary grief reaction once the child's lip is repaired and express that they miss the cleft (Curtin, 1990). A second adjustment to the new face is necessary and may take 1 to 2 weeks after surgery. Parents do not regret deciding to have the lip repair done, but rather it is a normal adjustment. Parents are reassured when the team providers give them anticipatory guidance about their feelings. The feelings of grief commonly experienced by parents at the birth of their child with a cleft can resurface at times of stress, such as hospitalization, initiation of speech, dental eruption, and school entry. It is important for parents to recognize that everyone copes with grief differently and not to expect other family members to be feeling the same emotions at the same time.

The health care provider can model acceptance of the child and encourage the parents to support their child's interests and talents in areas such as music, art, sports, or academia. One technique parents can use to communicate acceptance of their child with a cleft is to incorporate stories about the child's adventures as a baby going to the hospital for lip surgery with a positive outcome. That way, the cleft is part of the child, and the outcome is because of their innate characteristics. In the age of social media, #smileversary is a way to celebrate the anniversary of a child's cleft lip repair in a positive way.

Children in the preschool years gain an increased understanding of their birth defects as they develop a sense of self-awareness and experience teasing from peers. Simple explanations about the cleft can be reviewed, and strategies for deflecting the teasing can be suggested. A one-liner can be adopted by the child to provide a concise and simple description and deflect further questions or comments. School-age children may need support from counselors, school personnel, and their family to promote a positive self-image and to cope with teasing (Hunt et al., 2006). Teenagers can articulate their wishes and priorities in treatment planning and should participate in the decision-making process. Teenagers also have increased self-image concerns and may benefit from counseling services.

PROGNOSIS

The long-term prognosis for children with nonsyndromic cleft lip and palate is excellent. The goals of team management are to achieve good speech articulation, functional dental occlusion, normal hearing acuity, an acceptable appearance, and positive self-regard. In addition, children with Pierre Robin sequence have a goal of achieving adequate airway function. They are generally cared for in tertiary medical centers with cleft-craniofacial teams working with pediatric pulmonary or otolaryngology specialists to achieve adequate airway function.

The prognosis for development can vary from normal for a child with a nonsyndromic cleft to severely delayed for a child with a chromosomal defect causing the cleft. Therefore all infants with cleft lip and palate need to be examined by a geneticist before surgery (ACPA, 2004; Arosarena, 2007).

PRIMARY CARE MANAGEMENT

HEALTH CARE MAINTENANCE

Growth and Development

Growth and development are not affected in children with a nonsyndromic cleft lip and palate. In the past, infant feeding devices used to provide nutrition for neonates with a cleft palate were suboptimal. With the evolution of specialty bottles and the proliferation of team care and trained professionals to provide teaching, this aspect of management has improved. In addition, current postoperative feeding routines are simpler, and hospital stays are shorter, which all contribute to a more normalized nutritional status.

Infants with cleft lip and palate are expected to grow along the same parameters as infants without clefts. Once the feeding method has been taught by a member of the cleft-craniofacial team, the primary care provider will monitor the child's growth. All children with craniofacial abnormalities should be referred to a pediatric endocrinologist if short stature (other than constitutional) is identified. Children who have a known syndrome may have growth and developmental problems related to the syndrome.

Occasionally, infants with clefts do not grow along the expected norms. Extenuating psychosocial factors may challenge the parent or caretaker in feeding the infant. Initially, observation and review of the feeding method should be pursued along with a 24- to 72-hour diet record. Serial weight checks can provide both parents and health care providers reassurance. For the infant with Pierre Robin sequence, deceleration on the growth curve should prompt a careful reassessment of respiratory status and the probable finding of some degree of upper airway obstruction.

Diet

Mothers of infants with cleft palate can provide expressed breastmilk for their children. Hospital-grade electric pumps work the best and can be rented from a lactation consultant who is trained to provide education and support regarding long-term pumping and storage of breastmilk. Most mothers use a double pumping system attachment to decrease the amount of time spent pumping breastmilk. Mothers with low income may be able to procure an electric pump from their local Women, Infants, and Children agency.

Mothers pumping breastmilk four to six times per day and bottle feeding six to eight times per day need support and assistance from others. It is important to balance the needs of the mother and the family with the needs of the infant with a cleft in such a way that the mother not only feels encouraged to continue but also feels support if she decides to discontinue pumping. Mothers who are able to persevere with providing their infant expressed breastmilk will be encouraged by a study that linked breastmilk intake to a decreased incidence of otitis media, specifically in infants with clefts (Aniansson et al., 2002; Paradise et al., 1994).

Upright positioning of the infant during feeding will decrease the amount of nasal regurgitation. Parents should be reassured that a small amount of nasal regurgitation is expected and should be handled by simply wiping the nose of the infant with a cloth rather than interpreting it as a signal of a problem. Cleansing the nose and mouth with water or a cotton-tipped applicator or bulb syringe is not necessary because the mouth is self-cleaning, and the nasal secretions and breastmilk or formula will drain by gravity. The parent may need to be reassured about the anatomy of the cleft palate. The oral cavity and nasal cavity are continuous, and the parent may have an unspoken fear that the feeding will hurt the infant or that the nasal turbinates and the vomer represent brain tissue that can be injured with feeding. It is not unusual to see an ulcer on the vomer (bottom of nasal septum seen near the middle of the open cleft palate). This is caused by suckling or bottle feeding and goes away as the tissue toughens. The use of feeding plates has not been shown to improve feeding or nutritional status (Prahl et al., 2005).

The primary care provider can offer anticipatory guidance by discouraging the use of bottles in bed, especially when filled with formula, milk, or juice. This practice causes early childhood caries. The supine position favors the accumulation of fluid into the middle ear space when the eustachian tube is open in a population that is already at risk for recurrent otitis media.

For an infant who is 4 to 6 months old, the introduction of solid foods and progression to table foods is sequenced the same as for infants without clefts. There may be some nasal regurgitation as the infant learns this new skill. Nasal regurgitation of solids and purees is not harmful to the infant. Varying textures can sometimes alleviate this issue. Some parents require extra encouragement to proceed with the introduction of solid foods by spoon. Delayed initiation of this normal developmental skill can create negative feeding behaviors and may interfere with the normal oral motor development that is a precursor to speech development. Using a bottle type of infant feeder or enlarging nipple holes to accommodate solid foods also delays normal development. Messy spoon feedings are expected, and nasal reflux of solids should be handled calmly. Infants and children have only minor dietary restrictions. Some tricky foods for a child with an unrepaired cleft palate include peanut butter, soft cheese, and sweets, which are all gummy in texture. Avoiding foods that are a choking risk, such as peanuts, popcorn, and pellet candy, is advised because these foods can lodge in the nasal cavity.

Safety

In addition to routine anticipatory guidance on safety issues, the child may have some restrictions during the first 2 to 4 weeks following reconstructive surgical procedures. Elbow splints are generally used for 1 to 3 weeks after reconstructive surgery in the infant and toddler. Older preschool children may need the immobilizers at nap times and bedtime as reminders not to put their fingers in the mouth immediately postoperatively.

Dietary restrictions that are recommended postoperatively (e.g., avoidance of utensils, straws, and textured foods) are generally only necessary for about 2 to 3 weeks after surgery to allow for nontraumatic healing of the oral tissues. Some families may need encouragement and reassurance to advance to soft foods after the surgery and an unrestricted diet 1 month after the surgery.

Children need to avoid contact sports for 4 to 6 weeks after alveolar bone grafting procedures, nasal reconstruction, and midface jaw procedures to prevent disruption of the surgery before bone healing.

Infants with Pierre Robin sequence who require prone positioning for adequate respiration may need a car safety bed rather than a car seat when traveling in an automobile; these beds are available commercially (see Resources, later). A hospital's protocol will likely dictate the need for car seat testing or alternative travel options. The pediatric health care provider can further assist with this.

Immunizations

Infants and children with cleft lip and palate should receive all routine immunizations at the ages recommended by the American Academy of Pediatrics

(AAP) Committee on Infectious Diseases (Kimberlin et al., 2021). A planned surgical procedure is not a rationale for deferring routine immunizations; the child is better protected within the hospital setting when immunization status is current. Administration of immunizations within 72 hours of a planned surgical procedure is not advisable because a low-grade fever following vaccine administration may preclude surgery. Administration of the measles-mumps-rubella (MMR) or varicella vaccine within 1 week before scheduled surgery is not recommended for similar reasons. Administration of the pneumococcal vaccine is advocated for this population because of its protective effect in preventing some of the episodes of acute otitis media, although admittedly the vaccine's prime target is the more life-threatening meningitis risk (Overturf, 2000). Respiratory syncytial virus (RSV) immunoprophylaxis (Synagis) is recommended for children with conditions that compromise pulmonary function and congenital abnormalities of the airways, such as Pierre Robin sequence (Kimberlin et al., 2021). The surgical or anesthesia team may provide more specific or tailored guidance regarding vaccine timing in the perioperative period.

Screenings

Vision. Routine vision screening is recommended. Children with cleft palate alone should have pediatric ophthalmology dilated examination at approximately 1 year of age and again before school entry at age 4 or 5 years to screen for Stickler syndrome, which is associated with myopia and sometimes leads to retinal detachment (Jones, 2006).

Hearing. A high index of suspicion and prompt referral to an audiologist and otolaryngologist should be made if the child does not pass an audiologic screening in the school-age years. Detailed audiologic testing (see earlier) is done by the specialty center in the early years of life.

Dental. Routine screening is recommended for a child with an isolated cleft lip. Dental and orthodontic care is indicated for children with clefts of the alveolar ridge or the secondary palate. A pediatric dental provider is strongly advised—even if the family needs to travel some distance to obtain the service. The primary care provider should promote good oral hygiene practices, including initiation of tooth brushing or cleansing with a rough face cloth with the eruption of the first tooth. Parents must be counseled on the hazards of early childhood caries (Cheng et al., 2007).

Dental eruption may be slightly delayed in a child with a cleft. Many families may mistakenly believe that once their child starts orthodontic care, they no longer need to see a regular pediatric dentist. However, dental cleanings and topical fluoride treatment are even more important during active orthodontic management.

Blood pressure. Routine screening is recommended.

Hematocrit. Routine screening is recommended.

Urinalysis. Routine screening is recommended.

Tuberculosis. Routine screening is recommended.

Condition-specific screening. Children with cleft lip and palate require vigilance in vision, hearing, and dental screening (see earlier).

COMMON ILLNESS MANAGEMENT
Differential Diagnosis
Fever. The parents of a child with a cleft are alerted to the increased incidence of middle ear disease. The presence of a fever, increased irritability, tugging at the ears, and asking family members to repeat verbalizations all signal the need to have the ears examined for acute or serous otitis media.

Children with cleft palate are defined as an outlying population by the current AAP recommendations regarding middle ear disease, which means they favor ongoing monitoring of serous otitis media rather than aggressive surgical management (AAP & American Academy of Family Physicians [AAFP], 2004). Primary care providers are advised to refer these children to the otolaryngologist for a microscopic examination if they have persistent (≥3 months) middle ear fluid or recurrent (every 1–2 months) acute otitis media. Acute otitis media should be managed with the usual oral antibiotics. Prompt management is indicated for acute otitis media rather than the watch-and-wait approach currently in practice in the healthy child population because of the frequency of otitis media and the deleterious effects on hearing in an at-risk population. Prophylactic antibiotic use is not recommended because of the development of resistant pathogens (AAP & AAFP, 2004; Gungor & Bluestone, 2001) as well as its ineffectiveness in the management of chronic serous otitis media—the main problem in children with cleft palate.

Drug interactions. Medications are not required as part of the normal treatment regimen.

DEVELOPMENTAL ISSUES
Sleep Patterns
Infants and children with a unilateral cleft lip usually have a deviated nasal septum that causes noisy breathing during upper respiratory tract infections but does not negatively affect air exchange.

Children who have secondary palatal surgery to address nasal speech have a smaller upper airway space in the nasopharynx. A wide posterior pharyngeal flap works by narrowing the gap in the posterior pharynx to reduce nasality but carries with it the risk of obstructive sleep apnea. These children are particularly at risk for sleep state upper airway obstruction during the first 6 weeks following surgery when local edema is present. Symptoms may include chest wall retractions with or without partial ventilation, irregular snoring with pauses greater than 15 to 20 seconds, diaphoresis, nighttime waking (especially after an apnea episode), daytime somnolence, and enuresis (Muntz et al., 2008). The child's symptoms should be reported to the specialty center health care provider, who may be a pediatric pulmonologist or otolaryngologist. The severity of the symptoms will be assessed, and medical management (e.g., steroid administration or inpatient observation) may be warranted. Treatments can range from intranasal steroids (e.g., Flonase) to supplemental oxygen or positive pressure airway support. The surgical procedure rarely needs to be revised because the symptoms are usually temporary, and the desired outcome is to provide a decreased nasal airflow during speech without negatively affecting the ventilatory capabilities. However, persistent obstructive sleep apnea should be closely monitored to determine the need for revision.

An infant with Pierre Robin sequence may have a disrupted sleep experience because of obstructive sleep apnea. Careful history taking, evaluation, and management by the pediatric pulmonologist or otolaryngologist are appropriate. A formal overnight pediatric polysomnogram is often ordered. Ideally this test should be done with the infant in various sleep positions (prone, supine, side-lying, and while in the intended car seat) to document tolerance to position changes.

Sleep patterns are usually disrupted following hospitalizations because of upset routines and psychological distress. Families should be told of this probable change in sleeping pattern at both the preoperative and postoperative visits.

Toileting

There is no physiologic effect on toileting. The psychological impact of stressful surgeries and hospitalization experiences can temporarily delay the acquisition of toileting skills or result in regression of recently acquired skills.

Discipline

Parents of children with a congenital birth defect often feel guilty that they "caused" the problem in some way. This feeling can then translate into an altered perception of the child as being special and requiring extra attention to overcompensate for the guilt. In addition, parents are very saddened to learn of the initial surgeries that their child will require and the long-term management. Many parents report that they wish the treatment could be done on them rather than on the child. Because the initial surgeries are done in infancy, the psychological burden is thrust on the parents.

Parents must be encouraged to return to the infant's or child's normal routine following hospitalizations (Strauss, 2001). A routine is reassuring for the child and promotes normalcy and an earlier return to normal behavior. Parents who focus exclusively on the needs of the infant or child who is sick and cater to every whim soon find that this is not functional or pleasant for the child or the family. Symptoms of this phenomenon include the following: no structured feeding or meal routine; irregular nap times; nighttime waking; nighttime feedings; cosleeping in the parental bed (only if this is not the family's usual practice); excessive fussiness, irritability, or clinginess; loss of previously achieved developmental milestones; and inability to get along with others. These are all normal reactions to a stressful experience such as a hospitalization but usually do not persist beyond 2 to 6 weeks after a 24- to 48-hour hospital stay. Parents can benefit from anticipatory guidance and encouragement to promote normalcy, which initially may appear harsh and unsympathetic. However, most parents embrace the concept when it is presented as comforting for the child.

Issues of discipline arise again when a child with a cleft lip or palate enters school, especially if the child appears very different from peers and is teased. Overprotectiveness and lack of appropriate limits can exacerbate these problems. The child and family can often benefit from short-term counseling regarding self-image concerns and the development of skills to cope with teasing from others.

Child Care

Child care in a group day care setting can be stressful for parents of a child who is at risk for frequent ear infections. For this reason, some parents may choose a setting with a more limited number of children, especially during the winter months.

Once children are old enough to attend a Head Start program or structured preschool, they should. Such programs can be helpful as an adjunct to speech therapy because a child's peers will promote expressive language development. Peers usually do not understand the elaborate gesturing system and monosyllabic vocalizations that substitute for expressive language and may encourage children to expand their repertoire by modeling.

Schooling

Children with cleft palate are eligible for special education services (i.e., speech therapy) under the Individuals with Disabilities Education Act (IDEA) of 1991, amended in 2004. Parents should request in writing a speech evaluation focused on articulation when a child is 2 years of age. It is helpful if the parents provide medical information and any prior speech evaluations.

Peer teasing can occur as a child progresses through school because of speech and facial appearance issues (Millard & Richman, 2001). Some parents and children use the class presentation approach to explain the cleft, and teachers can incorporate this into their lesson plans about differences among people. A child rarely reports teasing and ridicule so severe that school phobia and frequent absences become an issue. It is important to query parents about these issues at primary care visits and offer supportive services and coordinated efforts between the primary care providers and the school system.

Children with cleft lip and palate may have learning disabilities, particularly in the areas affected by expressive language, such as reading problems (Endriga & Kapp-Simon, 1999). Children who have an isolated cleft palate that is part of a syndrome may have a lower intellectual potential that is specifically associated with the syndrome. These children should be evaluated by special education professionals as appropriate. Research has shown a higher than typical incidence of reading problems among school-aged children with cleft lip and cleft palate (Richman et al., 2012). This is thought to be related to subtle neuropsychological deficits.

Children with cleft lips and cleft palates may have a specialized IEP or 504 plan. IDEA covers school-aged children with designated disabilities such as specific learning disabilities, attention-deficit/hyperactivity disorder, hearing impairment, or intellectual disability. The disability must impact the child's learning performance and is addressed with the IEP. This is reviewed annually and reassessed every 3 years. Section 504 of the Rehabilitation Act of 1973 protects the educational rights of children with a physical or mental condition that affects their functioning in a major life activity such as hearing, speaking, or learning. The 504 plan allows accommodations for children for academic progress and are created by teachers and parents (Stock et al., 2020).

Sexuality

No special sexual problems are associated with cleft lip and palate. The obvious concerns about self-image may be exaggerated during adolescence.

When discussing reproductive issues, the risks of recurrence for clefting must be addressed. The rates quoted for nonsyndromic clefts are between 2% and 8% (CHOP, n.d.; Gorlin et al., 2001), depending on previous family history and severity of the cleft. A bilateral cleft lip is rare and more severe than a unilateral and has a slightly higher risk of recurrence. Other factors, such as sex, influence the recurrence risk as well. It is important to have a complete family history and a physical examination of an affected individual by a geneticist and a genetic counselor to provide the most accurate information.

Women with an increased risk of having a child with a cleft are eligible for a detailed ultrasound that has a better resolution of the facial features than the traditional ultrasound. Women of childbearing age are counseled to take increased folic acid and a multivitamin supplement 3 months before conception and during the first trimester in the hope of reducing the recurrence risk of a cleft condition (Prescott et al., 2002).

Transition to Adulthood

State funding for the care of children with cleft lip and palate is available to financially eligible children up to age 21 years through Medicaid. Most individuals can complete orthodontic and oral-maxillofacial surgical procedures by this age. Problems are encountered if there are treatment lapses or delays during crucial stages of dental development or orthodontic management that necessitate restarting the treatment. In addition, orthodontic interventions are effective during active treatment, and then the position of the teeth and the occlusion are often maintained with removable appliances (e.g., a retainer worn at night). Adolescents and their families often do not appreciate the need for these appliances, so relapse occurs. If relapse occurs before the insurance is terminated, some active management can be reinitiated. Otherwise, young adults must usually pay for these services as out-of-pocket expenses. It is difficult for young adults to gain third-party payment for some components of the revisional lip, nasal, or jaw surgery because such procedures are cosmetic by insurance carriers even though the treatment is for the reconstruction of a congenital birth defect.

Adolescent patients should be encouraged to participate in their visits in preparation for the transition of care. Their understanding of their previous treatment and diagnoses should be assessed. It is important to promote adherence to orthodontic care for potential orthognathic surgery at this age (Stock et al., 2020).

Family Concerns

Postpartum depression is not uncommon in the general population and is a treatable condition that may be overlooked when present in a mother who has just given birth to a child with a cleft lip and/or palate. Primary care providers should assess the mother for signs and symptoms of depression, such as persistent tearfulness, isolation, and lack of social support systems (Bennett & Indman, 2006).

Parents of children with cleft lip worry about their child's physical attractiveness to others, especially strangers. Parents are sensitive to the reactions and comments of professionals and their family and look at others' facial and emotional reactions when viewing their baby with a facial deformity. Fears of feeding or hurting the face and the mouth and concern that the cleft extends into the brain are common. Demonstrating feeding techniques and promoting normal infant care routines provide opportunities for learning and allaying anxieties.

Families who received a prenatal diagnosis of a cleft lip and/or palate report this allows for increased understanding of the diagnosis and associated challenges such as feeding (Stock et al., 2020). This also helps prepare them for a surgical timeline. This can lead them to have increased difficulties with coping with imagining what their baby will look like and the stress of planning for surgeries and multiple office visits.

It is beneficial to recommend that parents photograph their infant with a facial cleft. The provider can discuss with parents the usefulness of retaining a photograph that will be available for the child to view when older. If the parents are resistant, stating that they prefer to forget this time of sadness and wish to defer picture taking until after cleft lip repair, it may be prudent for a professional working with the family to take a photograph to keep in the infant's chart. Serial photographs are standard in most pediatric plastic surgery offices.

Families may verbalize concerns regarding oral, auditory, and dental problems in their children. These concerns and consequent stressors recur over time with multiple hospitalizations, tooth eruption, initial speech, school entry, and adolescent self-image concerns.

Orthodontic services are a crucial component of the rehabilitation process and are covered by the local, state, and federal funding programs for children with birth defects if a family is financially eligible. Families who do not meet the financial eligibility often find this care very expensive. Many insurance companies do not authorize treatment by nonmedical providers who render services such as dental, orthodontic, or prosthetic care, as well as speech and psychological care.

Special cultural issues affecting families with a child with a cleft lip and palate are mostly concerned with the etiology of the cleft condition. Superstitions about why clefts occur often originate in a family's country of origin. Hispanic and Filipino cultural folklores believe that clefting is related to the lunar cycle. A lunar eclipse or a crescent moon during a woman's pregnancy predisposes her unborn child to clefts. Some Asian cultural folklores relate construction, cutting, a fall, or moving the mother's bed during pregnancy with birth defects, especially clefting. In Chinese culture, the center of a person's face is very important and integral to that person's being (i.e., instead of the heart, which is common in Western culture). This view has implications for a cleft lip and palate deformity in its central location.

Most young parents acknowledge that such beliefs are part of cultural folklore and are explanations that their parents and grandparents provided for the untoward events that happened during pregnancy. Trying to disprove these theories is unnecessary because the etiology of clefts is unknown. It is more useful to focus on the common feeling of paternal and maternal guilt associated with a birth defect and work through the grief process over time.

Some families bring with them extreme fears of surgery and hospitalization, but fear usually seems to be experience related (i.e., a relative who died after a surgical procedure) rather than related to a specific cultural framework. The concept of health care in general, especially preventive health care (e.g., the routine dental care or anticipatory guidance needed to prevent speech articulation problems), is unfamiliar to some families. The very idea of seeking nonemergent health care services is particularly unknown in families who originate from other countries outside the United States that do not have many health care resources.

RESOURCES

ORGANIZATIONS

Ameriface (provides newsletter, information, and support): http://www.ameriface.org

American Cleft Palate-Craniofacial Association (referral to a local cleft-craniofacial team; written pamphlets and fact sheets in English and Spanish): https://acpa-cpf.org/ and www.cleftline.org

American Society of Plastic Surgeons (provides information about cleft lip and palate repairs): https://www.plasticsurgery.org

Changing Faces (support organization and publisher of child and adult books and material on the emotional and social aspects of living with a facial difference): www.changingfaces.co.uk

Children's Craniofacial Association (nonprofit organization, provides support to those with facial differences): https://ccakids.org

Cleft Advocate (support organization for families with children born with clefts and provides legislative advice and activity for obtaining insurance coverage for procedures): www.cleftadvocate.org

COSCO Safety 1st Shop (Dream Ride SE infant car bed/car seat in infants who require prone positioning): https://www.safety1st.com/us-en

FACES: The National Craniofacial Association (nonprofit organization, provides craniofacial support): https://www.faces-cranio.org

Let's Face It (comprehensive guide to support and information on craniofacial anomalies): www.dent.umich.edu/faceit

March of Dimes (supports research, education, and advocacy): https://www.marchofdimes.org/index.aspx

Philly Phaces (example of a local support organization; nonprofit organization in Philadelphia region for children with congenital facial differences): https://phillyphaces.org

Dr. Brown's (specialty feeding system): www.drbrownsbaby.com

Mead Johnson & Co., Nutritional Division (free booklet for cleft lip and palate nursers [*Your Cleft Lip and Palate Child: A Basic Guide for Parents*]): www.store.enfamil.com/bottles_and_nursers.html

Medela, Inc. (for breast pump rentals and Special-Needs Feeders [6000S]): www.medela.com

Wide Smiles (online support organization for families with children born with clefts): www.widesmiles.org

BOOKS FOR PARENTS

Berkowitz, S. (1994). *The cleft palate story*. Quintessence Publishing.

Bristow, L., & Bristow, S. (2007). *Making faces: Logan's cleft lip and palate story*. Pulsus Group Inc.

Charkins, H. (1996). *Children with facial difference: A parent's guide*. Woodbine House.

Moller, K.T., Starr, C.D., & Johnson, S.A. (1990). *A parent's guide to cleft lip and palate*. University of Minnesota Press.

 Summary

Primary Care Needs for the Child With Cleft Lip and Palate

HEALTH CARE MAINTENANCE

Growth and Development
- Expectations for physical growth and development are the same as those for the noncleft population.
- Syndromic clefts may be associated with poor growth and developmental delay.

Diet
- Use of a cleft palate nurser or special nipples enhances bottle feeding. Provision of expressed breastmilk with the use of an electric pump is desirable in infants with cleft palate.
- Introduction of solids by spoon is possible at the same time as in unaffected infants.
- Gummy or sticky foods or foods that can cause choking should be avoided.

Safety
- Elbow splints are needed following surgical procedures to prevent the baby's hands from disrupting repaired lip or palate.
- Avoidance of utensils, straws, and textured foods is recommended for approximately 2 weeks after surgical procedures to allow for nontraumatic oral healing.
- Contact sports should be avoided for 4 to 6 weeks after surgeries.
- Prone positioning for infants with Pierre Robin sequence may require a car safety bed vs. a car seat.

Immunizations
- All routine immunizations should be given on schedule.
- May elect not to administer DTaP within 72 hours of a surgical procedure and MMR/varicella 1 week before a surgery.
- Administer pneumococcal vaccine as additional protective effect in preventing otitis media.
- RSV immunoprophylaxis for children with Pierre Robin sequence under age 2 years per RSV eligibility guidelines.

Screening
- *Vision.* Routine screening is recommended. Children with isolated cleft palate or Pierre Robin sequence need a dilated eye examination by a pediatric ophthalmologist at 1 year of age and 4 to 5 years of age to rule out myopia, which is found in Stickler syndrome.
- *Hearing.* Audiology screening for children with cleft lip and alveolus is recommended with the same guidelines as for the unaffected population. Ongoing close monitoring for conductive hearing loss in children with cleft palate is required because of eustachian tube dysfunction.
- *Dental.* Screening for early childhood caries is important to preserve dentition and prevent alveolar bone loss. Routine pediatric dental care is given for children with cleft lip. In addition, children with cleft alveolus and palate need an orthodontic evaluation by age 5 to 7 years.
- *Blood pressure.* Routine screening is recommended.
- *Hematocrit.* Routine screening is recommended.
- *Urinalysis.* Routine screening is recommended.
- *Tuberculosis.* Routine screening is recommended.

COMMON ILLNESS MANAGEMENT

Differential Diagnosis
- *Fever.* Rule out acute otitis media. Chronic serous otitis media or recurrent acute otitis media must be aggressively treated.
- *Drug interactions.* There are no drug interactions.

DEVELOPMENTAL ISSUES

Sleep Patterns
- Unilateral cleft lip and palate and deviated septum result in noisy breathing, especially with an upper respiratory infection.
- There is an increased risk of sleep state obstructive apnea following secondary palatal surgical procedures.
- Disruption of sleep patterns may occur following surgical procedures and hospitalization.
- Signs of sleep state obstructive apnea require careful pulmonary and airway evaluation and management in infants with Pierre Robin sequence.

Toileting
- Temporary regression may occur following surgical procedures and hospitalization.

Discipline
- Discipline expectations are normal, with allowances during hospitalizations and 1 to 2 weeks after surgery.

Child Care
- Child care may need to be in a smaller group setting during the winter months because of the increased risk of otitis media.
- Speech therapy sessions need to be coordinated with child care arrangements.

Schooling
- Speech therapy may begin at age 3 years for children with cleft palate, and they require an IEP. They may also require assistance with expressive language development.
- Peer teasing may negatively affect performance.
- Teasing may occur because of lip, nose, and dentition appearance or speech articulation problems.

Sexuality
- Genetic counseling is recommended to discuss recurrence risks.
- It is recommended that women of childbearing age take folic acid in an attempt to reduce the recurrence risk of clefts.

Continued

- During pregnancy, a detailed level 2 ultrasound is available for women affected with a cleft condition to ascertain whether the fetus has a cleft lip. Further advanced imaging with a fetal MRI, fetal echo, and comprehensive ultrasound may also be needed.

Transition to Adulthood
- Treatment plan should be completed by the age 21 years.
- There is difficulty in procuring third-party payment for any orthodontic, oral-maxillofacial, or plastic surgical services in adulthood.

FAMILY CONCERNS
- There is a heightened awareness of physical appearance.
- Presurgical photographs are important.
- Speech, audiology, and dental issues are challenging for families.
- Orthodontic treatment may span over 10 years.
- Cultural superstitions are common regarding the etiology of clefts.
- Multiple surgical procedures during childhood are stressful for families.

REFERENCES

Agrawal, K., & Panda, K. (2006). Use of vomer flap in palatoplasty: Revisited. *The Cleft Palate-Craniofacial Journal, 43*(1), 30–37. doi:10.1597/04-034.1.

American Academy of Pediatrics (AAP), American Academy of Family Physicians (AAFP), Subcommittee on Management of Acute Otitis Media, (2004). Diagnosis and management of acute otitis media. *Pediatrics, 113,* 1451–1465.

American Cleft Palate–Craniofacial Association. (2004). Parameters for evaluation and treatment of patients with cleft lip/palate or other craniofacial anomalies. In *Official Publication of the American Cleft Palate–Craniofacial Association* (rev. ed.). Chapel Hill, NC: Author.

American Cleft Palate-Craniofacial Association (2014). *ACPA family services: Prenatal diagnosis.* Available at https://acpa-cpf.org/wp-content/uploads/2019/03/ACPA_booklet_prenatal.pdf. Retrieved on September 9, 2022.

American Cleft Palate-Craniofacial Association (2019). *Standards for approval of cleft palate and craniofacial teams.* Available at https://acpa-cpf.org/wp-content/uploads/2019/04/Standards-2019-Update.pdf. Retrieved September 9, 2022.

American Speech-Language-Hearing Association (n.d.). *Cleft lip and palate.* Available at www.asha.org/Practice-Portal/Clinical-Topics/Cleft-Lip-and-Palate. Retrieved September 9, 2022.

Anderson, K. D., Cole, A., Chuo, C. B., & Slator, R. (2007). Home management of upper airway obstruction in Pierre Robin sequence using a nasopharyngeal airway. *Cleft Palate Craniofacial Journal, 44*(3), 269–273.

Aniansson, G., Svensson, H., Becker, M., & Ingvarsson, L. (2002). Otitis media and feeding with breast milk of children with cleft palate. *Scandinavian Journal of Plastic and Reconstructive Surgery and Hand Surgery, 36*(1), 9–15. doi:10.1080/028443102753478318.

Arosarena, O. (2007). Cleft lip and palate. *Otolaryngologic Clinics of North America, 40,* 27–60.

Bender, P. L. (2000). Genetics of cleft lip and palate. *Journal of Pediatric Nursing, 15,* 242–249.

Bennett, S., & Indman, P. (2006). *Beyond the blues: A guide to understanding and treating prenatal and postpartum depression.* San Jose, CA: Moodswings Press.

Bluestone, C. D. (2004). Studies in otitis media: Children's Hospital of Pittsburgh–University of Pittsburgh progress report—2004. *Laryngoscope, 114,* 1–26.

Carbonell, R., & Ruiz-Garcia, V. (2002). Ventilation tubes after surgery for otitis media with effusion or acute otitis media and swimming. Systematic review and meta-analysis. *International Journal of Pediatric Otorhinolaryngology, 66*(3), 281–289.

Centers for Disease Control and Prevention (2020). *Cleft lip/cleft palate.* Available at https://www.cdc.gov/ncbddd/birthdefects/cleftlip.html. Retrieved September 9, 2022.

Charkins, H. (1996). *Children with facial differences: A parent's guide.* Bethesda, MD: Woodbine House.

Cheng, L., Moor, S., & Ho, C. (2007). Predisposing factors to dental caries in children with cleft lip and palate: A review and strategies for early prevention. *Cleft Palate Craniofacial Journal, 44*(1), 67–72.

Children's Hospital of Philadelphia (n.d.) *Cleft lip and palate repair surgery.* Available at https://www.chop.edu/treatments/surgical-repair-cleft-lip-and-palate. Retrieved September 9, 2022.

Craven, C., Cole, P., Hollier, L., & Stal, S. (2007). Ensuring success in alveolar bone grafting: A three-dimensional approach. *Journal of Craniofacial Surgery, 18*(4), 855–859.

Curtin, G. (1990). The infant with cleft lip or palate: More than a surgical problem. *Journal of Perinatal and Neonatal Nursing, 3,* 80–89.

Daskalogiannakis, J., Ross, R., & Tompson, B. (2001). The mandibular catch-up growth controversy in Pierre Robin sequence. *American Journal of Orthodontics and Dentofacial Orthopedics, 120*(3), 280–285.

El-Ashmawi, N., ElKordy, S., Salah Fayed, M., El-Beialy, A., & Attia, K. (2019). Effectiveness of gingivoperiosteoplasty on alveolar bone reconstruction and facial growth in patients with cleft lip and palate: A systematic review and meta-analysis. *The Cleft Palate-Craniofacial Journal, 56*(4), 438–453. doi:10.1177/1055665618788421.

Endriga, M. C., & Kapp-Simon, K. A. (1999). Psychological issues in craniofacial care, state of the art. *Cleft Palate Craniofacial Journal, 36*(1), 3–11.

ERAS Society (n.d.) *ERAS society guidelines.* Available at https://erassociety.org/guidelines. Retrieved September 9, 2022.

Fetal Medicine Foundation (2022). *Facial cleft.* Available at https://fetalmedicine.org/education/fetal-abnormalities/face/facial-cleft#:~:text=Unilateral%20in%2075%25%20of%20cases%20%28more%20common%20on,cavity%20or%20even%20the%20floor%20of%20the%20orbit. Retrieved September 9, 2022.

Gailey, D. G. (2016). Feeding infants with cleft and the postoperative cleft management. *Oral and Maxillofacial Surgery Clinics of North America, 28*(2), 153–159. doi: 10.1016/j.coms.2015.12.003. PMID: 27150302.

Goldstein, N. A., Mandel, E. M., Kurs-Lasky, M., Rockette, H. E., & Casselbrant, M. L. (2005). Water precautions and tympanostomy tubes: A randomized, controlled trial. *Laryngoscope, 115*(2), 324–330. doi:10.1097/01.mlg.0000154742.33067.fb.

Good, P., Mulliken, J., & Padwa, B. (2007). Frequency of LeFort I osteotomy after repaired cleft lip and palate or cleft palate. *Cleft Palate Craniofacial Journal, 44*(4), 396–401.

Gorlin, R. Y., Cohen, M. M., & Hennekam, R. C. (2001). Orofacial clefting syndromes: General aspects. In Gorlin, R. Y., Cohen, M. M., & Hennekam, R. C. (Eds.), *Syndromes of the head and neck* (4th ed.). New York: Oxford University Press.

Gungor, A., & Bluestone, C. D. (2001). Antibiotic theory in otitis media. *Current Allergy and Asthma Reports, 1*(4), 364–372.

Henningsson, G., Kuehn, D. P., Sell, D., Sweeney, T., Trost-Cardamone, J. E., & Whitehill, T. L.; Speech Parameters Group. (2008). Universal parameters for reporting speech outcomes in individuals with cleft palate. *Cleft Palate Craniofacial Journal, 45*(1), 1–17. doi:10.1597/06-086.1.

Houkes, R., Smit, J., Mossey, P., Don Griot, P., Persson, M., Neville, A., Ongkosuwito, E., Sitzman, T., & Breugem, C. (2023). Classification systems of cleft lip, alveolus and palate: Results of an international survey. *Cleft Palate Craniofacial Journal, 60*(2), 189–196. doi: 10.1177/10556656211057368. Epub 2021 Nov 23.

Hunt, O., Burden, D., Hepper, P., Stevenson, & M., Johnston, C. (2006). Self-reports of psychosocial functioning among children and young adults with cleft lip and palate. *Cleft Palate Craniofacial Journal, 43*(5), 598–605. doi:10.1597/05-080.

Isaac, K. & Chong, D. (2020). von Langenbeck palatoplasty. Available at https://plasticsurgerykey.com/von-langenbeck-palatoplasty/. Retrieved on September 9, 2022.

Jones, K. L. (2006). *Smith's recognizable patterns of human malformation* (6th ed.). Philadelphia: Elsevier Saunders.

Kimberlin, D., Barnett, E. D., Lynfield, R., & Sawyer, M. (2021). *Red book 2021: Report of the Committee on Infectious Diseases* (32nd ed.). American Academy of Pediatrics.

Klein, T., Pope, A. W., Getahun, E., & Thompson, J. (2006). Mothers' reflections on raising a child with a craniofacial anomaly. *Cleft Palate Craniofacial Journal, 43*(5), 590–597. doi:10.1597/05-117.

Koul, R. (2007). Describing cleft lip and palate using a new expression system. *Cleft Palate Craniofacial Journal, 44*(6), 595–597.

Kramer, F. J., Baethge, C., Swennen, G., Bremer, B., Schwestka-Polly, R., & Dempf, R. (2005). Dental implants in patients with orofacial clefts: A long-term follow-up study. *International Journal of Oral and Maxillofacial Surgery, 34*(7), 715–721. doi:10.1016/j.ijom.2005.04.014.

Krishnamurthy, S., Debnath, S., & Gupta, P. (2011). Breast feeding-associated hypernatremic dehydration: A preventable tragedy in newborn infants. *Journal of Case Reports*, 1–5. https://doi.org/10.17659/01.2011.0001.

Kurnik, N. M., Calis, M., Sobol, D. L., Kapadia, H., Mercan, E., & Tse, R. W. (2021). A comparative assessment of nasal appearance following nasoalveolar molding and primary surgical repair for treatment of unilateral cleft lip and palate. *Plastic and Reconstructive Surgery, 148*(5), 1075–1084. doi:10.1097/PRS.0000000000008462.

Lansdon, L. A., Dickinson, A., Arlis, S., Liu, H., Hlas, A., Hahn, A., Bonde, G., Long, A., Standley, J., Tyryshkina, A., Wehby, G., Lee, N. R., Daack-Hirsch, S., Mohlke, K., Girirajan, S., Darbro, B. W., Cornell, R. A., Houston, D. W., Murray, J. C., & Manak, J. R. (2023). Genome-wide analysis of copy-number variation in humans with cleft lip and/or cleft palate identifies Cobll1, ric1, and ARHGEF38 as clefting genes. *The American Journal of Human Genetics, 110*(1), 71–91. https://doi.org/10.1016/j.ajhg.2022.11.012.

Lin-Shiao, E., Lan, Y., Welzenbach, J., Alexander, K. A., Zhang, Z., Knapp, M., Mangold, E., Sammons, M., Ludwig, K. U., & Berger, S. L. (2019). p63 establishes epithelial enhancers at critical craniofacial development genes. *Science Advances, 5*(5), eaaw0946. doi:10.1126/sciadv.aaw0946.

Lous, J., Burton, M. J., Felding, J. U., Ovesen, T., Rovers, M. M., & Williamson, I. (2005). Grommets (ventilation tubes) for hearing loss associated with otitis media with effusion in children. *Cochrane Database of Systematic Reviews, 25*(1), CD011801. doi:10.1002/14651858. CD001801.pub2. Update in: Cochrane Database Syst Rev. 2010;(10):CD001801.

Masarei, A. G., Wade, A., Mars, M., Sommerlad, B. C., & Sell, D. (2007). A randomized control trial investigating the effect of presurgical orthopedics on feeding in infants with cleft lip and/or palate. *Cleft Palate Craniofacial Journal, 44*(2), 182–193. doi:10.1597/05-184.1.

Millard, T., & Richman, L. C. (2001). Different cleft conditions, facial appearance, and speech: Relationship to psychological variables. *Cleft Palate Craniofacial Journal, 38*(1), 68–75.

Moggi, L., Ventorutti, T., & Bennun, R. (2020). Cleft palate repair: A new maxillary nerve block approach. *Journal of Craniofacial Surgery, 31*(6), 1547–1550. doi:10.1097/SCS.0000000000006633.

Moller, K. T., Starr, C. D., & Johnson, S. A. (1990). *A parent's guide to cleft lip and palate*. Minneapolis: University of Minnesota Press.

Mulliken, J. (2004). The changing faces of children with cleft lip and palate. *New England Journal of Medicine, 351*(8), 745–747.

Muntz, H. R. (1993). An overview of middle ear disease in cleft palate children. *Facial and Plastic Surgery, 9*, 177–180.

Muntz, H., Wilson, M., Park, A., Smith, M., & Grimmer, J. F. (2008). Sleep disordered breathing and obstructive sleep apnea in the cleft population. *Laryngoscope, 118*(2), 348–353. doi:10.1097/MLG.0b013e318158195e.

Murray, J. C. (2002). Gene/environment causes of cleft lip and/or palate. *Clinical Genetics, 61*(4), 248–256.

MyFace (n.d.). *Cleft lip and/or palate*. Available at https://www.myface.org/craniofacial-conditions/cleft-lip-and-or-palate/?nowprocket=1#prevalence. Retrieved September 9, 2022.

Oberoi, S., Chigurupati, R., & Vargervik, K. (2008). Morphologic and management characteristics of individuals with unilateral cleft lip and palate who require maxillary advancement. *Cleft Palate Craniofacial Journal, 45*(1), 42–49.

Overturf, G. D. (2000). American Academy of Pediatrics Committee on Infectious Diseases technical report: Prevention of pneumococcal infections, including the use of pneumococcal conjugate and polysaccharide vaccines and antibiotic prophylaxis. *Pediatrics, 106*, 367–376.

Paradise, J. L., Elster, B. A., & Tan, L. (1994). Evidence in infants with cleft palate that breast milk protects against otitis media. *Pediatrics, 94*, 853–860.

Peterson-Falzone, S., Hardin-Jones, M., & Karnell, M. (2001). *Cleft palate speech* (3rd ed.). St. Louis: Mosby.

Prahl, C., Kuijpers-Jagtman, A. M., Van't Hof, M. A., & Prahl-Andersen, B. (2005). Infant orthopedics in UCLP: Effect on feeding, weight, and length: A randomized clinical trial (Dutchcleft). *Cleft Palate Craniofacial Journal, 42*(2), 171–177. doi:10.1597/03-111.1.

Prescott, N. J., Natalie, J., & Malcolm, S. (2002). Folate and the face: Evaluating the evidence for the influence of folate genes on craniofacial development. *Cleft Palate Craniofacial Journal, 39*(3), 327–331.

Reilly, S., Reid, J., Skeat, J., & Academy of Breastfeeding Medicine Clinical Protocol Committee. (2007). ABM protocols. *Breastfeeding Medicine, 2*(2), 243–248.

Richman, L. C., McCoy, T. E., Conrad, A. L., & Nopoulos, P. C. (2012). Neuropsychological, behavioral, and academic sequelae of cleft: Early developmental, school age, and adolescent/young adult outcomes. *Cleft Palate Craniofacial Journal, 49*(4), 387–396. doi:10.1597/10-237. PMID: 21905907; PMCID: PMC3408555.

Romitti, P. A., Sun, L., Honein, M. A., Reefhuis, J., Correa, A., & Rasmussen, S. A. (2007). Maternal periconceptional alcohol consumption and risk of orofacial clefts. *American Journal of Epidemiology, 166*(7), 775–785. doi:10.1093/aje/kwm146.

Sidman, J. D., Sampson, D., & Templeton, B. (2001). Distraction osteogenesis of the mandible for airway obstruction in children. *Laryngoscope, 111*, 1137–1146.

Sie, K. C., Tampakopoulou, D. A., Sorom, J., Gruss, J. S., & Eblen, L. E. (2001). Results with Furlow palatoplasty in management of velopharyngeal insufficiency. *Plastic and Reconstructive Surgery, 108*(1), 17–25, discussion 26-9. doi:10.1097/00006534-200107000-00004.

Singhal, M. (2022). Nutritional needs of cleft lip and palate child. *Journal of Cleft Lip Palate and Craniofacial Anomalies, 9*, 69–73.

Sitzman, T. J., Verhey, E. M., Kirschner, R. E., Pollard, S. H., Baylis, A. L., & Chapman, K. L. (2022). Cleft Outcomes Research NETwork (CORNET) Consortium. Cleft palate repair postoperative management: Current practices in the United States. *Cleft Palate Craniofacial Journal*, 10556656221146891. doi:10.1177/1055665221146891.

Smith, M. C., & Senders, C. W. (2006). Prognosis of airway obstruction and feeding difficulty in the Robin sequence. *International Journal of Pediatric Otorhinolaryngology, 70*(2), 319–324.

Stanier, P., & Moore, G. (2004). Genetics of cleft lip and palate: Syndromic genes contribute to the incidence of non-syndromic clefts. *Human Molecular Genetics, 13*(review issue 1), 73–81.

Stock, N. M., Marik, P., Magee, L., Aspinall, C. L., Garcia, L., Crerand, C., & Johns, A. (2020). Facilitating positive psychosocial outcomes in craniofacial team care: Strategies for medical providers. *Cleft Palate Craniofacial Journal, 57*(3), 333–343. doi:10.1177/1055665619868052. PMID: 31446785.

St. Hilaire, H., & Buchbinder, D. (2000). Maxillofacial pathology and management of Pierre Robin sequence. *Otolaryngology Clinics of North America, 33*(6), 1241–1258.

Strauss, R. P. (2001). "Only skin deep": Health, resilience, and craniofacial care. *Cleft Palate Craniofacial Journal, 38*(3), 226–230.

Swanson, J. W. (2022). *Global cleft care in low-resource settings.* Springer Nature.

Tse, R. (2012). Unilateral cleft lip: Principles and practice of surgical management. *Seminars in Plastic Surgery, 26*(4), 145–155. https://doi.org/10.1055/s-0033-1333884.

Valtonen, H., Dietz, A., & Qvarnberg, Y. (2005). Long-term clinical, audiologic, and radiologic outcomes in palate cleft children treated with early tympanostomy for otitis media with effusion: A controlled prospective study. *Laryngoscope, 115*(8), 1512–1516.

Vieira, A. (2008). Unraveling human cleft lip and palate research. *Journal of Dental Research, 87*(2), 119–125.

Wang, H., Zhang, T., Wu, T., Hetmanski, J. B., Ruczinski, I., Schwender, H., Liang, K. Y., Murray, T., Fallin, M. D., Redett, R. J., Raymond, G. V., Jin, S. C., Chou, Y. H., Chen, P. K., Yeow, V., Chong, S. S., Cheah, F. S., Jee, S. H., Jabs, E. W., ... Beaty, T. H. (2013). The FGF and FGFR gene family and risk of cleft lip with or without cleft palate. *Cleft Palate Craniofacial Journal, 50*(1), 96–103. doi:10.1597/11-132.

Wilkins-Haug, L. (2022). Etiology, prenatal diagnosis, obstetric management, and recurrence of cleft lip and/or palate. *UpToDate.* Available at: https://www.uptodate.com/contents/etiology-prenatal-diagnosis-obstetric-management-and-recurrence-of-cleft-lip-and-or-palate?search=cleft%20lip%20palate&source=search_result&selectedTitle=1~150&usage_type=default&display_rank=1. Retrieved September 9, 2022.

Willner, J. P. (2000). Genetic evaluation and counseling in head and neck syndromes. *Otolaryngology Clinics of North America, 33*(6), 1159–1169.

Ysunza, A., Pamplona, M. C., Mendoza, M., Molina, F., Martinez, P., García-Velasco, M., & Prada, N. (2001). Surgical treatment of submucous cleft palate: A comparative trial of two modalities for palatal closure. *Plastic and Reconstructive Surgery, 107*(1), 9–14. doi:10.1097/00006534-200101000-00002.

17

Congenital Adrenal Hyperplasia*

Teresa Whited

ETIOLOGY

Congenital adrenal hyperplasia (CAH) encompasses a family of autosomal recessive disorders involving impaired synthesis of cortisol by five enzymes in the adrenal cortex that causes an overproduction of androgens (Allis, 2021; Narasimhan & Khattab, 2018). The most common is 21-hydroxylase deficiency (21-OHD), accounting for 95% of all forms of CAH (Merke & Auchus, 2020; Narasimhan & Khattab, 2018). Other forms are rare and account for less than 5% of all cases, with presentation usually in adolescence and adulthood; these will not be discussed here (Auchus, 2022; Merke & Auchus, 2020).

The adrenal cortex synthesizes mineralocorticoids (mainly aldosterone), glucocorticoids (primarily cortisol), and androgens (male hormones) through three separate metabolic pathways (Fig. 17.1). Cortisol, aldosterone, and adrenal androgens play a crucial role in maintaining homeostasis by helping to regulate the body's blood pressure; glucose, sodium, and water levels; sexual development; and other metabolic processes (Allis, 2021; Narasimhan & Khattab, 2018) Cortisol is particularly crucial in the mediation of the body's response to stress. An adrenal crisis results in hypotension, shock, and electrolyte abnormalities, most commonly hypoglycemia, hyponatremia, and hyperkalemia (Yau et al., 2019).

A feedback system regulates the adrenal production of glucocorticoids in the hypothalamus and pituitary gland (Fig. 17.2). The hypothalamus secretes corticotropin-releasing factor, which causes the pituitary gland to produce adrenocorticotropic hormone (ACTH), which stimulates the adrenals to produce cortisol. Cortisol feeds back to the hypothalamus and pituitary, reducing the release of corticotropin-releasing hormone and ACTH and thus the level of adrenal stimulation. In CAH the block at 21-hydroxylase leads to decreased cortisol production, which means less feedback and therefore ever-increasing stimulation of the adrenals by ACTH, causing hypertrophy of the gland. Because the androgen pathway is upstream of the block, androgens (dehydroepiandrosterone, Δ4-androstenedione) are overproduced (Allis, 2021; Yau et al., 2019).

In severe cases of CAH, where the 21-hydroxylase enzyme is completely or nearly completely inactive, these high levels of androgens lead to in utero virilization of females, causing them to be born with ambiguous genitalia (Fig. 17.3). Males are generally normal in appearance. Without treatment in the first several weeks after birth, the lack of cortisol and aldosterone can result in salt loss, hypovolemic shock, and death (i.e., adrenal crisis) (Merke & Auchus, 2020).

CLASSIFICATION

21-OHD CAH occurs in classic and nonclassic forms. In the classic form, prenatal exposure to potent androgens such as testosterone and Δ4-androstenedione at critical stages of sexual differentiation virilizes the external genitalia of genetic females, often resulting in genital ambiguity at birth. The classic form is further divided into the simple virilizing form (~25%) and the salt-wasting form, in which aldosterone production is inadequate (~75%) (Carvalho et al., 2022).

Individuals with the nonclassic form of 21-OHD CAH have only mild to moderate enzyme deficiency and postnatally have signs of hyperandrogenism; females with the nonclassic form are not virilized at birth (New et al., 2019).

This classification system is somewhat arbitrary and misleading because it suggests a qualitative difference among the groups. In reality there is a continuum of severity, from mild to severe, based on the specific combination of 21-hydroxylase gene defects with variable phenotypic expression occurring based on the severity or type of genetic mutation (Merke & Auchus, 2020). The term non–salt wasting should be used with caution because it is now well appreciated that all affected children are salt wasters to some extent (Twayana et al., 2022). Neonatal mass screening has variable cutoffs from state to state and may not detect nonclassic CAH; most are found after puberty because of symptoms of androgen excess or in the course of family studies (Draznin et al., 2022; Edelman et al., 2020).

GENETIC ETIOLOGY

CAH is an autosomal recessive disease—two defective genes must be inherited (one from the mother, one from the father) for the disease to manifest. Most children with CAH are compound heterozygotes (Merke & Auchus, 2020; Narasimhan & Khattab, 2018), having

*The author gratefully acknowledges the contribution of Betty Flores, Judy Ruble, and Angelique M. Champeau, the authors of this chapter in previous editions.

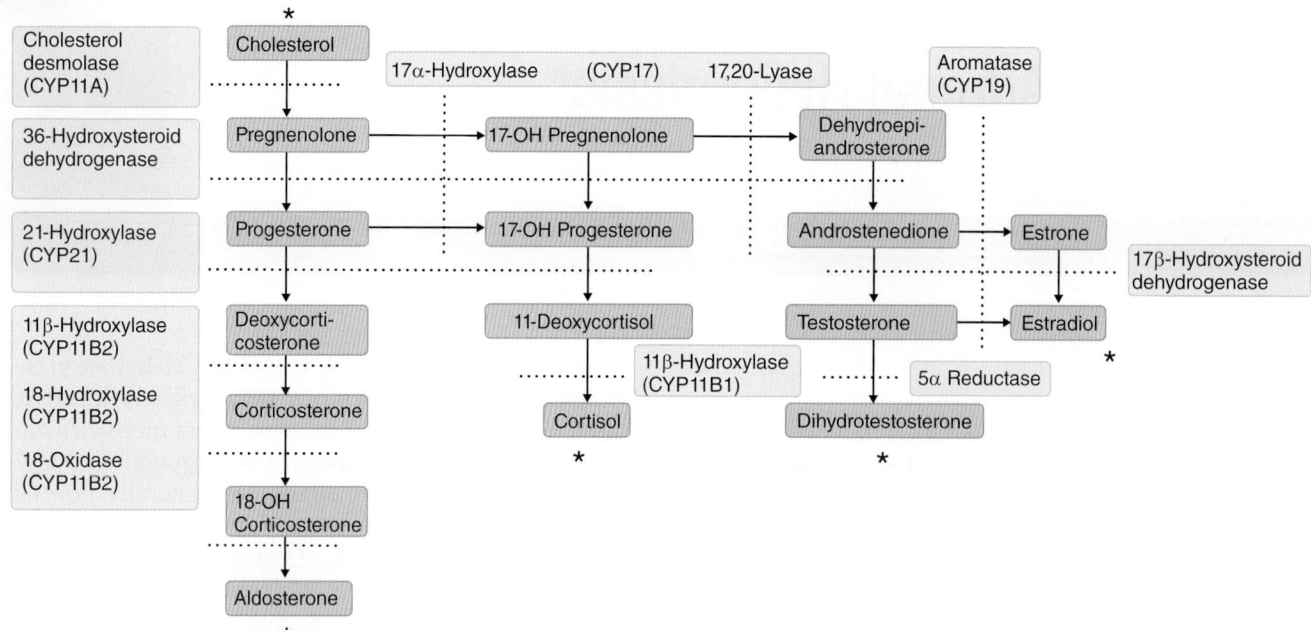

Fig. 17.1 Adrenal steroid pathway for mineralocorticoids, glucocorticoids, and androgens. (From Goldman L, Schafer AI, editors. *Goldman-Cecil Medicine*, 26th ed. Elsevier; 2020.)

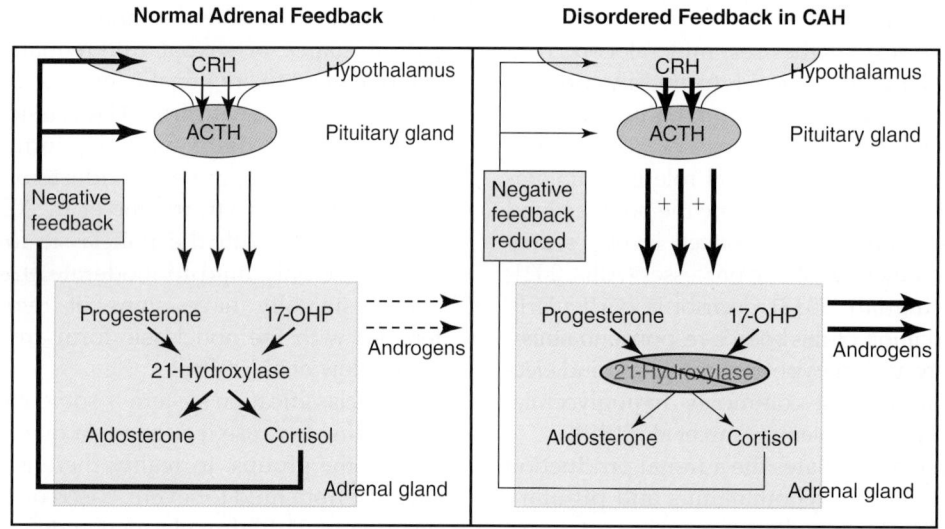

Fig. 17.2 Hypothalamic/pituitary/adrenal feedback loop in normal subjects and in those with congenital adrenal hyperplasia *(CAH)*. Note that in CAH, corticotropin-releasing hormone *(CRH)* and adrenocorticotropic hormone *(ACTH)* are increased because of decreased cortisol feedback. This leads to adrenal gland hypertrophy and a buildup of upstream steroids—progesterone and 17-hydroxyprogesterone *(17-OHP)*, which are then shunted toward androgen production.

inherited a different mutation from each of their parents. If a null or no enzyme activity mutation is inherited from both parents, usually from a large deletion or mutation, then the child will be severely affected (classic salt wasting). If two mild defects are inherited, then the child will be mildly affected (nonclassic). Those who inherit a null or no enzyme activity mutation from one parent and a less severe mutation from the other will fall somewhere in between, usually resulting in a simple virilizing form (Merke & Auchus, 2020).

The gene for adrenal 21-hydroxylase, *CYP21A2*, and a pseudogene, *CYP21A2p*, are located on chromosome 6p21.3 within the human leukocyte antigen gene cluster and are about 30 kb apart (Krone & Arlt, 2009). The major mechanism by which the active gene acquires defects is via the transfer of segments from the pseudogene to the active gene. To date, hundreds of different *CYP21* mutations have been reported that are mostly point mutations, but small deletions or insertions have also been described as well as complete gene deletions and complex gene rearrangements. Typically the

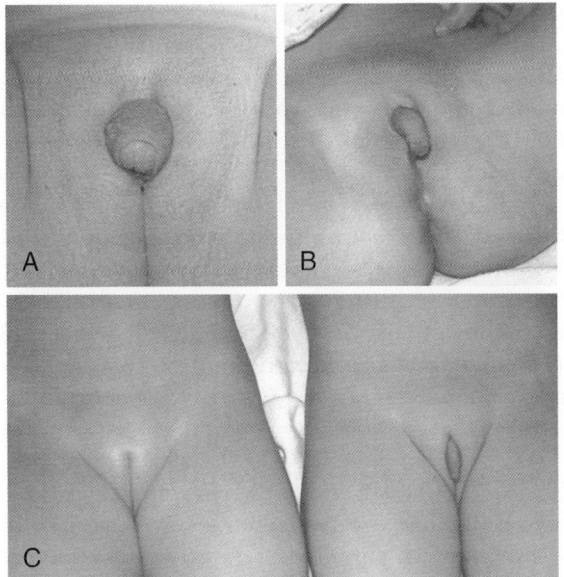

Fig. 17.3 Examples of ambiguous genitalia. (A) A female infant with congenital adrenal hyperplasia (CAH), and (B) a toddler with CAH. (C) Fraternal twins (age 3 years), one with CAH and the other unaffected, highlight the difference in clitoral development.

larger the deletion, the greater the impact on cortisol production (large deletions) versus pinpoint deletions, which can result in milder forms of the disease process (Karlsson et al., 2019; Narasimhan & Khattab, 2018).

Parents

Most parents are heterozygotes with one normal allele and one mutated allele. Heterozygotes are asymptomatic but may have slightly elevated 17-hydroxyprogesterone (17-OHP) levels when stimulated with ACTH, as compared with individuals with two normal alleles. Approximately 1% of mutations occur de novo, and thus 1% of affected children have only one parent who is heterozygous (Witchell, 2017). In some instances a parent who was previously not known to be affected may be found to have the nonclassic form of 21-OHD CAH. It is appropriate to evaluate both parents with molecular genetic testing and hormonal profiling to determine if either has nonclassic 21-OHD CAH when an offspring is affected by CAH.

Siblings

If the parents of an affected child are both heterozygotes, each sibling has a 25% chance of inheriting both altered alleles and being affected, a 50% chance of inheriting one altered allele and being an unaffected carrier, and a 25% chance of inheriting both normal alleles and being unaffected. Once an at-risk sibling is known to be unaffected, the risk of the sibling being a carrier is two-thirds. If one parent is heterozygous and the other has 21-OHD CAH, each sibling has a 50% chance of inheriting both mutated alleles and being affected and a 50% chance of inheriting one mutated allele and being a carrier.

Offspring of an Affected Individual

An affected individual transmits one disease-causing allele to each child. Given the high carrier rate for 21-OHD CAH, it is appropriate to offer molecular genetic testing of the *CYP21A2* gene to the reproductive partner of an affected individual. If the reproductive partner is determined not to be a carrier, the prospective child has a significantly decreased risk of having 21-OHD. If the reproductive partner is determined to be heterozygous for an identified mutation, then the risk to each prospective child of being affected is 50% (Gomes et al., 2019; New et al., 2019).

Carrier Detection

Carrier testing using molecular genetic testing of the *CYP21A2* gene is available to at-risk relatives when one or both disease-causing mutations have been identified in the affected individual.

INCIDENCE AND PREVALENCE

CLASSIC 21-HYDROXYLASE CONGENITAL ADRENAL HYPERPLASIA

The estimated incidence of classic CAH is between 1 in 9000 and 1 in 18,000 based on neonatal and national registry cases (Speiser et al., 2018; Navarro-Zambrana & Sheets, 2022). However, certain ethnic groups and regions have a higher incidence than those from the eastern Mediterranean and Southeast Asia, with the highest overall rates of CAH (Navarro-Zambrana & Sheets, 2022). Native Alaskans and the Canadian Yupik have the highest incidence of the classic form of CAH, with estimates of 1 in 282 (Speiser et al., 2018). The incidence is lower in Blacks (1 in 42,000) when compared to Whites (1 in 15,500) in the United States (Carvalho et al., 2022; Merke & Auchus, 2020).

NONCLASSIC 21-HYDROXYLASE CONGENITAL ADRENAL HYPERPLASIA

Nonclassic 21-OHD CAH is much more common, but data are more variable. It is estimated that nonclassic CAH is humans' most common autosomal recessive disease (Speiser et al., 2018). The prevalence of nonclassic 21-OHD CAH in the general heterogeneous population was estimated between 1 in 100 and 1 in 200 (Hannah-Shmouni et al., 2017; Speiser et al., 2018). Furthermore, the nonclassic prevalence was broken down, with the highest prevalence found in Ashkenazi Jews, with 3.7% affected and 30% as carriers (Hannah-Shmouni et al., 2017).

DIAGNOSTIC CRITERIA

A diagnosis of 21-OHD should be considered in any newborn infant with genital ambiguity, salt wasting, or hypotension (Speiser et al., 2018).

A multidisciplinary team of specialists in pediatric endocrinology, pediatric urology, medical genetics, and psychology is essential for diagnosing and managing an individual with ambiguous genitalia (Merke, 2021).

17-HYDROXYPROGESTERONE

Newborns with either form of classic CAH will have significantly elevated 17-OHP levels by 24 to 36 hours of age. False-positive results are possible in premature or low-birth-weight infants; therefore in these infants serial measurements of 17-OHP may be necessary (Draznin et al., 2022).

PLASMA RENIN

Plasma renin activity (PRA) is markedly elevated in individuals with salt-wasting 21-OHD and can be elevated in some with simple virilizing 21-OHD (Carvalho et al., 2022). Direct measurement of active renin can also be used. In salt-wasting 21-OHD, the serum concentration of aldosterone is inappropriately low compared with the degree of PRA elevation (Carvalho et al., 2022).

OTHER ADRENAL STEROIDS

Δ^4-Androstenedione and progesterone are increased in males and females. Serum concentrations of testosterone and adrenal androgen precursors are increased in affected females and prepubertal males (Allis, 2021).

ACTH STIMULATION TEST

The serum concentration of 17-OHP and Δ^4-androstenedione measured at baseline and 60 minutes after intravenous (IV) administration of a standard bolus of synthetic ACTH are plotted on a normogram. Although the ACTH stimulation test provides a far more reliable diagnosis of 21-OHD CAH than a test of baseline values alone, the results must be confirmed with molecular genetic testing (Yau et al., 2019).

ELECTROLYTES

Children with untreated or poorly controlled salt-wasting CAH may have decreased levels of sodium, chloride, and carbon dioxide; increased potassium; and an inappropriately increased urine concentration of sodium (Twayana et al., 2022).

KARYOTYPE

Females have normal 46,XX, and males have normal 46,XY chromosomes.

MOLECULAR GENETIC TESTING

Molecular genetic analysis is not essential for the diagnosis but may be helpful to confirm the basis of the defect, carrier testing, prenatal testing, genotype/phenotype correlation for management, preimplantation genetic diagnosis, and to establish the diagnosis in uncertain cases (Draznin et al., 2022; Speiser et al., 2018).

Genetic testing methods include targeted mutation analysis, deletion/duplication, and sequence analysis. In targeted mutation analysis, the *CYP21A2* gene is tested for a panel of common mutations and gene deletions. This detects 80% to 98% of disease-causing alleles in affected individuals (Narasimhan & Khattab, 2018). Deletion/duplication analysis detects about 20% of mutant alleles and uses Southern blot analysis to detect large deletions. Last, entire gene sequencing (sequence analysis) may detect rare alleles not detected by targeted mutation or deletion/duplication analysis (Baumgartner-Parzer et al., 2020).

GENOTYPE-PHENOTYPE CORRELATIONS

A strong correlation between the severity of the clinical disease and the mutation is generally observed. However, for reasons that are not understood, genotype does not always predict phenotype within mutation-identical groups or even within the same family (Narasimhan & Khattab, 2018) (Box 17.1).

Box 17.1 Evaluations at Initial Diagnosis to Establish the Extent of Disease

TO ASSESS FOR SALT WASTING
- Plasma renin activity or direct renin assay
- Serum electrolytes

TO DISTINGUISH CLASSIC AND NONCLASSIC FORMS OF 21-HYDROXYLASE DEFICIENCY CONGENITAL ADRENAL HYPERPLASIA
- Baseline 17-hydroxyprogesterone (17-OHP), Δ^4-androstenedione, cortisol, and aldosterone
- Adrenocorticotropic hormone stimulation test to compare the stimulated concentration of 17-OHP to the baseline level

TO ASSESS THE DEGREE OF PRENATAL VIRILIZATION IN FEMALES
- Careful physical examination of the external genitalia and its orifices
- Genitogram[a] to assess the anatomy of urethra, vagina, common urogenital sinus (high vs. low confluence)

TO ASSESS THE DEGREE OF POSTNATAL VIRILIZATION IN BOTH MALES AND FEMALES
- Bone maturation assessment by bone age
- Serum concentration of adrenal androgens (unconjugated dehydroepiandrosterone, Δ^4-androstenedione, and testosterone)

[a]A genitogram is a radiologic procedure that can help identify internal genital structures and define the level of the confluence (location where the urethra and vagina connect) of the common urogenital sinus in virilized females. If the confluence is closer to the bladder (high), the surgery to correct will be more complicated; if the confluence is closer to the perineum (low), the surgery will be less complicated. The evaluation of an infant with ambiguous genitalia includes a complete history, a physical examination, a reliable ultrasound of the internal genitalia and adrenals, and a genitogram; however, the diagnosis of 21-OHD CAH is made by biochemical findings.

PRENATAL SCREENING

As of December 2005, all 50 states within the United States, as well as Washington, DC, and Guam, are screening for CAH at birth (Edelman et al., 2020).

Neonatal mass screening for 21-OHD identifies both male- and female-affected infants, prevents incorrect sex assignment, and decreases mortality and morbidity rates; therefore newborn screening for CAH is beneficial and is recommended (Draznin et al., 2022; Edelman et al., 2020; Held et al., 2020).

Newborn screening is sufficiently specific and sensitive to detect almost all infants with classic CAH and some with nonclassic CAH. A sampling of blood spots should be performed, ideally between 48 and 72 hours of age, and sent to the screening laboratory without delay. At present, fluoroimmunoassay for 17-OHP is utilized in all states. The concentration of 17-OHP is measured on a filter paper blood-spot sample obtained by the heelstick technique as used for newborn screening for other disorders (Edelman et al., 2020).

The cost of screening is estimated to be about $150,000 per quality-adjusted life-year per case of CAH diagnosed, which is considered reasonable (Grosse & Vliet, 2020).

The infant mortality rate for CAH is estimated at 4% among those without newborn screening (Grosse & Vliet, 2020).

Only laboratories with excellent internal and external quality control that have demonstrated accuracy and a rapid turnaround time on a large number of samples should be used. The laboratory should report immediately any abnormal result to the practitioner responsible for the patient. A positive screening result needs to be confirmed.

There are potential false screening results. Samples taken in the first 24 hours of life are elevated in all infants and may give false positives. In addition, a false positive may occur in premature or low-birth-weight infants. Conversely, false negatives may occur in neonates receiving dexamethasone to manage unrelated problems. Some states require a second screen at 2 weeks of age to improve the detection of newborns (Edelman et al., 2020; Grosse & Vliet, 2020).

CLINICAL MANIFESTATIONS AT TIME OF DIAGNOSIS

The diagnosis of 21-OHD CAH is suspected in females who are virilized at birth (Fig. 17.4), who become virilized postnatally, or who have precocious puberty or adrenarche. In males, CAH is suspected with virilization in childhood and infants of either sex with a salt-wasting crisis in the first 4 weeks of life (Merke & Auchus, 2020).

 Clinical Manifestations at Time of Diagnosis

CLASSIC

Virilization
- Elevated 17-OHP (hydroxyprogesterone)

Electrolyte instability
- Vomiting, dehydration
- Failure to thrive
- Metabolic alkalosis

Adrenal crisis

NONCLASSIC

Female: virilization
Male: early beard growth, enlarged hallus with small testes
Both: accelerated growth, advanced bone age, premature adrenarche

CLASSIC SIMPLE VIRILIZING

Excess adrenal androgen production in utero results in genital virilization at birth in 46,XX females. In affected females the excess androgens result in varying degrees of enlargement of the clitoris, fusion of the labial scrotal folds, and formation of a common urogenital sinus (CUGS). A CUGS occurs when the vagina, because of internal fusion with the urethra, does not extend to the perineum. In males, antimüllerian hormone (AMH) is secreted by the testicles, preventing the development of internal female reproductive organs. In CAH there is no AMH secretion, and the müllerian ducts develop normally into the uterus and fallopian tubes. The examiner cannot differentiate between simple virilizing classic and salt-wasting classic CAH based on the degree of virilization at birth.

After birth, males and females with classic simple CAH who do not receive glucocorticoid replacement therapy develop signs of androgen excess, such as precocious development of pubic and axillary hair, acne, rapid linear growth, and advanced bone age. Untreated males have progressive penile enlargement and small testes. Untreated females have clitoral enlargement, hirsutism, male pattern baldness, menstrual abnormalities, and reduced fertility.

CLASSIC SALT-WASTING CONGENITAL ADRENAL HYPERPLASIA

Infants with renal salt wasting have poor feeding, weight loss, failure to thrive, vomiting, dehydration, hypotension, and hyponatremic-hyperkalemic metabolic acidosis progressing to adrenal crisis (azotemia vascular collapse, shock, and death). Adrenal crisis can occur as early as 1 to 4 weeks (Allis, 2021).

Affected males who are not detected in the newborn screening program are at high risk for a salt-wasting adrenal crisis because their normal genitalia does not alert medical professionals to their condition; they are often discharged from the hospital after birth without diagnosis and experience a salt-wasting crisis at home (Held et al., 2020). Conversely, the ambiguous genitalia of females with salt-wasting forms usually prompt diagnosis and treatment.

Prader scale

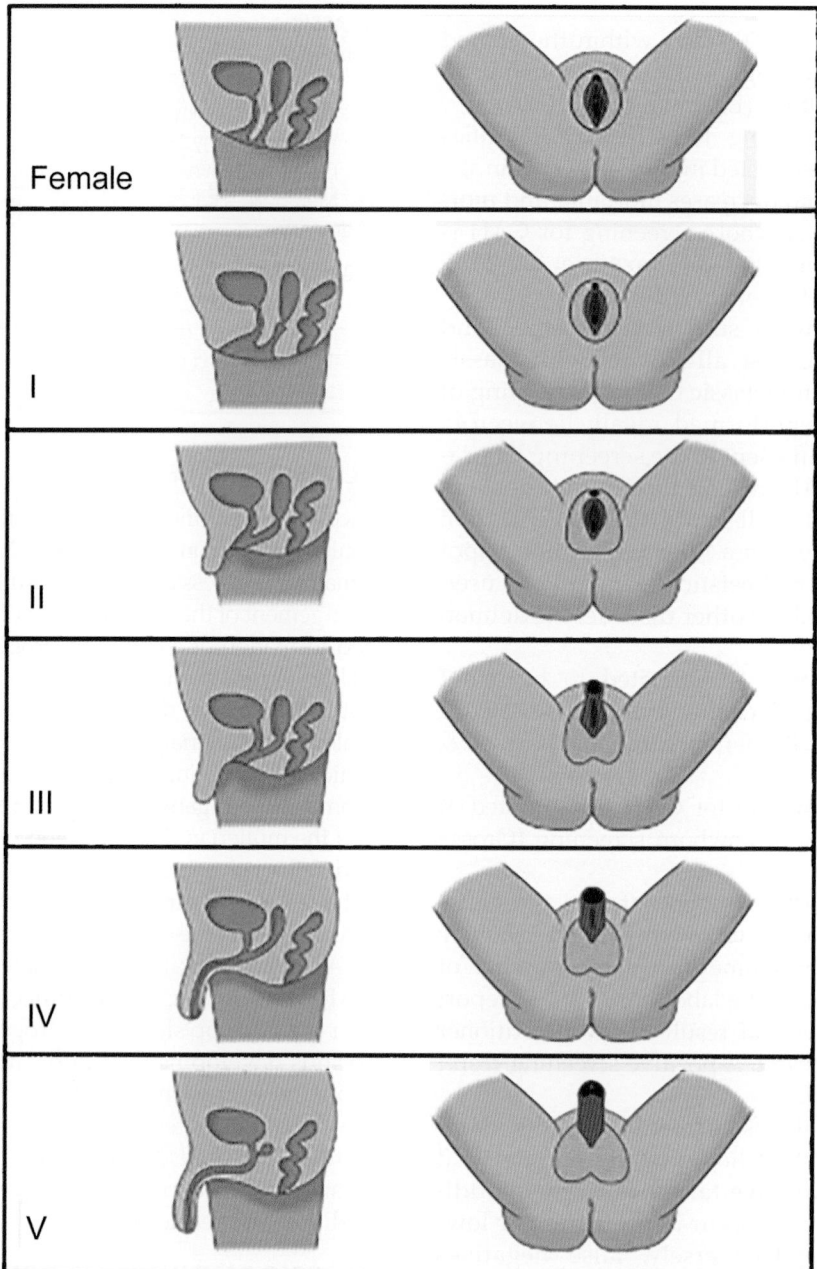

Fig. 17.4 **The continuum of virilization proposed by Prader.** Virilization ranges from mild clitoral enlargement (Prader I) to male-appearing phallus with penile urethra (Prader V). (From Obgyn Key. Operative concerns in patients with congenital anomalies of the reproductive tract and external genitalia for the obstetrician. Available at: https://obgynkey.com/operative-concerns-in-patients-with-congenital-anomalies-of-the-reproductive-tract-and-external-genitaliafor-the-obstetrician/).

NONCLASSIC CONGENITAL ADRENAL HYPERPLASIA

Nonclassic 21-OHD CAH may postnatally manifest with excess androgen symptoms, including acne, premature pubic hair, accelerated growth, and advanced bone age. These children may have reduced adult stature due to premature epiphyseal fusion.

Females with nonclassic CAH are born with normal genitalia; postnatal symptoms may include hirsutism, temporal baldness, delayed menarche, menstrual irregularities, and infertility. Among adult females with nonclassic CAH, about 60% have hirsutism only, about 10% have hirsutism and menstrual disorder, and 10% have menstrual disorder only. The fertility rate among untreated females is reported to be 50%. Many females with nonclassic forms develop polycystic ovaries (Haddad & Eugster, 2019; Livadas & Bothou, 2019; Neeman et al., 2019). Males with nonclassic CAH have early beard growth and enlarged phallus with relatively small testes. Mildly reduced cortisol synthesis is not clinically significant in nonclassic forms (Table 17.1).

		NEWBORN–2 YR (FEMALE)	
AGE AT DIAGNOSIS	**NEWBORN–6 MO**	**2–4 YR (MALE)**	**CHILD–ADULT**
Genitalia	Males normal Females ambiguous	Males normal Females ambiguous	Males normal Females virilized
Incidence	1:20,000	1:60,000	1:10,000
Hormones			
Aldosterone	Reduced	Normal	Normal
Renin	Increased	Normal or increased	Normal
Cortisol	Reduced	Reduced	Normal
17-OHP	>5000 nmol/L	2500–5000 nmol/L	500–2500 nmol/L (ACTH stimulation)
Growth	–2 to –3 SD	–1 to –2 SD	Probably normal
21-hydroxylase activity	0%	1–2%	20–60%

Table 17.1 Evaluation at Initial Diagnosis to Establish Extent of Condition

17-OHP, 17-hydroxyprogesterone; *ACTH*, adrenocorticotropic hormone; *SD*, standard deviation.
From Carvalho, B., Carvalho, F., & Carvalho, D. (2022). Congenital adrenal hyperplasia—the main effect of 21-hydroxylase deficiency. *Current Stages and New Perspectives on Disease Treatment*. https://www.intechopen.com/chapters/83494.

GROWTH

The initial growth in a child with CAH is rapid; however, potential height is reduced from premature epiphyseal fusion. Even if cortical replacement therapy is started at an early age and secretion of excess androgens is controlled, individuals do not usually achieve expected adult height. Actual bone age remains advanced compared with chronologic bone age (Haddad & Eugster, 2019; Yau et al., 2019).

PUBERTAL DEVELOPMENT

In males and females with proper therapy, puberty usually occurs at appropriate chronologic age. However, even when well controlled, there are exceptions. In some previously untreated children, starting glucocorticoid replacement therapy triggers true precocious puberty. This central precocious puberty may occur when glucocorticoid treatment releases the hypothalamic-pituitary axis from inhibition by estrogens derived from excess adrenal androgen secretion (Haddad & Eugster, 2019).

FERTILITY

Females may have issues with fertility because of elevated androgens leading to ovarian dysfunction, effects of genital surgery, progesterone hypersecretion, and less heterosexual partnerships (Gomes et al., 2019; Grinton et al., 2021; Reisch, 2019). Those affected by the nonclassic form are more likely to experience oligoovulation but may still benefit from glucocorticoid therapy (New et al., 2019). If pregnancy occurs, most are uneventful, but there is an increased risk of hypertension, gestational diabetes, and small for gestational age newborns (Badeghiesh et al., 2020).

In males the main cause of subfertility is the presence of testicular adrenal rest tumors, which are thought to originate from aberrant adrenal tissue and respond to treatment with glucocorticoids. Further, gonadotropic hypogonadism may result from the suppression of luteinizing hormone (LH) secretion by the pituitary by excessive adrenal androgens and their aromatization product (Reisch, 2019).

TREATMENT

 Treatment

CLASSIC
- Glucocorticoid replacement
- Mineralocorticoids and sodium chloride replacement
- Stress treatment
- Genital surgery
- Psychological assessment and support

NONCLASSIC
- Female: pregnancy

CLASSIC CONGENITAL ADRENAL HYPERPLASIA

The goal of treatment of classic 21-OHD CAH is to replace deficient steroids while minimizing adrenal sex hormone and glucocorticoid excess, preventing virilization, optimizing growth, and protecting potential fertility (Reisch, 2019). Treatment does not always mimic physiologic secretion, and the outcome is not always ideal.

Glucocorticoid Replacement

Treatment for CAH principally involves glucocorticoid replacement therapy usually in the form of hydrocortisone. Glucocorticoid therapy for children involves balancing suppression of adrenal androgen secretion against iatrogenic Cushing syndrome to maintain a normal linear growth rate and bone maturation. During infancy the initial reduction of markedly elevated adrenal sex hormones may require higher dosing.

Excessive doses, especially during infancy, may cause persistent growth suppression, obesity, and other cushingoid features (Merke, 2021). Therefore complete adrenal suppression should be avoided. Insufficient data exist to recommend higher morning or evening dosages. Overtreatment resulting in cushingoid features often occurs when the serum concentration of 17-OHP is reduced to the physiologic range for age. An acceptable range for serum concentration of 17-OHP in the treated individual is higher (100–1000 ng/dL) than normal provided androgens are maintained appropriately for gender and pubertal status.

Undertreatment will cause signs of adrenal insufficiency, impair the individual's response to stress, and lead to the overproduction of adrenal androgens, which will hasten epiphyseal maturation and closure, thus compromising ultimate adult height (Kim, 2022; Speiser et al., 2018).

During periods of stress (e.g., surgery, febrile illness, shock), all individuals with classic 21-OHD CAH require increased amounts of glucocorticoid. Typically, two to three times the normal dose is administered orally or by intramuscular (IM) injection when oral intake is not tolerated (Kim, 2022; Yau et al., 2019). Affected individuals should carry medical information regarding emergency steroid dosing.

Individuals with classic 21-OHD CAH require lifelong administration of glucocorticoids. After linear growth is complete, a more potent glucocorticoid (e.g., prednisone and dexamethasone) can be used. These should not be used in childhood because they tend to suppress growth. Prednisone and prednisolone need to be given twice daily. Prednisolone may be preferable because this is an active drug. Monitoring of these more potent glucocorticoids should include blood pressure, weight checks, and other clinical and laboratory variables. These steroids have minimal mineralocorticoid effects compared with hydrocortisone. In children with advanced bone age, such as in males with non–salt-losing CAH, initiation of therapy may precipitate central precocious puberty, requiring treatment with a gonadotropin-releasing hormone (GnRH) agonist (Merke, 2021; Speiser et al., 2018).

Mineralocorticoids and Sodium Chloride Replacement

Replacement therapy with mineralocorticoids is indicated for children with salt-losing CAH (Merke, 2021; Speiser et al., 2018). All children with classic CAH should be treated with fludrocortisones at diagnosis in the newborn period. Dosage requirements in early infancy may be higher than typical maintenance doses. The dose depends on the sodium intake. Such therapy will reduce vasopressin and ACTH levels and lower the dosage of glucocorticoid required. The need for continuing mineralocorticoid should be assessed based on PRA and blood pressure. Sodium chloride supplements are often needed in infancy and distributed in several feedings. Sodium chloride supplementation may not be necessary after infancy, and the amount of mineralocorticoid required daily may decrease with age.

Monitoring Treatment for Classic Congenital Adrenal Hyperplasia

Monitoring may be accomplished based on physical and hormonal findings suggestive of excessive or inadequate steroid therapy. Laboratory measurements may include serum/plasma electrolytes, serum 17-OHP, androstenedione and/or testosterone, and PRA or direct renin every 3 months during infancy and every 4 to 12 months after that. The time from the last glucocorticoid dose should be noted. The diurnal rhythm of the adrenal axis should be considered (Mallappa & Merke, 2022; Merke, 2021; Speiser et al., 2018).

Children receiving adequate replacement therapy may have hormone levels above the normal range. Alternative measurements include urinary metabolites (pregnanetriol) or filter paper blood and salivary hormones. Ideally, laboratory data will indicate a need for dosage adjustments before physical changes, growth, and skeletal maturation indicate inadequate or excessive dosing. Bone age to assess osseous maturation should be done at 12-month intervals beginning under the age of 2 years until near adult height is attained (Merke, 2021; Speiser et al., 2018).

Stress Treatment

Children with CAH should carry medical identification and information concerning therapy for stress. Caregivers should have an emergency supply of IM hydrocortisone or glucocorticoid suppositories. Because circulating cortisol levels normally increase during stress, children should be given increased doses of glucocorticoids during febrile illness (>38.5°C [>101°F]), when vomiting, or when unable to take oral feedings, after trauma, and before surgery. Participation in endurance sports may also require extra steroid dosing. Evidence has not shown that individuals need increased dosing for mental and emotional stress, such as school examinations. Stress dosing should be two to three times the maintenance glucocorticoid dose for children able to take oral medications. Glucose concentrations should be monitored, and IV sodium and glucose replacement may be required (Kim, 2022; Yau et al., 2019).

Genital Surgery

Deciding when, what type, and even if genital surgery should be performed in infants with genital ambiguity is the subject of continuing debate. Some adults with disorders of sexual development (not specific to 21-OHD CAH) who are unhappy with their gender assignment, as well as some medical professionals, advocate postponing genital surgery until the affected individual is able to provide informed consent. Others advocate that all children should have genital surgery early in life to match their gender of rearing and obviate any gender dysphoria (Almarsri et al., 2018; Speiser et al., 2018). Having better knowledge of the neuroanatomy of the genitalia and further knowledge about sexual function may provide an answer somewhere between these two views. It is important to remember that genital surgery is irreversible. Although concerns about undergoing irreversible genital surgery at a young age are valid, also valid are concerns regarding how families would accept raising a child with ambiguous genitalia and whether children reared as a gender not congruent with their external genitalia would be able to develop a clear gender identity.

It is recommended that parents be informed of surgical options, including the option to delay surgery until the child is older. Surgical decision making should be the family's prerogative and include joint decision making in older children. It is recommended in those with urogenital sinus or severely virilized females to repair the urogenital sinus. For those with whom surgery is chosen, the recommended procedure should be based on underlying anatomic structures but often includes vaginoplasty using urogenital mobilization and neurovascular-sparing clitoroplasty (Almarsri et al., 2018; Speiser et al., 2018).

Furthermore, each specific disorder of sexual differentiation has different levels of clarity with regard to future gender identity. Clinicians must be careful not to lump disorders of sexual development into one category when making decisions regarding genital surgery. In this chapter, 21-OHD CAH is discussed, which is, as mentioned, not only the most common form of CAH but also the most common cause of ambiguous genitalia. Because males born with this condition have normal anatomy, only virilized females with 21-OHD will be discussed with regard to genital surgery.

Most 46,XX females with 21-OHD CAH born with ambiguous genitalia grow up with fairly consistent female gender identity. However, data reveal gender dysphoria rates occur in 6.3% to 27.2% of CAH patients (Chawla et al., 2019; Seneviratne et al., 2021). It is hypothesized that nonheterosexual orientation and masculinized behavior in females with CAH may be related to high androgen exposure in fetal life (Seneviratne et al., 2021). In some cases the surgeon could recommend genital surgery to repair the CUGS and, at the same time, consider minor cosmetic surgery to hide an enlarged clitoris, preserving the erectile tissue and nerves of the clitoris. Later (in adulthood or adolescence), individuals who find the enlarged clitoris to be functionally problematic or are not happy with its appearance can choose to have the clitoris reduced. At the same time, in adolescence or adulthood, the individual can choose to have vaginoplasty if desired (Almarsri et al., 2018; Speiser et al., 2018).

The most difficult decision making lies with the 46,XX 21-OHD CAH females who are completely virilized (appear phenotypically male with bilateral undescended testicles). Though rare, these children have a much less clear course and outcome for two reasons: (1) Despite prenatal screening, some infants/children may present at a later age, having been reared male since birth; and (2) these individuals may have more gender identity issues than less virilized individuals (Seneviratne et al., 2021). These infants must be assessed and addressed case-by-case with an experienced team of experts familiar with Prader 5 (see Fig. 17.4). Consideration for sex reassignment must be undertaken only after a thorough psychological evaluation of the patient and family, and any surgery should be undertaken after endocrine treatment (Seneviratne et al., 2021; Speiser et al., 2018).

Psychological Assessment and Support

Females with CAH can show behavioral masculinization, most pronounced in gender role behavior, less in sexual orientation, and rarely in gender identity. Even in females with psychosexual problems, the general psychological adjustment seems similar to that of females without CAH (Sewell et al., 2021). Psychological assessment and support of patients and families should be a routine component of these patients' comprehensive care and management. Parents and patients should be offered the option of age- and sex-appropriate psychological counseling at the initial diagnosis. Counseling regarding sexual function, future surgeries, gender role, and issues related to living with a chronic disorder should be addressed (Speiser et al., 2018).

Gender Role Assignments

Prenatal exposure to androgens can correlate with a decrease in self-reported femininity by adult females but not an increase in self-reported masculinity by adult females. Changes in childhood play behavior correlate with reduced female gender satisfaction and reduced heterosexual interest in adulthood. In contrast, males with 21-OHD do not show an alteration in childhood play behavior or sexual orientation (Chawla et al., 2019; Seneviratne et al., 2021).

NONCLASSIC CONGENITAL ADRENAL HYPERPLASIA

Individuals with nonclassic 21-OHD CAH do not always require treatment. Many are asymptomatic throughout their lives, or symptoms may develop during puberty, after puberty, or postpartum. Treatment is only recommended for symptomatic patients: those with an advanced bone age coupled with a poor height prediction (compared with the family target height), hirsutism, severe acne, menstrual irregularities, testicular masses, and (in the young adult) infertility (Livadas & Bothou, 2019).

MANAGEMENT OF WOMEN WITH CONGENITAL ADRENAL HYPERPLASIA IN PREGNANCY

Pregnant women with CAH should be monitored and delivered in a tertiary center equipped and experienced to handle such pregnancies. These women are at increased risk for pregestational type 2 diabetes, obesity, and cardiovascular disease, so screening for complications should be done early in pregnancy. Glucocorticoids that do not cross the placenta, such as hydrocortisone and prednisolone, should be used. Dexamethasone should be avoided (except when used in prenatal therapy). Glucocorticoid doses should be adjusted to maintain maternal serum testosterone concentrations near the upper range of normal for pregnancy. When reconstructive surgery has been performed, an elective cesarean section should be considered if there is a risk to the genital tract. When the cesarean section is performed, the dosage of hydrocortisone has to be increased before and tapered after delivery. A pediatric health care provider should be present during delivery to care for the newborn and initiate diagnostic procedures when an affected child is expected, according to the results of prenatal testing (Badeghiesh et al., 2020; Speiser et al., 2018).

COMPLEMENTARY AND ALTERNATIVE THERAPIES

One alternative therapy that families might seek is Ashwagandha, a versatile herb with properties to increase cortisol levels and improved insulin sensitivity (Kalani et al., 2012). Other remedies may include chasteberry, thought to improve menstrual symptoms; black cohosh, thought to lower LH levels; and saw palmetto, which may affect testosterone levels (Lam, 2018). Spearmint tea, green tea, soy, flaxseed, and nettle root are all thought to lower testosterone levels and increase the binding of androgens (Lam, 2018). Multiple therapies are being investigated, mostly in nonclassic or adult patients, but insufficient evidence exists for recommending these treatment modalities.

ANTICIPATED ADVANCES IN DIAGNOSIS AND MANAGEMENT

PRENATAL TREATMENT

Prenatal treatment has been used since the 1980s for some fetuses at risk for classic 21-OHD CAH (Lajic et al., 2018). This involves dexamethasone treatment beginning at 6 weeks of gestation (Carvalho et al., 2022). However, the appropriateness, ethics, and outcomes of the prenatal treatment of CAH remain controversial. Multiple studies have shown mixed results and adverse outcomes related to this therapy. It is approximately 75% effective in minimizing the effects of genital virilization. However, some untoward effects may occur between the pregnant woman and the fetus (Carvalho et al., 2022). Some studies reveal negative effects on executive and cognitive functioning and potential impacts on social functioning, especially in females treated prenatally (Lajic et al., 2018). The maternal complications of prenatal management are variable and include striae, weight gain, and edema.

Most important, prenatal therapy does not cure the disease; it merely allows for decreased virilization, obviating the need for surgery. An extensive review of the risks and benefits must be done with the family, and informed consent must be obtained.

ADRENALECTOMY IN CONGENITAL ADRENAL HYPERPLASIA

Bilateral adrenalectomy by laparoscopy effectively decreases adrenal androgens and the likelihood of iatrogenic hypercortisolism. Proponents believe it should be considered in severe cases where conventional therapy is failing, whereas others believe it is too radical a step. A systematic review and meta-analysis by MacKay et al. (2018) revealed that the most common indication for surgery was the inability to control hyperandrogenism/virilization (Cushing syndrome). Most patients reported symptomatic improvement following the procedure with relatively low adverse outcomes; however, an Endocrine Society clinical practice guideline currently recommends against this management strategy (Speiser et al., 2018)

Although some patients have been managed with adrenalectomy, further data are needed before deciding whether it is a viable therapeutic alternative. The procedure should only be carried out where long-term follow-up is secured and in the form of ethically approved clinical studies. It should only be considered in severe cases that are refractory to standard treatment. Vigilance in maintaining regular substitution of hydrocortisone and fludrocortisone is mandatory, with the prompt institution of stress dosages at the onset of illness. Throughout life, the patient must be monitored for activation of ectopic adrenal rest tissue (MacKay et al., 2018).

ANDROGEN/ESTROGEN ANTAGONISTS AND SYNTHESIS INHIBITORS

In this approach, traditional physiologic replacement doses of glucocorticoid are used with a secondary therapy that inhibits androgen and estrogen production/action. The goal of this therapy is to normalize growth and development in children by reducing glucocorticoid exposure (Speiser et al., 2018).

GROWTH HORMONE AND GONADOTROPIN-RELEASING HORMONE INHIBITOR

Growth and short stature remain areas of concern in CAH despite good control of androgens and appropriate glucocorticoid therapy. To improve final adult height, studies have looked at the utilization of growth hormone and GnRH inhibitor to promote growth and prevent premature closure of epiphyseal plates. In three studies, researchers found that final adult height and growth were improved with this therapy (Merke, 2021).

GLUCOCORTICOID DELIVERY METHODS

This therapy aims to mimic the normal circadian rhythm of cortisol and limit daily dose exposure of glucocorticoids. In an effort to achieve this goal, new modalities are being explored, including infusion of hydrocortisone in a circadian fashion, modified release form of hydrocortisone, and subcutaneous hydrocortisone infusion. Each of these modalities is to mimic the physiologic diurnal cortisol secretion but is still experimental at this stage (Merke, 2021).

GENE THERAPY

Currently there is one study on gene therapy initiated in 2021 with multiple centers for CAH. This initial trial looks at dosing regimens, adverse effects, changes in 17-OHP levels, changes in endogenous cortisol levels, and androstenedione (Clinical Trials.gov, 2021). Gene therapy represents a potential cure for CAH. Preimplantation genetic diagnosis for CAH is possible, but further research is required to determine its utility (Speiser, 2019).

ADRENOMEDULLARY DYSFUNCTION/ EPINEPHRINE DEFICIENCY

Patients with CAH suffer from varying degrees of dysfunction of the adrenal medulla, primarily expressed by epinephrine deficiency. This may play a role in response to stress. More studies are needed on the risk of low blood glucose in CAH and the function of the adrenal medulla in patients with nonclassic CAH (Speiser, 2019).

CONGENITAL ADRENAL HYPERPLASIA AND THE BRAIN

A magnetic resonance imaging (MRI) study found that the structure and function of the amygdala (the part of the brain that regulates emotion and fear) is affected in patients with CAH (Merke & Auchus, 2020). The implications need to be further studied.

DNA BANKING

DNA banking stores deoxyribonucleic acid for possible future use. Understanding of the genetics of 21-OHD CAH will certainly improve in the future. Some consideration should be given to banking DNA of affected individuals.

ASSOCIATED PROBLEMS OF CONGENITAL ADRENAL HYPERPLASIA AND TREATMENT

The problems associated with CAH are limited to children receiving appropriate therapy. However, primary care providers must be aware of the potential for acute adrenal insufficiency, growth disorders, virilization, and problems surrounding issues of sexuality and cognitive function (Hamed et al., 2018; Merke & Auchus, 2020).

⇄ **Associated Problems of Congenital Adrenal Hyperplasia and Treatment**

- Acute adrenal insufficiency
- Accelerated growth and bone age
- Virilization
- Problems with sexual development
- Precocious puberty
- Reduced fertility
- Testicular masses
- Congenital anomalies

PRECOCIOUS PUBERTY

The true precocious puberty that may occur in 21-OHD CAH can be treated with analogs of LHRH (Haddad & Eugster, 2019; Neeman et al., 2019).

FERTILITY

For females treated, menses are normal, and pregnancy is possible. Overall, fertility rates are lower than the general population. Reported reasons include inadequate introitus, elevated androgens leading to ovarian dysfunction, and psychosexual behaviors around gender identity and selection of sexual partners (Gomes et al., 2019; New et al., 2019; Reisch, 2019; Seneviratne et al., 2021).

Studies have shown male subfertility arises from suppression of gonadotropins by adrenal testosterone, adrenal androgen excess driving gonadotropin suppression, and excessive ACTH drive resulting in testicular adrenal rest tumors (TART) with subsequent testicular failure (Reisch, 2019). Further, gonadotropic hypogonadism may result from suppressing the pituitary's LH secretion by excessive adrenal androgens and their aromatization product. It is important to discuss fertility, TART formation, and other issues with patients and considerations for sperm cryoconservation (Reisch, 2019).

CONGENITAL ANOMALIES

The incidence of congenital anomalies and small for gestational age is slightly increased over the general population with a risk of 2.7% compared to 0.4% and 8% compared to 2.2%, respectively, in females with CAH (Badeghiesh et al., 2020).

PROGNOSIS

The major risk for children with CAH is death from an unrecognized salt-losing crisis early in infancy or from inadequately treated acute adrenal insufficiency during stress. It is estimated that the increased risk of mortality is two- to fivefold compared to the general population (Lousada et al., 2021). Screenings of individuals with a family history of CAH for the carrier state, prenatal screenings, and routine neonatal screenings have the potential to greatly reduce the number of children who die of CAH (Draznin et al., 2022).

Nearly all female infants with classic CAH have morbidity associated with prenatal virilization and the surgical procedures necessary to correct it.

PRIMARY CARE MANAGEMENT

HEALTH CARE MAINTENANCE

Growth

Because abnormal linear growth indicates inappropriate treatment or poor compliance, careful monitoring of growth is essential; linear growth should be measured every 1 to 4 months for infants and every 3 to 6 months for children older than 2 years. These measurements should be done carefully, using an infantometer for length and a stadiometer for height. The standard scale-mounted measuring device is not accurate enough to detect slight variations in growth. Measurements should be plotted on a standardized growth chart and assessed for changes in growth rate.

Poor linear growth. Linear growth is acutely sensitive to excessive levels of hydrocortisone; therefore any decrease in height percentile on the growth chart should prompt a reassessment of the hydrocortisone dosage. A child's hydrocortisone therapy will occasionally be increased based on a high laboratory 17-OHP result when the result was high because of acute illness, stress from an unusually traumatic venipuncture, or frequently missed hydrocortisone doses before sampling. To avoid unnecessary and possibly harmful increases in hydrocortisone doses, clinicians must rule out these other causes of high 17-OHP values before increasing medication doses. Clinicians can do this by taking a careful history and comparing the prescribed dose of hydrocortisone with the established dose ranges. The primary care provider may be able to identify the problem and should contact the endocrinologist with this information.

Another cause of poor linear growth in children with CAH is chronically inadequate mineralocorticoid levels. An abnormally high PRA level indicates that a child needs additional mineralocorticoid or dietary sodium. A careful history and comparison with established dose ranges will determine if this problem is one of compliance or inadequately prescribed doses (Speiser et al., 2018).

A child with poorly controlled CAH or one not diagnosed until preschool or school age may have early cessation of growth because of premature closure of the epiphyses. If such premature closure is suspected, radiographic studies of bone age should be done to assess skeletal maturity.

Excessive growth. Inadequate hydrocortisone replacement will cause excessive androgen synthesis by the adrenals, resulting in accelerated linear growth. An elevated serum 17-OHP level or clinical findings of increased virilization (e.g., pubic and axillary hair, oily skin, acne, enlargement of the phallus) confirm the cause of excessive growth. Clinicians must carefully assess whether the inadequate hydrocortisone replacement is secondary to an inappropriate dose or poor adherence.

Excessive weight gain. Glucocorticoid replacement therapy—even at doses within the accepted therapeutic range—has been associated with obesity (Haddad & Eugster, 2019). Clinicians must closely monitor weight gain, avoid overtreatment with glucocorticoids, and encourage good dietary and activity habits to reduce any tendency toward obesity.

Development

Children with CAH diagnosed in infancy or early childhood and receiving consistently adequate treatment should develop normally (Messina et al., 2020). However, if the diagnosis of CAH is not made until late childhood, these children will be much taller and more mature looking than their peers. When they stop growing early because of premature epiphyseal closure, these children will go from being the tallest to the shortest in their peer group. Short stature affects behavior and social relationships and probably has an even greater effect on someone who spent early childhood as the tallest person in any group of peers (Sewell et al., 2021).

Parents, school personnel, child care workers, and others who regularly interact with these children should be given clear, frequently reinforced guidelines on age-appropriate expectations to avoid demanding too much of tall but immature children or too little of short adolescents.

Diet

The main modification to a normal diet is an allowance for adequate sodium intake. Although an appropriate dose of mineralocorticoid prevents significant sodium depletion in children with salt-losing CAH, these children should be offered salty foods and allowed to salt their food to taste. This recommendation also applies to children with non–salt-losing CAH because they may have a mild salt deficit when compared with unaffected children. As mentioned, good dietary habits are essential to reduce the tendency to gain excessive weight (Merke, 2021). The advice of a dietitian can help identify nutritionally dense foods that meet a child's dietary needs without excessive calories.

Safety

Children with CAH are not physically impaired or at increased risk for any of the usual physical hazards of childhood, but they are at risk of having their special needs neglected when away from home. Injuries such as a broken bone may not be recognized as potentially life threatening. Teachers, child care personnel, coaches, and others in regular contact with the child should have written information describing the condition and the need for prompt treatment in an emergency. The child should wear a medical alert bracelet with this information on it.

The decision to keep injectable hydrocortisone at home or with day care personnel depends on the situation and must be made on a case-by-case basis. Factors to consider are as follows: (1) Can the primary care provider or emergency department be reached in 5 to 10 minutes? (2) Is a parent always available at short notice? (3) Are trained personnel at the site willing to give an IM injection? (4) Does the child engage in activities with a high risk of serious injury?

Participation in sports is a normal part of childhood and should be encouraged. If possible, some believe children with CAH should be directed toward activities with a low risk of serious injury (e.g., swimming, track, tennis); however, this needs to be considered on a case-by-case basis, and ultimately the decision lies with the parents after risks and benefits have been explored. Minor injuries (e.g., bruises, mild or moderate sprains, abrasions) are not cause for special concern. If these children are involved in high-risk sports (e.g., football), parents should meet with the coach to explain their child's special needs in an emergency and provide appropriate written materials, instructions, and authorization for treatment. A parent or team clinician should ideally be present and have hydrocortisone for an IM injection during competition. Their presence should be mandatory if the activity takes place more than 15 minutes away from a source of emergency care.

Immunizations
Children with CAH are not immunosuppressed and should receive all standard immunizations at the usual ages (Centers for Disease Control and Prevention, 2021). There is currently no recommendation for or against giving additional immunizations, but the benefits of immunity to these diseases must be weighed against the possibility of adverse reactions to the vaccine. In weighing these factors, many clinicians believe that giving additional immunizations is worthwhile to reduce the risk of acute adrenal insufficiency triggered by illness.

Increasing the basal dose of hydrocortisone before immunizations are given is unnecessary unless there is a history of adverse reactions to previous immunizations with that vaccine. A common but discretionary recommendation is to give a child acetaminophen a few hours before giving an immunization that typically produces a rapid-onset febrile reaction and continue it for 24 to 48 hours afterward.

For new vaccines or new combinations of vaccines, the package insert should be referred to for information on the type and timing of possible reactions, and families should be counseled to observe their child closely on the days when reactions are likely to occur (e.g., 5–12 days after measles vaccination).

Stress doses of hydrocortisone should be given when a child develops a temperature of more than 38.4°C (101.1°F) or is fussy or lethargic after an immunization. Any immunization reaction should be documented so that stress doses of hydrocortisone can be given before subsequent immunizations with the same vaccine.

Screenings
Vision. Routine screening is recommended.

Hearing. Routine screening is recommended.

Dental. Routine screening is recommended.

Blood pressure. Blood pressure should be checked at each primary care visit. Every effort should be made to relax and quiet children so that readings are accurate.

Elevated blood pressure in a quiet child may indicate excessive mineralocorticoid or hydrocortisone dosage, whereas low blood pressure may indicate an inadequate mineralocorticoid or hydrocortisone dosage. Either situation should prompt an evaluation of the replacement therapy regimen and compliance.

Hematocrit. Routine screening is recommended.

Urinalysis. Routine screening is recommended.

Tuberculosis. Routine screening is recommended.

Condition-Specific Screening
Serum 17-OHP. Primary care providers may want to order additional screening tests to monitor the adequacy of replacement therapy more closely in children who have difficulty with adherence. The serum 17-OHP level is widely accepted as a measure of hydrocortisone therapy, even though it has the disadvantage of being influenced by temporary stress (e.g., traumatic venipuncture), the length of time since the last hydrocortisone dose, and diurnal fluctuations. To help evaluate the significance of 17-OHP results, clinicians should note on the specimen the time of day (i.e., preferably morning) and the time of the last dose of hydrocortisone (Speiser et al., 2018).

Androstenedione and testosterone levels can be evaluated along with 17-OHP to monitor the adequacy of hydrocortisone therapy. Some clinicians rely on 24-hour urinary 17-ketosteroid and pregnanetriol levels to monitor hydrocortisone therapy because of the lack of short-term fluctuations, despite the difficulty in collecting a 24-hour specimen. Serum 17-OHP levels should be no more than three times above normal (i.e., preferably <200 ng/dL). Urinary 17-ketosteroid and pregnanetriol levels should also be in the normal to near-normal range for age, as should PRA. Specimens ordered by the primary care provider should be coordinated with the endocrinologist and sent to the same laboratory to ensure consistency (Speiser et al., 2018).

Plasma renin activity. Mineralocorticoid therapy is monitored by measuring PRA levels. The primary care provider monitoring 17-OHP levels should include a PRA assay for individuals with salt-losing CAH (Speiser et al., 2018).

Bone age. The frequency of radiographic studies of bone age depends on the clinical course. Bone age evaluations are not helpful in newborns. Initial bone age should be determined early in childhood (i.e., at 2–3 years of age or at the time of diagnosis if the diagnosis is delayed) and can be used as a baseline for future studies. If a child is growing normally and has consistently acceptable 17-OHP and PRA levels, routine screening should not be necessary more than every few years.

If a child has growth acceleration, physical findings of increased virilization, or consistently high 17-OHP laboratory results, bone age should be determined to further assess the effects of androgen excess. If bone age is accelerated, this finding can help impress the family with the seriousness and permanent consequences of poor adherence. The same person should ideally read all bone age studies to avoid inconsistencies in interpretation.

Monitoring for testicular abnormalities in males. Periodic imaging of the testes, either by ultrasonography or MRI, should begin after puberty (Speiser et al., 2018).

COMMON ILLNESS MANAGEMENT

Children with CAH are not immunosuppressed, and their susceptibility to common childhood illnesses is no different from that of their peers; their ability to withstand the stress of illness is impaired. During periods of illness, these children must be observed closely; consultation with an endocrinologist is necessary if a child shows any signs or symptoms of acute adrenal insufficiency (Box 17.2).

The primary care provider caring for a child with CAH should keep injectable hydrocortisone in the office for emergencies. In addition to a medical alert bracelet or necklace, the child and family should carry written materials (e.g., a wallet card) with the diagnosis, a stress dose of hydrocortisone, indications for administering the stress dose, and the name and telephone number of the endocrinologist. This emergency information should be updated regularly.

Box **17.2**	**Signs and Symptoms of Acute Adrenal Insufficiency**

- Nausea or vomiting
- Pallor
- Cold, moist skin
- Weakness
- Dizziness or confusion
- Rapid heart rate
- Rapid breathing
- Abdominal, back, or leg pain
- Dehydration
- Hypotension

Upper Respiratory Infections and Allergies

If the symptoms are mild and the child does not have a fever or marked malaise, no specific treatment or increase in the basal dose of hydrocortisone is necessary for upper respiratory infections or allergies. Parents should watch for the worsening of symptoms, fever, or unusual lethargy, and school-age children should know to report these symptoms to their teacher and contact their parents. If symptoms worsen or complications develop, children should be promptly treated with a stress dose of hydrocortisone and seen by the primary care provider for assessment and specific therapy.

Acute Illnesses

Any known or suspected bacterial illness (e.g., acute otitis media, urinary tract infection, streptococcal pharyngitis, cellulitis) should be treated aggressively with the appropriate antibiotic and stress doses of hydrocortisone during the acute phase of the illness if fever, pain, and malaise are present. When the diagnosis is uncertain, or there is a significant risk for secondary infections or complications (e.g., a suspicious but not clearly inflamed tympanic membrane, viral pneumonia, prolonged or marked nasal congestion in a child with a history of frequent acute otitis media or sinusitis), it is wise to treat the child with antibiotics rather than wait for the situation to worsen. The child must be observed closely, with an initial office visit for diagnosis and assessment of the child's overall condition and daily telephone progress reports until the acute phase of the illness has passed. Follow-up office visits should be scheduled as for any other child.

Fever

Although fever is a physiologic response to illness, it is also a stress. Therefore fever in a child with CAH should be treated with the recommended dose for the age of antipyretics. Stress doses of hydrocortisone should be given. It is important to advise families that reducing the fever does not cure the illness and that other treatments (e.g., antibiotics and stress doses of hydrocortisone) should continue to be given as directed. The child must be observed closely (i.e., as described for bacterial and viral illnesses) until the illness has resolved (Kim, 2022).

Vomiting

If a child with CAH vomits once but otherwise appears well, three times the usual oral dose of hydrocortisone should be given about 20 minutes later, and the child should be closely observed. If a child appears weak or lethargic after vomiting once or vomiting more than once, the family should give injectable hydrocortisone IM and contact the endocrinologist immediately. If family members are not able to give injectable hydrocortisone, they must immediately take the child to the nearest emergency department to receive parenteral hydrocortisone and appropriate fluid and electrolyte therapy because this can be a life-threatening situation. The emergency department staff should contact the endocrinologist but should not delay hydrocortisone therapy while awaiting consultation. A wallet card or written information on the child's diagnosis, emergency treatment, and endocrinologist can facilitate prompt and appropriate care (Kim, 2022; Yau et al., 2019).

Injury

A child with a significant injury (e.g., fracture, concussion, injury from an automobile accident) should immediately be given hydrocortisone IM and evaluated further for acute adrenal insufficiency at an emergency department. Emergency department personnel should contact the endocrinologist but not delay hydrocortisone therapy while awaiting consultation (Yau et al., 2019).

Differential Diagnosis: Acute Adrenal Insufficiency

Acute adrenal insufficiency is a life-threatening situation. Symptoms of acute adrenal insufficiency include weakness, nausea, abdominal discomfort, vomiting, dehydration, and hypotension. These signs or symptoms in a child with CAH should be presumed to indicate acute adrenal insufficiency and be treated with hydrocortisone IV or IM at three to five times the basal dose. This administration should be done at home—or in the primary care setting if the child is there—instead of delaying initial treatment until the child arrives at an emergency department. Further, a workup can be done after the initial hydrocortisone treatment.

The diagnosis of acute adrenal insufficiency can be confirmed by laboratory values showing hyponatremia and hyperkalemia. Although consultation with an endocrinologist should be sought, treatment should not be delayed.

An IM injection of hydrocortisone or IV therapy in an emergency department is a frightening experience that no one wants to go through unnecessarily. In this type of situation, however, it is always best to err on the side of aggressive treatment (Kim, 2022; Yau et al., 2019).

Drug Interactions

Medications for CAH replace hormones normally present in the body; therefore concern about using other medications is limited to their effect on the absorption or rate of metabolism (Box 17.3).

Barbiturates (e.g., phenobarbital [Donnatal], phenytoin [Dilantin], and rifampin [Rifadin, Rifamate, Rimactane]) increase the rate of metabolism of glucocorticoids. Therefore children with CAH taking any of these medications for more than a few weeks may

---

Box 17.3 Drug Interactions

- Barbiturates
- Phenytoin
- Rifampin

---

require a higher dose of hydrocortisone for adequate cortisol replacement (Thijs et al., 2019). A serum 17-OHP level done approximately 2 weeks after starting any of the medications listed here will show if an adjustment in the hydrocortisone dose is necessary. Short-term use of barbiturates perioperatively or prophylactic use of rifampin for *Haemophilus influenzae* meningitis should not require a change in hydrocortisone dose.

Antibiotics, decongestants, antihistamines, cough preparations, analgesics, antipyretics, and topical preparations have no unusual adverse effects.

Varicella-Zoster Virus (Chickenpox)

Affected children who come down with varicella-zoster virus should still be given stress doses despite concerns with regard to steroid use in the presence of the virus. Complications of acute adrenal insufficiency outweigh concerns about steroid use in varicella-zoster virus infections. Prevention with immunization is the best defense.

DEVELOPMENTAL ISSUES

Sleep Patterns

Children with CAH do not differ from their peers in their sleep patterns or needs as long as their corticosteroid treatment is adequate. Unusual fatigue may indicate an illness or inadequate cortisol replacement and should be evaluated (Schröder et al., 2022).

Toileting

Children with obvious virilization of their external genitalia should be given privacy when using the toilet to avoid teasing. The initial corrective surgery for females who experience virilization is usually done at an early age to avoid problems related to looking different. However, some parents will postpone surgery until children are older and can give informed consent. In these cases, notes should be written for physical education classes that allow changing clothes privately and a private restroom. Although males who experience excessive virilization may have some regression in pubic hair and penile size once they establish consistently adequate treatment, they will be noticeably different from their peers until adolescence.

Females with a CUGS will be prone to vaginal voiding and vaginitis caused by vaginal voiding. Vaginal voiding is when, during urination, urine refluxes into the vagina because of the close proximity of the vagina and urethra. The symptoms are urinary leaking after voiding, mildly wet underwear, and smelly urine. Vaginal voiding can easily be treated with leg abduction with voiding (sitting backward on the toilet for younger females) and sitting on the toilet a few seconds after urination has stopped. The associated vaginitis can be treated with sitz baths and prevented with leg abduction with voiding. These children are otherwise no different in toileting readiness or skills than their peers and are not unusually prone to constipation, other types of incontinence, enuresis, polyuria, or other disorders related to toileting (Mehmood & Rentea, 2022).

Discipline

Children with CAH should be expected to behave appropriately for their age. The only special consideration has to do with children who appear older than their actual age. Parents, teachers, and others must be given clear guidelines on appropriate expectations for a child's developmental stage if it is different from the child's appearance.

Another area that raises disciplinary issues is adherence to taking medication, especially during toddlerhood and adolescence when children struggle with issues of dependency and autonomy. Parents should be advised from the beginning to use a matter-of-fact approach and avoid negotiating something that is nonnegotiable. Parents have full responsibility for giving medications during infancy and early school years. As children mature and are able to assume more responsibility, parents should encourage their child's active participation (e.g., by remembering when it is "pill time," marking off the calendar for each dose, or filling a pillbox). Adolescents should be primarily responsible for taking the medication, with the parents offering support. Using a watch with a beeper is helpful for adolescents, as is a pillbox, which also provides an unobtrusive way for a parent to see if the medication disappears on schedule.

Clinicians can help make older children and adolescents aware of the consequences of poor adherence by pointing out signs of virilization to females and slowed growth to both genders and emphasizing that it is within their power to return to normal. The risks of acute adrenal insufficiency and impaired fertility associated with poor adherence should also be discussed with adolescents, again emphasizing that such things are avoidable.

An adolescent will occasionally choose to make adherence to medications the focus of serious rebellion. Every effort should be made to explain the purpose and necessity of medication, and counseling should promptly be sought if the problem is severe or chronic.

Child Care

Parents should meet with child care personnel before enrollment to explain their child's special needs. Child care personnel do not require detailed knowledge of CAH but should be given a clear explanation that a child has a metabolic disorder that requires simple but important treatment.

Written information for the child care center should include authorization to give hydrocortisone orally with instructions on the dose, time, and purpose when to call parents, the telephone numbers where they can be reached, and what symptoms or events require emergency care. Information on where to take the child for care, authorization for treatment, and the name and telephone number of the primary care provider and endocrinologist is also important for the child care center. It is neither necessary nor desirable to have special rules or restrictions on activities at school or child care for children with CAH. The usual policies on safety and appropriate play are sufficient to avoid serious injury.

Because hydrocortisone is usually given every 8 hours, many children will need at least one dose while at day care. Mineralocorticoid is given once daily to children with salt-losing CAH and can be administered at home. Although most child care providers are conscientious, they may occasionally miss or delay doses of hydrocortisone if they do not understand its importance or are distracted by other demands. A routine that ties medication time to a regular activity (e.g., rest period or story time) can be established, or the child can wear a watch programmed to beep at the desired time. A letter from the primary care provider or the endocrinologist is helpful in making this invisible condition real to the people caring for these children.

Schooling

Children with CAH may have more absences than usual because they need close observation at home during acute illnesses. Concerns about excessive absences should be brought to the attention of the primary care provider, who can assess their appropriateness. Legitimate absences include any illness that would keep other children at home. In addition, symptoms such as a scratchy throat and malaise that might be ignored in other children should be initially observed at home.

Studies of cognitive abilities and school function in children with CAH have shown evidence of the importance of early diagnosis and early intervention. If treated early and consistently, normal intelligence and cognitive function have been identified (Messina et al., 2020). However, other studies have found lower-than-normal intelligence and cognitive deficits in those affected by CAH. Researchers hypothesize this is related to treatment with glucocorticoids, androgen excess, and the number of hyponatremic episodes (Hamed et al., 2018).

Although it is not possible to identify what influence CAH itself has on cognitive and educational function with the information currently available, it is clear that acute CAH crises have a deleterious effect. Not surprisingly, children who had episodes of acute adrenal insufficiency with hypoglycemia or convulsions have a significantly higher prevalence of learning difficulties than children—with or without

CAH—who did not experience such events (Hamed et al., 2018). Because hypoglycemia and convulsions are associated with learning difficulties, these findings may represent a complication of poor management rather than the biochemical abnormality inherent in CAH. A child with CAH with severe hypoglycemia and convulsions should be assessed for learning difficulties and referred for special education intervention if indicated.

It is essential to communicate emergency management guidance to the school setting for the child with CAH. If a child has a significant injury, illness, or fever, the child with CAH is at risk for an adrenal crisis, resulting in hypotension, shock, and electrolyte abnormalities. To prevent an adrenal crisis, the school nurse and other health care personnel should be educated on the signs and symptoms of an adrenal crisis, and the child should receive the stress dosing of corticosteroids. Solu-Cortef is a common medication for families to administer in these situations, with dosing for school-age children under 40 kg of 50 mg and 100 mg for those over 40 kg. Additionally, rehydration therapy with some type of glucose-containing beverage may be beneficial. The family should be notified immediately so sick management can be implemented at home, such as doubling or tripling the normal daily dose per endocrinology recommendations. All this should be communicated in writing and kept in the child's health plan to allow optimal management of these children in the school setting (Yau et al., 2019).

Sexuality

Because of the considerable attention paid to the genital examination during clinic visits, females with CAH may get the message that there is something wrong with them and that it has to do with their genitalia. It is important to reassure them that they have all the normal female organs, hormones, and chromosomes and that any surgeries are simply to correct a cosmetic mistake that happened before they were born. Frequent genital examinations in females, unless there is concern about poor control or to assess pubertal progression, should be limited, and genital photography should be done only with informed consent from the parents. Children with CAH should be regularly evaluated for premature sexual development to determine the adequacy of therapy. Clinicians should include appropriate counseling regarding sexual development for the child and family.

Menstrual irregularities caused by androgen excess are common in adolescent females with CAH. Androgen excess can also cause hirsutism and acne in children and adolescents of either gender and may contribute to impaired fertility (Haddad & Eugster, 2019; Neeman et al., 2019).

Gender role behavior and gender identity have been explored in females with CAH. It has been found that conventionally reared females may show more male-like behaviors and gender identity issues compared to the general population. Prenatal androgen exposure is considered to be a predisposing—rather than a causative—factor in gender behavior. Other factors to consider are male-rearing or sociocultural factors. All aspects of psychosocial development must be considered in caring for females with CAH (Seneviratne et al., 2021). Primary care providers must use caution when interpreting these data and base discussions of sexuality on an individualized assessment of each child and family.

Females with CAH—particularly those with the salt-losing form—may not have an adequate introitus for vaginal penetration. In spite of surgical intervention, inadequate reconstruction and poor compliance with therapy can result in fertility and sexual complication (New et al., 2019; Reisch, 2019). In addition, females who become pregnant may require cesarean delivery because of a small birth canal (Badeghiesh et al., 2020).

For treated females, menses are normal, and pregnancy is possible, but overall fertility rates are lower when compared to the general population. Reported reasons include inadequate introitus, elevated androgens leading to ovarian dysfunction, gender identity, and selection of sexual partners (Badeghiesh et al., 2020; Gomes et al., 2019; New et al., 2019; Reisch, 2019).

There are no published studies on the sexual function of females with classic CAH who did not have surgery. In addition, the surgery performed on females with CAH who are currently adults is very different from the surgical techniques performed on infants today, so the relevance of adult outcome studies to children with CAH is questionable. There is some optimism that the outcomes will be improved for today's infants when they reach adulthood; however, we will not know for another 20 or more years. Males with CAH generally do not have problems with erectile function or fertility. In males, the main cause of subfertility is the presence of testicular adrenal rest tumors, which are thought to originate from aberrant adrenal tissue and respond to treatment with glucocorticoids (Grinton et al., 2021; New et al., 2019).

Transition to Adulthood

Improved care for individuals with 21-OHD CAH has resulted in a good prognosis and normal life expectancy with the oldest individuals in their late 60s (Reisch, 2019). During the transition from adolescence into adulthood, youth with CAH assume the primary responsibility for managing the condition, and the medical issues change from a focus on growth and development to long-term health preservation. Sexuality and fertility issues become a focus. Educating the adolescent (not just the parent) on the principles of adrenal suppression and the diurnal rhythm of the adrenal glands requires time and encouragement. Consideration should be given to leaving parents in the waiting room for part or all of the visits. Transition affords the young adult the opportunity for an educational review of CAH. Management should involve a multidisciplinary team, including the patient, endocrinology, gynecology, urology, fertility specialists, dietitians, sex therapists, biochemists, geneticists, clinical psychologists, and nursing (Chawla et al., 2019; Livadas & Bothou, 2019).

Changes in Requirements for the Adolescent

Glucocorticoids. Glucocorticoid treatment in adolescence must be adjusted according to individual goals because there is no perfect regimen. In contrast to the pediatric agenda of optimizing final height, adult concerns relate to the long-term consequences of glucocorticoid use. A common strategy is to find the minimal effective glucocorticoid dose for adult maintenance based on a combination of clinical and biochemical markers. The goal is to achieve a glucocorticoid regimen that fails to fully suppress 17-OHP but maintains androgens in the midnormal range (Reisch, 2019).

Mineralocorticoids. Mineralocorticoids require precise monitoring in adulthood. The sensitivity to salt loss noted in childhood diminishes throughout the teen years, and salt wasting in adults is far less precarious. In addition, the tendency to develop hypertension with age means that many adults are better off on progressively lower doses of fludrocortisone. To avoid hypertension, one must use renin as a guide to fludrocortisone dosing adjustments (Reisch, 2019).

Males are often lost to follow-up during the transition, and permanent infertility may result from neglected care. As children with CAH approach adulthood, primary care providers need to help their families identify an internist or family practice provider to assume primary care responsibilities. If a child has had specialty care through a pediatric endocrinologist, the transition must also be made to adult endocrine care; the pediatric endocrinologist usually has a list of names available. Counseling for early prenatal care (i.e., prenatal screening, diagnosis, and potential treatment) should also be provided (Chawla et al., 2019).

Unfortunately, insurance may become a problem when children reach an age when they are no longer covered by government-sponsored insurance for children with disabilities or their parent's insurance. Medicaid—for those who meet the criteria—and group insurance through employment—for those with medical benefits—will cover care for CAH. Information about other programs and resources can be sought from county social services agencies, health departments, and state insurance commissions.

Family Concerns

The parents of an infant female with CAH must cope with the effect of ambiguous genitalia and possibly a delayed or incorrect gender assignment. The initial explanations and reassurances that health care personnel give to the family must be sensitive and accurate to prevent serious misperceptions of the child's condition and prognosis. Discussions with parents should focus on listening to the parents' concerns, reinforcing the normality of their daughter's internal female organs and chromosomes, and explaining that the appearance of the external genitalia is correctable and the underlying condition is treatable (Rautmann et al., 2023).

People tend to blame the occurrence of an abnormality in a baby on something the mother or father did. It is important to discuss this issue with the parents and the extended family and to repeatedly reinforce the lack of fault. Even after the best explanations and reassurances, these families have anxiety and guilt about their child's condition, so constant reinforcement and support are necessary (Rautmann et al., 2023).

Ongoing communication with the endocrinologist and other health care providers is essential to promote optimal management of steroid therapies and the multiple aspects of CAH care to prevent conflicts or miscommunication with the family or delays in care (Rautmann et al., 2023). Families should be encouraged to be assertive in communicating the urgency of their child's need for hydrocortisone to health care personnel who are unfamiliar with the child or CAH. Unfortunately, treatment can be delayed because of a lack of understanding of the implications of acute illness in children with CAH. Primary care providers can help avoid delays in treatment by alerting other health care personnel (e.g., call group, emergency department staff) to a child's special needs. The endocrinologist should be consulted for any questions about treatment. In addition, the child should wear a medical alert bracelet or necklace, and the family should carry written information on the child's condition (e.g., wallet card) to facilitate prompt treatment.

Parents might initially have difficulty believing the seriousness of CAH unless the diagnosis was made during an episode of acute adrenal insufficiency. Once parents experience the rapidity with which their child can change from being robustly healthy to being deathly ill, they may be fearful of future episodes. It is difficult for these parents to find a balance between protecting their child from serious harm and allowing the child to have an active, normal life. This balance must be assessed at each primary care visit by asking about the child's social and academic progress, outside interests and activities, and special concerns. Any problem areas should then be discussed (Rautmann et al., 2023).

Children with CAH may experience emotional disturbances related to multiple factors involved in having this chronic condition. Such factors include being concerned about sexuality and fertility; being perceived and treated as different by others, including their parents; receiving mixed or confusing messages from health care personnel; being overprotected by their parents; and dealing with their fears related to life-threatening crises they may have experienced. Psychotherapy is indicated for significant emotional disturbance and behavioral problems. Newborn siblings should be screened for CAH, and tests should be given to confirm if the screening results are positive. Because nonclassic CAH can cause virilization or accelerated growth, all older siblings with these findings should be screened. Although prenatal diagnosis and treatment are still being refined, they should be discussed in detail with parents. Testing for the carrier state is also available and should be explained to unaffected siblings and other first-degree relatives.

The effect of CAH on a family varies with their cultural beliefs about the cause of congenital disorders and their attitudes toward sexuality. Primary care providers must determine what these beliefs are to provide sensitive and successful care to the child and family. Families will usually tell providers their beliefs if asked. Individuals from cultures where sexual topics are not openly discussed can be expected to have difficulty asking questions about CAH. Primary care providers and endocrinologists are faced with the challenge of presenting information on a sensitive subject without offending a family's values. In some cultures it may be helpful to have a male health care provider speak to the males in the family and a female provider speak separately to the females in the family (Pellur et al., 2019; Rautmann et al., 2023).

Families may be afraid of giving their children steroids because of negative publicity in the popular press. It is important to stress to families that the hydrocortisone and fludrocortisone medications their child takes for CAH are replacing substances normally produced in the body, and the recommended doses are calculated to match normal blood levels as closely as possible. This differs from taking high doses of glucocorticoids to treat inflammatory diseases or deleterious reasons. Families may have read stories of athletes having severe side effects from using steroids to increase muscle mass, so they should be told that anabolic steroids are completely different from hydrocortisone in actions and side effects. Replacement therapy for CAH is also entirely different from taking a foreign substance such as an antibiotic.

RESOURCES

FOR FAMILIES

Cares Foundation (support groups for patients and families of CAH): https://caresfoundation.org/support

Children's Hospital of Philadelphia (discussion on CAH): https://www.chop.edu/conditions-diseases/congenital-adrenal-hyperplasia

Kids Health (information on CAH): https://kidshealth.org/en/parents/congenital-adrenal-hyperplasia.html

Living with CAH (support group): https://www.livingwithcah.com

National Organization of Rare Diseases: https://rarediseases.org/rare-diseases/congenital-adrenal-hyperplasia

National Organization of Rare Diseases (CAH support group): https://rarediseases.org/organizations/climb-cah-support-group

Welcome to Congenital Adrenal Hyperplasia: A Handbook for New CAH Families: https://www.amazon.com/Welcome-Congenital-Adrenal-Hyperplasia-Handbook-ebook/dp/B09J1TCLJX/ref=sr_1_2?crid=H632R2IVQRJJ&keywords=congenital±adrenal±hyperplasia±for±families&qid=1665932210&sprefix=congential±adrenal±hyperplasia±for±families%2Caps%2C103&sr=8-2#detailBullets_feature_div

MEDICATION INFORMATION

Endocrine Society: https://www.endocrine.org/patient-engagement/endocrine-library/congenital-adrenal-hyperplasia

Mayo Clinic: https://www.mayoclinic.org/diseases-conditions/congenital-adrenal-hyperplasia/diagnosis-treatment/drc-20355211

National Institutes of Health (treatments for CAH): https://www.nichd.nih.gov/health/topics/cah/conditioninfo/treatments

ORGANIZATIONS

CARES Foundation Inc. (nonprofit organization to educate the public, primary care providers, and legislators about CAH and provide support to families of children with CAH. Provides useful information about CAH and links to other related sites): www.caresfoundation.org

National Adrenal Diseases Foundation (nonprofit organization dedicated to providing support, information, and education to individuals with Addison disease and other diseases of the adrenal glands): https://www.nadf.us

Pediatric Endocrinology Nursing Society (lists professional members in many regions who are willing to speak to parents, schools, professionals, or other groups): www.pens.org

Summary

Primary Care Needs for the Child With Congenital Adrenal Hyperplasia

HEALTH CARE MAINTENANCE
- A temperature greater than 101.1°F (38.4°C), significant malaise, pain, lethargy, or persistent vomiting (regardless of cause) should be covered by stress doses of hydrocortisone in addition to appropriate specific therapy.
- If the child has hypertension, excessive dietary sodium intake and overtreatment with mineralocorticoids or glucocorticoids should be ruled out.
- If the child has hypotension, inadequate mineralocorticoid and glucocorticoid dosage should be ruled out.
- If the child has nausea or vomiting, pallor, cold moist skin, weakness, dizziness or confusion, rapid heart rate, rapid breathing, abdominal/back/leg pain, dehydration, or hypotension, acute adrenal insufficiency should be ruled out.

Growth and Development
- If CAH is diagnosed in infancy and adequately and consistently treated, growth and development are normal.
- Accelerated linear growth occurs if CAH is inadequately treated.
- Accelerated bone age advancement and early closure of epiphyses with reduced final adult height will occur if CAH is inadequately treated.
- Stunted linear growth will occur if CAH is overtreated with hydrocortisone.
- Precocious puberty may occur with improved treatment.

Diet
- Children should be allowed to salt food to taste and eat salty foods.
- Good dietary and activity habits are necessary to counteract the tendency for hydrocortisone therapy to promote excessive weight gain.

Safety
- These children have no increased susceptibility to injury.
- There is a risk of acute adrenal insufficiency with a serious injury (e.g., fracture, concussion).
- A medical alert bracelet or necklace should be worn, and written information should be carried stating the diagnosis, stress dosage of hydrocortisone, and the name and telephone number of the endocrinologist.

Immunizations
- Routine immunizations are recommended.
- Increased stress doses of hydrocortisone are not prophylactically necessary unless the child has a history of previous adverse reactions to the vaccine.
- Give increased stress dose of hydrocortisone for immunization reactions involving fever, unusual malaise, and lethargy.
- Giving acetaminophen before immunizations with a likelihood of febrile reaction is discretionary.

Screening
- *Vision*. Routine screening is recommended.
- *Hearing*. Routine screening is recommended.
- *Dental*. Routine screening is recommended.
- *Blood pressure*. Blood pressure should be checked at each visit (including for infants). Children with abnormal findings should be referred to an endocrinologist.
- *Hematocrit*. Routine screening is recommended.
- *Urinalysis*. Routine screening is recommended.
- *Tuberculosis*. Routine screenings is recommended.

Condition-Specific Screening
- Screening serum 17-OHP levels or 24-hour urine pregnanetriol values may be indicated and should be coordinated with the endocrinologist.
- Checking PRA levels may be indicated and should be coordinated with the endocrinologist.
- Bone age should be checked every 2 to 3 years or more often if there are indications of androgen excess.
- Imaging of tests by ultrasound or MRI should occur after puberty.

COMMON ILLNESS MANAGEMENT
- If the child has nausea or vomiting, pallor, cold moist skin, weakness, dizziness or confusion, rapid heart rate, rapid breathing, abdominal/back/leg pain, dehydration, or hypotension, acute adrenal insufficiency should be ruled out.
- A temperature greater than 101.1°F (38.4°C), significant malaise, pain, lethargy, or persistent vomiting (regardless of cause) should be covered by stress doses of hydrocortisone in addition to appropriate specific therapy.
- If the child has hypertension, excessive dietary sodium intake and/or overtreatment with mineralocorticoids or glucocorticoids should be ruled out.
- If the child has hypotension, inadequate mineralocorticoid and glucocorticoid dosage should be ruled out.

Drug Interactions
- Long-term use of barbiturates, phenytoin, or rifampin increases the rate of metabolism of glucocorticoids. Adjustments in dosage may be required.

DEVELOPMENTAL ISSUES
Sleep Patterns
- Unusual fatigue or lethargy may indicate the need for increased doses of hydrocortisone.

Toileting
- Increased vaginal voiding symptoms (e.g., urinary leaking after voiding and vaginitis) are easily treated with leg abduction with voiding and sitz baths. There is no impairment in readiness or functioning. Children with obvious virilization should be allowed privacy.

Discipline
- Expectations are normally based on age and developmental level.
- Physical appearance may differ from age and developmental level, leading to inappropriate expectations.

Child Care
- Child care providers must be aware of special needs with illness and injury and the importance of routine and stress medication.

Schooling
- Children with CAH who have a history of acute adrenal insufficiency or hypoglycemic seizures should be assessed for learning difficulties.
- School personnel should be aware of the special needs of the child's illness and injury.

Sexuality
- Virilization of infant females requires surgical correction.
- Inadequate treatment results in continued virilization, acne, hirsutism, menstrual irregularities, and infertility in females; eventually impairment of fertility occurs in males.
- Most children will be fertile.

Transition to Adulthood
- Transition to providers of adult primary care and endocrine care should be accomplished.
- Source of medical insurance must be identified.

Family Concerns
- Rapid onset of acute adrenal insufficiency is possible.

- Appropriate emergency treatment may be delayed because health care providers lack awareness or knowledge of CAH.
- The normality of females should be stressed.
- Others in the family may be affected (e.g., siblings, children of the affected child). Genetic counseling, prenatal screening, diagnosis, and treatment are available.
- Family members may have difficulty speaking openly about sexuality and genitalia.

REFERENCES

Allis, K. (2021). A broken pathway: Understanding congenital adrenal hyperplasia in the newborn. *Neonatal Network, 40*(5), 286–294. doi:10.1891/11-T-694.

Almarsri, J., Zaiem, F., Rodriguez-Gutierrez, R., et al. (2018). Genital reconstructive surgery in females with congenital adrenal hyperplasia: A systematic review and meta-analysis. *Journal of Clinical Endocrinology & Metabolism Disorders, 103*(11), 4089–4096. doi:10.1210/jc.2018-01863.

Auchus, R. (2022). The uncommon forms of congenital adrenal hyperplasia. *Current Opinion in Endocrinology, Diabetes and Obesity, 29*(3), 263–270. doi:10.1097/MED.0000000000000727.

Badeghiesh, A., Ismail, S., Baghlaf, H., Suarthana, E., & Dahan, M. (2020). Pregnancy, delivery and neonatal outcomes among women with congenital adrenal hyperplasia: A study of a large US database. *RBMO, 41*(6), 1092–1099. doi:10.1016/j.rbmo.2020.08.0361472-6483.

Baumgartner-Parzer, S., Witsch-Baumgartner, M., Hoeppner, W. (2020). EMQN best practice guidelines for molecular genetic testing and reporting of 21-hydroxylase deficiency. *European Journal of Human Genetics, 28*(10), 1341–1367. doi: 10.1038/s41431-020-0653-5. Epub 2020 Jul 2. PMID: 32616876; PMCID: PMC7609334.

Carvalho, B., Carvalho, F., & Carvalho, D. (2022). Congenital adrenal hyperplasia—the main effect of 21-hydroxylase deficiency. *Current Stages and New Perspectives on Disease Treatment.* https://www.intechopen.com/chapters/83494.

Centers for Disease Control and Prevention (CDC). (2021). Vaccines and immunizations. https://www.cdc.gov/vaccines/index.html.

Chawla, R., Rutter, M., Green, J., & Weidler, E. (2019). Care of the adolescent patient with congenital adrenal hyperplasia: Special considerations, shared decision making and transition. *Seminars in Pediatric Surgery, 28*, 150845. doi:10.1016/j.sempedsurg.2019.150845.

Clinical Trials.gov. (2021). A study of gene therapy for classic congenital adrenal hyperplasia (CAH). https://clinicaltrials.gov/ct2/show/NCT04783181.

Draznin, M., Borgohain, P., & Kanungo, S. (2022). Newborn screening in pediatric endocrine disorders. *Endocrines, 3*, 107–114. doi:10.3390/endocrines3010010.

Edelman, S., Desai, J., Pigg, T., Yusuf, C., & Ojodu, J. (2020). Landscape of congenital adrenal hyperplasia newborn screening in the United States. *International Journal of Neonatal Screening, 6*(3), 64–78. doi:10.3390/ijns6030064.

Gomes, L. G., Bachega, T. A. S. S., & Mendonca, B. B. (2019). Classic congenital adrenal hyperplasia and its impact on reproduction. *Fertility and Sterility, 111*(1), 7–12. https://doi.org/10.1016/j.fertnstert.2018.11.037.

Grinton, H., Stikkelbroeck, N., Falhammar, H., & Reisch, N. (2021). Gonadal dysfunction in congenital adrenal hyperplasia. *European Society of Endocrinology, 184*(3), R85–R97. doi:10.1530/EJE-20-1093.

Grosse, S., & Vliet, G. (2020). Challenges in assessing the cost-effectiveness of newborn screening: The example of congenital adrenal hyperplasia. *International Journal of Neonatal Screening, 82*(6), 1–19. doi:10.3390/ijns6040082.

Haddad, N., & Eugster, E. (2019). Peripheral precocious puberty including congenital adrenal hyperplasia: Causes, consequences, management, and outcomes. *Best Practice and Research in Clinical Endocrinology and Metabolism, 33*, 101273.

Hamed, S., Metwalley, K., & Faghaly, H. (2018). Cognitive function in children with classic congenital adrenal hyperplasia. *European Journal of Pediatrics, 177*, 1633–1640. doi:10.1007/s00431-018-3226-7.

Hannah-Shmouni, F., Morissette, R., Sinaii, N., Elman, M., Prezant, T. R., Chen, W., Pulver, A., & Merke, D. P. (2017). Revisiting the prevalence of nonclassic congenital adrenal hyperplasia in US Ashkenazi Jews and Caucasians. *Genetics in Medicine: Official Journal of the American College of Medical Genetics, 19*(11), 1276–1279. https://doi.org/10.1038/gim.2017.46.

Held, P., Bird, I., & Heather, N. (2020). Newborn screening for congenital adrenal hyperplasia: Review of factors affecting screening accuracy. *International Journal of Neonatal Screening, 67*(6), 1–17. doi:10.3390/ijns6030067.

Kalani, A., Bahtiyar, G., & Sacerdote, A. (2012). Ashwagandah root in the treatment of non-classical adrenal hyperplasia. *BMJ Case Reports*, 1–4. doi:10.1136/bcr-2012-006989.

Karlsson, L., de Paula Michelatto, D., Lusa, A. L. G., D'Almeida Mgnani Silva, C., Östberg, L. J., Persson, B., Guerra-Júnior, G., Valente de Lemos-Marini, S. H., Baldazzi, L., Menabó, S., Balsamo, A., Greggio, N. A., Palandi de Mello, M., Barbaro, M., & Lajic, S. (2019). Novel non-classic CYP21A2 variants, including combined alleles, identified in patients with congenital adrenal hyperplasia. *Clinical Biochemistry, 73*, 50–56. https://doi.org/10.1016/j.clinbiochem.2019.07.009.

Kim, M. (2022). *Treatment of adrenal insufficiency in children. UpToDate.* https://www.uptodate.com/contents/treatment-of-adrenal-insufficiency-in-children.

Krone, N., Arlt, W. (2009). Genetics of congenital adrenal hyperplasia. *Best Pract Res Clin Endocrinol Metab, 23*(2), 181–192. doi:10.1016/j.beem.2008.10.014.

Lajic, S., Karlsson, L., & Nordenstrom, A. (2018). Prenatal treatment of congenital adrenal hyperplasia: Long term effects of excess glucocorticoid exposure. *Hormone Research in Pediatrics, 89*, 362–371. doi:10.1159/000485100.

Lam, M. Remediation of congenital adrenal hyperplasia. 2018. https://www.drlamcoaching.com/blog/adrenal-hyperplasia-or-afs-part-3.

Livadas, S., & Bothou, C. (2019). Management of the female with non-classical congenital adrenal hyperplasia (NCCAH): A patient oriented approach. *Frontiers in Endocrinology, 10*, 366–376. doi:10.3389/fendo.2019.00366.

Lousada, L., Mendonca, B., & Bachega, T. (2021). Adrenal crisis and mortality rate in adrenal insufficiency and congenital adrenal hyperplasia. *Archives Endocrinology and Metabolic Disorders, 65*(4), 488–493. doi:10.20945/2359-3997000000392.

MacKay, D., Nordenstrom, A., & Falhammer, H. (2018). Bilateral adrenalectomy in congenital adrenal hyperplasia: A systematic review and meta-analysis. *Journal of Clinical*

Endocrinology and Metabolic Disorders, 103(5), 1767–1778. doi:10.1210/jc.2018-00217.

Mallappa, A., & Merke, D. (2022). Management challenges and therapeutic advantages in congenital adrenal hyperplasia. *Nature Reviews Endocrinology, 18,* 337–343. doi:10.1038/s41574-022-00655-w.

Mehmood, K., & Rentea, R. (2022). Ambiguous genitalia and disorders of sexual differentiation. *StatPearls.* https://www.ncbi.nlm.nih.gov/books/NBK557435.

Merke, D., & Auchus, R. (2020). Clinical manifestations and diagnosis of classic congenital adrenal hyperplasia due to 21-hydroxylase deficiency in infants and children. *UpToDate.* https://www.uptodate.com/contents/clinical-manifestations-and-diagnosis-of-classic-congenital-adrenal-hyperplasia-due-to-21-hydroxylase-deficiency-in-infants-and-children?search=clinical%20manifestations%20and%20diagnosis%20of%20classic%20congenital%20adrenal%20hyperplasia&source=search_result&selectedTitle=1~150&usage_type=default&display_rank=1.

Merke, D. (2021). Treatment of classic congenital adrenal hyperplasia due to 21-hydroxylase deficiency in infants and children. *UpToDate.* https://www.uptodate.com/contents/treatment-of-classic-congenital-adrenal-hyperplasia-due-to-21-hydroxylase-deficiency-in-infants-and-children.

Messina, V., Karlsson, L., Hirvikoski, T., Nordenstrom, A., & Lajic, S. (2020). Cognitive function of children and adolescents with congenital adrenal hyperplasia: Importance of early diagnosis. *Journal of Clinical Endocrinology and Metabolism, 105*(3), e683–e691. doi:10.1210/clinem/dgaa016.

Narasimhan, M., & Khattab, A. (2018). Genetics of congenital adrenal hyperplasia and genotype-phenotype correlation. *Fertility and Sterility, 111*(1), 24–29. doi:10.1016/j.fetnstert.2018.11.007.

National Organization for Rare Disorders (NORD). *Congenital adrenal hyperplasia.* 2021. https://rarediseases.org/rare-diseases/congenital-adrenal-hyperplasia.

Navarro-Zambrana, A., & Sheets, L. (2022). Ethnic and national differences in congenital adrenal hyperplasia incidence: A systematic review and meta-analysis. *Hormone Research in Paediatrics.* doi:10.1159/000526401.

Neeman, B., Bello, R., Lazar, L., Phillip, M., & Vries, L. (2019). Central precocious puberty as a presenting sign of nonclassical congenital adrenal hyperplasia: Clinical characteristics. *Journal of Clinical Endocrinology and Metabolic Disorders, 104*(7), 2695–2700. doi:10.1210/jc.2018-02605.

New, M., Ghizzoni, L., Meyer-Bahlburg, H., Khattab, A., Reichman, D., & Rosenwaks, Z. (2019). Fertility in patients with nonclassical congenital adrenal hyperplasia. *Fertility and Sterility, 111*(1), 13–20. doi:10.1016/j.fertnstert.2018.11.023.

Pellur, M., Narasimhan, H., & Mahadevan, S. (2019). Socio-cultural dimensions of congenital adrenal hyperplasia: An ethnographic study from Chennai, South India. *Indian Journal of Endocrinology and Metabolism, 23*(2), 227–231. doi:10.4103/ijem.IJEM_177_18.

Rautmann, L., Witt, S., Theiding, C., Odenwald, B., Nennstiel-Ratzel, U., Dörr, H. G., & Quitmann, J. H. (2023). Caring for a child with congenital adrenal hyperplasia diagnosed by newborn screening: parental health-related quality of life, coping patterns, and needs. *International Journal of Environmental Research and Public Health, 20*(5), 4493. https://doi.org/10.3390/ijerph20054493.

Reisch, N. (2019). Review of health problems in adult patients with classic congenital adrenal hyperplasia due to 21-hydroxylase deficiency. *Experimental and Clinical Endocrinology and Diabetes, 127,* 171–177. doi:10.1055/a-0820-2085.

Schröder, M. A. M., van Herwaarden, A. E., Span, P. N., van den Akker, E. L. T., Bocca, G., Hannema, S. E., van der Kamp, H. J., de Kort, S. W. K., Mooij, C. F., Schott, D. A., Straetemans, S., van Tellingen, V., van der Velden, J. A., Sweep, F. C. G. J., & Claahsen-van der Grinten, H. L. (2022). Optimizing the timing of highest hydrocortisone dose in children and adolescents with 21-hydroxylase deficiency. *The Journal of Clinical Endocrinology and Metabolism, 107*(4), e1661–e1672. https://doi.org/10.1210/clinem/dgab826.

Seneviratne, S., Jayarajah, U., Gunawardana, S., Samarasinghe, M., & Silva, S. (2021). Gender-role behaviour and gender identity in girls with classical congenital adrenal hyperplasia. *BMC Pediatrics, 21,* 262–267. doi:10.1186/s12887-021-02742-9.

Sewell, R., Buchanan, C. L., Davis, S., Christakis, D. A., Dempsey, A., Furniss, A., Kazak, A. E., Kerlek, A. J., Magnusen, B., Pajor, N. M., Pyle, L., Pyle, L. C., Razzaghi, H., Schwartz, B. I., Vogiatzi, M. G., & Nokoff, N. J. (2021). Behavioral health diagnoses in youth with differences of sex development or congenital adrenal hyperplasia compared with controls: A PEDSnet study. *The Journal of Pediatrics, 239,* 175–181.e2. https://doi.org/10.1016/j.jpeds.2021.08.066.

Speiser, P. W., Arlt, W., Auchus, R. J., Baskin, L. S., Conway, G. S., Merke, D. P., Meyer-Bahlburg, H. F. L., Miller, W. L., Murad, M. H., Oberfield, S. E., & White, P. C. (2018). Congenital adrenal hyperplasia due to steroid 21-hydroxylase deficiency: An Endocrine Society clinical practice guideline. *The Journal of Clinical Endocrinology and Metabolism, 103*(11), 4043–4088. https://doi.org/10.1210/jc.2018-01865.

Speiser, P. (2019). Emerging medical therapies for congenital adrenal hyperplasia. *F1000 Res, 8,* 363–369. doi:10.12688/f1000research.17778.1.

Thijs, E., Wierckx, K., Vandecasteele, S., & Bruel, A. (2019). Adrenal insufficiency, be aware of drug interactions. *Endocrinology, Diabetes and Metabolism Case Reports,* 19-0062. doi:10.1530/EDM-19-0062.

Twayana, A. R., Sunuwar, N., Deo, S., Tariq, W. B., Anjum, A., Rayamajhi, S., & Shrestha, B. (2022). Salt-wasting form of congenital adrenal hyperplasia: A case report. *Cureus, 14*(8), e27807. https://doi.org/10.7759/cureus.27807.

Witchell, S. (2017). Congenital adrenal hyperplasia. *Journal of Pediatric and Adolescent Gynecology, 30*(5), 52–534. doi:10.1016/j.jpag.2017.04.001.

Yau, M., Gujral, J., & New, M. (2019). Congenital adrenal hyperplasia: Diagnosis and emergency treatment. *Endotext.* https://www.ncbi.nlm.nih.gov/books/NBK279085.

Congenital Heart Disease

18

Julie Martin

ETIOLOGY

Congenital heart disease (CHD) results from the abnormal development of the heart or related vascular structures during the first 8 weeks of embryologic development. The heart is the first functional organ to be developed in vertebrate embryos through a process controlled by a gene regulatory network. CHD is one of the most frequent and severe types of congenital malformation and is the leading cause of neonatal mortality from a congenital malformation. The severity of the different types of CHD varies depending on the combination of associated anatomic defects (Diz et al., 2021). Although the etiology of CHD is largely unknown, it is presumed to have a multifactorial cause, with both genetic and environmental factors acting together during a vulnerable time of fetal cardiac development contributing to the formation of the disease (Diz et al., 2021; Saliba et al., 2020; Yasuhara & Garg, 2021; Zhang et al., 2021.

The recent advances in understanding the genetic causes and anatomic subtypes of cardiac defects have revealed links between genetic etiology, pathogenic mechanisms, and cardiac phenotypes (Calcagni et al., 2021) (Table 18.1). These genetic advancements have led to a greater understanding of the etiology of CHD. Presently a genetic etiology for CHD is identified in 20% to 30% of cases (Armstrong et al., 2008; Katz et al., 2022).

Environmental factors contribute to a 2% to 4% risk of CHD development (Mishra et al., 2020). Identified environmental risk factors include parental exposure to chemicals or toxins from organic solvents, pesticides, air pollution, carbon monoxide, and nitrous oxide (Upadhyay et al., 2019). Maternal medical conditions that are risk factors include diabetes, obesity, vaginal infection, fevers, viral infections (especially rubella virus, cytomegalovirus, and influenza virus during the first trimester), stress, or personal history of CHD (Dolk et al., 2020; Mishra et al., 2020) (Table 18.2). The maternal prenatal risk factors include ingestion of alcohol or prescription medications such as antiepileptic drugs (gabapentin, carbamazepine, phenytoin, phenobarbital, and sodium valproate), retinoic acid, lithium, nonsteroidal antiinflammatory drugs (NSAIDs), and angiotensin-converting enzyme (ACE) inhibitors, paroxetine, or tricyclic antidepressants (Dolk et al., 2020; Scott & Neal, 2021; Upadhyay et al., 2019.; Zhang et al.,

2021). Maternal cigarette smoking during pregnancy accounts for 1.4% of CHD cases (Mishra et al., 2020). Fertility procedures such as in vitro fertilization and intracytoplasmic sperm injection are reported risk factors (Giorgione et al., 2018; Mishra et al., 2020). The fewer identified paternal risk factors are age, smoking, and alcohol consumption. In addition, parental socioeconomic status, diet, education, and access to care can impact fetal and cardiac development and increase the risk of CHD development (Borjali et al., 2021; Dolk et al., 2020).

INCIDENCE AND PREVALENCE

CHD occurs in 0.8% to 1% of all live births. CHD represents 33% of all congenital malformations and is a leading cause of morbidity and mortality during childhood (Upadhyay et al., 2019). Most CHD cases occur as isolated malformations, but 25% to 30% are associated with extracardiac anomalies and genetic syndromes (Calcagni et al., 2021; Yasuhara & Garg, 2021). The reported prevalence of infants born with complex CHD is 25% (Glidewell et al., 2019; Reddy et al., 2022) (Table 18.3). Sex distribution has been studied. The distribution of CHD development is fairly equal, with males having a slightly greater incidence of CHD. In addition, there are sex-based cardiac disease tendencies. Females have more CHD defects involving cardiac inflow, such as patent ductus arteriosus (PDA), Ebstein anomaly, truncus arteriosus (TA), atrioventricular canal, atrioventricular septal defect (AVSD), and tetralogy of Fallot (TOF). Males have a higher incidence of left-sided heart lesions and transposition of the great arteries (TGA) (Bradley et al., 2019).

The risk of CHD recurring in the same family depends on several factors. The risk of recurrence of a nongenetic CHD is 3% to 7% in mothers with CHD. In comparison, the recurrence risk for the father is 2% to 3% and lower in siblings, although the rate of reoccurrence increases to 2% to 6% if more than one sibling has CHD (Donofrio et al., 2014). If the defect is associated with a syndrome or chromosomal abnormality, the cardiac lesion recurrence risk will reflect the identified risks for the syndrome or genetic finding. Genetic testing is beneficial and can identify a genetic cause of CHD in 31% to 46% of individuals with a known phenotype of familial CHD.

417

Table 18.1   Genetic Syndrome and/or Gene Variants Commonly Associated With Cardiac Malformations

CHROMOSOME (ASSOCIATED GENE[S]) INVOLVED	EXTRACARDIAC FINDINGS	ASSOCIATED CHD LESIONS	FREQUENCY OF CHD
Aneuploidies			
Trisomy 13	Cleft lip and palate, hypotelorism, coloboma, holoprosencephaly, deafness, severe intellectual disability, polydactyly, omphalocele, cryptorchidism	ASD, VSD, PDA, valve abnormalities	51–64%
Trisomy 18	Micrognathia, short sternum, rocker-bottom feet, omphalocele, renal anomalies, severe intellectual disability	ASD, VSD, PDA, TOF, DORV, TGA, valve abnormalities	80%
Trisomy 21	Facial features, short stature, hypotonia, intellectual disability, behavioral problems, small ears, upslanting palpebral fissures, epicanthal folds, duodenal atresia, imperforate anus, Hirschsprung disease, leukemia	AVSD, VSD, ASD, PDA, TOF	40–50%
Turner syndrome (XO)	Short stature, delayed puberty and menarche, anovulation and infertility, lymphedema, webbed neck, low posterior hairlines, cubitus valgus, skeletal anomalies in skeletal and renal, developmental delays nonverbal learning disabilities and behavioral problems	BAV, CoA, partial anomalous pulmonary venous return, HLH	20–40%
Copy Number Variants			
1p36 deletion	Dysmorphic facies, intellectual disabilities, hypotonia, seizures, structural brain anomalies, ophthalmologic and vision issues, hearing loss, skeletal anomalies, genitourinary anomalies, behavioral problems	ASD, VSD, valvular abnormalities, PDA, TOF, CoA, right ventricular infundibular stenosis, Ebstein anomaly, cardiomyopathy, LVNC, dilated cardiomyopathy	50%
1q21.1 deletion	Microcephaly, intellectual disability, mildly dysmorphic features, short stature, eye abnormalities, sensorineural hearing loss, skeletal malformation, genitourinary alterations, autism, ADHD	PDA, truncus arteriosus, VSD, ASD, TOF, BAV, dilation of the ascending aorta, AV insufficiency, IAA, anomalous origin of the right coronary artery, PVS, TA	20–40%
1q21.1 duplication (GAJR)	Hypospadias, clubbed feet, hemivertebrae, hip dysplasia, intellectual disabilities, developmental delays, expressive language delay, autism, ADHD	TOF, VSD, TGA, PVS	20–40%
8p23.1 deletion (GATA4)	Congenital diaphragmatic hernia, growth impairment, microcephaly, hyperactivity, impulsiveness, intellectual disability, developmental delays	ASD, AVSD, PVS, HRV, DORV, double inlet left ventricle	90%
22q11.2 deletion syndrome (formerly DiGeorge syndrome)	Dysmorphic facies, palatal malformation, learning disabilities, immunodeficiency, hypocalcemia, feeding/swallowing problems, constipation, anomalies (renal, nervous system, skeletal, ophthalmologic), hearing loss, growth hormone deficiency, laryngotracheoesophageal findings, enamel hypoplasia, behavioral and learning disabilities, autism, psychiatric disorders (schizophrenia), ADHD, anxiety	Conotruncal defects, IAA type B, aortic arch anomalies, ASD, PV stenosis, TOF, TA, VSD, HLHS, DORV, TGA, vascular rings, heterotaxy syndrome	74–85%

Table 18.1 Genetic Syndrome and/or Gene Variants Commonly Associated With Cardiac Malformations—cont'd

CHROMOSOME (ASSOCIATED GENE[S]) INVOLVED	EXTRACARDIAC FINDINGS	ASSOCIATED CHD LESIONS	FREQUENCY OF CHD
Jacobsen syndrome (11q terminal)	Dysmorphic features, growth retardation, insulin-like growth factor-1 deficiency, cognitive and behavioral dysfunction, thrombocytopenia, platelet dysfunction, immune deficiency, problems in ophthalmology, gastrointestinal, and genitourinary	Membranous VSD, LVOT defects, BAV, hypoplasia of the mitral valve, aortic valve or aorta, DORV, TGA, AVSDS, ASD, dextrocardia, aberrant right subclavian artery, PDA, persistent LSVC, TV atresia, IAA type B, PVS	>50%
Williams-Beuren syndrome (7q11.23 deletion)	Dysmorphic features, specific cognitive profile, unique social personality, growth abnormalities, connective tissue disorder, skeletal anomalies, endocrine abnormalities, feeding problems when young, overweight, DM, systemic HTN as adult	Supravalvular aortic stenosis, pulmonary artery stenosis, elastin arteriopathy, aortic and mitral valve defects	
Single Gene Variants			
Alagille syndrome (JAG 1, NOTCH2)	Bile duct paucity, posterior embryotoxon, butterfly vertebrae, renal defects	PPS, TOF, PA	>90%
Cardiofaciocutaneous (BRAF, KRAS, MAP2K1, MAP2K2)	Curly hair, sparse eyebrows, feeding problems, developmental delay, intellectual disability	PVC, ASD, HCM	75%
Cantu (ABCC9)	Hypertrichosis at birth, macrocephaly, narrow thorax, coarse facies, macroglossia, broad hands, advanced bone age	PDA, BAV, HCM, CoA, PE, AS	75%
Char (TFAP2B)	Wide-set eyes, down-slanting palpebral fissures, thick lips, hand anomalies	PDA, VSD	58%
CHARGE (CHD7)	Coloboma, choanal atresia, genital hypoplasia, ear anomalies, hearing loss, developmental delay, growth retardation, intellectual disability	TOF, PDA, DORV, AVSD, VSD	75–85%
Costello (HRAS)	Short stature, feeding problems, broad facies, bitemporal narrowing, redundant skin, intellectual disability, deep creases in hands	PVS, ASD VSD, HCM, arrhythmia	44–52%
Ellis-Van Creveld syndrome (EVC, EVC2)	Skeletal dysplasia, short limbs, polydactyly, short ribs, dysplastic nails, respiratory insufficiency	Common atrium	60%
Holt-Oram syndrome (TBX5)	Absent, hypoplastic, or triphalangeal thumbs; phocomelia; defects of radius; limb defects more prominent on left	VSD, ASD, AVSD, conduction defects	
Kabuki syndrome (MLL2, KMT2D, KDM6A)	Growth deficiency, wide palpebral fissures, large protuberant ears, fetal finger pads, intellectual disability, clinodactyly	CoA, BAV, ASD, VSD, TOF, TGA, HLHS	
Noonan syndrome (PTPN11, RAF1, KRAS, NRAS, RIT1, SHOC2, SOS2, BRAF)	Short stature, hypertelorism, down-slanting palpebral fissures, ptosis, low posterior hairline, pectus deformity, bleeding disorder, chylothorax, cryptorchidism	Dysplastic PVS, ASD, TOF, AVSD, HCM, VSD, PDA	60–90%
VACTERL association (unknown)	Vertebral anomalies, anal atresia, tracheoesophageal fistula, renal anomalies, radial dysplasia, thumb hypoplasia, single umbilical artery	VSD, ASD, HLHS, PDA, TGA, TOF, TA	53–80%
Carpenter syndrome (RAB23)	Craniosynostosis, brachydactyly, syndactyly, polydactyly, obesity	VSD, ASD, PDA, PS, TOF, TGA	50%

Continued

| Table 18.1 | Genetic Syndrome and/or Gene Variants Commonly Associated With Cardiac Malformations—cont'd |

CHROMOSOME (ASSOCIATED GENE[S]) INVOLVED	EXTRACARDIAC FINDINGS	ASSOCIATED CHD LESIONS	FREQUENCY OF CHD
Coffin-Siris syndrome (ARID 1B, SMARCB 1M, ARID 1A SMARCB 1, SMARCA 4, SMARCE 1)	Developmental delays, coarse facies, hypoplastic distal phalanges, short stature, intellectual disability	ASD, AVSD, VSD, MR, PDA, PS, DEX, AS	20–44%
Cornelia de Lange syndrome (NIPBL, SMC, SMC3)	Restricted growth, craniofacial abnormalities, hirsutism, gastroesophageal reflux disease, limb dysplasia, genitourinary malformations, heart defect	CoA, PS, TOF, ASD, VSD	33%
Goldenhar syndrome (unknown)	Hemifacial microsomia, epibulbar dermoids, microtia, hemivertebrae	VSD, PDA, TOF, CoA, conotruncal defect	32%
Mowat-Wilson syndrome (ZEB2)	Short stature, microcephaly, Hirschsprung disease, intellectual disability, seizures	VSD, CoA, ASD, PDA, PAS	54%
Rubinstein-Taybi syndrome (CBP, EP300)	Microcephaly, growth retardation, down-slanting palpebral fissures, low-set malformed ears, prominent or beaked nose, intellectual disability, broad thumbs and toes	PDA, VSD, ASD, HLHS, BAV	33%
Smith-Lemli-Opitz syndrome (DHCR7)	Microcephaly, ptosis, genital anomalies, renal anomalies, broad nasal tip with anteverted nostrils, intellectual disability, syndactyly	AVSD, HLHS, ASD, PDA, VSD	50%
Marfan syndrome (fibrillin)	Arm span to height >1.05, disproportionate tall stature, long narrow face, ectopia lentis, pectus excavatum, pectus carinatum, high-arched palate	Aortic aneurysm, mitral valve prolapses, dilated pulmonary artery	

AS, Aortic stenosis; *ASD,* atrial septal defect; *AVA,* aortic valve anomaly; *AVSD,* atrioventricular septal defect; *BAV,* bicuspid aortic valve; *BPV,* bicuspid pulmonary valve; *CFC,* cardiofaciocutaneous; *CHARGE,* coloboma, heart defects, choanal atresia, retarded growth and development, genital anomalies, and ear anomalies; *CM,* cardiomyopathy; *CoA,* coarctation of the aorta; *DEX,* dextrocardia; *DOLV,* double-outlet left ventricle; *DORV,* double-outlet right ventricle; *HCM,* hypertrophic cardiomyopathy; *HD,* heart disease; *HLHS,* hypoplastic left heart; *HRH,* hypoplastic right heart; *IAA,* interruption of aortic arch; *LVNC,* left ventricular noncompaction; *LVOT,* left ventricular outflow tract; *MR,* mitral regurgitation; *MVP,* mitral valve prolapse; *OFD,* oral-facial-digital; *PA,* pulmonary atresia; *PAS,* pulmonary artery stenosis; *PDA,* patent ductus arteriosus; *PE,* pericardial effusion; *PPS,* peripheral pulmonary stenosis; *PS,* pulmonary stenosis; *PVS,* pulmonary stenosis; *SVAS,* supravalvular aortic stenosis; *TA,* truncus arteriosus; *TGA,* transposition of great arteries; *TOF,* tetralogy of Fallot; *VACTERL,* association of vertebral defects, anal atresia, cardiac defects, tracheoesophageal fistula, renal and limb anomalies; *VR,* vascular ring; *VSD,* ventricular septal defect.

Modified from Diz, O.M., Campuzano, O., Toro, R., Cesar, S., Sarquella-Brugada, G., & Gomez, O. (2021). Personalized genetic diagnosis of congenital heart defects in newborns. *Journal of Personalized Medicine,* 11(6), 562.

| Table 18.2 | Maternal Medical Conditions and Environmental Risk Factors and Associated Congenital Heart Defects |

MATERNAL CONDITIONS	ASSOCIATED CARDIAC CONDITION(S)
ART/IVF	CHD major/minor
Connective tissue disorder	ASD, VSD, AVSD, conotruncal defect, heterotaxia
Febrile illness	ASD, RVOTO, conotruncal defect, VSD, TGA
Diabetes	ASD, TGA, VSD, AVSD, HLH, cardiomyopathy, LVOTO, TOF
Gestational diabetes	TOF
Gestational HTN	VSD
HTN	ASD, VSD, AVSD, conotruncal defects, heterotaxia
Influenza	TGA, VSD, TA, CoA, RVOTO, LVOTO
Rubella	PDA, ASD, VSD, PPS
Lupus erythematous	Heart block
Obesity	ASD, VSD, aortic arch defects, PDA, HLH, TOF, CoA, conotruncal defect, AVSD, RVOTO, heterotaxia
Phenylketonuria	TOF, PDA, VSD, CoA
Maternal Ingestions	
Air pollutants	ASD, VSD, CoA, TOF
Alcohol	ASD, VSD, AVSD, TGA, TOF, PVS, conotruncal defect

Table 18.2   Maternal Medical Conditions and Environmental Risk Factors and Associated Congenital Heart Defects—cont'd

MATERNAL CONDITIONS	ASSOCIATED CARDIAC CONDITION(S)
Amphetamine	VSD, PDA, ASD, TGA
Antihypertensive agent	ASD, VSD, CoA, PVS
Cocaine	Heterotaxy ASD, VSD
Fluconazole (first trimester)	Septal defects
Ibuprofen	VSD, TGA
Lithium	Ebstein anomaly
Marijuana	VSD, Ebstein anomaly
Nitrofurantoin	HLH, ASD
Organic solvents	TGA, TOF, PS
Phenytoin	CoA, AS, PS, PDA
Quinolones	Conotruncal, TOF
Retinoic acid	VSD, varied CHD
Sertraline	ASD, VSD, PDA, persistent fetal circulation
Smoking	ASD, VSD, AVSD, TGA, RVOTO, PVS, TA, TOF
SSRIs	ASD, VSD, RVOTO
Sulfonamide	HLH, CoA
Thalidomide	TOF, TA, VSD, ASD
Trimethadone	TOF, TGA
Valproic acid	TOF, VSD, AS, PS, RVOTO, LVOTO
Warfarin	TOF, VSD
ART/IVF	CHD, major/minor
Connective Tissue disorder	ASD, VSD, AVSD, conotruncal defect, heterotaxia
Febrile illness	ASD, RVOTO, conotruncal defect, VSD, TGA
Diabetes	ASD, TGA, VSD, AVSD, HLH, cardiomyopathy, LVOTO, TOF
Gestational diabetes	TOF
Gestational HTN	VSD
HTN	ASD, VSD, AVSD, conotruncal defects, heterotaxia
Influenza	TGA, VSD, TA, CoA, RVOTO, LVOTO
Rubella	PDA, ASD, VSD, PPS
Lupus erythematous	Heart block
Obesity	ASD, VSD, aortic arch defects, PDA, HLH, TOF, CoA, conotruncal defect, AVSD, RVOTO, heterotaxia
Phenylketonuria	TOF, PDA, VSD, CoA
Maternal ingestions	
Air pollutants	ASD, VSD, CoA, TOF
Alcohol	ASD, VSD, AVSD, TGA, TOF, PVS, conotruncal defect
Amphetamine	VSD, PDA, ASD, TGA
Anti-hypertensive agent	ASD, VSD, CoA, PVS
Cocaine	Heterotaxy ASD, VSD
Fluconazole 1st trimester	Septal defects
Ibuprofen	VSD, TGA
Lithium	Ebstein's anomaly
Marijuana	VSD, Ebstein's anomaly
Nitrofurantoins	HLH, ASD
Organic solvents	TGA, TOF, PS
Phenytoin	CoA, AS, PS, PDA
Quinolones	Conotruncal, TOF
Retinoic acid	VSD, varied CHD
Sertraline	ASD, VSD, PDA, persistent fetal circulation
Smoking	ASD, VSD, AVSD, TGA, RVOTO, PVS, TA, TOF
SSRIs	ASD, VSD, RVOTO

Continued

Table 18.2	Maternal Medical Conditions and Environmental Risk Factors and Associated Congenital Heart Defects—cont'd
MATERNAL CONDITIONS	**ASSOCIATED CARDIAC CONDITION(S)**
Sulfonamide	HLH, CoA
Thalidomide	TOF, TA, VSD, ASD
Trimethadone	TOF, TGA
Valproic acid	TOF, VSD, AS, PS, RVOTO, LVOTO
Warfarin	TOF, VSD

ART, Artificial productive technologies; *ASD*, atrial septal defect; *AVSD*, atrioventricular septal defect; *CoA*, coarctation of the aorta; *HLH*, hypoplastic left heart; *HTN*, hypertension; *IVF*, in vitro fertilization; *LVOTO*, left ventricular outflow tract obstruction; *PDA*, patent ductus arteriosus; *PPS*, peripheral pulmonary artery stenosis; *PS*, pulmonary stenosis; *PVS*, pulmonary valve stenosis; *RVOTO*, right ventricular outflow tract obstruction; *SSRI*, selective serotonin reuptake inhibitor; *TOF*, tetralogy of Fallot; *TGA*, transposition of the great arteries; *TA*, truncus arteriosus; *VSD*, ventricular septal defect.

Modified from Upadhyay, J., Rana, M., Joshi, A., Durgapal, S., & Bisht, S. (2019). Pathophysiology, etiology, and recent advancement in the treatment of congenital heart disease. *Journal of Indian College of Cardiology, 9*; Nie, X., Liu, X., Wang, C., et al. (2022). Assessment of evidence on reported non-genetic risk factors of congenital heart defects: The updated umbrella review. *BMC Pregnancy and Childbirth, 22*, 371; and Zhang, T.N., Wu, Q.J., Liu, Y.S., Lv, J.L., Sun, H., Chang, Q., Liu, C.F., & Zhao, Y.H. (2021). Environmental risk factors and congenital heart disease: An umbrella review of 165 systematic reviews and meta-analyses with more than 120 million participants. *Frontiers in Cardiovascular Medicine, 8*, 640729.

Table 18.3	Incidence of Congenital Heart Disease (CHD)
CHD SUBTYPE	**INCIDENCE (%)**
Ventricular septal defect	35.56
Atrial septal defect	15.37
Patent ductus arteriosus	10.17
Pulmonary stenosis	6.23
Tetralogy of Fallot	4.42
Atrioventricular septal defect	3.59
Coarctation of the aorta	3.57
Transposition of the great arteries	3.18
Pulmonary arteriosus aneurysm	2.97
Hypoplastic left heart syndrome	2.56
Aortic stenosis	2.33
Congenital heart block	2.32
Aortic valve insufficiency	2.31
Total anomalous pulmonary venous return	1.5
Mitral insufficiency	1.34
Double outlet right ventricle	1.3
Pulmonary atresia	1.3
Single ventricle	1.14
Tricuspid valve atresia/stenosis	1.07
Dextrocardia	1.03
Truncus arteriosus	0.98
Mitral stenosis	0.96
Interrupted aortic arch	0.61
Ebstein anomaly	0.53
Coronary artery aneurysm	0.42
Partial anomalous pulmonary venous return	0.31

From Liu, Y., Chen, S., Zühlke, L., Black, G.C., Choy, M.K., Li, N., & Keavney, B.D. (2019). Global birth prevalence of congenital heart defects 1970-2017: Updated systematic review and meta-analysis of 260 studies. *International Journal of Epidemiology, 48*(2), 455–463.

Advancements in the diagnosis of CHD, as well as in the medical treatments, interventional cardiac catheterization procedures, and surgery management of CHD, have resulted in increased survival rates of 85% to 90% for individuals with CHD (Gilljam et al., 2019; Givertz et al., 2019; Muthurangu, 2021; Reardon & Lin, 2021). It is estimated over 1.4 million US adults are living with CHD. The survivors of CHD require lifetime cardiac surveillance of the CHD, assessment for residual effects from the corrective surgery or procedure, and monitoring of possible cardiovascular complications (Apostolopoulou et al., 2020; Bradley et al., 2019).

PATHOPHYSIOLOGY

Alterations during embryology development result in cardiac malformation. Congenital cardiac malformations encompass multiple aspects of the heart, which may include anatomic, pathophysiology, vascular anomalies, and electrical conduction pathways or channelopathies. Structural CHD can be categorized in many ways, including simplex versus complex, acyanotic or cyanotic lesions, shunt lesions versus obstructive lesions, and ductal dependent versus nonductal dependent. Within these broad classifications, the pathophysiology and the hemodynamics of the cardiac defects need to be considered when managing an individual with CHD.

CHD often has intracardiac shunting lesion(s) (i.e., atrial septal defect [ASD], ventricular septal defect [VSD]). In normal cardiac physiology there is a complete separation of deoxygenated and oxygenated blood. These two circulations run in parallel, maintaining a one-to-one volume relationship in the pulmonary and systemic regions of circulation, each feeding the other. The deoxygenated blood returns to the right atrium (RA), is pumped to the right ventricle (RV), and then is pumped to the lungs as pulmonary blood flow. After oxygenation, the blood returns from the pulmonary veins to the left atrium (LA), is pumped to the left ventricle (LV), and then is pumped to the aorta as the systemic blood flow or cardiac output. The cardiac conduction system is responsible for the efficient contraction-relaxation cycle of the atria and ventricles (Buijtendijk et al., 2020).

A shunt refers to the abnormality in the flow of blood from one side of the circulation to the other side. In the left-to-right shunt, the oxygenated pulmonary venous blood returns directly to the lungs instead of being pumped into the body. Similarly, in the right-to-left shunt, the deoxygenated systemic venous blood returns, bypassing the lungs and returning directly to the body without becoming oxygenated. Circulation in each shunt becomes less efficient and increases the demand on the ventricles. In most cases, the severity of the symptoms is determined by the volume of shunted blood (Sommer et al., 2008; Upadhyay et al., 2019). Specific heart defects can result in obstruction of blood flow into the pulmonary or systemic circulation. With increased stenosis or obstructions, a greater pressure or volume load within the adjacent cardiac chambers may occur.

CONGENITAL HEART DISEASES

CHD may occur as an isolated finding (i.e., VSD) or may involve a combination of cardiac findings (i.e., a bicuspid aortic valve with coarctation of the aorta [CoA]). A child with CHD is managed by a cardiologist or an advanced provider, such as a nurse practitioner or physician assistant. The primary care provider should also possess an understanding of CHD, clinical findings associated with the specific cardiac findings, an awareness of potential concerns, and cardiac treatment options. This section of the cardiac chapter will discuss the more common CHDs.

LEFT-TO-RIGHT SHUNTS

Patent Ductus Arteriosus
Description
- The ductus arteriosus is a fetal vascular connection between the main pulmonary artery (PA) and the aorta, which during fetal life diverts blood away from the pulmonary bed and into the aorta.
- Functional closure of the ductus normally occurs after birth when the systemic arterial oxygen tension increases and the circulating prostaglandin level decreases, triggering ductal constriction.
- If the ductus remains patent after birth, the blood flow reverses, resulting in blood flow from the aorta into the pulmonary bed.

Natural history
- Spontaneous closure is expected within 48 hours.
- Premature infants have a greater incidence of persistent PDA.

Complications
- Heart failure
- Infective endocarditis
- Pulmonary hypertension (PH)

Treatment options
- Observe for spontaneous closure
- Pharmacologic therapy: inhibitors of prostaglandin synthesis (indomethacin, ibuprofen)
- Cardiac catheter device closure (coil, ductal occluder, vascular plug)
- Surgical ligation via left thoracotomy

Atrial Septal Defect
Description
- An abnormal opening between the right and left atria, which results from incomplete fusion of the atrial septum
- Three main types
  - Primum defects (septum primum does not fuse with endocardial cushions)
  - Secundum defects (located within fossa ovalis)
  - Sinus venosus defect (located at the entry of superior vena cava into the RA; may be associated with right upper pulmonary vein draining into the RA)

Natural history
- Small ASD; often closure is spontaneous during infancy
- Moderate or large ASD; unlikely to close spontaneously

Complications
- Pulmonary vascular disease
- Arrhythmias
- Heart failure

Management
- Diuretic therapy (rarely required)
- If evidence of right heart enlargement and pulmonary overcirculation, then cardiac intervention may be required

Treatment options
- Cardiac catheterization with device closure
- Surgical closure with primary (stitch) closure or patch closure

Ventricular Septal Defect
Description
- An abnormal opening between the RVs and LVs, which results from incomplete closure of the ventricular septum
- VSD can be located at the membranous, muscular, subaortic, subpulmonic (outlet), or AV canal (inlet) region

Natural history
- Muscular VSD; often closes spontaneously within the first 2 years of life
- Physiologic effects depend on the size of the defect and pulmonary vascular resistance

Complications
- Congestive heart failure (CHF)
- Endocarditis
- Aortic valve regurgitation

Treatment options
- Surgical options
  - PA band placement (temporary treatment)
  - Ventricular septal repair with primary (stitch) or patch closure
  - Cardiac catheterization
  - Transcatheter closure (generally reserved for VSD not amendable to surgical repair [i.e., muscular VSD])

Complete Atrioventricular Canal (Endocardial Cushion Defect)

Description
- Group of congenital cardiac defects involving the AV septum and valves (tricuspid valve and mitral valve)
- Occurs when there is a failure of fusion between the superior and inferior endocardial cushions
- Cardiac findings include an ostium primum ASD, inlet VSD, cleft in the mitral valve, and a large common AV valve instead of two separate AV valves

Natural history
- AV canal associated with 40% to 50% risk of trisomy 21
- Surgical intervention required

Complications
- CHF
- Pulmonary overcirculation
- PH
- AV valve regurgitation or stenosis
- Atrial arrhythmia
- Subaortic stenosis

Management
- Anticongestive management
  - Diuretics
  - Digoxin
  - ACE inhibitors
  - Optimized nutrition
- Cardiac catheterization may be completed preoperatively to assess pulmonary vascular resistance with concerns of PH.

Treatment options
- Surgical repair to include the closure of ASD, closure of VSD, and construction of two separate and competent AV valves

OBSTRUCTIVE LESIONS

Right Ventricular Outflow Tract Obstructions/ Pulmonary Stenosis

Description
- Right ventricular outflow tract (RVOT) obstructive lesions are characterized by obstruction to flow from the RV to the PAs.
- The obstruction or stenosis can occur at different levels and can be multiple, including valvular pulmonic stenosis (PS), subvalvar PS, supravalvar PS, and peripheral PS.
- The stenosis may be caused by thickened valve leaflets, hypoplasia of the pulmonary valve, or narrowing within the PA or PA branches.
- These lesions can occur in isolation or may be associated with other cardiac defects (i.e., TOF, tricuspid atresia).

Natural history
- Mild PV stenosis and peripheral stenosis may resolve without intervention.

- It may be associated with William, Noonan, and Alagille syndromes.

Complications
- RV hypertrophy
- RV dysfunction
- Arrhythmia

Management
- Monitor for clinical findings of oxygen desaturations, cyanosis, tachypnea, right-sided heart failure
- Surveillance echocardiograms and electrocardiography (ECG)

Treatment options
- Moderate to severe valvular PV stenosis may increase and require cardiac catheterization with balloon valvuloplasty or surgical repair (e.g., pulmonary valvotomy, Blalock-Thomas-Taussig shunt (BTT) placement, PV replacement).
- Cardiac surgery may be indicated for moderate to severe supravalvular PS (e.g., patch enlargement at the site of PS) and subvalvar PS (e.g., muscular resection, infundibular patch).

Aortic Stenosis

Description
- Aortic stenosis is characterized by obstruction of blood flow or stenosis located at the aortic valve, subvalvar, or supravalvar regions.
- Aortic valve stenosis (AVS) is often caused by the thickening and fusion of aortic valve cusps.
- May occur as an isolated finding or associated with the bicuspid aortic valve or other CHD.
- Subaortic stenosis caused by a fibrous ridge or membrane below the aortic valve resulting in left ventricular outflow tract (LVOT) obstruction.

Natural history
- Aortic stenosis ranges from mild to severe.
- Requires surveillance for increased stenosis, aortic valve insufficiency, aorta dilation.

Complications
- LV hypertrophy
- LV dysfunction
- Ventricular arrhythmia
- Decreased systemic output
- Aorta aneurysms
- Endocarditis
- Death

Management
- Monitor for clinical findings of poor systemic perfusion, left-sided CHF, pulmonary congestion, feeding intolerance, exercise intolerance
- Surveillance echocardiograms and ECGs

Table 18.4	Modified Ross Heart Failure Classification
Class I	Asymptomatic
Class II	Mild tachypnea or diaphoresis with feeding in infants, exertional dyspnea in older children
Class III	Marked tachypnea or diaphoresis with feeding in infants, marked exertional dyspnea, prolonged feeding time with failure of growth
Class IV	Tachypnea, grunting, retractions, sweating at rest

From Budakoty, S. (2020). Approach to a child with congestive heart failure. *Indian Journal of Pediatrics, 87,* 312–320.

Treatment options
- Cardiac catheterization with balloon valvuloplasty or angioplasty
- Cardiac surgery options
  - AVS: aortic valvotomy, aortic valve replacement, Ross procedure (Table 18.4)
  - Supravalvar stenosis: patch augmentation
  - Subaortic membrane resection

Coarctation of the Aorta
Description
- Characterized by narrowing within the aorta, typically located at the insertion of the ductus arteriosus just distal to the left subclavian artery
- May be associated with the bicuspid aortic valve and other CHDs

Natural history
- Coarctation obstruction ranges from mild to severe
- Requires surveillance for increased narrowing of the size of the aorta resulting in increased obstruction of blood flow
- Coarctation associated with Turner syndrome

Complications
- Systemic hypertension
- Left-sided heart failure
- LV hypertrophy
- Ventricular arrhythmia
- Aorta dilation/aneurysm
- Kidney dysfunction
- Abdomen/intestinal hypoperfusion

Management
- Monitor for clinical symptoms of decreased peripheral perfusion, coolness in lower extremities, weak or absent pulses in femoral or lower extremities, blood pressure discrepancy in upper and lower extremities, tachycardia, feeding intolerance, exercise intolerance

Treatment options
- Cardiac catheterization
  - Balloon angioplasty
  - Aortic stent placement
- Cardiac surgery for coarctation repair
  - Discrete CoA: resection with end-to-end anastomosis
  - Coarctation repair with patch augmentation

- Long segment CoA: subclavian flap aortoplasty
- Aortic arch reconstruction is required for hypoplastic aortic arch

Posttreatment: monitor for rebound hypertension or recurrent CoA. Recurrent CoA may require cardiac catheterization with balloon angioplasty and/or stent placement.

CYANOTIC LESIONS
Transposition of the Great Arteries
Description
- TGA is a ventriculoarterial discordant lesion in which the aorta arises from the RV carrying desaturated blood to the body, and the PA arises from the LV carrying oxygenated blood back to the lungs.
- There is a complete separation of the pulmonary and systemic circulations resulting in hypoxemic blood circulating throughout the body, and hyperoxygenated blood circulating in the lungs that is not compatible with survival. Defects that permit the mixing of the two circulations (i.e., ASD, VSD, PDA) are necessary for survival.

Natural history
- Unrepaired: progressive hypoxia, acidosis, and heart failure if left untreated

Management
- Presurgical repair
- Admit to intensive care unit or intensive cardiac care unit
- Prostaglandin infusion to maintain PDA
- May require cardiac catheterization for balloon atrial septostomy for improved intracardiac mixing of blood at the level of atrium septum

Treatment options
- Cardiac surgery
  - Arterial switch operation (ASO) is a procedure of choice. ASO surgery entails the following: The aorta and the PA are transected and transposed/switched in position and then sewn onto the opposite great vessel trunk. The coronary arteries are removed from the aortic trunk and then reimplanted onto the PA trunk. The ASD is closed. These interventions result in an anatomic correction.
  - Rastelli procedure may be performed in patients with VSD and severe PV stenosis. Rastelli procedures entail baffling the LVOT through the VSD, which closes the VSD and directs oxygenated blood from the LV into the aorta and placing a conduit from the RV to the PA. These interventions result in unoxygenated blood from the RV being sent through the conduit into the PA and oxygenated blood from the LV being sent into the aorta.

Chronic complications/concerns
- Monitor for atrial or ventricular arrhythmia, ventricular function

- Additional considerations
  - ASO: monitor for pulmonary stenosis, aorta stenosis, coronary artery insufficiency, neoaortic root dilation, neoaortic regurgitation
  - Rastelli: monitor for stenosis within the RV to PA conduit. The conduit will need replacement when the child outgrows the conduit, which does not grow over time

Tetralogy of Fallot
Description
- TOF includes four main abnormalities
  1. RV outflow obstruction
  2. VSD
  3. Overriding aorta
  4. RV hypertrophy
- The main and the branch PAs are variably hypoplastic in many patients.

Natural history
- Unrepaired: progressive cyanosis, polycythemia develops secondary to cyanosis, increased RVOT obstruction, increased RV hypertrophy

Management
- Presurgical repair
- Monitor for progressive oxygen desaturations, tachypnea, increased work of breathing, feeding difficulties, poor weight gain
- Assess for hypoxic (tet) spells especially during times of illness, fever, pain, hypovolemia
  - Clinical findings of cyanosis, rapid and deep respirations, fussiness, and decreased murmur intensity
  - Severe hypoxic spell can lead to limpness, convulsions, cerebrovascular accident, or death
- Tet spell treatment options: Calm infant. Hold child in the knee-chest position. Administer morphine. Administer oxygen. Administer intravenous fluid bolus. Beta-blocker therapy may be prescribed by a cardiologist.

Treatment options
- A minority of patients require palliative shunts, RVOT stents, or ductal stents prior to cardiac surgery. Reasons include severe RVOT obstruction, hypoplastic PAs, unusual coronary artery anatomy, or small patient size (e.g., prematurity).
- Most patients undergo complete TOF repair with patch closure of the VSD, widening of the RVOT by division and/or resection of infundibular tissue and muscle bundles, and pulmonary valvotomy or pulmonary transannular patch placement

Chronic complications/concerns
- Pulmonary valve regurgitation
- Pulmonary valve stenosis (PVS)
- RV enlargement
- RV dysfunction
- Ascending aorta dilation
- Arrhythmia (especially ventricular)
- Sudden death

Tricuspid Atresia
Description
- Characterized by tricuspid valve absence resulting in no communication between the RA and ventricle
- Associated cardiac defects of ASD, RV hypoplasia, VSD, pulmonary outflow obstruction
- Systemic venous blood flows into the RA. Blood moves across the ASD, mixes with oxygenated blood returning from the lungs, flows into the lungs, and then is propelled into the systemic circulations. The lungs receive blood flow from the PDA or VSD.
- Three types of tricuspid atresia
  - Type I (70–80%): normal anatomy of great arteries
  - Type II (12–25%): dextro-TGA (d-TGA)
  - Type III (3–6%): malposition of the great arteries other than d-TGA (TA, AVSD, double outlet RV)

Natural history
- Untreated: high mortality rate

Management
- Presurgical repair
- Admit to intensive care unit or cardiac care unit
- Initiate prostaglandin infusion if cyanotic
- Monitor for respiratory compromise, hypotension, poor perfusion, acidosis
- Cardiac catheterization with balloon atrial septostomy if ASD is small and restrictive

Treatment options
- Cardiac surgery management consists of three staged palliative surgical procedures
  1. Norwood procedure: systemic to PA shunt
  2. Glenn procedure
  3. Fontan procedure
See Hypoplastic Left Heart Syndrome (later) for staged surgery details.

Truncus Arteriosus
Description
- Characterized by a single arterial trunk with a truncal valve that leaves the heart and gives rise to pulmonary, systemic, and coronary circulation. Associated cardiac finding of VSD and aortic arch abnormalities.
- Different forms of TA: Collet and Edwards classifications
  - Type I: main PA arises from the left side of the truncal root
  - Type II: right and left branch PAs have two closely spaced but separate origins from the posterior aspect of the truncal root
  - Type II: branch PA origins are widely separated from the truncal root

Natural history
- Cyanosis was noted immediately after birth. CHF develops within several days to weeks after birth as the pulmonary vascular resistance decreases.
- High mortality if left untreated

Management
- Anticongestive management: diuretic
- Inotropic agents to improve myocardial contractility
- Angiotensin blockade reduces afterload
- Noninvasive positive pressure ventilation for respiratory distress

Treatment options
- Surgical repair
  - The PAs are moved from the truncus and reattached to the RV to the PA conduit
  - Opening and repair of truncus with a patch of pulmonary homograft material or pericardium
  - Closure of the VSD

Chronic complications/concerns
- Heart failure
- Conduit stenosis
- Arrhythmia

Anomalous Pulmonary Venous Return
Description
- Oxygenated blood returning from the lungs is carried abnormally to the right heart by one or more pulmonary veins emptying directly or indirectly through venous channels into the RA.
- Partial anomalous return of the pulmonary veins to the RA functions the same as an ASD.
- In total anomalous return of the pulmonary veins there are no pulmonary veins connected to the LA; an interatrial communication (e.g., PFO or ASD) is necessary for survival.
- Pulmonary veins may be unobstructed or develop obstruction.
- Types of total anomalous pulmonary venous return (TAPVR)
  - Supracardiac: pulmonary veins drain into the superior vena cava through a left vertical vein and left innominate vein.
  - Cardiac: pulmonary veins drain into the coronary sinus or into the RA.
  - Infracardiac: pulmonary veins drain below the diaphragm into the portal vein, ductus venosus, hepatic vein, or inferior vena cava.

Natural history
- Unobstructed pulmonary veins: mild cyanosis at birth
- Obstructed pulmonary veins: marked cyanosis and respiratory distress develop in the neonatal period. Pulmonary congestion and CHF develop with TAPVR with growth retardation. Without surgery, two-thirds of infants die before 1 year of age.

Management
- Unobstructed venous return: anticongestive medications (e.g., diuretics)
- Monitor for PA hypertension, progressive pulmonary venous congestion, hypoxemia, systemic hypoperfusion.
- A restrictive PFO or ASD may require cardiac catheterization and balloon atrial septostomy.

Treatment options
- Cardiac surgery is required to redirect pulmonary venous return to the LA.
- Specific types of anomalous venous return will influence the surgical approach.

Chronic complications/concerns
- Pulmonary venous stenosis/obstruction at the site of surgical anastomosis
- Arrhythmia, usually atrial

Hypoplastic Left Heart Syndrome
Description
- Characterized by a group of anomalies by hypoplasia of the LV, atresia or critical stenosis of the aortic valve and/or mitral valve, hypoplasia of the ascending aorta or the aortic arch. The LV is hypoplastic and nonfunctional or totally atretic.

Natural history
- If left untreated, pulmonary edema and CHF develops within the first week of life.
- Circulatory shock, progressive hypoxemia, and acidosis result in death, usually in the first month of life.

Management
- Infants with an unrestrictive ASD may have mild cyanosis at birth otherwise appear normal initially.
- When the PDA constricts, and pulmonary vascular resistance decreases, a decrease in systemic perfusion results. Clinical features of diminished peripheral pulses and increased pulmonary blood flow occur, which leads to hypotension, acidosis, tachypnea, respiratory distress, poor feeding, and cardiogenic shock. Symptoms can rapidly progress. Refer to cardiology immediately.
- Fetal ultrasounds can often diagnose hypoplastic left heart syndrome (HLHS).
- Neonate admitted to the intensive care unit
- Prostaglandin infusion to maintain PDA
- Preoperatively may require diuretic therapy, inotropic support, and possibly mechanical ventilation for ventricular support
- Balloon atrial septostomy may be necessary to help relieve left atrial pressure and improve oxygenation.

Treatment options
- Palliative staged surgeries completed
- Stage 1: Norwood procedure or Sano shunt completed within first 1 to 2 weeks of life

- Norwood procedure involves:
  1. Main PA divided, and the distal stump closed with a patch
  2. PDA is ligated and divided
  3. Placement of BTT shunt
  4. Atrium septum removed
  5. A neoaorta is created by sewing the hypoplastic ascending aorta to the main PA, which results in an aortic arch reconstruction and a single outflow tract to the systemic circulation from the RV.
- Sano shunt surgery involves:
  1. Creating a neoaorta (similar to Norwood). Blood flows from the RV out to the systemic circulation.
  2. Placement of homograft conduit between the RV and PA bifurcation to provide a source of pulmonary blood flow
- The RV sends blood flow into both the systemic and pulmonary circulations.
- Stage 2: bidirectional Glenn completed between 4 and 12 months of age
  - Surgery involves:
    1. Removal of BTT shunt
    2. A cavopulmonary shunt is created from an end-to-side anastomosis of the superior vena cava, typically to the right branch PA
  - The systemic venous blood flow continues to return to the inferior vena cava and into the RA
- Stage 3: Fontan procedure completed between 18 months and 3 years of age
  - Fontan procedure involves:
    1. Creation of connection vessel (i.e., extracardiac conduit or intraatrial tunnel) from the inferior vena cava to the PA
  - This connection directs all the returned systemic venous blood into the PA and into the lungs
  - Pulmonary venous blood from the lungs drains into the atrium, into the RV, and then across the neoaorta, which provides blood into the systemic circulation

Chronic complications/concerns
- Central shunt occlusion (stage I)
- Glenn or Fontan shunt stenosis
- CoA
- Thrombosis
- Heart failure
- Atrial arrhythmias
- Plastic bronchitis
- Protein-losing enteropathy
- Liver congestion, cirrhosis, increased risk of hepatocellular carcinoma
- Pulmonary thromboembolic event

DIAGNOSTIC CRITERIA

Early detection of CHD results in improved care, risk stratification, and earlier management initiation. The first opportunity for detection of CHD may occur when the mother is receiving prenatal care. Based on findings from the obstetric evaluation or the mother's predisposing conditions, a fetal echocardiogram and/or genetic testing may be ordered. A comprehensive fetal echocardiogram, which includes additional views of the cardiac structures and color Doppler imaging, can detect and diagnose 85% of cardiac anomalies (Reddy et al., 2022; Scott & Neal, 2021). Genetic testing with a microarray comparative genomic hybridization is recommended when sonographic abnormalities are detected. Positive genetic findings may help identify other structural anomalies or identify a genetic syndrome with CHD phenotypes (Diz et al., 2021; Geddes & Earing, 2018; Kowalczyk et al., 2021; Saliba et al., 2020).

The diagnosis of CHD often occurs prenatally or during the neonatal period and less frequently during the childhood or adult years. Neonates may develop clinical findings that are suggestive of underlying CHD within hours or days of life. A health care provider or a parent may identify signs and symptoms to include a murmur, cyanosis, coolness of the extremities, decreased perfusion, tachycardia, lower oxygen saturations, tachypnea, pulmonary congestion, or feeding difficulties in the infant with CHD. A referral to cardiology for formal consultation is recommended if there is a high suspicion of a CHD.

Methods of diagnosing CHD include thorough family history, patient history and physical examination, neonatal pulse oximetry screening, and cardiac tests and procedures. The echocardiogram is the most common imaging test completed for identifying cardiac malformations. Echocardiography provides data on cardiac morphology and structure, chamber volumes and diameters, septal and wall thickness, ventricular systolic and diastolic function, and pulmonary pressures. ECGs evaluate the cardiac conduction pathway, rhythm, and heart rate and assess for findings suggestive of atrial enlargement, ventricular hypertrophy, or cardiac strain. Additional imaging modalities such as cardiac magnetic resonance imaging (MRI), computed tomography (CT), and catheterizations provide further delineation of the vascular and intracardiac anatomy, hemodynamics, ventricular volumes, mass, and function. Three-dimensional (3D) images of the cardiac structures can be generated, which further enhance the detection of cardiac findings (Muthurangu, 2021). The combining or fusion of the different imaging morphologies is a recent advancement in cardiac assessment (Table 18.5).

CLINICAL MANIFESTATIONS AT TIME OF DIAGNOSIS

The clinical presentation of CHD noted in an individual will vary on pathophysiology of the specific defect, severity of the cardiac lesion, age of the person, chronicity of the CHD, and other extracardiac medical conditions (Kundan, 2020; Masarone et al., 2017; Rohit & Rajan, 2020; Spaziani et al., 2021).

Table **18.5**   Congenital Heart Disease and Physical Examination Findings

CONGENITAL HEART DEFECT	PHYSICAL EXAMINATION—COMMON FINDINGS
Left-to-Right Shunt Lesions	
Patent ductus arteriosus (PDA) 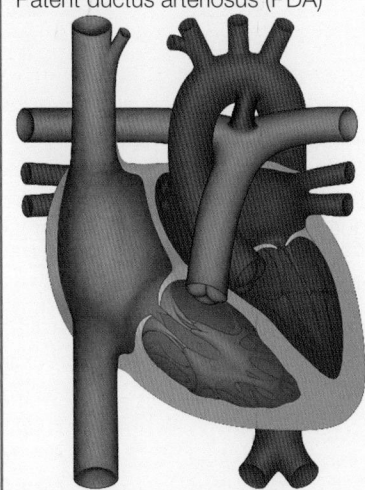	Tachycardia and tachypnea with a large shunt • Bounding peripheral pulses with wide pulse pressure • Precordium is hyperactive with a large shunt • Systolic thrill at upper left sternal border • Apical diastolic rumble may be heard P2 is normal, but accentuated with pulmonary hypertension Grade I–IV/VI continuous (machinery) murmur best heard at left infraclavicular area or left sternal border
Atrial septal defect (ASD) 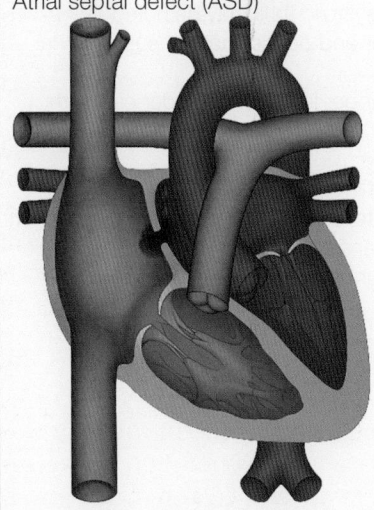	Widely split and fixed S_2 Grade II–III/VI systolic ejection murmur located over the pulmonic region (second intercostal space) Middiastolic rumble may be noted with a large ASD
Ventricular septal defect (VSD) 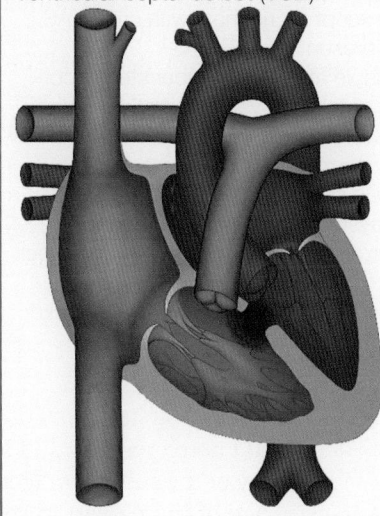	P2 normal with small VSD, moderately increased with large a shunt S_2 loud and single if there is pulmonary hypertension or pulmonary vascular obstructive disease Systolic thrill located at the left lower sternal border Precordial bulge and hyperactivity present with a large VSD Grade II–V/VI regurgitant systolic murmur located at lower sternal border Murmur may be holosystolic or early systolic Apical diastolic rumble present with moderate or large shunt

Continued

Table **18.5**	Congenital Heart Disease and Physical Examination Findings—cont'd

CONGENITAL HEART DEFECT	PHYSICAL EXAMINATION—COMMON FINDINGS
Complete atrioventricular canal (endocardial cushion) defect 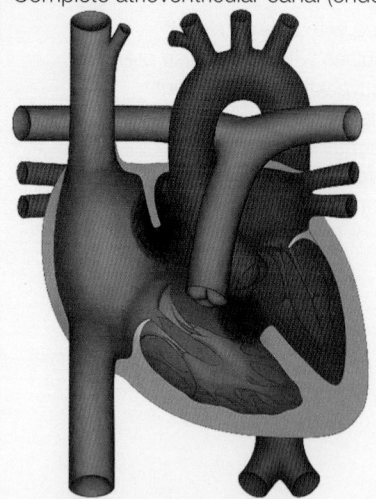	Tachycardia and tachypnea Hyperactive precordium with a systolic thrill at the lower left sternal border S_1 is accentuated S_2 narrowly split P2 increases in intensity Grade III–IV/VI holosystolic murmur heard at lower sternal border Systolic murmur may transmit to left axilla and apex with significant mitral valve regurgitation Middiastolic rumble possible at lower left sternal border or apex with stenosis of tricuspid or mitral valve

Obstructive Lesions

Pulmonary stenosis (PS) 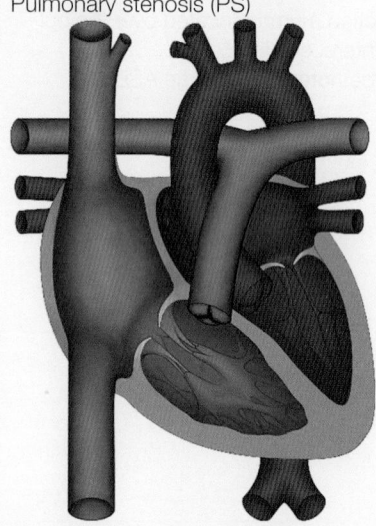	Right ventricular tap and systolic thrill may be noted at the upper left sternal border and occasionally at suprasternal notch Systolic ejection click at upper left sternal border only with valvular stenosis. S_2 may be split widely P2 diminished may be diminished Grade II–V/VI ejection systolic murmur heard best at upper left sternal border, which transmits well to the back Louder and longer murmur heard with more severe PS
Aortic stenosis (AS) 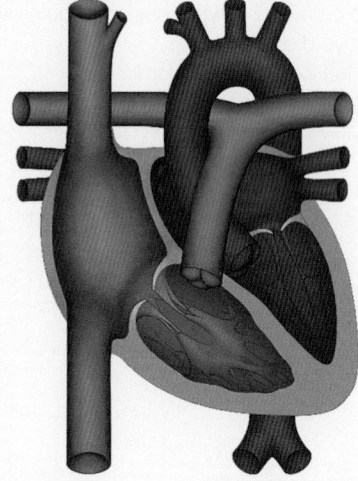	Normal blood pressures except for neonate with critical AS Narrow pulse pressure is present in severe AS Systolic thrill may be palpable at the right upper sternal border, in the suprasternal notch, or over the carotid arteries Ejection click noted with valvular AS S_2 splits normal or slightly narrowed S_2 may split paradoxically in severe AS Grade II–IV/VI harsh, midsystolic murmur heard best at second right or left intercostal space, transmits well to neck and apex High pitched early diastolic decrescendo murmur with aortic regurgitation

| Table 18.5 | Congenital Heart Disease and Physical Examination Findings—cont'd |

CONGENITAL HEART DEFECT	PHYSICAL EXAMINATION—COMMON FINDINGS
Coarctation of the aorta 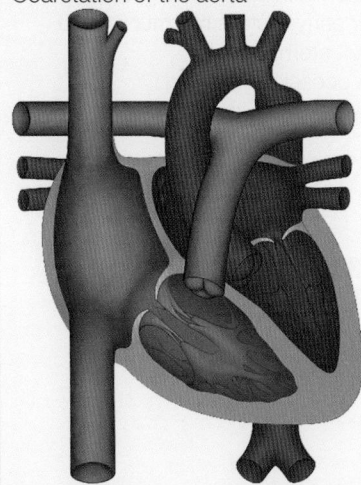	Peripheral pulses are weak and thready Blood pressure differential noted between upper and lower extremities Single S_2 and loud, loud S_3 usually present No murmur heard in 50% of sick infants Nonspecific ejection murmur is heard over the precordium
Cyanotic Lesions	
Transposition of the great arteries 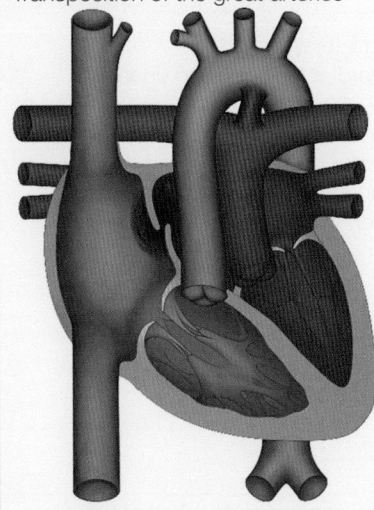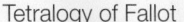	S_2 is single and loud No murmur is heard with an intact ventricular septum Early or holosystolic murmur of VSD may be audible in less cyanotic infants with associated VSD Soft midsystolic murmur of pulmonary stenosis (LVOTO) may be heard
Tetralogy of Fallot 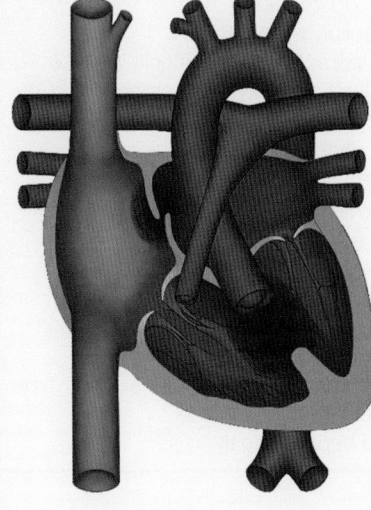	Right ventricular tap along left sternal border and systolic thrill at the upper and mid-left sternal borders are commonly noted Ejection click from the aorta may be heard Grade III–VI/VI long, loud ejection-type systolic murmur heard at mid- and upper left sternal borders from pulmonary stenosis The more severe the obstruction of the RVOT, the shorter and softer the systolic murmur

Continued

Table 18.5 | **Congenital Heart Disease and Physical Examination Findings—cont'd**

CONGENITAL HEART DEFECT	PHYSICAL EXAMINATION—COMMON FINDINGS
Tricuspid atresia 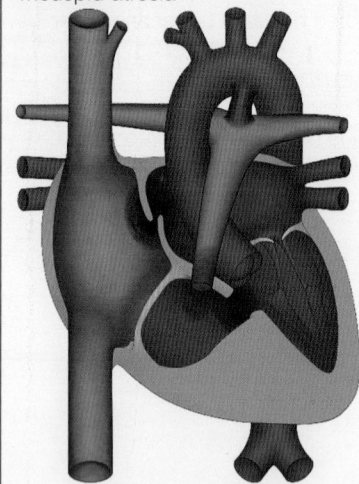	Systolic thrill is rarely palpable when associated with PS Grade II–III/VI holosystolic or early systolic murmur of VSD often heard at the lower left sternal border Continuous murmur of PDA occasionally heard Apical diastolic rumble rarely audible with large pulmonary blood flow
Truncus arteriosus 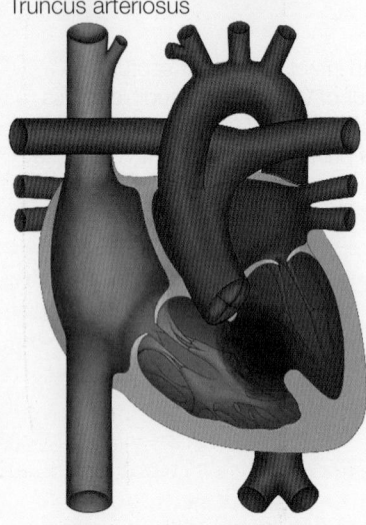	Varying degrees of cyanosis, tachypnea, dyspnea are present Peripheral pulses are bounding with a wide pulse pressure Precordium is hyperactive Apical impulse is displaced laterally Systolic click frequently heard at the apex and upper left sternal border S_2 is single Grade II–IV/VI systolic murmur may be heard from truncal stenosis or pulmonary artery branch stenosis Apical diastolic rumble when the pulmonary blood flow is large
Total anomalous pulmonary venous return 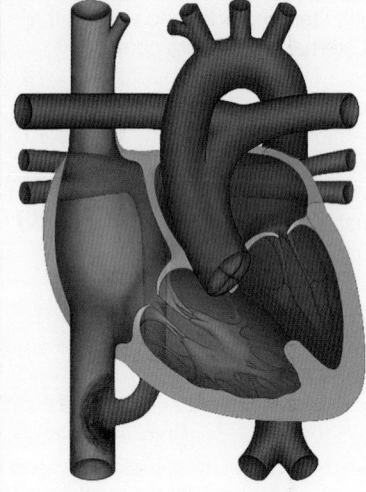	Clinical manifestations differ, depending on whether there is obstruction to the pulmonary venous return *Without pulmonary venous obstruction:* • Infant undernourished, mildly cyanotic • Precordial bulge with hyperactive right ventricle impulse • Cardiac impulse is maximal at the xyphoid process and lower left sternal border • Quadruple or quintuple rhythm is present • S_2 is widely split and fixed, P2 may be accentuated • Grade II–III/VI ejection systolic murmur heard at upper left sternal border • Middiastolic rumble present at lower left sternal border *With pulmonary venous obstruction:* • Marked cyanosis, respiratory distress develop in newborn • Loud, single S_2, and gallop rhythm are present • Heart murmur is usually absent, possible faint ejection-type systolic murmur at upper left sternal border • Pulmonary crackles and hepatomegaly

Table 18.5 Congenital Heart Disease and Physical Examination Findings—cont'd

CONGENITAL HEART DEFECT	PHYSICAL EXAMINATION—COMMON FINDINGS
Hypoplastic left heart 	Neonate becomes critically ill with the first 6–8 weeks of life Tachycardia, dyspnea, pulmonary crackles, weak peripheral pulses, and vasoconstricted extremities are characteristic Skin color may be gray-blue with poor perfusion S_2 is loud and single Absent heart murmur is common Occasional grade I–II/VI nonspecific ejection systolic murmur heard over the precordium

LVOTO, Left ventricular outflow tract obstruction; *RVOT,* right ventricular outflow tract; in figures: *blue color,* deoxygenated blood; *purple color,* mixing of deoxygenated and oxygenated blood; *red color,* oxygenated blood.

CONGESTIVE HEART FAILURE

CHF in patients with CHD is defined as a syndrome characterized by either or both pulmonary and systemic venous congestion and/or inadequate peripheral oxygen delivery at rest or during stress caused by cardiac dysfunction (Bigras, 2020). Heart failure results when the body is unable to maintain cardiac output to sustain the metabolic demands, which then leads to a chain reaction. The metabolic and neurohumoral mechanisms are activated. There is the activation of the sympathetic nervous system and the renin-angiotensin-aldosterone system. In response, sodium and fluid retention occurs in an attempt to sustain preload and cardiac output. Within the peripheral vasculature, vasoconstriction raises blood pressure for vital organ perfusion. In response to changes in afterload and wall stress there is myocardial cell growth and adaptation. These reactions lead to an increase in myocardial oxygen consumption, ventricular afterload due to eccentric hypertrophy, interstitial fibrosis, and reduction in capillary density. Direct cardiotoxicity results when there are changes in the gene expression involving calcium handling in the sarcoplasmic reticulum and contractile proteins (Watanabe & Shih, 2020).

There are multiple causes of heart failure in patients with CHD. CHD and cardiomyopathies are the most common cause of CHF in infants and children. Left-to-right shunts and valvular regurgitation can lead to volume overload. Obstructive lesions and valvular lesions can result in pressure overload. Myocardial dysfunction can cause ventricular failure. PH from CHD, ventricular dysfunction, or comorbidities such as obstructive sleep apnea and chronic lung disease result in a greater risk for right-sided heart failure. Systemic arterial hypertension from CoA, acquired renal disease, essential hypertension, anomalous coronary artery, or arteriosclerosis increases the risk for left-sided heart failure. Heart failure following cardiac surgery may be transient or chronic due to residual lesions, ventricular dysfunction, valvular regurgitation, or single ventricle physiology. Cardiac conduction abnormalities such as persistent tachycardia rhythm, symptomatic bradycardia, or complete heart block may result in decreased cardiac output.

The clinical manifestation of CHF presents differently in infants versus older children (Table 18.6). Neonates develop CHF in the presence of defects with large left-to-right shunt (i.e., PDA, AVSD, VSD) or complex CHD. The clinical manifestations may be gradual and increase after the pulmonary vascular resistance decreases during the first 6 to 8 weeks of life. Infants may develop feeding difficulties, tachycardia, tachypnea, increased work of breathing/grunting, color changes (i.e., pallor, cyanosis, or ashen color), cold extremities, delayed capillary refill, weak pulses, failure to thrive, increased napping, diaphoresis, hepatomegaly, ascites, and increased frequency of illness. Older children may have similar findings as the infant, as well as exercise intolerance, difficulties keeping up with their peers, chest pain/angina, orthopnea, abdominal pain, oliguria, orbital or peripheral edema, increased jugular venous pressures, palpitations, rhythm disturbances, or altered level of alertness with syncopal events (Kundan, 2020; Masarone et al., 2017; Reardon & Lin, 2021; Rohit & Budakoty, 2020; Spaziani et al., 2021).

Table 18.6   Congestive Heart Failure: Clinical and Physical Findings

KEY FINDINGS	SIGNS/SYMPTOMS	INFANT	CHILDREN/ADOLESCENCE
Pulmonary congestion	Tachypnea, wheeze, rales, grunt, cough	+	+
Systemic venous congestion	Hepatomegaly, ascites, pleural effusion, increased weight gain, elevated jugular venous pressure	+	+
Impaired cardiac output	Delayed capillary refill, decreased pulses, fatigue, pallor, sweating, poor weight gain, altered sensorium	+	+
Feeding problems	Fatigue with feedings, prolonged feeding durations, intolerance of diet, poor weight gain, gastric reflux	+	+
Exercise intolerance	Tires easily, unable to keep up with peers		+
Abdominal pain	Abdominal tenderness		+
Oliguria	Decreased urine output	+	+
Pitting peripheral edema	Prolonged skin indention, stretched or shiny skin over affected region		+

Severity can be classified on the basis of Ross modified criteria for younger children and New York Heart Association for older children.
From Kundan, M. (2020). Pediatric heart failure. *Journal of Pediatric Critical Care*, 7(3), 147–151.

HYPOXEMIA AND CYANOSIS

Hypoxemia is the presence of an arterial oxygen saturation that is below normal. Cyanosis is the blue coloration of the skin and mucous membranes caused by deoxygenated hemoglobin. Acrocyanosis is usually a benign finding and is secondary to peripheral vasoconstriction from the immature vascular tone or as a response to being cold. Discoloration is usually seen where the skin is thin, such as around the eyes, lips, and mouth, and within the hands and feet and their nailbeds. Central cyanosis occurs with a lower amount of oxygenated blood and is often associated with cardiac disease, intrinsic lung disease, or hematologic conditions. The cyanosis is seen in the oropharynx and on the head and truncal regions. Cyanotic cardiac defects may be secondary to right-to-left shunts, intracardiac mixing of oxygenated and deoxygenated blood, significant RV obstruction to blood flow, or ventricular dysfunction. Children with cyanotic CHD without heart failure are exposed to moderate but prolonged hypoxia until the time of correction or palliation of the defect following cardiac surgery. Children with cyanotic CHD and heart failure are exposed to both severe antenatal/postnatal hypoxia and cerebral hypoperfusion.

The clinical manifestations of cyanosis from CHD are dependent on the specific cardiac lesion and on the restrictive blood flow and intracardiac mixing of oxygenated and deoxygenated blood. Individuals with a cyanotic cardiac defect may present with tachypnea without distress, increased tachypnea with activity, feedings, or crying; feeding difficulties such as poor coordination of breathing, drinking, and swallowing; prolonged feeding times or frequent rest breaks during feedings; and tachycardia, fatigue, increased somnolence. With chronic cyanosis, additional findings occur, such as clubbing of the nail beds, increased fussiness with greater cyanosis/hypoxemia, slower weight gain, decreased exercise endurance requiring frequent rest breaks, tiredness with activity, and polycythemia as the body attempts to increase the oxygen-carrying capacity.

ARRHYTHMIA AND HEART BLOCK

Arrhythmias can be detected in individuals with CHD. The arrhythmias may occur from abnormal anatomy with displaced or malformed sinus nodes or AV conduction systems, abnormal hemodynamics, primary myocardial disease, hypoxic tissue injury, residual or postoperative sequelae, or genetic influence (European Society of Cardiology [ESC] Scientific Document Group et al., 2018). The incidence of arrhythmias generally increases as the patient ages. Specific cardiac malformations have a higher incidence of rhythm disturbances. Ebstein anomaly increases the risk of atrial tachycardias, AV reentry tachycardia, and rare ventricular tachycardia. Congenitally corrected TGA (levo-TGA [l-TGA]) has a greater risk for AV conduction abnormalities, which may progress to complete heart block. ASDs have increased the incidence of atrial arrhythmias. VSD, AVSD, and LVOT obstructions are at a greater risk of premature ventricular complexes and ventricular arrhythmias. Patients with TOF, especially following cardiac surgery, can present with ventricular arrhythmias, including premature ventricular complexes and ventricular tachycardia. Individuals with a history of Fontan procedure may develop atrial fibrillation and atrial tachycardias.

AV conduction abnormalities may occur in a structurally normal heart or in association with a variety of CHD, such as l-TGA, heterotaxy syndrome, single ventricle patients, and secundum ASDs, or as a postoperative finding, particularly after the closure of VSD, TOF repair, left-sided outflow tract region, and left-sided valve surgery.

Supraventricular tachycardia is the most common sustained tachyarrhythmia and may be seen during the neonatal period, postcardiac surgery, or later in life (Aljohani et al., 2021).

The clinical manifestation of an arrhythmia or heart block will be influenced by the heart rate, irregularity of the rhythm, frequency, duration of the arrhythmia, and underlying CHD. Individuals may complain of palpitations, tachycardia, bradycardia, dizziness, syncopal events, chest pain, shortness of breath, increased fatigue, decreased exercise tolerance, and cooler extremities. Potential clinical findings seen during the physical examination may include coolness and/or mottling of the skin, weak or thready pulses, hepatomegaly, pulmonary congestion, and increased lethargy.

TREATMENT

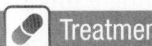 **Treatment**

- Corrective surgery
- Staged surgery
- Interventional cardiac catheterization
- Control of congestive heart failure
- Prevention of pulmonary hypertension

The goal of CHD management is to prevent CHF, ventricular dysfunction, and PH. There is an aim to maintain a balanced pulmonary-to-systemic blood flow. The management of CHD begins at the time of diagnosis, such as during the prenatal, neonatal, or childhood timeframe. When CHD is identified prenatally, management of the CHD begins then. Families can receive appropriate counseling from specialists in perinatology and cardiology, arrangements for delivery of the infant at a fetal health center can be secured, predelivery consultation with cardiology and/or cardiac surgeon is scheduled, and if indicated and safe fetal interventions are completed (Reddy et al., 2022; Waern et al., 2021). Studies have shown infants with ductal-dependent lesions or critical cardiac lesions who receive immediate life-sustaining medications

such as prostaglandin infusion or undergo cardiac surgery or cardiac catheterization interventions have increased neonatal survival, decreased morbidity, and better neurocognitive outcomes. The infant is exposed to fewer negative consequences of hypoxemia, myocardial strain, and pulmonary overcirculation.

The natural history of some CHDs, such as ASDs, VSDs, PDA, and mild PVS, may resolve spontaneously. CHD with significant valvular disease, larger septal defects, or moderate to complex lesions, however, will require cardiac surgery or interventional cardiac catheterization procedures. The timing of the intervention varies based on the underlying cardiac lesions, the patient's clinical symptoms, and the natural history of the progression of the CHD if left untreated. The performed cardiac surgeries are classified as corrective or palliative.

CORRECTIVE SURGERY

Corrective cardiac surgeries involve the repair of the cardiac lesion ranging from simple to complex CHD. The timing of the surgery is dependent on the lesion, the severity of the CHD, and the individual's clinical status. Although the goal is for a single cardiac surgery, the more complex cardiac lesions (e.g., AVSD, TGA, TOF, critical CoA) may require additional cardiac surgery or cardiac intervention. Potential causes for additional interventions may involve repair of residual defects, treatment of progressive valvular disease and/or vascular stenosis, or the need for replacement of conduits, grafts, or valves either from the patient outgrowing the initial surgery intervention or the development of stenosis, regurgitation, or calcification within the placed conduit or valve. A patient who has undergone cardiac surgery will require lifelong cardiac surveillance to monitor for residual defects, arrhythmias, or ventricular dysfunction.

STAGED SURGERY

The more complex and/or severe CHDs (e.g., HLHS, hypoplastic RV, pulmonary valve atresia [PVA] with multiple collaterals) often require cardiac surgeries as a staged repair. The patients may require multiple cardiac catheterizations or cardiac imaging with cardiac CT, cardiac MRI, or pulmonary perfusion lung scans to better delineate the cardiac structures and hemodynamics. A child with a single ventricle requires a series of palliative surgeries. The initial surgery may include a BTT shunt placement, a Norwood procedure, a Sano surgery, or a hybrid approach consisting of bilateral PA banding and ductal stenting to maintain a balanced pulmonary to systemic circulation. A Glenn procedure, where the superior vena cava is sewn into the PA, often occurs between 3 and 6 months of age. A Fontan surgery, where the blood from the inferior vena cava is directed into the PA via a conduit, is completed between 18 months and 3 years of age. An infant with a single ventricle is at a higher risk of interstage morbidity and mortality. Many pediatric cardiac centers have developed home monitoring programs to closely follow patients with a single ventricle for interstage medical concerns, which may include inappropriate weight gain, oxygen desaturations, pulmonary overcirculation, CHF, neurologic findings, or feeding difficulties.

Cardiovascular Surgery Postoperative Care

Optimal postoperative management begins immediately following the cardiovascular surgery, continues during the recovery phase within the hospital setting, and shifts to the primary care provider upon discharge to home. The child or adolescent who underwent cardiovascular surgical correction and parents will receive instructions prior to leaving the hospital. Topics discussed at the time of discharge may include the individual's activity restrictions, pain management, surgical incision care instructions, signs and symptoms of surgical site infection, immunization schedule adjustments, discharge medications, nutrition and diet recommendations, dental care and subacute bacterial endocarditis (SBE) recommendations, and the potential for a change in the individual's behavior and sleep pattern secondary to the hospitalization, altered daily routine, or possible night terrors.

The child or adolescent will have appointments scheduled within the cardiovascular surgery clinic and cardiology clinic for cardiac assessment, as well as follow-up care with the primary care provider within the first month of the surgery. Ideally, the primary care provider has knowledge of CHD and the type of cardiovascular surgery completed. During the initial clinic visit, the primary care providers should assess the individual's pain level, quality of sleep, nutritional intake, growth pattern, and behavior. In addition, the provider should evaluate for potential postoperative concerns such as residual cardiac defect, cardiac rhythm disturbance, pericardial effusion, pulmonary congestion, PH, cardiac dysfunction, chylothorax resulting in pleural effusion and edema, vocal cord paralysis or paresis, infections, and poor weight after cardiovascular surgery. If a medical concern is identified, a consultation with the primary cardiologist or cardiovascular surgeon is recommended.

INTERVENTIONAL CARDIAC CATHETERIZATION

Cardiac catheterization is an invasive procedure that serves two main purposes: obtaining diagnostic cardiac information and as an interventional modality. Over the last three decades, cardiac catheterization procedures have evolved along with other technologies. While fluoroscopy and standard angiography remain an important part of diagnostic cardiac catheterization, there are emerging imaging techniques such as 3D rotational angiography, multimodal image fusion, 3D printing, and holographic imaging, which can provide more detailed information of the cardiac anatomy, spatial vascular relationship, and surrounding structures of the trachea, bronchi, and pulmonary vasculature (Kang & Benson, 2018). Interventional cardiac catheter procedure advancements have significantly improved the management of CHD. Catheter-directed interventions can complete the primary repair of a CHD with device closure of defects (e.g., PDA, ASD, VSD) or balloon angioplasty for management of cardiac lesions, including pulmonary and aortic valvular stenosis and CoA. Interventional procedures have replaced the need for additional cardiac surgery with percutaneous placement of a Melody valve or Edwards Sapien valve within the pulmonary valve region for management of dysfunction within a RV to PA conduit, bioprosthetic valve, or homograft. Other unique cardiac catheterization interventions involve the interventional cardiologist and the surgeon working together to complete a hybrid procedure. Hybrid procedures include placement of a stent within the PDA for a palliative option for the cyanotic infant with a duct-dependent pulmonary circulation (e.g., HLHS, PVA) or stent implantation within the RVOT in a symptomatic neonate with TOF.

Cardiac catheterization procedures with an electrophysiology study and possible ablation are completed to identify and treat atrial and/or ventricular arrhythmias. Arrhythmias can develop with cardiac structural lesions, lethal rhythms secondary to channelopathies, long QT syndrome, and cardiomyopathy. Abnormal anatomy, surgical scarring, chronic hypoxemia, hemodynamic compromise, neurohormonal abnormalities, and genetic factors can contribute to creating a unique substrate for arrhythmia development.

Additional electrophysiology procedures are completed for cardioversion of atrial flutter/atrial fibrillation or insertion of cardiac devices such as a pacemaker, an implantable cardioverter-defibrillator, or a resynchronization device for initiation of cardiac resynchronization therapy. Like interventional cardiac catheterization, electrophysiology procedures incorporate more advanced technology to include 3D electroanatomic mapping systems to accurately detect the region of the arrhythmia and to apply more precise ablation strategies (ESC Scientific Document Group et al., 2018).

CONTROL OF CONGESTIVE HEART FAILURE

The management of CHD is based on pathophysiologic conditions, acquired heart disease, or abnormality within the cardiac conduction system. The goals of treatment are to improve cardiac hemodynamics and prevent the progression of heart failure. Control of CHF can be achieved with the use of diuretics (i.e., furosemide, bumetanide, spironolactone, or aldosterone), inotropes (i.e., digoxin), afterload reducing agents to include ACE inhibitors (i.e., captopril, enalapril, lisinopril), and beta-blockers (i.e., carvedilol, metoprolol) (Kundan, 2020; Masarone et al., 2017; Watanabe & Shih, 2020). Management of CHF secondary to PA hypertension requires additional medication therapy considerations, including bosentan, sildenafil, prostacyclin, and riociguat. Losartan is prescribed for patients with Marfan syndrome who have a dilated aorta to slow the progression of the dilation.

Individuals with CHF are at a greater risk of experiencing failure to thrive and malnutrition. Hypermetabolic state, swallowing difficulties, upper respiratory tract infections, gastroesophageal reflux, malabsorption, and genetic syndromes are important etiologic factors. Feeding support is a priority in management. Supportive measures may include limiting oral feeding durations to less than 30 minutes, increasing the caloric concentration of the formula, administering gavage feedings, and managing gastric reflux symptoms.

The population of patients with a single ventricle requiring staged palliative surgeries is clinically more fragile. Their delicate balance of remaining in a stable state can be disrupted by illnesses, fevers, dehydration, anemia, or changes within the surgically placed shunts. Parents must be vigilant in assessing the infant with CHD and communicate concerns to the interstage home monitoring program and cardiologist. Frequent clinic appointments within the primary care clinic and cardiology clinic are required to assess for subtle changes and prevent unexpected complications or sudden death.

PREVENTION OF PULMONARY HYPERTENSION

PH in children is defined as a mean PA pressure greater than 25 mmHg at rest. There are a variety of potential underlying causes, including cardiac disease; pulmonary, hematologic, rheumatologic abnormalities; and genetic syndromes. Regardless of the cause, for many patients the natural history of PH involves progressive elevation in PA resistance and pressure, RV dysfunction, and eventually heart failure (Frank & Ivy, 2018; Hansmann, 2017). The primary management focus is on the prevention of PH. Cardiac lesions with large left-to-right shunts can lead to irreversible pulmonary vascular disease. Cardiac surgery for repair of the CHD during the first year of life is recommended before permanent pulmonary vascular changes occur. Avoiding a thrombotic event, especially in cyanotic lesions, ventricular dysfunction, or secondary to thrombus development within a pulmonary shunt (e.g., BTT shunt, Sano shunt) or mechanical heart valves, is another preventive measure. These patients may require anticoagulation therapy, avoidance of dehydration, and close monitoring for clinical changes of increased cyanosis, tachypnea, tachycardia, hepatomegaly, and worsening systemic perfusion.

COMPLEMENTARY AND ALTERNATIVE THERAPIES

Complementary therapies and alternative therapies are used in conjunction with approved medical therapies. They are used by patients to prevent or treat illnesses, improve health, and reduce pain and anxiety. Examples of complementary therapies are homeopathy, yoga, meditation, massage, chiropractic therapy, or magnetic therapy. Other complementary therapies include herbal and dietary supplements. Parents need to be cautioned about some complementary therapies, which may interfere with prescribed medications to manage the heart condition. The herbal supplements of carnitine, coenzyme Q 10, garlic, gingko, and St. John's wort can interfere with warfarin. St. John's wort can decrease digoxin levels. Another potential concern with unregulated supplements is impurities, contaminants, and adulterants found in the products (Başaran et al., 2022).

An important responsibility of the cardiologist and cardiac providers is counseling the family on the specific CHD and the natural disease progression of the lesion. Parents may be hesitant to agree to cardiac surgery or intervention for a child who appears well. For many children with CHD there is no alternative therapy for correction of the CHD, which must be communicated to parents.

Parents should discuss these therapies with the cardiologist to ensure there are no risks associated with their use.

ANTICIPATED ADVANCES IN DIAGNOSIS AND MANAGEMENT

There have been major advancements in the diagnosis and treatment of CHD over the last 30 years. These advancements were applied to fetal cardiology, cardiac imaging, cardiac catheterizations, cardiac surgery, and cardiac devices (Upadhyay et al., 2019). The introduction of emerging advances in technology, genetics, and research will continue to benefit pediatric cardiology.

Anticipated advancements are seen in multiple fields of cardiology and cardiac surgery and include cardiac imaging modalities (echocardiogram, MRI, CT). Imaging advancements in real-time 3D rotational angiography with holography, 3D roadmap, and 3D printing will continue to evolve (Upadhyay et al., 2019)

1. Advancements continue to evolve in echocardiogram quality of the images and software programs to allow for more hemodynamic information, such as cardiac strain patterns, from the echocardiogram.
2. Advancements within cardiac catheterization procedures are expected (Kang & Benson, 2018):
   a. Radiation-free, real-time cardiac MRI with 3D soft tissue imaging and superior hemodynamic data have the potential to be the preferred catheterization laboratory imaging modality of the

future. Cardiac MRI is an appealing modality for CHD cardiac catheterization image guidance as it provides radiation-free 3D soft tissue visualization and additional hemodynamic data for complex congenital anatomy and interventions (Amin et al., 2022).

b. Advancements in catheters and devices, such as a microvascular plug (Medtronic Inc.) for PDA closure in extremely premature infants and microcatheters provide valuable results.

c. Stent implantation into the RVOT as a palliative procedure for cyanosis and PA growth

d. Ductal stenting for duct-dependent pulmonary circulation

e. Percutaneous pulmonary valve implantation in the RV to PA conduit and native outflow tract

f. Transcatheter tricuspid and mitral valve replacement

3. Electrophysiologic advancements in the ability to better identify conduction abnormalities and electrical pathways are expected. A process to complete electrophysiologic mapping-derived 3D print models, which can provide reliable representations of the electrical substrate with potential surgical applications to include support for VT ablation, minimizing trauma to the conduction system, and pacemaker leads for complex CHD is expected (Moore et al., 2020).

4. Fetal surgical interventions have the potential to alter the natural progression of CHD from earlier cardiac interventions aimed at optimizing the growth of cardiac structures. Fetal surgeries and prenatal interventions include ongoing advancement in valvuloplasty of AVS or PVS, balloon atrial septostomy, pulmonary valvuloplasty, and ex utero intrapartum procedures as palliative procedures for HLHS. Anticipated future procedures for the management of severe mitral valve stenosis with an intact atrium, absent pulmonary valve, restrictive PDA, and tachycardia management is expected (Stephens et al., 2021).

5. Surgery

a. Hybrid procedures involve cooperation between interventions and surgeons within a surgery where a cardiac intervention procedure is completed during a surgery procedure. Examples include the hybrid approach for (i) the management of HLHS and the placement of a stent within the arterial duct percutaneously and a surgical banding of the PA and (ii) VSD closure.

b. Tissue engineering of prosthetic valves and conducts allows, once implanted, the material to be gradually and fully integrated into the host tissue, promoting cellular and vascular regeneration and de novo formation of tissues similar to the native valve (Bielli et al., 2018).

c. New patch material, such as decellularized bovine pericardium

6. Advancement in technology or software programs allows information obtained from a cardiac imaging modality to be sent to a computer program followed by an actual 3D model. Future advancements in the current technology are expected and allow for additional developments in biologic engineering technology, materials science, biology, and computer science (Ma et al., 2021).

7. Currently, fetal echocardiography can accurately detect and diagnose approximately 85% of cardiac anomalies. Advancements in artificial intelligence (AI) is a field within computer science that focuses on the development of algorithms that learn, reason, and self-correct in a human-like fashion. When applied to fetal echocardiography, AI has the potential to improve image acquisition, image optimization, automated measurements, identification of outliers, classification of diagnoses, and prediction of outcomes (Reddy et al., 2022).

8. Increased emphasis is on radiation safety awareness and techniques to reduce the child's radiation exposure by using flat panel detector technology (which converts x-ray photon energy to digital signals more efficiently), a fusion of MRI/CT imaging with fluoroscopy, and transesophageal echocardiograms.

9. Stem cell therapy has been studied in heart muscle diseases such as ischemic heart disease and cardiomyopathy. The field of stem cell therapy is evolving and in the future may have a significant impact on the management of cardiac pathology and CHD. Stem cell transplants may result in the preservation of ventricular function and ventricular remodeling. In the future, stem cells may be used to create cellular grafts and structures that may be surgically implanted into the heart using bioengineering technology, which can revolutionize CHD management (Pincott & Burch, 2012).

10. Increased quality of care and improved outcomes in the management of children with CHD is expected from data collected and analyzed from the current pediatric research and quality improvement networks and multicenter registries, which have a collaborative focus on positive patient outcomes.

ASSOCIATED PROBLEMS OF CONGENITAL HEART DISEASE AND TREATMENT

Associated Problems

- Hematologic problems
- Infectious process
- Infective endocarditis
- Central nervous system (CNS) complications
- Arrhythmia/heart block
- Failure to thrive
- Obesity
- Slowed development
- Vulnerable child syndrome (VCS)

HEMATOLOGIC PROBLEMS

CHD may impose hematologic problems and risks, including polycythemia, thrombosis development, thrombocytopenia, platelet abnormalities, and coagulation problems (Mohammadi et al., 2022). Several cardiac conditions have a higher prevalence of polycythemia and include cyanotic heart lesions, single ventricle conditions, and TOF. Polycythemia develops to increase the oxygen-carrying capacity of the blood. If the hematocrit level is greater than 65%, there is increased viscosity of the blood and a greater risk of thrombus formation. Thrombosis may result from CHF secondary to a diminished ventricular force and stagnated blood within the heart chamber. Interventional stents or grafts, mechanical heart valves, frequent catheterization, residual lesions or shunts, presence of pacemaker leads, and vascular abnormalities also increase the risk of thrombosis in patients, especially if anticoagulation therapy is subtherapeutic (Bigras, 2020). Arrhythmias such as atrial flutter and atrial fibrillation may result in diminished atrial chamber contraction, which increases the risk of thrombus formation. Thrombocytopenia and platelet abnormalities impose the risk of increased incidence of bleeding, thromboembolism, and death in hypoxemic CHD patients (Mohammadi et al., 2022). The concerns with coagulopathy are the increased risk for both bleeding and thrombotic complications. An individual may develop a coagulopathy secondary to abnormal blood flow, endothelial dysfunction, reduced coagulation factors, low platelet count or function, or fibrinolysis. Bloodwork results may show prolongation of the prothrombin time and partial prothrombin times, decreased levels of fibrinogen, and factors V and VII. These individuals may bruise more easily and develop petechia, gingival bleeding, or epistaxis (Bigras, 2020; Candelino et al., 2022).

Anemia is seen in children and adults with CHD. These patients typically have multifactorial etiologies for anemia, including iron deficiency, bleeding, renal insufficiency, and anemia of chronic disease. In children with CHF, decreased hemoglobin may exacerbate myocardial strain. In those with cyanotic CHD, iron deficiency anemia is frequently missed because of elevated hemoglobin levels associated with cyanosis. Ideally, patients with cyanotic CHD are screened annually for iron deficiency with measurements of iron, ferritin, and transferrin saturation levels. Children should be monitored for fatigue, pallor, decreased exercise tolerance, and tachycardia.

Supplemental iron may be prescribed for the anemia. It is important to monitor the response to the iron supplement therapy to avoid undesirable high iron levels, thus increasing the blood viscosity, especially in children with cyanosis. Children should maintain an adequate hydration status to decrease the risk of hemoconcentration. Clinical symptoms of dehydration should be assessed, especially during times of fevers, exposure to hot weather, vomiting, diarrhea, or when receiving diuretic therapy.

INFECTIOUS PROCESSES

Children with congenital disease are at a higher risk of developing a variety of infections. Contributing factors for the increased illnesses include heart failure, malnourishment, immune system dysfunction in isolation or with genetic abnormalities with known autoimmune deficiency (e.g., trisomy 21, 22q11.2 deletion, Jacobson syndrome), neutropenia, and impaired T-cell function (Kavya et al., 2021).

Respiratory tract infections are especially common in cardiac lesions with increased pulmonary blood flow. Viral respiratory infections, including influenza and SARS-CoV-2 virus (the cause of COVID-19), impose a higher risk of mortality, a longer duration of hospitalization, and more complications and economic costs in children with CHD than in the general population. Aspiration pneumonia from gastric reflux disease or decreased muscle tone is another respiratory concern.

Bacterial sepsis may cause endocarditis (see Infective Endocarditis, later).

Infections within the CNS are relatively rare in children with CHD but are among the most serious given the associated life-threatening complications and long-term neurologic sequelae. In children with a cyanotic heart lesion related to a right-to-left intracardiac shunt, the normal effective phagocytic filtering action of the pulmonary bed is bypassed. Bacteria may enter directly into the cerebral circulation; this, combined with the increased blood viscosity, increases the risk for an infection and the development of a brain abscess (Chen & Jiang, 2021; Mameli et al., 2019). Other possible etiologies for the development of a CNS infection are infective endocarditis, cardiac shunt physiology, immune deficiencies, hypoxia, and surgical or interventional procedures, which pose an increased risk of systemic infection (Bagge et al., 2020).

An infection can impact the child with a CHD or CHF in the following ways: (1) Respiratory tract infections can result in an exacerbation of hypoxemia, (2) fever can increase the metabolic rate and oxygen demands, (3) dehydration can increase the risk of polycythemia or thrombus formation, (4) resulting tachycardia and/or tachypnea can be seen in the child, and (5) electrolyte imbalances can occur from vomiting, diarrhea, or poor oral intake during the illness, which potentially increases the risk of rhythm disturbances or digoxin toxicity.

Children with asplenia syndrome have a greater susceptibility to bacteremia and higher mortality rates. *Streptococcus pneumoniae, Neisseria meningitidis*, and *Haemophilus influenzae* are the most common pathogens. These individuals require special immunization considerations and management. The current vaccines recommended for patients with asplenia include pneumococcal vaccines (13-valent pneumococcal conjugate vaccine followed by the 23-valent pneumococcal polysaccharide vaccine), meningococcal vaccines (meningococcal conjugate vaccines for serogroups A, C, Y, and W-135 and serogroup B meningococcal vaccines), *H. influenzae* type b vaccines, and inactivated influenza vaccines. Ongoing booster doses are also recommended for pneumococcal and meningococcal vaccines to maintain protection (Lee, 2020). Routine immunizations are recommended, although mumps-measle-rubella and the varicella vaccine are not recommended if the child has a weakened immune system, while the zoster vaccine is recommended after 19 years of age if there is a weakened immune system. Daily antimicrobial prophylaxis against pneumococcal infection is recommended in children less than 5 years of age for at least 1 year after splenectomy and sometimes throughout childhood and adulthood. The recommended treatment for prophylaxis is oral penicillin V 125 twice a day for children under 5 years and penicillin V 250 mg twice a day for children older than 5 years.

INFECTIVE ENDOCARDITIS

Infective endocarditis is caused by bacteria that enter the bloodstream and settle in the endocardium of the heart. The most common causative organisms are *Streptococcus viridians* and *Staphylococcus aureus*. Other organisms that have been identified include *Klebsiella* species, *Pseudomonas aeruginosa*, and *Enterococcus* species. The incidence of infective endocarditis is rare but often with serious consequences. Studies have reported 40% to 50% of affected individuals will require valve surgery. The associated mortality rate is 20% to 25%. CHD is the biggest identifiable risk factor for infective endocarditis. Cardiac surgery and interventional cardiology procedures in which grafts, stents, mechanical valves, transcatheter valve implantation, intracardiac devices (both cardiovascular implantable electronic devices and LV assist devices), pacemaker, or implantable defibrillator are implanted all are potential causes of infection and bacterial endocarditis. Other risk factors include rheumatic fever, degenerative valve disease, indwelling catheters, nosocomial infection, and immunosuppression. Infective endocarditis can occur from random bacteremia for normal daily activities (e.g., chewing gum, brushing teeth) and with poor oral hygiene and periodontal diseases. Body art, including piercing and tattoos, may also impose a risk of infective endocarditis (Armstrong et al., 2008).

Prevention against infective endocarditis is vital. Cardiac providers and primary care providers need to emphasize to children and parents the importance of maintaining healthy teeth and gums to decrease the risk of bacterial infections and possible endocarditis. Individuals with CHD may have an abundance of bacteria present in the oral cavity, such as *Streptococcus*

species, *Lactobacillus salivarius*, *Solobacterium moorei*, and *Atopobium parvulum* (Schulz-Weidner et al., 2021). All individuals with CHD require meticulous oral care and regularly scheduled dental visits for assessment of gingivitis or dental caries as primary infective endocarditis prevention. In addition, a select group of cardiac lesions will require SBE prophylaxis with an antibiotic given 1 hour before dental or high-risk procedures.

The American Heart Association (AHA) made significant revisions to the SBE prophylaxis guidelines in 2007 and recommended only high-risk individuals receive prophylaxis antibiotics. In 2021 the AHA released a scientific statement that continued to support the 2007 guideline recommendations with a revision in which the administration of clindamycin as an alternative to amoxicillin or ampicillin was also no longer recommended for SBE prophylaxis.

The AHA (2021) currently recommends antibiotic prophylaxis only in patients with the following high-risk cardiac conditions: (1) prosthetic cardiac valves, (2) previous infective endocarditis, (3) cardiac transplant recipients with valve regurgitation due to a structurally abnormal valve, and (4) patients with CHD with (a) unrepaired cyanotic CHD, including palliative shunts and conduits, (b) a totally repaired congenital heart defect, repaired with prosthetic material or device that has been placed by surgery or catheter intervention during the first 6 months after the procedure, and (c) repaired CHD with residual defects at the site or adjacent to the site of a prosthetic patch or prosthetic device.

Patients with high-risk conditions should receive antibiotics for SBE prophylaxis for dental procedures that involve manipulating gingival tissue, manipulating the periapical region of teeth, or perforating the oral mucosa. The recommended regimen for patients with cardiac risk factors includes the use of antimicrobials administered as a single dose 30 to 60 minutes before the procedure, with the preferred pediatric regimen of oral amoxicillin dosed at 50 mg/kg. If the patient is unable to take oral medication, they may be given ampicillin (50 mg/kg IM or IV), cefazolin, or ceftriaxone (50 mg/kg IM or IV).

Alternative regimens in children with penicillin allergy include cephalexin 50 mg/kg, azithromycin or clarithromycin 15 mg/kg, or doxycycline 2.2 mg/kg in patients weighing less than 45 kg and 100 mg for patients weighing more than 45 kg. (Clindamycin is no longer recommended for antibiotic prophylaxis before dental procedures or oral surgery due to the high incidence of adverse events, such as *Clostridium difficile* colitis (Wilson, et al., 2007). This does not include (1) routine anesthetic injections through noninfected tissue, dental radiographs, placement or adjustment of orthodontic devices, or trauma to the lips and teeth; (2) invasive respiratory tract procedures that involve incision or biopsy of the respiratory mucosa (e.g., tonsillectomy, adenoidectomy);

and (3) procedures of infected skin, skin structures, or musculoskeletal tissue.

Prophylaxis against infective endocarditis is not recommended in other nondental procedures, such as a transesophageal echocardiogram, esophagogastroduodenoscopy, colonoscopy, or cystoscopy, in the absence of active infection (Box 18.1). Patients with implantable cardiovascular devices do not require prophylaxis except at the time of cardiovascular device implantation and any subsequent manipulation of the surgically created device pocket.

CENTRAL NERVOUS SYSTEM COMPLICATIONS

The presence of a CNS condition in patients with CHD is often multifactorial. Developmental dysfunction results from a complex interaction between patient-specific factors (genetic susceptibility, cardiac diagnosis, fetal development) and environmental factors (preoperative events, techniques of support during surgical repair, postoperative events, socioeconomic status). Prenatally a fetus that is exposed to an altered blood flow to the brain can be born with abnormal brain development, white matter injuries, stroke, or hemorrhages. There is mounting evidence obtained from neuroimaging studies to demonstrate delays in (micro)structural brain development, mainly in cortical folding and myelination, and associated acquired brain injury in CHD (Hermans et al., 2022). Cerebral ischemia can result from low oxygen delivery from decreased cardiac output, severe hypoxemia, severe anemia, or postcardiac arrest. Postoperative agitation, pain, and/or hyperthermia may increase

Box 18.1 Infective Endocarditis Prophylaxis

DENTAL PROCEDURES

Antibiotic prophylaxis is reasonable before dental procedures that involve manipulation of the gingival tissue, manipulation of the periapical region of teeth, or perforation of the oral mucosa in patients with valvular heart disease and congenital heart disease who have any of the following:

- Prosthetic cardiac valves, including transcatheter-implanted prostheses and homografts
- Prosthetic material used for cardiac valve repair, such as annuloplasty rings, chords, or clips
- Left ventricular assist devices or implantable heart
- Previous infective endocarditis
- Unrepaired cyanotic congenital heart defect (CHD) or repaired CHD[a] with:
  - Residual shunts or valvular regurgitation at the site of or adjacent to the site of a prosthetic patch or prosthetic device
  - Completed repaired congenital heart disease with prosthetic material or device, whether placed by surgeon or by transcatheter during the first 6 months after the procedure
  - Surgical or transcatheter pulmonary artery valve or conduit placement such as Melody valve or Contegra device
- Cardiac transplant with valve regurgitation due to a structurally abnormal valve

Antibiotic prophylaxis is *not* recommended for the following dental procedures or events:

- Routine anesthetic injections through noninfected tissue
- Taking dental radiographs
- Placement of removable prosthodontic or orthodontic appliances
- Adjustment of orthodontic appliances
- Placement of orthodontic brackets
- Shedding of deciduous teeth and bleeding from trauma to the lips or oral mucosa

NONDENTAL PROCEDURES

In patients with valvular heart disease or congenital heart disease who are at high risk of infective endocarditis, antibiotic prophylaxis is not recommended for nondental procedures (e.g., transesophageal echocardiogram, esophagogastroduodenoscopy, colonoscopy, or cystoscopy) in the absence of active infection.

OTHER PROCEDURES

Prophylaxis for procedures involving the respiratory tract, infected skin and skin structures, tissues just under the skin, or musculoskeletal tissue.

- Respiratory tract procedures. There is no direct evidence that bacteremia associated with respiratory tract procedures causes infective endocarditis. Antimicrobial prophylaxis is suggested only for procedures involving incision or biopsy of the respiratory tract mucosa; examples include tonsillectomy, adenoidectomy, or bronchoscopy with biopsy or with invasive respiratory tract procedure as part of treatment for an established infection.
- Skin or soft tissue procedures. Patients undergoing a surgical procedure for management of infected skin, skin structure, or musculoskeletal tissue should receive antibiotic therapy with activity against skin flora. If the pathogen is known, the antibiotic should be targeted; accordingly, if the pathogen is not known, empiric antibiotic therapy with activity against methicillin-resistant *Staphylococcus aureus* and beta-hemolytic streptococci should be administered.

[a]Except for the conditions listed above, antibiotic prophylaxis before dental procedures is not recommended for any other types of CHD.

From American College of Cardiology/American Heart Association. (2021). Guideline for the management of patients with valvular heart disease: A report of the ACC/AHA Joint Committee on Clinical Practice Guidelines. *Circulation, 143,* e72–e227.

the metabolic needs of the brain, resulting in worsening CNS injury. CHD may increase the risk for strokes from environmental factors, including cardiac surgery with cardiopulmonary bypass and deep hypothermic circulatory arrest, mechanical support extracorporeal membrane oxygenation (ECMO), or LV assist device (Wernovsky & Licht, 2016; Williams et al., 2021). There is an increased risk of thrombus development from hematologic findings of blood hemoconcentration, increased blood viscosity or coagulation abnormalities, arrhythmia resulting in poor atrial or ventricular contractility, or following surgically placed shunts. A child requiring a Glenn or Fontan procedure is at a higher risk of thrombus development secondary to a right-to-left shunt resulting from the inferior cava connection to the systemic atrium, a fenestrated Fontan, venovenous collaterals, or pulmonary arteriovenous malformations. In addition, the passive blood into the cavopulmonary connection can result in relative stasis, increasing the risk of thrombus development and a cerebrovascular accident (Lang et al., 2021). Intracranial hemorrhages can occur secondary to the immature brain, vascular abnormalities, or secondary to anticoagulation therapy with elevated therapeutic levels and/or head injury. The role of genetic polymorphisms in determining susceptibility to CNS injury in children with CHD is another possible risk factor for CNS complications. Recent studies suggest that polymorphisms of apolipoprotein E (ε2 polymorphism) may be predictors of adverse neurodevelopmental sequelae following infant cardiac surgery (Wernovsky & Licht, 2016).

ARRHYTHMIAS AND HEART BLOCK

Rhythm disturbances can occur in children and adults with CHD and generally increase as patients age. Predisposing risk for arrhythmias may include congenitally malformed or displaced conduction pathways, altered hemodynamics, hypoxic stress, primary myocardial disease, hypoxic tissue injury, residual or postoperative sequelae (e.g., surgical incisions or sutures near the conduction pathway, or injury to the sinus node or AV noted), and genetic influence (Arslani et al., 2018; ESC Scientific Document Group et al., 2018; Khairy & Balaji, 2009). Rhythm disturbances may also be noted with electrolyte disturbances, medication effects, or during times of illness and fever.

Atrial rhythms are more common than ventricular rhythm disturbances in children. The atrial rhythm may result in episodes of bradycardia, junctional tachycardia, atrial tachycardia, or atrial conduction abnormalities. The underlying CHD and the completed cardiac intervention may increase the risk of atrial arrhythmia. For example, postoperatively, atrial rhythm disturbances are more prevalent after surgical manipulation of the atrium (e.g., Fontan procedure, repair of TAPVR, ASD repair). Patients with congenitally corrected transposition of the greater arteries

(l-TGA) have fragile AV conduction and a greater risk for AV conduction abnormalities, including complete AV block and postoperative atrial tachycardia (ESC Scientific Document Group et al., 2018; Khairy & Balaji, 2009). Accessory pathways are noted with greater frequency in Ebstein anomaly with the tricuspid valve displacement, heterotaxy syndromes, AVSD, and single ventricular hearts.

Ventricular ectopy and ventricular tachycardia, although less common, have a higher risk of morbidity and mortality. Ventricular rhythm disturbances are thought to be the leading cause of sudden death in several subtypes of CHD (Khairy & Balaji, 2009). Potential causes for the development of a monomorphic ventricular arrhythmia are the underlying CHD, cardiac surgeries with ventricular incisions, placement of conduits or grafts, especially within the RVOT for the repair of TOF, or surgical scars. More serious polymorphic ventricular tachycardia can be seen in patients with severely diseased ventricular myocardium, significant fibrosis, or with specific CHD to include LVOT obstructive lesions, d-TGA after atrial switch procedure with failing systemic RV, TOF with significantly impaired RV function, Eisenmenger syndrome, and single ventricular hearts with a Fontan circulation (ESC Scientific Document Group et al., 2018).

AV conduction abnormalities may result from the underlying CHD lesion or as a consequence of open heart surgery repair (especially procedures involving the closure of VSD, TOF repair, AVSD repair) or interventional cardiac catheterization with device placement for closure of a VSD. Postprocedural AV blocks may be the result of inflammation near the conduction pathway and often are temporary. Persistent complete heart block will require an implantable pacemaker for management.

FAILURE TO THRIVE

Adequate nutrition is important for the child's physical growth and brain development. A child with CHD requires close monitoring for failure to thrive. Growth failure is a concern and observed in children with CHD, with a reported prevalence between 15% and 64% (Bigras, 2020; Diao et al., 2022). Often a child demonstrates slower growth in weight while maintaining the growth of height. The underlying causes for failure to thrive may be multifactorial. A child with CHF may have an inadequate daily intake of calories from increased metabolic demands for calories. Feeding difficulties are from poor coordination of breathing and swallowing due to tachypnea. Increased fatigue and reduced endurance result in prolonged feeding times of greater than 30 minutes and may result in increased caloric/energy expenditure. Other medical conditions such as ventricular dysfunction, decreased cardiac output, and PH can result in hypoperfusion of the peripheral tissues and organs, leading to impaired nutritional absorption within the intestinal tract, venous congestion, and decreased appetite. Gastroesophageal reflux is common in infants with CHD and may contribute to failure to thrive and an increased risk of aspiration. An infant with hemodynamically significant CHD may have greater energy need, which varies from 130 to 180 kcal/day depending on the type of CHD (Blue et al., 2017). Infants may require concentrated feedings or gavage feedings to optimize nutritional intake. Preoperatively improved nutrition may be fundamental to stimulate growth, wound healing, and myocardial and vascular function, decreasing the risk of nosocomial infections, improving neurodevelopmental outcomes, and reducing postoperative length of hospitalization (Blue et al., 2017).

During the early postoperative days, an infant or child may have additional risk factors for poor growth. Frequent interruption in feedings, loss of feeding skills, the presence of a chylothorax requiring a low-fat diet and/or fluid restrictions, and vocal cord dysfunction may contribute to poor growth. Fortunately, corrective cardiac surgery improves the infant's or child's hemodynamics and decreases metabolic needs, restoring a normal growth pattern.

OBESITY

Obesity is a concern with the general population as well as children with CHD. Studies confirm over 25% of children with CHD patients are overweight. The increased weight is often carried into the adult years, in which 22% to 53% of adults with CHD are overweight, and 7% to 26% are obese. Obesity is noted in patients with noncyanotic and cyanotic heart lesions. A child with complex CHD or cyanotic heart lesions often has a lower prevalence of overweight and obesity, possibly secondary to residual cardiac sequelae and ongoing complications from the underlying CHD.

The reasons for the development of obesity are complex. Proposed contributing factors for excessive caloric intake are learned behaviors and decreased calorie expenditure. The increased weight may be influenced by exposure to higher caloric feedings as an infant and young child, excessive eating, and unhealthy dietary behavior demonstrated by family members. The social and community environment may also have an influence. Limited exercise and physical activity can contribute to excessive weight gain. A child with CHD may be restricted from physical activity per the recommendations of the cardiac provider, secondary to the child's cardiac condition with increased cardiac risks during exercise. Frequently, though, the restricted physical activity is self-imposed, initiated by overprotective parents, or the result of the uncertainty as to which extent and intensity of physical exercise is recommended for the child. An individual with anxiety, depression, or lower self-esteem has an increased risk for obesity (Andonian et al., 2019; Willinger et al., 2021).

Excessive weight increases the individual risk of future medical conditions such as ischemic heart disease, coronary artery disease, heart failure, altered lipid profiles (high cholesterol/low-density lipoprotein/triglycerides), hypertension, or diabetes. In addition, the child or young adult may experience decreased exercise tolerance. These long-term consequences of obesity need to be addressed by the primary care provider and the cardiac health care provider to lower the risk of persistent obesity and future medical conditions. Children and adolescents may benefit from lifestyle interventions, such as dietary counseling, prescribed physical activity recommendations, psychological or behavioral counseling, and lipidemia prevention screening and prevention education (Andonian et al., 2019; Willinger et al., 2021).

SLOW DEVELOPMENT

Children with CHD, including complex heart lesions, are surviving into their adult years and living productive lives. A new focus on the neurodevelopment of CHD patients has emerged. One of the most concerning sequelae of CHD is an altered neurodevelopment. The impact of CHD on neurodevelopment is multifactorial with intrinsic, preoperative, perioperative, and postoperative risk factors. Infants with more complex cardiac lesions are most often affected.

Intrinsic risk factors include abnormal fetal cerebral blood flow, diminished oxygen delivery to the fetal brain, and associated genetic diagnosis. Neonatal risk factors include prematurity and low birth weight. Preoperative risks include abnormal neonatal transitional physiology and impaired cerebral autoregulation. Perioperative factors are deep hypothermic circulatory arrest, lower cerebral perfusion, acidosis, temperature dysregulation, hypoxia, ischemic reperfusion injury, embolism, and anesthesia (Ryan et al., 2019). Postoperative risk factors include low cardiac output, hypotension, hypoxemia, embolism, seizures, cardiac arrest, need for ECMO support, infections, sedation/analgesia, and nutritional deficits. A prolonged hospitalization can increase the stress level of the child due to an interrupted sleep pattern, loud noises, bright lights, or separation from family members. Posthospital risks include socioeconomic status, parental and family stress, medical comorbidities, and the need for additional surgical interventions (Howell et al., 2019; Scott & Neal, 2021).

Slow development may result from CHF, failure to thrive, increased tiredness with activity, or overprotective parents. The child's fine motor skills may be normal, whereas gross motor skills of sitting, crawling, and walking may be delayed. Early neurodevelopmental screening and initiation of interventions such as occupational therapy, physical therapy, feeding evaluation, speech therapy, and cognitive behavioral therapy are important to halt the progression of a neurodevelopmental concern.

Many studies have reported on neurologic deficits, which exist across a variety of domains and include cognitive impairment, difficulties with language, visual perception, executive functioning, impulsivity and hyperactivity, fine and gross motor skills, and psychosocial maladjustment (Ryan et al., 2019). These neurologic findings impact the individual's social adaptation, academic achievements, and quality of personal and family life even in adulthood.

VULNERABLE CHILD SYNDROME

VCS describes a phenomenon in which a child is perceived as being at higher risk for medical, behavioral, or developmental problems than is warranted by the child's current health. It most often occurs in children who have experienced a serious or life-threatening event or who have a chronic medical condition (Schmitz, 2019; Verbeek et al., 2021). Children with cardiac disease related to CHD or arrhythmias are at a higher risk for experiencing VCS. The parents develop greater fear and a heightened perception of the child's vulnerability, which leads to a pattern of overprotective parenting and extreme concerns (Hoge et al., 2021; Schmitz, 2019; Verbeek et al., 2021). Parents often are unable to set age-appropriate boundaries or trust others to care for their children. These parental perceptions of exaggerated risks may lead to the overuse of medical services and possible unnecessary interventions. The parent's behaviors may result in adverse neurodevelopmental and behavioral outcomes in their child. Children of overprotective parents are more likely to become overweight and obese from increased food offered by the parents or physical exercise restrictions initiated by the parents (Andonian et al., 2019). Feelings of sadness, depression, anxiety, or being overwhelmed may be present in the child and parent. The child may demonstrate separation anxiety, increased hyperactivity, aggression, sleeping problems, learning disabilities, missed school days, and other somatic symptoms.

PROGNOSIS

In the current era, greater than 85% of children with CHD survive into adulthood. Survival of infants with CDH depends on the severity of the cardiac lesion, timing of the diagnosis, and treatment received. Advancements in pharmacology options, imaging modalities, cardiac surgery, and cardiac catheter-based interventions have all contributed to higher survival rates. Many mild cardiac lesions may resolve spontaneously or require a single cardiac procedure. The more complex and critical CHD lesions often require surgery during the neonatal period or within the first year of life. There are several CHD lesions, such as hypoplastic LV syndrome, PVA, or TOF, that will require multiple cardiac surgeries and cardiac catheterizations for palliation of the CHD. According to the Centers for Disease Control and Prevention (CDC, 2022), 97% of infants born with a noncritical CHD are expected to survive to at least 1 year of age, while 95% of those infants will survive until at least 18 years of age; 75% of infants born with a critical CHD are expected to survive to at least 1 year of age, and 69% are expected to survive to at least 18 years of age. HLHS, although with better outcomes, continues to have a higher risk of morbidity and mortality.

The success of pediatric cardiac management and surgery is confirmed by the growing population of adults living with congenital heart defects. Adults with CHD will require lifelong cardiac care either with an adult cardiologist or an adult congenital heart cardiologist. This adult population has a higher prevalence of arrhythmias, cardiac failure, PH, myocardial infarctions, coronary artery disease, hypertension, and strokes (Gilljam et al., 2019; Givertz et al., 2019; Reardon & Lin, 2021). Cardiac surveillance will include a monitor for cardiac sequels, which may include arrhythmias, residual defects, outgrown prosthetic material, ventricular systolic or diastolic dysfunction, and infective endocarditis.

PRIMARY CARE MANAGEMENT

HEALTH CARE MAINTENANCE

Growth and Development

An infant or child with CHD often demonstrates delays in physical and neurodevelopmental growth. The frequency and severity of the growth restrictions tend to be noted with a greater prevalence in children with cyanotic and more severe forms of CHD, such as HLHS (Chinawa et al., 2021). Weight is usually more often affected than height, and the head circumference should not be affected. The growth of the infant and child should be monitored closely to ensure adequate nutrients are being delivered to promote physical growth and brain development. If a flattened growth curve is noted, the child should be referred to the cardiac provider for evaluation of CHF or worsening cardiac condition. Despite optimal cardiac management and appropriate caloric intake, a child with CHD may demonstrate slower weight gain because of increased caloric need or other associated hereditary or genetic conditions. The slower growth may be noted at the time of diagnosis, during cardiac management, and persist for months or several years following cardiac repair (Brief et al., 2022).

Another physical growth concern in children with CHD is the increased prevalence of excessive weight gain or obesity during later childhood. Children may need specific physical activity recommendations and nutrition counseling throughout childhood and adolescence. Overweight and obese children with CHD require screening for the development of associated comorbidities such as hypertension, diabetes, obstructive sleep apnea, and nonalcoholic fatty liver disease (Scott & Neal, 2021).

Infants and children with CHD should be able to meet their developmental milestones, albeit at slower rates of achievement. Following a hospitalization, an individual may display developmental regressions of previously achieved skills as an adaptation to the stress of the hospitalization, sedation, or prolonged bedrest. Parents may notice disturbances in the child's pattern of sleep, feeding, behavior, toilet training, or speech. The child may exhibit increased fussiness or anxiety when arriving at primary care clinic visits. Although these changes can be very concerning for parents, providers should reassure the parents the child's regressions often resolve within a few weeks. If, though, the child demonstrates other neurologic symptoms such as a change in the level of consciousness, seizures, weakness, or cardiac symptoms (e.g., decreased peripheral perfusion, unexplained tachycardia), the child should be examined and referred as needed.

In assessing the development of and emotional status of children with CHD, primary care providers must take into consideration the individual underlying CHD, the number of cardiac surgeries or catheterizations, the need for ECMO support, extended hospitalizations, preexisting conditions, genetic diagnosis, parental overprotection, and physical incapacity. Any child with complex CHD requiring cardiac surgery, ECMO support, or developmental concerns should be referred for formal developmental evaluation within a cardiac neurodevelopment program if available. These clinic providers are specially trained to focus specifically on the developmental risks associated with CHD.

Although major impairments are noted during early childhood, learning disabilities, attention deficits, hyperactivity, and executive functions may not be obvious until the secondary education years when school courses exceed the child's developmental abilities (Gaudet et al., 2021). Early detection of concerns and referrals to services such as occupational therapy, physical therapy, or early education intervention programs is necessary to implement intervention and improve the prognosis (Billotte et al., 2020). Assessing the mental well-being of a child and adolescent within the primary care office should occur during each visit. The CHD diagnosis, in addition to normal childhood social and academic challenges, may increase the risk of depression, anxiety, or maladaptive behaviors. When discussing developmental concerns with parents, the primary care provider should help the parents normalize their response to the child with a chronic condition. Parents should be encouraged to treat their children normally and allow them to participate in extracurricular activities, active play, and exercises. Providers can reassure parents that symptomatic children will self-limit naturally and not push themselves beyond their level of discomfort or physical capabilities.

Diet. Infants typically do best when fed more often (an on-demand schedule) and allowed to drink a varying volume with the feedings; these flexibilities include a child with CHD. Feedings are often a major problem with children with CHD, particularly if they have a complex defect or experiencing CHF. During feedings, symptomatic infants often have difficulties coordinating sucking, swallowing, and breathing. The infant may have difficulties completing a feeding within 30 minutes, resulting in increased fatigue and a calorie deficit. The distribution of the calories in most infants may be similar to the recommended dietary allowances, but the needs of symptomatic infants with failure to thrive may require 130 to 150 kcal/kg/day for adequate growth (Lantin-Hermoso et al., 2017). Fortified human milk or a high-calorie formula is a way to deliver more calories and nutrients without increasing the volume. Human milk is fortified with a human milk fortifier, glucose polymers, medium-chain triglyceride oil, or protein supplement. The concentrated formula may be made by adding extra powder or liquid concentrate to the standard base recipe of the formula. Parents should be advised to monitor their infant's feeding tolerance to the higher calories, which may result in osmotic diarrhea (Luca et al., 2022; Salvatori et al., 2022). Consulting a nutritionist and the cardiac provider is advised when higher-calorie formulas are required.

Breastfeeding is not contraindicated if growth is adequate. Human milk has protective properties, especially in infants with CHD who are at greater risk of necrotizing enterocolitis, and therefore should be encouraged. Human milk promotes the growth of healthy bacteria in the infant's gut, promotes gastric motility and maturity of the digestive tract, minimizes intestinal membrane permeability, and has an antiinflammatory effect on the digestive tract. Infants with CHD receiving human milk have demonstrated improved weight gain for age compared to infants receiving formula (Davis et al., 2019). All infants with CHD should be given the opportunity to breastfeed directly. Available research suggests direct breastfeeding causes less physiologic stress than bottle feeding and contributes to maternal-child bonding. Methods to decrease the work of the breast or bottle feedings include holding the infant at a 45-degree angle to minimize tachypnea, limiting the duration of the feedings to 30 minutes to minimize fatigue, allowing the infant to develop a rhythm of feeding and resting, and following cues from the infant for hunger, satiety, and tiring.

An infant or child with a complex CHD may struggle to gain weight despite optimizing cardiac management and increased caloric intake. These individuals may benefit from gavage feedings to minimize the calories used with feeding. Offering the infant a pacifier during the feeding helps develop a strong suck, facilitates the transition to oral feedings, and promotes future language development. A successful feeding plan safely provides adequate nutrition. Additionally, maintaining a pleasant feeding experience for the child may result in decreased feeding aversions or feeding difficulties in the future.

Children requiring cardiac surgery may develop a chylous pleural effusion secondary to damage to the thoracic duct or from physiologic changes associated with the specific CHD. Single-ventricle patients requiring staged cardiac surgeries have a greater incidence of pleural effusions and chylous effusions. A proposed mechanism of the effusion is the increase in hydrostatic capillary pressure resulting in excessive filtration in the interstitial space and overwhelming drainage into the lymphatic system (Lo Rito et al., 2018). The treatment options include temporary fluid restrictions, diuretic therapy, and a low-fat formula or diet. The child may be discharged to home with this regimen for days or weeks. Providers should assess the patient for potential electrolyte disturbances secondary to the diuretic therapy, slower weight gain, or poor wound healing.

Nutrition and growth represent one of the most stressful problems in these infants. Parents often need a tremendous amount of support to feed a child with CHD. Infant feeding times require energy and are anxiety provoking. Children with symptomatic CHD and tachypnea have difficulty consuming enough calories to satisfy hunger and may be irritable. The infant is less responsive to feeding cues and may need to be aroused when asleep and offered a feeding. The parent and child may exhibit less fostering behavior (e.g., eye contact, smiling, and cuddling) during feeding. Parents with a child with CHD may perceive pressure to get the infant to meet the weekly weight expectation for the child to reach a specific weight for surgery. The parent may feel significant stress and develop lower self-esteem. If a child has a nasogastric tube or gastric tube, additional concerns such as harming the child, embarrassment about using the feeding tube in public, and concerns of long-term consequences to the feeding tube can be noted (Tsintoni et al., 2020).

A primary care provider who understands the potential problems of feeding can be instrumental in fostering a positive feeding relationship by providing support and counseling. Identifying and managing an infant's gastric reflux symptoms can lessen esophageal irritation resulting in a less fussy infant. Primary care providers can offer clear nutrition instructions and appropriate weight goals to parents. The parent should receive ongoing support, which includes teaching the parents to be attentive to the infant's cues for hunger, satiety, and distress and reinforcing feeding skills. An emphasis on the positive aspects of building a relationship with their child, and the bonding experience during feeding, may help ease some of the parental anxiety or concerns.

Safety. In addition to the standard safety precautions, children with CHD have unique needs. Medications are often required for cardiac management.

There are special safety considerations with medications. Safe storage and administration of the medications are essential. The medication should be taken as prescribed to maintain a therapeutic level and prevent harm. For example, digoxin has properties that include a long half-life, a narrow therapeutic level, and additional medication interactions. Digoxin toxicity is a risk secondary to accidental or intentional ingestion or inappropriate medication administration. Digoxin toxicity should be suspected if a child presents with new-onset feeding intolerance, gastrointestinal upset, neurologic changes, and bradycardia/arrhythmias (Law & Raffini, 2015). Anticoagulants such as coumadin, low molecular heparin (Lovenox), clopidogrel (Plavix), and Xa inhibitors (rivaroxaban) increase the risk of gastrointestinal and intracranial bleeding with elevated levels, whereas a subtherapeutic level increases the risk of deep vein thrombosis, neurologic events, pulmonary emboli, or prosthetic heart valve dysfunction. In children, the use of warfarin poses significant challenges because changes in their diet, other medications, and illnesses may alter the international normalized ratio (INR) levels. Ideally, the child should maintain a consistent dietary intake of foods with vitamin K. Other challenges include possible altered absorption of the warfarin, the need for scheduled venipuncture for monitoring the INR level, and unknown optimal dosing (Law & Raffini, 2015). Health care providers can stress the importance of administering the appropriate dose of medication and medication compliance. Pharmacies may provide written and verbal instructions on the medications and dispense premarked syringes identifying the correct dose. Children prescribed anticoagulation should avoid activities or contact sports, which increase the risk of internal bleeding, and monitor for bleeding following dental care or excessive bleeding after falls resulting in disruption of the skin integrity.

Electrical safety and electronic considerations are necessary for children with permanent pacemakers or implantable defibrillators. Although contemporary pacemakers are less susceptible to interference than older models, electromagnetic energy can interfere in some cases. The child and parents should receive information on the pacemaker and possible outside sources of interference. Most household appliances such as microwave ovens, televisions, radios, toasters, and electric blankets are safe. Cellular phones with strong magnetic fields, such as wireless charging and magnetic accessories, including smartwatches, can affect the function of the device if patients are very close (<6 inches) to the device. Individuals are advised to use the cell phone at the ear on the side opposite the cardiac device and to carry the phone in a pocket or bag below the waist. Electromagnetic antitheft security systems used in the screening process in buildings are generally considered safe with minimal interference with a pacemaker. The child or adolescent should be aware of the antitheft systems and walk through them at a normal pace to avoid leaning or standing close to the system. Similarly, metal detectors at airports may result in limited interference, especially with a limited duration of exposure and greater distance between the security system and the pacemaker. Individuals are advised to carry the pacemaker identification card since the metal detector will likely be triggered by the pacemaker.

Surgery and procedures may interfere with pacemakers. The use of electrocautery can inhibit pacemaker function. The pacemaker pulse generator may require specific reprogramming before the procedure and programming back to its baseline condition after the procedure. MRI requires safety precautions that arise from the interaction with medical implants, such as a permanent pacemaker, implantable defibrillator, stents, or coils. There are risks secondary to electromagnetic interactions and heating. Large magnets directly over the pacemaker (especially the older generation of pacemakers) may temporarily change the device's function. Magnetic force of an MRI can damage the leads or device. In the past, an MRI procedure was a relative contraindication for patients with a pacemaker. However, with the introduction of specialized pacemakers that are MRI safe, such scans can be performed. Even patients with a standard pacemaker (i.e., not designated MRI safe) can often undergo MRI scans with careful monitoring and other appropriate precautions. Other procedures that interfere with pacemaker function are transcutaneous electrical nerve/muscle stimulators, diathermy, extracorporeal shockwave lithotripsy, and therapeutic radiation for cancer or tumors.

Children with CHD should consult with the cardiac provider to discuss exercise and sports participation and review the AHA (2021) recommendations for competitive and recreational sports activities. Besides the individual's underlying CHD, which may impose activity restrictions, other special considerations may be necessary. Individuals with an implantable pacemaker or automated implantable cardioverter defibrillator will be advised not to participate in contact sports or exercise activities that may result in trauma to the device and to avoid performing repetitive motions or exercise movements over the site of the pacemaker or lead to decrease the risk of lead fracture or lead displacement. A child receiving anticoagulation, which increases the risk of bleeding, will be restricted from sports or activities that may result in trauma, internal bleeding, or prolonged bleeding.

Air travel is often safe for an infant or a child with CHD. Commercial airplanes usually fly at an altitude between 6700 and 13,400 m, and the cabin pressure is kept constant at 8000 feet or less. The partial pressure of oxygen in the arterial blood at this altitude is 60 to 69 mmHg, and hypoxia at this level is often well tolerated.

Special air travel precautions may be required with CHD lesions with intracardiac shunts, PH, significant hypoxemia, and Eisenmenger syndrome because an increase in pulmonary vascular constriction may occur. Individuals are encouraged to maintain good hydration and avoid prolonged sitting and moving or walking in the aisle during longer flights. Oxygen therapy for air travel may be recommended by the cardiologist and require special preflight arrangement and approval from the airlines.

Long QT syndrome is a disorder of myocardial repolarization characterized by prolongation of the QTc interval. Ventricular arrhythmias and torsades de pointes may occur, resulting in collapse or death. Individuals are encouraged to make lifestyle changes to decrease the risk of repolarization abnormalities in response to autonomic change, particularly during sudden changes in the heart rate. Individuals may be advised to avoid swimming and other vigorous exercise, stressful situations, or situations of being startled (e.g., sudden loud noises such as alarms or when unexpectedly surprised by a noise or person). Primary care providers prescribing medications that can prolong the QTc interval should be avoided; or if prescribed, the patients should be closely monitored (Krahn et al., 2022).

Body art, including body piercing and tattoos, has grown in popularity. Infective endocarditis is a rare but dangerous complication of tattooing and body piercing. An individual with CHD and personal history of cardiac surgery, device placement (e.g., cardiac valves, stents, pacemakers), cardiac transplant, or underlying single-ventricle anatomy has a higher risk of infective endocarditis. The cardiologist may discourage body piercing or tattoos in adolescents or adults to decrease the risk of infective endocarditis. If, though, an individual makes a personal decision to have the body art completed, there is a strong recommendation the piercing or tattoo is completed at a licensed parlor by an artist using clean needles, and SBE prophylaxis is prescribed (Müller et al., 2021).

Preparing the family for medical emergency situations may be lifesaving. Cardiopulmonary resuscitation training for parents, teachers, and coaches may be effective and warranted for children with known CHD. Families may want to inquire if an automated external defibrillator is available at the child's school, sporting events, and community buildings in case the child collapses from an arrhythmia and needs immediate medical intervention.

Immunizations. The standard immunization protocol (including pneumococcal, meningococcal, and yearly vaccines) is recommended for children with CHD. Immunizations should be administered according to the standard protocols as much as possible. The administration of an immunization near the date of a scheduled cardiac surgery requires additional considerations. Although vaccines can be safely administered, concern for a potential febrile response or a decreased ability to mount an immune response after cardiopulmonary bypass may exist. Cardiac providers may recommend patients undergoing cardiopulmonary bypass avoid vaccine administration for 2 weeks before and 6 weeks after the surgery (Puri et al., 2017). Additional immunization considerations are required following the administration of blood products (e.g., whole blood, packed red blood cells, and plasma) and other antibody-containing blood products (e.g., immunoglobulin, hyperimmune globulin, and intravenous immunoglobulin), which can inhibit the immune response to measles and rubella vaccines for 3 months or longer. The CDC (2022) recommends following the administration of blood products; live vaccines such as varicella and measles are delayed for 6 to 7 months or until the passive antibody has degraded. There are no current recommendations for delays to Ty21a typhoid, yellow fever, live attenuated influenza vaccine, and rotavirus vaccine administration.

During respiratory syncytial virus (RSV) season, prophylaxis against RSV is recommended in infants with unrepaired cyanotic CHD, receiving anticongestive medications, and significant hemodynamic abnormalities. Primary care provider offices may be requested to prescribe Synagis, a manufactured antibody to RSV. Synagis is administered as a monthly intramuscular injection given during the early fall to late spring seasons. A subgroup of patients with CHD has additional immunization considerations. A child with functional asplenia should receive subsequent doses of the 23-valent polysaccharide vaccine, and a child with immune compromise should not receive live attenuated vaccines.

Screenings

Vision. Routine screening is recommended.

Hearing. Routine screening is recommended.

Dental. Schedule dental examination every 6 months.

- A child needs to perform meticulous oral hygiene care with daily teeth brushing and flossing to prevent dental caries and gum disease. Parental assistance with dental care may be necessary for younger children.
- Children with a high risk of infective endocarditis require SBE prophylaxis before a dental visit, which includes oral procedures (e.g., deep dental cleaning, drilling at the gum level, teeth extraction, dental implants, bone and gum grafting) to eliminate or reduce transient bacteremia caused by invasive dental procedures.
- Cardiology providers and primary care providers should educate the family on the concerns and risks of infective endocarditis.
- Wallet-sized SBE prophylaxis cards are available for references.

Blood pressure. Obtain blood pressure at least yearly during primary care provider visits and during each cardiology visit.

- Blood pressures should be obtained in the upper and lower extremities in infants or children with suspected or confirmed CoA, aortic arch anomalies, or following cardiac surgery or cardiac catheterization intervention for management of aortic arch anomalies. A discrepancy in the readings may indicate the progression of the heart lesion or a recurrent aortic arch obstruction.
- Hypertension may occur at an earlier age in children with CHD with a history of aortic arch anomalies or bicuspid aortic valves. Refer to cardiology for further assessment.
- A child who had a BTT shunt or a subclavian flap repair for CoA may have diminished blood pressure or absent pulse on the side of the cardiac surgery.

Hemoglobin/hematocrit. Obtain complete blood cell (CBC) count as clinically indicated.

- Inquire with family if recent bloodwork was obtained by the cardiologist to avoid duplicated/unnecessary bloodwork.
- Cyanotic CHD, single ventricles with palliative surgeries, or PH patients require at least a yearly CBC count to assess for secondary erythrocytosis and increased hemoglobin production resulting in iron deficiency anemia. Iron supplements should be prescribed for management of the anemia.
- CHD patients may develop anemia from a chronic medical condition, blood loss from frequent labs, and poor nutritional intake. Assess for associated clinical findings such as tachycardia, fatigue, pallor, and lower oxygen saturation.

Urinalysis. Routine screening is recommended.

- Urinalysis is used to assess for impaired renal function secondary to decreased cardiac output and medication side effects.

Tuberculosis. Routine screening is recommended

- CHD with associated immunology abnormality may be more susceptible to tuberculosis (TB) after contact with a person with active TB.

Lipid panel. Routine screening per universal serum lipid screening guidelines is recommended.

- The National Heart, Blood, and Lung Institute and American Academy of Pediatrics recommend universal serum lipid screening for children between ages 9 and 11 years and again when they reach ages 17 to 21 years.
- Targeted screening is recommended for children age 2 to 8 years and 12 to 16 years who have cardiovascular risk factors such as hypertension, obesity, or a family history of premature cardiovascular disease.

Psychosocial. Routine screening for anxiety, depression, and suicidal thoughts is recommended.

Neurodevelopmental

- Recommended for children requiring cardiac surgery, ECMO support, or with other special health needs.
- In screening for the developmental outcome, it is relevant to identify children with CHD with mild or emerging disorders to refer for developmental evaluation when identified and to initiate an early intervention for the child.

Condition-Specific Screenings

Drugs and electrolytes

- Digoxin: assess level as needed to ensure a therapeutic level or if toxicity is suspected.
- Warfarin: cardiology or hematology will obtain INR levels as needed to ensure a therapeutic level.
- Diuretics: electrolyte imbalance may occur with increased diuresis, during illness resulting in increased emesis or diarrhea, or when a child is prescribed multiple diuretics or frequent daily dosing.

COMMON ILLNESS MANAGEMENT

The primary care provider has an essential role in caring for children with CHD. Cardiology and other specialty providers will notify the primary care provider with updates and plans of care. Families will establish trust and a working relationship with their primary care provider. Parents may request their primary care provider to interpret procedures or test results or to reassure them about their child's health status. In addition, parents may need to hear from the primary care provider that their child is normal with special health care considerations. The primary care provider can help alleviate some of the parental concerns regarding the health of their child and build a rapport with the child. The child with CHD who has required hospitalization or surgery may present to the primary care provider clinic with hesitancy or fear of medical staff and may require more time to reestablish trust with the primary care provider before an examination can be completed.

A child with CHD requires routine well-child visits and vaccination administrations. The primary care provider handles the child's routine care and illness visits. A child with CHD may be susceptible to common pediatric problems and/or illness and present to the primary care provider with more severe symptoms than a child with no chronic medical condition. The primary care provider, with expertise in common childhood problems and cardiac knowledge, will be able to identify more subtle clinical symptoms in an infant or child, leading to prompt illness management and decreasing the risk of patient clinical deterioration or serious complications.

Differential Diagnosis

Fever. Although febrile illnesses can have serious consequences in children with CHD, an acute fever may be related to common, uncomplicated childhood illnesses. The primary care provider should complete a thorough history and physical examination of the child to assess for tachycardia, tachypnea, color changes, or decreased perfusion. If the child's examination is not significantly different from the child's norm, the primary care provider should investigate, identify the source of the fever, and recommend a treatment plan offered to another child of the same age. Parents should be informed to return to the primary care provider clinic if the child does not respond to the treatment plan. Antibiotics should be prescribed for a confirmed diagnosis, not as a prophylaxis against a specific disease. Overprescribing antibiotics can increase the risk of the patient developing antibiotic-resistant organisms.

A fever within a few weeks after heart surgery may be a sign of an operative infection or an inflammatory reaction that results in a postpericardiotomy syndrome or pericardial effusion. A careful and complete examination to identify the source of the fever should occur. If no focus of infection (e.g., ear infection, upper respiratory infection, or pharyngitis) is found, the cardiac provider or cardiac surgeon should be notified. If the surgical incision appears infected, the primary care provider should obtain a CBC count with differential, creatine-reactive protein (CRP), erythrocyte sedimentation rate (ESR), and blood culture before antibiotics are prescribed. Antibiotic therapy should be prescribed, and a close follow-up assessment should be arranged within the primary care provider or cardiology clinic. Other potential etiologies for fever postsurgery could be a postpericardiotomy syndrome or pericardial effusion. The child may present to the clinic 7 to 10 days after surgery with tachycardia, tachypnea, pericardial friction rub, muffled heart tones, pallor, mottled skin, irritability, and fatigue. The child may be more comfortable in an upright position or while leaning forward compared to a supine position. A chest radiograph may reveal an increased cardiac silhouette. A referral to cardiology is recommended. Possible treatment options include antiinflammatory agents (e.g., aspirin, NSAIDs, occasional steroids). Significant pericardial effusions may result in cardiac tamponade and require pericardiocentesis procedure.

Fevers may increase the metabolic demands, oxygen consumption, and workload of the heart. Children with more serious cardiac conditions and/or who have required staged and palliative surgery are at greater risk of developing CHF or clinical instability. A child with asplenia and fever requires an immediate evaluation and a complete workup from the primary care provider to identify the cause and initiate antibiotic therapy.

Infective endocarditis. Infective endocarditis, also known as bacterial endocarditis, is caused by bacteria that enter the bloodstream and settle in the endocardium of the heart (Lee, 2020). Infective endocarditis can occur from random bacteremia from normal daily activities (e.g., chewing gum, brushing teeth) and with poor oral hygiene and periodontal diseases. Older adolescents may develop infective endocarditis after body art, including piercing or tattoos, and intravenous drug abuse. Medical reasons for infective endocarditis development include a recent dental procedure or a surgery involving oral mucosa, implantable devices such as a pacemaker, stents, closure devices, damaged heart valves, or artificial heart valves. Although infective endocarditis is rare, there is an increased trend in occurrence (Lee, 2020).

Health care providers should be knowledgeable of infective endocarditis, which may present as an acute or subacute infection. Acute infections present as a rapidly progressive disease with high fevers, temperature instability, sepsis, and systemic complications. A new-onset murmur or an illness unresponsive to antibiotic therapy raises concern for infective endocarditis. In contrast, SBE diagnosis is often delayed and presents with non-specific symptoms such as weight loss, fatigue, muscle aches, and dyspnea over several weeks to months. Uncommon findings include skin findings of painless red, purple, or brown flat spots on the soles of the feet or the palms of the hands (Janeway lesions), painful red or purple bumps or patches of darkened skin (hyperpigmented) on the tips of the fingers or toes (Osler nodes), or petechia inside the mouth or sclera region (Wang et al., 2018).

Children presenting with fevers and findings suspicious of infective endocarditis should be referred to their cardiologist for evaluation. Diagnostic tests may include an echocardiogram to assess for valvular vegetation or ventricular dysfunction and an ECG to assess for arrhythmia. Additional imaging with cardiac CT and nuclear imaging may provide more definite findings. Blood cultures should be drawn before initiating antibiotics. Once infective endocarditis is established, antibiotic therapy needs to be initiated. A prolonged course of intravenous antibiotics of 4 to 8 weeks will be prescribed. Surgical intervention may be indicated in situations with insufficient antibiotic response, infected prosthetic cardiac valve or material, or prolonged clinical symptoms.

An emphasis on the prevention of infective endocarditis is important. Cardiology and primary care providers can educate the parents and child on the importance of daily oral hygiene, SBE prophylaxis recommendations, and the signs and symptoms of infective endocarditis that require immediate medical attention.

Respiratory compromise. The primary care provider evaluating a child with CHD and respiratory symptoms needs to consider several differential diagnoses, including decreased cardiac function, cardiac shunt stenosis, arrhythmia, aspiration pneumonia, or viral illness, before initiating treatment. A change in the child's baseline examination findings, such as adventitious breath sounds, tachycardia, sweating, slow weight gain, and increased pallor or cyanosis but with no symptoms of fevers or increased nasal congestion, may be suggestive of a cardiac cause for the respiratory compromise. Parental reports of observing heavier breathing, grunting, increased sleepiness, poor weight gain, increased feeding difficulties, and unexplained fussiness in their child may also support a cardiac source. A chest radiograph should be obtained; if cardiomegaly, increased pulmonary congestion, or diminished vascular markings from an occluded or narrowed shunt, are noted, a prompt referral to cardiology is recommended. On the other hand, a child with CHD, particularly with a left-to-right intracardiac shunt, a weakened immune system, failure to thrive, or CHF, may have an increased risk for upper and lower respiratory infections. The child may present with a productive cough, nasal congestion, fever, and radiographic findings of infiltrates, localized pneumonia, or pleural effusion from an upper or lower respiratory illness. The child's treatment plan will focus on managing the patient's respiratory disease, symptoms, and fever control. Close follow-up within the primary care provider clinic within 1 week of the initial symptoms should be arranged.

RSV can have serious effects on a child with symptomatic CHD, which may require hospitalization for the management of the respiratory illness. Any scheduled cardiac surgery or cardiac catheterization procedure should be postponed for at least 4 to 6 weeks to allow for pulmonary healing. An infection from RSV close to the time of surgery can increase the risk of PH, prolonged respiratory support, or slower surgical recovery.

Gastrointestinal symptoms. Children may present to the primary care office with symptoms of poor appetite, feeding intolerance, emesis, loose stools, or poor weight gain. The primary care provider should investigate for cardiac reasons such as CHF, decreased intestinal perfusion, electrolyte disturbance secondary to diuretic therapy, increased concentrated feedings leading to higher osmolarity, or digoxin toxicity. Evaluation for common childhood conditions such as gastroenteritis, food allergies, gastric reflux, or an underlying gastroenterology diagnosis should also be considered. Special attention for evidence of dehydration from emesis, diarrhea, anorexia, or decreased fluid intake is important. A child with CHD should be monitored closely for clinical concerns, including lethargy, decreased peripheral perfusion, tachycardia, and thrombus formation, especially in a cyanotic lesion or those with a central shunt (e.g., BTT shunt). Replacement fluids, referral to cardiology, or possible hospital admission may be warranted.

Neurologic symptoms. A child with unexplained fever, headache, focal neurologic signs, or seizures must be immediately referred to a medical center for evaluation. Neurologic concerns associated with CHD are brain abscesses in children younger than age 2 years or cerebral vascular disease in those older than 2 years.

Chest pain. Children will present to the primary care clinic and emergency room with complaints of chest pain. A complete history and physical examination are important to determine the possible source of chest pain. Fortunately, chest pain in children is rarely (1–6%) related to a serious or life-threatening etiology (e.g., cardiac condition, PH, pneumothorax, airway, foreign body, tumors, spinal cord compression), and ultimately a noncardiac cause is suspected (Barbut et al. 2020) (Box 18.2). A large percentage of the chest pain will be from an unclear or idiopathic pain, followed by musculoskeletal cause (e.g., costochondritis, chest wall pain, muscular strain, precordial catch syndrome, or trauma). Less common causes include asthma, pneumonia, gastric reflux disease, irritable bowel disease, anxiety, depression, or somatization. Cardiac etiologies of chest pain include pericarditis, aortic stenosis, obstructive hypertrophic cardiomyopathy, coronary artery ischemia, arrhythmia, or aortic aneurysm or dissection. Older children may present with chest pain after recreational drug use (e.g., cocaine, amphetamines, bath salts, marijuana, and synthetic cannabinoids) or associated with e-cigarette use.

Critical components in the child's history and associated symptoms may clarify the cause of the chest pain. A positive response to the following questions may raise concern for a cardiac issue and the need for cardiology referral: Have you ever fainted, passed out, or had a seizure suddenly and without warning, especially during exercise or in response to auditory triggers such as doorbells, alarm clocks, and ringing telephones? Have you experienced exercise-induced chest pain? Are you related to anyone with sudden, unexplained, or unexpected death before the age of 50 years? Are you related to anyone diagnosed with a predisposing heart condition such as hypertrophic cardiomyopathy, long QT syndrome, or catecholaminergic polymorphic ventricular tachycardia? Other specific questions to ask include: When did the pain start? How frequent is the pain? Where is the pain located? Is the chest pain related to exercise, eating, or breathing? Is there any associated dizziness,

---

Box 18.2   **Life-Threatening Chest Pain Conditions and Common Chest Pain Conditions**

LIFE-THREATENING CONDITIONS (PREVALENCE FOR CHEST PAIN 1–6%)

Cardiac conditions (prevalence 0.5–5%)
- Hypertrophic cardiomyopathy
- Aortic stenosis
- Coarctation of the aorta
- Coronary artery abnormalities (e.g., anomalous coronary artery, Kawasaki disease)
- Angina after recreational drug use (e.g., cocaine, amphetamines, bath salts, marijuana, synthetic cannabinoids)
- Classic angina (early atherosclerotic disease from hyperlipidemia or diabetes mellitus)
- Pericarditis
- Myocarditis
- Cardiomyopathies (dilated, restrictive, hypertrophic)
- Tachyarrhythmias
- Aortic aneurysm or dissection
- Ruptured sinus of Valsalva aneurysms
- Pericardial effusion with cardiac tamponade

Airway foreign body

Spontaneous pneumothorax

Pulmonary embolism

Sickle cell disease with acute chest pain syndrome

Tumor (chest wall, pulmonary, mediastinum)

Nontraumatic esophageal rupture (Boerhaave syndrome)

Spinal cord compression (tumor, vertebral collapse, epidural abscess)

COMMON CONDITIONS (PREVALENCE FOR CHEST PAIN 94–96%)

Idiopathic (prevalence 35–40%)

Muscular conditions (prevalence 5–30%)
- Muscle strain
- Costochondritis
- Slipping rib syndrome
- Precordial catch syndrome (Texidor twinge)
- Fibromyalgia
- Pectus excavatum or carinatum

Psychiatric conditions (prevalence 10–16%)
- Anxiety
- Panic disorder with or without hyperventilation syndrome
- Depression
- Recent stressor
- Hypochondriasis
- Somatization
- Functional neurologic disorder (conversion disorder)

Respiratory conditions (prevalence 2–11%)
- Pneumonia (possible life threatening)
- Asthma (possible life threatening)
- Chronic cough with muscle strain
- Spontaneous pneumomediastinum

Gastrointestinal conditions (prevalence 8–10%)
- Gastroesophageal reflux disease
- Esophageal foreign body
- Esophageal spams and achalasia
- Gastritis
- Peptic ulcer
- Irritable bowel disease
- Cholecystitis
- Pancreatitis

Breast (prevalence 1–5%)
- Male adolescents: gynecomastia
- Female adolescents: pregnancy, thelarche, mastitis, fibrocystic disease

lightheadedness, or syncope? Do you notice palpitations or tachycardia with chest pain? What alleviates the pain? What makes the pain worse? Does direct pressure or a deep breath increase the pain? Is the pain worse after eating, or do you have a bad taste in your mouth? Have you had a recent illness or trauma event or started a new exercise routine? Do you have chronic medical conditions? Have you experienced stressors, episodes of anxiety, or depression? Have there been any significant life events such as a change in living arrangement, school concerns, or social interactions? Are you well hydrated? How often do you drink caffeinated or energy drinks?

A careful history and physical examination can usually differentiate a benign condition from a dangerous one. An ECG and a referral to cardiology should occur if the primary care provider identifies chest pain in conjunction with syncope, dizziness, palpitations, dyspnea, easy fatigue, exertion, drug use, or associated medical condition (e.g., lupus erythematous, Marfan syndrome, Kawasaki disease, rheumatic fever, PH).

Syncope. Syncope is the transient loss of consciousness, usually from decreased cerebral blood flow. The most common cause of syncope in pediatrics involves the autonomic nervous system. These conditions may be caused by quick positional changes, orthostatic intolerance, emotional stress, breath-holding, hypovolemia, dehydration, or anemia. More concerning causes include arrhythmias, cardiac conduction abnormalities (e.g., long QT syndrome or Brugada syndrome), cardiac conditions (e.g., known congenital heart and history of cardiac surgery, hypertrophic cardiomyopathy, coronary artery anomalies), seizures, PH, hypercyanotic spells, or psychogenic reaction with associated hyperventilation or functional neurologic disorder (conversion disorder).

A thorough history and physical examination is the most important diagnostic assessment. Frequently the etiology can be identified from specific questions and answers. The primary care provider should pay attention to the activity, position, and precipitating events before the syncope as well as associated symptoms. Children with palpitations, tachycardia, chest pain, dizziness before a syncopal event, or exercise-induced syncope increase the possibility of a cardiac condition or a marker for sudden death. Family history of syncope, seizures, deafness, sudden death, long QT syndrome, Brugada syndrome, or cardiomyopathies could indicate a potential increased risk of a hereditary cause for the syncope. The physical examination should concentrate on the neurologic and cardiovascular systems. Diagnostic workup may include orthostatic vital signs, an ECG, and referral to cardiology for further evaluation if a cardiac concern is identified. A small percentage of children with syncope will require additional cardiac tests such as an echocardiogram, exercise stress test, Holter monitor, and rarely tilt-table test.

Drug interactions. Children with CHF or arrhythmias often receive combinations of digoxin, diuretics, and other medications. The addition of any drug to a child's cardiac medication regimen requires close attention and consultation with a pharmacist or cardiology provider if there are questions about interactions. Providers may also review information from evidence-based resources to determine adverse reactions, drug interactions, and drug compatibility. Coadministration of digoxin and quinidine, verapamil, or amiodarone may elevate digoxin plasma concentration. Aminoglycosides can affect renal function and alter the excretion of digoxin. Children have been prescribed ACE inhibitor (e.g., captopril, enalapril, lisinopril) to decrease cardiac afterload and for the management of CHF. These medications may increase serum potassium and require special caution and serum potassium levels obtained when potassium-sparing diuretics (e.g., spironolactone) are prescribed. The combination of adenosine and carbamazepine may act synergistically and cause heart block. Concurrent use of clonidine and verapamil may lead to severe hypotension or AV conduction block. There are well-documented interactions between cardiac and psychogenic drugs, and a consultation with the cardiologist is vital before prescribing these drugs.

Warfarin is prescribed to decrease the risk of thrombus formation, especially in children with increased clotting (e.g., those with prosthetic valves, PH, following Fontan completion). The underlying condition or indication for warfarin determines the ideal target ranges. Periodic warfarin levels, measured as an INR, are obtained to confirm therapeutic levels. The INR level can be altered with the concomitant use of warfarin and other medications. The child is encouraged to have a consistent dietary intake of food with higher amounts of vitamin K, which may be challenging in younger children. Since there are no interactions between immunizations and warfarin, there is no need to alter the immunization schedule.

Acquired heart disease. When obtaining the child's medical history, the provider should inquire about significant illnesses or events that may impact cardiac health. A child may present to the primary care clinic with an acquired heart disease such as Kawasaki disease with coronary involvement, rheumatic fever with heart valve damage, infectious myocarditis resulting in CHF, or chronic obstructive pulmonary disease with right-sided heart strain. These acquired cardiac diseases will require surveillance assessments within cardiology and the primary care clinic. During times in which there is a surge in community illnesses or a pandemic situation, a child may present to the primary care clinic with new cardiac symptoms, fever, and other associated general complaints. Increased awareness of a developing cardiac condition such as myocarditis, arrhythmia, pericardial effusion, or coronary artery disease may be necessary. Earlier detection of a cardiac disease process and initiation of management of an underlying cardiac condition are important to help resolve the cardiac symptoms and prevent the development of chronic cardiac disease. A cardiology referral in which cardiac tests such as an ECG, echocardiogram, Holter, or stress test may be warranted.

DEVELOPMENTAL ISSUES

Sleep Pattern

Sleep plays a crucial role in the development of infants and children. Quality sleep positively impacts alertness, cognitive performance, mood, learning, and memory. A child's sleep quality and pattern should be assessed during clinic visits. Early diagnosis and treatment of obstructive sleep apnea are crucial to improve the quality of life and potentially decreasing future cardiovascular risks (Drake et al., 2020). Parents should be strongly advised to establish healthy sleep habits for their child or adolescent. Adhering to a nightly routine, such as a set bedtime, the child sleeping in own bed, and no electronic use 1 hour before bed, may promote quality sleep.

Infants and children with CHD may experience an altered or obstructive sleep pattern from abnormal neurologic development, frequent interruptions during sleep for medical care, airway abnormalities associated with the genetic condition (e.g., 22q11.2 deletion, trisomy 21), or CHF resulting in episodes of fussiness and tachypnea. Infants with CHF are tachypneic, diaphoretic, and easily tired. They may be unable to satisfy their hunger and thus have a difficult time sleeping through the night from hunger. The child may be restless during sleep to find a position of comfort. There may be a preference to have the head of the bed raised to ease shortness of breath, tachypnea, or chest heaviness. A referral to cardiology is advised if the child is demonstrating increased CHF symptoms, poor sleep, and feeding difficulties.

A child with CHD may have a greater risk of experiencing a sudden cardiac arrest or respiratory deterioration during sleep compared to the general population. Potential etiologies for cardiac and/or respiratory deterioration include CHF, occlusions of cardiac placed pulmonary to aorta shunts, mechanical valve dysfunction, hypoxemia, aspiration, or arrhythmias. Individuals diagnosed with an electrical condition abnormality (e.g., Brugada syndrome, long QT syndrome, and polymorphic ventricular tachycardia) may be at risk for a sudden event during sleep (Mishra et al., 2020).

Toileting

Children receiving diuretics experience increased frequency and urgency from the response of the medication. A younger toddler may have more difficulties with toilet training; therefore parents may choose to delay toilet training until the diuretics are discontinued. If a child requires chronic diuretic therapy, the timing of the administration of the diuretic should be considered and adjusted to facilitate toilet training. Toilet training, as well as other developmental milestones, often show regression following hospitalization.

Discipline

Behavioral expectations of children with CHD should be similar to those of children without heart disease, and normal parenting skills and discipline behaviors are recommended. The diagnosis of CHD may result in changes in the family's approach and attitude to discipline not only for the child with CHD but other siblings as well. Parents may become overprotective and pamper the child with CHD. Out of fear of the CHD diagnosis, parents may respond too quickly to the cries of the infant or child, resulting in fewer opportunities for the child to learn the skills of self-soothing skills. Primary care providers play a role in reinforcing the importance of setting limits and disciplining children with consistency, as well as encouraging normal family dynamics. The coping skills of parents should be assessed specifically if the child is irritable, difficult to console, or difficult to feed. If parents report significant stress or poor coping skills, the child may be at a greater risk of poor parenting behaviors or possible abuse. Health care providers should offer community resources or support group recommendations to the parents.

Child Care

There are usually no contraindications to an infant or child with CHD attending a child care setting. Special considerations are required when the child has more complex medical needs (i.e., tracheostomy, feeding tube, oxygen), a weaker immunity, or greater developmental needs. These children require a child care setting with staff members trained in these needs. Children with asplenia or 22q11.2 deletion are at the highest risk of infection. For these children who are prone to infection, home or small group child care is advised. Although some parents choose to stay at home with their child with cardiac conditions, other parents continue to work. Several factors are considered with the parents' decision to return to work and include the following: (1) financial and emotional need to return to work, (2) parental anxiety about leaving the child, (3) increased incidence of infection for children in child care and the effect on infection on the child's cardiovascular status, and (4) parental confidence in a child care provider's ability to recognize symptoms, give medications properly, and respond to emergencies appropriately.

Before cardiac surgery or catheterization, parents may be counseled to take their child out of day care to avoid exposure to infection. After cardiac surgery, special chest precautions to avoid trauma or sternum instability are required for 6 weeks. The child should not be lifted under the arm but scooped or lifted while supporting the buttock region by caregivers. The child is instructed to avoid activities (e.g., climbing, heavy lifting, rough play, riding a bike or skateboard, jumping on a trampoline, or contact sports) that may cause strain or trauma to the sternum. Normal daily activities such as tummy time are allowed. Parents must communicate these restrictions to the child care provider to determine if there are concerns with the child returning to the child care with the recommended activity precautions.

Schooling

Children with CHD may attend school with their peers or be home schooled. Most children with a cardiac condition will be in the regular classroom, while some children benefit from special education services. The etiology of the child's limitations can be multifactorial and may be due to genetic or chromosomal abnormalities, abnormalities in the fetal brain, and perioperative factors, including single-ventricle physiology, hospital length of stay, and duration of cardiopulmonary bypass (Howell et al., 2019; Jonas, 2020). Although most children with CHD have cognitive skills comparable to their peers during early elementary school, recent studies have documented that children with CHD have a higher prevalence of cognitive and motor limitations, attention disorder, hyperactivity, lower academic achievement scores, and more school absenteeism compared to their peers (Nematollahi et al., 2020). During adolescence, a greater disparity in performance is noted. The adolescent may report learning difficulties, poor concentration, and exercise limitations. In addition, increased awareness of the surgical scar may influence body image.

Primary care providers should be alert to signs of learning disabilities in the child. When indicated, it is important to initiate early intervention, such as working with schools and other services (i.e., speech, occupational, or physical therapy), to prevent or mitigate further functional limitations in children with heart disease (Nematollahi et al., 2020). The provider can inquire about school absences to include the frequency and reason when appropriate home or hospital-based schooling for prolonged absences from schools may be necessary. If the absences are associated with the parental perception of the child's vulnerability or concerns about the child attending school, the primary care provider should acknowledge the parent's worries but offer reassurances and stress the importance of normal life experiences for the child.

Most children and adolescents with CHD may participate in physical education classes and extracurricular activities offered at school. Involvement in extracurricular activities and exercise is encouraged to normalize the child's school experience. Fewer activity restrictions were a change from past years when clinicians restricted physical activity for children with CHD because of concerns that increased activity might be dangerous. Currently there is a better understanding that promoting physical activity benefits the health and well-being of children and adults with CHD. In fact, regular exercise has been shown to be associated with many physiologic and psychological health benefits (i.e., decreased risk of stroke, coronary artery disease,

hypertension, diabetes, obesity, osteoporosis, depression, and anxiety) at any age and is recommended by the AHA (2021) and CDC (2022). For children age 6 to 17 years, the CDC (2022) recommends participating in at least 60 minutes of daily moderate-vigorous physical activity daily, and a greater volume of physical activity (i.e., aerobic physical activity, but also some strength training and bone-strengthening activity) is associated with greater health benefit. The cardiology provider will tailor exercise recommendations to each child depending on the clinical status, type of CHD, and arrhythmia risk to ensure safe participation in regular physical activity (Selamet Tierney, 2020). During exercise, children with CHD should monitor their exercise tolerance and modify the activity if clinical symptoms develop to prevent a medical crisis.

It is advisable the parents provide the school with a list of the child's medical conditions, medications, and exercise allowance to have on file in case of emergency. In addition, parents should inquire if the school has an automated cardioversion device available if a need arises.

Sexuality

Adolescents and adults with CHD are living longer, increasing the need for appropriate reproductive health care and services. The AHA (2021) recommends that clinic-based reproductive health counseling is introduced in early adolescence. The cardiac provider, primary care provider, and gynecologist (for females) are in the positions to provide education in areas of reproductive health, specifically CHD recurrence risk in offspring, possible cardiac complications during pregnancy, and appropriate use of contraception (Katz et al., 2022). Communication between these providers is important to share critical information about a young female's risk factors for contraception and pregnancy, given her cardiac condition.

In adolescence, menstrual irregularities, concerns about developing sexuality, self-image, and the risk of pregnancy are important topics of discussion. In females with CHD, menarche occurs later than in their peers. Females with acyanotic CHD, cyanotic CHD, and complex CHD experience their first menarche at 13, 13.9, and 14.5 years of age, respectively. In addition, adolescents may have a potentially higher frequency of menstrual irregularities or heavy bleeding, especially with prescribed anticoagulants (Haberer & Silversides, 2019).

Contraceptive counseling is an essential part of the care of adolescent and adult females with CHD because an unanticipated pregnancy may potentially have an adverse maternal and neonatal outcome. When considering contraception, a balanced choice needs to be made between effectiveness, safety, and personal preference. Contraception options include (1) barrier methods, such as a condom or a diaphragm, which are safe for females with CHD, but with failure rates of at least 13% to 17% depending on appropriate use. A barrier method is not recommended as the sole method of contraception. (2) Oral contraceptives include combined estrogen-progesterone and progesterone-only preparations. The combined formulations with higher proportions of estrogen may increase the risk of thromboembolic complications and therefore are not recommended in patients with Eisenmenger syndrome, prosthetic valves, ventricular dysfunction, or Fontan circulation. The oral progesterone-only formulations reduce the risk of thromboembolism but have a higher failure rate (7%) and are not advised for women in whom prevention of pregnancy is important. (3) Other forms of hormonal contraception, such as depot medroxyprogesterone acetate or progesterone-releasing intrauterine device (IUD), are often good alternatives for women with CHD. Vagal reactions can occur in women at the time of IUD insertion, and this can result in serious complications in those with Fontan circulation or pulmonary vascular disease. Antibiotic prophylaxis is not required before IUD insertion, but screening for sexually transmitted infections may be done in high-risk patients. (4) Irreversible options such as tubal occlusion or vasectomy may be considered for some high-risk females, although there is a generally increased operation risk, including postoperative infection.

Pregnant women with CHD may have a greater risk for adverse events during pregnancy and delivery, especially with coexisting morbidities (i.e., cardiomyopathy, valvular heart disease, PH, systemic hypertension, cardiac conduction disorder, anemia, and nongestational diabetes) (Haberer & Silversides, 2019; Ramlakhan et al., 2020; Schlichting et al., 2019). The modified World Health Organization (WHO) classification categorized patients into four pregnancy risk classes (I–IV) as determined by their medical condition and is useful for risk stratification. Class I consists of mild CHD, such as a small PDA, mitral valve prolapse, and repaired simple lesions. These lesions are not associated with a significant risk of morbidity or mortality compared with the general pregnant population. The risk of pregnancy gradually increases with an extremely high risk in modified WHO class IV, including women with PA dilatation, severe systemic ventricular dysfunction, or severe aortic dilatation. Pregnant women in class I can be cared for in a peripheral hospital, whereas those in class IV are advised against pregnancy. Classes II, II to III, and III include females at a mild-moderate increased risk, and evaluation and management during pregnancy are required accordingly in a tertiary center (Van Hagen et al., 2020). All females with CHD should receive normal prenatal care, while those with higher risks will require additional cardiac evaluation and tests. A multidisciplinary approach involving the cardiologist, high-risk obstetrician, and primary care providers is crucial for adolescents and women with CHD who are pregnant.

Males with CHD may present to the primary care clinic with sexual health questions and concerns, including a decreased sexual drive and erectile dysfunction.

The proposed causes for erectile dysfunction are extra-cardiac morbidities, endothelial dysfunction, exercise limitations, or perceived or actual malignant cardiac arrhythmia during exertion (Fischer et al., 2021).

Transition to Adulthood
Over the last decade, tremendous advances in diagnostic and therapeutic surgical techniques have resulted in increases in the survival of patients with CHD. Adolescents and emerging adults with CHD are estimated at 1.4 million, which comprises 15% to 20% of the overall population with CHD (Hayman & Martyn-Nemeth, 2022). Young adults with CHD and prior cardiac surgery often have special health care needs and require cardiology care throughout adulthood. Many pediatric hospitals and clinics have established a structured transitional process or program to optimize a successful transfer of care of the young adult with a CHD from the pediatric cardiology provider to an adult cardiologist. At the time of the transfer of care, a young adult with CHD is often referred to an adult CHD (ACHD) program. The ACHD program is staffed by a cardiologist, nurses, sonographers, and cardiovascular surgeons with specialized training in CHD, the impact of CHD on adult health, arrhythmia management, and cardiovascular disease.

According to the AHA (2021) transition statement, the goal of health care transition is to maximize lifelong functioning through developmentally appropriate health care services that empower patients as well as their caregivers in the process. Health care transition should be achieved through an organized clinical process with the goals of (1) improving adolescents' knowledge about their CHD, (2) supporting self-management and self-advocacy skills, (3) learning to navigate a complex medical system, and (4) coordinating integration into adult-centered care for both primary care and subspecialty care (Hayman & Martyn-Nemeth, 2022; John et al., 2022).

The transition process should begin in early adolescence and be completed by 18 years of age. Ideally, the CHD history and the normal teen anticipatory guidance information is presented to the adolescent, which is tailored to the age and the individual's developmental abilities. The adolescent will receive a progressive amount of detailed information on their CHD and their surgeries/cardiac interventions history during the cardiology clinic visits. The team of cardiac members will provide the adolescent with structured education about maintaining and protecting health, recognizing cardiac changes requiring intervention, and instructions on how to respond to symptoms of health deterioration. The complex physical and psychological needs of the young adult should be discussed. A successful transition process helps prepare a young adult for adulthood, promote self-management, and provide them with confidence in navigating the health care system. The adolescent's knowledge of CHD will be assessed throughout the transition process (Hays et al., 2020). For example, a 14-year-old's report of CHD may be, "I have a hole in my heart," whereas an 18-year-old may report, "I had a ventricular septal defect, which required cardiac surgery for a patch closure when I was 6 months old. I developed complete heart block after surgery and have a permanent pacemaker."

As young adults with CHD transition to adulthood it is important to know if they have attained the autonomy, abilities, and understanding needed for optimal self-care management. Neurodevelopmental and functional deficits are well documented in children with histories of cardiac surgeries and may have more difficulties with self-care (Farr et al., 2018). Individuals with more significant neurodevelopmental deficits, coexisting genetic syndromes, or limited cognitive abilities may require parental guardianship.

Facilitating the effective coordination of care from a pediatric to an adult health care provider is essential. If the young adult is transferred to an ACHD program, a protocol for sharing information may occur. A transition clinic appointment attended by the young adult with CHD and the ACHD team (i.e., cardiac provider, nurse coordinator, staff nurse, social worker) is sometimes included in the transfer process. During the transition clinic, topics of discussion may include cardiac education, medication management, barriers to health care, and surgical information. Communication with an additional adult specialist may be necessary. A formal cardiology clinic visit with the ACHD provider should be arranged to ensure a smooth transfer of care.

Family Concerns

Parents with an infant or child diagnosed with CHD will experience many emotions and stressful events. Often the parents are afraid of future and unknown events such as the seriousness of the cardiac condition, potential risks of cardiac surgery or cardiac intervention, the child's overall well-being, the effect the child's cardiac disease will have on the lives of their other sibling(s), and the economic impact from missed days of work, medical bills, or frequent doctor appointments.

The specific age of the child may result in different concerns from the parents. During infancy, parents may have questions about (1) the significance of the congenital diagnosis, extracardiac anomalies, or genetic findings, (2) the reason for the feeding difficulties or poor weight gain, (3) the appropriate weight gain for an infant with CHD, (4) the risk of sudden death, (5) the safety of immunizations, and (6) whether the family needs to restrict their life to keep the infant safe and avoid family gatherings, shopping, or community events. During the childhood years, parents may express concerns regarding the child's ability to notice cardiac symptoms and then express these to the parents, have play dates or sleepovers, participate in exercise, academically perform well in school, and travel for family vacations.

Parental concerns during the adolescent years will include additional worries related to CHD and the general teenage stressors. Anticipated concerns are (1) the need for additional cardiac surgery or cardiac intervention for residual cardiac lesions, (2) the adolescent's ability to complete the higher level classes in middle and high school, (3) the potential risk associated with strenuous activities (e.g., sports, dance, cheerleading, bicycling), amusement park rides, body piercing/tattoos, tobacco/e-cigarettes use, drinks with caffeine or stimulants, (4) the emotional well-being of an adolescent with increased stressors, anxiety, or depression, (5) the transition process and final readiness of the adolescent (and family) for the transfer of care from a pediatric to an adult provider, (6) the ability for the adolescent to obtain health insurance with an underlying CHD, and (7) future expectations for the young adult, such as long-term cardiac risks, life longevity, career and employment options, and the potential concerns of future offspring being diagnosed with CHD.

Parental concerns. Multiple studies have reported mothers and fathers of a child with CHD frequently develop posttraumatic stress syndrome, psychological distress, depression, and anxiety (Hoffman et al., 2020). The primary care provider is the ideal person to monitor the child and adolescent health as well as provide education, guidance, and support to the patient and the family.

ADDITIONAL SUPPORT

Parent support groups are valuable resources and provide an important network for families to receive helpful information and share mutual experiences. Newsletters, special interest groups, and social media sites often develop from parent networking. Many pediatric cardiology clinics and health care systems have cardiac support groups, which provide parental and patient educational symposiums, recommendations for school accommodations, and lists of available community resources. Public health and home health nursing agencies may be additional sources of support, especially for families learning to identify clinical symptoms, give multiple medications, provide nutritional support to a newly diagnosed infant with CHD, or care for a child with complex home health needs. Summer camps for children or adolescents with CHD are available in several locations across the country. Adolescents with CHD may seek out teen-based support groups with other teens with a chronic medical condition or cardiac-specific groups.

The internet has a wealth of information about heart defects, surgical procedures, and support for families or children with heart defects. Parents should be advised to use websites from the AHA (2021) and medical centers with pediatric cardiology subspecialty departments for medical information regarding their child's disease.

Informational Materials

The AHA website provides parents and adolescents access to cardiac information and specific topics pertinent to children with cardiac disease. The child's cardiology provider and clinic may also have resource booklets and pamphlets available for families.

Following are examples of information material available to family and health care providers from the AHA:

- Understanding the risk of congenital heart defects
- Symptoms and diagnosis of congenital heart defects
- Care and treatment of congenital heart defects
- Impact of congenital heart defects
- Infective endocarditis
- Your child's abnormal heart rhythm
- Feeding tips for your baby
- Special needs for children with a congenital heart defect
- Heart healthy recommendations
- Physical activity
- Heart murmurs
- Kawasaki disease

RESOURCES

Adult Congenital Heart Association: www.achaheart.org
American Academy of Pediatrics: www.aap.org
American Heart Association: www.heart.org
Children's Heart Foundation: www.childrensheartfoundation.org
Congenital Heart Public Health Consortium: www.aap.org/en/patient-care/congenital-heart-defects
Conquering CHD: www.conqueringchd.org
MedlinePlus (CHD information): www.medlineplus.gov
Mended Hearts: www.mendedhearts.org
National Heart, Lung, and Blood Institute: www.nhlbi.nih.gov
SADS Foundation (support for sudden arrhythmia death syndromes): www.sads.org

---

 Summary

Primary Care Needs for the Child With Congenital Heart Disease

HEALTH CARE MAINTENANCE
Growth and Development
- Delays in physical growth and neurodevelopmental growth may occur, especially with cyanotic and more severe forms of CHD.
- Significant delays in weight and less frequent height are common in children with symptomatic CHD preoperatively. Close monitoring of growth is necessary. Corrective surgery improves growth.
- Excessive weight gain or obesity in childhood or adolescence with CHD is a concern. Individuals require screening for the development of associated comorbidities such as hypertension, diabetes, obstructive sleep apnea, and nonalcoholic fatty liver disease.
- Infants and children with CHD should be able to meet their developmental milestones, albeit at slower rates of achievement.
- Intellectual development is significantly impaired by CHD; cyanosis, parental overprotection, and CHF may contribute to delayed development.
- Learning disabilities, attention deficits, hyperactivity, and executive functions may not be obvious until the secondary education years when school courses exceed the child's developmental abilities.
- Referral to a cardiac neurodevelopmental program is recommended for developmental screening.
- Behavioral regression during or after hospitalization is common.
- It is important to assess the well-being of a child and adolescent.

Diet
- Feeding is a major problem for children with CHD, especially for a child with CHF; required daily allowances are normal, but caloric needs may be higher.
- Breastfeeding is encouraged if growth is adequate.
- May need to concentrate formula or breastmilk if growth is inadequate. Gavage feeding may be necessary to conserve energy.
- Parents should be taught methods to decrease the work of feeding.
- Feeding is a major source of stress for parents, who will need much support.

- Children with a postcardiac surgery pleural effusion may require a special diet and fluid restriction, especially those with CHD with a single ventricle.

Safety
- Safe storage of medications is critical.
- Children on anticoagulants or with permanent pacemakers or implantable automatic defibrillators should avoid contact sports.
- For a child with a pacemaker, electrical safety is critical. There is no risk of damage with usual household appliances, including microwaves. Cellular phones with stronger magnetic fields can affect the function of the pacemaker if too close to the device. Surgery and procedures with electrocautery can inhibit pacemaker function. New-generation pacemakers may be safe during MRI but require careful monitoring and precautions.
- Air travel is often safe. Children with CHD lesions with intracardiac shunts, PH, or significant hypoxemia require special travel precautions and oxygen therapy during the flight.
- Children diagnosed with long QT syndrome may be advised to avoid swimming/vigorous exercise, stressful situations, or situations of being startled.
- Body art, including piercing and tattoos, may be discouraged to decrease the risk of infective endocarditis. If an adolescent or adult makes the personal decision to have body art completed, it is highly recommended the work is completed in a licensed parlor and SBE prophylaxis prescribed.

Immunizations
- Standard immunization protocol, including meningococcal, pneumococcal, and influenza vaccines, is recommended; delay should occur only around cardiac catheterization or surgery.
- Prophylaxis against the RSV is recommended in CHD infants/children with unrepaired cyanotic CHD, CHF, or significant hemodynamic abnormalities. Synagis is administered monthly during the early fall to the late spring season.
- Following blood product (e.g., whole blood, packed red blood cells, and plasma) administration, varicella and mumps vaccine should be delayed for 6 to 7 months.
- With asplenia syndrome, the child receives the full complement of the pneumococcal vaccine.

Continued

- Immune-compromised children should not receive live attenuated vaccines.

Screening

- Vision. Routine screening is recommended.
- Hearing. Routine screening is recommended
- Dental. Dental care is important to prevent caries, which predisposes a child to bacteriemia and endocarditis. Biannual dental examinations are recommended.
- Endocarditis prophylaxis is recommended for oral dental procedures (deep cleaning, drilling at the gum level, teeth extraction, dental implants, bone and gum grafting), although not required for routine adjustment of braces and shedding of deciduous teeth.
- Blood pressure. Check blood pressure in all upper and lower extremities for children with aortic abnormalities pre-operatively and postoperatively. Children with a BTT shunt or subclavian flap repair of CoA will have low or absent blood pressure values in the arm on the side of surgery.
- Hematocrit. A rise in hematocrit may indicate worsening cyanosis. Anemia is problematic in children with CHF or cyanosis. Monitor hemoglobin levels closely in coordination with the cardiologist.
- Urinalysis. Routine screening is recommended.
- TB. Routine screening is recommended.

CONDITION-SPECIFIC SCREENING

- Bloodwork may be required to assess digoxin level, INR to ensure therapeutic warfarin level, or electrolytes when diuretics are prescribed.
- Lipid panel is recommended per lipid screen guidelines.
- Psychosocial. Routine screening for anxiety, depression, suicidal thoughts is recommended.
- Neurodevelopmental assessment is recommended for children requiring cardiac surgery, ECMO support, or with other special health needs.

COMMON ILLNESS MANAGEMENT
Differential Diagnosis

- Fever. Postoperatively rule out (1) wound infection and (2) postpericardiotomy syndrome. If no focus is found, obtain a CBC, CRP, ESR, and blood culture and consult with the cardiologist. The child with asplenia with fever must be seen immediately. Fever may worsen CHF.
- Infective endocarditis. Increased risk of infective endocarditis with poor dental hygiene and periodontal diseases or following surgeries involving implantable devices. Symptoms may be acute or subacute; a high level of suspicion is needed for diagnosis. The child should be referred to the cardiologist for evaluation if infective endocarditis is suspected. Refer to the cardiologist if fever, malaise, anorexia, or unexplained skin findings.
- Respiratory compromise. Consider differential diagnoses to include decreased cardiac function, cardiac shunt stenosis, arrhythmia, aspiration pneumonia, or viral illness. Frequent or significant upper and lower respiratory infections may occur. An RSV infection can cause significant morbidity and/or require cardiac procedures or surgery postponed for 4 to 6 weeks.
- Gastrointestinal symptoms. Consider differential diagnoses from cardiac etiology (CHF, decreased intestinal perfusion, electrolyte disturbance secondary to diuretic therapy, increased concentrated feedings leading to higher osmolarity, or digoxin toxicity) and common childhood conditions such as gastroenteritis, food allergies, gastric reflux. Excessive fluid losses are dangerous in children who are cyanotic, taking diuretics and digoxin, or those with central shunts.

- Neurologic symptoms. Cyanotic children are at increased risk for brain abscess (if >2 years) or cerebrovascular accident (if <2 years); unexplained fever, headaches, seizures, or focal neurologic signs require immediate referral to a medical center. Children with CHD are at increased risk of neurologic abnormalities (e.g., seizures, muscle tone abnormalities, and motor asymmetry).
- Chest pain. Most chest pain is caused by noncardiac problems. A careful history and physical examination usually differentiate benign from dangerous conditions.
- Syncope. The differential diagnoses to be considered when completing syncopal evaluation include cardiology (arrhythmia, CHD, cardiomyopathy, coronary artery abnormalities, PH), neurology (seizures, dysautonomia, functional neurologic disorder), and other health conditions (orthostatic intolerance, emotional stress, breath holding, hypovolemia, dehydration, anemia). A thorough medical history and physical examination are important and often can identify the cause of the syncopal event. Obtain orthostatic vital signs. An ECG may be useful to rule out cardiac causes.

Drug Interactions

- The addition of any drug to a child's regimen should be preceded by consultation with a pharmacist or cardiologist.
- Important to review information from evidence-based resources to determine adverse reactions, drug interactions, and drug compatibility.
- Accurate administration of digoxin is critical. Many medications can alter plasma levels of digoxin.
- Digoxin or anticoagulant levels may need to be monitored.
- Children on warfarin (Coumadin) may have prothrombin time and INR altered when placed on antibiotics.
- Interactions between antiarrhythmic drugs and psychotropic drugs may occur.

ACQUIRED HEART DISEASE

- Inquire about illnesses and their potential impact on the cardiac health.
- Acquired cardiac heart disease may occur with Kawasaki disease, rheumatic fever, viral or bacterial infections, and PH.
- When a surge of community illnesses or a pandemic occurs, a child may present with new cardiac symptoms, fevers, and other associated general complaints. Consider cardiac conditions such as myocarditis, arrhythmia, pericardial effusion, or coronary artery disease.
- Early detection of acquired heart disease and management of the cardiac condition is important. Referral to cardiology is appropriate.

DEVELOPMENTAL ISSUES
Sleep

- A child's sleep quality and pattern should be assessed during clinic visits. Quality sleep positively impacts alertness, cognitive performance, mood, learning, and memory.
- Children may have altered sleeping secondary to CHF, tachypnea, obstructive sleep pattern, or hunger.
- Sudden cardiac arrest or respiratory deterioration can occur during sleep.

Toileting

- Toilet training children receiving diuretics may be difficult.
- Toilet training, as well as other developmental milestones, often show regression following hospitalization.

Discipline

- Normal behavior should be expected from children regardless of CHD. Parents often overprotect and pamper children with CHD.
- Primary care providers play a role in reinforcing the importance of setting limits and disciplining children

with consistency, as well as encouraging normal family dynamics.

Child Care
- There are usually no contraindications to an infant or child with CHD attending a child care setting.
- Infants with 22q11.2 deletion or asplenia syndrome are prone to infection, so home day care or small group day care is recommended.
- The child care provider must understand medications, be able to recognize symptoms, and know emergency procedures.
- Support the family's decision to either stay at home to care for the child or return to work.

Schooling
- Children with CHD may attend school with their peers or be home schooled.
- Special education services or accommodations may be required for some children.
- During adolescence, a greater disparity in academic performance and decreased ability to focus may emerge.
- Exercise and physical education classes are often permitted.
- The cardiology provider will tailor exercise recommendations to each child depending on the clinical status, type

of CHD, and arrhythmia risk to ensure safe participation in regular physical activity.

Sexuality
- Communication between these providers is important to share critical information about a young woman's risk factors for contraception and pregnancy, given her cardiac condition.
- Contraceptive counseling is required.
- Pregnant women with CHD may have a greater risk for adverse events during pregnancy and delivery, especially with coexisting morbidities.
- Males with CHD may present to the primary care clinic with sexual health questions and concerns, including a decreased sexual drive and erectile dysfunction.

Transition to Adulthood
- A structured transitional process to optimize a successful transfer of care of the young adult with a CHD from the pediatric cardiologist provider to an adult cardiologist is important for continuity of care. The transition process should begin in early adolescence and be completed by 18 years of age.
- Facilitating the effective coordination of care from a pediatric to an adult health care provider is essential
- During the transition clinic, topics of discussion may include cardiac education, medication management, barriers to health care, and surgical information.

REFERENCES

Aljohani, O. A., Herrick, N. L., Borquez, A. A., Shepard, S., Wieler, M. E., Perry, J. C., & Williams, M. R. (2021). Antiarrhythmic treatment duration and tachycardia recurrence in infants with supraventricular tachycardia. *Pediatric Cardiology, 42*(3), 716–720. https://doi.org/10.1007/s00246-020-02534-5.

American Heart Association. Young Hearts Rheumatic Fever, Endocarditis and Kawasaki Disease Committee of the Council on Lifelong Congenital Heart Disease and Heart Health in the Young; Council on Cardiovascular and Stroke Nursing; the Council on Quality of Care and Outcomes Research, Wilson, W. R., Gewitz, M., Lockhart, P. B., et al. Prevention of viridans group streptococcal infective endocarditis: A scientific statement from the American Heart Association. *Circulation,* 143(20), e963–e978. https://doi.org/10.1161/CIR.0000000000000969.

Amin, E. K., Campbell-Washburn, A., & Ratnayaka, K. (2022). MRI-guided cardiac catheterization in congenital heart disease: How to get started. *Current Cardiology Report, 24*(4), 419–429. https://doi.org/10.1007/s11886-022-01659-8.

Andonian, C., Langer, F., Beckmann, J., Bischoff, G., Ewert, P., Freilinger, S., et al. (2019). Overweight and obesity: An emerging problem in patients with congenital heart disease. *Cardiovascular Diagnosis & Therapy, 9*(Suppl 2), S360–S368. doi: 10.21037/cdt.2019.02.02.

Apostolopoulou, S., Brili, S., Sbarouni, E., Tousoulis, D., & Toutouzas, K. (2020). Acquired coronary artery disease in patients with congenital heart disease: Issues in diagnosis and management. *Congenital Heart Disease, 15*(5), 369–375. https://doi.org/10.32604/CHD.2020.012092.

Armstrong, M. L., DeBoer, S., & Cetta, F. (2008). Infective endocarditis after body art: A review of the literature and concerns. *Journal of Adolescent Health, 43*(3), 217–225. https://doi.org/10.1016/j.jadohealth.2008.02.008.

Arslani, K., Roffler, N., Zurek, M., Greutmann, M., Schwerzmann, M., Bouchardy, J., Rutz, T., Ehl, N. F., Jost, C. A., Tobler, D., & SACHER Investigators (2018). Patterns of incidence rates of cardiac complications in patients with congenital heart disease. *Canadian Journal of Cardiology, 34*(12), 1624–1630. https://doi.org/10.1016/j.cjca.2018.09.010.

Bagge, C. N., Smit, J., Madsen, N. L., & Olsen, M. (2020). Congenital heart disease and risk of central nervous system infections: A nationwide cohort study. *Pediatric Cardiology, 41*(5), 869–876. https://doi.org/10.1007/s00246-020-02324-z.

Barbut, G., & Needleman, J. P. (2020). Pediatric chest pain. *Pediatrics in Review, 41*(9), 469–480. https://doi.org/10.1542/pir.2019-0058.

Başaran, N., Paslı, D., & Başaran, A. A. (2022). Unpredictable adverse effects of herbal products. *Food and Chemical Toxicology: An International Journal Published for the British Industrial Biological Research Association, 159,* 112762.

Bielli, A., Bernardini, R., Varvaras, D., Rossi, P., Di Blasi, G., Petrella, G., Buonomo, O. C., Mattei, M., & Orlandi, A. (2018). Characterization of a new decellularized bovine pericardial biological mesh: Structural and mechanical properties. *Journal of the Mechanical Behavior of Biomedical Materials, 78,* 420–426. https://doi.org/10.1016/j.jmbbm.2017.12.003.

Bigras, J. (2020). Cardiovascular risk factors in patients with congenital heart disease. *Canadian Journal of Cardiology, 36*(9), 1458–1466. https://doi.org/10.1016/j.cjca.2020.06.013.

Billotte, M., Deken, V., Joriot, S., Vaksmann, G., Richard, A., Bouzguenda, I., Godart, F., Baudelet, J. B., Rakza, T., Nguyen The Tich, S., & Guillaume, M. P. (2021). Screening for neurodevelopmental disorders in children with congenital heart disease. *European Journal of Pediatrics, 180*(4), 1157–1167. https://doi.org/10.1007/s00431-020-03850-x.

Blue, G. M., Kirk, E. P., Giannoulatou, E., Sholler, G. F., Dunwoodie, R. P., & Winlaw, D. S. (2017). Advances in the genetics of congenital heart disease: A clinician's guide. *Journal of the American College of Cardiology, 69*(7), 859–870. https://doi.org/10.1016/j.jacc.2016.11.060.

Borjali, M., Amini-Rarani, M., Nosratabadi, M., & Chen, R. (2021). Nonmedical determinants of congenital heart diseases in children from the perspective of mothers: A qualitative study in Iran. *Cardiology Research and Practice, 2021,* 1–10. https://doi.org/10.1155/2021/6647260.

Bradley, E.A., Saraf, A., & Book, W. (2019). Heart failure in women with congenital heart disease. *Heart Failure Clinics, 15*(1), 87–96. https://doi.org/10.1016/j.hfc.2018.08.009.

Brief, F., Guimber, D., Baudelet, J., et al. (2022). Prevalence and associated factors of long term growth failure in infants with congenital heart disease who underwent cardiac surgery before the age of one. *Pediatrics Cardiology,* 1–7. https://doi.org/10.1007/s00246-022-02933-w.

Buijtendijk, M. F. J., Barnett, P., & van den Hoff, M. J. B. (2020). Development of the human heart. *American Journal of Medical Genetics. Part C: Seminars in Medical Genetics, 184*(1), 7–22. https://doi.org/10.1002/ajmg.c.31778.

Calcagni, G., Pugnaloni, F., Digilio, M. C., Unolt, M., Putotto, C., Niceta, M., Baban, A., Piceci Sparascio, F., Drago, F., De Luca, A., Tartaglia, M., Marino, B., & Versacci, P. (2021). Cardiac defects and genetic syndromes: Old uncertainties and new insights. *Genes, 12*(7), 1047. https://doi.org/10.3390/genes12071047.

Candelino, M., Tagi, V. M., & Chiarelli, F. (2022). Cardiovascular risk in children: A burden for future generations. *Italian Journal of Pediatrics, 48*(1), 1–9. https://doi.org/10.1186/s13052-022-01250-5.

Centers for Disease Control and Prevention (2022). *Data and statistics on congenital heart defects.* U.S. Department of Health and Human Services. https://www.cdc.gov/ncbddd/heartdefects/data.html.

Chen, K., & Jiang, P. (2021). Brain abscess associated with ventricular septal defect and Eisenmenger syndrome: A case report. *International Journal of Surgery Case Reports, 81*, 105799. https://doi.org/10.1016/j.ijscr.2021.105799.

Chinawa, A. T., Chinawa, J. M., Duru, C. O., Chukwu, BF, & Obumneme-Anyim, I. (2021). Assessment of nutritional status of children with congenital heart disease: A comparative study. *Frontiers in Nutrition, 8*, 644030. https://doi.org/10.3389/fnut.2021.644030.

Davis, J. A., Spatz, D. L., Spatz, D. L., & Spatz, D. L. (2019). Human milk and infants with congenital heart disease: A summary of current literature supporting the provision of human milk and breastfeeding. *Advances in Neonatal Care, 19*(3), 212–218. https://doi.org/10.1097/ANC.0000000000000582.

Diz, O. M., Toro, R., Cesar, S., Gomez, O., Sarquella-Brugada, G., & Campuzano, O (2021). Personalized genetic diagnosis of congenital heart defects in newborns. *Journal of Personalized Medicine, 11*(6), 562. https://doi.org/10.3390/jpm11060562.

Diao, J., Chen, L., Wei, J., Shu, J., Li, Y., Li, J., Zhang, S., Wang, T., & Qin, J. (2022). Prevalence of malnutrition in children with congenital heart disease: A systematic review and meta-analysis. *Journal of Pediatrics, 242*, 39–47.e4. https://doi.org/10.1016/j.jpeds.2021.10.065.

Dolk, H., McCullough, N., Callaghan, S., Casey, F., Craig, B., Given, J., Loane, M., Lagan, B. M., Bunting, B., Boyle, B., & Dabir, T. (2020). Risk factors for congenital heart disease: The Baby Hearts Study, a population-based case-control study. *PLoS One, 15*(2), e0227908. doi: 10.1371/journal.pone.0227908. PMID: 32092068; PMCID: PMC7039413.

Donofrio, M. T., Moon-Grady, A. J., Hornberger, L. K., Copel, J. A., Sklansky, M. S., Abuhamad, A., Cuneo, B. F., Huhta, J. C., Jonas, R. A., Krishnan, A., Lacey, S., Lee, W., Michelfelder, E. C., Sr, Rempel, G. R., Silverman, N. H., Spray, T. L., Strasburger, J. F., Tworetzky, W., Rychik, J., & American Heart Association Adults With Congenital Heart Disease Joint Committee of the Council on Cardiovascular Disease in the Young and Council on Clinical Cardiology, Council on Cardiovascular Surgery and Anesthesia, and Council on Cardiovascular and Stroke Nursing (2014). Diagnosis and treatment of fetal cardiac disease: A scientific statement from the American Heart Association. *Circulation, 129*(21), 2183–2242. https://doi.org/10.1161/01.cir.0000437597.44550.5d.

Drake, M., Ginde, S., Cohen, S., Bartz, P., Sowinski, J., Reinhardt, E., Saleska, T., & Earing, M. G. (2020). Prevalence, risk factors, and impact of obstructive sleep apnea in adults with congenital heart disease. *Pediatric Cardiology, 41*(4), 724–728. https://doi.org/10.1007/s00246-020-02289-z.

Farr, S. L., Downing, K. F., Riehle-Colarusso, T., Abarbanell, G., Downing, K. F., & Abarbanell, G. (2018). Functional limitations and educational needs among children and adolescents with heart disease. *Congenital Heart Disease, 13*(4), 633–639. https://doi.org/10.1111/chd.12621.

Fischer, A. J., Grundlach, C., Helm, P. C., Bauer, U. M., Baumgartner, H., Diller, G. P., & German Competence Network for Congenital Heart Defects Investigators (2022). Erectile dysfunction in men with adult congenital heart disease: A prevalent but neglected issue. *Korean Circulation Journal, 52*(3), 233–242. https://doi.org/10.4070/kcj.2021.0184.

Frank, B., & Ivy, D. (2018). Diagnosis, evaluation and treatment of pulmonary arterial hypertension in children. *Child, 5*(4), 44. https://doi.org/10.3390/children5040044.

Gaudet, I., Paquette, N., Bernard, C., Doussau, A., Harvey, J., Beaulieu-Genest, L., Pinchefsky, E., Trudeau, N., Poirier, N., Simard, M. N., Gallagher, A., & Clinique d'Investigation Neuro-Cardiaque (CINC) interdisciplinary team (2021). Neurodevelopmental outcome of children with congenital heart disease: A cohort study from infancy to preschool age. *Journal of Pediatrics, 239*, 126–135.e5. https://doi.org/10.1016/j.jpeds.2021.08.042.

Geddes, G. C., & Earing, M. G. (2018). Genetic evaluation of patients with congenital heart disease. *Current Opinions in Pediatrics, 30*(6), 707–713. https://doi.org/10.1097/MOP.0000000000000682.

Gilljam, T., Mandalenakis, Z., Dellborg, M., Lappas, G., Eriksson, P., Skoglund, K., & Rosengren, A. (2019). Development of heart failure in young patients with congenital heart disease: A nation-wide cohort study. *Open Heart, 6*(1), e000858. https://doi.org/10.1136/openhrt-2018-000858.

Giorgione, V., Parazzini, F., Fesslova, V., Cipriani, S., Candiani, M., Inversetti, A., Sigismondi, C., Tiberio, F., & Cavoretto, P. (2018). Congenital heart defects in IVF/ICSI pregnancy: Systematic review and meta-analysis. *Ultrasound in Obstetrics and Gynecology, 51*(1), 33–42. https://doi.org/10.1002/uog.18932.

Glidewell, J., Grosse, S. D., Riehle-Colarusso, T., Pinto, N., Hudson, J., Daskalov, R., Gaviglio, A., Darby, E., Singh, S., & Sontag, M. (2019). Actions in support of newborn screening for critical congenital heart disease – United States, 2011–2018. *MMWR, 68*(5), 107–111. https://doi.org/10.15585/mmwr.mm6805a3.

Givertz, M. M., DeFilippis, E. M., Landzberg, M. J., Pinney, S. P., Woods, R. K., & Valente, A. M. (2019). Advanced heart failure therapies for adults with congenital heart disease: JACC state-of-the-art review. *Journal of the American College of Cardiology, 74*(18), 2295–2312. https://doi.org/10.1016/j.jacc.2019.09.004.

Haberer, K., & Silversides, C. K. (2019). Congenital heart disease and women's health across the life span: Focus on reproductive issues. *Canadian Journal of Cardiology, 35*(12), 1652–1663. https://doi.org/10.1016/j.cjca.2019.10.009.

Hansmann, G. (2017). Pulmonary hypertension in infants, children, and young adults. *Journal of the American College of Cardiology, 69*(20), 2551–2569. https://doi.org/10.1016/j.jacc.2017.03.575.

Hayman, L. L., & Martyn-Nemeth, P. (2022). Transitioning adolescents and young adults with congenital heart disease to adult-centered care: Challenges and opportunities. *Journal of Cardiovascular Nursing, 37*(4), 310–311. https://doi.org/10.1097/JCN.0000000000000924.

Hays, L., McSweeney, J., Mitchell, A., Bricker, C., Green, A., & Landes, R. (2020). Self-management needs of adults with congenital heart disease. *Journal of Cardiovascular Nursing, 35*(6), E33–E43. https://doi.org/10.1097/JCN.0000000000000701.

Hermans, T., Thewissen, L., Gewillig, M., Cools, B., Jansen, K., Pillay, K., De Vos, M., Van Huffel, S., Naulaers, G., & Dereymaeker, A. (2022). Functional brain maturation and sleep organisation in neonates with congenital heart disease. *European Journal of Paediatric Neurology, 36*, 115–122. https://doi.org/10.1016/j.ejpn.2021.12.008.

Hernández-Madrid, A., Paul, T., Abrams, D., Aziz, P. F., Blom, N. A., Chen, J., Chessa, M., Combes, N., Dagres, N., Diller, G., Ernst, S., Giamberti, A., Hebe, J., Janousek, J., Kriebel, T., Moltedo, J., Moreno, J., Peinado, R., Pison, L., … ESC Scientific Document Group (2018). Arrhythmias in congenital heart disease: A position paper of the European Heart Rhythm Association (EHRA), Association for European Paediatric and Congenital Cardiology (AEPC), and the European Society of Cardiology (ESC) Working Group on Grown-up Congenital heart disease, endorsed by HRS, PACES, APHRS, and SOLAECE. *EP Europace, 20*(11), 1719–1753. https://doi.org/10.1093/europace/eux380.

Hoffman, M. F., Karpyn, A., & Christofferson, J. (2020). Fathers of children with congenital heart disease—sources of stress and opportunities for intervention. *Pediatric Critical Care Medicine: A Journal of the Society of Critical Care Medicine and the World Federation of Pediatric Intensive and Critical Care Societies, 21*(11), e1002–e1009.

Hoge, M. K., Heyne, E., Nicholson, T. F., Acosta, D., Mir, I., Brown, L. S., Shaw, R. J., Chalak, L., & Heyne, R. (2021). Vulnerable child syndrome in the neonatal intensive care unit: A review and a new preventative intervention with feasibility and parental satisfaction data. *Early Human Development, 154*, 105283. doi: 10.1016/j.earlhumdev.2020.105283.

Howell, H. B., Zaccario, M., Kazmi, S. H., Desai, P., Sklamberg, F. E., & Mally, P. (2019). Neurodevelopmental outcomes of children with congenital heart disease: A review. *Current Problems in Pediatric and Adolescent Health Care, 49*(10), 100685. https://doi.org/10.1016/j.cppeds.2019.100685.

John, A. S., Jackson, J. L., Moons, P., Uzark, K., Mackie, A. S., Timmins, S., Lopez, K. N., Kovacs, A. H., Gurvitz, M., & American Heart Association Adults With congenital Heart Disease Committee of the Council on Lifelong congenital Heart Disease and Heart Health in the Young and the Council on Clinical Cardiology; Council on Cardiovascular and Stroke Nursing; Council on Arteriosclerosis, Thrombosis and Vascular Biology; and Stroke Council (2022). Advances in managing transition to adulthood for adolescents with congenital heart disease: A practical approach to transition program design: A scientific statement from the American Heart Association. *Journal of the American Heart Association, 11*(7), e025278. https://doi.org/10.1161/JAHA.122.025278.

Jonas, R. A. (2020). Challenges for adult survivors of simple congenital heart disease. *Journal of the American Heart Association, 9*(11), e017210. https://doi.org/10.1161/JAHA.120.017210.

Kang, S.L., & Benson, L. (2018). Recent advances in cardiac catheterization for congenital heart disease. *F1000Research, 7*, 370. https://doi.org/10.12688/f1000research.13021.1.

Katz, A. J., Lyon, S., Farrell, A. G., Srivastava, N., Wilkinson, T. A., & Shew, M. L. (2022). Adolescent women with congenital heart disease: Self-reported reproductive health discussions with health care providers. *Journal of Pediatric and Adolescent Gynecology, 35*(3), 299–304. https://doi.org/10.1016/j.jpag.2021.12.013.

Khairy, P., & Balaji, S. (2009). Cardiac arrhythmias in congenital heart disease. *Indian Pacing and Electrophysiology Journal, 9*(6), 299–317.

Kowalczyk, K., Bartnik-Głaska, M., Smyk, M., Plaskota, I., Bernaciak, J., Kędzior, M., Wiśniowiecka-Kowalnik, B., Jakubów-Durska, K., Braun-Walicka, N., Barczyk, A., Geremek, M., Castañeda, J., Kutkowska-Kaźmierczak, A., Własienko, P., Dębska, M., Kucińska-Chahwan, A., Roszkowski, T., Kozłowski, S., Mikulska, B., Issat, T., … Nowakowska, B. A. (2021). Prenatal diagnosis by array comparative genomic hybridization in fetuses with cardiac abnormalities. *Genes, 12*(12), 2021. https://doi.org/10.3390/genes12122021.

Krahn, A. D., Laksman, Z., Sy, R. W., Postema, P. G., Ackerman, M. J., Wilde, A. A. M., & Han, H. C. (2022). Congenital long QT syndrome. *JACC, 8*(5), 687–706. https://doi.org/10.1016/j.jacep.2022.02.017.

Kundan, M. (2020). Pediatric heart failure. *Journal of Pediatric Critical Care, 7*(3), 147–151. doi:10.4103/JPCC.JPCC_78_20.

Lang, S. S., Valeri, A., Storm, P. B., Heuer, G. G., Tucker, A. M., Kennedy, B. C., Kozyak, B. W., Sinha, A., Kilbaugh, T. J., & Huh, J. W. (2021). Acute neurological injury in pediatric patients with single-ventricle congenital heart disease. *Journal of Neurosurgery: Pediatrics, 28*(3), 335–343. https://doi.org/10.3171/2021.2.PEDS2142.

Lantin-Hermoso, M. R., Berger, S., Bhatt, A. B., Richerson, J. E., Morrow, R., Freed, M. D., & Beekman, R. H., 3rd, Section on Cardiology, & Cardiac Surgery (2017). The care of children with congenital heart disease in their primary medical home. *Pediatrics, 140*(5), e20172607. https://doi.org/10.1542/peds.2017-2607.

Law, C., & Raffini, L. (2015). A guide to the use of anticoagulant drugs in children. *Pediatric Drugs, 17*(2), 105–114. https://doi.org/10.1007/s40272-015-0120-x.

Lee, G. M. (2020). Preventing infections in children and adults with asplenia. *Hematology. American Society of Hematology. Education Program, 2020*(1), 328–335. https://doi.org/10.1182/hematology.2020000117.

Lo Rito, M., Al-Radi, O. O., Saedi, A., Kotani, Y., Ben Sivarajan, V., Russell, J. L., Caldarone, C. A., Van Arsdell, G. S., & Honjo, O. (2018). Chylothorax and pleural effusion in contemporary extracardiac fenestrated fontan completion. *Journal of Thoracic and Cardiovascular Surgery, 155*(5), 2069–2077. https://doi.org/10.1016/j.jtcvs.2017.11.046.

Luca, A. C., Miron, I. C., Mîndru, D. E., Curpăn, A. Ş., Stan, R. C., Ţarcă, E., Luca, F. A., & Pădureţ, A. I. (2022). Optimal nutrition parameters for neonates and infants with congenital heart disease. *Nutrients, 14*(8), 1671. https://doi.org/10.3390/nu14081671.

Ma, Y., Ding, P., Li, L., Liu, Y., Jin, P., Tang, J., & Yang, J. (2021). Three-dimensional printing for heart diseases: Clinical application review. *Bio-design and Manufacturing, 4*(3), 675–687. https://doi.org/10.1007/s42242-021-00125-8.

Mameli, C., Genoni, T., Madia, C., Doneda, C., Penagini, F., & Zuccotti, G. (2019). Brain abscess in pediatric age: A review. *Child's Nervous System: ChNS: Official Journal of the International Society for Pediatric Neurosurgery, 35*(7), 1117–1128. https://doi.org/10.1007/s00381-019-04182-4.

Masarone, D., Valente, F., Rubino, M., Vastarella, R., Gravino, R., Rea, A., Russo, M. G., Pacileo, G., & Limongelli, G. (2017). Pediatric heart failure: A practical guide to diagnosis and management. *Pediatrics and Neonatology, 58*(4), 303–312. https://doi.org/10.1016/j.pedneo.2017.01.001.

Mishra, V., Zaidi, S., Axiaq, A., & Harky, A. (2020). Sudden cardiac death in children with congenital heart disease: A critical review of the literature. *Cardiology in the Young, 30*(11), 1559–1565. https://doi.org/10.1017/S1047951120003613.

Mohammadi, H., Mohammadpour Ahranjani, B., Aghaei Moghadam, E., Kompani, F., Mirbeyk, M., & Rezaei, N. (2022). Hematological indices in pediatric patients with acyanotic congenital heart disease: A cross-sectional study of 248 patients. *Egyptian Journal of Medical Human Genetics, 23*(1), 1–8. https://doi.org/10.1186/s43042-02200262-4.

Moore, J. P., Gallotti, R., Lecky, M. A., & Perens, G. (2020). Three-dimensional printing for electrophysiology procedures in congenital heart disease. *Journal of the American College of Cardiology, 75*(11), 577. https://doi.org/10.1016/S0735-1097(20)31204-3.

Müller, N., Breuer, J., Adler, K., & Freudenthal, N. J. (2021). "Body modification: Piercing and tattooing in congenital heart disease patients", decoration or disaster?—a narrative review. *Cardiovascular Diagnosis and Therapy, 11*(6), 1395–1402. https://doi.org/10.21037/cdt-21-458.

Muthurangu, V. (2021). Cardiovascular magnetic resonance in congenital heart disease: Focus on heart failure. *Heart Failure Clinics, 17*(1), 157–165. https://doi.org/10.1016/j.hfc.2020.08.012.

Nematollahi, M., Bagherian, B., Sharifi, Z., Keshavarz, F., & Mehdipour-Rabori, R. (2020). Self-care status in children with congenital heart disease: A mixed-method study. *Journal of Child and Adolescent Psychiatrics Nursing, 33*(2), 77–84. https://doi.org/10.1111/jcap.12265.

Pincott, E. S., & Burch, M. (2012). Potential for stem cell use in congenital heart disease. *Future Cardiology, 8*(2), 161–169. https://doi.org/10.2217/fca.12.13.

Puri, K., Allen, H. D., & Qureshi, A. M. (2017). Congenital heart disease. *Pediatrics in Review, 38*(10), 471–486. https://doi.org/10.1542/pir.2017-0032.

Ramlakhan, K. P., Johnson, M. R., & Roos-Hesselink, J. W. (2020). Pregnancy and cardiovascular disease. *Nature Reviews Cardiology, 17*(11), 718–731. https://doi.org/10.1038/s41569-020-0390-z.

Reardon, L., & Lin, J. (2021). Advanced heart failure and transplant in congenital heart disease. *Heart (British Cardiac Society), 107*(3), 245–253. https://doi.org/10.1136/heartjnl-2019316366.

Reddy, C. D., Van den Eynde, J., & Kutty, S. (2022). Artificial intelligence in perinatal diagnosis and management of congenital heart disease. *Seminars in Perinatology, 46*(4), 151588. https://doi.org/10.1016/j.semperi.2022.151588.

Rohit, M., & Budakoty, S. (2020). Approach to a child with congestive heart failure. *Indian Journal of Pediatrics, 87*(4), 312–320. https://doi.org/10.1007/s12098-020-03255.

Rohit, M., & Rajan, P. (2020). Approach to cyanotic congenital heart disease in children. *Indian Journal of Pediatrics, 87*(5), 372–380. https://doi.org/10.1007/s12098020-03274-3.

Ryan, K. R., Jones, M. B., Allen, K. Y., Marino, B. S., Casey, F., Wernovsky, G., & Lisanti, A. J. (2019). Neurodevelopmental outcomes among children with congenital heart disease: At-risk populations and modifiable risk factors. *World Journal for Pediatric & Congenital Heart Surgery, 10*(6), 750–758. https://doi.org/10.1177/2150135119878702.

Saliba, A., Figueiredo, A. C. V., Baroneza, J. E., Afiune, J. Y., Pic-Taylor, A., Oliveira, S. F., & Mazzeu, J. F. (2020). Genetic and genomics in congenital heart disease: A clinical review. *Jornal de Pediatria, 96*(3), 279–288. https://doi.org/10.1016/j.jped.2019.07.004.

Salvatori, G., De Rose, D. U., Massolo, A. C., Patel, N., Capolupo, I., Giliberti, P., Evangelisti, M., Parisi, P., Toscano, A., Dotta, A., & Di Nardo, G. (2022). Current strategies to optimize nutrition and growth in newborns and infants with congenital heart disease: A narrative review. *Journal of Clinical Medicine, 11*(7), 1841. https://doi.org/10.3390/jcm11071841.

Schlichting, L. E., Insaf, T. Z., Zaidi, A. N., Lui, G. K., & Van Zutphen, A. R. (2019). Maternal comorbidities and complications of delivery in pregnant women with congenital heart disease. *Journal of the American College of Cardiology, 73*(17), 2181–2191. https://doi.org/10.1016/j.jacc.2019.01.069.

Schmitz, K. (2019). Vulnerable child syndrome. *Pediatrics in Review, 40*(6), 313–315. https://doi.org/10.1542/pir.2017-0243.

Schulz-Weidner, N., Weigel, M., Turujlija, F., Komma, K., Mengel, J. P., Schlenz, M. A., Bulski, J. C., Krämer, N., & Hain, T. (2021). Microbiome analysis of carious lesions in pre-school children with early childhood caries and congenital heart disease. *Microorganisms, 9*(9), 1904. https://doi.org/10.3390/microorganisms9091904.

Scott, M., & Neal, A. E. (2021). Congenital heart disease. *Primary Care, 48*(3), 351–366. https://doi.org/10.1016/j.pop.2021.04.005.

Selamet Tierney, E. (2020). The benefit of exercise in children with congenital heart disease. *Current Opinions in Pediatrics, 32*(5), 626–632. https://doi.org/10.1097/MOP.0000000000000942.

Sommer, R. J., Hijazi, Z. M., Rhodes, J. F., Jr, & Sommer, R. J. (2008). Pathophysiology of congenital heart disease in the adult: Part I: Shunt lesions. *Circulation, 117*(8), 1090–1099. https://doi.org/10.1161/CIRCULATIONAHA.107.714402.

Spaziani, G., Bennati, E., & Marrone, C. (2021). Pathophysiology and clinical presentation of paediatric heart failure related to congenital heart disease. *Acta Paediatrica (Oslo, Norway: 1992), 110*(8), 2336–2343. https://doi.org/10.1111/apa.15904.

Stephens, E. H., Dearani, J. A., Qureshi, M. Y., Segura, L. G., Arendt, K. W., Bendel-Stenzel, E. M., & Ruano, R. (2021). Toward eliminating perinatal comfort care for prenatally diagnosed severe congenital heart defects: A vision. *Mayo Clinic Proceedings, 96*(5), 1276–1287. https://doi.org/10.1016/j.mayocp.2020.08.029.

Tsintoni, A., Dimitriou, G., & Karatza, A. A. (2020). Nutrition of neonates with congenital heart disease: Existing evidence, conflicts and concerns. *Journal of Maternal-Fetal Neonatal Medicine, 33*(14), 2487–2492. https://doi.org/10.1080/14767058.2018.1548602.

Upadhyay, J., Rana, M., Joshi, A., Durgapal, S., & Bisht, S. (2019). Pathophysiology, etiology, and recent advancement in the treatment of congenital heart disease. *Journal of Indian College of Cardiology, 9*(2), 67–77. https://doi.org/10.4103/JICC.JICC_11_19.

Van Hagen, I. M., Roos-Hesselink, J. W., & Van Hagen, I. M. (2020). Pregnancy in congenital heart disease: Risk prediction and counselling. *Heart, 106*(23), 1853–1861. https://doi.org/10.1136/heartjnl-2019-314702.

Verbeek, I. N. E., van Onzenoort-Bokken, L., & Zegers, S. H. J. (2021). Vulnerable child syndrome in everyday paediatric practice: A condition deserving attention and new perspectives. *Acta Paediatrica, 110*(2), 397–399. doi:10.1111/apa.15505. Epub 2020 Aug 11. PMID: 32726476.

Waern, M., Mellander, M., Berg, A., & Carlsson, Y. (2021). Prenatal detection of congenital heart disease – results of a Swedish screening program 2013–2017. *BMC Pregnancy and Childbirth, 21*(1), 579. https://doi.org/10.1186/s12884-021-04028-5.

Wang, A., Gaca, J. G., & Chu, V. H. (2018). Management considerations in infective endocarditis: A review. *JAMA, 320*(1), 72–83. https://doi.org/10.1001/jama.2018.7596.

Watanabe, K., & Shih, R. (2020). Update of pediatric heart failure. *Pediatric Clinics of North America, 67*(5), 889–901. https://doi.org/10.1016/j.pcl.2020.06.004.

Wernovsky, G., & Licht, D. J. (2016). Neurodevelopmental outcomes in children with congenital heart disease—what can we impact? *Pediatrics Critical Care Medicine, 17*(8 Suppl 1), S232–S242. https://doi.org/10.1097/PCC.0000000000000800.

Williams, J. L., Torok, R. D., D'Ottavio, A., Spears, T., Chiswell, K., Forestieri, N. E., Sang, C. J., Paolillo, J. A., Walsh, M. J., Hoffman, T. M., Kemper, A. R., & Li, J. S. (2021). Causes of death in infants and children with congenital heart disease. *Pediatric Cardiology, 42*(6), 1308–1315. https://doi.org/10.1007/s00246-021-02612-2.

Willinger, L., Brudy, L., Meyer, M., Oberhoffer-Fritz, R., Ewert, P., & Müller, J. (2021). Overweight and obesity in patients with congenital heart disease: A systematic review. *International Journal of Environmental Research and Public Health, 18*(18), 9931. https://doi.org/10.3390/ijerph18189931.

Wilson, W., Taubert, K. A., Gewitz, M., Lockhart, P. B., Baddour, L. M., Levison, M., Bolger, A., Cabell, C. H., Takahashi, M., Baltimore, R. S., Newburger, J. W., Strom, B. L., Tani, L. Y., Gerber, M., Bonow, R. O., Pallasch, T., Shulman, S. T., Rowley, A. H., Burns, J. C., Ferrieri, P., ... Durack, D. T. American Heart Association Rheumatic Fever, Endocarditis, and Kawasaki Disease Committee; American Heart Association Council on Cardiovascular Disease in the Young; American Heart Association Council on Clinical Cardiology; American Heart Association Council on Cardiovascular Surgery and Anesthesia; Quality of Care and Outcomes Research Interdisciplinary Working Group. (2007). Prevention of infective endocarditis: guidelines from the American Heart Association: a guideline from the American Heart Association Rheumatic Fever, Endocarditis, and Kawasaki Disease Committee, Council on Cardiovascular Disease in the Young, and the Council on Clinical Cardiology, Council on Cardiovascular Surgery and Anesthesia, and the Quality of Care and Outcomes Research Interdisciplinary Working Group. *Circulation, 116*(15), 1736–1754. doi: 10.1161/CIRCULATIONAHA.106.183095. Epub 2007 Apr 19. Erratum in: Circulation, 2007 Oct 9;116(15):e376-7. PMID: 17446442.

Yasuhara, J., & Garg, V. (2021). Genetics of congenital heart disease: A narrative review of recent advances and clinical implications. *Translational Pediatrics, 10*(9), 2366–2386. https://doi.org/10.21037/tp-21-297.

Zhang, T. N., Wu, Q. J., Liu, Y. S., Lv, J. L., Sun, H., Chang, Q., Liu, C. F., & Zhao, Y. H. (2021). Environmental risk factors and congenital heart disease: An umbrella review of 165 systematic reviews and meta-analyses with more than 120 million participants. *Frontiers in Cardiovascular Medicine, 8*, 640729. https://doi.org/10.3389/fcvm.2021.640729.

Cystic Fibrosis

Heather Thomas

19

ETIOLOGY

Cystic fibrosis (CF) is a progressive genetic disease that affects the lungs, pancreas, and other organs. In the United States, close to 40,000 children and adults live with CF (estimated 105,000 people with CF across 94 countries). CF affects people of every racial and ethnic group (Cystic Fibrosis Foundation [CFF], 2021c). When CF was first described in the 1930s, most children with CF died in infancy. Due to therapeutic gains, the median predicted survival age increased from 28 years in 1986 to 53.1 years in 2021 (Fig. 19.1). Now 52.7% of people living with CF are adults (Goetz & Ren, 2019). CFF's focus is on a path to a cure (CFF, 2021c).

After a succession of scientific breakthroughs in genetics in 1989, the CF gene was isolated on the long arm of chromosome 7, which encodes a protein called the cystic fibrosis transmembrane conductance regulator (CFTR) (Davis, 2006). More than 2010 unique mutations in the *CFTR* gene have been reported, the most common of which is F508del. This mutation accounts for approximately 85.5% of CF alleles (CFF, 2021b). Approximately 99.4% of individuals in the CFF Registry have been genotyped, and no other single CFTR variant is currently found in more than 5% of the population with CF (CFF, 2021b). CF genetic mutations are divided into five classes based on their influence on CFTR production and function at the cellular level. These defects include defective protein synthesis, defective protein procession, disordered regulation, defective chloride conductance, and accelerated channel turnover (Awatade et al., 2018). The specific class of defect, in part, may explain the phenotypic expression of the disease; however, the variability in disease severity is also influenced by the presence of environmental, therapeutic, and other gene modifiers (Davis, 2006). It is increasingly recognized that this classification schema is an oversimplification given that many variants lead to more than one defect in the CFTR function (CFF, 2021b).

The CFTR protein functions as a transmembrane cAMP-activated chloride channel. All mutations result in decreased chloride secretion and increased sodium resorption into the cellular space. The increased sodium reabsorption leads to increased water resorption and manifests as thicker mucous secretions on epithelial linings and more viscous secretions from exocrine tissues. Thickened mucous secretions in nearly every organ system involved in CF result in mucous plugging with obstruction pathologies (Yu, 2022). CF is considered a multisystem disease as it affects every organ in the body directly or indirectly, but the lungs and pancreas are the most directly affected.

INCIDENCE AND PREVALENCE

CF is inherited in an autosomal recessive mode, therefore each parent is an obligate carrier. It has historically been considered a disease of White newborns; however, it is now recognized in other racial populations in increasing frequency most likely due to the wider implementation of newborn screening (NBS). In the United States, CF affects approximately 1 in 4000 newborns (approximately 1 in 3200 White newborns, 1 in 10,000 Hispanic newborns, 1 in 15,000 Black newborns, and 1 in 30,000 Asian newborns) (Hamosh et al., 1998). With a carrier rate in White newborns of approximately 1 in 25, it is estimated that for 1 in 400 to 500 couples, both partners are asymptomatic carriers of this recessive trait, with a subsequent 1 in 4 risk of bearing a child with CF with each pregnancy (Langfelder et al., 2005). The 2021 CFF Patient Registry reported 32,100 individuals living with CF in the United States, with 779 newly diagnosed individuals that year (CFF, 2021b).

DIAGNOSTIC CRITERIA

NBS for CF has been universally implemented in every state and the District of Colombia since 2011. Every state screens for CF; the process is not the same in every state, however. All states screen for the immunoreactive trypsinogen (IRT) level in the blood, which is typically high in babies with CF; however, it can also be high in premature babies or those with a traumatic birth. Of note, the IRT level in babies with meconium ileus can be artificially low. Some states use the IRT/IRT method, and some use the IRT/DNA method. The IRT/IRT screening algorithm reduces the costs to laboratories and insurance companies but has more system failures. IRT/DNA offers other advantages, including fewer delayed diagnoses and lower out-of-pocket costs to families (Wells et al., 2012). The floating IRT cutoff improves sensitivity to as high as 96%, and this is the

463

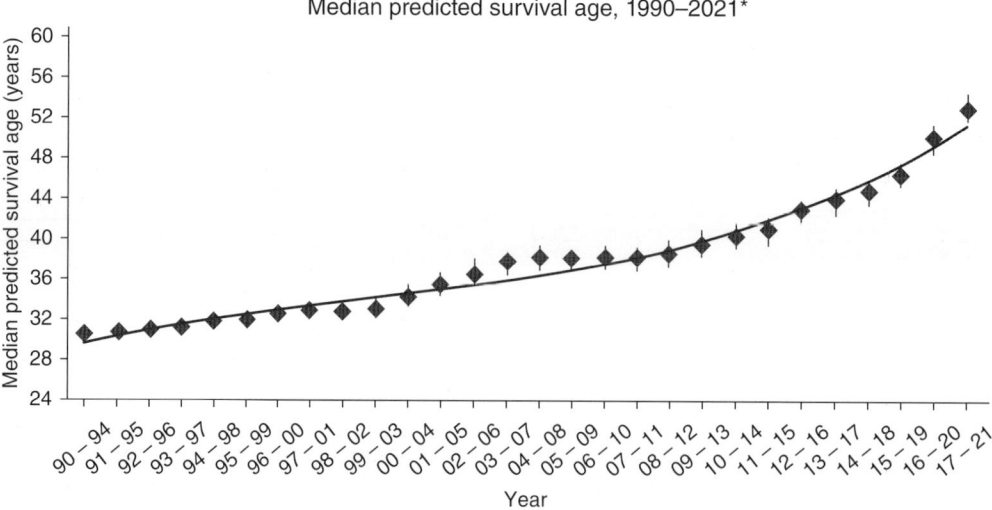

Median predicted survival age, 1990–2021*

*Using the currently recommended method for calculating median predicted survival. For more information about the methodology, see the Technical Supplement available at cff.org.

Fig. 19.1 **Median predicted survival in 5-year increments.** (From Cystic Fibrosis Foundation. [2021]. *Patient registry 2010 annual data report to the center directors.* Author.)

Box 19.1	Symptoms Suggestive of a Cystic Fibrosis (CF) Diagnosis That Should Be Screened With a Sweat Test

EAR/NOSE/THROAT	LUNGS/AIRWAYS	PANCREAS	GASTROINTESTINAL	OTHER
Pansinusitis	Cough	Steatorrhea	Constipation	Infertility
Chronic sinusitis	Recurrent bronchitis	Chronic pancreatitis	Rectal prolapse	Congenital absence vas
Nasal polyps	Recurrent pneumonia	Vitamin A, D, E, K	Gastroesophageal	deferens
	Airway obstruction	deficiency	reflux disease	Digital clubbing
	Bronchiectasis	CF-related diabetes	Distal intestinal obstruc-	Hyponatremic, hypo-
	Hemoptysis	Failure to thrive	tion syndrome	chloremic dehydration
	Pneumothorax		Meconium ileus	Aquagenic wrinkling of
			Cirrhosis	the skin
			Prolonged neonatal	Osteoporosis
			jaundice	Arthritis
			Liver failure	Anxiety/depression
				Salty tasting skin

method supported by the CFF. The DNA panels are state specific, with most screening between 23 and 40 CFTR mutations, and are reflective of the local population. A few states do full gene sequencing; however, this can increase the likelihood of finding mutations of uncertain significance, making diagnosis more complicated (Kharrazi et al., 2015). It is important to note that the health care professional who initially informs families of an abnormal NBS result is the primary care provider. Care should be taken to communicate the news confidently and compassionately. The primary care provider's responsibility is to refer the family to a CF-accredited center for further evaluation as soon as possible.

An expert panel was assembled in 2015 to review the diagnostic criteria for CF, given the implementation of NBS and an evolving understanding of CF genetics (Farrell et al., 2017). Prior to NBS, the diagnosis of CF relied primarily on a constellation of phenotypic features such as failure to thrive, malabsorption, respiratory infections, and male infertility (Box 19.1). While unscreened individuals who display symptoms consistent with CF should undergo a sweat test, most screened individuals are asymptomatic prior to diagnosis. The 2021 CFF Registry report showed NBS detected 64.4% of new diagnoses with an average age of 3 months (CFF, 2021b). Sweat testing by pilocarpine iontophoresis with quantitative sweat chloride analysis in a CFF-certified center is still considered the gold standard for diagnosis. A value greater than 60 mmol/L is diagnostic of CF (Farrell et al., 2017). A sweat test value less than 30 mmol/L in all ages is now considered normal, and CF is unlikely (Farrell et al., 2017).

Individuals who present with an abnormal NBS, symptoms or family history, and intermediate sweat chloride values (30–59 mmol/L) require further genetic testing, including full *CFTR* gene sequencing with deletion/duplication and poly-T variant detection. Newborns with an inconclusive diagnosis based on elevated IRT on NBS, intermediate sweat chloride values, and two possible disease-causing mutations fall into the CFTR-related metabolic syndrome (CRMS) or CF screen positive, inconclusive diagnosis (CFSPID) category. The two terms are considered identical, and the term *CRMS/CFSPID* should be used (Farrell et al., 2017). According to the 2021 CFF Registry, 130 individuals were diagnosed with CRMS/CFSPID in 2021. Individuals not newborn screened but with an inconclusive diagnosis fall into the category of CFTR-related disorder as CF cannot be excluded, and a single organ system may be affected. The CFF Registry reported 74 individuals who were diagnosed with CFTR-related abnormality in 2021 (CFF, 2021). Providers should avoid the terms *non-classic CF* or *atypical CF*. Genetic testing for all groups should be performed in a lab that screens for *CFTR* gene sequencing with del/dup and poly-T status. The genetic mutations can be confirmed as disease causing, of varying clinical consequence, mutation of unknown significance, or non-CF causing on the website CFTR2.org (CFF, 2021c). This website provides clinical information about genetic mutations to health care professionals, patients, and families. All individuals with a CF diagnosis require full genetic testing because these mutations dictate which CFTR modulator is indicated (Fig. 19.2).

CLINICAL MANIFESTATIONS

The pathophysiologic hallmarks of CF are pancreatic enzyme deficiency from duct blockage by viscous mucus, progressive chronic obstructive lung disease associated with viscous infected mucus and subsequent interstitial destruction, and sweat gland dysfunction resulting in abnormally high sodium and chloride concentrations in the sweat (Davis, 2006).

Since the implementation of NBS, the clinical presentation has been much different than in the past because most infants diagnosed with NBS are asymptomatic. In 2021 93.1% of infants were diagnosed with NBS or prenatal screening (CFF, 2021b). Historically, nutritional failure was the cause of death in infants with CF until pancreatic enzyme replacement therapy (PERT) and nutritional supplementation became available. Pancreatic insufficiency (PI) is present in 83.1% of individuals (CFF, 2021b). With earlier diagnosis and implementation of therapy, symptoms such as failure to thrive (6.9%), electrolyte imbalance (0.4%), and steatorrhea (7.7%) can be avoided; however, if present it should still raise the primary care provider's suspicion for CF (CFF, 2021c).

Meconium ileus or intestinal obstruction in the neonatal period can cause a false-negative NBS and should be presumed related to CF until excluded otherwise with a sweat test. In the CFF Registry, 11.2% of infants presented with meconium ileus as the initial

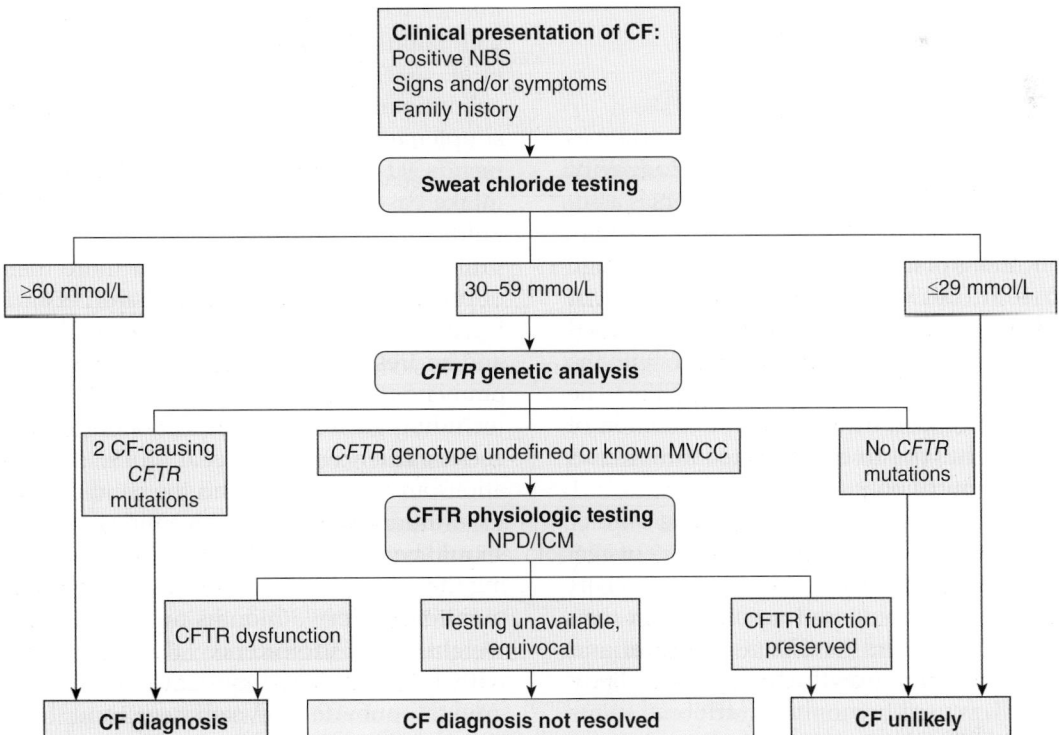

Fig. 19.2 Algorithm for diagnostic consideration of cystic fibrosis *(CF)*. All individuals with CF should have a sweat chloride test and genetic testing. This evaluation should occur in a CF-accredited center. *CF,* Cystic fibrosis; *CFTR,* cystic fibrosis transmembrane conductance regulator; *ICM,* intestinal current measurement; *MVCC,* mutation of varying clinical consequences; *NBS,* newborn screening; *NPD,* nasal potential difference. (From Farrell, P.M., White, T., Ren, C., et al. [2017]. Diagnosis of cystic fibrosis: Consensus guidelines from the Cystic Fibrosis Foundation. *Journal of Pediatrics, 181,* S7.)

presentation of CF (CFF, 2021a). Meconium ileus can be managed conservatively but often requires surgical intervention.

Recurrent respiratory infections in the upper and lower airways are common in those with CF, even those diagnosed via NBS. Manifestations include nasal polyps, chronic sinusitis, recurrent pneumonia, and bronchiectasis. Typical symptoms include a persistent chronic cough and hyperinflation noted on chest x-ray and pulmonary function tests consistent with obstructive airway disease. The presence of nasal polyps or chronic sinus infections should prompt suspicion of CF because 15.5% of individuals with CF had this on initial presentation (CFF, 2021c). Typical pathogens isolated in the respiratory tract include *Staphylococcus aureus*, *Pseudomonas aeruginosa*, and eventually other more difficult to treat gram-negative rods. Crackles and wheezing can be noted on physical exam, but the exam is frequently normal. These lung findings have occurred despite NBS diagnosis, suggesting that traditional pulmonary therapies are inadequate in preventing the progression of CF lung disease (Goetz & Ren, 2019).

CF is a multisystem disease, and the presentation may be variable and subtle; therefore it must be considered even if NBS is normal. Additionally, CF should be considered in older adolescents and adults who may not have undergone NBS for CF. Diagnostic delays may be decreased if primary care providers maintain a high level of suspicion of the various symptoms associated with CF even in the presence of a normal NBS.

TREATMENT

NUTRITIONAL MANAGEMENT

Optimal growth in individuals with CF is important as it is associated with improved lung function, longevity, and quality of life. Greater weight at age 4 years is associated with greater height, better pulmonary function, fewer complications of CF, and better survival through age 18 (Yen et al., 2013). Individuals with CF are at risk for malnutrition due to malabsorption, increased calorie needs, and reduced appetite; however, with the implementation of NBS and earlier diagnosis it may be possible to prevent malnutrition. The introduction of CFTR modulators has positively impacted individuals with CF and their nutritional status.

Growth charts are used as an objective measure of nutritional status. For children less than 2 years of age, the World Health Organization (WHO) growth chart is used, and for children and adolescents greater than 2 years of age, the Centers for Disease Control and Prevention (CDC; 2022a) growth chart is used. Body mass index (BMI) is used to monitor nutritional status for those 2 to 20 years of age and weight/length % for those less than 2 years of age. For children and adolescents aged 2 to 20 years, the CFF recommends that weight-for-stature assessment use the BMI percentile method and that children and adolescents maintain

a BMI at or above the 50th percentile (Stallings et al., 2008). According to the 2021 CFF Registry, the median BMI for those 2 to 19 years is 62.1 percentile. For adults age 20 years and older, the CFF recommends that weight-for-stature assessment use the BMI method and that females maintain a BMI at or above 22 kg/m^2 and males at or above 23 kg/m^2 (Stallings et al., 2008). According to the CFF Registry, the median BMI for those age 20 to 40 years is 23.4 kg/m^2 (CFF, 2021). For children diagnosed before age 2 years, the CFF recommends that children reach a weight-for-length status of greater than the 75th percentile by age 2 years using the WHO growth chart (Stallings et al., 2008). According to the CFF Registry, the median weight-for-length in those under 24 months is 62.8 percentile (CFF, 2021a).

Because NBS is used for most new CF diagnoses, monitoring weight starts early, and interventions are put into place proactively rather than reacting to growth failure. The CFF recommends that children (age >24 months) with CF be seen every 3 months, infants less than age 12 months be seen every month, and those age 12 to 24 months be seen every 2 to 3 months depending on clinical status (Borowitz et al., 2009). Some of the more frequent visits may occur with the primary care provider, depending on the distance to the CF center. Expected weight gain is based on age and on the expected rate of weight gain at the 50th percentile. Infants birth to 1 month of age should average 30 g/day weight gain; infants age 5 to 6 months should average 15 g/day. The CFF recommends infants who have weight loss or suboptimal weight gain should receive calorie-dense feedings (Borowitz et al., 2009). Preschool-age children (2–5 years) with suboptimal weight gain may require calorie-dense oral supplements rather than whole milk. The CFF recommends 90 to 110 kcal/kg/day or more and protein intake based on dietary reference intakes and dietary guidelines recommendations of more than 13 g/day of protein in 2- to 3-year-olds and more than 19 g/day of protein in 4- to 5-year-olds (Lahiri et al., 2019). During preschool, feeding behaviors should be monitored and addressed if interfering with intake. The CFF recommends an expanded evaluation of poor growth, including gastrointestinal, endocrine, behavioral, and social influences (Lahiri et al., 2019). If standard evaluations are unrevealing and the child does not respond to multidisciplinary interventions, enteral feedings should be strongly considered (Lahiri et al., 2019). During the school years (>6 years to puberty), children are monitored every 3 months unless there is suboptimal weight gain. Adolescence (11–18 years) is associated with high nutrient requirements due to accelerated growth, pubertal development, and high levels of physical activity (Stallings et al., 2008). CF adolescent pubertal development should reflect that of the general population; however, continued discussion about the need for optimal nutrition with the teen and parent is important.

PANCREATIC ENZYME REPLACEMENT THERAPY

Most individuals with CF are considered to have exocrine PI or PI. While PI is generally considered a lifelong condition, in some instances PI is delayed or prevented with the early initiation of CFTR modulator medications. Individuals with PI frequently report large bulky stools with oil or grease present. Once toilet trained, individuals with PI may report floating stools due to the high-fat content. The principal treatment for the resulting malabsorption in CF is oral pancreatic enzyme replacement. The CFF Registry showed 83.1% of the CF population required PERT in 2021 (CFF, 2021b). Pancreatic status is confirmed with a fecal elastase level (Taylor et al., 2015). PERT should not be delayed in those with two disease-causing mutations known to be associated with PI (Borowitz et al., 2009).

Enteric coating of enzyme preparations decreases the likelihood of inactivation by gastric acid, and doses may be adjusted to achieve weight gain and one to two formed stools per day. Most CF centers now use dosing guidelines of 500 to 2500 lipase units/kg/meal as a safe range. Fibrosing colonopathy is a rare but theoretic risk with doses between 2500 and 6000 lipase units/kg/meal (Stallings et al., 2008). Generic preparations of PERT should not be used (Borowitz et al., 2009). Older children and adults can swallow the pills. In infants and younger children, the capsule is opened, and the enzyme beads are given with soft acidic food, typically applesauce.

Any adjustment to PERT dosing should be monitored clinically for a response. Children often experience continued malabsorption despite reasonable PERT. Table 19.1 lists factors that contribute to a poor response to PERT. Initial assessment and intervention should address adherence, enzyme storage, and a child's eating habits (i.e., small frequent snacks or grazing without taking enzymes). Neutralizing gastric acid with antacids or inhibiting its production with histamine-receptor antagonists can improve the efficacy of the enzyme preparation. The CF dietitian is extremely helpful in managing PERT and malabsorption.

HIGH-CALORIE DIET

There is no perfect method to estimate the caloric needs of individuals with CF as it varies based on the severity of the disease, pancreatic status, and progression of the disease. It is known that there is a strong correlation between BMI at the 50th percentile for children 2 to 19 years of age and BMI of 22 kg/m² for females and 23 kg/m² for males 20 years and older with preservation of lung function (forced expiratory volume of 1 second [FEV$_1$]). The CFF recommends human milk or standard infant formula and feeding with solids be initiated at 4 to 6 months of age (Borowitz et al., 2009). If the weight trend is poor, the formula should be calorie condensed or added to breastmilk. In the preschool age group (2–5 years), the CFF recommends 90 to 110 kcal/kg with 13 g protein/day in 2- to 3-year-olds

Table 19.1	Factors Contributing to a Poor Response to Pancreatic Enzyme Replacement Therapy
Enzyme factors	Generic enzymes used Expired medications Not taking it before a meal Inappropriate dose Enzymes stored in heat
Dietary factors	Grazing eating behavior Higher-fat foods Taking with a hot drink Perception that therapy is not needed with certain foods (i.e., milk) Need to take with nutritional supplements
Poor adherence to prescribed enzyme regimen	Toddler's willful refusal Chaotic or multiple households Desire to be "normal" Embarrassment Too expensive or not approved by insurance Teenage females' desire to be thin
Acid intestinal environment	Presence of gastroesophageal reflux disease Poor dissolution of enteric coating Microcapsule contents are released all at once
Concurrent gastrointestinal disorder	Acute viral gastroenteritis Celiac disease Small bowel bacterial overgrowth

Modified from Borowitz, D., Grand, R.J., & Durie, P.R. (1995). Use of pancreatic enzyme supplements for patients with cystic fibrosis in the context of fibrosing colonopathy. *Journal of Pediatrics, 127*, 681–684.

and 19 g protein/day in 4- to 5-year-olds (Lahiri et al., 2019). In preschool-age children who are not meeting nutritional goals, the CFF recommends introduction of oral supplements and possible enteral feeds after other factors (i.e., behavioral, social, endocrine, gastrointestinal) for poor growth have been excluded (Lahiri et al., 2019). With the introduction of CFTR modulators, the nutritional status of individuals with CF has significantly improved and may alleviate the need for a high-calorie diet. In fact, 40.4% of individuals were classified as overweight and 11.7% as obese in the 2021 CFF Registry report, according to CDC (2022a) definitions.

VITAMIN, MINERAL, AND SODIUM SUPPLEMENTATION

Optimal dietary intake includes attention to fat-soluble vitamins, calcium, iron, zinc, and sodium in all age groups. The CFF recommends that blood levels of fat-soluble vitamins be screened for deficiencies regularly after starting vitamin supplementation and at least annually unless adjustments are made to dosing (Borowitz et al., 2009; Lahiri et al., 2019). All individuals with CF should take a multivitamin at the start of the diagnosis, designed to provide at least the recommended levels of vitamins A, D, E, and K (Borowitz et al., 2009).

Vitamin D deficiency is common in individuals with CF due to impaired absorption of fat-soluble vitamins, decreased sunlight exposure, and suboptimal intake of vitamin D–containing foods and/or supplements. Vitamin D deficiency has been associated with decreased bone mass in children, failure to achieve expected peak bone mass in young adults, and osteoporosis in mature adults (Tangpricha et al., 2012). The CFF recommends that all individuals with CF should be treated with vitamin D_3 (cholecalciferol) and have a 25-hydroxyvitamin D level measured at least annually, and that level should be at least 30 ng/mL. Infants from birth to 12 months should be treated with 400 to 500 IU vitamin D_3/day and 12 months to 10 years with 800 to 1000 IU vitamin D_3/day. If vitamin D levels remain low, the supplementation amount can be increased as high as 10,000 IU/day in close collaboration with the CF dietitian (Tangpricha et al., 2012).

Children with CF lose more salt in their sweat than other children because of the basic CF defect of chloride ion transport. Salt needs to be replaced through diet. It is recommended that infants from birth to 6 months receive 0.125 teaspoon salt/day and infants age 6 to 24 months receive 0.25 teaspoon salt/day (Borowitz et al., 2009). After 2 years of age it is recommended that individuals with CF use the saltshaker liberally (Lahiri et al., 2019). Individuals with CF need to have salt and adequate hydration when the weather is hot or when participating in sports or other activities that increase sweat.

RESPIRATORY MANAGEMENT

Although there has been significant improvement in survival and quality of life in the CF population, lung disease remains the leading cause of morbidity and mortality in individuals with CF. Interventions are designed to interrupt or slow lung damage by preventing abnormal airway secretions and lung infections or treating the existing infection and inflammation. Chronic therapies in CF aim to prevent the development of bronchiectasis or end-stage lung disease.

A multidisciplinary committee reviewed the 2007 chronic care guidelines put forth by the CFF and made new recommendations (Mogayzel et al., 2013). Table 19.2 reviews the new guidelines put forth and incorporates other newer therapies.

CFTR MODULATORS

This class of drugs acts by improving the production, intracellular procession, and function of the defective CFTR protein. Specific drugs are indicated for specific genetic mutations. Currently available in order of development are ivacaftor (Kalydeco), lumacaftor-ivacaftor (Orkambi), tezacaftor-ivacaftor (Symdeko), and elexacaftor-tezacaftor-ivacaftor (Trikafta). The potentiators (ivacaftor and elexacaftor) help open the CFTR channel and increase the movement of chloride and bicarbonate across the cell surface. The correctors (elexacaftor, tezacaftor, lumacaftor) help normalize the folding of defective CFTR protein. Not only do these medications provide significant improvement in lung function, pulmonary exacerbation rates, BMI, and sweat chloride values, but they are the first medications that target the basic defect rather than its consequences (Davies et al., 2013; Middleton & Taylor-Cousar, 2021; Taylor-Cousar et al., 2017; Wainwright et al., 2015).

Choosing which drug to start is dependent on genotype and age. Currently ivacaftor is US Food and Drug Administration (FDA) approved to age 4 months, lumacaftor-ivacaftor to age 1 year, tezacaftor-ivacaftor to age 6 years, and elexacaftor-tezacaftor-ivacaftor to 6 years (FDA approval received April 2023, for 2–5 years). Prior to starting the medication, an eye exam focusing on the presence of cataracts is necessary because in the research trials the incidence was increased in animals. Liver function tests are monitored at the initiation of therapy, every 3 months for the first year, then annually. Vertex, a drug manufacturer, provides a helpful tool on its website (https://www.vertextreatmentshcp.com/eligibility-tool), which can assist in choosing the appropriate modulator (Table 19.3). Approximately 10% of the CF population is not eligible for a CFTR modulator based on genotype. Patients with CF from minority groups have increased disease severity and earlier mortality and are less likely to be eligible for CFTR modulators based on genotype, thus further contributing to health disparities (McGarry & McColley, 2021).

AIRWAY CLEARANCE AND EXERCISE

Airway clearance can be accomplished with a variety of different devices. Airway clearance twice daily when well and four times daily when symptomatic is considered the standard of care to help relieve bronchial obstruction through clearance of pulmonary secretions. There is no evidence to suggest one method is superior to another, and the chosen method of airway clearance should be individualized based on the severity of the disease, age of the individual, quality of life, and individual choice. Insufficient data suggest exercise can replace an airway clearance session; however, the positive impacts are apparent (Flume, Robertson, et al., 2009). Different forms of airway clearance devices are listed in Box 19.2. According to CFF Registry data, 76.3% of individuals used a high-frequency chest wall oscillation vest after infancy (CFF, 2021a).

The CFF recommends that for infants under 2 years of age, airway clearance should be started in the first few months of life and include albuterol administration prior to percussion (Borowitz et al., 2009). For children age 2 to 5 years, the CFF recommends routine airway clearance twice daily and four times daily with exacerbation; however, it could not recommend routine use of a bronchodilator prior to airway clearance (Lahiri et al., 2019). Recommendations for those older than 5 years are the same. The CF center provider, respiratory therapist, and family/patient should work together to determine the best method that will lead to compliance with airway clearance.

Table 19.2 Recommended Chronic Pulmonary Therapies for Those With Cystic Fibrosis (CF)

THERAPY	INDICATION	COMMENTS
CFTR modulator	• 4 mo: ivacaftor • 1 yr: lumacaftor/ivacaftor • 6 yr: tezacaftor/ivacaftor • 6 yr: elexacaftor/tezacaftor/ivacaftor	Choice of a modulator is dependent on genotype (vertextreatments.com)
Airway clearance therapy	• Twice daily airway clearance in all with CF starting in infancy • Increase to four times daily with exacerbation	Choice of therapy should be individualized
Mucolytics		
Inhaled DNase	• May be used in symptomatic infants and preschool-age children • Recommended for those age ≥6 yr	Given once daily Pretreat with bronchodilator
Hypertonic 7% saline	• May be used in symptomatic infants and preschool-age children • Recommended for those age ≥6 yr	Given twice daily Pretreat with bronchodilator
Inhaled mannitol	• Recommended for those age ≥18 yr	Given twice daily First dose must be given in a clinical setting
Inhaled N-acetylcysteine	• Not recommended	
Antimicrobial Therapy		
Inhaled tobramycin	• After two *Pseudomonas aeruginosa (PA)* eradication attempts, chronic inhaled tobramycin should be used in infants • Preschool-age children colonized with *PA* should receive chronic inhaled tobramycin • Those colonized with *PA* age ≥6 yr should receive chronic inhaled tobramycin	Inhaled tobramycin should be used in *PA* eradication attempts
Inhaled aztreonam	• Recommended for those age ≥6 yr with *PA* colonized in the airways	Typically added in addition to inhaled tobramycin Given three times daily
Oral antibiotic	• Used to treat acute exacerbation	Chosen based on past respiratory cultures
Intravenous antibiotic	• Used to treat acute exacerbation after inhaled or oral antibiotics have failed • Used to treat severe exacerbation or respiratory failure	Chosen based on past respiratory cultures
Antiinflammatory Therapy		
Azithromycin	• Insufficient evidence to recommend for or against in infant and preschool-age child • Consider use in infant and preschool-age children who culture *PA* • Recommended for those age ≥6 yr who are colonized with *PA*	Dose is given three times a week Do not initiate in those with nontuberculous mycobacteria
Ibuprofen	• Insufficient evidence to recommend for or against in preschool-age children and those age >18 yr • For individuals age 6–17 yr, chronic high-dose ibuprofen is recommended	Rarely used because of side effect profile and need for monitoring drug levels in serum
Inhaled corticosteroids	• Recommend against routine use in all with CF unless symptoms of asthma or allergic bronchopulmonary aspergillosis (ABPA)	
Oral corticosteroids	• Recommend against routine use in all with CF unless symptoms of asthma or ABPA	
Other Therapies		
Immunizations	• Annual influenza vaccination starting at age 6 mo • Palivizumab is not routinely recommended unless other risk factors are present • Pneumovax starting at age 2 yr • COVID-19 vaccination starting at age 6 mo	Individuals with CF should receive all routine childhood immunizations as scheduled
Infection control measures	• Recommended for all with CF in all health care settings	Consists of a gown, gloves, mask, and hand hygiene

CFTR, Cystic fibrosis transmembrane conductance regulator.
From Mogayzel, P.J., Naureckas, E.T., Robinson, K.A., et al. (2013). Cystic fibrosis pulmonary guidelines. Chronic medications for maintenance of lung health. *American Journal of Respiratory and Critical Care Medicine, 187*(7), 680–689.

Table 19.3   CFTR Modulator Indications and Side Effects

DRUG	INDICATION	SIDE EFFECTS
Ivacaftor	Individuals with CF who are age ≥4 mo and have 1 of 97 eligible mutations (kalydeco.com)	Interactions with certain drugs Elevated liver tests Cataracts Headache Respiratory symptoms (i.e., URI) Abdominal pain, diarrhea, nausea Dizziness
Lumacaftor/ ivacaftor	Individuals with CF who are age ≥1 yr and have 2 copies of the F508del mutation	Elevated liver tests Cataracts Chest tightness when starting medication Elevated blood pressure Nausea, diarrhea, gas, stomach pain Fatigue Rash
Tezacaftor Ivacaftor	Individuals with CF who are age ≥6 yr and have 2 copies of F508del mutation or at least 1 other mutation that is responsive (symdeko.com)	Elevated liver tests Cataracts Headache Dizziness Nausea
Elexacaftor Tezacaftor Ivacaftor	Individuals with CF who are age ≥6 yr and have at least 1 copy of F508del mutation	Elevated liver tests Cataracts Headache Rash Abdominal pain, diarrhea

CF, Cystic fibrosis; *CFTR,* cystic fibrosis transmembrane conductance regulator; *URI,* upper respiratory infection.

Box 19.2   Airway Clearance Treatment Options

Palm cups
Chest physiotherapy (postural drainage and percussion)
High-frequency chest wall oscillating vest
Huff cough
Airway oscillating device (Aerobika)
Positive expiratory pressure (TheraPep)
Active cycle of breathing
Autogenic drainage
Exercise

MUCOLYTICS

Dornase alfa (DNase) cleaves extracellular DNA, which is present in high concentrations in purulent CF airway mucus, and reduces its viscosity to a more liquid form. Currently, the CFF recommends DNase be taken once daily in patients older than 2 years, regardless of symptoms or lung function (Lahiri et al., 2019). DNase was found to reduce the rate of acute exacerbations compared with a placebo or no treatment. The use of DNase for a 2-year period was associated with a reduction in the rate of lung function (FEV$_1$) decline (Konstan, Wagener, et al., 2011). The CFF Registry reported that 86.8% of individuals older than 6 years were prescribed DNase in 2021 (CFF, 2021a). The need for DNase in the era of highly effective CFTR modulators is uncertain and is being evaluated by the CFF.

Inhaled hypertonic saline (7%) (HTS) twice daily should be considered in all individuals with CF and may be used in symptomatic children younger than 5 years (Borowitz et al., 2009; Lahiri et al., 2019). The infant study of inhaled saline (ISIS) did not find a significant difference in the group of infants with HTS; however, a subsequent study showed preventive inhalation with 6% hypertonic saline in the first 4 months of life was safe and well tolerated and resulted in improvement in lung clearance index (LCI) and weight gain (Rosenfeld et al., 2012). It is thought that LCI is a more sensitive measurement of improvement in lung function (Stahl et al., 2019). Similar results were found in a study of 3- to 6-year-olds (Ratjen et al., 2019). The CFF Registry reported 72.9% of individuals older than 6 years received HTS in 2021 (CFF, 2021a). The need for HTS in the era of highly effective CFTR modulators is uncertain and is being evaluated by the CFF.

Inhaled mannitol received FDA approval in 2020 and is now considered a second-line treatment in adults older than 18 years. Due to concerns for bronchospasm, the first dose must be given in a health care setting, which can be prohibitive (Nevitt et al., 2018). Inhaled N-acetylcysteine is no longer recommended for use.

ANTIBIOTIC THERAPY

Most of the morbidity and mortality associated with CF is due to lung disease resulting from chronic respiratory infection or pulmonary exacerbations. The definition of pulmonary exacerbation generally includes an increase in cough and sputum production and a decline in lung function (FEV$_1$) by 10% predicted from baseline; however, a universal definition has been elusive (VanDevanter et al., 2021). There is a known association between viral and bacterial illnesses in individuals with CF. Along with directly causing severe respiratory symptoms in CF populations, the impact of respiratory viral infections may be more far reaching, indirectly promoting bacterial persistence and pathogenesis in the CF respiratory tract (Kiedrowski & Bomberger, 2018).

Frequent and early use of antibiotics is standard in the CF population, even if the illness is thought to be viral in nature. Prophylactic antibiotics are not recommended in individuals with CF. A Cochrane review of antistaphylococcal antibiotics evaluated four studies with 303 participants and concluded that the clinical significance of decreased *S. aureus* in treated children is unclear, especially given the potential for increased risk of *P. aeruginosa* infection (Smyth et al., 2020).

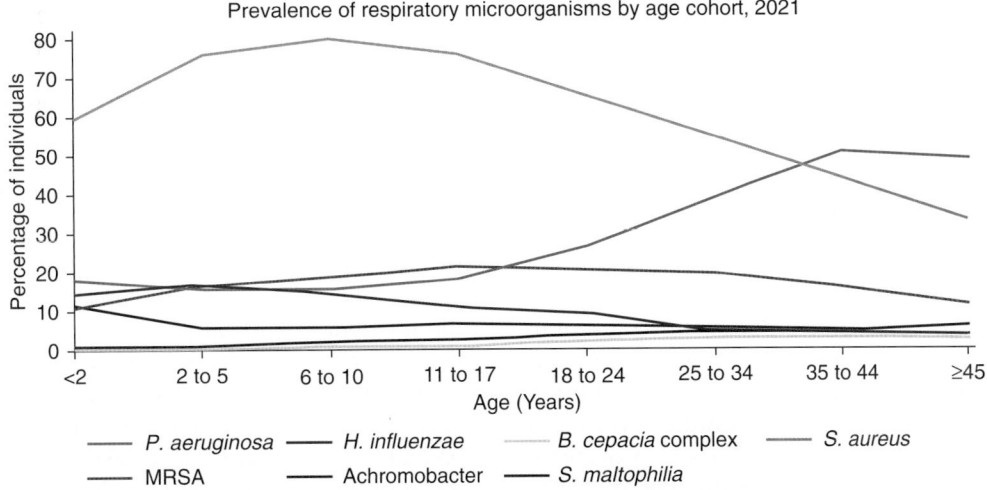

Fig. 19.3 Common pathogens found in cystic fibrosis airways by age cohort. (From Cystic Fibrosis Foundation. [2021]. *Patient registry 2010 annual data report to the center directors.* Author.)

It is recommended that individuals with CF have a sputum culture, typically an oropharyngeal swab, every 3 months (Borowitz et al., 2009; Goetz & Ren, 2019; Lahiri et al., 2019). The pathogens isolated and the sensitivity pattern can help the primary care provider choose an appropriate antibiotic. The appearance of different organisms in the sputum tends to vary by age, with *S. aureus* appearing first and eventually *P. aeruginosa* (CFF, 2021c) (Fig. 19.3). Until *P. aeruginosa* is isolated, the initial choice of antibiotic and dosage should provide broad-spectrum coverage specifically for *S. aureus, Streptococcus pneumoniae,* and *Haemophilus influenzae.*

Chronic colonization with *P. aeruginosa* is associated with a faster decline in lung function. An aggressive approach to eradication is now recommended. The CFF strongly recommends inhaled antibiotic therapy for the treatment of initial or new growth of *P. aeruginosa,* and the favored antibiotic regimen is inhaled tobramycin (300 mg twice daily) for 28 days (Mogayzel et al., 2013). Information is limited on treatment for patients who fail initial eradication therapy. Treatment with a second course of inhaled tobramycin for 28 days did not significantly decrease colonization, and many required intravenous (IV) antibiotic therapy (Blanchart et al., 2017). These measures are taken regardless of symptoms. The percentage of individuals with a positive culture for *P. aeruginosa* has continued to decline over time, with the largest decrease observed among individuals younger than 18 years; 44.6% had a positive culture in 2001 compared with 16.8% in 2021 (CFF, 2021b). Once an individual is deemed colonized, continuous alternating therapy with inhaled antibiotics should be considered. Current guidelines recommend inhaling tobramycin for individuals age 6 years or older with CF and persistent *P. aeruginosa* infection (Mogayzel et al., 2013).

Inhaled antibiotic therapy delivers high concentrations of antibiotics to the site of infection while decreasing the risk of systemic absorption. Tobramycin

inhalation solution (TIS) 300 mg twice daily for 28 days on and 28 days off is generally considered first-line therapy in those colonized with *P. aeruginosa* who are 6 years and older (Mogayzel et al., 2013). Often this same therapy is used in younger children even though not officially recommended. Tobramycin inhalation powder (TIP) has a safety and efficacy profile comparable with TIS and offers a far more convenient treatment option for *P. aeruginosa* lung infection (Konstan, Flume, et al., 2011). Inhaled aztreonam lysine is considered second-line therapy reserved for those who cannot tolerate TIS/TIP or as add-on therapy for continuous alternate therapy in those with declining lung function or advanced lung disease (Oermann et al., 2010). The CFF Registry reports 60% of eligible individuals are on TIS/TIP, and 37.7% are on inhaled aztreonam (CFF, 2021a).

When individuals with CF experience symptoms consistent with a pulmonary exacerbation despite oral and/or inhaled antibiotics, strong consideration is given to proceed with IV antibiotic therapy. The choice of antibiotics is based on previous sputum culture results and generally includes double coverage of *P. aeruginosa* (i.e., often an aminoglycoside with either a semisynthetic penicillin or third-generation cephalosporin) (Flume, et al., 2009). Often referred to as a "tune-up" or "clean out," the hospitalization for IV antibiotic therapy will also include physical therapy, increased airway clearance, and attention to nutritional status.

ANTIINFLAMMATORY THERAPY

The progressive inflammatory response of the CF airway begins early in life, becomes persistent, is excessive relative to the bacterial burden, impairs host defenses, worsens airway obstruction, causes structural damage to the airway wall architecture, and ultimately contributes to a progressive loss in lung function (Roesch et al., 2018). High-dose ibuprofen has been shown to slow inflammation in CF lung disease; however, it is rarely used because of potential side effects and drug-level monitoring challenges. The CFF recommends high-dose ibuprofen with serum levels of 50 to 100 μg/mL for children age 6 to 17 years; however, the certainty rating was moderate. The CFF found insufficient information to make a recommendation for those older than 18 years (Mogayzel et al., 2013). Azithromycin is a macrolide antibiotic that has antiinflammatory properties. It has been shown to slow lung function decline and decrease the frequency of exacerbations. Currently azithromycin is recommended by the CFF for individuals 6 years of age and older, with *P. aeruginosa* persistently present in cultures of the airways to improve lung function and reduce exacerbations (Mogayzel et al., 2013). In individuals not infected by *P. aeruginosa*, azithromycin should be considered because it has been shown to decrease pulmonary exacerbations by 50% (Saiman et al., 2010). The CFF recommends with high certainty of net benefit against oral or inhaled steroids for individuals older than 6 years who do not have asthma or allergic bronchopulmonary aspergillosis (Mogayzel et al., 2013).

LUNG TRANSPLANTATION

Although the CF population as a whole is considered healthier secondary to the advancement of highly effective CFTR modulators, there is still a subset of individuals with advanced lung disease as defined by FEV_1 less than 40% predicted, referred for a lung transplant, previous intensive care unit admission for respiratory failure, hypercarbia with $PaCO_2$ above 50 mm Hg, daytime oxygen requirement, pulmonary hypertension, or 6-minute walk test distance below 400 m (Kapnadak et al., 2020). Lung transplantation for individuals with CF and advanced lung disease is viable but must be considered early (Morrell & Pilewski, 2010). According to the 2019 CFF consensus guidelines, discussions about lung transplantation and possible referral to a transplant center should start to occur when the individual's FEV_1 is consistently less than 50% predicted. Nutritional status, CF-related diabetes, and mental health challenges should be addressed to optimize candidacy. Individuals are recommended to be referred to a transplant center with an accredited CF care center (Ramos et al., 2019). The number of lung transplants is declining according to the CFF Registry, with 226 transplants in 2015 compared with 54 lung transplants in 2021 (CFF, 2021b).

ASSOCIATED PROBLEMS OF CYSTIC FIBROSIS AND TREATMENT

Pancreatic Insufficiency

Most individuals with CF will develop PI over time, and many have evidence at birth. Approximately 83.1% of individuals in the CFF Registry take PERT, suggesting PI (CFF, 2021b). Symptoms of PI include poor weight gain, bulky, foul-smelling stools, oil/grease in the stool, floating stools, and abdominal distention. The diagnosis is confirmed with a stool fecal elastase level below 200 μg/g. Treatment of PI includes pancreatic enzyme replacement (500–2500 lipase units/kg) at a dose to control symptoms and allow for adequate growth. It is important to involve the CF dietitian in PERT management as there are nuances regarding administration and timing.

Rectal Prolapse

Rectal prolapse is a circumferential, full-thickness protrusion of the rectal wall through the anal orifice. With universal NBS and the implementation of PERT, the incidence of rectal prolapse has decreased. A retrospective review of children who presented to the Children's Hospital of Wisconsin with rectal prolapse between 2000 and 2010 revealed that 3.6% of patients had CF; conversely, 3.5% of the patients with CF had a rectal prolapse. Based on this, the authors recommend that a sweat test be performed on children with rectal prolapse with the understanding that it is a test with a low yield in the era of NBS (El-Chammas et al., 2015). The primary care provider may need to guide parents on how to gently reduce a prolapse by using a glove and lubricant jelly with the child side-lying.

Meconium Ileus and Distal Intestinal Obstruction Syndrome

Obstruction of the small intestine at the level of the terminal ileum with inspissated meconium is termed *meconium ileus*. While not overall common, affecting 11.2% of all individuals with CF, it is very specific to CF, and all infants with meconium ileus should have confirmatory sweat testing or genetic testing (CFF, 2021c). Meconium ileus can be treated surgically or nonsurgically. Contemporary series of noninvasive management with Gastrografin enema report success rates of 36% to 39%. The optimal surgical technique remains controversial, although primary anastomosis results in surgical complication rates between 21% and 31%, higher than those noted with delayed anastomosis (Carlyle et al., 2012). Complete or incomplete intestinal obstruction by viscid fecal material in the terminal ileum and proximal colon, distal intestinal obstruction syndrome (DIOS; previously known as meconium ileus equivalent), is a common complication in CF (Colombo et al., 2011). Symptoms include abdominal pain, decreased stool output, and right lower quadrant mass. It is important that the diagnosis be established by those familiar with CF care because the management is typically not surgical. Partial DIOS can be treated with rehydration and stool softeners (osmotic laxatives containing polyethylene glycol) or Gastrografin orally via a nasogastric tube or as an enema (Colombo et al., 2011).

Cystic Fibrosis–Associated Liver Disease

CF liver disease (CFLD) is a common complication of CF and often presents subclinically. The most common presentation of CFLD is hepatomegaly with or without change in liver function tests. Annual screening with physical examination, liver function tests, and abdominal ultrasound if concern exists is recommended (Debray et al., 2011). The CF team may consider starting ursodeoxycholic acid. Approximately 3.5% of individuals in the CFF Registry had identified liver disease, and 18 individuals received a liver transplant (CFF, 2021b).

Chronic Sinusitis

Chronic rhinosinusitis (CRS) is common in the CF population, with 37.3% of individuals affected (CFF, 2021c). Chronic congestion, frontal headaches, tenderness to palpation, and purulent nasal discharge are all reported symptoms. The CFF guidelines recommend all individuals with CRS be evaluated by an otolaryngologist and treated with nasal saline irrigation, topical nasal corticosteroids if allergic rhinitis is present, and if refractory to medical management, undergo endoscopic sinus surgery (Kimple et al., 2022). It is reasonable to assume highly effective CFTR modulators will positively impact CRS.

Anxiety and Depression

Symptoms of anxiety and/or depression symptoms are two to three times higher in individuals with CF and their caregivers compared to community samples. They are associated with decreased lung function, lower BMI, worse adherence, worse health-related quality of life, and more frequent hospitalizations (Quittner et al., 2016). In 2015 the CFF and European CF Society published guidelines recommending screening for anxiety (PHQ-9) and depression (GAD-7) in all caregivers and individuals with CF older than 12 years (Quittner et al., 2016). In the CFF Registry, 24.7% of all individuals screened positive for anxiety, and 25.2% screened positive for depression (CFF, 2021b). In those who screen positive it is recommended that referral to a licensed therapist occur. Many CF teams have a dedicated therapist as a part of the team

Osteoporosis and Bone Disease

As the life expectancy of individuals living with CF improves, there is a recognition of the importance of bone health (Stalvey & Clines, 2014). Almost 10.5% of individuals in the CFF Registry had osteopenia (CFF, 2021b). According to CFF guidelines, screening for osteopenia should start at age 18 years unless other risk factors (i.e., broken bones, frequent steroid use) are present. Individuals with normal bone mineral density should undergo dual-energy x-ray absorptiometry (DXA) every 5 years, those with z scores less than 1 but more than 2 every 2 to 4 years, and those with z scores less than 2 every year. Treatment recommendations focus on vitamin D and calcium supplementation while maintaining nutritional status (Aris et al., 2005).

Cystic Fibrosis–Related Diabetes

The incidence of CF-related diabetes (CFRD) is increasing as individuals with CF live longer. With 18.6% of individuals with CF reporting CFRD, it is the most common complication of CF (CFF, 2021b). The pathophysiology of CFRD is different than type 1 or 2 diabetes and may present differently. It is caused by slowly progressive insulin deficiency due to the destruction of pancreatic tissue. CFRD is associated with weight loss, protein catabolism, lung function decline, and increased mortality; thus regular screening is warranted. The CFF guidelines suggest screening for CFRD should start at age 10 years unless other risk factors are present. It is done using a 2-hour oral glucose tolerance test (OGTT). Glucola is dosed at 1.75 g/kg to a maximum dose of 75 g. Specific guidelines exist for normal glucose levels at different time points during the test (fasting and 2-hour glucose) (Moran et al., 2010). Individuals with CFRD should be seen quarterly by a specialized multidisciplinary team with expertise in CFRD. The primary care provider should maintain a high index of suspicion especially in adolescents and children with more severe diseases or nutritional problems.

Other Complications

CF is a multisystem disease with an increased risk of complication and morbidity with age and disease progression. The complications listed in Box 19.3 are more serious and require the expertise of the CF care team. Primary care providers should recognize the early signs and symptoms of these complications to make a timely referral for evaluation and treatment possible.

PROGNOSIS

Discovery of the *CFTR* gene on chromosome 7 in 1989 led to significant excitement in the CF community that a cure would be found. To date, that is not the case, but significant progress toward that goal has been made. Much research surrounds a cure for CF, and the CF community will not stop until CF stands for "cure found." For a child born between 2017 and 2021, the median predicted age of survival is 53 years, up from 38 years just a decade prior. Median lung function in children 10 years of age has improved from FEV_1 87% predicted to FEV_1 100% predicted over the past 20 years (CFF, 2021b). Currently there are more adults living with CF than children. Approximately 30.9% of adults are college graduates, 40% are employed full time, and 45% are married (CFF, 2021b).

PRIMARY CARE MANAGEMENT

HEALTH CARE MAINTENANCE

Growth and Development

With the universal adoption of NBS for CF, failure to thrive, vitamin and mineral deficiencies, stunting, and wasting are identified and managed early and potentially avoided. The infant diagnosed with CF through NBS should be seen at the CF center at 1 to 2 weeks of age, every month until 6 months, and then every 3 months if gaining weight well (Borowitz et al., 2009).

Box 19.3   Serious Complications of Cystic Fibrosis

Hemoptysis
Colonization with highly resistant bacteria
Fungal infections
Allergic bronchopulmonary aspergillosis
Pneumothorax
Pancreatitis
Hyponatremic dehydration
Hypertrophic pulmonary osteoarthropathy
Cor pulmonale
Respiratory failure
Death

The goal for infants with CF is for normal growth, and the CFF recommends that children reach a weight-for-length status of the 75th percentile by 2 years of age, though achieving this goal earlier in infancy is likely beneficial (Stallings et al., 2008). The goal for BMI after the age of 2 years is the 50th percentile. Communication with the primary care provider is very important as the nutritional goals for infants with CF are different ("slightly chubby") than for children without CF.

Visits to the CF center during infancy focus on growth, nutrition, disease understanding, and coping. Weight, length, and head circumference are measured at each visit. Weight in infants is measured without clothes and no or a dry diaper. Weights are plotted on the WHO growth chart until 2 years of age and then transitioned to the CDC (2022a) growth chart. Length is measured on a length board until 2 years of age and then standing without shoes on a stadiometer. Infants who do not achieve expected gains in weight and length or those who are less than the 25th percentile on the growth chart should be followed very closely with appropriate evaluations and interventions made (Borowitz et al., 2009) (Fig. 19.4).

The timing of puberty impacts linear growth, psychosocial well-being, body image, and bone density; therefore assessing pubertal development in a child with CF is important. Historically it was thought that individuals with CF have delayed puberty; however, that is no longer the case in the absence of CFRD, CFLD, and malnutrition (Goldsweig et al., 2019). Pubertal development should be assessed in individuals with CF starting at age 9 in females and age 12 in males. Delayed pubertal development in people with CF requires a full evaluation and referral to an endocrinologist and should not be attributed to CF alone (Goldsweig et al., 2019).

HEADSS Examination

A HEADSS (home, education/employment, activities, drugs, sexuality, suicide/depression) assessment in adolescents with CF should be performed as in the general population (Cohen et al., 1991). The assessment should be performed with the parent out of the room. Particular attention to the dangers of inhaling any kind of smoke should be emphasized because this could cause further progression of lung disease. Emphasizing alcohol avoidance in the CF population is important as many medications interact with alcohol and can further affect the liver. There are ample opportunities for the primary care provider and CF care team to discuss avoidance of high-risk behaviors with adolescents with CF because of their frequent visits to the clinic.

Diet

Individuals with CF maintain a high-calorie, high-fat, high-protein diet. Human breastmilk is recommended as the first choice for nutrition, and if a formula is utilized it should be a cow milk–based formula (Borowitz et al., 2009). Often the formula is underdiluted to allow for higher calories per ounce. Introducing solid foods is the same as in the non-CF population; however, calorie-condensing cereal (i.e., add peanut butter or oil) may be necessary. Infant formula or breastmilk should be continued until 12 months of age, and if growing well the infant could be transitioned to whole milk. A higher-calorie toddler formula is considered if the infant is not meeting expected growth goals.

Attention to abnormal behavioral eating patterns is important during the toddler and preschool years. The CFF recommends for children 2 to 5 years of age that the CF team set energy-intake goals and assess progress on a regular basis. Regular assessment for the presence of mealtime behavior challenges and, if present, referral to a behavioral feeding specialist is recommended (Lahiri et al., 2019). The primary care provider can help families set limits, encourage child feeding autonomy, and avoid grazing between meals.

School-age children should have a basic understanding of the importance of PERT and eating high-calorie foods. Notes to the school can be written to allow for second portions of school lunch by the CF team or primary care provider. Schools do not allow for a long lunchtime, which can be confounded by the child going to the nurse's office for PERT. School-age children often experience taste fatigue with oral supplements and do not want to take their PERT in front of their peers.

Adolescence is a time of rapid growth and may require more attention to diet. It is also a time of more independence, increased activity, and a decline in health. Nutritional counseling will be more effective if directed at the adolescent and parents (Borowitz et al., 2009). The goal for males with CF is a BMI of 23 kg/m², and for females the goal is 22 kg/m².

In the era of highly effective CFTR modulators, obesity is becoming an issue in the CF population. In the CFF Registry, 37% of adults have a BMI in the range categorized by the CDC (2022a) as overweight (26.7%) or obese (10.3%), with a higher prevalence in males (41.3%) than females (32.4%). The percentage of adults who are overweight or obese has more than doubled in the past 20 years (14.3% in 2000) (CFF, 2021b). The causes of excess weight gain in CF are likely multifactorial, including adherence to the high-fat legacy diet, reduced exercise tolerance, therapeutic advances, and

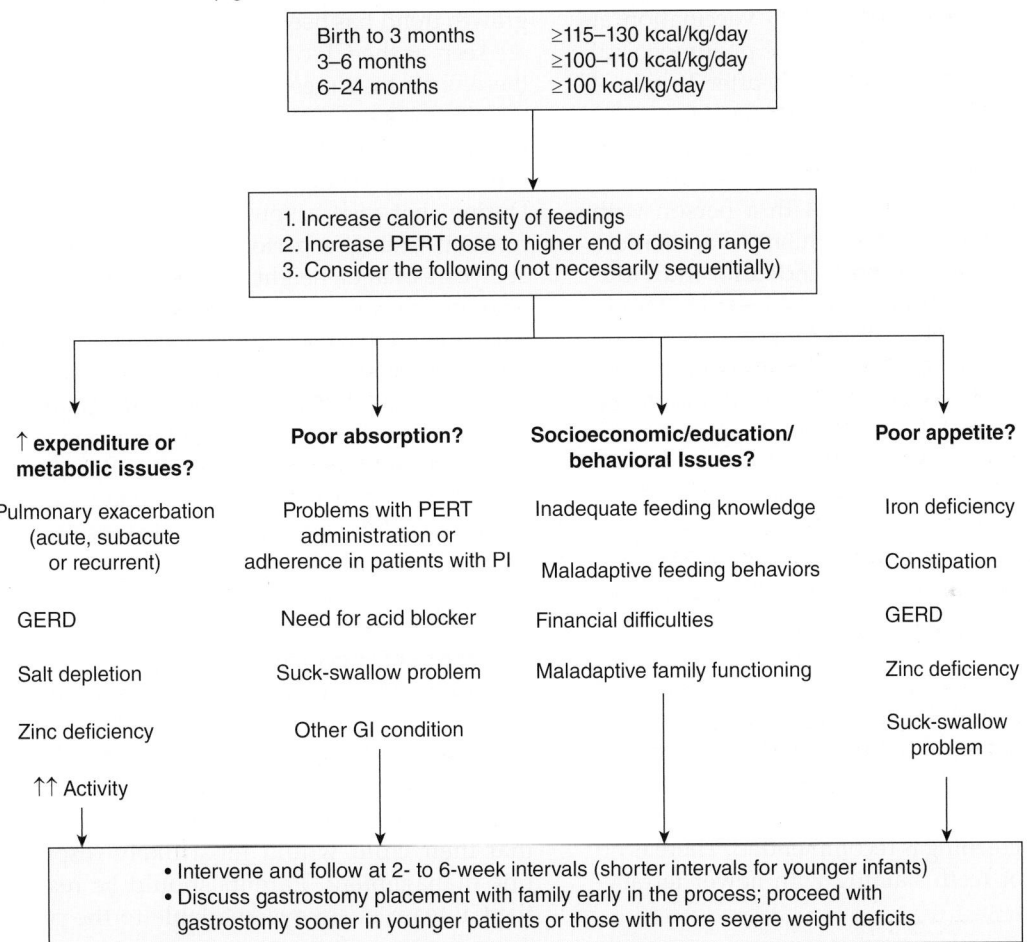

Calculate average daily weight gain since last visit and compare to expected*

Age range	Males (gm/day)	Females (gm/day)	Age range	Males (gm/day)	Females (gm/day)
Birth–1 month	30	26	4–5 months	17	16
1–2 months	35	29	5–6 months	15	14
2–3 months	26	23	6–9 months	10–13	10
3–4 months	20	19	9–24 months	7–10	7–10

Expected weight gain not achieved: refer for dietitian evaluation and assess intake**

Values for weight gain and intake are based on term, well-nourished infants; increased intakes and rates of weight gain are needed for catch-up growth.

Birth to 3 months	≥115–130 kcal/kg/day
3–6 months	≥100–110 kcal/kg/day
6–24 months	≥100 kcal/kg/day

1. Increase caloric density of feedings
2. Increase PERT dose to higher end of dosing range
3. Consider the following (not necessarily sequentially)

↑ expenditure or metabolic issues?

Pulmonary exacerbation (acute, subacute or recurrent)

GERD

Salt depletion

Zinc deficiency

↑↑ Activity

Poor absorption?

Problems with PERT administration or adherence in patients with PI

Need for acid blocker

Suck-swallow problem

Other GI condition

Socioeconomic/education/ behavioral Issues?

Inadequate feeding knowledge

Maladaptive feeding behaviors

Financial difficulties

Maladaptive family functioning

Poor appetite?

Iron deficiency

Constipation

GERD

Zinc deficiency

Suck-swallow problem

- Intervene and follow at 2- to 6-week intervals (shorter intervals for younger infants)
- Discuss gastrostomy placement with family early in the process; proceed with gastrostomy sooner in younger patients or those with more severe weight deficits

Fig. 19.4 Evaluation of infants with weight loss of inadequate weight gain. *GERD,* Gastroesophageal reflux disease; *GI,* gastrointestinal; *PERT,* pancreatic enzyme replacement therapy; *PI,* pancreatic insufficiency. *Based on expected rate of weight gain at the 50th percentile for age from Guo et al. (1991). *Journal of Pediatrics, 119,* 355–362. **Intake values from Beal, V. A. (1970). In McCammon (Ed.). *Human Growth and Development* (pp. 63–100). Charles C. Thomas. (From Borowitz, D., Robinson, K., Rosenfeld, M., et al. [2009]. Cystic Fibrosis Foundation evidence-based guidelines for management of infants with cystic fibrosis. *Journal of Pediatrics, 155,* 30.)

general population trends. Treating obesity in people with CF requires carefully weighing the metabolic risks of overnutrition with the impact of low or falling BMI on lung function (Kutney et al., 2021).

Infection Prevention and Control

Individuals with CF should receive the same age-appropriate anticipatory guidance as their non-CF peers. Special considerations for individuals with CF include infection prevention and control, and there are special considerations for CF. While in the health care setting, all people with CF are in contact isolation regardless of pathogens (gown, glove), should wear a mask outside the clinic room, and minimize the time in common areas outside the CF clinic (Saiman et al., 2014). When in the community, individuals with CF should always stay 6 feet apart, only one person with CF may attend an indoor CFF function, should not be in the same classroom, and practice hand hygiene with alcohol-based hand rub or antimicrobial soap and water when hands could be potentially contaminated with pathogens (Saiman et al., 2014). All CF summer camps, once held solely for individuals with CF, have been closed due to infection prevention concerns.

Immunizations

Infants and children should receive all routine vaccinations at the ages recommended by the CDC (2023). There is no evidence to support a delay in immunizations or avoidance of immunizations. In addition to the routine childhood vaccinations, individuals with CF should receive the Pneumovax-23 vaccination at least 8 weeks after their last dose of the pneumococcal conjugate vaccine (Prevnar 13), usually after 2 years of age. Annual influenza vaccination starting at 6 months is recommended for individuals with CF. Two doses are necessary with the first vaccine and then annually in the fall. Individuals who live with a person with CF should also receive annual influenza vaccination. The COVID-19 vaccine is recommended for individuals with CF older than 6 months and all eligible family members (Lahiri et al., 2019). The American Academy of Pediatrics does not recommend palivizumab prophylaxis for infants with CF; however, it should be considered in infants with evidence of lung disease or nutritional compromise (Fink et al., 2019).

Screenings

Vision. Routine screening is recommended. Before initiating CFTR modulator therapy, a baseline eye exam for cataracts is recommended.

Hearing. Routine screening is recommended. CFF guidelines recommend hearing screening prior to initiation and annually for individuals exposed to ototoxic medications (i.e., aminoglycosides) (Kimple et al., 2022).

Dental. Routine screening is recommended. There is no longer concern for teeth staining with newer tetracycline medications.

Blood pressure. Routine screening is recommended.

Hematocrit. Routine screening is recommended. If abnormal, further studies may be warranted to differentiate between iron deficiency and anemia of chronic illness.

Tuberculosis. Routine screening is no longer recommended for all children with CF unless other risk factors (i.e., homelessness, incarceration, travel to endemic areas) are present.

Condition-Specific Screenings

Individuals with CF should maintain a primary care provider as it is recommended that they receive all routine health care maintenance and developmental assessments that may fall outside the CF center. Routine pediatric visits are at age 1 to 2 weeks and 2, 4, 6, 9, and 12 months in the first year of life; CF center visits should be monthly for the first 6 months and every 1 to 2 months in the second 6 months of life (Borowitz et al., 2009). Collaboration among the family, primary care provider, and a CF-accredited care center is essential, and information about CF and the child's CF care should be provided to the primary care provider (Lahiri et al., 2019). The CFF recommends the primary care provider contact the CF center with any pulmonary or gastrointestinal symptoms.

Typically after reaching 1 year of age, if an acceptable growth trend has been established, individuals with CF are seen at the CF care center every 3 months. During these visits they meet with the multidisciplinary team, which consists of a pharmacist, nurse, respiratory therapist, physical therapist, dietitian, social worker, genetic counselor, psychologist, and primary care provider. During that visit a sputum culture is collected, lung function testing is performed if available (i.e., usually at 5 years of age), height and weight are measured, and ongoing education on their disease is provided. Individuals with CF have an annual visit that includes bloodwork (complete blood count (CBC); comprehensive metabolic panel (CMP); gamma-glutamyl transferase (GGT); immunoglobulin E (IgE) after age 6 years; vitamin A, D, and E levels; prothrombin time/international normalized ratio) and a two-view chest x-ray. At age 10 years, an OGTT is performed, and at age 18 years a DXA scan is performed (Table 19.4).

COMMON ILLNESS MANAGEMENT
Differential Diagnosis

Children with CF will experience symptoms associated with common pediatric illnesses; however, some of these symptoms may be specific to CF and treated differently. Parents should be educated on some common pediatric illnesses and reassured that their child would most likely respond to routine management. Parents should be reassured that the CF team is always available to the primary care provider, and after a thorough history and physical examination the primary care provider will consult with the CF team.

Gastrointestinal Symptoms

Abdominal pain is a common complaint, especially in children with CF. The most common causes of abdominal pain in children include constipation, viral gastroenteritis, or functional abdominal pain; however, in CF, DIOS should also be considered as it is unique to CF. DIOS is complete or incomplete intestinal obstruction by viscid fecal material in the terminal ileum and proximal colon (Colombo et al., 2011). It typically presents with cramping abdominal pain in the right lower quadrant, abdominal distention, weight loss, and poor appetite. Preventing dehydration and optimizing

PERT may decrease the recurrence. The differential diagnosis of DIOS should include chronic constipation, intussusception, appendicitis, volvulus, and fibrosing colonopathy (Colombo et al., 2011). Gastroesophageal reflux disease (GERD) is more common in the CF population, with 36.8% reported (CFF, 2021). Symptoms of GERD are similar in the general and CF populations and include regurgitation, heartburn, and emesis. The diagnosis is generally made clinically. Treatment should initially focus on nonpharmacologic interventions such as thickened feedings, positioning, and timing of chest percussion. The head-down position in infant and child chest percussion should not be used. Dietary changes have a very limited role in managing

---

Table 19.4   Clinical Care Schedule for Newborns to 5-Year-Olds With Cystic Fibrosis

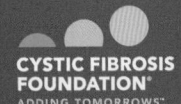

CLINICAL CARE SCHEDULE
FOR NEWBORNS TO 5 YEAR OLDS WITH CYSTIC FIBROSIS

CYSTIC FIBROSIS FOUNDATION®
ADDING TOMORROWS™

Clinical care guidelines for the management of both infants and preschoolers with cystic fibrosis have been published.[1, 2] This table combines the recommended care management schedules from those publications. Please note while this schedule is intended as a guide, individual circumstances will dictate the timing and care provided.

[1] *Infant Care Guidelines:* Cystic Fibrosis F, Borowitz D, Robinson KA, et al. Cystic Fibrosis Foundation evidence-based guidelines for management of infants with cystic fibrosis. The Journal of pediatrics. 2009;155(6 Suppl):S73-93.

[2] *Preschool Guidelines:* Lahiri T, Hempstead SE, Brady C, et al. Clinical Practice Guidelines From the Cystic Fibrosis Foundation for Preschoolers With Cystic Fibrosis. Pediatrics. 2016;137(4).

KEY: ● Do   ○ Consider   ◆ Attempt   ■ Perform Quarterly   Perform at one of these visits

DATE DONE →

AGE AT VISIT	DAY OF SWEAT TEST	24-48 HOURS OF DX	1WK LATER OR AGE 1 MO	2 MO	3 MO	4 MO	5 MO	6 MO	8 MO	10 MO	1 YR	EVERY 2-3 MO. IN THE 2ND YR OF LIFE	2 YR	3 YR	4 YR	5 YR
CARE ISSUES																
Discuss diagnosis			●	○	○	○					●	●	●	●	●	●
NUTRITION																
Assess weight gain, caloric intake, and PERT dosing and CF specific vitamin use		Start PERT and CF specific vitamins	●	●	●	●	●	●	●	●	●	■	■	■	■	
Encourage human milk feeding			●	●	●	●					●					
Salt supplementation	1/8 tsp salt							● Increase to 1/4 tsp salt				● Continue supplement				
History and physical with weight, length, OFC			●	●	●	●	●	●	●	●	●	■	■	■	■	
PULMONARY																
Airway clearance, review airway clearance techniques			● Teach & initiate airway clearance								○	● Assess annually and review technique				
Introduce chronic Dornase Alfa and/or Hypertonic Saline													○	○	○	○
Seasonal influenza vaccination								●	●	●	●	●	●	●	●	●

*Annual labs include: Vitamin levels A,D, E, prothrombin time, serum electroytes BUN creatine glucose, complete blood count, AST/ALT/GGT/ Bili, albumin, ALP

Continued

From CFF.

Table 19.4 Clinical Care Schedule for Newborns to 5-Year-Olds With Cystic Fibrosis—cont'd

KEY: ● Do   ○ Consider   ◆ Attempt   ■ Perform Quarterly   [shaded] Perform at one of these visits

DATE DONE →

AGE AT VISIT	DAY OF SWEAT TEST	24-48 HOURS OF DX	1WK LATER OR AGE 1 MO	2 MO	3 MO	4 MO	5 MO	6 MO	8 MO	10 MO	1 YR	EVERY 2-3 MO. IN THE 2ND YR OF LIFE	2 YR	3 YR	4 YR	5 YR
TESTING AND ASSESSMENTS																
Sweat test and genotyping confirmed documentation	●	○	All 1st° siblings										●	○	○	○
Annual labs*											●		●	●	●	●
NUTRITION/GI																
Pancreatic functional status testing	[shaded]	[shaded]	[shaded]	○	○	○	○	○	○	○	○	○	○	○	○	○
Abdominal pain assessment													■	■	■	■
Set energy and caloric goals and assess progress													●	●	●	●
PULMONARY																
Respiratory culture			●		●			●			●	●	■	■	■	■
Chest radiograph or CT				[shaded]	[shaded]	[shaded]	[shaded]	[shaded]			●		●	○	●	○
Spirometry														◆	◆	■
BEHAVIOR																
Assess ability to sustain daily care				○	○	○	○	○	○	○	○	○	○	○	○	○
Assess for presence of mealtime behavior challenges and provide proactive behavioral assistance						Anticipatory guidance	Anticipatory guidance	Anticipatory guidance	Anticipatory guidance		Anticipatory guidance	Anticipatory guidance	●	●	●	●
EDUCATION																
Teach and assess infection control			●	●	●			●			●		●	●	●	●
Fill out "who to call-where to go" sheet			[shaded]													
Consent and document CFF patient registry				●	●	●	●	●	●	●	●	●	●	●	●	●
Discuss clinical research		○		○	○	○					○		○	○	○	○
Tobacco smoke exposure avoidance education		●	●	●	●	●	●	●	●	●	●	●	●	●	●	●
Genetic counseling	[shaded]	[shaded]	[shaded]	[shaded]				○			○			●	●	●

*Annual labs include: Vitamin levels A,D, E, prothrombin time, serum electroytes BUN creatine glucose, complete blood count, AST/ALT/GGT/ Bili, albumin, ALP

For questions, call 1-800-FIGHT-CF (800-344-4823) or email info@cff.org.

GERD, and the benefits of a high-calorie, high-fat diet in the CF population are well established. The initiation of a proton pump inhibitor (PPI) to suppress gastric acid secretion is an appropriate treatment strategy for those with CF. Often PPIs are also used to help optimize PERT and fat absorption. The need for PPI should be reassessed regularly as there are increasing concerns about side effects, including their effect on bones, pulmonary health, and vitamin B_{12} deficiency. Surgical management (i.e., fundoplication) of GERD in the CF population should be considered after other diagnoses have been excluded, including gastroparesis, CFRD, small intestine bacterial overgrowth, and others. The use of fundoplication in the CF population may not control ongoing GERD or lead to improved nutritional or pulmonary outcomes (Boesch & Acton, 2007).

Fever

Fever associated with pulmonary exacerbations in CF is relatively rare. Fever in the CF population should be evaluated and managed in the general population with antipyretics and hydration with electrolyte-balanced clear liquids. Viral illnesses are detected in many cases of acute exacerbations and may be associated with declining pulmonary function (Asner et al., 2012). In the general population, antibiotic therapy is not considered if the fever is secondary to a viral illness; however, in the CF population, antibiotics are regularly prescribed even if the trigger is thought to be viral (Asner et al., 2012). The typical treatment regimen consists of increased airway clearance and targeted antibiotic therapy based on known organisms from prior respiratory cultures. A viral panel should be obtained if influenza or COVID-19 is suspected. Individuals with CF are at a higher risk for severe disease secondary to influenza or COVID-19 infection, and appropriate antiviral treatment should be strongly considered. Influenza can be treated with oseltamivir in those over 2 weeks of age (CDC, 2022b). COVID-19 can be treated with Paxlovid or bebtelovimab in those over age 12 years and weighing more than 40 kg or remdesivir in those 28 days to 12 years (CDC, 2022b).

Chest Pain

Chest pain is a common complaint in the general and CF populations, which should be evaluated to ensure pneumothorax is not present. Typically pneumothorax is associated with sudden onset of stabbing pain, and frequently a "pop" is experienced. It is diagnosed with clinical history, physical exam, and chest x-ray. Management is stabilization with a chest tube or thoracentesis as needed and consultation with the CF team. Pleurodesis should be cautiously considered in individuals with recurrent pneumothorax as it could make lung transplantation more difficult.

Other causes of chest pain include costochondritis, which is a musculoskeletal cause of chest pain. It is classically reproduced with palpation of the chest wall.

It is treated with antiinflammatory medications, heat packs, and rest. Chest pain secondary to pleural inflammation during an acute exacerbation is not uncommon. This pain is typically worse with deep inspiration and is not reproducible with palpation. Individuals often endorse an increase in cough and sputum production. Treatment aims to treat the underlying cause with increased airway clearance and oral or inhaled antibiotics. The primary care provider should involve the CF team when making decisions about the etiology and treatment of chest pain in individuals with CF.

Cough

Cough is often considered the hallmark of CF lung disease and is caused by thick and sticky mucus that is not cleared from the lower airways. When cough presents, it is different in all individuals with CF and should always be treated aggressively with increased airway clearance and antibiotics targeted at pathogens in the sputum. The CF center should be notified whenever a cough develops, and treatment initiated. With earlier diagnosis by NBS and implementation of CFTR modulators, it is possible to prevent a chronic cough. Based on a questionnaire, individuals treated with elexacaftor/tezacaftor/ivacaftor showed a 63% decrease in pulmonary exacerbations and respiratory symptoms (Sutharsan et al., 2022). Individuals with CF should be encouraged to cough, and cough suppressants should never be used to mask cough. It is important for the primary care provider to notify the CF team anytime an individual with CF develops a new or increased cough.

Wheezing

Wheezing in infants and toddlers is very common in the general and CF populations and is often triggered by a viral infection. Evidence is insufficient to recommend for or against the chronic use of inhaled bronchodilators; however, the routine use of inhaled corticosteroids is not recommended (Lahiri et al., 2019). If a significant family history of asthma, personal atopy, or significant response to a bronchodilator is present, it is reasonable to treat it with a bronchodilator and/or inhaled steroids. The CFF Registry reports 25.9% are younger than 18 years, and 30.8% of the entire CF population have asthma diagnoses (CFF, 2021). As in the general population, other causes of wheezing must be considered, such as foreign body aspiration, bronchiolitis, tracheobronchomalacia, recurrent aspiration, and GERD.

DEVELOPMENTAL ISSUES
Sleep Patterns

Sleep is an important component of general health and normal development in children, and insufficient sleep, sleep disruption, and sleep-disordered breathing have physical and psychological consequences. Many factors can be disruptive for individuals with

CF, including chronic cough, GERD, abdominal pain, frequent stooling, and medication side effects. Objective and subjective measurements can indicate reduced sleep efficiency, such as the time spent asleep as the percentage of time spent in bed, in children with CF compared to children without CF (Reiter et al., 2017). Also, children with CF are expected to complete at least 30 minutes of treatments prior to starting their day, resulting in an earlier wakeup time. The severity of lung disease is closely associated with poorer sleep quality. With the progression of lung disease, a low threshold for noninvasive nighttime respiratory support should be considered. If a clinical history of snoring is obtained, a diagnosis of obstructive sleep apnea should be explored with a sleep study and referral to otolaryngology for consideration of tonsillectomy and adenoidectomy. Consideration of anxiety and/or depression should be assessed in the individual with poor sleep. It is important to help families maintain a consistent bedtime ritual appropriate for their developmental stage at home and in the hospital if hospitalized.

Toileting

Toilet training should begin when clear signs of readiness are present. These signs may include pulling at a wet or dirty diaper, hiding poop, showing interest in others' use of the toilet, or having a dry diaper for a longer time. Most children show signs of bowel and bladder awareness between 18 and 24 months, but most are not ready to be toilet trained until closer to 24 to 36 months. Children with CF may be delayed in toilet training as they may have more frequent and runnier stools even with adequate PERT. Children with CF who require high-calorie supplements before bed or nighttime enteral feedings will have a harder time staying dry during the night. When the child with CF starts school, permission for unrestricted and possibly private bathroom privileges should be put into place as stools may be excessive, urgent, malodorous, and an embarrassment for children and adolescents with CF.

In adolescent and adult females with CF, urinary incontinence is common secondary to progressive pelvic floor muscle weakness and recurrent coughing episodes. Often symptoms are not reported due to embarrassment and a lack of knowledge of treatment options. In individuals with CF age 6 to 21 years, 56.3% report symptoms of urinary incontinence, 12.5% report fecal incontinence, and 31.2% report combined symptoms (Neemuchwala et al., 2020). Most CF care teams include a physical therapist, with exercises directed at strengthening the pelvic muscles, which should be implemented. Primary care providers should assess the degree of incontinence because it can cause anxiety and embarrassment for individuals with CF.

Discipline

Most CF diagnoses are through NBS, with a median age of diagnosis at 3 months and frequently much earlier (CFF, 2021c). One of the main developmental

goals during infancy is the attachment between parent and child. The quality of the attachment can predict important psychosocial factors, such as emotional and behavioral regulation, social skills, and the inability to manage stress (Ernst et al., 2010). During this time, it is important to screen parents for symptoms of depression and help implement developmentally appropriate effective routines around both general daily activities and CF-specific treatment tasks.

During the preschool developmental stage, children become more verbal and may start to resist therapies. The increased opportunities for parent/child conflict may alter parenting strategies such that parents may become more authoritative or more permissive due to parenting resources stretched thin by a chronic illness or overprotection (Ernst et al., 2010). It is important for parents to use the same parenting style with children with and without CF and not allow the non-CF child to feel left out. Problematic behavioral issues surrounding mealtime may present during this time, and behavioral therapy should be instituted by the team psychologist early (Borowitz et al., 2009). Helping families maintain healthy family dynamics despite the treatment burden is a priority for children at this age.

The school-age period is characterized by evolving cognitive skills and an increased emphasis on peer relationships. It is essential that children's sense of ownership and control over their chronic illness be encouraged during this period to develop skills and self-efficacy related to self-management throughout their lifespan (Ernst et al., 2010). During this time, children generally engage in sports, dance, and other activities that make for a hectic home life, making completing CF care more challenging. It is important not to make the child with CF feel different or miss out on activities due to the need for therapies. Screening for anxiety and depression should start in this age group, and behavioral and cognitive-behavioral therapies should be instituted if it is identified. Normalizing parental thoughts that their child with CF is vulnerable, encouraging developmentally appropriate behavior expectations, and allowing children to learn from their mistakes, is important (Ernst et al., 2010).

Adolescence is a time of rapid social, cognitive, and physiological changes, and the proportion of time spent with peers increases relative to family time, with peers also becoming more influential (Ernst et al., 2010). While parents try to encourage more independence with therapies, they are often frustrated and anxious because this is when disease progression may start; however, this is uncertain in the era of highly effective CFTR modulator therapies. Teens who generally feel well may not see the long-term benefit of airway clearance and other therapies and may start to skip therapies or shorten treatment time. Generally, therapies with more short-term consequences (i.e., PERT) are easier for the adolescent to maintain compliance. During this time, most CF care centers have a transition clinic where the adolescent is seen without their parent present, which can cause some anxiety on the part of the parent. It is important for the CF team and primary care provider to start addressing the adolescent rather than the parent. The CF team and primary care provider need to address high-risk behaviors such as drinking, drugs, smoking, and sexual intercourse and the consequences on their health.

Child Care

Parents of children with CF often struggle with child care decisions. The primary care provider and CF team should discuss options with families, including day care centers, in-home day care, and nannies. The family's financial status and what is available in the community may impact the decision. The biggest concern most family members express is exposure to germs and infections (CFF, 2021c). The primary medication the care provider will need to be educated about is PERT. Communication with the child care center is important because measures (i.e., hand sanitizer, frequent hand washing, physical distance from others with symptoms) can be implemented to minimize exposures. It is important to discuss any guilt parents may have with putting their child in child care and normalize that feeling. Once parents see their child with CF thriving in child care, those feelings are often lifted.

Schooling

Individuals with CF are not affected cognitively and should be encouraged to attend school; however, certain accommodations may need to be considered. For this reason, parents should disclose the diagnosis with school officials, teachers, principals, coaches, and school nurses. It is helpful for the student to have an individualized education plan (IEP) or 504 plan in place so others understand what accommodations should exist.

Many students with CF will need to take PERT with meals and snacks and have access to snacks during the school day as well as seconds at lunchtime. It is helpful for students with CF to self-administer PERT when old enough so they do not miss out on activities or lunchtime. Students with CF need to have access to water or electrolyte-containing drinks, especially with exercise. It is not necessary to restrict these students during physical education class or other activities, and they should be encouraged to participate. Unrestricted bathroom access is important for students with CF as the urge to stool is sometimes urgent. Access to a private bathroom (i.e., in the nurse's office) should be considered, as the stools and gas associated with CF can be foul smelling. Teachers and families should be aware that a child with CF who has issues with flatulence may be the target of bullying. If bullying does occur, it should be dealt with immediately.

Students with CF may be fatigued due to early-morning treatments and may be absent more than others due to illness or clinic visits. Teachers should provide accommodation for absenteeism and help these students make up work. If individuals with CF are hospitalized, they may miss up to 2 weeks of school. It is important for the hospital teacher to collaborate with the schoolteacher and obtain work while in the hospital.

A main concern parents of children with CF have when entering school is germs. There are recommendations from the CFF regarding hand hygiene with soap and water or hand sanitizer. Students should avoid sharing personal items such as straws and eating utensils. Teachers should encourage students to cover their cough or sneeze with a tissue or inner elbow. Teachers need to understand that individuals with CF will intermittently cough; however, it is not contagious, and they do not need to be sent home from school. This was a big concern during the COVID-19 pandemic, and families of children with CF had to educate teachers on the issue. While lung infections in people with CF pose no danger to the public, they do pose a significant danger to others with CF. If there is more than one student with CF at the school (not siblings), they should maintain at least a 6-foot distance from each other. Ideally, they should be in different classrooms.

Sexuality

Males with CF have normal male characteristics and sexual function; however, it is estimated that 98% of males with CF are infertile due to azoospermia related to the complete or partial agenesis of the vas deferens. Adolescent and young adult males must understand that infertility does not affect sexual function or potency. It is also important to emphasize to males that reproductive technology can help them have a biological child. Evidence suggests adolescents and young adult men are underinformed and want more information about the assessment and management of infertility as well as sexually transmitted infections (STI). Although infertility is a common finding in males with CF, there have been reports of males with normal semen analysis; therefore it is recommended that contraception should be used during sexual intercourse to avoid unwanted pregnancy and STI (Tsang et al., 2010).

Females with CF generally have reproductive anatomy like those without CF, but abnormal CFTR function can lead to viscous, pH-imbalanced cervical secretions that lead to subfertility in some females. With the substantial gains in health experienced by people with CF over the last 20 years, the number of females who desire families and are becoming pregnant is increasing. It is likely that CFTR modulators increase fertility in females with CF, but the safety of their use in pregnancy and lactation is understudied. A CFF therapeutics–funded study, Maternal and Fetal Outcomes in the Era of Modulators (MAYFLOWERS), will prospectively evaluate the impact of this class of drugs on the health of females with CF and their infants (Taylor-Cousar, 2020). The number of pregnancies in females with CF increased from 210 in 2011 to 675 in 2021 (CFF, 2021b). Given these numbers, the primary care provider needs to counsel females with CF about birth control measures.

Females with CF who pursue pregnancy should be counseled on the effect of pregnancy on their health. The future father should undergo genetic screening for CF so the risk of having a baby with CF is fully understood because the baby will be an obligate carrier. In addition to routine pre-pregnancy care, it is imperative in the CF pregnancy that careful attention is given to maintaining pulmonary health and nutrition, medications administered during pregnancy, and surveillance and treatment of diabetes. The pregnant females with CF must be cared for by an interdisciplinary team, including the CF care team, a high-risk obstetrician, and the primary care provider. It is extremely important for good communication among team members (Geake et al., 2014).

Transition to Adulthood

Earlier diagnosis through NBS and advances in CF treatment have led to significantly improved outcomes and greater life expectancy. Currently 58.3% of individuals living with CF are older than 18 years (CFF, 2021a). Recognizing the unique needs of adults with CF, the CFF convened a consensus conference in 1999 to address care standards for adults with CF. CFF-sponsored benchmarking studies of high-performing adult and pediatric CF programs found that patient outcomes were more closely related to care systems, attitudes, practices, patient/family involvement, and improvement projects than to any specific care elements (Boyle et al., 2014). The CFF consensus guidelines suggest the concept of transition should be introduced early, and at many centers this is part of the initial visit during infancy. A successful transition requires effective communication between the pediatric and adult care teams to achieve a thorough understanding of the patient prior to transfer. Many CF centers have a specific transition clinic that allows adolescents to be seen without a parent present with the goal of assuming more and more responsibility and independence for self-care and decision making, health education, and training (CFF, 2021c). The CFF recommends that all individuals with CF should be cared for in an adult center by age 21 but recognizes that this can be individualized and may happen earlier. CF RISE (responsibility, independence, self-care, education) is a tool endorsed by the CFF that is available to help the transitioning individual become more independent (Baker et al., 2015).

Family Concerns

Caring for a child with CF can be difficult and time consuming. Parents experience stress and anxiety at every new disease milestone, including diagnosis, first exacerbation, weight loss, first hospitalization, and starting new medications. It is important to incorporate the care required into everyday life and not exclude an individual with CF from activities because of therapies. Offering a CF mentor to a newly diagnosed family can help normalize the diagnosis and allow for support from someone further along in the CF journey. The care team needs to acknowledge the stress and possibly anxiety or depression experienced by caregivers of those with CF. The CFF recommends screening all caregivers of those with CF annually (Quittner et al., 2016). It is important for families to feel they can have open and honest conversations with the CF care team and the primary care provider.

People living with CF and their families face complicated issues related to getting the care they need. Many of the newer medications are expensive and cause financial burdens for families. Navigating insurance coverage and the language associated with insurance (e.g., copayment, deductible, preferred provider organization, health maintenance organization) make understanding difficult. The CFF (n.d.) has a resource tool called CF Foundation Compass, which provides one-on-one service for people living with CF. Families are paired with a case manager who helps with complex challenges, including understanding insurance basics, troubleshooting insurance coverage issues, seeking financial assistance for medical care and other living expenses, and finding answers to legal questions related to work, school, disability/government benefits, and much more (see Resources). The CF team social worker is also an invaluable resource for families.

Although the life expectancy of those living with CF has dramatically improved with the use of CFTR modulators, it is still considered a life-shortening disease, and end-of-life issues may need to be addressed. A committee to look at the use of palliative care in the CF population established the following definition: "Palliative care focuses on reducing physical and emotional symptoms and improving quality of life for people with CF throughout their lives. Palliative care occurs alongside usual treatments and is individualized according to the unique goals, hopes, and values of each person with CF" (Kavalieratos et al., 2021). The CFF recommends for individuals with CF ages 12 years to adulthood the integrated palliative care outcome scale (IPOS) be administered annually and at disease milestones. For children with CF under age 12 years, the IPOS should guide conversations with children and caregivers annually and at disease milestones. The IPOS allows the care teams to explore problems related to physical and psychological symptoms, social and spiritual issues, communication, information needs, and practical concerns. Together, primary care providers and the CF care team can help prepare individuals and their families for the decisions they will face at the end of life.

RESOURCES

Cystic Fibrosis Foundation: www.cff.org
CF Foundation Compass: www.cff.org/support/get-help-cf-foundation-compass
National CFF Chapter of Maryland: www.cff.org/chapters/maryland-chapter
North American Cystic Fibrosis Conference: nacfconference.org

Summary

Primary Care Needs for the Child With Cystic Fibrosis

HEALTH CARE MAINTENANCE
Growth and Development
- Malnutrition and growth delay are common complications, but catchup growth can be achieved with proper nutritional therapy and treatment for pulmonary complications.
- Careful surveillance of growth is essential.
- Pubertal development is often delayed.
- Pubertal development should be assessed in those with CF: females at age 9 years and males at age 12 years.
- Assessment of bone health is essential, especially for those with specific risk factors.

Diet
- Goal is to promote normal growth.
- Breastfeeding is encouraged.
- Diet is well-balanced, high-protein, high-calorie plan with unrestricted fat that promotes 110% to 200% of recommended dietary allowances.
- Important to play close attention to abnormal behavioral eating patterns.
- Nutritional issues correlate with age of the child and severity of the child's disease.

Safety
- Emphasize safe storage of multiple medications.
- Use sunscreen or avoid sun when on antibiotics.
- Perform hand hygiene at routine times, such as before and after coughing, as well as with therapies that expose others with CF.

Immunizations
- All routine immunizations should generally be given on schedule.
- Influenza vaccine should be given annually per CDC (2023) guidelines, internasal vaccine is not recommended.
- RSV immunizations for those with additional risk factors should be used in CF.
- Pneumococcal vaccine should be administered to all children with CF age 2 years and older.
- COVID-19 vaccination should be started at 6 months of age.

Screenings
- *Vision.* Routine screening is recommended. Before initiating CFTR modulator therapy, a baseline eye exam for cataracts is recommended.
- *Hearing.* Routine screening is recommended. Hearing screening prior to initiation and annually for individuals exposed to ototoxic medications.
- *Dental.* Routine care and screening. No longer concerns for teeth staining with newer tetracycline medications.
- *Hematocrit.* Routine screening is recommended with full review of iron status as indicated.
- *Blood pressure.* Measure at every visit for those on corticosteroids.
- *Tuberculosis.* Routine screening is no longer recommended. Screen only those who are at increased risk of acquiring tuberculosis.
- *Condition-specific screening.* Pulmonary function test, chest roentgenography, sputum culture with antibiotic sensitivities, blood, and urine assays of liver and renal function, DXA bone scan, OGTT, complete blood count, and serum and anthropometric measures of nutritional status are monitored at routine CF center visits.

- Screening for those with CF who are older than 12 years for anxiety is recommended (PHQ-9) and for depression (GAD-7).
- Screening for CFRD should begin at age 10 years.

COMMON ILLNESS MANAGEMENT
Differential Diagnosis
- *Constipation or diarrhea.* Rule out DIOS.
- *Abdominal pain.* Rule out DIOS, gallstones, pancreatitis, appendicitis, intussusception, fibrosing colonopathy, volvulus.
- *Fever.* Prevention of hyponatremia and dehydration. A viral panel should be obtained if influenza or COVID-19 is suspected.
- *Chest pain.* Rule out pneumothorax, musculoskeletal strain, pleural inflammation, GERD.
- *Cough/wheezing.* Differentiation between asthma, exacerbation of CF, rhinitis, and/or sinusitis will help select treatment.

Drug Interactions/Substance Abuse
- *Corticosteroids.* Increased risk for gastrointestinal ulceration with high-dose nonsteroidal antiinflammatory drugs (e.g., ibuprofen). Itraconazole and ketoconazole can decrease clearance of steroids.
- *Ciprofloxacin.* Avoid antacids, zinc, or calcium supplements concurrently. Avoid ultraviolet exposure.
- *Herbal supplements.* Many can have potential side effects or interactions.
- *Tobacco smoke.* Those with chronic respiratory disease are most vulnerable to passive smoke.
- *Alcohol.* Detrimental effects if abused, especially because people with CF have increased liver disease and malnutrition.

DEVELOPMENTAL ISSUES
Sleep Patterns
- Sleep patterns may be altered with acute exacerbation or progression of disease because of increased cough and decreased oxyhemoglobin saturation.
- Early-morning routines may require adjustment of bedtime.
- Difficulty falling asleep may be a sign of depression.
- Snoring may be related to obstructive sleep apnea.

Toileting
- Delayed bowel training may occur, secondary to increased frequency of stools and associated abdominal cramping.
- Provide privacy for toileting.
- Stress urinary incontinence is common in CF.

Discipline
- Expectation should be normal with allowances during periods of acute illnesses.
- Encourage independence in CF management with child/adolescent having some control over treatment choices.
- Individual and family counseling are indicated when needed.

Child Care
- Assist parents in making appropriate child care choices and educational providers.
- In-home or small group child care is preferred to reduce exposure to infectious diseases.

Continued

Schooling

- Education of school officials is imperative. Development of an IEP or 502 plan is beneficial.
- Allow child to carry own enzymes, if possible.
- School schedule may need to be altered as the disease progresses.
- Unrestricted bathroom access (i.e., the nurse's office) is needed.
- Provide privacy for coughing episodes.
- A child with CF may be a target for bullying (this needs to be dealt with immediately).
- Avoid dehydration with physical activities and sports.
- School performance may be affected by fatigue and coughing related to impending pulmonary exacerbation.
- CF does not affect one's intellectual/academic performance.

Sexuality

- It is estimated that 98% of males are infertile; sperm count recommended for males.
- Provide education about STI and prevention.
- Genetic counseling for anyone with CF considering having a biological child.
- Females contemplating pregnancy need counseling regarding their and their child's risks.
- Frequent use of antibiotics can cause fungal vaginitis.

Transition to Adulthood

- Prepare for transition by increasing independence and self-management in pre- and adolescence.
- Transition to adult primary care provider and CF care center is recommended by age 21 years.

Family Concerns

- Despite a multitude of special concerns, including the stress of its prognosis, financial burden, and uncertainty of illness, most families adjust well.
- Provide open and honest communication.
- Provide multidisciplinary team support.
- End-of-life care often is a mix of preventive, therapeutic, and palliative treatments.

REFERENCES

Aris, R. M., Merkel, P. A., Bachrach, L. K., Borowitz, D. S., Boyle, M. P., Elkin, S. L., Guise, T. A., Hardin, D. S., Haworth, C. S., Holick, M. F., Joseph, P. M., O'Brien, K., Tullis, E., Watts, N. B., & White, T. B. (2005). Guide to bone health and disease in cystic fibrosis. *Journal of Clinical Endocrinology and Metabolism, 90*(3), 1888–1896. doi:10.1210/jc.2004-1629. Epub 2004 Dec 21. PMID: 15613415.

Asner, S., Waters, V., Solomon, M., Yau, Y., Richardson, S. E., Grasemann, H., Gharabaghi, F., & Tran, D. (2012). Role of respiratory viruses in pulmonary exacerbations in children with cystic fibrosis. *Journal of Cystic Fibrosis, 11*(5), 433–439. doi:10.1016/j.jcf.2012.04.006. Epub 2012 May 10. PMID: 22579414; PMCID: PMC7105203.

Awatade, N. T., Wong, S. L., Hewson, C. K., Fawcett, L. K., Kicic, A., Jaffe, A., & Waters, S. A. (2018). Human primary epithelial cell models: Promising tools in the era of cystic fibrosis personalized medicine. *Frontiers in Pharmacology, 9*, 1429. doi:10.3389/fphar.2018.01429. PMID: 30581387; PMCID: PMC6293199.

Baker, A., Riekert, K., Sawicki, G., & Eakin, M. (2015). CF RISE: Implementing a clinic-based transition program. *Pediatric Allergy, Immunology, and Pulmonology, 28*(4).

Blanchart, A. C., Horton, E., Stanojevic, S., Taylor, L., Waters, V., & Ratjen, F. (2017). Effectiveness of a stepwise *Pseudomonas aeruginosa* eradication protocol in children with cystic fibrosis. *Journal of Cystic Fibrosis, 16*(3), 395.

Boesch, R., & Acton, J. (2007). Outcomes of fundoplication in children with cystic fibrosis. *Journal of Pediatric Surgery, 42*(8), 1341.

Borowitz, D., Robinson, K. A., Rosenfeld, M., Davis, S. D., Sabadosa, K. A., Spear, S. L., Michel, S. H., Parad, R. B., White, T. B., Farrell, P. M., Marshall, B. C., & Accurso, F. J. (2009). Cystic Fibrosis Foundation evidence-based guidelines for management of infants with cystic fibrosis. *Journal of Pediatrics, 155*(6 Suppl), S73–93. doi:10.1016/j.jpeds.2009.09.001. PMID: 19914445; PMCID: PMC6324931.

Boyle, M. P., Sabadose, K. A., Quinton, H. B., Marshall, B. C., & Schechter, M. S. (2014). Key findings of the US Cystic Fibrosis Foundations' clinical practice benchmarking project. *BMJ Quality Safety, 23*, i15–i22.

Carlyle, B. E., Borowitz, D. S., & Glick, P. L. (2012). A review of pathophysiology and management of fetuses and neonates with meconium ileus for the pediatric surgeon. *Journal of Pediatric Surgery, 47*(4), 772–781.

Centers for Disease Control and Prevention. (2022a). Growth charts. https://www.cdc.gov/growthcharts/.

Centers for Disease Control and Prevention. (2022b). Influenza antiviral medications: Summary for clinicians. https://www.cdc.gov/flu/professionals/antivirals/summary-clinicians.htm.

Centers for Disease Control and Prevention. (2023). Immunization schedules. https://www.cdc.gov/vaccines/schedules/index.html.

Cohen, E., Mackenzie, R., & Yates, G. (1991). HEADSS, a psychosocial risk assessment instrument: Implications for designing effective intervention programs for runaway youth. *Journal of Adolescent Health, 12*(7), 539–544.

Colombo, C., Ellemunter, H., Houwen, R., Munck, A., Taylor, C., & Wilschanski, M.: ECFS. (2011). Guidelines for the diagnosis and management of distal intestinal obstruction syndrome in cystic fibrosis patients. *Journal of Cystic Fibrosis, 10*(Suppl 2), S24.

Cystic Fibrosis Foundation. (2021a). *Patient registry 2010 annual data report to the center directors.* Bethesda, MD: Author.

Cystic Fibrosis Foundation. *Patient registry highlights 2021b.* Bethesda, MD: Author.

Cystic Fibrosis Foundation. About cystic fibrosis. 2021c. https://www.cff.org/What-is-CF/About-Cystic-Fibrosis. Accessed October 19, 2022.

Cystic Fibrosis Foundation. (n.d.). CF Foundation compass. https://www.cff.org/support/get-help-cf-foundation-compass.

Davies, J. C., Wainwright, C. E., Canny, G. J., Chilvers, M. A., Howenstine, M. S., Munck, A., Mainz, J. G., Rodriguez, S., Li, H., Yen, K., Ordoñez, C. L., & Ahrens, R.; VX08-770-103 (ENVISION) Study Group. (2013). Efficacy and safety of ivacaftor in patients aged 6 to 11 years with cystic fibrosis with a G551D mutation. *American Journal of Respiratory and Critical Care Medicine, 187*(11), 1219–1225. doi:10.1164/rccm.201301-0153OC. PMID: 23590265; PMCID: PMC3734608.

Davis, P. B. (2006). Cystic fibrosis since 1938. *American Journal of Respiratory and Critical Care Medicine, 173*, 475–482.

Debray, D., Kelly, D., Houwen, R., Strandvik, B., & Colombo, C. (2011). Best practice guidance for the diagnosis and management of cystic fibrosis-associated liver disease. *Journal of Cystic Fibrosis, 10*(Suppl 2), S29–S36.

El-Chammas, K., Rumman, N., Goh, V., Quintero, D., & Goday, P. (2015). Rectal prolapse and cystic fibrosis. *Journal of Pediatric Gastroenterology and Nutrition, 60*(1), 110–112.

Ernst, M. M., Johnson, M. C., & Stark, L. J., (2010). Developmental and psychosocial issues in CF. *Child and Adolescent Psychiatric Clinics of North America, 19*(2), 263–283.

Farrell, P. M., White, T. B., Ren, C. L., Hempstead, S. E., Accurso, F., Derichs, N., Howenstine, M., McColley, S. A., Rock, M., Rosenfeld, M., Sermet-Gaudelus, I., Southern, K. W., Marshall, B. C., & Sosnay, P. R. (2017). Diagnosis of cystic fibrosis: Consensus guidelines from the cystic fibrosis foundation. *Journal of Pediatrics, 181S,* S4–S15.e1. doi:10.1016/j.jpeds.2016.09.064.

Fink, A., Graff, G., Byington, C., Loeffler, D., Rosenfeld, M., & Saiman, L. (2019). Palivizumab and long-term outcomes in cystic fibrosis. *Pediatrics, 144*(1), e20183495.

Flume, P. A., Mogayzel, P. J. Jr., Robinson, K. A., Goss, C. H., Rosenblatt, R. L., Kuhn, R. J., & Marshall, B. C.; Clinical Practice Guidelines for Pulmonary Therapies Committee. (2009). Cystic fibrosis pulmonary guidelines: Treatment of pulmonary exacerbations. *American Journal of Respiratory and Critical Care Medicine, 180*(9), 802–808. doi:10.1164/rccm.200812-1845PP. Epub 2009 Sep 3. PMID: 19729669.

Flume, P. A., Robinson, K. A., O'Sullivan, B. P., et al. (2009). Cystic fibrosis pulmonary guidelines: Airway clearance therapies. *Respiratory Care, 54*(4), 522–537.

Geake, J., Tay, G., Callaway, L., & Bell, S. (2014). Pregnancy and cystic fibrosis: Approach to contemporary management. *Obstetric Medicine, 7*(4), 147–155.

Goetz, D., & Ren, C. (2019). Review of cystic fibrosis. *Pediatric Annals, 48*(4).

Goldsweig, B., Kaminski, B., Sidhaye, A., Blackman, S., & Kelly, A. (2019). Puberty in cystic fibrosis. *Journal of Cystic Fibrosis, 18,* S88–S94.

Hamosh, A., FitzSimmons, S., Macek, M., Knowles, M., Rosenstein, B., & Cutting, G. (1998). Comparison of the clinical manifestations of cystic fibrosis in black and white patients. *Journal of Pediatrics, 132*(2), 255–259.

Kapnadak, S. G., Dimango, E., Hadjiliadis, D., et al. (2020). Cystic Fibrosis Foundation consensus guidelines for the care of individuals with advanced cystic fibrosis lung disease. *Journal of Cystic Fibrosis, 19*(3), 344.

Kavalieratos, D., Georgiopoulos, A. M., Dhingra, L., Basile, M. J., Rabinowitz, E., Hempstead, S. E., Faro, A., & Dellon, E. P. (2021). Models of palliative care delivery for individuals with cystic fibrosis: Cystic Fibrosis Foundation evidence-informed consensus guidelines. *Journal of Palliative Medicine, 24*(1), 18–30. doi:10.1089/jpm.2020.0311. Epub 2020 Sep 16. PMID: 32936045; PMCID: PMC7757696.

Kharrazi, M., Yang, J., Bishop, T., Lessing, S., Young, S., Graham, S., Pearl, M., Chow, H., Ho, T., Currier, R., Gaffney, L., & Feuchtbaum, L.; California Cystic Fibrosis Newborn Screening Consortium. (2015). Newborn screening for cystic fibrosis in california. *Pediatrics, 136*(6), 1062–1072. doi:10.1542/peds.2015-0811. Epub 2015 Nov 16. PMID: 26574590.

Kiedrowski, M., & Bomberger, J. (2018). Viral-bacterial co-infections in the cystic fibrosis respiratory tract. *Frontiers in Immunology, 9,* 3067.

Kimple, A. J., Senior, B. A., Naureckas, E. T., Gudis, D. A., Meyer, T., Hempstead, S. E., Resnick, H. E., Albon, D., Barfield, W., Benoit, M. M., Beswick, D. M., Callard, E., Cofer, S., Downer, V., Elson, E. C., Garinis, A., Halderman, A., Hamburger, L., Helmick, M., ... Lee, S. E. (2022). Cystic Fibrosis Foundation otolaryngology care multidisciplinary consensus recommendations. *International Forum of Allergy and Rhinology, 12*(9), 1089–1103. doi:10.1002/alr.22974. Epub 2022 Feb 22. PMID: 35089650; PMCID: PMC9545592.

Konstan, M. W., Flume, P. A., Kappler, M., Chiron, R., Higgins, M., Brockhaus, F., Zhang, J., Angyalosi, G., He, E., & Geller, D. E. (2011). Safety, efficacy and convenience of tobramycin inhalation powder in cystic fibrosis patients: The EAGER trial. *Journal of Cystic Fibrosis, 10*(1), 54–61. doi:10.1016/j.jcf.2010.10.003. Epub 2010 Nov 12. PMID: 21075062; PMCID: PMC4086197.

Konstan, M. W., Wagener, J. S., Pasta, D. J., Millar, S. J., Jacobs, J. R., Yegin, A., & Morgan, W. J.; Scientific Advisory Group and Investigators and Coordinators of Epidemiologic Study of Cystic Fibrosis. (2011). Clinical use of dornase alpha is associated with a slower rate of FEV1 decline in cystic fibrosis. *Pediatric Pulmonology, 46*(6) 545–553. doi:10.1002/ppul.21388. Epub 2011 Mar 24. PMID: 21438174; PMCID: PMC4109161.

Kutney, K., Sndouk, Z., Desimone, M., & Moheet, A. (2021). Obesity in cystic fibrosis. *Journal of Clinical and Translational Endocrinology, 26,* 100276.

Lahiri, T., Hempstead, S. E., Brady, C., Cannon, C. L., Clark, K., Condren, M. E., Guill, M. F., Guillerman, R. P., Leone, C. G., Maguiness, K., Monchil, L., Powers, S. W., Rosenfeld, M., Schwarzenberg, S. J., Tompkins, C. L., Zemanick, E. T., & Davis, S. D. (2016). Clinical practice guidelines from the cystic fibrosis foundation for preschoolers with cystic fibrosis. *Pediatrics, 137*(4), e20151784. doi:10.1542/peds.2015-1784. Epub 2016 Mar 23. PMID: 27009033.

Langfelder-Schwind, E., Kloza, E., Sugarman, E., & Pettersen, B. (2005). NSGC Subcommittee on Cystic Fibrosis Carrier Testing. Cystic fibrosis prenatal screening in genetic counseling practice: Recommendations of the National Society of Genetic Counselors.

McGarry, M. E., & McColley, S. A. (2021). Cystic fibrosis patients of minority race and ethnicity less likely eligible for CFTR modulators based on CFTR genotype. *Pediatric Pulmonology, 56*(6), 1496.

Middleton, P. G., & Taylor-Cousar, J. L. (2021). Development of elexacaftor-tezacaftor-ivacaftor: Highly effective CFTR modulation for the majority of people with cystic fibrosis. *Expert Review of Respiratory Medicine, 15*(6), 723.

Middleton, P. G., Mall, M. A., Dřevínek, P., Lands, L. C., McKone, E. F., Polineni, D., Ramsey, B. W., Taylor-Cousar, J. L., Tullis, E., Vermeulen, F., Marigowda, G., McKee, C. M., Moskowitz, S. M., Nair, N., Savage, J., Simard, C., Tian, S., Waltz, D., Xuan, F., Rowe, S. M., & Jain, R.; VX17-445-102 Study Group. (2019). Elexacaftor-Tezacaftor-Ivacaftor for Cystic Fibrosis with a Single Phe508del Allele. *New England Journal of Medicine, 381*(19), 1809–1819. doi:10.1056/NEJMoa1908639. Epub 2019 Oct 31. PMID: 31697873; PMCID: PMC7282384.

Mogayzel, P. J. Jr., Naureckas, E. T., Robinson, K. A., Mueller, G., Hadjiliadis, D., Hoag, J. B., Lubsch, L., Hazle, L., Sabadosa, K., & Marshall, B.; Pulmonary Clinical Practice Guidelines Committee. (2013). Cystic fibrosis pulmonary guidelines. Chronic medications for maintenance of lung health. *American Journal of Respiratory and Critical Care Medicine, 187*(7), 680–689. doi:10.1164/rccm.201207-1160oe. PMID: 23540878.

Moran, A., Brunzell, C., Cohen, R. C., Katz, M., Marshall, B. C., Onady, G., Robinson, K. A., Sabadosa, K. A., Stecenko, A., & Slovis, B.; CFRD Guidelines Committee. (2010). Clinical care guidelines for cystic fibrosis-related diabetes: A position statement of the American Diabetes Association and a clinical practice guideline of the Cystic Fibrosis Foundation, endorsed by the Pediatric Endocrine Society. *Diabetes Care, 33*(12), 2697–2708. doi:10.2337/dc10-1768. PMID: 21115772; PMCID: PMC2992215.

Morrell, M. R., & Pilewski, J. M. (2010). Lung transplantation for cystic fibrosis. *Clinics in Chest Medicine, 37*(1), 127–138.

Neemuchwala, F., Ahmed, F., & Nasr, S. (2020). Prevalence of pelvic incontinence in patients with cystic fibrosis. *Journal of Clinical Medicine, 9*(9), 2706.

Nevitt, S., Thornton, J., Murray, C., & Dwyer, T. (2018). Inhaled mannitol for cystic fibrosis. *Cochrane Database Systematic Reviews, 2*(2).

Oermann, C. M., Retsch-Bogart, G. Z., Quittner, A. L., Gibson, R. L., McCoy, K. S., Montgomery, A. B., & Cooper, P. J. (2010). An 18-month study of the safety and efficacy of repeated courses of inhaled aztreonam lysine in cystic fibrosis. *Pediatric Pulmonology, 45*(11), 1121–1134. doi:10.1002/ppul.21301. PMID: 20672296; PMCID: PMC3867945.

Quittner, A. L., Abbott, J., Georgiopoulos, A. M., Goldbeck, L., Smith, B., Hempstead, S. E., Marshall, B., Sabadosa, K. A.,

& Elborn, S.; International Committee on Mental Health; EPOS Trial Study Group. (2016). International Committee on Mental Health in Cystic Fibrosis: Cystic Fibrosis Foundation and European Cystic Fibrosis Society consensus statements for screening and treating depression and anxiety. *Thorax*, 71(1), 26–34. doi:10.1136/thoraxjnl-2015-207488. Epub 2015 Oct 9. PMID: 26452630; PMCID: PMC4717439.

Ramos, K. J., Smith, P. J., McKone, E. F., Pilewski, J. M., Lucy, A., Hempstead, S. E., Tallarico, E., Faro, A., Rosenbluth, D. B., Gray, A. L., & Dunitz, J. M.; CF Lung Transplant Referral Guidelines Committee. (2019). Lung transplant referral for individuals with cystic fibrosis: Cystic Fibrosis Foundation consensus guidelines. *Journal of Cystic Fibrosis*, 18(3), 321–333. doi:10.1016/j.jcf.2019.03.002. Epub 2019 Mar 27. PMID: 30926322; PMCID: PMC6545264.

Ratjen, F., Davis, S. D., Stanojevic, S., Kronmal, R. A., Hinckley Stukovsky, K. D., Jorgensen, N., & Rosenfeld, M.; SHIP Study Group. (2019). Inhaled hypertonic saline in preschool children with cystic fibrosis (SHIP): A multicentre, randomised, double-blind, placebo-controlled trial. *Lancet Respiratory Medicine*, 7(9), 802–809. doi:10.1016/S2213-2600(19)30187-0. Epub 2019 Jun 6. PMID: 31178421.

Reiter, J., Breuer, O., Cohen-Cymberknoh, M., Forno, E., & Gileles-Hillel, A. (2017). Sleep in children with cystic fibrosis: More under the covers. *Global Pediatric Health*, 4, 2333794x17743424.

Roesch, E. A., Nichold, D. P., & Chmiel, J. F. (2018). Inflammation in cystic fibrosis: An update. *Pediatric Pulmonology*, 53(S3).

Rosenfeld, M., Ratjen, F., Brumback, L., Daniel, S., Rowbotham, R., McNamara, S., Johnson, R., Kronmal, R., & Davis, S. D.; ISIS Study Group. (2012). Inhaled hypertonic saline in infants and children younger than 6 years with cystic fibrosis: The ISIS randomized controlled trial. *JAMA*, 307(21), 2269–2277. doi:10.1001/jama.2012.5214. PMID: 22610452; PMCID: PMC3586815.

Saiman, L., Anstead, M., Mayer-Hamblett, N., Lands, L. C., Kloster, M., Hocevar-Trnka, J., Goss, C. H., Rose, L. M., Burns, J. L., Marshall, B. C., & Ratjen, F.; AZ0004 Azithromycin Study Group. (2010). Effect of azithromycin on pulmonary function in patients with cystic fibrosis uninfected with *Pseudomonas aeruginosa*: A randomized controlled trial. *JAMA*, 303(17), 1707–1715. doi:10.1001/jama.2010.563. PMID: 20442386.

Saiman, L., Siegel, J. D., LiPuma, J. J., Brown, R. F., Bryson, E. A., Chambers, M. J., Downer, V. S., Fliege, J., Hazle, L. A., Jain, M., Marshall, B. C., O'Malley, C., Pattee, S. R., Potter-Bynoe, G., Reid, S., Robinson, K. A., Sabadosa, K. A., Schmidt, H. J., Tullis, E., ... Weber, D. J.; Cystic Fibrous Foundation; Society for Healthcare Epidemiology of America. (2014). Infection prevention and control guideline for cystic fibrosis: 2013 update. *Infection Control & Hospital Epidemiology*, 35(Suppl 1), S1–S67. doi:10.1086/676882. Epub 2014 Jul 1. PMID: 25025126.

Smyth, A., & Rosenfeld, M. and Cochrane Cystic Fibrosis and Genetic Disorders Group. (2020). Prophylactic anti-staphylococcal antibiotics for cystic fibrosis. *Cochrane Database Systematic Reviews*, 2017(4).

Stahl, M., Wielpütz, M. O., Ricklefs, I., Dopfer, C., Barth, S., Schlegtendal, A., Graeber, S. Y., Sommerburg, O., Diekmann, G., Hüsing, J., Koerner-Rettberg, C., Nährlich, L., Dittrich, A. M., Kopp, M. V., & Mall, M. A. (2019). Preventive inhalation of hypertonic saline in infants with cystic fibrosis (PRESIS). A randomized, double-blind, controlled study. *American Journal of Respiratory and Critical Care Medicine*, 199(10), 1238–1248. doi:10.1164/rccm.201807-1203OC. PMID: 30409023.

Stallings, V. A., Stark, L. J., Robinson, K. A., Feranchak, A., & Quinton, H. (2008). Evidence-based practice recommendations for nutrition-related management of children and adults with cystic fibrosis and pancreatic insufficiency: Results of a systematic review. *Journal of the American Dietetic Association*, 108, 832.

Stalvey, M., & Clines, G. (2014). Cystic fibrosis-related bone disease: Insights into a growing problem. *Current Opinion in Endocrinology, Diabetes, and Obesity*, 20(6), 547–552.

Sutharsan, S., McKone, E. F., Downey, D. G., Duckers, J., MacGregor, G., Tullis, E., Van Braeckel, E., Wainwright, C. E., Watson, D., Ahluwalia, N., Bruinsma, B. G., Harris, C., Lam, A. P., Lou, Y., Moskowitz, S. M., Tian, S., Yuan, J., Waltz, D., & Mall, M. A.; VX18-445-109 study group. (2022). Efficacy and safety of elexacaftor plus tezacaftor plus ivacaftor versus tezacaftor plus ivacaftor in people with cystic fibrosis homozygous for F508del-CFTR: A 24-week, multicentre, randomised, double-blind, active-controlled, phase 3b trial. *Lancet Respiratory Medicine*, 10(3), 267–277. doi:10.1016/S2213-2600(21)00454-9. Epub 2021 Dec 20. PMID: 34942085.

Tangpricha, V., Kelly, A., Stephenson, A., Maguiness, K., Enders, J., Robinson, K. A., Marshall, B. C., & Borowitz, D.; Cystic Fibrosis Foundation Vitamin D Evidence-Based Review Committee. (2012). An update on the screening, diagnosis, management, and treatment of vitamin D deficiency in individuals with cystic fibrosis: Evidence-based recommendations from the Cystic Fibrosis Foundation. *Journal of Clinical Endocrinology and Metabolism*, 97(4), 1082–1093. doi:10.1210/jc.2011-3050. Epub 2012 Mar 7. PMID: 22399505.

Taylor, C. J., Chen, K., Horvath, K., Hughes, D., Lowe, M. E., Mehta, D., Orabi, A. I., Screws, J., Tomson, M., Van Biervliet, S., Verkade, H. J., Husain, S. Z., & Wilschanski, M. (2015). ESPGHAN and NASPGHAN report on the assessment of exocrine pancreatic function and pancreatitis in children. *Journal of Pediatric Gastroenterology and Nutrition*, 61(1), 144–153.

Taylor-Cousar, J. L., Munck, A., McKone, E. F., van der Ent C. K., Moeller, A., Simard, C., Wang, L. T., Ingenito, E. P., McKee, C., Lu, Y., Lekstrom-Himes, J., & Elborn, J. S. (2017). Tezacaftor-ivacaftor in patients with cystic fibrosis homozygous for Phe508del. *New England Journal of Medicine*, 377(21), 2013–2023. doi:10.1056/NEJMoa1709846. Epub 2017 Nov 3.

Taylor-Cousar, J. (2020). CFTR modulators: Impact on fertility, pregnancy, and lactation in women with cystic fibrosis. *Obstetric Medicine*, 7(4), 147–155.

The Clinical and Functional TRanslation of CFTR (CFTR2); available at http://cftr2.org. @ Copyright 2011 US CF Foundation, Johns Hopkins University, The Hospital for Sick Children.

Tsang, A., Moriarty, C., & Towns, S. (2010). Contraception, communication and counseling for sexuality and reproductive health in adolescents and young adults with CF. *Paediatric Respiratory Reviews*, 11(2), 84–89.

VanDevanter, D. R., Hamblett, N. M., Simon, N., McIntosh, J., & Konstan, M. W. (2021). Evaluating assumptions of definition-based pulmonary exacerbation endpoints in cystic fibrosis clinical trials. *Journal of Cystic Fibrosis*, 20(1), 39.

Wainwright, C. E., Elborn, J. S., Ramsey, B. W., Marigowda, G., Huang, X., Cipolli, M., Colombo, C., Davies, J. C., De Boeck, K., Flume, P. A., Konstan, M. W., McColley, S. A., McCoy, K., McKone, E. F., Munck, A., Ratjen, F., Rowe, S. M., Waltz, D., & Boyle, M. P.; TRAFFIC Study Group; TRANSPORT Study Group. (2015). Lumacaftor-Ivacaftor in patients with cystic fibrosis homozygous for Phe508del CFTR. *New England Journal of Medicine*, 373(3), 220–231. doi:10.1056/NEJMoa1409547. Epub 2015 May 17. PMID: 25981758; PMCID: PMC4764353.

Wells, J., Rosenberg, M., Hoffman, G., Anstead, M., & Farrell, P. M. (2012). A decision-tree approach to cost comparison of newborn screening strategies for cystic fibrosis. *Pediatrics*, 129(2), e339–e347.

Yen, E., Quinton, H., & Borowitz, D. (2013). Better nutritional status in early childhood is associated with improved clinical outcomes and survival in patients with cystic fibrosis. *Journal of Pediatrics*, 162, 530.

Yu, E. (2022). Cystic fibrosis. *National Library of Medicine*. StatPearls [Internet].

Diabetes Mellitus (Types 1 and 2)

20

Elizabeth A. Doyle, Devyn R. Thurber

ETIOLOGY

Diabetes mellitus was first described in the Egyptian Ebers Papyrus in 1500 BCE. Type 1 diabetes mellitus (T1D) most commonly occurs in young people and is characterized by beta-cell failure. Type 2 diabetes mellitus (T2D) (formerly known as adult-onset diabetes) individuals are often overweight and usually more than 30 years of age, overproduce insulin, and have a receptor-site defect. In recent years, however, T2D has become increasingly common in children and youth. Individuals with T2D can often be treated with oral medications and other treatments, although those with T1D must be treated with insulin for their lifetime.

The cause of T1D is unknown, but many factors have been hypothesized to contribute to the cause of the disease. T1D is an autoimmune disease. In autoimmunity, self-antigens are no longer recognized as such, so a self-destructive process occurs. Islet cell antibodies can be detected in a majority of individuals newly diagnosed with T1D, and evidence of an autoimmune response may be present up to 9 years before the onset of clinical symptoms (Bingley et al., 1993). Genetic susceptibility is a necessary precursor to the development of T1D. Certain human leukocyte antigen (HLA) genes are thought to play a role in the genetic inheritance of the tendency to develop T1D. Individuals with T1D have an increased frequency of HLA genes *B8, B15, DR3,* and *DR4.* The *HLA-DR* genes are known to be associated with autoimmunity. Evidence of autoimmunity is necessary but not sufficient for the development of T1D. It is hypothesized that other factors will not initiate the autoimmune process without genetic susceptibility. Other factors (e.g., host and environmental factors) may influence the development of the condition because the concordance rate is only 50% in identical twins. Such factors include stress and infectious agents (Leslie & Elliot, 1994).

The genetic and pathologic processes leading to the development of T2D are multiple and not yet well defined. There is an interplay of genetic and environmental factors, with a significant hereditary component that appears to be polygenic. In the SEARCH for Diabetes in Youth study, 83% of children with T2D had a positive family history (Gilliam et al., 2007). It is not clear, however, how genetic factors work in T2D. Other factors are also associated with higher risk: obesity (especially central obesity), sedentary lifestyle, a diet high in fat and low in fiber, minority group, family history of T2D, use of psychotropic drugs, insulin resistance, puberty, and female gender (Pihoker et al., 1998). Those most likely to be affected include Indigenous, Black, and Hispanic children (Mayer-Davis et al., 2017). Peripheral insulin resistance is the primary metabolic defect associated with T2D, hyperinsulinemia, glucose intolerance, nonalcoholic fatty liver, and dyslipidemia. Insulin resistance is also associated with acanthosis nigricans, a thickening and darkening of skin usually seen on the neck and axilla. Insulin resistance is an independent risk factor for developing T2D, hypertension, and atherosclerosis. The combination of obesity, insulin resistance, hypertension, dyslipidemia, and atherosclerosis is metabolic syndrome (Pinhas-Hamiel & Zeitler, 2007). In addition, insulin resistance is associated with polycystic ovary syndrome (PCOS) and infertility. Of concern, studies by the TODAY (Treatment Options for Type 2 Diabetes in Adolescents and Youth) Study Group (2012) have demonstrated T2D to be a more aggressive disease in childhood, with a greater degree of beta-cell decline than previously published in adults. Furthermore, more recent studies by the TODAY Study Group (2021) have demonstrated that youth with T2D develop complications earlier in the course of the disease, including a cumulative incidence rate of 80.1% for any microvascular disease with 15 years of duration. A comparison of T1D and T2D is shown in Table 20.1.

INCIDENCE AND PREVALENCE

T1D is the most common metabolic disorder in childhood, affecting about 244,000 children and adolescents in the United States in 2019. In 2014–15, the annual incidence rate of the diagnosis of diabetes in the United States was 18,200 for T1D and 5800 for T2D (American Diabetes Association [ADA], 2022b). The incidence is on the rise for both T1D and T2D. The SEARCH trial (Mayer-Davis et al., 2017) has demonstrated that incidence rates of T1D have increased by 1.4% annually from 2002–03 to 2011–12, and the increase was greater among Hispanic compared to non-Hispanic Whites (4.2% vs. 1.2%). The incidence rate for T2D in children has increased by 7.1% annually. The relative increase was lower among non-Hispanic Whites compared with

Table 20.1	Comparison of Type 1 and Type 2 Diabetes in Youths		
AGE	**THROUGHOUT CHILDHOOD**	**PUBERTY**	
Onset	Acute, severe	Mild to severe, often insidious	
Insulin secretion	Very low	Variable	
Insulin dependence	Permanent	Variable	
Genetics	Polygenic	Polygenic	
Race/ethnic distribution	All	All	
ASSOCIATION			
Obesity	No	Strong	
Acanthosis nigricans	No	Yes	
Autoimmunity	Yes	Unclear	

other ethnicities/races (non-Hispanic Black, Hispanic, Asian or Pacific Island, and Indigenous, with the greatest rates seen in Indigenous children (3.1% in 2002–03 vs. 8.9% in 2011–12) (Mayer-Davis et al., 2017). The average age of onset of T2D in youths is 12 to 14 years, but cases have been reported in children as young as 5 years of age (Glaser, 1997).

DIAGNOSTIC CRITERIA

Diabetes can be diagnosed based on three different parameters: fasting plasma glucose (FPG), 2-hour plasma glucose (2-h PG), or hemoglobin A1c (ADA, 2022a). A patient is diagnosed with diabetes if one of the following criteria is met: FPG is greater than or equal to 126 mg/dL (7 mmol/L), 2-h PG is greater than or equal to 200 mg/dL (11.1 mmol/L), A1c is greater than or equal to 6.5% (48 mmol/L), or a random plasma glucose is greater than or equal to 200 mg/dL (11.1 mmol/L) with classic symptoms of hyperglycemia or hyperglycemic crisis (ADA, 2022a). In the absence of a clear clinical picture of diabetes, diagnosis requires two abnormal screening test results, either from the same or two separate samples (ADA, 2022a). A1c is often preferred over FPG and 2-h PG because it is more convenient and less affected by day-to-day variations in blood glucose levels. However, it is important to use a method certified by the National Glycohemoglobin Standardization Program and standardized to the Diabetes Control and Complications Trial (DCCT) reference assay. Point-of-care A1c assays are not recommended for the diagnosis of diabetes (ADA, 2022a).

Determining whether a patient has T1D or T2D is not always straightforward at diagnosis but is important for establishing the best course of treatment. The pattern of T1D presenting only in children and T2D only in adults no longer stands, as both types can present in either age group. Additionally, while patients with T1D traditionally have a normal or underweight body mass index (BMI) at diagnosis, it is also possible

for them to be overweight or obese. For patients without traditional risk factors for T2D or younger at diagnosis, testing for diabetes autoantibodies can help exclude the diagnosis of T1D (ADA, 2022a).

CLINICAL MANIFESTATIONS AT TIME OF DIAGNOSIS

Although the autoimmune process may be long-standing before the diagnosis of T1D is made, the signs and symptoms of T1D are usually present for a short time. Once the autoimmune process has destroyed enough of the pancreatic beta (islet) cells to produce clinical evidence of diabetes, the classic symptoms (i.e., polydipsia, polyuria, polyphagia) of diabetes occur. As seen in Fig. 20.1, the lack of insulin production leads to disturbances in the metabolism of carbohydrates, protein, and fat.

◎ Clinical Manifestations at Time of Diagnosis

Type 1 diabetes
- Polydipsia
- Polyuria
- Polyphagia

Sometimes weight loss or lack of weight gain
Sometimes abdominal pain, nausea, vomiting
Sometimes Kussmaul respirations

Type 2 diabetes
- Obesity
- Acanthosis nigricans
- Polydipsia
- Polyuria
- Polyphagia

The hormone insulin, produced by the pancreatic beta cells (i.e., islets of Langerhans), is responsible for glucose in the cell. In the absence of insulin there are three general alterations: (1) reduced entry of glucose into the cell, (2) unavailability of carbohydrate as a substrate for energy needs, and (3) the cell's use of alternate substrates (i.e., fatty acids derived from adipose stores and amino acids from body protein). Thus when there is a lack of insulin, glucose cannot be used in the cell for energy, and hyperglycemia results. The extraordinary glucose concentration in the blood promotes osmotic diuresis, producing large amounts of urine. This osmotic diuresis is responsible for the symptom of polyuria, and as the body struggles to maintain homeostasis polydipsia ensues.

If glucose is not available as an energy source, alternative sources must be used. The body relies on lipolysis as well as proteolysis. When this occurs, polyphagia becomes prominent as the body tries to avoid starvation. If these symptoms go uncorrected, hyperglycemia and ketonemia secondary to increased lipolysis will progress to severe levels, and diabetic ketoacidosis (DKA) will occur.

The primary defect in T2D is peripheral insulin resistance, with obesity and a sedentary lifestyle

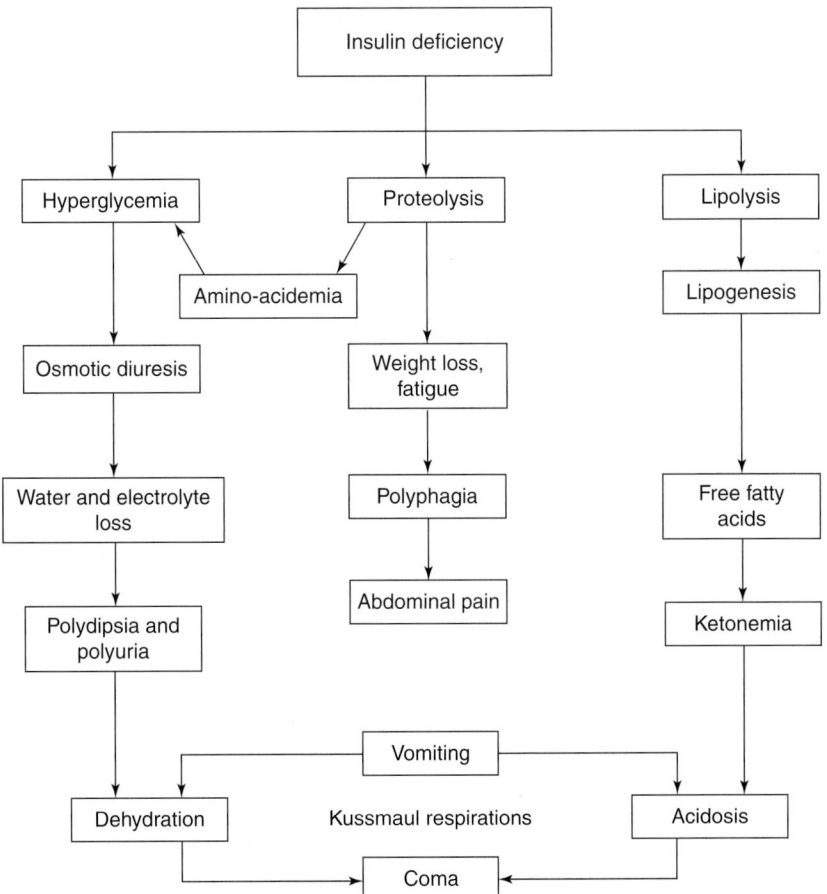

Fig. 20.1 Signs and symptoms of type 1 diabetes mellitus.

contributing to its development. Weiss (2007) demonstrated that severe obesity contributes to insulin resistance partially because of abnormalities in lipid partitioning, with greater fat deposition in intramyocellular and intraabdominal compartments. Once there is insulin resistance, there is initially a compensatory increase in insulin secretion and a decrease in the first-phase insulin response when chronic hyperglycemia ensues. Inappropriate hepatic gluconeogenesis causes fasting hyperglycemia that worsens peripheral insulin resistance and beta-cell function. Most affected individuals have marked peripheral insulin resistance with high serum insulin levels, but they are insufficient to maintain normoglycemia (Callahan & Mansfield, 2000). Pancreatic beta-cell function eventually declines, and insulin secretion decreases. Because the onset of T2D is gradual and insidious compared with T1D, the condition may go undetected for months or years. Clinical manifestations that suggest T2D include obesity and acanthosis nigricans, in addition to polydipsia and polyuria. Providers should consider screening youth who are overweight (≥85th percentile) or who have obesity (≥95th percentile) and who have at least one of the following risk factors for T2D: maternal history of gestational diabetes or diabetes during the specific child's gestation, first- or second-degree family member with T2D, specific race/ethnicity including

Black, Indigenous, Latino, Pacific Islander, or Asian, and/or signs of insulin resistance or its associated conditions, including hypertension, lipid abnormalities, acanthosis nigricans, PCOS, or small for gestational age birth weight. T2D screening should be with a FPG, an A1C test, or an oral glucose tolerance test (ADA, 2022a). The criteria for diagnosis of diabetes are described previously and shown in Box 20.1. If a child meets the criteria for impaired glucose tolerance (or prediabetes), then refer for intensive lifestyle management to prevent T2D from developing. If symptoms of diabetes occur, they will be similar to those of T1D, including polyphagia, polydipsia, and polyuria.

| Box 20.1 | Diagnostic Criteria for Diabetes Mellitus |

- Random plasma glucose ≥200 mg/dL in a patient with classic symptoms of hyperglycemia or hyperglycemic crisis
  OR
- Fasting plasma glucose ≥126 mg/dL. Fasting is defined as no caloric intake for at least 8 hr.
  OR
- 2-hr plasma glucose ≥200 mg/dL, using 75 g anhydrous glucose dissolved in water.

From American Diabetes Association. (2022). Clinical practice recommendations 2022. *Diabetes Care, 45*(Suppl 1).

TREATMENT

TYPE 1 DIABETES

Diabetes Control and Complications Trial

The DCCT was a multicenter, randomized clinical trial of 1441 people with T1D designed to compare intensive diabetes therapy with conventional therapy to determine its effects on the development and progression of early microvascular and neurologic complications of T1D (DCCT Research Group, 1993b). The goals of intensive therapy are to reduce glucose to the normal range and keep glycosylated hemoglobin in the normal range. Intensive therapy consisted of insulin pump therapy (otherwise known as continuous subcutaneous insulin infusion [CSII]) of three or more injections per day with frequent blood glucose monitoring; conventional therapy consisted of one or two insulin injections per day.

Study results showed that in the group without retinopathy, the risk for developing it decreased by 76% with intensive therapy; in the secondary prevention group, the progression of retinopathy was slowed by 54%. Further, microalbuminuria was reduced by 39%, albuminuria by 54%, and clinical neuropathy by 60%. Intensive therapy, however, was associated with a two- to threefold increase in severe hypoglycemia and clinically significant weight gain. Based on this landmark finding, researchers and the ADA recommended that for individuals with T1D, "a primary treatment goal should be blood glucose control at least equal to that achieved in the intensively treated cohort" (ADA, 1993, p. 1555).

 Treatment

Type 1 Diabetes
- Insulin to achieve near-normal blood glucose
- Diet and activity for glucose control and growth
- Monitoring of blood glucose 6–10 times daily
- Continuous glucose monitoring
- Monitoring by the diabetic treatment team with use of glycosylated hemoglobin (A1c)

Type 2 Diabetes
- Initial treatment to correct diabetic ketoacidosis
- Lifestyle intervention
- Diet lower in fats and calories
- Decreased sedentary activity
- Pharmacologic treatment
- Insulin
- Metformin
- Glucagon-like peptide-1

The current ADA (2022a) guidelines recommend that the blood glucose level be normalized using intensive treatment regimens as the goal of treatment for children and adolescents. Insulin doses are often adjusted according to frequent blood glucose monitoring (i.e., 6–10 times/day or through the analysis of continuous glucose data), monitored dietary intake, and anticipated exercise. Treatment goals may be slightly

more relaxed in children who cannot detect symptoms of hypoglycemia if they have hypoglycemic unawareness or lack access to analog insulins and/or continuous glucose monitoring (CGM) devices (ADA, 2022a). These regimens require frequent and careful monitoring by the diabetes team (i.e., primary care provider, nurse, dietitian, behaviorist) and are difficult to accomplish in a primary care setting.

Insulin Therapy

There are many approaches to providing insulin to children and adolescents with T1D. The appropriate regimen should be determined with involvement from the child and the family. Multiple insulin types with different peak actions can be combined to create a regimen that fits the child's lifestyle and the provider's and family's goals. Genetically engineered human insulin preparations are utilized, with most children using insulin analogs.

Insulin replacement results in a dramatic reversal of diabetes symptoms. At diagnosis, most children are hospitalized to correct their metabolic derangement. A recent international study (Cherubini et al., 2020) has shown that the adjusted prevalence rate of children with DKA at diagnosis was 29.9. However, another important purpose of this hospitalization is for education in managing the condition; therefore children, even those not in DKA, are often hospitalized. Many centers have moved to provide follow-up education in an ambulatory setting. Once any acidosis is corrected, subcutaneous treatment with insulin is the mainstay of therapy. The initial regimen must be carefully chosen on an individual basis after a discussion with the family. Many children start on a basal-bolus regimen where they take a quick-acting analog insulin before meals, based on the planned carbohydrate intake and current blood glucose level, and an injection of basal (18–24-hour) insulin once per day. Other children who may be reluctant to take an insulin injection during school (or if a school nurse is not available) may instead start on an injection of intermediate insulin (i.e., NPH) and an injection of quick-acting insulin in the morning, so a lunch injection is not required, and then injections of quick-acting insulin and basal insulin in the evening. These injections are typically given with insulin pens, which can be easier for families to use and provide more accuracy in dosing. Two ultrarapid insulins were recently approved, which have a quicker onset than the original rapid analogs. One example is Fiasp (insulin aspart), where ʟ-arginine and niacinamide (vitamin B$_3$) are added to insulin aspart, facilitating a more rapid movement of insulin through the capillaries, leading to a slightly quicker onset of action. Another approved similar ultrarapid insulin is lispro-aabc injection (Lyumjev). While both insulins have been approved for use in insulin pumps, only Fiasp is US Food and Drug Administration (FDA) approved for use in children. The dose is titrated based on the blood glucose response to achieve blood glucose levels as close to normal as possible.

Shortly after the diagnosis is made, many children experience a significant reduction in insulin requirement because of incomplete destruction of islet cells. Commonly, the doses of quick insulin are sharply reduced during this time. The insulin requirement eventually returns, and children should be cautioned that this honeymoon period (the duration of which is highly variable) does not indicate that the diabetes has gone away. Once the destruction of the beta cells is complete—usually within 2 years of diagnosis—most children will require insulin replacement of approximately 1 U/kg of body weight per day, although 2 U/kg of body weight or more may be necessary, particularly in adolescents.

Once the honeymoon phase is over, it is difficult to achieve optimal metabolic control without using flexible insulin regimens. These regimens consist of three or more daily injections or an insulin pump. Multiple daily injection regimens usually consist of rapid-acting insulin (aspart or lispro) before meals and a long-acting basal analog insulin once or twice a day. There are now three basal insulin options: glargine, degludec (both used once per day), and detemir (usually used twice per day). When these peakless, long-acting insulins are used, quick-acting insulin is taken before each meal and large snack, based on the carbohydrate amount in the meal and the current glucose level. Such regimens mimic the body's normal response to a carbohydrate meal. These regimens are referred to as basal-bolus therapies.

Insulin pump therapy (i.e., CSII) is the other option for flexible therapy. The pumps are battery powered and are small enough to fit in a pocket. There are two broad types of pumps: a pump with tubing or a tubeless pod pump. For the pumps with tubing, a reservoir containing quick-acting insulin is inserted into the pump and connected to fine tubing, connected to an infusion set that is inserted into the hip or the abdomen area every 2 to 3 days. Multiple different infusion sets are available for use. Most sets are inserted at a 90-degree angle with an inserter, and the cannula through which the insulin is delivered comes in different lengths; shorter cannulae seem to work better for very young children and those with very little subcutaneous fat. These infusion sets are inserted with a spring-loaded device, making insertion easy for the parent or older child. They also have disconnect mechanisms that allow the pump to be easily removed for bathing, sports, and so on while leaving the catheter under the skin. Additionally, other sets use a very small (6 mm) needle inserted at 90 degrees and left in place. These have worked very well for toddlers and young children who experience problems with even the smaller cannulas crimping because of little subcutaneous fat.

The other main type of insulin pump is the tubeless pod pump, specifically the Omnipod (Insulet, Bedford, MA). The Omnipod system consists of a lightweight, self-enclosed, watertight pod filled with quick-acting insulin. It is disposable and has a spring-loaded automated cannula insertion. The pod delivers insulin according to preprogrammed instructions that are wirelessly transmitted from a handheld device. The device calculates meal and correction doses similarly to the other pumps and communicates this information to the pod for insulin delivery. All pumps deliver small amounts of quick-acting insulin at a basal rate, which can be varied throughout the 24-hour day based on personal needs, and larger bolus doses are programmed in by the child or family to cover all meals and snacks. Bolus doses are varied based on the amount of carbohydrates in the planned meal or snack, current blood glucose level, and any anticipated exercise.

Pump technology has been advancing rapidly, with different infusion sets and smaller pumps on the market. However, one of the most promising advances came in 2016 with the approval of the first insulin pump hybrid closed-loop system (FDA, 2016). These pumps are worn along with a specific continuous glucose sensor (see later). With these systems (three are available now on the market), the pump will automatically give either less or more insulin in very small doses based on current and/or predicted sensor glucose levels. The use of these devices has resulted in an improvement in A1c levels and less hypoglycemia. These devices are an excellent option for children and have been approved for those as young as 6 years of age.

Although less frequently used by children in the past, many more primary care providers are recommending pump therapy for children and adolescents. Many studies have demonstrated that both traditional pumps (Ahern et al., 2002; Boland et al., 1999; Buckingham et al., 2001; Fox et al., 2005; Philip et al., 2007; Tubiana-Rufi et al., 1996; Weinzimer et al., 2004; Wilson et al., 2005) and the hybrid closed loop (HCL) systems (Adolfsson et al., 2022, Buckingham et al., 2021) are safe and effective for children. The T1D Exchange is a registry that has demonstrated the greatest increase in pump use from 2010–12 to 2016–18 was in children age 6 years and under (50–60% of participants) and those age 6 to 12 years (58–68%) (Foster et al., 2019).

Diet and Activity

Because insulin replacement does not mimic the minute-to-minute response to blood glucose, attention to diet and activity helps minimize variations in blood glucose levels. Routine activity should be encouraged for all children, including those with T1D. However, insulin doses often have to be adjusted, or an extra snack may be necessary to help prevent hypoglycemia, which can occur with prolonged activity.

Children with T1D—unlike individuals with T2D—are often slender, particularly at the time of diagnosis. Therefore, dietary therapy aims to provide sufficient calories for normal growth and development. Initially, a meal plan based on an individual's usual intake pattern is used to integrate insulin therapy into typical eating and exercise patterns. Such a meal plan helps avoid hyperglycemia, prevent hypoglycemia, and maintain metabolic balance. As discussed in the later section on diet, carbohydrate counting is an approach that allows for more flexibility in dietary management.

Daily caloric requirements can be estimated to be 1000 calories for the first year of life, with approximately 100 calories added each year until age 10 to 12. After that, unless they are exceptionally active on a regular basis, females may need their total calories reduced to the common adult level of 1400 to 1600 calories daily. Males, however, will continue to need approximately 2000 calories daily. Shortly after diagnosis, children may need an additional 200 to 700 kcal daily to compensate for the negative energy balance at diagnosis.

Glucose Monitoring

Maintenance of near-normal or normal blood glucose levels requires constant self-monitoring. The goal of therapy is to maintain blood glucose levels as close to the normal range as possible. Self-monitored blood glucose (SMBG) levels let children know exactly what their blood glucose level is at any moment and adjust the insulin dose in response to their actual blood glucose level.

It is recommended that most children test their blood 6 to 10 times daily (ADA, 2022a), at various times throughout the day, and when symptoms are present. The results of SMBG testing are used to identify asymptomatic hypoglycemia, determine patterns in insulin action, and appropriately alter the insulin dose. For example, if a child consistently has high blood glucose levels before lunch, the morning intermediate-acting insulin (i.e., NPH) is increased to prevent this effect. If the child is using a basal-bolus therapy regimen, the morning quick-acting insulin may need to be increased to normalize the lunch values.

Continuous glucose monitoring. Real-time CGMs have revolutionized diabetes care in individuals of all ages, particularly children. They measure interstitial glucose levels and are inserted just under the skin with a spring-loaded device and changed periodically (every 10–14 days, dependent on the sensor used). The sensor is plugged into a small transmitter taped to the skin that communicates glucose data wirelessly to a receiver, an insulin pump display, and/or an application on the phone. The receiver emits alarms when the glucose levels go above or below the targets set by the user to alert the user to hyperglycemia and hypoglycemia. With some devices, a user can also share the data with other people; for example, parents could be alerted on their phone when their child's sensor glucose value is above or below the threshold chosen. This can be especially helpful to parents at night or when their child is away from home.

Many children now are using these devices, and children often like eliminating most fingerstick blood glucose tests. For example, in 2018, 51% of the participants were under the age of 6 years, 37% were between the ages of 6 and 13 years, and 24% of those 13 to 18 years were using a CGM device. CGMs also provide essential real-time data for children and their families to help them manage their diabetes and prevent hypoglycemia. Moreover, a tremendous amount of data is available that guides caregivers in management decisions. Families must remember that CGM readings are delayed by about 5 minutes, and high or low blood glucose levels should be confirmed with a fingerstick check before making treatment decisions. For children who wear this device, primary care providers use the time in range (70–180 mg/dL) on the CGM for the last 2 weeks and the A1c to assess diabetes control (see later).

Monitoring by the diabetes treatment team. Children and adolescents with diabetes are evaluated at least every 3 months by the diabetes treatment team. Quarterly visits correspond to the rate at which the glycosylated hemoglobin levels can be expected to change. Glycosylated hemoglobin (A1c) is a measure of the attachment of glucose to the circulating hemoglobin molecule. In individuals without diabetes, A1c makes up 3% to 6% of the total hemoglobin; those with diabetes, however, have levels above 6% that vary in proportion to the blood glucose levels. The A1c level reflects the average blood glucose level over the most recent 3 months because the lifespan of the hemoglobin molecule is approximately 90 to 120 days. This level is not affected by short-term fluctuations and is considered an objective and accurate measure of long-term diabetes control (ADA, 2022a; Goldstein et al., 1995). For people using a CGM, clinicians should also use the time in range (70–180 mg/dL) to assess metabolic control, with the goal of having 70% of sensor glucose values within this range in a 14-day period. For children, many primary care providers will utilize a more conservative goal of 60% (Battelino et al., 2019).

TYPE 2 DIABETES

Initial Treatment

Youth with T2D may have DKA at diagnosis, but much less commonly. Many are asymptomatic at diagnosis, and elevated A1c levels are commonly discovered on routine screening for overweight or obesity during regular well checks. If children with T2D have DKA at the time of diagnosis, they may need insulin initially to correct the metabolic derangement at diagnosis.

Treatment with insulin, as with T1D, rapidly improves the symptoms of diabetes. Pancreatic autoantibodies should be drawn at diagnosis to confirm that the child does not have T1D (Arslanian et al., 2018).

Lifestyle Intervention

Because the underlying pathology is insulin resistance, the initial approach to treatment focuses on improving insulin sensitivity. The cornerstone of treatment for T2D in youth is an intensive lifestyle intervention that focuses on decreasing adiposity, increasing activity, and behavior change approaches to improve these lifestyle behaviors. Demonstrable improvement in insulin sensitivity occurs with moderate, gradual weight loss (Ludwig & Ebbeling, 2001; Pinhas-Hamiel & Zeitler, 2007). It is believed that modest weight loss or weight maintenance as a child grows, with improvement in physical fitness, can delay or prevent the need for pharmacologic treatment (Upchurch et al., 1999).

Lifestyle interventions should be developmentally and culturally appropriate. Youth should be encouraged to participate in 60 minutes of moderate-intense physical activity daily and receive nutritional counseling from a dietitian focusing on healthy eating behaviors, emphasizing nutrient-dense, high-quality foods, and particularly avoiding sugar-added beverages (ADA, 2022b).

Pharmacologic Treatment

Metformin is the preferred initial treatment for youth with T2D who are metabolically stable at diagnosis (Arslanian et al., 2018). Metformin has been approved for use in children age 10 and older (Jones, 2002; Soliman et al., 2020). Metformin improves metabolic control by reducing hepatic glucose production, increasing insulin sensitivity, and reducing intestinal glucose absorption without increasing insulin secretion. Metformin has been found to significantly improve metabolic control compared with a placebo and does not have a negative effect on body weight or lipid profiles. Further, the rates of adverse events in children (mostly gastrointestinal symptoms, especially diarrhea) were consistent with those reported in adults and tended to decrease over the first few weeks of treatment (Jones et al., 2002; Soliman et al., 2020).

If the A1c is below 8.5% at diagnosis and no acidosis/ketosis is present, then metformin should be initiated in children age 10 years and older with T2D and titrated up to 2000 mg/day as tolerated. If the A1c is 8.5% or more without acidosis/ketosis, then in addition to the metformin youth should be treated with basal insulin starting at 0.5 units/kg/day and titrated based on self-monitoring of blood glucose (Arslanian et al., 2018). When glucose stability is achieved, insulin may no longer be necessary, at least for a time (Arslanian et al., 2018). Limited data suggest that youth with T2D who initially had to be treated with insulin because of DKA, ketosis, or acute hyperglycemia

could be initially treated with metformin alone successfully once glucose stability was achieved after a short course of insulin. Demonstrated in a large multi-center (TODAY) study, more than 90% of the subjects initially screened for participation were able to achieve adequate control on metformin for a period of time regardless of their initial treatment of T2D (Kelsey et al., 2016).

Unfortunately, the TODAY Study Group (2012) demonstrated that youth with T2D have a greater degree of beta-cell decline than adults experience, and 45% had a loss of glycemic control while on metformin and needed to start insulin (medium time to failure of metformin treatment was 11.5 months). Thus additional treatment is often eventually necessary. Basal insulin is usually added if children or adolescents with T2D are no longer meeting A1c goals. Recently the FDA approved two medications from a different class called glucagon-like peptide receptor agonists (GLP-1 agonists) for treating T2D in children and adolescents age 10 years and older with T2D. These medications are either daily (liraglutide) or weekly (exenatide) injections. The Ellipse Trial demonstrated that a 26-week treatment with liraglutide reduced A1c compared to a placebo group treated with a stable dose of metformin with or without basal insulin.

Interestingly, a significant decrease in BMI was not seen in the liraglutide group, as in previous studies in adults. However, the authors attribute this to the possible fact that some of these subjects were still growing, and only 50% of the subjects were able to get to the full 1.8-mg dose suggested. The side effects of liraglutide in this study of children were mostly gastrointestinal, and the most common were nausea (Tamborlane et al., 2019). If A1c goals are still not met with the addition of basal insulin and/or a GLP-1 agonist if tolerated, then typically prandial insulin is added (Arslanian et al., 2018). Research is ongoing with other oral medications currently approved in adults for T2D, so there may be other options for youth with T2D in the future to best tailor their treatment.

T1D AND T2D COMPLEMENTARY AND ALTERNATIVE THERAPIES

Type 1 Diabetes

Although insulin is necessary for the treatment of T1D, there is some suggestion that additional behavioral, biofeedback-assisted relaxation may help improve glucose control (McGrady et al., 1991). The rationale is that stress can raise glucose levels, so therapies aimed at decreasing stress may help overall glucose control. Additionally, Usla and Bayat (2018) completed a review of studies regarding complementary and alternative medicine (CAM) for children with T1D. They found that the most often used therapies included herbal therapies, vitamins/minerals, nutritional/dietary supplements, prayer/spiritual practices, homeopathy, and/or acupuncture. These authors concluded that these therapies were not effective in reducing A1c levels in children.

Type 2 Diabetes

Although adults commonly use complementary therapies such as hypnosis with diabetes to achieve weight loss, minimal literature supports their use in children and adolescents. One study, which included a small percentage of youth with T2D, demonstrated that using CAM was not associated with significantly increased or decreased quality of life in these youth (McCarty et al., 2010). Families may also resort to fad diets (e.g., keto diet) to help youth with T2D lose weight. This diet is particularly risky for youth with T1D because it may increase their risk of developing DKA.

RECENT AND ANTICIPATED ADVANCES IN DIAGNOSIS AND MANAGEMENT

Insulin delivery and glucose sensor technology have rapidly progressed over the last 20 years, which has led to the development and successful use of HCL insulin delivery systems (see earlier). Studies are ongoing to improve these systems, and more recent research has focused on creating a system where the user would no longer have to enter the carbohydrates for the meals consumed. For example, researchers have coupled a current HCL model pump with a smartwatch that detected eating hand gestures, and during a 5-day period where subjects did not enter any carbohydrate doses there was no difference in the time in range of sensor glucose values and the time in the hypoglycemia range, compared with when they entered the carbohydrates (Roy et al., 2022). Cohen et al. (2022) demonstrated that with the use of an insulin pump with a dual delivery of Fisap insulin and pramlintide (an amylin analog that slows the food passage through the stomach) and a simple meal announcement, adolescent and adult subjects could avoid carbohydrate counting, without sacrificing glucose control. These advancements may improve the quality of life for people with diabetes, making treatment less cumbersome while maintaining glycemia.

Transplantation of beta cells or the whole pancreas has reduced insulin requirements for people with diabetes (Sutherland & Gruessner, 1997). The first attempted whole pancreas transplantation was in 1966, with early dismal results, but the advances in surgical technique, immunosuppression, and management have considerably improved the safety and efficacy of this approach (McCall & Shapiro, 2014). Pancreas transplants alone or combined with a kidney have been successful in adults but rarely used in children because of the procedure's risks and the following immunosuppression (Dholakia et al., 2016). Islet-cell transplantation in adults advanced considerably in the first decade of the 21st century, but the

first recorded attempt in children occurred in 1893, with a 13-year-old dying from diabetes. A UK surgeon implanted minced pieces of a sheep's pancreas in an attempt to reverse the child's ketoacidotic state. Since then, we have seen an increased understanding of the optimal selection of pancreas donors, thus making dramatic differences in outcomes (McCall & Shapiro, 2014). With the ultimate goal of islet transplantation to be insulin independence (normal blood glucose levels without the need for exogenous insulin therapy) and continued research and improvement in surgical technique, we will see growth in this area for the pediatric population and improved outcomes. While this is a simpler surgical procedure, isolation and refinement of islet cells remain a limiting factor without the complications of solid-organ transplantation. Over 1 million islets are needed for a single transplant, which requires up to six purified pancreata (Dholakia et al., 2016). Advances over the last few years have suggested that functional beta cells generated from stem cells may be a possible treatment strategy in the future (Dholakia et al., 2016). Further research to determine effective, safe immunosuppressive therapies, as well as these and other potential sources for insulin-producing cells, is needed so that islet cell transplantation may result in an eventual cure for T1D.

New pharmacologic treatments for T2D are currently being evaluated in children. While the medication has had some efficacy for adults, studies using a dipeptidyl peptidase 4 inhibitor (sitagliptin) did not show improvements in A1c levels in pediatric patients age 10 to 18 years when used as an initial treatment for T2D (Shankar et al., 2022). Other authors have demonstrated that adding this medication to metformin does not improve metabolic control for youth with T2D (Julaudin et al., 2022). In a study of 72 youth age 10 to 24 years with T2D, the use of a sodium-glucose transport protein 2 inhibitor (dapagliflozin) as directed (subjects nonadherent with the treatment were filtered out) had a significant decrease in A1c (0.51%) compared to the placebo when added to a treatment regimen of metformin alone or metformin with insulin. Side effects were reported as mild (Tamborlane et al., 2022). Further research is needed with this class of medication with a larger sample. In addition, advances in the pharmacologic and surgical treatment of obesity will likely affect treatment for T2D in children and adolescents.

ASSOCIATED PROBLEMS OF DIABETES MELLITUS (T1D AND T2D) AND TREATMENT

Diabetic Ketoacidosis

A physiologic process results in DKA when there is a lack of insulin (see Fig. 20.1). Any potential stressor (e.g., illness, fever, injury, psychosocial stress) can increase the risk of metabolic derangement caused by disturbances in counterregulatory hormones and lead to DKA. Any stressor in a child with diabetes must be managed with care.

It should be noted that children with T2D can have DKA, but once they are stabilized after diagnosis DKA becomes rare in these children (Rewers et al., 2008). What can occur is nonketotic severe hyperglycemia (nonketotic hyperosmolar coma), which is usually associated with significant dehydration and is characterized by very high plasma glucose levels (>750 mg/dL) without ketosis or ketoacidosis. Treatment with intravenous hydration and insulin is required.

Hypoglycemia

Children with diabetes occasionally experience hypoglycemia episodes, especially when treated with insulin. Because the symptoms of hyperglycemia and hypoglycemia can sometimes be confused, they are compared in Box 20.2. Hypoglycemia may be caused by too much insulin, too little food, too much activity, or a combination of these. Although hypoglycemia is easily treated, prevention is the best approach. Again, SMBG determination is helpful, along with using a continuous glucose sensor. With SMBG testing or sensor use, children can identify patterns of lower blood glucose levels that may indicate periods of increased risk. During these periods, the insulin dose can be altered to prevent hypoglycemia. If a child anticipates unusual physical activity, both insulin and diet can be adjusted to prevent low glucose levels. Hypoglycemia can also occur with sulfonylureas, an older treatment for T2D; however, this is rarely used in children with this condition today.

Box **20.2**	Comparison of Hyperglycemia and Hypoglycemia

DIABETIC KETOACIDOSIS (HYPERGLYCEMIA)
- Slow onset
- Increased thirst and urination
- High blood and urine glucose levels
- Urinary ketones
- Weakness and abdominal pain
- Heavy, labored breathing
- Anorexia
- Nausea and vomiting
- Monilial vaginitis

HYPOGLYCEMIA
- Rapid onset
- Excessive sweating
- Fainting
- Headache
- Trembling and shaking
- Hunger
- Unable to wake
- Irritability
- Personality change

Associated Problems

Diabetes Mellitus and Treatment

	TYPE 1	TYPE 2
Diabetic ketoacidosis or nonketotic severe hyperglycemia	Yes	Sometimes
Hypoglycemia	Common	Rare
Monilial vaginitis	Yes	Yes
Cardiovascular complications		
Hyperlipidemia	Yes	Yes
Hypertension	Yes	Yes
Nonalcoholic fatty liver disease	Rare	Yes
Polycystic ovary syndrome	Rare	Yes
Long-term complications		
Renal failure	Yes	Yes
Retinopathy	Yes	Yes
Neuropathies	Yes	Yes
Vascular insufficiency	Yes	Yes
Depression/psychosocial problems	Yes	Yes

Hypoglycemia presents particular problems at different ages. Infants and toddlers are unable to express the feelings associated with hypoglycemia, so they must be observed for listlessness, sleepiness, or irritability. Parents should be instructed that unusual behavior at any time is an indication for blood glucose levels to be measured. If the result is less than 70 mg/dL, a conscious infant should be given 2 to 4 oz of sweet liquids or a small amount of cake frosting (gel), and an unconscious or convulsing infant should be given 0.25 to 0.5 mL of glucagon by injection. Older children can be taught the symptoms of hypoglycemia (i.e., shakiness, tremors, sweatiness, nervousness) and how to prevent its occurrence. They should also be instructed to carry high-sugar foods with them at all times. The goal is to treat any hypoglycemic event with oral carbohydrates while the symptoms are still mild. Typically, children are advised to take 15 g of quick-acting sugar and recheck their glucose 15 minutes later. If their glucose is still below their low threshold, this process is repeated every 15 minutes until blood glucose is normalized—a process known as the rule of 15s.

Occasionally, severe hypoglycemia (unconscious or seizure) events can occur if a mild event is not treated appropriately with glucagon either by injection (based on weight) or by nasal route. Glucagon is the antagonist hormone to insulin and releases glycogen from the liver. When glucagon is administered by intramuscular injection to rapidly raise blood glucose, the dose is 0.5 mg (0.5 mL) for infants or toddlers and 1 mg (1 mL) for older children. Baqsimi is the first (and only) dry nasal spray approved by the FDA (in 2019) to treat severe hypoglycemia for children and adults age 4 years and older. Studies (Sherr et al., 2016) have demonstrated this nasal delivery of glucagon was as effective as the injectable formulation. Many families will call emergency personnel (911) once the child is treated since this is such a fearful event to witness. All children with diabetes should wear medical identification so that they can be diagnosed and treated appropriately if they lose consciousness while away from home. Some substances can increase the likelihood of hypoglycemia. Adolescents need to know that alcohol augments the glucose-lowering effects of insulin and that the symptoms of alcohol intoxication and hypoglycemia are similar. Low blood glucose levels can increase the body's sensitivity to alcohol, and many experimenting teenagers have found themselves in the emergency department with profound hypoglycemia. Stimulants such as amphetamines and cocaine may increase metabolism and decrease appetite, so hypoglycemia may occur.

Monilial Vaginitis
Once healthy females are toilet trained, monilial infections of the perineum are rare until adolescence when the estrogeneration of the vagina provides a potential environment for the growth of candida. Hyperglycemia also leads to increased glucose levels in vaginal secretions, providing an ideal medium for candida. Females with poorly controlled diabetes (either T1D or T2D) are at increased risk for monilial vaginitis, any vaginal discharge, and itching and should be investigated and treated appropriately.

Cardiovascular Complications
Because diabetes predisposes people to the development of accelerated arteriosclerosis, all patients, including children with diabetes, must be screened for both hyperlipidemia and hypertension (ADA, 2022a).

Hyperlipidemia. For children with T1D, the ADA (2022a) recommends that the initial lipid testing be done when glycemic control is obtained after diagnosis and the child is 2 years or older. If the initial low-density lipoprotein (LDL) is below 100 mg/dL, the child should be tested again at age 9 to 11 years; as long as the LDL remains below 100 mg/dL, a lipid panel should be repeated every 3 years until adulthood. Statin therapy may be considered for children at least 10 years of age who, despite medical and nutritional therapy and lifestyle changes, have an LDL above 160 mg/dL (or >130 mg/dL with one or more cardiovascular risk factors). Reproductive counseling is necessary for all females requiring treatment because of the teratogenic effects of statins (ADA, 2022a).

For children with T2D, the ADA (2022a) recommends that blood lipids (total cholesterol, LDL, high-density lipoprotein [HDL], triglycerides) should be measured once initial glycemic control is obtained and then yearly. Goals include an LDL below 100 mg/dL, HDL above 35 mg/dL, and triglycerides below 150 mg/dL. If lipid levels are elevated, initial therapy should include optimizing metabolic control and medical and nutritional therapy. If the LDL is still above 130 mg/dL after 6 months of treatment, statin therapy should be initiated (after reproductive counseling in females). If the triglycerides are above 400 mg/dL fasting or above 1000 mg/dL nonfasting, then glycemia should be optimized and a fibrate initiated to decrease the fasting triglycerides to below 400 mg/dL to reduce the risk of pancreatitis (ADA, 2022a).

Hypertension. Blood pressure should be recorded at every quarterly visit, as hypertension is common in children with diabetes, especially those with T2D. Elevated blood pressure readings should be confirmed on three separate days. Initial treatment for elevated blood pressure readings (systolic blood pressure >90th–95th percentile or in adolescents age ≥13 years, systolic blood pressure 120–129 mm Hg with diastolic measurements <80 mm Hg) includes dietary and lifestyle interventions. If hypertension is confirmed (systolic or diastolic blood pressure consistently >95th percentile or >140/90 mm Hg in adolescents aged ≥13 years), pharmacologic treatment should be considered concomitant with an evaluation of renal function (ADA, 2022a). Guidelines suggest that angiotensin-converting enzyme inhibitors in children 13 years and older to help achieve and maintain normotension may also decrease the risk for microvascular kidney complications (Clarke et al., 2001).

Nonalcoholic Fatty Liver Disease
Nonalcoholic fatty liver disease (NAFLD) is a long-term complication of obesity, hyperlipidemia, and diabetes. Elevations in liver enzymes, especially alanine aminotransferase (ALT), may indicate NAFLD. Children and youth with NAFLD are usually asymptomatic. Liver enzymes should be done at diagnosis and then yearly after that, and a referral should be made to gastroenterology if the levels are persistently elevated or worsen (ADA, 2022a).

Polycystic Ovary Syndrome
Insulin resistance and T2D are also associated with PCOS in females. This disorder is associated with increased ovarian or adrenal androgen production. Symptoms include menstrual irregularities and evidence of hyperandrogenism, especially hirsutism and acne. Females with PCOS should be referred to a reproductive endocrinologist for care. Treatment with

low-dose birth control pills may be necessary. Metformin may also be used to control hyperglycemia and, in addition to lifestyle modifications, may improve menstrual cycle irregularity and hyperandrogenism (ADA, 2022a).

LONG-TERM COMPLICATIONS

Diabetes is the seventh leading cause of death in the United States (ADA, 2022b). For the most part, this high mortality rate results from the condition's long-term complications. Between 2000 and 2016 there was a 5% increased risk of early mortality (before the age of 70) if someone was diagnosed with diabetes (World Health Organization, 2022). Because diabetes treatment and technology are continuing to improve, there is hope that children diagnosed more recently will have lower rates of long-term complications and therefore a better prognosis.

Long-term complications of T1D (renal failure, eye degeneration, neuropathies, vascular insufficiency) are well known. Unfortunately, recent data suggest that complications in T2D in youth follow a more rapid trajectory than in adults. The TODAY Study Group (2021) published long-term follow-up data of a large national cohort of youth with T2D, demonstrating that the cumulative incidence of any microvascular complication was 80.1% after 15 years with the condition. Thus it is recommended by the ADA (2022) to aggressively achieve both glycemic and blood pressure control in youth with both T1D and T2D and screen for microvascular complications.

Complications can range from asymptomatic mild proteinuria to blindness, renal failure, painful neuropathies, cardiovascular disease, and death. Hyperglycemia is a necessary—but not sufficient—factor for developing complications. In addition to hyperglycemia, genetic factors seem to influence the development of complications.

In the United States, diabetes remains the leading cause of new cases of blindness. Diabetes is also the leading cause of end-stage kidney disease. Based on 2017–2020 data, 39.2% of patients with diabetes age 18 years and older had chronic kidney disease (CKD) (stages 1–4), with 15.7% having moderate-severe CKD (stages 3–4) (Centers for Disease Control and Prevention [CDC], 2022). Although the DCCT showed that improvement in metabolic control to near-normal levels delayed the onset or progression of complications, complications were not eliminated. It is clear, however, that the better the metabolic control, the better the chance of avoiding complications. In the long-term follow-up of the TODAY study it was found that the cumulative incidence of any microvascular disease was 80.1% in the 15 years subjects were followed. Hypertension (cumulative incidence 67.5%) and kidney disease (cumulative incidence 54.8%) were the two most common complications. Thus aggressive blood glucose control, blood

pressure control, and lifestyle change are essential in youth with T2D.

PSYCHOSOCIAL COMPLICATIONS

Research has shown that more than one-third of youth with T1D age 11 to 25 years screened positive for depression, 21.3% for anxiety, and 20.7% for disordered eating. Furthermore, those who screened positive for one of these disorders had twice the odds of having high A1c levels (Bernstein et al., 2013). Of further concern, studies have shown youth and young adults with T1D endorse suicidal/death ideation, and 16% of those studied had made a previous attempt (Majidi et al., 2020). Studies have shown that compared with their peers without diabetes, adolescents with T1D are 1.7 times more likely to attempt suicide, sometimes with deliberate overdosing of insulin (Butwicka et al., 2015). It is not surprising that the ADA (2022) recommends periodic screening for these psychosocial complications. Although a smaller percentage of adolescents with diabetes manifest significant psychiatric problems, many have difficulty in psychosocial adjustment. The presence of diabetes in adolescence may hinder normal adolescent development by limiting the development of independence. One small study examined the personal meaning and perceived impact of diabetes on 54 adolescents and found that youth felt that diabetes controlled or limited their freedom and independence (Kyngas & Barlow, 1995).

Furthermore, a meta-analysis by Rechenberg et al. (2017) revealed that anxiety is common among youth with T1D and is associated with higher A1c levels, a lower frequency of glucose monitoring, depressive symptoms, fears of hypoglycemia, and less optimal coping behaviors in self-management skills. Interventions such as coping skills training (Grey et al., 2000) and parent-child conflict prevention (Anderson et al., 1999) may help reduce these problems. Appropriate referral to behavioral treatment should not be delayed if problems in adjustment are suspected.

Research on the psychosocial consequences of T2D in youth is limited, although studies have demonstrated that almost one-fifth of youth diagnosed with T2D have neuropsychiatric problems at the time of diagnosis (Levitt Katz et al., 2005). Interestingly, in the SEARCH for Diabetes in Youth Study, the incidence of depression was higher in males with T2D than in males with T1D (Lawrence et al., 2006). Additionally, youth with T2D who exhibit binge eating have a higher incidence of extreme obesity, depressed mood, and impaired quality of life (Wilfley et al., 2011). It is recommended that youth with T2D be screened for mental/behavioral health conditions, particularly depression and disordered eating, and be referred to mental health providers as indicated (ADA, 2022a).

PRIMARY CARE MANAGEMENT

HEALTH CARE MAINTENANCE

Growth and Development

Because T1D is a metabolic disorder affecting metabolism, growth and sexual development may be slowed. Children and adolescents whose diabetes is less well controlled may fail to grow normally. Therefore accurate measurements of height and weight and comparison with growth norms are imperative.

Even when children have normal linear growth there may be delays in the onset and progression of puberty if glycemic control is inadequate. At each visit, Tanner stages should be assessed and recorded. Any deviation from the normal pattern should be investigated. In females, menarche may be delayed. Loss of regular menses once cycling has been established may indicate a further degeneration in metabolic control and should be investigated.

Obesity can occur in children and adolescents with T1D, especially those on flexible regimens. Management of this obesity should be done carefully, with attention to the need to maintain self-monitoring because glucose levels may change dramatically when a weight loss program is followed. Another concern is adolescents who manipulate weight by overeating or reducing or omitting insulin. Deliberate insulin omission leads to hyperglycemia and glycosuria, resulting in weight loss. This dangerous practice has been seen in up to 34% of adolescent and young adult females with T1D (Rodin et al., 2002). Adolescent and young adult females with T1D are twice as likely to develop eating disorders compared with their nondiabetic peers (Rodin et al., 2002). Similarly, up to 20% of patients with T2D also have eating disorders, the most common of which is binge eating disorder (Harris et al., 2021). For this reason, the clinician should have a high index of suspicion for eating disorders in any patient with diabetes who is experiencing rapid weight changes, growth difficulties, or consistently poor glycemic control.

In T2D, obesity is often associated with early puberty and accelerated linear growth. Height and weight should be measured at each visit, and BMI should be calculated. BMI should be plotted and followed as an indicator of the effectiveness of treatment. Tanner staging should be completed at each visit, and unusually rapid progression should be noted and referred to endocrinology. Calculation of BMI z score, which shows how far above or below normal the BMI is at every primary care visit, can be used to help prevent obesity and the development of T2D.

Diet

Although insulin therapy is the cornerstone of treatment for T1D, a dietary plan is important in maintaining near-normoglycemia without wide swings in blood glucose levels. Long-term adherence to the dietary plan is probably the most difficult aspect of management for families.

All dietary management plans for T1D aim to provide adequate calories and nutrients for normal growth and maintain blood glucose as normal as possible. The consistency of daily intake with regular meals and snacks is important. In consultation with the diabetes team, families should select the appropriate meal plan because they are in the best position to judge the approach that will work. Imposing a rigid approach on an unwilling family only leads them not to adhere to the diet. In addition, most children will not adhere without question to a diet perceived as different from that of peers. Thus primary care providers must understand their approach and work with families to ensure as much dietary consistency as possible.

Most diabetes clinicians advocate carbohydrate counting for dietary management. The family is taught which foods have carbohydrates and reading nutrition labels to determine the carbohydrate count for different foods. If the child is using a fixed insulin regimen, the dietitian and family will determine specific amounts of carbohydrates the child should consume at meals and snacks. The child can vary the kinds of carbohydrates at a particular meal as long as the total number remains constant.

A more flexible carbohydrate counting approach is used most frequently by those on flexible insulin regimens (DCCT Research Group, 1993a). This method provides more flexibility in the diet by providing varying amounts of carbohydrates at meals and snacks with appropriate coverage with rapid-acting insulin. Protein and fat intake are not controlled, but efforts to stay within low-fat guidelines are encouraged. For example, adolescents who choose to eat a second sandwich at lunch (i.e., 30 g of extra carbohydrate in the bread) may need to take 5 to 10 units of rapid-acting insulin before the meal, depending on their regimen.

The wide availability of artificially sweetened foods and drinks has eased some of the difficulties children with diabetes face in following the meal plan. Parents sometimes express concern that extensive use of artificial sweeteners will be problematic for their children. The FDA has approved six nonnutritive sweeteners in the United States: saccharin, aspartame, sucralose, acesulfame potassium, neotame, and advantame. For these and all other additives, the FDA determines an acceptable daily intake (ADI) (i.e., the amount that can be safely consumed daily over a person's lifetime without any adverse effects), which includes a 100-fold safety factor. The average intake is much less than the ADI. While sugar-free alternatives may reduce the amount of insulin needed at a given meal, it is important to note that research has shown artificial sweeteners to be implicated in longer-term insulin resistance for patients with diabetes (Mathur et al., 2020).

As noted, dietary management is the cornerstone of treatment for T2D. A multidisciplinary approach involving dietary modification, increased physical activity, decreased sedentary time, and behavior modification offers the best hope for a successful outcome. Traditionally, dietary approaches have emphasized individualization and reduction in dietary carbohydrate intake. Often, reducing calories from sodas and fruit drinks can result in substantial improvement. Carbohydrate counting can help children prevent hyperglycemia after meals as well.

Physical activity is encouraged for all children irrespective of diabetes type. Children should aim for 60 minutes of moderate-vigorous intensity aerobic exercise each day and muscle- and bone-strengthening activities at least three times per week (ADA, 2022a). Regular exercise and active participation in organized sports positively affect the psychosocial and physical well-being of children with T1D. Parents and their children should be advised that different types of exercise may affect blood glucose levels. For example, sports that involve short bursts of activity may increase glucose levels, whereas a more prolonged activity is more likely to decrease blood glucose levels. Parents and their children also need to be warned that a prolonged physical activity session during the day may lead to hypoglycemia while the child is sleeping during the night, and therefore an extra bedtime snack or a change in the evening insulin may be necessary. Additionally, if the blood glucose level before exercise is greater than 240 mg/dL, urinary ketones should be checked; if they are present, the child should not exercise because the presence of ketones means the child has considerably insufficient insulin levels.

For children with T2D, physical activity is strongly encouraged to enhance weight management. Activities that decrease sedentary behavior and increase aerobic capacity (McMurray et al., 2000) have been demonstrated to lower insulin and glucose levels. Physical activity should be aimed at establishing lifelong habits rather than youth sports alone. Encouraging families to participate in activities together may help establish an exercise habit.

Safety

The safety issues faced by families with a child or adolescent with diabetes are twofold. As discussed earlier, hypoglycemia is a significant risk for all affected children on insulin, so families and others in a child's social sphere should be prepared to respond appropriately. Children should wear medical identification so proper treatment can be instituted quickly. Older children need to know how to prevent severe hypoglycemia especially when exercising. Children should be taught to eat a snack of complex carbohydrates and protein (e.g., peanut butter and crackers) before exercise, not to inject insulin into an exercising muscle, and to always carry glucose and glucagon with them. When traveling or on school day trips, children or their parents should carry the supplies with them—not in checked baggage—and always have food available

in case a meal is delayed. Airlines require insulin and syringes to be carried in a box with the pharmacy label to bring them on board an airplane. Another important safety issue is the proper disposal of syringes. Children and parents must be taught the importance of properly disposing of syringes to reduce the risk of injury to themselves and others.

Care should be taken for youth with T2D on oral medications to ensure that medications are taken as prescribed. As with all medications, safety containers should be used so that young children do not accidentally ingest them. Should accidental ingestion occur, children should be watched for hypoglycemia, and a poison control center should be contacted at (800) 222–1222.

Immunizations

Routine immunizations are recommended. Children with diabetes are potentially at an increased risk for developing complications from influenza and COVID-19; therefore they should receive a yearly influenza vaccination after the age of 6 months (ADA, 2022a) and be up to date on COVID vaccinations per CDC recommendations. Some providers also recommend that youth with diabetes receive the 23-valent pneumococcal vaccine, but with improved metabolic control there is less risk for overwhelming infection.

Screenings

Children with diabetes should undergo the same regular screenings as their nondiabetic peers, as outlined annually by the American Academy of Pediatrics. These include but are not limited to vision, hearing, growth, development, and tuberculosis. Additionally, they require regular condition-specific screenings.

Hypertension. Blood pressure screening should be performed at each visit. Elevated blood pressure and hypertension have been reported in approximately 30% of children and adolescents with T1D and in about 25% with T2D (Cioana et al., 2021). Aggressive blood pressure control may significantly improve the long-term outcome for children with both types of diabetes.

Dyslipidemia. Individuals with T1D and T2D are at increased risk for lipid metabolism disorders, which may increase the risk of macrovascular complications. Children with T1D should be screened for dyslipidemia with a lipid panel (preferably fasting) soon after diagnosis once glycemia has improved if the child is 2 years or older (ADA, 2022a). If LDL cholesterol is 100 mg/dL or below, the ADA (2022) recommends repeating at age 9 to 11 years and then every 3 years after that. More frequent screenings may be needed for children with LDL above 130 mg/dL. For children with T2D, lipid screening is recommended soon after diagnosis and annually after that (ADA, 2022a).

Nephropathy. Diabetes puts children at increased risk for kidney complications, especially in the context of poor glycemic control. Children with T1D should be screened with an albumin-to-creatinine ratio from a random urine sample once they start puberty or turn 10 years old (whichever happens earlier) if they have had diabetes for at least 5 years (ADA, 2022a). For children with T2D, this ratio is initially checked at diagnosis (ADA, 2022a). For both diabetes types, this screening is repeated annually if normal; if abnormal, it is repeated with confirmation of two of three samples over 6 months (ADA, 2022a).

Retinopathy. Vision screening is particularly important in children with diabetes because visual problems are common. A few children develop cataracts early in the course of the condition; therefore observing the normalcy of the red reflex during the ophthalmic examination is very important. Fluctuations in blood glucose levels can also affect visual acuity. Children experiencing hypoglycemia may complain of visual disturbances, and those with hyperglycemia may also complain of blurred vision. Thus it is important to relate the results of routine visual screening to the level of metabolic control because improvement in metabolic control may improve the results of the visual testing.

Parents and children are often most concerned about the risk of diabetic retinopathy. Retinopathy of diabetes is the leading cause of blindness. The ADA (2022) recommends dilated fundoscopic exam every 2 years once the child reaches puberty or 11 years of age (whichever is earlier) if the child has had diabetes for at least 3 years. If normal, the frequency can be decreased to every 4 years if A1c is less than 8% and the ophthalmologist agrees (ADA, 2022a). For children with T2D, the dilated fundoscopic exam is recommended with diagnosis and then annually after that (ADA, 2022a).

Neuropathy. Children with T1D should be screened for diabetic neuropathy with a monofilament foot exam once they start puberty or turn 10 years old (whichever is earlier) once they have had diabetes for at least 5 years. Children with T2D should start this screening at diagnosis. For both types of diabetes, this screening should be completed at least annually if normal (ADA, 2022a).

Dental caries. Dental cleanings and exams are recommended every 6 months. If metabolic control is poor, children may experience increased dental caries and gingivitis caused by increased glucose in saliva. Thus those with poorer control should have frequent dental screenings and appropriate treatment.

Depression. Due to the increased incidence of depression or anxiety in children and adolescents with diabetes, they should be screened regularly for mental health concerns or symptoms.

T1D and T2D Condition-Specific Screening

Type 1 diabetes. Because T1D is an autoimmune disease it is associated with other autoimmune diseases. For this reason, it is important to screen regularly for other immune-mediated conditions.

Thyroid disorder. Hashimoto thyroiditis is a common immune-mediated disease that often occurs with T1D. At diagnosis, children with T1D should be screened for thyroid peroxidase and thyroglobulin antibodies. Thyroid-stimulating hormone (TSH) should be measured after glucose control has been established, and if normal they should be rechecked every 1 to 2 years (ADA, 2022a). Children and adolescents who show any change in growth pattern or develop signs and symptoms of hypothyroidism (e.g., fatigue, dry skin, constipation) or hyperthyroidism (e.g., heat intolerance, tremor, diarrhea) should be tested with thyroid function studies sooner.

Celiac disease. Celiac disease is another immune-mediated condition that is seen in increased frequency with T1D. Symptoms include diarrhea, weight loss, poor weight gain or growth, abdominal pain, fatigue, malnutrition, and unexplained hypoglycemia or erratic blood glucose control. Children with T1D should be screened for celiac disease soon after diagnosis by measuring tissue transglutaminase immunoglobulin A (IgA) levels (with documentation of normal serum IgA levels). If IgA is deficient, deaminated gliadin antibodies should be checked. If the child screens positive for celiac disease, then refer to a gastroenterologist for evaluation. Once the diagnosis is confirmed, the child should be placed on a gluten-free diet, and the family should be referred to a nutritionist for guidance (ADA, 2022a). If the test is negative, the screening should be repeated within 2 years and then 5 years after diagnosis or sooner if symptoms present (ADA, 2022a).

Type 2 diabetes. Most children with T2D are overweight or obese, which puts them at increased risk for other conditions.

Nonalcoholic fatty liver disease. Many obese adolescents with T2D have elevated liver enzymes, suggesting NAFLD. Obese children with T2D should be screened for NAFLD by checking aspartate transaminase (AST) and ALT levels at diagnosis and then annually after that. Children with persistently elevated levels should be referred to a gastroenterologist for evaluation (ADA, 2022a).

Polycystic ovary syndrome. Children with T2D should be screened for symptoms of PCOS (menstrual irregularities, facial hair, acne) at diagnosis and every follow-up visit. If positive, a laboratory workup should be completed (ADA, 2022a).

Obstructive sleep apnea. Children with T2D should be screened for symptoms of obstructive sleep apnea (excessive daytime sleepiness, snoring, apneic events while sleeping, morning headache) at diagnosis and every follow-up visit after that. If positive, they should be referred to a sleep specialist for a polysomnogram (ADA, 2022a).

COMMON ILLNESS MANAGEMENT

Differential Diagnosis

Management of vomiting and diarrhea and prevention of DKA. Provided that their diabetes is under reasonable metabolic control, children and adolescents with diabetes are not at higher risk than their nondiabetic peers for most common infectious diseases of childhood. Because any stressor may lead to DKA in a child with T1D, infections and other stressors must be managed with care.

Regardless of the stress, there are several important principles for management; the need to continue to take insulin even when unable to eat a normal diet is of utmost importance because the excess of counterregulatory hormones released in response to the stressor will more than offset the decreased oral intake. Thus even though dietary intake may be decreased, the insulin requirement may be increased.

🔍 Differential Diagnosis

- Stressors, including illness, can lead to DKA.
- Sick day management is needed for common illnesses and stress.
- It is important to maintain hydration during illness.
- Vaginal discharge may be monilial infection.
- Skin manifestations may require referral.
- Weight loss may indicate poor metabolic control.
- Gastroparesis may be the cause of prolonged vomiting.

The principles of management include monitoring glucose and ketone levels, maintaining hydration, preventing hypoglycemia, and preventing DKA and nonketotic hyperosmolar coma. For these principles to work effectively, the child and family must know that any illness or insult involving fever, gastrointestinal symptoms, congestion in the head or chest, or urinary symptoms should be managed as a sick day. Once a day is identified as such, the usual rules for self-monitoring are altered to reflect the need for closer monitoring. Blood glucose levels should be tested every 1 to 4 hours, and individuals should check their urine ketone at least once daily (even if blood glucose levels are normal). Blood glucose levels above 400 mg/dL on two or more determinations, moderate or large ketone levels in the urine that do not decrease with additional insulin, or any persistent vomiting regardless of the blood glucose level should be viewed as an indication that the child should be seen and evaluated by either the primary care provider or the specialist.

Maintaining hydration is important to help clear extra glucose and ketones, and hydration must be carefully monitored if vomiting or diarrhea is present. If children cannot eat their usual diet, a large fluid intake should be maintained. This amount should be more than 8 oz of fluid in adolescents hourly. Such fluids should contain adequate carbohydrates (i.e., 50–75 g in 6–8 hours) to maintain the usual caloric intake. Children often drink regular (i.e., not diet) sodas, flavored gelatin water, or suck on ice pops when ill. If a child is vomiting or has diarrhea, broth or electrolyte solutions help replace sodium losses.

A child with T1D may need additional insulin to prevent DKA, and a child with T2D may need insulin to treat DKA or to prevent nonketotic hyperosmolar coma when sick. If the urine ketones are moderate or higher, the family should also check the glucose level and consult their diabetes provider for treatment modifications to help lower the ketone levels and prevent DKA. If the blood glucose level is above the target range, a correction dose of 110% the usual dose should be given. If urine ketones are large and the blood glucose level is above the target range, 120% the usual correction dose should be given. If a child has moderate or large ketones, the blood glucose level is in the target range.

Box 20.3 lists the indications for which children or adolescents should be seen and evaluated. Most important is the need for children with any alteration in mental status to be evaluated. Primary care providers should never assume that sleepiness in children with diabetes is merely the result of the fatigue associated with an illness or that vomiting is simply the result of gastroenteritis

Other conditions

Vaginal discharge. Young females with diabetes are prone to monilial infections when glucose control is inadequate. Treatment with an antifungal agent is warranted in young females if vaginal discharge with itching exists without evidence of sexual activity. If there has been sexual contact of any kind, the external vagina may be examined, and testing for other infections (e.g., *Chlamydia* or *Gonorrhea*) should be performed.

Box 20.3 | Indications for Evaluation by a Primary Care Provider

- Vomiting for >6 hr or >5 diarrheal stools in 1 day
- Any change in mental status
- Syncope
- Temperature >102.2°F (38.9°C) for 12 hr
- Blood glucose levels >400 mg/dL that do not decrease with insulin intake after 2 hr
- Moderate or high ketone levels that do not decrease with extra insulin intake
- Dysuria or other symptoms of urinary tract infection
- Decreased urinary output

Other skin manifestations. Children and adolescents with diabetes may develop skin lesions associated with diabetes (e.g., necrobiosis diabeticorum). If scaly lesions develop—usually on extensor surfaces—treatment by a dermatologist is warranted. Children with thyroid disease may have alopecia.

Acanthosis nigricans is a marker for insulin resistance. If acanthosis is present, the child should receive laboratory screening for diabetes. Females with PCOS often have hirsutism. Treatment with combined oral contraceptive pills (OCPs) or spironolactone will often correct the hirsutism.

Weight loss. The most common cause of weight loss in youth with T1D is worsening metabolic control. Therefore weight loss evaluation should include an assessment of overall glucose control. If control is inadequate and attempts to improve control are unsuccessful, then deliberate withholding of insulin for weight control should be investigated. Weight loss could also be related to the development of celiac disease, so this should be considered. Individuals with diabetes may also develop bulimic characteristics as a method of weight control, but vomiting and abdominal distress in youth with long-standing diabetes may also be a symptom of diabetic gastroparesis. Evaluation for gastroparesis includes radiographic gastric emptying studies that should be done under the direction of a specialist.

Medication Considerations

Many over-the-counter medications and antibiotics contain glucose, and some contain alcohol or traces of gluconeogenic substances, such as sorbitol or glycerin (Kumar et al., 1991). These compounds may raise blood glucose levels slightly in the amounts usually ingested but should not markedly impair metabolic control. Similarly, inhaled corticosteroids, commonly used to control asthma, have not been shown to cause significant increases in blood glucose levels (Faul et al., 2009). On the other hand, short courses of oral steroids are known to cause spikes in blood glucose levels, and patients/families should contact their diabetes provider for advice regarding short-term insulin management changes.

DEVELOPMENTAL ISSUES AND FAMILY CONCERNS

Sleep Patterns

Children with diabetes whose metabolic control is good should have no problems sleeping. Those who are hyperglycemic overnight, however, will have difficulty sleeping because of the recurrent need to urinate. This problem can be managed by improving metabolic control.

Nighttime hypoglycemia is a concern of parents of children on insulin. A child may not wake with the usual early signs and symptoms; the first sign may be a severe event with nightmares or seizures. Therefore, it is important to prevent nighttime hypoglycemia by appropriately adjusting the evening insulin dose and offering a bedtime snack with carbohydrates, protein, or fat. Parents should also be instructed to use the counterregulatory hormone glucagon in case the child cannot be aroused.

Nightmares are common in young children and may be caused by hypoglycemia. Parents should determine the blood glucose level before assuming the cause of a nightmare. If the cause is hypoglycemia, treatment includes the administration of glucose. If the nightmares are not related to hypoglycemia, appropriate comfort measures should be instituted. Prevention is the key; however, significant nighttime hypoglycemia must be avoided as much as possible by carefully adjusting diet and insulin.

Toileting

Several issues related to toileting are important in managing diabetes in children. Many children have secondary enuresis at the time of diagnosis. It is important to tell children who were previously dry that diabetes is the cause of their enuresis and that the enuresis should diminish once the diabetes is adequately controlled. Enuresis can occur, however, with well-controlled diabetes as well. Other methods of diagnostic confirmation and treatment should be explored with these families.

Although testing urine for glucose is not as critical to management as before SMBG testing was available, urinary ketone levels are important indicators of status when a child with diabetes is ill. Parents should know how to obtain such samples from infants and toddlers. Cotton balls tucked into a diaper can provide an adequate sample for use on a dipstick to determine ketone levels in children who are not yet toilet trained. Urine is readily obtainable when a child uses a potty chair during toilet training and when children begin to use the bathroom commode, parents need to teach them to urinate into a paper cup so that the urine can be tested. If taught when a child is feeling well, this task can be made into a game so that, when necessary, the behavior has been learned.

Discipline

Although the issues related to discipline of a child with diabetes are not different from those of all children with a chronic condition, parents of children with diabetes often report discipline as a concern in follow-up visits. Parents often worry that a hypoglycemic episode will be missed by attributing the unruly behavior to a lack of discipline. It is appropriate for parents to test the blood glucose level at any time hypoglycemia is suspected; if the result is within the normal range, the child can be appropriately disciplined. Blood testing should be performed matter-of-factly so that children do not misinterpret the test as a punishment. Some parents also worry that the stress of imposed discipline will raise the blood glucose level because of counterregulatory hormones. Although severe stressors may increase blood glucose levels, no evidence suggests that usual disciplinary measures increase blood glucose levels or worsen metabolic control.

Child Care

Toddlers and preschoolers with diabetes benefit from the socialization of preschool programs, as do all children, and they do not need specialized medical day care. Preschool teachers should be informed of parental expectations, such as blood glucose testing and insulin administration. Snack and lunch intake are very important, so preschool teachers must know what the child needs to eat and what should be served at each mealtime. They should be aware of appropriate food substitutions when food is refused. All caregivers should be told how to manage the symptoms of hypoglycemia. Emergency telephone numbers should always be available and include parents' telephone numbers, another emergency contact, the primary care provider, and the diabetes specialists. The ADA (2022) has specific guidelines for diabetes care in the school and day care setting in its standards of care document, which is updated annually and is an excellent resource for parents and school personnel.

Parents of children with diabetes often express concerns about the abilities of babysitters or day care workers to manage a young child's T1D. Parents of young children can begin by leaving the child for only short periods of time, thus reassuring themselves that the sitter can successfully care for the child. Clear instructions on the child's meal plan and management of hypoglycemia should be provided in writing. Parents should be encouraged to train sitters in blood glucose monitoring and recognizing hypoglycemic symptoms. Remote monitoring with a CGM has also helped to ease these stresses for parents.

Schooling

Children whose diabetes is adequately controlled should attend school regularly and participate in any activities for which they are otherwise suited. Parents should be encouraged to inform the school nurse and the child's teachers when diabetes is diagnosed. It is important that school personnel are knowledgeable about the child's care so that hypoglycemia or illness can be appropriately managed. The need for other involvement (e.g., SMBG testing or injections) depends on the child's usual regimen. For youth with T2D, the school can be invaluable in providing support and follow-up in a weight loss program.

With older children, providers need to work with the child, family, and school personnel to arrange a school schedule that fits the child's diabetes regimen. For example, a child who has had regular and NPH insulin at 7:00 a.m. should probably have a snack before a gym class that precedes a late lunch period. Arrangements must be made so the child can always access glucose-containing foods or tablets in case of a hypoglycemic episode. The child should always have food available on field trips. A sack lunch with all food groups is a substitute if a meal is unexpectedly delayed.

Sports are encouraged. For youth with T1D, coaches should be aware of the diabetes and keep foods containing glucose on hand. Depending on the degree of exercise on extra-activity days, the insulin dose may be lowered, the diet increased, or both to prevent hypoglycemia. Hypoglycemia following exercise may occur up to 12 hours after the event, so children should be carefully monitored when any new activity is undertaken. Children should be advised that insulin is absorbed more rapidly from exercising muscle; therefore if a muscle is to be exercised, insulin should be injected into another site. For example, if a child runs track, the insulin could be administered in the arm or the abdomen instead of the leg. For youth with T2D, physical activity is crucial to improving outcomes. These youth should be encouraged to participate in physical activities at school and home.

Children with T1D or T2D whose diabetes is in poor control may experience difficulties in school performance. Because hypoglycemia can cause a child to lose the ability to concentrate when the blood glucose level is low, learning can be a problem. When the blood glucose level is consistently too high, many children experience difficulties concentrating, and their grades may suffer. Any child with diabetes whose school performance changes should be carefully assessed for alterations in metabolic control. Unless there are other problems, children with diabetes should not require special education or an individual learning plan. Indeed, several class action suits have been brought against school districts that required otherwise well children with diabetes to attend special education classes.

However, children with diabetes are encouraged to set up an individualized 504 plan (pursuant to Section 504 of the Rehabilitation Act of 1973). This type of plan helps ensure they are medically safe at school and have other accommodations related to their diabetes to ensure they can thrive in the school setting. Some examples of items included in 504 plans include but are not limited to extra trips to the restroom, the ability to carry snacks/sugar on their person throughout the school day, and permission to retake an exam if they experience a low blood sugar while testing.

Because children and adolescents with diabetes are encouraged to participate fully in sports and other activities, they may also be encouraged to go to camp. Specialized camps for children with diabetes may help young people learn about their diabetes and meet peers who also have diabetes. Children and adolescents with diabetes may also safely attend regular camps. Whether the camp is a diabetes-specific camp or not, care should be taken to adjust the insulin dose and food intake to account for the markedly increased physical activity at camp. Extra blood glucose monitoring may be necessary.

As with all children with chronic conditions, emphasis should be on the normality of the child, not on the diabetes. Such an approach helps minimize the sense of being different that all affected children can experience.

Sexuality

Achievement of normal growth and development is a goal of therapy for T1D. If the diabetes is adequately controlled, sexual development should be normal. However, if sexual development is delayed, normal concerns about self-adequacy and physical adequacy may be amplified. Primary care providers must carefully monitor secondary sexual development in children with diabetes, and any deviation from normal should be investigated. Tightening the metabolic control often improves growth. If not, the cause should be investigated further.

All sexually active teenagers need information about birth control. Such information is especially important for those with either type of diabetes because the risks for complications of pregnancy are at least five times greater for adolescents with diabetes than for their nondiabetic peers. Because of the risk for sexually transmitted infections (STIs), many providers encourage condoms in combination with other birth control methods. Unfortunately, as with all teenagers, proper and consistent use of condoms is variable. Other barrier methods (e.g., diaphragms, foams, and creams) may also be used by those with diabetes but share the same disadvantages as condoms and do not prevent STIs.

Teenagers with diabetes who are or plan to be sexually active should be encouraged to start birth control like their nondiabetic peers. Earlier versions of combined OCPs carried risks for cerebral ischemia, myocardial infarction, and rapid progression of retinopathy and were not recommended for adolescents with diabetes. Newer OCPs, however, seem to be well tolerated. Since the risk of pregnancy is much greater than those associated with taking any available contraceptive methods, sexually active teenagers with T1D should be encouraged to be on the form of birth control with which they are likely to be the most compliant to prevent pregnancy. Teenagers with T2D should avoid the contraceptive patch if they are obese since it is contraindicated in obesity. It is also well known that the Depo-Provera shot can lead to a 15- to 20-lb weight gain and should be avoided in teenagers with T2D who are trying to lose weight. Teenagers with T2D and concurrent PCOS may benefit from combined OCPs to help regulate their periods, improve their acne, and manage their hirsutism.

Although avoidance of adolescent pregnancy is clearly preferred for youth with either type of diabetes, some teenagers express the desire to become pregnant. However, it has been clearly demonstrated that pregnancy outcomes can be dramatically improved if euglycemia is maintained both in the months preceding conception and throughout the pregnancy. Therefore female adolescents at risk for pregnancy or contemplating pregnancy should receive preconception counseling.

Male adolescents often express concern about the well-known complication of impotence in adult males. Impotence is thought to result from vascular and neurologic compromise in those with long-standing diabetes. Fortunately impotence caused by diabetes is very rare in adolescence, so most of these individuals can be reassured.

Transition to Adulthood

The transition from pediatric to adult diabetes care is a high-risk time. During this phase, individuals often assume responsibility for their diabetes care and become more self-sufficient concerning their housing, work, social, and financial situations, including health insurance coverage and copayments. These competing demands often interrupt diabetes care, leading to poorer glycemic control and increased risk for acute complications. This interruption to diabetes care is compounded by increased rates of depression and substance use during this period, which can also negatively impact glycemic control (Peters & Laffel, 2011).

For these reasons, assisting teenagers with diabetes with this transition is important to ensure they are prepared and not lost to follow-up. Although scientific evidence is still limited (especially for T2D), the ADA (2022) recommends that pediatric health care providers start this transition in early adolescence and at least 1 year before the official transition occurs. For many practices, this transition happens around 22 years or sometimes later if teenagers remain on their parents' insurance through 25 years. In preparing these patients for this transition, it is important to gradually transfer diabetes self-care tasks from the parent to the youth. This includes medical tasks, such as insulin administration and glucose analysis and adjustment, but it also includes peripheral tasks around diabetes, such as scheduling appointments, navigating the nuances of insurance coverage, and ordering supplies (Peters & Laffel, 2011). This process should also include screening for depression, anxiety, substance abuse, and eating disorders that could put these transitioning youth at greater risk for noncompliance with their diabetes care and follow-up visits.

Social Determinants of Health

Social determinants of health (SDOH) can significantly impact glycemic control for children with diabetes. SDOH often fall into five major categories: socioeconomic status (SES), neighborhood and physical environment, food environment, health care, and social context. Children from lower SES have been shown to have poorer glycemic control and be at greater risk for complications from their diabetes than their higher SES peers (Zuijwijk et al., 2013). One study suggests that Hispanic youth with T1D are at greater risk for poor glycemic control because of their low SES rather than their ethnicity (Gallegos-Macias et al., 2003). This relationship between SES and diabetes outcomes is often multifactorial. Children with diabetes from lower SES backgrounds, for instance, may not have consistent insurance coverage or may be on an insurance that is less likely to approve advanced diabetes technologies, such as insulin pumps and CGMs, which have been shown to improve glycemic control. Children from lower SES backgrounds may also have parents with lower educational attainment and occupational status or language barriers. This can mean decreased health and math literacy for those family members involved in the child's day-to-day diabetes care. It may also be difficult for these family members to miss time from work to attend diabetes follow-up visits for the child.

Lower SES can also result in housing instability. Unstable housing can make it difficult for families to engage in consistent routines for diabetes management, store diabetes medications safely, have regular access to healthy foods, and find safe spaces for physical activities (Hill-Briggs et al., 2021). Families without consistent transportation rely heavily on food sources within walking distance of their homes. In lower SES neighborhoods, convenience stores and fast-food restaurants are often more accessible than grocery stores. This often means that families consume more foods with higher carbohydrate and fat content. In a national study of food environments, limited access to healthy food was associated with higher rates of T2D (Ahern et al., 2011). Limited access to safe spaces for physical activity is concerning for children with T2D who need regular physical activity to lose weight and improve their insulin resistance to improve their glycemic control.

Children with diabetes from lower SES may also have limited access to affordable and high-quality health care. Although federally qualified health centers have improved access to primary care services for underserved populations across the country in recent years, access to pediatric endocrinology specialists continues to vary substantially by state and county in the United States (Lu et al., 2015). Families living in more rural parts of the country may not have the transportation or financial means to travel for routine specialty care. While expanding telehealth services during the COVID-19 pandemic helped with this temporarily, many specialty offices have returned to seeing their patients in person preferentially. For adolescents with diabetes, not having a usual provider (primary care or diabetes specialist) translates to higher A1c levels and greater use of urgent care centers for acute diabetes complications (Liese et al., 2019). It is important for pediatric primary care providers to familiarize themselves with the basics of managing T1D and T2D discussed herein to help bridge the gap with diabetes specialty care for all of their patients with diabetes, especially those from lower SES backgrounds.

Support

Three national organizations provide help for families coping with diabetes in a child: the ADA, the Juvenile Diabetes Research Foundation (JDRF), and Beyond Type 1 (see Resources). The ADA is the largest organization, composed of lay individuals and professionals. The ADA supports research, education, fundraising, and camps and provides lobbying efforts related to diabetes. It publishes several pamphlets and books for families to use in understanding diabetes. Many affiliates provide support and educational programs for families and children at the local level. The ADA deals with all types of diabetes, not only T1D.

Research toward a cure for T1D is the primary focus of JDRF. The organization provides some support for families, but its major effort is devoted to fundraising for research to find a cure for T1D. Some families find that working toward the cure helps them deal with the condition in their family. Beyond Type 1 funds advocacy, education, and cure research and aims to unite the global diabetes community around improving the everyday lives of those with diabetes.

RESOURCES

American Diabetes Association: www.diabetes.org
Beyond Type 1: https://beyondtype1.org
Centers for Disease Control and Prevention (diabetes home page): www.cdc.gov/Diabetes
Children with Diabetes: www.childrenwithdiabetes.com
College Diabetes Network: https://collegediabetesnetwork.org
Diabetes Book Store: www.members.aol.com/healthbook/diabetes
Juvenile Diabetes Research Foundation: www.jdrf.org
National Institute of Diabetes and Digestive and Kidney Disease: www.nih/niddk.gov
News and Chat Groups: misc.health.diabetes (the place to find people to talk with about diabetes); alt.support.diabetes.kids (a support group for parents with children with diabetes)

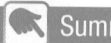 Summary

Primary Care Needs for the Child With Diabetes Mellitus (Types 1 and 2)

HEALTH CARE MAINTENANCE
Growth and Development
- Height and weight are normal in type 1 unless diabetes control is less than adequate.
- Secondary sexual development may be delayed.
- Rapid weight gain may require intervention.
- Weight loss usually indicates poor control or insulin omission.
- Weight and BMI are elevated in T2D.
- Secondary sexual development may be accelerated in T2D with hirsutism if PCOS is present.

Diet
- Maintenance of normoglycemia is critical.
- Stress the importance of regular distribution of meals and snacks.
- In T1D, sufficient calories for growth is paramount.
- In T2D, reducing calories and fat is a cornerstone of treatment to reduce obesity.
- Physical activity is encouraged in T1D with modification of insulin as needed.
- Increasing aerobic capacity while decreasing sedentary behaviors is the focus in children with T2D.
- Celiac disease is more common in children with T1D.

Safety
- Prevent hypoglycemia with careful monitoring; be sure a glucose source is always available.
- Dispose of syringes properly.
- Use glucagon for severe hypoglycemic episodes.
- Ensure safe storage of oral medications.
- Medical identification should be worn to ensure appropriate prompt treatment.

Immunizations
- Routine immunizations are recommended.
- Yearly influenza vaccine is recommended.
- COVID vaccine is recommended.

Screening
- *Vision.* Routine screening is recommended.
- *Hearing.* Routine screening is recommended.
- *Tuberculosis.* Routine screening is recommended.
- *Hypertension.* Blood pressure should be checked at each visit. Hypertension should be aggressively managed.
- *Dyslipidemia.* For T1D, lipid screening should be done at diagnosis and once glycemia is improved if child is 2 years and older. For LDL at or below 100 mg/dL, it should be repeated at 9 to 10 years of age and every 3 years after that. More frequent screenings may be needed for LDL above 130 mg/dL. For T2D, lipid screening should be done at diagnosis and annually.
- *Nephropathy.* For T1D, albumin-to-creatinine ratio should be checked once they start puberty or turn 10 years old and have had diabetes for at least 5 years. It should be repeated annually if normal and more frequent if abnormal. For T2D, it should be checked at diagnosis and annually after that.
- *Retinopathy.* For T1D, dilated fundoscopic exam should be completed every 2 years once the child starts puberty or turns 11 years old and has had diabetes for at least 3 years. If normal, intervals between screenings can be extended to every 4 years. For T2D, the exam should be completed at diagnosis and annually.
- *Neuropathy.* For T1D, monofilament exam should be completed once the child starts puberty or turns 10 years old once they have had diabetes for 5 years. For T2D, monofilament exam should be completed at diagnosis. If normal, it should be repeated at least annually for both.
- *Dental.* Dental cleanings and exams are recommended every 6 months. Caries should be aggressively managed.
- *Depression.* Routine screening is recommended.

Condition-Specific Screening
Type 1 Diabetes
- *Thyroid disorder.* TPO and thyroglobulin antibodies should be checked at diagnosis. TSH should be checked after glucose control is established and every 1 to 2 years after that or sooner if symptoms start.
- *Celiac disease.* Tissue transglutaminase–IgA (and IgA levels) should be checked at diagnosis. If negative, it should be repeated in 2 years, then every 5 years.

Type 2 Diabetes
- *NAFLD.* AST and ALT levels should be checked at diagnosis and annually after that.
- *PCOS.* Symptoms screening should occur at every visit and a lab workup completed if positive.
- *Obstructive sleep apnea.* Symptoms should be screened for at every visit and referral to sleep specialist made if positive.

COMMON ILLNESS MANAGEMENT
Differential Diagnosis
- Common illnesses and stress require sick day management.
- It is important to maintain hydration during illness.
- It is most important to evaluate for hypoglycemia with changes in mental status.
- Monilial vaginal infections are more common in adolescent females.
- Skin lesions must be evaluated.
- Weight loss in T1D and weight gain in T2D may indicate poor metabolic control.
- Diabetic gastroparesis may cause vomiting or abdominal pain.

Drug Interactions
- Beware that many over-the-counter medications and antibiotics contain glucogenic substances or alcohol.
- Oral steroids can cause hyperglycemia.

DEVELOPMENTAL ISSUES AND FAMILY CONCERNS
Sleep Patterns
- Prevention of nighttime hypoglycemia is important.
- Nightmares may be the result of hypoglycemia.

Toileting
- Enuresis may be present when control is poor.
- Measurement of urinary ketones is important when blood glucose levels are high or when the child is ill.

Discipline
- Unruly behavior may be caused by hypoglycemia.
- The potential for conflict over diet, blood testing, and insulin administration should be recognized.
- Stress associated with discipline should not elevate blood glucose.

Child Care
- Teachers and babysitters need training in management of dietary needs and hypoglycemia.

Schooling
- Full attendance and participation are expected.
- School personnel must be aware of the child's special needs.
- If metabolic control is poor, performance may be affected.

Sexuality
- If diabetes is adequately controlled, sexual development should be normal.
- Pregnancy prevention is very important because of combined risks of diabetes and adolescent pregnancy.

- Pregnancy outcomes are dramatically improved if euglycemia is maintained preceding and during pregnancy.
- Impotency caused by long-term vascular and neurologic compromise is a rare problem during adolescence.

Transition to Adulthood
- The transition from pediatric to adult diabetes care should start in early adolescence and at least 1 year before the official transition occurs.

Social Determinants of Health
- Lower SES is associated with poorer glycemic control and increased risk for diabetes complications.

REFERENCES

Adolfsson, P., Björnsson, V., Heringhaus, A., & Sjunnesson, K. (2022). A prospective controlled study evaluating the long-term outcomes on glucose control, sleep, and health economy after implementation of tandem control-IQ technology in a pediatric population with relatively good glucose control already at start. In: *Poster presented at 15th Annual International Conference on Advanced Technologies & Treatments for Diabetes (ATTD)*; Barcelona, Spain.

Ahern, J. A., Boland, E. A., Doane, R., Ahern, J. J., Rose, P., Vincent, M., & Tamborlane, W. V. (2002). Insulin pump therapy in pediatrics: A therapeutic alternative to safely lower HbA1c levels across all age groups. *Pediatr Diabetes, 3*(1), 10–15. doi: 10.1034/j.1399-5448.2002.30103.x. PMID: 15016169.

Ahern, M., Brown, C., & Dukas, S. (2011). A national study of the association between food environments and county-level health outcomes. *Journal of Rural Health, 27*, 367–379.

American Diabetes Association. (1993). Position statement: Implications of the diabetes control and complications trial. *Diabetes, 42*, 1555–1558.

American Diabetes Association. (2022a). Clinical practice recommendations. *Diabetes Care, 45*(Suppl 1), entire issue.

American Diabetes Association. (2022b). Diabetes facts. Available at www.diabetes.org. Retrieved June 8, 2022.

Anderson, B. J., Brackett, J., Ho, J., & Laffel, L. M. (1999). An office-based intervention to maintain parent-adolescent teamwork in diabetes management. Impact on parent involvement, family conflict, and subsequent glycemic control. *Diabetes Care, 22*(5), 713–21. doi:10.2337/diacare.22.5.713. PMID: 10332671.

Arslanian, S., Bacha, F., Grey, M., Marcus, M. D., White, N. H., & Zeitler, P. (2018). Evaluation and management of youth-onset type 2 diabetes: A position statement by the American Diabetes Association. *Diabetes Care, 41*(12), 2648–2668. https://doi.org/10.2337/dci18-0052.

Battelino, T., Danne, T., Bergenstal, R. M., Amiel, S. A., Beck, R., Biester, T., Bosi, E., Buckingham, B. A., Cefalu, W. T., Close, K. L., Cobelli, C., Dassau, E., DeVries, J. H., Donaghue, K. C., Dovc, K., Doyle, F. J. 3rd, Garg, S., Grunberger, G., Heller, S., ... Phillip, M. (2019). Clinical targets for continuous glucose monitoring data interpretation: Recommendations from the international consensus on time in range. *Diabetes Care, 42*(8), 1593–1603. doi:10.2337/dci19-0028. Epub 2019 Jun 8. PMID: 31177185; PMCID: PMC6973648.

Bernstein, C. M., Stockwell, M. S., Gallagher, M. P., Rosenthal, S. L., & Soren, K. (2013). Mental health issues in adolescents and young adults with type 1 diabetes: Prevalence and impact on glycemic control. *Clinical Pediatrics, 52*(1), 10–15. https://doi.org/10.1177/0009922812459950.

Bingley, P. J., Bonfacio, E., & Gale, E. A. M. (1993). Can we really predict IDDM? *Diabetes, 42*, 213–220.

Boland, E. A., Grey, M., Oesterle, A., Fredrickson, L., & Tamborlane, W. V. (1999). Continuous subcutaneous insulin infusion.

A new way to lower risk of severe hypoglycemia, improve metabolic control, and enhance coping in adolescents with type 1 diabetes. *Diabetes Care, 22*(11), 1779–1784. doi:10.2337/diacare.22.11.1779. PMID: 10546007.

Buckingham, B. A., Paguntalan, H., Fassl, B., et al. (2001). Continuous subcutaneous insulin infusion (CSII) in children under five years of age. *Diabetes, 50*(Suppl 2), A107.

Buckingham, B. A., Forlenza, G. P., Criego, A. B., Hansen, D. W., Bode, B. W., Brown, S. A., MacLeish, S. A., Pinsker, J. E., DeSalvo, D. J., Sherr, J. L., Mehta, S. N., Laffel, L. M., Bhargava, A., & Ly, T. T. (2021). Safety evaluation of the Omnipod® 5 automated insulin delivery system over three months of use in children with type 1 diabetes (T1D). *Journal of the Endocrine Society, 5*(Suppl 1), A454. doi:10.1210/jendso/bvab048.927. PMCID: PMC8090047.

Butwicka, A., Frisén, L., Almqvist, C., Zethelius, B., & Lichtenstein, P. (2015). Risks of psychiatric disorders and suicide attempts in children and adolescents with type 1 diabetes: A population-based cohort study. *Diabetes Care, 38*(3), 453–459.

Callahan, S. T., & Mansfield, M. J. (2000). T2D in adolescents. *Current Opinions in Pediatrics, 12*, 310–315.

Centers for Disease Control and Prevention (2022). National diabetes statistics report. https://www.cdc.gov/diabetes/data/statistics-report/index.html. Accessed June 16, 2022.

Cherubini, V., Grimsmann, J. M., Åkesson, K., Birkebæk, N. H., Cinek, O., Dovč, K., Gesuita, R., Gregory, J. W., Hanas, R., Hofer, S. E., Holl, R. W., Jefferies, C., Joner, G., King, B. R., Mayer-Davis, E. J., Peña, A. S., Rami-Merhar, B., Schierloh, U., Skrivarhaug, T., ... Dabelea, D. (2020). Temporal trends in diabetic ketoacidosis at diagnosis of paediatric type 1 diabetes between 2006 and 2016: results from 13 countries in three continents. *Diabetologia, 63*(8), 1530–1541. doi:10.1007/s00125-020-05152-1. Epub 2020 May 8. PMID: 32382815; PMCID: PMC7351855.

Cioana, M., Deng, J., Hou, M., Nadarajah, A., Qiu, Y., Chen, S. S. J., Rivas, A., Banfield, L., Chanchlani, R., Dart, A., Wicklow, B., Alfaraidi, H., Alotaibi, A., Thabane, L., & Samaan, M. C. (2021). Prevalence of hypertension and albuminuria in pediatric type 2 diabetes: A systematic review and meta-analysis. *JAMA Network Open, 4*(4), e216069. doi:10.1001/jamanetworkopen.2021.6069. Erratum in: JAMA Netw Open. 2023 Oct 2;6(10):e2341796. PMID: 33929524; PMCID: PMC8087958.

Clarke, P., Gray, A., Adler, A., Stevens, R., Raikou, M., Cull, C., Stratton, I., & Holman, R.; UKPDS Group. (2001). United Kingdom prospective diabetes study. Cost-effectiveness analysis of intensive blood-glucose control with metformin in overweight patients with type II diabetes (UKPDS No. 51). *Diabetologia, 44*(3), 298–304. doi:10.1007/s001250051617. PMID: 11317659.

Cohen, E., Tsoukas, M., Oettingen, J. E., Yale, Y., et al. (2022). A randomised controlled trial to alleviate carbohydrate counting in type 1 diabetes with automated Fiasp and pramlintide closed-loop delivery. *Diabetes, 71*(Suppl 1) 290-OR. https://doi.org/10.2337/db22-290-OR.

Dholakia, S., Oskrochi, Y., Easton, G., & Papalois, V. (2016). Advances in pancreas transplantation. *Journal of the Royal Society of Medicine, 109*(4), 141–146.

Diabetes Control and Complications Trial Research Group. (1993a). Expanded role of the dietitian in the DCCT: Implications for clinical practice. *Journal of the American Dietetic Association, 93*, 758–767.

Diabetes Control and Complications Trial Research Group. (1993b). The effect of intensive treatment of diabetes on the development and progression of long-term complications in insulin-dependent diabetes mellitus. *New England Journal of Medicine, 329*, 435–459.

Faul, J. L., Wilson, S. R., Chu, J. W., Canfield, J., & Kuschner, W. G. (2009). The effect of an inhaled corticosteroid on glucose control in type 2 diabetes. *Clinical Medicine & Research, 7*(1–2), 14–20. doi:10.3121/cmr.2009.824. Epub 2009 Feb 26. PMID: 19251584; PMCID: PMC2705276.

Foster, N. C., Beck R. W., Miller, K. M., Clements, M. A., Rickels, M. R., DiMeglio, L. A., Maahs, D. M., Tamborlane, W. V., Bergenstal, R., Smith, E., Olson, B. A., & Garg, S. K. (2019). State of type 1 diabetes management and outcomes from the T1D exchange in 2016–2018. *Diabetes Technol Ther, 21*(2), 66–72. doi: 10.1089/dia.2018.0384. Epub 2019 Jan 18. Erratum in: Diabetes Technol Ther. 2019 Apr;21(4):230.

Fox, L. A., Buckloh, L. M., Smith, S. D., Wysocki, T., & Mauras, N. (2005). A randomized controlled trial of insulin pump therapy in young children with type 1 diabetes. *Diabetes Care, 28*(6), 1277–1281. doi:10.2337/diacare.28.6.1277. PMID: 15920039.

Gallegos-Macias, A. R., Macias, S. R., Kaufman, E., Skipper B., & Kalishman, N. (2003). Relationship between glycemic control, ethnicity and socioeconomic status in Hispanic and white non-Hispanic youths with type 1 diabetes mellitus. *Pediatr Diabetes, 4*(1), 19–23. doi: 10.1034/j.1399-5448.2003.00020.x.

Gilliam, L. K., Liese, A. D., Bloch, C. A., Davis, C., Snively, B. M., Curb, D., Williams, D. E., & Pihoker, C.; SEARCH for Diabetes in Youth Study Group. (2007). Family history of diabetes, autoimmunity, and risk factors for cardiovascular disease among children with diabetes in the SEARCH for Diabetes in Youth Study. *Pediatric Diabetes, 8*(6), 354–361. doi:10.1111/j.1399-5448.2007.00241.x. PMID: 18036060.

Glaser, N. S. (1997). Non-insulin-dependent diabetes mellitus in childhood and adolescence. *Pediatric Clinics of North America, 44*, 307–333.

Goldstein, D. E., Little, R. R., Lorenz, R. A., Malone, J. I., Nathan, D., & Peterson, C. M. (1995). Tests of glycemia in diabetes. *Diabetes Care, 18*(6), 896–909. doi:10.2337/diacare.18.6.896. PMID: 7555528.

Grey, M., Boland, E. A., Davidson, M., Li, J., & Tamborlane, W. V. (2000). Coping skills training for youth with diabetes mellitus has long-lasting effects on metabolic control and quality of life. *Journal of Pediatrics, 137*(1), 107–113. doi:10.1067/mpd.2000.106568. PMID: 10891831.

Grey, M., & Tamborlane, W. V. (2003). Behavioral and family aspects of treatment of children and adolescents with type 1 diabetes. In Porte, D., Sherwin, R. S., & Baron, A. (Eds.), *Ellenberg and Rifkins diabetes mellitus.* McGraw-Hill.

Harris, S., Carrillo, M., & Fjioka, K. (2021). Binge-eating disorder and type 2 diabetes: A review. *Endocrine Practice, 27*, 158–164.

Hill-Briggs, F., Adler, N. E., Berkowitz, S. A., Chin, M. H., Gary-Webb, T. L., Navas-Acien, A., Thornton, P. L., & Haire-Joshu, D. (2020). Social determinants of health and diabetes: A scientific review. *Diabetes Care, 44*(1), 258–279. doi:10.2337/dci20-0053. Epub ahead of print. PMID: 33139407; PMCID: PMC7783927.

Jalaludin, M. Y., Deeb, A., Zeitler, P., Garcia, R., Newfield, R. S., Samoilova, Y., Rosario, C. A., Shehadeh, N., Saha, C. K., Zhang, Y., Zilli, M., Scherer, L. W., Lam, R. L. H., Golm, G. T., Engel, S. S., Kaufman, K. D., & Shankar, R. R. (2022). Efficacy and safety of the addition of sitagliptin to treatment of youth with type 2 diabetes and inadequate glycemic control on metformin without or with insulin. *Pediatric Diabetes, 23*(2), 183–193. doi:10.1111/pedi.13282. Epub 2021 Dec 20. PMID: 34779103.

Jones, K. L. (2002). Treatment of type 2 diabetes mellitus in children. *JAMA, 287*, 716.

Jones, K. L., Arslanian, S., Peterokova, V. A., Park, J. S., & Tomlinson, M. J. (2002). Effect of metformin in pediatric patients with type 2 diabetes: a randomized controlled trial. *Diabetes Care, 25*(1), 89–94. doi:10.2337/diacare.25.1.89. PMID: 11772907.

Kelsey, M. M., Geffner, M. E., Guandalini, C., Pyle, L., Tamborlane, W. V., Zeitler, P. S., & White, N. H.; Treatment Options for Type 2 Diabetes in Adolescents and Youth Study Group. (2016). Presentation and effectiveness of early treatment of type 2 diabetes in youth: Lessons from the TODAY study. *Pediatric Diabetes, 17*(3), 212–221. doi:10.1111/pedi.12264. Epub 2015 Feb 17. PMID: 25690268; PMCID: PMC4539288.

Kumar, A., Weatherly, M., & Beaman, D. C. (1991). Sweeteners, flavorings, and dyes in antibiotic preparations. *Pediatrics, 87*, 352–360.

Kyngas, H., & Barlow, J. (1995). Diabetes: An adolescent's perspective. *Journal of Advanced Nursing, 22*, 941–947.

Lawrence, J. M., Standiford, D. A., Loots, B., et al. (2006). Prevalence and correlates of depressed mood among youth with diabetes: The SEARCH for Diabetes in Youth Study. *Pediatrics, 117*(4), 1348–1358. https://doi.org/10.1542/peds.2005-1398.

Leslie, D. G., & Elliot, R. G. (1994). Early environmental events as a cause of IDDM: Evidence and implications. *Diabetes, 43*, 843–850.

Levitt Katz, L. E., Swami, S., Abraham, M., Murphy, K. M., Jawad, A. F., McKnight-Menci, H., & Berkowitz, R. (2005). Neuropsychiatric disorders at the presentation of type 2 diabetes mellitus in children. *Pediatric Diabetes, 6*(2), 84–89. doi:10.1111/j.1399-543X.2005.00105.x. PMID: 15963035.

Liese, A. D., Ma, X., Reid, L., Sutherland, M. W., Bell, B. A., Eberth, J. M., Probst, J. C., Turley, C. B., & Mayer-Davis, E. J. (2019). Health care access and glycemic control in youth and young adults with type 1 and type 2 diabetes in South Carolina. *Pediatric Diabetes, 20*(3), 321–329. doi:10.1111/pedi.12822. Epub 2019 Feb 19. PMID: 30666775; PMCID: PMC6456401.

Lu, H., Holt, J. B., Cheng, Y. J., Zhang, X., Onufrak, S., & Croft, J. B. (2015). Population-based geographic access to endocrinologists in the United States, 2012. *BMC Health Services Research, 15*, 541. doi:10.1186/s12913-015-1185-5. PMID: 26644021; PMCID: PMC4672571.

Ludwig, D. S., & Ebbeling, C. B. (2001). Type 2 diabetes mellitus in children: Primary care and public health considerations. *JAMA, 286*, 1427–1430.

Majidi, S., O'Donnell, H. K., Stanek, K., Youngkin, E., Gomer, T., & Driscoll, K. A. (2020). Suicide risk: Assessment in youth and young adults with type 1 diabetes. *Diabetes Care, 43*(2), 343–348. https://doi.org/10.2337/dc19-0831.

Mathur, K., Agrawal, R. K., Nagpure, S., & Deshpande, D. (2020). Effect of artificial sweeteners on insulin resistance among type-2 diabetes mellitus patients. *J Family Med Prim Care, 9*(1), 69–71. doi: 10.4103/jfmpc.jfmpc_329_19.

Mayer-Davis, E. J., Lawrence, J. M., Dabelea, D., Divers, J., Isom, S., Dolan, L., et al. For SEARCH for Diabetes in Youth Study (2017). Incidence trends of type 1 and type 2 diabetes among youths: 2002–2012. *New England Journal of Medicine, 376*, 1419–1427.

McCall, M., & Shapiro, J. (2014). Islet transplantation. *Diapedia,* https://doi.org/10.14496/dia.

McCarty, R. L., Weber, W. J., Loots, B., Breuner, C. C., Vander Stoep, A., Manhart, L., & Pihoker, C. (2010). Complementary and alternative medicine use and quality of life in pediatric diabetes. *Journal of Alternative & Complementary Medicine, 16*(2), 165–173. doi:10.1089/acm.2008.0566. PMID: 20180689; PMCID: PMC3110095.

McGrady, A., Bailey, B. K., & Good, M. P. (1991). Controlled study of biofeedback-assisted relaxation in type 1 diabetes. *Diabetes Care, 14,* 360–365.

McMurray, R. G., Bauman, M. J., Harrell, J. S., Brown, S., & Bangdiwala, S. I. (2000). Effects of improvement in aerobic power on resting insulin and glucose concentrations in children. *Eur J Appl Physiol, 81*(1–2), 132–9. doi: 10.1007/PL00013786.

Peters, A., & Laffel, L. (2011). Diabetes care for emerging adults: Recommendations for transition from pediatric to adult diabetes care systems. *Diabetes Care, 34,* 2477–2485.

Phillip, M., Battelino, T., Rodriguez, H., Danne, T., & Kaufman, F.; European Society for Paediatric Endocrinology; Lawson Wilkins Pediatric Endocrine Society; International Society for Pediatric and Adolescent Diabetes; American Diabetes Association; European Association for the Study of Diabetes. (2007). Use of insulin pump therapy in the pediatric age-group: Consensus statement from the European Society for Paediatric Endocrinology, the Lawson Wilkins Pediatric Endocrine Society, and the International Society for Pediatric and Adolescent Diabetes, endorsed by the American Diabetes Association and the European Association for the Study of Diabetes. *Diabetes Care, 30*(6), 1653–1662. doi:10.2337/dc07-9922. Epub 2007 Mar 19. PMID: 17372151.

Pihoker, C., Scott, C. R., Lensing, S. Y., Cradock, M. M., & Smith, J. (1998) Non-insulin dependent diabetes mellitus in African-American youths of Arkansas. *Clinical Pediatrics (Phila), 37*(2), 97–102. doi:10.1177/000992289803700206. PMID: 9492117.

Pinhas-Hamiel, O., & Zeitler, P. (2007). Clinical presentation and treatment of type 2 diabetes in children. *Pediatr Diabetes, 8*(Suppl 9), 16–27.

Rechenberg, K., Whittemore, R., & Grey, M. (2017). Anxiety in youth with type 1 diabetes. *Journal of Pediatric Nursing, 32,* 64–71. https://doi.org/10.1016/j.pedn.2016.08.007.

Rewers, A., Klingensmith, G., Davis, C., Petitti, D. B., Pihoker, C., Rodriguez, B., Schwartz, I. D., Imperatore, G., Williams, D., Dolan, L. M., & Dabelea, D. (2008). Presence of diabetic ketoacidosis at diagnosis of diabetes mellitus in youth: The search for diabetes in youth study. *Pediatrics, 121*(5), e1258–e1266. doi:10.1542/peds.2007-1105. PMID: 18450868.

Rodin, G., Olmsted, M. P., Rydall, A. C., Maharaj, S. I., Colton, P. A., Jones, J. M., Biancucci, L. A., & Daneman, D. (2002). Eating disorders in young women with type 1 diabetes mellitus. *Journal of Psychosomatic Research, 53*(4), 943–949. doi:10.1016/s0022-3999(02)00305-7. PMID: 12377307.

Roy, A., Grosman, B., Miller, D., Engel, T., Cohen, O., Shalit, R., Shalem, S., Hirsh, M. L., Cohen, Y., & Tirosh, A. (2022). 287-or: Eliminating manual meal bolusing: A feasibility trial using minimed 780G and hand gesture algorithms. *Diabetes, 71*(Supplement_1). https://doi.org/10.2337/db22-287-or.

Shankar, R. R., Zeitler, P., Deeb, A., Jalaludin, M. Y., Garcia, R., Newfield, R. S., Samoilova, Y., Rosario, C. A., Shehadeh, N., Saha, C. K., Zhang, Y., Zilli, M., Scherer, L. W., Lam, R. L., Golm, G. T., Engel, S. S., & Kaufman, K. D. (2021). A randomized clinical trial of the efficacy and safety of Sitagliptin as initial oral therapy in youth with type 2 diabetes. *Pediatric Diabetes, 23*(2), 173–182. https://doi.org/10.1111/pedi.13279.

Sherr, J. L., Ruedy, K. J., Foster, N. C., Piché, C. A., Dulude, H., Rickels, M. R., Tamborlane, W. V., Bethin, K. E., DiMeglio, L. A., Fox, L. A., Wadwa, R. P., Schatz, D. A., Nathan, B. M., Marcovina, S. M., Rampakakis, E., Meng, L., & Beck, R. W; T1D exchange intranasal glucagon investigators. (2016). Glucagon nasal powder: A promising alternative to intramuscular glucagon in youth with type 1 diabetes. *Diabetes Care, 39*(4), 555–562. doi: 10.2337/dc15-1606. Epub 2016 Feb 16.

Soliman, A., De Sanctis, V., Alaaraj, N., & Hamed, N. (2020). The clinical application of metformin in children and adolescents: A short update. *Acta Biomedica, 91*(3), e2020086.

10.23750/abm.v91i3.10127. PMID: 32921782; PMCID: PMC7717009.

Sutherland, D. E. R., & Gruessner, R. W. G. (1997). Current status of pancreas transplantation for the treatment of type 1 diabetes mellitus. *Clinical Diabetes, 15,* 152–156.

Tamborlane, W. V., Barrientos-Pérez, M., Fainberg, U., Frimer-Larsen, H., Hafez, M., Hale, P. M., Jalaludin, M. Y., Kovarenko, M., Libman, I., Lynch, J. L., Rao, P., Shehadeh, N., Turan, S., Weghuber, D., & Barrett, T.; Ellipse Trial Investigators. (2019). Liraglutide in children and adolescents with type 2 diabetes. *New England Journal of Medicine, 381*(7), 637–646. doi:10.1056/NEJMoa1903822. Epub 2019 Apr 28. PMID: 31034184.

Tamborlane, W. V., Laffel, L. M., Shehadeh, N., Isganaitis, E., Van Name, M., Ratnayake, J., Karlsson, C., & Norjavaara, E. (2022). Efficacy and safety of dapagliflozin in children and young adults with type 2 diabetes: A prospective, multicentre, randomised, parallel group, phase 3 study. *Lancet Diabetes and Endocrinology, 10*(5), 341–350. doi:10.1016/S2213-8587(22)00052-3. Epub 2022 Apr 1. PMID: 35378069.

Today Study Group. (2021). Long-term complications of youth-onset type 2 diabetes. *New England Journal of Medicine, 385*(5), 416–426.

Today Study Group. (2012). A clinical trial to maintain glycemic control in youth with type 2 diabetes. *New England Journal of Medicine, 366*(24), 2247–2256.

Tubiana-Rufi, N., de Lonlay, P., Bloch, J., & Czernichow, P. (1996). Disparition des accidents hypoglycémiques sévères chez le très jeune enfant diabétique traité par pompe sous-cutanée [Remission of severe hypoglycemic incidents in young diabetic children treated with subcutaneous infusion]. *Archives in Pediatrics, 3*(10), 969–976. French. doi:10.1016/0929-693x(96)81717-9. PMID: 8952790.

Upchurch, S. L., Anding, R., & Brown, S. A. (1999). Promoting weight loss in persons with type 2 diabetes: What do we know about the most effective dietary approaches? *Practical Diabetology, 18*(9), 22–28.

US Food and Drug Administration. (2016). FDA approves first automated insulin delivery device for type 1 diabetes. https://www.fda.gov/news-events/press-announcements/fda-approves-first-automated-insulin-delivery-device-type-1-diabetes. Retrieved June 30, 2022.

Uslu, N., & Bayat, M. (2018). The use of complementary and alternative medicine in children with type 1 diabetes mellitus. *Journal of Traditional Medicine & Clinical Naturopathy, 07*(01). https://doi.org/10.4172/2573-4555.1000265.

Weinzimer, S. A., Ahern, J. H., Doyle, E. A., Vincent, M. R., Dziura, J., Steffen, A. T., & Tamborlane, W. V. (2004) Persistence of benefits of continuous subcutaneous insulin infusion in very young children with type 1 diabetes: A follow-up report. *Pediatrics, 114*(6), 1601–1605. doi:10.1542/peds.2004-0092. Erratum in: Pediatrics. 2005 Feb;115(2):518. PMID: 15574621.

Weiss, R. (2007). Impaired glucose tolerance and risk factors for progression to type 2 diabetes in youth. *Pediatric Diabetes, 8*(Suppl 9), 70–75.

Wilfley, D., & Berkowitz, R., TODAY Study Group. (2011). Binge eating, mood, and quality of life in youth with type 2 diabetes: Baseline data from the TODAY study. *Diabetes Care, 34*(4), 858–860. https://doi.org/10.2337/dc10-1704.

Wilson, D. M., Buckingham, B. A., Kunselman, E. L., Sullivan, M. M., Paguntalan, H. U., & Gitelman, S. E. (2005). A two-center randomized controlled feasibility trial of insulin pump therapy in young children with diabetes. *Diabetes Care, 28*(1), 15–19. doi:10.2337/diacare.28.1.15. PMID: 15616227.

World Health Organization. (2022). *Diabetes.* World Health Organization. https://www.who.int/health-topics/diabetes.

Zuijwijk, C. S., Cuerden, M., & Mahmud, F. H. (2013). Social determinants of health on glycemic control in pediatric type 1 diabetes. *Journal of Pediatrics, 162,* 730–735.

21 Down Syndrome

Teresa Whited

ETIOLOGY

Down syndrome, first described by Jean Etienne Esquirol in 1838 and promulgated by John Langdon Down in 1866, is a condition associated with a recognizable phenotype and intellectual disabilities because of extra chromosome 21 material. It is the most frequent autosomal chromosomal anomaly and the primary chromosomal cause of intellectual and developmental disabilities associated with 80+ phenotypic traits (Rafferty et al., 2021). Chromosome 21 was the second chromosome to be completely mapped with the DNA sequence fully determined and is the smallest chromosome (Moyer et al., 2020). The long arm of chromosome 21 contains over 500 genes, but two theories exist regarding expression of the Down phenotype: One is overexpression, and the other is a subset of these genes that has been designated the Down syndrome critical region, located at 21q22-qter (Mowery et al., 2018). However, until the functions of each gene and protein are understood, the pathology of Down syndrome remains unknown.

NONDISJUNCTION

Nondisjunction of chromosome 21 is responsible for the majority of cases (~95%) of trisomic Down syndrome, with approximately 90% of maternal meiotic origin; this form is not inherited (Atli, 2021). Paternal nondisjunction is mainly a meiosis II error and has a higher male gender selection (Atli, 2021). Nondisjunction (i.e., the uneven division of chromosomes) can occur during anaphase 1 or 2 in meiosis (i.e., reduction and division of germ cells) or in anaphase of mitosis (i.e., somatic cell division). In nondisjunction, the pair of chromosomes fails to separate and migrate properly during cell division. When this occurs in meiosis, the haploid number for the respective daughter cells is unequal. If the cell receiving 24 rather than 23 chromosomes is fertilized, a trisomic zygote results (Fig. 21.1). Mosaicism, though associated with fewer phenotypic features and defined by the presence of a percentage of cell lines with trisomy 21, is also most often caused by maternal mitotic nondisjunction (see Fig. 21.1) (Atli, 2021; Bull et al., 2022).

The recurrence risk for nondisjunction Down syndrome is approximately 1%. For older mothers, the risk is 1% plus the percentage of risk for chronologic age with risks as high as 1 in 32 for mothers 45 years of age (Antonarakis et al., 2020; Seshadri et al., 2021).

TRANSLOCATION

In Down syndrome caused by translocation (~4–5% of cases), there are also three copies of chromosome 21. The third copy does not occur independently but is attached to another chromosome—usually to one of the D or G group. Robertsonian translocations, where the long arms of chromosome 21 attach to the long arms of chromosome 14, 21, or 22, are the most common translocations, although other forms can occur (Atli, 2021; Hines & Simmons, 2022).

The total chromosome count in Down syndrome is 46, even though material for 47 chromosomes is present. Although the phenotype for Down syndrome caused by translocation is the same as that for nondisjunction, the inheritance pattern is quite different. With translocation, the disorder may recur in future pregnancies. If one parent has 45 chromosomes—including a translocation of chromosome 21—the gametes produced could result in a trisomic zygote. Although six combinations are theoretically possible, three are nonviable. Of the three that are viable, one is normal (i.e., $N = 46$), one results in a balanced translocation (i.e., $N = 45$), and one is an unbalanced translocation resulting in Down syndrome (i.e., $N = 46$) (Fig. 21.2). The recurrence risk for a second child with translocation Down syndrome (usually 14:21) is approximately 10% at the lowest probable maternal age and very low for the mother older than 35 years. If the translocation carrier is the father, the risk is approximately 5% (Antonarakis, et al., 2020; Atli, 2021; Hines & Simmons, 2022). If the translocation involves both copies of chromosome 21 (21:21), the recurrence risk is 100% (Atli, 2021).

A variety of hypotheses as to the cause of Down syndrome have been offered over the years, including the following: (1) a genetic predisposition to nondisjunction; (2) autoimmunity; (3) hormonal alterations in aging women; (4) advanced age of the maternal grandmother; (5) environmental and chemical factors such as irradiation before conception, smoking, and drug exposure; (6) chromosomal damage; (7) gestational diabetes; and (8) maternal socioeconomic status (Antonarakis et al., 2020). No one factor has been confirmed, although new genetic findings suggest that the cause is probably multifactorial.

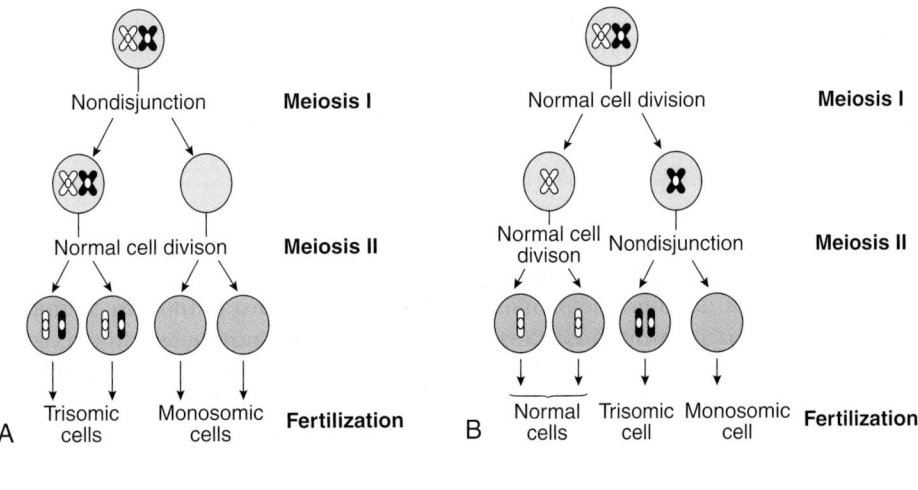

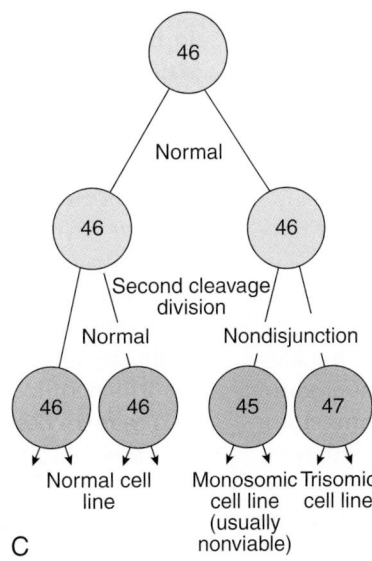

Fig. 21.1 (A) Nondisjunction during meiosis I. (B) Nondisjunction during meiosis II. (C) Nondisjunction following fertilization, during mitosis, resulting in mosaicism. (From Hockenberry, M.J. [2002]. *Wong's nursing care of infants and children* [7th ed.]. Mosby.)

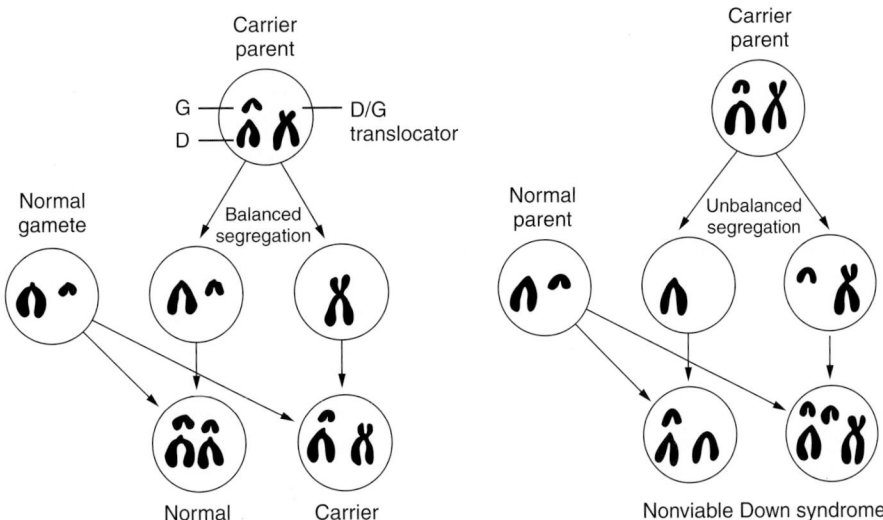

Fig. 21.2 Possible zygotes from the union of a somatically normal carrier of D/G translocation and a genetically and somatically normal individual. (From Wong, D. L., Hockenberry, M. J., Wong, D., Wilson, D., Winklestein, M., Ahmann, E., & Divito-Thomas, P. [1999]. *Whaley and Wong's nursing care of infants and children* [6th ed.]. Mosby.)

INCIDENCE AND PREVALENCE

The prevalence rate for Down syndrome is 1 per 700 births per year, with the incidence rate at around 6000 children born each year with Down syndrome in the United States (Centers for Disease Control and Prevention [CDC], 2020). Prenatal diagnosis of women of advanced maternal age explains this difference over time. Prevalence rates vary by inheritance pattern. Nondisjunction is found in the majority of Down syndrome conceptions. Approximately 90% of these cases are of maternal meiotic causation, with 75% of this number occurring at maternal meiosis I. Only about 8% of total cases of nondisjunction are of paternal origin. Translocation occurs in about 4% to 5% of cases, and mosaicism occurs in approximately 2% of cases (Bull et al., 2022).

Down syndrome caused by translocation is independent of parental age. The incidence is also stable across age cohorts, although one-third of the cases of translocation Down syndrome are inherited from parents (Bull et al., 2022).

For females in their early 20s, the incidence of having a child with Down syndrome is approximately 1 in 1300 births. The incidence rises gradually until maternal age surpasses 35 years and then climbs to approximately 1 in 30 live births for 45-year-old females (Thompson, 2019). Advanced paternal age (≥45 years) has also been shown to affect the incidence of nondisjunction Down syndrome (Thompson, 2019). Although the extra chromosome is paternal in origin, nondisjunction still occurs after fertilization. Because an overwhelming percentage of cases of Down syndrome are caused by nondisjunction, parental age directly affects the overall incidence (Fig. 21.3).

Down syndrome is found in all races and ethnic groups. Although the incidence rates of Down

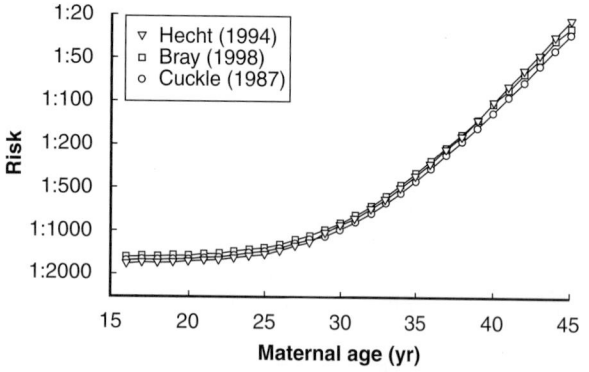

Fig. 21.3 Age-specific risks for Down syndrome from three different studies. (From Spencer, K., Crossley, J. A., Aitken, D. A., Nix, A. B., Dunstan, F. D., & Williams, K. [2002]. Temporal changes in maternal serum biochemical markers of trisomy 21 across the first and second trimester of pregnancy. *Ann Clin Biochem, 39*(Pt 6), 567–576. doi: 10.1177/000456320203900604. Prenatal screening for neural tube defects and aneuploidy. In D.L. Rimoin, et al. [Eds.], *Emory and Rimoin's principles and practices of medical genetics* [4th ed., pp. 763–801]. Churchill Livingstone.)

syndrome vary little among White, Black, and Hispanic infants born to mothers under 35 years of age, rates are significantly higher in Hispanic infants and moderately higher in Black infants born to mothers over 35 years of age (Chaiken et al., 2022; Khoshnood et al., 2000).

DIAGNOSTIC CRITERIA

Prenatal screening through maternal plasma cell-free DNA and ultrasound of the nuchal translucency in the first and second trimesters can be done through noninvasive methods (Bull et al., 2022; Messerlian et al., 2022). However, diagnosis of Down syndrome is most often through karyotyping of fetal cells after chorionic villus sampling or amniocentesis after positive screening results (Benn, 2021; Bull et al., 2022). Karyotyping can also be done postnatally if either the prenatal screening produced a false-negative result or no prenatal screening or testing was done. In such cases with infants of color or those born very prematurely, diagnosis may be delayed because the clinical features may not be as clearly recognized. Although more than 50 physical characteristics can be identified at birth, no one feature is considered diagnostic. Features vary in their expression and are not always present. Some of the most associated features include generalized hypotonia, brachycephaly, epicanthal folds, palpebral fissures, single transverse palmar creases, incurved fifth finger, neck skinfold, and widely spaced first and second toes (c; Ostermaier, 2022).

CLINICAL MANIFESTATIONS AT TIME OF DIAGNOSIS

A variety of congenital anomalies are commonly associated with Down syndrome. Congenital heart disease is seen in approximately 60% of children with Down syndrome, with endocardial cushion defects accounting for about 42% and ventricular septal defects making up another 22% of cardiac malformations Another cardiac manifestation can include pulmonary hypertension, which occurs as high as 44.8% of the time in children with congenital heart disease and 34% of the time in children without congenital heart disease (Lagan et al., 2020). Gastrointestinal malformations are seen in 13% of children with Down syndrome; among the most common problems are duodenal or esophageal atresia, congenital megacolon (Hirschsprung disease), imperforate anus, tracheoesophageal fistula, and pyloric stenosis (Lagan et al., 2020). Anomalies can usually be surgically corrected in the neonatal period. Although many children experience total correction of the anomaly, others will experience untoward sequelae throughout their lifetime.

TREATMENT

No treatment can eliminate the chromosomal defect that causes Down syndrome. Extensive interdisciplinary services and research have, however, transformed society's view of children with Down syndrome and accepted treatment protocols. Accepted approaches include genetic counseling, prompt referral for surgical correction of congenital anomalies, prevention of secondary conditions, enrollment in an early intervention program, and inclusion from preschool through higher education.

GENETIC COUNSELING

Pregnant females are given the option of prenatal screening. Current practice for the prenatal screening for Down syndrome consists of an ultrasound to measure nuchal translucency and maternal bloodwork for free beta–human chorionic gonadotropin and pregnancy-associated plasma protein at 10 to 13 weeks of gestation (American College of Obstetricians and Gynecologists [ACOG], 2022). Further bloodwork can be done during the second trimester, or diagnostic testing can be done. ACOG (2022) suggests that first-trimester positive results be diagnostically tested and those females with borderline results undergo further bloodwork, ultrasound testing, and diagnostic testing during the second trimester. Although this validation will not affect a child's treatment or prognosis, it has significant implications for the genetic counseling of family members. Because translocation is the cause of about 5% of cases, parents and siblings must be tested to determine their carrier status and have the risk of recurrence in future pregnancies carefully explained to them. Genetic counseling of the family regarding this pregnancy and future pregnancies is essential to prenatal testing.

Clinical Manifestations at Time of Diagnosis

SKULL
- False fontanel
- Flat occipital area
- Brachycephaly
- Separated sagittal suture
- Hypoplasia of midfacial bones
- Reduced interorbital distance
- Underdeveloped maxilla
- Obtuse mandibular angle

EYES
- Oblique narrow palpebral fissures
- Epicanthal folds
- Brushfield spots
- Strabismus
- Nystagmus
- Myopia
- Hypoplasia of the iris

EARS
- Small, shortened ears
- Low and oblique implantation
- Overlapping helices
- Prominent antihelix
- Absent or attached earlobes
- Narrow ear canals
- External auditory meatus
- Structural aberrations of the ossicles
- Stenotic external auditory meatus

NOSE
- Hypoplastic
- Flat nasal bridge
- Anteverted, narrow nares
- Deviated nasal septum

MOUTH
- Prominent, thickened, and fissured lips
- Corners of the mouth turned downward
- High-arched, narrow palate
- Shortened palatal length
- Protruding, enlarged tongue
- Papillary hypertrophy (early preschool)
- Fissured tongue (later school years)
- Periodontal disease
- Partial anodontia
- Microdontia
- Abnormally aligned teeth
- Anterior open bite
- Mouth held open

NECK
- Short, broad neck
- Loose skin at nape

CHEST
- Shortened rib cage
- Twelfth rib anomalies
- Pectus excavatum or carinatum
- Congenital heart disease

ABDOMEN
- Distended and enlarged abdomen
- Diastasis recti
- Umbilical hernia
- Muscle tone and musculature
  - Hyperflexibility
  - Muscular hypotonia
  - Generalized weakness
- Integument
  - Skin appears large for the skeleton
  - Dry and rough
  - Fine, poorly pigmented hair

EXTREMITIES
- Short extremities
- Partial or complete syndactyly
- Clinodactyly
- Brachyclinodactyly

UPPER EXTREMITIES
- Short, broad hands
- Brachyclinodactyly
- Single palmar transverse crease
- Incurved, short fifth finger
- Abnormal dermatoglyphics

Continued

Clinical Manifestations at Time of Diagnosis—cont'd

LOWER EXTREMITIES
- Short and stubby feet
- Gap between first and second toes
- Plantar crease between first and second toes
- Second and third toes grouped in a forklike position
- Radial deviation of the third to fifth toes

PHYSICAL GROWTH AND DEVELOPMENT
- Short stature
- Increased weight in later life

OTHER FINDINGS SEEN IN NEWBORNS
- Enlarged anterior fontanel
- Delayed closing of sutures and fontanels
- Open sagittal suture
- Nasal bone not ossified, underdeveloped
- Reduced birth weight

Treatment
- Genetic counseling
- Surgical correction of anomalies
- Prevention or treatment of secondary conditions
- Early intervention programs
- Choosing appropriate educational settings (e.g., inclusion)

SURGERY

Surgical corrections of most major cardiac, gastrointestinal, and genitourinary anomalies are now performed routinely, although not without risk. The risk for upper airway compromise during and after surgery is increased in Down syndrome because of clinical features such as subglottic stenosis, smaller middle and lower face skeleton, adenoid and tonsil volume, tracheal stenosis, hypotonia, and a narrow nasopharyngeal inlet. Atlantoaxial instability also poses a surgical risk, and it is recommended that the necks of all children with Down syndrome, with or without normal cervical spine radiographs, should be treated carefully when undergoing surgical procedures. A smaller sized endotracheal tube than normal for the child's age should be used for children with Down syndrome (Delany et al., 2021). Further, bradycardia, airway obstruction, pulmonary hypertension, and postextubation stridor (Borland et al., 2004; Delany et al., 2021; Mundakel, 2022) are common, and a longer hospital stay may be required for children with Down syndrome.

In addition to lifesaving surgeries, some children with Down syndrome also undergo plastic surgery to alter their phenotypic appearance. As these children continue to become more integrated into society, they may be stigmatized because of their physiognomy. Some parents, concerned about their child's social acceptance, seek plastic surgery for the child (e.g., partial glossectomies, neck resections, silastic implants for the chin and nose, and reconstruction of dysplastic helices). Better articulation of speech, less mouth breathing, fewer and less severe upper respiratory tract infections, and improved mastication and swallowing may be realized, especially if a pathologic condition exists that warrants corrective surgery. The degree of success, however, may be small or nonexistent. There are surgical risks, surgery is expensive, and it is often not covered by insurance. Any parents or children with Down syndrome wanting to undergo plastic surgery should talk at length with their primary care provider and surgeon before the procedure so they understand the risks.

PREVENTION AND TREATMENT OF SECONDARY CONDITIONS

Children with Down syndrome are susceptible to a number of secondary conditions, including but not limited to feeding problems, vision and hearing abnormalities, constipation, upper respiratory infections, thyroid disorders, and skin problems. Regular visits to the primary care provider, a Down syndrome clinic (if available), or specialists and comprehensive anticipatory guidance can help prevent these problems. If they do occur, intervention and treatment should begin early. Referring the family to a support group composed of other families with a child with Down syndrome can also provide a means for information and support to prevent such conditions.

EARLY INTERVENTION

Infant stimulation programs and continued early childhood education are designed to optimize a child's development rate and minimize the developmental lag between children with Down syndrome and their developmentally normal peers. In addition to developmental delays, children with Down syndrome are at increased risk for autism spectrum disorders, often requiring early and intensive therapies (Bull et al., 2022). Specific therapeutic exercises are devised to stimulate an infant's cognitive, social, motor, and language domains. These exercises are incorporated in the individualized family service plan mandated by the Individuals with Disabilities Education Improvement Act (IDEA) of 2004 (Public Law [PL] 108-446). Researchers have found motor and cognitive improvement in infants after their participation in an early intervention program (Arslan et al., 2022; Bull et al., 2022). Parents are usually taught these skills by special education teachers, physical therapists, occupational therapists, and speech pathologists so that therapy can be conducted at home. However, timing seems to be a critical factor, with earlier interventions correlated with greater developmental gains. These children will later be referred to a specialized program designed to continue these intervention strategies and then integrated into generic child care or school.

INCLUSION

With inclusion, children age 3 to 21 years are included in the regular classroom, including preschool programs, under IDEA (2004). The individualized education program developed by the child (if age appropriate), parents, and the school's interdisciplinary team gives direction to the child's preferences, interests, and academic and developmental needs (Sanderson & Goldman, 2022). The family, primary care provider, and school personnel should collaborate to improve their partnership in the care of the child (Sanderson & Goldman, 2022).

COMPLEMENTARY AND ALTERNATIVE THERAPIES

Therapies that have been reported to be used by children with Down syndrome are nutritional supplements, herbal therapies, massage therapy, and diet modifications (Lewanda et al., 2018). Lewanda et al. (2018) found approximately 50% of parents in their study utilized supplements in the care of the child with Down syndrome with the goal of improving health and intellectual function. Field (2019) reviewed literature that massage therapy was utilized for muscle tone disorders such as Down syndrome to increase vagal activity and reduce stress hormones. Individuals with Down syndrome have a long-term risk of low bone mineral density and fracture in later adult years; therefore it is proposed to promote physical activity and supplementation with calcium and vitamin D if deficiencies exist to promote optimal bone mineralization (LaCombe & Roper, 2019). Providers need to discuss potential alternative therapies and counsel families appropriately regarding these therapies.

ANTICIPATED ADVANCES IN DIAGNOSIS AND MANAGEMENT

Many advances in the genetic understanding of Down syndrome from human and animal models continue to occur as genomic research progresses. Areas under investigation continue in regard to early brain development, long-term management of the disorder, dementia care, and other long-term outcomes of Down syndrome as more patients are living into their 60s or beyond (Baburamani et al. 2019; Bull et al., 2022; Godfrey & Lee, 2018). Additional research is warranted in all areas to promote recommendations for general practice.

ASSOCIATED PROBLEMS OF DOWN SYNDROME AND TREATMENT

INTELLECTUAL AND DEVELOPMENTAL DISABILITIES

The intellectual capabilities of children with Down syndrome vary dramatically. Most of these children have moderate intellectual limitations (i.e., intelligence quotient [IQ] of 40–55, standard deviation [SD] of 15), but a small percentage are either mildly affected (i.e., IQ 56–69, SD 15) or severely impaired (i.e., IQ 39, SD 15). For a few children, their IQs are inconsistent with a diagnosis of an intellectual and developmental disability. Known correlates to children's intelligence and adaptive behavior skills are their physical condition, home environment, and individualized early intervention. Unfortunately, cognitive function often deteriorates with age, and significant losses in intelligence, memory, and social skills are seen earlier (i.e., often by age 40 years) than in persons without Down syndrome (Godfrey & Lee, 2018).

Associated Problems
Down Syndrome and Treatment

Intellectual and developmental disabilities
Cardiac defects
Gastrointestinal tract anomalies
Musculoskeletal and motor abilities
Immune system deficiency
Sensory deficits
Vision problems
Hearing loss
Growth delay
Altered respiratory function
Thyroid dysfunction
Malignancies
Leukemia
Tumors
Celiac disease
Sleep-disordered breathing
Skin conditions
Dental changes
Seizure disorders

Behavior disorders may also be present, such as social withdrawal, noncompliance, aggression, inattention, hyperactivity, or a thought disorder. The prevalence of mood disorders such as depression, anxiety, personality disorders, and others may be higher in persons with Down syndrome (Rivelli et al., 2022). Depression, autistic behavior, and psychotic episodes have been reported. Neurologic deterioration, disturbed family life, and stress may affect the mental health of children with Down syndrome.

CARDIAC DEFECTS

Approximately 50% of children with Down syndrome have congenital heart defects. In order of decreasing frequency, the most common heart anomalies include atrioventricular septal defect (i.e., endocardial cushion defect and atrioventricular canal defect), ventricular septal defect, mitral valve abnormalities, patent ductus arteriosus, and atrial septal defect. Other heart or cardiac-associated conditions that may occur in Down syndrome include tetralogy of Fallot, coarctation of the aorta, tricuspid valve abnormalities, rare single-ventricle anomalies, and pulmonary artery hypertension (Bull et al., 2022; Delany et al., 2021).

Children with Down syndrome often require early cardiac surgery to prevent long-term issues with cardiac function and pulmonary hypertension. Bacterial endocarditis is a risk for children with residual cardiac defects, and the guidelines for endocarditis prophylaxis should be utilized for prevention (Wilson et al., 2021). The use of echocardiography and a cardiac evaluation during the prenatal and newborn periods have greatly enhanced detection rates, early management, and survival rates (Lagan et al., 2020).

GASTROINTESTINAL TRACT ANOMALIES

Approximately 3% to 13% of infants have gastrointestinal atresia (Bull et al., 2022; Lagan et al., 2020). Common congenital gastrointestinal tract anomalies include tracheoesophageal fistula, Hirschsprung disease, pyloric stenosis, duodenal atresia, annular pancreas, aganglionic megacolon, and imperforate anus. The most common being duodenal atresia and imperforate anus (Lagan et al., 2020). Most of these anomalies require immediate surgical correction and careful follow-up throughout life.

MUSCULOSKELETAL AND MOTOR ABILITIES

Orthopedic problems are common among children with Down syndrome. Flaccid muscle tone and ligamentous laxity occur to some extent in all children with Down syndrome (Foley & Killeen, 2019; Lagan et al., 2020). Among these conditions are pes planus, patellar subluxation, scoliosis, dislocated hips, atlantoaxial subluxation, joint and muscle pain, and rapid muscle fatigue. Children and adults are at increased risk for inflammatory arthritic conditions with approximately 7% of children affected by these concerns (Foley & Killeen, 2019). These problems may occur throughout a child's life, and the primary care provider should carefully screen for them at each visit.

Another significant disorder associated with Down syndrome is atlantoaxial instability. Atlantoaxial instability results from a so-called loose joint between C1 and C2 and increased space between the atlas and odontoid process and affects approximately 10% to 30% of children with Down syndrome (Shimony, 2022). At least 98% to 99% of affected children are asymptomatic. Subluxation or dislocation may result, and early manifestations may include neck pain, torticollis, deteriorating gait, or changes in bowel or bladder function. If left untreated, symptoms may progress to frank neurologic findings associated with spinal cord compression, which occurs in about 2% of children and may require surgical or other interventions, but exact timing and need for surgery remain controversial (Shimony, 2022). Providers should be aware of these concerns when clearing for sports participation, especially in sports with high risk for head or neck injury.

IMMUNE SYSTEM DEFICIENCY

Children with Down syndrome have altered immune function. Immune system deficits directly contribute to the increased incidence and severity of numerous other conditions, including but not limited to periodontal disease, respiratory problems, thyroid disorders, lymphocytic thyroiditis, leukemia, diabetes mellitus, alopecia areata, adrenal dysfunction, vitiligo, and joint problems (Bull et al., 2022; Lagan et al., 2020). Immune dysregulation with reduced ranges of T- and B-cell lymphocytes, potential suboptimal antibody response to vaccines, and proinflammatory cytokine dysregulation can lead to many of the immunologic disorders in children with Down syndrome (Lagan et al., 2020). Diabetes type 1, autoimmune thyroid diseases, and other autoimmune disorders have been identified in individuals with Down syndrome and should be considered when screening for concerns (Bull et al., 2022; Whooten et al., 2018). Some children with Down syndrome will require immunoglobulin or other immunotherapies to improve the immune dysfunction.

SENSORY DEFICITS

Vision Problems

An increased prevalence of numerous ocular deviations is associated with Down syndrome and occurs in approximately 60% to 80% of these children, with most experiencing more than one ocular problem. The most commonly occurring abnormalities are, in order of decreasing frequency, slanted palpebral fissures, spotted irises, refractive errors, strabismus, nystagmus, cataracts, blepharitis, pseudopapilledema, keratoconus, and abnormalities in the optic nerve head (Postolache, 2019). A significant loss in visual acuity will result if many of these conditions are not diagnosed and treated in early childhood. Moreover, visual problems—especially refractive errors—increase with age (Postolache, 2019) and may interfere with cognitive development. It is essential to screen for visual issues starting at birth throughout the lifetime of the individual with Down syndrome.

Hearing Loss

The incidence of hearing loss in children with Down syndrome is approximately 40% to 75%. Structural deviations of the skull, foreface, external auditory canal, middle and inner ears, and throat accompanied by eustachian tube dysfunction are associated with congenital and acquired hearing loss that can be sensorineural or conductive or both and occur unilaterally or bilaterally (Lagan et al., 2020). Hearing loss may greatly affect speech and cognitive development if not treated promptly and correctly.

GROWTH ABNORMALITIES

At birth, infants with Down syndrome weigh less, are typically shorter, and have smaller occipital-frontal circumferences than unaffected children. The velocity of linear growth is also reduced, with the most marked reductions between 6 and 24 months of age. This reduction in velocity recurs during adolescence, when the growth spurt—less vigorous than would normally be expected—occurs earlier in adolescents with Down syndrome (Ostermaier, 2022). Other causes for the reduction in linear growth may be congenital heart disease, hypothalamic dysfunctions, thyroid disorders, and nutrition problems, and each should be evaluated if suspected (Bull et al., 2022; Cohen, 1999; Lagan et al., 2020).

Children with Down syndrome tend to be overweight. Beginning around 3 to 4 years of age, these children often have untoward weight gain that persists throughout their lives. One study found that approximately 51.6% of males and 40% of females with Down syndrome met the criteria for obesity (O'Shea et al., 2018). Regular nutritional guidance, promotion of physical activity, and monitoring of weight are essential in the long-term health of individuals with Down syndrome.

ALTERED RESPIRATORY FUNCTION

Combined with a compromised immune system, pulmonary hypertension and hyperplasia, fewer alveoli, a decreased alveolar blood capillary surface area, aspiration, sleep disordered breathing, and associated upper airway obstruction (e.g., lymphatic hypertrophy in the Waldeyer ring) predispose children with Down syndrome to respiratory tract infections (Santoro et al., 2020). If recurrent severe respiratory tract infections occur, they may require frequent and prolonged hospitalizations resulting in effects on the child's development and potential increased risks for mortality (Santoro et al., 2020). In a meta-analysis, Beckhaus and Castro-Rodriguez (2018) identified the presence of Down syndrome as a risk for respiratory syncytial virus (RSV) bronchiolitis and found that if children with this condition needed to be hospitalized, their conditions were much worse than other children, with increased mortality in children 2 years and younger. Prophylaxis for this condition should be considered for children with Down syndrome.

THYROID DYSFUNCTION

Thyroid dysfunction in Down syndrome can be associated with congenital hypothyroidism, or thyroid autoimmunity, and occurs more often than in the general population (Whooten et al., 2018). The recommendation is to have thyroid screening beginning at birth and throughout childhood (Bull et al., 2022). Appropriate management and consultation with a pediatric endocrinologist should occur if abnormalities are found in screening labs.

MALIGNANCIES

Leukemia

Children with Down syndrome have an approximate 10- to 20-fold greater incidence of leukemia than the general population. Under the age of 5 years, children with Down syndrome are at greatest risk for acute myeloid leukemia (AML) and acquired acute megakaryoblastic leukemia (AMKL). Across all ages, children with Down syndrome are at increased risk for acute lymphoblastic leukemia (ALL) compared with children without Down syndrome (Marlow et al., 2021). The increased risk for preleukemic and leukemia cells begins prenatally and has been linked to distinct chromosome microRNAs and overexpression of genes associated with a mutation of *GATA1* (Wagenblast et al., 2021). The focus of current research continues to be on the epidemiology, genetics, and pathogenesis of leukemia in Down syndrome.

Children with Down syndrome require treatment with leukemia protocols specific to Down syndrome to minimize treatment toxicities and optimize outcomes for these patients (Laurent et al., 2020). Most children with Down syndrome and AML appear to have a better clinical outcome than children without Down syndrome with AML. However, if relapse or treatment failure occurs, they have a higher risk of mortality related to bone marrow transplant and other therapies (Laurent et al., 2020). Today, children with Down syndrome with ALL survive at similar rates as children without Down syndrome with this condition; this was not always the case and is largely due to improvements in treatment and making changes based on biologic differences (Laurent et al., 2020). A final form of leukemia, transient leukemia or transient abnormal myelopoiesis (TAM), occurs most often in infants with Down syndrome (~10%). This form of leukemia occurs during the newborn period and usually resolves spontaneously within the first 3 months. Rarely does it cause complications or death in less than 10% of patients. Approximately 20% of these patients go on to develop AMKL before the age of 4 years (Watanabe, 2018).

Tumors

Individuals with Down syndrome appear to be at lower risk of developing solid tumors, although the incidence of testicular germ cell tumors may be increased in young males with Down syndrome. Because they can occur at an early age, ongoing assessment of the gonads is warranted (Bull et al., 2022; Rethore et al., 2020).

CELIAC DISEASE

The frequency of celiac disease in children with Down syndrome is approximately 5%, which is higher than the general population (1–3%) (Ostermaier et al., 2022). Because Down syndrome is an at-risk condition for celiac disease, it is recommended that children with Down syndrome be screened and evaluated at every well-child visit (Bull et al., 2022). Evaluation for celiac disease can include tissue transglutaminase–immuno-globulin A (TTG-IgA) test, endomysial antibody IgA test, total IgA test, and biopsy (Sahin, 2021).

SLEEP-DISORDERED BREATHING

Anatomic and physiologic differences (e.g., midfacial hypoplasia, glossoptosis) predispose children with Down syndrome to obstructive sleep apnea and other sleep-disordered breathing problems. This may occur in all children with Down syndrome. Discussion with parents regarding this issue should occur within the first 6 months, and all children with symptoms of sleep-disordered breathing problems should be evaluated by an expert in pediatric sleep disorders (Bull et al., 2022).

SKIN CONDITIONS

Several skin conditions, especially infectious, inflammatory, autoimmune, and connective tissue disorders are common in individuals with Down syndrome. The most diagnosed condition is atopic dermatitis. Other conditions include hidradenitis suppurativa, fissured tongue, lichen nitidus, psoriasis, alopecia areata, calcinosis cutis, dermatofibroma, melanoma, syringomas, elastosis perforans serpiginosa, seborrheic dermatitis, xerosis, ichthyosis, and vitiligo (Desingu et al., 2019; Lam et al., 2022).

DENTAL CHANGES

Children with Down syndrome seem to develop caries less often than unaffected children. However, numerous other dental problems (e.g., bruxism, malocclusion, defective dentition, microdontia, periodontal disease) are more prevalent in these children because of anatomic anomalies of the oral cavity and immunologic anomalies and dysfunction (Desingu et al., 2019; Silva et al., 2020). Primary teeth can stay in place until the child reaches age 14 or 15 years. Children with Down syndrome have higher concentrations of the salivary *Streptococcus mutans*–specific IgA than children without Down syndrome, and this may be the reason why these children have fewer caries (Silva et al., 2020). Mouth breathing and consumption of a diet high in soft foods—two common occurrences in children with Down syndrome—also contribute to their dental problems (Desingu et al., 2019; Silva et al., 2020).

SEIZURE DISORDERS

Children with Down syndrome have an increased frequency of seizure disorders, with the risk for epilepsy increasing with age (Altuna et al., 2021). The distribution of the onset of seizures is trimodal, occurring before age 3 years, after 9 years, and late onset around 40 years (Bösebeck, 2022). Of the affected children, 40% begin to have seizures (i.e., generally infantile spasms and generalized tonic-clonic seizures) before 1 year of age (Rahman & Fatema, 2019). Adult-onset seizures tend to be tonic-clonic seizures and partial simple and partial complex seizures. Seizures in adulthood can be indicative of Alzheimer disease or dementia (Altuna et al., 2021).

PROGNOSIS

Individuals with Down syndrome have an average life expectancy of 60 years, which is about 28 years younger than the general population. With improved care and change in interventional care from the 1980s, life expectancy has improved from an average 25 years of age to the now 60 years. In a systematic review, O'Leary et al. (2018) found the leading causes of death were congenital heart disease and respiratory conditions. Other causes of early mortality include comorbidities, low birth weight, minority ethnicity, younger maternal age, and low parental education. Because Down syndrome is associated with numerous anatomic and physiologic aberrations, life expectancy is reduced, with approximately a 6% to 8% mortality rate in the first year of life that increases to 12% by 20 years of age (CDC, 2020; O'Leary et al., 2018). The number and severity of congenital anomalies significantly decrease life expectancy for some of these children. As persons with Down syndrome age, comorbidities of early Alzheimer disease, dementia, worsening seizure disorders, and premature aging may reduce life expectancy for adults (Priebe et al., 2020). With correct medical, educational, and social interventions, most individuals live well into adulthood and have satisfying, productive lives. Successful outcomes heavily depend on the early interventions children and their families receive. If children with Down syndrome are to reach their full potential, aggressive and interdisciplinary management is paramount.

PRIMARY CARE MANAGEMENT

HEALTH CARE MAINTENANCE

Primary care providers are encouraged to consult the American Academy of Pediatrics (AAP) *Health Supervision for Children and Adolescents with Down Syndrome 2022 Revision* (Bull et al., 2022) (Tables 21.1 and 21.2).

Growth and Development

Evaluating the growth of children with Down syndrome is a detailed process. When linear growth is assessed, primary care providers must consider the variations in velocity. Whereas growth adequacy is often determined by maintaining a particular percentile rank, variations in growth velocity affect the growth curves of these children during early childhood. Growth velocities for

Table **21.1**	Recommendations for Prenatal and Neonatal Care Based on the American Academy of Pediatrics (AAP) Guidelines for Health Supervision for Children and Adolescents With Down Syndrome
VISIT (AGE)	**AAP RECOMMENDATIONS**
Prenatal	• Prenatal testing and confirm diagnosis • Meet with family regarding diagnosis, plan for delivery and neonatal care • Connect family with resources • Refer for genetic counseling
Birth–1 mo	• Confirm or make diagnosis (depending on prenatal testing) • Discuss diagnosis with family with supportive measures in place • Echocardiogram (50% risk of heart defects) • Identify and address feeding problems with possible dysphagiogram • Full examination to identify anomalies (e.g., cataracts, gastrointestinal defects, cardiac defects, airway anomalies, Hirschsprung disease) • Hearing screen to identify congenital hearing loss • Car safety seat evaluation for apnea, bradycardia, or deoxygenation • Obtain complete blood count by 3 days of life to identify transient abnormal myelopoiesis, polycythemia, leukocytosis, or other hematologic abnormalities • Obtain a thyroid-stimulating hormone or newborn screening for hypothyroidism • Discuss and refer to early intervention services • Evaluate comorbidities and health status • Discuss cervical spine–positioning precautions • Consider possibility of renal or urinary tract anomalies and educate families on signs and symptoms of urinary issues • If tympanic membrane cannot be visualized, refer to otolaryngology

(Bull et al., 2022)

Table **21.2**	Recommendations for 1 Month to 5 Years of Age Based on the American Academy of Pediatrics (AAP) Guidelines for Health Supervision for Children and Adolescents With Down Syndrome
VISIT (AGE)	**AAP RECOMMENDATIONS**
1 mo–1 yr	• Review newborn screening, if normal then rescreen in 6 mo • Monitor for otitis media with effusion and stenotic canals with referral to otolaryngology as needed • Refer to pediatric ophthalmologist in first 6 mo • If thyroid-stimulating hormone (TSH) is normal at birth, rescreen at 6 mo and 12 mo • If cardiac disease, monitor signs and symptoms of congestive heart failure and pulmonary hypertension • Complete blood count (CBC) with differential and ferritin and C-reactive protein (CRP) or serum iron and total iron binding capacity (TIBC) at age 1 yr • Closely monitor for signs and symptoms of leukemia especially in the first 5 yr of life • Begin conversations about obstructive sleep apnea • Review early intervention services and ongoing needs • Clarify recurrence risk and offer genetic counseling referral
1–5 yr	• If TSH normal, screen annually • Monitor for hearing loss risk and screen every 6 mo until age 4 yr, then subsequent behavioral hearing tests annually • Vision evaluation annually or more frequently based on visual needs • Discuss atlantoaxial instability and symptoms of spinal compression. If symptomatic, radiologic evaluation and if abnormal referral to neurosurgery/orthopedic surgeon • Discuss signs and symptoms of sleep apnea or other sleep disorders; referral for sleep study by age 3–5 yr • CBC with differential and ferritin and CRP or serum iron and TIBC annually • Discuss body mass index/obesity and risk for complications and diet/exercise considerations • Discuss self-help skills and counseling to prevent wandering • Discuss behavioral concerns and behavior management. Refer children for evaluation for autism, attention-deficit/hyperactivity disorder, or other behavioral concerns • Discuss transition from early intervention to preschool/school-based services by age 3 yr • Reassure parents about delayed and irregular dental eruption patterns and ongoing dental care • Appropriate terminology for genitalia and prevention of sexual exploitation

(Bull et al., 2022)

children with and without Down syndrome are similar during the school-age period; however, stability is seen in the percentile curves.

Measurements should be plotted on growth charts with specific norms for children with Down syndrome (Figs. 21.4 to 21.9, Table 21.3, Box 21.1). The specialty charts, in which all percentiles for stature are less than their analogous percentiles on the National Center for Health Statistics charts, provide an excellent reference point for comparing growth among children with Down syndrome and determining those at risk for failure to thrive or obesity. The growth charts are easily accessed on the CDC website (https://www.cdc.gov/ncbddd/birthdefects/downsyndrome/growth-charts.html).

Interventions for weight management may be introduced as necessary. Caloric reduction and increased

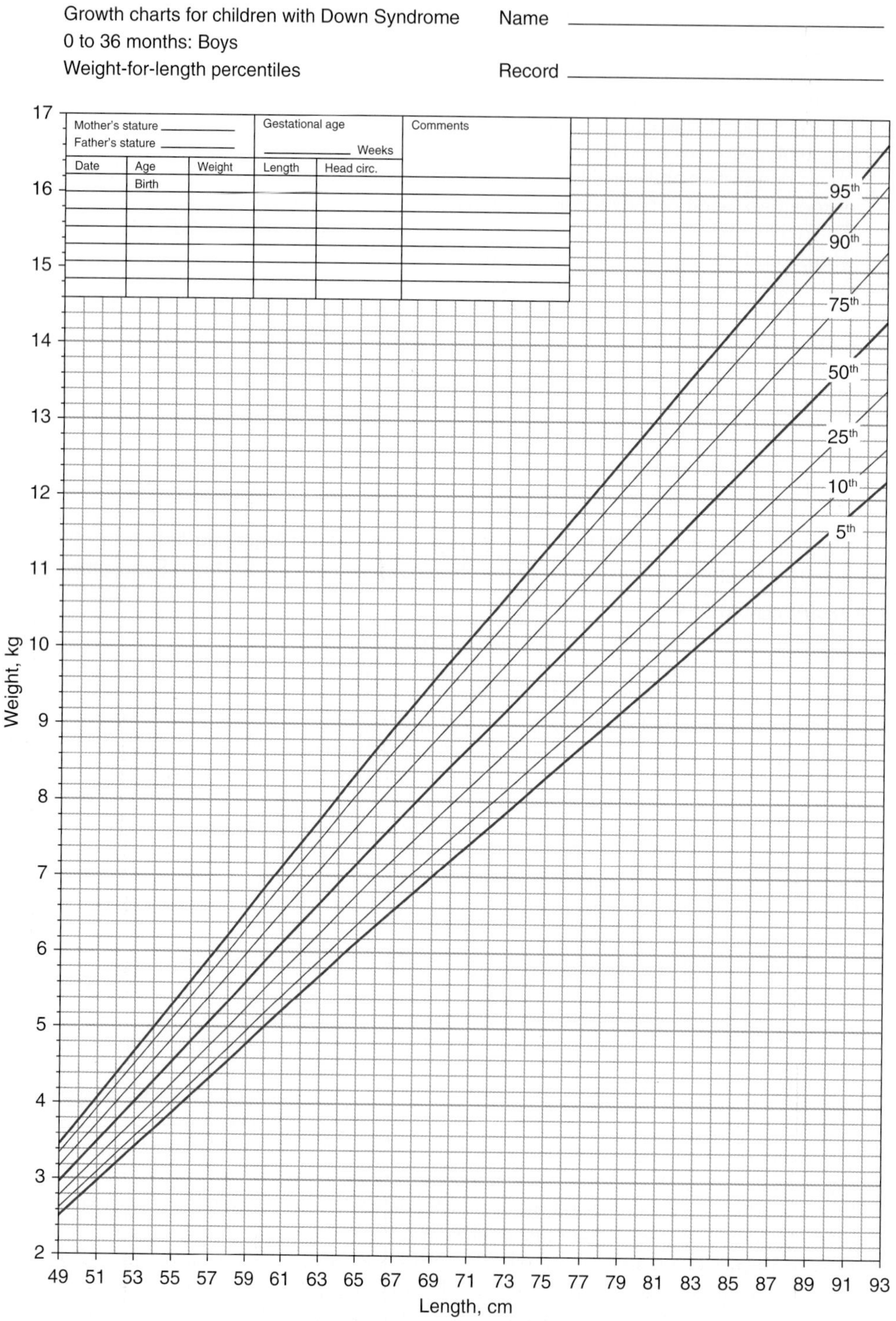

Fig. 21.4 Males with Down syndrome: Physical growth 0 to 36 months. (From Zemel, B.S., Pipan, M., Stallings, V.A., Hall, W., Schgadt, K., Freedman, D.S., & Thorpe, P. [2015]. *Growth charts for children with Down syndrome in the US pediatrics*. Centers for Disease Control and Prevention. https://www.cdc.gov/ncbddd/birthdefects/downsyndrome/documents/DS_Boys_WeightLength_Birthto36mo.pdf.)

Growth charts for children with Down Syndrome
0 to 36 months: Girls
Weight-for-length percentiles

Name _____

Record _____

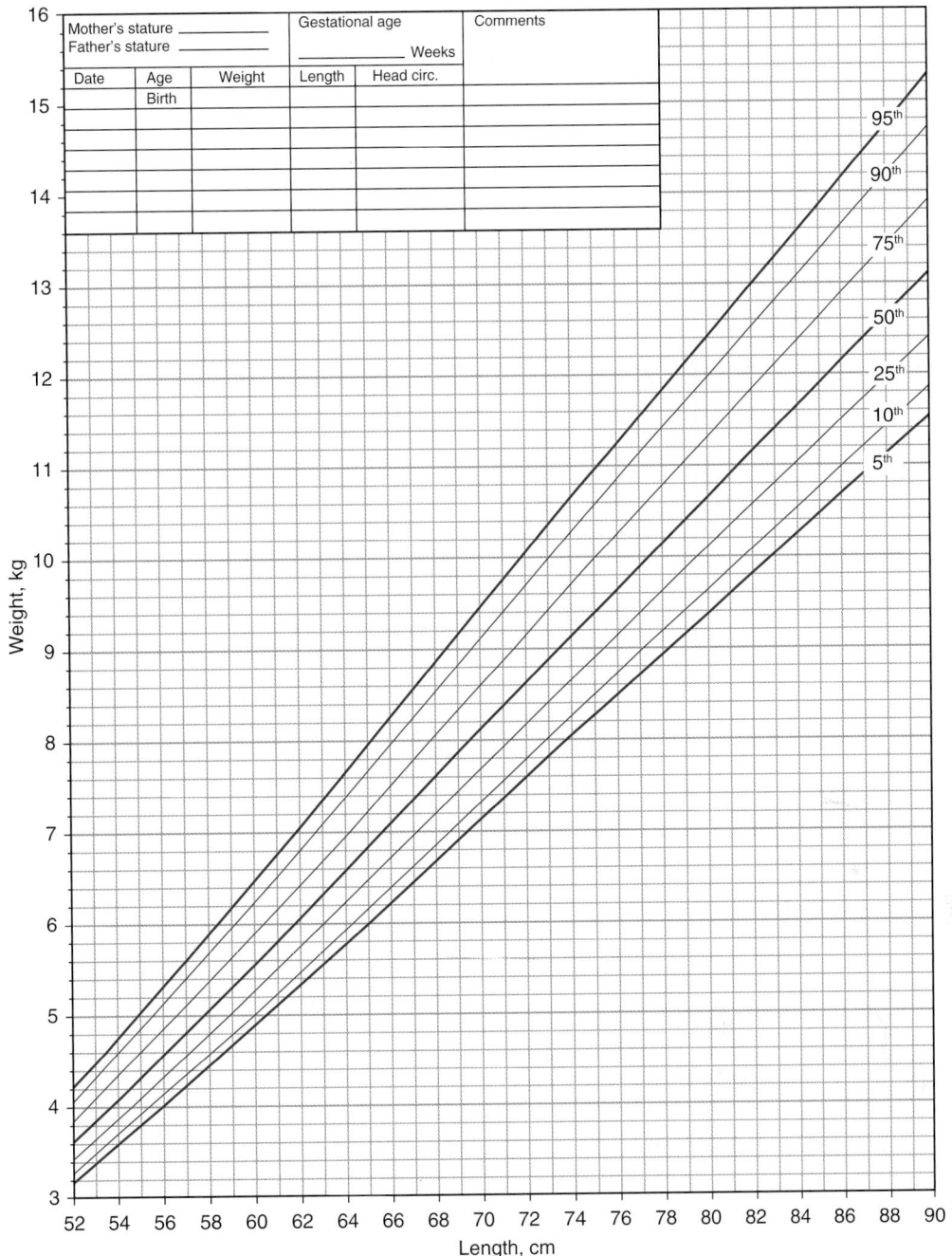

Fig. 21.5 Females with Down syndrome: Physical growth 0 to 36 months. (From Zemel, B.S., Pipan, M., Stallings, V.A., Hall, W., Schgadt, K., Freedman, D.S., & Thorpe, P. [2015]. *Growth charts for children with Down syndrome in the US pediatrics*. Centers for Disease Control and Prevention. https://www.cdc.gov/ncbddd/birthdefects/downsyndrome/documents/DS_Girls_WeightforLength_Birthto36mo.pdf.)

exercise incorporated into a behavior management program are likely to be the most effective approach to decrease cardiovascular risk factors of obesity, hypertension, and other issues associated with a sedentary lifestyle (Barnard et al., 2019; Bull et al., 2022).

Virtually all children will have an intellectual and developmental disability; the most difficult is language development, especially with expressive language. Males appear to have more difficulties, and language development issues persist into adolescence (Soriano et al., 2020). Both receptive and expressive language development are delayed, but expressive language tends to lag more significantly (Soriano et al., 2020). Hearing impairments also affect speech-language development in children

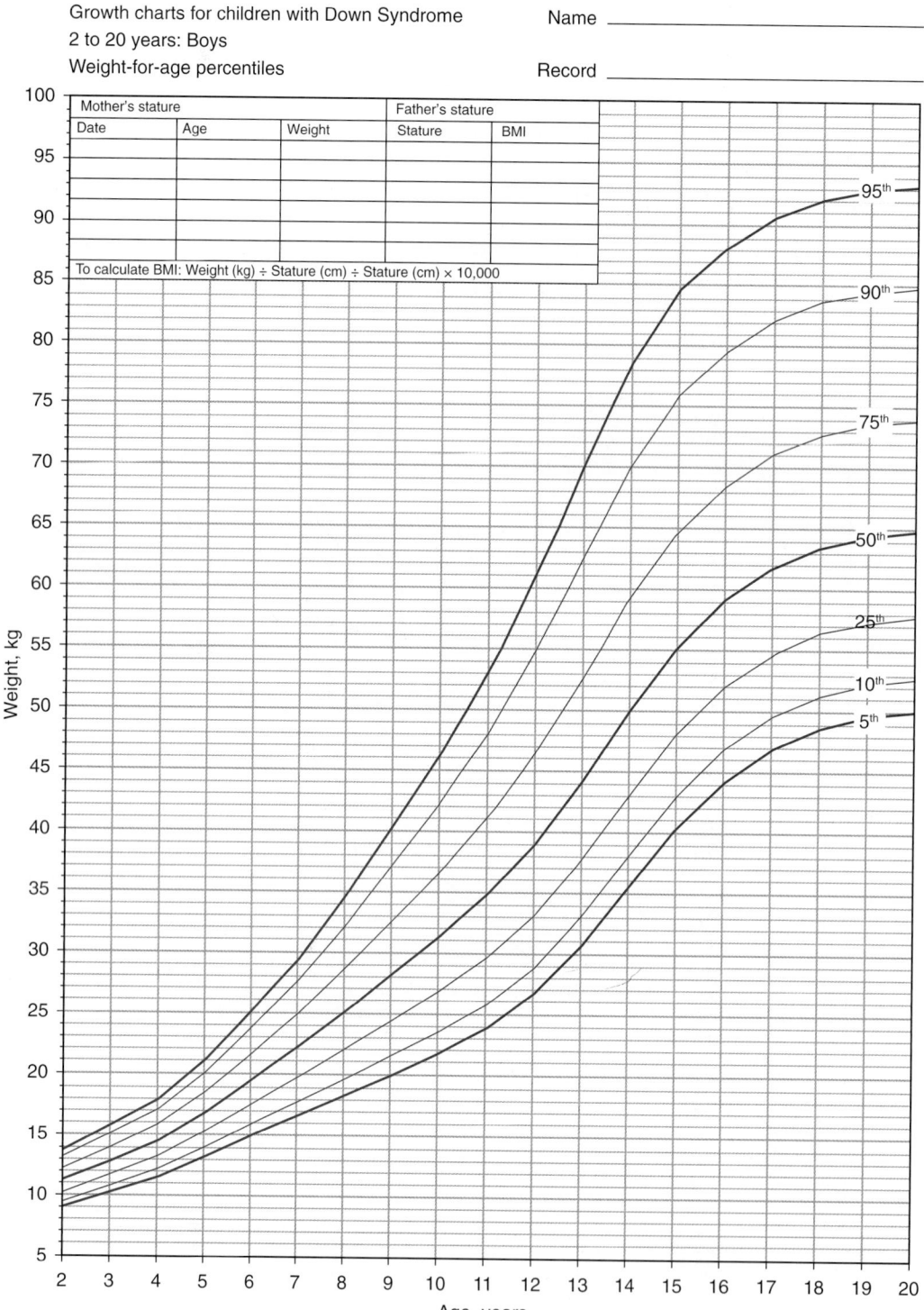

Growth charts for children with Down Syndrome
2 to 20 years: Boys
Weight-for-age percentiles

Name _____

Record _____

To calculate BMI: Weight (kg) ÷ Stature (cm) ÷ Stature (cm) × 10,000

Fig. 21.6 Males with Down syndrome: Weight 2 to 20 years. From Zemel, B.S., Pipan, M., Stallings, V.A., Hall, W., Schgadt, K., Freedman, D.S., & Thorpe, P. [2015]. *Growth charts for children with Down syndrome in the US pediatrics.* Centers for Disease Control and Prevention. https://www.cdc.gov/ncbddd/birthdefects/downsyndrome/documents/DS_Boys_Weight_2-20years.pdf.)

with Down syndrome. O'Toole et al. (2018) found parents significantly impact communication abilities in children with Down syndrome. Soriano et al. (2020) found in adolescents that communication increases, but quality of communication does not always occur. Therefore children with Down syndrome should have their language skills frequently assessed across all domains and all age ranges (Soriano et al., 2020). Success has been found with high-frequency, naturalistic settings and delivered in conjunction with parents in which the child with Down syndrome is taught to interact with gestures, eye contact, and vocalizations; parents are instructed on how to respond to their child's words, sounds, and communicative gestures (Seager et al., 2022). Further research is needed to

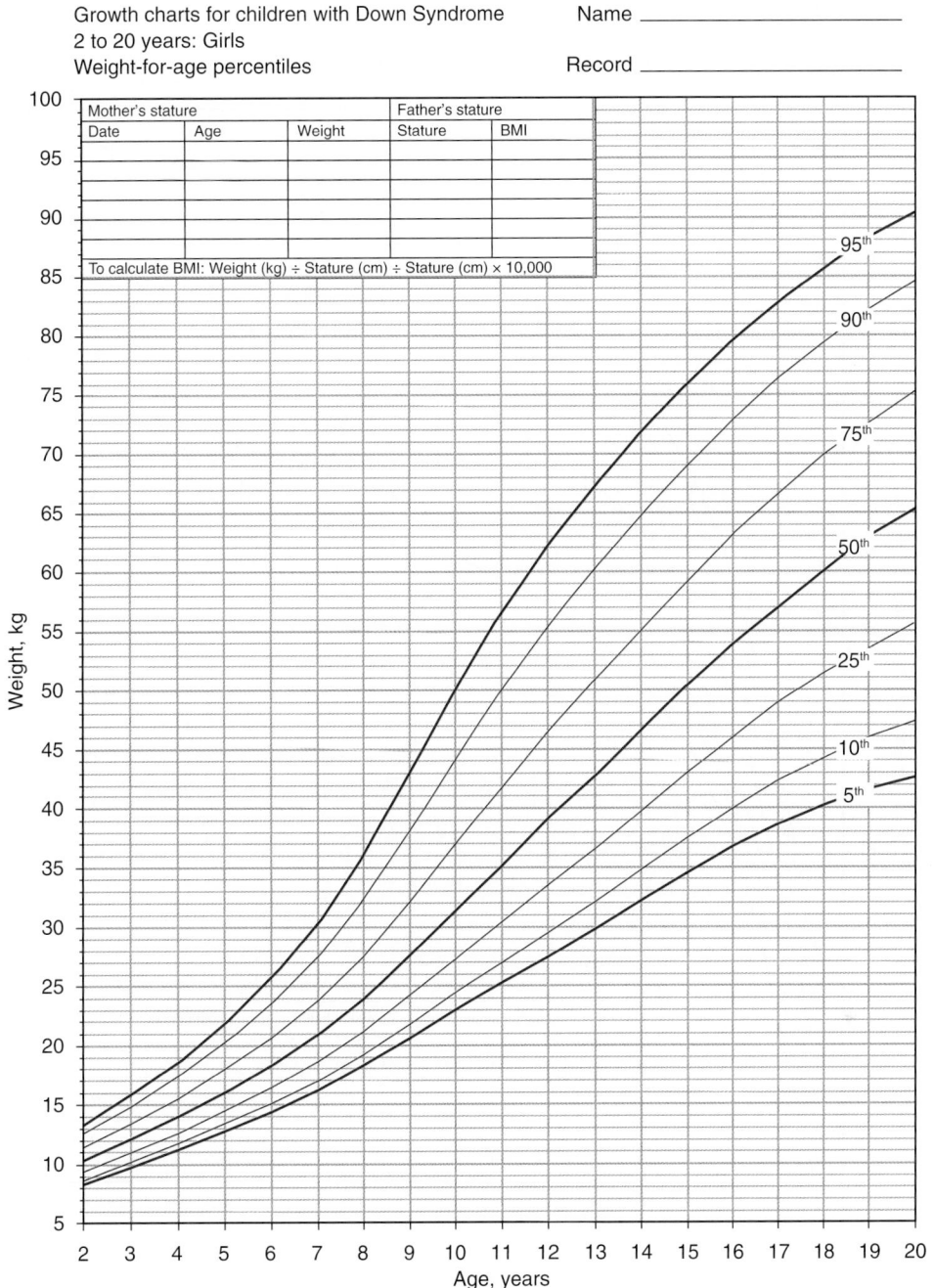

Fig. 21.7 Females with Down syndrome: Weight 2 to 20 years. (From Zemel, B.S., Pipan, M., Stallings, V.A., Hall, W., Schgadt, K., Freedman, D.S., & Thorpe, P. [2015]. *Growth charts for children with Down syndrome in the US pediatrics*. Centers for Disease Control and Prevention. https://www.cdc.gov/ncbddd/birthdefects/downsyndrome/documents/DS_Girls_Weight_2to20years.pdf.)

identify the oral motor patterns and examine the progression of gestures and vocalizations to speech-language in children with Down syndrome.

Children with Down syndrome will pass through the normal developmental milestones at a much slower rate than expected. The primary care provider can assist in a child's development by referring the family to an early intervention program as soon as possible after the child's birth. As the child grows older, a variety of activities that are known to assist in

development (e.g., Special Olympics, summer camps) can be encouraged. If a child has significant congenital anomalies, program personnel will need guidance regarding the intensity of activity the child is allowed. A child's progress should be carefully documented on standardized developmental schedules at each primary care visit. Because Down syndrome is associated with global developmental delay, most children with Down syndrome will have IQs below the second standard deviation on standardized tests, such as the Wechsler

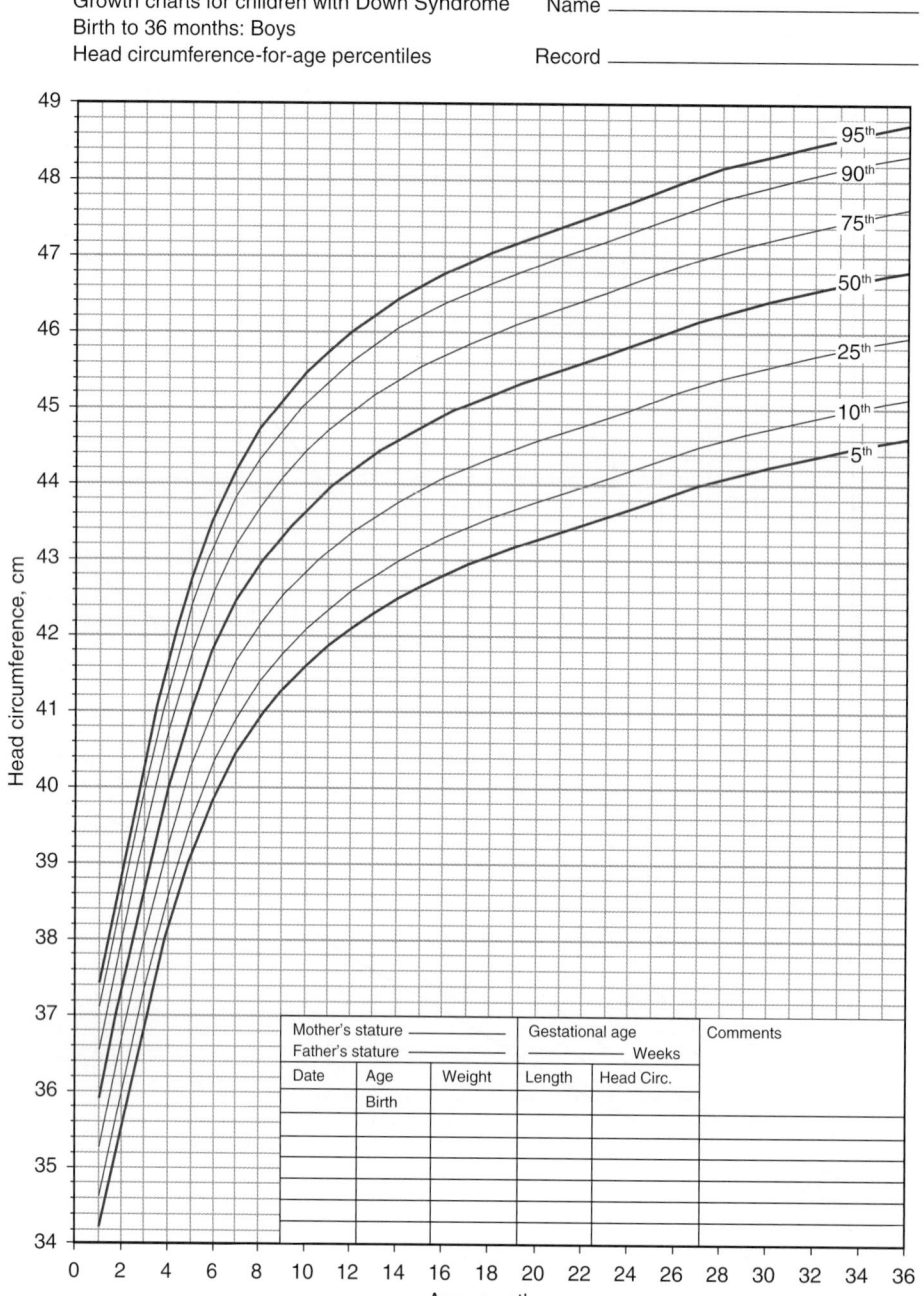

Fig. 21.8 Head circumference growth curves for males with Down syndrome. (From Zemel, B.S., Pipan, M., Stallings, V.A., Hall, W., Schgadt, K., Freedman, D.S., & Thorpe, P. [2015]. *Growth charts for children with Down syndrome in the US pediatrics.* Centers for Disease Control and Prevention. https://www.cdc.gov/ncbddd/birthdefects/downsyndrome/documents/DS_Boys_HeadCirc_Birthto36mo.pdf.)

Intelligence Scale for Children–Revised or the Bayley Scales of Infant Development (Lee et al., 2023).

Normal childhood and adolescent stressors are also of concern. For example, adolescents with Down syndrome often desire to date other adolescents of normal intelligence. If rejected, along with their inability to drive to social events, adolescents with Down syndrome can become depressed. Therefore social setbacks, behavioral concerns, and social determinants

of health should be assessed and addressed at each health care visit.

Diet

Among the most significant concerns are feeding difficulties in young children and obesity in older children. Feeding problems may be encountered because of the disproportionately large tongue, muscle flaccidity, poor coordination, significantly delayed social

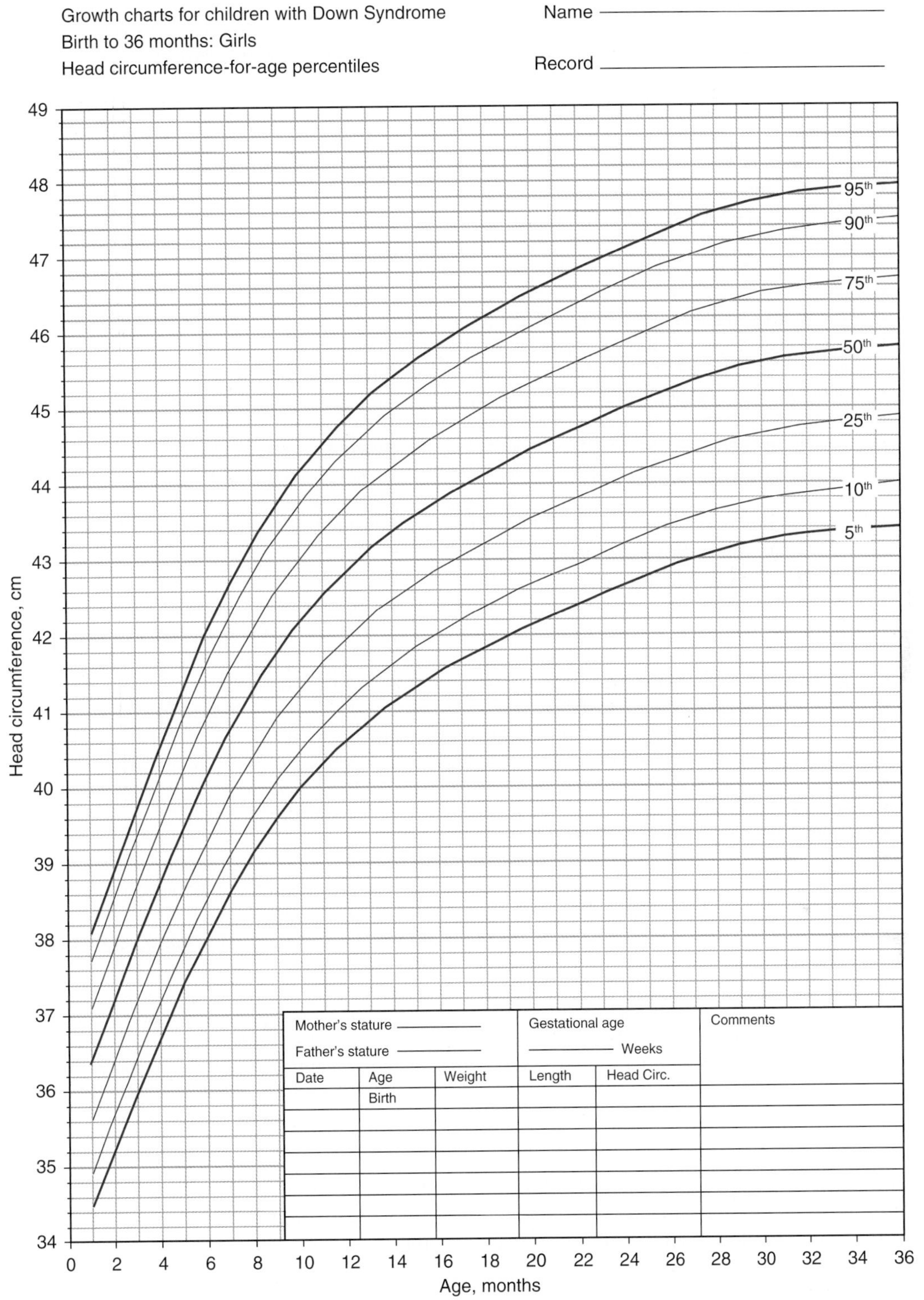

Growth charts for children with Down Syndrome
Birth to 36 months: Girls
Head circumference-for-age percentiles

Name _____

Record _____

Fig. 21.9 Head circumference growth curves for females with Down syndrome. (From Zemel, B.S., Pipan, M., Stallings, V.A., Hall, W., Schgadt, K., Freedman, D.S., & Thorpe, P. [2015]. *Growth charts for children with Down syndrome in the US pediatrics*. Centers for Disease Control and Prevention. https://www.cdc.gov/ncbddd/birthdefects/downsyndrome/documents/DS_Girls_HeadCircumference_Birthto36mo.pdf.)

maturation, thyroid or pituitary disorders, and congenital heart disease.

For infants, breastfeeding should be encouraged. The immunogenic qualities of breastmilk offer additional protection against upper respiratory tract infections, leukemia, and bowel problems (Ravel et al., 2020). The extra effort required of breastfeeding infants also helps them develop orofacial muscles and tongue control and promotes greater jaw stability. Breastfeeding may take longer at first, and mothers will need to be encouraged in

Table **21.3**	Recommendations for 5 Years to 21 Years of Age Based on the American Academy of Pediatrics (AAP) Guidelines for Health Supervision for Children and Adolescents With Down Syndrome
VISIT (AGE)	**AAP RECOMMENDATIONS**
5–12 yr	• Begin transition discussion at age 10 yr and ongoing for subsequent visits from then on • Annual audiology evaluation • Discuss body mass index (BMI)/obesity and risk for complications and diet/exercise considerations • Thyroid-stimulating hormone (TSH) annually • Annual vision evaluation with ophthalmology • Complete blood count (CBC) with differential and ferritin and C-reactive protein (CRP) or serum iron and total iron binding capacity (TIBC) annually • Palpate testes to monitor for testicular cancer • Review celiac disease symptoms and test if symptomatic • Review atlantoaxial instability symptoms and test if symptomatic • Discuss skin, hair, and scalp care; make dermatology referral as needed • Encourage self-help skills, developmental, behavioral, and school/home function • Monitor medications and alternative therapies • Discuss sleep and neurologic issues, and monitor for disorders to refer if appropriate • Discuss school transitions and school placement, including individualized education plan (IEP) and other resources • Discuss hygiene, pubertal changes, birth control, sexually transmitted infection (STI) prevention, etc.
12–21 yr	• Continue transition discussions with family and patient • Annual audiology evaluation • Discuss BMI/obesity and risk for complications and diet/exercise considerations • TSH annually • Annual vision evaluation with ophthalmology • CBC with differential and ferritin and CRP or serum iron and TIBC annually • Palpate testes to monitor for testicular cancer • Review celiac disease symptoms and test if symptomatic • Review atlantoaxial instability symptoms and test if symptomatic • Discuss skin, hair, and scalp care; make dermatology referral as needed • Encourage self-help skills, developmental, behavioral, and school/home function • Monitor medications and alternative therapies • Discuss sleep and neurologic issues and monitor for disorders to refer if appropriate • Discuss school transitions and school placement, including IEP and other resources • Discuss hygiene, pubertal changes, birth control, STI prevention, etc. • Monitor for behavioral concerns and social status and refer patients with depression or other behavioral health concerns • Evaluate annually for acquired mitral or aortic valve disease • Discuss issues related to adulthood, including work, independence, goals, and medical care; discuss guardianship and long-term financial planning from early adolescent as needed • Discuss recurrence risk should pregnancy occur in the adolescent/adult with Down syndrome

(Bull et al., 2022)

their efforts. The La Leche League International (2022) has materials on breastfeeding infants with Down syndrome.

Blended and chopped foods and shallow-bowl, latex-covered spoons may help children who are learning to eat solids. Infants with Down syndrome are at increased risk for aspiration, gastroesophageal reflux, masticatory dysfunction, and other feeding issues (Ravel et al., 2020). Early intervention with speech, occupational, physical, and other therapies should be initiated within the first 6 months of life (Bull et al., 2022).

There are no routine dietary restrictions for older children. Care should be taken to avoid excessive caloric intake if inappropriate weight gain is a problem. A balanced diet, physical exercise program, and vitamin and mineral supplementation are recommended as necessary (Bull et al., 2022). The only dietary restriction for children with Down syndrome is for those diagnosed with celiac disease or other food allergies/intolerances.

Safety

Safety issues for children with Down syndrome are the same as for their developmental, not chronologic, peers. Primary care providers must adjust their normal schedule for providing anticipatory guidance to the development of children with Down syndrome. If information is given too far in advance of a child's developmental progression, parents may forget or find the information to be a painful reminder that their child is progressing more slowly than unaffected children.

Children with Down syndrome are more likely to sustain joint injuries as a result of their joint laxity and

| Box **21.1** | Recommendations Across All Visits Based on the American Academy of Pediatrics (AAP) Guidelines for Health Supervision for Children and Adolescents With Down Syndrome |

- Thorough history and physical exam, including cardiac, neurologic, dermatologic, and other concerns
- Monitor growth and weight on Down syndrome–specific charts
- Ongoing developmental evaluation
- Ongoing feeding and evaluation for deficiencies in iron or other vitamins/minerals
- Ongoing visual and hearing evaluation
- Administer immunizations per Centers for Disease Control and Prevention guidelines unless specific contraindications
- Ongoing follow-up with subspecialist (e.g., cardiology, neurology)
- Safety discussions, including trampoline, contact sports, and other items specific to neurologic, development, and health concerns
- Encourage participation in Special Olympics and other activities that support children with intellectual disabilities
- Evaluate the emotional status of families, caregivers, and educational needs
- Provide support to family regarding resources and needs
- Encourage conversation regarding how to discuss Down syndrome and their child
- Promote positive family experiences and discuss the strengths of the child and resilience factors
- Encourage participation in support groups, provide reading materials, and connect with the community and financial resources
- Discuss complementary alternative therapies and safety
- Ongoing discussion of future pregnancy and recurrence risks with genetic counseling as needed
- Transition planning and long-term care specific to patient/family needs

(Bull et al., 2022)

hypermobility (Lagan et al., 2020). For children with atlantoaxial instability or those who have not yet been adequately evaluated, contact sports, somersaults, or other activities that may result in cervical injury should be restricted (Bull et al., 2022). The child without symptoms of atlantoaxial instability does not require routine radiologic evaluations; however, if there are symptoms of atlantoaxial instability, plain cervical spine radiography is recommended in the neutral position (Bull et al., 2022). When significant abnormalities are present, the child should be referred to neurosurgery or orthopedic surgery to manage this condition (Bull et al., 2022). Documentation of physical examination, including evaluation for symptoms of atlantoaxial instability, is required for participation in Special Olympics.

Immunizations

All routine immunizations should be given in children with Down syndrome unless there are specific contraindications. Reasons to not vaccinate might include severely immunocompromised patients (live vaccines) or severe allergic reaction (only the specific immunization) (Bull et al., 2022; CDC, 2022).

It is recommended that children with Down syndrome with a qualifying heart disease, chronic lung disease, airway clearance issues, or prematurity of less than 29 weeks of gestation should receive palivizumab (Synagis) injections monthly during RSV season in the first 2 years (AAP Committee on Infectious Diseases, 2021).

Screenings

Vision. Because of the large number of ocular defects associated with Down syndrome, all children should be evaluated by an ophthalmologist by 6 months of age, and vision should be evaluated at every visit using age/developmental-appropriate tools (Bull et al., 2022). Early referral is critical considering the synergistic effects that diminished vision and hearing have on development. Many of the conditions leading to visual impairment are correctable, including strabismus, cataracts, and myopia (Bull et al., 2022). Future screening recommendations should be determined in conjunction with the ophthalmologist according to the status of the child's eyes. At minimum, the primary care provider should screen for visual problems at each well-child visit. Such screening should include testing acuity, examining the red reflex and optic fundi, and checking alignment and oculomotor functions. Because children with Down syndrome may have difficulty using a Snellen or lazy E chart, acuity screening performed with the Titmus picture test or Teller acuity cards will yield more valid results.

Many children with Down syndrome have difficulty keeping their glasses in place, so parents should be counseled that purchasing glasses with lightweight plastic lenses and using an elastic strap around the child's occiput to secure them will help correct this problem. Contact lenses are not routinely recommended but may be appropriate for children with keratoconus.

Hearing. Because good hearing is required for cognitive, social, and language development, and these children are at high risk for conductive hearing loss, careful assessment is necessary. The health care provider should use the smallest size speculum (2 mm) for the examination because of typically tiny ear openings. It is recommended that all infants be evaluated for auditory brainstem responses or otoacoustic emission during the first month of life and rescreened at 6 months if they passed newborn hearing screenings (Bull et al., 2022). Ear-specific exams every 6 months should continue until normal hearing is established bilaterally (usually age >4 years), and then behavioral audiograms should take place every 1 year thereafter (Bull et al., 2022). Because of the importance of early intervention, infants between 9 and 12 months of age should be referred for microotoscopy if examination is difficult. When middle ear disease occurs, it deserves aggressive intervention and close follow-up if further developmental insult is to be prevented. Therefore referral to an otolaryngologist should take place (Bull et al., 2022).

If hearing aids are required, those that fasten onto the earpiece of eyeglasses may be better than ear molds. Hearing aids dependent on ear molds are hard to fit for children who are just beginning to wear them. These children often do not like the increased sound. Parents may need help finding methods (e.g., behavior management) to help improve their child's compliance for leaving the hearing aid in place. Parents must also be cautioned to devise mnemonic cues for remembering to change the batteries routinely because it is unlikely that their child will be able to realize that the hearing aid is malfunctioning.

Dental. Delayed and irregular eruption of teeth is common along with high prevalence of dental problems in young children (Bull et al., 2022). Therefore regular dental care is necessary. Primary care providers must document and carefully observe the dental problems of these children. All children with Down syndrome should be evaluated by 12 months of age or within 6 months of the first tooth eruption by a dentist or pedodontist skilled in caring for children with developmental disabilities. Locating such dentists is often difficult for parents, and specific referrals to professionals may be warranted.

Good dental hygiene—including twice-daily brushing and flossing—is indicated to reduce the amount of periodontal disease. Using a Water Pik or an electric toothbrush should be considered if good dental hygiene is difficult to achieve. Effective toothbrushing techniques may be difficult to achieve because of the child's limited manual dexterity, enlarged tongue, and small mouth. Close supervision is required, and independent toothbrushing and mouth care may not be feasible until the child is at least of preschool age.

Weaning children from a bottle by age 12 months and diets that contain low-sugar, crunchy foods (e.g., fresh vegetables) also help deter dental deterioration and should be encouraged. In areas where the water supply is nonfluoridated, fluoride treatment and fluoride toothpaste are recommended. For children with congenital heart disease, prophylactic antibiotics may be warranted for dental interventions (Wilson et al., 2021).

Blood pressure. Routine screening is recommended. If there is a history of cardiac disease or a positive family history of cardiac disease or hypertension, more careful assessment is required. However, compared to the general population, there is a lower incidence of hypertension in people with Down syndrome (Lagan et al., 2020). However, a cardiac evaluation, including an echocardiogram, is warranted during infancy to rule out congenital heart disease or cardiac defects (Bull et al., 2022).

Hematocrit. Routine screening is recommended. All infants should have a complete blood count (CBC), and all neonates with Down syndrome, within 3 days of birth because TAM, leukocytosis, polycythemia, and other hematologic disorders can be present (Bull et al., 2022; Marlow et al., 2021).

Urinalysis. Routine screening is recommended.

Tuberculosis. Routine screening is recommended. No special precautions must be taken unless the child is or has been institutionalized.

Condition-Specific Screenings

Thyroid dysfunction. Because the abnormalities seen in Down syndrome are similar to some seen in thyroid dysfunction, it is difficult to diagnose thyroid problems by clinical examination. Thyroid-stimulating hormone levels should be assessed at birth and every 5 to 7 months until 1 year of age and then annually after that (Bull et al., 2022). If antithyroid antibodies are present, then every 6-month screening should continue (Bull et al., 2022). If any signs or symptoms are suggestive of thyroid dysfunction, a complete thyroid panel should be drawn.

Atlantoaxial instability. Primary care providers must appraise the risk of atlantoaxial subluxation for all children with Down syndrome who are planning to engage in physical activity, the Special Olympics, or undergo surgical or rehabilitative procedures. Only patients with symptoms should undergo routine radiologic evaluation (Bull et al., 2022).

Hip dislocation. Hip instability can occur throughout the lifespan. Assessing for hip instability early and throughout childhood is important because early detection (i.e., before the dislocation is fixed and acetabular dysplasia occurs) allows for optimal surgical correction (Maranho et al., 2018). Early signs of habitual dislocation are an increasing limp, decreasing activity, and an audible click. Pain does not usually occur unless the dislocation is acute. In older children, radiographic studies may be necessary for assessment.

Mitral valve prolapse. Mitral valve prolapse or long-term complications related to the underlying congenital heart disease can occur as the child ages. Therefore cardiac-specific screenings and echocardiograms may be required with regular care by a cardiologist (Bull et al., 2022).

Celiac disease. Although screening is not mandatory for individuals with Down syndrome, increased attention has been brought to the incidence of celiac disease in this population. The primary care provider should review for symptoms of celiac disease in those whose diet contains gluten (Bull et al., 2022). TTG-IgA and quantitative IgA should be drawn, and those referred with abnormal labs (Bull et al., 2022).

COMMON ILLNESS MANAGEMENT
Differential Diagnosis
Immune dysfunction. The significant changes in the immune systems of children with Down syndrome have significant implications for primary care providers. Specifically, all infections must be treated aggressively because negative sequelae are more likely to develop. The incidence of many autoimmune diseases (including insulin-dependent diabetes mellitus and chronic arthritis) is also much greater in this population. A thorough evaluation is indicated if a child exhibits signs and symptoms compatible with a diagnosis of any of these diseases. Parents must be educated about the signs and symptoms of conditions and the need to seek medical advice promptly.

> ### 🔍 Differential Diagnosis
>
> - Infectious diseases require aggressive treatment due to underlying immune dysfunction.
> - Upper respiratory tract infections and sequelae are common.
> - Behavioral changes may have physical cause.
> - Gastrointestinal symptoms in infants may be due to congenital anomalies.
> - Leukemia is 18 to 20 times more likely to be acquired than in the general population.

Upper respiratory tract infections. Children with Down syndrome are prone to upper respiratory tract infections. These infections should be managed aggressively because untoward sequelae, including otitis media and pneumonia, are apt to develop. Children with congenital heart disease should be examined at the first signs of illness because they are more likely to develop secondary problems, and parents may confuse an upper respiratory tract infection with early congestive heart failure. These children

may also need to be given subacute bacterial endocarditis prophylaxis.

Behavioral changes. Behavioral changes may be caused by a variety of physiologic and psychological problems, including the following: thyroid dysfunction, obstructive sleep apnea, neurodegeneration (primarily in older individuals), declining physical competence (e.g., congestive heart failure), disturbed home environment, and overstimulation. Cause-specific interventions are necessary. Trials with stimulants, antidepressants, or antipsychotic drugs may be indicated in some cases after a thorough evaluation, although diagnosis of mental illness should not be given based solely on the fact that the child has Down syndrome.

Gastrointestinal symptoms. Because pyloric stenosis and Hirschsprung disease are more common in children with Down syndrome, primary care providers should carefully pursue reports of persistent vomiting, constipation, or chronic diarrhea in infants.

Leukemia. Children with Down syndrome acquire leukemia 18 to 20 times as often as other children. Easy bruising, unusual pallor, or listlessness must be fully evaluated. Parents must be alerted to seek health care for their child immediately if any of these signs or symptoms develop.

Drug Interactions
Because children with Down syndrome are at risk for health problems affecting any organ or system of their body, they may often be taking medications. It is important that family members understand how to administer the medications, what the side effects are, and to report any allergic reactions to the primary care provider. Over-the-counter medications are often ineffective (e.g., with skin problems), and prescription medications may be needed.

DEVELOPMENTAL ISSUES
Sleep Patterns
Sleep disorders are common in children with Down syndrome, except for obstructive sleep apnea and related conditions. Anatomic and immunologic differences predispose school-age children in particular to this condition. The primary care provider should have a high index of suspicion if the child has a history of snoring, restless sleep, abnormal sleep positions, being awake for hours during the night, night terrors, or daytime somnolence, as well as if failure to thrive, pulmonary hypertension, or behavioral problems are present. As a result, a thorough history and physical examination are warranted, especially an examination of the oral and nasal passages. Referral to a sleep laboratory for periodic overnight polysomnography evaluation may be warranted. Options for

treatment may include saline spray, oxygen at night, or continuous positive airway pressure also delivered at night. Surgical treatment can range from tonsillectomy and adenoidectomy to a combination of skeletal and soft tissue alterations to eliminate the specific cause of obstruction. It is recommended that a sleep study be conducted after recovery from surgery to verify that the cause of obstruction was eliminated. It is important to address sleep disorders because sleep problems can significantly affect the child's behavior, learning, and quality of life (Horne et al., 2019).

Toileting

The median age for toilet training children with Down syndrome is approximately 3.4 years with completion by 6.6 years (Dreher et al., 2022). Parents must be advised of this to reduce frustrations associated with unrealistic expectations. Routine toilet training techniques are effective. It takes longer to train a child with Down syndrome, and additional positive reinforcement is necessary.

Constipation, a common problem, may also be related to inadequate peristalsis, poor diet, lack of exercise, or thyroid dysfunction. The cause of constipation must be assessed to initiate the correct interventions. It is important for the child to maintain a healthy diet with fruits and vegetables, to exercise regularly, and use an osmotic agent such as polyethylene glycol if needed (Mulhem et al., 2022).

Discipline

Children with Down syndrome are usually not more difficult to discipline than other children. Parents must be encouraged to remember that discipline needs to be appropriate for the child's developmental, not chronologic, age. Children with Down syndrome should not receive special compensation just because they have Down syndrome. Parental expectations should be consistent, and limits should be set for all children in the family. Behavior management programs can be developed for specific discipline problems when a child has not been responsive to the parents' usual methods.

Child Care

Day care should provide appropriate social, cognitive, and physical stimulation for a child with Down syndrome. When selecting the type of day care setting, parents should be encouraged to consider the child's personality and medical needs and their own philosophy about inclusion. Many generic day care centers include children with Down syndrome into their programs and are sufficiently staffed to provide an excellent experience for these children. Specialized day care, often available through the school system, may be a better option if a child has significant medical problems. If a child is highly susceptible to infections,

a home care setting (i.e., with fewer than six children) is recommended. Primary care providers should be aware of resources in their community to assist parents with day care placement. Local parent groups for children with Down syndrome, as well as the local affiliates of the Arc of the United States (see Resources, later) and other specialty agencies, may also help with placement.

Schooling

A variety of options—from total inclusion to residential placement—for academic placement exist. If circumstances permit, children with Down syndrome do best in an environment fully integrated with nondisabled peers. However, children with Down syndrome need support from their families while dealing with being exceptional and social pressures from peers. Parents and teachers working together to create a supportive environment can ensure that a child has some social and academic successes. Otherwise, the child may become frustrated and demoralized, leading to disruptive behavior and poor self-esteem.

Families may need assistance in choosing the school setting they deem most appropriate for their child. Primary care providers can be instrumental in helping families locate appropriate community services to assist in educational placement. All children with Down syndrome are eligible for educational provisions under PL 108-446 (IDEA, 2004). Parents should be encouraged to contact their social worker or local office of intellectual disabilities shortly after the child's birth so that they can receive the educational, vocational, and supportive services for which the child is eligible.

Sexuality

Pubertal changes in adolescents with Down syndrome occur approximately the same as in their unaffected peers. Accompanying these physical changes, adolescents will have social interests and biologic drives similar to those of their chronologic-age peers and must be given the opportunity to participate in social activities with their peers. For highly protective parents, the social education and sexual education that accompany their child's increasing independence are often difficult and sensitive issues (Bull et al., 2022). Primary care providers need to help parents recognize their responsibility in ensuring that children can handle themselves in a socially and sexually appropriate manner.

Individualized instruction about self-care skills, biologic changes, social implications, and contraception is paramount to minimizing the appearance of sexual impropriety and the risk of being sexually exploited. Routine pelvic examination is not recommended for females unless specific concerns arise until adulthood. Genetic counseling for both the parents and the child is necessary. Both males and females with Down syndrome can reproduce (Whooten et al., 2018). Planned Parenthood, the Arc of the United States, and parent support groups offer printed and audiovisual materials specifically designed for use with these families.

The age at onset of menses for females is similar to that of their mothers. Handling pubertal changes is difficult for some female adolescents. Family members must be helped to recognize the behavior changes that may be related to normal hormonal cycles. For females who are menstruating and are unable to manage their hygienic care, parents and other caregivers must follow universal precautions. Decisions concerning birth control, sterilization, and other reproductive issues should include the parents, patient, and health care provider team with patient-centered approach to decision making.

Transition to Adulthood

The life expectancy for individuals with Down syndrome has increased dramatically with most living well into middle age, creating the need to address independent living, sexuality, vocational choices, and health maintenance in adulthood and older adulthood.

Individuals with Down syndrome vary in their abilities to live independently; some require ongoing, consistent supervision, and others merely need minimal guidance with complex tasks. Some individuals remain at home until a crisis forces different arrangements. Because individuals with Down syndrome often have aged parents, families can help plan for a smooth transition to a different living situation within the context of normal development. For example, some parents may help their child move to a group home at about the same age as their other children leave for college. Recreational activities such as bowling, swimming, and dancing are encouraged because they promote social relationships and physical fitness. Registering to vote is also an important function of adulthood.

Vocational choices are directed by an individual's cognitive abilities, social skills, and adaptive abilities. Many persons with Down syndrome can seek competitive employment in custodial work, offices, housekeeping, restaurants, landscaping, or other occupations where the required skills are not too difficult and are repetitive, and there is ongoing supervision. The skills necessary to survive in the workforce (e.g., basic money management, telling time, using public transportation) must be mastered before such positions are sought. Working in sheltered workshops is a better option for others because this type of job requires fewer adaptive abilities.

Generally, the overall health of most individuals with Down syndrome is good. Premature aging may occur as early as the 20s with dental changes often seen first. Dermatologic, thyroid, cardiac, and sensory problems are the most troublesome and worsen with age. Changes in mental health may also be a concern after children complete formal schooling at 21 years of age. Depression and obsessive-compulsive behaviors continue to be seen in adulthood. Of concern is Alzheimer disease, which occurs in a sizable proportion of adults (~40%) with Down syndrome over 40 years of age (Matthews et al., 2018). The actual percentage differs among studies, approximately 50% by age 50 or older. The incidence rises as the person ages. IQ levels and adaptive functioning also decline over time. Further longitudinal study of adults with Down syndrome, especially documentation of health status changes, is warranted.

Family Concerns

Parents of children with Down syndrome will experience joy and pride in their child, although they will be faced with many challenges throughout their child's life. Most parents meet these challenges with resilience and adaptive functioning (Pruktarat et al., 2021). For some parents, however, raising these children can become overwhelming. Locating and coordinating acceptable medical, educational, and ancillary personnel may produce stress. Primary care providers may greatly assist them in identifying appropriate resources (e.g., respite care) and helping parents become their child's best lifelong advocate. Mothers (in particular) may find it difficult to balance their time and responsibilities among their children and spouse. One of the greatest unmet parental needs is information about special services and programs, friends for their child with Down syndrome, and getting a break from responsibilities.

Down syndrome parent support groups have also been invaluable to families, especially in the first year after a child with Down syndrome is born.

Siblings are also important members of any family, and their adjustment to a child with Down syndrome has been researched over the past several years. Overall, researchers have found their adjustment to be primarily positive, and their own development has not been negatively influenced by having a brother or sister with Down syndrome. However, there can be issues with siblings that arise, such as resentment, maladjustment, self-esteem, and feelings of loneliness (Takataya et al., 2019). It is recommended that parents maintain honest and open communication about the child with Down syndrome and explain the condition to their other children as soon as possible, encourage expression of feelings, recognize that all interactions will not be positive (as with any siblings), reduce the amount of time that the sibling has to care for the child with Down syndrome, recognize each child's uniqueness, and offer informal or formal support when needed for the sibling(s) without Down syndrome.

Although many concerns are similar for all families who have a child with special needs, one notable issue for families of children with Down syndrome is the need for long-range planning. Most individuals with Down syndrome never become totally self-sufficient, and families must plan for a child's lifetime through, for example, estate planning and custody arrangements. They must also enroll an adult child to receive Supplemental Security Income. However, other individuals with Down syndrome may marry and live somewhat independent lives. The degree of the child's limitations, the internal strengths of the family, and the support from extended family and community networks all affect a family's adjustment.

INFORMATIONAL MATERIALS

Caring for a child with Down syndrome is a complex task because of the physical, cognitive, and social concerns that must be addressed. Additional resources for professionals and parents of children with Down syndrome are vital. These following printed materials provide parents with valuable information (also see Resources):

Jacob, J., & Sikora, M. (2015). *The parent's guide to Down syndrome: Advice, information, inspiration, and support for raising your child from diagnosis through adulthood.* Adams Media.

Pueschel, S.M. (2001). *A parent's guide to down syndrome: Toward a brighter future.* Brookes Publishing.

Skallerup, S.J. (2009). *Babies with Down syndrome: A new parents guide* (3rd ed.). Woodbine House.

RESOURCES

The Arc of the United States: www.thearc.org

Canadian Down Syndrome Society: www.cdss.ca

Commission on Mental and Physical Disability Law: www.americanbar.org/groups/diversity/disabilityrights

Down Syndrome Diagnosis Network: www.dsdiagnosisnetwork.org

National Down Syndrome Society: www.ndss.org

 Summary

Primary Care Needs for the Child With Down Syndrome

HEALTH CARE MAINTENANCE

Growth and Development

- Children usually have a shorter stature and increased weight (after infancy).
- Children should have height and weight measured at each visit and plotted on CDC growth charts for children with Down syndrome.
- Caloric reduction and increased exercise are recommended with untoward weight gain.
- Virtually all children will have an intellectual and developmental disability.
- Expressive language problems are common.
- Normal progression of developmental milestones occurs but at a slower rate.
- Early intervention programs are recommended.

Diet

- Feeding support is needed in infancy to ensure adequate weight gain. Problems with dysphagia, reflux, and hypotonia may result in inadequate weight gain.
- Breastfeeding is encouraged in infancy.
- Adaptive equipment and occupational therapy may be needed when teaching feeding skills.
- Diets may need to be tailored to help correct constipation or obesity in childhood and adulthood.
- Vitamin D supplementation is recommended in all children, but some may require additional vitamin and mineral supplementation based on deficiencies.
- Children with celiac disease require a gluten-free diet.

Safety

- Anticipatory guidance needs to be based on a child's developmental, not chronologic, age.
- There is an increased incidence of musculoskeletal or joint injuries from laxity.
- Atlantoaxial instability is a hazard and must be assessed for before active sports programs.

Immunizations

- Routine immunizations are recommended.
- Live viral vaccines may be contraindicated in children with immunodeficiency disorders.
- RSV immunoprophylaxis should be considered in the first 2 years with other comorbidities such as congenital heart disease, chronic lung disease, or prematurity.

Screening

- *Vision.* The incidence of ocular defects is high. All infants should be evaluated by an ophthalmologist by 6 months of age and then regularly throughout childhood.
  - Acuity and alignment testing and examination of the red reflex and optic fundi should be done at each visit.
- *Hearing.* Anatomic abnormalities of the ears are common.
  - Auditory brainstem response or otoacoustic emission testing is recommended by 1 month of age.
  - Behavioral audiograms are recommended every 6 months until age 4 years and then annually.
  - Tympanometry is often a useful adjunct over 1 year of age.
  - Evaluation by a specialist is recommended every 6 months until age 4 years and then annually.
  - Cerumen impaction and otitis media are common.
  - A majority of children have hearing loss. Many will require hearing aids.
- *Dental.* Dental screening should be done a minimum of every 6 months within 6 months of first tooth eruption or by 12 months of age because of the high incidence of periodontal disease.
  - Good dental hygiene is important. Fluoride treatment in the primary care office and use of fluoride toothpaste are recommended.
  - Children should be weaned from the bottle by 12 months to prevent dental deterioration.

- Children with congenital heart disease may require antibiotic prophylaxis to prevent endocarditis.
- *Blood pressure.* Routine screening is recommended.
  - A full cardiac evaluation with echocardiogram should be done by 1 month of age.
- *Hematocrit.* Routine screening is recommended. A CBC in the first 3 days of life to assess for neutrophilia, polycythemia, and thrombocytopenia is recommended.
- *Urinalysis.* Routine screening is recommended.
- *Tuberculosis.* Routine screening is recommended.

Condition-Specific Screening
- Obtain karyotype in neonatal period if prenatal diagnostic tests for Down syndrome are not done.
- Thyroid-stimulating hormone levels should be checked at 5 to 7 months to 1 year of age and then annually if normal antibodies.
- Atlantoaxial instability risk should be assessed before surgery or athletic involvement.
- Screening for hip dislocation is necessary whenever a gait abnormality occurs.
- Screening for mitral valve prolapse should start in adolescence.
- Screening for celiac disease should be done with TTG-IgA and quantitative IgA.

COMMON ILLNESS MANAGEMENT
Differential Diagnosis
- *Immune dysfunction.* Children with Down syndrome are more susceptible to infections and autoimmune disorders.
- *Upper respiratory tract infections.* These are often associated with otitis media and pneumonia and should be managed aggressively, especially when a child has congenital heart disease.
- *Behavioral changes.* Thyroid dysfunction, obstructive sleep apnea, neurodegeneration, declining physical functioning, disturbed home environment, and overstimulation should be ruled out as a cause for behavioral changes.
- *Gastrointestinal symptoms.* Pyloric stenosis and Hirschsprung disease should be ruled out.
  - Constipation is a common problem and may be due to decreased peristalsis, poor diet, lack of exercise, or thyroid dysfunction.
- *Leukemia.* Unusual pallor, easy bruising, and listlessness should be fully evaluated.

Drug Interactions
- Children may be taking different medications for different conditions, so primary care providers should be aware of drug interactions and side effects and inform family members who are administering the medications.

DEVELOPMENTAL ISSUES
Sleep Patterns
- Obstructive sleep apnea may occur. Surgical intervention may be necessary. Refer for periodic overnight polysomnography if history warrants further assessment.

Toileting
- Delayed bowel and bladder training may occur as a result of developmental lag; constipation is common because of low activity level, decreased peristalsis, and poor diet.

Discipline
- Discipline must be developmentally appropriate; behavior management programs are often successful.

Child Care
- Small group day care lessens the risk of repeated infections.
- Children may be eligible for specialized day care programs; infants up to 3 years of age may be eligible for early intervention programs.

Schooling
- Children and youth are eligible for special education services through PL 108-446 (IDEA, 2004).

Sexuality
- Sex education must be taught so that children with Down syndrome are not abused and do not display inappropriate sexual behaviors.
- Females may need assistance with menstrual hygiene.
- Both males and females are able to reproduce, and fertility issues should be discussed.

Transition to Adulthood
- Emphasis should be on independent living, vocational skills, and health maintenance.
- Premature aging is present, and signs appear in the 20s with dental changes.
- Mental health problems (e.g., depression, obsessive-compulsive disorder, Alzheimer disease) may be problematic.

FAMILY CONCERNS
- Special family concerns may include long-term care and prolonged adaptation to the diagnosis.

REFERENCES

Altuna, M., Giménez, S., & Fortea, J. (2021). Epilepsy in down syndrome: A highly prevalent comorbidity. *J Clin Med, 10*(13), 2776. doi: 10.3390/jcm10132776.

American College of Obstetricians and Gynecologists (ACOG). NIPT summary of recommendations. 2022. https://www.acog.org/advocacy/policy-priorities/non-invasive-prenatal-testing/current-acog-guidance.

AAP Committee on Infectious Diseases Immunizations and Down syndrome. Publications.aap.org. (2021). https://publications.aap.org/aapbooks/book/663/Red-Book-2021-Report-of-the-Committee-on.

Antonarakis, S. E., Skotko, B. G., Rafii, M. S., Strydom, A., Pape, S. E., Bianchi, D. W., Sherman, S. L., & Reeves, R. H. (2020). Down syndrome. *Nature Reviews Disease Primers, 6*(9), 9. doi:10.1038/s41572-019-0143-7.

Arslan, F. N., Dogan, D. G., Canaloglu, S. K., Baysal, S. G., Buyukavci, R., & Buyukavci, M. A. (2022). Effects of early physical therapy on motor development in children with Down syndrome. *North Clin Istanb, 9*(2), 156–161. doi: 10.14744/nci.2020.90001.

Atli, E. (2021). What causes down syndrome? In Dey, S. K. (Ed.), *Down syndrome and other chromosome abnormalities.* IntertechOpen.

Baburamani, A., Patkee, P., Arichi, T., & Rutherford, M. (2019). New approaches to studying early brain development in Down syndrome. *Developmental Medicine and Child Neurology, 61*(8), 867–879. doi:10.1111/dmcn.14260.

Barnard, N. D., Goldman, D. M., Loomis, J. F., Kahleova, H., Levin, S. M., Neabore, S., & Batts, T. C. (2019). Plant-based diets for cardiovascular safety and performance in endurance sports. *Nutrients, 11*(1), 130. doi: 10.3390/nu11010130.

Beckhaus, A., & Castro-Rodriguez, J. (2018). Down syndrome and the risk of severe RSV infection: A meta-analysis. *Pediatrics, 142*(3), e20180225. doi:10.1542/peds.2018-0025.

Benn, P. (2021). Prenatal diagnosis of chromosome abnormalities through chorionic villus sampling and amniocentesis. In Milunsky, A., & Milunsky, J. M. (Eds.), *Genetic disorders and the fetus: Diagnosis, prevention, and treatment* (8th ed.). Wiley & Sons.

Borland, L. M., Colligan, J., & Brandom, B. W. (2004). Frequency of anesthesia-related complications in children with down syndrome children under general anesthesia for noncardiac procedures. *Pediatr Anesth, 14*, 733–738.

Bösebeck, F. (2022). Epilepsy and other comorbidities in down syndrome. *Zeitschrift Für Epileptologie, 35*(3), 235–241. https://doi.org/10.1007/s10309-022-00506-8.

Bull, M., Trotter, T., Santoro, S., Christensen, C., & Grout, R., The Council on Genetics. (2022). Health supervision for children and adolescents with Down syndrome. *Pediatrics, 149*(5), e2022057010. doi:10.1542/peds/2022-057010.

Centers for Disease Control and Prevention (CDC). Contraindications and precautions. 2022. https://www.cdc.gov/vaccines/hcp/acip-recs/general-recs/contraindications.html.

Centers for Disease Control and Prevention (CDC). Data and statistics on Down syndrome. 2020. https://www.cdc.gov/ncbddd/birthdefects/downsyndrome/data.html.

Chaiken, S., Susich, M., Doshi, U., Packer, C., Garg, B., & Caughey, A. (2022). Down syndrome trends by race/ethnicity in the United States from 2012–2018. *American Journal of Obstetrics and Gynecology, 226*(1), s481–s482. doi:10.1016/j.ajog.2021.11.797.

Cohen, W. I., (Ed.). (1999). Health care guidelines for individuals with Down syndrome: 1999 revision. *Down Syndr Q, 4*, 1–16.

Delany, D. R., Gaydos, S. S., Romeo, D. A., Henderson, H. T., Fogg, K. L., McKeta, A. S., Kavarana, M. N., & Costello, J. M. (2021). Down syndrome and congenital heart disease: Perioperative planning and management. *Journal of Congenital Cardiology, 5*(1). https://doi.org/10.1186/s40949-021-00061-3.

Desingu, V., Adapa, A., & Devi, S. (2019). Dental anomalies in down syndrome individuals: A review. *Journal of Scientific Dentistry, 9*(1), 6–8. https://doi.org/10.5005/jp-journals-10083-0902.

Dreher, T., Wolter-Warmerdam, K., Holland, S., Katz, T., & Patel, L. (2022). Toilet training in children and adolescents with Down syndrome. *J Dev Behav Pediatr, 43*(6), e381–e389. doi:10.1097/DBP.0000000000001058. Epub 2022 Jan 12.

Field, T. (2019). Pediatric massage therapy research: A narrative review. *Multidisciplinary Digital Publishing Institute Journal, 6*(5), 78.

Foley, C., & Killeen, O. (2019). Musculoskeletal anomalies in children with Down syndrome: An observational study. *Archives of Disease in Childhood-BMJ, 104*, 482–487. doi:10.1136/archdischild-2018-315751.

Godfrey, M., & Lee, N. (2018). Memory profiles in Down syndrome across development: A review of memory abilities throughout the lifespan. *Journal of Neurodevelopmental Disorders, 10*(5), 1–94. doi:10.1186/s11689-017-9220-y.

Hines, C., & Simmons, S. (2022). Down syndrome: A review of the key perioperative implications. *Association of Perioperative Registered Nurses Journal, 116*(1), 5–20. doi:10.1002/aorn.13712.

Horne, R., Wijayaratne, P., Nixon, G., & Walter, L. (2019). Sleep and sleep disordered breathing in children with Down syndrome: Effects on behavior, neurocognition and the cardiovascular system. *Sleep Medicine Reviews, 44*, 1–11. doi:10.1016/j.smrv.2018.11.002.

Individuals with Disabilities Education Act, (2004). Public Law 108-446. Washington, DC: U.S. Government Printing Office.

Khoshnood, B., Pryde, P., & Wall, S. (2000). Ethnic differences in the impact of advanced maternal age on birth prevalence of Down syndrome. *Am J Public Health, 90*, 1778–1781.

La Leche League International. My new baby was born with special needs. Can I still breastfeed? 2022. https://www.llli.org/breastfeeding-info/special-needs/.

LaCombe, J., & Roper, R. (2019). Skeletal dynamics of Down syndrome: A developing perspective. *Bone, 133*, 115215. doi:10.1016/j.bone.2019.115215.

Lagan, N., Huggard, D., Mc Grane, F., Leahy, T. R., Franklin, O., Roche, E., Webb, D., O' Marcaigh, A., Cox, D., El-Khuffash, A., Greally, P., Balfe, J., & Molloy, E. J. (2020). Multiorgan involvement and management in children with Down syndrome. *Acta Paediatrica (Oslo, Norway: 1992), 109*(6), 1096–1111. https://doi.org/10.1111/apa.15153.

Lam, M., Lu, J. D., Elhadad, L., Sibbald, C., & Alhusayen, R. (2022). Common dermatologic disorders in Down syndrome: Systematic review. *JMIR Dermatology, 5*(1). https://doi.org/10.2196/33391.

Laurent, A., Kotecha, R., & Malinge, S. (2020). Gain of chromosome 21 in hematological malignancies: Lessons from studying leukemia in children with Down syndrome. *Leukemia, 34*, 1984–1999.

Lee, K., Cascella, M., & Marwaha, R. (2023). Intellectual Disability. In: StatPearls [Internet]. Treasure Island (FL): StatPearls Publishing; 2023 Jan–. PMID: 31613434.

Lewanda, A., Gallegos, M., & Summar, M. (2018). Patterns of dietary supplement use in children with Down syndrome. *Journal of Pediatrics, 201*, 100–105.e30. doi:10.1016/j.jpeds.2018.05.022.

Maranho, D., Fush, K., Kim, Y., & Novais, E. (2018). Hip instability in patients with Down syndrome. *Journal of the American Academy of Orthopedic Surgery, 26*(13), 455–462. doi:10.5435/JAAOS-D-17-00179.

Marlow, E. C., Ducore, J., Kwan, M. L., Cheng, S. Y., Bowles, E. J. A., Greenlee, R. T., Pole, J. D., Rahm, A. K., Stout, N. K., Weinmann, S., Smith-Bindman, R., & Miglioretti, D. L. (2021). Leukemia risk in a cohort of 3.9 million children with and without Down syndrome. *The Journal of Pediatrics, 234*, 172–180.e3. https://doi.org/10.1016/j.jpeds.2021.03.001.

Matthews, T., Allain, D., Matthews, A., Mitchell, A., Santoro, S., & Cohen, L. (2018). An assessment of health, social, communication, and daily living skills of adults with Down syndrome. *American Journal of Medical Genetics. Part A., 176*(6), 1389–1397. doi:10.1002/ajmg.a.38721.

Messerlian G., Halliday J., Palomaki G. (2022). Down syndrome: Overview of prenatal screening. *UpToDate.* https://www.uptodate.com/contents/down-syndrome-overview-of-prenatal-screening.

Mowery, C. T., Reyes, J. M., Cabal-Hierro, L., Higby, K. J., Karlin, K. L., Wang, J. H., Kimmerling, R. J., Cejas, P., Lim, K., Li, H., Furusawa, T., Long, H. W., Pellman, D., Chapuy, B., Bustin, M., Manalis, S. R., Westbrook, T. F., Lin, C. Y., & Lane, A. A. (2018). Trisomy of a down syndrome critical region globally amplifies transcription via HMGN1 overexpression. *Cell Reports, 25*(7), 1898–1911.e5. https://doi.org/10.1016/j.celrep.2018.10.061.

Moyer, A., Gardiner, K., & Reeves, R. (2020). All creatures great and small: New approaches for understanding down syndrome genetics. *Trends in Genetics, 37*(1), 444–459. doi:10.1016/j.tig.2020.09.017.

Mulhem, E., Khondoker, F., & Kandiah, S. (2022). Constipation in children and adolescents: Evaluation and treatment. *American Family Physician, 105*(5), 469–478.

Mundakel, G. (2022). Down syndrome treatment and management. *Medscape.* https://emedicine.medscape.com/article/943216-treatment#d8.

O'Leary, L., Hughes-McCormack, L., Dunn, K., & Cooper, S. (2018). Early death and cause of death of people with Down syndrome: A systematic review. *Journal of Applied Research in Intellectual Disabilities, 31*, 687–708. doi:10.1111/jar.12446.

O'Shea, M., O'Shea, C., Gibson, L., Leo, J., & Carty, C. (2018). The prevalence of obesity in children and young people with Down syndrome. *Journal of Applied Research in Intellectual Disabilities, 31*(6), 1225–1229. doi:10.1111/jar.12465.

O'Toole, C., Lee, A., Gibbon, F., Bysterveldt, A., & Hart, N. (2018). Parent-mediated interventions for promoting communication and language development in young children with Down syndrome. *Cochrane Database Systematic Reviews*, 1–46. doi:10.1002/14651858.CD012089.pub2.

Ostermaier K. (2022). Down syndrome: Clinical features and diagnosis. *UpToDate*. https://www.uptodate.com/contents/down-syndrome-clinical-features-and-diagnosis/print.

Postolache, L. (2019). Abnormalities of the optic nerve in Down syndrome and associations with visual acuity. *Frontiers, 14*, 1–34. doi:10.3389/fneuro.2019.00633.

Priebe, G., & Kanzawa, M. (2020). Reducing the progression of Alzheimer's disease in Down syndrome patients with micro-dose lithium. *Medical Hypotheses, 137*, 109573. doi:10.1016/j.mehy.2020.109573.

Pruktarat, W., Prasopkittikun, T., Sitthimomgkol, Y., & Vongsirimas, N. (2021). Factors including family functioning related to pre-school children with Down syndrome. *Pacific Rim International Journal of Nursing Research, 25*(4), 505–676.

Rafferty, K., Archer, K., Turner, K., Brown, R., & Jackson-Cook, C. (2021). Trisomy 21-associated increases in chromosomal instability are unmasked by comparing isogenic trisomic/disomic leukocytes from people with mosaic Down syndrome. *PLOS One, 16*(7), 1–18. doi:10.1371/journal.pone.0254806.

Rahman, M. M., & Fatema, K. (2019). Seizures in down syndrome: An update. *Mymensingh Medical Journal: MMJ, 28*(3), 712–715. PMID: 31391451.

Ravel, A., Mrcher, C., Rbillat, S., Cieuta-Walti, C., & Megarbane, A. (2020). Feeding problems and gastrointestinal disease in Down syndrome. *Archives de Pediatrie, 27*(1), 53–60. doi:10.1016/j.arcped.2019-11.008.

Rethoré, M. O., Rouëssé, J., & Satgé, D. (2020). Cancer screening in adults with down syndrome, a proposal. *Eur J Med Genet, 63*(4), 103783. doi: 10.1016/j.ejmg.2019.103783. Epub 2019 Oct 9.

Rivelli, A., Fitzpatrick, V., Chaudhari, S., Chicoine, L., Jia, G., Rzhetsky, A., & Chicoine, B. (2022). Prevalence of mental health conditions among 6078 individuals with down syndrome in the united states. *Journal of Patient-Centered Research and Reviews, 9*(1), 58–63. https://doi.org/10.17294/2330-0698.1875.

Sahin, Y. (2021). Celiac disease in children: A review of the literature. *World J Clin Pediatr, 10*(4), 53–71. doi: 10.5409/wjcp.v10.i4.53.

Sanderson, K., & Goldman, S. (2022). Factors associated with parental IEP satisfaction. *Remedial and Special Education*. https://journals.sagepub.com/doi/pdf/10.1177/07419325221111571.

Santoro, S. L., Chicoine, B., Jasien, J. M., Kim, J. L., Stephens, M., Bulova, P., & Capone, G. (2021). Pneumonia and respiratory infections in Down syndrome: A scoping review of the literature. *American Journal of Medical Genetics. Part A, 185*(1), 286–299. https://doi.org/10.1002/ajmg.a.61924.

Seager, E., Sampson, S., Sin, J., Pagnamenta, E., & Stojanovik, V. (2022). A systematic review of speech, language and communication interventions for children with Down syndrome from 0 to 6 years. *International Journal of Language & Communication Disorders, 57*(2), 441–463. doi:10.1111/1460-6984.12699.

Seshadri, S., Morris, G., Serhal, P., & Saab, W. (2021). Assisted conception in women of advanced maternal age. *Best Practice and Research in Clinical Obstetrics and Gynecology, 70*, 10–20. doi:10.1016/j.bpobgyn.2020.06.012.

Shimony N. (2022) Atlantoaxial instability in Down syndrome. *Medscape*. https://emedicine.medscape.com/article/1180354-overview.

Silva, M. C., Lyra, M. C., Almeida, H. C., Alencar Filho, A. V., Heimer, M. V., & Rosenblatt, A. (2020). Caries experience in children and adolescents with Down Syndrome: A systematic review and meta-analysis. *Archives of Oral Biology, 115*, 104715. https://doi.org/10.1016/j.archoralbio.2020.104715.

Soriano, L., Thurman, A., Harvey, D., Kover, S., & Abbeduto, L. (2020). Expressive language development in adolescents with Down syndrome and fragile X syndrome: Change over time and the role of family-related factors. *Journal of Neurodevelopmental Disorders, 12*(18), 1–76.

Spencer, K., Crossley, J. A., Aitken, D. A., Nix, A. B., Dunstan, F. D., & Williams, K. (2002). Temporal changes in maternal serum biochemical markers of trisomy 21 across the first and second trimester of pregnancy. *Ann Clin Biochem, 39*(Pt 6), 567–576. doi: 10.1177/000456320203900604.

Takataya, K., Mizuno, E., Kanzaki, Y., Sakai, I., & Yamazaki, Y. (2019). Feelings of siblings having a brother/sister with Down syndrome. *Archives of Psychiatric Nursing, 33*(4), 337–346. doi:10.1016/j.apnu.2019.01.001.

Thompson, J. (2019). Disentangling the roles of maternal and paternal age on birth prevalence of Down syndrome and other chromosomal disorders using a Bayesian modeling approach. *BMC Medical Research Methodology, 19*(82), 1–8. doi:10.1186/s12874-019-0720-1.

Wagenblast, E., Araújo, J., Gan, O. I., Cutting, S. K., Murison, A., Krivdova, G., Azkanaz, M., McLeod, J. L., Smith, S. A., Gratton, B. A., Marhon, S. A., Gabra, M., Medeiros, J. J. F., Manteghi, S., Chen, J., Chan-Seng-Yue, M., Garcia-Prat, L., Salmena, L., De Carvalho, D. D., … Lechman, E. R. (2021). Mapping the cellular origin and early evolution of leukemia in Down syndrome. *Science (New York, N.Y.), 373*(6551), eabf6202. https://doi.org/10.1126/science.abf6202.

Watanabe, K. (2018). Recent advances in the understanding of transient abnormal myelopoiesis in down syndrome. *Pediatrics International, 61*(3), 222–229. https://doi.org/10.1111/ped.13776.

Whooten, R., Schmitt, J., & Schwartz, A. (2018). Endocrine manifestations of Down syndrome. *Current Opinion in Endocrinology, Diabetes, and Obesity, 25*(1), 61–66. doi:10.1097/MED.0000000000000382.

Wilson, W. R., Gewitz, M., Lockhart, P. B., Bolger, A. F., DeSimone, D. C., Kazi, D. S., Couper, D. J., Beaton, A., Kilmartin, C., Miro, J. M., Sable, C., Jackson, M. A., Baddour, L. M., & American Heart Association Young Hearts Rheumatic Fever, Endocarditis and Kawasaki Disease Committee of the Council on Lifelong Congenital Heart Disease and Heart Health in the Young; Council on Cardiovascular and Stroke Nursing; and the Council on Quality of Care and Outcomes Research (2021). Prevention of viridans group streptococcal infective endocarditis: A scientific statement from the American Heart Association. *Circulation, 143*(20), e963–e978. https://doi.org/10.1161/CIR.0000000000000969.

Eating Disorders

Laura White, Julie Prasad Dunne

"My child wants macaroni and cheese every night." "She refuses to eat spinach." "I don't like that!" "This is what we eat in my family." Pediatric primary care providers often hear parental concerns regarding feeding issues. Eating patterns in childhood and adolescence vary widely; however, growth and development have predictable trajectories that reflect adequate energy intake and nutrition. Feeding issues such as picky eating, decreased or increased appetite, and food jags are common, and feeling dissatisfaction while judging oneself in relation to peers may be a typical expectation (Andersen, 2022). However, when alterations in feeding and eating are associated with significant psychosocial distress or impairment in developmentally and culturally typical functioning, an eating disorder may be suspected (American Psychiatric Association [APA], 2013, 2022). Eating disorders are chronic conditions typically developing during childhood or adolescence, putting the individual at risk for developmental delay, psychosocial challenges, suicidality, and dangerous physical sequelae associated with increased mortality (van Hoeken & Hoek, 2020).

The *Diagnostic and Statistical Manual of Mental Disorders* (5th ed., revised text [DSM-V-TR]; APA, 2022) provides a classification and criteria for the diagnosis of mental disorders and classifies feeding and eating disorders into six categories: pica, rumination disorder, avoidant/restrictive food intake disorder (ARFID), anorexia nervosa, bulimia nervosa, and binge eating disorder. Presentations that do not meet the criteria for these recognized diagnoses but exhibit patterns of behaviors consistent with a feeding or eating problem, distress, or functional impairment may be diagnosed with other specified feeding or eating disorder or unspecified feeding or eating disorder.

Individuals with anorexia nervosa typically present with low weight or failure to gain weight for age, height, and gender, along with inadequate energy intake by restrictive eating or behaviors that control weight (i.e., overexercise). In contrast, individuals with bulimia nervosa may be at or above the typically expected weight but experience recurrent binging episodes followed by compensatory behaviors such as self-induced vomiting and laxative and diuretic use to control weight. Binge eating disorder is a newly recognized diagnostic disorder in the DSM-V (2013) manifested by recurrent episodes of binging behaviors without the compensatory mechanisms present with bulimia nervosa leading to weight exceeding the expectations for age, height, and gender. Similar to anorexia nervosa, individuals with ARFID present with restriction, weight loss, or failure to gain adequate weight, but these children may be younger and do not share the fear of gaining weight. Individuals with ARFID typically desire weight gain.

The impact of eating disorders may have a particularly deleterious effect on a child's developing brain, and early recognition and treatment of eating disorders are paramount to improving long-term outcomes (Golden et al., 2015). However, the presentation of eating disorder may be surreptitious and requires a high index of suspicion. Pediatric primary care providers are often the first to detect the signs and symptoms of eating disorders and have the therapeutic relationship to facilitate patient disclosure and initiate the multidisciplinary team required for early treatment. Because nutrition assessment, counseling, and anticipatory guidance are a focus of routine health care maintenance, pediatric primary care providers are also in a position to prevent eating disorders and recognize suspicious behavior prior to advancing to the full eating disorder criteria. Throughout treatment, the care provider remains an active participant in the treatment team and may manage the medical sequelae and ensure routine health care maintenance, which is integral to the optimal growth and development of the child and facilitates healthy family functioning.

ETIOLOGY

A variety of theories exist about the etiology of eating disorders. Overall, the development of these disorders is considered multifaceted rather than having a single cause. This section reviews some of the major theories related to the development of an eating disorder. It is useful to remember that most studies have been conducted in adult populations and may not be entirely generalizable to children and adolescents.

PSYCHOLOGICAL THEORIES

Psychological theories have focused on underlying psychological conflicts. The role of inconsistent and negative mother-child interactions was considered part of the psychological underpinning of an eating disorder (Bruch, 1982). While there is support for the impact of early life experiences and relationships on eating disorders, current understanding goes well beyond solely the role of the mother. Contemporary research considers overall family dynamics and relationships, including with peers, teachers, and coaches (Le Grange et al., 2010; Marcos et al., 2013). These theories underscore the importance of eating disorder behaviors to cope and control one's environment and highlight the lack of healthy self-concept and identity that may result from an eating disorder.

Psychological theories have also focused on the potential role of childhood trauma, including neglect and physical or sexual abuse. This relationship spans all types of eating disorders, with trauma histories being most common in individuals with bulimia nervosa, followed by binge eating disorder, then anorexia nervosa (Mitchell et al., 2021). Trauma may lead to characteristics such as self-criticism, low self-worth, anxiety, depression, emotion dysregulation, and impulsivity, resulting in a higher likelihood of developing an eating disorder (Mitchell et al., 2021). These theories have been an area of debate in the literature with regard to the specificity of a cause-and-effect relationship, with research suggesting the role of abuse as a nonspecific risk factor (Brewerton, 2007; Hilbert et al., 2014; Mitchell et al., 2021).

FAMILY THEORIES

In the classic work by Minuchin et al. (1975), the child's eating disorder symptoms were viewed as psychosomatic, playing a homeostatic role in a system of family conflict. Families of a child with anorexia nervosa were characterized as overly involved, intrusive, or lacking boundaries. Often the parents and child were seen as being overprotective of each other, rigid, and limited in conflict resolution (Minuchin et al., 1975). The child's disorder enables family members to avoid underlying family issues. Researchers have tried to discern the extent to which these types of interactions are unique to families of a person with anorexia nervosa or reflect families of a person with a psychiatric illness in general. However, there is no consistent evidence for a specific pattern of dysfunction even within the same diagnostic category (Erriu et al., 2020).

More recent studies show lower levels of healthy family functioning among the interactions and roles of all family members in persons with an eating disorder. For example, low family cohesion, poor communication, and high family achievement orientation are associated with eating disorder symptoms (Holtom-Viesel & Allan, 2014). Similarly, families that emphasize dieting or engage in weight-related teasing may increase the likelihood of developing an eating disorder. Prioritizing eating meals together and modeling healthy eating habits may be protective factors (Golden et al.,

2016). These family dynamics may help explain adaptive or problematic behaviors in general, including those related to eating.

The American Academy of Eating Disorders cautions against placing too much emphasis on family functioning as the etiology of an eating disorder and especially advises against blaming parents or guardians for the illness (Le Grange et al., 2010). Today the role of the family in recovery from an eating disorder is well established, with family-based therapy being at the forefront of treatment options.

SOCIOCULTURAL THEORIES

Emphasis on thinness in Western cultural standards has been theorized in the development of an eating disorder. The roots of Western beauty standards and antifatness can be attributed to racist policies (e.g., literature that supports slavery and racial hierarchy based on physical attributes), religious teachings (e.g., body size as a sign of morality), and even more recent medical education (e.g., weight bias and an emphasis on the obesity epidemic) (Strings, 2023). Across studies, factors such as internet and social media use (Rodgers & Melioli, 2016) and the level of acculturation toward Western body ideals (Rikani et al., 2013) appear to influence the development of an eating disorder.

The role of subcultures that idealize thinness may also play a role in developing eating disorders. For example, athletes, including ballet dancers, jockeys, and wrestlers, exhibit a higher risk for disordered eating (Bratland-Sanda & Sundgot-Borgen, 2013). Subscribers of niche pro-anorexia and pro–eating disorder websites or bloggers are other groups at increased risk (Mento et al., 2021).

Sexual orientation and gender identity are other factors associated with the risk of an eating disorder. Individuals identifying as sexual minorities are more likely than heterosexual individuals to have an eating disorder, including anorexia nervosa, bulimia nervosa, and binge eating disorder (Nagata et al., 2020). Similarly, transgender individuals are more likely to develop an eating disorder than their cisgender counterparts (Feder et al., 2017; Nagata et al., 2020). Minority stress and discrimination faced by sexual and gender minority groups may perpetuate disordered eating and prevent access to appropriate care.

The COVID-19 pandemic has been associated with new-onset, relapse, and exacerbation of eating disorders. Devoe et al. (2022) noted that symptoms and hospital admissions increased, especially during the pandemic periods of lockdown, which may have been attributed to a lack of access to routine care and social isolation. However, mixed results showed that symptoms improved for some individuals with eating disorders (Devoe et al., 2022). These inconsistencies may be related to individual differences in terms of the effect of school and home environments.

BIOLOGIC THEORIES

The role of neurobiology in the maintenance and recovery of an eating disorder continues to be an area of growth in research. Genetics and neurobiology are evolving due to global cooperation on genome-wide studies, neuroimaging, and animal models (Bulik et al., 2022).

Familial aggregation studies suggest a biologic heritability of eating-related psychopathology. Family members of people diagnosed with anorexia nervosa, bulimia nervosa, or binge eating disorder are 2 to 11 times more likely to have an eating disorder than families in which no family member has an eating disorder (Trace et al., 2012). Twin studies, which provide an opportunity to examine genetic and environmental effects, suggest a heritability of approximately 28% to 88% for anorexia nervosa, 59% to 83% for bulimia nervosa, and 41% to 57% for binge eating disorder (Trace et al., 2012).

The role of neurobiology in the onset, maintenance, and recovery of an eating disorder has been an area of intense investigation. Studies have focused on the role of neurotransmitters, particularly serotonin, because of their involvement in appetite regulation. Serotonin 1A-receptor binding appears to be state independent in anorexia nervosa and bulimia nervosa; serotonin 2A-receptor binding showed dynamic variations (e.g., normal in anorexia nervosa participants during acute illness, but lower after recovery) (Frank et al., 2019). Related to serotonin function is the role of dietary intake (or lack thereof) on neurotransmitter functioning. Dieting in healthy women has been shown to decrease the availability of the essential amino acid tryptophan (Wolfe et al., 1997). Plasma tryptophan competes with other large neutral amino acids for transport into the central nervous system (CNS), where it is converted into the neurotransmitter serotonin. Thus severe dietary restrictions in persons with eating disorders may influence CNS serotonin and subsequent appetite regulation. Beyond serotonin, in individuals with bulimia nervosa, decreased striatal dopamine release was linked to higher binge eating frequency (Frank et al., 2019).

In addition to neurotransmitter systems, other biologic substrates involved in regulating feeding behavior have been implicated. For example, leptin and ghrelin, peptides that regulate food intake and energy expenditure, appear to be altered during acute stages of anorexia nervosa, bulimia nervosa, and obesity. Such alterations may stimulate or diminish brain dopamine response, which could alter the approach to food intake (Frank et al., 2019). Cytokines, particularly tumor necrosis factor-alpha, have also been elevated in persons with anorexia nervosa, no alterations have been found in bulimia nervosa, and no data exist for binge eating disorder (Dalton et al., 2018). The individual microbiome may also play a role in eating disorders, but data are still emerging. Decreased diversity of gut microbiota was noted in anorexia nervosa, while bulimia nervosa and binge eating disorder were associated with antimicrobial medication use (Frank et al., 2019). However, the microbiome normalizes with weight recovery, indicating no clear causal relationship with eating disorders.

Neuroanatomic and neurofunctional studies have been yet another source of investigation into the cause of eating disorders. Findings during active illness may be related to a host of factors, including hydration and body mass index (BMI), which render it difficult to determine whether they are antecedents or consequences of the disorder. Additional studies, including those in anorexia nervosa and other eating disorders, have found mixed results, and no consensus exists. Fractional anisotropy tends to be lower in anorexia nervosa and bulimia nervosa but also normalizes during weight recovery (Frank et al., 2019). Across studies, executive function, reward processing, and perception (including interoception) have been implicated in eating disorder behavior (Frank et al., 2019).

INCIDENCE AND PREVALENCE

The lifetime prevalence of eating disorders provides a crude index of the lifetime occurrence of the disorder. The lifetime prevalence for anorexia nervosa is estimated to be 0.3% in adolescents and 0.8% in adults; the prevalence of bulimia nervosa is approximately 0.9% in adolescents and 0.3% in adults, and the prevalence of binge eating disorder is 1.6% in adolescents and 0.85% in adults (Udo & Grilo, 2019). Data on young children are lacking. Across eating disorders, the average age of onset is typically around 12 years. However, the disorders and prodromal symptoms can occur earlier or later.

Prevalence rates are typically higher in females than males, although found similar rates of anorexia nervosa across adolescent males and females (Gorrell & Murrary, 2019). Very limited data exist on gender minority groups. However, the lifetime prevalence of eating disorders appears to be higher in gender-minority populations (Nagata 2020). In transgender youth, growth charts based on sex may present a unique challenge in diagnosis.

There are mixed results related to differences in the prevalence of eating disorders by ethnoracial groups. More individuals who identify as non-Hispanic and White reported having anorexia nervosa, while there were significantly higher rates of bulimia nervosa among Hispanic-identifying adolescents but not adults (Udo & Grilo, 2019). No significant differences were noted in binge eating disorder, but there was a trend toward ethnic minority adolescents more often having this disorder. Evidence should be interpreted with caution as eating disorders in historically marginalized populations are understudied and often misdiagnosed or undertreated (Goel et al., 2022). Further, misdiagnosis due to clinician bias related to gender minorities and ethnoracial stereotypes may play a role (Gorrell & Murrary, 2019).

DIAGNOSTIC CRITERIA

ANOREXIA NERVOSA

The cardinal features of anorexia nervosa include a restriction of energy intake resulting in weight loss or failure to thrive based on developmental needs (APA, 2013). Severe or dangerous weight loss or the refusal to maintain a healthy weight is common. The severity of anorexia nervosa is based on BMI for adults and BMI percentile for children; however, it is important to note that individuals with a normal BMI may still meet the criteria for a diagnosis of anorexia nervosa. For example, individuals with BMI 17 kg/m^2 or above meet the criteria for mild severity of anorexia nervosa or atypical anorexia nervosa (see Other Feeding and Eating Disorders, later). More significant weight loss is classified as moderate (BMI 16–16.99 kg/m^2), severe (BMI 15–15.99 kg/m^2), or extreme (BMI <15 kg/m^2) severity. Additional features of anorexia nervosa are a fear of weight gain or persistent behavior that interferes with weight gain and body image disturbance (APA, 2013).

Anorexia Nervosa Specifiers

Individuals who struggle with anorexia nervosa are classified into one of two subtypes: restricting and binge eating/purging. Those with the restricting subtype engage in severe dieting, fasting, and excessive exercise. Those who binge or purge regularly engage in self-induced vomiting, abuse of laxatives or diuretics, and use of enemas after eating (APA, 2013). Individuals with this subtype may purge after binge eating episodes and after small meals.

BULIMIA NERVOSA

Bulimia nervosa is classified by recurrent episodes of binge eating and inappropriate compensatory or purging behaviors (e.g., self-induced vomiting, misuse of laxatives, diuretics or other medications, fasting, or excessive exercise) (APA, 2013). Binge eating episodes entail eating a quantity of food larger than most other individuals would eat in a designated period (e.g., 2 hours). Loss of control overeating is essential to a binge eating episode (APA, 2013). Importantly, bulimia nervosa, including binging and purging behaviors, occurs outside the context of a diagnosis of anorexia nervosa. The severity of bulimia nervosa is based on the average number of episodes of compensatory behaviors occurring each week, with 1 to 3 weekly episodes being classified as mild, 4 to 7 weekly episodes being classified as moderate, 8 to 13 episodes being classified as severe, and 14 or more weekly episodes being classified as extreme (APA, 2013). Bulimia nervosa may

be difficult to identify because of extreme secrecy, and affected children and adolescents may be of normal weight for their age and height, with some individuals above a normal weight range (Hay & Claudino, 2012). Thus obtaining a thorough history from the child and family is particularly important. Similar to persons with anorexia nervosa, these individuals experience body dissatisfaction and place great importance on their body weight and shape.

BINGE EATING DISORDER

Much like bulimia nervosa, binge eating disorder is marked by recurrent episodes of binge eating (e.g., consuming objectively large quantities of food in a designated period and loss of control overeating). However, binge eating disorder is not associated with compensatory behaviors, and diagnostic features occur outside a diagnosis of bulimia nervosa or anorexia nervosa. Episodes of binge eating in this disorder are often associated with eating quickly, eating until physically uncomfortable, eating despite not being hungry, and eating alone or in secret due to feeling embarrassed and disgusted, or guilty (APA, 2013). Individuals with binge eating disorder experience emotional and physical distress from binge eating. The level of severity of binge eating disorder is based on the average number of binge eating episodes occurring each week, with 1 to 3 weekly episodes being classified as mild, 4 to 7 weekly episodes being classified as moderate, 8 to 13 episodes being classified as severe; and 14 or more weekly episodes being classified as extreme (APA, 2013). Binge eating disorder is often associated with negative affect and depression, and these mood states or other stressful situations may trigger episodes of binge eating (Leehr et al., 2015).

OTHER FEEDING AND EATING DISORDERS

Outside of anorexia nervosa, bulimia nervosa, and binge eating disorder, the DSM-V (APA, 2013) also describes other eating disorders. One such disorder, ARFID, is sometimes seen in childhood and is characterized by a lack of interest in food, avoidance of food due to sensory issues, or fear of the consequences of eating (e.g., choking) (APA, 2013). ARFID may result in weight loss, nutritional deficiencies, and issues with psychosocial functioning making it distinct from developmentally normative picky eating in children. It is not associated with any body image disturbance, anorexia nervosa, bulimia nervosa, or another medical conditions. Rumination disorder and repeated food regurgitation may also occur during childhood (APA, 2013). Rumination disorder is not attributable to a gastrointestinal (GI) or other medical condition, anorexia nervosa, bulimia nervosa, binge eating disorder, or ARFID, and occurs across the life span, including in infants as young as 3 months. Pica is another disorder that may impact children. The cardinal feature of pica is the consumption of nonnutritive, nonfood substances (APA, 2013). Importantly, pica includes only abnormal consumption outside developmental norms (e.g., infants and toddlers mouthing objects as a means of exploration) and cultural or social practices. Atypical anorexia nervosa, in which an individual is of normal or above average weight but meets all other criteria of anorexia nervosa, and night eating syndrome are considered to be other specified types of eating disorders (APA, 2013). An individual may have an unspecified feeding and eating disorder not classified by the DSM that still causes clinically significant distress and impairment.

CLINICAL MANIFESTATIONS AT TIME OF DIAGNOSIS

A high index of suspicion and knowledge of the early manifestations of eating disorders are paramount to early recognition and treatment and improved outcomes (Golden et al., 2015). A delay in diagnosis and treatment may hinder the full growth potential and limit the linear catchup growth of children (Tanner & Spaulding-Barclay, 2022). However, eating disorders are surprisingly difficult to recognize and differ in presentation depending on the specific eating disorder behaviors.

Individuals with eating disorders, unless very low weight with anorexia nervosa or ARFID or very high weight in binge eating disorder, may not appear to be malnourished. Individuals with eating disorders also may be hesitant to disclose their behaviors and may present as high functioning and appearing to meet measurable developmental achievements. Adolescents may hide their restricting behaviors by starting special diets such as vegetarianism. Stressful events may also precipitate changes in eating behaviors, and pediatric primary care providers should assess eating behaviors in the context of a stressful event or trauma.

The COVID-19 pandemic required social isolation and quarantine, cancellation of in-person social events, and change to online virtual or hybrid (part virtual/part in-person) schooling. A significant rise during the pandemic in mental health and eating disorders in children and adolescents (Graell et al., 2020; Robertson et al., 2021), along with related hospitalizations (Otto et al., 2021), suggests that social isolation may have a role in onset of eating disorders. This rise led the American Academy of Pediatrics (AAP) (2021), American Academy of Child and Adolescent Psychiatry (AACAP), and the Children's Hospital Association to declare a national emergency in child and adolescent mental health, citing the effects of decreased family safety and stability.

Children with eating disorders may not present the same as adults, thus increasing the risk of missed diagnoses. It is important to understand the growth and development of the child at the time of the presentation because eating disorders may vary by the child's age. Rather than weight loss and medical sequelae commonly seen in adolescents or emerging adults, children may present with failure to achieve expected growth or pubertal milestones (Tanner & Spaulding-Barclay, 2022). The primary care provider needs to consider eating disorders in any context of change in growth trajectory or delayed puberty.

Further complicating early diagnosis is the tendency for individuals with eating disorders to conform to rigid patterns and rituals and remain secretive regarding their behaviors. Identification with the eating disorder may lead to limited insight into the seriousness of the disorder and health status and may contribute to resistance to change. The clinical presentation in anorexia nervosa and ARFID reflects starvation, bulimia nervosa reflects dehydration and purging effects, and binge eating disorder reflects problems with excess energy and weight.

ANOREXIA NERVOSA

The fear of gaining weight drives behaviors restricting energy intake, manifesting as weight loss, or decreased expected gain (APA 2013, 2022). Children with anorexia nervosa may demonstrate behaviors of excessively cutting food, chewing, and unusual food combinations, which should be explored during routine primary care visits. The clinical manifestations of anorexia nervosa affect the whole body and reflect chronic energy deficiency, malnutrition, and starvation leading the body to prioritize vital functions by slowing metabolism (Table 22.1) (Gaudiani, 2019; Mehler, 2022; Westmoreland et al., 2016). However, losing weight to a dangerously low range with associated symptoms may not alter the self-perception of an individual with anorexia nervosa due to a distorted body image (APA, 2022). In children with eating disorders, failure to gain weight as expected may be considered weight suppression (Tanner & Spaulding-Barclay, 2022).

Puberty, sexual maturity rating (SMR), weight, height, and orthostatic signs need to be closely monitored, and bone age and hormone levels may be considered. Although many clinical findings of eating disorders are evident at any age, many eating disorder medical checklists may not identify such findings in children. Children and teens may report feeling tired, cold, dizzy, or lightheaded with moving from sitting to standing (orthostasis), shortness of breath, heart palpitations, or chest pain. GI complaints reflect a slowed digestive system manifesting as abdominal pain, bloating, early satiety, and constipation. The last menstrual period should be recorded with consideration for primary or secondary amenorrhea or delayed puberty. The absence of a menstrual period is no longer required for a diagnosis of anorexia nervosa due to the lack of consistency in the relationship with nutritional status. A history of multiple fractures may reflect low bone mineral density.

Physical exam findings resulting from insufficient energy intake include cognitive slowing noted by a

Table 22.1 **Clinical Manifestations at Time of Diagnosis: Signs (Symptoms)**

	ANOREXIA NERVOSA	BULIMIA NERVOSA	BINGE EATING DISORDER
Growth: Measured on appropriate growth charts (height, weight, BMI)	Loss of weight trajectory	May be the typical weight for age	Deviation from growth, increased weight
Vital signs	Temperature <36°C (<96.8°F) Bradycardia Hypotension Orthostasis (HR increase >20 BPM or BP decreased by >10 mm Hg) Syncope	Orthostatic signs	Elevated BP or hypertension
General	Cachexia, flat affect, weakness, dehydration (fatigued, apathetic, irritable, cold intolerance, hot flashes)	Weakness Syncope	
Hair, skin, nails	Thin or dull hair, lanugo on the body, brittle nails, decreased turgor, carotenemia, pallor, scars or lesions related to self-injury, acrocyanosis, brittle nails	Bruising or hyperemia over vertebral processes from excessive exercise, Russell sign (abrasions on knuckles), poor turgor, edema	Acanthosis nigricans, acne, hirsutism
HEENT	Dysphagia	Angular stomatitis, erythematous, scratched posterior pharynx, palatal petechiae, dental erosion particularly on the posterior surface, parotid, submandibular salivary gland enlargement (pharyngeal pain, heartburn)	
Chest	Delayed SMR, dyspnea		Premature/advanced SMR
Cardiac	Murmur associated with mitral valve prolapse, arrhythmia, acrocyanosis, prolonged capillary refill (>3 s), cool extremities (dizziness, chest pain, palpitations, faintness)	Arrhythmia (dizziness, faintness, palpitations)	
Abdominal	Scaphoid, stool mass lower left quadrant, distension (nausea, bloating, pain, early satiety, constipation)	Epigastric tenderness (nausea, abdominal discomfort, constipation, diarrhea if laxatives)	Hepatomegaly
Genital/reproductive	Delayed SMR, vaginal dryness, small testes, amenorrhea (low libido)	Rectal prolapse (low libido)	Premature puberty or advanced SMR
Musculoskeletal, spine, extremities	Decreased muscle mass, weakness, edema, stress fractures (bone pain)	Edema with refeeding (bone pain, paresthesia)	Tenderness
Neurologic	Poor concentration, slow to answer questions or follow directions, seizure if severe	Seizure if severe (headache, lightheaded, dizzy)	

BMI, Body mass index; *BP*, blood pressure; *BPM*, beats per min; *HEENT*, head, eyes, ears, nose, throat; *HR*, heart rate; *SMR*, sexual maturing rating.

delay in answering questions. Vital signs are significant for lower than normal temperature, bradycardia, hypotension, or orthostasis. An adolescent may appear cachexic or emaciated, with flat affect and signs of dehydration on examination. Hair may appear dull

and thin with lanugo on the body as an adaptation to low body temperature and brittle nails.

The skin may show evidence of exercise with bruising over the vertebral processes, as with bulimia nervosa. A murmur consistent with mitral valve prolapse may be noted with acrocyanosis from poor perfusion and brady-cardia. The abdomen may appear scaphoid, flat, or distended due to gastric dilation with possible palpable stool from constipation. Growth may be affected by a delayed SMR. The extremities may appear cool to the touch with slow capillary refill and edema (Gaudiani, 2019; Mehler & Andersen, 2022; Rome & Strandjord, 2016, Rosen & Committee on Adolescence, 2010; Walsh & Mehler, 2022).

Atypical anorexia nervosa is a variation of anorexia nervosa with significant weight loss but a weight that remains in the typical range for height, age, and gender (APA, 2013, 2022). Despite the appearance of normal weight, losing weight remains a risk for the same dangerous mental and physical health sequelae and requires the same level of vigilance in early detection, evaluation, and treatment.

BULIMIA NERVOSA

Individuals with bulimia nervosa may maintain their growth along their growth charts without evidence of significant weight changes. The bingeing episodes are characterized by a feeling of loss of control and subsequent feelings of guilt and shame, which prompt compensatory behaviors (APA, 2013). The compensatory purging may lead to chronic dehydration, and potential electrolyte disturbances manifested as dizziness, faintness, and fatigue. Repeated self-induced vomiting may cause dental pain, pharyngeal pain, heart palpitations, heartburn, reflux, nausea, abdominal pain, constipation, and diarrhea (if using laxatives).

The physical effects of repetitive purging may present with dehydration and orthostatic vital signs, muscle weakness, poor skin turgor and prolonged capillary refill time, scratched posterior pharynx and palatal petechiae and dental erosion, enlarged parotid and submandibular salivary glands, and epigastric tenderness. The skin may show evidence of exercise with bruising over the vertebral and calluses over the dorsum of the hands over the metacarpophalangeal joints (Russell sign). Rectal prolapse and edema of the extremities may be noted particularly if the laxatives were recently stopped (Gaudiani, 2019; Mehler & Andersen, 2022; Rome & Strandjord, 2016, Rosen & Committee on Adolescence, 2010) and hemorrhoids (Walsh & Mehler, 2022).

BINGE EATING DISORDER

The diagnosis of binge eating disorder was new to the DSM-5 in 2013 and includes the primary behavior of binging without the compensatory purging behaviors leading the individual to present with weight gain or increased weight trajectory. While the long-term diagnosis may lead to the health problems associated with excess energy intake, in children the long-term health effects may not be evident due to the relative length of the disease state. Elevated blood pressure may be noted, and findings are consistent with excess weight, such as hyperglycemia, insulin resistance, and premature pubertal development. Physical exam findings may be significant for acanthosis nigracans, hirsutism, acne, polycystic ovarian syndrome, hepatomegaly, and advanced SMR (Hornberger et al., 2021; McCuen-Wurst et al., 2018).

When taking the history, assess night eating syndrome in which an individual ingests a large caloric intake during the nighttime, associated with insomnia, weight gain, and a higher risk of diabetes and metabolic problems and may be comorbid with mood and anxiety disorders (McCuen-Wurst et al., 2018).

AVOIDANT-RESTRICTIVE FOOD AND INTAKE DISORDER

Children with ARFID may present with insufficient energy intake leading to malnutrition and weight loss but do not share a distorted body image as in anorexia nervosa (APA, 2013, 2022). Similar to anorexia nervosa, these children may have growth and pubertal delay and manifestations of malnutrition; however, the heterogeneous presentation of food avoidance associated with this diagnosis suggests the need for further study (Bourne et al., 2020). Children with ARFID present at an earlier age and tend to be male and have a disturbance in feeding and eating, such as food avoidance, low appetite or disinterest, and reliance on enteral or oral supplements for nutrients (Seetharama & Fields, 2020). Individuals with ARFID often have had a workup for failure to thrive and relay a history of choking or vomiting as a precipitating factor for the onset of the disorder. They may present with severe nutrient deficiency leading to rickets or scurvy (Tanner & Spaulding-Barclay, 2022). Assessment for ARFID should be considered with children with underlying risk factors. Feeding problems and GI problems are common in children with Down syndrome (Ravel et al., 2020), and food avoidance is common with autism spectrum disorder, obsessive-compulsive disorder, anxiety, and learning disabilities (Tanner & Spaulding-Barclay, 2022).

PHYSICAL HEALTH ASSESSMENT

The evaluation of eating disorders requires a head-to-toe physical exam focusing on the signs of malnutrition, dehydration, and purging, as discussed. The general appearance focuses on the individual's engagement, energy, and affect, noting thinning hair or alopecia, lanugo, dry skin, brittle nails, cracked lips, scars suggesting self-injury, Russell sign, and carotenemia. Petechiae may be noted on the face or palate related to self-induced vomiting, dental erosion to the posterior teeth may be secondary to the acid of gastric contents, along with an assessment of thyromegaly and nodules. The cardiac exam includes the evaluation of new murmurs particularly related to the mitral valve. A careful abdominal exam should note shape, distention, and tenderness, particularly over the gastric area. The stool may be palpated in the left lower quadrant. The extremities should be examined for temperature, acrocyanosis, turgor, pulses, and edema, particularly after the cessation of chronic laxative abuse. The rate and tone of voice, ability to follow directions, balance, and complete neurologic exam are recommended. A more focused exam is needed to address the specific problems associated with eating disorder behaviors (see Associated Problems of Eating Disorders and Common Illness Management, both later).

TREATMENT

Several levels of psychiatric care are available for children and adolescents with an eating disorder, including outpatient psychotherapy, intensive outpatient day or partial hospitalization programs, residential programs, and hospitalization. The level of care needed is largely determined by the child's medical stability, the risk for suicide, the percent of ideal body weight, coexisting conditions, and motivation for recovery. Hospitalization should be considered for children and adolescents who are not medically stable, as well as for those who are suicidal, severely depressed, at low body weight, and in need of nutritional stabilization or a highly structured environment to contain the level of symptomatology (APA, 2006). Specialized inpatient units are preferred but are not always geographically available. Outpatient therapy involves individual, group, or family psychotherapy with a mental health care specialist. Inpatient and outpatient treatment can involve adjunct therapies, including nutritional counseling, medications, and supportive therapies. In addition, primary health care monitoring is often a key component during outpatient treatment, particularly for individuals susceptible to weight loss and medical instability. The least restrictive environment is the preferred level of care for children and adolescents that can optimally meet their medical, psychological, and safety needs.

PSYCHOTHERAPY

Anorexia Nervosa

Treatment of children and adolescents with anorexia nervosa can be particularly challenging. Although there is a consensus that psychotherapy is valuable, some forms of psychotherapy may be more promising at different stages of illness. For example, cognitive-behavioral or mindfulness-based therapies may be less effective during the acute stage of illness when the child is likely to have greater cognitive impairment.

Although a wide range of therapies exists, family therapy is most often recommended and is the most heavily researched form of psychotherapy for children and adolescents (Zeeck et al., 2018). Family therapy is more helpful than individual therapy in adolescents at 6- and 12-month follow-ups (Lock et al., 2010). Variations in family therapy include the duration of intervention, meeting with patients and parents together or separately, and using single- or multifamily groups.

The amount of research in this area has grown over the past years, but there is still a need for more high-powered studies and independent replication of findings (Zeeck et al., 2018).

Bulimia Nervosa

Similar to anorexia nervosa, it can be challenging to engage children and adolescents with bulimia nervosa in therapy. Also, like anorexia nervosa, family therapy is often recommended and is useful. Although cognitive-behavioral therapy (CBT) is typically recommended for adults with anorexia nervosa, family therapy was related to higher rates of abstinence from binge eating and purging in adolescents with bulimia nervosa compared to CBT (Le Grange et al., 2015). CBT, which focuses on restructuring illogical thought patterns (cognitions) that lead to maladaptive behaviors, is effective in adolescents with bulimia nervosa when adapted to fit their developmental needs, age, and specific triggers (e.g., peer interaction and influence), and when paired with parental monitoring of behaviors in the early stages (Schapman-Williams et al., 2006).

Binge Eating Disorder

Treatment of patients with binge eating disorder is not as well researched as other eating disorders. Moreover, little is known about the best approach for treating binge eating disorder in adolescents and children. However, as with other child and adolescent eating disorders, family involvement and family therapy are likely beneficial (Iacovino et al., 2012).

CBT and interpersonal therapy (IPT) are effective therapies in the adult population (Miniati et al., 2018). IPT addresses social and emotional problems that may foster binge eating as a coping mechanism. These findings can guide treatment for younger patients with binge eating disorder, although further studies on adapting these therapies to children and adolescents are needed.

PSYCHOPHARMACOLOGIC INTERVENTIONS

Most studies on psychopharmacologic interventions have been conducted with adults, and there is a dearth of knowledge on prescribing for eating disorders in children and adolescents. Therefore prescribing is often off label, which can be risky particularly with young children. It is very important to be cognizant of the medical instability that often cooccurs with eating disorders and to be aware of the potential adverse effects of different drugs in persons with these disorders.

Anorexia Nervosa

There are no Food and Drug Administration (FDA)–approved medications for anorexia nervosa, although medications may be helpful as an adjunct intervention in treatment. Sometimes drugs may help treat cooccurring disorders. When medications are used in anorexia nervosa they are often prescribed in lower doses (APA, 2006). Given that affected individuals typically have low body weight and malnutrition, they are at greater risk for side effects and possibly a lowered seizure threshold (APA, 2006).

Second-generation antipsychotic agents (e.g., olanzapine) have been studied in adults with anorexia nervosa and are thought to be mildly helpful with some symptoms, such as BMI and level of depression (Lebow et al., 2013). Results are mixed in adolescent populations (Golden et al., 2011; Kafantaris et al., 2011). Antipsychotic agents have significant side effects that merit serious consideration before use in vulnerable populations such as children and adolescents. These effects include extrapyramidal symptoms, prolonged QTc interval, and hyperlipidemia.

Other medications include selective serotonin reuptake inhibitors (SSRIs) for depression, although target symptoms typically remit with weight restoration. Anxiolytic drugs (e.g., lorazepam or hydroxyzine) may be used on a short-term basis and are generally given immediately before meals, as they may help prevent excessive anxiety triggered by eating. Special care is essential in treating individuals with coexisting attention-deficit/hyperactivity disorder (ADHD) with medications because stimulant abuse may result from desired drug-induced weight loss. Bupropion is contraindicated as it may lower the seizure threshold.

Bulimia Nervosa

Unlike anorexia nervosa, there is more empiric support for pharmacologic interventions in adults with bulimia nervosa, with promising evidence in children and adolescents. In bulimia nervosa, various antidepressants have been shown to reduce the frequency of binge eating and purging, as well as to help alleviate comorbid depressive symptoms (Broft et al., 2010). Despite decades of treatment development research in bulimia nervosa, fluoxetine 60 mg/day holds promise in treatment for adolescents (Hagan & Walsh, 2021). It is preferred over other antidepressant agents because of its more favorable side effect profile and is FDA approved for treating depression in children and adolescents. Antidepressants are accompanied by an FDA black box warning regarding an increased risk for suicidal thoughts and behavior in children and adolescents. Any antidepressant use should be monitored closely. As with anorexia nervosa, bupropion should not be used due to the risk of seizures.

Tricyclic drugs and monoamine oxidase inhibitors (MAOIs), at doses similar to those used for depression, have been shown to decrease bulimia nervosa symptoms in adults, but they are rarely used because of their side effect profiles. MAOIs are risky because following the specific dietary restrictions required on this drug regimen (e.g., low-tyramine diet) can be particularly difficult for the patient with bulimia nervosa. Ondansetron may help reduce binge and purge episodes in adults, but there is limited research, and it is not typically used in children (Golden & Attia, 2011).

Binge Eating Disorder

Treatment for binge eating disorder, much like that for bulimia nervosa, has not been specifically tested in adolescents and children. However, lisdexamfetamine is FDA approved for binger eating disorder in adults (Heo & Duggan, 2017) and is approved for the treatment of ADHD in children and could be useful for individuals with overlapping disorders (Guerdjikova et al., 2019). SSRIs have been shown to reduce the frequency of binge eating and symptoms of depression. Further understanding of the neurobiology of binge eating disorder in both children and adults will promote the development of targeted pharmacotherapies. Growing research suggests that medications with anorectic or weight loss effect may be helpful for patients with binge eating disorder.

COMPLEMENTARY AND ALTERNATIVE THERAPIES

Other psychotherapy modalities may be beneficial and are receiving more attention, even among child and adolescent populations. Mindfulness-based interventions, yoga, art therapy, psychodrama, and occupational therapy have recently gained popularity. These forms of therapy may be especially beneficial when used as adjunctive practices in treatment (Couturier et al., 2020; Godsey, 2013). More research is needed to understand the usefulness of therapies with the pediatric population.

ANTICIPATED ADVANCES IN DIAGNOSIS AND MANAGEMENT

The DSM-V (APA, 2013) was created to guide diagnoses toward evidence-based treatment for optimally informed practice. It is a fluid document, and changes are made with each version to reflect the latest advances in diagnoses and treatment of psychiatric disorders. The lack of research on eating disorders in children and adolescents leaves room for many advances in diagnosing and managing these disorders.

An area needing further examination is the extent to which eating disorder diagnostic criteria are age, gender, and culture sensitive. For example, it is unclear how a child expresses the fear of fat or defines distorted body image when, developmentally, the child may not yet fully understand the experiences and the labels attributed to them. Similarly, it is unclear whether parental observations might be accepted for endorsing a child's preoccupation with weight and shape rather than assuming that the child will be able to verbalize self-evaluation to others (Bravender et al., 2010). In terms of gender sensitivity, most research is limited to cisgendered females, which creates issues in terms of identification and management of individuals who do not fall into this category (e.g., male, trans, and nonbinary individuals) (Jones & Morgan, 2010). Recognition of the role of culture in eating disorders is underscored as all variants of these are prevalent across diverse racial and ethnic groups with evidence of increasing eating disorders in non-White individuals (Acle et al., 2021). Addressing culture in eating disorders is imperative due to the differences in clinical presentations as well as the variances in seeking and receiving treatments.

ASSOCIATED PROBLEMS OF EATING DISORDERS

Eating disorders are associated with coexisting conditions that occur with increased frequency in this population. Depression is common across eating disorders (APA, 2013). Mood symptoms such as social withdrawal, irritability, and insomnia may be related to malnutrition, weight changes, and self-esteem issues. The increased risk for depression makes the need for assessment of suicidal ideation critically important. Anxiety disorders, including social anxiety and substance use disorders (e.g., stimulant use disorder, alcohol use disorder), are also seen across the spectrum of eating disorders (APA, 2013). Often noted in persons with anorexia nervosa are obsessive-compulsive behaviors, both related and unrelated to food (Boileau, 2022). Current research also shows the correlation between binge eating disorder and dyslipidemia and diabetes (Mitchell, 2016; Winston, 2020).

The treatment of coexisting conditions typically occurs concurrently with the treatment of the eating disorder. The exception is if the individual's safety is compromised (e.g., suicidal ideation) or the severity of symptoms requires immediate, intense treatment (e.g., detoxification from substance dependence). Some coexisting psychiatric symptoms in children and adolescents with anorexia nervosa tend to improve with weight recovery (e.g., depression).

Associated physical findings include all body systems reflecting the effects of malnutrition and starvation (anorexia nervosa, ARFID), dehydration and electrolyte abnormalities (bulimia nervosa), or excess weight (binge eating disorder). Many of the physical sequelae of eating disorder behaviors may be reversed with adequate nutrition. However, low bone mineral density (BMD) may persist regardless of nutritional rehabilitation (Workman et al., 2020). Additional unique health problems may present during the cessation of purging, nutritional rehabilitation, and treatment. The pediatric primary care provider may be responsible for evaluating and managing the physical health complaints of children and adolescents particularly for individuals treated as outpatients.

In addition to the findings in Table 22.1, common presentations involve the GI, cardiac, and endocrine systems. Common GI problems related to eating disorders are primarily due to slowed metabolism or purging and include constipation, gastroparesis, gastroesophageal reflux (purging), gastric dilation, abdominal pain, and bloating. Cardiac problems may include dysrhythmias related to electrolyte abnormalities (purging), bradycardia related to slowed metabolism, mitral valve prolapse, and decreased cardiac deconditioning due to muscle wasting with malnutrition. The endocrine system is affected by eating disorders with changes in thyroid, gonadotropins, oxytocin, sodium, and cortisol affecting puberty and reproductive and bone health.

GASTROINTESTINAL

The GI system is affected by both the slowed metabolism of restriction and the recurrent purging of bulimia nervosa. The slowed metabolic rate slows the GI tract leading to gastroparesis, gastric dilation, reflux, and constipation. In bulimia nervosa, vomiting may be associated with heartburn, dental pain, erosion, hoarse voice, sore throat, and hematemesis. Laxative use is associated with diarrhea, constipation, abdominal pain, and hematochezia (Gibson et al., 2022).

Gastroparesis, a delay in gastric emptying, may present with a complaint of bloating, nausea, vomiting, postprandial fullness, upper abdominal pain, and early satiety (Camilleri et al., 2013) that worsens with high fiber intake and is associated with reflux and vomiting (Gibson et al., 2022). Treatment includes limiting fiber and smaller, high-calorie frequent meals. Metoclopramide may be considered to increase transit time (Camilleri et al., 2013; Gaudiani, 2019). Left upper quadrant pain, vomiting, early satiety, and abdominal distension may warrant an abdominal radiograph for gastric dilation.

Gastroesophageal reflux and disease (GERD) may result from gastroparesis in anorexia nervosa but are also due to the recurrent purging behaviors that weaken the lower esophageal sphincter leading to heartburn and spontaneous vomiting (Gibson et al., 2022). Notation of blood in the emesis (hematemesis) may suggest an esophageal tear (Mallory-Weiss tear) and require urgent assessment. A hoarse voice may result from the gastric acid on the vocal cords. Prolonged or increasing symptoms of GERD increase the risk of precancerous Barrett esophagitis diagnosed by upper endoscopy (Pacciardi et al., 2015). Reflux symptoms may require treatment with proton pump inhibitors (Maret-Ouda et al., 2020). A referral to a gastroenterologist should be considered for persistent vomiting, severe reflux, or dysphagia.

Constipation is a common complaint and may be related to a slowed colon, loss of function due to chronic stimulant laxative use, dehydration, medication side effects, or poor oral intake. Assessment of a history of constipation and bowel movement pattern prior to the onset of the eating disorder and a careful medication and laxative use history should be reviewed, and impaction and rectal prolapse should be considered (Sato & Fukudo, 2015). Constipation may also be a risk factor for the development of disordered eating, and children and adolescents with constipation may be screened and monitored for eating disorders

(Wiklund et al., 2019). The definition of constipation should be considered with the current Rome IV criteria (Rome IV criteria 2023).

Treatment includes education regarding normal bowel patterns, increasing fluids, weight restoration with emotional support, and using a footstool during defection. Polyethylene glycol, an osmotic laxative, may increase bowel movements and require higher twice-daily dosing (Gaudiani, 2019). An alternative is a lactulose which, despite the sweet taste, is not absorbed. If an individual presents with use or abuse, the stimulants should be discontinued without a taper, and osmotic laxatives should be considered (Roerig et al., 2010).

Diffuse abdominal pain is common and most likely related to malnutrition, eating disorder behaviors, or nutritional rehabilitation (treatment with adequate nutrition). However, acute infectious or inflammatory etiologies need to be considered. Abdominal pain with constipation and then diarrhea should prompt consideration for impaction, celiac disease, or inflammatory bowel disease (with blood). Pain that resolves with defecation with various stool patterns prompts the consideration for irritable bowel syndrome. Diarrhea with fever suggests an infectious etiology, and vomiting with right upper quadrant pain suggests cholelithiasis. A rare cause of abdominal pain, vomiting, and upper quadrant pain after meals in a malnourished individual is superior mesenteric artery (SMA) syndrome—trapping of the duodenum between the aorta and the SMA diagnosed by abdominal computed tomography (Gibson et al., 2022; Sato & Fukudo, 2015).

CARDIOVASCULAR

Cardiac sequelae include bradycardia, autonomic dysfunction, and QT dispersion. A prolonged QTc interval was initially thought to be associated with eating disorder; however, rather than assuming the eating disorder as the etiology, a family history for prolonged QT syndrome should be obtained, and a review of adverse reactions to medication should be considered (Sachs et al., 2022). Bradycardia is associated with an athlete's healthy conditioned heart muscle and the deconditioned decreased heart muscle of malnutrition. While an athlete's heart rate may be low when getting up and moving, there is usually not a large change in heart rate as is seen with a malnourished heart. An electrocardiogram (ECG) will show normal voltage in the healthy heart of an athlete and loss of voltage with a malnourished deconditioned heart muscle (Rome & Strandjord, 2016).

ENDOCRINE

The endocrine system is also affected by malnourishment and dehydration. Thyroid studies may demonstrate nonthyroidal illness syndrome with a low-normal thyroid stimulating hormone (TSH) and low total thyroxine (TT_4), and low triiodothyronine (T_3) as an adaptation to chronic starvation. Subclinical hypothyroidism (elevated TSH, normal T_4) with positive antithyroid antibody tests may be related, and treatment may not be necessary unless TSH levels exceed 10 mU/L (Mehler, 2022).

Changes in thyroid, estrogen, and glucocorticoids may be associated with an elevated cholesterol level, which is usually of no clinical significance if attributed to elevated high-density lipoproteins. The low levels of sex hormones associated with amenorrhea suppress bone resorption and formation particularly dangerous during a time of expected bone formation and thus increases the risk of low BMD (Schorr & Miller, 2016; Workman et al., 2020). Assessing a history of multiple broken bones or stress fractures may suggest low BMD. Dual-energy x-ray absorptiometry (DEXA) scan should be considered for anyone with a 9- to 12-month history of amenorrhea with follow-up every 2 years (Mehler, 2022). A DEXA scan may also be considered in males. The z score should be used to interpret the results. No treatment for osteopenia or osteoporosis is supported at this time. Treatment includes weight gain, the return of menses, vitamin D (600 IU), and calcium supplementation (Hornberger et al., 2021). Treatment is also guided by serum vitamin D (25-hydroxy) and recommended replacement. Any consideration of estrogen or testosterone use needs to consider the SMR and level of epiphysis ossification. While weight restoration and nutrition are the more efficacious treatment for bone health, a low BMI may persist regardless of the recovery status (Schorr & Miller, 2016), highlighting the importance of early intervention, supplementation, and recovery.

The dehydration from chronic purging causes the kidney to upregulate aldosterone, which remains active after purging, leading to sodium and water retention and potassium and hydrogen excretion, which may lead to hypokalemia, metabolic alkalosis, and pseudo-Bartter syndrome. Cessation of laxatives or purging or rapid infusions of liquids in increased aldosterone activity may lead to accumulation of sodium and water and fluid retention and edema (Mascolo et al., 2012; Ragunathan et al., 2021). The weight gain and appearance of edema may be particularly upsetting for a person struggling with an eating disorder.

REFEEDING SYNDROME

During the first weeks of nutritional replenishment for someone chronically malnourished or with acute food refusal, the life-threatening physiologic response of refeeding syndrome needs to be monitored and prevented. While thought to be primarily a disruption of phosphorus levels, the American Society for Parenteral and Enteral Nutrition consensus definition is a measurable fall in levels of phosphorus, potassium, magnesium, or signs of thiamin deficiency developing hours to days after restarting feeding to someone with a "substantial period of undernourishment" (da Silva et al., 2020, p. 188). During starvation with no glucose intake, insulin is reduced, and fat is metabolized. During refeeding, the increased glucose leads to increased insulin that causes sodium retention (edema) and transcellular shifts of glucose, potassium, and magnesium (Boateng et al., 2010). These deficiencies are associated with arrhythmias and phosphorus depletion leading to anemia, muscle weakness, rhabdomyolysis, and dyspnea. Lab values need to be monitored daily with phosphorus and thiamine supplementation and refeeding starting as an inpatient for individuals who are severely malnourished.

PROGNOSIS

Overcoming an eating disorder is a difficult and sometimes lifelong battle. Eating disorders are considered one of the deadliest psychiatric disorders (Campbell & Peebles, 2014); in addition to life-threatening medical complications, the risk of suicide is greater in persons with eating disorders (Mandelli et al., 2019). Psychiatric illness, including anxiety or depression, may persist over time.

Although the majority of individuals with an eating disorder achieve recovery (e.g., 50–80% across studies), these rates are most typically observed longitudinally after 10 or more years, and about 20% remain significantly impaired (Rosen & Committee on Adolescence, 2010). Additionally, it is not uncommon for individuals with eating disorders to relapse or switch between diagnostic categories (e.g., anorexia nervosa to bulimia nervosa). Individuals recovering from anorexia nervosa often report experiencing bulimia nervosa–like symptoms on the way to weight recovery while learning to readapt to normal amounts of food intake and hunger and satiety cues.

Factors associated with prognosis have not always led to consistent findings. Studies suggest that younger age of onset, shorter duration of symptoms, and a more positive parent-child relationship are associated with a better outcome, whereas purging behavior, significant weight loss, and chronic duration of illness have been associated with less favorable outcomes (Rosen & Committee on Adolescence, 2010). Adolescents with a diagnosed eating disorder generally have a better long-term prognosis than their adult counterparts (Miller & Golden, 2010). Early detection and intervention for an eating disorder that begins in childhood or adolescence are associated with a better prognosis for an otherwise potentially chronic condition (Austin et al., 2021).

PRIMARY CARE MANAGEMENT

Eating disorders may present in late childhood and early adolescence, and early evaluation and treatment improve outcomes (Golden et al., 2015; Le Grange et al., 2014; Treasure & Russell, 2011) and improve the chance for catchup growth (Tanner & Spaulding-Barclay, 2022). The ability to prevent, recognize, and collaborate with treatment is a mental health competency in pediatric primary care (Foy et al., 2019). Feeding and eating problems such as picky eating or pediatric feeding disorders are complex and lack a unified conceptual definition, but they also require early identification and multidisciplinary treatment (Goday et al., 2019; Sharp et al., 2017; Taylor et al., 2015). Pediatric primary care providers are in a position to prevent/identify risk factors, screen for eating disorders, and assess for physiologic stability.

Any presentation for unexplained significant weight loss or gain, depression, anxiety, obsessive-compulsive disorder (OCD), self-injury, signs or symptoms of eating disorder, or indication of dissatisfaction with body weight and shape should prompt the consideration of an eating disorder (see Table 22.1). Evaluation for food allergies or GI conditions should be reserved for those children with a suspicious history, and no child should be prescribed an elimination diet in lieu of an appropriate referral for targeted evaluation (Tanner & Spaulding-Barclay, 2022). Reviewing the diagnostic criteria with the individual's presentation helps rule in the diagnosis of an eating disorder rather than excluding multiple medical differentials (Andersen, 2022). A careful review of the growth parameters and changes in trajectory should be noted. If an eating disorder is suspected, a medical and psychiatric evaluation should begin.

SCREENING TOOLS AND TARGETED QUESTIONS

Using a screening tool such as the SCOFF (Morgan et al., 1999) or the Screening for Disordered Eating (SDE) (Maguen et al., 2018) may guide discussion (Box 22.1). The SCOFF is not a reliable and validated tool for ARFID or binge eating disorder (Kutz et al., 2019). Some behaviors may not be relevant for younger teens and children, and qualifying the question with a statement highlighting the undesirable effect of the behavior is recommended. An example by Rome and Stranjorn (2016) is to phrase a question regarding intentional vomiting as: "Individuals who vomit intentionally may not realize that this behavior can result in long-term weight gain because your body thinks it has to 'store up nuts for the winter' to survive future episodes of vomiting" (p. 325). After interviewing the adolescent or child, collateral information is required from the family and relevant contacts.

Targeted questions to clarify eating patterns, body image disturbance, and patterns are listed in Box 22.2. The priority of care is assessing medical stability with targeted laboratory tests (Box 22.3). At a minimum, laboratory values are needed to guide the decision for hospital admission (Box 22.4). Although a laboratory assessment focusing on electrolytes is needed to evaluate medical stability, normal laboratory values

Box 22.1   Screening for Eating Disorders

SCREEN FOR DISORDERED EATING

1. Do you often feel the desire to eat when you are emotionally upset or stressed?
2. Do you often feel that you can't control what or how much you eat?
3. Do you sometimes make yourself throw up (vomit) to control your weight?
4. Are you often preoccupied with a desire to be thinner?
5. Do you believe yourself to be fat when others say you are thin?

SCOFF SCREEN

1. Do you make yourself sick because you feel uncomfortably full?
2. Do you worry you have lost control over how much you eat?
3. Have you recently lost more than one stone (14 lb) in a 3-month period?
4. Do you believe yourself to be fat when others say you are too thin?
5. Would you say that food dominates your life?
   (≥2 suggests anorexia nervosa or bulimia nervosa)

From Maguen, S., Hebenstreit, C., Li, Y., Dinh, J., Donalson, R., Dalton, S., Rugin, E., & Masheb, R. (2018). Screen for disordered eating: Improving the accuracy of eating disorder screening primary care. *General Hospital Psychiatry, 50*, 20–25; Morgan, J.F., Reid, F., & Lacey, J.H. (1999). The SCOFF questionnaire: Assessment of a new screening tool for eating disorders. *BMJ, 319*(7223), 1467–1468.

Box 22.2   Targeted Eating Disorder Questions

DIETARY AND NUTRITION PATTERNS AND INTAKE

Did you have any feeding problems as an infant?
Have you ever had a fearful episode of choking, etc.?
How many meals and snacks do you usually eat in a day (e.g., 3 meals, 2 snacks)?
Do you ever skip meals?
Are there certain foods you avoid, and why?
Do you have any food allergies?
Over the past week, how many times have you eaten breakfast, lunch, dinner?
What did you eat yesterday?
Do you count calories? If so, how many calories do you consume in a day?
Do you follow any special diets?
Have you ever had a binge episode?
Is there anything that triggers eating for you?
Ever feel like your eating has been out of control?

WEIGHT HISTORY

What is the most you have weighed in the past month? Past 3 months? Past 6 months?
What is the least you have weighed in the past month? Past 3 months? Past 6 months?
Are you trying to lose weight?

BODY IMAGE

How do you view your body and shape? Do you compare yourself to others?
What weight would you like your body to be? What is too high? What is too low?
Are you currently trying to lose weight? If so, how much and how?

PURGING

Do you do anything specific to maintain your weight or lose weight?
What kind of movement do you enjoy? How often? How intense do you work out?
Do you ever feel like you need to earn meals or work off calories through exercise?
Do you vomit? How often? How soon after eating?
Do you use laxatives, diuretics, diet pills, or caffeine? What types? How many? How often?

do not preclude serious disease. Individuals and families must be reminded that the child may be at risk for serious short- and long-term health problems despite normal lab values.

A targeted review of symptoms/systems followed by a complete physical exam with vital orthostatic signs is needed to assess the severity and to support the decision for hospitalization (see Box 22.4). Despite the reported symptoms and findings on the complete physical exam, the individual may lack insight into the magnitude or presence of the eating disorder and may self-identify with the disorder. This is especially important during adolescence when identity formation is a developmental task. Starvation may also account for cognitive slowing manifested by delayed responses. Building a therapeutic alliance with nonjudgment is balanced with stating concern for the facts of what the primary care provider is observing.

PREVENTION

The pediatric primary care provider is responsible for using the longitudinal therapeutic family relationship to prevent eating disorders through thoughtful anticipatory guidance. Language should remain nonjudgmental and culturally sensitive while avoiding stigmatizing language such as "obese," "fat," or "judging based on appearance." Health care providers need to reframe their approach to a philosophy that supports multiple body shapes and avoid associating standard ideas of physical health with actual health status (AAP, 2021). Demonstrating and discussing respect for all body types (Andersen, 2022) sets the groundwork to prevent the body image distortions of eating disorders. Routine media use counseling and the need for parental supervision include awareness of electronic and social media that supports dysfunctional eating disorder behaviors.

Referral

Consultation with an eating disorder specialist and team is preferable. The eating disorder treatment team, at the minimum, includes a nutritionist, medical provider, and psychiatric provider. A program or therapist familiar with family-based treatment/therapy (FBT) is preferred, particularly with younger adolescents and children.

Box 22.3	Laboratory Evaluation

- Complete blood count with differential (anemia, leukopenia in anorexia nervosa [AN])
- Electrolytes (hyponatremia, hypokalemia, hypomagnesemia)
- Calcium, magnesium, phosphorus (hypomagnesemia, hypophosphatemia in AN)
- Serum glucose (hypoglycemia in AN)
- Liver transaminases, alkaline phosphatase, bilirubin
- Thyroid stimulating hormone (TSH) with reflex to free thyroxine (low T_4, low TSH in AN)
- Vitamin B_{12}, vitamin D (25-hydroxy), iron studies, zinc
- Urinalysis
- Pregnancy test (urine or serum)
- Prolactin, serum gonadotropins, estrogen, testosterone (if amenorrhea) (AN)
- Serum amylase (salivary) and lipase if purging (in bulimia nervosa)
- Stool occult blood if abdominal pain or anemia
- Lipid panel (hypercholesterolemia in AN)

Box 22.4	Indications Supporting Hospitalization in an Adolescent With an Eating Disorder

ONE OR MORE OF THE FOLLOWING JUSTIFY HOSPITALIZATION

1. ≤75% median BMI for age and sex (percent median BMI calculated as patient BMI/50th percentile BMI for age and sex in reference population × 100)
2. Dehydration
3. Electrolyte disturbance (hypokalemia, hyponatremia, hypophosphatemia)
4. ECG abnormalities (e.g., prolonged QTc or severe bradycardia)
5. Physiologic instability:
   a. Severe bradycardia (HR <50 beats per min daytime; <45 beats per min at night)
   b. Hypotension (90/45 mm Hg)
   c. Hypothermia (body temperature <96°F [35.6°C])
   d. Orthostatic increase in pulse (>20 beats per min) or decrease in BP (>20 mm Hg systolic or >10 mm Hg diastolic)
6. Arrested growth and development
7. Failure of outpatient treatment
8. Acute food refusal
9. Uncontrollable binge eating and purging
10. Acute medical complications of malnutrition (e.g., syncope, seizures, cardiac failure, pancreatitis)
11. Comorbid psychiatric or medical condition that prohibits or limits appropriate outpatient treatment (e.g., severe depression, suicidal ideation, obsessive-compulsive disorder, type 1 diabetes mellitus)

BMI, Body mass index; *ECG*, electrocardiogram; *HR*, heart rate; *QTc*, corrected QT interval.

From Society for Adolescent Health and Medicine. (2015). Position paper of the Society for Adolescent Health and Medicine: Medical management of restrictive eating disorders in adolescents and young adults. *Journal of Adolescent Health, 56*, 124.

HEALTH MAINTENANCE

The primary care provider is responsible for ensuring that all children and adolescents reach their optimal health and potential and continue routine health care maintenance and eating disorder–related screenings.

Growth and Development

Growth and developmental assessment and stimulation are prioritized in pediatric primary care, with height, weight, and BMI measured and plotted onto an appropriate growth chart, and BMI z score obtained. The measures for children less than 2 years of age should be plotted on the World Health Organization (WHO) charts, and for children older than 2 years on the Centers for Disease Control and Prevention (CDC) chart (https://www.cdc.gov/growthcharts/clinical_charts.htm). The BMI z score may be obtained at https://www.cdc.gov/growthcharts/growthchart_faq.htm or calculated with www.peditools.org.

Children with growth and pubertal delay due to eating disorder may not catch up to their potential linear growth, and early diagnosis and intervention are needed to mitigate long-term effects on growth potential (Tanner & Spaulding-Barclay, 2022). If an eating disorder is suspected, the most accurate weight would be obtained in the morning in a gown after voiding and after a jumping jack to release any possible weights.

Because children and adolescents are growing, an ideal or expected weight is difficult to identify and implies that one weight is the target. Rather, discuss an individual healthy weight range, nutrition, and development. To assess the degree of malnutrition, the BMI z score, premorbid growth patterns, weight at optimal health (i.e., menstruation), percent of weight lost, rate of weight loss, and percent median BMI can be used to identify a target weight with the caveat that this is not one number and will change with growth. The percent median BMI is calculated: (current BMI/50th percentile BMI for age and sex) × 100.

The percentage of weight loss may be calculated: initial weight lost/initial weight (Tanner & Spaulding-Barclay, 2022). The percent of expected body weight may also be used to assess malnutrition and is calculated: (BMI/50th percentile BMI for age, height, and sex) × 100 (Le Grange et al., 2012).

During eating disorder treatment, showing children or adolescents their weight is an individual decision, and nonjudgement and thoughtful terminology should be used. The primary care provider should be vigilant for atypical anorexia nervosa, which may present with a decreased weight trajectory but remain in the normal range. Failure to gain weight at the expected trajectory should be assessed as weight suppression and an evaluation regardless of any signs or symptoms of an eating disorder (Tanner & Spaulding-Barclay, 2022).

Nutrition

Assessing food insecurity, as recommended by Bright Futures (Hagan et al., 2017), is part of routine health care maintenance and is associated with eating disorders (Becker et al., 2017). Nutrition counseling in childhood may prevent later eating disorders and sets developmental expectations and long-term nutritional patterns. A conceptual approach understands family roles; the caregiver of a young child chooses the food and the preparation, considering the presentation of the food, and the child decides how much and whether to eat. This approach assumes that children can regulate their food intake, and mealtimes may be pleasant, setting the stage for a healthy relationship with food (Satter, 1987).

When assessing nutrition, the primary care provider should be thoughtful about unconscious bias through language and reconsider terminology such as "obesity," "needing to lose weight," or "diet." Saying "nutrition" rather than "diet" is more consistent with what primary care providers are evaluating. Shifting the approach from weight focused to health focused requires rethinking the relationship between adiposity and morbidity and fostering body acceptance, supporting intuitive and mindful eating, while recognizing the ethnic and genetic variabilities that support health at every size (Penney & Kirk, 2015). The Health at Every Size program is endorsed by the Association for Size Diversity and Health (https://asdah.org/health-at-every-size-haes-approach/). Any weight maintenance or weight loss interventions may focus on a healthy lifestyle rather than only weight loss, body size, and shape. Providers may also be thoughtful regarding comments they may make regarding their appearance or attempts at dieting and be role models for a positive self-image. Besides the developmentally appropriate routine questions recommended in Bright Futures (Hagan et al., 2017), a targeted eating disorder tool such as the SCOFF or SDE may be considered.

The primary care provider must recognize children and teens at greater risk for eating disorders, including LGBTQ, who are more likely to experience body dissatisfaction (McClain & Peebles, 2016; Milano et al., 2020; Nagata, 2020); children with type 1 diabetes mellitus (Coleman & Caswell, 2020); participants in sports, particularly elite athletes (Carvalhais et al., 2019; Giel et al., 2016; Joy et al., 2015); or activities that require a specific weight or shape, such as gymnastics (Oon et al., 2016) or ballet. However, research is not conclusive, and in some cases nonathletes may endorse disordered eating behaviors (Petisco-Rodríguez et al., 2020). Exercise and nutrition should be balanced with excessive exercise leading to weight loss (Milano et al., 2020). Individuals with anorexia nervosa will continue exercising without concern for severe weight loss (Walsh & Mehler, 2022) and may not appreciate this as a health risk. Males and females in sports may present with a relative energy deficiency in sports (REDS), affecting bone health, menstruation in females, BMI, immunity, and cardiovascular health (Mountjoy et al., 2018). Although no clear guidelines exist regarding

safe return to play or risk stratification (De Souza et al., 2014), tools such as the REDS Clinical Assessment Tool may help guide the decision for a safe return to strenuous activity (Mountjoy et al., 2014, 2018).

Safety

Age-related safety and anticipatory guidance, according to the AAP Bright Futures guidelines (Hagan et al., 2017), are relevant to children and adolescents with eating disorder. The most serious threat to safety is medical instability related to severe malnutrition, restriction, or electrolyte imbalance, as well as assessment for head injury related to syncope, infection from self-injurious behavior, and suicidality. Assessment of weight, behaviors, body image, vital orthostatic signs, and criteria for hospitalization (see Box 22.4) are assessed at each interaction. The most serious psychological risk is the increased risk of suicidality, and formal screening is needed during routine visits.

Immunizations

The current routine immunization schedule outlined by the CDC is recommended and available at https://www.cdc.gov/vaccines/schedules/hcp/imz/child-adolescent.html.

Screenings

Routine child and adolescent screenings are recommended by the AAP Bright Futures guideline (Hagan et al., 2017).

Vision. Routine screening is recommended; however, psychotropic medication use must be considered in evaluating vision regarding side effects or adverse reactions.

Hearing. Routine screening is recommended. Individuals with severe malnutrition may report autophony, an abnormal hyperperception of breathing or talking related to a patulous eustachian tube (Hollis et al., 2022).

Dental. Dental erosion may result from recurrent gastric acid related to recurrent self-induced emesis. Until the cessation of the self-induced vomiting, the mouth may be rinsed with water and fluoridated wash mouth after vomiting and may need medicated fluoride toothpaste and specialized dental care. Referral to a dentist experienced with eating disorders may be considered.

Blood pressure. Orthostatic vital signs should be measured at each visit after rest to avoid artificially elevated blood pressure or pulse from exercise immediately before measurement. Bradycardia, hypotension, and orthostatic vital signs may indicate a higher level of medical care and hospitalization.

Hematocrit/hemoglobin. See Condition-Specific Screening.

Condition-Specific Screening

A comprehensive review of systems, vital signs, physical exam, and laboratory evaluation should be done to assess medical stability and appropriate level of care. Common symptoms may include headache, fatigue, temperature instability, dizziness, lightheadedness, heart palpitations, heartburn, hematemesis (esophageal tear), abdominal pain, early satiety or bloating, constipation, leg cramps, extremity paresthesia, cold hands or feet, blue lips or fingers, joint pain, and irregular or absent menstrual periods (see Table 22.1). Routine laboratory tests assess the effects of malnutrition and electrolyte imbalances. The effects of binge eating disorder are not typically evident in childhood or early adolescence, but medical sequelae of elevated weight should be considered along with the effects of atypical antipsychotic medications.

Laboratory. Malnutrition may be associated with anemia, leukopenia, and thrombocytopenia (Hutter et al., 2009). Macrocytosis is more common than microcytosis (Walsh et al., 2020).

Chemistry. A comprehensive metabolic profile, including electrolytes, glucose, magnesium, phosphorus, liver, and renal function studies, helps assess physical health. A particular focus is on low electrolytes. Hypokalemia, hypophosphatemia, hypochloremia, and increased sodium bicarbonate may be associated with self-induced emesis (alkalosis). Reduced sodium bicarbonate may be related to laxative abuse and acidosis. An elevated blood urea nitrogen (BUN) or BUN/creatinine ratio may be associated with dehydration. Hypoglycemia may be associated with starvation or refeeding with the reintroduction of carbohydrates. Elevated aminotransferases are common. Elevations of amylase may suggest purging, and elevated lipase may suggest pancreatitis.

Urinalysis. Baseline and routine weight checks are recommended. A urinalysis positive for ketones suggests starvation and glucose, and ketones suggest diabetes. The specific gravity may indicate dehydration or deliberate excessive water intake prior to a weight check (water loading).

Endocrine. As discussed previously, thyroid studies may be affect-ed by malnutrition. Biological females with secondary amenorrhea or adolescents of any gender with pubertal delay should have a human chorionic gonadotropin (HCG) test to exclude pregnancy, TSH, prolactin (especially if taking an atypical antipsychotic medication), estrogen, testosterone, FSH, and luteinizing hormone (LH) from an experienced laboratory. A baseline vitamin D (25-hydroxy) should be obtained for all children and adolescents, treating insufficiency and deficiency. A bone density examination should be considered for anyone with greater than 6 months of amenorrhea, malnutrition with multiple fractures, or evidence of puberty delay.

Cardiology. An ECG is recommended for anyone with severe malnutrition, bradycardia, abnormal cardiac exam, suspected electrolyte imbalance, family history, or medications that may prolong the QTc interval.

COMMON ILLNESS MANAGEMENT

Differential diagnoses for the common eating disorder–related presentations are summarized in Box 22.5. Common illness presentations in which eating disorder should be suspected or treatment modified are subconjunctival hemorrhages (emesis), sore throat from emesis, or after nasogastric tube insertion with treatment. A heart rate within the normal range in a severely malnourished child with bradycardia may indicate infection, and a thorough physical exam and review of systems are required. A history of constipation or diarrhea suggests the need for an assessment of nutrition intake, medications, treatment history, and careful examination to rule out impaction. A hoarse voice in the absence of upper respiratory symptoms or scratches on the palate with a sore throat may suggest self-induced emesis. As previously discussed, a child or adolescent presenting with dehydration requiring fluid resuscitation may need it at a slower rate in consideration of pseudo-Bartter syndrome.

DEVELOPMENTAL ISSUES

Sleeping

A careful sleep history and routine sleep assessment are needed to consider feeding and eating nighttime behaviors, psychological comorbidities, posttraumatic stress disorder, or medication side effects. Daytime fatigue may be related to malnutrition and poor sleep quality at night. The eating disorder may not affect sleep; however, night eating syndrome should be assessed in the history of sleeping (McCuen-Wurst et al., 2018). Other factors specific to eating disorders impacting sleep quality may be night sweating, comorbid depression or posttraumatic stress disorder, or medication side effects.

Toileting

Constipation and diarrhea with disordered eating may predate the onset of eating disorder. Children with a history of constipation in childhood were more likely to present with disordered eating in adolescence, although some confounding familial variables were limiting the findings (Wiklund et al., 2019). Incontinence may be associated with children meeting the criteria for obesity, and children may refuse food or fear going out (Wagner et al., 2015).

Box 22.5	Differential Diagnoses for Eating Disorder Clinical Presentations

SYMPTOMS OF ANOREXIA NERVOSA (WEIGHT LOSS)
Drug use
Acquired immunodeficiency syndrome
Chronic infection
Addison disease
Diabetes mellitus
Hyperthyroidism
Malignancy
Irritable bowel syndrome
Malabsorption
Inflammatory bowel disease
Parasitic intestinal infection
Chronic pancreatitis
Cystic fibrosis
Superior mesenteric artery syndrome
Psychiatric disorders associated with weight loss (depression, obsessive-compulsive disorder, body dysmorphic disorder, schizophrenia, social anxiety disorder)

SYMPTOMS OF BULIMIA NERVOSA (PURGING)
Connective tissue disorders with gastrointestinal involvement
Gastroenteritis
Eosinophilic esophagitis (vomiting)
Inflammatory bowel disease
Malabsorptive states
Gastroesophageal disorder
Cyclic vomiting, migraine
Bowel obstruction
Esophageal stricture
Peptic ulcer disease
Gastric outlet syndrome
Parasitic intestinal infection
Chronic pancreatitis
Diabetes
Hypothalamic lesion or tumor
Hydrocephalus
Pseudotumor cerebri
Zenker diverticulum
Food allergy
Kleine-Levin syndrome
Depression, borderline personality disorder

WEIGHT GAIN
Hypothyroid, hypercortisolism
Medication side effect
Prader-Willi syndrome
Kleine-Levin syndrome
Obesity
Depression, bipolar disorder, borderline personality disorder

Discipline

Effective discipline principles focus on developmentally appropriate teaching, emotional regulation, and safety (Sege et al., 2018). Prevention of eating problems may be related to avoidance of using food as a reward or punishment. Struggles and shifts of independence and control between caregivers and children and young teens may be exacerbated by FBT, which shifts the responsibility of meals to parents at a time when teens are developing independence. Participation in sports, active hobbies, sleep-away camp, etc., may be used as a contingency for adequate nutrition intake that may be associated with family struggles.

Child Care

Young children with feeding and eating problems may require collaboration and education with child care providers to ensure the plan of care and nutrition and avoid feeding struggles.

Schooling

Individuals with eating disorder may be high achievers, but treatment of the disorder may be related to higher grades (Claydon & Zullig, 2020). Educational achievement and perfectionism are considered attributes of individuals with eating disorder; however, Schilder et al. (2021) found that students with eating disorders may demonstrate high educational achievement but have a lower IQ than normative data suggesting that it is the self-oriented perfectionism associated with educational achievement.

Children and teens may need to leave school to enter a higher level of care, and coordination with the school adjustment counselor or teacher may be needed to prevent losing grade progression or falling behind in academic performance. A child with a behavioral or mental disorder or issue may require a 504 plan that may be modified throughout treatment. Interventions to increase the knowledge of school-based personnel are needed to enhance recognition of eating disorder behaviors and their role in the treatment plan. Many school health personnel lack the knowledge and awareness of eating disorders (Knightsmith et al., 2020), thus highlighting a role for the primary care provider to collaborate with the school nurse and behavioral health staff. School-based interventions may also play a role in early diagnosis (Wolter et al., 2021) or prevention (Harrer et al., 2020). School factors affect the needs of children with eating disorders, especially children with special needs or lower socioeconomic status with constipation or reflux (Kabasakal et al., 2020).

Sexuality

Delayed puberty, lack of social interaction, and gender dysphoria affect psychosocial development. Despite no menstrual period, sexual activity may lead to pregnancy, and contraception should be considered as well as routine safer sex counseling. However, considerations of low BMD may limit some hormonal contraception. Sexual minority youth are at particular risk for disordered eating and weight control behaviors, and the primary care provider must remain vigilant in screening for eating disorder behaviors and body image as well as ensuring a safe and welcoming environment (McClain & Peebles, 2016; Milano et al., 2020; Nagata et al., 2020). Using the standard growth charts based on sex assigned at birth for a transgender teen is a clinical problem (Nagata et al., 2020). Further research is needed to explore the intersection of sexual and ethnic identities to create and evaluate early recognition, treatment, and prevention (Calzo et al., 2017).

Transition to Adulthood

The period of emerging adulthood is the period between ages 18 and 25 years, an interplay between adolescence and young adulthood. Interventions adapted to the needs of this age are more effective than usual treatment (Potterton et al., 2020). This is a time of planning for college and vocation; however, the eating disorder may disrupt life plans, and many colleges are ill equipped to work with students with such disorders (Webb & Schmidt, 2021).

Collaboration between the primary care provider and college health services may facilitate the successful transition to school. Some adolescents with eating disorders may be unable to attend college or move away from their families due to medical instability. Some students may decide on a gap year to focus on medical and psychological stabilization (Derenne, 2019). This may in some cases be used as a motivation for nutritional replenishment and adherence to treatment. More research is needed to meet the needs of this developmental period effectively.

Difficulties may arise when the adolescent turns 18 and becomes a legal adult. Parents who were able to mandate treatment now lose power in health care. The emerging adult may discontinue treatment or go to college, and eating disorder behaviors may resume. Guardianship may be considered if an adolescent is medically compromised, and cognitive or self-care ability or safety is a concern (Cook-Cottone, 2016).

Family Concerns

The diagnosis of an eating disorder in a child affects the whole family. The family structure and relationships affect the onset and maintenance of eating disorder behaviors (Erriu et al., 2020; Gilbert et al., 2000; Hillege, 2006). An older qualitative exploration of families' stories of living with a child with an eating disorder described the overarching themes of financial burden, lack of understanding, inconsiderate or thoughtless comments from significant relations, and social isolation partially related to a perceived negative view of them by health care professions and social relations.

The diagnosis of an eating disorder affects the entire family and may lead to parental confusion over the diagnosis, how to best help the affected child, and how to find treatment. Siblings report anger at the family disruption and resent parental attention targeted to the affected sibling and siblings trying to be supportive or protective. The greatest predictors of family relationship changes were found to be the age of the daughter (18–22 years), feeling confused and not knowing how to help, leading to frustration, and a change in family leisure activities associated with emotional exhaustion and fear to travel or leave the daughter home alone. The diagnoses studied only included mothers of daughters diagnosed with anorexia nervosa, bulimia nervosa, and other-specified eating disorders. Positive affective relationships, communication, resiliency, and vulnerability may affect the onset and maintenance of an eating disorder. Family functioning, relationships, emotional involvement, communication, and organization need to be explored further to understand the role of the family context, risk, and protective factors (Erriu et al., 2020).

The recommended treatment of eating disorder for children and adolescents is family focused with FBT as the main therapeutic approach, particularly in anorexia nervosa (Hornberger et al., 2021; Golden et al., 2015; Lock et al., 2015; Resmark et al., 2019). The responsibility for treatment is on the family and the parent or caregiver to oversee a teen's meals, especially one who refuses to eat, making it stressful and inconsistent with family role expectations.

Parents with disordered eating patterns may now be confronted with their own challenges and relationships. Once the child reaches legal age or leaves home for college, stress and fear of relapse may remain even with the resolution of eating disorder behaviors. Families may continue to monitor the individual's behavior long after the resolution of the eating disorder, which may also contribute to relationship strains.

Families from cultures in which food is related to love or health may be particularly challenged to understand their child who will not eat. The difficulty of observing a child or sibling visibly losing weight or purging after meals is stressful, worrying, and frustrating. Family life may completely change to accommodate the eating disorder behaviors, which may increase the very behaviors they are trying to change (Anderson et al., 2021). Parents may be encouraged to use leverage for desired expectations, such as not paying for school or lifestyle. This tough behavior is associated with a better chance for recovery but is very difficult and may affect family relationships (Gaudiani, 2019).

RESOURCE

National Eating Disorders Association: www.nationaleatingdisorders.org

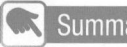 Summary

Primary Care Needs for the Child or Adolescent With an Eating Disorder

HEALTH CARE MAINTENANCE
Growth and Development
Height, weight, and BMI are measured and plotted onto an appropriate growth chart, and BMI z score is obtained (https://www.cdc.gov/growthcharts/growthchart_faq.htm).

Measures for children younger than 2 years should be plotted on the WHO charts, and children older than 2 years on the CDC chart (https://www.cdc.gov/growthcharts/clinical_charts.htm).

To assess the degree of malnutrition:
- Use the BMI z score
- Premorbid growth patterns
- Weight at optimal health (i.e., menstruation)
- Percent of weight lost
- Rate of weight loss

Percent median BMI can be used to identify a target weight with the caveat that this is not one number and will change with growth.

The percent median BMI is calculated: (current BMI/50th percentile BMI for age and sex) × 100.

Nutrition
Assess for food insecurity.

Say "nutrition" rather than "diet."

Shift from a weight-focused approach to a health focus requires rethinking the relationship with adiposity and morbidity and fostering body acceptance, supporting intuitive and mindful eating while recognizing ethnic and genetic variabilities.

Assess for atypical growth trajectories even if within a normal weight range (atypical anorexia nervosa).

Safety
Medical instability is a risk.

Monitor vital signs, bradycardia, and orthostasis.

Laboratory monitoring (electrolyte imbalances, cardiac dysrhythmias) is recommended.

Assess for criteria for hospitalization.

Assess for suicidality (https://www.nimh.nih.gov/research/research-conducted-at-nimh/asq-toolkit-materials).

Immunizations
Routine immunizations are recommended.

Screening
Vision. Routine screening is recommended.

Hearing. Routine screening is recommended. Autophony may present with severe anorexia nervosa.

Dental. Examine every visit for dental erosion and the need to prescribe fluoridated toothpaste.

Blood pressure. Routine (see Condition-Specific Screening).

Hematocrit/hemoglobin. Routine (see Condition-Specific Screening).

Condition-Specific Screening (Note Criteria for Hospitalization)
Vital signs. Take orthostatic blood pressure and heart rate after a period of rest each visit.

Complete blood count with differential. Check for normocytic anemia, leukopenia, and thrombocytopenia.

Electrolytes, magnesium, phosphorus. Check for hypoglycemia, hyponatremia, hypophosphatemia, and hypomagnesemia.

Renal function tests. Check for elevated BUN/creatinine ratio (dehydration).

Liver function tests. Aminotransferases are elevated during eating disorder and refeeding.

Amylase and lipase. Elevated salivary amylase indicates purging. Lipase is elevated in pancreatitis.

Lipid profile. Check for hypercholesterolemia (elevated high-density lipoprotein [HDL] in anorexia nervosa). Note atypical antipsychotic use (elevated triglycerides, low HDL).

Endocrine. Check for abnormal thyroid function tests, FSH, LH, low estrogen, low testosterone, HCG, prolactin.

Bone mineral density. Check if amenorrhea is a factor.

ECG. Check if bradycardia or medications may prolong the QTc interval.

COMMON ILLNESS MANAGEMENT
Differential Diagnosis
Rule in an eating disorder rather than rule out medical conditions.

Weight changes may be a symptom of autoimmune deficiency disorders, malignancy, GI, and endocrine disorders.

Weight gain is characteristic of Kleine-Levin syndrome, Prader-Willi syndrome, and some brain tumors.

Other mental health disorders may include depression, bipolar disorder, schizophrenia, body dysmorphic disorder, and OCD.

DEVELOPMENTAL ISSUES
Sleeping Patterns
Changes in sleep patterns may be associated with depression or posttraumatic stress disorder.

Note night sweating and night eating syndrome.

Toileting
Constipation may precede an eating disorder.

Incontinence may occur with children meeting the criteria of obesity.

Note medication side effects affecting enuresis.

Not using the bathroom after meals to assess for purging is recommended.

Stimulant laxative abuse should be stopped, and osmotic laxatives started.

Discipline
Avoid using food as a reward.

Struggles may occur during mealtimes, and parents need support with FBT.

Participation in sports and hobbies may be used as motivation or contingency for healthy nutrition.

Altering family plans to accommodate the child may increase eating disorder behaviors.

Child Care
Educate and collaborate with child care providers to prevent food struggles.

Schooling
Although it may demonstrate academic achievement and perfectionism, IQ may not match academic leveling.

Collaboration with school nurse and staff for academic accommodations and education regarding eating disorders is recommended.

An academic plan may be needed for residential level of treatment.

Children with larger bodies may be bullied.

Sexuality

Puberty may be delayed in all genders, and females may have primary or secondary amenorrhea.

Amenorrhea may cooccur with low BMD, and DEXA scan should be considered.

Sexual minority youth are at greater risk for eating disorders.

Transition to Adulthood

Plans for college and vocation may be disrupted.

Referral to the university health service for medical and psychiatric care should be arranged prior to the start of the school year.

Note the need for care during times of transitions and stress and possible exacerbation of eating disorder behaviors.

Enhance motivation for recovery prior to adulthood.

Facilitate transition to adult care starting prior to adulthood.

Family Concerns

Eating disorders may disrupt family structure and relationships.

Family-based treatment is difficult with teens trying to achieve independence and shift the responsibility for eating to parents.

Parents may not understand the refusal to eat and need support dealing with comments made by family and friends.

Siblings' needs should be addressed. Siblings report feeling angry, resentful, and protective.

Positive affective relationships, communication, resiliency, and vulnerability may affect the onset and maintenance of eating disorders.

Alterations in family leisure activities are stress related to the eating disorder. Assisting families to maintain enjoyed activities and share attention with all children (siblings) may enhance family relationships and functioning.

REFERENCES

Acle, A., Cook, B. J., Siegfried, N., & Beasley, T. (2021). Cultural considerations in the treatment of eating disorders among racial/ethnic minorities: A systematic review. *Journal of Cross-Cultural Psychology, 52*(5), 468–488. https://doi.org/10.1177/00220221211017664.

American Academy of Pediatrics. (2021). AAP-AACAP-CHA declaration of a national emergency in child and adolescent mental health. https://www.aap.org/en/advocacy/child-and-adolescent-healthy-mental-development/aap-aacap-cha-declaration-of-a-national-emergency-in-child-and-adolescent-mental-health/.

American Psychiatric Association Workgroup on Eating Disorders (2006). *Practice guideline for the treatment of patients with eating disorders* (3rd ed.). Author.

American Psychiatric Association. (2013). *Diagnostic and statistical manual of mental disorders* (5th ed.). Author. https://doi.org/10.1176/appi.books.9780890425596.

American Psychiatric Association. (2022). *Diagnostic and statistical manual of mental disorders* (5th ed. text rev.). Author.

Andersen, A. (2022). Diagnosis and treatment of the eating disorders spectrum in primary care medicine. In Mehler, P. S., & Andersen, A. E. (Eds.), *Eating disorders: A comprehensive guide to medical care and complications* (4th ed., pp. 1–106). Johns Hopkins University Press.

Anderson, L., Smith, K., Nuñez, M., & Farrell, N. (2021). Family accommodation in eating disorders: A preliminary examination of correlates with familial burden and cognitive-behavioral treatment outcome. *International Journal of Eating Disorders, 29*(4). https://doi.org/10.1080/10640266.2019.1652473.

Austin, A., Flynn, M., Richards, K. L., Sharpe, H., Allen, K. L., Mountford, V. A., Glennon, D., Grant, N., Brown, A., Mahoney, K., Serpell, L., Brady, G., Nunes, N., Connan, F., Franklin-Smith, M., Schelhase, M., Jones, W. R., Breen, G., & Schmidt, U. (2021). Early weight gain trajectories in first episode anorexia: Predictors of outcome for emerging adults in outpatient treatment. *J Eat Disord, 9*(1), 112. doi:10.1186/s40337-021-00448-y.

Becker, C. B., Middlemass, K., Johnson, R., & Gomez, F. (2017). Food insecurity and eating disorder pathology. *International Journal of Eating Disorders, 50*(9), 1031–1040. https://doi.org/10.1002/eat.22735.

Boateng, A. A., Sriram, K., Meguid, M., & Crook, M. (2010). Refeeding syndrome: Treatment considerations based on collective analysis of literature case reports. *Nutrition, 26,* 156–167.

Boileau, B. (2022). A review of obsessive-compulsive disorder in children and adolescents. *Dialogues in Clinical Neuroscience.*

Bourne, L., Bryant-Waugh, Cook, J., & Mandy, W. (2020). Avoidant/restrictive food intake disorder: A systematic scoping review of the current literature. *Psychiatry Research, 288.* https://doi.org/10.1016/j.psychres.2020.112961.

Bratland-Sanda, S., & Sundgot-Borgen, J. (2013). Eating disorders in athletes: overview of prevalence, risk factors and recommendations for prevention and treatment. *European Journal of Sport Science, 13*(5), 499–508.

Bravender, T., Bryant-Waugh, R., Herzog, D., Katzman, D., Kriepe, R. D., Lask, B., Le Grange, D., Lock, J., Loeb, K. L., Marcus, M. D., Madden, S., Nicholls, D., O'Toole, J., Pinhas, L., Rome, E., Sokol-Burger, M., Wallin, U., & Zucker, N.; Workgroup for Classification of Eating Disorders in Children and Adolescents. (2010). Classification of eating disturbance in children and adolescents: Proposed changes for the DSM-V. *Eur Eat Disord Rev, 18*(2), 79–89. doi:10.1002/erv.994.

Brewerton, T. D. (2007). Eating disorders, trauma, and comorbidity: Focus on PTSD. *Eating Disorders, 15,* 285–304.

Broft, A., Berner, L. A., & Walsh, B. T. (2010). Pharmacotherapy for bulimia nervosa. *The treatment of eating disorders: A clinical handbook,* 388–401. Publisher: The Guilford Press.

Bruch, H. (1982). Anorexia nervosa: Therapy and theory. *American Journal of Psychiatry, 139,* 1531–1538.

Bulik, C. M., Coleman, J. R. I., Hardaway, J. A., Breithaupt, L., Watson, H. J., Bryant, C. D., & Breen, G. (2022). Genetics and neurobiology of eating disorders. *Nature Neuroscience, 25*(5), 543–554. doi: 10.1038/s41593-022-01071-z. Epub 2022 May 6. PMID: 35524137; PMCID: PMC9744360.

Calzo, J., Blashill, A., Brown, T., & Argenal, R. (2017). Eating disorders and disordered weight and shape control behaviors in sexual minority populations. *Current Psychiatry Report, 19*(8). https://doi.org/10.1007/s11920-017-0801-y.

Camilleri, M., Parkman, H., Shafi, M., Abell, T., & Gerson, L. (2013). Clinical guideline: Management of gastroparesis. *American Journal of Gastroenterology, 108,* 18–37. https://doi.org/10.1038/ajg.2012.373.

Campbell, K., & Peebles, R. (2014). Eating disorders in children and adolescents: state of the art review. *Pediatrics, 134*(3):582–592. doi:10.1542/peds.2014-0194. PMID: 25157017.

Carvalhais, A., Araújo, J., Jorge, R., & Bø, K. (2019). Urinary incontinence and disordered eating in female elite athletes. *Journal of Science and Medicine in Sport, 22*, 140–144.

Claydon, E., & Zullig, K. (2020). Eating disorders and academic performance among college students. *Journal of American College Health, 68*(3), 320–325. https://doi.org/10.1080/07448481.2018.1549556.

Coleman, S., & Caswell, N. (2020). Diabetes & eating disorders: An exploration of diabulimia. *BMC Psychology, 8*, 101. https://doi.org/10.1186/s40359-020-00468-4.

Cook-Cottone, C. (2016). Embodied self-regulation and mindful self-care in the prevention of eating disorders. *Eating Disorders, 24*(1), 98–105.

Couturier, J., Isserlin, L., Norris, M., Spettigue, W., Brouwers, M., Kimber, M., … & Pi-lon, D. (2020). Canadian practice guidelines for the treatment of children and adolescents with eating disorders. *Journal of Eating Disorders, 8*(1), 1–80.

da Silva, J., Seres, D., Sabino, K., Adams, S., Berdahl, G., Wolfe, S., Cover, M., Evans, D., Greaves, J., Gura, K., Michalski, A., Plogsted, S., Sacks, G., Tucker, A., Worthington, P., Walker, R., Ayers, P., & Parenteral Nutrition Safety and Clinical Practice Committees, American Society for Parenteral and Enteral Nutrition (2020). ASPEN consensus recommendations for refeeding syndrome. https://doi./10.1002/ncp.10474

Dalton, B., Bartholdy, S., Robinson, L., Solmi, M., Ibrahim, M. A., Breen, G., … & Himmerich, H. (2018). A meta-analysis of cytokine concentrations in eating disorders. *Journal of Psychiatric Research, 103*, 252–264.

Derenne, J. (2019). Eating disorders for transitional age youth. *Child and Adolescent Psychiatric Clinics of North America, 28*, 567–572. https://doi.org/10.1016/j.chc.2019.05.010.

De Souza, M., Nattiv, A., Joy, E., Misra, M., Williams, N., Mallinson, R., Gibbs, J., Olmsted, M., Goolsby, M., & Matheson, G. (2014). 2014 Female Athlete Triad coalition consensus statement on treatment and return to play of the female athlete triad: 1st International Conference held in San Francisco, California, May 2012 and 2nd International Conference held in Indianapolis, Indiana, May 2013. *British Journal of Sports Medicine, 48*, 289. https://doi.org/10.1136/bjsports-2013-093218.

Devoe, D., Han, A., Anderson, A., Katzman, D. K., Patten, S. B., Soumbasis, A., Flanagan, J., Paslakis, G., Vyver, E., Marcoux, G., & Dimitropoulos, G. (2023). The impact of the COVID-19 pandemic on eating disorders: A systematic review. *Int J Eat Disord, 56*(1), 5–25. doi:10.1002/eat.23704. Epub 2022 Apr 5.

Erriu, M., Cimino, S., & Cerniglia, L. (2020). The role of family relationships in eating disorders in adolescents: A narrative review. *Behavioral Sciences, 10*(4), 7. https://doi.org/10.3390/bs10040071.

Feder, S., Isserlin, L., Seale, E., Hammond, N., & Norris, M. L. (2017). Exploring the association between eating disorders and gender dysphoria in youth. *Eating Disorders, 25*(4), 310–317.

Foy, J., Green, C., Earls, M., & Committee on Psychosocial Aspects of Child and Family Health, Mental Health Leadership Work Group, American Academy of Pediatrics. (2019). Mental health competencies for pediatric practice. *Pediatrics, 44*(5), e20192757. https://doi.org/10.1542/peds.2019-2757.

Frank, G. K., DeGuzman, M. C., & Shott, M. E. (2019). Motivation to eat and not to eat–the psycho-biological conflict in anorexia nervosa. *Physiology & Behavior, 206*, 185–190.

Gaudiani, J. (2019). *Sick enough*. Taylor & Francis.

Gibson, D., Puckett, L., & Mehler, P. (2022). Gastrointestinal complaints. In Mehler, P. S., & Andersen, A. E. (Eds.), *Eating disorders: A comprehensive guide to medical care and complications* (4th ed., pp. 194–216). Johns Hopkins University Press.

Giel, K., Hermann-Werner, A., Mayer, J., Diehl, K., Schneider, S., Thiel, N., & Zipfel, S., for the GOAL Study Group. (2016). Eating disorders pathology in elite adolescent athletes. *International Journal of Eating Disorders, 49*, 553–562.

Gilbert, A., Shaw, S., & Notar, M. (2000). The impact of eating disorders on family relationships. *Eating Disorders, 8*(4), 331–345. https://doi.org/10.1080/10640260008251240.

Goday, P., Huh, S., Silverman, A., Lukens, C., Dofrill, P., Cohen, S., Delaney, A., Feuling, M., Noel, R., Gisel, E., Kenzer, A., Kessler, D., Carmargo, Kraus de, Browne, J., & Phalen, J. (2019). Pediatric feeding disorder—consensus definition and conceptual framework. *Nutrition, 68*(1), 124–129. https://doi.org/10.1097/MPG.0000000000002188.

Godsey, J. (2013). The role of mindfulness-based interventions in the treatment of obesity and eating disorders: An integrative review. *Complementary Therapies in Medicine, 21*(4), 430–439.

Goel, N. J., Mathis, K. J., Egbert, A. H., Petterway, F., Breithaupt, L., Eddy, K. T., Franko, D. L., & Graham, A. K. (2022). Accountability in promoting representation of historically marginalized racial and ethnic populations in the eating disorders field: A call to action. *Int J Eat Disord, 55*(4), 463–469. doi:10.1002/eat.23682. Epub 2022 Jan 29.

Golden, N. H., Schneider, M., Wood, C., Daniels, S., Abrams, S., Corkins, M., … & Slusser, W. (2016). Preventing obesity and eating disorders in adolescents. *Pediatrics, 138*(3).

Golden, N. H., & Attia, E. (2011). Psychopharmacology of eating disorders in children and adolescents. *Pediatric Clinics, 58*(1), 121–138.

Golden, N. H., Katzman, D. K., Sawyer, S. M., Ornstein, R. M., Rome, E. S., Garber, A. K., Kohn, M., & Kreipe, R. W. (2015). Update on the medical management of eating disorders in adolescents. *Journal of Adolescent Health, 56*(4). https://doi.org/10.1016/j.jadohealth.2014.11.020.

Gorrell, S., & Murray, S. (2019). Eating disorders in males. *Child and Adolescent Psychiatric Clinics of North America, 28*, 641–651. https://doi.org/10.1016/j.chc.2019.05.012.

Graell, M., Morón-Nozaleda, M. G., Camarneiro, R., Villaseñor, A., Yáñez, S., Muñoz, R., Martínez-Núñez, B., Miguélez-Fernández, C., Muñoz, M., & Faya, M. (2020). Children and adolescents with eating disorders during COVID-19 confinement: Difficulties and future challenges. *European Eating Disorders Review, 28*(6), 864–870. https://doi.org/10.1002/erv.2763.

Guerdjikova, A. I., Mori, N., Casuto, L. S., & McElroy, S. L. (2019). Update on binge eating disorder. *Medical Clinics, 103*(4), 669–680.

Hagan, J., Shaw, J., & Duncan, P. (Eds.). (2017). *Bright futures guidelines for health supervision of infants, children, and adolescents* (4th ed.). American Academy of Pediatrics.

Hagan, K. E., & Walsh, B. T. (2021). State of the art: The therapeutic approaches to bulimia nervosa. *Clinical Therapeutics, 43*(1), 40–49. https://doi.org/10.1016/j.clinthera.2020.10.012.

Harrer, M., Adam, S., Mag, E-M., Baumeister, H., Cuijpers, P., Bruffaerts, R., Auerbach, R., Kessler, R., Jacobi, C., Tayler, C., & Ebert, D. (2020). Prevention of eating disorders at universities: A systematic review and meta-analysis. *International Journal of Eating Disorders, 53*, 813–833.

Hay, P. J., & de Claudino, A. (2012). Evidence-based treatment for the eating disorders. *Oxford Handbooks Online*. https://doi.org/10.1093/oxfordhb/9780195373622.013.0025.

Heo, Y. A., & Duggan, S. T. (2017). Lisdexamfetamine: A review in binge eating disorder. *CNS Drugs, 31*(11), 1015–1022.

Hilbert, A., Pike, K. M., Goldschmidt, A. B., Wilfley, D. E., Fairburn, C. G., Dohm, F. A., … & Weissman, R. S. (2014). Risk factors across the eating disorders. *Psychiatry Research, 220*(1-2), 500–506.

Hillege, S. (2006). Impact of eating disorders on family life: Individual parents' stories. *Journal of Clinical Nursing, 15*, 1016–1022.https://doi.org/10.1111/j.1365-2702.2006.01367.x.

Hollis, J., Man, S., Watters, A., Oakes, J., & Mehler, P. (2022). Autophony in inpatients with anorexia nervosa or avoidant restrictive food intake disorder. *International Journal of Eating Disorders, 55*, 388–392. https://doi.org/10.1002/eat.23667.

Holtom-Viesel, A., & Allan, S. (2014). A systematic review of the literature on family functioning across all eating disorder diagnoses in comparison to control families. *Clinical Psychology Review, 34*(1), 29–43.

Hornberger, L. L., Lane, M., & A. AAP The Committee on Adolescence. (2021). Identification and management of eating disorders in children and adolescents. *Pediatrics, 147*(1). https://doi.org/10.1542/peds.2020-040279O.

Hutter, G., Ganepola, S., & Hofmann, W. K. (2009). The hematology of anorexia nervosa. *International Journal of Eating Disorders, 42*, 293–300.

Iacovino, J. M., Gredysa, D. M., Altman, M., & Wilfley, D. E. (2012). Psychological treatments for binge eating disorder. *Current Psychiatry Reports, 14*(4), 432–446.

Jones, W., & Morgan, J. (2010). Eating disorders in men: A review of the literature. *Journal of Public Mental Health, 9*(2), 23–31.

Joy, E., Kussman, A., & Nattiv, A. (2015). 2016 update on eating disorders in athletes: A comprehensive narrative review with a focus on clinical assessment and management. *British Journal of Sports Medicine, 50*, 154–162. https://doi.org/10.1136/bjsports-2015-095735.

Kabasakal, E., Özcebe, H., Arslan, & Umut, E. A. (2020). Eating disorders and needs of disabled children at primary school. *Child Care Health Development, 46*, 637–643. http://dx.doi.org/10.1111/cch.12788.

Kafantaris, V., Leigh, E., Hertz, S., Berest, A., Schebendach, J., Sterling, W. M., … & Malhotra, A. K. (2011). A placebo-controlled pilot study of adjunctive olanzapine for adolescents with anorexia nervosa. *Journal of Child and Adolescent Psychopharmacology, 21*(3), 207–212.

Knightsmith, P., Treasure, J., & Schmidt, U. (2020). Spotting and supporting eating disorders in school: Recommendations from school staff. *Health Education Research, 28*, 1004–1013. https://doi.org/10.1093/her/cyt080.

Kutz, A., Marsh, A., Gunderson, C., Maguen, S., & Masheb, R. (2019). Eating disorder screening: A systematic review and meta-analysis of diagnostic test characteristics of the SCOFF. *Journal of General Internal Medicine, 35*(3), 885–893. http://dx.doi.org/10.1007/s11606-019-05478-6.

Lebow, J., Sim, L. A., Erwin, P. J., & Murad, M. H. (2013). The effect of atypical antipsychotic medications in individuals with anorexia nervosa: A systematic review and meta-analysis. *International Journal of Eating Disorders, 46*(4), 332–339.

Leehr, E. J., Krohmer, K., Schag, K., Dresler, T., Zipfel, S., & Giel, K. E. (2015). Emotion regulation model in binge eating disorder and obesity-a systematic review. *Neuroscience & Biobehavioral Reviews, 49*, 125–134.

Le Grange, D., Accurso, E. C., Lock, J., Agras, S., & Bryson, S. W. (2014). Early weight gain predicts outcome in two treatments for adolescent anorexia nervosa. *International Journal of Eating Disorders, 47*(2), 124–129. https://doi.org/10.1002/eat.22221. PMID: 24190844.

Le Grange, D., Lock, J., Loeb, K., & Nicholls, D. (2010). Academy for eating disorders position paper: The role of the family in eating disorders. *International Journal of Eating Disorders, 43*(1), 1.

Le Grange, D. L., Doyle, P. M., Swanson, S. A., Ludwig, K., Gluna, C., & Kreipe, R. (2012). Calculation of expected body weight in adolescents with eating disorders. *Pediatrics, 129*(2), e438–e446. https://doi.org/10.1542/peds.2011-1676.

Le Grange, D., Lock, J., Agras, W. S., Bryson, S. W., & Jo, B. (2015). Randomized clinical trial of family-based treatment and cognitive-behavioral therapy for adolescent bulimia nervosa. *Journal of the American Academy of Child & Adolescent Psychiatry, 54*(11), 886–894.

Lock, J., Le Grange, D., Agras, W. S., Moye, A., Bryson, S. W., & Jo, B. (2010). Randomized clinical trial comparing family-based treatment with adolescent-focused individual therapy for adolescents with anorexia nervosa. *Archives of General Psychiatry, 67*(10), 1025–1032.

Lock, J., La Via, M., & the American Academy of Child and Adolescent Psychiatry (AACAP) Committee on Quality Issues (CQI). (2015). Practice parameter for the assessment and treatment of children and adolescents with eating disorders. *Journal of the American Academy of Child and Adolescent Psychiatry, 54*(5), 412–425.

Maguen, S., Hebenstreit, C., Li, Yo, Dinh, Jl, Donalson, R., Dalton, S., Rugin, E., & Masheb, R. (2018). Screen for disordered eating: Improving the accuracy of eating disorder screening primary care. *General Hospital Psychiatry, 50*, 20–25. http://dx.doi.org/10.1016/j.genhosppsych.2017.09.004.

Mandelli, L., Arminio, A., Atti, A. R., & Ronchi, D. D. (2019). Suicide attempts in eating disorder subtypes: A meta-analysis of the literature employing DSM-IV, DSM-5, or ICD-10 diagnostic criteria. *Psychol Med, 49*(8), 1237–1249. doi:10.1017/S0033291718003549. Epub 2018 Nov 29. PMID: 30488811.

Maret-Ouda, J., Markar, S., & Lagergren, J. (2020). Gastroesophageal reflux disease: A review. *JAMA, 324*(24), 2536–2547. https://doi.org/10.1001/jama.2020.21360.

Marcos, Y. Q., Sebastián, M. Q., Aubalat, L. P., Ausina, J. B., & Treasure, J. (2013). Peer and family influence in eating disorders: A meta-analysis. *European Psychiatry, 28*(4), 199–206.

Mascolo, M., Trent, S., Colwell, C., & Mehler, P. (2012). What the emergency department needs to know when caring for your patients with eating disorders. *International Journal of Eating Disorders, 45*, 977–981.

McClain, Z., & Peebles, R. (2016). Body image and eating disorders among lesbian, gay, bisexual and transgender youth. *Pediatric Clinics of North America, 63*, 1079–1090. http://dx.doi.org/10.1016/j.pcl.2016.07.008.

McCuen-Wurst, C., Ruggieri, M., & Allison, K. (2018). Disordered eating and obesity: associations between binge-eating disorder, night-eating syndrome, and weight-related comorbidities. *Annals of the New York Academy of Sciences, 1411*, 96–105. https://doi.org/10.1111/nyas.13467.

Mehler, P. (2022). General endocrinology. In Mehler, P. S., & Andersen, A. E. (Eds.), *Eating disorders: A comprehensive guide to medical care and complications* (4th ed., pp. 134–216). Johns Hopkins University Press.

Mehler, P., & Andersen, A. (Eds.). (2022). *Eating disorders: A comprehensive guide to medical care and complications* (4th ed.). Johns Hopkins University Press.

Mento, C., Silvestri, M. C., Muscatello, M. R. A., Rizzo, A., Celebre, L., Praticò, M., … & Bruno, A. (2021). Psychological impact of pro-anorexia and pro-eating disorder websites on adolescent females: A systematic review. *International Journal of Environmental Research and Public Health, 18*(4), 2186.

Milano, W., Ambrosio, P., Carizzone, F., De Biasio, V., Foggia, G., & Capasso, A. (2020). Gender dysphoria, eating disorders and body image: An overview. *Endocrine, Metabolic & Immune Disorders-Drug Targets, 20*, 1–7. https://doi.org/10.2174/1871530319666191015193120.

Miller, C. A., & Golden, N. H. (2010). An introduction to eating disorders: clinical presentation, epidemiology, and prognosis. *Nutr Clin Pract, 25*(2), 110–115. doi:10.1177/0884533609357566.

Miniati, M., Callari, A., Maglio, A., & Calugi, S. (2018). Interpersonal psychotherapy for eating disorders: Current perspectives. *Psychol Res Behav Manag, 11*, 353–369. doi:10.2147/PRBM.S120584.

Minuchin, S., Baker, L., Rosman, B. L., Liebman, R., Milman, L., & Todd, T. C. (1975). A conceptual model of psychosomatic illness in children. Family organization and family therapy. *Archives of General Psychiatry, 32*(8), 1031–1038. doi: 10.1001/archpsyc.1975.01760260095008. PMID: 808191.

Mitchell, J. E. (2016). Medical comorbidity and medical complications associated with binge-eating disorder. *International Journal of Eating Disorders, 49*(3), 319–323.

Mitchell, K. S., Scioli, E. R., Galovski, T., Belfer, P. L., & Cooper, Z. (2021). Posttraumatic stress disorder and eating disorders: Maintaining mechanisms and treatment targets. *Eating Disorders, 29*(3), 292–306.

Morgan, J. F., Reid, F., & Lacey, J. H. (1999). The SCOFF questionnaire: Assessment of a new screening tool for eating disorders. *British Medical Journal, 319*(7223), 1467–1468. https://doi.org/10.1136/bmj.319.7223.1467.

Mountjoy, M., Sundgot-Borgen, J., Burke, L., Carter, S., Constantini, N., Lebrun, D., Meyer, N., Sherman, R., Steffen, K., Budgett, R., Ljungqvist, A., & Ackerman, K. (2014). RED-S CAT™ relative energy deficiency in sport (RED-S) clinical assessment tool (CAT*). British Journal of Sports Medicine, 49*, 421–423. https://doi.org/10.1136/bjsports-2014-094559.

Mountjoy, M., Sundgot-Borgen, J., Burke, L., Carter, S., Constantini, N., Lebrun, D., Meyer, N., Sherman, R., Steffen, K., Budgett, R., Ljungqvist, A., & Ackerman, K. (2018). Consensus statement on relative energy deficiency in sport (RED-S): 2018 update. *British Journal of Sports Medicine, 52*, 687–697. https://doi.org/10.1136/bjsports-2018-099193.

Nagata, J. (2020). Eating disorders in adolescent boys and young men: An update. *Current Opinion in Pediatrics, 32*(4), 476–481.

Nagata, J., Ganson, K., & Austin, B. (2020). Emerging trends in eating disorders among sexual and gender minorities. *Current Opinion in Psychiatry, 33*(6), 562–567. https://doi.org/10.1097/YCO.0000000000000645.

Oon, J., Calitri, R., Bloodworth, A., & McNamee, M. (2016). Understanding eating disorders in elite gymnastics: Ethical and conceptual challenges. *Clinics in Sports Medicine, 35*(2), 275–292. http://dx.doi.org/10.1016/j.csm.2015.10.002.

Otto, A. K., Jary, J. M., Sturza, J., Meller, C., Prohaska, N., Bravender, T., & Van Huysse, J. (2021). Medical admissions among adolescents with eating disorders during the COVID-19 pandemic. *Pediatrics, 148*(4), e2021052201. https://doi.org/10.1542/peds.2021-052201.

Pacciardi, B., Cargioli, C., & Mauri, M. (2015). Barrett's esophagus in anorexia nervosa: A case report. *International Journal of Eating Disorders, 48*, 147–150. https://doi.org/10.1002/eat.22288.

Penney, T. L., & Kirk, S. F. (2015). The Health at Every Size paradigm and obesity: Missing empirical evidence may help push the reframing obesity debate forward. *American Journal of Public Health, 105*(5), e38–e42. https://doi.org/10.2105/AJPH.2015.302552.

Petisco-Rodríguez, C., Sánchez-Sánchez, L., Fernández-García, R., Sánchez-Sánchez, J., & Garcia-Montes, J. (2020). Disordered eating attitudes, anxiety, self-esteem and perfectionism in young athletes and non-athletes. *International Journal of Environmental Research in Public Health, 17*, 6754. https://doi.org/10.3390/ijerph17186754.

Potterton, R., Richards, K., Allen, K., & Schmidt, U. (2020). Eating disorders during emerging adulthood: A systematic scoping review. *Frontiers in Psychology, 10*, 1–16. https://doi.org/10.3389/fpsyg.2019.03062.

Ragunathan, A, Singh, P, Gosal, K., Schibelli, N., & Collier, V. (2021). Laxative abuse cessation leading to severe edema. *Cureus, 13*(6), e15847. https://doi.org/10.7759/cureus.15847.

Ravel, A., Mircher, C., Rebillat, A.-S., Cieuta-Walti, C., & Megarbane, A. (2020). Feeding problems and gastrointestinal diseases in Down syndrome. *Archives de Pediatrie, 27*, 53–60. https://doi.org/10.1016/j.arcped.2019.11.008.

Resmark, G., Herpertz, S., Herpertz-Dahlmann, B., & Zeeck, A. (2019). Treatment of anorexia nervosa—new evidence-based guidelines. *Journal of Clinical Medicine, 8*, 153. https://doi.org/10.3390/jcm8020153.

Rikani, A. A., Choudhry, Z., Choudhry, A. M., Ikram, H., Asghar, M. W., Kajal, D., … & Mobassarah, N. J. (2013). A critique of the literature on etiology of eating disorders. *Annals of Neurosciences, 20*(4), 157.

Robertson, M., Duffy, F., Newman, E., Prieto Bravo, C., Ates, H. H., & Sharpe, H. (2021). Exploring changes in body image, eating and exercise during the COVID-19 lockdown: A UK survey. *Appetite, 159*, 105062. https://doi.org/10.1016/j.appet.2020.105062.

Roerig, J., Steffen, K., Mitchell, J., & Sunker, C. (2010). Laxative abuse: Epidemiology, diagnosis and management. *Drugs, 70*(12), 1487–1503. https://doi.org/10.2165/11898640-000000000-00000.

Rodgers, R. F., & Melioli, T. (2016). The relationship between body image concerns, eating disorders and internet use, part I: A review of empirical support. *Adolescent Research Review, 1*(2), 95–119.

Rome, E., & Strandjord, S. (2016). Eating disorders. *Pediatrics in Review, 37*(8), 323–336.

Rome IV criteria. Rome Foundation. (2023, March 6). https://theromefoundation.org/rome-iv/rome-iv-criteria/.

Rosen, D. & the Committee on Adolescence. (2010). Identification and management of eating disorders in children and adolescents. *Pediatrics, 126*, 1240–1253. http://pediatrics.aappublications.org/content/126/6/1240.full.html.

Sachs, K., Mehler, P., & Krantz, M. (2022). Cardiac abnormalities and their management. In Mehler, P. S., & Andersen, A. E. (Eds.), *Eating disorders: A comprehensive guide to medical care and complications* (4th ed., pp. 217–236). Johns Hopkins University Press.

Satter, E. (1987). *How to get your kid to eat…but not too much*. Bull Publishing Company.

Sato, Y., & Fukudo, S. (2015). Gastrointestinal symptoms and disorders in patients with eating disorders. *Clinical Journal of Gastroenterology, 8*, 255–263. https://doi.org/10.1007/s12328.

Schapman-Williams, A. M., Lock, J., & Couturier, J. (2006). Cognitive-behavioral therapy for adolescents with binge eating syndromes: A case series. *International Journal of Eating Disorders, 39*, 252–255.

Schilder, C., Sternheim, L., Aarts, E., van Elburg, A., & Danner, U. (2021). Relationships between educational achievement, intelligence, and perfectionism in adolescents with eating disorders. *International Journal of Eating Disorders, 54*, 794–801. https://doi.org/10.1002/eat.23482.

Schorr, M., & Miller, K. (2016). The endocrine manifestations of anorexia nervosa: Mechanisms and management. *Nature, 13*, 174–186. https://doi.org/10.1038/nrendo.2016.175.

Seetharama, S., & Fields, E. (2020). Avoidant/restrictive food intake disorder. *Pediatrics in Review, 41*(12), 613–622.

Sege, R., Siegel, B., & Council on child Abuse and Neglect, Committee on Psychosocial Aspects of Child and Family Health. (2018). Effective discipline to raise healthy children. *Pediatrics, 142*(6), e20183112. https://doi.org/10.1542/peds.2018-3112.

Sharp, W., Volkert, V., Scahill, L., McCracken, E., & McElhanon, B. (2017). Systematic review and meta-analysis of intensive multidisciplinary intervention for pediatric feeding disorders: How standard is the standard of care? *Journal of Pediatrics, 181*, 116–124.

Strings, S. (2023). How the use of BMI fetishizes white embodiment and racializes fat phobia. *AMA J Ethics, 25*(7), E535–539. doi:10.1001/amajethics.2023.535.

Tanner, A., & Spaulding-Barclay, M. (2022). Special considerations for eating disorders in children and young adolescents. In Mehler, P. S., & Andersen, A. E. (Eds.), *Eating disorders: A comprehensive guide to medical care and complications* (4th ed., pp. 134–216). Johns Hopkins University Press.

Taylor, C. M., Wernimont, S. M., Northstone, K., & Emmett, P. M. (2015). Picky/fussy eating in children: Review of definitions, assessment, prevalence and dietary intakes. *Appetite, 95*, 349–359. doi:10.1016/j.appet.2015.07.026.

Trace, S. E., Thornton, L. M., Root, T. L., Mazzeo, S. E., Lichtenstein, P., Pedersen, N. L., & Bulik, C. M. (2012). Effects of reducing the frequency and duration criteria for binge eating on lifetime prevalence of bulimia nervosa and binge eating disorder: Implications for DSM-5. *International Journal of Eating Disorders, 45*(4), 531–536.

Treasure, J, & Russell, G. (2011). The case for early intervention in anorexia nervosa: Theoretical exploration of maintaining factors. *British Journal of Psychiatry, 99*(1), 5–7. https://doi.org/10.1192/bjp.bp.110.087585.

Udo, T., & Grilo, C. M. (2019). Psychiatric and medical correlates of DSM-5 eating disorders in a nationally representative sample of adults in the United States. *International Journal of Eating Disorders, 52*(1), 42–50.

van Hoeken, D., & Hoek, H. W. (2020). Review of the burden of eating disorders: Mortality, disability, costs, quality of life, and family burden. *Current Opinion in Psychiatry, 33*(6), 521–527. https://doi.org/10.1097/YCO.0000000000000641.

Wagner, D., Equit, M., Niemczyk, J., & von Gontard, A. (2015). Obesity, overweight, and eating problems in children with incontinence. *Journal of Pediatric Urology, 11*, 202–207. http://dx.doi.org/10.1016/j.jpurol.2015.05.019.

Walsh, K., & Mehler, P (2022). Medical evaluation of patients with eating disorders. In Mehler, P. S., & Andersen, A. E. (Eds.), *Eating disorders: A comprehensive guide to medical care and complications* (4th ed., pp. 134–216). Johns Hopkins University Press.

Walsh, K., Blalock, D. V., & Mehler, P. S. (2020). Hematologic findings in a large sample of patients with anorexia nervosa and bulimia nervosa. *American Journal of Hematology, 95*(4), E98–E101. doi:10.1002/ajh.25732.

Webb, H., & Schmidt, U. (2021). Facilitators and barriers to supporting young people with eating disorders during their transition to, and time at, university: An exploration of clinicians' perspectives. *European Eating Disorders Review, 23*, 443–457. https://doi.org/10.1002/erv.2795.

Westmoreland, P., Krantz, M., & Mehler, P. (2016). Medical complications of anorexia nervosa and bulimia. *American Journal of Medicine, 129*, 30–37. http://dx.doi.org/10.1016/j.amjmed.2015.06.031.

Wiklund, C., Kuja-Halkola, R., Thornton, L., Hübel, C., Leppä, V., & Bulik, C. (2019). Prolonged constipation and diarrhea in childhood and disordered eating in adolescence. *Journal of Psychosomatic Research, 126*, 1–8.

Winston, A. (2020). Eating disorders and diabetes. *Current Diabetes Reports, 20*, 32. https://doi.org/10.1007/s11892-020-01320-0.

Wolfe, B. E., Metzger, E. D., & Stollar, C. (1997). The effect of dieting on plasma tryptophan concentration and food intake in healthy women. *Physiology & Behavior, 61*, 537–541.

Wolter, W., Hammerle, F., Buerger, A., & Ernst, V. (2021). Prevention of eating disorders—efficacy and cost-benefit of a school-based program ("MaiStep") in a randomized controlled trial (RCT). *International Journal of Eating Disorders, 54*, 1855–1864. https://doi.org/10.1002/eat.23599.

Workman, C., Blalock, D., & Mehler, P. (2020). Bone density status in a large population of patients with anorexia nervosa. *Bone, 131*, 1–6. https://doi.org/10.1016/j.bone.2019.115161.

Zeeck, A., Hartmann, A., Wild, B., De Zwaan, M., Herpertz, S., & Burgmer, M., … & Antop Study Group. (2018). How do patients with anorexia nervosa "process" psychotherapy between sessions? A comparison of cognitive–behavioral and psychodynamic interventions. *Psychotherapy Research, 28*(6), 873–886.

Seizures result from the hypersynchronous neuronal activity and may be provoked (head trauma, fever, drugs) or unprovoked. The International League Against Epilepsy (ILAE) defines epilepsy as two or more seizures occurring greater than 24 hours apart or one unprovoked seizure with an electroencephalogram (EEG) suggesting an increased risk for additional seizures (Fisher et al., 2014). Based on this definition, about 0.6% of children in the United States have active epilepsy (Zack & Kobau, 2017).

While the neurology specialist will manage much of the care of children with epilepsy, primary care providers significantly impact the care, health, and support of children with epilepsy and their families. Given the frequency of epilepsy, primary care providers must be well versed in the disease process and treatment.

EPIDEMIOLOGY

Incidence of seizures and epilepsy varies in childhood with a bimodal distribution, with peaks in infancy and in adolescence. Epilepsy will affect 1 in 26 people (4%), reflective of varying etiology, with 3.4 million persons having active epilepsy in the United States (Zack & Kobau, 2017).

Febrile seizures occur in 2% to 4% of children before the age of 5 years (Seinfeld et al., 2017). While febrile seizures are provoked and do not meet clinical criteria for epilepsy, they are frequently occurring episodes seen in pediatrics and may also be seen in children with epilepsy.

ETIOLOGY

The etiology of epilepsy varies, and it is important to note that a diagnosis of epilepsy does not describe its etiology. While diagnosis and treatment of epilepsy are essential, care should be taken to assess for etiology of epilepsy as this may result in changes to treatment recommendations.

Provoked seizures are those occurring near a neurologic insult. These may include febrile, trauma, acute hypoxic-ischemic encephalopathy, hypertension, metabolic abnormalities, hypocalcemia, hypoglycemia, electrolyte imbalance, infection, drug withdrawal, pyridoxine dependency, and toxins. Causes of unprovoked seizures or epilepsy include genetic, structural-metabolic, and unknown causes.

PATHOPHYSIOLOGY

Children have a higher propensity to develop seizures than their adult counterparts. In immature brains there are higher levels of excitatory N-methyl-D-aspartate (NMDA) receptor transmission in animal models, which may contribute to epileptogenicity (Awin, 2017). Postnatally gamma-aminobutyric acid (GABA) also has excitatory effects in the hippocampus, cerebral cortex, cerebellum, and spinal cord (Awin, 2017). The net excitation develops in parallel with excitation synapses, while inhibition synapse development lags, resulting in an overall increase in excitation without appropriate inhibition.

The substantia nigra pars reticulata, superior colliculus, subthalamic nucleus, pedunculopontine nucleus, anterior thalamus, and area tempestas likely play a role in the control and propagation of seizures; however, evidence is currently strongest for the substantia nigra pars reticulata (Awin, 2017).

SEIZURE CLASSIFICATION

Seizures are classified and described based on terminology agreed upon by the ILAE. Based on ILAE criteria, seizures fall into one of three categories: focal, generalized, and unknown onset (Fisher et al., 2017). All seizures are classified based on how they start. After classification in one of these categories, the seizures are then further classified and described based on clinical features associated with the seizure.

Focal seizures originate in a limited location, which may be very limited or have a wider distribution across a single hemisphere; however, children with focal epilepsy may have more than one seizure foci. Since this seizure does not initially involve the entire cortex, it is important to assess for awareness of these seizures. The ILAE describes two categories for this feature, focal awareness or focal with impaired awareness. Focal aware seizures may be motor or nonmotor, but the distinctive feature is that the person experiencing the seizure has retained awareness and the ability to interact with the environment at baseline. For example, a child may experience a focal aware nonmotor seizure and

Table 23.1 Seizure Classification

	CLASSIFICATION	SEIZURE TYPE	FEATURES
Motor	Both	Epileptic spasms	Flexion or extension of body/extremities
		Atonic	Loss of tone
		Clonic	Rhythmic jerking
		Tonic	Stiffening
		Myoclonic	Jerk
	Generalized	Tonic-clonic	Stiffening followed by rhythmic jerking
		Myoclonic-tonic-clonic	Jerk followed by stiffening and rhythmic jerking
		Myoclonic-atonic	Jerk followed by loss of tone
	Focal	Hyperkinetic	Rapid, unorganized movements
		Automatisms	Nonpurposeful movements, typically of hands
Nonmotor	Generalized (absence)	Typical	Behavior arrest, staring, associated electroencephalogram (EEG) findings
		Atypical	As above, but longer in duration, variation in EEG findings, changes in tone
		Myoclonic	Associated muscle jerking causing abduction of upper extremities
		Eyelid myoclonia	Absence seizure with eye deviation up and eyelid flutter
	Focal	Autonomic	Heart rate changes, flushing, nausea, piloerection
		Behavior arrest	Paucity in movement
		Cognitive	Aphasia, déjà vu, jamais vu, memory impairment
		Emotional	Anxiety, crying, laughing
		Sensory	Changes in smell, taste, seeing colorful balls in vision

describe a metallic taste in the mouth. Focal aware seizures often evolve to focal with impaired awareness or even to bilateral tonic-clonic seizures, which is why they are often called an aura or seen as a warning to families of an imminent seizure. Focal seizures with impaired awareness, in contrast, are seizures that involve alteration in the child's ability to engage in the environment. This alteration may range from repetitive, nonsensical speech to unresponsiveness when asked questions. Unilateral movement, forced eye deviation, or asymmetry characterize this seizure's semiology of motor features.

Generalized seizures originate from a broad focus across the cortex and involve both hemispheres. They therefore by nature involve impaired awareness. Since awareness does not need to be considered in this semiology, the major assessment is between motor and nonmotor seizures, also known as absence seizures. Motor features of these seizures will be characterized by bilateral synchronous movement.

Seizures with unknown onset are patterns that do not fit into the other categories or seizures presenting insufficient information to allow categorization. Unknown onset seizure is not a true classification but a temporary description for seizures that cannot be further classified at the time. This may be used in situations where the clinical findings are unclear, an EEG was nondiagnostic, or the onset of the seizure has not been witnessed for clinical classification.

Seizures are further described by the clinical features associated with the seizure (Table 23.1). As more information is collected about a patient, a more precise classification can be provided about their seizures.

While febrile seizures are provoked and not epilepsy, it is essential to discuss classifications of febrile seizures as they can be associated with an increased risk for epilepsy. These are typically seen between 6 months and 5 years of age; however, they may be seen outside of this range (Seinfeld et al., 2017). Febrile seizures are broken into two categories, simple and complex. Simple febrile seizures are characterized by a single, generalized seizure lasting less than 15 minutes. Complex febrile seizures are characterized by multiple seizures within 24 hours, focal features of seizures, or prolonged seizures. Fever may be noted at the time of seizure or shortly thereafter. In addition to complex febrile seizures, neurodevelopmental abnormalities, family history of epilepsy, and those with seizures shortly after fever development have higher risks of epilepsy (Seinfeld et al., 2017). However, interventions are rarely needed for febrile seizures, and treatment is supportive management, specifically fever management and emergency medications for prolonged seizures. In some instances, medications may be recommended for those with higher risk factors or prolonged, frequent febrile seizures, but this is done at the discretion of the neurology provider.

DIAGNOSIS

Seizures and epilepsy are clinical diagnoses. While it may be helpful to obtain specific testing, the primary diagnosis is made with history and physical examination. Primary care providers and caregivers are the first to witness events concerning seizures, and appropriate

Box 23.1 History Questions

- What does the child do?
- Is there one type of event, or multiple types?
- Is the child aware of having events? If so, what is the child's experience?
- Where does it happen?
- When does it happen?
- Does anything make it more likely to happen (e.g., sleep deprivation, stress, menstruation, illness)?
- How have symptoms changed since the onset?
- Are the child's eyes open or closed?
- How have you tried interacting with the child during these (e.g., verbal or tactile stimulation)?
- Has the child had any injuries related to these?
- Has the child had any changes in cognition/school performance?
- Has the child suffered any loss of developmental milestones?
- Has there been an increase in daytime fatigue?

referral is important to the ongoing diagnosis and care of a child with epilepsy.

When obtaining a history, it is important to be as specific as possible (Box 23.1). Videos of the events are also helpful in allowing the provider to assess semiology appropriately. Identifying what side of the body moves, how the body moves, and what caregivers have done to assess responsiveness help identify awareness, onset, and motor versus nonmotor seizures. Encourage families to demonstrate how the child's body moves instead of just using descriptive words such as "shaking," as this can be interpreted in multiple ways. In addition, seizures will typically worsen in frequency and intensity when not treated, so assessing how symptoms have changed since onset is also helpful in developing a differential diagnosis. It is important to assess for any injuries related to the events and bowel or bladder continence loss. While this is not necessary for a seizure diagnosis, it is helpful in assessing and planning safety measures. Identify when seizures occur and if there are any triggers related to seizures. Stress can reduce the seizure threshold further for someone with epilepsy and increase the likelihood of experiencing seizures. Common triggers include sleep deprivation, stress, illness, menstruation, hyperventilation, and flashing lights.

Assess for provoking factors, commonly fever, acute head injury, or recent medication changes. Remember that provoked seizures do not meet the clinical criteria for epilepsy; however, additional evaluation may be recommended for those with focal features. In addition, assess for any risk factors for epilepsy, such as trisomy 21, stroke, cerebral palsy, other neurologic symptoms, and family history of seizures. When possible, it is important to assess why family members have seizures/epilepsy, as many etiologies do not represent a genetic predisposition.

Physical examination interpretation will depend on if the examination is ictal (during the seizure), interictal

(between seizures), or postictal (during seizure recovery). Without an underlying structural cause or previous abnormalities on examination, most children will have a normal neurologic examination interictally. During an interictal assessment, some findings may indicate specific etiologies or the need for additional testing. Therefore a complete examination is needed (Table 23.2). If you are examining the child ictally, assess for responsiveness, provide a cue word such as "purple elephant," and following the seizure ask if the child recalls the word. Look for changes in tone and any asymmetry on examination. Postictally, assess for localizing signs such as weakness on one side of the body. For children where the absence seizures are a concern, it can be useful to have the child complete hyperventilation in the clinic. This may occur in a safe location, typically seated in a chair next to an adult, and have the child hyperventilate by blowing on a pinwheel or bubble wand for no more than 3 minutes. This may provoke seizures in some children with absence and is diagnostic of absence seizures in those children. However, the absence of a hyperventilation-induced seizure does not preclude the diagnosis of absence epilepsy, and a routine EEG should still be completed. Hyperventilation should be avoided in children with poorly controlled asthma, sickle cell disease, or sickle cell trait.

The differential diagnosis for seizures may vary depending on the presentation. Common diagnoses in the differential include syncope, arrhythmias, migraine, stroke, functional neurologic disorder, sleep disorders, staring, attention-deficit/hyperactivity disorder (ADHD), and dystonia. Based on features, additional testing may be considered.

DIAGNOSTIC TESTING

Diagnostic testing can be used to support decision making and clinical diagnosis. EEG is the most common testing done in children with concerns for seizures. This involves the placement of electrodes on the scalp to record electrical activity. While some EEG findings are consistent with epilepsy, such as epileptiform discharges, specifically sharps and spikes, other EEG findings are nonspecific, such as slowing. It is also important to note that some children with epilepsy may have a normal EEG, and those without epilepsy may have abnormalities seen on EEG (Box 23.2). Overall, EEGs can be used in conjunction with the history and physical findings to assess for epilepsy.

The majority of EEGs are interictal (occur between seizures). The EEG study is to assess for any abnormal brainwave activity that is consistent with an increased risk for seizures, such as sharps or spikes. In addition, this activity's location or pattern can help further classify seizures. Routine EEGs are typically brief, lasting about 30 minutes, and capture both wake and sleep. When more information is needed on EEG, prolonged EEGs may be considered. Prolonged EEGs are useful when additional clarification of the epilepsy diagnosis

Table **23.2**   Physical Assessment

BODY SYSTEM	NORMAL FINDINGS	NOTABLE FINDINGS	RATIONALE
Head, eyes, ears, nose, throat	Atraumatic, normocephalic with moist mucous membranes with neck supple	Microcephaly Macrocephaly	Abnormal head size/shape may indicate underlying structural abnormalities
Heart	Regular rhythm and rate; no murmurs or additional sounds	Abnormal rate/rhythm, murmurs	Underlying cardiac abnormalities may result in syncope, a common seizure mimic
Abdomen	Soft, nontender and nondistended	Organomegaly	May be associated with metabolic storage disease
Skin	No erythema or skin rash; no hyper- or hypopigmentation	Hamartomas, six or more café-au-lait spots, intertriginous freckles, portwine stain	Multiple neurocutaneous syndromes associated with seizures
Neurologic examination	Awake, alert, and oriented to place and people Speech clear/age appropriate Cranial nerves 2–12 intact with pupils equal, round, and reactive to light Extraocular movements intact with grossly intact facial sensations and grossly intact hearing Face symmetric with palate symmetrically upgoing and tongue midline Can move tongue side to side Optic fundi revealed sharp optic discs and normal venous pulsations	Alterations in cognition, speech Abnormalities in cranial nerves	Abnormalities in the neurologic examination may help identify focality, structural abnormality, or etiology
Motor	Normal tone and muscle bulk with normal and symmetric strength bilaterally Sensations were grossly intact for tactile and painful stimulations Deep tendon reflexes were 2+ throughout over brachioradialis, biceps, patellae, Achilles tendons, with toes downgoing bilaterally on plantar reflex Reaching for objects without signs of dysmetria or past pointing No ataxia or tremors Normal base and stance for age Can tandem walk heel/toe walk without problem Negative Romberg test	Hypo/hypertonia, abnormalities in movement, and hyper/hyporeflexia	Tone and motor abnormalities indicate underlying neurologic dysfunction and may indicate etiology or risk for additional seizures

Box **23.2**   **Electroencephalogram Considerations**

Are there fish in the pond?

If you ask me if there are fish in the pond, I may respond by saying, "let's go fishing and find out." If we fish for 30 minutes and don't come up with anything, that doesn't mean there are no fish in the pond.

Maybe we didn't use the right bait, we weren't in the right spot, or we didn't give the fish enough time. On the other hand, if we catch a fish, all we can say with confidence is that there was one fish, not that there are more.

Electroencephalograms (EEGs) are similar to going fishing. An abnormal EEG, in the appropriate clinical context, can support a diagnosis of epilepsy but is only a snapshot in time. Conversely, a normal EEG does not rule out the possibility of seizures. Sometimes it is important to complete longer studies where seizures/events can be captured.

is required, to evaluate medication efficacy, and for localization of seizure onset for surgical planning. These studies may last several hours to weeks, based on the need of the study.

Due to the nature of the study, sedation is rarely used as it can falsely normalize an EEG. Therefore additional planning may be needed for children with sensory needs. The family can practice with a comb and have the child lie flat on a bed while brushing the hair. A cotton-tipped applicator can be used to gently rub the scalp, and a hairdryer can be blown on the head to mimic the sensations of electrode placement (Box 23.3).

Magnetic resonance imaging (MRI) of the brain is recommended for those with focal features during the seizure (including those with complex febrile seizures), focal findings on examination, or known focal

Box 23.3	Preparing a Patient for an Electroencephalogram

Glue or paste will be used to place electrodes.
Hair should be clean and dry.
Scalp should be free of nits or lice.
The patient may be directed to alter sleep prior to the study.
No trimming/shaving of hair is required.
Continue all medications unless directed otherwise.

epilepsy. This is important to evaluate for any structural abnormalities that may put the child at risk for seizures. These structural malformations may include congenital anomalies, stroke, mesial temporal sclerosis, or space-occupying lesions.

Genetic testing is not necessary for diagnosing epilepsy but is extremely valuable in evaluating the child's etiology, prognosis, and treatment planning. Genetics can aid in classifying a specific epilepsy syndrome, such as Dravet syndrome, which is associated with a mutation in the *SCN1A* gene. Some genetic etiologies of epilepsy require specific treatment, such as mutations associated with *SLC2A* that result in glucose transporter deficiency, requiring treatment with a ketogenic diet. Recommended genetic testing may vary based on presentation but typically include chromosomes, microarray, and exome or next-generation sequencing as available.

Additional testing may be needed for children with refractory epilepsy, particularly those being evaluated for epilepsy surgery. This may include functional MRI, neuropsychological evaluation, Wada, single-photon emission computed tomography scans, and magnetoencephalography. Testing for these children is individualized based on seizure focus and surgical planning needs.

EPILEPSY SYNDROMES

Epilepsy syndromes may involve multiple seizure types and have a variety of prognoses and other associated features. Syndromes are defined as "a characteristic cluster of clinical and EEG features, often supported by specific etiological findings" (Wirrell et al., 2021). These may have an age-dependent presentation and may be associated with resolution at specific ages. Given the age of onset association, these are typically grouped by the age of onset and further defined by seizure semiology (Wirrell et al., 2021). A wide spectrum of features and even etiology is also associated with some syndromes with a clinical diagnosis, such as Lennox-Gastaut syndrome. However, genetic epilepsy syndromes, such as frontal lobe epilepsy associated with a mutation at *CHRNA4*, are associated with a wide range of impairments. Further specifying epilepsy as a syndrome can help identify prognostic information but may also direct treatment. Table 23.3 outlines features of select epilepsy syndromes from the ILAE.

TREATMENT

Initiation of daily antiseizure medications should be considered for children following their second unprovoked seizure or based on EEG findings, those that meet the criteria for a diagnosis of epilepsy. Treatment following a single unprovoked seizure does not reduce the recurrence risk; therefore the risks outweigh the benefits in this case. Medications may be held if seizures remain rare in epilepsy syndrome with infrequent seizures, such as self-limited epilepsy with centrotemporal spikes (SeLECTS).

The treatment goals will vary based on etiology, seizure type, and epilepsy syndrome, with the typical goal being zero seizures and zero side effects. However, some children will continue to have seizures despite treatment with two or more appropriately chosen and dosed antiseizure medications. These children have refractory or drug-resistant epilepsy. The number of children with drug-resistant epilepsy varies, but based on a recent systemic review and meta-analysis is reported at 25% of children with epilepsy (Sultana et al., 2021). For these children, while the goal is still improved seizure control, a larger focus shifts to quality of life and balance between medication side effects and seizures. In addition, while medications are still utilized in this population, consideration should be given to nonpharmacologic treatment, which will be discussed later.

Medications are chosen based on seizure types and epilepsy syndrome (Table 23.4). In addition, consideration is given to the mechanism of action when utilizing polypharmacy to maximize benefit. While many medications have US Food and Drug Administration (FDA) indications in pediatrics, off-label usage by epilepsy providers may be based on the most recent literature. Dosing ranges will also change based on updated guidelines and literature and should be reviewed frequently.

Most seizure medications are titrated over several weeks; however, there are some exceptions, such as lamotrigine, which must be titrated over a longer period due to the risk of Stevens-Johnson syndrome. During the titration of medications it is important to monitor for medication side effects. Additionally, during this time, breakthrough seizures are not uncommon. Given the long half-life of many medications, it can take several days to weeks on a dose prior to assessing efficacy.

During medication titration, common side effects to assess include fatigue, nausea, and mood changes. Several antiseizure medications also have a warning regarding the risk of suicidal thoughts and behaviors, and patients should be monitored for worsening depression, suicidal thoughts or behavior, and mood changes.

It is recommended that children remain on medication until seizure free for approximately 2 years,

| Table **23.3** | Select Epilepsy Syndromes | | |

EPILEPSY SYNDROME	TYPICAL AGE OF ONSET	COMMON FEATURES	CLINICAL COURSE
Self-limited epilepsy with centrotemporal spikes (previously known as benign Rolandic)	School age, 4–12 yr	Focal seizures in sleep, typically within hours of falling asleep or waking Infrequent seizures	Seizures typically resolve by puberty
Self-limited epilepsy with autonomic seizures (previously known as Panayiotopoulos syndrome)	3–6 yr	One-quarter will only have one seizure Seizures characterized by retching, vomiting, flushing, abdominal pain	Resolves typically within 3 yr of onset
Epilepsy with eyelid myoclonia (previously known as Jeavons syndrome)	6–8 yr	Frequent eyelid myoclonia with or without absence seizures, induced by eye closer and photic zone Tonic-clonic seizures not uncommon	Commonly drug resistant, but tonic-clonic seizures improve with medications
Epilepsy with myoclonic atonic seizures (previously known as Doose syndrome)	2–6 yr	Males more commonly Myoclonic-atonic is primary seizure feature	Seizures are commonly drug resistant but improve after 3 yr for majority Due to atonic seizures, may require a helmet for safety
Lennox-Gastaut syndrome	3–5 yr	Multiple drug-resistant seizures, one of which must be tonic Cognitive and behavioral impairments Specific electroencephalogram (EEG) findings (diffuse slow spike-and-wave and generalized paroxysmal fast activity)	Wide range of etiologies from genetic to structural Syndrome is defined as drug-resistant epilepsy Children typically have a significant disability
Childhood absence epilepsy	4–10 yr	Frequent absence seizures Generalized spike-wave seen on EEG with hyperventilation-induced seizures	Majority (60%) will resolve by puberty
Juvenile myoclonic epilepsy	10–24 years	Myoclonic seizures, worse upon waking Generalized tonic-clonic seizures common Generalized spike-wave on EEG may have photic-induced myoclonic seizures	Many have a history of febrile seizures Commonly need lifelong treatment of seizures
Infantile epileptic spasms syndrome	1–24 mo (may occur later and would be known as epileptic spasms)	Flexor, extensor, or mixed epileptic spasms Seizures occur in clusters, commonly upon waking Development regression/slowing after onset	Extensive testing recommended to determine etiology Frequently evolves into other epilepsy, particularly Lennox-Gastaut

Modified from Hirsch, E., French, J., Scheffer, I., et al. (2022). ILAE definition of the idiopathic generalized epilepsy syndromes: Position statement by the ILAE Task Force on Nosology and Definitions. *Epilepsia, 63,* 1475–1499; Specchio, N., Wirrell, E., Scheffer, I., et al. (2022). International League Against Epilepsy classification and definition of epilepsy syndromes with onset in childhood: Position paper by the ILAE Task Force on Nosology and Definitions. *Epilepsia, 63,* 1398–1442; Zuberi, S.M., Wirrell, E., Yozawitz, E., et al. (2022). ILAE classification and definition of epilepsy syndromes with onset in neonates and infants: Position statement by the ILAE Task Force on Nosology and Definitions. *Epilepsia, 63,* 1349–1397.

although recommendations may vary in cases where etiology is known. For example, a child with childhood absence epilepsy who has gone through puberty may be considered for early weaning given the typical offset of this syndrome. Of those who have been seizure free for 2 years, 60% to 75% will remain seizure free when medications are discontinued (Gloss et al., 2021). The highest risk for the recurrence of seizures is within the first 6 months, when approximately half of the recurrence occurs. It is important to note that

in rare instances, seizure recurrence after medication weaning can develop drug-resistant epilepsy (Gloss et al., 2021). Careful counseling of these risks is important when considering medication weaning.

In addition to daily medications, children with epilepsy should have a plan in place in the event of a prolonged seizure or prolonged cluster of seizures. While there is no standard definition for a seizure cluster, this typically represents an increase in seizure frequency above baseline or repetitive brief seizures occurring

Table 23.4   Daily Medications

MEDICATION	INDICATION	PROPOSED MECHANISM OF ACTION	DOSAGE RANGE	SIDE EFFECT PROFILE	CONSIDERATIONS
Adrenocorticotropic hormone	Monotherapy for epileptic spasms age <2 yr	Increases cortisol secretion	7.5 IU/m² IM BID × 2 wk, then taper	Increased risk for infections, adrenal insufficiency, Cushing syndrome, decreased growth, gastric ulcers, bleeding, weight gain, behavior/mood disturbances	Do not administer with live or live attenuated vaccines Caution in children with cardiac abnormalities
Brivaracetam	Focal epilepsy age ≥4 yr	Inhibits synaptic vesicle SV2A protein	25–100 mg BID	Sedation, nausea/vomiting, dizziness, suicidal thoughts, anger, psychosis	Interacts with enzyme-inducing medications
Cannabidiol	Seizures associated with Lennox-Gastaut syndrome (LGS) or Dravet age ≥2 yr	Unclear	10–20 mg/kg/day divided BID	Somnolence, sedation, decreased appetite, weight loss, diarrhea, rash	Monitor with medications utilizing CYP3A4 or 2C19 pathways Commitment use with clobazam will result in increased plasma levels of clobazam Artisanal formulation of cannabidiol is not biopharmaceutically equivalent
Carbamazepine	Focal epilepsy, generalized tonic-clonic seizures	Enhance rapid inactivation of sodium (Na+) channels	2 mg/kg/day divided BID, max dose 2400 mg daily	Sedation, diplopia, ataxia, dizziness, blurred vision, hyponatremia, nausea, vomiting	Enzyme inducer, monitor interactions with other medications Risk for Stevens-Johnson syndrome (SJS) and drug reaction with eosinophilia and systemic symptoms (DRESS)
Cenobamate	Focal epilepsy in adults	Inhibits voltage-gated sodium channels, a positive allosteric modulator of GABA_A ion channels	200–400 mg once daily	QT shortening, dizziness, fatigue, headache, ataxia	Moderate CYP2C19 inhibitor Risk for DRESS
Clobazam	Adjunctive treatment of seizures associated with LGS in age ≥2 yr	GABA_A receptor agonist	≤30 kg 5 mg BID–10 mg BID >30 kg up to 20 mg BID	Sedation, fever, upper respiratory infection, drooling, constipation, insomnia, irritability	SJS reported Cannabidiol inhibits metabolism
Clonazepam	LGS, myoclonic, absence seizures	GABA_A receptor agonist	≤30 kg = 0.1–0.2 mg/kg/day divided TID >30 kg maximum daily dose 20 mg/day	Sedation, dizziness, drooling, respiratory depression, anger, irritability	May impact tone in children with an underlying hypotonia
Eslicarbazepine acetate	Focal seizures, ≥4 yr	Enhances Na+ rapid inactivation; blocks HCav3.2, calcium (Ca²⁺); enhance potassium (K+) conductance	11–21 kg = 400–600 mg/day 22–31 kg = 500–800 mg/day 31–38 kg = 600–900 mg/day 39+ kg = 800–1600 mg/day	Hyponatremia, dizziness, sedation, headache, ataxia, tremor	Risk for SJS

Table 23.4 Daily Medications—cont'd

MEDICATION	INDICATION	PROPOSED MECHANISM OF ACTION	DOSAGE RANGE	SIDE EFFECT PROFILE	CONSIDERATIONS
Ethosuximide	Absence	Impacts slow T-Ca^{2+} thalamic current	20 mg/kg/day Adult: 1500 mg divided BID or TID	Nausea, vomiting, abdominal pain, weight loss, sedation, decreased white blood cells	Risk for SJS, DRESS Monitor complete blood count (CBC) and comprehensive metabolic panel (CMP)
Everolimus	Adjunctive for tuberous sclerosis focal seizures in age ≥2 yr	mTOR inhibitor	Initial: 5 mg/m^2 daily, then titrated based on drug levels	Stomatitis, infection, thrombocytopenia, neutropenia	Monitor other antiepileptic drugs (clobazam, carbamazepine, oxcarbazepine)
Felbamate	Refractory focal epilepsy and LGS in age ≥2 yr	Enhance Na^+ inactivation, blocks Ca^{2+}, inhibits NMDA, potentiates, $GABA_A$	45–60 mg/kg/day Divided BID or TID Max dose 1200 mg TID	Headache, insomnia, anorexia, anxiety, tremor	Risk for aplastic anemia; monitor CBC and CMP Hepatic enzyme inhibitor will require adjustments to carbamazepine, phenytoin, phenobarbital, or valproic acid
Fenfluramine	Seizures associated with Dravet syndrome or LGS age ≥2 yr	Unknown increase extracellular serotonin, agonist of the 5HT-2 receptor	0.4–0.7 mg/kg/day divided twice daily Maximum daily dose 26 mg/day	Aortic insufficiency, mitral valve insufficiency, weight loss, anorexia, diarrhea, drowsiness	Dose adjustments for patients on stiripentol Restricted use by risk evaluation and mitigation strategy (REMS) due to risk for valvular heart disease
Gabapentin	Adjunctive for focal seizures age ≥3 yr	Ca^{2+} modulation decreases glutamate	Age 3–4 yr: 40 mg/kg/day divided TID Age 5–11 yr: 25–35 mg/kg/day divided TID Age ≥12 yr: 600 mg TID	Drowsiness, sedation, ataxia, dizziness	Risk for DRESS and neuropsychiatric changes
Lacosamide	Focal seizures ≥1 month Adjunctive generalized tonic-clonic age ≥4 yr	Enhances Na^+ slow inactivation	6–12 mg/kg/day 200 mg BID maximum	Dizziness, ataxia, diplopia, headache, prolonged PR	Risk for cardiac arrhythmias, SJS, and DRESS
Lamotrigine	Focal seizures age ≥16 yr Adjunctive for LGS, focal, tonic-clonic in age ≥2 yr	Enhances Na^+ slow inactivation Inhibits Ca^{2+}, activates postsynaptic HCN	5–15 mg/kg/day divided BID Range varied by serum levels	Dizziness, headache, diplopia, nausea	Dosing adjustments are needed when used with valproic acid and with enzyme inducers Risk for SJS
Levetiracetam	Focal ≥1 mo, adjunctive myoclonic, juvenile myoclonic epilepsy age 12 yr, tonic-clonic age ≥6 yr	Inhibits synaptic vesicle SV2A	30–50 mg/kg/day divided BID 3000 mg/day maximum	Fatigue, irritability, psychosis, ataxia	Medication should be discontinued for significant behavioral changes
Methsuximide	Refractory absence	Slow T-Ca^{2+} thalamic currents	5–30 mg/kg/day divided BID-TID 1200 mg/day maximum	Nausea, vomiting, abdominal pain, anorexia, ataxia	Risk for SJS, DRESS Monitor CBC and CMP

Continued

Table 23.4	Daily Medications—cont'd				
MEDICATION	**INDICATION**	**PROPOSED MECHANISM OF ACTION**	**DOSAGE RANGE**	**SIDE EFFECT PROFILE**	**CONSIDERATIONS**
Oxcarbazepine	Focal seizures age ≥4 yr, adjunctive age ≥2 yr	Enhances Na+ inactivation	20–45 mg/kg/day divided BID 2400 mg BID	Dizziness, nausea, headache, hyponatremia	Risk for SJS CYP3A4 inducer
Perampanel	Focal seizures and adjunctive for tonic-clonic age ≥12 yr	Selective noncompetitive antagonist AMPA glutamate	4–12 mg daily	Dizziness, somnolence, fatigue, aggression, anger	Homicidal ideation reported
Phenobarbital	Focal and generalized seizures	Nonspecific GABAA receptor binding	5–8 mg/kg/day	Sedation, cognitive slowing, headache, depression, confusion, hepatic dysfunction	Risk for SJS, DRESS Strong CYP3A4 inducer Monitor CBC and CMP levels
Phenytoin	Focal and generalized seizures	Enhances rapid inactivation of Na+	5–9 mg/kg/day	Nystagmus, ataxia, dysarthria, cognitive slowing	Risk for SJS Monitor medication interactions
Pregabalin	Adjunctive focal seizures ≥1 mo	Presynaptic Ca2+	2.5–14 mg/kg/day Not to exceed 600 mg daily	Dizziness, dry mouth, edema, somnolence	Risk for angioedema
Rufinamide	Adjunctive for LGS age ≥1 yr	Enhances Na+ rapid inactivation	10–45 mg/kg/day divided BID Max 3200 mg/day	Leukopenia, shortening of QT, dizziness	Risk for DRESS CYP3A4 inducer
Stiripentol	Adjunctive treatment of seizures associated with Dravet syndrome age ≥2 yr	Unknown, may impact GABAA	50–100 mg/kg/day divided BID Max 4000 mg/day	Drowsiness, agitation, nausea, neutropenia, weight loss	Adolescents may need lower dosing Monitor CBC and CMP
Tiagabine	Adjunctive focal seizures age ≥12 yr	Selective GABA reuptake inhibitor	32–56 mg/day divided BID	Dizziness, nausea, vomiting, somnolence, fatigue, tremor, cognitive slowing	Higher doses when on enzyme inducers May worsen generalized seizures
Topiramate	Focal and generalized tonic-clonic age ≥2 yr, adjunctive for LGS age ≥2 yr	Inhibits Na+ channels, carbonic anhydrase inhibitor	5–12 mg/kg/day divided BID Max 400 mg/day	Paresthesia, anorexia, weight loss, speech and cognitive disturbances, fatigue, hypohidrosis	Risk for acute myopia with secondary angle closure glaucoma
Valproic acid	Focal and absence age ≥10 yr, mixed seizure types adjunctive	Inhibits Na+ channels and Ca2+	25–60 mg/kg/day divided BID	Hyperammonemia, encephalopathy, thrombocytopenia, somnolence, abdominal pain, alopecia, dizziness	Monitor for hepatotoxicity Risk for DRESS Monitor valproic acid levels
Vigabatrin	Epileptic spasms 1 mo–2 yr Refractory focal epilepsy adjunctive age ≥2 yr	Inhibits GABA	Epileptic spasms: 150 mg/kg/day divided BID Focal: 20–60 mg/kg/day Max 2000 mg BID	Somnolence, nystagmus, tremor, tremor, ataxia,	Restricted use by REMS due to the risk of peripheral vision loss Abnormal magnetic resonance imaging signal changes
Zonisamide	Adjunctive for focal seizures age ≥16 yr	Inhibits Na+ channels, carbonic anhydrase inhibitor	400–600 mg/day *Limited evidence for doses >400 mg	Somnolence, fatigue, anorexia, weight loss, dizziness, kidney stones	Risk for SJS, DRESS

BID, 2 times/day; *GABA*, gamma-aminobutyric acid; *HCN*, hyperpolarization-activated cyclic nucleotide gated; *NMDA*, N-methyl-D-aspartate; *TID*, 3 times/day.
Data from Lexicomp. (2022). Pediatric and neonatal Lexi-drugs online, from UpToDate, Inc.

Table 23.5 | **Commonly Used Medications for Rescue Therapy**

MEDICATION	ROUTE	ONSET	AGE	DOSE WEIGHT (KG)	DOSE MG
Diazepam	Rectal	5–30 min	2–5 yr (0.5 mg/kg)	6–10	5
				11–15	7.5
				16–20	10
				21–25	12.5
				26–30	15
				31–35	17.5
				36–44	20
			6–11 yr (0.3 mg/kg)	10–16	5
				17–25	7.5
				26–33	10
				34–41	12.5
				42–50	15
				51–58	17.5
				59–74	20
			≥12 yr	14–25	5
				26–37	7.5
				38–50	10
				51–62	12.5
				63–75	15
				76–87	17.5
				88–111	20
	Intranasal	3–5 min	6–11 yr	10–18.9	5
				19–37.9	7.5
				38–55.9	15
				56–74	20
			≥12 yr	14–27.9	5
				28–51	7.5
				51–75.9	15
				≥76	20
Midazolam	Intranasal	3–5min	≥12 yr	5 mg nasal, may repeat in 10 min if seizure does not abate	
Clonazepam	Buccal	Up to 15 min		"Height of Man Rule" (Troester et al., 2010) Crawling child: 0.25 mg Knee height as compared to adult: 0.5 mg Waist height as compared to adult or <50 kg: 1 mg Shoulder height as compared to adult or >50 kg: 2 mg	

Data from Lexicomp. (2022). Pediatric and neonatal Lexi-drugs online, from UpToDate, Inc.

over 20 minutes. There are clearer guidelines for treating a prolonged seizure; commonly, 5 minutes is the threshold at which medications are administered. All emergency medications should be tailored to the individual child, seizure history, and previous response to emergency medications.

Benzodiazepines are used as rescue therapy for children experiencing prolonged seizures or seizure clusters. Formulation, route, and dose should be carefully considered based on age, weight, history of status epilepticus, and previous response to medications (Table 23.5).

In addition to medications, there are several non-pharmacologic treatments for epilepsy. While these are traditionally considered for children with drug-resistant epilepsy, they may also be considered first-line treatment for some epilepsy etiologies or syndromes. Non-pharmacologic therapies include epilepsy surgery and diet therapy.

SURGICAL

Epilepsy surgery may be considered for children with medication-resistant epilepsy or those with focal onset epilepsy. While it may be considered earlier in children with structural abnormalities or space-occupying lesions on MRI, it can be considered for a number of children with focal epilepsy, even when the MRI is found to be normal. Surgeries can be described in several ways, but perhaps the best way to discuss them is to divide them into the intention to cure epilepsy or as a palliative measure.

Curative surgeries are resections, typically of one seizure focus, with the reasonable belief that it will result in the cessation of seizures. The goal is seizure free and eventually to wean off medications. Lesionectomoy is utilized when there is a localized area of the seizure focus. These may be seen on MRI or only under microscopy and involve a range of causes, including focal cortical dysplasia, low-grade tumors, and vascular malformations (Dallas et al., 2020). Results of lesionectomy are variable based on location and lesion. Another common epilepsy surgery is a temporal lobectomy, most commonly the anterior temporal lobectomy. This is beneficial for children with temporal lobe epilepsy and can be achieved with several different surgical techniques, including some minimally invasive techniques. Temporal lobectomy has positive surgical outcomes, with 76% being seizure free after surgery (Dallas et al., 2020). While temporal lobe epilepsy is most common in adults, extratemporal epilepsy is more common in children. Outcomes from extratemporal resection are lower and varied based on location. Extratemporal resections are more likely to be limited by the eloquent cortex, resulting in incomplete resection of the epileptogenic zone and suboptimal response to surgery. For some children, a hemispheric resection or disconnection may be recommended for seizure control. While there are different approaches and techniques to hemispherotomy, these are typically discussed as anatomic hemispherectomy, full resection of the hemisphere, versus functional hemispherotomy, where disconnection is complete but some structures remain intact, which may reduce complications (Dallas et al., 2020). Surgical success is commonly graded on the Engle classification, which describes seizure reduction and surgical outcomes.

Palliative surgeries cross a number of surgical interventions, including resections, callosotomy, and neuromodulation. Any curative surgery procedure can be considered palliative in the case of a child with multiple seizure foci or multiple seizure types, where surgery may be focused on just one seizure type or seizure reduction. In addition, corpus callosotomy is often considered for those with atonic or other drop seizures (Dallas et al., 2020). For these children, seizures often cause significant injury, and corpus callosotomy can reduce seizures significantly, with 55.3% becoming free of drop seizures following surgery (Dallas et al., 2020).

Another umbrella under palliative surgery is neuromodulation. This is a growing field and includes the utilization of vagus nerve stimulation (VNS), responsive nerve stimulation (RNS), and deep brain stimulation (DBS). Despite the breadth of neuromodulation used, little is known about the mechanism of action, although it is believed that the stimulation may increase activity in the nucleus tractus solitarius, causing increases in norepinephrine and serotonin (Starnes et al., 2019). The risks and benefits of each neuromodulation option vary based on center and technique, but reported infection rates for VNS are the lowest and range from 3% to 9% (Panov et al., 2020). In comparison, DBS placement for epilepsy has infection rates reported at 12.7%, with 7% requiring explanation (Panov et al., 2020).

VNS is the oldest type of neuromodulation for epilepsy, having been approved in 1997 for intractable focal epilepsy (Starnes et al., 2019). Since then, it has been utilized for children with various seizures, including generalized seizures. VNS has several modes that help reduce seizures. Programming can be completed in the neurology office by a trained nurse or provider, and the varying modes are adjusted based on seizure types and needs. VNS has a maintenance mode that provides a scheduled stimulation onto the vagus nerve at programmed intervals.

Additionally, for some patients, an autostimulation feature can be utilized that will trigger a stimulation when the heart rate reaches a preprogrammed increase from baseline, helping abort seizure activity. The final mode is the magnet mode, triggered by either the patient or caretaker swiping a strong magnet over the device, triggering a more intense impulse to stop seizure activity. Not all patients will use all the modes of the device based on seizure activity; for example, someone with nonmotor seizures is unlikely to trigger the autostimulation because there is rarely a heart rate change associated with these seizures.

RNS varies from VNS as it responds to changes in EEG and does not provide a maintenance dosing stimulation. This device is paired with intracranial EEGs that monitor activity and, following programming, detect seizure activity. The stimulation is then provided in that localized region by the device. Unlike VNS, which widely provides stimulation, RNS utilizes small electrodes to stimulate the seizure focus. This provides a unique opportunity for prolonged EEG monitoring of seizure foci in patients with epilepsy. RNS is currently FDA approved to be used as adjunctive therapy in adults with refractory focal epilepsy. Its use in pediatrics remains off-label; however, evidence continues to grow regarding its safety and utilization in this population. Special consideration has been given to placement as RNS is placed into the outer skull table. Therefore skull size and thickness changes must be considered for appropriate placement in pediatrics. Early data on RNS placement demonstrate improvement in seizures, with 13% achieving a greater than 90% improvement in seizures and 35% having a greater than 50% improvement in seizures (Nagahama et al., 2021).

DBS, similar to RNS, is FDA approved for adults with refractory epilepsy. DBS involves stimulation of the anterior nucleus of the thalamus for seizure reduction. Stimulation is provided at programmed intervals without responsive or seizure-abortive options. This population has demonstrated an average seizure reduction of 69% (Starnes et al., 2019). The most common adverse events with DBS implantation include implantation site pain (23.6%), paresthesias (22.7%), and site infection (12.7%) (Salanova et al., 2015). DBS adverse events are notable for depression, even in patients without a prior history, as well as suicidal ideation. While these may be multifactorial, they are important considerations when counseling patients on their treatment options.

Patients with RNS or VNS may still undergo MRI, although some restrictions and recommendations do apply.

Expected recovery from epilepsy surgery is varied, but for children with resective surgeries, school accommodations will likely be needed as they recover. Some medication changes may be made initially, but many children will continue without changes in their medications for 3 to 6 months postsurgical procedure to reduce any kindling of remaining epileptogenic zones. Neurologic deficits may be expected in some epilepsy surgeries, and these risks are discussed in depth with the family before surgery. For example, hemiplegia is an expected outcome following hemispherotomy, but in the setting of Rasmussen epilepsy (progressive epilepsy), if the epilepsy is left untreated the child will sustain hemiplegia and continued seizures.

Evaluation for epilepsy surgery may be extensive based on seizures, surgical planning, EEG findings, and neuropsychological evaluations. Overall, the goal of evaluation is to determine surgical planning and possible surgical outcomes. Some children may undergo several stages of surgery based on their testing outcomes.

There are significant disparities noted in the evaluation and completion of epilepsy surgery in pediatrics. These are not limited to access, although it is noted that access to a large epilepsy center that completes complex surgeries is a significant limitation. Families with limited English proficiency report a longer wait time for surgery, nearly four times as compared to those with English proficiency (Armour et al., 2021). In addition, even when adjusting for sociodemographic factors, Black patients with epilepsy are less likely to obtain surgery (Armour et al., 2021). In addition to racial and ethnic disparities, disparities exist based on socioeconomic status. Children with public insurance are less likely to undergo epilepsy surgery (Armour et al., 2021).

KETOGENIC DIET

The ketogenic diet is a medically prescribed diet that results in the child utilizing dietary fat as the primary energy source, also known as ketosis. The ketogenic diet used for epilepsy therapy should not be confused with the ketogenic diet utilized by the public for weight loss, as these are not interchangeable. While there are some differences in how sugar alcohols may be counted, the goals and structure are markedly different.

This therapy is considered for children with refractory epilepsy, those with epilepsy syndrome known to be responsive to the ketogenic diet, or those with GLUT1 transporter deficiency, for whom the ketogenic diet is the recommended primary therapy (Kossoff et al., 2018). While the mechanism of action of the ketogenic diet is not fully understood, it is believed to work in several ways to reduce both the frequency of seizures and epileptic discharges in the brain (Martin et al., 2016). The ketogenic diet is typically an adjunctive therapy to reduce the frequency of seizures; in some children, medication discontinuation may be possible, but most will continue on antiseizure medications.

The ketogenic diet is a strict diet where children are required to eat a portion of carbohydrates, fat, and protein at each meal in accordance with their prescription. A ketogenic diet can be used for children who eat by mouth and tube feeding (gastrostomy, nasogastric, or jejunostomy). This requires families to carefully weigh or measure out components of their meals and snacks. Each meal or snack is maintained in the same ratio. The restrictive nature of the diet requires close supervision by a skilled team, including ketogenic dietitians. This team will also recommend supplements to meet daily needs, including a multivitamin, vitamin D, and calcium (Kossoff et al., 2018). Routine labs monitor side effects, including hyperlipidemia, acidosis, and osteopenia. Urine ketones may be monitored at home to assess for adequate ketosis.

For children on a ketogenic diet, all sources of carbohydrates are monitored. This includes all other medications, specifically liquid medications that commonly contain a significant amount of carbohydrates. Therefore, for children on the ketogenic diet, most medications will be transitioned to low carbohydrate forms, specifically tablets, to reduce the carbohydrates per day. This includes over-the-counter medications, such as acetaminophen and antibiotics, even if only used for a short duration.

Adverse effects of the ketogenic diet are experienced by up to 50% of children, including constipation, emesis, and abdominal pain (Kossoff et al., 2018). Constipation management and adequate hydration can be important to adherence to the ketogenic diet. Additional side effects include hyperlipidemia, renal calculi, abnormal growth, cardiac abnormalities, osteopenia, and pancreatitis.

The ketogenic diet may be discontinued based on patient response and quality of life, but it is recommended that children without apparent improvement after 6 months be considered for discontinuation (Kossoff et al., 2018). For those with significant improvement, weaning or discontinuing the diet may be considered after 2 years or longer based on their response and consideration for side effects and epilepsy etiology (Kossoff et al., 2018).

COMORBIDITIES

Seizures are just one component of managing patients with epilepsy as they deal with a number of comorbid conditions. Using the example of an iceberg is very well suited to epilepsy diagnosis, where the visible portion of the iceberg is the seizures and the multiple challenges, including comorbid conditions, that children and their families must face. It is important to treat epilepsy with this in mind to work and improve the quality of life for those impacted.

SUDDEN UNEXPECTED DEATH IN EPILEPSY

Sudden unexpected death in epilepsy (SUDEP) is a significant cause of mortality for children with epilepsy. SUDEP is defined as the "sudden, unexpected, witnessed, or unwitnessed, nontraumatic, and nondrowning death in patients with epilepsy, with or without evidence for seizures, and excluding documented status epilepticus in which postmortem examination does not reveal a toxicological or anatomical cause for death" (Maguire et al., 2016). The incidence reported is variable based on studies; however, it is consistently reported to occur at a lower frequency than in adults. Most recently, the risk of SUDEP for children was reported at 0.22/1000 patient-years (95% confidence interval) (Harden et al., 2017).

While the exact mechanism is poorly understood, the proposed mechanisms are cardiac, respiratory, or central/autonomic dysregulation, likely following a seizure (Ryvlin et al., 2013). Those deemed at the highest risk are those with poorly controlled tonic-clonic seizures in sleep; however, it is important to note that any person with epilepsy is at risk for SUDEP (Sveinsson et al., 2020). In addition, those with intellectual disabilities and intractable epilepsy are also at higher risk for SUDEP. Investigation into genetic predispositions has yet to demonstrate a single gene that may contribute to SUDEP risk (Abdel-Mannan et al., 2019).

SUDEP prevention is focused mainly on reducing risks, including improved seizure control and medication adherence. Additional mechanisms to manage seizures should be considered, including VNS and the ketogenic diet. Persons with epilepsy should be encouraged to avoid sleeping in a prone position, as this has been associated with an increased risk (Shmuely et al., 2016). In addition, items that may increase the risk of suffocation, such as stuffed animals, should be removed from the bed. Nighttime supervision has been associated with a reduced risk of SUDEP (Sveinsson et al., 2020). When near-SUDEP has occurred, and cardiopulmonary resuscitation is initiated quickly, patients have been successfully resuscitated, underlying the importance of discussing with families and reviewing emergency action plans (Wicker & Cole, 2021). While some wearable monitoring devices are available, these have not yet demonstrated a significantly decreased risk for SUDEP or near-SUDEP in pediatrics (Wicker & Cole, 2021). All patients with epilepsy should be carefully counseled on the risk for SUDEP as well as prevention measures that are most applicable to them.

MENTAL HEALTH

Mental health is a significant factor for children with epilepsy. The umbrella of mental health disorders is broad, but here we will talk about some of the most common diagnoses for children and youth with epilepsy. This includes depression, anxiety, ADHD, and functional neurologic disorder. Overall, the increased risk for these disorders is present even when seizures are well controlled, and regular assessment or screening should be done for all children with epilepsy.

A negative perception of epilepsy and mental health by the patient and family has also been associated with an increased risk for depression as well as the patient's willingness to obtain mental health services (Dunn et al., 1999; Vona et al., 2009). Providing families with routine education about mental health and available services may positively improve their attitude toward mental health (Vona et al., 2009).

Depression and Anxiety

As with other mental health comorbidities, depression in this population represents a complex and multifaceted disorder that is impacted by patients' underlying neurologic disorder, the social stigma associated with epilepsy, patient perception of seizures, seizure frequency, and the impact of antiepileptic drugs on suicidal ideation and mood changes. It is important to note that while depression can negatively impact the quality of life, it can also impact seizure control, resulting in those experiencing depression having a higher risk for breakthrough seizures (Guilfoyle et al., 2015).

Adolescents with epilepsy have higher rates of depression as compared to their peers without epilepsy (Engel et al., 2021). Frequency varies, but one study looking at anxiety and depressive symptoms in youth with epilepsy demonstrated that 36% of those with epilepsy had symptoms of depression or anxiety (Engel et al., 2021). Implementation of standardized depression screening identified that 15% of patients with epilepsy, able to participate in self-report screenings, had results consistent with a likely depression diagnosis (Fecske et al., 2020). The reported frequency is likely low due to inconsistent screening and multiple tools utilized in the literature. Depression is also a significant risk factor for suicide, with one study reporting that 11.9% of patients with epilepsy and depression had suicidal ideation within the past 2 weeks (Hecimovic et al., 2012). For patients with epilepsy, diagnosis of depression is made more difficult as many side effects of seizure medications may mimic symptoms of depression, specifically fatigue, sleep disturbance, and mood lability (Kanner et al., 2012).

Routine screening tools and practice guidelines are recommended to support identifying depression in adolescents (Zuckerbrot et al., 2018). While several screening tools may be utilized, including Patient Health Questionnaire-2 (PHQ-2) and PHQ-9, consideration should be given to the utilization of a population-specific screening tool, such as Neurological Disorders Depression Inventory for Epilepsy (NDDI-E) and its youth counterpart NDDI-E-Y. These tools screen for depressive symptoms in patients with epilepsy while reducing the impact medication side effects, specifically fatigue and appetite changes, may have on screening (Wagner et al., 2016). In addition, NDDI-E-Y, as well as the PHQ-9, screen for suicidality. Given the increased risk for suicidality in patients with epilepsy, 1.8-fold increase, choosing a tool that screens for suicidality is important (Hesdorffer et al., 2016). Those screened as positive for suicidal thoughts or those at risk of harm should complete a safety evaluation and safety planning at the time of screening.

For those with epilepsy and depression, consider appropriate treatment based on the Guidelines for Adolescent Depression in Primary Care (GLAD-PC). Cognitive-behavioral therapy (CBT) should be utilized where available. GLAD-PC recommended fluoxetine as a first-line treatment for depression, and evidence demonstrates no increase in seizures for those with epilepsy (Cheung et al., 2018). Bupropion should be avoided in this population as it increases the risk of seizures. Notable barriers to accessing mental health care for children and youth with epilepsy include accessing CBT, patient resistance, and lack of appropriately trained therapists (Gandy et al., 2021). This may explain why more children are started on medication rather than receiving the recommended CBT.

Children with epilepsy have been reported to experience higher anxiety rates than those peers of the same age (Wang et al., 2019). It is important to assess if anxiety is periictal versus interictal to provide appropriate treatment. Anxiety associated with seizure activity, particularly noted for those with temporal lobe epilepsy, will need to be addressed in conjunction with seizures. However, interictal anxiety may persist despite seizure control and must be managed independently. Interictal anxiety may present in several different ways. Specifically, generalized anxiety, separation anxiety, social anxiety, and panic disorder may be present in those with epilepsy (Table 23.6). As with depression, a number of screening tools can be utilized to assist in identifying those with anxiety. The Hospital Anxiety and Depression Scale and the Generalized Anxiety Disorder 7-Item Scale can be utilized to screen for anxiety; however, as with depression, it is beneficial to consider a population-specific screening tool (Wang et al., 2019).

Anxiety can be managed utilizing recommendations from the American Academy of Child and Adolescent Psychiatry (Walter et al., 2020). This includes CBT as well as pharmaceutical management. Care should be given to current medications, as benzodiazepines are often used as emergency medications in children with epilepsy.

While many screening tools require a child to report symptoms, it is important to assess for mental health comorbidities in children and youth with cognitive impairments. In most instances, parent reports or specific parental report screening tools may be utilized to screen this population.

ATTENTION-DEFICIT/HYPERACTIVITY DISORDER

Children with epilepsy have higher rates of ADHD, which is 2.54 times more common in children with epilepsy, without a significant gender bias (Auvin et al., 2018). In addition, ADHD is often underdiagnosed in this population as behavioral challenges and attention difficulties are attributed to epilepsy or seizures and not to a comorbid condition; however, these behavioral difficulties often predate seizure onset. In addition to epilepsy being a risk for ADHD development, children with frequent seizures or breakthrough seizures carry an increased risk for ADHD (Auvin et al., 2018). Routine screening for ADHD should be completed for all children with epilepsy.

It can be difficult for children with absence epilepsy to distinguish seizures from ADHD. Common features of inattention that are less likely to be absence seizures include events that occur more often during difficult tasks, less often seen during play, often noted by school/teachers, and children responsive to tactile stimulation (Auvin et al., 2018).

Valproic acid has been associated with increased attention issues, topiramate, and zonisamide, so careful consideration should be given to medication influence on attention issues (Auvin et al., 2018). While polytherapy has also been reported to be associated with an increased risk for attention issues, this is more likely related to the refractory nature of epilepsy that needs multiple medications and less likely related to the medications.

Much concern and debate have revolved around using stimulant medications in children with epilepsy, given that this medication has a presumed increased risk for seizures. Several studies have demonstrated that methylphenidate is likely safe in this population. One study (Brikell et al., 2019) looked at 995 individuals with ADHD and epilepsy, and seizure frequency was monitored pre- and poststimulant medication intervention with no statistically significant difference in seizure frequency reported. When a seizure increase was seen, it was often transient, rarely resulting in the discontinuation of medications (Auvin et al., 2018). Therefore seizure frequency should be monitored when starting any stimulant, and medication may be discontinued if an increase in seizures is noted, but stimulants can be used in this population for the treatment of ADHD.

Table 23.6	Diagnosis of Interictal Anxiety
INTERICTAL ANXIETIES	**FEATURES**
Generalized anxiety	Excessive anxiety not focused on a single trigger with symptoms present most days >6 mo with ≥3 of the following symptoms: • Restlessness • Easily fatigued • Difficulty concentrating • Irritability • Muscle tension • Sleep disturbance
Panic disorder with or without agoraphobia	Recurrent and unexpected panic attacks and ongoing fear of panic attacks Abrupt surge of intense fear/discomfort peaking within minutes and including ≥4 of the following symptoms: • Palpitations, pounding heart, or accelerated heart rate • Sweating • Trembling/shaking • Sensation of shortness of breath • Feeling of choking • Chest pain or discomfort • Nausea or abdominal distress • Feeling dizzy, unsteady, lightheaded, or faint • Derealization or depersonalization • Fear of losing control • Fear of dying • Paresthesia • Chills or hot flashes
Specific phobia	Fear or anxiety about the presence of a specific object or situation (i.e., seizures) present for ≥6 mo
Social phobia	Fear of social situations and perceived scrutiny from others occurring for ≥6 mo. Fear is out of proportion to the actual threat. May avoid situations out of fear.
Separation anxiety	Excessive fear, anxiety, or distress regarding separation from a place (home) or people lasting at least 4 wk in children. Includes ≥3 of the following: • Recurrent excessive distress when anticipating or experiencing separation from home or from major attachment figure • Persistent and excessive worry about losing major attachment figures or possible harm to them • Persistent and excessive worry about experiencing an untoward event that causes separation • Persistent reluctance or refusal to go out away from home, to school, to work, or elsewhere because of fear of separation • Persistent and excessive fear of or reluctance about being alone or without major attachment figures • Persistent reluctance or refusal to sleep away from home or to go to sleep without being near a major attachment figure • Repeated nightmares involving the theme of separation • Repeated complaints of physical symptoms when separation occurs or is anticipated

FUNCTIONAL NEUROLOGIC DISORDER

Functional neurologic disorder (FND), previously known as conversion disorder in the DSM-5, is associated with abnormal movements or alterations in awareness without associated changes on EEG. FND is a large diagnosis that can cover numerous abnormal movements; however, in relation to children with epilepsy, we will specifically focus on functional seizures. Many terms have been used to describe these; however, there are currently two accepted terms: psychogenic nonepileptic seizures and functional seizures. The terms pseudoseizure, hysterical seizure, and pseudoepileptic seizure are outdated and should no longer be used, as they carry a significant stigma. Significant misnomers exist about FND, particularly that this occurs in the setting of abuse history and that persons experiencing this disease are faking it. While this population has a high rate of positive adverse childhood experiences, this includes a wide range of challenges and cannot fully explain the development of FND (Pal et al., 2022). In addition, FND is distinct from malingering and factitious disorder, and it is important to note that these symptoms are not intentionally produced (Espay et al., 2018).

Functional seizures can be seen in children with and without epilepsy, with studies demonstrating that between 5% and 20% of those with functional seizures have epilepsy (Operto et al., 2019). For those children with epilepsy, care should be taken to differentiate the clinical features of their epileptic seizures versus functional seizures. Prolonged video EEG monitoring can be useful in having a better understanding of seizure types. The typical age of presentation ranges from 10 to 13 years and has female predominance (Operto et al., 2019). Children often present with several different functional seizure types, commonly with motor involvement (Operto et al., 2019).

For children with a seizure diagnosis, consideration should be given to FND when seizures do not respond to antiseizure medications or have features uncharacteristic of their epilepsy (e.g., reports of retained awareness with bilateral movements).

Diagnosis is made based on history, physical exam, testing, and several positive signs of FND. Treatment of FND relies on collaboration between neurology and psychiatry, specializing in the care of FND. CBT and behavioral-informed psychotherapy are recommended for FND (Espay et al., 2018). Comorbid anxiety and depression can also be treated pharmaceutically as needed.

For children with FND it is important that the family understand the diagnosis and treatment recommendations. Access to psychiatry services may be limited even further when considering specialists aware of FND. However, many patients have resolution of symptoms within a few months of diagnosis (Pal et al., 2022).

NEURODEVELOPMENTAL DISORDERS

Neurodevelopmental disorders are not uncommon in children with epilepsy, and these children should be regularly screened. Neurodevelopmental disorders include autism, learning disorders, auditory processing disorder, dyslexia, and cognitive impairment. This can be seen in children with drug-resistant epilepsy and well-controlled epilepsy; however, it is seen more commonly in children with the former (Eom et al., 2014). Therefore it is important to note that all children with epilepsy should be carefully monitored for neurodevelopmental disorders, regardless of their seizure control. The Ages and Stages Questionnaire, Modified Checklist for Autism in Toddlers, and Social Communication Questionnaire can be utilized to screen for developmental concerns (Eom et al., 2014). Children with abnormal screening should be referred to appropriate specialty care for additional support and interventions. Specialized neuropsychology testing may be utilized in children for whom screening does not provide an adequate picture or who continue to struggle despite current interventions.

SLEEP

Sleep problems are another common challenge in persons with epilepsy. This may be related to factors dependent on the child's epilepsy and etiology. However, nocturnal seizures may be associated with changes to sleep structures, increase nocturnal arousals, and cause daytime fatigue. Those with epilepsy are also at higher risk for obstructive sleep apnea, with 20% having the condition (Tsai et al., 2019). Antiseizure medications may also cause daytime fatigue, further disrupting expected sleep patterns for the child. In addition to the direct impact of epilepsy on their sleep, children with epilepsy experience a higher rate of sleep-associated anxiety that can cause delayed onset of sleep (Tsai et al., 2019).

Consideration should also be given to behavioral sleep disturbances in the family unit. Specifically, when counseling on SUDEP risk and recommendations for nocturnal supervision, help the family identify ways to support this without cosleeping or decreasing sleep quality for the child or caregivers.

For children with sleep complaints, consideration should be given to behavioral versus medical causes and appropriate referrals completed. Poor sleep can be associated with breakthrough seizures, so it is important to address these concerns.

INJURIES

Persons with epilepsy are at increased risk for injuries associated with their seizures. Risk varies based on the individual's seizure types, size, and activity levels. Injuries may include bruising, tooth fractures, shoulder dislocations, head injuries, drowning, and muscle strains. Following seizures, the child and caregiver must assess for injuries. Seizure precautions are recommended for children and youth with epilepsy to reduce the risk of injuries and to protect to the best of their ability.

Seizure precautions include avoidance of heights, driving restrictions (based on individual state laws), caution around heating elements and power tools, and supervision around water. While children with epilepsy typically shower independently, any baths or swimming should be supervised.

PRIMARY CARE MANAGEMENT

GROWTH AND DEVELOPMENT

Based on an epilepsy syndrome or specific diagnosis, you may be able to provide additional information to the family about expectations for growth and development. Both should be monitored closely, as changes to these may indicate a change in their epilepsy and should be communicated to their neurology provider.

Diet

Except for children on the ketogenic diet or other medically prescribed diet, no changes to diet are recommended for children with epilepsy. For children on the ketogenic diet, support family in the management, identification of side effects, and communication with other care team members about the diet's restrictions, needs, and purpose.

Seizure Action Plans

Ensure that all children with epilepsy have a seizure action plan. Their school, day care, and caregivers can utilize this to outline recommendations for seizure emergencies. A seizure action plan should include daily medications, typical seizure semiology, rescue medications, and indications of a seizure emergency. Seizure action plans should be reviewed and updated annually, with changes to their medication recommendations.

Seizure Restrictions

Participation in sports is a common question for children with epilepsy. Recommendations may vary based on the provider; overall, the ILAE has categorized sports into three activities based on risk: group 1 sports, with no significant risk; group 2 sports, with moderate risk to the person with epilepsy but not increased risk to bystanders; and group 3, with a high risk for the person with epilepsy and potential risk for bystanders (Capovilla et al., 2016). Sports in group 1 include most athletics, specifically wrestling, baseball, football, dancing, golf, and bowling. Group 2 includes activities with an increased risk of injury, such as cycling, gymnastics, ice hockey, and archery. Group 3 sports include diving, climbing, motorsports, and scuba diving. Participation may be considered based on the type and frequency of seizures and provider discretion. Children who have been seizure free for 12 months or more are commonly permitted to participate in all sports and activities. Other restrictions may be needed based on the specific seizure and triggers (e.g., if a child has hyperventilation-induced seizures, then soccer may need to be avoided until the seizures are better controlled). For each sport, it is important to discuss with the child and family the risks and benefits of participation concerning specific seizures, current seizure control, and known triggers.

For adolescents with epilepsy, driving may be a significant concern. Each state has its own legislation about when persons with epilepsy may drive, and it is important to assess your state restrictions to understand the child's responsibility as well as your responsibility as a provider. States typically outline a period of seizure freedom (3–12 months) prior to driving. Even for those who are legally able to drive, caution should be utilized when they are under significant stress, around typical triggers, or during medication changes. Many children with epilepsy have common triggers for their seizures, such as sleep deprivation, flashing lights, and illness. Additional restrictions may be implemented for those children to support their seizure control.

School Support

Academic needs and support will vary based on each individual child; however, 504 plans or an individualized education plan (IEP) can help provide the appropriate learning environment and curriculum. A 504 plan is typically utilized when a child needs adjustments to the learning environment but not the curriculum. Common modifications include additional time for testing and attendance modifications in the event of appointments or seizures. Consideration can be given to additional modifications based on the child. For example, a child with frequent seizures first thing in the morning may benefit from a delayed start to the day. Children with concerns for cognitive limitations and learning difficulties will benefit from neuropsychological testing to determine the best support that can be provided in their IEP. In addition, all children attending school should have a seizure action plan, and staff should be aware of the child's diagnosis and know how to appropriately and safely respond to a seizure.

Immunizations

Routine immunizations are recommended for children with epilepsy. However, children treated with adrenocorticotropic hormone (ACTH) or prednisone should avoid immunizations during therapy. The immunization schedules can be resumed following therapy. For children with a history of seizures following immunizations or at high risk for seizures during that time, consideration may be given to treatment with clonazepam around immunizations.

Bone Density

Children with epilepsy are at increased risk for decreased bone density (Shellhaas & Joshi, 2010). Those who are nonambulatory are at the highest risk for decreased bone mineral density. Some epilepsy therapies, such as valproic acid and the ketogenic diet, are also associated with an increased risk (Shellhaas & Joshi, 2010). While there is currently no specific treatment or screening guideline, monitoring of vitamin D and bone density may be considered in children with multiple risk factors.

Mental Health

Regular screening for mental health comorbidities is important for children and youth with epilepsy. Provide resources and discuss common symptoms of these disorders with the family and child—review treatment options when needed, including medications. For children with ADHD, as previously discussed, stimulant medications can be utilized while monitoring seizure frequency.

Drug Interactions

All new prescriptions should be reviewed for potential drug-drug interactions. Care should be given to seizure medications, which can change the efficacy of other medications. Interaction reviews should also include any supplements that the child may be taking.

In addition to prescribed or over-the-counter medications, care should be taken to review illicit drug and alcohol use in children with epilepsy. Not only can these interact with their antiseizure medications, but some substances, such as alcohol and marijuana, can reduce the seizure thresholds, making them more likely to experience breakthrough seizures.

Epilepsy in Females

Special considerations are needed for females with epilepsy. Some experience worsening of their seizures in relation to their menstrual cycles, which have been reported to occur during the perimenstrual phase most commonly but may also occur during ovulation or throughout the luteal phase (Pennell, 2017). In addition, oral contraceptives, while not associated with the worsening of seizures, are less effective in patients taking enzyme-inducing antiseizure medications (Pennell, 2017). It is therefore important to counsel women with epilepsy regarding the risk of contraceptive failure and recommend barrier method contraception in addition to hormonal contraception.

Due to the increased risk for fetal malformations associated with antiseizure medications, supplementation with folic acid is recommended for any person with childbearing potential.

Children Undergoing Gender-Affirming Hormone Therapy

Limited literature is available on the care of the transgender epilepsy population; however, similar to oral contraception, enzyme-inducing seizure medications may impact gender-affirming hormone therapy (Waldman & Benson, 2022). Seizures should be monitored with treatment and care closely coordinated with the neurologist to support the child's overall health and well-being during the transition.

Referrals

Children with epilepsy, or concerns about epilepsy, should be referred to a neurologist for additional evaluation. When children continue to have seizures despite current therapies, consideration should be given to a referral to a National Association of Epilepsy Center–designated level IV epilepsy center, which can provide care to children with complex epilepsy and medical needs.

In addition, referrals should be provided based on the presentation of comorbid conditions, such as psychiatry, psychology, and early intervention services.

RESOURCES

American Academy of Pediatrics National Coordinating Center for Epilepsy https://www.aap.org/en/patient-care/epilepsy
Centers for Disease Control and Prevention (Epilepsy) https://www.cdc.gov/epilepsy/index.html
Danny Did Foundation https://www.dannydid.org
Epilepsy Foundation https://www.epilepsy.com
   3540 Crain Highway, Ste. 675
   Bowie, MD 20716
   United States
   Phone:(301) 459-3700
   Toll Free:(800) 332-1000
HealthyChildren.org   https://www.healthychildren.org/English/health-issues/conditions/seizures/Pages/default.aspx_gl=1*acc7r6*_ga*MjE1ODQ2NTEzLjE3MDIyNTg0Nzg.*_ga_FD9D3XZVQQ*MTcwMjI1ODQ3OC4xLjEuMTcwMjI1ODgwNS4wLjAuMA uMA

 Summary

Primary Care Needs for the Child With Epilepsy and Seizures

Epilepsy is a commonly occurring neurologic disorder in children and represents recurrent unprovoked seizures.

DIAGNOSIS
- Clinical diagnosis and history will be key.
- EEG and MRI can assist in the diagnosis.
- Diagnosis of epilepsy may be further defined by the location of seizure onset or epilepsy syndrome.

TREATMENT
- Treatment is directed by the neurology provider.
- Seizure medications are utilized to manage seizures and control seizures for approximately two-thirds of persons with epilepsy.
- Nonpharmacologic management may include medical diet therapies and surgical options.

COMORBIDITIES
- Routine assessment and education on risk for comorbid conditions is recommended.
- Risk for premature death (SUDEP) is a factor.

- Increased risks for the neurodevelopmental disorder, sleep disorders, mental health disorders, and injuries are factors.

GROWTH AND DEVELOPMENT
- Growth should be closely monitored as medications are dosed based on weight, and adjustments may be needed for growth.
- Monitor for developmental changes.

DIET
- Closely monitor and restrict for patients on a ketogenic diet.
- For patients on medical diets, monitor growth and side effects.

SEIZURE ACTION PLANS
- Ensure all patients have an updated seizure action plan.

SEIZURE RESTRICTIONS
- Restrictions will vary based on seizure type and control.
- Assess physical activities and review risk with patient.
- Review and counsel on driving restrictions based on individual state laws.

Continued

SCHOOL
- Ensure all patients have a seizure action plan at school.
- Counsel on the need for 504 or IEP to support children.

IMMUNIZATIONS
- Delay immunizations for those receiving ACTH or steroid therapy.
- Consider benzodiazepine bridge for patients with seizures following immunizations.

BONE DENSITY
- Children with epilepsy are at increased risk for decreased bone density.
- Consider vitamin D monitoring for patients with multiple risk factors.

MENTAL HEALTH
- Routine screening for mental health comorbidities (depression, anxiety, ADHD) is recommended.

- Initiate treatment as indicated, including stimulant medications when needed.

DRUG INTERACTIONS
- Counsel patients on interactions with over-the-counter medications.

SPECIAL POPULATIONS
- Assess for changes in seizures around menstrual cycles.
- Counsel patients on the teratogenic effects of medications.
- Monitor for medication interactions for patients on hormone therapy.

REFERRALS
- Consider referral to a level IV epilepsy center for patients with continued seizures.

REFERENCES

Abdel-Mannan, O., Taylor, H., Donner, E. J., & Sutcliffe, A. G. (2019). A systematic review of sudden unexpected death in epilepsy (SUDEP) in childhood. *Epilepsy & Behavior, 90*, 99–106. doi:10.1016/j.yebeh.2018.11.006.

Armour, E. A., Yiu, A. J., Shrey, D. W., & Reddy, S. B. (2021). Underrepresented populations in pediatric epilepsy surgery. *Seminars in Pediatric Neurology, 39*, 100916. doi:10.1016/j.spen.2021.100916.

Auvin, S., Wirrell, E., Donald, K. A., Berl, M., Hartmann, H., Valente, K. D., Van Bogaert, P., Cross, J. H., Osawa, M., Kanemura, H., Aihara, M., Guerreiro, M. M., Samia, P., Vinayan, K. P., Smith, M. L., Carmant, L., Kerr, M., Hermann, B., Dunn, D., & Wilmshurst, J. M. (2018). Systematic review of the screening, diagnosis, and management of ADHD in children with epilepsy. Consensus paper of the Task Force on Comorbidities of the ILAE Pediatric Commission. *Epilepsia, 59*(10), 1867–1880. doi: 10.1111/epi.14549. Epub 2018 Sep 3.

Awin, S. (2017). Pathophysiology of seizures in the developing brain. In Pellock, J. M., Nordili, D., Sankar, R., & Wheless, J. W. (Eds.), *Pellock's pediatric epilepsy diagnosis and therapy* (4th ed., pp. 3–20). Demos Medical.

Brikell, I., Chen, Q., Kuja-Halkola, R., D'Onofrio, B. M., Wiggs, K. K., Lichtenstein, P., Almqvist, C., Quinn, P. D., Chang, Z., & Larsson, H. (2019). Medication treatment for attention-deficit/hyperactivity disorder and the risk of acute seizures in individuals with epilepsy. *Epilepsia, 60*(2):284–293. doi: 10.1111/epi.14640. Epub 2019 Jan 25. PMID: 30682219; PMCID: PMC6365170.

Capovilla, G., Kaufman, K. R., Perucca, E., Moshé, S. L., & Arida, R. M. (2016). Epilepsy, seizures, physical exercise, and sports: A report from the ILAE Task Force on Sports and Epilepsy. *Epilepsia, 57*(1), 6–12. doi:10.1111/epi.13261.

Cheung, A. H., Zuckerbrot, R. A., Jensen, P. S., Laraque, D., & Stein, R. E. K. (2018). Guidelines for adolescent depression in primary care (GLAD-PC): Part II. Treatment and ongoing management. *Pediatrics, 141*(3). doi:10.1542/peds.2017-4082.

Dallas, J., Englot, D. J., & Naftel, R. P. (2020). Neurosurgical approaches to pediatric epilepsy: Indications, techniques, and outcomes of common surgical procedures. *Seizure, 77*, 76–85. doi:10.1016/j.seizure.2018.11.007.

Dunn, D. W., Austin, J. K., & Huster, G. A. (1999). Symptoms of depression in adolescents with epilepsy. *Journal of the American Academy of Child and Adolescent Psychiatry, 38*(9), 1132–1138. doi:10.1097/00004583-199909000-00017.

Engel, M. L., Shanley, R., Scal, P. B., & Kunin-Batson, A. (2021). Anxiety and depressive symptoms in adolescents and young adults with epilepsy: The role of illness beliefs and social factors. *Epilepsy & Behavior, 116*, 107737. doi:10.1016/j.yebeh.2020.107737.

Eom, S., Fisher, B., Dezort, C., & Berg, A. T. (2014). Routine developmental, autism, behavioral, and psychological screening in epilepsy care settings. *Developmental Medicine and Child Neurology, 56*(11), 1100–1105. doi:10.1111/dmcn.12497.

Espay, A. J., Aybek, S., Carson, A., Edwards, M. J., Goldstein, L. H., Hallett, M., LaFaver, K., LaFrance, W. C., Jr., Lang, A. E., Nicholson, T., Nielsen, G., Reuber, M., Voon, V., Stone, J., & Morgante, F. (2018). Current concepts in diagnosis and treatment of functional neurological disorders. *JAMA Neurology, 75*(9):1132–1141. doi:10.1001/jamaneurol.2018.1264. PMID: 29868890; PMCID: PMC7293766.

Fecske, E., Glasier, P., Vargas Collado, L. M., & Rende, E. (2020). Standardized screening for depression in pediatric epilepsy. *Journal of Pediatric Health Care, 34*(1), 47–53. doi:10.1016/j.pedhc.2019.07.004.

Fisher, R. S., Acevedo, C., Arzimanoglou, A., Bogacz, A., Cross, J. H., Elger, C. E., Engel, J., Jr., Forsgren, L, French, J. A., Glynn, M., Hesdorffer, D. C., Lee, B. I., Mathern, G. W., Moshé, S. L., Perucca, E., Scheffer, I. E., Tomson, T., Watanabe, M., & Wiebe, S. (2014). ILAE official report: A practical clinical definition of epilepsy. *Epilepsia, 55*(4):475–482. doi:10.1111/epi.12550. Epub 2014 Apr 14. PMID: 24730690.

Fisher, R. S., Cross, J. H., French, J. A., Higurashi, N., Hirsch, E., Jansen, F. E., Lagae, L., Moshé, S. L., Peltola, J., Roulet Perez, E., Scheffer, I. E., & Zuberi, S. M. (2017). Operational classification of seizure types by the International League Against Epilepsy: Position paper of the ILAE Commission for Classification and Terminology. *Epilepsia, 58*(4):522–530. doi:10.1111/epi.13670. Epub 2017 Mar 8. PMID: 28276060.

Gandy, M., Modi, A. C., Wagner, J. L., LaFrance, W. C. Jr., Reuber, M., Tang, V., Valente, K. D., Goldstein, L. H., Donald, K. A., Rayner, G., & Michaelis, R. (2021). Managing depression and anxiety in people with epilepsy: A survey of epilepsy health professionals by the ILAE Psychology Task Force. *Epilepsia Open, 6*(1):127–139. doi:10.1002/epi4.12455. PMID: 33681656; PMCID: PMC7918327.

Gloss, D., Pargeon, K., Pack, A., Varma, J., French, J. A., Tolchin, B., Dlugos, D. J., Mikati, M. A., & Harden, C; AAN Guideline Subcommittee. (2021). Antiseizure medication withdrawal in seizure-free patients: Practice advisory update summary: Report of the AAN Guideline Subcommittee. *Neurology,*

97(23):1072-1081. doi:10.1212/WNL.0000000000012944. PMID: 34873018.

Guilfoyle, S. M., Monahan, S., Wesolowski, C., & Modi, A. C. (2015). Depression screening in pediatric epilepsy: Evidence for the benefit of a behavioral medicine service in early detection. *Epilepsy & Behavior, 44*, 5–10.

Harden, C., Tomson, T., Gloss, D., Buchhalter, J., Cross, J. H., Donner, E., French, J. A., Gil-Nagel, A., Hesdorffer, D. C., Smithson, W. H., Spitz, M. C., Walczak, T. S., Sander, J. W., & Ryvlin, P. (2017). Practice guideline summary: Sudden unexpected death in epilepsy incidence rates and risk factors: Report of the Guideline Development, Dissemination, and Implementation Subcommittee of the American Academy of Neurology and the American Epilepsy Society. *Neurology, 88*(17):1674-1680. doi:10.1212/WNL.0000000000003685. Erratum in: Neurology. 2019 Nov 26;93(22):982. Erratum in: Neurology. 2020 Mar 3;94(9):414. PMID: 28438841.

Hecimovic, H., Santos, J. M., Carter, J., Attarian, H. P., Fessler, A. J., Vahle, V., & Gilliam, F. (2012). Depression but not seizure factors or quality of life predicts suicidality in epilepsy. *Epilepsy & Behavior, 24*(4):426–429. doi:10.1016/j.yebeh.2012.05.005. Epub 2012 Jun 8. PMID: 22683245; PMCID: PMC3408833.

Hesdorffer, D. C., Ishihara, L., Webb, D. J., Mynepalli, L., Galwey, N. W., & Hauser, W. A. (2016). Occurrence and recurrence of attempted suicide among people with epilepsy. *JAMA Psychiatry, 73*(1):80–86. doi:10.1001/jamapsychiatry.2015.2516. PMID: 26650853.

Hirsch, E., French, J., Scheffer, I. E., Bogacz, A., Alsaadi, T., Sperling, M. R., Abdulla, F., Zuberi, S. M., Trinka, E., Specchio, N., Somerville, E., Samia, P., Riney, K., Nabbout, R., Jain, S., Wilmshurst, J. M., Auvin, S., Wiebe, S., Perucca, E., ... Wirrell, E. C. (2022). ILAE definition of the Idiopathic Generalized Epilepsy Syndromes: Position statement by the ILAE Task Force on Nosology and Definitions. *Epilepsia, 63*(6), 1475–1499. doi:10.1111/epi.17236. Epub 2022 May 3.

Kanner, A. M., Schachter, S. C., Barry, J. J., Hesdorffer, D. C., Mula, M., Trimble, M., Hermann, B., Ettinger, A. E., Dunn, D., Caplan, R., Ryvlin, P., Gilliam, F., LaFrance, W. C., Jr. (2012). Depression and epilepsy, pain and psychogenic non-epileptic seizures: clinical and therapeutic perspectives. *Epilepsy & Behavior, 24*(2):169–181. doi:10.1016/j.yebeh.2012.01.008. Erratum in: Epilepsy Behav. 2014 Mar;32:171. LaFrance, W Curt Jr [added]; Hersdorffer, Dale C [corrected to Hesdorffer, Dale C]. PMID: 22632407.

Kossoff, E. H., Zupec-Kania, B. A., Auvin, S., Ballaban-Gil, K. R., Christina Bergqvist, A. G., Blackford, R., Buchhalter, J. R., Caraballo, R. H., Cross, J. H., Dahlin, M. G., Donner, E. J., Guzel, O., Jehle, R. S., Klepper, J., Kang, H. C., Lambrechts, D. A., Liu, Y. M. C., Nathan, J. K., Nordli, D. R. Jr., ... Wirrell, E. C; Charlie Foundation; Matthew's Friends; Practice Committee of the Child Neurology Society. (2018). Optimal clinical management of children receiving dietary therapies for epilepsy: Updated recommendations of the International Ketogenic Diet Study Group. *Epilepsia Open, 3*(2):175–192. doi:10.1002/epi4.12225. PMID: 29881797; PMCID: PMC5983110.

Lexicomp Online. (2022). *Pediatric and neonatal Lexi-drugs online.* Waltham, MA: UpToDate, Inc https://online.lexi.com.

Maguire, M. J., Jackson, C. F., Marson, A. G., & Nolan, S. J. (2016). Treatments for the prevention of sudden unexpected death in epilepsy (SUDEP). *Cochrane Database Systematic Review, 7*(7), Cd011792. doi:10.1002/14651858.CD011792.pub2.

Martin, K., Jackson, C. F., Levy, R. G., & Cooper, P. N. (2016). Ketogenic diet and other dietary treatments for epilepsy. *Cochrane Database Systematic Review, 2*, Cd001903. doi:10.1002/14651858.CD001903.pub3.

Nagahama, Y., Zervos, T. M., Murata, K. K., Holman, L., Karsonovich, T., Parker, J. J., Chen, J. S., Phillips, H. W., Fajardo, M., Nariai, H., Hussain, S. A., Porter, B. E., Grant, G. A., Ragheb, J., Wang, S., O'Neill, B. R., Alexander, A. L., Bollo, R. J., & Fallah A. (2021). Real-world preliminary experience with responsive neurostimulation in pediatric

epilepsy: A multicenter retrospective observational study. *Neurosurgery, 89*(6):997-1004. doi:10.1093/neuros/nyab343. PMID: 34528103; PMCID: PMC8637802.

Operto, F. F., Coppola, G., Mazza, R., Pastorino, G. M. G., Campanozzi, S., Margari, L., Roccella, M., Marotta, R., & Carotenuto, M. (2019). Psychogenic nonepileptic seizures in pediatric population: A review. *Brain and Behavior, 9*(12):e01406. doi:10.1002/brb3.1406. Epub 2019 Sep 30. PMID: 31568694; PMCID: PMC6908892.

Pal, R., Romero, E., He, Z., Stevenson, T., & Campen, C. J. (2022). Pediatric functional neurological disorder: Demographic and clinical factors impacting care. *Journal of Child Neurology,* 8830738221113899. doi:10.1177/08830738221113899.

Panov, F., Ganaha, S., Haskell, J., Fields, M., La Vega-Talbott, M., Wolf, S., McGoldrick, P., Marcuse, L., & Ghatan, S. (2020). Safety of responsive neurostimulation in pediatric patients with medically refractory epilepsy. *Journal of Neurosurgery: Pediatrics, 26*(5):525–532. doi:10.3171/2020.5.PEDS20118. Epub 2020 Jul 31. PMID: 33861559.

Pennell, P. (2017). The female patient and epilepsy. In Pellock, J. M., Nordili, D., Sankar, R., & Wheless, J. W. (Eds.), *Pellock's pediatric epilepsy diagnosis and therapy.* Demos Medical.

Ryvlin, P., Nashef, L., Lhatoo, S. D., Bateman, L. M., Bird, J., Bleasel, A., Boon, P., Crespel, A., Dworetzky, B. A., Høgenhaven, H., Lerche, H., Maillard, L., Malter, M. P., Marchal, C., Murthy, J. M., Nitsche, M., Pataraia, E., Rabben, T., Rheims, S., ... Tomson, T. (2013). Incidence and mechanisms of cardiorespiratory arrests in epilepsy monitoring units (MORTEMUS): A retrospective study. *Lancet Neurology, 12*(10):966–977. doi:10.1016/S1474-4422(13)70214-X. Epub 2013 Sep 4. PMID: 24012372.

Salanova, V., Witt, T., Worth, R., Henry, T. R., Gross, R. E., Nazzaro, J. M., Labar, D., Sperling, M. R., Sharan, A., Sandok, E., Handforth, A., Stern, J. M., Chung, S., Henderson, J. M., French, J., Baltuch, G., Rosenfeld, W. E., Garcia, P., Barbaro, N. M., ... Fisher, R.; SANTE Study Group. (2015). Long-term efficacy and safety of thalamic stimulation for drug-resistant partial epilepsy. *Neurology, 84*(10):1017–1025. doi:10.1212/WNL.0000000000001334. Epub 2015 Feb 6. PMID: 25663221; PMCID: PMC4352097.

Seinfeld, S., Glauser, T., & Shinnar, S. (2017). Febrile seizure. In Pellock, J. M., Nordili, D., Sankar, R., & Wheless, J. W. (Eds.), *Pellock's pediatric epilepsy diagnosis and therapy* (4th ed., pp. 505–516). Demos Medical.

Shellhaas, R. A., & Joshi, S. M. (2010). Vitamin D and bone health among children with epilepsy. *Pediatric Neurology, 42*(6), 385–393. doi:10.1016/j.pediatrneurol.2009.12.005.

Shmuely, S., Surges, R., Sander, J. W., & Thijs, R. D. (2016). Prone sleeping and SUDEP risk: The dynamics of body positions in nonfatal convulsive seizures. *Epilepsy & Behavior, 62*, 176–179. doi:10.1016/j.yebeh.2016.06.017.

Specchio, N., Wirrell, E. C., Scheffer, I. E., Nabbout, R., Riney, K., Samia, P., Guerreiro, M., Gwer, S., Zuberi, S. M., Wilmshurst, J. M., Yozawitz, E., Pressler, R., Hirsch, E., Wiebe, S., Cross, H. J., Perucca, E., Moshé, S. L., Tinuper, P., & Auvin, S. (2022). International League Against Epilepsy classification and definition of epilepsy syndromes with onset in childhood: Position paper by the ILAE Task Force on Nosology and Definitions. *Epilepsia. 63*(6):1398–1442. doi:10.1111/epi.17241. Epub 2022 May 3. PMID: 35503717.

Starnes, K., Miller, K., Wong-Kisiel, L., & Lundstrom, B. N. (2019). A review of neurostimulation for epilepsy in pediatrics. *Brain Science, 9*(10). doi:10.3390/brainsci9100283.

Sultana, B., Panzini, M. A., Veilleux Carpentier, A., Comtois, J., Rioux, B., Gore, G., Bauer, P. R., Kwon, C. S., Jetté, N., Josephson, C. B., & Keezer, M. R. (2021). Incidence and prevalence of drug-resistant epilepsy: A systematic review and meta-analysis. *Neurology, 96*(17):805–817. doi:10.1212/WNL.0000000000011839. Epub 2021 Mar 15. PMID: 33722992.

Sveinsson, O., Andersson, T., Mattsson, P., Carlsson, S., & Tomson, T. (2020). Clinical risk factors in SUDEP: A nationwide population-based case-control study. *Neurology, 94*(4), e419–e429. doi:10.1212/wnl.0000000000008741.

Troester, M. M., Hastriter, E., & Ng, Y-T. (2010). Dissolving oral clonazepam wafers in the acute treatment of prolonged seizures. *Journal of Child Neurology*, 25.

Tsai, S. Y., Lee, W. T., Jeng, S. F., Lee, C. C., & Weng, W. C. (2019). Sleep and behavior problems in children with epilepsy. *Journal of Pediatric Health Care, 33*(2), 138–145. doi:10.1016/j.pedhc.2018.07.004.

Vona, P., Siddarth, P., Sankar, R., & Caplan, R. (2009). Obstacles to mental health care in pediatric epilepsy: Insight from parents. *Epilepsy & Behavior, 14*(2), 360–366. doi:10.1016/j.yebeh.2008.11.014.

Wagner, J. L., Kellermann, T., Mueller, M., Smith, G., Brooks, B., Arnett, A., & Modi, A. C. (2016). Development and validation of the NDDI-E-Y: A screening tool for depressive symptoms in pediatric epilepsy. *Epilepsia, 57*(8):1265–1270. doi:10.1111/epi.13446. Epub 2016 Jun 29. Erratum in: Epilepsia. 2018 Oct;59(10):2004. PMID: 27354177.

Waldman, G., & Benson, R. (2022). Epilepsy care in transgender patients. *Current Neurology and Neuroscience Reports*, 22.

Walter, H. J., Bukstein, O. G., Abright, A. R., Keable, H., Ramtekkar, U., Ripperger-Suhler, J., & Rockhill, C. (2020). Clinical practice guideline for the assessment and treatment of children and adolescents with anxiety disorders. *Journal of the American Academy of Child and Adolescent Psychiatry, 59*(10):1107–1124. doi:10.1111/epi.13446. Epub 2020 May 18. PMID: 32439401.

Wang, Z., Luo, Z., Li, S., Luo, Z., & Wang, Z. (2019). Anxiety screening tools in people with epilepsy: A systematic review of validated tools. *Epilepsy & Behavior, 99*, 106392. doi:10.1016/j.yebeh.2019.06.035.

Wicker, E., & Cole, J. W. (2021). Sudden unexpected death in epilepsy (SUDEP): A review of risk factors and possible interventions in children. *Journal of Pediatric Pharmacology and Therapeutics, 26*(6), 556–564. doi:10.5863/1551-6776-26.6.556.

Wirrell, E. C., Nabbout, R., Scheffer, I. E., Alsaadi, T., Bogacz, A., French, J. A., Hirsch, E., Jain, S., Kaneko, S., Riney, K., Samia, P., Snead, O. C., Somerville, E., Specchio, N., Trinka, E., Zuberi, S. M., Balestrini, S., Wiebe, S., Cross, J. H., ... Tinuper, P. (2022). Methodology for classification and definition of epilepsy syndromes with list of syndromes: Report of the ILAE Task Force on Nosology and Definitions. *Epilepsia, 63*(6):1333–1348. doi:10.1111/epi.17237. Epub 2022 May 3. PMID: 35503715.

Zack, M., & Kobau, R. (2017). National and state estimates of the numbers of adults and children with active epilepsy—United States. *MMWR*. Retrieved from http://dx.doi.org/10.15585/mmwr.mm6631a1.

Zuberi, S. M., Wirrell, E., Yozawitz, E., Wilmshurst, J. M., Specchio, N., Riney, K., Pressler, R., Auvin, S., Samia, P., Hirsch, E., Galicchio, S., Triki, C., Snead, O. C., Wiebe, S., Cross, J. H., Tinuper, P., Scheffer, I. E., Perucca, E., Moshé, S. L., & Nabbout, R. (2022). ILAE classification and definition of epilepsy syndromes with onset in neonates and infants: Position statement by the ILAE Task Force on Nosology and Definitions. *Epilepsia, 63*(6), 1349–1397. doi:10.1111/epi.17239. Epub 2022 May 3.

Zuckerbrot, R. A., Cheung, A., Jensen, P. S., Stein, R. E. K., & Laraque, D. (2018). Guidelines for adolescent depression in primary care (GLAD-PC): Part I. Practice preparation, identification, assessment, and initial management. *Pediatrics, 141*(3). doi:10.1542/peds.2017-4081.

24

Fragile X Syndrome

Randi J. Hagerman

ETIOLOGY

GENETICS

Fragile X syndrome is a genetic disorder that causes cognitive impairment ranging from mild learning disabilities to severe intellectual impairment. This condition derives its name from the presence of a fragile site or break in the X chromosome at Xq27.3 (Fig. 24.1), which is identifiable by chromosome analysis. Because of the phenotypic variability among children with fragile X syndrome and because this condition was only recently discovered, most individuals with fragile X syndrome remain undiagnosed.

Fragile X syndrome is caused by a mutation in the gene called the fragile X messenger ribonucleoprotein 1 gene *(FMR1)*, which is located at Xq27.3. The *FMR1* gene was discovered and sequenced in 1991 by an international collaborative effort (Verkerk et al., 1991). The *FMR1* gene has a unique trinucleotide expansion located within the gene. This expansion is the source of the mutation that causes fragile X syndrome. All individuals have the *FMR1* gene, but when the trinucleotide repeat expansion (CGG)n increases in size dramatically, this expansion causes the silencing of the gene, which leads to a deficiency or lack of the *FMR1* protein. Normal individuals in the general population have between 6 and 44 CGG repeats within their *FMR1* gene. Individuals who are carriers of fragile X syndrome have an expansion of the CGG repetitive sequence from 55 to 200. This change in the DNA is called a premutation and causes an increased instability of this region and an elevation of the messenger RNA (mRNA); this sometimes can lead to clinical involvement in premutation carriers, including premature ovarian failure that has been renamed the fragile X–associated primary ovarian insufficiency (FXPOI) and the fragile X–associated tremor/ataxia syndrome (FXTAS) (Amiri et al., 2008; Wittenberger et al., 2007). Most recently, a common problem in premutation carriers includes psychiatric problems such as anxiety and depression, and these have been named fragile X–associated neuropsychiatric disorders (FXAND) (Hagerman et al. 2018). Further expansion can occur when this premutation is passed on to the next generation through a female carrier. Individuals significantly affected by fragile X syndrome have more than 200 repeats (i.e., full mutation). This full mutation is usually associated with methylation, a process of silencing the gene so that no *FMR1* protein (FMRP) is produced from a full mutation. The absence of FMRP production causes the physical, behavioral, and cognitive problems that comprise fragile X syndrome.

Fragile X syndrome is inherited in an X-linked fashion. Males are typically affected by any deleterious gene they carry on the X chromosome. On the other hand, females are usually less affected because the normal gene compensates for the abnormal gene on one X chromosome on the other X chromosome. Heterozygous females have a 50% chance of passing the abnormal gene to their children. However, males who carry the fragile X gene mutation will pass the premutation to their daughters but none of their sons. Males who are carriers have the premutation, which is a CGG repeat between 55 and 200. When males pass on this premutation to all their daughters, only minimal changes occur in the CGG repeat number, and it never increases to the full mutation. All sperm of affected males have only the premutation. When a female passes on the premutation, however, there is a high probability that the premutation will increase to a full mutation in the offspring who inherit the fragile X chromosome. The larger the size of the premutation in the carrier mother, the greater the chance that expansion will progress to a full mutation. In females with a premutation of 100 CGG repeats or larger, the expansion to the full mutation occurs 100% of the time when the fragile X chromosome is passed on to the next generation (McConkie-Rosell et al., 2007).

INCIDENCE AND PREVALENCE

Fragile X syndrome is the most common cause of inherited intellectual disability known. Down syndrome, which rarely is inherited, has an incidence of approximately 1 per 1000. In comparison, fragile X syndrome causes intellectual disability in approximately 1 per 3600 to 5000 individuals in the general population (Crawford et al., 2002; Turner et al., 1996). Studies by Dombrowski et al. (2002) have shown that approximately 1 in 250 females and 1 in 800 males in the general population carry the premutation. Other studies have found a frequency of 1 in 130 females and 1 in 250 males with the premutation (Hagerman, 2008). In some countries there can be a genetic cluster of individuals with fragile

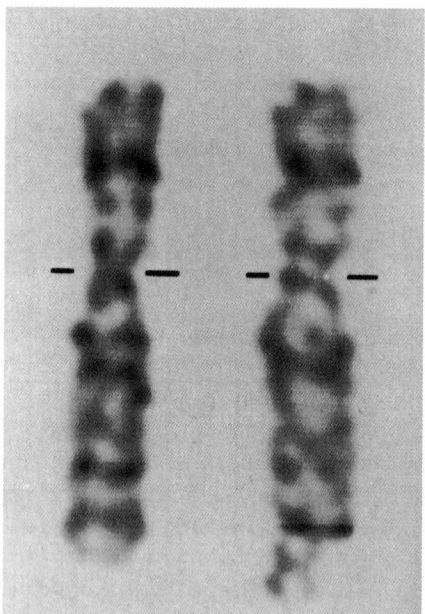

Fig. 24.1 A normal X chromosome and a fragile X chromosome demonstrating the fragile X site at Xq27.3.

X syndrome because of a founder effect; that is, carriers were founders of a population such that subsequent offspring had a high prevalence of fragile X syndrome (Saldarriaga et al., 2018). Screenings of individuals with intellectual disabilities in institutional and other residential settings have shown that 2% to 10% (Sherman, 2002) of this high-risk population have fragile X syndrome as the cause of their mental impairment. Screenings of individuals with autism find approximately 2% to 6% with fragile X syndrome, making fragile X the most common single-gene cause of autism (Hagerman et al., 2008). Testing for fragile X with *FMR1* DNA testing is recommended for all children with autism or autism spectrum disorders.

DIAGNOSTIC CRITERIA

When most health care providers hear "syndrome," they think of someone who appears phenotypically abnormal. Similarly, most syndromes have consistent cognitive and physical features that succinctly describe the clinical manifestations (see box in Clinical Manifestations, later). Although most individuals with fragile X syndrome share certain clinical findings, there is much variability. Health care providers should note that children with this syndrome may not be immediately recognizable by their phenotype.

To improve the diagnosis of fragile X syndrome, primary care providers must be familiar with the characteristic gestalt that defines this common condition. Individually, none of the physical, behavioral, or psychological characteristics is diagnostic of fragile X syndrome. However, the finding of one or more of the typical features, such as prominent ears, hyperextensible finger joints, and poor eye contact, in combination

Table 24.1 Fragile X Checklist

| | SCORE | | |
SYMPTOM	0 (NOT PRESENT)	1 (BORDERLINE OR PRESENT IN THE PAST)	2 (DEFINITELY PRESENT)
Intellectual disability			
Perseverative speech			
Hyperactivity			
Short attention span			
Tactile defensiveness			
Hand flapping			
Hand biting			
Poor eye contact			
Hyperextensible finger joints			
Large or prominent ears			
Large testicles			
Simian crease or Sydney line			
Family history of intellectual disability			
TOTAL SCORE:			

From Hagerman, R.J. (1987). Fragile X syndrome. *Current Problems in Pediatrics*, 17, 621–674.

with developmental delay or intellectual disability of unknown cause, should alert the clinician to order a DNA study for the *FMR1* mutation.

The fragile X syndrome checklist (Table 24.1) was designed to assist primary care providers in screening children with developmental delays or intellectual disabilities. A child receives a score of 0 for each feature not present, 1 point for those present in the past or questionably present, and 2 points for those definitely present; thus the higher the score, the greater the risk for fragile X syndrome (Hagerman, 2002b).

CLINICAL MANIFESTATIONS AT TIME OF DIAGNOSIS

MALES

Most males with fragile X syndrome have an intelligence quotient (IQ) in the mild to moderate range of intellectual disability. A significantly smaller percentage of affected males have severe to profound disabilities. Approximately 13% of males with fragile X syndrome have an IQ above 70 and therefore are not intellectually disabled (Bennetto & Pennington, 2002; Hagerman, 2002b). Most of these males have a variant pattern on DNA testing, including a lack of complete methylation of the full mutation or a mosaic pattern, some cells with the premutation, and some cells with the full mutation. The cognitive profile of males with fragile X syndrome includes difficulty with abstract reasoning, math, and attention.

◎ Clinical Manifestations at Time of Diagnosis

MALES
- Severe learning disabilities or intellectual disability
- Delayed onset of language
- Long or narrow face
- Prominent or cupped ears
- Enlarged testicles from puberty onward
- Hyperextensible finger joints, pes planus
- Hyperactivity or attention-deficit/hyperactivity disorder
- Perseveration in speech

FEMALES
- Mild cognitive deficits to intellectual disability
- Language delays
- Shyness, social anxiety
- Prominent ears
- Long, narrow face or high-arched palate
- Hyperextensible finger joints, pes planus
- Attentional problems but less prominent hyperactivity than in males

Delayed onset of language skills is present in approximately 85% of males with fragile X syndrome. In some children, particularly females or males with normal IQ, difficulties are only evidenced by language problems related to weaknesses in abstract reasoning. Other children as young as 18 months have delayed speech and significant deficits in receptive and expressive language (Roberts et al., 2008). Perseveration and echolalia (i.e.,

repetitive speech) are common speech characteristics of individuals with fragile X syndrome. A fast rate of speech, cluttering, mumbling, rambling, and poor topic maintenance are also frequent findings (Bennetto & Pennington, 2002; Scharfenaker et al., 2002).

The three classic physical features associated with the fragile X syndrome phenotype are a long and narrow face, prominent or large ears, and (in males) enlarged testicles. Approximately 80% of males with fragile X syndrome exhibit one or more of these features (Hagerman, 2002b). A long and narrow face is a common feature in adults and less common in young children. Large ears (i.e., >2 SD above the norm) are seen in 50% of males with fragile X syndrome (Fig. 24.2). Prominent or cupped ears are often a more useful discriminating feature among this younger group. This finding is observed in 60% to 70% of males and is often the only obvious physical feature associated with fragile X syndrome (Hagerman, 2002b).

Enlarged testicles are often seen in males with intellectual disability; 80% to 90% of males with fragile X syndrome have a testicular volume greater than 30 mL (Hagerman, 2002b). An orchidometer (Fig. 24.3) consisting of varying-sized ellipsoid shapes is useful for measuring testicular volume. However, most young children with fragile X syndrome do not have enlarged testicles. Macroorchidism begins to develop between 8 and 10 years of age; the largest testicle size is reached in late puberty with a mean volume of 50 mL (Lachiewicz & Dawson, 1994).

Other more subtle physical features noted in the population with fragile X syndrome include a prominent jaw, prominent forehead, and long palpebral fissures

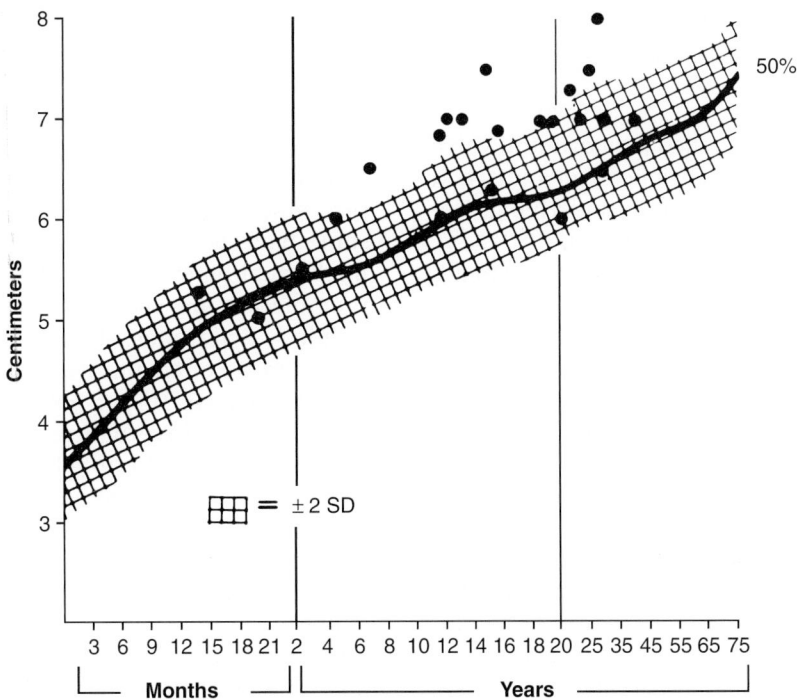

Fig. 24.2 Mean ear length. (From Hagerman, R., Smith, A.C., & Manner, R. [1983]. Clinical features of the fragile X syndrome. In *The fragile X syndrome: Diagnosis, biochemistry and intervention*. Spectra.)

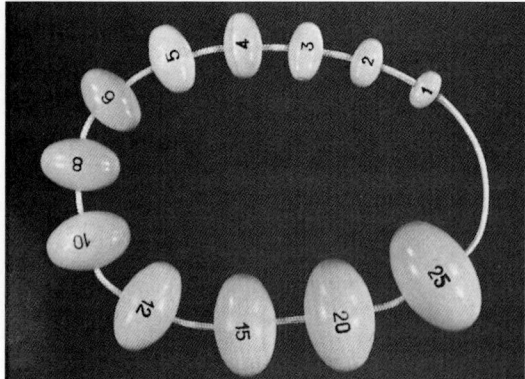

Fig. 24.3 Prader orchidometer used to measure testicular volume.

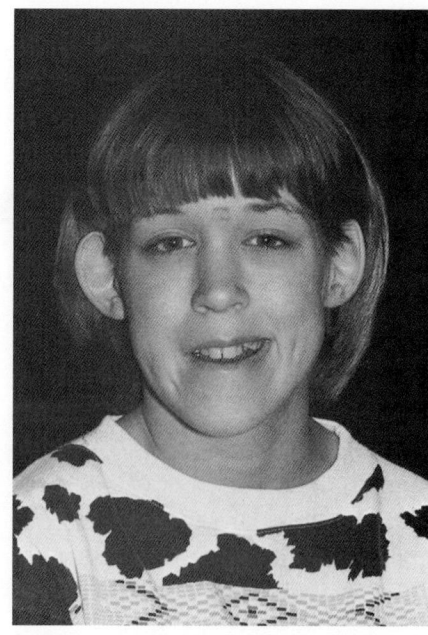

Fig. 24.5 Young heterozygous female with fragile X syndrome who is affected physically and cognitively by fragile X.

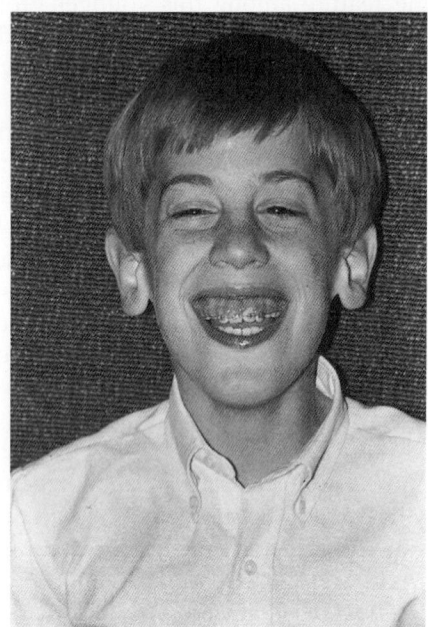

Fig. 24.4 Prepubertal male with fragile X syndrome.

(Hagerman, 2002b). A high-arched palate, mitral valve prolapse, hypotonia, hyperextensible finger joints, and flat feet suggest the possibility of an underlying connective tissue disorder (Hagerman, 2002b).

It is important to recognize that the majority of males with fragile X syndrome—especially younger males—appear physically normal (Fig. 24.4). Behavioral characteristics are often of more concern to parents. Hyperactivity is observed in more than 70% of boys with fragile X syndrome, but it frequently disappears after puberty. Poor attention span, often combined with impulsivity, is also problematic for all males with fragile X syndrome regardless of the level of cognitive functioning (Cornish et al., 2004; Sullivan et al., 2006). Approximately 90% have poor eye contact, and 60% to 70% display unusual hand mannerisms, including hand flapping and hand biting (Hagerman, 2002b).

Males with the premutation typically have a normal IQ, but attention problems, anxiety, shyness, and social deficits are relatively common (Farzin et al.,

2006). Occasionally a premutation carrier has features of fragile X syndrome, including full autism and intellectual disability (Hagerman, 2006). FXAND occurs in approximately 40% to 50% of young and old carriers, and these psychiatric problems include anxiety, depression, insomnia, chronic fatigue, chronic pain, obsessive-compulsive disorder, social deficits, and even autism spectrum disorders. FXTAS is seen in approximately 40% to 70% of older male carriers and about 8% to 16% of older female carriers (Coffey et al., 2008; Jacquemont et al., 2007). The tremor in FXTAS is typically an action tremor, and the ataxia is often characterized by frequent falling. These symptoms are usually slowly progressive and may include a cognitive decline in the 60s or 70s.

FEMALES

Overall, females affected by fragile X syndrome display milder phenotypic features than males, although some have been described with moderate or severe intellectual deficits (Fig. 24.5). Females who carry the premutation are usually unaffected intellectually by fragile X syndrome. However, females with the full mutation are often affected to a mild or severe degree. Approximately 70% of females with the full mutation have cognitive deficits, including borderline IQ or mild to moderate intellectual disability (Bennetto et al., 2001; de Vries et al., 1996). Executive function deficits—including attention and organizational difficulties—are common in most females with the full mutation but with an overall normal IQ. In addition, math difficulties, shyness, social anxiety, and poor eye contact are also common in females with the full mutation (Braden, 2002; Hagerman, 2002b).

The physical characteristics in females are less obvious than those for males with fragile X syndrome.

Prominent ears, a long and narrow face, a prominent forehead and jaw, and hyperextensible finger joints have been described (Hagerman, 2002b). The degree of involvement in individuals with the full mutation correlates to the level of FMRP (Loesch et al., 2004).

TREATMENT

Few health care professionals are knowledgeable about the diagnosis and treatment of fragile X syndrome. It is not uncommon, however, for a child with undiagnosed fragile X syndrome to be seen by the primary care provider for one of several associated medical problems, including repeated ear infections, strabismus, hyperactivity, delayed language, tantrums, violent outbursts, seizures, or hypotonia. Although much of the medical intervention is approached as it would be with any child, certain treatment options specific to the diagnosis of fragile X syndrome can significantly improve the developmental outcome for these children (Hagerman, 2006).

 Treatment

- Medications for hyperactivity
  - Methylphenidate (Ritalin, Concerta, Metadate, Daytrana)
  - Dextroamphetamine (Dexedrine) or dextroamphetamine/amphetamine (Adderall, Vyvanse)
  - Clonidine (Catapres) or guanfacine (Tenex; Intuniv)
- Medications for aggression or severe mood lability
  - Atypical antipsychotics: aripiprazole (Abilify) and risperidone (Risperdal)
  - Anticonvulsants: carbamazepine (Tegretol), or valproic acid and derivatives (Depakote)
  - Selective serotonin reuptake inhibitors (sertraline, fluoxetine)
- Special education support, including speech-language therapy, occupational therapy, and assistive technology therapy
- Genetic counseling for all extended-family members at risk

Any signs that indicate developmental delay, sensory integration dysfunction, or language delays deserve immediate and aggressive treatment in a child with fragile X syndrome. All areas of a child's presenting signs and symptoms should be addressed, and thus a multidisciplinary approach to evaluation and therapy is essential.

PHARMACOLOGIC THERAPY

Management of hyperactivity and attentional problems with medication can augment learning and behavioral management at home and in school. Central nervous system (CNS) stimulant medication has proved the most reliable, improving as many as two-thirds of affected children (Hagerman, 2002a). No single drug is effective for all children. Methylphenidate (Ritalin, Concerta, Quillivant XR, Metadate) is most prescribed,

but dextroamphetamine (Dexedrine) or dextroamphetamine/amphetamine equivalents (Adderall or Vyvanse) are also beneficial (Berry-Kravis & Potanos, 2004; Hagerman, 2002a).

Clonidine (Catapres) has been beneficial in approximately 80% of children with fragile X syndrome who have significant hyperactivity. Clonidine and guanfacine are antihypertensive medications that lower plasma and CNS norepinephrine levels and have an overall calming effect on attention-deficit hyperactivity disorder (ADHD) symptoms. These medications can be particularly helpful for children with severe hyperactivity, overexcitability, and aggression, which are typical problems in fragile X syndrome, so guanfacine, which is less sedating than clonidine, is often used before stimulants, particularly for children under 5 years of age because stimulants are rarely given in children that young (Berry-Kravis et al., 2017). Clonidine can be very helpful for sleeping problems because of its sedating effects, particularly in children under 5 years of age (Berry-Kravis & Potanos, 2004; Hagerman, 2002a).

Individuals with significant mood lability, mood instability, or aggression may benefit from the mood-stabilizing effects of aripiprazole (Abilify), an atypical antipsychotic (Hagerman, 2006), or an anticonvulsant (e.g., carbamazepine [Tegretol] or valproic acid and derivatives [Depakote]) (Hagerman, 1999, 2002a). In our clinical experience, gabapentin has not been helpful for individuals with fragile X syndrome.

Aggression in childhood or adolescence may be related to anxiety; the use of a selective serotonin reuptake inhibitor (SSRI) (e.g., fluoxetine [Prozac], sertraline [Zoloft], escitalopram [Lexapro], or citalopram [Celexa]) has been helpful in fragile X syndrome (Berry-Kravis & Potanos, 2004). SSRIs are widely known as antidepressant medications but may also help decrease obsessive-compulsive behavior and anxiety. The side effects of fluoxetine can include gastrointestinal upset or nausea and an activation effect, which can sometimes exacerbate hyperactivity. Rarely a child may experience an increase in obsessive-compulsive behavior, aggression, or suicidal ideation while taking an SSRI. For this reason, close follow-up is recommended in children who start taking this medication.

EDUCATIONAL INTERVENTION

Whenever possible, children should be mainstreamed into a regular school classroom and receive speech-language and occupational therapy as well as special education support on an individual basis (see Schooling, later). Studies have indicated that IQ declines with age in children with fragile X syndrome (Bennetto & Pennington, 2002). However, follow-up in some males whose IQs have remained stable over time has shown that occasionally IQ may remain within the normal range. This finding has been associated with a novel pattern revealed by DNA testing: an unmethylated or

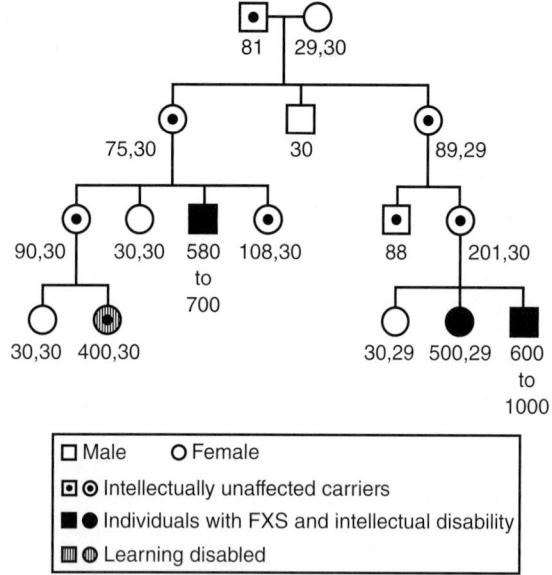

□ Male   ○ Female

▣ ⊙ Intellectually unaffected carriers

■ ● Individuals with FXS and intellectual disability

▥ ◍ Learning disabled

Fig. 24.6 A family tree with individuals affected by fragile X syndrome (FXS). The numbers underneath the circles and squares represent the CGG repeat number in the *FMR1* gene.

partially unmethylated full mutation that produces a significant level of FMRP (Loesch et al., 2004). Individuals with fragile X syndrome tend to perform better on some academic tests than their IQs would predict. Children with fragile X syndrome are typically better visual than auditory learners, which may be related to their ADHD symptoms. Significant memory abilities and well-developed skills in recognizing visual gestalts make reading, spelling, and vocabulary obvious areas of strength for many (Braden, 2002; Roberts et al., 2007, 2008; Scharfenaker et al., 2002).

Because children with fragile X syndrome are easily overstimulated, occupational therapy should be geared toward helping them reorganize, interpret, and adjust to sensory stimulation. For this reason, sensory integration therapy is the method of choice for these children. When this form of treatment is used, improvements should be noticeable in motor skills, balance, coordination, movement, sequencing, and attention (Scharfenaker et al., 2002).

GENETIC COUNSELING

Fragile X syndrome affects generation after generation; many families have two or more children affected by this condition (Fig. 24.6). Early diagnosis can provide relatives with important information about fragile X inheritance, recurrence risks, carrier testing, and family planning options (Gane & Cronister, 2002; McConkie-Rosell et al., 2007).

Because fragile X syndrome is inherited, obtaining a thorough family history or pedigree is essential. Questions about intellectual deficits, learning disabilities, emotional problems, and physical features associated with fragile X syndrome should be asked. Any relative with positive findings should be suspected as either

a carrier or an affected individual. Questions regarding premutation-specific conditions, including FXPOI, FXAND, and FXTAS problems, including tremors, ataxia, neuropathy, or cognitive decline, should also be asked (McConkie-Rosell et al., 2007).

Prenatal diagnosis is available to all families with a confirmed diagnosis of fragile X syndrome or with a history of intellectual disability. This testing includes amniocentesis (performed at 14–18 weeks of gestation), chorionic villus sampling (performed at 9.5–12 weeks of gestation), and percutaneous umbilical blood sampling (performed at 18–22 weeks of gestation). Each procedure has specific benefits and drawbacks that should be carefully discussed with a genetic counselor before pregnancy or testing is pursued (Gane & Cronister, 2002; McConkie-Rosell et al., 2007). The accuracy of prenatal diagnostic testing has improved significantly (i.e., >98% accurate) with DNA-*FMR1* studies. All family members at risk of carrying either the premutation or the full mutation should have DNA testing done by blood sampling. DNA testing is available internationally throughout the United States and at large genetic centers. Contact the National Fragile X Foundation for a list of laboratories that can perform DNA testing for fragile X syndrome (see Resources, later).

COMPLEMENTARY AND ALTERNATIVE TREATMENTS

Folic acid therapy appears to be helpful for approximately 50% of prepubertal boys with fragile X, although the reason for this is unknown (Hagerman, 2002a). Its use is controversial, however, and several studies have shown a lack of efficacy. Other studies have shown noticeable improvements in activity level, attention span, unusual mannerisms, and coping skills. The mechanism of action of folate is unclear, but it does not appear specific to fragile X syndrome. Because harmful side effects are rare, many families request folic acid as a trial. A prepubescent child can use a regimen of 10 mg/day (i.e., divided twice daily) for 3 to 6 months. Regardless of the dosage, careful follow-up is warranted to monitor vitamin B_6 and zinc serum levels, which may become deficient. The clinician should consider an alternative treatment if improvements are not noticeable within the trial period. According to parental reports, acetylcarnitine has been helpful for ADHD symptoms in children with fragile X syndrome (Torrioli et al., 2008).

ANTICIPATED ADVANCES IN DIAGNOSIS AND MANAGEMENT

Advances in the neurobiology of fragile X syndrome have demonstrated that the metabotropic glutamate 5 system (mGluR5) and many other pathways are upregulated without FMRP that normally inhibits these pathways. The enhanced mGluR5 activity leads to weakened synaptic connections and cognitive deficits in fragile X syndrome (Bear et al., 2004). The use of a mGluR5 antagonist should be helpful in the treatment for fragile X syndrome, and benefits have been seen in animal models of fragile X with such intervention (Dolen et al., 2007), but human studies have not demonstrated benefits in patients with fragile X syndrome (reviewed in Berry-Kravis et al., 2017). Many other targeted treatments for fragile X syndrome have not shown efficacy, but new treatments such as metformin (to downregulate the mTOR pathway that is too high in fragile X syndrome) (Biag et al., 2019; Protic et al., 2022), topical cannabidiol rubbed on the shoulders twice a day, and most recently a phosphodiesterase inhibitor (PDE4D) that upregulates cyclic adenosine monophosphate levels that are too low in fragile X syndrome have shown benefits in cognition and behavior (Berry-Kravis et al. 2021). Within the next few years gene therapy will be a reality in fragile X syndrome after animal studies demonstrate efficacy (Hagerman & Hagerman, 2021).

ASSOCIATED PROBLEMS OF FRAGILE X SYNDROME AND TREATMENT

SPEECH-LANGUAGE DIFFICULTIES

Both males and females with a full mutation have noted speech and language difficulties. Although more work is needed in this area, receptive and expressive language deficits (i.e., difficulties with auditory processing, inappropriate and tangential speech, poor topic maintenance, and written language difficulties) have been reported (Bennetto & Pennington, 2002; Roberts et al., 2007; Scharfenaker et al., 2002).

⇄ Associated Problems

Fragile X Syndrome and Treatment

- Speech-language difficulties
- Otitis media
- Connective tissue problems
  - Pes planus
  - Scoliosis
  - Mitral valve prolapse
- Vision problems
  - Strabismus
  - Nystagmus
- Seizures
- Oral problems; dyspraxia
- Autistic-like features (e.g., hand flapping, hand biting)
- Psychiatric manifestations, including anxiety and mood instability
- Sensory integration difficulties

OTITIS MEDIA

Recurrent otitis media has been reported in 45% to 60% of all children with fragile X syndrome. Approximately 40% of these children will require myringotomy tube insertions (Hagerman, 2002b). There has been some speculation that an unusual angle or collapsibility of the eustachian tube may cause this. Appropriate intervention for recurrent otitis media infections is critical to avoid conductive hearing loss, which could add to the language deficits typical of fragile X syndrome.

CONNECTIVE TISSUE PROBLEMS

Of all individuals with fragile X syndrome, 50% have pes planus. In addition, joint laxity is seen in approximately 70% of children 10 years or younger (Hagerman, 2002b). Rarely an individual with a clubfoot has been reported, which may be related to hypotonia in utero (Hagerman, 2002b). For reasons not clearly understood, hypotonia tends to disappear with age. Scoliosis may be present, and hernias appear to be more common in children with fragile X syndrome than in the general population. Gastroesophageal reflux is also common in infancy and is thought to be attributed to an underlying connective tissue disorder (Hagerman, 2002b). Routine intervention is recommended.

Cardiac problems have also been noted in individuals with fragile X syndrome and may be secondary to a connective tissue disorder. Mitral valve prolapse has been diagnosed in 22% to 55% of affected adult individuals, but it is rarely seen in children (Hagerman, 2002b). Although usually benign, mitral valve prolapse can predispose a person to arrhythmias, and prophylactic antibiotics before surgery or dental procedures may be recommended. Mild dilation of the base of the aorta has also been observed with ultrasound studies in as many as 50% of this population, but the dilation does not appear to be progressive except in rare individuals.

VISION PROBLEMS

Strabismus (i.e., either esotropia or exotropia) may be present in approximately 8% to 30% of those with fragile X syndrome. Other eye problems, such as myopia, nystagmus, and ptosis, have been observed with and without strabismus (Hagerman, 2002b).

SEIZURES

Seizures have been documented in approximately 20% of individuals with fragile X syndrome. Generalized seizures and partial complex seizures have been reported (Berry-Kravis, 2002). A careful history should be obtained; if clinical seizures are present, then treatment with an anticonvulsant such as carbamazepine or valproic acid is warranted (Hagerman, 2002a).

ORAL PROBLEMS

A high-arched palate is seen with greater frequency among the fragile X population and can explain the increased incidence of dental malocclusion. Several reports of Pierre Robin syndrome (micrognathia and cleft palate) have also been noted in combination with fragile X syndrome (Hagerman, 2002b).

AUTISTIC-LIKE TENDENCIES

An association between autism and fragile X syndrome has been mentioned frequently. Studies have estimated that approximately 60% of individuals with fragile X syndrome meet the *Diagnostic and Statistical Manual of Mental Disorders (DSM-V)* criteria for autism (Hagerman et al., 2008; Hatton et al., 2006; Kaufmann et al., 2004; Loesch et al., 2007). The other 40% of individuals, however, are interested in social interactions but have autistic-like features, such as poor eye contact, unusual hand mannerisms, tactile defensiveness, and obsessive interests. Those with autism and fragile X syndrome have a lower IQ, more severe language deficits, and a history of more frequent secondary medical problems, including seizures (Garcia-Nonell et al., 2008; Loesch et al., 2007). Anxiety can also interfere with social interactions, and social anxiety is obvious at times in most children with fragile X syndrome (Sullivan et al., 2007). However, many children with fragile X syndrome can be quite sociable intermittently, demonstrating a spontaneous and natural sense of humor (Hagerman et al., 2008; Hagerman & Hagerman, 2020).

PSYCHIATRIC MANIFESTATIONS

Researchers have only recently investigated the psychiatric manifestations of the fragile X gene in females. Social anxiety is a common complaint for males with fragile X syndrome. Many affected girls appear shy, withdrawn, and have poor eye contact (Franke et al., 1998; Hagerman, 2002b). Females with normal cognition occasionally recall that their childhood was burdened by similar types of problems. Poor self-image, schizotypal features, and depression have also been described (Franke et al., 1998; Hagerman, 2002b). The schizotypal features appear to be related to the executive function or frontal deficits present in most females with the full mutation (Bennetto & Pennington, 2002; Bennetto et al., 2001).

SENSORY INTEGRATION DIFFICULTIES

Other behavioral concerns include a child's inability to calm oneself when overstimulated or overwhelmed. New stimuli or novel situations can be frightening. Many parents describe their child as being hypersensitive to touch or tactilely defensive. An enhanced sympathetic response to a variety of sensory stimuli has been documented in research studies (Miller et al., 1999; Roberts et al., 2001). Sensory integration difficulties are evidenced by an inability to screen out noises, lights, or confusion. Common responses to sensory overload can include tantrums or outbursts, aggressive behavior, and emotional instability (Hagerman, 2002b; Scharfenaker et al., 2002). These problems are related to the underactivity of the gamma-aminobutyric acid (*GABA*) (inhibitory) system in the CNS; therefore individuals are not able to habituate to sensory stimuli, so over time the stimuli are become overactivating, leading to aggression or other behavior problems (Hagerman & Hagerman, 2020).

PROGNOSIS

Individuals with fragile X syndrome are expected to live a normal lifespan regardless of their intellectual functioning. However, reports of sudden death have occurred and may be related to rare cardiac arrhythmias (Hagerman, 2002b; Sabaratnam, 2000).

PRIMARY CARE MANAGEMENT

HEALTH CARE MAINTENANCE

Growth and Development

Growth parameters usually fall within the normal range, although head circumference greater than 75% has been reported (Hagerman, 2002b). Large heads in early childhood are more common in children who have both fragile X syndrome and autism (Chiu et al., 2007). Sometimes the large head circumference may lead to a misdiagnosis of Sotos syndrome.

In addition to deficits in cognitive functioning and speech, children with fragile X syndrome may be delayed in meeting other age-appropriate developmental milestones. Hypotonia is usually obvious in infancy. Developmental delay is evident with early developmental testing, such as the Bayley Scales of Infant Development. Other early warning signs are clumsiness and poor balance. Toe walking, unusual gait, lack of flow of movement, and trouble with motor planning may also occur secondary to hypotonia, joint laxity, and sensory integration difficulties (Scharfenaker et al., 2002). These children are easily overstimulated, and tantrums are common particularly during shopping or visiting a mall. Children usually like to watch their favorite videotapes over and over again.

Diet

Obsessive-compulsive behavior can be seen in children with fragile X syndrome and may involve food cravings. Obesity has been a problem for a small subgroup of children with fragile X syndrome, which may be secondary to perseverative eating or hypothalamic dysfunction. A subgroup of children with fragile X syndrome may have a Prader-Willi–like phenotype or general overgrowth (Nowicki et al., 2007). The Prader–Willi–like phenotype of fragile X syndrome is associated with a low level of a related protein expression called CYFIP (cytoplasmic *FMR1* interacting protein). Parents of obese children should be encouraged to use appropriate diets for their children coupled with intensive behavioral programs regarding food intake, as has been done with Prader-Willi syndrome (Hagerman et al., 2009). Exercise programs and videos may also benefit older children because they encourage them to use their visual and mimicking abilities. Failure to thrive is not uncommon in infants with fragile X syndrome but may result from gastroesophageal reflux, aversion to some food textures, frequent infections, or problematic mothering skills (i.e., if the mother herself is affected by the syndrome) (Hagerman, 2002b).

Safety
Families and educators should not expect every child with fragile X syndrome to be able to learn age-appropriate safety; this depends on each child's individual strengths and weaknesses. Many children can be taught to follow safety tips with strong visual and mimicking abilities and through the use of repetition.

Hyperactivity may lead to increased accidents, so affected children should be monitored closely. Home safety precautions, such as safety cabinet latches and switch-plate covers, should be based on the child's developmental rather than chronologic age. Because children with fragile X syndrome can be overstimulated by their environment, the home setting—particularly the child's playroom and bedroom—should be a calm and uncluttered environment. The use of beanbag chairs, vibrating pillows, musical tapes, and appropriate environmental changes can be discussed with an occupational therapist (Miller, 2006; Scharfenaker et al., 2002). The use of tools and motorized equipment requires additional precautions.

Parents also may be concerned about their child's safety if self-injurious behavior is displayed. Head banging is rare but can be harmful to the child; hand biting usually causes a callus and rarely scarring. Behavior management therapies to decrease the frequency of these behaviors are often helpful (Hills-Epstein et al., 2002; Scharfenaker et al., 2002). Safety issues are a concern when the parents are also affected. Recommendations in such situations include referral to a public health nurse and early infant stimulation programs to get professionals into the home to evaluate safety. Parents and professionals should also be advised of possible seizure activity and taught appropriate intervention.

Immunizations
The vaccination regimen is the same as for any infant or child (Centers for Disease Control and Prevention, 2009). Prevnar (for *Pneumococcus*) can decrease otitis media by 8% to 20%, which is important in patients with fragile X syndrome because of the increased frequency of otitis. The presence of intellectual disability increases the risk for oral and fecal contamination, so immunization for hepatitis A and B is important. If a child has a seizure disorder, the American Academy of Pediatrics (AAP; 2006) guidelines for administering pertussis and measles vaccinations to those with seizures should be followed.

Screenings
Vision.   An eye examination is recommended as early as possible after fragile X syndrome is diagnosed to rule out strabismus and the less-frequent findings of myopia,

hyperopia, astigmatism, nystagmus, and ptosis. The evaluation should include a complete case history, visual acuity evaluation, refractive error determination, oculomotor assessment, and funduscopy. Other testing may include an assessment of focusing function and visual developmental-perceptual skills. Yearly screening is sufficient unless visual difficulty is suspected. Early intervention is encouraged to prevent the development of blurred vision, amblyopia, or diplopia as a result of an uncorrected refractive error or strabismus. Treatment for many of the ophthalmologic problems includes corrective lenses, patching, or both (i.e., relatively inexpensive and noninvasive treatment). For some cases of strabismus, however, surgery may be the treatment of choice. Corrected vision maximizes a child's learning potential.

SCREENINGS FOR FRAGILE X SYNDROME
- Vision
- Hearing
- Dental
- Cardiac examination
- Speech-language delays
- Connective tissue problems
- Seizures

Hearing.   Because of the increased risk of recurrent ear infections, hearing evaluations are strongly recommended in newly diagnosed children. Audiometry testing is usually sufficient to assess hearing. Any child with a history of recurrent ear infections is best referred to an ear, nose, and throat specialist (otorhinolaryngologist) to determine whether pressure-equalizing tubes are warranted.

Dental.   Routine dental screening by the practitioner may reveal a high-arched palate, rare cleft palate, or dental malocclusion, all of which compound speech problems. Although it is not always possible, families should be referred to a pediatric dentist experienced in working with children who are developmentally delayed or hyperactive.

Blood pressure.   Routine screening is recommended.

Hematocrit.   Routine screening is recommended.

Urinalysis.   Routine screening is recommended.

Tuberculosis.   Routine screening is recommended.

Condition-Specific Screening
Cardiac examination: mitral valve prolapse.   Children with fragile X syndrome are at increased risk of mitral valve prolapse. Careful auscultation for a click or murmur is essential to detect this problem or any other cardiac involvement. Any child or adult with an abnormal cardiac examination should be referred to a cardiologist for formal evaluation.

Speech-language delays. Some children have early speech delays that are so subtle that they go undetected by parents or teachers. An early and annual speech-language evaluation should be performed to detect any speech-language deficits that can be improved through early intervention. Because of the diversity of speech-language difficulties in children with fragile X syndrome, no single screening tool is recommended. Each child should be approached on an individual basis. Children identified with fragile X syndrome should have a formal evaluation by a licensed speech-language pathologist, preferably one who is experienced with fragile X syndrome. Speech evaluation should be included in each individualized education plan to determine speech therapy's benefit.

Connective tissue problems. Early detection of scoliosis can often prevent further sequelae. Screening should also include a careful examination for excessive joint laxity and other complications of loose connective tissue (e.g., hernias).

Seizures. When clinical history suggests seizures, an electroencephalogram is indicated. Unusual findings can include a slow background rhythm and spike-wave discharges, which often resemble rolandic spikes (Berry-Kravis, 2002). Any child who appears to be having seizures should be treated with anticonvulsant medication with close follow-up by a pediatric neurologist (Hagerman, 2002a). If a child is taking medication to control seizures, anticonvulsant serum levels should be monitored.

COMMON ILLNESS MANAGEMENT
Differential Diagnosis
Recurrent otitis media. Children with fragile X syndrome must be vigorously monitored and treated for recurrent otitis media to avoid sequelae that could further compromise language development and learning. Parents of young children may not recognize otitis as the cause of their child's irritability. It may be helpful to inform parents of children with fragile X that recurrent otitis media is a common problem and review signs or symptoms that indicate infection (Hagerman, 2002a).

Differential Diagnosis
- Attention-deficit/hyperactivity disorder
- Autism
- Pervasive developmental disorder, not otherwise specified
- Sotos syndrome or cerebral gigantism
- Prader-Willi syndrome
- X-linked intellectual disability
- Fetal alcohol syndrome
- Tourette syndrome

Families of a child with a new diagnosis of fragile X syndrome should be referred to a health care team with expertise in fragile X syndrome for a thorough evaluation and consultation. Such referral will best determine a child's individualized medical management.

Drug interactions. Carbamazepine is a commonly prescribed anticonvulsant that is also used to control behavior problems (e.g., violent outbursts, aggression, and self-injurious behavior). Concurrent treatment with macrolide antibiotics (azithromycin [Zithromax], erythromycin), cimetidine (Tagamet), propoxyphene (Darvon), and isoniazid (INH) can interfere with the breakdown of carbamazepine, causing nausea, vomiting, and lethargy. Carbamazepine interacts with oral contraceptive pills and renders them ineffective. Folic acid therapy may worsen seizure frequency in children with epilepsy when coprescribed with aripiprazole (Abilify), so the dosage of aripiprazole should be increased. Aripiprazole also interacts with oral antifungal medications and the SSRI fluoxetine, and doses of aripiprazole should be reduced when prescribing these medications concurrently.

DEVELOPMENTAL ISSUES
Sleep Patterns
Frequent wakefulness in early childhood is a common problem in children with fragile X syndrome. Overstimulation can often interfere with sleep, and calming techniques (e.g., music) are useful in quieting the child in preparation for bedtime. Melatonin also helps sleep disturbances in a dose of 1 to 3 mg at bedtime. Behavioral interventions can also be helpful for sleep disturbances (Weiskop et al., 2005).

Toileting
Parents of children with fragile X syndrome often need help setting realistic expectations about toilet training. Some children achieve this milestone on time, but delayed training is more common. Parents should not be discouraged if a child takes longer to learn self-toileting. Establishing a predictable routine and consistent positive reinforcement are general principles that are helpful for children with fragile X syndrome (Crepeau-Hobson & O'Connor, 2002). Parents of any child having toilet-training difficulties are discouraged from being overly critical or reprimanding.

Discipline
Children with fragile X syndrome are especially noncompliant in response to an unexpected event or change in routine and therefore require a highly structured environment. Sending the child to school the same way each day, eating meals on a scheduled basis, and using the same nightly routines are encouraged. Behavior problems should be anticipated if a child is faced with an unexpected event. The prevention of

unpredictable events in the home or at school is an unrealistic expectation and should not be overemphasized. On the other hand, change and transitions should be gradually programmed into the child's learning and home environment. Setting limits, giving the child timeouts, and being consistent are appropriate responses when disciplinary action is required (Hills-Epstein et al., 2002; Reiss & Hall, 2007).

Child Care

Issues related to child care are common concerns for parents of a child with fragile X syndrome. Because of the short attention span and hyperactivity of children with fragile X syndrome, their child care providers should be knowledgeable about behavior modification techniques. The environment in which a child is placed is also important. Colors, noise levels, and the amount of light can be altered to avoid overstimulation both at home and in a child care setting. New events can be programmed slowly but gradually into a child's day. Setting a common time each week to introduce a new game, playing in a new space, or meeting a new day care provider can help a child anticipate and deal more effectively with change. If these aspects of day care are well managed, nothing precludes placing a child with fragile X syndrome in full-day or half-day programs. Placement with unaffected children helps model appropriate behavior. Children also can be mainstreamed in preschool programs, but providers should be experienced in specialized education. Children with fragile X syndrome are eligible for early intervention from birth to age 3 years, in addition to special education from age 3 years onward, so preschool programs affiliated with a school system should be able to provide special services such as speech-language and occupational therapy.

Schooling

Most children with fragile X syndrome who have been identified are receiving special education (Roberts et al., 2008). Inclusion is a potential goal (see Treatment, earlier). Speech therapy, occupational therapy, learning assistance, and psychological counseling can all be accessed through special education. A program that provides for individualized attention and a high teacher–student ratio is best. The success of any approach depends on several factors specific to each child, including the child's level of cognitive functioning, distractibility, impulsivity, class structure, classroom environment, and appropriate role models. All children with fragile X syndrome need a consistent routine and help with transitions in school (Braden, 2002). Sometimes their behavior problems require taking medication (e.g., stimulants or guanfacine) during school hours. It is important for the school nurse to be familiar with these medications and their use in children with fragile X syndrome (Hagerman, 2002a; Hagerman & Hagerman, 2020).

Because few educators are knowledgeable about fragile X syndrome, the health care professional can play an active role in helping families educate teachers and therapists about the specialized needs of an affected child and why an integrative approach that emphasizes a child's overall strengths and remediates weaknesses is essential for effective learning. Parents should be encouraged to become actively involved in their child's programs. Frequent visits to the classroom and observing therapy sessions help establish open communication among parents, teachers, and support personnel.

A child's overall intellectual abilities must be considered when developing an educational program. Inclusion is a realistic goal for some children, but others may need a more structured and specialized program. Children with fragile X syndrome will experience more significant improvement if they are shown appropriate role models. Educational intervention strategies should emphasize a child's strengths (e.g., imitating abilities, memory, computer skills, visual skills, and vocabulary). The curriculum should focus on areas of a child's interest (Braden, 2002; Scharfenaker et al., 2002). Logo reading is an example of a learning tool developed to capitalize on a child's strength for incidentally acquired knowledge (Braden, 2002). This concept uses logos from popular television commercials and advertisements as the basis for a sight word vocabulary. The logos are gradually faded away so that only the word, phrase, or number remains.

Another successful learning tool is the use of computers for learning enhancement. This medium may enhance language ability and academic progress in reading, spelling, and math. Computers can improve visual matching skills and help focus attention with colorful programs (Braden, 2002). Computer learning programs can enhance academic progress. Word prediction programs, such as Write: Out Loud or Co: Writer, can enhance written language on the computer for children and adults with fragile X syndrome (Greiss-Hess et al., 2009).

Speech, language, and occupational therapy interventions are critical components of the education program and are recommended for all children with fragile X syndrome. Therapy is most effective when it incorporates a child's primary areas of interest. When possible, speech-language therapy sessions should include one or two other children who function at a higher level. Again, early intervention and vigorous treatment can optimize a child's speech-language abilities (Scharfenaker et al., 2002).

Sexuality

Masturbation and other forms of self-stimulatory behavior are common among individuals with intellectual impairment and are sometimes problematic for adolescents with fragile X syndrome. Families can be supportive by providing appropriate sex education and talking openly about sexuality issues. Family or individual counseling can also meet this need (Hills-Epstein et al., 2002). Counseling or therapy can also train new behaviors that can replace socially inappropriate behavior (e.g., masturbation in public). Most important, counseling provides adolescents a place to discuss and deal with issues of sexuality in a supportive environment. See the National Fragile X Foundation's Adolescent and Adults Program (www.fragilex.org) for guidance specific to therapists and parents for sexuality education.

Fertility is usually normal in men with fragile X syndrome, although reproduction is rare because of cognitive deficits (Hagerman, 2002b). Most males with fragile X syndrome are not sexually active but may obsess over females they like and can become physically aggressive toward them on rare occasions. All female children of males with fragile X syndrome will have the premutation because only the premutation—not the full mutation—is carried in the sperm. Ovarian problems and premature menopause have been reported in females with the premutation (Wittenberger et al., 2007). Females with the full mutation are more likely to reproduce than males because they have higher cognitive abilities. However, unlike males, they have an approximately 50% risk of having a child affected by fragile X syndrome or a carrier. Sex education and genetic counseling should be available to them (McConkie-Rosell et al., 2007).

Transition to Adulthood

Transitioning to adulthood is usually difficult for adolescents with fragile X syndrome because living independently is a problem due to intellectual disability. Adequate vocational training is important for adolescents. Most individuals affected by fragile X syndrome can perform jobs in the community that are consistent with their level of mental functioning. Many individuals require a job trainer who can work with them for the first several days or weeks when a new job is started. Focusing on daily living skills is also critical for young adults with fragile X syndrome if they can successfully live independently or semi-independently. Individuals with mild or moderate intellectual disability can learn to use public transportation and successfully perform activities in the home, including laundry, self-care, and cooking. Most adults affected by fragile X syndrome do well with limited supervision in an apartment setting.

Females affected by fragile X syndrome have greater difficulty trying to raise their children who are affected by fragile X syndrome. This role can be extremely stressful and may overwhelm their limited resources, particularly if the mother is mildly impaired. Additional help from family or social services agencies is usually necessary. Affected mothers should be referred to a public health nurse and parenting classes, and their children affected by fragile X should have intervention from birth onward. Adults with fragile X syndrome

should also have protection under the Americans with Disabilities Act for employment and housing issues.

The connective tissue problems associated with fragile X syndrome usually improve in adulthood, and medical complications are uncommon. Hernia and mitral valve prolapse are more common in adulthood than in childhood. Follow-up with a cardiologist is recommended. Most adults with fragile X syndrome and cognitive deficits can receive Supplemental Social Security income and therefore can obtain health care and counseling through Medicaid, Medicare, or both programs. Such coverage is important for ongoing care and medication.

Approximately 30% of young adults—particularly males—with fragile X syndrome may have difficulty with episodic outbursts and behavior. This behavior should be treated with medications (such as SSRIs with or without atypical antipsychotic agents) in addition to counseling. Remarkable benefits have been seen with the use of a new atypical drug, aripiprazole (Abilify), at low doses (i.e., 2–5 mg/day) (Hagerman, 2006; Hagerman et al., 2009). Counseling can help develop calming techniques and recognize environmental situations that can lead to outburst behavior (Hills-Epstein et al., 2002). The occupational therapist can also help with calming techniques in adults with fragile X syndrome.

Family Concerns

Perhaps the most frustrating aspect of having a child with fragile X syndrome is realizing that few professionals understand this disorder and how it can affect a child and other family members. As a consequence, many parents become their child's primary advocates in both educational and medical settings. Health care professionals who are unfamiliar with fragile X syndrome should make every effort to listen carefully to families. It is also the parent's responsibility to educate themselves about this unique disorder so that they can appreciate the specialized needs of these children and their own needs if they require additional support because they may also be affected by the fragile X mutation.

Fragile X syndrome occurs in all ethnic and racial groups that have been studied. No evidence exists of increased prevalence in any individual group. In some cultural groups, such as certain Asian populations, genetic counseling in extended family members can be difficult because of the negative cultural implications of knowing about a genetic disorder that affects many members within the extended family. When such cultural concerns exist, permission is often denied to inform extended family members about this genetic disorder. It is helpful to write an explanatory letter about fragile X syndrome that the immediate family can distribute to other family members who may be affected or be carriers for fragile X syndrome (McConkie-Rosell et al., 2007).

The National Fragile X Foundation was established to educate parents, professionals, and the public on the diagnosis and treatment of fragile X syndrome; extensive treatment information can be found at www.fragilex.org. All parents with a child diagnosed with fragile X syndrome would benefit from local contact with another family affected by fragile X syndrome. This information can be found through the foundation, which has established parent support groups throughout the United States and internationally.

RESOURCES

Foundations

National Fragile X Foundation (sign-up for newsletter, other information): www.fragilex.org

FRAXA Research Foundation (sign-up for newsletter, other information): www.fraxa.org

Fragile X Research Foundation of Canada: www.fragile-x.ca (email)

The Fragile X Society (England): www.fragilex.org.uk

The International Fragile X Alliance (Australia): www.ifxa.net

Fragile X Association of Australia, Inc.: www.fragilex.org.au

READING FOR CHILDREN

Heyman, C. (2003). *My extra special brother.* Fragile X Association of GA. 404-778-8524.

O'Connor, R. (1995). *Boys with fragile X syndrome.* National Fragile X Foundation. 800-688-8765.

Steiger, C. (1998). *My brother has fragile X syndrome.* Avanta Publishing. 800-434-0322.

 Summary

Primary Care Needs for the Child With Fragile X Syndrome

HEALTH CARE MAINTENANCE

Growth and Development
- Physical growth is usually within normal limits, although often tall in childhood and short in adulthood.
- Some children, particularly those with autism, are reported to have large heads for body size.
- Deficits in cognitive function and speech are common.
- Developmental delays in gross motor and fine motor skills are common.

Diet
- Obsessive eating may result in obesity in older children.
- Stuffing of the mouth with food is common.
- Infants may have failure to thrive related to reflux or recurrent emesis.

Safety
- Cognitive dysfunction may limit these children's awareness of safety issues.
- Hyperactivity may make these children more accident prone.
- Self-injurious behavior may occur; parents can be taught behavior management therapies.
- If seizures are present, seizure precautions are necessary.
- Home safety may be further compromised if the parents also have fragile X syndrome.

Immunizations
- Routine immunizations are recommended.
- AAP guidelines for immunizations in children with seizures should be followed where indicated.

Screening
- *Vision.* Eye examination for strabismus, refractive errors, and visual perceptual skills is recommended at the time of diagnosis. If no problems are found, annual vision screening is recommended.
- *Hearing.* An increased risk of otitis media warrants audiometric testing. A child may need referral to an ear, nose, and throat specialist for pressure-equalizing tubes.
- *Dental.* Screening for palate and dental abnormalities is recommended. If mirtal valve prolapse is present, prophylactic antibiotics will be needed for dental work or other surgery.

- *Blood pressure.* Routine screening is recommended.
- *Hematocrit.* Routine screening is recommended.
- *Urinalysis.* Routine screening is recommended.
- *Tuberculosis.* Routine screening is recommended.

Condition-Specific Screening
- *Cardiac examination: Mitral valve prolapse.* If cardiac examination is abnormal, mitral valve prolapse must be evaluated by a cardiologist.
- *Speech and language.* Speech and language evaluation should be done annually, with early intervention if a problem is detected.
- *Connective tissue problems.* Children should be screened for flat feet, scoliosis, hernias, and excessive joint laxity.
- *Seizures.* A clinical history suggestive of seizures should be evaluated by electroencephalography. If a child is taking anticonvulsants, blood levels must be monitored.

COMMON ILLNESS MANAGEMENT

Differential Diagnosis
- Recurrent otitis media is common.

Drug Interactions
- Carbamazepine is altered by macrolide antibiotics, cimetidine, propoxyphene, and isoniazid. Carbamazepine interacts with oral contraceptives and makes them ineffective.
- Aripiprazole doses should be increased if the child is taking carbamazepine and should be reduced if oral antifungal medications or fluoxetine are being used.

DEVELOPMENTAL ISSUES

Sleep Patterns
- Frequent wakefulness in early childhood is not uncommon.
- Overstimulation should be avoided.

Toileting
- Delayed continence is not uncommon.

Discipline
- Children behave better in highly structured environments.
- Consistent limit setting is beneficial.
- Positive reinforcement is essential.

Continued

Child Care
- Short attention span and hyperactivity may be modified by subdued environments.
- New activities must be introduced slowly.

Schooling
- Most children receive special education services. The provider can help educate the school system personnel on condition and treatment.

Sexuality
- Self-stimulatory behaviors are common. Counseling may help decrease inappropriate behavior.
- Fertility is normal in males, but reproduction is rare because of cognitive delay.
- Carrier females may experience premature menopause.
- Sex education, birth control, and genetic counseling are necessary.

Transition to Adulthood
- Living independently is difficult; individuals will likely need support from others. Housing and employment opportunities are protected under the Americans with Disabilities Act.
- Connective tissue problems usually improve.
- Outburst behavior may be a problem and should be treated with medication and counseling.

FAMILY CONCERNS
- Families may have difficulty adjusting to the diagnosis; parents may also be affected.
- Genetic counseling is warranted.
- Because the condition is not well known, care may be nonspecific.

REFERENCES

American Academy of Pediatrics. (2006). In Pickering, L. K. (Ed.), *Red book: 2006 report of the Committee on Infectious Diseases* (27th ed.). Elk Grove Village, IL: American Academy of Pediatrics.

Amiri, K., Hagerman, R. J., & Hagerman, P. J. (2008). Fragile X-associated tremor/ataxia syndrome: An aging face of the fragile X gene. *Archives in Neurology, 65*, 19–25.

Bear, M. F., Huber, K. M., & Warren, S. T. (2004). The mGluR theory of fragile X mental retardation. *Trends in Neuroscience, 27*, 370–377.

Bennetto, L., & Pennington, B. F. (2002). Neuropsychology. In Hagerman, R. J., & Hagerman, P. J. (Eds.), *Fragile X syndrome: Diagnosis, treatment, and research* (3rd ed.). Baltimore: Johns Hopkins University Press.

Bennetto, L., Pennington, B. F., Porter, D., Taylor, A. K., & Hagerman, R. J. (2001). Profile of cognitive functioning in women with the fragile X mutation. *Neuropsychology, 15*(2), 290–299.

Berry-Kravis, E. (2002). Epilepsy in fragile X syndrome. *Developmental Medicine and Child Neurology, 44*, 724–728.

Berry-Kravis, E., & Potanos, K. (2004). Psychopharmacology in fragile X syndrome—present and future. *Mental Retardation and Developmental Disabilities Research Reviews, 10*, 42–48.

Berry-Kravis, E. M., Lindemann, L., Jonch, A. E., Apostol, G., Bear, M. F., Carpenter, R. L., Crawley, J. N., Curie, A., Des Portes, V., Hossain, F., Gasparini, F., Gomez-Mancilla, B., Hessl, D., Loth, E., Scharf, S. H., Wang, P. P., Von Raison, F., Hagerman, R., Spooren, W., & Jacquemont, S. (2017). Drug development for neurodevelopmental disorders: Lessons learned from fragile X syndrome. *Nature Reviews Drug Discovery.* doi:10.1038/nrd.2017.221. [Epub ahead of print]. PMID: 29217836.

Berry-Kravis, E. M., Harnett, M. D., Reines, S. A., Reese, M. A., Ethridge, L. E., Outterson, A. H., Michalak, C., Furman, J., & Gurney, M. E. (2021). Inhibition of phosphodiesterase-4D in adults with fragile X syndrome: A randomized, placebo-controlled, phase 2 clinical trial. *Nature Medicine, 27*(5), 862–870. doi:10.1038/s41591-021-01321-w. Epub 2021 Apr 29. PMID: 33927413.

Biag, H. M. B., Potter, L. A., Wilkins, V., Afzal, S., Rosvall, A., Salcedo-Arellano, M. J., Rajaratnam, A., Manzano-Nunez, R., Schneider, A., Tassone, F., Rivera, S. M., & Hagerman, R. J. (2019). Metformin treatment in young children with fragile X syndrome. *Molecular Genetics & Genomic Medicine, 7*(11), e956. doi:10.1002/mgg3.956. Epub 2019 Sep 14. PMID: 31520524; PMCID: PMC6825840.

Braden, M. (2002). Academic interventions in fragile X. In Hagerman, R. J., & Hagerman, P. J. (Eds.), *Fragile X syndrome: Diagnosis, treatment, and research* (3rd ed.). Baltimore: The Johns Hopkins University Press.

Centers for Disease Control and Prevention. (2009). Recommendations and guidelines: 2009 child and adolescent immunization schedules for persons aged 0–6 years, 7–18 years, and "catch up" schedule. Available at www.cdc.gov/vaccines/recs/schedules/child-schedule.htm. Retrieved March 16, 2009.

Chiu, S., Wegelin, J. A., Blank, J., Jenkins, M., Day, J., Hessl, D., Tassone, F., & Hagerman, R. (2007). Early acceleration of head circumference in children with fragile X syndrome and autism. *Journal of Developmental and Behavioral Pediatrics. 28*(1):31–35. doi:10.1097/01.DBP.0000257518.60083.2d. PMID: 17353729.

Coffey, S. M., Cook, K., Tartaglia, N., Tassone, F., Nguyen, D. V., Pan, R., Bronsky, H. E., Yuhas, J., Borodyanskaya, M., Grigsby, J., Doerflinger, M., Hagerman, P. J., & Hagerman, R. J. (2008). Expanded clinical phenotype of women with the FMR1 premutation. *American Journal of Medical Genetics. 146A*(8), 1009–1016. doi:10.1002/ajmg.a.32060. PMID: 18348275; PMCID: PMC2888464.

Cornish, K. M., Turk, J., Wilding, J., Sudhalter, V., Munir, F., Kooy, F., & Hagerman, R. (2004). Annotation: Deconstructing the attention deficit in fragile X syndrome: a developmental neuropsychological approach. *Journal of Child Psychology and Psychiatry, 45*(6), 1042–1053. doi:10.1111/j.1469-7610.2004.t01-1-00297.x. PMID: 15257661.

Crawford, D. C., Meadows, K. L., Newman, J. L., Taft, L. F., Scott, E., Leslie, M., Shubek, L., Holmgreen, P., Yeargin-Allsopp, M., Boyle, C., & Sherman, S. L. (2002). Prevalence of the fragile X syndrome in African-Americans. *American Journal of Medical Genetics, 110*(3), 226–233. doi:10.1002/ajmg.10427. PMID: 12116230.

Crepeau-Hobson, F., & O'Connor, R. (2002). Appendix 4. Toilet training the child with fragile X syndrome. In Hagerman, R. J., & Hagerman, P. J. (Eds.), *Fragile X syndrome: Diagnosis, treatment, and research* (3rd ed.). Baltimore: Johns Hopkins University Press.

de Vries, B. B., Wiegers, A. M., Smits, A. P., Mohkamsing, S., Duivenvoorden, H. J, Fryns, J. P., Curfs, L. M., Halley, D. J., Oostra, B. A., van den Ouweland, A. M., & Niermeijer, M. F. (1996). Mental status of females with an FMR1 gene full mutation. *American Journal of Human Genetics, 58*(5), 1025–1032. PMID: 8651263; PMCID: PMC1914633.

Dölen, G., Osterweil, E., Rao, B. S., Smith, G. B., Auerbach, B. D., Chattarji, S., & Bear, M. F. (2007). Correction of fragile X syndrome in mice. *Neuron, 56*(6), 955–962. doi:10.1016/j.neuron.2007.12.001. PMID: 18093519; PMCID: PMC2199268.

Dombrowski, C., Lévesque, S., Morel, M. L., Rouillard, P., Morgan, K., & Rousseau, F. (2002). Premutation and intermediate-size FMR1 alleles in 10572 males from the general population: Loss of an AGG interruption is a late event in the generation of fragile X syndrome alleles. *Human Molecular Genetics, 11*(4), 371–378. doi:10.1093/hmg/11.4.371. PMID: 11854169.

Farzin, F., Perry, H., Hessl, D., Loesch, D., Cohen, J., Bacalman, S., Gane, L., Tassone, F., Hagerman, P., & Hagerman, R. (2006). Autism spectrum disorders and attention-deficit/hyperactivity disorder in boys with the fragile X premutation. *Journal of Developmental and Behavioral Pediatrics, 27*(2 Suppl), S137–S144. doi:10.1097/00004703-200604002-00012. PMID: 16685180.

Franke, P., Leboyer, M., Gänsicke, M., Weiffenbach, O., Biancalana, V., Cornillet-Lefebre, P., Croquette, M. F., Froster, U., Schwab, S. G., Poustka, F., Hautzinger, M., & Maier, W. (1998). Genotype-phenotype relationship in female carriers of the premutation and full mutation of FMR-1. *Psychiatry Research, 80*, 113–127. doi:10.1016/s0165-1781(98)00055-9. PMID: 9754690.

Gane, L., & Cronister, A. (2002). Genetic counseling. In Hagerman, R. J., & Hagerman, P. J. (Eds.), *The fragile X syndrome: Diagnosis, treatment, and research* (3rd ed.). Baltimore: Johns Hopkins University Press.

García-Nonell, C., Ratera, E. R., Harris, S., Hessl, D., Ono, M. Y., Tartaglia, N., Marvin, E., Tassone, F., & Hagerman, R. J. (2008).Secondary medical diagnosis in fragile X syndrome with and without autism spectrum disorder. *American Journal of Medical Genetics. Part A, 146A*(15), 1911–1916. doi:10.1002/ajmg.a.32290. PMID: 18627038; PMCID: PMC4097171.

Greiss-Hess, L., Lemons-Chitwood, K., Harris, S., Borodyanskaya, M., Hagerman, R., Bodine, C., & Guralnick, M. (2009). Assistive technology to promote occupation and reduce mouthing by three boys with Fragile X Syndrome. *The American Occupational Association, 9*(1).

Hagerman, P. J. (2008). The fragile X prevalence paradox. *Journal of Medical Genetics, 45*, 498–499.

Hagerman, R. J. (1999). Psychopharmacological interventions in fragile X syndrome, fetal alcohol syndrome, Prader-Willi syndrome, Angelman syndrome, Smith-Magenis syndrome, and velocardiofacial syndrome. *Mental Retardation and Developmental Disabilities Research Reviews, 5*, 305–313.

Hagerman, R. J. (2002a). Medical follow-up and pharmacotherapy. In Hagerman, R. J., & Hagerman, P. J. (Eds.), *Fragile X syndrome: Diagnosis, treatment, and research* (3rd ed.). Baltimore: Johns Hopkins University Press.

Hagerman, R. J. (2002b). Physical and behavioral phenotype. In Hagerman, R. J., & Hagerman, P. J. (Eds.), *Fragile X syndrome: Diagnosis, treatment, and research* (3rd ed.). Baltimore: Johns Hopkins University Press.

Hagerman, R. J. (2006). Lessons from fragile X regarding neurobiology, autism, and neurodegeneration. *Journal of Developmental and Behavioral Pediatrics, 27*, 63–74.

Hagerman, R. J., Berry-Kravis, E., Kaufmann, W. E., Ono, M. Y., Tartaglia, N., Lachiewicz, A., Kronk, R., Delahunty, C., Hessl, D., Visootsak, J., Picker, J., Gane, L., & Tranfaglia, M. (2009). Advances in the treatment of fragile X syndrome. *Pediatrics, 123*(1), 378–390. doi:10.1542/peds.2008-0317. PMID: 19117905; PMCID: PMC2888470.

Hagerman, R. J., & Hagerman, P. J. (Eds.). (2020). *Fragile X syndrome and premutation disorders*. MacKeith Press.

Hagerman, R. J., & Hagerman, P. J. (2021). Fragile X syndrome: Lessons learned and what new treatment avenues are on the horizon. *Annual Review of Pharmacology and Toxicology*. doi:10.1146/annurev-pharmtox-052120-090147. PMID: 34499526.

Hagerman, R. J., Protic, D., Rajaratnam, A., Salcedo-Arellano, M. J., Aydin, E. Y., & Schneider, A. (2018). Fragile X-associated neuropsychiatric disorders (FXAND). *Frontiers in Psychiatry, 9*, 564. doi:10.3389/fpsyt.2018.00564. eCollection 2018. Review. PMID: 30483160.

Hagerman, R. J., Rivera, S. M., & Hagerman, P. J. (2008). The fragile X family of disorders: A model for autism and targeted treatments. *Current Pediatric Reviews, 4*, 40–52.

Hatton, D. D., Sideris, J., Skinner, M., Mankowski, J., Bailey, D. B. Jr., Roberts, J., & Mirrett, P. (2006). Autistic behavior in children with fragile X syndrome: prevalence, stability, and the impact of FMRP. *American Journal of Medical Genetics, 140A*(17), 1804–1813. doi: 10.1002/ajmg.a.31286. PMID: 16700053.

Hills-Epstein, J., Riley, K., & Sobesky, W. (2002). The treatment of emotional and behavioral problems. In Hagerman, R. J., & Hagerman, P. J. (Eds.), *Fragile X syndrome: Diagnosis, treatment, and research* (3rd ed.). Baltimore: Johns Hopkins University Press.

Jacquemont, S., Hagerman, R. J., Hagerman, P. J., & Leehey, M. A., (2007). Fragile-X syndrome and fragile X-associated tremor/ataxia syndrome: two faces of FMR1. *Lancet Neurology, 6*(1), 45–55. doi:10.1016/S1474-4422(06)70676-7. PMID: 17166801.

Kaufmann, W. E., Cortell, R., Kau, A. S., Bukelis, I., Tierney, E., Gray, R. M., Cox, C., Capone, G. T., & Stanard, P. (2004). Autism spectrum disorder in fragile X syndrome: communication, social interaction, and specific behaviors. *American Journal of Medical Genetics, 129A*(3), 225–234. doi:10.1002/ajmg.a.30229. PMID: 15326621.

Lachiewicz, A. M., & Dawson, D. V. (1994). Do young boys with fragile X syndrome have macroorchidism? *Pediatrics, 93*(6 Pt 1), 992–995.

Loesch, D. Z., Bui, Q. M., Dissanayake, C., Clifford, S., Gould, E., Bulhak-Paterson, D., Tassone, F., Taylor, A. K., Hessl, D., Hagerman, R., & Huggins, R. M. (2007). Molecular and cognitive predictors of the continuum of autistic behaviours in fragile X. *Neuroscience and Biobehavioral Reviews, 31*(3), 315–326. doi:10.1016/j.neubiorev.2006.09.007. Epub 2006 Nov 9. PMID: 17097142; PMCID: PMC2145511.

Loesch, D. Z., Huggins, R. M., & Hagerman, R. J. (2004). Phenotypic variation and FMRP levels in fragile X. *Mental Retardation and Developmental Disabilities Research Reviews, 10*, 31–41.

McConkie-Rosell, A., Abrams, L., Finucane, B., Cronister, A., Gane, L. W., Coffey, S. M., Sherman, S., Nelson, L. M., Berry-Kravis, E., Hessl, D., Chiu, S., Street, N., Vatave, A., & Hagerman, R. J. (2007). Recommendations from multi-disciplinary focus groups on cascade testing and genetic counseling for fragile X-associated disorders. *Journal of Genetic Counselors, 16*(5), 593–606. doi:10.1007/s10897-007-9099-y. Epub 2007 May 12. PMID: 17497108.

Miller, L. J. (2006). *Sensational kids: Hope and help for children with sensory processing disorder*. London: Penguin Books.

Miller, L. J., McIntosh, D. N., McGrath, J., Shyu, V., Lampe, M., Taylor, A. K., Tassone, F., Neitzel, K., Stackhouse, T., & Hagerman, R. J. (1999). Electrodermal responses to sensory stimuli in individuals with fragile X syndrome: A preliminary report. *American Journal of Medical Genetics, 83*(4), 268–279. PMID: 10208160.

Nowicki, S. T., Tassone, F., Ono, M. Y., Ferranti, J., Croquette, M. F., Goodlin-Jones, B., & Hagerman, R. J. (2007). The Prader-Willi phenotype of fragile X syndrome. *Journal of Developmental and Behavioral Pediatrics, 28*(2), 133–138. doi:10.1097/01.DBP.0000267563.18952.c9. PMID: 17435464.

Protic, D. D., Aishworiya, R., Salcedo-Arellano, M. J., Tang, S. J., Milisavljevic, J., Mitrovic, F., Hagerman, R. J., & Budimirovic, D. B. (2022). Fragile X syndrome: From molecular aspect to clinical treatment. *International Journal of Molecular Sciences, 23*(4), 1935. doi:10.3390/ijms23041935. PMID: 35216055; PMCID: PMC8875233.

Reiss, A. L., & Hall, S. S. (2007). Fragile X syndrome: Assessment and treatment implications. *Child and Adolescent Psychiatry Clinics of North America, 16*, 663–675.

Roberts, J. E., Boccia, M. L., Bailey, D. B. Jr., Hatton, D. D., & Skinner, M. (2001). Cardiovascular indices of physiological arousal in boys with fragile X syndrome. *Developmental Psychobiology, 39*(2), 107–123. doi:10.1002/dev.1035. PMID: 11568881.

Roberts, J. E., Chapman, R. S., & Warren, S. F. (2008). *Speech and language development and intervention in Down syndrome and fragile X syndrome*. Baltimore: Paul H. Brookes.

Roberts, J., Price, J., Barnes, E., Nelson, L., Burchinal, M., Hennon, E. A., Moskowitz, L., Edwards, A., Malkinm, C., Anderson, K., Misenheimer, J., & Hooper, S. R. (2007). Receptive vocabulary, expressive vocabulary, and speech production of boys with fragile X syndrome in comparison to boys with down syndrome. *American Journal of Mental Retardation, 112*(3), 177–193. doi:10.1352/0895-8017(2007)112[177:RVEVAS]2.0. CO;2. PMID: 17542655.

Sabaratnam, M. (2000). Pathological and neuropathological findings in two males with fragile X syndrome. *Journal of Intellectual Disabilities Research, 44*, 81–85.

Saldarriaga, W., Forero-Forero, J. V., González-Teshima, L. Y., Fandiño-Losada, A., Isaza, C., Tovar-Cuevas, J. R., Silva, M., Choudhary, N. S., Tang, H. T., Aguilar-Gaxiola, S., Hagerman, R. J., & Tassone, F. (2018). Genetic cluster of fragile X syndrome in a Colombian district. *Journal of Human Genetics, 63*(4), 509–516. doi:10.1038/s10038-017-0407-6. Epub 2018 Jan 29. PMID: 29379191.

Scharfenaker, S., O'Connor, R., Stackhouse, T., et al. (2002). An integrated approach to intervention. In Hagerman, R. J., & Hagerman, P. J. (Eds.), *Fragile X syndrome: Diagnosis, treatment, and research* (3rd ed.). Baltimore: Johns Hopkins University Press.

Sherman, S. (2002). Epidemiology. In Hagerman, R. J., & Hagerman, P. J. (Eds.), *Fragile X syndrome: Diagnosis, treatment, and research* (3rd ed.). Baltimore: Johns Hopkins University Press.

Sullivan, K., Hatton, D., Hammer, J., Sideris, J., Hooper, S., Ornstein, P., & Bailey, D. Jr. (2006). ADHD symptoms in children with FXS. *American Journal of Medical Genetics. 140*(21), 2275–2288. doi: 10.1002/ajmg.a.31388. PMID: 17022076.

Sullivan, K., Hooper, S., & Hatton, D. (2007). Behavioural equivalents of anxiety in children with fragile X syndrome: Parent and teacher report. *Journal of Intellectual Disabilities Research, 51*(Pt 1), 54–65.

Torrioli, M. G., Vernacotola, S., Peruzzi, L., Tabolacci, E., Mila, M., Militerni, R., Musumeci, S., Ramos, F. J., Frontera, M., Sorge, G., Marzullo, E., Romeo, G., Vallee, L., Veneselli, E., Cocchi, E., Garbarino, E., Moscato, U., Chiurazzi, P., D'Iddio, S., ... M., Neri, G. (2008). A double-blind, parallel, multicenter comparison of L-acetylcarnitine with placebo on the attention deficit hyperactivity disorder in fragile X syndrome boys. *American Journal of Medical Genetics. Part A, 146A*(7), 803–812. doi:10.1002/ajmg.a.32268. PMID: 18286595.

Turner, G., Webb, T., Wake, S., & Robinson, H. (1996). Prevalence of fragile X syndrome. *American Journal of Medical Genetics, 64*(1), 196–197. doi:10.1002/(SICI)1096-8628(19960712)64:1<196::AID-AJMG35>3.0.CO;2-G. PMID: 8826475.

Verkerk, A. J., Pieretti, M., Sutcliffe, J. S., Fu, Y. H., Kuhl, D. P., Pizzuti, A., Reiner, O., Richards, S., Victoria, M. F., & Zhang, F. P., (1991). Identification of a gene (FMR-1) containing a CGG repeat coincident with a breakpoint cluster region exhibiting length variation in fragile X syndrome. *Cell, 65*(5), 905–914. doi:10.1016/0092-8674(91)90397-h. PMID: 1710175.

Weiskop, S., Richdale, A., & Matthews, J. (2005). Behavioural treatment to reduce sleep problems in children with autism or fragile X syndrome. *Developmental Medicine and Child Neurology, 47*, 94–104.

Wittenberger, M. D., Hagerman, R. J., Sherman, S. L., McConkie-Rosell, A., Welt, C. K., Rebar, R. W., Corrigan, E. C., Simpson, J. L., & Nelson, L. M. (2007). The FMR1 premutation and reproduction. The *FMR1* premutation and reproduction. *Fertility and Sterility, 87*(3), 456–465. doi:10.1016/j.fertnstert.2006.09.004. Epub 2006 Oct 30. PMID: 17074338.

Human Immunodeficiency Virus Infections and Acquired Immunodeficiency Syndrome

Nellie R. Lazar

25

EPIDEMIOLOGY

Treatment and prevention of human immunodeficiency virus (HIV) infections have led to a dramatic decline in the number of new pediatric cases in the United States since the early 1990s (Centers for Disease Control and Prevention [CDC], 2020), with rates now less than 1% in the United States (Fig. 25.1). Despite these improvements, disproportionate rates of HIV infection among Black children remain. A total of 32 children were infected with HIV in the most recent year due to perinatal transmission, and most were Black (Fig. 25.2).

The reduction in new HIV infections due to perinatal infection is a result of universal HIV screening recommendations for pregnant patients, treatment of those who are infected with antiretroviral therapy (ART) regimens during pregnancy, intravenous (IV) administration of ART during labor, scheduled cesarean delivery for females with plasma HIV RNA above 1000 copies/mL near delivery, ART administered to the infant for 6 weeks after delivery, and avoidance of breastfeeding. The American Academy of Pediatrics (AAP) and the CDC recommend universal opt-out HIV testing early in pregnancy as key to primary prevention of perinatal transmission (Havens, 2008). Some states promote universal HIV testing for all pregnant women, and universal testing varies by state prenatal testing coverage (Salvant Valentine & Poulin, 2018). In the United States, approximately 20% to 34% of infants with perinatal HIV exposure were born to people whose HIV diagnosis was unknown before pregnancy (Nesheim et al., 2019).

In the United States, adolescents and young adults (AYA) between the ages of 13 and 24, especially among Black males who have sex with males (MSM), represent one of the fastest growing HIV-positive groups. The most common mode of transmission among adolescents is male-to-male sexual transmission (Fig. 25.3). AYA aged 13 through 24 comprised 21% of all new HIV infections (CDC, 2021). AYA may engage in behaviors such as unprotected sex that put them at risk for HIV acquisition. HIV prevention challenges for young MSM include inadequate HIV prevention education, lack of appropriate and inclusive sex education programs, limited awareness of infection, low perception of risk, alcohol and drug use, and feelings of rejection and isolation (CDC, 2021).

Many inequalities result in poor outcomes for children living with HIV in resource-limited countries. The number of new HIV infections among children worldwide has declined by more than half (54%) from 2010 to 2020 because of expanded treatment to reduce perinatal transmission, but the momentum has slowed in parts of Africa (United Nations AIDS [UNAIDS], 2021). The 2021 UNAIDS report estimated 150,000 children younger than 15 years of age would become infected with HIV in 2020. Most of these infections were due to limited access to ART during pregnancy or breastfeeding. In addition, the number of children on treatment has declined since 2019, leaving almost 800,000 children (aged 0–14 years) living with HIV not on ART in 2020 (UNAIDS, 2021). This continuing problem in resource-limited countries is primarily caused by a lack of general resources and health care infrastructures and exceeds the scope of this chapter (Fig. 25.4).

PATHOGENESIS AND TRANSMISSION

HIV is a retrovirus member of the *Lentivirus* genus. This virus selectively infects the T-helper (Th) (i.e., CD4) subset of the T lymphocytes. Other cells that express CD4 (e.g., monocytes, macrophages, and glial cells) and some cells with detectable cell surfaces can also become infected. Early detection and treatment have significantly decreased morbidity and mortality in children and adults, and HIV is now a manageable chronic infection. If HIV infection is undetected and untreated, HIV infection can progress to acquired immunodeficiency syndrome (AIDS).

Through reverse transcription, HIV integrates itself into the genetic material of the organism it infects. HIVs bind to CD4 and chemokine coreceptors (CCR5 or CXC4), enabling the HIV genome and protein-containing capsid to enter the cell. The shell of the capsid disintegrates, and the HIV protein called reverse transcriptase transcribes the viral RNA into DNA. The viral DNA is transported across the nucleus, where the HIV protein integrates with the host DNA. Transcription creates multiple copies of new HIV RNA, some of which become the genome of a new virus and other copies of the RNA to make new HIV proteins. The immature virus is ultimately released from the cell,

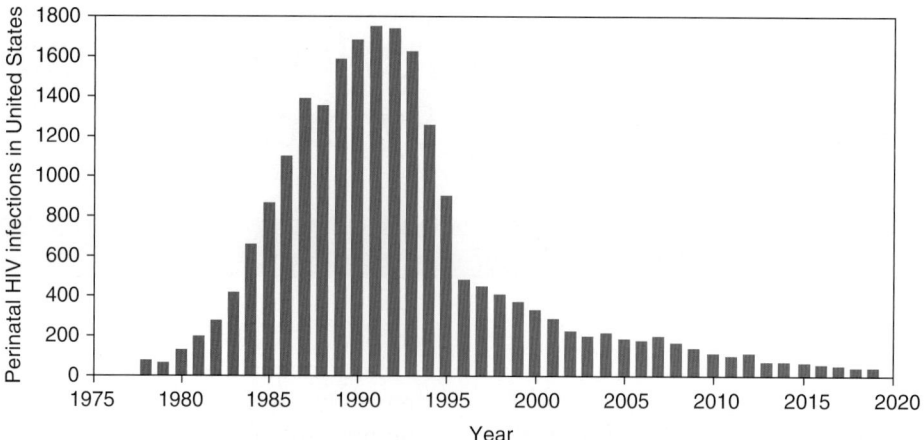

Fig. 25.1 Perinatal human immunodeficiency virus *(HIV)* infections in the United States.

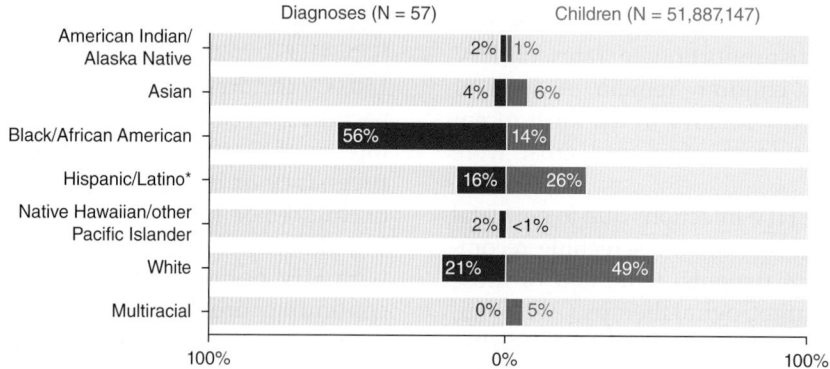

Fig. 25.2 Percentages of diagnoses of human immunodeficiency virus infection and population among children, by race/ethnicity, 2020 (COVID-19 pandemic)—United States. (From Centers for Disease Control and Prevention. Health disparities. Centers for Disease Control and Prevention. [2020]. Retrieved August 16, 2022, from https://www.cdc.gov/healthyyouth/disparities/index.htm. Note: Data for 2020 should be interpreted with caution due to the impact of the COVID-19 pandemic on access to HIV testing, care-related services, and case surveillance activities in state/local jurisdictions. *Hispanic/Latino persons can be of any race.)

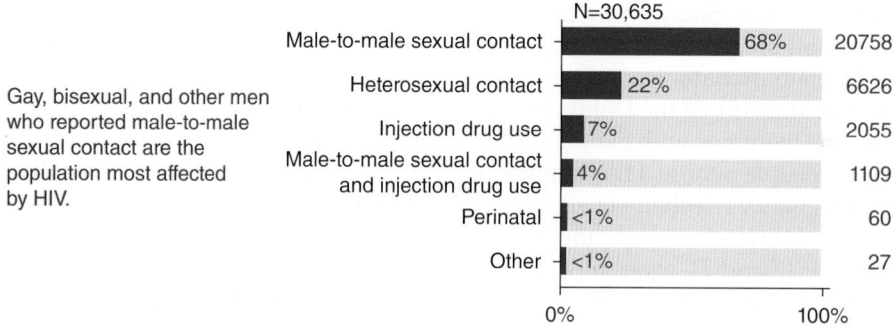

Fig. 25.3 Differences in new human immunodeficiency virus diagnoses by transmission category among people age >13 years. Transmission category is classified based on a hierarchy of risk factors most likely responsible for HIV transmission. Classification is determined based on the person's sex assigned at birth. Data have been statistically adjusted to account for missing transmission category. Note: Data for 2020 should be interpreted with caution due to the impact of the COVID-19 pandemic. For more information, view the report commentary section. (From Centers for Disease Control and Prevention. [2021]. Diagnoses of HIV infection in the United States and dependent areas. *HIV Surveillance Report, 33.*)

and the HIV protease protein facilitates the maturation of an infectious virus. HIV then causes immunodeficiency that destroys the host's ability to withstand infection. The latent HIV reservoir is a collection of infected cells in the tissues that remain hidden from

immune elimination. It is resistant to ART and clearance by the immune system.

HIV is transmitted to infants through maternal-to-child transmission in various modes. This may occur transplacentally in utero (vertically to the fetus), during

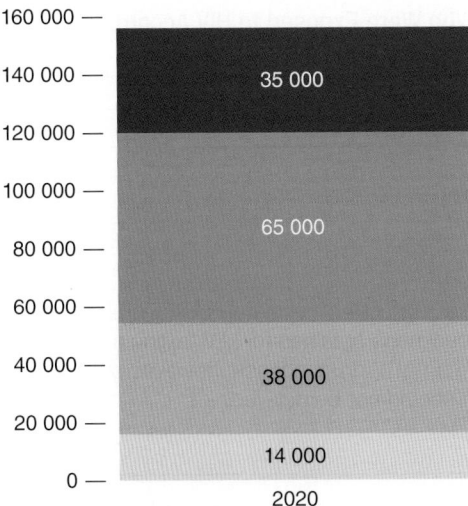

- ■ Mother acquired HIV during pregnancy or breastfeeding
- ■ Mother did not receive antiretroviral therapy during pregnancy or breastfeeding
- ■ Mother did not continue with treatment during pregnancy or breastfeeding
- ■ Mother was on antiretroviral therapy but not virally suppressed

Fig. 25.4 New vertical human immunodeficiency virus *(HIV)* infections by cause of transmission, global, 2020. (From United Nations AIDS. [2021]. UNAIDS epidemiological estimates, 2021. https://aidsinfo.unaids.org/.)

delivery by exposure to infected blood and vaginal secretions, and by breastfeeding (CDC, 2021). Many factors (i.e., fetal, viral, placental, obstetric, neonatal) influence perinatal HIV transmission. The course of infection and response to treatment differ dramatically depending on the timing and potentially the route of infection (Semrau & Aldrovandi, 2021).

Fetus and infants have an immature, developing immune system with a well-developed T-cell (cell-mediated) immune system and an immature B-cell (humoral-mediated) immune system. As a result, they are more susceptible to bacterial infections. T-cell defects allowing for opportunistic infections (OIs), such as *Pneumocystis jirovecii* pneumonia (PCP), are also often seen in young infants. In addition, infants' degree of lymphopenia, percentage of CD4 cells, absolute CD4 count, and degree of reversal of the helper-suppressor (T4/T8) ratio are more variable. Depletion of T-cell numbers and inversion of helper/suppressor ratio generally occur later in the disease in children than in adults. Another significant difference between adults and children with HIV is that the time from infection to developing signs and symptoms is shorter in children.

Early in HIV infection seroconversion, acute retroviral syndrome, when symptomatic, can mimic other viral illnesses, including malaise, fevers, lymphadenopathy, oral ulcers, leukopenia, and, occasionally, aseptic meningitis. This can often be a missed opportunity for HIV testing and should be considered in children and AYA.

DIAGNOSTIC CRITERIA

In the United States, HIV nucleic acid (DNA and RNA) assays are used most widely for the diagnosis of HIV infection in infancy. HIV can be diagnosed definitively by virologic testing (i.e., HIV RNA or HIV DNA nucleic acid tests [NATs]) in most nonbreastfed infants with perinatal HIV exposure by age 1 to 2 months and in almost all infants with HIV by age 4 to 6 months. It is important to note that the results of plasma HIV RNA or HIV DNA NAT can be affected by ART administered to the infant as prophylaxis or presumptive HIV therapy (Puthanakit et al., 2020). Antibody tests, including the antigen/antibody combination immunoassays, should not be used, as they do not establish the presence of HIV in infants because of the transplacental transfer of maternal HIV antibodies. An assay that detects HIV non-B subtype viruses or group O infections (e.g., an HIV RNA NAT or a dual-target total DNA/RNA test) is recommended for use in infants and children who were born to mothers with known or suspected non-B subtype virus or group O infections. If clinicians do not have access to virologic testing, children should be referred to a pediatric HIV specialty center.

The recommendations and timing of virologic diagnostic testing for infants are based on HIV transmission risk (Table 25.1). A positive virologic test should be confirmed as soon as possible by a repeat virologic test. Definitive exclusion of HIV infection in nonbreastfed infants is based on two or more negative virologic tests, with one negative test obtained at age 1 month or older and one at age 4 months or older, or two negative HIV antibody tests from separate specimens that were obtained at age 6 months or older.

HIV antibody and antigen/antibody tests should be used for diagnosis in children age 24 months or older. It is now possible to detect HIV earlier, and the performance time for laboratory-based assays is less than 1 h. The (CDC, 2014b) Laboratory Testing for the Diagnosis of HIV Infection recommends that clinicians initiate HIV testing with an immunoassay that is capable of detecting HIV-1 antibodies, HIV-2 antibodies, and HIV-1 p24 antigen (referred to as an antigen/antibody combination immunoassay). Individuals with a reactive antigen/antibody test should be further tested with an HIV-1/HIV-2 antibody differentiation assay (referred to as supplemental testing). Individuals with a reactive antigen/antibody combination immunoassay and a nonreactive differentiation test should be tested with an HIV RNA assay to establish a diagnosis of acute HIV infection.

In early infection before seroconversion, the antigen-antibody will be negative, and the HIV RNA assay will be positive. The test combination of a positive antigen-antibody screen, negative antibody differentiation assay or supplemental testing, and positive HIV RNA assay can also be seen in early HIV infection. If someone has symptoms consistent with acute HIV infection or a

Table 25.1	Recommended Virologic Testing Schedules for Infants Who Were Exposed to HIV According to Risk of Perinatal HIV Acquisition[a]

INFANTS AT HIGH RISK	
CRITERIA	**AGE AT HIV NAT TESTING**
Infants born to mothers with HIV who:	Birth[b]
• Did not receive prenatal care	14–21 days
• Received no antepartum ARVs or only intrapartum ARV drugs	1–2 mo
	2–3 mo[b]
• Initiated ART late in pregnancy (during the late second or third trimester)	4–6 mo
• Received a diagnosis of acute HIV infection during pregnancy or in labor; and/or	All infants at high risk of perinatal HIV transmission should have specimens obtained for HIV testing at birth before initiating an ARV drug regimen; however, presumptive HIV therapy should not be delayed.
• Had detectable HIV viral loads (≥50 copies/mL) close to the time of delivery, including those who received ART but did not achieve sustained viral suppression	

INFANTS AT LOW RISK	
CRITERIA	**AGE AT HIV NAT TESTING**
Infants born to mothers who:	14–21 days
• Received ART during pregnancy	1–2 mo[c]
• Had sustained viral suppression (usually defined as <50 copies/mL); *and*	4–6 mo
• Were adherent to their ARV regimens	

ART, Antiretroviral therapy; *ARV*, antiretroviral; *HIV*, human immunodeficiency virus; *NAT*, nucleic acid test.
[a]This table summarizes standard time points for HIV virologic diagnostic testing of infants who are not breastfeeding. For information about HIV testing time points for infants born to women with HIV who opt to breastfeed after comprehensive counseling, see Breastfeeding subsection of this chapter and Counseling and Managing Individuals with HIV in the United States Who Desire to Breastfeed.
[b]For high-risk infants, virologic diagnostic testing is recommended at birth. For infants treated with multiple ARVs in the first 2–4 wk of life, additional virologic testing is recommended 2–6 wk after ARV drugs are discontinued (i.e., at 8–12 wk of life).
[c]For low-risk infants, test may be timed to occur at least 2 wk after cessation of ARV prophylaxis.
From HIV.gov. (2023). Recommendations for the use of antiretroviral drugs during pregnancy and interventions to reduce perinatal HIV transmission in the United States (table 10). https://clinicalinfo.hiv.gov/en/guidelines/perinatal.

Table 25.2	HIV Infection Stage[a] Based on Age-Specific CD4+ T-lymphocyte Count or CD4+ T-lymphocyte Percentage of Total Lymphocytes

	AGE ON DATE OF CD4+ T-LYMPHOCYTE TEST					
	<1 YR		**1–5 YR**		**≥6 YR**	
STAGE	**CELLS/μL**	**%**	**CELLS/μL**	**%**	**CELLS/μL**	**%**
1	≥1500	≥34	≥1000	≥30	≥500	≥26
2	750–1499	26–33	500–999	22–29	200–499	14–25
3	<750	<26	<500	<22	<200	<14

[a]The stage is based primarily on the CD4+ T-lymphocyte count; the CD4+ T-lymphocyte count takes precedence over the CD4 T-lymphocyte percentage, and the percentage is considered only if the count is missing. There are three situations in which the stage is not based on this table: (1) If the criteria for stage 0 are met, the stage is 0 regardless of criteria for other stages (CD4 T-lymphocyte test results and opportunistic illness diagnoses); (2) if the criteria for stage 0 are not met and a stage 3–defining opportunistic illness has been diagnosed, then the stage is 3 regardless of CD4 T-lymphocyte test results; or (3) if the criteria for stage 0 are not met and information on the abovementioned criteria for other stages is missing, then the stage is classified as unknown.

recent high-risk exposure, the patient should have an HIV RNA ordered with an HIV antigen/antibody test. IV intrapartum zidovudine (ZDV) is recommended to prevent perinatal transmission of HIV pending results. Results of maternal HIV testing should be documented in the newborn's medical record and communicated to the newborn's primary care provider.

AIDS is an advanced stage of HIV infection when CD4+ T-lymphocyte values are usually persistently depressed. The case definition is used for purposes of surveillance and reporting and is not used for clinical decisions for individual patients. In 2014 the CDC revised and combined the surveillance case definitions for HIV infection into a single case definition for persons of all ages (CDC, 2014a). A confirmed case can be classified in one of five HIV infection stages (0, 1, 2, 3, or unknown); early infection, recognized by a negative HIV test within 6 months of HIV diagnosis, is classified as stage 0, and AIDS is classified as stage 3 (Table 25.2).

CLINICAL MANIFESTATIONS AT TIME OF DIAGNOSIS

HIV infection is a multisystem condition. The clinical manifestations during early infection are often nonspecific and frequently like a viral illness and may be missed. When not diagnosed early and symptomatic, infants and children with HIV present to care with a wide range of signs and symptoms. In most children and adolescents, the diagnosis of HIV infection is made early, before any signs and symptoms of illness, with rapid initiation of ART. Routine opt-out testing during pregnancy and adolescence has improved the early detection of HIV. These advances have contributed to the dramatic reduction in pediatric HIV cases in Western and European countries and the transition of HIV from an acute illness to a chronic condition.

TREATMENT

HIV infection is a chronic, manageable condition. ART is standard therapy and has demonstrated long-term safety and effectiveness in children (Szpak et al., 2022).

Currently the initiation of ART regimens includes three drugs from two differing classes. Mortality has declined significantly with the introduction of ART for the treatment of pediatric HIV. The advances in ART have provided substantial clinical benefits to children with HIV with immunologic or clinical symptoms of the disease. Studies have shown definite improvements in neurodevelopment, growth, and immunologic or virologic status, as well as improved quality of life with ART. Treatments are potent and can reduce viral load to undetectable, meaning that the virus is unable to be transmitted and is important for treatment and prevention (Eisinger et al., 2019; Sibiude et al., 2023).

Treatment should be initiated as soon as possible following diagnosis (Boxes 25.1 and 25.2). Early treatment in infants has the potential to greatly shrink the reservoir of cells that might permit virus replication and is associated with better outcomes for therapeutic intervention and a healthier immune system. Early initiation has been associated with the preservation of HIV-specific T-cell immune response, reduced immune activation (Rinaldi et al., 2020), and better immune reconstitution (Muenchhoff et al., 2019). Early initiation of ART is the most efficient therapeutic intervention to limit the seeding of HIV reservoirs. In 2013, the "Mississippi baby" was the first infant living with HIV reported to be undetectable for 27 months without

Box 25.1 Antiretroviral (ARV) Management of Newborns With Perinatal HIV Exposure to Prevent Mother-to-Child Transmission

- Newborn antiretroviral therapy (ART) regimens at doses for the infant's gestational age should be initiated within 6 h of delivery.
- Newborn ART regimen should be determined based on maternal and infant factors that influence the risk of perinatal transmission of human immunodeficiency virus (HIV):
  - **ART prophylaxis:** The administration of one or more ART drugs to a newborn without documented HIV infection to reduce the risk of perinatal acquisition of HIV.
  - **Presumptive HIV therapy:** The administration of ART to newborns who are at highest risk of perinatal acquisition of HIV. Presumptive HIV therapy is intended to be preliminary treatment for a newborn who is later documented to have HIV, but it also serves as prophylaxis against HIV acquisition for those newborns who are exposed to HIV in utero, during the birthing process, or during breastfeeding and who do not acquire HIV.
  - **HIV therapy:** The administration of ART at treatment doses to newborns with documented HIV infection.
- A 4-wk zidovudine ARV prophylaxis regimen can be used in newborns whose mothers received ART during pregnancy and had viral suppression within 4 wk prior to delivery.
- Newborns at high risk of perinatal acquisition of HIV should begin presumptive HIV therapy. Newborns at high risk of HIV acquisition include those born to people with HIV who:
  - Have not received antepartum ARV drugs, or
  - Have received only intrapartum ARV drugs, or
  - Have received antepartum ARV drugs but who did not achieve viral suppression (defined as a confirmed HIV RNA level <50 copies/mL) within 4 wk of delivery, or
  - Have primary or acute HIV infection during pregnancy.

Box 25.2 Panel's Recommendations for Intrapartum Care for People With HIV

ANTIRETROVIRAL MANAGEMENT OF PREGNANT PEOPLE WITH HIV TO PREVENT MOTHER-TO-CHILD TRANSMISSION
- Females with human immunodeficiency virus (HIV) who are receiving antiretroviral therapy (ART) and who present for pregnancy care should continue their ART during pregnancy.
- For females with HIV RNA >1000 copies/mL or unknown HIV RNA near the time of delivery (within 4 wk of delivery)
  - Intrapartum intravenous zidovudine (IV ZDV) should be administered in the following situations based on laboratory and clinical information near the time of delivery: (a) HIV RNA >1000 copies/mL, (b) unknown HIV RNA, (c) known or suspected lack of adherence since the last HIV RNA result, or (d) a positive expedited antigen/antibody HIV test result during labor. Begin IV ZDV when patients present in labor or at least 3 h prior to scheduled cesarean delivery.
  - When HIV RNA is >1000 copies/mL or is unknown near the time of delivery, scheduled cesarean delivery at 38 wk of gestation is recommended to minimize perinatal HIV transmission, irrespective of administration of antepartum ART.
  - IV ZDV is **not** required for people who meet **all** three of the following criteria: (1) are receiving ART, (2) have HIV RNA <50 copies/mL within 4 wk of delivery, and (3) are adherent to their ARV regimen.

Table 25.3 What to Start: Regimens Recommended for Initial Therapy of Antiretroviral-Naive Children

	PREFERRED REGIMEN BY AGE, WEIGHT, AND DRUG CLASS			
	BIRTH TO <14 DAYS OF AGE	AGE ≥14 DAYS AND ≥2 KG TO <4 WK	AGE ≥4 WK AND ≥3 KG TO <6 YR	AGE ≥6 YR AND ≥25 KG
INSTI-based regiments	Two NRTIs *plus* RAL			
				Two NRTIs *plus* BIC
			Two NRTIs *plus* DTG	
NNRTI-based regiments	Two NRTIs *plus* NVP			
PI-based regiments		Two NRTIs *plus* LPV/r		

BIC, Bictegravir; *DTG*, Dolutegravir; *INSTI*, Integrase Strand Transfer Inhibitor; *LPV/r*, Lopinavir/ritonavir; *NNRTIs*, Non-Nucleoside Analogue Reverse Transcriptase Inhibitors; *NRTI*, Nucleaotide Reverse Transcriptase Inhibitors; *NVP*, nevirapine; *PI*, Protease Inhibitors; *RAL*, Raltegravir.
From HIV.gov. (2023). Guidelines for the use of antiretroviral agents in pediatric HIV infection (figure 1). https://clinicalinfo.hiv.gov/en/guidelines/pediatric-arv.

Table 25.4 What to Start: Regimens Recommended for Initial Therapy of Antiretroviral-Naive Children

ANTIRETROVIRAL REGIMENS RECOMMENDED FOR INITIAL THERAPY FOR HIV INFECTION IN CHILDREN		
Newborns age birth to <14 days	None	Two NRTIs **plus** NVP
	≥2 kg	Two NRTIs **plus** RAL
Neonates age ≥14 days to <4 wk	None	Two NRTIs **plus** LPV/r
	≥2 kg	Two NRTIs **plus** RAL
Infants and children age ≥4 wk	3 kg	Two NRTIs **plus** DTG
		Two NRTIs **plus** DTG
Children age ≥2 yr	≥14 kg	Two NRTIs **plus** BIC
Adolescents age ≥12 yr with SMRs of 4 or 5	Refer to the *Adult and Adolescent Antiretroviral Guidelines*	

BIC, Bictegravir; *DTG*, Dolutegravir; *LPV/r*, Lopinavir/ritonavir; *NNRTIs*, Non-Nucleoside Analogue Reverse Transcriptase Inhibitors; *NVP*, nevirapine; *RAL*, Raltegravir; *SMR*, Sexual Maturity Rate.

ART. ART was started in the first 30 hours of life and continued until 18 months of life when there was a treatment interruption (Persaud et al., 2013). Despite a reported detectable viral load later in 2014, this gave hope that when ART is started early, it may take a longer time for viral rebound (Luzuriaga et al., 2015).

Presumptive HIV therapy is intended to be an early treatment for a newborn who is later documented to have acquired HIV, but it also serves as ART prophylaxis against HIV acquisition for those newborns who are exposed to HIV in utero, during the birthing process, or during breastfeeding and who do not acquire HIV (Tables 25.3 and 25.4). All newborns who were perinatally exposed should receive ART as soon as possible, preferably within 6 h, after delivery. A complete blood count (CBC) and differential should be performed before initiating ART in newborns who were exposed to HIV. ZDV can be used for 4 weeks as a prophylaxis regimen in newborns whose mothers received ART during pregnancy and had viral suppression within 4 weeks prior to delivery (defined as a confirmed HIV RNA level <50 copies/mL) and for whom maternal adherence is not of concern. Prophylaxis is the administration of ART to a newborn without documented HIV infection to reduce the risk of HIV acquisition. If possible, newborns who are at high risk for HIV acquisition should receive ZDV for 6 weeks. The Pediatric AIDS Clinical Trials Group (PACTG) 076 study (Connor et al., 1994) first found that prenatal, intrapartum, and neonatal ZDV reduced the incidence of perinatal HIV transmission. The risk

of HIV acquisition in newborns born to females who received ART during pregnancy and labor, which had undetectable viral load near or at the time of delivery, and avoided breastfeeding is now less than 1%.

The following include goals for treating pediatric patients with HIV infection from the Panel on Antiretroviral Therapy and Medical Management of HIV-Infected Children:

- Reducing HIV-related mortality and morbidity
- Restoring or preserving immune function
- Maximally and durably suppressing viral replication
- Minimizing drug-related toxicity
- Maintaining normal physical growth and neurocognitive development
- Improving the quality of life

Although the pathogenesis of HIV infection and the general virologic and immunologic principles for the use of ART are similar for all individuals with HIV, there are unique considerations for their use in infants, children, and adolescents. These considerations include the following: (1) perinatal transmission; (2) in utero, intrapartum, and neonatal postpartum exposure to ART; (3) differences in diagnostic evaluations in perinatal infection; (4) differences in immunologic markers in young children; (5) changes in pharmacokinetics with age caused by the continuing development and maturation of organ systems involved in the drug metabolism and clearance; (6) difference in the clinical and virologic manifestations of perinatal HIV infection in relation to the occurrence of primary infection in growing, immunologically immature bodies; and (7) special issues associated with treatment adherence for children and adolescence (CDC, 2022a).

Preexposure prophylaxis (PrEP) is also now available and recommended for uninfected individuals who are trying to conceive or are pregnant, postpartum, or breastfeeding to prevent HIV acquisition (Hsu & Rakhmanina, 2021). PrEP is available as a daily pill or to be used on demand in the form of a pill or long-acting injectable to prevent HIV acquisition. Postexposure prophylaxis is also available in the prevention of HIV and includes the administration of three-drug ART administered within 72 hours of a high-risk exposure (e.g., unprotected sex, sexual assault, or IV drug use) and continued for 28 days.

Children with HIV are treated with comprehensive, multidisciplinary care, including prompt diagnosis and prompt initiation of ART (see Table 25.4). Although systemic bacterial infections can occur, which can progress to pneumonia, meningitis, and sepsis, these are becoming less frequent in children with HIV infections. Although bacterial infection contributes greatly to morbidity, it is potentially preventable and treatable. The treatment strategy focuses on the early initiation of ART to help preserve the child's immune system, as well as clinical and antimicrobial interventions to reduce the frequency and intensity of bacterial infections.

Children with HIV can live healthy, normal lives if they start early on treatment and are provided support for medication adherence. They may take medications and spend time in the hospital and outpatient clinics, but they also attend day care, school, and college and engage in many after school activities. It is important for primary care providers to remember that these children will develop common childhood illnesses and that all symptoms are not necessarily related to HIV. Children with HIV, however, must be quickly assessed and aggressively managed when the possibility of concurrent illness or complications related to their ART treatment occurs. Children with HIV and their families must develop strong partnerships with their primary care providers and HIV specialists to ensure prompt evaluation and treatment. Infants, children, and adolescents with HIV are best treated by pediatric and adolescent HIV specialists. Effective management requires a multidisciplinary team approach of providers, including nurses, primary care providers, dentists, nutritionists, psychologists, social workers, pharmacists, and community outreach workers (CDC, 2022a). Treatment centers ensure access to clinical trials and the most up-to-date information and expertise, as well as to other children and families living with this condition. Clear lines of responsibility and access to the primary care provider and the center team must be developed for each family.

Adult treatment guidelines are appropriate for adolescents who have been infected by sexual activity or needle-sharing behaviors because their clinical course is more like that of adults than that of children who were perinatally infected (CDC, 2022a). Adolescents who are long-term survivors of perinatal HIV infection or transfusion-related infection as young children, however, may have a unique clinical course. Dosages of medications for HIV infection and OI should be based on Tanner staging of puberty rather than age; adolescents in early puberty should be given dosages based on pediatric schedules, and those in late puberty should follow adult dosing schedules (CDC, 2022a).

HIV EXPOSED AND UNINFECTED INFANTS

There is evidence to suggest that HIV-exposed and uninfected infants may be at higher risk for adverse outcomes such as increased susceptibility to infections, immunologic dysfunction, growth and metabolic abnormalities, and impaired neurodevelopment (Ruck et al., 2016; Wedderburn et al., 2019). Current ART has not been linked to teratogenic risk and is closely monitored by the Antiretroviral Pregnancy Registry, but studies suggest that specific ART may adversely affect neurologic development (Toledo et al., 2021). As research emerges to determine the physical factors that may cause growth, language, and behavioral problems in HIV-exposed and uninfected children, primary care providers should document exposure to ART in the problem list (Emmanuel et al., 2022).

COMPLEMENTARY AND ALTERNATIVE MEDICINE

Complementary and alternative medicine (CAM) for HIV is frequently used in combination with ART. Forms of therapy include massage, acupuncture, exercise, dietary and vitamin supplements, and mindfulness. Studies have shown the use of CAM is common in pediatric populations and few with negative effects (Ang et al., 2005; Oshikoya et al., 2014). CAM is often underreported by patients and their families, and the provider should assess its use. In a randomized control trial of mindfulness-based stress reduction (MBSR) with adolescents, MBSR was associated with improved emotional regulation and improved HIV viral load (Webb et al., 2017).

CONDITIONS ASSOCIATED WITH HIV INFECTION

Early identification and advances in treatment have improved outcomes in children living with HIV, increasing survival rates and quality of life. All conditions associated with HIV infection are more common in resource-limited settings and are related to the availability of testing and treatment.

FAILURE TO THRIVE

Hospitalizations due to failure to thrive have decreased dramatically, and significant improvements in nutritional status have occurred in children living with HIV. Despite these advancements, many infants and children living with HIV demonstrate poor weight gain and often fall below the 5th percentile on the National Center for Health Statistics growth curves for weight. Nutrition continues to be a significant problem for children with HIV, particularly those with chronic diarrhea and *Candida* spp. esophagitis.

The gastrointestinal (GI) tract is a major target for HIV because it constitutes 60% of all the lymphocytes in the body, causing an alteration in the microbiota (Basile et al., 2021). Malabsorption, malnutrition, immunodeficiency, and enteric infections appear to be interrelated (Melvin et al., 2017). Children living with HIV can experience malabsorption and may have malnutrition-induced immunodeficiency, which creates an environment for enteric pathogens such as *Cryptosporidium*, *Giardia*, and *Mycobacterium avium*-intracellulare (MAI) spp., leading to chronic infectious diarrhea. Many children living with HIV also have chronic diarrhea, affecting their quality of life, and a specific cause is not found. A stepwise approach with nonpharmacologic interventions such as hydration and electrolyte supplementation and dietary optimization with increased consumption of fibers is recommended. Some older medications have significant associated GI side effects and cardiometabolic problems. Prevention and appropriate surveillance and intervention in terms of nutrition, diet, and exercise are standards of care for all children.

NEUROLOGIC MANIFESTATIONS

HIV can affect neurologic function by directly invading glial cells in the developing brain that protect neurons and causing chronic inflammation that can result in developmental delay, cognitive impairment, and behavioral concerns. Early ART initiation has decreased many concerns, but continued viral replication in the central nervous system (CNS) and ongoing neuroinflammation persist (Crowell et al., 2015).

Those who experience a severe early illness are most at risk for significant impairment and may have irreversible CNS injury prior to ART initiation. The degree of neurologic deficit is variable and related to an individual's age at the first symptom, stage of disease and rate of disease progression, and current age (Crowell et al., 2015). Computed tomography scanning and magnetic resonance imaging often show impaired brain growth with diffuse cortical atrophy and basal ganglia calcifications in severely affected children. Cerebrospinal fluid (CSF)—even if positive for HIV culture—usually shows normal glucose and protein levels and normal cell count. Children and youth living with HIV are at risk for depression. The neurobiologic effects of HIV on the brain can cause chronic neuroinflammation and changes in neurotransmitters such as dopamine, leading to cognitive dysfunction and depression (Molinaro et al., 2021). Furthermore, perinatally infected children and youth living with HIV are at an increased risk for depression due to adverse childhood events, stigma, and neurobiologic effects.

Adolescents living with HIV infected through sexual transmission are at additional risk due to stigma and social minority stress.

OPPORTUNISTIC INFECTIONS

Among children with HIV in the United States, rates of all OIs decreased during 1997 to 2016. Earlier, OI rates were highest among non–US-born children but were later compared with those among US-born children for all OIs except tuberculosis (TB) (Nesheim et al., 2021). OIs continue to be the presenting symptom of HIV infection among children whose HIV exposure status is unknown usually because of a lack of maternal antenatal HIV testing or unrecognized acquisition of HIV infection during adolescence. For infants and children with known HIV infection, barriers such as inadequate medical care, lack of availability of suppressive ART regimens in the face of extensive prior treatment and drug resistance, caregiver substance abuse or mental illness, and multifactorial adherence difficulties may hinder effective HIV treatment and put patients at risk of OIs even in the ART era.

The natural history of OIs in children is different than that among adults with HIV; adults generally reactivate a previously acquired OI disease, whereas children more often have a primary infection with a pathogen. Additionally, children with perinatally acquired HIV infection probably become infected with the opportunistic pathogen after HIV infection has been established and the child is immunocompromised. The scenario can lead to manifestations of infection that are different than those in adults. Laboratory diagnosis can be difficult in children because of several factors, including issues of interpretation of maternal antibodies and the child's developmental capacity to describe symptoms of the infection.

OI is rarely the presenting illness for a child who was not identified as infected at birth. Management and treatment of OIs continue to be critical. The treatment and prevention of OIs is an ever-evolving science, and new agents and data analyses may improve therapeutic options and preferences. Initial and secondary prophylaxis with the use of systemic antifungal, antiviral, and antimicrobials is commonly indicated to prevent disease in children with moderate-severe immunosuppression.

PULMONARY DISEASE

Pulmonary disease and resultant respiratory disease contribute significantly to the morbidity and mortality of HIV infection in children. Despite successful trends in the treatment of HIV disease, chronic lung disease (CLD) is common in older children and adolescents living with HIV (Rylance et al., 2016). Constrictive obliterative bronchiolitis is the leading cause of CLD in children and adolescents with HIV (Price et al., 2021). Increasing evidence shows that HIV-infected children and adolescents have a high prevalence of lung function impairment, predominantly irreversible lower airway obstruction, and reduced aerobic function (Githinji et al., 2018). PCP accounts for approximately one-half of all AIDS-defining conditions diagnosed during the first year of life. Symptoms are likely to be acute with fever, dyspnea, dry cough, cyanosis, and hypoxemia. Treatment of acute infection usually begins with trimethoprim/sulfamethoxazole (TMP-SMX [Bactrim, Septra]) and corticosteroids. Prophylaxis, both primary and secondary, with oral TMP-SMX is extremely effective. TB is the most common OI in HIV-infected people worldwide. HIV-positive children are at risk of diagnostic error as well as delayed diagnosis of TB because of overlapping clinical and radiographic features with other lung diseases. Other pathogens that cause pulmonary infection include cytomegalovirus (CMV), respiratory syncytial virus, *Mycobacterium avium* complex, rubeola, varicella, and other viral, fungal, and bacterial sources.

PANCYTOPENIA

In cases of delayed diagnosis, children can have thrombocytopenia, an immune response to circulating platelets. Intravenous immunoglobulin (IVIG) is sometimes effective in raising platelet count. An alternative treatment is administering pulses of high-dose corticosteroids. Platelet transfusions are rarely required. Anemias of chronic disease and iron deficiency are common in this population and often require iron supplementation. Abnormalities of the white blood cell line (i.e., neutropenia, lymphocytopenia, leukopenia) are also often noted (Cao et al., 2022).

FUNGAL INFECTIONS

The most common fungal infections in children with HIV infection are caused by *Candida*. Localized disease caused by *Candida* results in oral thrush and diaper dermatitis, occurring in 50% to 85% of children with HIV infection. Oropharyngeal candidiasis (OPC)

continues to be one of the most frequent OIs in children with HIV infection. Invasive candidiasis is less frequent; however, it can result from dissemination from the esophagus when coinfected with other organisms, such as herpes simplex virus or CMV.

First-line treatments for OPC usually include oral nystatin (Mycostatin) and clotrimazole (Mycelex) oral troches. Infants can be treated either by placing the suppository into the nipple of a bottle, allowing the infant to suck formula through it, or by dissolving the suppository in warm water and swabbing the mouth. Older children can suck the suppositories. Oral fluconazole is more effective than nystatin suspension for the initial treatment of infants, easier to administer to children than topical therapies, and is the recommended treatment when systemic therapy is needed in more moderate-severe cases. Both nystatin and clotrimazole creams are available for skin infections.

PRENATAL AND PERINATAL SUBSTANCE USE EXPOSURE

Children with HIV born to mothers with HIV who have had drug or alcohol exposure are often premature, small for gestational age, and have very immature immune systems. Their development is often delayed, and learning and behavioral differences are common.

PROGNOSIS

There has been a steep decrease in morbidity and mortality among children and adolescents living with HIV. Perinatally infected children and adolescents infected through sexual transmission are living longer with HIV/AIDS (CDC, 2022b; Cantos et al., 2021). Although the prognosis initially was an average of 10 years from diagnosis of HIV infection to AIDS-related death, long-term prognosis and length of life are improved due to rapidly changing medical treatments and their improved effectiveness (Fig. 25.5).

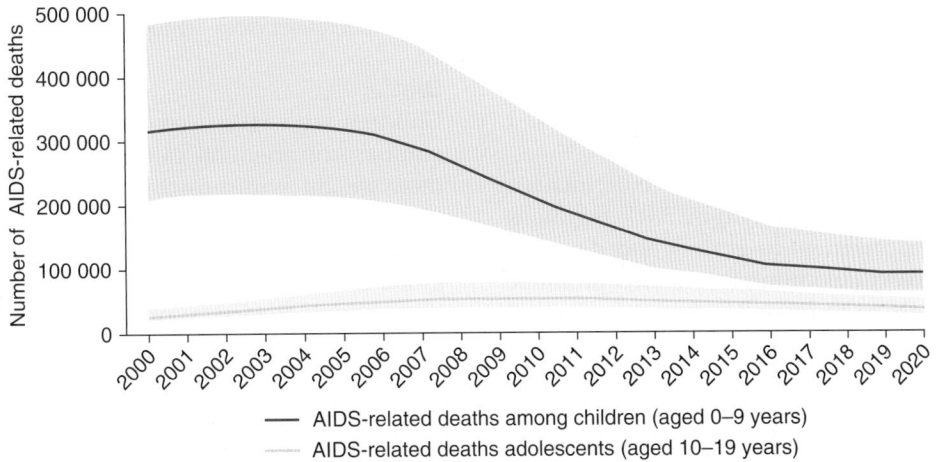

Fig. 25.5 Acquired immunodeficiency syndrome *(AIDS)*–related deaths among children (age 0–9 years) and adolescents (age 10–19 years), global, 2000–2020. (From United Nations AIDS. [2021]. UNAIDS epidemiological estimates, 2021. https://aidsinfo.unaids.org/.)

Pediatric HIV infection in resource-rich countries is now a chronic manageable condition. Since 2010, new HIV infections among children have declined by 52%. However, progress against HIV has been uneven. In resource-limited countries, pediatric HIV disease continues, with females in sub-Saharan Africa at a higher risk of HIV infection due to gender inequality and gender-based violence. Recent estimates from UNAIDS suggest that 90% of the estimated 2.1 million children younger than age 15 who have HIV live in sub-Saharan Africa (UNAIDS, 2021).

ADOLESCENTS

In the United States, 21% of new HIV diagnoses in 2019 were among young people age 13 to 24 years. The HIV epidemic disproportionately impacts Black MSM and transgender females. Eighty-eight percent of youth who received a new HIV diagnosis were young males, and 12% were young females, the majority Black. In addition, as the management and therapeutic treatments for children with perinatally acquired HIV infection continue to improve, when infected children reach adolescence they will need continuing care throughout these years and into adulthood.

PRIMARY CARE MANAGEMENT

HEALTH CARE MAINTENANCE

All children, including children treated at HIV centers, must also have a primary care provider. HIV specialty care providers and primary care providers must work together, collaborating with the child and family to provide the highest level of care.

Long-term morbidities for children and adolescents treated for HIV include the following:
- Mental health concerns (anxiety, mood, substance abuse disorders)
- Dyslipidemia
- Cardiovascular complications (cardiomyopathy, accelerated atherosclerosis)
- Insulin resistance and diabetes mellitus
- Decreased bone mineral
- Density renal disease

Growth and Development

Among HIV-infected children and adolescents, increasing the use of effective combination ART regimens has resulted in improvement in growth and development. The poor growth of children with symptomatic HIV disease appears to be related more to the general failure to thrive associated with HIV infection when untreated than to specific problems with calorie intake or GI losses. When ART is initiated at less than 1 year of age, catchup growth is usually associated with the achievement of normal height.

A health care practitioner or a skilled assistant should carefully measure height, weight, and body mass index at least monthly and plot the findings on the child's individual National Center for Health Statistics growth chart. The same scale should be used at each visit if possible.

Adequate nutrition is required for the healthy development of all children. Poor nutrition further compromises the immune system of a child with HIV and can lead to increased disease progression and the development of OIs. The metabolic needs of a child's body may also be higher because of the physiologic stress of HIV infection. Untreated HIV and immunosuppression have also been linked to delayed puberty.

Developmental delay is common in HIV-infected children and may have worse neurodevelopmental outcomes compared with uninfected children (McHenry et al., 2018). Early intervention in young children seems to produce significant results, and therefore a skilled clinician must regularly assess children as part of the comprehensive team approach. Older children and adolescents are at risk for impaired working memory, processing speed, and executive function. It is important for the primary care provider and the clinician to discuss the developmental assessments and formulate a collaborative action plan. In a recent study that examined developmental screenings for early treated HIV-infected and HIV-exposed and uninfected children, all children had worse developmental outcomes compared with HIV-uninfected and HIV-unexposed children. There are increasing concerns with outcomes in those who are exposed to ART and ultimately uninfected. Some researchers suggest that HIV-exposed and uninfected children may also have poorer development compared with their unexposed peers (McHenry et al., 2018).

Early intervention strategies can change a development path and improve outcomes. Infant stimulation programs that focus on motor and language skills and additional specialties (e.g., physical, occupational, and speech therapy) can be provided at home, in the hospital, or in the clinic or group settings. Preschool and school-aged children can attend general education programs with special services added (Zinyemba et al., 2019).

Diet

Children with HIV need a well-balanced diet with an emphasis on adequate calories to maintain and increase their weight with growth. Nutritionists must be part of the multidisciplinary primary care team to obtain dietary histories and perform nutritional assessments to guide clinical decisions. HIV infection does not involve any special dietary recommendations or restrictions. Because failure to thrive is common in infected children, however, early nutritional intervention before wasting occurs is important. Severe acute malnutrition is associated with increased microbial translocation, immune activation, immune exhaustion, and worse prognosis and impaired immune recovery in HIV-infected children on ART (Muenchhoff et al., 2018).

Dietary supplementation and special formulas are often beneficial for weight stabilization and potential gain. Enteral feedings and IV alimentation may be used acutely, intermittently, or chronically for children with severe anorexia, vomiting, diarrhea, or other GI problems. Families should regularly consult the primary care provider regarding the child's particular needs. Oral megestrol (Megace) has increased appetite in some children (Clarick et al., 1997; Samour et al., 2003).

In the United States, the most recent AAP policy statement, "Breastfeeding and the Use of Human Milk" (Meek & Noble, 2022), recommends that mothers in the United States living with HIV should not breastfeed or feed expressed milk to their infants. In resource-limited settings, the benefits of breastfeeding outweigh the risks, and evidence is increasingly clear that the risk of transmission is low if exclusively breastfeeding. In the United States, supporters of breastfeeding have published a consensus statement in which they "[a]ssert the need for parents living with HIV to have access to the information, support, and tools necessary to make informed infant-feeding decisions." More information can be found at The Well Project (https://www.thewellproject.org/hiv-information/expert-consensus-statement-breastfeeding-and-hiv-united-states-and-canada) (Agwu, 2022).

Safety

Primary care providers must teach safety precautions for children with neutropenia and thrombocytopenia, as well as how to evaluate a child with neutropenia for signs and symptoms of infection. Caretakers may benefit from education on infectious disease transmission and control (e.g., the need for frequent hand washing and avoiding people with known contagious infections). Children with HIV and their household contacts must learn universal/standard blood and body substance precautions; day care and school personnel also must be knowledgeable regarding infection control issues. Several prospective studies of family and school contacts have found no evidence of the spread of HIV within these settings (CDC, 2022b; Courville et al., 1998). Although HIV has been isolated in a variety of body fluids (including blood, CSF, pleural fluid, breast milk, semen, cervical secretions, saliva, and urine), only blood, semen, cervical secretions, and human milk have been implicated in its transmission. Children with HIV may be developmentally delayed or exhibit neurologic regression as the infection progresses, and safety precautions must be adjusted accordingly. If an HIV-infected parent cares for the child, the parent's ability to provide safe care must be frequently assessed because of cognitive changes that can be associated with HIV infections in adults.

Immunizations

In the past, live virus vaccines were not recommended for children with congenital or drug-induced immunodeficiencies because of the concern that live attenuated vaccine viruses may produce infection in an immunocompromised host. Prospective studies, however, failed to reveal such problems in children with HIV (CDC, 2021).

In addition, the dysfunction of the B-cell system typical of infants with HIV disease, which includes markedly elevated immunoglobulins, reflects nonspecific stimulations that are suggestive of a poor immune response to antigens and therefore to vaccines. This immunologic dysfunction may lower the immunogenicity and efficacy of vaccines in infected children. In general, children with symptomatic HIV infections have poor immunologic responses to vaccines and therefore should be considered susceptible regardless of the history of vaccination. They should receive passive immunoprophylaxis if indicated when they are exposed to a vaccine-preventable disease such as measles or tetanus (CDC, 2021).

For older children and adolescents diagnosed with HIV, immunity should be checked with titers at diagnosis, and vaccines should be administered to those who were not previously vaccinated and nonimmune.

The routine immunization schedule for infants and children continues to be the standard of care. Most immunizations follow the standard pediatric schedule without regard for the child's HIV status in terms of stage of infection and symptoms with specific considerations, and few immunizations are contraindications. Current recommendations are as follows (CDC, 2023) (Fig. 25.6):

- *Hepatitis B virus.* Routine immunizations are recommended.
- *Rotavirus.* Routine immunizations are recommended. Practitioners should consider the potential risks and benefits of administering *Rotavirus* to infants with known or suspected altered immunocompetence. Consultation with an immunologist or infectious disease specialist is advised, particularly for infants with HIV infection who have a low CD4 cell percentage or count. Limited safety and efficacy data are available for the administration of *Rotavirus* to infants who are potentially immunocompromised, including those with HIV infection. However, the following considerations support the vaccination of infants who are HIV exposed or infected:
  - In infants born to mothers with HIV, an HIV diagnosis may not be established before the age of the first *Rotavirus* dose.
  - Vaccine strains of *Rotavirus* are considerably attenuated.
- *DTaP, Dt, Tdap.* Routine immunizations recommended. Children with HIV should receive tetanus immunoglobulin (TIG) regardless of vaccine status after an injury that places them at risk for tetanus infection.
- *Haemophilus influenzae type B (Hib).* Routine immunization recommended. *H. influenzae* organisms are

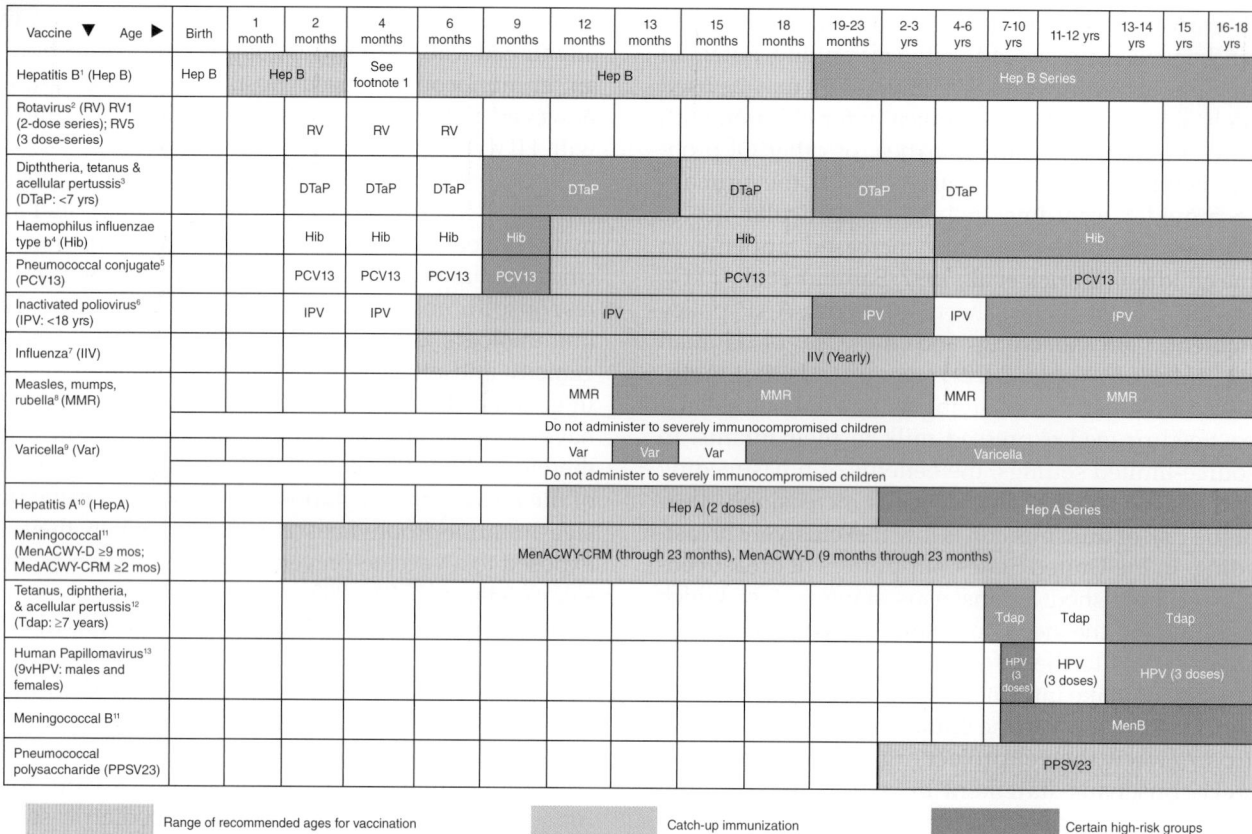

Range of recommended ages for vaccination   Catch-up immunization   Certain high-risk groups

(Last updated October 25, 2019: last reviewed October 25, 2019)

Fig. 25.6 Recommended immunization schedule for children with human immunodeficiency virus infection age 0 through 18 years; United States, 2019. (From Siberry, G.K., Abzug, M.J., Nachman, S., Brady, M.T., Dominguez, K.L., Handelsman, E., Mofenson, L.M., Nesheim, S., Panel on Opportunistic Infections in HIV-Exposed and HIV-Infected Children, National Institutes of Health, Centers for Disease Control and Prevention, HIV Medicine Association of the Infectious Diseases Society of America, Pediatric Infectious Diseases Society, & American Academy of Pediatrics. [2013]. Guidelines for the prevention and treatment of opportunistic infections in HIV-exposed and HIV-infected children. *Pediatric Infectious Disease Journal, 32*, Si–SKK4.)

common and serious pathogens in children with HIV. Even children who have had one or more episodes of documented infections with *H. influenzae* before 2 years of age may not produce enough antibodies, making vaccinations critical. Prophylaxis with rifampin (Rifadin) is required even if vaccinated if there is a known contact with Hib (CDC, 2021).

- *Pneumococcal conjugate vaccine* (13-valent [PCV13], 15-valent [PCV15], 20-valent [PCV20]) and pneumococcal polysaccharide vaccine (23-valent [PPSV23]) are recommended as routine immunizations. Pneumococci are prevalent pathogens in children with HIV. PCV13 should be given to infants on schedule. Children age 2 years and above also should receive PPSV23 8 weeks after their last PCV13 dose. A second dose of PPSV23 should be administered 5 years after the first dose of PPSV23. Adults should also receive catchup vaccines with PCV15 or PCV20 if never immunized as well as two PPSV23 vaccines.
- *Inactivated polio.* Routine immunization is recommended.
- *Influenza.* Routine immunization is recommended. Inactivated influenza vaccine is recommended for

children with HIV. Administer two doses (separated by at least 4 weeks) to children less than 9 years of age per current influenza vaccine recommendations. Caretakers and primary care providers must remember to have the child receive annual influenza vaccine as soon as available to provide prolonged protection. In addition, all people who have contact with individuals with HIV infection should be strongly encouraged to receive annual influenza vaccination to limit the exposure of persons with compromised immune systems to influenza. Primary care providers should ensure that children with HIV and their caretakers receive the influenza vaccine as soon as it is available each year.

- *Measles, mumps, rubella (MMR).* Routine immunization is recommended except for children who are severely immunocompromised (CDC, 2022). Two doses of MMR vaccine are also recommended for all individuals with HIV infection 12 months of age and older who do not have evidence of current severe immunosuppression. The first dose should be administered at age 12 to 15 months, and the second dose at age 4 through 6 years (or as early as 28 days after the first dose). Regardless of vaccination status, children should receive prophylaxis with immunoglobulin after exposure to measles. Immunoglobulin prophylaxis may help prevent or minimize measles if it is administered within 6 days of exposure. It is also indicated for household contacts of children with HIV disease who are measles susceptible, especially infants younger than 12 months. Immunoglobulin may be unnecessary if a child is receiving regular IVIG infusions and the last dose was within 3 weeks of exposure.

- *Varicella (VZV).* Routine immunization is recommended except for children who are severely immunocompromised (CDC, 2022). Varicella poses significant risks for dissemination, encephalitis, and pneumonia in children who are immunosuppressed. Single-antigen varicella vaccine should be considered for children and adolescents with HIV infection with CD4 percentages of 15% or above. Children with HIV who are susceptible to varicella and have had significant exposure to varicella or herpes zoster, and are severely immune compromised, should receive varicella zoster immunoglobulin as soon as possible within the first 10 days after exposure. MMR vaccine has not been studied in children or adolescents with HIV infection and should not be substituted for the single-antigen varicella vaccine.
- *Hepatitis A virus.* Routine immunization is recommended.
- *Meningococcal.* Routine immunization is recommended.
- *Meningococcal B.* Young adults age 16 through 23 years (preferred age range is 16–18 years) may be vaccinated with either a two-dose series of Bexsero or a three-dose series of Trumenba vaccine to provide short-term protection against most strains of serogroup B meningococcal disease.
- *Tdap.* Routine immunization is recommended. Administer one dose of the Tdap vaccine to pregnant adolescents during each pregnancy (preferred early during 27–36 weeks of gestation) regardless of the time since prior Td or Tdap vaccination.
- *Human papillomavirus (HPV).* Routine immunization is recommended. The 9vHPV is not a live virus vaccine and can therefore be administered safely regardless of immune status. The immune response and vaccine efficacy, however, in immunosuppressed individuals may be decreased. HPV vaccines are most effective for both males and females when given before exposure to HPV through sexual contact. Administer the first dose at age 11 or 12 years (CDC, 2022).
- *SARS-CoV-2.* Routine immunization is recommended. The immune response and vaccine efficacy, however, in immunosuppressed individuals may be decreased.

Screenings

Vision. Primary care providers must elicit a thorough visual history and provide a careful visual and funduscopic examination due to a potential risk for CMV retinitis in children living with HIV. Comprehensive pediatric HIV centers may recommend that all children living with HIV be referred to a knowledgeable pediatric ophthalmologist for baseline screening and annual follow-up. If the findings are normal, the primary care provider can then continue to provide regular follow-ups.

Hearing. Because of frequent acute suppurative otitis media (OM) in children living with HIV and the possibility of hearing loss, periodic audiometry and tympanometry should be performed. Children who require myringotomy tube placement must use specific precautions for swimming and showers (e.g., regular use of well-fitting earplugs). Children with severe neurologic disease, some children with chronic OM, and those receiving maintenance aminoglycoside therapy need baseline brainstem, auditory-evoked response hearing testing if routine acuity testing cannot be done or test results are abnormal.

Dental. Early screening (i.e., starting at 2–3 years of age) is strongly recommended because dental caries can create a focus on infection. Fluoride treatments are recommended if the community water supply does not contain adequate amounts to protect enamel. Severe dental caries and gingivitis, as well as dental abscesses, are reported in some infected children (Ramos-Gomez & Folayan, 2013). Clinicians must educate families regarding appropriate oral hygiene and encourage regular dental care. Liquid medications contain sweeteners to increase drug palatability, which also increases the risk of caries.

Blood pressure. Blood pressure measurements should be taken every 3 to 6 months unless changes warrant more frequent measurements. Increased blood pressure can indicate renal disease.

Hematocrit. Routine screening is deferred because of the need for frequent assessment of complete blood cell counts.

Urinalysis. Children with HIV require urinalysis with a microscopic examination at least every 6 months because urine abnormalities can be the first sign of illness. Findings can include hematuria and proteinuria and can result in azotemia and nephrotic syndrome.

Tuberculosis. Yearly screening is strongly advised. Because many individuals infected with HIV demonstrated anergy to skin testing, close surveillance of families may include regular chest radiographic studies. Diagnostic methods for latent TB infection include the tuberculin skin test (TST) or interferon-gamma release assays (IGRA). TST is preferred over IGRA in children younger than 5 years of age.

Condition-Specific Screening

Vital signs. Vital signs should be assessed and documented at each visit. Children can be asymptomatic yet febrile, needing a workup. Elevations in heart and respiratory rates can indicate pulmonary or cardiac dysfunction.

Complete blood count. Because of bone marrow suppression caused by HIV and some OIs, children with HIV require regular CBCs with differential and platelet counts. Asymptomatic children should have a CBC performed every 3 to 6 months; symptomatic children usually need them at least monthly. This bloodwork can be performed by the primary care provider or at the pediatric HIV center. If anemia is present, its cause should be investigated because children with iron-deficiency anemia usually benefit from oral iron supplementation. A specific cause, however, is not often discovered. CBCs are usually performed every 2 weeks for the first 2 months and then done every 3 months if the children are stable.

Immunologic markers. Absolute CD4 T-lymphocyte cell count should be measured at the time of HIV diagnosis. T-cell subset values and T4/T8 ratios are usually checked every 3 to 6 months. Clinicians must consider age as a variable in interpreting immunologic markers for children. These markers are used in conjunction with other markers to guide primary PCP and other OIs after 1 year of age.

HIV viral load. The viral burden can be determined by using a quantitative HIV RNA viral load assay of peripheral blood. During primary infection in adults and adolescents, the HIV RNA viral load rises to peak levels and then—coinciding with the body's humoral and cell-mediated immune response—declines to a stable lower level 6 to 12 months later. This leveling reflects the balance (steady state) between ongoing viral production and immune elimination (CDC, 2022). This pattern differs in perinatally infected infants in that high HIV RNA levels usually persist during the first year of life and then gradually decline over the next few years. This pattern may reflect an immature but developing immune system's lower efficiency in containing viral replication and more HIV-susceptible cells. Trends in HIV RNA levels are helpful in determining the response to ART and when agents should be changed. Because of the complexities of testing and the age-related changes in values, interpretation of HIV RNA levels for clinical decision making should

be made by or in consultation with pediatric HIV experts. The message of undetectable = untransmittable (U=U) is based on a large body of research in which no transmitted HIV infections were transmitted when the viral load was below detection (Eisinger, 2019). U=U is a critical tool in counseling children and adolescents living with HIV regarding treatment as prevention.

Chemistry panel. Routine serum chemistry panels (including electrolytes, blood urea nitrogen, creatinine, glucose, hepatic transaminases, calcium, phosphorus), pancreatic enzyme evaluations, and serum lipid evaluations should be obtained every 3 to 6 months and more often for some symptomatic children or those taking medications that might affect liver or kidney function. Many children with HIV have elevated baseline liver function test results, often with aspartate aminotransferase and alanine aminotransferase enzyme levels two to three times normal levels. Children taking some older medications must be monitored for additional side effects, and providers can consult the HIV treatment guidelines or an HIV provider.

Pulmonary function. Children with CLD need baseline pulmonary function testing with oxygen saturation and regular serial testing based on disease severity. When available, pulse oximetry (a noninvasive technique) is used in place of arterial blood gas sampling. A baseline radiograph is useful as a comparison study for later pulmonary complaints. Children with either acute infection or chronic pneumonitis often have no adventitious sounds. Pulmonary consultation is a useful adjunct for the primary care provider in the follow-up of these children.

Antiretroviral medication adherence assessment. Medication adherence is fundamental to the success of ART. The degree of viral suppression achieved and the restoration of the immune system are related to early initiation and degree of medication adherence (Uprety et al., 2017). Adherence is a complex issue that is influenced by many factors (e.g., age, ability to swallow, behavioral factors), family issues (supportive or distant), and characteristics of the health care providers (supportive and engaging or distant and prescriptive). Multiple methods to assess adherence are recommended. These include a self-report, verbal description of medication regiment, pill counts, checking pharmacy refills, and use of electronic monitoring devices. A nonjudgmental attitude and trusting relationship are the most valuable tools for all providers (CDC, 2022).

COMMON ILLNESS MANAGEMENT
Differential Diagnosis
Fever. Fever is often a sign in children with HIV disease and can be caused by the HIV itself or can

indicate a separate infectious process. Practitioners must ensure that families have a thermometer that they can use accurately, in addition to clear guidelines about when to contact their primary care provider. Whenever a child's temperature is 101°F (38.5°C) or higher, the child needs to be examined and a treatment plan initiated based on objective and subjective findings. A thorough interval history and complete physical examination are the most important part of the workup of a febrile child with HIV. Some children will have OM, sinusitis, pneumonia, or sepsis. Others will have a common cold and other viral infections that can be traced to school or household contacts. In consultation with the infectious disease specialist or the HIV center, the primary care provider can order cultures of blood and other body fluids as indicated for aerobic, anaerobic, and fungal organisms. Cultures are essential to identifying the infectious process. Cultures are often negative—even in seriously ill children—but positive cultures will determine specific antibiotic therapy. Chest radiographic studies may be an important part of the workup of a febrile child with HIV.

Respiratory distress. A variety of respiratory conditions may occur in children with HIV. History and physical examination are paramount to differential diagnosis. A dry hacking cough is common in interstitial pneumonia but could also be a sign of PCP. Children with cardiac disease occasionally have respiratory symptoms and need cardiologic consultation and diagnosis. Children with known reactive airway disease may benefit from equipment and medications for aerosol delivery at home. The primary care provider must evaluate the family's ability to provide assessment and treatment and can be taught the necessary skills.

Otitis media. OM is one of the most common infectious diseases in children with HIV and is often diagnosed on routine physical examination when no pain or fever is present, even when the tympanic membrane may be ruptured with pus filling the external canal. Children with presumptive infection, rather than noninfectious effusion, should be promptly treated with antibiotics using standard treatment. Follow-up must be done after treatment is completed because the OM may not resolve, and complications may occur. Children who have persistent and refractory OM should be referred to an ear, nose, and throat specialist for evaluation for placement of myringotomy tubes.

Sinusitis. Although sinusitis is uncommon in children, it is common in children with HIV disease and often occurs after a viral respiratory tract infection. Primary care providers can teach families to report changes in nasal mucus from clear or white to yellow or green, which may indicate infection; other signs and symptoms may include fever, headache, facial pain, and prolonged nasal discharge and congestion. If not appropriately treated, sinusitis can lead to mastoiditis and directly extend into the brain, causing meningitis.

Varicella-Zoster virus. The incidence of varicella and its associated morbidity and mortality have decreased by 88% or more because of universal vaccination. Varicella vaccination is also associated with a decrease in herpes zoster in children living with HIV. Children living with HIV who are susceptible to varicella and have had significant exposure to varicella or herpes zoster, and are severely immunocompromised, should receive varicella zoster immunoglobulin as soon as possible within the first 10 days after exposure. Oral therapy with acyclovir for 7 to 10 days is recommended for children living with HIV with herpes zoster, although longer therapy duration should be considered when lesions are slow to resolve. Initial IV administration is recommended for children living with HIV with severe immunosuppression, extensive multidermatomal herpes zoster, disseminated infection, visceral involvement, or otherwise complicated herpes zoster. With this treatment few children progress to disseminated disease, and most go home within 5 days of starting therapy, continuing with oral therapy to complete a 7- to 10-day course.

Drug Interactions
Antiretroviral drugs. The antiretroviral medications used in children living with HIV are listed in Box 25.3. Many of these drugs have significant drug interactions. It is best to identify the specific potential interactions of every drug to be prescribed in primary care before prescribing the medication. The primary care provider can contact the HIV treatment center for consultation if questions regarding medication prescription arise.

TMP-SMX. Major adverse effects of TMP-SMX are a rash, GI complaints, and renal and hematologic problems. Children receiving PCP or treatment regimens in whom persistent neutropenia develops secondary to TMP-SMX treatment either alone or with azidothymidine (AZT) must often discontinue TMP-SMX treatment. Dapsone, atovaquone, and IV or aerosolized pentamidine can be used as alternatives in older children. Allergic reactions to sulfa are not uncommon, and primary care providers must teach families how to recognize the symptoms of skin rash and hives as part of the reaction complex. Based on adult randomized clinical trials, unless the reaction has been life threatening, TMP-SMX PCP can be resumed in children, preferably by beginning with low desensitizing daily doses and gradually increasing to

Box 25.3 **HIV Medication**

INTEGRASE INHIBITORS
Bictegravir
Cabotegravir
Dolutegravir
Elvitegravir
Raltegravir

NUCLEOSIDE AND NUCLEOTIDE ANALOGUE REVERSE TRANSCRIPTASE INHIBITORS
Abacavir
Emtricitabine
Lamivudine
Tenofovir alafenamide
Tenofovir disoproxil fumarate
Zidovudine

NONNUCLEOSIDE ANALOGUE REVERSE TRANSCRIPTASE INHIBITORS
Doravirine
Efavirenz
Etravirine
Nevirapine
Rilpivirine

PROTEASE INHIBITORS
Atazanavir
Darunavir
Lopinavir/ritonavir

therapeutic dosing. The overall frequency of adverse reactions appears to be lower in HIV-infected children than in adults.

Intravenous immunoglobulin. There is no specific drug interaction noted with IVIG. Allergic reactions have been documented but appear to be rare.

DEVELOPMENTAL ISSUES

Sleep Patterns
ART is generally given during waking hours. Frequent dosing is no longer required as was necessary for the early days of ART. Many regimens are available as single-tablet therapy. Other medications may require night dosing schedules that interrupt sleep; however, children whose normal sleeping hours must be interrupted for treatment may have trouble returning to sleep. Therefore parents may need to try a variety of schedules to find one that works best for them and their child to minimize interruptions in their child's sleeping.

Toileting
Children with HIV who are in diapers may experience diaper dermatitis, which is often associated with candidiasis and with chronic and cyclic diarrhea. Impeccable perineal care, including frequent diaper changes, exposure of the perineum to air, and the use of topical medications, can significantly reduce morbidity. When the perineum is bloody or the child has hematuria or diarrhea, caretakers should wear gloves and protect themselves during diapering. Neurologic deterioration can lead to incontinence in children who have previously stopped using diapers.

Discipline
Discipline is often difficult for the family of a child with a chronic, life-threatening condition. Some parents are unable to set developmentally appropriate and necessary limits and need guidance and information from their primary care provider. Discipline needs and appropriate expectations will vary as the illness progresses; if neurologic and motor deterioration occur, caretakers must be given anticipatory guidance in these areas. Other factors (i.e., mental health, homelessness, parental illness) can make consistent discipline difficult. Practitioners may need to help families and caregivers understand the child's needs for safety and limits.

Child Care
Child care, respite care, and preschool placement are difficult issues for families of children with HIV. Primary care providers must advise parents that children in group settings are at increased risk for exposure to infectious diseases and common childhood illnesses compared with children who stay at home. The particular care setting must be individualized for each child based on the child's and the family's needs and resources. Practitioners can provide education on universal infection control and infectious disease guidelines for these agencies.

Child care and respite care are important resources for families of children with chronic conditions. Some foster families have access to respite hours through their social services division, but others do not. The regular availability of respite care and other support services may allow many infected mothers to continue caring for their children. It is important to note that uninfected parents and caregivers also need respite care. Head Start, a federal preschool program that provides preschool for economically disadvantaged children, is specifically mandated to enroll children with HIV.

Because day care and preschool are not legal requirements for children, individual day care providers may develop their own policies in accordance with local, state, and federal regulations. Parents/guardians of a child with HIV are not required to reveal that their child is infected with HIV. They may choose to share the information confidentially so they can ask the program to observe the child more closely than other children for signs of illness that might require medical attention. If parents/guardians share the HIV status of their children, this information is not to be disclosed to staff members without written permission of the parents/guardians. Only the child's parents/guardians and health professionals have an absolute need to know the child is infected with HIV. Some families choose to conceal the diagnosis of HIV in their family, but other families openly discuss it. Clinicians have an important role in helping families decide how, when, and to whom information about HIV disease should be disclosed.

Schooling

School is critically important for children living with HIV. It is normalizing and imperative for socialization and a sense of belonging. It can result in the development of healthy self-esteem. The major school issues faced by children living with HIV are related to concerns about confidentiality, information sharing, and infection control. These issues have created strife in many communities nationwide. Zinyemba et al. (2019), in a systematic review, found the following ways HIV affects children's education attainment: sickness of the child and orphanhood, effects on gender gaps, and intergenerational transmission of education due to parental illness.

Public Law 101-476 supports the attendance of children living with HIV in public schools. No child with HIV should be denied access to school or the ability to be involved in contact sports. Psychoeducational testing should be completed for special education services. Primary care providers can help families secure appropriate services.

The legal duty to inform school officials about an HIV diagnosis varies from state to state. As more children are aware of their own HIV infection, discussion among children may ensue, resulting in increased awareness in the school and larger community that a child with HIV is in attendance. The provider should be available to the school (i.e., students, faculty, parents) for education and discussion sessions.

Teenagers living with HIV often have difficulty in school. Social determinants of health, such as parental drug abuse, lack of social support, parental illness and death, or changes in living circumstances, all play a role in school functioning (van Opstal et al., 2021).

Primary care providers can support their teenage clients by helping them gain more knowledge and determine with whom they might trust this sensitive information. It may be helpful for infected teens to meet in face-to-face groups and online groups to work together on developing strategies for dealing with school-based problems. Referral to the school nurse or counselor may be appropriate. The risk of blood contamination during sports, particularly contact sports, as well as related to accidents, is an issue to consider for children and adolescents with HIV. Universal precautions should be stressed so that infected children can lead healthy, active lives both in and out of school.

Sexuality

Children and adolescents with HIV need to learn about all modes of HIV transmission, with an emphasis on sexual, IV drug use, and perinatal transmission. Adolescence is the time for sexual experimentation and the emergence of sexual identity; sexual activity increases steadily throughout these years, and many adolescents living with HIV will become sexually active. Children and adolescents living with HIV may have difficulty attaining a healthy, integrated sexual identity because of the concerns of sexual transmission and disclosure (Flynn & Abrams, 2019; Tassiopoulos, 2013). Teens with cognitive delays stemming from the neurologic effects of HIV may have a particularly difficult time understanding transmission risks. Primary care providers must discuss medication adherence in the context of U=U and other sexual risk reduction strategies, including PrEP for partners, as well as demonstrate the proper use of barrier methods. Health care providers must be able to have regular discussions about adolescent risk-taking behaviors with their patients.

Schools should provide health education to students, families, and staff. Educating students can help reduce the prevalence of sexual risk behaviors among teens, while appropriate school health policies can help protect the rights and health of students with HIV infection and staff members and reduce the probability of HIV transmission to others (CDC).

Transition to Adulthood

Adolescents living with HIV will continue to need a vast array of medical and psychosocial services throughout their childhood and transition to adulthood (Flynn, 2019). At year-end 2020, in the United States and six dependent areas, there were 12,588 persons living with diagnosed perinatally acquired HIV infection (CDC, 2021).

Children born to mothers with HIV are at risk of losing their mothers, as well as other infected family members, to HIV while they are young. Adult caretakers may not be available to help assist the adolescent into adulthood.

Transition is a time when 10% to 25% of youth living with HIV are at risk of dropping out of care (Flynn & Abrams, 2019). Many who are eventually engaged in an adult care environment have long gaps between their last appointment in pediatric and the first one in adult services. Knowledge of one's HIV status can affect the transition of care. It has also been observed that increases in mortality can occur shortly after transition, with increasing mortality rates depending on age and type of clinic. Outcomes are dependent on when and where they were born. In high- and middle-income countries there have been steep declines every year in morbidity and mortality rates since the late 1980s due to the availability of more effective ART and early treatment initiation (Flynn & Abrams, 2019).

Children and teenagers who are infected with HIV have many other concerns to face in their transmission to adulthood. Survival times have continued to increase; there are now long-term survivors among children who were perinatally infected (CDC, 2021). Some issues facing these children include the risk of sexual transmission, intimacy, and stigma. As HIV infection becomes a more chronic, life-threatening disease integrated into the mainstream of health care, these special issues may gradually decline. Facilitating a smooth transition for adolescents with HIV to adult care facilities can be complicated. Pediatric HIV care models are family centered, with input from a multidisciplinary team of providers. The relationships of these providers with the adolescent with HIV are typically long-standing and include the adolescent and family members. Adult HIV care facilities tend to provide more individual-centered care and can be busier and less inviting and comfortable for adolescents. General guidelines for transitional plans and the benefits of using them are available to assist primary providers (Flynn & Abrams, 2019).

Family Concerns

Many children living with HIV have mothers living with HIV who may be ill or deceased, and they also may have an infected father and siblings. Mothers who transmit HIV to their children may experience tremendous guilt. The physical and emotional burden of caring for a child who requires frequent medical and supportive treatments and who may have a developmental delay is enormous for all parents and caregivers, regardless of whether the adults are infected.

The most significant psychosocial issue facing children with HIV and their families is the social stigmatization associated with the condition. Many families initially feel isolated and unable to rely on their usual support systems for fear of rejection and retaliation. Fears of transmission by casual contact continue despite scientific knowledge to the contrary, and these fears affect the stigma associated with HIV.

Intervention by health care personnel can help educate and allay family fears, and information about transmission prevention is a useful and important component of anticipatory guidance for adolescents. Infected families may also lack other resources because the majority of those infected are historically disenfranchised and minoritized. With support, affected families may reach out to extended family, friends, and community agencies. Noninfected parents and caregivers also need support in caring for their children and in obtaining the available community support. During the early years of the HIV epidemic, many children were not told of their diagnosis because of family concerns that the child would become depressed and angry or might tell others and expose the family to discrimination or stigmatization. Now that infected children are surviving into adolescence and adulthood, disclosure is becoming a more common clinical issue. Recommendations and guidelines for disclosure are available through the AAP and national AIDS groups (Elizabeth, 2020). The process of disclosure should consider the child's age, psychosocial maturity, and family dynamics. Most recommend a gradual process of giving children age-appropriate information about their illness with complete disclosure of the diagnosis when the child has the cognitive and emotional maturity to process the information, usually in late childhood.

Family and caregivers must understand the importance of pharmacotherapy adherence, and interventions to support the successful transition of medication responsibility from family and caregivers to older children and youth are imperative in improving health outcomes (MacDonell et al., 2015). Among 381 children and adolescents with perinatally acquired HIV, the prevalence of nonadherence increased from 31% to 50% ($p < 0.001$), and the prevalence of unsuppressed viral loads increased from 16% to 40% ($p < 0.001$) between preadolescence and late adolescence/young adulthood (Kacanek et al., 2019). Regimen, patient/family, and health care–related medication adherence strategies all have found promise in improving adherence.

Most children who were perinatally infected with HIV are Black or Hispanic. Some children are placed in foster or adoptive care after birth if their birth mother is unable to care for them. Others are later placed with caregivers outside the home when resources cannot support their parents' ability to care for them. Foster and adoptive parents need considerable support (i.e., ongoing education, financial support, respite care, emotional support and counseling, and social support and legal counseling) to provide optimal care for children with HIV. Because children in foster care are wards of the juvenile court, the decision about consent for investigational drugs and experimental protocols, as well as do-not-resuscitate orders, must be court ordered. Working relationships among the primary care provider, HIV center, and social services must be developed and maintained to ensure that children with HIV receive optimal care in the child's welfare system. Support groups are invaluable resources for networking, keeping current, and decreasing social isolation. Most pediatric HIV/AIDS comprehensive treatment centers offer such groups on an ongoing basis.

RESOURCES

Elizabeth Glaser Pediatric AIDS Foundation: www.pedaids.org

National Center for Youth Law: www.youthlaw.org

Office of AIDS Research, National Institutes of Health (clinical guidelines): https://clinicalinfo.hiv.gov/en/guidelines

Summary

Primary Care Needs for the HIV Infections and AIDS

HEALTH CARE MAINTENANCE
Growth and Development
- Growth in both weight and height should be measured and plotted quarterly; if below the 5th percentile on the growth curve, measure and plot monthly.
- Body composition surveillance is needed.
- Careful developmental screening (with serial screening) and collaboration with a psychologist as needed are recommended.
- Early intervention programs are recommended to maximize developmental potential.

Diet
- A balanced high-calorie diet should be emphasized.
- Nutritionist to collaborate in the care.
- Nutritional supplements and medications to increase appetite are often beneficial.

Safety
- If immunocompromised, the risk of infection is increased. Frequent hand washing and avoiding people with known infections are recommended.
- Bleeding can be increased if thrombocytopenia is present.
- Universal/standard blood and body substance precautions should be taught to the family and caregivers.
- Safe storage of medication in the home is important.
- Developmental delay or regression may alter safety requirements.
- Parents may benefit from a home evaluation, especially as medications/treatments become more complex.

Immunizations
- Routine vaccine schedules are recommended for all vaccines if immunocompetent.
- If immunocompromised, wait to administer live vaccines such as varicella and MMR.
- See Fig. 25.6 and follow CDC guidelines for up-to-date recommendations.
- Passive immunoprophylaxis may be indicated when exposure occurs.
  - Give immunoglobulin within 6 days of measles exposure to prevent or modify the course unless the child has received IVIG within the previous 3 weeks.
  - Known exposure to Hib requires prophylaxis with rifampin.
  - Varicella-zoster immunoglobulin (VZIG) is recommended within 96 hours of varicella exposure.

Screening
- *Vision.* Consider baseline funduscopic examination by an ophthalmologist with practitioner follow-up every 3 to 6 months; consider ophthalmologist follow-up every 1 to 2 years.
- *Hearing.* Periodic audiometry and tympanometry screenings are recommended. Frequent acute OM and treatment with aminoglycosides may affect hearing. A brainstem evoked-response hearing test should be given to children with chronic OM or abnormal screening.
- *Dental.* Early screening is recommended to prevent dental infections; it should be followed up at least every 6 months to prevent and/or treat dental caries.
- *Blood pressure.* Measure every 3 to 6 months. Increased blood pressure may indicate renal disease.
- *Hematocrit.* Routine screening is deferred because of the need for frequent CBCs.
- *Urinalysis.* Urinalysis with microscopic examination should be done at least every 3 months to rule out renal disease; monthly for children taking indinavir (Crixivan).
- *Tuberculosis.* Yearly screening is recommended. Chest radiographic studies may be needed if a child is anergic. MAI infections are responsible for significant morbidity.

Condition-Specific Screening
- *Vital signs.* Temperature, heart rate, and respiratory rate should be checked at each visit.
- *Complete blood cell count.* A CBC should be assessed at baseline and then every 3 to 6 months if a child is asymptomatic; those who are stable on ART may require only quarterly blood counts.
- *Immunologic markers.* CD4 count (total and %) should be checked every 3 to 6 months.
- *HIV markers.* HIV RNA viral load assays are taken at baseline and quarterly to determine disease progression and response to ART.
- *Chemistry panel.* Serum chemistry panels should be obtained at baseline and then every 3 to 6 months if the child is asymptomatic/stable.
  - CD4 count, CBC, and chemistries can be monitored less frequently (every 6–12 months) in children and youth who are adherent to therapy, who have CD4 count values that are well above the threshold for opportunistic infection risk, and who have had sustained virologic suppression and stable clinical status for more than 2 to 3 years.
- *Pulmonary function.* Baseline pulmonary function testing, including pulse oximetry if available, is recommended for children with lung disease.
- *ART adherence assessment.* Adherence, toxicity, and efficacy assessments need to be done at least quarterly, including blood counts, chemistry panels, CD4 count/percentage, and HIV viral load. Some medications require additional regular monitoring.

COMMON ILLNESS MANAGEMENT
Differential Diagnosis
- *Fever.* Rule out bacterial, viral, fungal infections, and OIs.
- *Respiratory distress.* Rule out PCP, other respiratory diseases, and cardiac disease.
- *Otitis media.* Rule out tympanic membrane perforation.
- *Sinusitis.* Rule out bacterial sinusitis, mastoiditis, and meningitis.
- *Varicella.* Use VZIG as primary prevention and acyclovir as secondary prevention even with the history of varicella vaccine.

Drug Interactions
- *ART medications.* Determine drug interactions and adverse reactions known with each prescribed drug.
- *TMP-SMX.* Bone marrow suppression (neutropenia, thrombocytopenia) and allergic reactions may occur.
- *IVIG.* No specific drug interactions, and allergic reactions are rare.

Continued

DEVELOPMENTAL ISSUES
Sleep Patterns
- Sleep patterns may be disturbed because of medications needed around the clock.

Toileting
- Impeccable perineal care is necessary to reduce the morbidity of diaper dermatitis. Caretakers should use gloves for blood or diarrhea. Neurologic deterioration can lead to incontinence.

Discipline
- Help caregivers to develop appropriate expectations of the child and refer as necessary to therapy for support.

Child Care
- Participation in child care and preschool increases the risk of infections. The child care program should be individualized to meet the child's and family's needs.
- IDEA 2004 (IDEA ensures that children with disabilities receive an appropriate education) and the Lanterman Act (covers early intervention services; all babies born to infected mothers are potentially at risk and qualify for services until the age of 3 years).
- Head Start is mandated to enroll children with HIV.
- Child care personnel need education on standard precautions.

Schooling
- Public Law 101-476 aids public school attendance.
- There is no duty to inform school officials of a child's HIV status.

- The school community may benefit from education.
- Children are allowed to engage in contact sports.
- Teens may need extra support from the school nurse or counselor.

Sexuality
- Children, adolescents, and families need to understand sexual and perinatal transmission risks.
- Safer sex techniques, including the use of condoms, barrier methods, and PrEP, should be provided and discussed.
- An undetectable viral load means someone living with HIV cannot transmit the virus to another person via sexual transmission.

Transition to Adulthood
- With improved treatment, HIV disease has become a chronic condition.
- Care and attention need to be given to preparing the adolescent for transition to adult HIV care.

FAMILY CONCERNS
- HIV infection may be present in multiple family members.
- Many families have been marginalized; as a result they lack adequate social resources and support systems.
- HIV is an enormous physical and emotional burden.
- Stigmatization continues as a major issue.
- Many children with HIV are placed in foster or adoptive homes.
- Counseling regarding death, dying, and bereavement is helpful.

REFERENCES

Agwu S on D. J. Expert consensus statement on breastfeeding and HIV in the United States and Canada. The Well Project. 2022. Retrieved August 23, 2022, from https://www.thewellproject.org/hiv-information/expert-consensus-statement-breastfeeding-and-hiv-united-states-and-canada#:~:text=Breastfeeding%20is%20the%20standard%20of,parent%20has%20sustained%20viral%20suppression.

Ang, J. Y., Ray-Mazumder, S., Nachman, S. A., Rongkavilit, C., Asmar, B. I., & Ren, C. L. (2005). Use of complementary and alternative medicine by parents of children with HIV infection and asthma and well children. *Southern Medical Journal, 98*(9), 869–875. https://doi.org/10.1097/01.smj.0000173089.51284.69.

Basile, F. W., Fedele, M. C., & Lo Vecchio, A. (2021). Gastrointestinal diseases in children living with HIV. *Microorganisms, 9*(8), 1572. https://doi.org/10.3390/microorganisms9081572.

Cantos, K., Franke, M. F., Tassiopoulos, K., Williams, P. L., Moscicki, A. B., & Seage, G. R. (2021). Inconsistent sexual behavior reporting among youth affected by perinatal HIV exposure in the United States. *AIDS Behavior, 25*(10), 3398–3412. https://doi.org/10.1007/s10461-021-03268-y.

Cao, G., Wang, Y., Wu, Y., Jing, W., Liu, J., & Liu, M. (2022). Prevalence of anemia among people living with HIV: A systematic review and meta-analysis. *eClinical Medicine, 44*, 101283. https://doi.org/10.1016/j.eclinm.2022.101283.

Centers for Disease Control and Prevention. (2014a). Revised surveillance case definition for HIV infection—United States, 2014. *MMWR Recommendations and Reports.* 2014. Retrieved January 8, 2023.

Centers for Disease Control and Prevention. (2014b). Technical update: Use of the determine HIV 1/2 ag/ab combo test with serum or plasma in the laboratory algorithm for HIV diagnosis. Retrieved August 16, 2022, from https://stacks.cdc.gov/view/cdc/48472.

Centers for Disease Control and Prevention. (2020). Health disparities. Retrieved August 16, 2022, from https://www.cdc.gov/healthyyouth/disparities/index.htm.

Centers for Disease Control and Prevention. (2022a). HIV Basics. Retrieved August 16, 2022, from https://www.cdc.gov/hiv/basics/index.html.

Centers for Disease Control and Prevention. (2022b). HIV surveillance. Retrieved August 16, 2022, from https://www.cdc.gov/hiv/library/reports/hiv-surveillance.html.

Centers for Disease Control and Prevention. (2023). Vaccine recommendations and guidelines of the ACIP. Retrieved August 23, 2023, from https://www.cdc.gov/vaccines/hcp/acip-recs/general-recs/contraindications.html.

Clarick, R. H., Hanekom, W. A., Yogev, R., & Chadwick, E. G. (1997). Megestrol acetate treatment of growth failure in children infected with human immunodeficiency virus. *Pediatrics, 99*(3), 354–357. https://doi.org/10.1542/peds.99.3.354.

Connor, E. M., Sperling, R. S., Gelber, R., Kiselev, P., Scott, G., O'Sullivan, M. J., VanDyke, R., Bey, M., Shearer, W., & Jacobson, R. L. (1994). Reduction of maternal-infant transmission of human immunodeficiency virus type 1 with zidovudine treatment. Pediatric AIDS Clinical Trials Group Protocol 076 Study Group. *New England Journal of Medicine, 331*(18), 1173–1180. doi:10.1056/NEJM199411033311801. PMID: 7935654.

Courville, T. M., Caldwell, B., & Brunell, P. A. (1998). Lack of evidence of transmission of HIV-1 to family contacts of HIV-1 infected children. *Clinical Pediatrics (Phila), 37*(3), 175–178. doi: 10.1177/000992289803700303.

Crowell, C. S., Huo, Y., Tassiopoulos, K., Malee, K. M., Yogev, R., Hazra, R., Rutstein, R. M., Nichols, S. L., Smith, R. A.,

Williams, P. L., Oleske, J., & Muller, W. J.; PACTG 219C Study Team and the Pediatric HIVAIDS Cohort Study (PHACS). (2015). Early viral suppression improves neurocognitive outcomes in HIV-infected children. *AIDS, 29*(3), 295–304. doi:10.1097/QAD.0000000000000528. PMID: 25686678; PMCID: PMC4332557.

Eisinger, R. W., Dieffenbach, C. W., & Fauci, A. S. (2019). HIV viral load and transmissibility of HIV infection. *JAMA, 321*(5), 451. https://doi.org/10.1001/jama.2018.21167.

Elizabeth Glaser Pediatric AIDS Foundation. (2020). Disclosure of HIV status toolkit for pediatric and adolescent populations. Retrieved August 16, 2022, from https://www.pedaids.org/resource/disclosure-of-hiv-status-toolkit-for-pediatric-and-adolescent-populations/.

Emmanuel, P. J., Mansfield, J., & Siberry, G. K. (2022). Human immunodeficiency virus infection: An update for pediatricians. *Pediatrics in Review, 43*(6), 335–346. https://doi.org/10.1542/pir.2020-001644.

Flynn, P. M., & Abrams, E. J. (2019). Growing up with perinatal HIV. *AIDS, 33*(4), 597–603. https://doi.org/10.1097/qad.0000000000002092.

Githinji, L. N., Gray, D. M., & Zar, H. J. (2018). Lung function in HIV-infected children and adolescents. *Pneumonia, 10*(1). https://doi.org/10.1186/s41479-018-0050-9.

Havens, P. (2008). HIV testing and prophylaxis to prevent mother-to-child transmission in the United States, Committee on Pediatric AIDS. *Pediatrics, 122*(5), 1127–1134. https://doi.org/10.1542/peds.2008-2175.

Hsu, K. K., & Rakhmanina, N. Y. (2021). Adolescents and young adults: The pediatrician's role in HIV testing and pre- and postexposure HIV prophylaxis. *Pediatrics, 149*(1). https://doi.org/10.1542/peds.2021-055207.

Kacanek, D., Huo, Y., Malee, K., Mellins, C. A., Smith, R., Garvie, P. A., Tassiopoulos, K., Lee, S., Berman, C. A., Paul, M., Puga, A., & Allison, S.; Pediatric HIV/AIDS Cohort Study. (2019). Nonadherence and unsuppressed viral load across adolescence among US youth with perinatally acquired HIV. *AIDS, 33*(12), 1923–1934. doi:10.1097/QAD.0000000000002301. PMID: 31274538; PMCID: PMC6776473.

Luzuriaga, K., Gay, H., Ziemniak, C., Sanborn, K. B., Somasundaran, M., Rainwater-Lovett, K., Mellors, J. W., Rosenbloom, D., & Persaud, D. (2015). Viremic relapse after HIV-1 remission in a perinatally infected child. *New England Journal of Medicine, 372*(8), 786–788. doi:10.1056/NEJMc1413931. PMID: 25693029; PMCID: PMC4440331.

MacDonell, K. K., Jacques-Tiura, A. J., Naar, S., & Isabella Fernandez, M. (2015). Predictors of self-reported adherence to antiretroviral medication in a multisite study of ethnic and racial minority HIV-positive youth. *Journal of Pediatric Psychology, 41*(4), 419–428. https://doi.org/10.1093/jpepsy/jsv097.

McHenry, M. S., McAteer, C. I., Oyungu, E., McDonald, B. C., Bosma, C. B., Mpofu, P. B., Deathe, A. R., & Vreeman, R. C. (2018). Neurodevelopment in young children born to HIV-infected mothers: A meta-analysis. *Pediatrics, 141*(2), e20172888. doi:10.1542/peds.2017-2888. PMID: 29374109; PMCID: PMC5810606.

Meek, J. Y., & Noble, L. (2022). Policy statement: Breastfeeding and the use of human milk. *Pediatrics, 150*(1). https://doi.org/10.1542/peds.2022-057988.

Melvin, A. J., Warshaw, M., Compagnucci, A., Saidi, Y., Harrison, L., Turkova, A., & Tudor-Williams, G.; PENPACT-1 (PENTA 9/PACTG 390/ANRS 103) Study Team. (2017). Hepatic, renal, hematologic, and inflammatory markers in HIV-infected children on long-term suppressive antiretroviral therapy. *Journal of Pediatric Infectious Diseases Society, 6*(3), e109–e115. doi:10.1093/jpids/pix050. PMID: 28903520; PMCID: PMC5907869.

Molinaro, M., Adams, H. R., Mwanza-Kabaghe, S., Mbewe, E. G., Kabundula, P. P., Mweemba, M., Birbeck, G. L., & Bearden, D. R. (2021). Evaluating the relationship between depression and cognitive function among children and adolescents with HIV in Zambia. *AIDS and Behavior, 25*(9), 2669–2679. doi:10.1007/s10461-021-03193-0. Epub 2021 Feb 25. PMID: 33630200; PMCID: PMC8456506.

Muenchhoff, M., Healy, M., Singh, R., Roider, J., Groll, A., Kindra, C., Sibaya, T., Moonsamy, A., McGregor, C., Phan, M. Q., Palma, A., Kloverpris, H., Leslie, A., Bobat, R., LaRussa, P., Ndung'u, T., Goulder, P., Sobieszczyk, M. E., & Archary, M. (2018). Malnutrition in HIV-infected children is an indicator of severe disease with an impaired response to antiretroviral therapy. *AIDS Research and Human Retroviruses, 34*(1), 46–55. doi:10.1089/AID.2016.0261. Epub 2017 Sep 6. PMID: 28670966; PMCID: PMC5771534.

Muenchhoff, M., Adland, E., Roider, J., Kløverpris, H., Leslie, A., Boehm, S., Keppler, O. T., Ndung'u, T., & Goulder, P. J. R. (2019). Differential pathogen-specific immune reconstitution in antiretroviral therapy-treated human immunodeficiency virus-infected children. *Journal of Infectious Diseases, 219*(9), 1407–1417. doi:10.1093/infdis/jiy668. PMID: 30624717; PMCID: PMC6467189.

Nesheim, S. R., FitzHarris, L. F., Mahle Gray, K., & Lampe, M. A. (2019). Epidemiology of perinatal HIV transmission in the United States in the era of its elimination. *Pediatric Infectious Disease Journal.* Retrieved August 16, 2022, from. https://pubmed.ncbi.nlm.nih.gov/30724833/.

Nesheim, S. R., Balaji, A., Hu, X., Lampe, M., & Dominguez, K. L. (2021). Opportunistic illnesses in children with HIV infection in the United States, 1997–2016. *Pediatric Infectious Disease Journal, 40*(7), 645–648. https://doi.org/10.1097/inf.0000000000003154.

Oshikoya, K. A., Oreagba, I. A., Ogunleye, O. O., Hassan, M., & Senbanjo, I. O. (2014). Use of complementary medicines among HIV-infected children in Lagos, Nigeria. *Complementary Therapies in Clinical Practice, 20*(2), 118–124. https://doi.org/10.1016/j.ctcp.2013.12.001.

Persaud, D., Gay, H., Ziemniak, C., Chen, Y. H., Piatak, M. Jr., Chun, T. W., Strain, M., Richman, D., & Luzuriaga, K. (2013). Absence of detectable HIV-1 viremia after treatment cessation in an infant. *New England Journal of Medicine, 369*(19), 1828–1835. doi:10.1056/NEJMoa1302976. Epub 2013 Oct 23. PMID: 24152233; PMCID: PMC3954754.

Price, A., McHugh, G., Simms, V., Semphere, R., Ngwira, L. G., Bandason, T., Mujuru, H., Odland, J. O., Ferrand, R. A., & Rehman, A. M. (2021). Effect of azithromycin on incidence of acute respiratory exacerbations in children with HIV taking antiretroviral therapy and co-morbid chronic lung disease: A secondary analysis of the breathe trial. *eClinical Medicine, 42,* 101195. https://doi.org/10.1016/j.eclinm.2021.101195.

Puthanakit, T., Ananworanich, J., & Akapirat, S. (2020). Pattern and frequency of seroreactivity to routinely used serologic tests in early-treated infants with HIV. *Journal of Acquired Immune Deficiency Syndrome, 83*(3), 260–266. https://pubmed.ncbi.nlm.nih.gov/31917751/.

Ramos-Gomez, F. J., & Folayan, M. O. (2013). Oral health considerations in HIV-infected children. *Current HIV/AIDS Report, 10*(3), 283–293. https://doi.org/10.1007/s11904-013-0163-y.

Rinaldi, S., Pallikkuth, S., Cameron, M., de Armas, L. R., Cotugno, N., Dinh, V., Pahwa, R., Richardson, B., Saini, S. R., Rocca, S., Lain, M. G., Williams, S. L., Palma, P., & Pahwa, S. (2020). Impact of early antiretroviral therapy initiation on HIV-specific CD4 and CD8 T cell function in perinatally infected children. *Journal of Immunology, 204*(3), 540–549. doi:10.4049/jimmunol.1900856. Epub 2019 Dec 30. PMID: 31889024; PMCID: PMC6981070.

Ruck, C., Reikie, B. A., Marchant, A., Kollmann, T. R., & Kakkar, F. (2016). Linking susceptibility to infectious diseases to immune system abnormalities among HIV-exposed uninfected infants. *Frontiers in Immunology, 7.* https://doi.org/10.3389/fimmu.2016.00310.

Rylance, J., Mchugh, G., Metcalfe, J., Mujuru, H., Nathoo, K., Wilmore, S., Rowland-Jones, S., Majonga, E., Kranzer, K., & Ferrand, R. A. (2016). Chronic lung disease in HIV-infected children established on antiretroviral therapy. *AIDS, 30*(18), 2795–2803. doi:10.1097/QAD.0000000000001249. PMID: 27662546; PMCID: PMC5106089.

Salvant Valentine, S., & Poulin, A. (2018). Consistency of state statutes and regulations with Centers for Disease Control and Prevention's 2006 perinatal HIV testing recommendations. *Public Health Reports, 133*(5), 601–605. https://doi.org/10.1177/0033354918792540. Epub 2018 Aug 10.

Samour, P., Helm, K., & Lang, C., (2003). *Handbook of Pediatric Nutrition.* Boston: Jones and Barlett.

Semrau, K., & Aldrovandi, G. M. (2021). MTCT HIV-1 transmission update: Transmission routes and mechanisms. *Encyclopedia AIDS,* 1377–1382. https://doi.org/10.1007/978-1-4939-7101-5_132.

Siberry, G. K., Abzug, M. J., Nachman, S., Brady, M. T., Dominguez, K. L., Handelsman, E., Mofenson, L. M., Nesheim S; Panel on Opportunistic Infections in HIV-Exposed and HIV-Infected Children; National Institutes of Health, Centers for Disease Control and Prevention, HIV Medicine Association of the Infectious Diseases Society of America, Pediatric Infectious Diseases Society, American Academy of Pediatrics. (2013). Guidelines for the prevention and treatment of opportunistic infections in HIV-exposed and HIV-infected children: recommendations from the National Institutes of Health, Centers for Disease Control and Prevention, the HIV Medicine Association of the Infectious Diseases Society of America, the Pediatric Infectious Diseases Society, and the American Academy of Pediatrics. *The Pediatric Infectious Disease Journal, 32* Suppl 2(02), i-KK4. doi:10.1097/01.inf.0000437856.09540.11.

Sibiude, J., Le Chenadec, J., Mandelbrot, L., Hoctin, A., Dollfus, C., Faye, A., Bui, E., Pannier, E., Ghosn, J., Garrait, V., Avettand-Fenoel, V., Frange, P., Warszawski, J., & Tubiana, R. (2023). Update of perinatal human immunodeficiency virus type 1 transmission in france: Zero transmission for 5482 mothers on continuous antiretroviral therapy from conception and with undetectable viral load at delivery. *Clinical Infectious Diseases, 76*(3), e590–e598. doi:10.1093/cid/ciac703.

Szpak, R., Lombardi, N. F., Dias, F. A., Borba, H. H., Pontarolo, R., & Wiens, A. (2022). Safety of antiretroviral therapy in the treatment of HIV/AIDS in children: Systematic review and meta-analysis. *AIDS Reviews, 3*(4). https://doi.org/10.24875/aidsrev.200001071.

Tassiopoulos, K., Moscicki, A. B., Mellins, C., Kacanek, D., Malee, K., Allison, S., Hazra, R., Siberry, G. K., Smith, R., Paul, M., Van Dyke, R. B., & Seage, G. R. 3rd; Pediatric HIV/AIDS Cohort Study. (2013). Sexual risk behavior among youth with perinatal HIV infection in the United States: Predictors and implications for intervention development. *Clinical Infectious Diseases, 56*(2), 283–290. doi:10.1093/cid/cis816.

Toledo, G., Côté, H. C., Adler, C., Thorne, C., & Goetghebuer, T. (2021). Neurological development of children who are HIV-exposed and uninfected. *Developmental Medicine and Child Neurology, 63*(10), 1161–1170. https://doi.org/10.1111/dmcn.14921.

United Nations AIDS. UNAIDS 2021 report. (2021). Retrieved August 16, 2022, from https://www.unaids.org/sites/default/files/media_asset/2021-global-aids-update_en.pdf.

Uprety, P., Patel, K., Karalius, B., Ziemniak, C., Chen, Y. H., Brummel, S. S., Siminski, S., Van Dyke, R. B., Seage, G. R., & Persaud, D.; Pediatric HIV/AIDS Cohort Study (PHACS). (2017). Human immunodeficiency virus type 1 DNA decay dynamics with early, long-term virologic control of perinatal infection. *Clinical Infectious Diseases, 64*(11), 1471–1478. doi:10.1093/cid/cix192. Erratum in: Clin Infect Dis. 2017 Oct 15;65(8):1431–1433.

van Opstal, S. E. M., Wagener, M. N., Miedema, H. S., Utens, E. M. W. J., Aarsen, F. K., van der Knaap, L. C., van Gorp, E. C. M., van Rossum, A. M. C., & Roelofs, P. D. D. M. (2021). School functioning of children with perinatal HIV-infection in high-income countries: A systematic review. *PLoS One, 16*(6), e0252746. doi:10.1371/journal.pone.0252746. PMID: 34086807; PMCID: PMC8177442.

Webb, L., Perry-Parrish, C., Ellen, J., & Sibinga, E. (2017). Mindfulness instruction for HIV-infected youth: A randomized controlled trial. *AIDS Care, 30*(6), 688–695. https://doi.org/10.1080/09540121.2017.1394434.

Wedderburn, C. J., Yeung, S., Rehman, A. M., Stadler, J. A. M., Nhapi, R. T., Barnett, W., Myer, L., Gibb, D. M., Zar, H. J., Stein, D. J., & Donald, K. A. (2019). Neurodevelopment of HIV-exposed uninfected children in South Africa: Outcomes from an observational birth cohort study. *Lancet Child and Adolescent Health, 3*(11), 803–813. doi:10.1016/S2352-4642(19)30250-0. Epub 2019 Sep 9. PMID: 31515160; PMCID: PMC6876655.

Zinyemba, T., Pavlova, M., & Groot, W. (2019). Effects of HIV/AIDS on children's educational attainment: A systematic literature review. *Journal of Economic Surveys, 34*(1), 35–84. https://doi.org/10.1111/joes.12345.

Hydrocephalus

Cathy C. Cartwright

ETIOLOGY

Hydrocephalus is a chronic condition resulting from an increase in cerebrospinal fluid (CSF) in the brain because of an imbalance in the production and absorption of CSF (Nielsen & Breedt, 2017). This increase in CSF causes ventriculomegaly, increased intracranial pressure (ICP), and an abnormally increasing head size (Fig. 26.1B). Hydrocephalus is a symptom of an underlying condition and occurs when there is poor absorption, obstruction to flow, or (rarely) overproduction of CSF. The usual rate of CSF production is 0.35 mL/min (~400–500 mL/day), with the total volume being 65 to 140 mL in children and 90 to 150 mL in adults (Abou-Hamden & Drake, 2015). CSF is a clear, colorless fluid that provides buoyancy to the brain and removes waste products. CSF also functions as a shock absorber to protect the brain and spinal cord. The majority of CSF (50–80%) is thought to be produced by the choroid plexus located in the ventricles, with other production in subarachnoid sites (Abou-Hamden & Drake, 2015).

CSF flows from the lateral ventricles through the foramen of Monro to the third ventricle, through the aqueduct of Sylvius, and into the fourth ventricle. CSF exits the fourth ventricle via the foramen of Luschka and Magendie and travels around the brainstem and spinal cord, over the surface of the brain, and then flows into the subarachnoid spaces and basilar cisterns before absorption into the large intracranial sinuses at the arachnoid villi (Fig. 26.2). Minor pathways have been proposed where CSF absorption also occurs along nerve root sleeves and lymphatics (Abou-Hamden & Drake, 2015). Alternate pathways for CSF absorption may come into play when ICP is increased.

Occasionally the terms *internal hydrocephalus* and *external hydrocephalus* are used. Internal hydrocephalus refers to ventricular enlargement due to the accumulation of CSF and commonly describes the condition of hydrocephalus. External hydrocephalus is the accumulation of CSF in the subdural or subarachnoid spaces, shown radiographically as enlarged frontal subarachnoid spaces (Nielsen & Breedt, 2017). CSF mixed with blood in the subdural space requires further investigation and treatment as it may be related to nonaccidental trauma.

Hydrocephalus has been generally categorized into two types, communicating and noncommunicating (previously referred to as nonobstructive and obstructive). The latter two terms are no longer used, as most hydrocephalus is thought to be obstructive at some point along the pathway. Communicating hydrocephalus occurs when CSF flows freely through the normal pathways but cannot be absorbed through the subarachnoid spaces, the basal cisterns, or the arachnoid villi. Common causes of communicating hydrocephalus are meningitis, intrauterine infection, intraventricular hemorrhage (IVH), trauma, or congenital malformation of the subarachnoid spaces. Rarely, communicating hydrocephalus may be related to an overproduction of CSF, which occurs because of a choroid plexus papilloma or carcinoma (Nielsen & Breedt, 2017).

Noncommunicating hydrocephalus is characterized by the failure of CSF to flow through its normal pathways from one ventricle to another or from the ventricles to the subarachnoid cisterns. CSF therefore does not reach the arachnoid villi where it would normally be absorbed. This results in an enlargement of the ventricles proximal to the site of the obstruction. An example of noncommunicating hydrocephalus would be an obstruction of the aqueduct of Sylvius in which the lateral and third ventricles are enlarged, but the fourth ventricle is normal sized.

Noncommunicating hydrocephalus can be further classified as congenital or acquired. Conditions that occur congenitally include Chiari malformation, aqueductal stenosis, Dandy-Walker malformation, X-linked hydrocephalus, arachnoid cysts, tumors, vascular malformations, encephalocele, and prenatal infections such as cytomegalovirus and rubella (Nielsen & Breedt, 2017). Congenital hydrocephalus is present at birth and accounts for approximately 55% of all cases of hydrocephalus (Abou-Hamden & Drake, 2015). Many of these can be diagnosed prenatally during routine maternal ultrasonography and follow-up fetal magnetic resonance imaging (MRI). Five percent of all congenital hydrocephalus is due to primary aqueductal stenosis (Patel et al., 2021). Other causes of aqueductal stenosis can be attributed to infection, tumor blocking the aqueduct of Sylvius, or hemorrhage. The most common inherited form of congenital hydrocephalus is the X-linked gene *L1CAM*, with 10% of those cases occurring in males (Adle-Biassette et al., 2013). Primary care practitioners should recommend

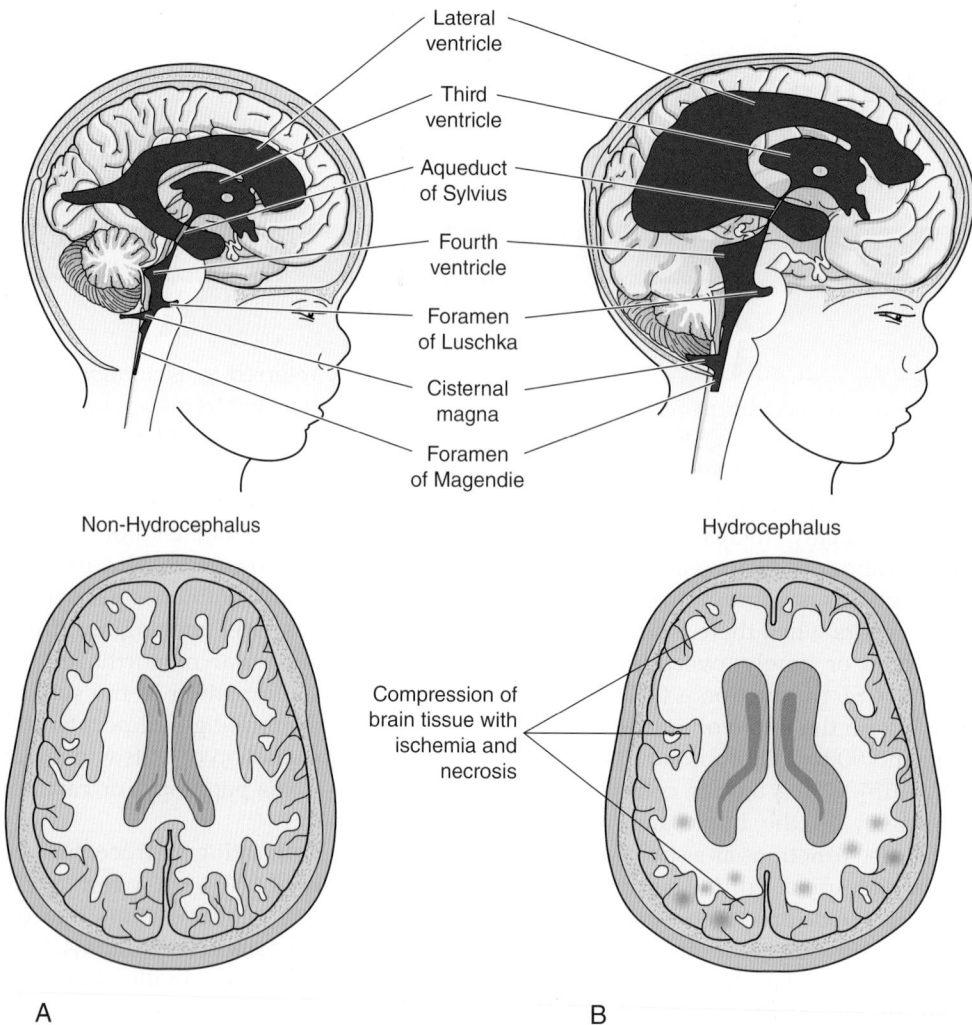

Fig. 26.1 **Illustration of intracranial ventricles.** (From Huether, S.E., & McCance, K.L. [2020]. *Understanding pathophysiology* [7th ed.]. Mosby.)

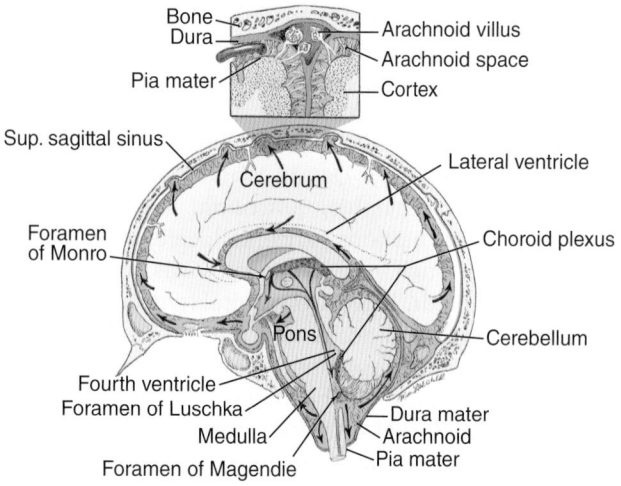

Fig. 26.2 **Sagittal view of the brain.** *Arrows* indicate cerebrospinal fluid flow. (From Elisha, S. [2022]. *Nurse anesthesia* [7th ed.]. Saunders.)

genetic counseling to couples with one child with hydrocephalus before they attempt to conceive a second child. Those couples who have conceived should be offered prenatal diagnosis in the second trimester for all subsequent pregnancies.

Acquired hydrocephalus can be caused by infection or parasitic disease, such as cysticercosis, causing obstruction in the ventricular system. It can also be caused by hemorrhage as a result of IVH from prematurity, head injury, or rupture of an intracranial blood vessel or vascular malformation (Abou-Hamden & Drake, 2015). The post-IVH flow and absorption of CSF are impaired due to fibrosing arachnoiditis, meningeal fibrosis, and subependymal gliosis (Abou-Hamden & Drake, 2015).

INCIDENCE AND PREVALENCE

The overall incidence of hydrocephalus is difficult to determine because the condition can occur alone or in association with other diseases. However, hydrocephalus is believed to occur globally at 88 per 100,000 and is the most common condition treated by pediatric neurosurgeons, costing almost $2 billion per year in the United States (Isaacs et al., 2018; Simon et al., 2008). The incidence of primary congenital hydrocephalus is 0.2 to 0.8 per 1000 live births (Faria et al., 2015). Hydrocephalus can be caused antenatally by

Box 26.1 Clinical Manifestations of Hydrocephalus at Time of Diagnosis

INFANTS	TODDLERS	CHILDREN AND ADOLESCENTS
Macrocephaly	Macrocephaly	Headache
Bradycardia (neonates)	Headache	Nausea/vomiting
Apnea (neonates)	Vomiting	Irritability
Full or tense fontanel	Irritability	Sleepiness
Splayed cranial sutures	Lethargy	Declining school performance
Prominent scalp veins	Developmental delays	Gait disturbance
Sunsetting eyes	Sunsetting eyes	Sunsetting eyes
Poor feeding	Parinaud syndrome	Memory loss
Vomiting		Papilledema
Parinaud syndrome		Parinaud syndrome
Drowsiness		
Irritability		

infections, trauma, hemorrhage, tumors, neural tube defects, X-linked recessive disorders, or other brain malformations (Faria et al., 2015). Hydrocephalus occurs in approximately 80% to 85% of infants born with myelomeningocele (Nielsen & Breedt, 2017). The etiology correlates with the child's age. Hydrocephalus in children from birth to 2 years of age is usually caused by perinatal hemorrhage, meningitis, or developmental abnormalities, whereas in older children (age 2–10 years), hydrocephalus is caused by a posterior fossa tumor or aqueductal stenosis (Abou-Hamden & Drake, 2015). Hydrocephalus is often associated with neural tube defects, and 70% to 90% of children diagnosed with spina bifida will also have hydrocephalus.

DIAGNOSTIC CRITERIA

Neuroimaging of the brain is essential for the diagnosis and management of hydrocephalus. The most used neuroimaging techniques for diagnosing and monitoring hydrocephalus are ultrasonography, computed tomography (CT), and MRI. Prenatal ultrasound can be used to diagnose ventriculomegaly in a fetus as early as the first trimester. Cranial ultrasound is a screening tool often used on infants with an open anterior fontanel to visualize the lateral and third ventricles and intraventricular clots. Serial cranial ultrasounds are helpful in following ventriculomegaly or a resolving clot without exposing the infant to radiation or the need for sedation.

CT scans are quick, readily available, and frequently used to visualize ventricular size, blood, calcifications, and shunt hardware, particularly in emergencies. However, because CT scans use ionizing radiation, and children are more sensitive to radiation than adults, they should be used judiciously because children with hydrocephalus face a lifetime of neuroimaging. It is important for radiologists to follow the ALARA (as low

as reasonably achievable) dosing principle to obtain necessary imaging (Strauss & Kaste, 2006). To minimize exposure to ionizing radiation from CT scanning, a half-Fourier single-shot turbo spin-echo (HASTE) MRI is a limited T2 study that provides good visualization of ventricular anatomy (Nielsen & Breedt, 2017). A HASTE MRI is quick and does not require sedating the child. Although the cost may be more than a head CT, limiting lifetime exposure to radiation may justify this expense (O'Neill et al., 2013).

An MRI provides detail of brain anatomy in the axial, sagittal, and coronal planes and can be useful in determining the cause of hydrocephalus. The aqueduct of Sylvius can be visualized, as well as loculations or membranes that may obstruct the flow of CSF. A CSF flow study is a cine-phase MRI used to demonstrate flow through the aqueduct or a third ventriculostomy. Because a brain MRI takes longer than a head CT, and the patient must be still to obtain the best images, children often need to be sedated. The MRI is a magnet and can affect some programmable shunt valves, so it is important to notify the neurosurgery provider before the MRI if the child has a programmable valve because it may need to be reprogrammed after the scan. There are other neuroimaging modalities, such as plain radiographs and nuclear medicine studies, but the neurosurgery provider usually determines the need for those.

CLINICAL MANIFESTATIONS AT TIME OF DIAGNOSIS

CLINICAL MANIFESTATIONS IN INFANCY

The signs and symptoms of hydrocephalus depend on the age of the child, how quickly the skull expands, and whether the cranial sutures are still open (Box 26.1). Fetal ultrasound and fetal MRI can diagnose hydrocephalus prenatally, allowing elective cesarean section for infants with cephalopelvic disproportion. Rapidly increasing head circumference in the premature or term infant should strongly suggest the diagnosis of hydrocephalus. Normal head circumference at birth is 34 to 36 cm within the 25% to 75% range (Disabato & Daniels, 2017). During the first few weeks of life, a newborn may have enlarged ventricles without exhibiting an increase in head size or signs and symptoms of increased ICP (Volpe, 2008). The infant skull and sutures can expand to accommodate increasing ventricular size, thereby minimizing an elevation in ICP. If the accumulation of excessive CSF occurs slowly, an infant or young child may be asymptomatic until the hydrocephalus is advanced.

The anterior fontanel closes between 6 and 18 months of age. For some infants, the anterior fontanel may appear closed upon palpation, but this could be a normal finding if the head is not misshapen (normocephalic), the head circumference falls within normal limits on the head circumference chart, and the infant is doing well developmentally. Continue to monitor the head circumference and developmental progress.

A newborn with a head circumference greater than the 95th percentile should be evaluated promptly for hydrocephalus. In a newborn with suspected hydrocephalus, the head circumference should be measured at least daily with rapid increases evaluated by ultrasonography. Neonates may have spells of apnea or bradycardia, a full fontanel, and increasing head circumference that crosses percentiles on growth charts. Infants may also present with a tense or bulging anterior fontanel that is nonpulsatile. As the hydrocephalus progresses, the cranial sutures may be splayed, the scalp veins appear prominent, and the eyes have a sun-setting appearance or upward gaze palsy (Parinaud syndrome). Lethargy, irritability, vomiting, poor feeding, poor head control, and seizures are also symptoms of hydrocephalus and should be investigated.

Macrocephaly is an occipitofrontal circumference (OFC) at least 2 SDs above normal or 0.5 cm above the 97th percentile (Bryant et al., 2021). OFC is measured from the most prominent points on the front and back of the skull, glabella to the opistocranium (Winden et al., 2015). Normally, the head circumference increases approximately 2 cm per month the first 3 months after birth, 1.5 cm for the next 2 months, and 0.5 cm for months 6 to 12, for a total of 12 cm the first year.

CLINICAL MANIFESTATIONS IN CHILDREN

Children greater than 2 years of age may have more acute signs and symptoms of increased ICP as the cranial sutures are closed, and accommodation for increasing ventricular size has decreased. Macrocephaly is not necessarily a component of the presentation in older children. For this reason, the presentation of hydrocephalus in older children is typically acute.

Box 26.2	Treatment

SURGICAL
Shunt placement
- Ventriculoperitoneal
- Ventriculoatrial
- Ventriculopleural

Endoscopic third ventriculostomy
- Choroid plexus cauterization

Temporary cerebrospinal fluid diversion
- Shunt tap
- Reservoir tap
- External ventricular drain
- Externalized shunt
- Subgaleal shunt

COMPLICATIONS
- Shunt failure
- Infection

Hydrocephalus in children beyond infancy is usually associated with a neoplasm, a mass secondary to obstruction of CSF flow, or a history of traumatic brain injury. Younger children may present with headache, vomiting, irritability, and visual or gait disturbance. Symptoms in older children may be acute or subtle and can range from headache, visual disturbance, nausea, vomiting, sleepiness, and irritability to declining school performance. They can present with papilledema or Parinaud syndrome and gait disturbances.

TREATMENT

The ultimate goal of the treatment for hydrocephalus is to prevent or reverse the neurologic damage caused by the distortion of the brain from increased ICP and accumulation of CSF (Box 26.2). Intermediate goals include allowing the actual brain tissue volume to increase and reconstitution of the cortical mantle.

PHARMACOLOGIC TREATMENT

Historically, acetazolamide and Lasix were used as temporizing measures but have not been shown to be safe or effective medical treatment options for hydrocephalus.

SURGICAL TREATMENT

Surgical treatment for hydrocephalus is directed at restoring CSF flow by either removing the obstruction to CSF flow or creating a new CSF pathway. In most cases, the obstruction to CSF flow cannot be effectively or safely removed; therefore surgical shunting is required. Surgical placement of a shunt is the standard treatment to divert the excess accumulation of CSF from the ventricles to a distal space in the body, usually the peritoneum, with a ventriculoperitoneal (VP) shunt. No single type of shunt is superior to another. The choice of shunt type is the preference of the neurosurgeon based on training, personal experience, and

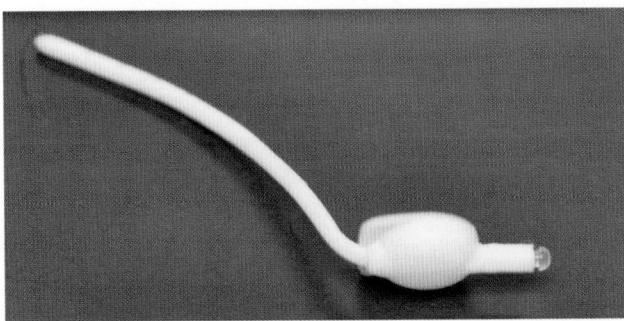

Fig. 26.3 McComb reservoir. When a shunt is not an option, a reservoir can be surgically placed in a neonate for temporary removal of cerebrospinal fluid by tapping the reservoir.

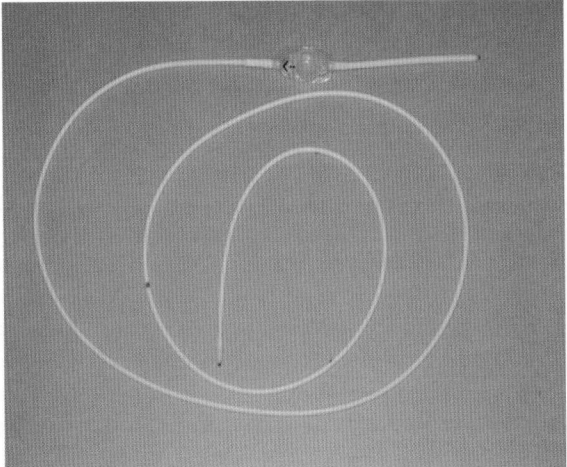

Fig. 26.4 Shunt system. A shunt system has three parts: The proximal catheter is placed in the ventricle, the valve regulates the flow of cerebrospinal fluid (CSF), and the distal catheter drains CSF to an area with optimum absorption.

patient needs. No data exist to support a recommendation of one shunt design over another.

In some cases of neonatal hydrocephalus, the infant may be too small (<2 kg) for a VP shunt placement or have other comorbidities, and a reservoir is placed as a temporizing measure to allow for serial taps to decrease the amount of CSF in the ventricles (Fig. 26.3). Another temporizing measure used in small neonates is the ventriculosubgaleal shunt. The proximal end of the shunt catheter is placed in the ventricle, and the distal portion is placed in the subgaleal space under the scalp, allowing passive drainage of CSF. This can cause a fluctuant mass to appear in the neonate's skull as the CSF collects in the subgaleal space until it is absorbed.

There are three parts to a shunt system: the proximal end, which is placed in the ventricle; the valve, which controls the amount of CSF drained; and the distal end (Fig. 26.4). Shunt catheters are made of silastic material; some are impregnated with antibiotics to lessen the chance of a shunt infection. Although placing the distal catheter in the peritoneal cavity is preferred, that may not be possible due to infection, adhesions, inadequate absorption, or other abdominal hardware. The distal catheter can be placed in the pleural space (ventriculopleural shunt), into the right atrium of the heart (ventriculoatrial [VA] shunt) via the superior vena cava, or (less commonly) the gall bladder (Fig. 26.5). The proximal catheter is usually inserted into the ventricle through a burr hole via a frontal or occipital parietal approach and through the nondominant right cerebral hemisphere. The distal catheter of a VP shunt is tunneled under the skin to the designated location, where a small incision is made, and the shunt is inserted through the abdomen into the peritoneal cavity. The VA shunt is inserted through the neck into the superior

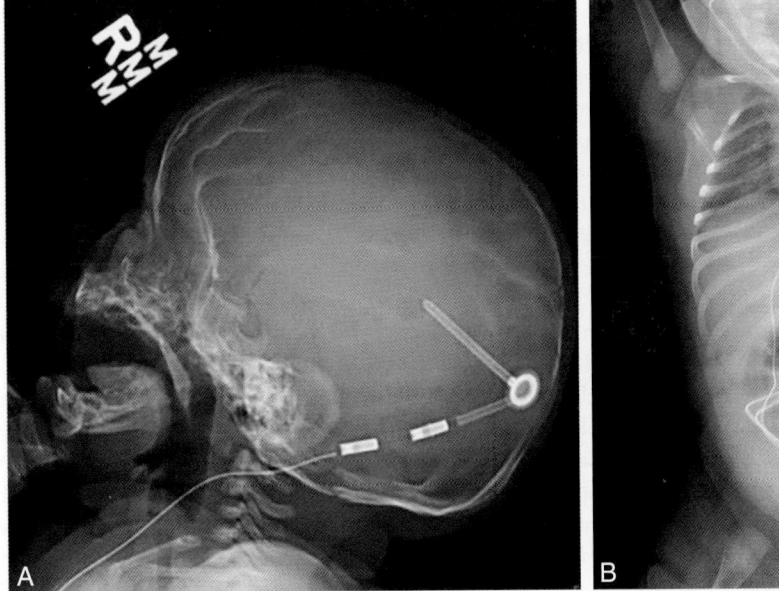

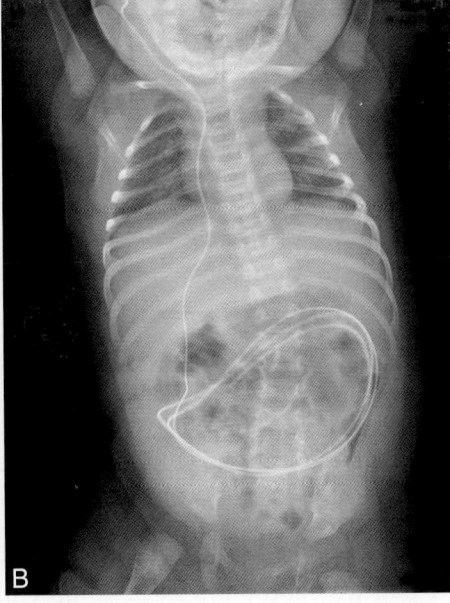

Fig. 26.5 Shunt series (A). X-ray image of ventriculoperitoneal shunt location in an infant **(B)**.

vena cava and into the right atrium. The distal end of the ventriculopleural shunt is guided subcutaneously to an area just below the nipple, where an incision is made, and the tube is inserted into the pleural space.

Lumboperitoneal (LP) shunts are less commonly used in children. The proximal catheter of the LP shunt is placed in the lumbar intradural space and tunneled under the skin so the distal catheter drains into the peritoneum.

Reservoirs are part of the valve or may be added after the proximal catheter exits the skull through the burr hole. Reservoirs are used for tapping with a small needle to obtain CSF if an infection is suspected or for emergent aspiration of CSF. They can also be used to inject radioisotopes for shunt flow studies called shunt-o-grams. The reservoir and tubing for the shunt are palpable under the skin from the burr hole in the skull to the tube's insertion into either the abdomen or chest. Identifying and accessing the shunt reservoir is important in evaluating shunt infection and/or malfunction.

CSF shunts regulate flow by means of a one-way valve. Valves can be grouped into four general design categories: differential pressure valves, siphon-resisting valves, flow-regulating valves, and adjustable valves. Differential pressure valves are considered standard and have been used for decades. These valves simply open or close depending on the pressure across them. The pressure at which they open is termed the *opening pressure*; typically, they have designations of low, medium, and high corresponding to 5, 10, and 15 cm of H_2O pressure (Nielsen & Breedt, 2017). Siphon-resisting valves are designed to reduce the flow of CSF when the patient is upright. Flow-regulating valves maintain constant flow regardless of patient position or changing pressures. Programmable valves allow the opening pressure of the valves to be adjusted externally with a magnet instead of undergoing another surgery to replace the valve as the child's pressure needs to change. Care must be taken around strong magnetic sources, and valve manufacturers' recommendations should be consulted. Because the strong MRI magnet can change some programmable valves, the neurosurgery provider should be notified before and after an MRI if the valve needs to be reprogrammed (Fig. 26.6).

Improvements in neuroendoscopy have allowed for the increased use of endoscopic third ventriculostomy (ETV) as an alternative for shunt placement in select patients with noncommunicating hydrocephalus. The patients that benefit from ETV are those with obstruction of CSF flow from the ventricles into the subarachnoid space and normal absorption from the subarachnoid space into the venous system (Nielsen & Breedt, 2017). The neurosurgeon uses an endoscope to visualize intraventricular anatomy while making an opening in the floor of the third ventricle. This creates a new pathway and allows CSF to flow into the subarachnoid spaces, bypassing the obstruction

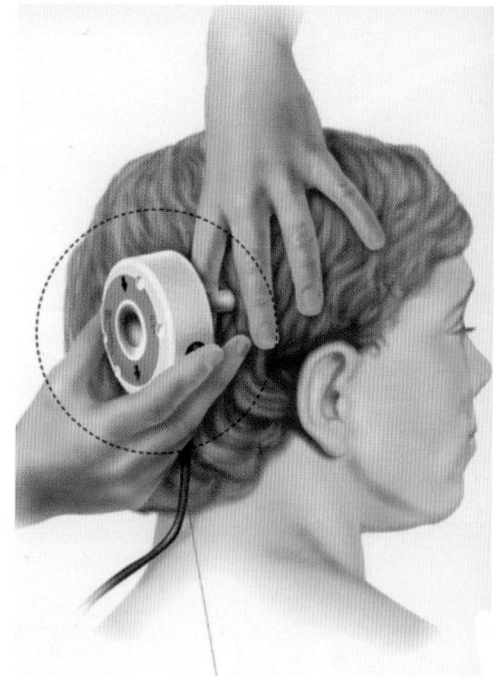

Fig. 26.6 Programming a shunt valve. Illustration demonstrates use of the Codman programmer to externally adjust the pressure setting on the valve. (Courtesy Integra LifeSciences Corporation, Princeton, NJ.)

(Fig. 26.7). The ETV success score is a guide to selecting the best candidates for an ETV instead of a shunt by scoring their age, etiology of hydrocephalus, and whether they had a previous shunt (Kulkarni et al., 2010).

Choroid plexus cauterization can be done at the same time as the ETV, cauterizing the choroid plexus within the lateral ventricles to decrease the amount of CSF produced. Patients who have undergone ETV to treat hydrocephalus continue to need neurosurgical follow-up because the ETV can fail at any time. Patients whose ETV has failed will exhibit signs and symptoms of increased ICP and may require another ETV or shunt placement.

Complications of Surgical Treatment

Shunt failure. Although CSF shunting has dramatically improved the prognosis for children with hydrocephalus, shunts still have inherent problems: malfunction, infection, and over- and underdrainage. Almost 20,000 hospitalizations each year are related to pediatric shunt surgeries (Simon et al., 2008). Shunt complications may occur at any time, from immediately after shunt placement to years later, leading to shunt failure. Children under 2 years of age are at a higher risk of failure than older children, with a shunt failure rate of 30% to 40% within the first year (Kalra & Kestle, 2011). The incidence of shunt failure is greater if revised within 6 months of a previous shunt revision. Complication rates after VP shunt placement have been reported to be between 17% and 33% (Merkler et al., 2017).

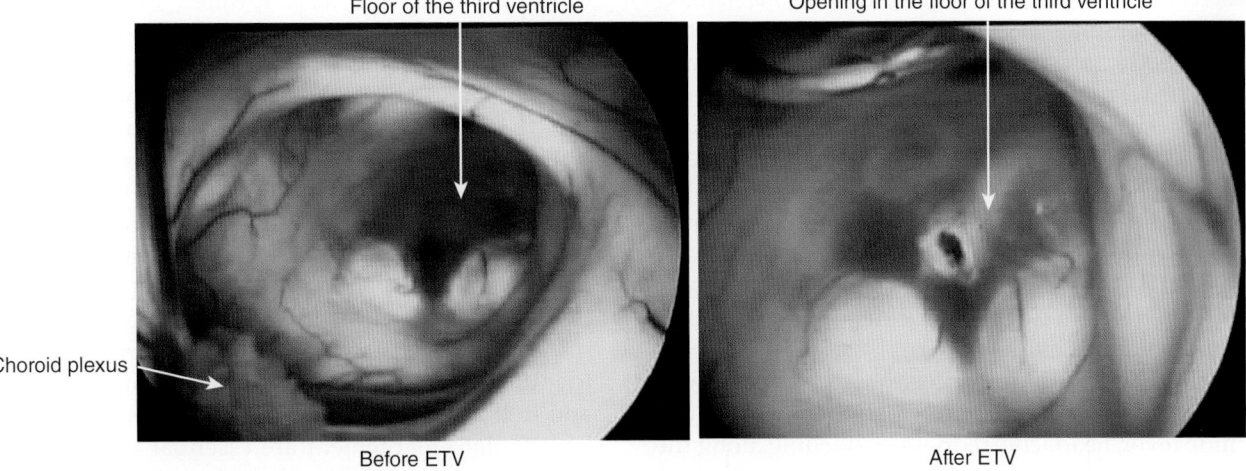

Floor of the third ventricle

Choroid plexus

Opening in the floor of the third ventricle

Before ETV

After ETV

Fig. 26.7 Endoscopic third ventriculostomy *(ETV)* as seen through an endoscope. *(Left)* An intact floor of the third ventricle. *(Right)* Surgical opening for cerebrospinal fluid to drain into the subarachnoid space.

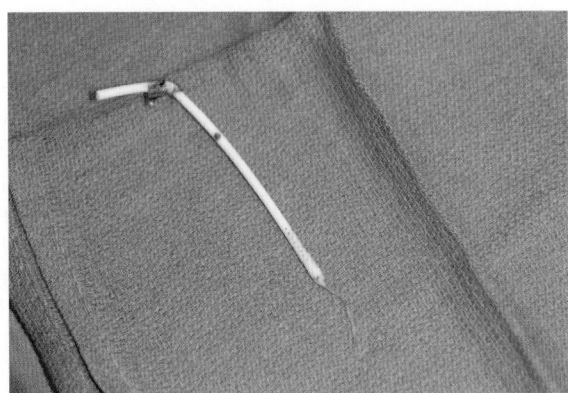

Fig. 26.8 Ventricular catheter removed from child with shunt failure. Note the openings occluded by debris blocking drainage of cerebrospinal fluid.

Shunt occlusion. The most common shunt complication in the pediatric population is shunt occlusion, usually involving the proximal catheter. Shunt revisions are sometimes necessary for children who have shunted hydrocephalus. Shunt obstruction may occur because of chronic or acute inflammation, overgrowth of the choroid plexus, accumulation of cellular debris or blood, or displacement of either the distal or proximal end of the shunt because of the child's growth (Fig. 26.8).

Overdrainage of CSF can decompress the ventricles too much or too rapidly so that subdural fluid collections, such as subdural hematomas or slit ventricle syndrome (SVS), can occur (Nielsen & Breedt, 2017). SVS usually occurs in a delayed fashion after shunt placement, with the patient experiencing severe headache and slit ventricles on CT scan (Nielsen & Breedt, 2017). Programmable shunt valves can help prevent too rapid decompression of the ventricles by allowing the provider to control the flow of CSF by using an external programmer to slowly decrease the valve pressure over time.

CT and MRI studies evaluate shunt failure and the need for shunt revision. These scans must be compared with prior imaging studies and reviewed in conjunction with clinical findings of probable shunt failure, as assessed by an experienced clinician. In some cases, ventricular enlargement is noted only when the latest imaging is compared with prior studies. CT imaging may not show increased ventricle size in every child with a possible shunt malfunction. A shunt series, or plain x-rays, consisting of an anterior-posterior (AP) skull x-ray and a chest and abdomen AP x-ray, can rule out shunt position, disconnection or migration, and type of valve. Primary care providers must remember that negative or stable CT scan findings do not rule out shunt malfunction.

Other diagnostic tools to evaluate shunt function include radionuclide CSF shunt studies, shunt tap to obtain CSF for culture, and ICP monitoring. Measurement of ICP can be obtained either intermittently via the shunt reservoir or by the placement of an ICP monitor. Keeping in mind the morbidity associated with delayed diagnosis of a shunt malfunction, primary care providers must have a low threshold for ordering a CT scan or referring a child to a neurosurgeon when symptoms of increased ICP or shunt infection are apparent.

Shunt infection. The second most frequent shunt complication is an infection, with the greatest incidence in the first year after placement (Nielsen & Breedt, 2017). Over two-thirds of shunt infections are diagnosed within 2 months of surgery (Thompson & Hartley, 2015). Shunt infections are serious complications and account for more than 2000 hospitalizations per year (Simon et al., 2008). Shunt infections, especially resulting from gram-negative organisms, can have significant detrimental effects on cognition in the host.

It is believed that the infecting organism is introduced at the time of surgery (Simon et al., 2019). The most common causative organisms are *Staphylococcus* spp., including *S. aureus,* and coagulase-negative staphylococci, accounting for 50% to 80% of shunt infections (Dawod et al., 2016). Because a shunt is a foreign body, biofilm can grow on the inner and outer shunt surfaces, allowing a child to be susceptible to infection of the shunt and CSF (Dawod et al., 2016). Some studies show that antibiotic impregnated shunt material can decrease the rate of infection (Kalra & Kestle, 2011). There seems to be a consensus that very young children have a higher incidence of shunt infection than older individuals.

A child with a shunt infection can appear well or seriously ill. Symptoms of a shunt infection can include fever, headache, redness or swelling along the shunt track, or redness or drainage at the incision site. The shunt may fail as well, and the child may exhibit symptoms of shunt malfunction, such as headache, vomiting, and excessive sleepiness. Abdominal pain can be a symptom of a pseudocyst, where the distal catheter is walled off in the abdomen due to an inflammatory response to infected CSF (Yuh & Vassilyadi, 2012).

A positive CSF culture is definitive of a shunt infection and should be obtained when possible before initiating antibiotics and after other sources for fever or infection have been excluded (Thompson & Hartley, 2015). A positive blood culture in a child with a VA shunt indicates shunt infection (Simon et al., 2014). Treatment of a shunt infection requires the child to be hospitalized between 7 and 21 days with the removal of the shunt and administration of intravenous antibiotics. An external ventricular drain provides temporary drainage of CSF until cultures are sterile before a new shunt system can be placed.

Prevention of shunt infections is key to improving outcomes in children with shunted hydrocephalus and decreasing the cost of their care. Using a standardized shunt surgery protocol has decreased infection rates (Kestle et al., 2011). Perioperative systemic antibiotics, meticulous intraoperative aseptic technique, and attention to postoperative wound care are accepted ways to minimize the risk of infection (Nielsen & Breedt, 2017).

COMPLEMENTARY AND ALTERNATIVE TREATMENTS

No evidence is available in the current literature regarding complementary or alternative treatment of hydrocephalus.

ANTICIPATED ADVANCES IN DIAGNOSIS AND MANAGEMENT

Advances in obstetric and neonatal intensive care have decreased the incidence of hydrocephalus due to IVH and meningitis. In addition, nutritional guidelines recommending supplementation of folic acid in females

of childbearing age have lowered the incidence of hydrocephalus by decreasing the number of children born with myelomeningocele and other neural tube defects. The Centers for Disease Control and Prevention (CDC, 2022) recommends that females of reproductive age receive 400 µg of folic acid each day along with consuming food with folate.

Neural tube defects may be identified by fetal ultrasound and elevated levels of maternal alpha-fetoprotein (AFP). Prenatal evaluation (i.e., including high-resolution ultrasound scanning and measures of AFP) has increased the number of fetal anomalies identified. Assessment for other congenital anomalies and follow-up ultrasound scans to detect progressive ventricular enlargement are essential when counseling families. If severe brain dysfunction or other congenital anomalies are suspected, parents may decide to terminate the pregnancy. Otherwise, pregnancy can be continued as close to term as possible, and a shunt or ventricular access device can be placed soon after birth.

Fetal surgery continues to be explored as a treatment for congenital hydrocephalus, particularly with myelomeningocele. The Management of Myelomeningocele Study (MOMS) demonstrated that intrauterine closure of a myelomeningocele resulted in less need for a shunt for infants at 1 year of age as compared to the postnatal closure, as well as a better composite score for mental and motor function at 30 months (Adzick et al., 2011). Tulipan et al. (2015) revised the criteria for in utero closure of myelomeningocele and found similar results for the revised outcome. The revised criteria may be useful for treating hydrocephalus prenatally. Elbabaa et al. (2017) found that ETV could be an alternative to VP shunt placement in infants with hydrocephalus following prenatal myelomeningocele closure.

ASSOCIATED PROBLEMS OF CONDITION AND TREATMENT

Associated problems of hydrocephalus include intellectual deficits, ocular abnormalities, motor disabilities, and seizures. Each of these problems is discussed in this section.

INTELLECTUAL DEFICITS

The intellectual function is difficult to predict early after diagnosis of hydrocephalus. Cognitive function depends on the cause of hydrocephalus, age of onset, promptness of treatment, comorbidities, and history of shunt infection, particularly with gram-negative organisms. Increased ICP and ventriculomegaly cause damage to the white matter structure of the brain and are risk factors that affect cognition (Yuan et al., 2015). In a meta-analysis of neurodevelopmental outcomes after VP shunt placement in children with noninfectious hydrocephalus (S-NIH), Sobana et al. (2021) found that children with S-NIH had a higher risk of mental developmental delay compared to normal children. The younger the individual is when hydrocephalus is diagnosed, the greater the risk for intellectual impairment. Children in whom hydrocephalus is diagnosed in utero have the poorest outcome intellectually. In a study by Lindquist et al. (2005), approximately 33% of the children with hydrocephalus had intelligence quotients (IQs) in the normal range (>85), 33% had mild-moderate intellectual deficit (IQs 70–84), and 33% had severe intellectual deficit (IQs <70). An increased risk of intellectual deficit has been associated with gestational age and hydrocephalus at birth (Lindquist et al., 2005).

Radiographic studies cannot predict future cognitive function, as some children with normal neuroimaging can have severe cognitive dysfunction (Nielsen & Breedt, 2017). Some infants with severe hydrocephalus and virtually no cortical mantle visible on the initial imaging studies have experienced normal growth and development.

OCULAR ABNORMALITIES

Vision loss, oculomotor problems, visual field deficits, and visual-perceptive deficiencies can affect up to 83% of patients (Andersson et al., 2006). Children with hydrocephalus had a higher incidence of ocular abnormalities compared with an age- and sex-matched group (Aring et al., 2007).

Abnormalities in vision are associated with lower intelligence scores and may help identify children at risk for cognitive delay. These children may eventually require the use of large-print and increased-contrast work materials, as well as placement of work items within their visual field. Correctable visual problems should be addressed as soon as possible so that poor vision does not interfere with learning potential.

MOTOR DISABILITIES

Children with S-NIH have a significantly higher risk of motor development delay than normal children and an eight times higher risk for cerebral palsy (Sobana et al., 2021). As many as 60% of children with hydrocephalus have some form of motor disability (Hoppe-Hirsch et al., 1998). These disabilities vary from severe paraplegia to mild imbalance or weakness. Delayed walking (at age 16–22 months) is not unusual in children with infantile hydrocephalus (Persson et al., 2006). The severity of the motor deficit is most often related to the diagnosis; conditions such as porencephaly, Dandy-Walker malformation, and myelomeningocele portend more serious motor defects than simple congenital hydrocephalus. About half of the children with myelomeningocele need wheelchair assistance by adolescence (Persson et al., 2006). Hydrocephalus also affects fine motor control. The kinesthetic-proprioceptive abilities of the hands are often negatively affected and—coupled with the impaired bimanual manipulation and frequent visual deficits—make it difficult for children with hydrocephalus to perform well on time-limited, nonverbal intelligence tests.

SEIZURES

Since the introduction of shunting for individuals with hydrocephalus, controversies have arisen regarding the likelihood of the development of epileptic seizures because of the shunting itself and/or its complications. Hydrocephalus is not commonly recognized as a cause of seizures in general, although epilepsy is reported to be frequently associated with shunt-treated hydrocephalus, especially in children. Children with S-NIH have a 15.75 times higher risk than other children of acquiring seizures/epilepsy (Sobana et al., 2021).

The insult to the brain at the time of ventricular catheter insertion, the presence of the shunt tube itself as a foreign body, the burr hole location, the number of shunt revisions after a malfunction, associated infection, the cause of hydrocephalus, and associated developmental delay are thought to be related to the risk of epilepsy. Age at the time of initial shunt placement also seems to be an important factor. Early shunting is a well-known determinant of risk in shunt obstruction, and children younger than age 2 years are consequently at a higher risk of developing epilepsy than older children. It is reported that antiepileptic drug treatment is not as efficacious as might be expected in such children. Routine electroencephalogram recordings in children treated with antiepileptic medications may be beneficial during follow-up. Although VP shunts have been the standard treatment for hydrocephalus for decades, the long-term morbidity, including postshunt epileptic seizures, must be seriously considered.

PROGNOSIS

Hydrocephalus is the result of some event on the nervous system. A child's prognosis is ultimately determined by the underlying cause of hydrocephalus, the severity of symptoms, the age of onset, and the time between diagnosis and treatment (American Association of Neurological Surgeons, 2022). Although developing brains can recover due to their plasticity, the prognosis is worse for those with the in utero or perinatal onset of hydrocephalus (McAllister, 2012). Untreated hydrocephalus has a mortality rate of 50% to 60% (Nielsen & Breedt, 2017). However, the overall prognosis for successful management of hydrocephalus is excellent. Shunt dependency may carry a mortality rate as high as 1% per year, with most of the mortality related to delays in accessing a responsive system in time to prevent death. Primary care providers should remember that children with hydrocephalus are at risk for increased morbidity and early mortality after years of excellent progress and shunt function. Early detection and treatment of shunt malfunction and complications can reduce morbidity and mortality significantly.

PRIMARY CARE MANAGEMENT

HEALTH CARE MAINTENANCE

Growth and Development

Measurements of children seen in a primary care practice are typically done by minimally trained office or clinic personnel. If a child is suspected of having hydrocephalus or is known to have hydrocephalus, the primary care provider should measure the head circumference and plot it on a chart appropriate for age. Head circumference is a major diagnostic tool in evaluating a child's condition until the cranial sutures are completely fused, which is often delayed in these children. Normal head circumference at birth is 33 to 36 cm. During the first year, the head circumference increases by 9 cm during the first 6 months and 3 cm from 9 to 12 months. A diagnosis of hydrocephalus is indicated more by increases across growth percentiles than by a normal rate of growth paralleling the 95th percentile. Increasing head circumference from hydrocephalus is usually associated with a full fontanel, splayed sutures, prominent scalp veins, and frontal bossing.

Once the diagnosis of hydrocephalus has been made and a shunt inserted, head circumference may decrease by 1 to 2 cm as the pressure is relieved. The sutures may become overriding and the fontanel sunken. After this initial decrease, the head should grow only in proportion to the child's body. Therefore a newborn whose weight and height are in the 50th percentile for age and whose head size is 40 cm when a shunt is placed shortly after birth may not resume head growth for 2 to 4 months. The resumption of growth before that time might indicate shunt malfunction. The significance of head size measurements in a child with a shunt cannot be overestimated, and daily measurements may be necessary during the evaluation of shunt-dependent infants for possible shunt malfunction. Weight gain must be assessed carefully because the increasing weight of the head of the infant with hydrocephalus may mask failure to thrive.

Endocrine abnormalities can occur in children with hydrocephalus due to a disturbance of the gonadostimulin axis (Vinchon et al., 2012). Precocious puberty is fairly common in children with hydrocephalus. It is thought to be caused by chronic or intermittent increased ICP affecting the hypothalamus and pituitary gland, which is responsible for the timing and release of gonadotropins and sex hormones (Nielsen & Breedt, 2017). Precocious puberty is eight times more frequent in females than in males and is defined for females as the appearance of secondary sex characteristics before 8 years of age (Sultan et al., 2018). Precocious puberty is a concern because premature closing of the long bones results in short stature, and there is a risk of pregnancy in children with cognitive and behavioral difficulties (Nielsen & Breedt, 2017). Treatment is available, and the primary care practitioner should refer the child to a pediatric endocrinologist should a question of precocious puberty arise.

The standard early infant developmental assessment tools used in primary care practice (e.g., Denver Developmental Screening Test II) are of little help in assessing infants with hydrocephalus. Tasks that require head control (e.g., elevating the head while the child is in the prone position, rolling over, pulling to a sitting position without head lag, and even sitting unassisted) will be delayed in infants with macrocrania. It is important for primary care providers to interpret developmental findings in light of other clinical observations to help parents set reasonable expectations for their infant.

Other motor delays can be expected during infancy and childhood, given that approximately 60% of children with hydrocephalus have some form of motor disability. For children younger than age 3 years, referral to an early intervention program is often appropriate to evaluate and treat motor delays. Primary care providers must carefully document motor skill acquisition, even in older school-age children, because a loss of skill may indicate shunt malfunction or progression of the primary cause. Ataxia, slurred speech, lack of progression in school, incontinence, or other regression in developmental ability may indicate a deterioration in neurologic status and a need for further evaluation.

Long-term cognitive outcomes depend on the cause of the hydrocephalus and other comorbidities, but cognition is the area most severely affected in children with hydrocephalus (Kahle et al., 2016). Verbal skills are usually commensurate with intellectual abilities, and these children perform better on verbal tests than on fine motor–visual perception tests. Primary care providers must assess speech carefully with each health care visit. These children often benefit from infant stimulation programs and speech therapy. Primary care providers should become familiar with the program offerings in the family's community to help them identify the most beneficial services for their child.

Diet

Children with hydrocephalus have no special dietary requirements. Many parents become overly concerned about the episodes of regurgitation or vomiting that are common in all infants, and clarification as to what is considered normal and what is pathologic vomiting should be made soon after the diagnosis of hydrocephalus. Parents may be hesitant to burp their infant because of poor head control or concern over dislodging the shunt. Alternate positions for burping can be demonstrated. If repeated regurgitation occurs, parents should be advised on how to use an infant seat for postfeeding positioning and introducing solids (if age appropriate). The primary care provider can be supportive of the parents of a child with newly diagnosed hydrocephalus by reassuring them that their concerns are valid and helping clarify symptoms common in newborns, which may indicate increased ICP or some other condition, such as gastroesophageal reflux. Neurosurgical practitioners reassure these same parents that it is better to notify early and too often regarding a symptom of possible shunt malfunction than to miss something and cause the child harm. Eventually, the majority of parents that have children with shunted hydrocephalus become experts at recognizing shunt problems. Narayan et al. (2015) found that parents accurately recognized shunt failure 57% of the time.

Safety

Primary care providers play a major role in educating parents and children about safety. Families may be so overwhelmed with the task of parenting a child with a chronic condition that routine safety measures are overlooked. Children with hydrocephalus may have trouble with head control as a result of low motor tone, which predisposes these children to head injury. If an infant has poor head control and is unable to sit unsupported, it may be necessary to use a rear-facing convertible car seat so that the infant's head is maintained in a reclined position. The health care provider plays a crucial role in helping families choose the best safety seat for their children. Hospitals should have a child passenger safety program that can advise on the proper car seat, and this should be part of the child's safety plan (O'Neil et al., 2019).

As the child grows, activities should be limited as little as possible to encourage normal development and peer relationships. Many parents of children with shunted hydrocephalus become overly concerned about head injuries. Parents may ask about the child wearing a helmet at all times to protect the shunt in the event of a fall or head injury. Children with shunts need to wear helmets for the same reasons all children should wear helmets (while riding scooters, bicycles, skateboards, etc.) unless they have difficulty with head control or seizures. It is important for the primary care provider to encourage parents not to be overly protective of their child with shunted hydrocephalus. Hydrocephalus or spina bifida camps provide opportunities for children to participate in activities and make friends with others with similar health care needs.

A child's neurologic disabilities and visual perceptual integration may make competitive sports difficult and the operation of motor vehicles hazardous. Few sports are contraindicated in children with hydrocephalus. Contact sports such as wrestling, tackle football, and hockey might increase the risk of shunt damage or head trauma, so participation in these sports may need to be restricted. Each individual's ability must be regularly assessed to determine the risks and benefits of activities.

Physical activity is important for the child's growth and development, even those with hydrocephalus. In a study of 110 children under 18 years of age with shunted hydrocephalus, Stanuszek et al. (2021) found that children with shunted hydrocephalus could safely engage in physical education and after-school sports. However, neurologic deficits before and after treatment and comorbidities can put the child at risk, and those children may not be able to return to play (Stanuszek et al., 2021). Blount et al. (2004) surveyed 92 providers, of whom 77% had never observed a sport-related shunt complication; they found the incidence of sport-related CSF complications was less than 1%. Ninety percent of pediatric neurosurgeons do not restrict their patients from noncontact sports.

Immunizations

Routine immunizations are recommended (CDC, 2020). Some precautions should be considered before administering diphtheria and tetanus toxoids and the acellular pertussis vaccine (DTaP). According to the CDC, acellular pertussis-containing vaccines are contraindicated if the child experiences an episode of encephalopathy within 7 days of a previous dose of DTP, DTaP, or Tdap (CDC, 2024). Precaution is recommended for the DTaP and Tdap vaccines in children with progressive neurologic disorders, and the decision to administer those vaccines should be made individually with the provider (CDC, 2021).

Generally, infants and children with stable neurologic conditions should be vaccinated, including well-controlled seizures and/or developmental delays. Seizures may be present in the infant with hydrocephalus, and it may be difficult to determine which of these infants has a progressive neurologic disorder. An infant's neurologic status should be evaluated at each primary care visit to determine whether the DTaP vaccine is contraindicated. The acellular pertussis vaccine is associated with fewer neurologic side effects and is recommended for children with hydrocephalus. Because pertussis outbreaks still occur in the United States, deferral of the vaccine must be weighed against the potential for disease and disease-related complications. Children in day care, attending special developmental programs, or receiving care in residential centers are exposed to other children who may not be immunized and are at increased risk for developing pertussis. In such difficult situations, consultation with the child's neurosurgeon or neurologist may help assess the child's seizure potential. If the primary care provider, with parental consent, decides early in infancy that the pertussis immunization will be withheld, diphtheria and tetanus vaccines should be given on schedule.

Screenings

Vision. Because of the high incidence of visual defects in children with hydrocephalus, practitioners must pay particular attention to visual screening. The Hirschberg light reflex, cover test, tracking, and funduscopic examinations should be performed at each office visit, and the results should be carefully documented in the child's record. At approximately 6 months of age, the child should be referred to a pediatric ophthalmologist for a thorough examination. Yearly examinations should be scheduled after that. Children with hydrocephalus often need surgery on their eye muscles to correct esotropia or exotropia. Practitioners can be instrumental in completing preoperative examinations and preparing the families for surgery. The primary care provider must remember that alterations in the funduscopic examination, eye muscle control, or visual ability may be associated with shunt malfunction and should be evaluated carefully when shunt malfunction or infection is part of the differential diagnosis. Referral to a neurologist or neurosurgeon for evaluation of an infant or young child for papilledema or evidence of increased pressure may help differentiate benign headache from that caused by shunt malfunction.

Hearing. In addition to routine newborn and office screening for hearing acuity, brainstem auditory evoked responses should be ordered if an infant has a history of central nervous system (CNS) infection or antibiotic treatment with aminoglycosides. Subsequent shunt malfunctions or CNS infections require a reassessment of hearing. Periodic evaluation by an audiologist is recommended.

Dental. Routine dental care is recommended. If a child takes phenytoin (Dilantin) for seizure control, more frequent dental care may be needed because of hyperplasia of the gums. Poor dental hygiene and periodontal disease may produce bacteremia—even without dental procedures (Wolf et al., 2004). Because intravascular foreign bodies are susceptible to bacterial colonization, any episode of transient bacteremia places a child with a VA shunt at risk for infection. Antibiotic prophylaxis is not recommended for children with VP shunts prior to dental care but is recommended for children with VA shunts (Ramasamy, 2018).

Blood pressure. Blood pressure readings should be recorded at each clinic or office visit. Elevations in blood pressure with a widening pulse pressure are a late sign of increased ICP. An established baseline reading can help the practitioner assess a child for possible shunt malfunctions or progression of the disease process.

Hematocrit. Routine screening is recommended.

Urinalysis. Routine screening is recommended.

Tuberculosis. Routine screening is recommended.

Condition-Specific Screening

Head circumference. Head circumference measurements should be taken at every clinic or office visit until a child's sutures are completely fused.

COMMON ILLNESS MANAGEMENT

Differential Diagnosis

Many shunt malfunction or infection symptoms are the same as those commonly found with routine childhood illnesses (Box 26.3). It is important to remember that children with hydrocephalus experience otitis media, gastrointestinal (GI) illnesses, headaches, and viral infections with fever, just like their unaffected peers. Primary care providers must approach these children as they would children without hydrocephalus. A calm manner and a thorough history and examination are reassuring to parents and productive for the primary care provider.

Shunt malfunction. The most frequent symptoms of shunt malfunction include irritability, headache, nausea, vomiting, lethargy, and delays or loss of developmental milestones. Other symptoms include personality changes, diplopia, new seizures or a change in seizure pattern, worsening school performance, decreased level of consciousness, loss of upward gaze, nuchal rigidity, sixth nerve palsy, papilledema, and hemiparesis or loss of coordination and balance. If the shunt is infected, it may continue to work properly, and therefore the child may not exhibit signs of increased ICP. Children with shunt infections may present with low-grade and intermittent fevers, redness, tenderness, swelling along the shunt tract, abdominal pain, nuchal rigidity, headache, and seizures. Infections associated with VA shunts may present with glomerulonephritis (Duhaime, 2006).

Box 26.3	Signs and Symptoms of Common Shunt Illnesses

SHUNT MALFUNCTION
1. Irritability
2. Headache
3. Nausea/vomiting
4. Lethargy
5. Personality changes
6. Loss of developmental milestones
7. Worsening school performance
8. Enlarging hernia

SHUNT INFECTION
1. Low-grade or intermittent fevers
2. Fever
3. Redness, tenderness, and swelling along the shunt tract
4. Abdominal pain
5. Headache
6. Scalp infections or breaks in the skin around shunt tubing or valve

Fever. There is no characteristic combination of signs and symptoms of shunt infections. Perhaps the most important clinical aspect of identifying a shunt infection is understanding that the presentation is highly variable, and keen observation is required to diagnose. Early in an infant's first year, when shunt infections are most common, parents should be encouraged to consult the primary care provider whenever the infant has a temperature above 101.3°F (38.5°C). The practitioner, with the consulting primary care provider, can evaluate the child early in the course of illness and note the progression of symptoms. If a focus of infection other than the shunt is identified, it should be treated appropriately. No studies indicate that frequent antibacterial therapy for illnesses of questionable origin reduces the incidence of shunt malfunction. Children being treated for bacterial infections (e.g., otitis media, pneumonia, or streptococcal sore throat) should be carefully reassessed in the office or clinic 24 to 48 hours after the treatment is initiated. Continued or worsening symptoms may indicate the progression of the infection into bacteremia or a CNS infection caused by the increased susceptibility resulting from the shunt. The primary care provider should obtain a complete blood cell (CBC) count, urinalysis, and blood cultures if a shunt infection is suspected and immediately consult the child's neurosurgeon.

If a child has a mild-moderate fever of unknown origin with other symptoms compatible with a common childhood illness and no obvious signs of shunt malfunction, the primary care provider can adopt a wait-and-see attitude. Arrangements for telephone follow-up or a return appointment in 24 hours should be made. The parents must be instructed to report symptoms such as lethargy, confusion, or recurrent vomiting (more than three times within 24 hours) immediately if they occur.

In children with very high temperatures (i.e., >101.3°F [38.5°C]) and symptoms of moderate-severe illness, a shunt infection must be assumed until proven otherwise. Consultation with the neurosurgeon is advised. Blood cultures for aerobic and anaerobic organisms should be obtained, although results often are not initially positive. A CBC count is also indicated, but minimal leukocytosis does not rule out shunt infection. The neurosurgeon may obtain CSF for culture through the shunt reservoir. Although a shunt infection can be present despite normal CSF cell count, Lan et al. (2003) found several factors predictive of shunt infection; these include an increased C-reactive protein level, CSF leukocytosis (>100/mm³), CSF neutrophils (>10%), decreased CSF glucose level, and increased CSF protein level. Shunt aspiration should be done with a meticulous aseptic technique so as not to contaminate a sterile shunt system or introduce a second organism into an already infected shunt. A lumbar puncture is not advised in a child with a shunt because of the possibility of downward brain herniation and death if ventriculomegaly with increased ICP is present.

A chest radiograph and urine culture are recommended to rule out pneumonia or urinary tract infection. However, these may be omitted if the history and physical findings strongly suggest shunt involvement. Include all test results and radiographs obtained for the current workup if the child is transferred to a hospital. Throughout the workup for the source of the fever, the primary care practitioner should be in close communication with the primary neurosurgeon.

Gastrointestinal symptoms. Nausea and vomiting are common clinical symptoms during childhood and often accompany such diverse conditions as influenza, otitis media, and urinary tract infections. Diarrhea and abdominal pain are also frequent complaints in childhood. Children with hydrocephalus can be expected to have these common complaints as often as other children. When a child has mild GI symptoms, the practitioner must consider the presence or absence of other symptoms and the history of exposure to GI illness. The diagnostic workup should include an evaluation for shunt infection and GI disease. The primary care provider must recognize that abdominal symptoms may be the presenting symptom of peritoneal shunt malfunction or an acute condition in the abdomen in children with shunts (Kim et al., 2006). Children with shunt-dependent hydrocephalus should follow a regimen to maintain normal bowel movements since chronic constipation has been shown to lead to distal shunt obstruction (Muzumdar & Ventureyra, 2007).

Children with a peritoneal shunt infection may have mild-moderate fever, abdominal pain, anorexia, nausea, vomiting, and diarrhea. They may guard their abdomen and be unwilling to ambulate. Swelling, redness, or inflammation along the catheter tract or at the incision site is highly suggestive of shunt involvement. Abdominal ultrasound and CSF cultures should help differentiate between an acute condition in the abdomen and a shunt infection. A CT scan of the abdomen can demonstrate specific signs of appendicitis, but identification of an abdominal pseudocyst is more characteristic of a distal shunt infection (Browd et al., 2006). Abdominal pseudocysts may develop around the peritoneal end of the VP shunt and usually result from past or current shunt infection. A history of recent or recurrent shunt revisions also substantially increases the risk of infection. The primary care practitioner may not be able to differentiate the symptoms of an acute condition in the abdomen from a peritoneal shunt malfunction. Consultation with and referral to the attending neurosurgeon is advised.

Another abdominal concern relates to infants with inguinal or umbilical hernias and the potential for

CSF or shunt tubing to migrate into the hernia. If this occurs, the hernia becomes enlarged with a collection of CSF. Treatment includes repair of the hernia and possible shunt revision.

Extraneural spread of CNS malignancies implicating VP shunts has been reported; however, in a review of the literature by Narayan et al. (2015), only 28 cases were found in patients less than 18 years of age. This side effect must be considered when a differential diagnosis is made in children with chronic or recurring abdominal symptoms if these children also have a history of brain tumor. An appropriate referral is required to rule out this possibility after more common reasons for the complaint have been eliminated.

Headache. Children often report headaches, which can also occur in children with a shunt and may have the same origin as in children without hydrocephalus. If routine treatment of headache with mild analgesics and rest does not relieve the symptom, or if the headaches become frequent, affect school attendance, or are associated with lethargy or irritability, then evaluation by the neurologist and/or neurosurgeon is required. Repetitive and vigorous investigation of shunt malfunction may not be necessary in the absence of other symptoms.

Shunt malfunction can be partial or variable, depending on cerebral blood flow, CSF production, and a child's activity, and may result in periodic episodes of increased ICP and headaches. Children with shunts occasionally experience headache and vomiting in the early morning after sleeping all night. These symptoms may be caused by temporary partial blockage of the shunt from cellular debris, inactivity, and the horizontal sleeping position, negating gravity's beneficial effect on ventricular drainage. These symptoms usually subside after children have been up for a few hours. If these episodes are infrequent and self-limited, they do not require treatment other than acetaminophen or ibuprofen for pain. Parents should be instructed to call the primary care provider if these symptoms continue for more than 6 hours or are associated with a decrease in the child's level of consciousness or loss of motor ability.

Scalp infections. A thin layer of skin covers the shunt reservoir on the scalp. If the skin around the shunt reservoir becomes infected, the integrity of the skin barrier may be broken, and infection of the shunt is possible. The primary care provider should manage scalp infections aggressively in collaboration with the neurosurgeon. Any break in the skin on or around the shunt tubing or valve, especially if the shunt hardware is exposed, should prompt a call to the neurosurgery provider, as there is a potential for a shunt infection (Fig. 26.9).

Alterations in behavior. All children experience mood swings and temporary behavior changes. Parents of

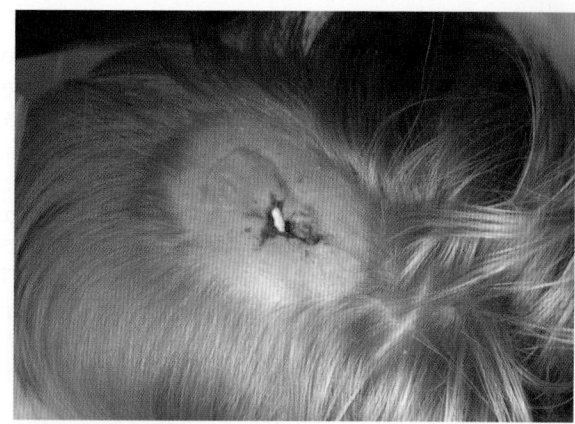

Fig. 26.9 Exposed shunt hardware due to skin breakdown in the scalp. An exposed shunt is a pathway for infection and necessitates a call to the neurosurgery provider.

children with hydrocephalus may comment on them not being themselves, school performance may falter, normal interest in activities may dwindle, and lethargy or irritability may develop. If these changes persist beyond a few days, a child should be seen by the neurosurgeon for an evaluation. Subtle changes in behavior, cognition, or motor ability may be symptoms of shunt malfunction.

Drug interactions. No routine medications are prescribed for children with hydrocephalus.

DEVELOPMENTAL ISSUES

Sleep
Parents may be concerned about their infant or child sleeping in a position that might adversely affect the shunt. During the immediate period after shunt placement, these children should be positioned off the reservoir site to avoid skin breakdown. With the exception of this brief period after shunt placement or revision, parents and caretakers must be reassured that their child can sleep in any comfortable position without fear of affecting the shunt. Infants and young children should be encouraged to assume a normal sleep pattern at night. Children who seem to be sleeping or napping more than usual should be evaluated for possible increased ICP.

Toileting
Children with neurologic deficits associated with hydrocephalus may have a delayed ability to develop bowel and bladder control. Parents need to be counseled on the possibility of this difficulty, and the toilet training methods should be reviewed. The neurologist, neurosurgeon, and physiatrist (if applicable) monitoring a child's development should be consulted about the child's neurologic capability to attain satisfactory toilet training. Chronic constipation may exert pressure on the peritoneal shunt, resulting in a malfunction. Maintenance of regular stool patterns may prevent unnecessary hospitalization and the need for

shunt revision. Special bowel training and clean intermittent catheterization education should be provided if necessary. These techniques can usually be obtained through referral to a pediatric urologist or physiatrist.

Discipline

Discipline for children with hydrocephalus should be managed as for other children, recognizing the limitations of cognitive and motor development of the individual child. Some parents may have difficulty understanding the discrepancy between their child's verbal and performance skills or have expectations that are too high for the child to attain, which may lead to inappropriate discipline. On the other hand, parents may be afraid to discipline their children and must be encouraged to set appropriate limits.

Practitioners must always be concerned with the increased possibility of child abuse in children with chronic conditions. Head and abdominal injuries are common in child abuse and may result in further brain injury or shunt malfunction in children with hydrocephalus.

Child Care

Most parents work outside the home. Child care and preschool placement are major issues for all working parents but are even more problematic when a child has a chronic condition. Fortunately, the current shunt systems are self-maintained and do not require special care (e.g., pumping periodically) throughout the day. Children with hydrocephalus have no special care needs unless other disabilities (e.g., cerebral palsy with spasticity or dystonia, seizures, or developmental delay) are present. If a child has significant disabilities, child care arrangements must be evaluated for their ability to meet the child's needs. Public Law (PL) 108-446 (Individuals with Disabilities Education Improvement Act, 2004) extends services to children with disabilities from birth to school entry, so federally funded programs are accessible to children with disabilities. Parents of children with disabilities such as spina bifida and hydrocephalus may visit the website http://idea.ed.gov/ for more information about the law and current amendments.

Schooling

Children with hydrocephalus have a greater risk of cognitive delays, including learning disabilities (Nielsen & Breedt, 2017). Primary care providers can help families plan their child's individualized education program (IEP) to ensure appropriate interventions for the child. Although PL 108-446 requires the school district to assess a child's needs, the district's financial constraints may limit neuropsychological testing. Therefore the results of any testing before the child attends school may be beneficial and should be forwarded to the school district. Parents may need help obtaining medical records to facilitate the formulation of their child's IEP, and the primary care practitioner can assist the family during this process.

Some children with hydrocephalus qualify for separate special education classes because of physical or intellectual limitations. Other children can be mainstreamed into regular classrooms and receive special services (e.g., adaptive physical education to help with motor control and balance, occupational therapy to assist with kinesthetic-proprioceptive deficits, speech therapy, or psychological counseling to address emotional issues). As these children reach middle and high school, some limitations may be made on competitive, high-impact sports. If a child has mild-moderate neuromotor deficits, an evaluation by a sports medicine professional may help identify sports activities that the child can successfully perform. Involvement in sports activities or formal group activities such as scouting is often beneficial to a child's self-esteem and encourages peer relationships, both of which may be problematic areas for children with hydrocephalus.

Children with less severe disabilities may experience psychosocial struggles because they may have a difficult time fitting in with nondisabled peers but also do not fit in with those children with more disabilities. Their disabilities may not be recognized by teachers and peers unable to understand why these individuals have difficulty in school or sports. Adolescents who are trying to blend in may not disclose their learning or motor deficits but will not be able to successfully compete with unaffected peers. The resulting incongruity between expectations and ability can lead to a sense of failure and lowered self-esteem.

Primary care providers should routinely ask parents and children about school progress. If academic difficulties develop, these children should be referred for repeat neuropsychological testing to rule out medical reasons for these problems. Shunt malfunction may result in gradual changes in cognition, fine motor abilities, or personality and must be ruled out as a contributing factor. If difficulties are assessed to be more emotional, which often happens during adolescence when children struggle with their body image and identity, children should be referred for counseling. This referral should be made to a professional experienced in working with children with disabilities.

Sexuality

As previously mentioned, delayed or precocious puberty may occur in children with hydrocephalus. Their progression through puberty must be assessed and monitored; counseling may be indicated to support them during this period. Children with precocious puberty may have lowered self-esteem, poor peer relationships, and a higher incidence of sexual abuse than normally developing children. Sexuality and reproductive issues should be managed the same as with other children. Female adolescents receiving anticonvulsant therapy should be informed of the possible teratogenic effects of their medications. It is universally recommended that all females of child-bearing age take 400 µg of folic acid daily to help prevent serious birth defects (CDC, 2022). Adolescents with associated motor disabilities may have additional needs.

Transition to Adulthood

Since the 1970s, improvements in shunt techniques and management of shunt complications have dramatically increased the survival of individuals with hydrocephalus. Unique issues have arisen as young people with hydrocephalus make their transition into adulthood. These individuals and their families now find themselves dealing with vocational training, career placement, sexuality, and family roles. Social outcomes are often highly influenced by one's associated disabilities, especially developmental delay and motor handicaps. Many adults who were shunted during childhood have achieved full-time employment and successful personal relationships because either their disabilities were minor or they were able to overcome them.

The care given by pediatric providers and children's hospitals often ends when youth reach the age of 18 years. Hydrocephalus care continues during the adult years, yet many have a difficult time finding an adult neurosurgical provider. Guaranteed access to a responsive system is not a good idea for people with hydrocephalus; it is a matter of life and death because shunt malfunction can result in death if not treated early and appropriately. Primary care providers must be advocates for the continued care of children as they transition into adolescent and adult care. Transition to adult health care must start early in the teen years, with the youth taking on more responsibility as they are cognitively and physically able. Got Transition is a federally funded site with information for providers, parents, and youth to help youth transition to adult care (see Resources, later).

A supportive climate that encourages independence, maturity, and responsibility is essential if young adults with hydrocephalus are to complete school, maintain employment, and function as adults. Professional guidance is often necessary to create this environment. Health care professionals should emphasize a positive approach for young adults with hydrocephalus. Parents must be prepared to face the normal problems of adolescence and let their young children develop independence. The goals of the health care transition are to enable youth to use health care services and manage their health to the best of their ability (Williams et al., 2019).

Young adults dependent on a shunt should be cautious about living alone because they could become acutely ill, confused, or even comatose during a shunt malfunction. These individuals should form a buddy system to ensure their well-being, minimizing their risk of permanent brain injury from an unrecognized shunt malfunction. Vocational training and special education resources are also available at the college level to help young adults prepare for job placement.

Hydrocephalus alone should not interfere with a female's ability to conceive, but approximately 50% of pregnant females with shunted hydrocephalus will experience antepartum complications, with increased ICP being the most common (Al-Saadi et al., 2020). As the pregnancy progresses, intraabdominal pressure increases, which may result in increased ICP for females with VP shunts. Prenatal counseling and assessment should include genetic counseling and a review of family history for neural tube defects. A complete assessment of shunt function by the neurosurgery provider should be obtained if pregnancy is being considered. In addition, maternal supplementation with folic acid significantly diminishes the number of infants born with neural tube defects. Therefore females of childbearing age must be strongly encouraged to supplement their folic acid intake before conception.

Family Concerns and Resources

Parents of children with hydrocephalus constantly worry about continued shunt function. With every malfunction there is the need for surgery and the perceived threat of further brain damage. Listening carefully to parents' concerns is important as they know their child best. They may simply need reassurance; however, they may also describe a situation where the child is deteriorating.

The constant anxiety and the daily responsibility of caring for a child who may have multiple medical problems are stressful for families. The financial strain from numerous medical visits or surgical procedures may deplete a family's financial reserves. Private insurance may not be obtainable unless offered through a large group employment policy. Concern about a child's future ability to be self-supporting and independent is also an issue for parents as their child grows into adolescence and adulthood.

Traveling far from the child's neurosurgery provider can be a concern that limits family vacations and the child's ability to participate in activities such as summer camps and trips to see grandparents or other friends who live at a distance. Parents should be encouraged to locate the nearest neurosurgery provider and emergency contact information when planning the travel event. The HydroAssist app is a helpful tool to store treatment information about the child's hydrocephalus (e.g., neuroimaging, type of shunt, surgical history) (see Resources, later). This information can be readily provided to the neurosurgeon should there be a suspected shunt malfunction during travel.

Magnetic Field Interference

Programmable shunts are adjusted by the neurosurgery provider using a magnetic device. Parents should be aware that children may be inadvertently exposed to magnetic fields that could interfere with the valve setting on programmable valves. This inadvertent exposure can come from the many electronic devices available today, such as cell phones, magnetic toys, iPads, refrigerator door magnets, earbuds, and headphones (Fujimura et al., 2018). Even Vocera badges were found to change the valve setting when a child with a programmable valve was held for feeding by the nursing staff (Fujimura et al., 2018). Parents should be aware of their child's programmable shunt manufacturers' warnings regarding inadvertent exposure to magnetic fields.

Parent-to-parent support groups can offer support by publishing newsletters and hosting major medical conferences for health professionals and parents. These organizations also provide a network for children with hydrocephalus, offering them the opportunity to make new friends, develop peer support, and exchange knowledge. Support groups are now readily available online for adolescents with hydrocephalus and their parents (see Resources, later). Primary care providers should become familiar with the organizations in the community and web connections so that appropriate referrals can be made. It is better to make such referrals soon after a child's diagnosis than to wait to see how the parents cope. All parents need support above and beyond what is reasonable for a primary care provider or nurse to provide.

RESOURCES

Center for Parent Information & Resources (c/o SPAN): https://www.parentcenterhub.org/disability-landing
Got Transition: https://www.gottransition.org
HydroAssist Mobile Application: https://www.hydroassoc.org/hydroassist
Hydrocephalus Association: https://www.hydroassoc.org/about-us
Spina Bifida Association: https://www.spinabifidaassociation.org

 Summary

Primary Care Needs

HEALTH CARE MAINTENANCE
Growth and Development
- The head should be measured at each visit until the sutures are fused.
- If an enlarged head size is diagnosed in infancy and a shunt is placed, then head size should follow the normal growth curve.
- Carefully assess weight gain at each visit, as a larger head size may mask failure to thrive.
- Evaluate for signs of central early puberty (the most common endocrine disorder).
- Standard infant development tests may indicate delay because of poor head control.
- Sixty percent of all children with hydrocephalus will have some motor disability.
- Verbal skills are usually higher than performance skills.
- Cognitive ability varies and is determined by the cause and treatment of hydrocephalus.
- Early stimulation/intervention programs are recommended.

Diet
- A normal diet is indicated.
- Assessment of infant vomiting as normal or as a sign of increased ICP may be difficult.

Safety
- The risk of head injury is increased because of poor head control.
- A rear-facing car seat should be recommended until a child can sit unsupported.
- A helmet should be used for bicycle and skateboard riding.

- Neurologic deficits may make competitive sports difficult or unadvisable and the operation of motor vehicles hazardous.

Immunizations
- Routine immunizations are recommended.
- Pertussis vaccine may be deferred in infants with a progressive neurologic disorder or history of encephalopathy after previous DTaP dose.
- *Haemophilus influenzae* type B conjugated vaccine and pneumococcal conjugate vaccines are strongly recommended.

Screenings
- *Vision.* Hirschberg examination, cover test, ability to track, and funduscopic examination should be done at each visit. Children should be examined by an ophthalmologist at 6 months of age and then yearly thereafter.
- Alterations in eye examination may be associated with shunt malfunction.
- *Hearing.* A routine office screening is recommended. An auditory evoked response test should be given to children with a history of CNS infection or those who have been treated with aminoglycosides. Periodic screening by an audiologist is recommended.
- *Dental.* Routine dental care is recommended.
- Dental hygiene is important to reduce the risk of bacteremia.
- Antibiotic prophylaxis is not recommended for dental work for patients with VP shunts.
- Children receiving phenytoin therapy require more frequent dental care.
- *Blood pressure.* Record at each visit.

Continued

- Blood pressure increases with increased ICP.
- *Hematocrit.* Routine screening is recommended.
- *Urinalysis.* Routine screening is recommended.
- *Tuberculosis.* Routine screening is recommended.

Condition-Specific Screening

- *Head circumference.* Measure at each visit until the sutures are completely fused.

COMMON ILLNESS MANAGEMENT
Differential Diagnosis

- *Shunt malfunction.* Shunt malfunction needs to be ruled out acutely.
- *Fever.* Shunt or CNS infection should be ruled out.
- *GI symptoms.* Increased ICP with nausea and vomiting should be ruled out.
- Shunt infection caused by an abdominal infection should be ruled out.
- Constipation should be ruled out as a cause of shunt malfunction.
- Metastatic abdominal tumors should be ruled out in children with primary brain tumors and VP shunts.
- *Headache.* Shunt malfunction should be ruled out as the cause of acute or chronic headache.
- *Scalp infections.* Possible infection spread to the shunt reservoir should be ruled out.
- *Alterations in behavior.* Rule out as a symptom of shunt malfunction.

Drug Interactions

- No routine medications are prescribed.

DEVELOPMENTAL ISSUES
Sleep Patterns

- Standard developmental counseling is advised.

Toileting

- Delayed bowel and bladder training may occur because of a neurologic deficit.
- Constipation may cause peritoneal shunt malfunction.

Discipline

- Expectations are normal with recognition of the possible discrepancy between verbal and motor abilities. Physical punishment is a hazard because it may cause head or abdominal injury.

Child Care

- No special care needs are required except when a child has a severe motor disability or seizures.

- Home care or small day care programs are recommended during a child's first 2 years of life to reduce exposure to infections.

Schooling

- Associated problems are often covered by PL 108-446 (IDEA).
- Families should be assisted in IEP hearings.
- Children may have possible adjustment problems during adolescence.
- Children may need psychometric testing for poor school performance.
- Low-impact sports should be selected to prevent head trauma and abdominal injury.
- Minor, unseen disabilities should not be overlooked.

Sexuality

- Children should be evaluated for delayed or precocious puberty.
- Standard developmental counseling is advised unless associated problems warrant additional care.

Transition to Adulthood

- Research has identified difficulty with vocational training, career, sexuality, and family roles associated with hydrocephalus and mental retardation, and motor handicaps.
- Independence must be fostered from an early age to prepare young adults for independence.
- Shunt-dependent individuals should develop a buddy system to ensure that shunt malfunction leading to acute illness, confusion, or coma does not go unrecognized.
- Pregnancy may interfere with peritoneal shunt drainage. Securing independent health and life insurance may be difficult for individuals with hydrocephalus.

FAMILY CONCERNS

- Families are concerned about continued shunt function and the possibility of brain damage caused by shunt failure or infection.
- If travel is planned, locate emergency contact information for the neurosurgeon near the destination and store the child's hydrocephalus information on the HydroAssist app.

RED FLAGS

- Box 26.4 provides findings that require immediate attention.

Box 26.4   Red Flags

The following findings require immediate attention and consult with a neurosurgery provider:

- Rapidly increasing head circumference, jumping isocurves
- Bulging fontanel
- Change in level of consciousness
- Persistent vomiting

- Redness or swelling along the shunt tract
- Scalp rash, or skin opening near shunt valve or tubing
- Exposed shunt valve or tubing
- Cerebrospinal fluid leak
- Redness or drainage at the incision site
- Fever unexplained by common childhood illnesses

REFERENCES

Abou-Hamden, A., & Drake, J. M. (2015). Hydrocephalus. In Albright, A. L., Pollack, I. F., & Adelson, P. D. (Eds.), *Principles and practice of pediatric neurosurgery* (3rd ed., pp. 89–99). Thieme Medical Publishers, Inc.

Adle-Biassette, H., Saugier-Veber, P., Fallet-Bianco, C., Delezoide, A. L., Razavi, F., Drouot, N., Bazin, A., Beaufrère, A. M., Bessières, B., Blesson, S., Bucourt, M., Carles, D., Devisme, L., Dijoud, F., Fabre, B., Fernandez, C., Gaillard, D., Gonzales, M., Jossic, F., ... Laquerrière, A. (2013). Neuropathological review of 138 cases genetically tested for X-linked hydrocephalus: evidence for closely related clinical entities of unknown molecular bases. *Acta Neuropathologica, 126*(3), 427–442. doi:10.1007/s00401-013-1146-1. Epub 2013 Jul 3.

Adzick, N. S., Thom, E. A., Spong, C. Y., Brock, J. W., 3rd., Burrows, P. K., Johnson, M. P., Howell, L. J., Farrell, J. A., Dabrowiak, M. E., Sutton, L. N., Gupta, N., Tulipan, N. B., D'Alton, M. E., Farmer, D. L., & MOMS Investigators (2011). A randomized trial of prenatal versus postnatal repair of myelomeningocele. *The New England Journal of Medicine, 364*(11), 993–1004. https://doi.org/10.1056/NEJMoa1014379.

Al-Saadi, T. D., Glisic, M., Al Sharqi, A., Al Kharosi, S., Al Shaqsi, M., Al Jabri, N., & Al Sharqi, J. (2020). Safety of Pregnancy in Ventriculoperitoneal Shunt Dependent Women: Meta-analysis and Systematic Review of the Literature. *Neurology India, 68*(3), 548–554. https://doi.org/10.4103/0028-3886.288995.

American Association of Neurological Surgeons (AANS). (2022). Neurosurgical conditions and treatments. *Hydrocephalus.* https://www.aans.org/en/Patients/Neurosurgical-Conditions-and-Treatments/Hydrocephalus.

Andersson, S., Persson, E. K., Aring, E., Lindquist, B., Dutton, G. N., & Hellström, A. (2006). Vision in children with hydrocephalus. *Developmental Medicine & Child Neurology, 48*(10), 836–841. https://doi.org/10.1017/S0012162206001794.

Aring, E., Andersson, S., Hård, A. L., Hellström, A., Persson, E. K., Uvebrant, P., Ygge, J., & Hellström, A. (2007). Strabismus, binocular functions and ocular motility in children with hydrocephalus. *Strabismus, 15*(2), 79–88. https://doi.org/10.1080/09273970701405305.

Blount, J. P., Severson, M., Atkins, V., Tubbs, R., Smyth, M., Wellons, J., Grabb, P., & Oakes, W. (2004). Sports and pediatric cerebrospinal fluid shunts: Who can play? *Neurosurgery, 54*(5), 1190–1198. https://doi.org/10.1227/01.neu.0000119236.08000.49.

Browd, S. R., Ragel, B. T., Gottfried, O. N., & Kestle, J. R. (2006). Failure of cerebrospinal fluid shunts: Part I: Obstruction and mechanical failure. *Pediatric Neurology, 34*(2), 83–92. https://doi.org/10.1016/j.pediatrneurol.2005.05.020.

Bryant, J., Hernandez, N. E., & Niazi, T. N. (2021). Macrocephaly in the primary care provider's office. *Pediatric Clinics of North America, 68*, 759–773.

Centers for Disease Control and Prevention. (2020). Vaccines and preventable diseases. Diphtheria, tetanus, and pertussis vaccine recommendations. https://www.cdc.gov/vaccines/vpd/dtap-tdap-td/hcp/recommendations.html.

Centers for Disease Control and Prevention. (2021). Guidance for immunization. Epidemiology and prevention of vaccine-preventable diseases. *Pink Book,* https://www.cdc.gov/vaccines/pubs/pinkbook/chapters.html.

Centers for Disease Control and Prevention. (2022). Folic acid recommendations. https://www.cdc.gov/ncbddd/folicacid/recommendations.html.

Centers for Disease Control. (2024). Child and adolescent immunization schedule by medical indication. https://www.cdc.gov/vaccines/schedules/hcp/imz/child-indications.html.

Dawod, J., Tager, A., Darouiche, R. O., & Al Mohajer, M. (2016). Prevention and management of internal cerebrospinal fluid shunt infections. *Journal of Hospital Infection, 93*(4), 323–328. doi:10.1016/j.jhin.2016.03.010.

Disabato, J. A., & Daniels, D. A. (2017). Neurological assessment of the neonate, infant, child, and adolescent. In Cartwright, C. C., & Wallace, D. C. (Eds.), *Nursing care of the pediatric neurosurgery patient* (3rd ed., pp. 39–89). Springer International Publishing https://doi.org/10.1007/978-3-319-49319-0.

Duhaime, A. (2006). Evaluation of management of shunt infections in children with hydrocephalus. *Clinical Pediatrics, 45*(8), 705–713.

Elbabaa, S. K., Gildehaus, A. M., Pierson, M. J., Albers, J. A., & Vlastos, E. J. (2017). First 60 fetal in-utero myelomeningocele repairs at Saint Louis Fetal Care Institute in the post-MOMS trial era: Hydrocephalus treatment outcomes (endoscopic third ventriculostomy versus ventriculo-peritoneal shunt). *Child's Nervous System, 33*(7), 1157–1168. https://doi.org/10.1007/s00381-017-3428-8.

Faria, C. C., Terakawa, Y., & Rutka, J. T. (2015). Congenital and developmental cerebral disorders. In Albright, A. L., Pollack, I. F., & Adelson, P. D. (Eds.), *Principles and practice of pediatric neurosurgery* (3rd ed., pp. 89–99). Thieme Medical Publishers, Inc.

Fujimura, R., Lober, R., Kamian, K., & Kleiner, L. (2018). Maladjustment of programmable ventricular shunt valves by inadvertent exposure to a common hospital device. *Surgical Neurology International, 9*, 51. https://doi.org/10.4103/sni.sni_444_17.

Hoppe-Hirsch, E., Laroussinie, F., Brunet, L., Sainte-Rose, C., Renier, D., Cinalli, G., Zerah, M., & Pierre-Kahn, A. (1998). Late outcome of the surgical treatment of hydrocephalus. *Child's Nervous System, 14*(3), 97–99. https://doi.org/10.1007/s003810050186.

Individuals with Disabilities Education Act. (2004). https://sites.ed.gov/idea/

Isaacs, A. M., Riva-Cambrin, J., Yavin, D., Hockley, A., Pringsheim, T. M., Jette, N., Lethebe, B. C., Lowerison, M., Dronyk, J., & Hamilton, M. G. (2018). Age-specific global epidemiology of hydrocephalus: Systematic review, metanalysis and global birth surveillance. *PloS One, 13*(10), e0204926. https://doi.org/10.1371/journal.pone.0204926.

Kahle, K. T., Kulkarni, A. V., Limbrick, D. D., Jr, & Warf, B. C. (2016). Hydrocephalus in children. *Lancet (London, England), 387*(10020), 788–799. https://doi.org/10.1016/S0140-6736(15)60694-8.

Kalra, R. R., & Kestle, J. (2011). Treatment of hydrocephalus with shunts. In Albright, A. L., Kestle, J. R., Riva-Cambrin, J., Wellons, J. C., III, et al. A standardized protocol to reduce cerebrospinal fluid shunt infection: The Hydrocephalus Clinical Research Network quality improvement initiative. *Journal of Neurosurgery: Pediatrics, 8*(1), 22–29. https://doi.org/10.3171/2011.4.PEDS10551.

Kim, T. Y., Stewart, G., Voth, M., Moynihan, J. A., & Brown, L. (2006). Signs and symptoms of cerebrospinal fluid shunt malfunction in the pediatric emergency department. *Pediatric Emergency Care, 22*(1), 28–34. https://doi.org/10.1097/01.pec.0000195764.50565.8c.

Kulkarni, A. V., Drake, J. M., Kestle, J. R., Mallucci, C. L., Sgouros, S., Constantini, S., & Canadian Pediatric Neurosurgery Study Group (2010). Predicting who will benefit from endoscopic third ventriculostomy compared with shunt insertion in childhood hydrocephalus using the ETV Success Score. *Journal of Neurosurgery: Pediatrics, 6*(4), 310–315. https://doi.org/10.3171/2010.8.PEDS103.

Lan, C. C., Wong, T. T., Chen, S. J., Liang, M. L., & Tang, R. B. (2003). Early diagnosis of ventriculoperitoneal shunt infections and malfunctions in children with hydrocephalus. *Journal of Microbiology, Immunology and Infection, 36*(1), 47–50.

Lindquist, B., Carlsson, G., Persson, E. K., & Uvebrant, P. (2005). Learning disabilities in a population-based group of children with hydrocephalus. *Acta Paediatrica, 94*(7), 878–883. https://doi.org/10.1111/j.1651-2227.2005.tb02005.x.

McAllister, J. P., II. (2012). Pathophysiology of congenital and neonatal hydrocephalus. *Seminars in Fetal and Neonatal Medicine, 17*(5), 285–294. https://doi.org/10.1016/j.siny.2012.06.004.

Merkler, A. E., Ch'ang, J., Parker, W. E., Murthy, S. B., & Kamel, H. (2017). The rate of complications after ventriculoperitoneal shunt surgery. *World Neurosurgery, 98*, 654–658. https://doi.org/10.1016/j.wneu.2016.10.136.

Muzumdar, D., & Ventureyra, E. C. (2007). Transient ventriculoperitoneal shunt malfunction after chronic constipation: Case report and review of literature. *Child's Nervous System, 23*, 455–458.

Narayan, A., Jallo, G., & Huisman, T. A. (2015). Extracranial, peritoneal seeding of primary malignant brain tumors through ventriculo-peritoneal shunts in children: Case report and review of the literature. *Neuroradiology Journal, 28*(5), 536–539. https://doi.org/10.1177/1971400915609348.

Nielsen, N., & Breedt, A. (2017). Hydrocephalus. In Cartwright, C. C., & Wallace, D. C. (Eds.), *Nursing care of the pediatric neurosurgery patient* (3rd ed., pp. 39–89). Springer International Publishing https://doi.org/10.1007/978-3-319-49319-0.

O'Neil, J., & Hoffman, B. Council on Injury, Violence, and Poison Prevention. (2019). Transporting children with special health care needs. *Pediatrics, 143*(5), e20190724.

O'Neill, B. R., Pruthi, S., Bains, H., Robison, R., Weir, K., Ojemann, J., Ellenbogen, R., Avellino, A., & Browd, S. R. (2013). Rapid sequence magnetic resonance imaging in the assessment of children with hydrocephalus. *World Neurosurgery, 80*(6), e307–e312. https://doi.org/10.1016/j.wneu.2012.10.066.

Patel, S. K., Tari, R., & Mangano, F. T. (2021). Pediatric hydrocephalus and the primary care provider. *Pediatric Clinics of North America, 68*(4), 793–809. https://doi.org/10.1016/j.pcl.2021.04.006.

Persson, E. K., Hagberg, G., & Uvebrant, P. (2006). Disabilities in children with hydrocephalus—a population-based study of children aged between four and twelve years. *Neuropediatrics, 37*(6), 330–336.

Ramasamy, C. (2018). Relationship between dental procedures and shunt infections in hydrocephalic patients: A narrative review. *Journal of Clinical Pediatric Dentistry, 42*(1), 67–71. doi:10.17796/1053-4628-42.1.12.

Simon, T. D., Butler, J., Whitlock, K. B., Browd, S. R., Holubkov, R., Kestle, J. R., Kulkarni, A. V., Langley, M., Limbrick, D. D., Jr., Mayer-Hamblett, N., Tamber, M., Wellons, J. C., 3rd, Whitehead, W. E., Riva-Cambrin, J., & Hydrocephalus Clinical Research Network (2014). Risk factors for first cerebrospinal fluid shunt infection: findings from a multi-center prospective cohort study. *The Journal of Pediatrics, 164*(6), 1462–8.e2. https://doi.org/10.1016/j.jpeds.2014.02.013.

Simon, T. D., Riva-Cambrin, J., Srivastava, R., Bratton, S. L., Dean, J. M., Kestle, J. R., & Hydrocephalus Clinical Research Network (2008). Hospital care for children with hydrocephalus in the United States: Utilization, charges, comorbidities, and deaths. *Journal of Neurosurgery: Pediatrics, 1*(2), 131–137. https://doi.org/10.3171/PED/2008/1/2/131.

Simon, T. D., Schaffzin, J. K., Stevenson, C. B., Willebrand, K., Parsek, M., & Hoffman, L. R. (2019). Cerebrospinal fluid shunt infection: Emerging paradigms in pathogenesis that affect prevention and treatment. *Journal of Pediatrics, 206*, 13–19. https://doi.org/10.1016/j.jpeds.2018.11.026.

Sobana, M., Halim, D., Aviani, J. K., Gamayani, U., & Achmad, T. H. (2021). Neurodevelopmental outcomes after ventriculoperitoneal shunt placement in children with non-infectious hydrocephalus: a meta-analysis. *Child's Nervous System, 37*(4), 1055–1065. https://doi.org/10.1007/s00381-021-05051-9.

Stanuszek, A., Bębenek, A., Milczarek, O., & Kwiatkowski, S. (2021). Return to play in children with shunted hydrocephalus. *Journal of Neurosurgery in Pediatrics, 29*(1), 1–9. https://doi.org/10.3171/2021.7.PEDS21127.

Strauss, K. J., & Kaste, S. C. (2006). The ALARA (as low as reasonably achievable) concept in pediatric interventional and fluoroscopic imaging: Striving to keep radiation doses as low as possible during fluoroscopy of pediatric patients—a white paper executive summary. *Radiology, 240*(3), 621–622. https://doi.org/10.1148/radiol.2403060698.

Sultan, C., Gaspari, L., Maimoun, L., Kalfa, N., & Paris, F. (2018). Disorders of puberty. Best practice & research. *Clinical Obstetrics & Gynaecology, 48*, 62–89. https://doi.org/10.1016/j.bpobgyn.2017.11.004.

Thompson, D. N. P., & Hartley, J. C. (2015). Shunt infections. In Albright, A. L., Pollack, I. F., & Adelson, P. D. (Eds.), *Principles and practice of pediatric neurosurgery* (3rd ed., pp. 1010–1022). Thieme Medical Publishers, Inc.

Tulipan, N., Wellons, J. C., 3rd, Thom, E. A., Gupta, N., Sutton, L. N., Burrows, P. K., Farmer, D., Walsh, W., Johnson, M. P., Rand, L., Tolivaisa, S., D'alton, M. E., Adzick, N. S., & MOMS Investigators (2015). Prenatal surgery for myelomeningocele and the need for cerebrospinal fluid shunt placement. *Journal of Neurosurgery: Pediatrics, 16*(6), 613–620. https://doi.org/10.3171/2015.7.PEDS15336.

Vinchon, M., Baroncini, M., & Delestret, I. (2012). Adult outcome of pediatric hydrocephalus. *Child's Nervous System, 28*(6), 847–854. https://doi.org/10.1007/s00381-012-1723-y.

Volpe, J. J. (2008). *Neurology of the newborn* (5th ed.). Saunders.

Williams, M. A., van der Willigen, T., White, P. H., Cartwright, C. C., Wood, D. L., & Hamilton, M. G. (2018). Improving health care transition and longitudinal care for adolescents and young adults with hydrocephalus: report from the Hydrocephalus Association Transition Summit. *Journal of Neurosurgery*, 1–9. Advance online publication. https://doi.org/10.3171/2015.7.PEDS15336.

Winden, K. D., Yuskaitis, C. J., & Poduri, A. (2015). Megalencephaly and macrocephaly. *Seminars in Neurology, 35*, 277–287.

Wolf, H. F., Rateitschak-Pluss, E. M., Rateitschak, K. H., & Hassell, T. (2004). *Color atlas of periodontology (color atlas of dental medicine)* (3rd ed.). Thieme.

Yuan, W., Holland, S. K., Shimony, J. S., Altaye, M., Mangano, F. T., Limbrick, D. D., Jones, B. V., Nash, T., Rajagopal, A., Simpson, S., Ragan, D., & McKinstry, R. C. (2015). Abnormal structural connectivity in the brain networks of children with hydrocephalus. *NeuroImage. Clinical, 8*, 483–492. https://doi.org/10.1016/j.nicl.2015.04.015.

Yuh, S. J., & Vassilyadi, M. (2012). Management of abdominal pseudocyst in shunt-dependent hydrocephalus. *Surgical Neurology International, 3*, 146. https://doi.org/10.4103/2152-7806.103890.

27

Inflammatory Bowel Disease

Megan Canavan

Inflammatory bowel disease (IBD) is a chronic condition of the gastrointestinal (GI) tract, classically characterized by intestinal inflammation and intermittent periods of symptoms throughout the lifespan. There is significant heterogeneity in disease presentation and severity, especially in the pediatric population. IBD management has been revolutionized in recent years due to advances in science and paradigm shifts in therapy. Although IBD is a lifelong condition with no known cure to date, with precise treatment and close medical care individuals with IBD should be able to live a full life.

IBD is an umbrella term that can be segmented into different categories of disease types, including Crohn disease (CD), ulcerative colitis (UC), IBD unclassified (IBD-U), and very early onset IBD (VEO-IBD). The disease presents in unique ways with varying degrees of symptom severity and disease penetrance from person to person. Particularly in pediatrics it is paramount to recognize that IBD does not look or act the same way in every patient. Therefore clinicians must have an astute understanding of the variety of ways that IBD presents in children to properly diagnose and treat the disease. The management of pediatric IBD demands a specialized approach tailored to the patient's specific disease phenotype.

This chapter will highlight the current diagnostic approaches and treatment styles available for infants, children, adolescents, and young adults with IBD.

ETIOLOGY

The etiology of IBD is not fully understood. The current theory supports that IBD is caused by an abnormal immune system response to environmental exposures in a genetically suspectable host. Twin-twin studies indicate concordance rates in monozygotic twins of 10% to 15% in UC and 30% to 35% in CD, suggesting IBD is influenced by both genetic predisposition and something in the person's environment (Kaplan, 2015). Population studies show immigrants quickly develop the risk profile of their new region, suggesting a strong environmental influence on disease development (Sýkora et al., 2018). Environmental exposures include everything persons encounter within a lifetime, such as where they live, what germs and illnesses they encounter, and what they eat, drink, and breathe.

Environmental exposures constantly interact with and between all the microorganisms that make up the intestinal gut flora (i.e., microbiome). The microbiome is a living universe of trillions of microbes (bacteria, viruses, fungi, protozoa) residing in the GI tract, which interfaces with our environment and genes and evolves over time (Nishida et al., 2018).

The complex relationship between a person's microbiome, immune system, environment, and genes is the basis of IBD pathogenesis. Trillions of communities of organisms in the microbiome interplay with the body's environmental exposures and genetic makeup, which impacts how the body functions and develops. This fluid interaction is thought to program the body's immune system. Evidence suggests that a disruption in the harmony of the microbes in the gut, often referred to as intestinal dysbiosis, contributes to the expression of IBD by the immune system in a genetically susceptible person (Lane et al., 2017).

Exciting advances in gene sequencing technology and bioinformatics have greatly influenced research capabilities to better understand IBD. Next-generation DNA sequencing, including whole exome sequencing, is used to study underlying genetic influences on IBD. To date, over 200 loci have been identified as risk factors for adult IBD (Huang et al., 2017). In pediatrics, gene sequencing has been instrumental in identifying and understanding the youngest cohort of patients who develop IBD as neonates, infants, or children less than 6 years of age. This disease entity is VEO-IBD. At present there is a consensus of at least 75 causative genes identified in VEO-IBD, many associated with inborn errors of immunity and epithelial barrier function (Nambu et al., 2022).

INCIDENCE AND PREVALENCE

IBD has become a common chronic medical condition in the developed world. Data from a US National Health Interview Survey in 2015 estimated that 3.1 million adults are affected by IBD (Dahlamer et al., 2016). The overall incidence of IBD in North America in adults is estimated to be 249 per 100,000 persons for UC and 319 per 100,000 persons for CD (Molodecky et al., 2012).

Approximately 25% of all cases of IBD occur in childhood (Kaplan, 2015). Pediatric IBD incidence and prevalence vary among geographic, racial, and ethnic trends. The incidence of IBD in children and adolescents has undoubtedly increased. Estimates comparing prevalence from 2007 to 2016 show an increase of 133% (Ye et al., 2020). In 2016, 1 in 1299 children age 2 to 17 years was diagnosed with IBD. IBD was more prevalent in males than females, and CD was twice as prevalent as UC. Epidemiologic trends also demonstrate the highest increase in IBD cases is in those under 5 years of age (Benchimol et al., 2017).

Worldwide the highest rates of pediatric IBD are found in the Northern Hemisphere and industrialized regions of the world. Multiple studies demonstrate the highest incidence and prevalence in Northern Europe and North America and the lowest in Southern Europe, Asia, and the Middle East. Nationally, the study shows regional variation within the United States as well, with pediatric IBD to be increased in the Northeast compared to the West. Interestingly, recent data show IBD occurs in regions where it was not previously reported. There continues to be a need for further investigation on this topic, particularly in developing and newly developed parts of the world (Kappelman et al., 2013; Kuenzig et al., 2022; Sýkora et al., 2018).

Studies reviewing IBD prevalence and incidence in immigrant children suggest a relationship between geography, environment, and IBD development. Evidence suggests children who emigrate from less developed countries with a low incidence of IBD to westernized, more developed countries inherit an increased risk of developing IBD. The younger the child is at the time of emigration to a developed country, the more likely the child is to develop IBD (Benchimol et al., 2015).

In the past, IBD was thought to primarily affect those of European descent, but this is no longer the framework of thinking. Although historically IBD was reported to be less common in a non-White population, the paucity of heterogenous population studies questions the validity of the available data. The incidence of IBD is rising in non-White populations (Molodecky et al., 2012). IBD is a heterogeneous disease, and it is imperative that future research is conducted with diverse populations to better understand the disease process for all people affected by IBD.

Disease location and IBD phenotype have been shown to differ among racial and ethnic groups (Barnes et al., 2021). For instance, CD is two to four times more prevalent in the Ashkenazi Jewish population (Rivas et al., 2018). In Black pediatric patients, a more complex disease phenotype has been reported (Kugathasan, 2017). Comparisons between IBD characteristics in Black and non-Black patients show Black patients were more likely to present with a CD phenotype, were more likely to present at older ages, and were more likely to have lower hemoglobin at diagnosis (White et al., 2008). A study of IBD in Hispanic and Asian patients shows disease phenotype tends

to favor UC versus CD (Abramson et al., 2010; Hattar et al., 2012). In the South Asian patient population, the study shows a higher proportion of UC, shorter symptom duration at diagnosis, more extensive colonic disease, and an increased likelihood of therapy escalation compared to non–South Asian patients (Carroll et al., 2016).

There is a need for further research on IBD that is inclusive and diverse in regard to patient age, geographic location, race, and ethnicity. The vast majority of epidemiologic and research studies on IBD come from developed countries, many published by European and North American countries. It is critical to learn more about disease differences to treat all patients equally.

DISEASE CLASSIFICATION AND DIAGNOSTIC CRITERIA

Historically, IBD was divided into two distinct categories: ulcerative colitis and Crohn disease. With recent advances in understanding IBD, the disease is now further categorized into distinct subtypes based on the location and characteristics of disease penetration in the body. This includes the diagnosis of IBD-U and VEO-IBD.

CROHN DISEASE

CD is a chronic inflammatory disease of the bowel that may involve any portion of the GI tract. CD can be characterized by the location of disease activity and disease behavior. CD is described where the disease is present within the GI tract, anywhere from the mouth, the start of the upper GI tract, to the anus. Additionally, CD is described by how the disease process primarily acts, such as inflammatory, penetrating (fistulizing), stricturing, or perianal disease phenotype. Characteristics of pediatric CD are notoriously dynamic. Disease location and phenotype often evolve and overlap.

CD is characterized by inflammation that is transmural (extending through the entire wall of the intestine). It may begin as a mild superficial disease that extends from the intestinal mucosal lining through the serosal layer over time. Extensive transmural inflammation can lead to complications such as fistulae or abscess formation. Perianal skin tags, fistulae, or abscesses may be present. In severe cases, CD occurs in both the small and large intestines. Endoscopically, visual findings of CD are diseased segments of the bowel bordering segments of healthy tissue, giving it an uneven appearance with skip lesions. On biopsy, histologic findings of noncaseating epithelioid granulomas are diagnostic (though not mandatory) for CD.

Data show pediatric-onset CD has variable distributions of where the disease presents, with the most common disease presentation being ileocolonic, and the least common presentation being upper tract disease only (de Bie et al., 2013; Van Limbergen et al., 2008).

The way CD affects pediatric patients often evolves over time. Children often present with an inflammatory phenotype but may change phenotypes as they age. About 25% to 30% develop perianal disease with associated skin tags, fissures, and/or fistulae (Abraham et al., 2012).

CD is two times more common than UC in pediatric IBD. The average age of onset for CD in children is 10 to 12 years. Children and adolescents with CD often experience a more aggressive and severe disease course than adult-onset CD. Subsequently, pediatric-onset CD is associated with higher morbidity than adult-onset CD. Often children with CD will require higher immunosuppressive therapy compared to adults. Treatment goals are to find a therapy that is well tolerated and will minimize inflammation, heal intestinal mucosa, and prevent complications while allowing children to grow and develop (Mitchel & Rosh, 2022).

ULCERATIVE COLITIS

UC is characterized by inflammation that is confluent and limited to the colonic mucosa. Typically, the inflammation begins in the rectum and extends proximally in an uninterrupted pattern to involve parts of or all the large intestine (colon). The disease is localized to the large bowel only, except for possible findings of backwash ileitis. Backwash ileitis is nonspecific inflammation at the terminal ileum, without ileocecal valve changes, found in UC patients with pancolitis. There are no histologic findings of granulomas with UC.

UC can be described by the area of the colon most affected. Inflammation limited to the rectum may be called ulcerative proctitis. Inflammation primarily found in the sigmoid and descending colon, distal to the splenic flexure, is termed *left-sided colitis*. Inflammation involving the entire colon, from the cecum to the rectum, is described as pancolitis.

As with CD, pediatric UC may present differently and evolve over time. There are variable data available on the natural history of pediatric UC. A review of 115 pediatric patients with UC demonstrated the mean age at diagnosis to be about 11 years. Twenty percent of patients experienced extraintestinal (EI) symptoms, most commonly arthritis (48%), sclerosing cholangitis (35%), and aphthous stomatitis (17%). Studies estimate pediatric UC presents with left-sided colitis in about 22% to 40% of cases, pancolitis in about 34% to 66% of cases, and localized proctitis in 25% to 29% of cases. Rectal sparing was found in 15% of cases and correlated to a younger age (Aloi et al., 2013). Children with UC reported to present with rectal sparing should be interpreted cautiously, as the children may have Crohn colitis (Abramson et al., 2010; Dubinsky, 2008; Malaty et al., 2013).

INFLAMMATORY BOWEL DISEASE UNCLASSIFIED

Children with disease limited to the colon but whose condition cannot be categorized as CD or UC have been described in a separate category of IBD, now unclassified. Terms used synonymously with IBD-U include *indeterminate colitis, uncertain colitis*, and *idiopathic chronic colitis*. The 2014 Porto Criteria and European Crohn's and Colitis Organisation (ECCO) guidelines provide criteria for categorizing IBD as IBD-U. Criteria recommend a full evaluation with upper GI endoscopy and ileocolonoscopy for all pediatric patients with suspected IBD, including small bowel imaging. Pediatric patients present differently and dynamically, often making the diagnosis of IBD-U temporary until the disease declares itself as CD or UC with repeat evaluations over time (Levine et al., 2014).

VERY-EARLY-ONSET INFLAMMATORY BOWEL DISEASE

VEO-IBD is a new category of IBD characterized by disease onset at less than 6 years of age. VEO-IBD makes up an estimated 6% to 15% of pediatric-onset IBD cases (Benchimol et al., 2017). VEO-IBD is a heterogeneous subtype of IBD in infants, toddlers, and young children who often (but not always) experience more severe and aggressive disease activity. Disease distribution tends to be colonic but is highly variable. Patients with VEO-IBD have been found to have an increased risk of therapy failure, hospital readmission, growth failure, and surgical intervention compared to older children with IBD. The etiology of VEO-IBD is strongly associated with genetic and immunologic dysfunction.

In some cases that are called monogenic VEO-IBD, a singular gene defect is discovered that is causative for disease expression and can be specifically targeted for treatment. Given the young age of disease presentation, environmental contributors are thought to play a less instrumental part in disease presentation, and immunodeficiencies and genetic defects are often the key drivers of disease. Diagnostic evaluation for VEO-IBD must include evaluation of the immune system and genes at play, in addition to the standard evaluation for IBD (Kelsen et al., 2020).

DIAGNOSTIC EVALUATION

A diagnostic evaluation for IBD includes a thorough history and exam, evaluation of screening laboratory testing (including bloodwork and stool testing), small bowel imaging, and full endoscopy. Endoscopy should be total colonoscopy with ileal intubation and upper endoscopy (esophagogastroduodenoscopy) with multiple biopsies, as recommended by the North American Society for Pediatric Gastroenterology Hepatology and Nutrition (NASPGHAN), Crohn's and Colitis Foundation (CCF), and European Society for Pediatric Gastroenterology, Hepatology and Nutrition (ESPGHAN).

HISTORY

The symptoms of IBD in a pediatric patient can be missed without a complete evaluation. The diagnosis of IBD is often difficult or delayed because of the subtle manner in which it presents itself. Children and adolescents may present with vague or nonspecific symptoms (i.e., stomachaches, abdominal discomfort), and clinicians must elucidate a detailed history to not miss signs of early or evolving pediatric IBD. Presenting symptoms often mimic many other disease entities that prompt referrals to different pediatric specialists: the endocrinologist for growth or pubertal delay, the rheumatologist for joint swelling or pain; the hematologist for iron deficiency anemia, and the dermatologist for rashes (Fish & Kugathasan, 2004). An in-depth history of each of these symptoms may reveal important information to differentiate UC from CD and other diseases that resemble IBD.

A detailed history should include an evaluation of constitutional symptoms such as fevers, weight loss, night sweats, poor appetite, fatigue, or behavior change. History of GI symptoms may point to disease location. Symptoms of upper tract disease include oral ulcers, dysphagia, dyspepsia, early satiety, bloating, or abdominal pain. Symptoms of increased stool frequency, urgency, hematochezia, and painful defecation (tenesmus) indicate rectal involvement with inflammation (proctitis). Perianal pain, discharge, or skin tags point to perianal CD (De Zoeten et al., 2013). Overt GI symptoms such as vomiting, diarrhea, constipation, or anorexia may or may not be present. Diarrhea is common but may not be present, especially if the disease is localized to the small intestine. History should specifically evaluate for other symptoms as well, including visual problems, oral pain or ulcers, changes in hair or skin, rashes, joint swelling, fatigue, behavior change, and changes in appetite. The younger the child is, the more important it is to look for signs of immunologic or genetic disorders associated with VEO-IBD. This includes asking about fevers and recurrent or unusual infections, such as repeated infections requiring antibiotics, intravenous (IV) antibiotics, or hospitalization. Failure to thrive, food intolerance, food allergies, and anemia at routine screenings during infancy may also raise suspicion of IBD. Family history should be evaluated, especially with respect to any findings of immunologic childhood diseases. Evaluating for familial consanguinity is necessary to help identify genetic risk (Rivas et al., 2018). Evaluating for any recent travel, sick contact exposure, and pet/animal exposure will help clinicians rule out infectious conditions that may mimic or coincide with IBD presentation.

PHYSICAL EXAM

Obtaining vital signs and growth parameters is an important part of an evaluation for IBD. Changes in heart rate and blood pressure can reveal evidence of severe dehydration or malnutrition. Tachycardia or hypoxia are worrisome signs that may be indicative of significant anemia.

Growth parameters, including weight and height, should be plotted on pediatric growth charts. Growth assessment should look for trends in growth curves, specifically for signs of weight loss, growth plateau, and height velocity with respect to age and midparental height potential. Growth failure in stature and concomitant delay in sexual maturation may precede the development of overt intestinal manifestations by years in children with CD. At the time of initial diagnosis, 85% of children with CD and 65% of children with UC have lost weight (Kugathasan et al., 2007). A deceleration in linear growth may be the only clinical finding in children and adolescents with CD (Fish & Kugathasan, 2004).

A head-to-toe physical examination should be performed with consideration to the signs and symptoms of IBD's GI and EI manifestations. Physical exam assessment should look for signs of oral ulcers, abnormal dentition, oral cheilitis, pallor, murmur, digital clubbing, joint swelling, limpness, and hair and skin abnormalities, including alopecia and the presence of a rash. The abdomen exam should include inspection for distention or bloating, auscultation for bowel sounds, percussion for evidence of masses (such as hepatosplenomegaly, abscess, or fecal mass), and palpation for masses and tenderness. Perianal and digital exams are critical to assess for evidence of external skin tags, fissures, fistulas and/or abscesses, internal lesions, including anal stenosis, and the presence or absence of blood. Exams should include an assessment of Tanner staging to evaluate for signs of delayed puberty (Rufo et al., 2012).

LABORATORY EVALUATION

Laboratory assessment of bloodwork and stool studies is necessary for patients with suspected IBD. Infectious stool studies must be evaluated in patients with diarrhea. Infectious conditions of the GI tract, such as *Salmonella, Shigella, Campylobacter, Yersinia, Aeromonas, Escherichia coli* O157/H7, and *Clostridium difficile*, and the parasite *Entamoeba histolytica,* can mimic IBD and must be ruled out. Testing includes stool culture, specific *C. difficile* toxin testing, and ova and parasite testing, including for cryptosporidium and giardia. A positive infectious stool finding does not rule out the possibility of IBD but warrants appropriate treatment and further investigation. Blood testing to look for evidence of chronic intestinal inflammation is necessary. However, it is important to know that normal bloodwork also does not rule out the possibility of IBD (Mitchel & Rosh, 2022).

Laboratory findings help guide clinical management; key findings are highlighted in Table 27.1. Common laboratory findings associated with IBD include increased erythrocyte sedimentation rate (ESR) and C-reactive protein (CRP) (both nonspecific measures of inflammation), thrombocytosis, low serum iron level, low hematocrit value, and low hemoglobin level.

Table 27.1	Laboratory Evaluation of Suspected Inflammatory Bowel Disease
TESTING	**POSSIBLE SIGNS OF ACTIVE IBD**
ESR	High CRP, ESR, or calprotectin
CRP	Leukocytosis
Fecal calprotectin	Microcytic anemia
CBC	Thrombocytosis
CMP	Increased serum urea nitrogen to creatinine ratio
	Acidosis
	Hypoalbuminemia
	Elevated ALT, AST, GGT
	Elevated calprotectin indicated intestinal inflammation

ALT, Alanine aminotransferase; *AST*, aspartate aminotransferase; *CBC*, complete blood count; *CMP*, complete metabolic panel; *CRP*, C-reactive protein; *ESR*, erythrocyte sedimentation rate; *GGT*, gamma-glutamyltransferase; *IBD*, inflammatory bowel disease; *MCV*, mean corpuscular volume; *WBC*, white blood cell.

Hypoalbuminemia and a decreased total serum protein may also be noted, particularly in CD that affects the small bowel and in moderate-severe UC (Mack et al., 2007).

Fecal calprotectin testing is a noninvasive laboratory test that may be used to monitor IBD activity (Imondi et al., 2021). Calprotectin is a protein that may be present in the intestinal lumen as a byproduct of neutrophil activity. When there is active inflammation in the intestinal tract, fecal calprotectin levels may be detected as abnormally high. Fecal calprotectin testing is an objective measure that may be useful in conjunction with clinical history, assessment, and diagnosis. Particularly, periodically trending fecal calprotectin levels over time may be a useful adjunct to disease assessment. It is important to note that elevated fecal calprotectin detects nonspecific findings of an inflammatory process. There is variation in the specificity and sensitivity of calprotectin testing, and normative values vary from lab to lab, along with a variation in the normal level of calprotectin present throughout the lifespan.

Elevated calprotectin levels are sometimes detected in healthy children less than 4 years of age and infancy. Fecal calprotectin will reflect colonic inflammation better than small bowel disease (Imondi et al., 2021). Results can be increased with the use of nonsteroidal antiinflammatory drugs (NSAIDs). Results are also increased if blood is present in the stool and in circumstances of infectious enteritis, inflammatory polyps, and oncologic processes (D'Arcangelo et al., 2021).

When assessing a child's IBD, it is critical to use fecal calprotectin testing as only one piece of the puzzle. A full history, exam, bloodwork, endoscopy, and biopsy are necessary to fully assess a child's disease process (Koninckx et al., 2021).

ENDOSCOPY AND SMALL BOWEL IMAGING

The ESPGHAN, NASPGHAN, and CCF recommend a full upper (esophagogastroduodenoscopy) and lower (ileocolonoscopy) endoscopy with ileal intubation with biopsies and small bowel exploration to diagnosis IBD (Ardura et al., 2016). Colonoscopy and upper GI endoscopy can identify mucosal inflammation, assess the extent of the disease, and permit mucosal biopsies to obtain a histologic assessment to help differentiate UC from CD. Endoscopic evidence of ulcers, erythema, loss of vascular pattern, friability (spontaneous bleeding), pseudopolyps, continuous disease from the rectum extending more proximally, biopsies showing crypt distortion, and abscess is consistent with a diagnosis of UC. Visual findings of cobblestoning (nodularity) or linear ulceration in the ileum, or skip lesions throughout the colon, can be seen in CD (Levine et al., 2014).

Small bowel imaging is necessary to fully evaluate the intestinal tract, including the area of small bowel that endoscopy does not routinely capture. Small bowel imaging will also discover evidence of complicated diseases such as strictures or fistulae. Multiple modalities are available for bowel assessment; the upper GI study with small bowel follow-through has fallen out of favor due to low sensitivity and specificity and significant exposure to ionizing radiation. Now, magnetic resonance enterography of the abdomen and pelvis has become the preferred imaging due to high specificity and sensitivity without ionizing radiation exposure. Computed tomography enterography may be useful to delineate small intestinal wall thickening, fistulization to adjacent structures, and the presence of abscesses. A wireless video capsule may be used for in-depth visualization of small bowel in some older patients without concern for structuring disease. Bowel ultrasound with contrast may also be helpful; however, at this time there are no standard practice norms (Anupindi et al., 2014).

Clinicians should understand the diagnostic workup for IBD is multifactorial and includes procedures that may require sedation, intubation, and anesthesia.

CLINICAL MANIFESTATIONS

Clinical manifestations of IBD span a wide spectrum of severity and look different from patient to patient, depending on disease classification and activity. Even within the same patient, clinical manifestations change throughout the lifespan. Individuals experience periods of no symptoms when in clinical remission and periods of symptom exacerbations. An exacerbation of CD or UC sometimes is preceded by a concomitant illness or emotional stress or may occur for no apparent reason. Intercurrent GI infections may also trigger an exacerbation of disease activity, with *C. difficile* and viral infections often implicated. Change in diet is not considered a cause of disease exacerbation because it is not accompanied by changes in histologic, radiographic, or laboratory parameters; however, individuals may correlate foods with symptoms.

CROHN DISEASE

Common manifestations of CD are abdominal pain, weight loss, and diarrhea. Other symptoms of CD are fevers, rectal bleeding, anorexia, lethargy, mouth sores, perianal disease, anorexia, nausea/vomiting, and joint pain. Red flags that warrant close attention include rectal bleeding, nocturnal stooling, fecal urgency, tenesmus, vomiting, and weight loss (Rosen et al., 2015).

CD may have an insidious onset with abdominal pain and weight loss that may contribute to a delay in diagnosis. Nonspecific symptoms of abdominal pain, anorexia, weight loss, delayed sexual maturation, and decreased linear growth may or may not all be present or not immediately recognized to prompt a workup for IBD (Diefenbach & Breuer, 2006; Ponsky et al., 2007). If chronic diarrhea or rectal bleeding is present, diagnosis may be more expeditious (Diefenbach & Breuer, 2006). Abdominal pain is the most common symptom at presentation: It is most often periumbilical but may localize to the right lower quadrant or diffuse in the lower abdomen. Diarrhea may not be present if the disease is confined to the small intestine.

Important findings strongly suggesting CD include cobblestoning skip legions, segmental colitis, ileal stenosis and ulceration, perianal disease, and granulomas in the small bowel or colon.

ULCERATIVE COLITIS

The most common presenting symptoms of UC are diarrhea, abdominal pain, and rectal bleeding with blood and mucus. Red flags that warrant investigation include blood in stool, tenesmus, urgency and nighttime awakening to stool, fevers, weight loss, decreased height velocity, abdominal tenderness, peritoneal signs, palpable mass, perianal fistulae, abscesses, rectal stricture, mouth ulcers, cardiac flow murmur,

hepatomegaly, joint erythema or effusion, skin nodules, or ulcerations (Conrad & Rosh, 2017). Children with UC may present differently depending on the extent and severity of mucosal inflammation. Physical examination may reveal abdominal tenderness, and stool analysis will show various amounts of blood. The pediatric ulcerative colitis activity index (PUCAI) score is a validated measure for disease activity in patients with colitis. Scoring is based on symptoms and is used to provide objective data on clinical disease activity (Turner et al., 2009).

Severe colitis with an acute, fulminant presentation (i.e., acute severe colitis) is seen in 10% to 20% of pediatric cases, although data are limited. These children appear moderately to severely toxic and have more than six bloody stools per day with cramping abdominal pain, fever, anemia, leukocytosis, and hypoalbuminemia. Physical examination may reveal diffuse tenderness and distention. Serious complications, such as toxic megacolon, life-threatening hemorrhage, and perforation, are rare in the pediatric population (Turner et al., 2009).

When evaluating for suspected IBD in pediatric patients, the following findings are diagnostic clues pointing to UC: colonic symptoms of bloody diarrhea, tenesmus, nocturnal stools, and endoscopic findings of continuous diffuse inflammation (pancolitis).

It is important to recognize that patients with UC may have findings that lead clinicians to consider changing their disease classification to CD. However, features of backwash ileal inflammation, histologic gastritis, periappendiceal inflammation, and relative rectal sparing at disease presentation do not warrant changing patient diagnosis from UC to CD. Table 27.2 emphasizes the key differentiations between UC and CD.

Table 27.2 Differentiating Findings Characteristic of Crohn Disease vs. Ulcerative Colitis

	CROHN DISEASE	ULCERATIVE COLITIS
Clinical signs	Weight loss and/or growth failure Pubertal delay Abdominal pain Perianal skin tags, fissures, abscesses/fistulae Fever Diarrhea Abdominal pain	Diarrhea Blood in stool Abdominal pain, cramping, tenesmus
Labs	Hypoalbuminemia Micronutrient deficiencies	Anemia
Imaging	Abscesses Strictures Fistulae	Toxic megacolon in severe cases
Endoscopy	Skip legions Cobblestoning Aphthous ulcers	Friable erythema Loss of vascular markers Spontaneous bleeding Severe ulcers
Biopsy	Granulomas Transmural inflammation	Inflammation confined to mucosa

EXTRAINTESTINAL MANIFESTATIONS OF IBD

Studies estimate symptoms outside of the GI tract are present in up to a third of patients with pediatric IBD (Greuter et al., 2017). EI manifestations of IBD have been found in almost every organ system. The most common target organs are the skin, joints, bones, liver, and eyes. In children, EI manifestations may precede the onset of GI disease by years (Diefenbach & Breuer, 2006).

The pathogenic mechanisms of EI manifestations are not clearly understood. Some propose that an immune response from underlying IBD activity triggers EI symptoms. Many EI manifestations are hypothesized to be due to immune reactions, intestinal bacteria, or genetic factors (Hedin et al., 2019).

EI symptoms in pediatric patients have been associated with a more severe disease course (Dotson et al., 2010). In a study of 333 patients with pediatric-onset IBD, those patients exhibiting EI disease symptoms and patients with UC were found to have an increased risk of requiring biologic therapy or surgery, and patients with CD required increased therapy escalation compared to patients who did not experience EI symptoms (Breton et al., 2020; Jansson et al., 2020).

Musculoskeletal manifestations are the most common EI manifestation in IBD. Arthritis is the most common EI manifestation, occurring in 7% to 26% of children with IBD (Jose et al., 2009). Two types of arthritis are described: peripheral form and axial form. The peripheral form, sometimes referred to as colitis arthritis, affects large joints such as knees, hips, wrists, and elbows. The axial form affects the axial spine and sacroiliac joints and includes ankylosing spondylitis or sacroiliitis (Jose & Heyman, 2008). Peripheral arthritis tends to track the bowel disease and can respond to medical or surgical treatment of IBD, whereas axial form arthritis does not seem to remit with the treatment of IBD (Ephgrave, 2007). Arthritis is commonly observed when the colon is affected for unknown reasons (Fish & Kugathasan, 2004). Symptoms include pain/discomfort, redness, swelling, and heat at the joint, especially of the hips, knees, and ankles, and are typically asymmetric. Unlike the other musculoskeletal manifestations of IBD, arthritic symptoms may fluctuate with the activity of the bowel disease and response to treatment of the disease. Although usually avoided in patients with IBD, NSAIDs may be used to treat refractory joint complaints, but sparingly and with caution due to their potential GI side effects.

The most common dermatologic manifestations of IBD are erythema nodosum and pyoderma gangrenosum. Erythema nodosum prevalence rates in IBD are estimated to be about 10%, with an increase associated with CD compared to UC. Erythema nodosum presents as raised, red, tender nodules that appear primarily on the anterior surfaces of the leg. The rash may be mistaken for painful bruises on a child's shins. Sometimes erythema nodosum presents on the foot, back of the leg, or arm, but this is less common. It usually occurs when the intestinal disease is active but does not indicate severity (Griffiths & Buller, 2004). Therapy involves treating the underlying bowel disease (Diaconescu et al., 2020).

Pyoderma gangrenosum is a rare but serious disease manifestation of IBD. A recent meta-analysis showed pyoderma gangrenosum incidence to be 0.6% to 2.6%. Previously pyoderma gangrenosum was thought to be more common in UC; however, evidence is conflicting as new research reports show an increased incidence in CD (States et al., 2020). Pyoderma gangrenosum has been associated with female gender, erythema nodosum, and ocular EI manifestations of IBD. Pyoderma gangrenosum presents with a chronic, painful ulcerating legion. It may appear on the anterior aspect of the lower leg as erythematous pustules or nodules that spread rapidly to adjacent skin and develop into burrowing ulcers with dark red or purple borders surrounding deep skin ulcerations with necrotic centers. Pyoderma gangrenosum can also present as a peristomal complication or complication of a surgical wound. Lesions may develop at any time. Pyoderma gangrenosum is recurrent and challenging to treat. Immunosuppressive therapies are used for treatment. Arthritis develops in about 40% of individuals with IBD and pyoderma gangrenosum (Jose & Heyman, 2008; Plumptre et al., 2018).

Other skin manifestations of IBD include perianal and peristomal ulcers and fistulae, vulvar legions, and aphthous stomatitis. Aphthous ulceration in the mouth is the most common oral manifestation of CD, occurring in 20% to 30% of children with CD and 5% to 10% of those with UC (Jose & Heyman, 2008). Rare dermatologic manifestations of IBD include pyostomatitis vegetans, metastatic CD, epidermolysis bullosa acquisita, and Sweet syndrome. Psoriasis has been observed in patients on antitumor necrosis factor (anti-TNF) therapy. Psoriasis commonly presents on the scalp and skinfolds and may lead to alopecia. Onset is at any time during anti-TNF therapy, but it is often during times of IBD remission and often necessitates therapy change (Diaconescu et al., 2020).

TREATMENT

GOALS

The goal of the treatment of IBD is to induce and maintain clinical remission and achieve mucosal healing on biopsy (Cholapranee et al., 2017). Successful treatment with histologic remission is shown to decrease the risk of complications, including growth failure, hospitalizations, surgical interventions, and malignancy. Integral to treatment goals is utilizing the best therapy individualized to the patient's disease, with the least possible adverse effects and the best quality of life. Treatment demands a holistic approach to caring for a child with IBD, including the expertise of multiple specialists. The care team is expansive and diverse and includes a pediatric gastroenterologist, pediatric surgeon, health care provider, psychologist, nurse, nutritionist, social worker, and specialists catered to the disease demands, such as pediatric immunologists and geneticists. A hot topic is defining predictive tools that discover which therapy choice is best for each patient.

Treatment of pediatric IBD poses unique challenges given the complex, evolving, and aggressive phenotype found in pediatrics. The disease course is shown to be especially severe and refractory in the youngest cohort of pediatric IBD, VEO-IBD. The characteristics, coupled with the importance of meeting time-sensitive growth and development milestones and the limited availability of US Food and Drug Administration (FDA)–approved therapies in pediatrics, make treatment challenging and highlight the critical need for more pediatric study and research.

TREATMENT MODALITIES

Treatment of IBD is based on nutritional, pharmacologic, and surgical therapies. Probiotics, prebiotics, complementary and alternative therapies, and integrative medicine practices are new areas of interest. Treatment regimens vary by the individual clinician and are reliant on clinical practice guidelines, clinical judgment, experience, and observed patient response.

PHARMACOLOGIC THERAPY

Pharmacologic therapy is the primary treatment for the induction and maintenance of remission of IBD. As previously detailed, UC and CD have distinct pathophysiology and disease penetration. Therefore pharmacologic therapy varies between the approach of treatment for UC and CD. Therapy includes antiinflammatory agents, antibiotics, immunomodulators, and biologic and small molecule agents.

Historically, treatment began with locally acting agents, such as nutritional therapy, 5-aminosalicylic acid (5-ASA), or antibiotics, followed by steroids, and then escalated to immunomodulators, biologics, and surgery. In many cases, recent literature demands treatment take a top-down approach and begin therapy with immune-modifying therapy (Conrad & Rosh, 2017). Biologic therapy has revolutionized the treatment and progression of IBD (Breton et al., 2020; Conrad & Kelsen, 2020). In 2006, infliximab (Remicade) became the first genetically engineered product approved by the FDA for pediatric CD. At present, infliximab and adalimumab (Humira) are now FDA approved in pediatrics for both UC and CD (Croft et al., 2021). The landmark REACH trial first demonstrated clinical response and remission with infliximab therapy in children with CD (Hyams et al., 2008). Since then, several pediatric

landmark studies have shown evidence to support anti-TNF therapy in children with IBD. Infliximab or adalimumab are shown to achieve clinical remission, reduce surgical risk, and improve growth outcomes in pediatric UC and CD (Aloi et al., 2018; Hyams et al., 2012a & b; Turner et al., 2018). Several large-scale, multicenter pediatric studies are available for specialists to help create the best therapy plan for the patient.

Anti-TNF therapy has been used with other agents to treat IBD and provide better treatment outcomes (Qiu, 2017). There is limited pediatric data on combination therapy in IBD, and more study on this topic is needed.

Biosimilars are biologic products that are used in place of brand name or generic biologics. Biosimilars are increasingly being approved in the United States for the treatment of IBD since the Affordable Care Act and the Biologics Price Competition and Innovation Act of 2009 (Rudrapatna & Velayos, 2019). This decreases the costs of treatments, making them more affordable for all patient populations.

Consensus guidelines recommend specific treatment depending on disease phenotype and severity. Table 27.3 categorizes the pharmacologic agents available to treat IBD and summarizes the rationale and clinical implications for their use (Breton et al., 2019; Chavannes et al., 2019; Herfarth et al., 2016; Moore et al., 2021; Rosh, 2021; Singh et al., 2016; Turner et al., 2018).

Therapy regimens require meticulous care to achieve optimal outcomes. Clinical response and tolerance are frequently assessed. Monitoring therapeutic drug levels and trending biomarkers of disease activity, such as fecal calprotectin, is necessary. Table 27.4 summarizes suggested dosing schedules, common side effects, clinical monitoring, and considerations for using pharmacologic agents in practice (Chavannes et al., 2019; Church et al., 2019).

Prior to initiation of immunosuppressive therapy, baseline immune screening is needed to ascertain the risk of reactivation of underlying dormant infectious process (i.e., latent tuberculosis) and establish the patient's immunity to vaccine-preventable illnesses (i.e., varicella, hepatitis B). For patients presenting less than 6 years of age with VEO-IBD, the mechanism of the disease is particularly unique and may stem from primary immunodeficiencies. For these patients, baseline immunologic evaluation should also include dihydrorhodamine testing to rule out chronic granulomatous disease (CGD). Anti-TNF therapy is contraindicated in patients with CGD due to the increased risk of poor complications, including serious infections and death (Kelsen et al., 2020).

Immunosuppressive therapy requires clinicians to weigh the risks and benefits of all medical decision making and share the rationale with patients and their families. Many therapies are parental formulations, and children will need counseling and preparation for regular injections or IVs. IV infusions

Table **27.3**	Pharmacologic Therapy for Pediatric Inflammatory Bowel Disease: Therapeutic Options and Key Clinical Implications

ANTIINFLAMMATORY AGENTS		
THERAPEUTIC AGENTS	**ACTION AND USE**	**CLINICAL IMPLICATIONS**
5-Aminosalicylic Acid Preparations		
Oral agents: • Sulfasalazine (Azulfidine) • Olsalazine disodium (Dipentum) • Balsalazide (Colazal) • Mesalamine (Asacol, Pentasa, Lialda, Apriso, Delzicol)	• Locally acting antiinflammatory treatment • Primarily used in ulcerative colitis (UC) to treat colonic mucosa; only indicated in Crohn disease (CD) for select patients with extremely mild, uncomplicated disease with a primary colonic distribution.	• Oral and rectal preparation used concomitantly is more effective than oral therapy alone. • Rectal therapy with suppositories or enemas is used to target distal colonic disease. • Sulfasalazine contains sulfapyridine, which can cause significant allergic reactions in some patients. • Sulfapyridine interferes with folate absorption and can lead to megaloblastic anemia. All patients should be prescribed 1 mg folic acid daily for prevention.
Rectal agents: • Enema: Rowasa • Suppository: Canasa		
Corticosteroids: • Prednisone • Prednisolone • Methylprednisolone • Hydrocortisone • Oral budesonide • Corticosteroid suppositories, foams, and enemas are also available to deliver the corticosteroid directly to the rectum, sigmoid, and left colon providing relief of tenesmus and urgency associated with distal colitis	• Antiinflammatory • Broad immunosuppression • Primarily used short term to rescue patients with severe disease until long-term maintenance therapy is established (e.g., short intravenous [IV] course indicated in hospitalized patients with acute severe colitis) • Not recommended for maintenance therapy	• Limited indications for pediatric inflammatory bowel disease (IBD) • Clinical response is often rapid • Significant side effect profile • Long-term risks greatly outweigh its benefits • Oral budesonide may be preferred due to low bioavailability with subsequent less systemic glucocorticoid exposure • Side effects particularly troublesome in pediatrics: growth failure, bone demineralization, adrenal insufficiency, acne, emotional lability, and increased risk of infection • Other undesirable side effects include moon facies, weight gain, fluid retention with hypertension, hyperglycemia, striae, and hirsutism. • Long-term effects include growth retardation, calcium depletion, osteoporosis, immunosuppression, cataract formation, glaucoma, and aseptic necrosis of the hip or knees. • Adrenal suppression persists for 6–12 mo after corticosteroid therapy has been completed, therefore do not stop abruptly to prevent adrenal crisis, which presents with fever, hypotension, dehydration, vomiting, electrolyte abnormalities, hypoglycemia, severe abdominal pain, and lethargy; requires referral to emergency department for IV steroids and fluid resuscitation. • Adrenally insufficient patients need stress dosing for accidents, major illnesses, and surgery.
Antibiotic Therapy		
Amoxicillin Doxycycline Metronidazole Ciprofloxacin Azithromycin Rifaximin	• Affects intestinal dysbiosis thought to contribute to the pathogenesis of IBD • One or a combination of antibiotics acts on the enteric immune system's delicate balance of intestinal gut flora. • Used for perianal disease for patients with CD	• Limited data available, findings suggest it is effective as a steroid-sparing rescue therapy in severe IBD. • Metronidazole side effects to consider include gastrointestinal upset, metallic taste, dose-dependent peripheral neuropathy, and disulfiram-like effect if taken with alcohol. • Long-term impact of chronic antibiotic exposure must be considered.

Continued

Table 27.3	Pharmacologic Therapy for Pediatric Inflammatory Bowel Disease: Therapeutic Options and Key Clinical Implications—cont'd

Immunomodulators

Thiopurines:		
• 6-mercaptopurine and azathioprine	• Due to its potential side effect profile, specifically the increased risk of non-Hodgkin lymphoma and hepatosplenic T-cell lymphoma found particularly in adolescent males, as well as the increased support of biologic therapy, thiopurine monotherapy is no longer a mainstay IBD treatment in the United States.	• When used, response time averages 3–4 mo • Side effects include leukopenia and abnormal liver function; therefore routine lab screening of blood counts and liver enzymes is necessary throughout the duration of treatment time. • Monitoring thiopurine metabolites can help assess response and guide therapy.
• Methotrexate	• Folic acid derivative that interferes with DNA synthesis and induces the production of antiinflammatory cytokines and lymphocyte apoptosis • Used in conjunction with antitumor necrosis factor (anti-TNF) agents to sustain therapeutic drug levels	• Teratogenic • Causes nausea, which may be severe and treatment limiting • Supplement with 1 mg folic acid daily to mitigate side effects • Premedicate with ondansetron, especially in the first 8 wk of treatment, for tolerance • Other side effects: vomiting, diarrhea, stomatitis, rash, arthralgias, leukopenia, hepatotoxicity; requires monitoring of labs
• Tacrolimus (Prograf) • Cyclosporine (Sandimmune)	• Inhibitors of cell-mediated immunity are only used in select severe and refractory IBD for temporizing bridge therapy • Allow other therapeutic agents time to reach efficacy or allows the patient and family to prepare for surgical invention	• Tacrolimus is preferred due to the inconsistent response of cyclosporine and its risk for drug toxicity. • Side effects: hypertension, tremor, paresthesia, hirsutism, seizures, nausea and vomiting, multiple drug interactions, potential for renal insufficiency and infection • Prophylaxis with oral trimethoprim-sulfamethoxazole is used if taking another immunosuppressive therapy. • Frequent monitoring of vital signs, serum laboratory studies (including blood urea nitrogen and creatinine), and drug levels is mandatory.

Biologics and Small Molecule Therapy

Anti-TNF therapy:		
• Infliximab (Remicade) • Adalimumab (Humira)	• Monoclonal antibodies that neutralize the proinflammatory cytokine TNF	• Patients with acute severe colitis experience a high inflammatory burden and low albumin levels, which influence drug absorption and therefore often require dose escalation. • Monitoring therapeutic drug levels and biomarkers of disease activity, such as serial fecal calprotectin, helps guide dosing. • Adalimumab is shown to have better outcomes in infliximab-naïve patients. • About one-third of patients do not respond to anti-TNF therapy, and about another one-third lose response at 1-year follow-up. • All patients on anti-TNF therapy should be counseled on side effects and safety. • Infusion reaction secondary to autoimmune antibodies may occur in cases of immunogenicity, particularly with infliximab. Infusion reaction is not typical with adalimumab because it is a humanized drug. • There have been reports of increased risk for malignancy, such as lymphoma; however, the DEVELOP study supports that infliximab treatment was not likely associated with an increased risk of malignancy or hemophagocytic lymphohistiocytosis. Thiopurines, rather than anti-TNF agents, showed an increased risk of malignancy. • In pediatrics, the overall rate of serious infection is low.

Table 27.3	Pharmacologic Therapy for Pediatric Inflammatory Bowel Disease: Therapeutic Options and Key Clinical Implications—cont'd	
• Ustekinumab (Stelara)	• Monoclonal antibody that binds with proinflammatory interleukins IL-12 and IL-13 to neutralize their effect.	• Robust adult research supports efficacy induction and maintenance therapy in CD. • Pediatric data limited but mimic results in adult studies. • Ustekinumab is approved for psoriasis use in children but not approved for pediatric IBD. • Used off label for select cases of refractory disease • Safety profile is favorable in the adult population. Data from use in psoriasis suggest there is no increased risk of serious infection, malignancy, or mortality.
• Vedolizumab (Entyvio)	• Humanized antiintegrin receptor molecule that targets a specific integrin, $\alpha_4\beta_7$, to prevent T lymphocytes from entering the endothelial cells of the intestinal barrier and thus downregulate inflammation.	• The adult literature supports safety and efficacy in treating IBD. • Used off label for select cases of refractory disease • In the limited pediatrics studies available, shown to be safe and effective for UC and CD; however, results show better remission rates in UC. • Onset of action is longer than other biologics, such as anti-TNF, and must be considered. • Highly desirable safety profile. Side effects are uncommon and include nasopharyngitis, arthralgia, and nausea. • The mechanism of action is gut specific and does not cross the blood-brain barrier. Cases of progressive multifocal leukoencephalopathy due to John Cunningham virus infection have not been reported as with previous antiintegrin biologics.
• Tofacitinib (Xeljanz)	• Small molecule inhibitor that interferes with Janus kinase (JAK) 1 and 3 are involved in downstream cytokine receptor signaling	• Approved in adults with refractory UC. • Formation is oral as opposed to parental biologics available. • Off label rare use in pediatrics for select cases of refractory disease. • Serious potential side effects found in adult literature must be considered, including increased zoster reactivation, hyperlipidemia, thromboembolic events, and increased overall all-cause mortality, including sudden cardiac death.

and doctor's appointments may sometimes cause children to miss school or extracurricular activities. Frequent collaboration and discussion between the clinician and the patient and/or the patient's family are paramount. Involving child life specialists, nurses, social workers, and psychologists for support is critical.

SURGERY

Surgical intervention is indicated when medical therapies do not adequately control symptoms or in the event of IBD complications such as toxic megacolon, severe hemorrhage, bowel perforation, strictures leading to obstruction, fistulas, or abscesses. Surgical interventions are often used in conjunction with pharmacologic therapies (Kelay et al., 2019). The risk of surgical complications and disease recurrence must be considered for each patient (Abdelaal & Jaffray, 2016). Steroid exposure should be minimized prior to surgery, and anti-TNF therapy should be held in the immediate perioperative period to decrease the risk of surgical

infection. Optimizing nutritional status and correcting anemia when possible prior to surgery is recommended to decrease the risk of surgical complications (Amil-Dias et al., 2017). Despite the risks, surgery is still an attractive option for some children to allow for normal growth and development and to improve their quality of life.

Surgical interventions vary from temporary interventions used to allow pharmacologic therapies to reach efficacy, such as diverting ileostomy, to life-altering procedures, such as colectomy (Baillie & Smith, 2015; Maxwell et al., 2017). Table 27.5 summarizes surgical procedures children with IBD may undergo (Diederen et al., 2017; Gu et al., 2016; Maxwell et al., 2017).

NUTRITIONAL THERAPY

Exclusive enteral nutrition (EEN) is an intervention where formula, given orally or via a feeding tube, provides 80% to 100% of caloric needs to patients for about 8 weeks. The goal is to decrease intestinal inflammation by altering the gut microbiome and restoring the

Table 27.4	Pharmacologic Therapy Dosing, Side Effects, and Clinical Monitoring	
MEDICATION	**DOSING**	**SIDE EFFECTS, MONITORING, AND SPECIAL CONSIDERATIONS**
5-aminosalicylate (mesalamine)	Oral mesalamine: 50–100 mg/kg/day, max 4 g/day *Rectal mesalamine preparations:* Rowasa: 4 g/60 mL rectal enema given nightly Canasa: 500 mg suppository given twice daily or 1000 mg nightly	Headache, nausea, vomiting, abdominal pain, bloody diarrhea. Side effects may look similar to inflammatory bowel disease (IBD) symptoms. Rare, serious side effects: interstitial nephritis, pancreatitis, pericarditis, bone marrow suppression, allergic reaction Labs: blood count, liver chemistries, blood urea nitrogen (BUN), creatine. Check creatinine every 6 mo, obtain urinalysis if abnormal.
Sulfasalazine	Induction: 40–100 mg/kg/day Maintenance: 30–70 mg/kg/day Max dose: 4 g/day Oral	Headache, nausea, vomiting, abdominal pain, bloody diarrhea. Side effects may look similar to IBD symptoms. Rare, serious side effects: interstitial nephritis, pancreatitis, pericarditis, bone marrow suppression, allergic reaction Labs: blood count, liver chemistries, BUN, creatine. Check creatinine every 6 mo, obtain urinalysis if abnormal. Administer with 1 mg folic acid daily Males: causes oligospermia and reversible infertility
Thiopurine analogs	Azathioprine: 2–3 mg/kg/day 6-mercaptopurine: 1–1.5 mg/kg/day Oral	Myelosuppression, pancreatitis, lymphoma Discuss cancer risk with all patients. Association with lymphoma must be considered. Avoid in EBV negative patients and adolescent males given reports of malignancy. Labs: CBC and LFTs at weeks 1, 4, 8 and then every 3–4 mo Signs of toxicity: cytopenia, elevated LFTs
Methotrexate	15 mg/m^2 once a week Oral or subcutaneous injection	Nausea, malaise, fatigue, headache, myelosuppression, hepatotoxicity, pulmonary fibrosis Labs: CBC, LFTs (CMP) 1–2, 4, 8 wk after starting and then every 3–4 mo Consider premedication with ondansetron (Zofran) to prevent related nausea Teratogenic, persists 6 mo after discontinuation
Prednisone	1–2 mg/kg/day Max: 40 mg/day Oral or intravenous	Infection, secondary adrenal insufficiency, growth suppression, bone demineralization, mood lability, sleep disturbance, acne Patients with history of recurrent steroid use are at risk of adrenal insufficiency and should not stop steroids abruptly Use with caution due to side effects and impact on growth Not used for maintenance therapy
Budesonide	3–9 mg/day Oral	Possible similar effects as prednisone Need to swallow capsule
Infliximab	*Standard dosing:* 5 mg/kg at weeks 0, 2, 6 induction, followed by 5 mg/kg every at 8 wk maintenance dosing *Intravenous:* Interval shortened and/or dose increased based on clinical response and/or therapeutic drug monitoring of trough levels	Infection, psoriasis, allergic reaction, lymphoma, immunogenicity Prior to initiation: TB, hepatitis B, and varicella screening Labs: CBC, CMP every 3–4 mo. Trough levels at least by week 14 and every 6–12 mo if stable. Goal trough levels 6–10 µg/mL associated with mucosal healing. Higher troughs are associated with better outcomes in perianal phenotype. Risks for difficulty sustaining therapeutic trough levels: hypoalbuminemia, male gender, obesity Initiation of therapy at higher doses (10 mg/kg) needed in acute severe colitis, severe pancreatic disease, VEO-IBD

Table 27.4   Pharmacologic Therapy Dosing, Side Effects, and Clinical Monitoring—cont'd

MEDICATION	DOSING	SIDE EFFECTS, MONITORING, AND SPECIAL CONSIDERATIONS

Adalimumab	*CD dosing:*
	<40 kg:
	  Induction: 80 mg day 1, 40 mg day 15, 20 mg day 29
	  Maintenance (beginning day 29): 20 mg every 2 wk
	>40 kg:
	  Induction: 160 mg day 1, 80 mg day 15, 40 mg day 29
	  Maintenance (beginning day 29): 40 mg every 2 wk
	UC dosing:
	<40 kg:
	  Induction: 80 mg day 1, 40 mg day 8, 40 mg day 15
	  Maintenance (beginning day 29): 40 mg every 2 wk (or 20 mg weekly)
	>40 kg:
	  Induction: 160 mg day 1, 80 mg day 8, 80 mg day 15
	  Maintenance (beginning day 29): 80 mg every 2 wk (or 40 mg weekly
	Subcutaneous injection
		Infection, psoriasis, allergic reaction, lymphoma, immunogenicity
		Prior to initiation: TB, hepatitis B, and varicella screening
		Labs: CBC, CMP every 3–4 mo. Monitoring of trough levels to maintain goal trough levels >7.5 ng/mL, higher trough levels associated with mucosal healing.
		Interval may be shortened and/or dose increased based on clinical response and/or therapeutic drug monitoring of trough levels.

Vedolizumab	<40 kg: 5 mg/kg week 0, 2, 6, followed by maintenance 5 mg/kg every 8 wk beginning at week 14 >40 kg: 300 mg at week 0, 2, 6, followed by maintenance 300 mg every 8 wk beginning at week 14 Intravenous	Infection, allergic reaction Prior to initiation: TB, hepatitis B, and varicella screening Labs: CBC, CMP every 3–4 mo. Drug monitoring goals of trough levels not established. Off label use, no FDA approval for IBD in pediatrics

Ustekinumab	Intravenous induction dose given once
	Subcutaneous maintenance dosing every 8 wk
	Induction:
	  <40 kg: 6–9 mg/kg/dose
	  40–55 kg: 260 mg
	  56–85 kg: 390 mg
	  86 kg: 520 mg
	Maintenance:
	  <20 kg: 2 mg/kg every 8 wk
	  20–40 kg: 45 mg every 8 wk
	  40 kg: 90 mg every 8 wk
		Infection, allergic reaction
		Prior to initiation: TB, hepatitis B, and varicella screening
		Labs: CBC, CMP every 3–4 months. Drug monitoring goals of trough levels not established.

CBC, Complete blood count; *CD,* Crohn disease; *CMP,* comprehensive metabolic panel; *EBV,* Epstein-Barr virus; *FDA,* Food and Drug Administration; *LFT,* liver function test; *TB,* tuberculosis; *VEO-IBD,* very-early-onset inflammatory bowel disease; *UC,* ulcerative colitis.

intestinal bacterial flora, mucous layers, and tight epithelial junctions. EEN was previously thought to be more effective in patients with small bowel disease; however, evidence supports that EEN may be effective as induction therapy in patients with luminal disease regardless of the site of inflammation (Ruemmele et al., 2014).

The appeal of a nonpharmacologic intervention may entice patients and families. Education on EEN regarding its lifestyle implications is very important. The feasibility of EEN may be very challenging in practice.

PROBIOTICS AND PREBIOTICS

Prebiotics and probiotics target the interaction between the gut microbiota and the immune system. Sometimes thought of as healthy bacteria or microbes, probiotics theoretically alter the enteric microflora to downplay pathogenic bacteria and maintain the integrity of the intestinal immune system's mucosal barrier (Abraham & Quigley, 2017; Cremonini et al., 2006). Prebiotics are nondigestible fermentable fibers that travel undigested through the small bowel and then reach the colon, where they stimulate the growth of beneficial bacteria, such as bifidobacteria and lactic acid

Table 27.5 **Surgical Interventions for Inflammatory Bowel Disease**

SURGERY	USE AND RATIONALE	KEY POINTS
Intestinal resection	• In patients with Crohn disease (CD), a diseased intestinal segment is resected with primary anastomosis, most commonly ileocecal resection.	• Rates of disease recurrence after surgical resection are significant. • Disease recurs endoscopically before clinical symptoms are apparent, therefore endoscopy should be repeated within 6–12 mo postoperatively.
Diverting ileostomy	• In patients with severe, refractory colonic CD or perianal disease, an ileostomy is created to limit inciting disease activity in the affected colon by stopping exposure of the fecal stream to the diseased bowel.	• Surgery is meant as a temporary intervention to allow pharmacologic therapy time to treat the colon or perianal disease. • Surgery is reversible and therefore may be indicated for patients with unclear disease phenotypes, such as in IBD-U and VEO-IBD.
Perianal surgery	• In patients with perianal CD, an outlet thread, called a seton, is placed to drain perianal abscesses, allow for healing, and avoid premature closure of fistulae.	• Perianal skin tags should not be removed surgically. • Fistulotomy is not recommended and leads to a high rate of disease recurrence, risk of poor healing, and significant wound complications.
Colectomy	• In a patient within severe, refractory, transfusion-dependent, or steroid-dependent ulcerative colitis (UC), the colon is removed. Colectomy with end ileostomy may also be an elective procedure to improve the quality of life and growth in pediatric patients and can be curative in UC. • Elective surgery is also indicated in circumstances of colonic dysplasia.	• Different surgical options are available. In pediatrics, restorative proctocolectomy with ileal pouch-anal anastomosis (RPC-IPAA) is preferred. • RPC-IPAA is typically staged in two to three surgical procedures to take down the ileostomy and create an ileal pouch-anal anastomosis, commonly the J-pouch. • RPC-IPAA offers an alternative to a permanent ostomy, preserves body image, and allows somewhat normal bowel function. Stool incontinence and frequency typically improve within 3–12 mo postop. • Postop complications include symptoms similar to colitis secondary to inflammation of the pouch, called pouchitis, as well as small bowel obstruction, stricture, fistulae, anastomotic leak, abscess, wound infection, and pouch failure. • Long-term surveillance endoscopy of the pouch is needed to assess for dysplasia. • The previous practice of straight ileoanal pull-through or ileorectal anastomosis is no longer recommended.

IBD-U, Inflammatory bowel disease unclassified; *VEO-IBD*, very-early-onset inflammatory bowel disease.

bacteria (Guandalini, 2014). The role of prebiotics and probiotics in pediatric IBD requires further study. Currently there is insufficient evidence to support their use (Mishra et al., 2022).

INTEGRATIVE HEALTH

Complementary and alternative medicine (CAM) is an umbrella term for a broad range of health modalities or philosophies centered on holistic and integrative care for any number of health concerns. CAM includes therapies that incorporate chiropractic, homeopathy, naturopathy, acupuncture, aromatherapy, massage, biofeedback, probiotics, herbal medicines, dietary supplements, mindfulness, yoga, and more.

Many patients utilize CAM and integrative health techniques with or without the collaboration of their health care providers. A recent pediatric survey showed that 84% of patients used CAM therapy. Only 24% of the patients considered the interventions CAM therapy. The most common therapies were vitamins/

supplements, stress management techniques, and dietary changes. Patients with a history of side effects from conventional therapies and worse IBD were more likely to use CAM therapy (Serpico et al., 2016).

Clinicians benefit from engaging all patients in a discussion about any additional interventions used for their IBD, such as supplements or diet changes, and keeping an open dialogue with patients to foster transparency and safe outcomes. When used safely and in conjunction with conventional IBD therapy, CAM and integrative health interventions are an excellent way to help children and adolescents live full lives unencumbered by their IBD.

IBD-ASSOCIATED PROBLEMS

GROWTH FAILURE, DELAYED PUBERTY, AND BONE HEALTH

Growth failure and delayed puberty are associated with IBD, affecting children with CD more than those with

UC. The deceleration in linear growth or the absence of clinical signs of puberty, including delayed thelarche, menarche, or lack of testicular enlargement, may be the only presenting symptom of CD. A recent study of 161 pediatric patients with CD compared differences in height gain across sexes. Results showed that males with CD have more frequent growth impairment, and females with pediatric CD more frequently experience delayed puberty (Gupta et al., 2020).

Growth failure stems from multiple possible etiologies, including increased energy expenditure and metabolic needs secondary to chronic inflammation, decreased nutritional intake, and malabsorption (Sanderson, 2014). Decreased intake is seen from anorexia caused by circulating proinflammatory cytokines such as TNF-alpha. Ongoing inflammation with the release of specific cytokines that suppress growth factors is a key determinant of growth failure. Evidence reveals that interleukin-6 mediates growth failure in children with CD by suppressing insulin-like growth factor 1 (IGF-1) production at the hepatocyte level (Dubinsky, 2008). In some children, poor intake may also be secondary to food-related fears due to the association of eating with exacerbation of GI symptoms such as pain or diarrhea. Undernutrition delays the epiphyseal fusion of long bones and progression through puberty. Delay in the onset and progression through puberty may deleteriously affect the normal pubertal growth spurt and contribute to deficits in final adult heights. Prolonged corticosteroid exposure also has a deleterious impact on growth (Diefenbach & Breuer, 2006; Fish & Kugathasan, 2004).

Healthy bone formation and growth are dependent on the growth hormone (GH) IGF-1 axis. Previously, children with stunted growth in IBD were thought to be GH resistant; however, literature has demonstrated normal GH concentrations in IBD. Evidence supports that GH's mechanism on IGF-1 and, subsequently, bone growth falls along a spectrum of dysfunction rather than total resistance (Wong et al., 2010). Further research is needed on this topic.

Osteoporosis and decreased bone mineral density are frequent in children with IBD—up to 41% with CD and 25% with UC (Jose & Heyman, 2008). Children experience increased fracture risk and poor linear growth without attaining peak bone mass. Decreased bone mineral density can be caused by malabsorption of calcium and vitamin D, macronutrient and micronutrient deficiencies, decreased levels of physical activity, estrogen deficiency in females, and corticosteroid use (Dubinsky, 2008). Bone formation is inhibited by proinflammatory cytokine activity seen in IBD. Malnutrition causes low serum IGF-1 levels (Griffiths & Buller, 2004).

A patient's disease severity, diet, vitamin D and calcium intake, physical activity, and medication exposure all impact bone health. Those with a low body mass index (BMI), severe inflammatory activity, and low serum albumin are at particular risk for low bone mass and require a dual energy x-ray absorptiometry (DEXA) scan to evaluate bone age health.

In a study of 127 pediatric patients with CD, 81% were vitamin D deficient (serum 12-OH D level <20) (Jin et al., 2021). Vitamin D levels should be evaluated annually, typically in the spring, when levels are at risk of being the lowest. Vitamin D supplementation is recommended to maintain serum 25-OH D levels at or greater than 30 ng/mL. Adequate intake of calcium in the diet is also needed for healthy bone growth. Although there is no evidence recommending avoiding dairy products in IBD, patients' dietary habits, preferences, or lactose intolerance can lead to insufficient calcium intake. Clinicians should work closely with patients and families to assess a detailed diet history and incorporate the expertise of registered dieticians whenever possible to optimize nutritional health. Patients with osteoporosis, abnormal bone age, vitamin deficiencies, or a history of prolonged steroid exposure benefit from endocrinology evaluation.

DEXA scans are recommended for patients with IBD at diagnosis and then every 1 to 2 years for follow-up. Bone density is measured using DEXA scanning. DEXA scans are widely available and provide a very small amount of radiation exposure (~1/20 that of a chest x-ray). Results are reported in z scores to indicate the patient's bone density deviation from the mean bone density norms adjusted for age and sex (Rufo et al., 2012). Osteopenia is defined as a z score of -1 to -2.5, and osteoporosis is a z score lower than -2.5. Results should be interpreted using bone age or height age, not chronologic age, which overestimates the extent of bone disease (Pappa et al., 2011).

HEPATOBILIARY COMPLICATIONS

Hepatobiliary involvement is a particularly troublesome EI manifestation of IBD. Hepatobiliary complications include small bile duct and large bile duct inflammation; chronic active hepatitis, drug-induced hepatitis, granulomatous hepatitis; cirrhosis, cholangiocarcinoma; fatty liver, amyloidosis, hepatic abscess, and cholelithiasis (Jose & Heyman, 2008).

Hepatobiliary disease, both intra- and extrahepatic, is relatively common and is among the more serious EI manifestations of IBD. Liver disorders may be present before or during active disease, or they may even develop after surgical resection of the diseased bowel. One hepatic manifestation, primary sclerosing cholangitis (PSC), is seen more commonly in patients with UC. Up to 90% of children with PSC eventually have a diagnosis of IBD (Jose & Heyman, 2008). The incidence and prevalence of PSC in children with IBD are 0.2/100,000 and 1.5/100,000, respectively (Saubermann et al., 2017).

Periodic screening of serum aminotransferases (aspartate transaminase [AST], alanine transaminase [ALT]), alkaline phosphatase, gamma-glutamyltransferase (GGT), and bilirubin is necessary to detect asymptomatic patients. The frequency of screening is recommended at least once or twice a year; however, depending on a patient's medical therapy regimen, screening may be more frequent. Physical examination should be carefully monitored for signs of liver disease, including hepatic enlargement and/or portal hypertension (Rufo et al., 2012).

Mildly elevated liver enzymes are very common in children with IBD. Mild elevations in liver enzymes (<2 x upper limit of normal [ULN]) may be transient and can be monitored and reassessed by rechecking the ALT and GGT in about 2 weeks. Persistent elevations in liver enzymes, especially ALT, increased by greater than twice the ULN (>2 x ULN), and significantly high GGT (>252 U/L) warrants referral to pediatric hepatology for suspected PSC and autoimmune sclerosis cholangitis (ASC) (Valentino et al., 2015). Immunization history and history of immunosuppressive therapy posing a potential risk of reactivation of hepatitis must be taken into consideration (Saubermann et al., 2017).

Persistently abnormal liver enzyme tests are found in 20% to 30% of people with IBD. These findings can be categorized into three groups: a sign of EI IBD disease (i.e., PSC, autoimmune hepatitis [AIH], thrombotic disorder), a result of medication toxicity, or a result of an underlying primary hepatic disorder (i.e., gall stones, viral hepatitis, nonalcoholic fatty liver disease) (Saubermann et al., 2017).

PSC is a chronic inflammatory disorder of both the intra- and extrahepatic bile ducts, leading to bile duct stenosis and liver fibrosis. In some children, disease features include inflammation of the portal tract that extends into the lobules of the liver, as seen in AIH. This phenomenon is termed *PSC-AIH overlap syndrome* or ASC.

PSC-IBD has a distinct phenotype, usually presenting with mild disease activity, rectal sparing, backwash ileitis, colorectal dysplasia, and pouchitis following colectomy with ileal pouch-anal anastomosis. PSC may be diagnosed before IBD in many instances. Given the high frequency of asymptomatic colitis, rectal sparing, and colonic dysplasia, all patients with PSC warrant surveillance colonoscopy with extensive biopsy to diagnose IBD and detect dysplasia (Sinakos et al., 2013). More research is needed on the treatment of pediatric PSC. Medical therapy options include ursodeoxycholic acid and oral vancomycin. Immunosuppressive and biologic agents have not been shown to be of benefit for the treatment of PSC, regardless of their effect on IBD or AIH. Patients who present with symptoms of biliary obstruction require magnetic resonance cholangiopancreatography (MRCP) to relieve obstruction from strictures. MRCP is also used to diagnose and evaluate suspected cholangiocarcinoma (Laborda et al., 2019).

Both PSC and ASC are associated with morbidity and mortality. Without intervention, sclerosing cholangitis is known to progress and leads to liver cirrhosis and portal hypertension, requiring a liver transplant.

Within 10 years of diagnosis, 50% of children with PSC will experience complications, and 30% will require a liver transplant. Complications include cholangiocarcinoma affecting 1% of children. In cases of progressive PSC, the only definitive long-term treatment is liver transplantation (Deneau et al., 2017).

Abnormal liver enzymes in pediatric IBD without PSC/ASC are commonly associated with the medical therapies used to treat IBD. Many of the medical therapies for IBD put children at risk for developing elevated liver enzymes. These therapies include corticosteroids, antibiotics, methotrexate, thiopurine analogs, and anti-TNF biologics. Nutritional therapy with EEN is also associated with elevated liver enzymes (Valentino et al., 2015). Often it is unclear if the association between therapies and elevated liver enzymes is related to the effects of uncontrolled inflammation on the liver or medication hepatotoxicity (Saubermann et al., 2017).

Cholelithiasis and gallstones are found in 13% to 34% of individuals with IBD, with increased incidence in those with CD compared with UC. Gallstones seem to be related to the malabsorption of bile salts with subsequent cholesterol precipitation and calculus formation in the biliary system (Jose & Heyman, 2008). Patients present with symptoms of biliary colic, such as right upper quadrant intermittent abdominal pain with or without nausea. Symptoms worsen after meals high in fat content (Saubermann et al., 2017).

RENAL COMPLICATIONS

Renal complications in IBD include nephrolithiasis (kidney stones), tubulointerstitial nephritis, glomerulonephritis, and amyloidosis. In a review of 50 cases of pediatric renal complications in patients with IBD, 58% suffered from nephrolithiasis, 30% developed tubulointerstitial nephritis, 10% glomerulonephritis, and 2% amyloidosis (Domenico & Romano, 2016).

Glomerulonephritis has been observed in both UC and CD. Glomerulonephritis is directly related to intestinal disease, and renal function improves with IBD remission.

Renal calculi may complicate the course of individuals with IBD as a result of calcium oxalate or uric acid precipitation. These have been reported in 1% to 2% of children with IBD—the highest incidence occurring in children in CD after small bowel resection or ileostomy, possibly secondary to frequent episodes of dehydration (Jose & Heyman, 2008). Children with severe ileal disease or resection of the ileum are at risk for the formation of calcium oxalate stones. Sudden onset of severe abdominal, back, or flank pain in children or adolescents with IBD should lead to the investigation of stones (Jose & Heyman, 2008).

Tubulointerstitial nephritis has been observed in IBD, particularly with the use of 5-ASA, cyclosporine, and anti-TNF therapy. It is unclear whether tubuloint-erstitial nephritis is a manifestation of IBD or the effect of therapy. Amyloidosis is a rare but serious complication seen in patients with IBD that is more common in CD than in UC. Amyloidosis usually presents as proteinuria and nephrotic syndrome and can lead to kidney failure. Early detection of amyloidosis improves prognosis (Domenico & Romano, 2016).

FULMINANT COLITIS OR TOXIC MEGACOLON

Fulminant colitis presents with grossly bloody diarrhea, fever, tachycardia, abdominal pain with distention, decreased bowel sounds, and abnormal laboratory findings. When a markedly distended colon accompanies these symptoms on radiographs, toxic megacolon should be suspected (Benchimol et al., 2008; Leichtner & Higuchi, 2004). Fulminant colitis and toxic megacolon are medical emergencies, and many individuals eventually require a colectomy. Toxic megacolon is reported in up to 5% of children and adolescents with UC and less often in CD (Benchimol et al., 2008; Leichtner & Higuchi, 2004).

HEMATOLOGIC PHENOMENA: ANEMIA AND HYPERCOAGULOPATHY

Children with IBD often experience significant anemia. The prevalence of iron deficiency in children at diagnosis is significant. A recent study found 76.8% of pediatric patients diagnosed with IBD to be iron deficient and 43.5% to exhibit iron deficiency anemia (Carvalho et al., 2017).

The etiology of anemia in IBD is multifactorial and impacted by malnutrition, malabsorption, and chronic blood loss. Additionally, some IBD therapies, such as sulfasalazine, methotrexate, and thiopurine analog, have a myelosuppressive effect, further contributing to anemia. Treatment of anemia depends on the underlying cause. If anemia is left untreated, children suffer from symptoms that impact the critical skills needed for healthy growth and development in childhood. For instance, patients may experience poor cognitive skills, behavior change, and sleep disturbances. Patients with severe anemia may experience acute symptoms that warrant the emergent evaluation, such as dizziness, syncope, and tachycardia (Mattiello et al., 2020).

All patients with IBD require routine surveillance monitoring for anemia. A complete blood count, CRP, and ferritin should be obtained at diagnosis and every 3 months during active IBD periods and every 6 to 12 months during inactive IBD periods. Folic acid and vitamin B_{12} should be assessed annually. Patients with primarily small bowel disease or bowel resection are at increased risk for vitamin deficiency and require more frequent folic acid and B_{12} screening (Goyal et al., 2020).

Treatment of anemia is dependent on the etiology and severity of anemia. Daily supplementation with folic acid is recommended for children receiving sulfasalazine. Iron supplementation is recommended for children with iron deficiency. In severe cases of anemia, a blood transfusion is necessary. In mild iron deficiency without anemia, oral iron supplementation may be adequate. Often, oral iron preparations may be difficult for children with IBD to tolerate. Fortunately, recent research supports the safety and efficacy of IV iron replacement (Goyal et al., 2020).

Adults with IBD have associated hypercoagulable states manifested by thrombosis and blood tests revealing thrombocytosis, low prothrombin time, and low partial thromboplastin time. In children, thromboembolism and thrombosis are less frequently reported (Jose & Heyman, 2008). A recent multicenter, large cohort study in children with IBD found the incidence of venous thromboembolism to be 3.72/100,000, which was 14 times higher than that in the general pediatric population (Aardoom et al., 2022).

MALIGNANCY AND MORBIDITY

Though rare, there is an increased risk of malignancy associated with IBD. The epidemiologic data in the pediatric population is variable. A recent meta-analysis showed a 2.4-fold increased rate of cancer in patients with pediatric IBD, primarily from GI cancers (Elmahdi et al., 2022). Standardized incidence ratios (SIRs) show malignancy occurs 2.6 to 3.3 times more often in those with pediatric CD than in individuals without IBD (Mitchel & Rosh, 2022). In pediatric UC, SIRs were highly variable, from 1.16 to 37.9 (Fumery et al., 2016).

Malignancy risks in pediatric IBD include colorectal, lymphoma, and nonmelanoma skin cancer. Disease duration is linked to higher risk, which is important to consider for patients with VEO-IBD and pediatric-onset IBD. The increased risk of colorectal cancer in pediatric IBD is isolated to patients with ileocolonic and colonic diseases (Nasiri et al., 2017).

Non-Hodgkin lymphoma and hepatosplenic T-cell lymphoma have been associated with IBD and the use of thiopurines and possibly anti-TNF agents (Kotlyar, 2015). A review of these cases found lymphomas have a significant risk with thiopurine use in male patients younger than 35 years. It is recommended that patients and their families are counseled about the risks of using thiopurines as monotherapy or combination therapy (Hyams et al., 2017). Nonmelanoma skin cancers are associated with adult IBD in those exposed to thiopurines. In pediatrics, the association has been reported but is not widely known.

Increased malignancy rates in pediatric-onset IBD and VEO-IBD implicate the importance of endoscopic surveillance screening with colonoscopy. Pediatric consensus guidelines are lacking. Historically, colonoscopy screening for colorectal cancer has been recommended starting about 8 years after diagnosis and then annually or biannually (Leichtner & Higuchi,

2004; Stucchi et al., 2006). Currently, VEO-IBD and pediatric-onset IBD cancer screening guidelines are the same for adults and do not account for increased risk in the younger age of onset. Surveillance endoscopy screening should start earlier and occur at more frequent intervals than in adults. More research is needed to establish updated pediatric guidelines given the rise in early-onset IBD and increased risk of malignancy over time in pediatric IBD (El-Matary & Bernstein, 2020).

Data on mortality findings in pediatric IBD are limited. A survey study among pediatric gastroenterologists in Europe and Israel reports rare instances of mortality in pediatric IBD. Cases were related to infections, particularly in patients with two or more immunosuppressive drugs, cancer, and uncontrolled disease (de Ridder et al., 2014). In a pediatric study of 698 patients, 2 patients with CD and 1 patient with UC expired from IBD-related causes. IBD-related mortality was not increased compared to the reference population (Peneau et al., 2013).

PSYCHOSOCIAL ISSUES

Children and adolescents with IBD are at risk for mental and behavioral health disorders from their chronic diseases. IBD has the potential to impact social functioning and self-esteem development. The relapsing and remitting nature of the disease must also be considered (Mackner & Crandall, 2007). Research shows that pediatric IBD impacts the quality of life and overall well-being. Depressive disorders are shown to be more prevalent in patients with IBD compared to other chronic illnesses. Impacts on growth, such as short stature and delayed puberty, may impact self-acceptance. Practical implications of unpredictable symptoms can be associated with challenges in psychosocial adjustment (Greenley et al., 2010). Evidence in adolescents with CD shows that more severe disease is correlated with increased parental stress and affects the patient's quality of life (Gray et al., 2015).

Because of the relapsing and remitting course of IBD, lifestyle changes can occur unexpectedly due to disease exacerbation. Difficulty interacting with peers may result from school absenteeism, low self-esteem because of delayed growth and development (symptoms that can be embarrassing and limit social activities), and appearance-altering side effects from medications. Adolescents are particularly vulnerable because belonging to a particular social group and peer acceptance are important to their identity (Mackner & Crandall, 2007). Mackner and Crandall (2007) found significantly impaired social functioning in 35% of those with the disease diagnosed during adolescence compared with 5% of those diagnosed earlier in childhood.

A qualitative study of patients and their families provided evidence that anticipatory guidance to decrease the anxiety of the unknown and cognitive behavioral strategies to manage emotions support patients coping and adaptation to the new norm. Challenges identified include the unpredictable nature of IBD, disruptions in normalcy, treatment decisions, managing relationships, and life transitions. Practical challenges were identified, including pain and anxiety surrounding IV placement for infusions. Clinicians can create health care delivery systems within their teams to incorporate these considerations into IBD management.

Age and stages of psychosocial development also affect the ability of children with IBD to understand and participate in their care and impact adherence to the medical regimen prescribed by their pediatric gastroenterologist. Compliance rates for medications, especially during remission, are an ongoing problem. Adolescents have the lowest rate of adherence (50%) (Dubinsky, 2008). Family dysfunction and poor child coping strategies were associated with worse adherence (Dubinsky, 2008). This reinforces the need to address IBD's psychological and psychosocial impact on the pediatric population and their families. Support groups, the internet, and camps specifically for children with IBD are additional resources for improved psychosocial functioning.

PROGNOSIS AND FUTURE ADVANCES

New and emerging research is designed to identify prognostic factors in IBD. Clinicians and families alike strive to predict outcomes for patients. Although the era of biologic and small molecule therapy has made dramatic treatment advances in IBD care, uncertainty in ascertaining therapy responses and disease progression remains. Recent consensus guidelines provide risk stratification recommendations to identify the best medical decisions for each patient and thus prevent disease progression and complications.

For patients with UC, disease extent, PUCAI score, hemoglobin, hematocrit, and albumin at diagnosis may predict the chances of colectomy. In addition, a family history of UC and the presence of EI manifestations may predict colectomy, whereas PSC may be protective against colectomy. Acute severe colitis may be predicted by disease severity at onset and hypoalbuminemia. In cases of ASC, a higher PUCAI score and CRP on days 3 and 5 of hospital admission predict failure of IV steroids. The risk factors for malignancy for pediatric UC are a concomitant diagnosis of PSC, long-standing colitis (>10 years), male sex, and younger age at diagnosis (Orlanski-Meyer et al., 2021).

In CD, predictive considerations for surgery included diagnosis during adolescence, growth impairment, *NOD2/CARD15* polymorphisms, disease behavior, and positive anti–*Saccharomyces cerevisiae* antibody status. The isolated colonic disease has been associated with fewer surgeries. Risk factors to predict penetrating or stenotic disease include older age at presentation, small bowel disease, serology (anti–*S. cerevisiae* antibody, antiflagellin, *ompC*), *NOD2/CARD15* polymorphisms, perianal disease, and ethnicity. Growth impairment can be predicted with the following findings: male sex, young age at onset, small bowel disease, more active disease, and diagnostic delay. Additionally, malnutrition and higher disease activity were associated with reduced bone density (Ricciuto et al., 2021).

The recent paradigm shifts in IBD treatment objectives to achieve intestinal mucosa healing may modify the natural history of the disease and possibly decrease the chances of developing the perforating disease (fistulas and abscesses) and fibrostenosis, especially in CD. Emerging genetic factors may help predict individuals likely to have a more severe disease course, and the development of safer therapies that individualize strategies will be a critical part of the future management of pediatric IBD.

PRIMARY CARE MANAGEMENT

HEALTH CARE MAINTENANCE

Growth and Development

Children with IBD should have growth parameters (height, weight, BMI, Tanner staging) measured and assessed at each primary care visit. For children with recently diagnosed IBD, a review of the previous visit records to assess growth in the years prior may identify any deceleration in growth rate. Continued careful measurement and graphing of growth parameters are essential. Catchup growth is considered adequate if children return to their preillness growth percentiles. Patients with VEO-IBD may have impacts on meeting developmental milestones. Development must be carefully assessed with validated objective measures. Delays warrant prompt referral to early intervention services such as speech-language pathology, physical therapy, occupational therapy, or feeding skills. Healthy development in pediatric IBD is fostered by implementing school-based services, including a 504 plan, to provide supplementary support so that children with IBD can thrive and learn. Child life specialists, licensed social workers, and psychologists are used to help children and adolescents grow and develop to their maximum potential.

Diet

Diet and nutritional concerns for families of children and adolescents with IBD are extremely common. Careful attention to the child's diet is important, as there is no single diet plan that helps everyone with IBD; recommendations must be individualized depending on the type and location of the disease. Disease and/or inflammation of the large intestine should allow for normal digestion and absorption in the small intestine. The disease of the small intestine can affect the absorption of all nutrients, in particular carbohydrates, lipids, and micronutrients such as vitamin B_{12}, iron, and calcium. During periods of active disease, many children may feel more comfortable consuming a low-roughage diet. Narrowing of the small bowel or stricture formation may necessitate a low-residue diet and restriction of nuts, seeds, popcorn, and vegetables that are difficult to digest. The most important advice is to eat a well-balanced diet of proteins, calories, and nutrients. It should be stressed to the child's family that good nutrition is one of the ways the body restores itself to health. This is especially true with delayed growth when IBD is diagnosed before the onset of puberty.

Some individuals may identify foods that make them feel better or worse. Malabsorption, especially of carbohydrates, lactose, and fructose, may induce diarrhea and gas symptoms. If lactose intolerance is suspected, a hydrogen breath test can be performed for a definitive diagnosis. The prevalence of lactose intolerance does not appear to be any greater in children with CD and UC than in those in the general population. During periods of active disease, some children with IBD may experience temporary symptoms of lactose intolerance, including bloating, abdominal cramping, and diarrhea related to the intake of dairy products (Heyman & Committee on Nutrition, 2006). Without a definitive history of lactose intolerance, eliminating dairy products from the diet is not recommended. There is no evidence to suggest that routine avoidance of dairy products will decrease mucosal inflammation or clinical outcome in patients with IBD (Rufo et al., 2012).

Clinicians must be aware that concerned parents, who can attribute symptoms to multiple foods, may overly restrict the diet and make it much more difficult to achieve balanced nutritional goals. Such overrestriction may result in a diet that is unappealing to the child and too restrictive to provide enough calories for growth and development. Sometimes even junk food, which may be more appealing to children and adolescents, can have nutritious benefits when ingested in limited amounts (e.g., pizza, cheeseburgers, milkshakes). A nutritional assessment with a dietitian can assess a child's intake and nutritional status and, if necessary, counsel the child and family regarding augmentation of caloric and other nutrient intake. Supplements are recommended for specific clinical indications. Iron and vitamin D should be repleted if lab values show deficiency. Vitamin B_{12} deficiency is common with small bowel resection and may need to be repleted if levels are low. Folic acid should be supplemented in individuals taking sulfasalazine. Calcium is the most common mineral deficiency seen in IBD, mostly because of the limited dietary intake of dairy products related to lactose intolerance or long-term corticosteroid use. Calcium supplementation may be needed if dietary requirements fail to be enough. Nutritional supplementation with high-caloric formulas or an enriched diet is necessary for some patients. These can be delivered orally or by nasogastric or gastrostomy tube. Total parenteral nutrition administered through an IV catheter into a large blood vessel is indicated in severe malnutrition. Severe malnutrition requires hospitalization for safety and monitoring of refeeding syndrome when enteral feeding is gradually introduced. Children or adolescents (i.e., before epiphyseal closure) may recover lost growth with adequate calories.

Safety

Children with IBD require no special restrictions on activities. They should be encouraged to participate in all activities they enjoy, including extracurricular activities such as sports, dance, and swimming. Vigorous activities should pose no problem for children in remission.

Children and adolescents with IBD who plan to travel may need to make some special modifications. Consultation with a travel clinic may be beneficial when travel abroad is planned. General considerations include the purity of the water supply, exposure to ova and parasites, and proper immunization.

Alcohol consumption by adolescents with IBD who are in remission is of the same concern as alcohol consumption by their unaffected peers. Alcohol ingestion may cause discomfort for some individuals with IBD. If so, these individuals should limit intake. Individuals taking metronidazole should be informed that alcohol intake can induce a disulfiram (Antabuse) type of reaction, primarily nausea and vomiting.

Children who are immunosuppressed or adrenally insufficient should establish an easily identifiable means of communicating this fact to emergency medical personnel for instances of emergency. Patients and families should be educated on the risks of immunosuppression. Fever in patients on immunosuppressive therapy requires medical attention. Patients should notify their health care team of any fever, and a clinical assessment is required. Primary care providers should perform a history and physical exam and contact the patient's GI team with any concerns. Adrenally insufficient patients should receive teaching on how to start a stress dose of steroids in circumstances such as fever or vomiting. Education should be provided with clearly prescribed instructions, written and verbal, and include having patients and their families return demonstration learning skills. Interpreter services should be utilized for any language barriers.

Immunizations

At diagnosis, children and adolescents should have a complete reconciliation of their immunization history to ensure immunizations are up to date, and if not, they should be immunized before immunosuppressive therapy is initiated if possible. Immunosuppressive therapy is defined as high-dose systemic corticosteroids (≥2 mg/kg/day of prednisone or its equivalent or ≥20 mg/day of prednisone or its equivalent for ≥14 days), cyclosporine or tacrolimus, immunomodulatory agents, or biologic therapy (Rufo et al., 2012).

Children and adolescents with IBD are at higher risk for developing vaccine-preventable illnesses, such as influenza, pneumococcal pneumonia, and hepatitis B virus. Furthermore, IBD treatment with immunosuppressive therapy increases the risk of infections. There have been fatal reports of patients on biologic immunosuppressive therapy from vaccine-preventable illnesses, including pneumococcal pneumonia and hepatitis B infection. Educating and counseling families on the risks of immunosuppression and the rationale for immunization recommendations is critical (Reich et al., 2016).

The recommended immunizations include diphtheria, pertussis, acellular tetanus, hepatitis B virus, *Haemophilus* influenzae, inactivated polio, influenza, pneumococcus, and hepatitis A virus vaccinations in early childhood, as well as immunizations against human papillomavirus and meningococcal diseases during school age and adolescence. Pneumococcal immunization for all patients with IBD requires the 13-valent pneumococcal conjugate vaccine (PCV13) in addition to the 23-valent pneumococcal polysaccharide vaccine (PPSV23). The PCV13 should be administered once, followed by a dose of the PPSV23 after 8 weeks in immunosuppressed patients or after a minimum of 12 months in immunocompetent patients. A second dose of PPSV23 should be administered 5 years after the first dose. All patients with IBD should receive nonlive annual influenza immunization.

Patients on immunosuppressive therapy cannot receive live immunizations; however, they can and should receive all nonlive immunizations according to guidelines from the Advisory Committee on Immunization Practices (ACIP) and the American Academy of Pediatrics (AAP). This means patients on immunosuppressive therapy, which includes the use of steroids, immunomodulators, and biologics, cannot receive rotavirus, measle-mumps-rubella, and varicella vaccines until a safe time is established to implement a drug holiday for vaccine catchup (Reich et al., 2016). Exposure to varicella infection in those who have not been vaccinated nor had prior varicella infection and who are immunosuppressed warrants the administration of varicella-zoster immunoglobulin within 48 hours of exposure.

Screenings

Vision. Annual ophthalmic examinations are necessary to screen for ocular manifestations of IBD. Many individuals with ophthalmologic complications are asymptomatic, especially early in the disease course. Steroids increase the risk of ophthalmologic problems.

Hearing. Routine screening is recommended for all patients with IBD. In VEO-IBD, monogenic defects are observed that may present with hearing loss. Newborn hearing screening records should be reviewed, and findings of hearing loss in a patient with suspected VEO-IBD increase clinical suspicion and support the importance of timely genetic evaluation.

Dental. Children with IBD require proper dental hygiene. At each well-child visit, the primary care provider should ascertain patients are receiving regular dental care. Children who are being treated with cyclosporine are at risk for gingival hyperplasia. Oral iron supplements are associated with teeth discoloration. Antibiotic therapy can also impact oral health, including teeth discoloration and black hairy tongue.

Blood pressure. Blood pressure should be measured and recorded at every visit. Children who are taking cyclosporine or corticosteroids are at increased risk for hypertension. Evidence of hypertension should be reported to the gastroenterology team.

Tuberculosis. Prior to initiation of immunosuppressive therapy, all patients must undergo screening for latent tuberculosis and hepatitis, and varicella immune status should be determined.

Drug interactions. A meticulous reconciliation of a patient's current medications and supplements, prescribed or otherwise, must be evaluated to screen for drug interactions. Drugs used to treat IBD, as well as drugs used to treat other conditions in individuals with IBD, can cause a wide range of potentially serious interactions (Irving et al., 2007).

Condition-Specific Screenings
Regular follow-up is needed with the patient's gastroenterology team. Established, asymptomatic children and adolescents should be evaluated by their gastroenterology team at a visit every 6 months. Patients on immunosuppressive therapy should be evaluated more frequently (every 3–4 months). During these visits, condition-specific screening studies may be obtained, including blood count, chemistries, and inflammatory markers. Primary care practitioners must be aware that these studies are routinely evaluated. In some circumstances the primary care setting may be the most convenient or appropriate place to monitor these values. For patients receiving biologic therapy, labs are coordinated to be drawn at the time of the infusion if possible.

Laboratory screening for patients with IBD depends on disease severity and activity, as well as the risk of potential side effects associated with their specific therapy regimen. Routine surveillance labs include blood count evaluation, a liver and kidney metabolic panel, and inflammatory markers (ESR, CRP, calprotectin). The screening frequency varies depending on clinical circumstances, but it is often every 3 to 6 months for established patients. Laboratory assessment is done more often for patients undergoing therapy induction or change.

COMMON ILLNESS MANAGEMENT
The symptoms of IBD and its associated problems vary. Symptoms of common childhood illnesses such as acute gastroenteritis or influenza-like illnesses may be difficult to differentiate from exacerbations of a child's underlying disease process. A thorough history and physical exam are critical to rule out acute emergencies such as a surgical abdomen, severe dehydration, or sepsis.

Symptoms of diarrhea warrant infectious stool studies to be obtained because infections (e.g., with rotavirus, norovirus, *Yersinia*, *Campylobacter*, *Shigella*, and *C. difficile*) may mimic IBD. Any child with prolonged symptoms, including bloody diarrhea (with no identified pathogen) or weight loss, should be referred to the gastroenterology team. Children with abdominal pain should be examined for changes that might indicate a disease progression, fulminant colitis, or an obstruction. These children should be questioned about the similarity of their current pain to the pain experienced as a part of the IBD. A child who appears ill with acute pain should be immediately referred for emergent evaluation.

Vomiting in children with IBD, especially CD, could indicate an obstruction. The history and physical examination should elicit information about distention, associated pain, and its relation to meals and the nature of the emesis (bilious, nonbilious, bloody, coffee ground). As always, information about the child's bowel pattern and the nature of the stools should be gathered.

Children with IBD, especially those receiving corticosteroid therapy, are at increased risk for osteoporosis, aseptic necrosis of the hip or knee joints, and spinal fractures. Children with IBD who report back or hip pain require a radiologic examination to adequately assess these symptoms. When children with IBD report joint pain, they should be questioned about the presence of erythema or swelling. Children with symptoms suggesting joint involvement should also be assessed for increased disease activity.

Intercurrent illnesses, such as viral or bacterial gastroenteritis or another illness that must be treated with antibiotics, may contribute to a child's IBD flareups. Antibiotic use should be judicious. Empiric antibiotic treatment is not recommended. Antibiotic exposure impacts the intestinal flora and can lead to illness from the alteration of the normal flora of the bowel (e.g., *C. difficile*) after antibiotic therapy.

DEVELOPMENTAL CONCERNS
Sleep Patterns
Sleep may be disturbed due to nocturnal stooling or early morning awakening due to symptoms seen in active IBD. With the proper IBD therapy, nighttime

awakenings should not occur. Sleep hygiene is of utmost importance for healthy growth and development. Patients on enteral feeding therapy often receive tube feedings at nighttime to allow normalcy during the daytime routine. The feeding regimen should be carefully designed in collaboration with the patient, family, and (if possible) a registered dietician to create a well-tolerated schedule that optimizes success.

Toileting

For children who are not yet toilet trained, it is preferable to wait to start toilet training until IBD is in clinical remission and the character of bowel movements is as close to normal as possible. For children who are continent, episodes of incontinence can occur depending on disease activity. In the context of an overview of a child's condition and its implications, the possibility of incontinence should be shared with the school nurse and classroom teachers, who can make plans to ensure that incidents will be handled with sensitivity and that the child may retain as much control and dignity as possible. Management styles vary among practitioners with respect to the use of antispasmodic agents for the relief of chronic diarrhea in children with mild IBD. Drugs such as loperamide (Imodium) should be used cautiously to control symptoms during daytime activity.

Behavior, Child Care, and School

Behavioral expectations for children with IBD are similar to those of their unaffected peers. Parenting a child with IBD should be as close as possible to parenting styles for a child without IBD. Parents of children with IBD should be encouraged to use the same guidelines for choosing child care arrangements as for their well children. The overriding philosophy is not to unduly isolate a child from the normal activities of daily living. Children with CD and UC are as able to achieve in the classroom as their unaffected peers. Similar to many children with chronic conditions, children with IBD must juggle treatment schedules and cope with stigma, pain, fatigue, and (occasionally) frequent or prolonged school absences. An established relationship with the child's school nurse and a 504 plan is needed so that children reach peak outcomes.

Sexual and Reproductive Health

Adolescence is a time when concerns about body image, interpersonal relationships, and plans for the future are commonplace. It is not unusual that adolescents or young adults with IBD are concerned about the possible disease impact on sexual and reproductive health.

Physical findings associated with IBD, such as delayed puberty and growth, ostomies, or perianal disease, may impact acceptance of self and identity. Peer support groups may provide patients and their families opportunities to obtain support and acceptance. Involving a GI psychologist in the care of patients with IBD is highly important at varying stages of development. In

adolescence and the transition to adulthood, incorporating the multidisciplinary team is necessary for anticipatory guidance and support. Summer camp programs are now available for children with IBD. The goals of these camp programs are to allow children to participate in normal camp activities surrounded by their peers dealing with similar childhood issues (Dubinsky, 2008). A bonus of IBD camps is an increase in self-esteem, altered perceptions and attitudes toward illness, and the knowledge that they are not alone.

Patients may be inquisitive about the impact of their disease on reproductive health and fertility. Old reports of decreased fertility did not consider the circumstances of individuals choosing not to reproduce. Findings show that the overall fertility rates in females with UC are similar to that of the general population. Surgical resection may increase the risk of adhesions and impair tubal function in females. In a meta-analysis of eight studies, Waljee et al. (2006) found a 50% increased risk of infertility after colectomy with a J-pouch. However, a more recent study shows decreased fertility rates in females with IBD, demonstrating a history of surgery did not impact in vitro fertilization success compared to the general infertility population (Pabby et al., 2015).

Neither UC nor CD increases infertility in women with inactive diseases. Some studies have indicated that women with CD have higher rates of infertility than control populations. It is believed that the most common cause of infertility in women with CD is the activity of the disease. Other factors include poor nutritional status, rectovaginal fistulas, and fear of becoming pregnant (Leichtner & Higuchi, 2004).

In males, sulfasalazine is known to cause decreased sperm count and dysmotility, and sperm malformation. These effects are reversible, however, when they stop taking sulfasalazine for 3 months (Physician's Desk Reference, 2008). In females, methotrexate is a known teratogen and is contraindicated in those with childbearing potential.

Pregnancy does not increase the likelihood of relapse of either UC or CD, but if UC is active at conception, the course of disease activity may be worse during the pregnancy. The outcome of pregnancy in women with IBD approximates that of the general population, but some researchers have found a somewhat higher incidence of prematurity in infants born to mothers with IBD than in the general population (Leichtner & Higuchi, 2004).

Transition to Adulthood

Specialized programs to transition adolescents with IBD to adult care are greatly important. Many primary care providers have an informal policy of caring for their adolescent clients with IBD until they have weathered most of the anticipated developmental crises of late adolescence. However, incorporating the patient and multidisciplinary team to begin the transition to adulthood should begin years before the transfer of care. To facilitate this transition, the pediatric gastroenterologist should begin seeing affected adolescents without their parents in the examination room to build a relationship that promotes independence and self-reliance and resembles, in part, the relationship they will have with their internist-gastroenterologist (Afzali & Wahbeh, 2017; Baldassano et al., 2002; Dubinsky, 2008). The young adult and parents should be made aware of the need for a primary care provider who has expertise in IBD and in adult-type problems such as pregnancy, fertility, cancer surveillance, and common health problems of adulthood (Afzali & Wahbeh, 2017; Baldassano et al., 2002). It is important to identify the internist-gastroenterologist who recognizes that the young adult with IBD who was diagnosed in childhood may have a different set of expectations than the young adult with a recent diagnosis (Afzali & Wahbeh, 2017; Baldassano et al., 2002). It is not unusual for the transition process to be more difficult for the parents than for the child.

Family Concerns

IBD has a significant impact on the patient's family. It takes a collaborative approach that is sensitive and respectful of the patient's needs. IBD symptoms can be challenging for families to manage and discuss. GI psychology, social work, nursing, and child life specialists are integral to the care team and help connect families with the support and resources to cope and succeed. IBD care is individualized to the specific needs of each patient and family.

RESOURCES

ORGANIZATIONS

Crohn's & Colitis Foundation: https://www.crohnscolitisfoundation.org

Healthy Children (from American Academy of Pediatrics): https://healthychildren.org

North American Society for Pediatric Gastroenterology, Hepatology & Nutrition: https://naspghan.org/about

Pediatric IBD Foundation: https://pedsibd.org/contact-us

BOOKS

Oliva-Hemker, M. (2017). *Your child with inflammatory bowel disease: A family guide for caregiving.* Johns Hopkins Press.

 Summary

Primary Care Needs for the Inflammatory Bowel Disease

HEALTH CARE MAINTENANCE
Growth and Development
- Growth failure is a common problem for children with IBD but is more commonly seen in CD than UC.
- Growth parameters are important to measure and chart at each primary care visit.
- Cognitive abilities are unimpaired by IBD.
- Assessment of developmental milestones with validated objective measures helps identify delays associated with early-onset disease.

Diet
- Highly restrictive diets are not recommended in the pediatric population.
- Nutritional assessment by a registered dietician is recommended. Adequate caloric intake is essential for growth. Supplemental diet preparations may be beneficial in select patients.

Safety
- Immunosuppressed and adrenally insufficient children should carry medical identification.
- Fever in an immunosuppressed patient warrants medical evaluation, often by the primary care provider.
- Adrenally insufficient patients require stress dose steroids.
- Individuals taking metronidazole should be cautioned about an Antabuse-type reaction to alcohol.
- Take caution with travel, especially to tropical areas. Ova, parasites, and purity of water should be a concern.
- Children and families should be educated on the hazards of discontinuing treatment.

Immunizations
- Patients are high risk for vaccine-preventable diseases.
- Patients on immunosuppressive therapy cannot receive live immunizations.
- It is critically important patients are immunized according to established ACIP and American Academy of Pediatrics guidelines and recommendations and receive all recommended nonlive immunizations, including hepatitis A, human papillomavirus, annual influenza, and PPSV23 vaccinations.
- Prophylactic immunoglobulin may be used with exposures to varicella in nonimmune patients.

Screenings
- *Vision*. Annual ophthalmic examination is necessary at each visit. Twice-yearly ophthalmologist visits are recommended for a child taking maintenance doses of corticosteroids.
- *Hearing*. Routine screening is recommended.
- *Dental*. Routine care is recommended.
- *Blood pressure*. Routine screening is recommended; if a child is taking cyclosporine or corticosteroids, blood pressure should be measured at every visit.
- *Bone mineral density*. DEXA scan is recommended at diagnosis.

COMMON ILLNESS MANAGEMENT
Differential Diagnosis
- *Diarrhea*. Rule out flareups of disease, obtain cultures.
- *Abdominal pain*. Rule out flareups of disease, gastritis, fulminant colitis, and obstruction.

Continued

- *Vomiting.* Rule out flareups of disease and gastritis; assess for obstruction.
- *Skeletal complaints.* Rule out arthritic manifestations of the disease (i.e., sacroiliitis, ankylosing spondylitis, peripheral arthritis), aseptic necrosis of the femoral head, vertebral compression fractures, and osteoporosis.

DEVELOPMENTAL ISSUES

Sleep Patterns

- Children with IBD generally have no special needs; children receiving an evening dose of corticosteroids may have some difficulty sleeping. These children may also have some nighttime stooling, which interrupts sleep.

Toileting

- In patients who have not yet toilet trained, disease activity should be quiescent prior to instituting.
- For older children with active disease, occasional incontinence may be an issue.
- Antispasmodics may be used cautiously for daytime incontinence.

Behavior, Child Care, and Schooling

- Standard developmental counseling is advised.
- Participation in peer and parent support groups is recommended.

- Children with IBD are as able to achieve in the classroom as their unaffected peers.
- Frequent or prolonged absences may interfere with the school routine.
- School personnel must be educated about special issues related to IBD, and a 504 plan should be established.

Sexuality and Reproductive Health

- Self-esteem and body image issues are important to adolescents with IBD.
- Adolescents may have late-onset puberty because of growth delay.
- Sulfasalazine may cause infertility in males while they are taking the drug.
- Pregnancy outcomes are similar to those of the general population.

Transition to Adulthood

- Self-care responsibilities may be gradually assumed by adolescents.
- The transition to adult care is a collaborative process between the patient, family, and care team and should begin early.

Family Concerns

- IBD care is individualized to the specific needs of each patient and family.

REFERENCES

Aardoom, M. A., Klomberg, R. C. W., Kemos, P., & Ruemmele, F. M.; PIBD-VTE Group; van Ommen CHH, de Ridder L, Croft NM; PIBD-SETQuality Consortium. (2022). The incidence and characteristics of venous thromboembolisms in paediatric-onset inflammatory bowel disease: A prospective international cohort study based on the PIBD-SETQuality safety registry. *Journal of Crohn's and Colitis, 16*(5), 695–707. doi:10.1093/ecco-jcc/jjab171. PMID: 34599822; PMCID: PMC9228884.

Abdelaal, K., & Jaffray, B. (2016). Colonic disease site and perioperative complications predict need for later intestinal interventions following intestinal resection in pediatric Crohn's disease. *Journal of Pediatric Surgery, 51,* 272–276.

Abraham, B. P., Mehta, S., & El-Serag, H. B. (2012). Natural history of pediatric-onset inflammatory bowel disease: A systematic review. *Journal of Clinical Gastroenterology, 46*(7), 581–589. doi:10.1097/MCG.0b013e318247c32f.

Abraham, B. P., & Quigley, E. M. M (2017). Probiotics in inflammatory bowel disease. *Gastroenterology Clinics of North America, 46*(4), 769–782. doi:10.1016/j.gtc.2017.08.003.

Abramson, O., Durant, M., Mow, W., Finley, A., Kodali, P., Wong, A., Tavares, V., McCroskey, E., Liu, L., Lewis, J. D., Allison, J. E., Flowers, N., Hutfless, S., Velayos, F. S., Perry, G. S., Cannon, R., & Herrinton, L. J. (2010). Incidence, prevalence, and time trends of pediatric inflammatory bowel disease in Northern California, 1996 to 2006. *The Journal of Pediatrics, 157*(2), 233–239.e1. https://doi.org/10.1016/j.jpeds.2010.02.024.

Afzali, A., & Wahbeh, G. (2017). Transition of pediatric to adult care in inflammatory bowel disease: Is it as easy as 1, 2, 3? *World Journal of Gastroenterology, 23*(20), 3624–3631. doi:10.3748/wjg.v23.i20.3624.

Aloi, M., Bramuzzo, M., Arrigo, S., Romano, C., D'Arcangelo, G., Lacorte, D., Gatti, S., Illiceto, M. T., Zucconi, F., Dilillo, D., Zuin, G., Knafelz, D., Ravelli, A., Cucchiara, S., Alvisi, P., & SIGENP IBD Working Group (2018). Efficacy and safety of adalimumab in pediatric ulcerative colitis: A real-life experience from the SIGENP-IBD registry. *Journal of Pediatric Gastroenterology and Nutrition, 66*(6), 920–925. https://doi.org/10.1097/MPG.0000000000001883.

Aloi, M., D'Arcangelo, G., Pofi, F., Vassallo, F., Rizzo, V., Nuti, F., Di Nardo, G., Pierdomenico, M., Viola, F., & Cucchiara, S. (2013). Presenting features and disease course of pediatric ulcerative colitis. *Journal of Crohn's & Colitis, 7*(11), e509–e515. https://doi.org/10.1016/j.crohns.2013.03.007.

Amil-Dias, J., Kolacek, S., Turner, D., Pærregaard, A., Rintala, R., Afzal, N. A., Karolewska-Bochenek, K., Bronsky, J., Chong, S., Fell, J., Hojsak, I., Hugot, J. P., Koletzko, S., Kumar, D., Lazowska-Przeorek, I., Lillehei, C., Lionetti, P., Martin-de-Carpi, J., Pakarinen, M., Ruemmele, F. M., … IBD Working Group of ESPGHAN (IBD Porto Group) (2017). Surgical management of crohn disease in children: guidelines from the paediatric IBD Porto Group of ESPGHAN. *Journal of Pediatric Gastroenterology and Nutrition, 64*(5), 818–835. https://doi.org/10.1097/MPG.0000000000001562.

Anupindi, S. A., Grossman, A. B., Nimkin, K., Mamula, P., & Gee, M. S. (2014). Imaging in the evaluation of the young patient with inflammatory bowel disease: What the gastroenterologist needs to know. *Journal of Pediatric Gastroenterology and Nutrition, 59*(4), 429–439. https://doi.org/10.1097/MPG.0000000000000475.

Ardura, M. I., Toussi, S. S., Siegel, J. D., Lu, Y., Bousvaros, A., & Crandall, W. (2016). NASPGHAN clinical report: Surveillance, diagnosis, and prevention of infectious diseases in pediatric patients with inflammatory bowel disease receiving tumor necrosis factor-α inhibitors. *Journal of Pediatric Gastroenterology and Nutrition, 63*(1), 130–155. https://doi.org/10.1097/MPG.0000000000001188.

Baillie, C. T., & Smith, J. A. (2015). Surgical strategies in paediatric inflammatory bowel disease. *World Journal of Gastroenterology, 21*(20), 6101–6116. doi:10.3748/wjg.v21.i20.610.

Baldassano, R., Ferry, G., Griffiths, A., Mack, D., Markowitz, J., & Winter, H. (2002). Transition of the patient with inflammatory bowel disease from pediatric to adult care: Recommendations of the North American Society for Pediatric Gastroenterology, Hepatology and Nutrition. *Journal of Pediatric Gastroenterology and Nutrition, 34*(3), 245–248. doi:10.1097/00005176-200203000-00001.

Barnes, E. L., Loftus, E. V., & Kappelman, M. D. (2021). Effects of race and ethnicity on diagnosis and management of inflammatory bowel diseases. *Gastroenterology, 160*(3), 677–689. doi:10.1053/j.gastro.2020.08.064.

Benchimol, E. I., Bernstein, C. N., Bitton, A., Carroll, M. W., Singh, H., Otley, A. R., Vutcovici, M., El-Matary, W., Nguyen, G. C., Griffiths, A. M., Mack, D. R., Jacobson, K., Mojaverian, N., Tanyingoh, D., Cui, Y., Nugent, Z. J., Coulombe, J., Targownik, L. E., Jones, J. L., Leddin, D., … Kaplan, G. G. (2017). Trends in epidemiology of pediatric inflammatory bowel disease in canada: Distributed network analysis of multiple population-based provincial health administrative databases. *American Journal of Gastroenterology, 112*(7), 1120–1134. https://doi.org/10.1038/ajg.2017.97.

Benchimol, E. I., Mack, D. R., Guttman, A., Nguyen, G. C., To, T., Mojaverian, N., Quach, P., & Manuel, D. G. (2015). Inflammatory bowel disease in immigrants to Canada and their children: A population-based cohort study. *American Journal of Gastroenterology, 110*(4), 553–563. doi:10.1038/ajg.2015.52.

Benchimol, E. I., Turner, D., Mann, E. H., Thomas, K. E., Gomes, T., McLernon, R. A., & Griffiths, A. M. (2008). Toxic megacolon in children with inflammatory bowel disease: Clinical and radiographic characteristics. *American Journal of Gastroenterology, 103*(6), 1524–1531. https://doi.org/10.1111/j.1572-0241.2008.01807.x.

Bousvaros, A., Antonioli, D. A., Colletti, R. B., Dubinsky, M. C., Glickman, J. N., Gold, B. D., Griffiths, A. M., Jevon, G. P., Higuchi, L. M., Hyams, J. S., Kirschner, B. S., Kugathasan, S., Baldassano, R. N., & Russo, P. A. (2007). North American Society for Pediatric Gastroenterology, Hepatology, and Nutrition, Colitis Foundation of America. Differentiating ulcerative colitis from Crohn disease in children and young adults: report of a working group of the North American Society for Pediatric Gastroenterology, Hepatology, and Nutrition and the Crohn's and Colitis Foundation of America. *Journal of Pediatric Gastroenterology and Nutrition, 44*(5), 653–674. https://doi.org/10.1097/MPG.0b013e31805563f3.

Breton, J., Kastl, A., Conrad, M. A., & Baldassano, R. N. (2020). Positioning biologic therapies in the management of pediatric inflammatory bowel disease. *Gastroenterology & Hepatology, 16*(8), 400–414.

Breton, J., Kastl, A., Hoffmann, N., Rogers, R., Grossman, A. B., Mamula, P., Kelsen, J. R., Baldassano, R. N., & Albenberg, L. (2019). Efficacy of combination antibiotic therapy for refractory pediatric inflammatory bowel disease. *Inflammatory Bowel Disease, 25*(9), 1586–1593. doi:10.1093/ibd/izz006.

Carroll, M. W., Hamilton, Z., Gill, H., Simkin, J., Smyth, M., Espinosa, V., Bressler, B., & Jacobson, K. (2016). Pediatric inflammatory bowel disease among South Asians living in British Columbia, Canada: A distinct clinical phenotype. *Inflammatory Bowel Diseases, 22*(2), 387–396. doi:10.1097/MIB.0000000000000651.

Carvalho, F. S. G., de Medeiros, I. A., & Antunes, H. (2017). Prevalence of iron deficiency anemia and iron deficiency in a pediatric population with inflammatory bowel disease. *Scandinavian Journal of Gastroenterology, 52*(10), 1099–1103. doi:10.1080/00365521.2017.1342137.

Chavannes, M., Martinez-Vinson, C., Hart, L., Kaniki, N., Chao, C. Y., Lawrence, S., Jacobson, K., Hugot, J. P., Viala, J., Deslandres, C., Jantchou, P., & Seidman, E. G. (2019). Management of paediatric patients with medically refractory Crohn's disease using ustekinumab: A multi-centred cohort study. *Journal of Crohn's & Colitis, 13*(5), 578–584. https://doi.org/10.1093/ecco-jcc/jjy206.

Cholapranee, A., Hazlewood, G. S., Kaplan, G. G., Peyrin-Biroulet, L., & Ananthakrishnan, A. N. (2017). Systematic review with meta-analysis: comparative efficacy of biologics for induction and maintenance of mucosal healing in Crohn's disease and ulcerative colitis controlled trials. *Alimentary Pharmacology & Therapeutics, 45*(10), 1291–1302. https://doi.org/10.1111/apt.14030.

Church, P. C., Ho, S., Sharma, A., Tomalty, D., Frost, K., Muise, A., Walters, T. D., & Griffiths, A. M. (2019). Intensified infliximab induction is associated with improved response and decreased colectomy in steroid-refractory paediatric ulcerative colitis. *Journal of Crohn's & Colitis, 13*(8), 982–989. doi:10.1093/ecco-jcc/jjz019.

Conrad, M. A., & Kelsen, J. R. (2020). The treatment of pediatric inflammatory bowel disease with biologic therapies. *Current Gastroenterology Reports, 22*(8), 36. doi:10.1007/s11894-020-00773-3.

Conrad, M. A., & Rosh, J. R. (2017). Pediatric inflammatory bowel disease. *Pediatric Clinics, 64*(3), 577–591.

Croft, N., Faubion, W. A., & Kugathasan, S. (2021). Efficacy and safety of adalimumab in paediatric patients with moderate-to-severe ulcerative colitis (ENVISION I): A randomized, controlled, phase 3 study. *Lancet Gastroenterology & Hepatology, 6*(8), 616–627. https://doi.org/10.1016/S2468-1253(21)00142-4.

Dahlamer, J. M., Zammitti, E. P., Ward, B. W., & Wheaton, A. (2016). Prevalence of inflammatory bowel disease among adults aged >18 years—United States, 2015. *MMWR, 65*, 1166–1169. doi:10.15585/mmwr.mm6542a3.

D'Arcangelo, G., Imondi, C., Terrin, G., Catassi, G., & Aloi, M. (2021). Is fecal calprotectin a useful marker for small bowel Crohn disease? *Journal of Pediatric Gastroenterology and Nutrition, 73*(2), 242–246. doi:10.1097/MPG.0000000000003151.

Deneau, M. R., El-Matary, W., Valentino, P. L., Abdou, R., Alqoaer, K., Amin, M., Amir, A. Z., Auth, M., Bazerbachi, F., Broderick, A., Chan, A., Cotter, J., Doan, S., El-Youssef, M., Ferrari, F., Furuya, K. N., Gottrand, M., Gottrand, F., Gupta, N., Homan, M., … Jensen, M. K. (2017). The natural history of primary sclerosing cholangitis in 781 children: A multicenter, international collaboration. *Hepatology, 66*(2), 518–527. https://doi.org/10.1002/hep.29204.

de Bie, C. I., Paerregaard, A., Kolacek, S., et al. (2013). Disease phenotype at diagnosis in pediatric Crohn's disease: 5-year analyses of the EUROKIDS registry. *Inflammatory Bowel Diseases, 19*(2), 378–385. https://doi.org/10.1002/ibd.23008.

de Ridder, L., Turner, D., Wilson, D. C., Koletzko, S., Martin-de-Carpi, J., Fagerberg, U. L., Spray, C., Sladek, M., Shaoul, R., Roma-Giannikou, E., Bronsky, J., Serban, D. E., Cucchiara, S., Veres, G., Ruemmele, F. M., Hojsak, I., Kolho, K. L., Davies, I. H., Aloi, M., Lionetti, P., … Porto IBD Working Group of ESPGHAN (2014). Malignancy and mortality in pediatric patients with inflammatory bowel disease: A multinational study from the porto pediatric IBD group. *Inflammatory Bowel Diseases, 20*(2), 291–300. https://doi.org/10.1097/01.MIB.0000439066.69340.3c.

de Zoeten, E., Pasternak, B., & Mattei, P. (2013). Diagnosis and treatment of perianal Crohn disease: NASPGHAN Clinical Report and Consensus Statement. *Journal of Pediatric Gastroenterology and Nutrition, 57*(3), 401–412. doi:10.1097/MPG.0b013e3182a025ee.

Diaconescu, S., Strat, S., Balan, G. G., Anton, C., Stefanescu, G., Ioniuc, I., & Stanescu, A. M. A (2020). Dermatological manifestations in pediatric inflammatory bowel disease. *Medicina (Kaunas), 56*(9), 425. doi:10.3390/medicina56090425.

Diederen, K., de Ridder, L., van Rheenen, P., Wolters, V. M., Mearin, M. L., Damen, G. M., de Meij, T. G., van Wering, H., Tseng, L. A., Oomen, M. W., de Jong, J. R., Sloots, C. E., Benninga, M. A., & Kindermann, A. (2017). Complications and disease recurrence after primary ileocecal resection in pediatric crohn's disease: A multicenter cohort analysis. *Inflammatory Bowel Diseases, 23*(2), 272–282. https://doi.org/10.1097/MIB.0000000000000999.

Diefenbach, K., & Breuer, C. K. (2006). Pediatric inflammatory bowel disease. *World Journal of Gastroenterology, 12*, 3204–3212.

Domenico, C., & Romano, C. (2016). Renal involvement in inflammatory bowel diseases. *Journal of Crohn's and Colitis*, 10(2), 226–235. https://doi.org/10.1093/ecco-jcc/jjv138.

Dotson, J. L., Hyams, J. S., Markowitz, J., LeLeiko, N. S., Mack, D. R., Evans, J. S., Pfefferkorn, M. D., Griffiths, A. M., Otley, A. R., Bousvaros, A., Kugathasan, S., Rosh, J. R., Keljo, D., Carvalho, R. S., Tomer, G., Mamula, P., Kay, M. H., Kerzner, B., Oliva-Hemker, M., Langton, C. R., … Crandall, W. (2010). Extraintestinal manifestations of pediatric inflammatory bowel disease and their relation to disease type and severity. *Journal of Pediatric Gastroenterology and Nutrition*, 51(2), 140–145. https://doi.org/10.1097/MPG.0b013e3181ca4db4.

Dubinsky, M. (2008). Special issues in pediatric inflammatory bowel disease. *World Journal of Gastroenterology*, 14, 413–420.

Elmahdi, R., Lemser, C. E., Thomsen, S. B., Allin, K. H., Agrawal, M., & Jess, T. (2022). Development of cancer among patients with pediatric-onset inflammatory bowel disease: A meta-analysis of population-based studies. *JAMA Network Open*, 5(3), e220595. doi:10.1001/jamanetworkopen.2022.0595.

El-Matary, W., & Bernstein, C. N. (2020). Cancer risk in pediatric-onset inflammatory bowel disease. *Frontiers in Pediatrics*(8). doi:10.3389/fped.2020.00400.

Ephgrave, K. (2007). Extra-intestinal manifestations of Crohn's disease. *Surgical Clinics of North America*, 87, 673–680.

Fish, D., & Kugathasan, S. (2004). Inflammatory bowel disease. *Adolescent Medical Clinics*, 15.

Fumery, M., Duricova, D., Gower-Rousseau, C., Annese, V., Peyrin-Biroulet, L., & Lakatos, P. L. (2016). Review article: The natural history of paediatric-onset ulcerative colitis in population-based studies. *Alimentary Pharmacology & Therapeutics*, 43(3), 346–355. doi:10.1111/apt.13478.

Goyal, A., Zheng, Y., Albenberg, L. G., Stoner, N. L., Hart, L., Alkhouri, R., Hampson, K., Ali, S., Cho-Dorado, M., Goyal, R. K., & Grossman, A. (2020). Anemia in children with inflammatory bowel disease: A position paper by the IBD Committee of the North American Society of Pediatric Gastroenterology, Hepatology and Nutrition. *Journal of Pediatric Gastroenterology and Nutrition*, 71(4), 563–582. https://doi.org/10.1097/MPG.0000000000002885.

Gray, W. N., Boyle, S. L., Graef, D. M., Janicke, D. M., Jolley, C. D., Denson, L. A., Baldassano, R. N., & Hommel, K. A. (2015). Health-related quality of life in youth with Crohn disease: Role of disease activity and parenting stress. *Journal of Pediatric Gastroenterology and Nutrition*, 60(6), 749–753. doi:10.1097/MPG.0000000000000696.

Greenley, R. N., Hommel, K. A., Nebel, J., Raboin, T., Li, T., Simpson, P., & Mackner, L. (2010). A meta-analytic review of the psychosocial adjustment of youth with inflammatory bowel disease. *Journal of Pediatric Psychology*, 35(8), 857–869. doi:10.1093/jpepsy/jsp120.

Greuter, T., Bertoldo, F., & Rechner, R. on behalf of the Swiss IBD Cohort Study Group. (2017). Extraintestinal manifestations of pediatric inflammatory bowel disease: Prevalence, presentation, and anti-TNF treatment. *Journal of Pediatric Gastroenterology and Nutrition*, 65(2), 200–206. doi:10.1097/MPG.0000000000001455.

Griffiths, A. M., & Buller, H. B. (2004). Inflammatory bowel disease. In Walker, W. A., Durie, P. R., & Hamilton, J. R. et al (Eds.), *Pediatric Gastrointestinal Disease*. BC Decker.

Gu, J., Remzi, F. H., Lian, L., & Shen, B. (2016). Practice pattern of ileal pouch surveillance in academic medical centers in the United States. *Gastroenterology Reports (Oxford)*, 4(2), 119–124. doi:10.1093/gastro/gov063.

Guandalini, S. (2014). Are probiotics or prebiotics useful in pediatric irritable bowel syndrome or inflammatory bowel disease? *Frontiers in Medicine*, 1. doi:10.3389/fmed.2014.00023.

Gupta, N., Lustig, R. H., Andrews, H., Sylvester, F., Keljo, D., Goyal, A., Gokhale, R., Patel, A. S., Guthery, S., & Leu, C. S. (2020). Introduction to and screening visit results of the multicenter pediatric Crohn's disease growth study. *Inflammatory Bowel Disease*, 26(12), 1945–1950. doi:10.1093/ibd/izaa023.

Hattar, L. N., Abraham, B. P., Malaty, H. M., Smith, E. O., & Ferry, G. D. (2012). Inflammatory bowel disease characteristics in Hispanic children in Texas. *Inflammatory Bowel Disease*, 18(3), 546–554. doi:10.1002/ibd.21698.

Hedin, C. R. H., Vavricka, S. R., Stagg, A. J., Schoepfer, A., Raine, T., Puig, L., Pleyer, U., Navarini, A., van der Meulen-de Jong, A. E., Maul, J., Katsanos, K., Kagramanova, A., Greuter, T., González-Lama, Y., van Gaalen, F., Ellul, P., Burisch, J., Bettenworth, D., Becker, M. D., Bamias, G., … Rieder, F. (2019). The pathogenesis of extraintestinal manifestations: implications for IBD research, diagnosis, and therapy. *Journal of Crohn's & Colitis*, 13(5), 541–554. https://doi.org/10.1093/ecco-jcc/jjy191.

Herfarth, H. H., Kappelman, M. D., Long, M. D., & Isaacs, K. L. (2016). Use of methotrexate in the treatment of inflammatory bowel diseases. *Inflammatory Bowel Diseases*, 22(1), 224–233. doi:10.1097/MIB.0000000000000589.

Heyman, M. B. & Committee on Nutrition. (2006). Lactose intolerance in infants, children and adolescents. *Pediatrics*, 118, 1279–1286.

Huang, H., Fang, M., Jostins, L., Umićević Mirkov, M., Boucher, G., Anderson, C. A., Andersen, V., Cleynen, I., Cortes, A., Crins, F., D'Amato, M., Deffontaine, V., Dmitrieva, J., Docampo, E., Elansary, M., Farh, K. K., Franke, A., Gori, A. S., Goyette, P., Halfvarson, J., … Barrett, J. C. (2017). Fine-mapping inflammatory bowel disease loci to single-variant resolution. *Nature*, 547(7662), 173–178. https://doi.org/10.1038/nature22969.

Hyams, J., Crandall, W., Kugathasan, S., Griffiths, A., Olson, A., Johanns, J., Liu, G., Travers, S., Heuschkel, R., Markowitz, J., Cohen, S., Winter, H., Veereman-Wauters, G., Ferry, G., Baldassano, R., & REACH Study Group (2007). Induction and maintenance infliximab therapy for the treatment of moderate-to-severe Crohn's disease in children. *Gastroenterology*, 132(3), 863–1166. https://doi.org/10.1053/j.gastro.2006.12.003.

Hyams, J., Damaraju, L., Blank, M., Johanns, J., Guzzo, C., Winter, H. S., Kugathasan, S., Cohen, S., Markowitz, J., Escher, J. C., Veereman-Wauters, G., Crandall, W., Baldassano, R., Griffiths, A., & T72 Study Group (2012a). Induction and maintenance therapy with infliximab for children with moderate to severe ulcerative colitis. *Clinical Gastroenterology and Hepatology*, 10(4), 391–9.e1. https://doi.org/10.1016/j.cgh.2011.11.026.

Hyams, J. S., Dubinsky, M. C., Baldassano, R. N., Colletti, R. B., Cucchiara, S., Escher, J., Faubion, W., Fell, J., Gold, B. D., Griffiths, A., Koletzko, S., Kugathasan, S., Markowitz, J., Ruemmele, F. M., Veereman, G., Winter, H., Masel, N., Shin, C. R., Tang, K. L., & Thayu, M. (2017). Infliximab is not associated with increased risk of malignancy or hemophagocytic lymphohistiocytosis in pediatric patients with inflammatory bowel disease. *Gastroenterology*, 152(8), 1901–1914.e3. https://doi.org/10.1053/j.gastro.2017.02.004.

Hyams, J. S., Griffiths, A., Markowitz, J., Baldassano, R. N., Faubion, W. A., Jr, Colletti, R. B., Dubinsky, M., Kierkus, J., Rosh, J., Wang, Y., Huang, B., Bittle, B., Marshall, M., & Lazar, A. (2012). Safety and efficacy of adalimumab for moderate to severe Crohn's disease in children. *Gastroenterology*, 143(2), 365–74.e2. https://doi.org/10.1053/j.gastro.2012.04.046.

Imondi, C., Terrin, G., Catassi, G., & Aloi, M. (2021). Is fecal calprotectin a useful marker for small bowel Crohn disease? *Journal of Pediatric Gastroenterology and Nutrition*, 73(2), 242–246.

Irving, P., Shanahan, F., & Rampton, D. S. (2007). Drug interactions in inflammatory bowel disease. *American Journal of Gastroenterology*, 102, 1–13.

Jansson, S., Malham, M., Paerregaard, A., Jakobsen, C., & Wewer, V. (2020). Extraintestinal manifestations are associated with disease severity in pediatric onset inflammatory bowel disease. *Journal of Pediatric Gastroenterology and Nutrition, 71*(1), 40–45. doi:10.1097/MPG.0000000000002707.

Jin, H. Y., Lim, J. S., Lee, Y., Choi, Y., Oh, S. H., Kim, K. M., Yoo, H. W., & Choi, J. H. (2021). Growth, puberty, and bone health in children and adolescents with inflammatory bowel disease. *BMC Pediatrics, 21*(1), 35. https://doi.org/10.1186/s12887-021-02496-4.

Jose, F. A., Garnett, E. A., Vittinghoff, E., Ferry, G. D., Winter, H. S., Baldassano, R. N., Kirschner, B. S., Cohen, S. A., Gold, B. D., Abramson, O., & Heyman, M. B. (2009). Development of extraintestinal manifestations in pediatric patients with inflammatory bowel disease. *Inflammatory Bowel Disease, 15*(1), 63–68. doi:10.1002/ibd.20604.

Jose, F., & Heyman, M. (2008). Extraintestinal manifestation of inflammatory bowel disease. *Journal of Pediatric Gastroenterology and Nutrition, 46*, 124–133.

Kaplan, G. (2015). The global burden of IBD from 2015-2025. *Nature Reviews Gastroenterology and Hepatology, 12*(12), 720–727.

Kappelman, M. D., Moore, K. R., Allen, J. K., & Cook, S. F. (2013). Recent trends in the prevalence of Crohn's disease and ulcerative colitis in a commercially insured US population. *Digestive Disease and Sciences, 58*(2), 519–525. doi:10.1007/s10620-012-2371-5.

Kelay, A., Tullie, L., & Stanton, M. (2019). Surgery and paediatric inflammatory bowel disease. *Translational Pediatrics, 8*(5), 436–448. doi:10.21037/tp.2019.09.01.

Kelsen, J. R., Sullivan, K. E., Rabizadeh, S., Singh, N., Snapper, S., Elkadri, A., & Grossman, A. B. (2020). North American Society for Pediatric Gastroenterology, Hepatology, and Nutrition position paper on the evaluation and management for patients with very early-onset inflammatory bowel disease. *Journal of Pediatric Gastroenterology and Nutrition, 70*(3), 389–403. doi:10.1097/MPG.0000000000002567.

Koninckx, C. R., Donat, E., Benninga, M. A., Broekaert, I. J., Gottrand, F., Kolho, K. L., Lionetti, P., Miele, E., Orel, R., Papadopoulou, A., Pienar, C., Schäppi, M. G., Wilschanski, M., & Thapar, N. (2021). The use of fecal calprotectin testing in paediatric disorders: A position paper of the European Society for Paediatric Gastroenterology and Nutrition Gastroenterology Committee. *Journal of Pediatric Gastroenterology and Nutrition, 72*(4), 617–640. https://doi.org/10.1097/MPG.0000000000003046.

Kuenzig, M. E., Fung, S. G., Marderfeld, L., Mak, J. W. Y., Kaplan, G. G., Ng, S. C., Wilson, D. C., Cameron, F., Henderson, P., Kotze, P. G., Bhatti, J., Fang, V., Gerber, S., Guay, E., Kotteduwa Jayawarden, S., Kadota, L., Maldonado D, F., Osei, J. A., Sandarage, R., Stanton, A., ... Benchimol, E. I. (2022). Twenty-first century trends in the global epidemiology of pediatric-onset inflammatory bowel disease: Systematic review. *Gastroenterology, 162*(4), 1147–1159.e4. https://doi.org/10.1053/j.gastro.2021.12.282.

Kugathasan, S., Denson, L. A., Walters, T. D., Kim, M. O., Marigorta, U. M., Schirmer, M., Mondal, K., Liu, C., Griffiths, A., Noe, J. D., Crandall, W. V., Snapper, S., Rabizadeh, S., Rosh, J. R., Shapiro, J. M., Guthery, S., Mack, D. R., Kellermayer, R., Kappelman, M. D., Steiner, S., ... Dubinsky, M. C. (2017). Prediction of complicated disease course for children newly diagnosed with Crohn's disease: A multicentre inception cohort study. *Lancet (London, England), 389*(10080), 1710–1718. https://doi.org/10.1016/S0140-6736(17)30317-3.

Kugathasan, S., Nebel, J., Skelton, J. A., Markowitz, J., Keljo, D., Rosh, J., LeLeiko, N., Mack, D., Griffiths, A., Bousvaros, A., Evans, J., Mezoff, A., Moyer, S., Oliva-Hemker, M., Otley, A., Pfefferkorn, M., Crandall, W., Wyllie, R., Hyams, J., Wisconsin Pediatric Inflammatory Bowel Disease Alliance, ... Pediatric Inflammatory Bowel Disease Collaborative Research Group (2007). Body mass index in children with newly diagnosed inflammatory bowel disease: Observations from two multicenter North American inception cohorts. *Journal of Pediatrics, 151*(5), 523–527. https://doi.org/10.1016/j.jpeds.2007.04.004.

Laborda, T. J., Jensen, M. K., Kavan, M., et al. (2019). Treatment of primary sclerosing cholangitis in children. *World Journal of Hepatology, 11*(1), 19–36. doi:10.4254/wjh.v11.i1.19.

Lane, E. R., Zisman, T. L., & Suskind, D. L. (2017). The microbiota in inflammatory bowel disease: Current and therapeutic insights. *Journal of Inflammation Research, 10*, 63–73. doi:10.2147/JIR.S116088.org.

Leichtner, A. M., & Higuchi, L. (2004). Ulcerative colitis. In Walker, W. A., Goulet, O., & Kleinman R.E., et al. (Eds.), *Pediatric Gastrointestinal Disease*. BC Decker.

Levine, A., Koletzko, S., Turner, D., Escher, J. C., Cucchiara, S., de Ridder, L., Kolho, K. L., Veres, G., Russell, R. K., Paerregaard, A., Buderus, S., Greer, M. L., Dias, J. A., Veereman-Wauters, G., Lionetti, P., Sladek, M., Martin de Carpi, J., Staiano, A., Ruemmele, F. M., Wilson, D. C., ... European Society of Pediatric Gastroenterology, Hepatology, and Nutrition (2014). ESPGHAN revised porto criteria for the diagnosis of inflammatory bowel disease in children and adolescents. *Journal of Pediatric Gastroenterology and Nutrition, 58*(6), 795–806. https://doi.org/10.1097/MPG.0000000000000239.

Mack, D. R., Langton, C., Markowitz, J., LeLeiko, N., Griffiths, A., Bousvaros, A., Evans, J., Kugathasan, S., Otley, A., Pfefferkorn, M., Rosh, J., Mezoff, A., Moyer, S., Oliva-Hemker, M., Rothbaum, R., Wyllie, R., delRosario, J. F., Keljo, D., Lerer, T., Hyams, J., ... Pediatric Inflammatory Bowel Disease Collaborative Research Group (2007). Laboratory values for children with newly diagnosed inflammatory bowel disease. *Pediatrics, 119*(6), 1113–1119. https://doi.org/10.1542/peds.2006-1865.

Mackner, L. M., & Crandall, W. V. (2007). Psychological factors affecting pediatric inflammatory bowel disease. *Current Opinion in Pediatrics, 19*(5), 548–552. doi:10.1097/MOP.0b013e3282ef4426.

Malaty, H. M., Abraham, B. P., Mehta, S., Garnett, E. A., & Ferry, G. D. (2013). The natural history of ulcerative colitis in a pediatric population: A follow-up population-based cohort study. *Clinical and Experimental Gastroenterology, 6*, 77–83. doi:10.2147/CEG.S40259.

Mattiello, V., Schmugge, M., Hengartner, H., von der Weid, N., Renella, R., & SPOG Pediatric Hematology Working Group (2020). Diagnosis and management of iron deficiency in children with or without anemia: Consensus recommendations of the SPOG Pediatric Hematology Working Group. *European Journal of Pediatrics, 179*(4), 527–545. https://doi.org/10.1007/s00431-020-03597-5.

Maxwell, E. C., Dawany, N., Baldassano, R. N., Mamula, P., Mattei, P., Albenberg, L., & Kelsen, J. R. (2017). Diverting ileostomy for the treatment of severe, refractory, pediatric inflammatory bowel disease. *Journal of Pediatric Gastroenterology and Nutrition, 65*(3), 299–305. doi:10.1097/MPG.0000000000001498.

Michailidou, M., & Nfonsam, V. N. (2018). Preoperative anemia and outcomes in patients undergoing surgery for inflammatory bowel disease. *American Journal of Surgery, 215*, 78–81.

Mishra, J., Stubbs, M., Kuang, L., Vara, N., Kumar, P., & Kumar, N. (2022). Inflammatory bowel disease therapeutics: A focus on probiotic engineering. *Mediators of Inflammation, 2022*, 9621668. doi:10.1155/2022/9621668.

Mitchel, E. B., & Rosh, J. R. (2022). Pediatric management of Crohn's disease. *Gastroenterology Clinics of North America, 51*(2), 401–424. doi:10.1016/j.gtc.2021.12.013.

Molodecky, N. A., Soon, I. S., Rabi, D. M., Ghali, W. A., Ferris, M., Chernoff, G., Benchimol, E. I., Panaccione, R., Ghosh, S., Barkema, H. W., & Kaplan, G. G. (2012). Increasing incidence and prevalence of the inflammatory bowel diseases with time, based on systematic review. *Gastroenterology, 142*(1), 46–e30. https://doi.org/10.1053/j.gastro.2011.10.001.

Moore, H., Dubes, L., & Fusillo, S. (2021). Tofacitinib therapy in children and young adults with pediatric-onset medically refractory inflammatory bowel disease. *Journal of Pediatric Gastroenterology and Nutrition, 73*(3), e57–e62. doi:10.1097/MPG.0000000000003190.

Nambu, R., Warner, N., Mulder, D. J, Kotlarz, D., McGovern, D. P. B., Cho, J., Klein, C., Snapper, S. B., Griffiths, A. M., Iwama, I., & Muise, A. M. (2022). A systematic review of monogenic inflammatory bowel disease. *Clinical Gastroenterology and Hepatology, 20*(4), e653–e663. doi:10.1016/j.cgh.2021.03.021.

Nasiri, S., Kuenzig, M. E., & Benchimol, E. (2017). Long-term outcomes of pediatric inflammatory bowel disease. *Seminars in Pediatric Surgery, 26*(6), 398–404. doi:10.1053/j.sempedsurg.2017.10.010.

Nishida, A., Inoue, R., Inatomi, O., Bamba, S., Naito, Y., & Andoh, A. (2018). Gut microbiota in the pathogenies of inflammatory bowel disease. *Clinical Journal of Gastroenterology, 11*(1), 1–10. doi:10.1007/s12328-017-0813-5.

Orlanski-Meyer, E., Aardoom, M., Ricciuto, A., Navon, D., Carman, N., Aloi, M., Bronsky, J., Däbritz, J., Dubinsky, M., Hussey, S., Lewindon, P., Martin De Carpi, J., Navas-López, V. M., Orsi, M., Ruemmele, F. M., Russell, R. K., Veres, G., Walters, T. D., Wilson, D. C., Kaiser, T., ... Turner, D. (2021). Predicting outcomes in pediatric ulcerative colitis for management optimization: Systematic review and consensus statements from the Pediatric Inflammatory Bowel Disease-Ahead Program. *Gastroenterology, 160*(1), 378–402.e22. https://doi.org/10.1053/j.gastro.2020.07.066.

Pabby, V., Oza, S. S., Dodge, L. E., Hacker, M. R., Moragianni, V. A., Correia, K., Missmer, S. A., Fox, J. H., Ibrahim, Y., Penzias, A., Burakoff, R., Cheifetz, A., & Friedman, S. (2015). In vitro fertilization is successful in women with ulcerative colitis and ileal pouch anal anastomosis. *American Journal of Gastroenterology, 110*(6), 792–797. https://doi.org/10.1038/ajg.2014.400.

Pappa, H., Thayu, M., Sylvester, F., Leonard, M., Zemel, B., & Gordon, C. (2011). A clinical report on skeletal health of children and adolescents with inflammatory bowel disease. *Journal of Pediatric Gastroenterology and Nutrition, 53*(1), 11–25. doi:10.1097/MPG.0b013e31821988a3.

Peneau, A., Savoye, G., Turck, D., Dauchet, L., Fumery, M., Salleron, J., Lerebours, E., Ligier, K., Vasseur, F., Dupas, J. L., Mouterde, O., Spyckerelle, C., Djeddi, D., Peyrin-Biroulet, L., Colombel, J. F., & Gower-Rousseau, C. (2013). Mortality and cancer in pediatric-onset inflammatory bowel disease: A population-based study. *American Journal of Gastroenterology, 108*(10), 1647–1653. https://doi.org/10.1038/ajg.2013.242.

Plumptre, I., Knabel, D., & Tomecki, K. (2018). Pyoderma gangrenosum: A review for the gastroenterologist. *Inflammatory Bowel Disease, 24*(12), 2510–2517. doi:10.1093/ibd/izy174.

Physicians' desk reference. (2008). Medical Economics Data Production.

Ponsky, T., Hindle, A., & Sandler, A. (2007). Inflammatory bowel disease in the pediatric patient. *Surgical Clinics of North America, 87*, 643–658.

Qiu, Y., Chen, B. L, Mao, R., Zhang, S. H., He, Y., Zeng, Z. R., Ben-Horin, S., & Chen, M. H. (2017). Systematic review with meta-analysis: Loss of response and requirement of anti-TNFα dose intensification in Crohn's disease. *Journal of Gastroenterol, 52*(5), 535–554. doi:10.1007/s00535-017-1324-3.

Reich, J., Wasan, S., & Farraye, F. A. (2016). Vaccinating patients with inflammatory bowel disease. *Gastroenterology and Hepatology, 12*(9), 540–546.

Ricciuto, A., Aardoom, M., & Orlanski-Meyer, E., Pediatric Inflammatory Bowel Disease–Ahead Steering Committee. (2021). Predicting outcomes in pediatric Crohn's disease for management optimization: Systematic review and

consensus statements from the Pediatric Inflammatory Bowel Disease-Ahead Program. *Gastroenterology, 160*(1), 403–436. doi:10.1053/j.gastro.2020.07.065. e26.

Rivas, M. A., Avila, B. E., Koskela, J., Huang, H., Stevens, C., Pirinen, M., Haritunians, T., Neale, B. M., Kurki, M., Ganna, A., Graham, D., Glaser, B., Peter, I., Atzmon, G., Barzilai, N., Levine, A. P., Schiff, E., Pontikos, N., Weisburd, B., Lek, M., ... Daly, M. J. (2018). Insights into the genetic epidemiology of Crohn's and rare diseases in the Ashkenazi Jewish population. *PLoS Genetics, 14*(5), e1007329. https://doi.org/10.1371/journal.pgen.1007329.

Rosen, M. J., Dhawan, A., & Saeed, S. A. (2015). Inflammatory bowel disease in children and adolescents. *JAMA Pediatrics, 169*(11), 1053–1060. doi:10.1001/jamapediatrics.2015.1982.

Rosh, J. R., Turner, D., Padgett, L., Cohen, S. A., Jacobstein, D., Adedokun, O. J., Padgett, L., Terry, N. A., O'Brien, C., & Hyams, J. S. (2021). Ustekinumab in paediatric patients with moderately to severely active Crohn's disease: Pharmacokinetics, safety, and efficacy results from UniStar, a phase 1 study. *Journal of Crohn's & Colitis, 15*(11), 1931–1942. doi:10.1093/ecco-jcc/jjab089.

Rudrapatna, V. A., & Velayos, F. (2019). Biosimilars for the treatment of inflammatory bowel disease. *Practical Gastroenterology, 43*(4), 84–91.

Ruemmele, F. M., Pigneur, B., & Garnier-Lengliné, H. (2014). Enteral nutrition as treatment option for Crohn's disease: In kids only? In *Nutrition, gut microbiota and immunity: Therapeutic targets for IBD* (pp. 115–123). Karger Publishers.

Rufo, P. A., Denson, L. A, Sylvester, F. A., Szigethy, E., Sathya, P., Lu, Y., Wahbeh, G. T., Sena, L. M., & Faubion, W. A. (2012). Health supervision in the management of children and adolescents with IBD: NASPGHAN recommendations. *Journal of Pediatric Gastroenterology and Nutrition, 55*(1), 93–108. doi:10.1097/MPG.0b013e31825959b8.

Sanderson, I. (2014). Growth problems in children with IBD. *Nature Reviews Gastroenterology and Hepatology, 11*, 601–610. https://doi.org/10.1038/nrgastro.2014.102.

Saubermann, L. J., Deneau, M., Falcone, R. A., Murray, K. F., Ali, S., Kohli, R., Ekong, U. D., Valentino, P. L., Grossman, A. B., Rand, E. B., Jonas, M. M., Saeed, S. A., & Kamath, B. M. (2017). Hepatic issues and complications associated with inflammatory bowel disease: A clinical report from the NASPGHAN Inflammatory Bowel Disease and Hepatology Committees. *Journal of Pediatric Gastroenterology and Nutrition, 64*(4), 639–652. https://doi.org/10.1097/MPG.0000000000001492.

Serpico, M. R., Boyle, B. M., Kemper, K. J., & Kim, S. C. (2016). Complementary and alternative medicine use in children with inflammatory bowel diseases: A single-center survey. *Journal of Pediatric Gastroenterology and Nutrition, 63*(6), 651–657. doi:10.1097/MPG.0000000000001187.

Sinakos, E., Samuel, S., Enders, F., et al. (2013). Inflammatory bowel disease in primary sclerosing cholangitis: A robust yet changing relationship. *Inflammatory Bowel Diseases, 190*(5), 1004–1009. https://doi.org/10.1097/MIB.0b013e3182802893.

Singh, N., Rabizadeh, S., Jossen, J., Pittman, N., Check, M., Hashemi, G., Phan, B. L., Hyams, J. S., & Dubinsky, M. C. (2016). Multi-center experience of vedolizumab effectiveness in pediatric inflammatory bowel disease. *Inflammatory Bowel Diseases, 22*(9), 2121–2126. https://doi.org/10.1097/MIB.0000000000000865.

States, V., O'Brien, S., Rai, J. P., Roberts, H. L., Paas, M., Feagins, K., Pierce, E. J., Baumgartner, R. N., & Galandiuk, S. (2020). Pyoderma gangrenosum in inflammatory bowel disease: A systematic review and meta-analysis. *Digestive Disease and Sciences, 65*(9), 2675–2685. doi:10.1007/s10610-019-05999-4.

Stucchi, A. F., Aarons, C. B., & Becker, J. M. (2006). Surgical approaches to cancer in patients who have inflammatory bowel disease. *Gastroenterology Clinics of North America, 35*, 641–673.

Sýkora, J., Pomahačová, R., Kreslová, M., Cvalínová, D., Štych, P., & Schwarz, J. (2018). Current global trends in the incidence of pediatric-onset inflammatory bowel disease. *World Journal of Gastroenterology, 24*(25), 2741–2763. doi:10.3748/wjg.v24.i25.2741.

Turner, D., Hyams, J., Markowitz, J., Lerer, T., Mack, D. R., Evans, J., Pfefferkorn, M., Rosh, J., Kay, M., Crandall, W., Keljo, D., Otley, A. R., Kugathasan, S., Carvalho, R., Oliva-Hemker, M., Langton, C., Mamula, P., Bousvaros, A., LeLeiko, N., … Pediatric IBD Collaborative Research Group. (2009). Appraisal of the pediatric ulcerative colitis activity index (PUCAI). *Inflammatory Bowel Disease, 15*(8), 1218–1223. doi:10.1002/ibd.20867.

Turner, D., Levine, A., Kolho, K. L., Shaoul, R., & Ledder, O. (2014). Combination of oral antibiotics may be effective in severe pediatric ulcerative colitis: A preliminary report. *Journal of Crohn's & Colitis, 8*(11), 1464–1470. https://doi.org/10.1016/j.crohns.2014.05.010.

Turner, D., Ruemmele, F. M., Orlanski-Meyer, E., Griffiths, A. M., de Carpi, J. M., Bronsky, J., Veres, G., Aloi, M., Strisciuglio, C., Braegger, C. P., Assa, A., Romano, C., Hussey, S., Stanton, M., Pakarinen, M., de Ridder, L., Katsanos, K., Croft, N., Navas-López, V., Wilson, D. C., … Russell, R. K. (2018). Management of paediatric ulcerative colitis, part 1: Ambulatory care-an evidence-based guideline from European Crohn's and Colitis Organization and European Society of Paediatric Gastroenterology, Hepatology and Nutrition. *Journal of Pediatric Gastroenterology and Nutrition, 67*(2), 257–291. https://doi.org/10.1097/MPG.0000000000002035.

Valentino, P. L., Feldman, B. M., Walters, T. D., Griffiths, A. M., Ling, S. C., Pullenayegum, E. M., & Kamath, B. M. (2015). Abnormal liver biochemistry is common in pediatric inflammatory bowel disease: Prevalence and associations. *Inflammatory Bowel Diseases, 21*(12), 2848–2856. doi:10.1097/MIB.0000000000000558.

Van Limbergen, J., Russell, R. K., Drummond, H. E., Aldhous, M. C., Round, N. K., Nimmo, E. R., Smith, L., Gillett, P. M., McGrogan, P., Weaver, L. T., Bisset, W. M., Mahdi, G., Arnott, I. D., Satsangi, J., & Wilson, D. C. (2008). Definition of phenotypic characteristics of childhood-onset inflammatory bowel disease. *Gastroenterology, 135*(4), 1114–1122. https://doi.org/10.1053/j.gastro.2008.06.081.

Waljee, A., Waljee, J., Morris, A. M., & Higgins, P. D. (2006). Threefold increased risk of infertility: A meta-analysis of infertility after ileal pouch anal anastomosis in ulcerative colitis. *Gut, 55*(11), 1575–1580. https://doi.org/10.1136/gut.2005.090316.

White, J. M., O'Connor, S., Winter, H. S., Heyman, M. B., Kirschner, B. S., Ferry, G. D., Cohen, S. A., Baldassano, R. N., Smith, T., Clemons, T., & Gold, B. D. (2008). Inflammatory bowel disease in African American children compared with other racial/ethnic groups in a multicenter registry. *Clinical Gastroenterology and Hepatology, 6*(12), 1361–1369. doi:10.1016/j.cgh.2008.07.032.

Wong, S. C., Smyth, A., McNeill, E., Galloway, P. J., Hassan, K., McGrogan, P., & Ahmed, S. F. (2010). The growth hormone insulin-like growth factor 1 axis in children and adolescents with inflammatory bowel disease and growth retardation. *Clinical Endocrinology, 73*(2), 220–228. https://doi.org/10.1111/j.1365-2265.2010.03799.x.

Ye, Y., Manne, S., Treem, W. R., & Bennett, D. (2020). Prevalence of inflammatory bowel disease in pediatric and adult populations: Recent estimates from large national databases in the United States, 2007–2016. *Inflammatory Bowel Diseases, 26*(4), 619–625. doi:10.1093/ibd/izz182.

28 Juvenile Idiopathic Arthritis

Tedra S. Smith

ETIOLOGY

Juvenile idiopathic arthritis (JIA) is the most common chronic rheumatic disease in childhood (Spiegel et al., 2015). JIA has the potential to affect joints located in any part of the body. The etiology is unknown; however, it is considered genetic in nature and highly affected by environmental triggers that lead to an autoimmune response (McKeever & Kelly, 2015). JIA is divided into several subtypes based on symptoms, treatment, and prognosis. An interprofessional team is employed for efficient treatment.

Over the past few years many researchers have studied the genetic and environmental factors related to JIA. The etiology of chronic arthritis in childhood is unknown. This condition is not a single disease entity but represents a heterogeneous group of phenotypes with several modes of onset (Giancane et al., 2016). Differences in onset and clinical course should be considered when researching causation and treatment. Current hypotheses focus on inflammatory and immune dysregulation, infection, psychological stress, trauma, and hormonal factors as potential contributing factors in a child with a genetic predisposition. Inflammation in JIA results from the interaction of different cell types (myeloid, lymphoid, and stromal) and the mediators they release (Barut et al., 2017; Zaripova et al., 2021). Research has shown that children with chronic arthritis have elevated levels of numerous cytokines, including tumor necrosis factor-alpha (TNF-alpha), macrophage inhibitory factor, interleukin (IL), interferon-gamma, and several chemokines with different profiles among the different JIA onset types (Barut et al., 2017; Zaripova et al., 2021). Epidemiologic studies have shown familial, seasonal, geographic, and ethnic differences among the subtypes of chronic childhood arthritis, suggesting environmental and genetic factors (Zaripova et al., 2021).

A complex interaction of genetic and environmental factors determines susceptibility to JIA. JIA does not tend to occur in multiple family members. The observation that even identical twins do not have a high concordance for JIA suggests that other influences, such as environment and chance, are important. The division of JIA into different subtypes based on clinical characteristics has been reflected in differences in genetic associations among the subtypes. However, even within one subtype of JIA, multiple genes are involved.

Certain subtypes of JIA are associated with human leukocyte antigen (HLA) alleles (i.e., pauciarticular JIA with alleles of HLA-DR5). JIA subtypes with early onset are associated with the HLA-A2 allele (Rigante et al., 2015). DR5, DR8, and HLA-A2 are often associated with oligoarticular JIA, and DRB1*08 and DPBI*03 with rheumatoid factor (RF)–negative polyarticular arthritis (Rigante et al., 2015). In addition to HLA genes, some other individual genes associated with JIA susceptibility include tumor necrosis factor (TNF), macrophage migration inhibitory factor, IL-2, IL-10, and IL-6 (Zaripova et al., 2021).

CLINICAL MANIFESTATIONS

INCIDENCE AND PREVALENCE

The estimated incidence and prevalence of childhood chronic arthritis differ markedly across a range of studies, in part because of the discrepancies in classification criteria. One study reported that the prevalence of JIA in children and adolescents is 70/100,000 (Schmidt et al., 2022). According to a systematic review, the incidence varies worldwide, ranging from 1.6 to 23 per 100,000 (Marzetti et al., 2017). The prevalence in the same article reported 3.8 to 400 per 100,000 (Marzetti et al., 2017).

DIAGNOSTIC CRITERIA

By definition JIA in children and adolescents begins before the age of 16 years (National Institute of Arthritis and Musculoskeletal and Skin Diseases [NIAMS], 2021). Diagnostic criteria for JIA are determined by subtypes. Misdiagnosis of JIA results when the following four key points are missed: (1) Arthralgia (joint pain) alone is not sufficient to make the diagnosis; arthritis must be present. (2) Arthritis must persist for at least 6 weeks. (3) All other causes of chronic arthritis in children must be excluded. These causes include but are not limited to other pediatric rheumatic diseases such as lupus, dermatomyositis, vasculitis, sarcoidosis, scleroderma, and periodic fever syndromes. In addition, nonrheumatic causes of arthritis must be ruled out, including metabolic, infectious, neoplastic, congenital, traumatic, and degenerative causes. (4) There are no signs, symptoms, or results of laboratory investigations pathognomonic for JIA. Imaging such as x-rays and magnetic resonance imaging may be used to aid in diagnosis. Children should be referred to a pediatric rheumatologist when the clinician suspects an underlying rheumatic, inflammatory, or autoimmune disorder.

CLINICAL MANIFESTATIONS AT TIME OF DIAGNOSIS

A joint with arthritis exhibits one or more of the following signs of inflammation: swelling, warmth, redness, pain or tenderness, and/or reduced range of motion. Swelling results from an intraarticular effusion or hypertrophy (thickening) of the synovial membrane. Synovitis may develop insidiously and exist for months or years without causing detectable joint damage or may damage cartilage, subchondral bone, or other joint structures in a relatively short time (Mueller, 2015). Clinical features range from mild synovitis in one joint with no systemic symptoms to moderate-severe disease in many joints.

Common clinical manifestations, in addition to synovial inflammation, include morning stiffness and stiffness after a period of inactivity. Mild stiffness resolves within a few minutes of walking; however, severe stiffness may take several hours to dissipate. Many children present with painless joint effusions or mandibular asymmetry (Momah & Ray, 2019), and some may have joint contractures. However, because these children are able to maintain normal activity levels, the diagnosis is often delayed.

History and physical examination are key to the diagnosis of chronic inflammatory arthritis. Paradoxically, children whose chief complaint is musculoskeletal pain alone are highly unlikely to have chronic inflammatory arthritis. Another pitfall in the diagnosis of JIA is the erroneous belief that antinuclear antibody (ANA) and/or RF are sensitive and specific for diagnosis. At least 10% of healthy children have a positive ANA result, with a higher percentage in children who have relatives with autoimmune diseases. Therefore the rate of false-positive ANA results is too high for this test to be a good predictor of JIA. RF is rarely positive in healthy children but is present in only a small proportion of children with JIA. Therefore the utility of RF as a screening tool is very limited. This test should generally be ordered for prognostic value after a diagnosis of inflammatory arthritis is made clinically. The primary care provider must remember that childhood arthritis, except for polyarticular RF-positive JIA, is a different disease entity with different clinical and diagnostic parameters from the adult form of rheumatoid arthritis.

TYPES OF ONSET

Manifestations at the time of onset and throughout the first 6 months of the disease determine classification into one of seven major subtypes. These subtypes are defined by the number of joints involved and extraarticular features. They are characterized by differences in patterns in the severity of joint disease, immunogenetics, age at onset, and sex of the child (McKeever & Kelly, 2015). JIA typically manifests exacerbations (flares) followed by periods of improvement. Exacerbations may occur during episodes of acute illness or stress. The frequency and duration of flares are unpredictable but are easily recognized and should be rapidly treated. Children with systemic JIA may also experience constitutional symptoms, such as fever, anorexia, weight loss, growth failure, and fatigue.

Subtypes of Juvenile Idiopathic Arthritis

Oligoarthritis. Oligoarthritis typically affects the elbow, knee, and ankle joints. It occurs in four or less joints and affects more females than males. It is the most common and mildest subtype of JIA that may go into remission by adulthood. Onset is usually between the ages of 2 and 4 years. This subtype can be further divided into persistent and expanded oligoarthritis. About 50% of the cases of JIA are of this type (NIAMS, 2021). Uveitis, chronic inflammation of the anterior part of the eye, is a major complication in this group. Patients with this type should be evaluated by an ophthalmologist at the onset.

Polyarthritis (rheumatoid factor negative). Polyarthritis with RF negative affects five or more joints during the first 6 months and is usually bilateral. The RF result will be negative. Age of onset is typically between 2 and 4 years or late onset between 6 and 12 years of age. Females are generally more commonly affected than males.

Polyarthritis (rheumatoid factor positive). Those in the small subgroup with polyarticular JIA and RF positivity are more likely to have early onset of erosive arthritis, rheumatoid nodules, and a chronic course persisting into adulthood (McKeever & Kelly, 2015). Extraarticular manifestations can include fatigue, low-grade fevers, anemia, osteopenia, mild lymphadenopathy, and rheumatoid nodules. Laboratory findings in polyarticular JIA include elevated or normal erythrocyte sedimentation rate (ESR), leukocyte count, and platelet count. Onset is late childhood or adolescence.

Psoriatic arthritis. Psoriatic arthritis is diagnosed when there is a diagnosis of arthritis and psoriasis or a diagnosis of arthritis and at least two of the following: nail pitting, dactylitis, onycholysis, psoriasis in a first-degree relative. Females are more commonly affected than males.

Enthesitis-related arthritis. Enthesitis-related arthritis was previously known as spondyloarthropathy. The spine, hips, and entheses (points where tendons and ligaments attach to the bone) are often affected. It is not uncommon for acute uveitis to occur in patients with this subtype. Males are affected more than females. Diagnosis is determined by at least two of the following: sacroiliac joint pain, anterior uveitis, Reiter syndrome, the onset of JIA in males over 6 years of age, HLA-B27 antigen present, sacroiliitis with inflammatory bowel disease (McKeever & Kelly, 2015).

Systemic arthritis. Systemic arthritis may also be referred to as Still disease. This subtype may affect the entire body or many body systems. Symptoms often include a daily fever that lasts for 2 weeks or more and accompanied by an erythematous rash, lymph node enlargement, hepatomegaly, splenomegaly, or serositis. The diagnostic hallmark of this type of arthritis is the fever pattern. The fevers are characterized by daily or twice-daily spiking temperatures higher than 102°F (38.8°C), with a rapid return to normal or below the baseline. The fever usually occurs in the late afternoon or evening in conjunction with the classic systemic JIA rash. The rash consists of discrete, small (2–6 mm), evanescent (fleeting), salmon-pink, and generally circumscribed macular lesions (Giancane et al., 2016). This rash may become confluent, with larger lesions developing pale centers and pale peripheries. It is seen mostly on the trunk, extremities, and overpressure areas, but the face, palms, and soles also may be involved. The rash is most prominent during fever spikes and may be visible only after the skin is rubbed or scratched. Males and females are affected equally.

Undifferentiated arthritis. Arthritis symptoms, primarily inflammation, do not meet the criteria for any other subtype and are persistent for at least 6 weeks.

TREATMENT

Management of chronic arthritis in childhood is most successful with early diagnosis and institution of early aggressive treatment with targeted interventions. The cornerstones of treatment are antiinflammatory and disease-modifying medication, with newer, more effective treatments recently emerging. Interdisciplinary, family-centered treatment interventions incorporate the team approach, including the family and child, pediatric rheumatologist, advanced practice nurse, clinic nurse, primary care provider, physical therapist, occupational therapist, and social worker. Consultations with the ophthalmologist, orthopedist,

psychologist, dietitian, orthodontist, interventional radiologist, and other pediatric specialists are sought as indicated.

PHARMACOLOGIC THERAPY

Treatment of chronic arthritis in childhood has made great strides in the past 50 years. At one time, aspirin was the only antiinflammatory medication used, and many children with chronic arthritis eventually required wheelchairs or were blinded by uveitis. The pace of development of new therapies has increased most dramatically in the past 10 years.

Specific pharmacologic agents used to treat JIA are identified in Table 28.1. Nonsteroidal antiinflammatory drugs (NSAIDs) remain one of the cornerstones of treatment for JIA (Onel et al., 2022a); naproxen and ibuprofen are the most used (Giancane et al., 2016). Pediatric rheumatologists may trend toward less frequent use of NSAIDs in favor of intraarticular corticosteroids (IACs) and early aggressive treatment (Giancane et al., 2016).

IAC injections are a commonly used treatment of JIA and specifically for oligoarthritis; triamcinolone hexacetonide is considered the most effective (Giancane et al., 2016). Potential complications from using IACs include skin changes at the injection site, septic arthritis, and synovitis (Giancane et al., 2016).

Conventional synthetic disease-modifying antirheumatic drugs (DMARDs) are more aggressive treatment than NSAIDs and may be used either initially or after NSAID failure. Methotrexate is the most common DMARD for all forms of JIA based on its high efficacy to side effect profile in children (Onel et al., 2022a) and is commonly used in combination with other agents. Methotrexate may also be used for uveitis control when topical glucocorticoids are used and the patient is not currently on systemic therapy (Angeles-Han et al., 2019). Methotrexate may be given orally or subcutaneously; the latter is associated with better absorption and fewer gastrointestinal (GI) side effects. Folic acid should be used in conjunction with methotrexate to improve the tolerability of folate deficiency caused by methotrexate (Onel et al., 2022a). For the sickest children, particularly those with systemic-onset JIA, systemic glucocorticoids are often necessary to control disease activity. The steroids are usually given daily oral doses and weekly to monthly IV boluses. Unfortunately, systemic corticosteroids are associated with many adverse effects, including an increased risk of sepsis, fracture, and venous thromboembolism (Dvorin & Ebell, 2020). More aggressive therapy may be necessary to limit steroid usage to the shortest possible duration.

The introduction of biologic response modifiers, which inhibit cytokines or cellular immune responses, has been revolutionary for treating JIA. These medications are generally becoming more common in patients

Table 28.1 Pharmacologic Therapy for Juvenile Idiopathic Arthritis

DRUG	TRADE NAME	DOSING	SIDE EFFECTS	LABORATORY MONITORS
Nonsteroidal Antiinflammatory Drugs (NSAIDs)[a]				
Naproxen[b]	Anaprox DS Naprosyn Aleve (OTC)	10–20 mg/kg/day bid (PO)	*For all NSAIDs:* abdominal pain, dizziness, drowsiness, fluid retention, gastric ulcers and bleeding, greater susceptibility to bruising or bleeding, heartburn, indigestion, lightheadedness, nausea, rash, reduction in kidney function, anemia, increase in liver enzymes, behavioral changes *For naproxen and some others:* pseudoporphyria with sun exposure	CBC with differential, UA, BUN, creatinine, and LFTs initially, at 6 wk then every 6–12 mo
Ibuprofen[b]	Advil (OTC) Motrin IB (OTC) Motrin (Rx)	30–40 mg/kg/day (PO)	Same as all NSAIDs	Sane as Naproxen
Indomethacin[b]	Indocin Tivorbex	1–2 mg/kg/day bid-qid Max dose: the lesser of 4 mg/kg/24 hr or 200 mg/2 hr	*For Indomethacin:* depression, severe headaches, dizziness	
COX-2 Inhibitor				
*Celecoxib	Celebrex	≥10 kg to ≤25 kg: 50 mg bid >25 kg: 100 mg bid	Same as traditional NSAIDs, but less likely to cause gastric ulcers, bleeding, and bruising *Cautions:* sensitivity to sulfonamides or allergies to aspirin or other NSAIDs	CBC periodically
Disease Modifying Antirheumatic Drugs (DMARDs)				
*Methotrexate (MTX)	RediTrex Trexall	0.5 mg/kg once weekly (Max initial dose 15 mg/dose) (Oral and SQ)	Nausea, vomiting, mouth sores, increased liver enzymes, myelosuppression, hair loss *Cautions:* abnormal blood count, liver or lung disease, active infection or fever; NO alcohol; causes birth defects if taken during pregnancy	CBC with differential and platelets, serum creatinine, LFTs every month ×3 mo, then every 3–6 mo: Eye exam within 1 month of starting and every 3 months during active disease
Sulfasalazine	Azulfidine Azulfidine EN-Tabs	40–50 mg/kg/24 hr. (Mild) 5–75 mg/kg/24 hr. (Moderate/severe) Maximum 4 g/24 hr	Stomach upset, diarrhea, dizziness, headache, light sensitivity, itching, rash, loss of appetite, nausea, vomiting, increased liver enzymes, lowered blood count *Cautions:* allergy to sulfa or aspirin; kidney, liver, or blood disease; avoid prolonged sun exposure; take with food; do not take with Maalox or Mylanta-type antacids	CBC with differentials, serum creatinine, LFTS baseline then every 2–4 weeks for 3 mo after initiation and dose changes then every 12 weeks for 6 mo

[a]Pediatric dose of NSAIDs based on mg/kg should not exceed adult dose. Do not take NSAIDs with other OTC NSAIDs. Always take NSAIDs with food. Remind parents that NSAIDs are mainly to treat chronic inflammation and are to be continued as prescribed even if child does not complain of pain.
[b]Available as suspension.
BID, twice daily; *BP,* blood pressure; *BUN,* blood urea nitrogen; *CBC,* complete blood count; *LFTs,* liver function tests; *PO* by mouth, *SQ,* subcutaneously; *TB,* tuberculosis; *UA,* urinalysis.
From Kleinman, K., McDaniel, L., & Molloy, M. (2021). *The Harriet Lane Handbook* (22nd ed.). Elsevier.
*Methotrexate Drug Information (2023). Up To Date. Lexicomp.
*Celecoxib Drug Information (2023). Up To Date. Lexicomp.

with JIA to reach disease remission. Etanercept and adalimumab, administered by subcutaneous injection, inhibit TNF-alpha, a potent proinflammatory cytokine. Etanercept was the first available biologic agent for JIA and is safe and effective in the treatment of polyarticular JIA unresponsive to methotrexate (Vanoni et al., 2017). Adalimumab was approved by the US Food and Drug Administration (FDA) in 2009 for treatment of JIA (Vanoni et al., 2017). Infliximab injection has been effective in improving the status of patients with polyarticular JIA when combined with methotrexate (Vanoni et al., 2017). Abatacept, an inhibitor of lymphocyte activation by the costimulatory blockade, is FDA approved and often used to treat systemic JIA when it is TNF unresponsive (McKeever & Kelly, 2015). Anakinra (Kineret), an IL-1 receptor antagonist, has been useful in treating systemic JIA when administered in daily subcutaneous injections (Vanoni et al., 2017). Tocilizumab (Actemra), an IL-6 receptor antagonist given via intravenous infusion, is approved for children 2 years and older with polyarticular JIA and systemic JIA. Cosentyx (secukinumab), an IL-17A antagonist, decreases inflammation in the treatment of psoriatic arthritis and enthesitis-related arthritis in children. Stelara (ustekinumab) targets IL-2 and IL-3 and is used to treat psoriatic JIA in children 6 years and older. Screening for hepatitis B, human immunodeficiency virus infection, hepatitis C, and tuberculosis is important prior to starting biologics (Momah & Ray, 2019).

EXERCISE AND THERAPY

Studies have shown that children and adolescents with JIA have impaired aerobic and anaerobic exercise capacity (Bayraktar et al., 2018). Existing evidence does demonstrate that individualized conditioning programs, such as aerobic exercise and aquatic training, have both physical and psychological benefits. These programs can increase aerobic capacity, muscular strength, endurance, and stamina for daily activities without aggravating joint disease (Kuntze et al., 2018). Physical therapy goals include the following: (1) increasing range of motion, endurance, strength, and conditioning; (2) teaching principles of joint protection and energy conservation; (3) using appropriate splints; (4) recommending modalities and assistive devices; and (5) improving the performance of activities of daily living (NIAMS, 2021). Early aggressive pharmacotherapy has helped decrease the number of children with arthritis who require physical therapy or splints. Unfortunately, if treatment is delayed for a child with persistently swollen joints, the child may hold the joints comfortably, usually in flexion. This position contributes to a flexion contracture with decreased joint mobility and causes joint malalignment. Such a child may require therapy and splinting to reduce residual limitations after the institution of medications. Occupational therapists usually evaluate and fabricate splints for the upper extremities, whereas physical

therapists construct splints for the lower extremities, including foot orthotics. Splints can be useful adjuncts to therapy to regain motion in an involved joint or to rest a joint experiencing a disease flare. Resting splints are used during active disease. Night resting splints place the wrist in a cockup position (i.e., 20 degrees of wrist extension) and are the most common. Corrective splints include both serial casting and dynamic splints.

NUTRITIONAL COUNSELING

Nutritional counseling is recommended, particularly for children who are underweight, overweight, systemically ill, or receiving long-term steroid therapy. Nutritional education and dietary changes are necessary to minimize weight gain associated with long-term treatment with corticosteroids (see Primary Care Management, later).

SOCIAL SUPPORT

The chronicity and unpredictability of childhood arthritis and the necessary lifestyle changes lead to many situations in which psychological support is helpful. Counseling, support groups, and peer activities, such as camps for children with chronic diseases, are helpful adjuncts to care.

SURGERY

Orthopedic surgery plays a very limited but important role in correcting joint deformities or replacing joints entirely (Boyd & Moore, 2019). Arthroscopy is rarely performed for synovial biopsy or synovectomy. Synovectomy may be beneficial in select cases for pain relief and to improve range of motion but does not alter the long-term outcome (Boyd & Moore, 2019). For a child with functional impairment or secondary mechanical problems, soft tissue releases, osteotomies, posterior capsulotomy, and tendon lengthening may be performed (Boyd & Moore, 2019). Total joint replacements are beneficial in adolescents with marked disability and pain secondary to joint destruction (Boyd & Moore, 2019). As a child approaches adulthood and reaches bone maturity, reconstructive surgery plays a more vital role. Preoperative considerations for joint surgery and other surgical procedures are osteoporosis, contractures, the need for prostheses, and technical challenges related to small bone size (Boyd & Moore, 2019). NSAIDs inhibit platelet aggregation and should be withheld at least 3 days before surgery. Biologics and DMARDs can be taken as usual prior to surgery, but DMARDs can be restarted 1 to 3 days after, and biologics should be restarted after wound healing is complete, around 2 weeks (Boyd & Moore, 2019).

COMPLEMENTARY AND ALTERNATIVE THERAPIES

Complementary and alternative medicine (CAM) is often used because of fear of side effects from conventional medications and the perception that the child's condition is not improving. Commonly used products include vitamins, minerals, copper bracelets, herbal remedies, and fish oil; services are provided by chiropractors, homeopaths, manual healers, and other practitioners. Massages, hot paraffin, and splinting are also used for pain relief. Because parents are often reluctant to divulge their usage of CAM to the primary care provider, it is important to create an accepting environment where frustrations with conventional treatment can be aired and unproven remedies openly discussed. Many patients have reported pain relief and anxiety reduction with cannabidiol (CBD). CBD does have antiinflammatory properties; however, studies have not been validated in humans. The Arthritis Foundation has guidelines for CBD use in adults, but it is recommended that use in children wait until there has been more research. The primary rheumatologist should be consulted before recommending CBD for patient treatment. Primary care providers can help families differentiate between harmless and potentially harmful interventions. Warn parents to be wary of any product labeled as a cure, and discuss any additional treatments with the rheumatology team. Referral for counseling for the child and parent may be necessary to combat psychological stressors caused by JIA (Boyd & Moore, 2019).

ASSOCIATED PROBLEMS OF JUVENILE IDIOPATHIC ARTHRITIS AND TREATMENT

UVEITIS

Uveitis (i.e., iridocyclitis) is one of the most devastating complications associated with JIA and remains one of the major causes of visual impairment in children (Angeles-Han et al., 2019). Uveitis of JIA is a chronic anterior inflammation that primarily affects the anterior part of the eye, iris, and adjacent tissue (Wing et al., 2021). Persistent uveitis can lead to multiple ocular complications, such as glaucoma, cataracts, band keratopathy, posterior synechiae, ocular hypertension, macular edema, and loss of vision (Acharya et al., 2019). Risk factors associated with developing uveitis include female gender, young age (<16 years), ANA positive, and oligoarthritis subtype (Wing et al., 2021). Uveitis is generally asymptomatic; therefore regular screening with a slit-lamp examination, preferably by a pediatric ophthalmologist, is required for early detection (Table 28.2). When uveitis is symptomatic, the child may experience ocular pain, redness, vision change, photophobia, and headache. Children and adolescents with JIA are more likely to develop uveitis than adults diagnosed with arthritis during middle age or older (Cunningham et al., 2016).

Research studies vary on the prevalence of JIA, reporting between 10% and 38% (Angeles-Han et al., 2019; Ramana et al., 2017). Early, aggressive treatment of uveitis with topical corticosteroid drops with or without a mydriatic drug has been effective in preserving the vision of children without advanced disease (Hersh et al., 2018). Low-dose weekly methotrexate, subcutaneous, is preferred over oral and is considered the drug of choice for treating uveitis resistant to topical corticosteroids (Acharya et al., 2019; Angeles-Han et al., 2019). Cataracts and glaucoma are associated with topical corticosteroid drops, and therefore oral or subcutaneous methotrexate is being used more frequently and earlier during uveitis therapy (Angeles-Han et al., 2019). Over the past few years, infliximab and adalimumab have been used effectively for treatment-resistant uveitis (Angeles-Han et al., 2019). Children with JIA may develop symptomatic iritis manifested by acute onset of eye pain, redness, and photophobia. With acute iritis, ophthalmology evaluation and treatment are required only when the eye symptoms are present. Therefore the child with JIA does not need more than routine eye screening.

SKELETAL AND GROWTH ABNORMALITIES

Inflammatory conditions such as JIA are often associated with growth failure (D'Angelo et al., 2021). Disease severity is a crucial factor in the association between skeletal abnormalities, bone mineralization, and impaired bone formation (D'Angelo et al., 2021). Each subtype of JIA affects growth differently. Children with oligoarthritis

| Table 28.2 | Ophthalmologic Screening Schedule |

JRA SUBTYPE AT ONSET	ARTHRITIS ONSET <6 YR OF AGE			ARTHRITIS ONSET >6 YR OF AGE	
	FIRST 4 YR AFTER ONSET, EXAMINE EVERY:	NEXT 3 YR AFTER ONSET, EXAMINE EVERY:	AFTER 7 YR FROM ONSET, EXAMINE EVERY:	FIRST 4 YR AFTER ONSET, EXAMINE EVERY:	AFTER 4 YR FROM ONSET, EXAMINE EVERY:
Pauci-ANA-positive	3 mo	6 mo	12 mo	6 mo	12 mo
Pauci-ANA-negative	6 mo	6 mo	12 mo	6 mo	12 mo
Poly-ANA-positive	3–4 mo	6 mo	12 mo	6 mo	12 mo
Poly-ANA-negative	6 mo	6 mo	12 mo	6 mo	12 mo
Systemic	12 mo	12 mo	12 mo	12 mo	12 mo

ANA, Antinuclear antibody; *JRA,* juvenile rheumatoid arthritis.
From Cassidy, J., Kivlin, J., Lindsley, C., & Nocton, J.; Section on Rheumatology; Section on Ophthalmology. (2006). Ophthalmologic examinations in children with juvenile rheumatoid arthritis. *Pediatrics, 117*(5), 1843–1845. doi:10.1542/peds.2006-0421.

and those requiring long-term steroid therapy may experience growth failure more than children with other types of onsets and therapy (D'Angelo et al., 2021). Factors contributing to short stature and growth abnormalities are largely a result of poor disease control, including undertreatment, side effects of corticosteroids, and poor nutritional status (D'Angelo et al., 2021).

Temporomandibular joint (TMJ) involvement may lead to growth aberrations of the mandible and destruction of the condyle of the mandible, causing micrognathia, which has dental, nutritional, hygienic, speech, and cosmetic consequences. TMJ rarely exhibits signs of inflammation, and imaging rarely correlates with reported symptoms (Schmidt et al., 2022). With destructive TMJ disease, combined orthodontic and reconstructive surgery may improve function, decrease pain, and improve appearance (Schmidt et al., 2022).

Characteristic abnormalities of the cervical spine in JIA include apophyseal joint space narrowing, irregularity and undergrowth of the vertebral bodies, fusion (especially at C1-C2), and atlantoaxial subluxation or instability leading to impingement on the spinal cord and brainstem (Kotecki et al., 2021).

Hip pathology occurs in 20% to 50% of children with chronic arthritis. It is almost always associated with early-onset systemic subtype arthritis or enthesitis (Giancane et al., 2016). The majority develop irreversible hip changes within 5 years of diagnosis (Shelmerdine, 2018). A compensatory lumbar lordosis can occur with a hip contracture. Flexion contractures of the knees are common. Subtalar joint involvement often results in a valgus deformity or (rarely) in a varus deformity.

ANEMIA OF CHRONIC DISEASE

The anemia most often seen in JIA is a result of the anemia of chronic disease and is more severe in systemic JIA. Its pathogenesis is unclear, but its severity correlates with underlying disease activity and inflammation. The anemia of systemic JIA usually presents with inflammatory markers, elevated ESR, and C-reactive protein (Albokhari & Muzaffer, 2021). In children with poor nutrition or NSAID-induced GI manifestations, however, iron deficiency anemia and impaired vitamin B_{12} absorption may develop (Albokhari & Muzaffer, 2021).

SYSTEMIC DISEASE

Systemic JIA can include significant extraarticular manifestations, including hepatosplenomegaly, lymphadenopathy, pericarditis, pleuritis, or other serositis (Kimura, 2022). Nutritional problems, in particular protein-energy malnutrition, are common in systemic JIA.

MENTAL HEALTH DISTURBANCES

Children with chronic diseases are at increased risk for mental illness when compared with the general population (Stein, 2022). Researchers noted that children with a chronic condition are 62% more likely to receive a mental illness diagnosis than a child without a chronic condition (Suryavanshi & Yang, 2016). Many children with JIA may experience low self-esteem, depression, and anxiety due to physical disabilities and psychological symptoms caused by JIA (Min et al., 2021). These factors may greatly impact the overall quality of life. Symptoms of mental illness will vary from emotional distress to withdrawn behavior based on the developmental age of the patient (Stein, 2022). A mental health screening should be conducted regularly for all children, especially those with chronic health conditions.

PROGNOSIS

The prognosis for children with chronic arthritis depends on the disease type and course, symmetry of joint involvement, early hip joint involvement, duration of ESR elevation, RF positivity, and use of biologics for treatment (Momah & Ray, 2019). Patients with JIA have a relatively favorable prognosis, with only about one-third requiring rheumatology care in adulthood (Momah & Ray, 2019). Children with polyarthritis RF positive typically have more erosion and aggressive disease (Mahmud & Binstadt, 2019).

PRIMARY CARE MANAGEMENT

HEALTH CARE MAINTENANCE

Growth and Development

Linear growth may be retarded or delayed during periods of active disease, resulting in shorter stature in children with chronic arthritis than in healthy children (D'Angelo, 2021). Therefore monitoring height and weight via the National Center for Health Statistics growth chart is important. Factors contributing to the development of low bone mineral density include a longer duration of disease, a higher number of active and mobility-restricted joints, high ESRs, glucocorticoid use, and decreased weightbearing activities (Maresova, 2011). Therefore assessment and recommendation of adequate calcium and vitamin D intake by foods, milk, and/or supplementation are crucial. Children with arthritis have higher calcium needs than healthy children, and children receiving long-term steroid treatment have an even higher requirement (up to 1800 mg calcium/day). Excessive weight gain may also occur due to decreased activity, depression, poor nutrition, or corticosteroid usage.

Children with chronic arthritis generally do not have any cognitive or language delay; however, they may have a delay in fine and gross motor skills. Fine motor skills are less likely to be delayed if the young child is provided with toys and activities that encourage hand manipulation. Limited mobility and decreased opportunities to actively interact with their peer group place the child at risk for both motor and social delays. In these areas, the child's interprofessional team of providers can be valuable resources for primary care providers (McKeever & Kelly, 2015).

The acquisition of independence and self-care skills may be delayed in children with JIA. Certain skills, such as transitioning from a bottle to a cup or toilet training, should be postponed during diagnosis or active disease periods. Due to inflammatory symptoms, children with severe JIA often fall behind in acquiring hygiene, toileting, dressing, feeding, and handwriting skills. Regression in the performance of these skills is common during acute illness and may be sustained during remissions as a result of lowered parental expectations and continued reinforcement of a child's dependent behaviors. Adaptive clothing (e.g., shoes with Velcro closures, elastic waistband on pants) and dressing aids can facilitate activities of daily living. Every office visit can be an opportunity to discuss and promote independence in a child with arthritis. Educational materials are available for parents of children with arthritis regarding growth and development (see Resources, later). Moreover, developmentally appropriate functional assessment and quality-of-life measures for children with arthritis exist. These include the following standard and validated tools: the Childhood Health Assessment Questionnaire, the Juvenile Arthritis Functional Assessment Scale (JAFAS) and Report (JAFAR), and the Juvenile Arthritis Self-Report Index.

Diet

Nutritional problems are common in JIA. Factors contributing to the occurrence of these problems include increased inflammatory activity, anorexia, GI side effects of medication, physical limitations, depression, poor food choices, and limited movement of the TMJ (NIAMS, 2021). In addition, increased weight gain can occur with corticosteroid use as a result of increased appetite and fluid retention.

Alternative diets and dietary supplements have long been popular with people with rheumatic disease. Currently, no data support any type of special diet for JIA patients (NIAMS, 2021). Given the current knowledge of childhood arthritis and diet, educating families about proper nutrition for a growing child with a chronic condition and evaluating potentially harmful dietary manipulations, especially those involving nutrient restrictions, are important responsibilities of the primary care provider. Nutritional education and referral to a dietitian may be indicated.

Safety

Education about medication safety is an important responsibility of the primary care provider. All medications must be kept in childproof containers out of reach of young children, which is especially important when older children assume responsibility for self-care. Because of their limited grip strength, special grippers may be used to open containers. Children taking long-term immunosuppressive drugs are encouraged to wear a medical alert bracelet or necklace. Photosensitive skin reactions may occur with several JIA medications, including naproxen and other NSAIDs, methotrexate, sulfasalazine (Azulfidine), and hydroxychloroquine (Plaquenil). Therefore hypoallergenic sunblock lotion with a minimum sun protection factor of 30 or higher should be used routinely on exposed skin and reapplied every 30 minutes after swimming or sweating. Children on these medications should avoid direct sun exposure between 11 a.m. and 4 p.m. when ultraviolet exposure is highest.

Orthotic appliances are often recommended to prevent or correct deformities. Important safety issues related to splint wearing include care of the splint to maintain integrity, proper skin care, signs and symptoms of a poorly fitted splint (e.g., potential pressure points), and proper splint application. The splint should be adjusted to maintain correct function and ensure that the child has not outgrown it. Superficial heat and cold modalities are often recommended to relieve joint pain and stiffness. Determining the type of applications used by the family and reviewing safety precautions specific to each type of application is important. Some children with JIA use adaptive equipment to minimize joint stress and increase independence. Adaptive equipment should be evaluated for the safety of all family members. Bath safety can be improved using safety strips, rubber mats, wall grab bars, and tub chairs. As with all family members, a home fire safety plan should include a specific plan for the child with JIA.

Immunizations

Children with chronic arthritis in disease remission who are not taking immunosuppressive medications can receive all routine immunizations. If possible, children with arthritis should be immunized on schedule. Typically, children with JIA should receive live attenuated and inactivated vaccinations when not prescribed immunosuppressive treatment (methotrexate or biologics) (Onel et al., 2022a). Research supports the use of live attenuated vaccines such as measles-mumps-rubella (MMR) and MMR-varicella for children with JIA on immunosuppressive medications; however, the primary care provider and rheumatologist must discuss the best option prior to administering the vaccine (Rath, 2021). Children on immunosuppressive medications should get the pneumococcal polysaccharide and pneumococcal 13-valent conjugate vaccines as they are at higher risk for pneumococcal bacterial infections (Onel et al., 2022a; Rath, 2021). All children with chronic arthritis should receive the current recommended influenza vaccine each year. Overall, there has been widespread concern about the possibility of immunizations causing a flare of the underlying disease or immunologic disorder in chronic arthritis. Anecdotal experience views this as a potential problem, but scientific data to support this theory do not exist (Alfayadh et al., 2020). These concerns should not discourage primary care providers from immunizing children with chronic arthritis.

Screenings

Vision. A thorough funduscopic examination and visual acuity screening should be performed at each routine office visit. At the time of diagnosis, every child must be examined for uveitis by an ophthalmologist. Frequent ophthalmologic examinations are recommended for children at risk for uveitis, glaucoma, and cataracts. Young children with ANA-positive arthritis are at the greatest risk for developing ocular inflammation. The College of Rheumatoid/Arthritis Foundation (Angeles-Han et al., 2019) recommends an ophthalmic screening every 3 months in children with JIA at high risk for uveitis. More frequent follow-up is needed for children with active uveitis. Medications such as corticosteroids can cause glaucoma or cataracts. Children taking hydroxychloroquine (Plaquenil) should have a baseline and yearly ophthalmologic examination that includes visual field determinations.

Hearing. Routine office screening is recommended.

Dental. Dental visits should occur at least every 6 months and more frequently if malocclusions, crowded teeth, and dental caries result from TMJ disease. Orthodontic referrals are made as needed. Current research indicates that the incidence of dental caries in children with JIA is no different than in children without JIA (Gil et al., 2021). The side effects of medications used to treat JIA, such as DMARDs, may negatively impact oral hygiene and dietary habits (Gil et al., 2021). Children with JIA should be checked for bleeding gums and poor dental hygiene. In these situations, consultation with the pediatric rheumatology team and the dentist is necessary. Orthodontic referrals are made as needed. Individuals with joint replacements should receive prophylactic antibiotics before dental work.

Blood pressure. Routine screening is recommended. Mild hypertension may occur in children taking NSAIDs. Steroid-induced hypertension can occur, although it is less frequent when lower doses are prescribed (Zaripova et al., 2021).

Hematocrit. Hematologic testing is frequently ordered by the rheumatologist to screen for disease activity and medication toxicity, so routine screening may not be required in the primary care office.

Urinalysis. Routine urinalyses are generally checked at least every 6 months by the rheumatologist to screen for disease activity and medication toxicity.

COMMON ILLNESS MANAGEMENT
Differential Diagnosis
Children with an established diagnosis of chronic arthritis will seek care for common childhood illnesses from the primary care provider. Several signs and symptoms of common illnesses must be differentiated from a potential arthritis flare or from arthritis treatment, side effects, or toxicity.

Fever. The fever of systemic JIA is easily differentiated from the fever of an infectious process because of the characteristic pattern with normal or below-normal temperature most of the day with once- or twice-daily high spikes. In addition, children with systemic JIA often appear toxic and have a pronounced classic rash during the febrile spikes but are relatively well when afebrile. A careful history and complete physical examination usually determine the source of the fever.

Dermatologic symptoms. Primary care providers should be familiar with the classic rash associated with systemic JIA—a salmon-pink, evanescent, macular rash typically appearing on the trunk and extremities that coincides with fever spikes. Other types of rashes are rarely seen as part of the JIA condition and should be assessed and treated for children without JIA.

Photosensitive skin reactions may occur with medications used to treat JIA, including naproxen, methotrexate, sulfasalazine, and hydroxychloroquine. The most common rash is pseudoporphyria associated with naproxen (Naprosyn, Anaprox) and other NSAIDs (Emlets, 2022).

Otologic symptoms. TMJ arthritis may cause referred pain to the ear, which should be considered when evaluating children for otitis media.

Respiratory symptoms. Cricoarytenoid arthritis (i.e., laryngeal arthritis) can cause stridor, dyspnea, and cyanosis in JIA. Pleuritis and pericarditis can occur in systemic JIA. Very rarely, methotrexate therapy may lead to hypersensitivity pneumonitis within the first few weeks to months of starting the medication (Salehi et al., 2017).

Gastrointestinal symptoms. GI symptoms commonly occur in children with JIA who take NSAIDs and/or glucocorticoids. Although peptic ulcers are rare in children receiving NSAID treatment, they may present as chronic anemia secondary to occult blood loss.

The classic peptic ulcer symptom of epigastric pain that improves with eating and worsens with an empty stomach is more common in adolescents and is virtually absent in young children. A fecal calprotectin test can be used to screen for inflammatory bowel disease and ongoing inflammation of the digestive tract, followed by a referral to gastroenterology for further evaluation. A careful history and physical examination, as well as consultation with the pediatric rheumatologist and gastroenterologist as needed, will help the primary care provider evaluate the differential diagnoses.

Renal. Urinary tract infection versus renal toxicity from medications must be considered with abnormal urinalysis results.

Drug interactions. Potential interactions exist between medications commonly used to treat JIA and over-the-counter or prescription drugs used to manage common pediatric conditions. Major drug interactions of concern to primary care providers are identified in Box 28.1. Generally, providers should not discontinue a child's condition-specific medications without consulting the pediatric rheumatologist. Conditions warranting temporary cessation of arthritis medications may include the following: (1) exposure to chickenpox in unimmunized children; (2) significant bleeding of the nose, gums, or GI tract; and (3) significant emesis and dehydration as a result of infectious illness. Immunosuppressant medication should be held when a patient has a fever. On the other hand, children taking long-term corticosteroids may need increased steroid supplementation at times of significant illness. Communication with the rheumatology team is essential in these circumstances.

DEVELOPMENTAL ISSUES

Sleep Patterns
Sleep abnormalities are common in children with JIA (Saidi et al., 2022). They may also fatigue more readily during flares and require periods of rest during the day. Teaching a child to recognize body signals, set limits and priorities, pace activities, and plan ahead will help conserve energy. The severity and duration of morning stiffness increase with increased disease activity. Recommendations to alleviate morning stiffness include administration of medications 30 to 60 minutes before rising and stretching in a warm bath or shower before starting daily activities. In addition, the use of flannel sheets, thermal underwear, warmed clothing, and a sleeping bag may decrease morning stiffness.

Toileting
The acquisition of self-care skills may be delayed in children with JIA. Toilet training should be postponed during periods of active disease because a child may lack the motivation and physical capability to perform tasks necessary for successful toileting. Limitations in the upper and lower extremities may make it difficult for children to transfer on and off the toilet, manage toilet paper, and undress. Safety bars and elevated toilet seats are reliable assistive devices for children with lower extremity involvement. For children with upper extremity limitations, effective aids for wiping after toileting can be obtained from occupational therapists. Adaptive clothing and dressing aids can facilitate toileting. In severely affected children, bedpans, urinals, and commodes may also be required at night if pain and stiffness limit mobility.

Discipline
Parents of children with arthritis may have difficulty dealing with their guilt and concern over their child's condition. They may become overprotective and not handle behavioral issues as firmly as they would if the child was not sick. In addition, overindulgence during periods of active disease alternating with normalization of discipline practices during remissions fosters inconsistent limit setting. The primary care provider can reinforce normalcy in childhood expectations, responsibilities, chores, appropriate behavioral expectations, and discipline.

Child Care
Parents of children who are taking medications may have difficulty locating child care providers who are willing to administer medications. For caregivers who accept this responsibility, parents can prepare a list that

---

Box 28.1 Drug Interactions

- Concurrent use of nonsteroidal antiinflammatory drugs (NSAIDs) and glucocorticoids may increase risk of gastrointestinal (GI) side effects.
- Antacids may alter the absorption rate of NSAIDs and glucocorticoids, resulting in subtherapeutic levels.
- Methotrexate concentrations are increased by NSAIDs, which is generally not a concern in weekly low-dose methotrexate therapy.
- Concomitant use of methotrexate and alcohol may increase the risk of GI and hepatic side effects.
- Sulfonamides may displace or be displaced by other highly protein-bound drugs (e.g., NSAIDs, methotrexate). Monitor children for increased effects (i.e., increased hepatotoxicity) of highly bound drugs when sulfonamides (e.g., trimethoprim/sulfamethoxazole [Bactrim]) are added.
- Estrogen-based oral contraceptives may decrease the clearance and increase the serum concentration and toxic effects of corticosteroids and cyclosporine.
- NSAIDs plus acetaminophen increase the risk of adverse hepatic side effects.
- NSAIDs displace anticoagulants from protein-binding sites.

includes the name, dose, time, and method of administration, as well as the side effects of each medication. Caregivers need to understand that chronic arthritis is characterized by disease activity and symptom fluctuations. Therefore a child's functional capacity, energy level, and developmental progress may change on different days. Education about the child's abilities, limitations, disease, and treatments is likely to decrease anxiety among caregivers and promote appropriate interactions among caregivers, children, and families. Infants and young children with chronic arthritis may be eligible for special education and related services.

Schooling

Children with chronic arthritis can participate fully in school, physical education, and extracurricular activities with certain interventions and adaptations listed in Table 28.3. Many children have special needs that must be communicated to the school by verbal and written communication and addressed in an individualized educational plan (IEP). Most pediatric rheumatology centers have a standard letter for school personnel that describes the condition and recommended adjustments. Educating school personnel about morning stiffness and the variability of clinical manifestations is very important (Min et al., 2021). Severe disease flares or surgery may necessitate temporary home instruction and should be planned for in a child's IEP. Primary care providers can periodically question children and parents about school-related problems such as fatigue, distractibility, limited mobility, absences, and medications. The provider may interface with the family, school staff, and pediatric rheumatology team to identify and remedy problems before or when they occur. The student can participate in school athletic programs with modifications as necessary. Swimming as a sport is strongly encouraged because it strengthens muscle groups around joints, provides a good range of motion therapy, is less stressful on joints than weightbearing activities of contact sports, and promotes aerobic fitness.

Sexuality

Sexual maturation may be delayed in adolescents with chronic arthritis, especially those with systemic disease. Contraceptive advice is important and should include a discussion of interactions between arthritis medications and various oral contraceptives and any potential effects of arthritis medications on fetal development. Fertility is not impaired in females with JIA, but the rate of preeclampsia and preterm birth is higher than in healthy controls (Chen et al., 2013). Because of these factors, early referral to an obstetrician for females with JIA who are pregnant is very important.

Transition to Adulthood

Thoughtful planning for the transition into adulthood is necessary and useful. The optimal goal of health care

Table 28.3	Common School Problems for Students With Chronic Arthritis
PROBLEM	**INTERVENTION STRATEGIES**
Difficulty climbing stairs/walking long distance	Elevator permit Schedule classes to decrease walking and climbing Two sets of books: keep one in appropriate class, other at home Wheelchair if needed Proper footwear: supportive sneakers
Inactivity, stiffness as a result of prolonged sitting	Move! Change position every 20 min Sit to the side or back of the room to allow for standing or walking without disturbing the class Ask to be assigned jobs that permit walking (pass/collect papers)
Difficulty carrying books/cafeteria tray	Accessible desk Rolling backpack for books Two sets of books Determine cafeteria assistance plan or pack lunch (helper, reserved seat, wheeled cart)
Handwriting problems (slow, messy, painful)	Use "fat" pen/pencil, crayon or pencil/pen grips Felt tip pen Stretch hands about every 10 min Tape recorder for notetaking Computer for reports Alternatives for timed tests (oral test, extra time, computer) Educate teacher; messy writing may be unavoidable at times
Difficulty with shoulder movement, dressing, putting on coat, boots, tying shoes	Loose-fitting clothing, without buttons or zippers Velcro closures Adaptive equipment from an occupational therapist Assistance may be needed for some things, especially on "stiff days"
Reaching locker, opening locker	Locker modification/alternative place for storage Two lockers Key for locker instead of combination
Raising hand	Devise alternative signaling method

transition planning for the teenager with arthritis is to provide coordinated, uninterrupted care. The primary care provider can promote the transition process for the teenager in many ways. Health care providers can help the family identify a local adult rheumatologist, encourage independence in self-care, address adolescent developmental issues, counsel parents and teens, refer to community programs as needed, and collaborate with the interdisciplinary team (McKeever & Kelly, 2015). A coordinated transition program for adolescents with JIA improves adolescent health-related quality of life, adolescent and parent knowledge and satisfaction, and prevocational readiness (McKeever & Kelly, 2015). Adolescents must be counseled on the need for insurance coverage and the cost of treatment as they transition to adult care.

Economic Burden

Pharmacologic treatment of active JIA is associated with a high cost to families. Treatment may also include several specialists, such as physical therapy, nutrition, and psychological. Treatment may cost over $1000 per month, depending on the type of treatment and insurance coverage. Patients on biologics have significantly higher costs than those on nonbiologics (Marshall et al., 2019). Primary care providers should counsel families on appropriate insurance coverage and copay assistance resources for JIA treatment.

Family Concerns

Raising a child with chronic arthritis can be difficult. There are many misconceptions about arthritis. Families must repeatedly explain and educate others that arthritis is not just a problem to be quickly remedied by the multitude of treatments offered in television advertisements and magazines. Others often believe that arthritis is a condition that affects only the elderly and are often in disbelief when children discuss their arthritis. After hearing about the diagnosis of arthritis, well-meaning family and friends sometimes tend to overwhelm the family with information about the diagnosis and so-called cures they have heard or read about. Children with arthritis often appear healthy, which makes it difficult to explain their need for modifications at school and work. They have appropriate concerns about school attendance, sports participation, growth, and any limitations that make them feel different. Parents are concerned about long-term side effects of medications (e.g., fertility), whereas children are more concerned about the short-term effects (e.g., cushingoid facies with corticosteroids).

Children are asked to engage in several treatment regimens, such as medications, exercise, lifestyle changes, and added appointments with the primary care provider, rheumatologist, ophthalmologist, and other specialists. The child, adolescent, or parent may decide not to comply with the recommendations. Families and older children need to be aware of treatment risk/benefit ratios and the consequences of poor adherence to treatment regimens. Teaching problem-solving and decision-making skills and using contracts are helpful strategies to use with the adolescent. Key family resources and programs are available through several organizations. Families of children with chronic arthritis are strongly encouraged to use these educational and support services.

RESOURCES

American Juvenile Arthritis Organization (AJAO, a council of the Arthritis Foundation): www.arthritis.org
Juvenile Arthritis Research https://www.jarproject.org/home
National Institute of Arthritis, Musculoskeletal and Skin Diseases https://www.niams.nih.gov/health-topics/juvenile-arthritis

ACKNOWLEDGMENT

The authors acknowledge the work by Gail R. McIlvain-Simpson, Patricia M. Reilly, Patricia A. Rettig, Stephanie L. Merhar, and Randy Q. Cron on previous editions of this chapter.

 Summary

Primary Care Needs for the Child with Juvenile Idiopathic Arthritis

HEATLH CARE MAINTENANCE
Growth and Development
- Linear growth may be delayed during active systemic disease.
- Catchup growth occurs with disease control or during remission.
- Increased calcium needs as children may be osteopenic.
- Corticosteroids may suppress growth at doses above 0.15 mg/kg/day.
- Poor weight gain may be a result of systemic disease.
- Excessive weight gain may occur as a result of decreased activity, depression, poor nutrition, or corticosteroid usage.
- Gross motor delays and temporary regressions are not uncommon during periods of flares/active disease.
- Fine motor skills are less likely to be affected.
- Developmentally appropriate quality-of-life assessments are needed.

Diet
- Nutritional problems are common.
- Increased inflammatory activity, anorexia, GI side effects of medication, physical limitations, depression, corticosteroid usage, poor food choices, and limited movement of TMJ may contribute to nutritional problems.
- Daily vitamins should be added when warranted by the medication therapy.
- "Arthritis diets" should be evaluated for nutritional adequacy, and families should be educated about proper nutrition for a growing child with a chronic disease.

Safety
- Childproof containers should be used for medications.
- Children taking immunosuppressive agents should wear a medical alert bracelet or necklace.
- Sunblock should be used on exposed skin because of photosensitive skin reactions with some medications.

Continued

- Safety issues related to splint wear, heat and cold applications, and adaptive equipment should be reviewed.

Immunizations

- Children who are not taking immunosuppressive drugs or experiencing systemic disease symptoms should be routinely immunized.
- Coronavirus vaccination can be given before immunosuppressive therapy is started if biologic treatment can wait to be started or wait 3 months after immunosuppressive therapy has ended.
- In the absence of neurologic symptoms, a child with classic, intermittent JIA fever can be immunized during febrile episodes.
- All children with chronic arthritis should receive the current recommended influenza vaccine annually.

Screening

- *Vision*: A funduscopic examination and acuity screening should be performed at each visit. Children should be examined by an ophthalmologist for uveitis.
- *Hearing*: Routine visits are recommended.
- *Dental*: Children with TMJ involvement should have frequent dental visits (at least every 6 months).
- *Blood pressure*: Routine screening is recommended.
- *Hematocrit*: CBC, differential, ESR, C-reactive protein, platelet count, and liver function tests are routinely ordered by the rheumatologist to monitor disease activity, response to therapy, drug toxicity, and assess for anemia of chronic disease.
- *Urinalysis*: Urinalysis is routinely ordered by the rheumatologist to monitor disease-related factors
- *Tuberculosis*: Routine screening is recommended.

COMMON ILLNESS MANAGEMENT
Differential Diagnosis

- *Fever*: Classic, intermittent JIA fever should be differentiated from infectious process.
- *Dermatologic*: Rheumatoid rash should be ruled out in systemic JIA. Drug-related photosensitivity skin reactions should be ruled out.
- *Otologic*: TMJ arthritis with referred ear pain should be differentiated from otitis media.
- *Respiratory*: Colds and flu may cause arthritis flareups. Infectious process must be differentiated from pleuritis or cricoarytenoid arthritis.
- *Gastrointestinal*: Drug-related GI symptoms should be differentiated from a gastroenteritis infection.
- *Renal*: Urinary tract infection should be distinguished from medication toxicity.

DEVELOPMENTAL ISSUES
Sleep Patterns

- Fatigue associated with disease flares may necessitate rest periods during the day.
- Recommendations to promote comfort and sleep and to alleviate morning stiffness (e.g., use of an electric blanket with timer and morning bath or shower) should be discussed with the family.

Toileting

- Training should be postponed during periods of active disease.
- Assistive devices may be needed with individuals with severe disease, joint deformities, and limited mobility.

Discipline

- Overprotection, overindulgence, and inconsistent limit setting should be identified. Reinforce the need for consistent expectations (e.g., daily chores). Discuss impact of chronic arthritis on age-specific developmental tasks so parents have a framework for decision making about discipline.

Child Care

- Caregivers need to be knowledgeable of medications, the use of assistive devices, and applying splints.
- Parents should provide caregivers with information about the child's medications.
- Caregivers should be educated on the effect of JIA on a child's functional capacity, energy level, and developmental progress.
- Home-based, single-provider day care setting rather than group child care is recommended for children taking steroids or immunosuppressants.

Schooling

- Individuals with Disabilities Education Improvement Act (IDEA) entitles most students with JIA to occupational therapy, physical therapy, adaptive physical education, and transportation between school, home, and facilities where services are provided (see Table 28.3).
- Most students with JIA can participate in modified school athletic programs to their own tolerance level.
- Disease flares or surgery may necessitate home instructions for a brief period.
- Teaching families about their educational rights and how to advocate for their children in school is important.

Sexuality

- Discussion of puberty, sexual activity, appropriate contraception, and pregnancy is imperative with all adolescents.
- Medication modifications (i.e., methotrexate is an abortifacient and is teratogenic) must be made before planning a pregnancy.

Transition to Adulthood

- Adolescents can be referred to the state office of vocational rehabilitation for assistance with postsecondary educational opportunities.
- Primary care providers can assist the family with decisions regarding health care, psychosocial, vocational, financial, and family issues.
- Adolescents are advised to avoid drinking any alcohol. Alcohol significantly increases the risk of liver toxicity when taking methotrexate.

Economic Burden

- Counsel adolescents on the importance of obtaining insurance coverage, especially if JIA treatment includes biologics

Family Concerns

- Family frustration and concern over the lack of a cure and the unpredictability of the illness should be acknowledged.
- The impact of the illness on the child's ability to fully participate in school, sports, and social activities raises concerns for parents.
- Multiple treatment regimens and concern about side effects may lead to nonadherence.
- Referral for psychosocial and family issues may be necessary.

REFERENCES

Acharya, N. R., Patel, S., Homayounfar, G., Enanoria, W. T. A., Shakoor, A., Chakrabarti, A., & Goldstein, D. A. (2019). Relapse of juvenile idiopathic arthritis-associated uveitis after discontinuation of immunomodulatory therapy. *Ocular Immunology & Inflammation, 27*(4), 686–692. doi:10.1080/09273948.2018.1424341.

Albokhari, S. M., & Muzaffer, M. (2021). Anemia in juvenile idiopathic arthritis (JIA) and other pediatric rheumatologic diseases: A retrospective study. *Open Journal of Rheumatology and Autoimmune Diseases, 11*(4), 188–202. https://doi.org/10.4236/ojra.2021.114019.

Alfayadh, N. M., Gowdie, P. J., Akikusa, J. D., Easton, M. L., & Buttery, J. P. (2020). Vaccinations do not increase arthritis flares in juvenile idiopathic arthritis: A study of the relationship between routine childhood vaccinations on the Australian immunization schedule and arthritis activity in children with juvenile idiopathic arthritis. *International Journal of Rheumatology, 2020*(1078914). https://doi.org/10.1155/2020/1078914.

Angeles-Han, S. T., Ringold, S., Beukelman, T., Lovell, D., Cuello, C. A., Becker, M. L., Colbert, R. A., Feldman, B. M, Holland, G. N., Ferguson, P. J, Gewanter, H., Guzman, J., Horonjeff, J., Nigrovic, P. A., Ombrello, M. J., Passo, M. H., Stoll, M. L., Rabinovich, C. E., Sen, H. N., Schneider, R., … Reston, J. (2019). 2019 American college of rheumatology/arthritis foundation guideline for the screening, monitoring, and treatment of juvenile idiopathic arthritis-associated uveitis. *Arthritis Care Res (Hoboken), 71*(6), 703–716. doi:10.1002/acr.23871. Epub 2019 Apr 25. PMID: 31021540; PMCID: PMC6777949.

Barut, K., Adrovic, A., Sahin, S., & Kasapcopur, O. (2017). Juvenile idiopathic arthritis. *Balkan Medical Journal, 34*(2), 90–101. doi:10.4274/balkanmedj.2017.0111.

Bayraktar, D., Savci, S., Altug-Gucenmez, O., Manci, E., Makay, B., Ilcin, N., & Unsal, E. (2018). The effects of 8-week water-running program on exercise capacity in children with juvenile idiopathic arthritis: A controlled trial. *Rheumatology International, 39*(2019), 59–65. https://doi.org/10.1007/s00296-018-4209-8.

Boyd, K. M., & Moore, M. D. (2019). Juvenile idiopathic arthritis for the pediatric orthopedic surgeon. *Orthopedic Clinics of North America, 50*(4), 471–488. https://www-doi-org.ezproxy3.lhl.uab.edu/10.1016/j.ocl.2019.06.003.

Chen, J. S., Ford, J. B., Roberts, C. L., Simpson, J. M., & March, L. M. (2013). Pregnancy outcomes in women with juvenile idiopathic arthritis: A population-based study. *Rheumatology, 52*(6), 1119–1125. https://doi.org/10.1093/rheumatology/kes428.

Cunningham, E. T. Jr., Smith, J. R., Tugal-Tutkun, I., Rothova, A., & Zierhut, M. (2016). Uveitis in children and adolescents. *Ocular Immunology and Inflammation, 24*(4), 365–371. doi:10.1080/09273948.2016.1204777.

D'Angelo, D. M., Donato, G. D., Breda, L., & Chiarelli, F. (2021). Growth and puberty in children with juvenile idiopathic arthritis. *Pediatric Rheumatology, 19*(28). https://doi.org/10.1186/s12969-021-00521-5.

Dvorin, E. L., & Ebell, M. H. (2020). Short-term systemic corticosteroids: Appropriate use in primary care. *American Family Physicians, 101*(2), 89–94.

Emlets, C. A. (2022). *Pseudoporphyria.* UpToDate. Topic 13748 Version 14.0.

Giancane, G., Consolaro, A., Lanni, S., Davi, S., Schiappapietra, B., & Ravelli, A. (2016). Juvenile idiopathic arthritis: Diagnosis and treatment. *Rheumatology and Therapy, 2016*(3), 187–207. doi:10.1007/s40744-016-0040-4.

Gil, E. G., Åstrøm, A. N., Lie, S. A., Rygg, M., Fischer, J., Rosén, A., Bletsa, A., Luukko, K., Shi, X. Q., Halbig, J., Frid, P., Cetrelli, L., Tylleskär, K., Rosendahl, K., & Skeie, M. S. (2021). Dental caries in children and adolescents with juvenile idiopathic arthritis and controls: a multilevel analysis. *BMC Oral Health, 21*(1), 417. doi:10.1186/s12903-021-01758-y. PMID: 34433437; PMCID: PMC8390188.

Hersh, A. O., Cope, S., Bohnsack, J. F., Shakoor, A., & Vitale, A. T. (2018). Use of immunosuppressive medications for treatment of pediatric intermediate uveitis. *Ocular Immunology & Inflammation, 26*(4), 642–650. doi:10.1080/09273948.2016.1255340.

Kimura, Y. (2022). Systemic juvenile idiopathic arthritis: Clinical manifestations and diagnosis. *UpToDate.* Retrieved on September 18, 2022, from. https://www.uptodate.com/contents/systemic-juvenile-idiopathic-arthritis-clinical-manifestations-and-diagnosis.

Kotecki, M., Gietka, P., Posadzy, M., & Sudoi-Szopinska, I. (2021). Radiographs and MRI of the cervical spine in juvenile idiopathic arthritis: A cross-sectional retrospective study. *Journal of Clinical Medicine, 10*(24), 5798. https://doi.org/10.3390/jcm10245798.

Kuntze, G., Nesbitt, C., Whittaker, J. L., Nettel-Aguirre, A., Toomey, C., Esau, S., Doyle-Baker, P. K., Shank, J., Brooks, J., Benseler, S., & Emery, C. A. (2018). Exercise therapy in juvenile idiopathic arthritis: A systematic review and meta-analysis. *Archives of Physical Medicine and Rehabilitation, 99*(1), 178–193. https://doi.org/10.1016/j.apmr.2017.05.030.

Mahmud, S. A., & Binstadt, B. A. (2019). Autoantibodies in the pathogenesis, diagnosis, and prognosis of juvenile idiopathic arthritis. *Frontiers in Immunology, 9*(3168). https://doi.org/10.3389/fimmu.2018.03168.

Maresova, K. B. (2011). Secondary osteoporosis in patients with juvenile idiopathic arthritis. *Journal of Osteoporosis.*(569417). https://doi.org/10.4061/2011/569417.

Marshall, A., Gupta, K., Pazirandeh, M., Bonafede, M., & McMorrow, D. (2019). Treatment patterns and economic outcomes in patients with juvenile idiopathic arthritis. *ClinicoEconomics and Outcomes Research*(11), 361–371. https://doi.org/10.2147/CEOR.S197117.

Marzetti, V., Breda, L., Miulli, E., Filippetti, F., Mancini, C., Chiarelli, F., & Altobelli, E. (2017). Clinical characteristics of juvenile idiopathic arthritis in an area of central Italy: A population-based study. *Ann Ig, 29*(4), 281–292. doi:10.7416/ai.2017.2152.

McKeever, A., & Kelly, M. M. (2015). Growing up with juvenile idiopathic arthritis. *The American Journal of Maternal/Child Nursing, 40*(1), 8–15. doi:10.1097/NMC.0000000000000096.

Min, M., Hancock, D. G., Aromataris, E., Crotti, T., & Boros, C. (2021). Experiences of living with juvenile idiopathic arthritis: A qualitative systematic review. *JBI Evidence Synthesis, 20*(1), 60–120. doi:10.11124/JBIES-21-00139.

Momah, T., & Ray, L. (2019). Juvenile idiopathic arthritis: Old disease, new tactics. *The Journal of Family Medicine, 68*(2), E8–E13.

Mueller, L. O., Humphries, P., & Rosendahl, K. (2015). The joints in juvenile idiopathic arthritis. *Insights Imaging, 6*(3), 275–284. https://doi.org/10.1007/s13244-015-0406-0.

National Institute of Arthritis and Musculoskeletal and Skin Diseases. (2021, May). Juvenile idiopathic arthritis. https://www.niams.nih.gov/health-topics/juvenile-arthritis/diagnosis-treatment-and-steps-to-take.

Onel, K. B., Horton, D. B., Lovell, D. J., Shenoi, S., Cuello, C. A., Angeles-Han, S. T., Becker, M. L., Cron, R. Q., Feldman, B. M., Ferguson, P. J., Gewanter, H., Guzman, J., Kimura, Y., Lee, T., Murphy, K., Nigrovic, P. A., Ombrello, M. J., Rabinovich, C. E., … Reston, J. T. (2022a). 2021 American College of Rheumatology guideline for the treatment of juvenile idiopathic arthritis: Therapeutic approaches for oligoarthritis, temporomandibular joint arthritis, and systemic juvenile idiopathic arthritis. *Arthritis & Rheumatology, 74*(4), 553–569. doi:10.1002/art.42037.

Onel, K. B., Horton, D. B., Lovell, D. J., Shenoi, S., Cuello, C. A., Angeles-Han, S. T., Becker, M. L., Cron, R. Q., Feldman, B. M., Ferguson, P. J., Gewanter, H., Guzman, J., Kimura, Y., Lee, T., Murphy, K., Nigrovic, P. A., Ombrello, M. J., Rabinovich, C. E., ... Reston, J. T. (2022b). 2021 American College of Rheumatology guideline for treatment of juvenile idiopathic arthritis: Recommendations for nonpharmacologic therapies, medication monitoring, immunizations, and imaging. *Arthritis & Rheumatology, 74*(4), 570–585. doi:10.1002/art.42036.

Ramana, A. V., Dick, A. D., Jones, A. P., McKay, A., Williamson, P. R., Compeyrot-Lacassagne, S., Hardwick, B., Hickery, H., Hughes, D., Woo, P., Benton, D., & Edelsten, C. (2017). Adalimumab plus methotrexate for uveitis in juvenile idiopathic arthritis. *New England Journal of Medicine.*(376), 1637–1646. doi:10.1056/NEJMoa1614160.

Rath, L. (2021, October 27). Vaccinations for kids on biologics. Arthritis Foundation. https://www.arthritis.org/health-wellness/treatment/treatment-plan/ja-medical-decisions/vaccinations-for-kids-with-arthritis.

Rigante, D., Bosco, A., & Esposito, S. (2015). The etiology of juvenile idiopathic arthritis. *Clinical Reviews in Allergy Immunology,* (49), 253–261. https://doi.org/10.1007/s12016-014-8460-9.

Saidi, O., Rochette, E., Bourdier, P., Ratel, S., Merlin, E., Pereira, B., & Duche, P. (2022). Sleep in children and adolescents with juvenile idiopathic arthritis: A systematic review and meta-analysis of case-control studies. *Sleep, 45*(2). https://doi.org/10.1093/sleep/zsab233.

Salehi, M., Miller, R., & Khaing, M. (2017). Methotrexate-induced hypersensitivity pneumonitis appearing after 30 years of use: A case report. *Journal of Medical Case Reports, 11*(174). https://doi.org/10.1186/s13256-017-1333-0.

Schmidt, C., Ertel, T., Arbogast, M., Hugle, B., von Kalle, T., & Neff, A. (2022). Clinical practice guideline: The diagnosis and treatment of rheumatoid and juvenile idiopathic arthritis of the temporomandibular joint. *Deutsches Arzteblatt International,* (119), 47–54. doi:10.3238/arztebl.m2021.0388.

Shelmerdine, S. C., Di Paolo, P. L., Rieter, J. F. M. M., Malattia, C., Tanturri de Horatio, L., & Rosendahl, K. (2018). A novel radiographic scoring system for growth abnormalities and structural change in children with juvenile idiopathic arthritis of the hip. *Pediatric Radiology, 48*(8), 1086–1095. doi:10.1007/s00247-018-4136-6. Epub 2018 May.

Spiegel, L., Kristensen, K. D., & Herlin, T. (2015). Juvenile idiopathic arthritis characteristics: Etiology and pathophysiology. *Seminars in Orthodontics, 21*(2), 77–83.

Stein, R. (2022). Mental health concerns and childhood chronic physical health conditions: A narrative review. *Pediatric Medicine, 5*(5). http://dx.doi.org/10.21037/pm-2.

Suryavanshi, M., & Yang, Y. (2016). Clinical and economic burden of mental disorders among children with chronic physical conditions, United States, 2008-2013. *Preventing Chronic Disease, 2016*(13). http://dx.doi.org/10.5888/pcd13.150535.

Vanoni, F., Minoia, F., & Malattia, C. (2017). Biologics in juvenile idiopathic arthritis: A narrative review. *European Journal of Pediatrics, 2017*(176), 1147–1153. doi:10.1007/s00431-017-2960-6.

Wing, J., Wu, H., Liu, X., Jia, H., & Lu, H. (2021). Effect of LPS on cytokine secretion from peripheral blood monocytes in juvenile idiopathic arthritis-associated uveitis patients with positive antinuclear antibody. *Journal of Immunology Research,* 6691681. https://www-doi-org.ezproxy3.lhl.uab.edu/10.1155/2021/6691681.

Zaripova, L. N., Midgley, A., Christmas, S. E., Beresford, M. W., Baildam, E. M., & Oldershaw, R. A. (2021). Juvenile idiopathic arthritis: From aetiopathogenesis to therapeutic approaches. *Pediatric Rheumatology, 2021*(19), 135. https://doi.org/10.1186/s12969-021-00629-8.

Kidney Disease, Chronic

Kathleen F. Mallett

ETIOLOGY

Causes of chronic kidney disease (CKD) in children are varied and complex, the extent of which is beyond the scope of this chapter, but causes should be initially categorized as glomerular or nonglomerular (Table 29.1). This distinction is important to determine because the risk factors associated with progression may be different between the two causes (Atkinson et al., 2021). Progression to end-stage kidney disease (ESKD) may occur from either cause, but it is known to occur more rapidly in patients with glomerular diseases (Atkinson et al., 2021; Warady et al., 2015). Hypertensive nephrosclerosis and diabetic nephropathy, the most common causes of kidney failure in adults, are rare in children.

Congenital abnormalities of the kidney and urinary tract (CAKUT) account for the majority of pediatric ESKD and are classified as nonglomerular causes. CAKUT diagnoses include renal dysplasia/hypoplasia/aplasia, obstructive uropathies, reflux nephropathy, and cystic disorders (Talati et al., 2019; Warady et al., 2015). An environmental component (i.e., teratogenic medications in utero) causes some CAKUT, and genetic abnormalities are being discovered more often (Talati et al., 2019; Torra et al., 2021), yet some do not have identifiable causes.

Glomerulonephritis (GN) is responsible for most of the glomerular diseases and is classified as primary (within the kidney) or secondary (outside the kidney). Examples include but are not limited to steroid-sensitive nephrotic syndrome, focal segmental glomerular sclerosis (FSGS), immunoglobulin A (IgA) nephropathy, and Alport syndrome. As with CAKUT, the genetic origins of these diseases are being studied. Autoimmune diseases such as systemic lupus erythematosus (SLE) nephritis can have significant kidney involvement and are considered secondary causes of GN that lead to ESKD (Almaani et al., 2017).

INCIDENCE AND PREVALENCE

The US Renal Data System (USRDS) collects, analyzes, and distributes information about CKD and ESKD from all age groups in the United States. According to the 2021 USRDS annual report, the incidence of pediatric CKD in the United States is low (0.5%). Prevalence was highest in Black adolescents compared to their White or Hispanic ethnicity counterparts (USRDS, 2021b). In terms of ESKD, incidence fell from 12 per million population (pmp) in 2009 to 11 pmp in 2019. However, this rate has not changed significantly since 2014. The incidence of ESKD is highest among children less than 1 year and 13 to 17 years of age. Although nonglomerular and glomerular causes may occur at any age, some general trends are worth noting. Nonglomerular origins are responsible for most cases of pediatric kidney disease, but especially in children less than 5 years of age. In the United States, 54.9% of children less than 1 year of age with ESKD have a CAKUT diagnosis, but this has become less common in older children (USRDS, 2021b). Glomerular kidney disease is most often diagnosed in older children, especially preadolescents and adolescents (USRDS, 2021b). Combined, primary and secondary causes of GN comprise the majority of ESKD (38.5%) in the 13- to 17-year age group (USRDS, 2021b). Black and Hispanic children demonstrate a higher adjusted incidence of ESKD compared to their White, Asian, or "other" counterparts, and males have a significantly higher incidence of ESKD compared with their female counterparts (USRDS, 2021b).

DIAGNOSTIC CRITERIA

ESTIMATED GLOMERULAR FILTRATION RATE

Estimating Equations

The estimated glomerular filtration rate (eGFR) is the most important test to determine kidney function. The CKiD U 25 GFR, a new estimating equation for children, went live in September 2021 and is calculated using the enzymatic creatinine level, sex, age, and height in centimeters (Pierce et al., 2021). This new equation is the preferred method to calculate eGFR for patients 1 to 25 years of age, as it has been shown to remove the bias in prior equations at either end of the age spectrum and accounts for the changes in eGFR that can occur with puberty. The CKiD U25 GFR estimating equation was created and internally validated within the CKiD study, a national study that followed children with CKD through adulthood. The CKiD U25 GFR equation can be found online at https://ckid-gfrcalculator.shinyapps.io/eGFR/#, or in the QxMD calculator smartphone app.

Assays. It is important to note that two main assays are used by US laboratories: enzymatic and Jaffe. The preferred assay is the enzymatic assay, and it is the one with which current estimating equations are validated.

Table 29.1   Classification of Chronic Kidney Disease Diagnoses

GLOMERULAR	NONGLOMERULAR
Chronic glomerulonephritis	Aplastic/hypoplastic/dysplastic kidneys
Congenital nephrotic syndrome	Autosomal dominant polycystic kidney disease
Denys-Drash syndrome	Autosomal recessive polycystic kidney disease
Familiar nephritis	Branchio-oto-renal
Focal segmental glomerulosclerosis	Cystinosis
Hemolytic uremic syndrome	Medullary cystic disease/juvenile nephronophthisis
Henoch-Schönlein nephritis	Obstructive uropathy
Idiopathic crescentic glomerulonephritis	Oxalosis
Immunoglobulin A nephropathy	Pyelonephritis/Interstitial nephritis
Membranoproliferative glomerulonephritis types I and II	Reflux nephropathy
Membranous nephropathy	Renal infarct
Sickle cell nephropathy	Syndrome of agenesis of abdominal musculature
Systemic immunologic disease (including systemic lupus erythematosus)	Wilms tumor

Warady, B. A., Abraham, A. G., Schwartz, G. J., Wong, C. S., Muñoz, A., Betoko, A., Mitsnefes, M., Kaskel, F., Greenbaum, L. A, Mak, R. H., Flynn, J., Moxey-Mims, M. M., & Furth, S. (2015). Predictors of Rapid Progression of Glomerular and Nonglomerular Kidney Disease in Children and Adolescents: The Chronic Kidney Disease in Children (CKiD) Cohort. American Journal of Kidney Diseases, 65(6):878–888. doi:10.1053/j.ajkd.2015.01.008. Epub 2015 Mar 19.

Unfortunately, because of the cheaper cost, many labs still use the Jaffe assay. Creatinine levels using Jaffe may be falsely elevated by as much as 20% due to protein interference, especially in neonates and infants, and Jaffe values cannot be formally recommended for use in the current estimating equations.

Race variable removed. In September 2021, the NKF and American Society of Nephrology joint task force recommended using a new estimating equation: the CKD-EPI 2021, thus removing the race variable (Delgado et al., 2022). Prior equations used to estimate GFR in adults have included race, as it had been thought to biologically impact kidney function. Race has since been shown to be a social construct, not a physiologic variable, in determining kidney function. Including race in eGFR, results were confusing for those who identified as multiracial and did not account for the diversity within communities of color. Race inclusion within the prior eGFR equations may have adversely affected accurate diagnosis and subsequent health care in the Black population, overestimating kidney function. The updated calculator and those used for pediatric patients no longer include the race variable.

Special considerations. For patients who are obese or have decreased muscle mass, a cystatin C level, along with an enzymatic creatinine level, should be obtained. While the cystatin C lab test is not widely used due to availability and cost, it can be helpful in accurately determining kidney function. Creatinine alone can overestimate kidney function in these patients because it is influenced by nutrition, puberty, and muscle mass, whereas cystatin C is not. Cystatin C can be entered into the CKiD U25 equation, thus providing a more accurate estimation of kidney function.

STAGING KIDNEY DISEASE

The Kidney Disease Outcomes Quality Initiative (KDOQI) guidelines define CKD as abnormalities of kidney structure or function, present for more than 3 months, with implications for health (Inker et al., 2014). Once an accurate eGFR is calculated, the kidney function can be tracked over a 3-month timeframe, and kidney disease can be staged to guide diagnosis and management. There are five stages of kidney disease (Table 29.2), where stage 1 represents relatively normal function with eGFR greater than 90 mL/min/1.73 m², and stage 2 is a milder disease with eGFR 60 to 89 mL/min/1.73 m². There are few signs or symptoms noted in these first two stages. Stage 3 is considered a moderate disease with eGFR between 30 and 59 mL/min/1.73 m². The physiologic changes that cause long-term effects often begin in this stage but are not yet appreciated fully in labs and clinical presentations. This is the stage when, if identified, a referral should be made to the nephrology team. Stage 4 represents moderate-severe disease, with an eGFR of 16 to 29 mL/min/m², and lab abnormalities such as electrolyte disturbances, metabolic acidosis, bone mineral changes, and anemia begin to manifest. Radiologic abnormalities may also be present. Patients may have more overt symptoms of poor appetite and neurocognitive dysfunction. Stage 5 represents kidney failure with an eGFR of less than 15 mL/min/1.73 m². About 75% of children require dialysis at this time if a preemptive transplant cannot be arranged (Mitsnefes et al., 2013). While some children may have significant symptoms, some are functioning well enough to forgo dialysis initiation if lab values can be managed medically with diet restrictions and medications. Note that stage 3 is divided into 3a (45–59 mL/min/1.73 m²) and 3b (30–44 mL/min/1.73 m²) (Kirsztajn et al., 2009). This controversial recommendation was made to minimize late referral to a nephrologist and subsequent distress to patients who might have benefited from earlier interventions as it relates to the possibility of fast progression of kidney disease, especially within stage 3 CKD. Although albuminuria is factored into CKD staging for adults, this practice is

Table 29.2 Stages of Kidney Disease

GFR CATEGORY	GFR (mL/min/1.73 m²)	TERMS
G1	≥90	Normal or high
G2	60–89	Mildly decreased[a]
G3a	45–59	Mildly to moderately decreased
G3b	30–44	Moderately to severely decreased
G4	15–29	Severely decreased
G5	<15	Kidney failure

In the absence of evidence of kidney damage, neither GFR category G1 nor G2 fulfill the criteria for CKD.
[a]Relative to young adult level.
CKD, Chronic kidney disease; *GFR*, glomerular filtration rate.
From Inker, L. A., Astor, B. C., Fox, C. H., Isakova, T., Lash, J. P., Peralta, C. A., Kurella Tamura, M., & Feldman, H. I. (2014). KDOQI US commentary on the 2012 KDIGO clinical practice guideline for the evaluation and management of CKD. *American Journal of Kidney Diseases, 63*(5), 713–735.

not common in pediatric CKD. Children under 2 years of age do not fit within the above classification system because they normally have a low GFR even when corrected for body surface area (BSA) (Srivastava & Warady, 2021).

CLINICAL MANIFESTATIONS AT TIME OF DIAGNOSIS

In the primary care setting, CKD can be difficult to fully appreciate until later stages. Kidneys work under normal conditions to create homeostasis. The underlying kidney disease and amount of residual kidney function will impact the timing and severity of symptom presentation. However, recalling the basic functions of the kidney can offer some clues along the way, prompting the primary care provider to have CKD on the differential list. Although not exhaustive, Table 29.3 provides basic tasks performed by the kidney and associated manifestations of dysfunctional kidneys.

Clinical Manifestations at Time of Diagnosis

- Fluid and electrolyte and acid-base abnormalities
  - Hyperkalemia
  - Sodium imbalance
  - Fluid volume overload
- Metabolic abnormalities
  - Alterations in calcium and phosphorus
  - Increased secretion of parathyroid hormone
- Anemia
  - Decreased production of erythropoietin
  - Inadequate iron stores or blockage of uptake
  - Decreased uptake of growth hormone leading to poor growth
  - Blood pressure possibly elevated
- Uremia
  - Decreased energy, increased fatigue
  - In severe uremia: congestive heart failure, pericarditis, gastrointestinal bleeding, and encephalopathy may occur
- Growth failure
- Proteinuria
- Hematuria

FLUID AND ELECTROLYTE ABNORMALITIES

As renal function decreases, solute and toxins accumulate in the blood (i.e., uremia), and in most cases fluid retention also occurs. Hyperkalemia occurs because of excessive potassium intake and reduced renal excretion, metabolic acidosis, and—if untreated—can lead to fatal cardiac arrhythmias. Over 90% of potassium excretion occurs in the kidneys. Hypokalemia is a less common disturbance but may occur with tubular disorders or in children receiving intensive dialysis regimens (Desloovere et al., 2021).

Maintaining sodium and water balance is crucial for growth, neurocognitive development, and acid-base homeostasis. Depending on the underlying disease and severity, hyponatremia may or may not be present on lab work. Children with renal tubular disorders have abnormal salt wasting because it is not appropriately reabsorbed in the tubules. However, most children retain the ability to maintain sodium and water balance through compensatory mechanisms (Kleta & Bockenhauer, 2018). Additionally, as kidney function continues to decline, fluid is not removed appropriately and accumulates, contributing to hyponatremia, hypertension, or edema, often as the result of the osmotic gradient due to protein losses in the urine (proteinuria) (Hoenig & Hladik, 2022).

METABOLIC AND ACID-BASE ABNORMALITIES

Alterations in calcium, phosphorus, and acid-base metabolism begin to develop in the child with CKD as early as stage 2 before overt signs and symptoms are appreciated (Wesseling-Perry et al., 2012). Impairment of bicarbonate resorption and decreased acid and ammonia excretion lead to metabolic acidosis, evidenced by low bicarbonate (CO_2) levels on serum metabolic panels. Uncorrected metabolic acidosis will impair growth. Low bicarbonate levels also contribute to CKD progression (Brown et al., 2020).

The bone mineral axis becomes disrupted, exhibiting either poor bone turnover (mineralization), which puts children at risk for fractures with minor injuries, or disproportionate bone turnover with excessive

Table 29.3	Comparison of Basic Tasks of Healthy Kidneys and Associated Manifestations From Unhealthy or Absent Kidneys	

TASKS PERFORMED BY HEALTHY KIDNEYS	MANIFESTATIONS OF UNHEALTHY OR ABSENT KIDNEYS
Fluid and electrolyte management	Abnormal electrolytes Hypervolemia
Blood pressure control	Hypertension due to renin-angiotensin-aldosterone system disruption and hypervolemia
Growth	Abnormal bone metabolism Abnormal use of endogenous growth hormone leads to short stature
Red blood cell production	Anemia
Acid-base balance	Poor growth or weight gain Neurocognitive delays
Removal of waste products	Neurocognitive delays Gastrointestinal disturbances in appetite, nausea, vomiting lead to poor weight gain

phosphorus contributing to calcifications in the cardio-vascular system (McAlister et al., 2020). This dysregu-lation further compounds the cardiovascular disease risk in this population (Khouzam et al., 2015). Routine monitoring of serum levels of calcium, phosphorus, parathyroid hormone (PTH), vitamin D, and CO_2 is recommended at stage 3 (Ketteler et al, 2018).

Along with excessive intake of phosphorus-con-taining foods, decreased kidney function results in the retention of phosphorus, demonstrated by elevated serum phosphorus levels. In pediatric CKD, phos-phate retention leads to 1,25-dihydroxyvitamin D deficiency and hypocalcemia, which in turn causes secondary hypoparathyroidism. Increased bone turn-over and abnormalities in bone morphology are the results of secondary hyperparathyroidism (Srivastava & Warady, 2021).

Disturbance in the calcium-phosphorus-bone metab-olism relationship causes abnormal bone strength and structure and impairs growth. Previously referred to as renal osteodystrophy (ROD), in 2006 the Kidney Disease: Improving Global Outcomes group recom-mended using the term *chronic kidney disease–mineral bone disorder* (CKD-MBD) to describe the abnormalities associated with this complex relationship (Srivastava & Warady, 2021). In children, CKD-MBD resembles rick-ets because of the vitamin D disturbances. Bone defor-mities, bone pain, growth retardation (Shroff et al., 2017), muscle weakness, slipped capital femoral epiph-yses (SCFE), and subperiosteal resorption of bone with the widening of the metaphyses are common (Vogt & Avner, 2007).

ANEMIA

Many physiologic factors influence anemia, including various hormones, nutritional deficiencies, and meta-bolic dysfunction. Erythropoietin (EPO) is a hormone produced in the kidney that contributes to the produc-tion of red blood cells (RBCs). Consequently, as kidney function declines, anemia becomes more prevalent. Anemia is a known risk factor for increased cardiovas-cular disease progression, hospitalization, and mor-tality (Atkinson & Warady, 2018). In utero, the liver is the primary source for EPO production. After birth, peritubular interstitial cells in the kidney assume this function, but when these cells are injured or abnormal they are unable to produce EPO. Another indepen-dent factor of anemia is that of hypoxia-induced fac-tor, which becomes dysregulated and causes a relative excess of oxygen, thereby causing a decreased produc-tion of EPO (Koury & Haase, 2015) and a dispropor-tionate presentation of anemia. In kidney failure, the GFR is reduced, and the resulting uremia leads to the decreased lifespan of RBCs.

Additionally, the anemia associated with CKD may demonstrate functional iron deficiency where iron stores are adequate, but a hormone, hepcidin, blocks the appropriate use and transport of iron into the reticuloendothelial system to aid in erythropoiesis production (Berns, 2022). Additional factors for ane-mia include iron deficiency, nutritional deficiencies of vitamin B_{12}, folate, carnitine, vitamin C, and cop-per, and hyperparathyroidism (Atkinson & Warady, 2018). Initial abnormal lab results may include low hemoglobin and hematocrit levels, serum iron, ferritin, transferrin saturation, reticulocyte counts, or low lev-els of the nutritional vitamins and minerals mentioned previously.

UREMIA

The inability of the kidneys to adequately rid the body of nitrogenous wastes leads to a syndrome called ure-mia (Table 29.4). Uremia is defined as severely ele-vated concentrations of creatinine, blood urea, and other nitrogenous end products of protein and amino acid metabolism, which are usually excreted in the urine (Inker & Levey, 2023). These symptoms may be difficult to appreciate initially and can often be non-specific and vague. As kidney function decreases, the symptoms become more pronounced. For instance, a child with CKD may initially exhibit a loss of nor-mal energy and increased fatigue on exertion, prefer-ring sedentary activities to active play, which may evolve to disinterest in play. Children with taste dis-turbances and nausea may demonstrate low appetite or changes in food preferences, often labeled as picky

Table 29.4 Features of Uremia

METABOLIC/ENDOCRINE	NEUROMUSCULAR
Sexual dysfunction	Sleep disturbances
Amenorrhea	Restless legs
Protein/muscle catabolism increases	Decreased mental acuity
Resting energy expenditure decreases	Loss of energy
Insulin resistance	Peripheral neuropathy
Vomiting[a]	Taste and smell defects
Other	Anorexia and nausea
Platelet dysfunction	Muscle membrane potential reduced
Decreased red blood cell survival	Seizures[a]
Pruritis	Coma[a]
Oxidant stress	

[a]Much less commonly seen with advancements in recognition and treatment.
From Meyer, T. W., & Hostetter, T. H. (2014). Approaches to uremia. *JASN*, 25(10), 2151–2158.

eaters. Secondary weight loss often occurs concomitant with uremia severity (Ku et al., 2018a). Schoolwork or household chores may become more difficult to accomplish due to the impact of uremia on attention span and memory (Harshman et al., 2019). Sleep disturbances also exacerbate this presentation. Sexual development, including amenorrhea, can be common in adolescent females (Meyer & Hostetter, 2014). Symptoms of severe uremia can include congestive heart failure, pericarditis, uremic pleuritis, encephalopathy, and abnormal bleeding and require immediate hospitalization and kidney replacement therapy (Brophy & Muff-Luett, 2022).

GROWTH FAILURE

Growth failure is a significant consequence of CKD in children and is a symptom that occasionally leads to the diagnosis of kidney disease. Persistent growth failure is defined as height below the 3rd percentile and height velocity below the 25th percentile beyond a period of 3 months in infants or 6 months in children and adolescents (Drube et al., 2019). Growth failure is associated with an increased risk of death and poorer health-related quality-of-life scores and affects up to 35% of the pediatric CKD population (Brown et al., 2022). Growth failure is multifactorial and includes CKD-MBD, malnutrition, metabolic acidosis, electrolyte loss, intrauterine growth restriction, and disturbances of the somatotropic and gonadotropic hormone axes. Additionally, it is important to note that in CKD there is not a deficiency of growth hormone (GH); rather, it is insensitivity to circulating GH levels due to dysregulation of the insulin-like growth factor (IGF) process (Drube et al., 2019). Weight loss has been found to accelerate once eGFR is less than 35 mL/min/1.73 m^2 and is more highly associated with glomerular causes of CKD in children and adolescents (Ku et al., 2018a). However, children with nonglomerular diseases such as CAKUT also

present with slow growth and weight gain. Often, they receive nutritional support with specialized formulas via gastrointestinal or gastrojejunostomy tubes.

PROTEINURIA, BLOOD PRESSURE, AND CKD PROGRESSION

Proteinuria, especially in the nephrotic range (>2 mg/mg), is the strongest predictor of kidney disease progression regardless of glomerular or nonglomerular disease origin (Bokenkamp, 2020). In adults, albuminuria is the most utilized study to determine progression; its use has been primarily used in the setting of diabetes mellitus. In children, however, a urine protein–creatinine (UP/C) ratio demonstrates similar outcomes; thus it is utilized as a predictor of disease progression instead of a urine albumin–creatinine ratio (Fuhrman et al., 2017), especially since diabetes is not a significant cause of pediatric CKD (Atkinson et al., 2021). Proteinuria is often associated with elevated blood pressure and hypoalbuminemia (serum albumin <3.8 g/dL) in both glomerular and nonglomerular diseases as a risk factor for progression, although, as stated previously, it is most rapid in glomerular diseases. In addition to proteinuria, elevated blood pressure and hypoalbuminemia, dyslipidemia, male sex, and anemia have been identified as risk factors for disease progression in nonglomerular diseases (Atkinson et al., 2021).

Blood pressure may be the presenting sign or may develop because of CKD in the pediatric population. Depending on the stage of CKD, the causes for hypertension are varied but may include overcorrection of anemia, dysregulation of the renin-angiotensin-aldosterone system, renal vascular causes, including narrowed renal arteries, obesity, or other pre-existing cardiovascular causes.

HEMATURIA

Hematuria can be a nonspecific finding with benign and serious causes and may be macroscopic or microscopic. In contrast with other countries such as Israel and Japan, urinalysis is not used as a screening tool in the healthy population, so hematuria is often noted on a urinalysis when investigating the illness; in a majority of children this will be an isolated finding (Kallash & Rheault, 2020). However, for children with a higher risk for CKD, such as those with a history of acute kidney injury (AKI), CAKUT, hypertension, active nephritis or systemic disease, prematurity, intrauterine growth retardation, or a family history of kidney disease, a urinalysis to look for microscopic hematuria is warranted (American Academy of Pediatrics, 2022). Occasionally, hematuria may present along with proteinuria (Kallash & Rheult, 2020). Associated causes of hematuria related to CKD will be discussed later in this chapter.

TREATMENT

Treatment goals include restoring and maintaining the child's health and improving growth and developmental level of function to the highest degree possible. As significant psychosocial, emotional, and financial stressors accompany chronic medical conditions, the child and family should be provided with psychological and emotional support from a specialized and multidisciplinary kidney team. Treatment is based on the severity of the clinical manifestations of CKD. Approaches include conservative medical management and (eventually) renal replacement therapy (RRT).

 Treatment

- Conservative management
  - Fluid and electrolyte control
  - Metabolic control and calcium and phosphate homeostasis
  - Anemia management
  - Managing growth retardation
  - Proteinuria control
  - Blood pressure management
- Renal replacement therapy
  - Peritoneal dialysis (continuous ambulatory peritoneal dialysis, continuous cycling peritoneal dialysis, or nighttime intermittent peritoneal dialysis)
  - Hemodialysis
  - Transplantation

CONSERVATIVE MANAGEMENT

Fluid and Electrolyte Management

Early recognition and management of biochemical imbalances may prevent adverse consequences. Fluid overload and hypertension may be controlled by limiting total fluid intake to total urine output volume plus insensible losses, restricting salt intake, and using diuretic and antihypertensive medications. Thiazide and loop diuretics help control volume-dependent hypertension in CKD; although thiazides are effective only in children with a GFR greater than 45 mL/min/m², loop diuretics should be used in later stages because thiazides become ineffective in stages 4 and 5 (Warady et al., 2021). Mild hyperkalemia should be trended, critical levels should be repeated immediately to rule out hemolysis or other nondietary causes, and appropriate intervention should be provided. Hyperkalemia can be controlled through dietary restriction of high-potassium foods' use of bicarbonate (sodium citrate [Bicitra] or sodium bicarbonate) for intracellular mobilization and acidosis prevention. Potassium binders such as sodium polystyrene sulfonate (Kayexalate) and patiromer (Veltassa) have been recommended to remove potassium from the body. Sodium polystyrene sulfonate is not recommended for long-term management due to the potential for bowel necrosis, high rates of constipation, and low tolerability. Patiromer

is not currently approved for pediatric use, but studies are ongoing. For young adults over age 18 years, it can be useful, but constipation and hypomagnesemia are common side effects (Desloovere et al., 2021). Careful attention should be paid to salt substitutes as they often replace sodium chloride with potassium chloride. Additionally, processed foods may use potassium salts to preserve shelf life, with a bioavailability of up to 90% to 100%, which may be a hidden source of potassium. Careful education and monitoring should be provided (Desloovere et al., 2021). Consultation with a renal dietitian can improve adherence to a low-potassium diet as they can provide cooking strategies and counsel patients and families on how to read labels.

Metabolic Abnormalities

Metabolic acidosis may be controlled with alkalinizing medications (e.g., sodium citrate [Bicitra] or sodium bicarbonate tablets). Target serum bicarbonate levels should be greater than 22 mEq/L to help slow the progression of CKD (Brown et al., 2020). To prevent calcifications that contribute to CVD in children with CKD (Khouzam et al., 2015), ROD, and secondary hyperparathyroidism, conservative management of hyperphosphatemia includes limiting phosphorus-containing foods and utilizing vitamin D therapy such as calcitriol (Rocaltrol) and paricalcitol (Zemplar) (Shroff et al., 2017). Similar to potassium restrictions, modifying diet can be challenging due to the amount of phosphorus used as a preservative in processed foods and dairy, favorites of children and adolescents. In addition to dietary counseling and restriction, phosphorus binders such as calcium carbonate and sevelamer (Renvela, Renagel) can be used to manage phosphorus levels as part of the regimen to balance the mineral-bone dynamic. Calcium carbonate is an over-the-counter medication, and although it both increases serum calcium levels and binds to phosphorus to aid in excretion, total calcium daily recommended intake (DRI) should be considered when prescribing this for hyperphosphatemia. Sevelamer is available by prescription only and comes in powder and tablet form, allowing for flexibility for children receiving parenteral nutrition with a GI tube. The tablets should not be broken or crushed as they will expand and create a potential esophageal obstruction. Both calcium carbonate and sevelamer should be taken away from other medications if possible due to the possible binding and excretion of concomitant medications.

Anemia Management

Treatment is aimed at increasing RBC production and decreasing RBC loss. The administration of an EPO-stimulating agent (ESA) along with iron supplementation is a cornerstone for the treatment of anemia associated with CKD. Recombinant human EPO (rHuEPO) and darbepoetin (Aranesp) are the most common ESAs prescribed, although biosimilar ESAs are being used more commonly (Atkinson & Warady, 2018). Depending on the drug used, the current stage of renal failure, and desired hematocrit level, ESA dosing can be given one to three times per week for EPO and one to four times per month for darbepoetin. Both are available in subcutaneous or intravenous forms, the latter used for hemodialysis patients. The dose must be carefully titrated to prevent a rapid rise in hematocrit (>1–2 g/dL over 2–4 weeks) and possible hypertensive crisis. For dose titration of ESAs, laboratory monitoring is not recommended more often than every 2 to 4 weeks depending on the agent being administered. No specified Hgb level triggers ESA initiation, although clinically a level less than 10 g/dL is often the threshold. With the advent of rHuEPO replacement, blood transfusions are rarely recommended. Risks associated with blood transfusions are increased risk of acquiring viral or bacterial infections, hemolytic transfusion reactions, and allosensitization, which can negatively impact the opportunity for a well-matched kidney transplant (Atkinson & Warady, 2018).

As the desired erythropoiesis is achieved, iron stores become depleted. Iron supplementation is usually required to maximize the response to ESA therapy (Atkinson & Warady, 2018). The current goal of iron therapy is to maintain transferring saturation levels above 20% and serum ferritin at over 100 ng/mL. Oral therapy is often the initial route of iron supplementation, but a lack of therapeutic response secondary to decreased poor absorption, poor medication adherence, and GI side effects may warrant a change to intravenous iron supplementation.

Growth Failure

Growth failure is a significant consequence of CKD in children and is a symptom that occasionally leads to the diagnosis of renal disease. As discussed previously, the imbalance of circulating GH in relation to IGF-1 is thought to be integral in the reduction of linear bone growth, leading to growth impairment. Also observed are abnormalities in the gonadotropic hormones, which likely contribute to the suboptimal pubertal growth and development that has been noted in pediatric CKD (Mahan & Warady, 2006).

Pediatric nephrology teams will use recombinant human growth hormone (rhGH) to improve growth in children with CKD. This long-term therapy has been shown to safely and effectively result in catchup growth, possibly leading to a final (adult) height within the normal range. Before rhGH therapy is started, optimal nutritional management and dialysis efficacy should be achieved; the PTH level should be normal or reduced if very high. Baseline parameters should be established for funduscopic examinations, pubertal stage, thyroid function (thyroid-stimulating hormone, free thyroxine [T_3]), IGF-1 levels, bone age x-rays to evaluate for open epiphyses (which indicate room for growth), and bilateral hip x-rays to rule out SCFE, a complication of rhGH use. Avoid the use of rhGH if any of the following are present: within the first year posttransplant, severe elevation of PTH levels, closed epiphyses on bone age x-rays, hip pain or abnormal ambulation is noted (an indication of SCFE), or vomiting and headaches are reported (signs of increased intracranial hypertension) (Drube et al., 2019).

Proteinuria

As previously discussed, proteinuria is an independent risk factor for the progression of CKD in children and must be adequately managed to preserve renal function. Children with CKD and hypertension should have an evaluation for proteinuria that includes a urinalysis and UP/C ratio (Flynn et al., 2017). Ratios greater than 2 mg/mg place the patient with CKD at high risk for rapid progression to ESKD. Clinical practice guidelines for chronic kidney disease in children and adolescents published by the National Kidney Foundation (2015) recommend that simple spot urine samples should be used to detect and monitor proteinuria in children and adolescents. These are widely accepted as they can be performed randomly. Obtaining a timed urine collection is not usually necessary; although 24-hour urine collections remain the gold standard, they have proven difficult to obtain especially in the pediatric population (Noone & Langlois, 2016). Causes of proteinuria should be identified and appropriate treatment initiated as soon as possible. Optimal treatment depends on the underlying cause and is managed by the pediatric nephrology team but often includes corticosteroids, angiotensin-converting enzyme inhibitors (ACEIs)/angiotensin II receptor blockers (ARBs), and immunosuppressive medications.

RENAL REPLACEMENT THERAPY

As CKD progresses into stage 5, conservative management is no longer adequate, and treatment with either dialysis or transplantation is typically required. More frequent follow-up is required with the nephrology team, who will be responsible for ongoing discussions about the future and options for dialysis and transplantation with the child (if of suitable age) and parents. Family education regarding the different therapy modalities should commence while the child's CKD is in stage 4. Touring the pediatric dialysis center and introducing the child and parent to one or more well-adjusted families with a child treated with dialysis or who has experienced a transplant are helpful ways to prepare children and families.

Kidney function alone is not an indicator of dialysis initiation. Higher mortality was noted in children who initiated dialysis with higher eGFRs, although no randomized control trials have occurred to validate this finding (Zahr et al., 2021). Indications for the timing of RRT are individualized, with consideration given to the following clinical and psychosocial factors: fluid status, electrolyte imbalances, growth failure, acidosis, or uremic symptoms, including nausea and vomiting, anorexia, and poor school performance. Absolute indicators include uncontrollable hypertension, nephrectomies, pulmonary edema, uremic encephalopathy and pericarditis, refractory nausea, and emesis (Zahr et al., 2021), and the need for severe fluid restriction that will not allow for proper nutrition (Warady et al., 2014) (Box 29.1).

All treatment modalities have both positive and negative aspects. Initiation of dialysis or transplantation is traumatic for the child and family, even with pre-ESKD counseling, but the stress is worse if the child is very ill. However, denial is a strong coping mechanism and is enabled when a child feels well despite a significantly elevated creatinine level. The many special needs of children help determine the modality of RRT selected. Because of the problems associated with small blood vessels for vascular access, hemodialysis in young children may not be practical. Many adolescents begin hemodialysis due to having easier access to an adult dialysis center compared to pediatric centers. Peritoneal dialysis is the preferred dialysis modality for most children; however, many medical and psychosocially variables must be considered (Warady et al., 2014; Zahr et al., 2021). Most pediatric dialysis centers (65%) choose peritoneal dialysis as the initial modality for children and adolescents compared to adult centers (45%). Both modalities require a multidisciplinary approach that includes pediatric nephrologists and the specialized skills of nurses, social workers, and nutritionists. Transplantation is the RRT of choice due to the improved quality of life in the psychosocial and medical realms (Warady et al., 2014). Improved technology, surgical techniques, and more effective medications promote better survival (i.e., of both child and graft) with transplantation and offer the child and family greater potential to live a less restricted life (Hebert et al., 2017). The child and family must understand

that a kidney transplant is not a cure for CKD but is another treatment approach and can be successful only through carefully guided immunosuppression management with frequent clinical assessments. It also surprises some families to hear that they or their child will need more than one kidney transplant in their lifetime, but counseling from the nephrology team and reinforcement by the primary care team should occur.

Peritoneal Dialysis

As mentioned, peritoneal dialysis is the most common dialysis modality utilized in pediatric centers. Peritoneal dialysis uses the peritoneal membrane as a filtering membrane to remove waste products and excess fluid from the vascular system. Access to the peritoneal membrane is through a catheter placed in the child's abdomen. Two types of peritoneal dialysis catheters are used: acute and chronic. Acute peritoneal catheters are fairly rigid and are either straight or slightly curved. They are made to be placed at bedside. Because of technical and infectious complications associated with acute catheters, chronic catheters are most frequently used. Chronic peritoneal catheters are created with either silicone or polyurethane and have one or two polyethylene terephthalate (Dacron) cuffs, which elicit an inflammatory response in the tissue to form granulation tissue. This tissue secures the catheter in place and prevents bacterial migration into the peritoneum. Techniques and preferred catheter types have been outlined by both the International Society for Peritoneal Dialysis (ISPD) and Standardizing Care to Optimize Pediatric End Stage Kidney Disease (SCOPE) collaborative and recommend that downward pointing, double cuffed, swan neck, coiled catheters be placed to minimize complications associated with infection and dialysis delivery (Sethna et al., 2016; Warady et al., 2012). General recommendations are to allow the peritoneal dialysis catheter site to heal approximately 2 weeks before using it for dialysis due to the risk of leaking and subsequent infection, although data are mixed. In some scenarios, the peritoneal dialysis catheter needs to be used within hours or days of insertion. This is possible with close monitoring for leaking and signs of infection (Warady & Andrews, 2021).

For the peritoneal dialysis treatment, a prescribed volume of sterile solution (dialysate) of electrolytes and glucose is instilled through the catheter into the peritoneal space and allowed to dwell for a prescribed amount of time. The size of the peritoneal membrane correlates with the child's BSA. As a result, volume calculations should be based on BSA and age rather than weight and should consider any residual renal function a child may have (Warady et al., 2014). Diffusion removes waste particles from the blood across the peritoneal membrane, and excess water is removed (ultrafiltration) by osmosis. The amount of glucose regulates ultrafiltration in the dialysis solution in concentrations

---

Box **29.1**	**Timing for Initiating Renal Replacement Therapy**

RELATIVE INDICATORS
- Age of child
- Glomerular filtration rate <10%
- Primary renal disease and comorbid conditions
- Failure to thrive
- Developmental delay
- Inability to function at school
- Inadequate electrolyte and metabolic control
- Poor nutritional status

ABSOLUTE INDICATORS
- Pulmonary edema
- Uncontrollable hypertension
- Pericarditis
- Uremic encephalopathy
- Refractory nausea and emesis

of 1.5%, 2.5%, and 4.25%, and is dependent on the transport characteristics of the peritoneal membrane, classified as high, high-average, low-average, or low. The amount and duration of cycles prescribed are individualized for each child according to transport classification. In other words, a child who is a high transporter would benefit from short, frequent cycles; a low transporter would benefit from longer and fewer cycles (Warady et al., 2014). Infants and children are typically considered high transporters (Verrina & Harshman et al., 2019).

There are generally two types of peritoneal dialysis: manual and automated. Continuous ambulatory peritoneal dialysis (CAPD) is a manual dialysis regimen that delivers three to five dialysate bag exchanges daily into the peritoneum, with dwell times of 3 to 4 hours during the day and a long dwell overnight. CAPD affords greater freedom because no machine is required. Performing three to five exchanges during the day is time consuming, however, and inconvenient at work or school. Additionally, because of the long exchanges, this is not well suited for younger children due to the generally high permeability of the peritoneal membrane. Continuous cycling peritoneal dialysis (CCPD) involves a similar concept but uses an automated cycler; all exchanges can be performed at night while the child and parents sleep, so the daytime is free of exchanges. This is the most common type of peritoneal dialysis utilized for infants, children, and adolescents. After the last cycle is completed, the peritoneum is filled with dialysate (the last fill) that may or may not be exchanged throughout the day. It is generally half the volume instilled during the usual cycles and may be the same concentration as the last bag of dialysate used for the treatment. For patients who are absorbing the last fill, inadequate ultrafiltration (fluid removal) and inappropriate weight gain occur. These patients require a solution (icodextrin) that is not reabsorbed to allow for better weight management both from hypervolemia and caloric exposure from the dialysate and may help optimize blood pressure management secondary to hypervolemia. Patients who require abdominal imaging or procedures may need to have the last fill drained to obtain optimal results. Consultation with the nephrology team is highly recommended to avoid complications or suboptimal results. Nighttime intermittent peritoneal dialysis (NIPD) is similar to CCPD except no dialysate is left in the peritoneum at the end of the treatment.

Meticulous care is crucial with CAPD, NIPD, and CCPD to prevent contamination and infection at the catheter exit site and within the peritoneum. Current data show that this infection, called peritonitis, occurs more frequently in CAPD than in CCPD or NIPD, and infectious complications are the most common cause of death in children receiving long-term peritoneal dialysis. Exit site and catheter tunnel infections, as well as poor connection techniques, are risk factors for peritonitis. Case studies also describe the role pets, especially cats, may have as a risk factor for peritonitis due to chewing on tubing or other peritoneal dialysis supplies. Care should be taken to avoid allowing pets to be in the room during any portion of the home peritoneal dialysis procedure or treatment (Poliquin et al., 2015). The SCOPE collaborative, drawing primarily from the ISPD guidelines, has seen a remarkable reduction in peritonitis episodes among centers that are successfully using the standardized peritoneal dialysis bundle that includes many aspects of peritoneal dialysis care, from catheter insertion to long-term management (Sethna et al., 2016). Home training for caregivers and patients providing peritoneal dialysis care includes education on proper hand hygiene, aseptic technique, appropriate use of antibiotics and/or transfer set change following touch contamination, and routine exit site monitoring for early detection and treatment of an exit site infection (Warady et al., 2014). Still, peritonitis episodes are highest in individuals up to 1 year of age and decrease in frequency with age (Chadha et al., 2010). The key features of peritonitis include abdominal pain, cloudy effluent with white blood cell count greater than $100/mm^3$ and 50% neutrophils, and positive Gram stain or positive culture of microorganism(s) (Warady et al., 2012). Bacteria are the primary cause of peritonitis, with less than 5% of episodes attributed to fungal infections (Neu et al., 2016). Antibiotics used for common infections, but especially those used to treat frequent bacterial peritonitis episodes, are a major risk factor for fungal peritonitis (Warady et al., 2012). While nephrology teams will manage treatment for exit site or tunnel infections and peritonitis, they should be alerted when a patient has been prescribed antibiotics for infections unrelated to peritonitis so they can provide guidance for antifungal prophylaxis.

Staphylococcus aureus infection continues to be the most common cause of peritonitis but has fallen in adults and children likely due to prophylactic efforts like those related to the nasal carriage. Indeed, gram-positive bacteria (*S. aureus* and coagulase-negative *Staphylococcus*) are identified in over 60% of peritonitis episodes in children (Warady et al., 2012). *Pseudomonas* species are the most common gram-negative organism cultured in the United States and are becoming increasingly common (Neu et al., 2016). Effective treatment of peritonitis relies on extended antibiotic exposure to the site of infection—in this case, the peritoneal membrane. Early use of intraperitoneal antibiotics for suspected peritonitis usually resolves the infection without catheter replacement, with cefepime being the antibiotic of choice due to its coverage of both gram-positive and -negative organisms. However, careful selection of the appropriate antibiotic for either empiric or treatment is essential based on center- or regional-specific antibiograms (Warady et al., 2012). The SCOPE collaborative guidelines recommend daily dosing of intraperitoneal antibiotics for 14 to 21 days, depending on the causative organism (Neu et al., 2016). Repeated or persistent peritonitis can result in catheter colonization and require catheter replacement. While most episodes are treated successfully, and peritoneal dialysis can be continued, peritonitis from gram-negative and fungal causes is the most common reason for modality failure and a subsequent transition to hemodialysis (Chadha et al., 2010) due to the loss of membrane permeability by scarring. Other clinical problems associated with peritoneal dialysis include hernia development, leaking, catheter exit site or tunnel infection, catheter migration, cuff extrusion, and catheter outflow obstruction by the omentum or other intraabdominal structures (Warady & Andrews, 2021).

Peritoneal dialysis has many advantages over hemodialysis. Because peritoneal dialysis is performed continuously (as in CAPD) or overnight (with CCPD or NIPD), better control of blood pressure and volume status can be maintained with fewer dietary restrictions, leading to better growth and development. Because peritoneal dialysis is done in the home, caregivers must be taught to technically perform dialysis; however, it is a relatively simple procedure. The home environment must also be assessed for barriers that would increase the risk of complications for this method. Treating a child with home peritoneal dialysis also offers educational and psychological advantages. The most attractive feature of this method is it interferes less with normal daily activities and offers more control to the child and family. A child who uses peritoneal dialysis can attend school every day with little or no interruption, and family vacations are easier to arrange. There is, however, a downside: A common reason for failure is family burnout from the repetitive daily regimen of peritoneal dialysis. When follow-up care and competencies were reevaluated every 6 months per the SCOPE collaborative follow-up bundle, a reduction in peritonitis rates was observed, demonstrating that the nephrology team and the patient/family must work closely to stay competent and proficient in providing this home dialysis modality (Neu et al., 2016). Providing respite care may provide a solution in some cases. Nonadherence is common, particularly in the adolescent population. The presence of an external catheter can affect body image. In children with excessive glucose absorption, obesity further complicates self-esteem issues. By preventing peritonitis and exit site infections, promoting good nutrition, and assisting with the psychosocial aspects of chronic peritoneal dialysis, this method can be considered a potential long-term therapy.

Hemodialysis

Hemodialysis, which is usually performed three or four times per week, offers the advantage of more rapid correction of fluid, electrolyte, and metabolic abnormalities over peritoneal dialysis. Hemodialysis requires vascular access, a dialyzer, bloodlines; a delivery system with a blood pump and many monitoring devices; and heparin to prevent clotting. As the blood passes through the filtering membrane, waste particles diffuse across the membrane from the blood while excess water is removed (called ultrafiltration) by negative pressure into the waste dialysate. The 3- to 5-hour process is constantly monitored for pressure changes, air detection or leaks, chemical imbalance, temperature, and the child's vital signs. Blood flow rates, medications, and fluid volumes are calculated based on the weight of the child (refer to the Hemodialysis Adequacy sections of the NKF's [2015] KDOQI guidelines). Complications associated with hemodialysis include dialysis disequilibrium syndrome, blood and circuit component reactions, air embolism, hemolysis, blood leaks, access thrombosis, headache, nausea, vomiting, cramping, hypotension, hypertension, and infections (Borzych-Duzalka & Harvey, 2021).

Maintaining patent and infection-free vascular access is the greatest challenge for hemodialysis. Internal or external vascular access is necessary to deliver blood to the extracorporeal dialysis circuit for solute and fluid removal (Figs. 29.1 and 29.2). Currently, access is categorized into two types: permanent and temporary. Permanent access is created surgically and includes the arteriovenous fistula (AVF) (Fig. 29.3), arteriovenous graft (AVG), and cuffed venous catheters (CVC). Temporary hemodialysis catheters, which do not have Dacron cuffs, may be placed in some situations for immediate and short-term use. The decision for which access is best depends on the age, size, diagnosis, procedural risks, probability of long-term patency, and likelihood of transplantation (Boehm et al., 2021). KDOQI guidelines recommend a fistula-first approach, placing this permanent access in children weighing more than 20 kg for whom transplant is not imminent. Although this is widely accepted as the ideal approach, in a North American Pediatric Renal Trials and Collaborative Studies (NAPRTCS) consortium, as many as 78.7% of pediatric hemodialysis patients had a CVC as their primary access vs. 11.8% using an AVF, and the USRDS database also suggested CVC was the primary access in 87.6% of pediatric patients (Boehm et al., 2021). A maturation time of at least 2 weeks for a graft or 6 weeks to 4 months for a fistula is required before the access can be used; thus planning for vascular access should be discussed 6 to 12 months before the planned dialysis begins (Boehm et al., 2021). After adequate time has been given for healing, the fistula or graft is accessed through special fistula-needle cannulation. An internal fistula is preferred for children because it has excellent primary patency and low complication rates compared with CVC access. Unfortunately, the option for an AVF in children weighing 10 to 20 kg is limited because this requires specific surgical skills, and only a few pediatric centers have vascular surgeons

Although high morbidity and mortality exist, even very small infants can successfully undergo hemodialysis using specialized equipment and supplies adaptable to neonatal volume requirements (Swartz & Paglialonga, 2021). All medications and fluid volumes in pediatric hemodialysis are calculated based on a child's weight and medical condition. Pediatric hemodialysis should be performed in a pediatric dialysis center. If the distance to a pediatric dialysis center is problematic, adolescents can receive dialysis in adult centers but risk the lack of comprehensive assessment and therapies provided by a pediatric center. Child life specialists and art/music therapists who provide emotional support and teach coping skills by instituting play, art, or musical therapy, and social workers who give emotional and financial family counseling, are important members of the treatment team. On an individual basis, older children in very stable conditions might be considered for home hemodialysis. This is a unique situation and depends on the family's availability to undergo extensive training, home water systems, adaptability, and space for the machine and supplies. As with home peritoneal dialysis, the nephrology team authorizes and manages this scenario.

Kidney Transplantation

Kidney transplantation is the preferred treatment for CKD because it can restore normal kidney function. This eliminates many signs and symptoms of significantly impaired kidney function (Warady et al., 2014), improving neurocognitive development and academic performance, growth, and better quality of life compared with children treated with dialysis (Fernandez & Foster, 2022). Transplant evaluation is multidisciplinary and, in addition to transplant nephrologists, includes nurses, advanced practice providers (APPs), social workers, psychologists, pharmacists, and transplant surgeons experienced in transplant care. With CAKUT being the leading cause of ESKD in this population, pediatric urologists also should be available for formal evaluation and correction of bladder dysfunction and other urinary tract abnormalities (Warady et al., 2014). Preemptive transplants may allow patients to avoid dialysis therapy and account for approximately 25% of pediatric kidney transplants (NAPRTCS, 2014). As of 2022, 105,921 adult and pediatric patients are waiting for a transplant, with 89,964 needing a kidney (United Network for Organ Sharing [UNOS], 2021). Adult kidneys may be transplanted into small children with intraabdominal placement. Because transplantation is the preferred option and donor kidneys are scarce, eligible donors include live immediate family members, live related donors outside the immediate family, and live unrelated donors. Live related donor sources accounted for 50% of all pediatric transplants reported in the NAPRTCS group from 1987 to 2013, and parents are the majority of live donors (78.5%) for

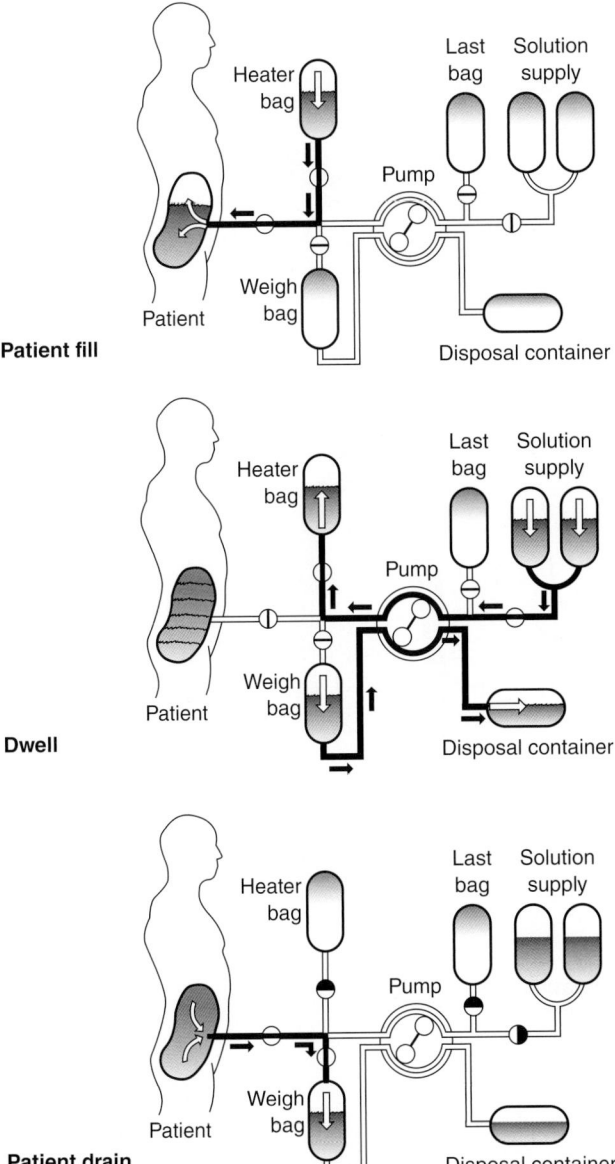

Fig. 29.1 An example of a system used for cycler-assisted peritoneal dialysis. The solution is heated before use and weighed after use. The last bag of solution may have a different concentration to last throughout the day. (From National Institutes of Health, National Institute of Diabetes and Digestive and Kidney Diseases. [2001]. *Treatment methods for kidney failure: Peritoneal dialysis*. Pub No. 01-4688.)

with expertise in microsurgical techniques (Swartz & Pagialonga, 2021). Thus central venous catheter may be the only option for dialysis access. Failure of access, external or internal, is common secondary to infection. Other complications include obstruction of the access device secondary to fibrin sheath formation around an external catheter, thrombosis, or vascular stenosis (Boehm et al., 2021). Access sites are at a premium and must be preserved because these children eventually require multiple vascular accesses. Potential problems warrant early assessment and intervention. Preservation of potential access sites should begin at the time of CKD diagnosis and are discussed in detail later in this chapter.

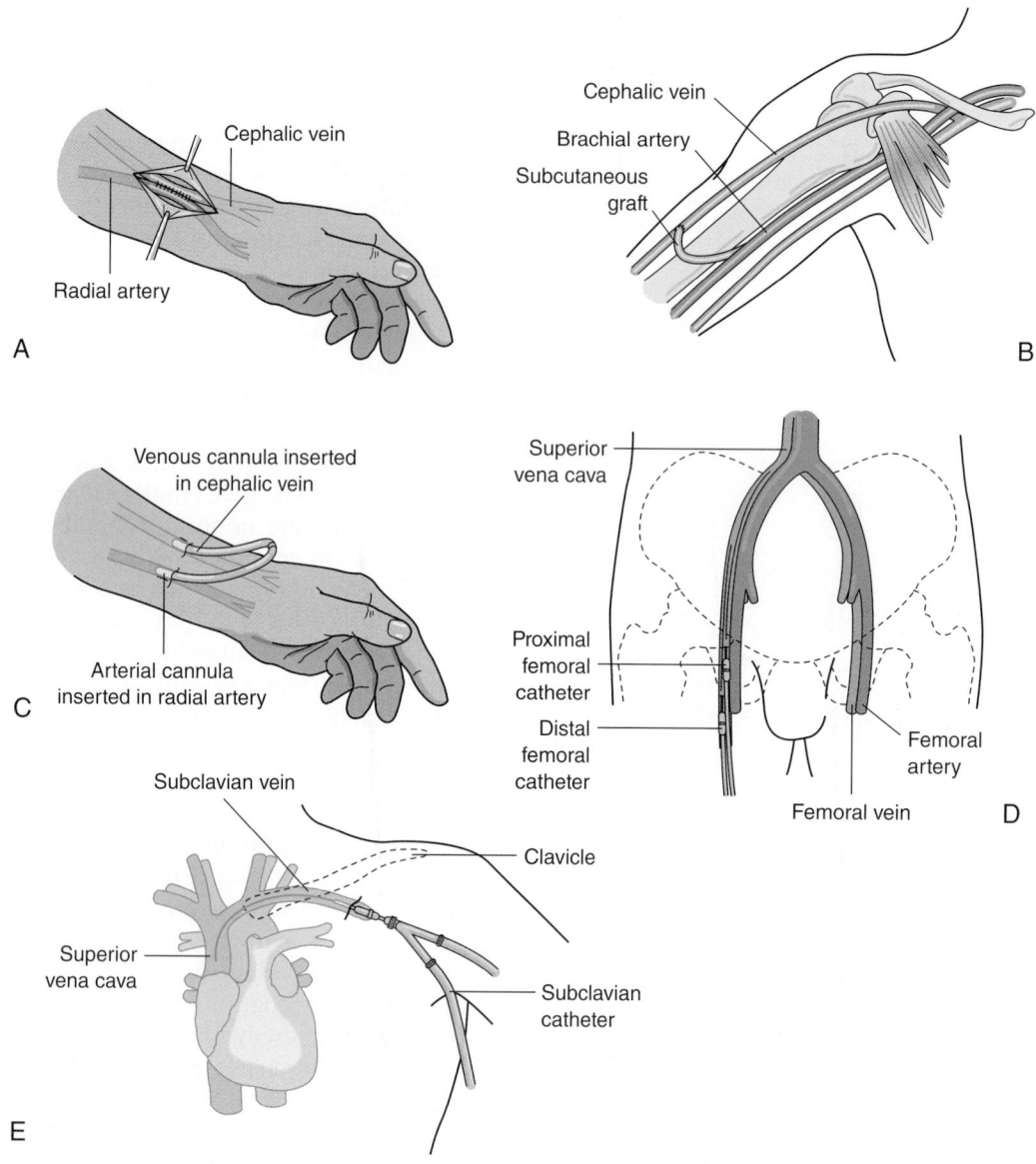

Fig. 29.2 Frequently used methods for gaining vascular access for hemodialysis. (A) Arteriovenous fistula, (B) arteriovenous graft, (C) external arteriovenous shunt, (D) femoral vein catheterization, and (E) subclavian vein catheterization. (From Phipps, W. J., Sands, J. K., & Mack, J. F. [1999]. *Medical-surgical nursing: Concepts and clinical practice* [6th ed.]. Mosby.)

pediatric recipients (NAPRTCS, 2014). Children will need more than one transplant in their lifetime, and the two highest risk periods of their transplant journey (early posttransplant and adolescence) can make finding a quality match challenging (Fernandez & Foster, 2022). Sixty-four confirmed transplants across ABO-compatible barriers have been done to date. This area of inquiry merits further study as early data suggest that graft outcomes are satisfactory in those recipients whose anti-A titer history is low (1:4) (NAPRTCS, 2014). Laparoscopic nephrectomy (living donation) can allow live donors to return to work and regular activities sooner and may increase the overall use of live donors. Aside from surgical techniques, careful medical management is the key to maintaining a successful kidney transplant.

COMPLEMENTARY AND ALTERNATIVE THERAPIES

Many complementary and alternative therapies are being explored for pediatric CKD patients, which is beyond the scope of this chapter. The most common complementary therapy used in renal diseases is fish oil (omega-3 fatty acid [O3FA]) to treat IgA nephropathy. IgA nephropathy is one of the most common types of GN and can result in proteinuria, hematuria, elevated serum creatinine level, and/or hypertension (Kallash & Rheault, 2020). It is thought that O3FA has an antiinflammatory effect. The use of O3FA in adults with IgA nephropathy is based on small clinical trials and is not ready to be extrapolated into the pediatric population. However, this therapy could be considered if dosed per current recommendations in the young adult

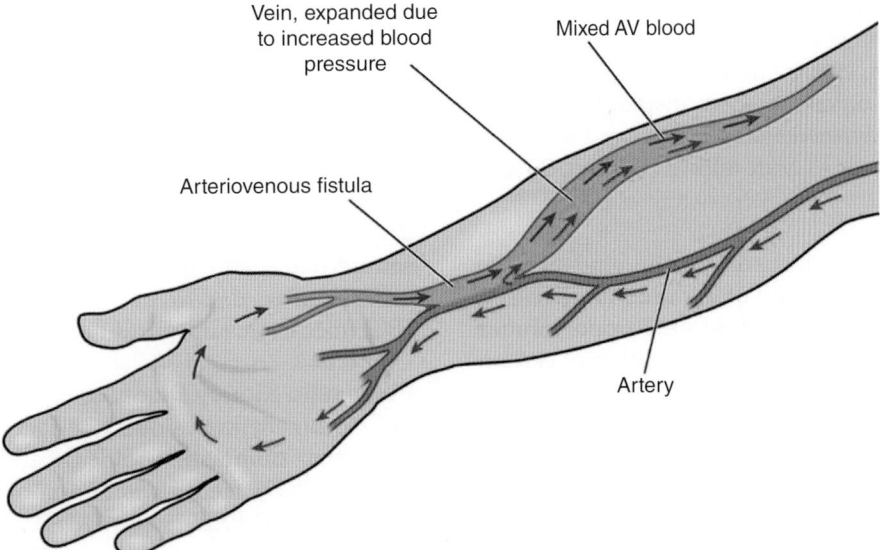

Fig. 29.3 Illustration of radiocephalic arteriovenous *(AV)* fistula. (From Singh, N. S., Grimes, J., Gregg, G. K., et al. [2021]. "Save the vein" initiative in children with CKD: A quality improvement study. *American Journal of Kidney Diseases,* 78(1), 96–102.e1.)

population. Daily doses should not exceed 3 g/day to avoid prolonged bleeding times. O3FA has also been suggested to mitigate increased levels of inflammatory markers associated with hemodialysis; however, larger and more robust studies are needed to support this in practice (Bukutu & Vohra, 2016).

Although no comprehensive studies have been completed, preliminary evidence suggests that a diet rich in phytoestrogens, such as soy protein and flaxseed, can slow the progression of renal disease. The mechanism of action is unknown, but the theory is that phytoestrogens may act as antioxidants, reduce proteinuria and hyperlipidemia, and stabilize GFR (Joshi et al., 2021).

Not all complementary therapies are considered beneficial, and some are potentially harmful to individuals with CKD. Emphasis on probiotics for gut regulation or urinary tract infection (UTI) prevention has been ongoing. Many underlying kidney diseases have some association with GI dysfunction, and probiotics may be appealing. Some have been deemed safe in healthy children at appropriate doses. However, case reports exist that describe fungemia, bacteremia, endocarditis, and other life-threatening complications associated with probiotic use. Patients with indwelling medical devices or immunosuppressive medications should avoid probiotics due to the high risk of infectious complications (Bukutu & Vohra, 2016).

Drug-herb interactions are abundant and usually unknown to the individual seeking alternative therapy. Garlic, ginseng, and ginkgo biloba can potentiate the effects of anticoagulants such as aspirin and warfarin. Grapefruit is known to interact with many drugs, especially those metabolized on the CYP3A4 pathway (Ainslie et al., 2014). In transplant patients who take tacrolimus, drug levels may be elevated if grapefruit

in any form is consumed. St. John's wort affects the metabolism of antidepressants, digoxin, warfarin, and cyclosporin. Much study is needed in this area to provide safe choices for treating the effects of CKD.

ANTICIPATED ADVANCES IN DIAGNOSIS AND MANAGEMENT

OVERVIEW

The primary care provider's early detection of potential renal problems and referral of the child to a pediatric nephrologist often can prevent irreversible renal damage and is recommended at stage 3a or 3b. Significant technical advances in the treatment of infants and children with CKD have occurred over the past decade. More children are receiving dialysis or transplant for ESKD, surviving longer, and living with a higher quality of life. This longevity and improved quality can be credited to some of the following developments: the use of rHuEPO and their biosimilar counterparts, as well as longer-acting epogens (continuous EPO receptor activators [Mircera]) (Chanu et al., 2020); greater compliance to kinetic modeling calculations with immunosuppression medications such as mycophenolate (CellCept), biochemical parameters, and clinical responses to individually tailor the adequacy of dialysis and improve efficiency; early and aggressive correction of electrolyte and metabolic imbalances; and prevention of associated consequences of ESKD. New medications that bind potassium are utilized in adolescents and young adults with advanced CKD for whom dietary restrictions are problematic. Technologic advances in kidney replacement therapies, such as cloud-based home peritoneal dialysis machines, continuous kidney replacement therapies (CKRT) for infants as small as 2.5 kg, and strategies to safely ultrafiltrate excess volume during hemodialysis while mitigating cardiac stress, have also become commonplace. In terms of transplants, epitope matching for living donation has improved outcomes for transplant recipients by reducing antibody-mediated rejection and reducing sensitization that leads to graft failure (Tambur, 2016).

GENETICS

Academic research has focused on the study of the genetic origin and expression of a variety of diseases. Genetic research aims to provide new opportunities for the diagnosis, treatment, and prevention of certain medical conditions. Ethical considerations surrounding the outcomes of genetic testing continue to evolve and present challenges, as well as exciting discoveries that will continue to impact our ability to identify and treat pediatric CKD (Wong et al., 2019). Monogenic diseases are thought to account for 70% of the causes of pediatric CKD. Currently, massive-parallel sequencing (MPS) techniques can identify about 30% of those CKD causes, with some diseases specifically having higher yields (i.e., Alport 55–80%, renal tubulopathies ~64%) (Knoers et al., 2022). MPS techniques allow for specific exome sequencing or complete genome sequencing, and careful pre- and posttest genetic counseling should be performed (Knoers et al., 2022). Although genetic testing is not common practice at the time of this publication, the practice is picking up momentum as more is discovered and insurance coverage is increasing. Examples of pediatric kidney diseases on which genetic research has been focused include but are not limited to the following: Wilms tumor, FSGS, polycystic kidney disease (PKD), Alport syndrome, CAKUT, and pharmacogenetics.

Wilms Tumor

Wilms tumor is the most common malignant kidney tumor in childhood, most commonly affecting children younger than 6 years. Thankfully, survival is ~90%. However, about 15% of children will relapse, which has prompted further work to develop insights into those patients and prevent complications. A prognostic marker emerging from the research is 1q gain. Further study of this marker will hopefully create more opportunities for the precision treatment of Wilms tumor (Nelson et al., 2021).

Focal Segmental Glomerulosclerosis

FSGS is a major cause of the idiopathic steroid-resistant nephrotic syndrome and often progresses to ESKD within 5 to 10 years of diagnosis (Gbadegesin et al., 2016; Trautmann et al., 2020). FSGS is categorized as primary or secondary. Primary FSGS is characterized by hematuria, hypertension, significant proteinuria, decreased serum albumin levels, elevated cholesterol and triglyceride levels, normal C3 and C4 complement levels, and edema. Secondary causes include obesity or human immunodeficiency virus (HIV) infection and

may have a less severe presentation and slower progression. Genetic testing is valuable when there is a family history or neither a primary nor secondary cause can be easily identified (Fervenza & Sethi, 2020). Monogenic causes are highly likely in neonates and infants but less likely in older children and adolescents. There may or may not be a family history of this disease. Blacks are disproportionately affected compared to their White counterparts, and this could be linked to the higher prevalence of *APOL1* polymorphisms associated with FSGS (Sethna & Gipson, 2014).

Polycystic Kidney Disease

PKD is a genetic disorder that takes two major forms: autosomal dominant (ADPKD) and autosomal recessive (ARPKD). ADPKD is caused by a mutation in one of two genes, *PKD-1* and *PKD-2*. ARPKD occurs less frequently and is caused by mutations in a single gene: polycystic kidney and hepatic disease 1 *(PKHD-1)* (Knoers et al., 2022). Both forms can result in pediatric renal failure as a result of cyst formation; however, ADPKD typically occurs later in life. ARPKD, which affects both the liver and kidney, is typically diagnosed in infancy or early childhood, and approximately 50% of affected children who survive the neonatal period progress to ESKD within the first decade of life (Sweeney & Avner, 2014). The identification of a gene mutation in a patient with polycystic kidneys can identify which form of the disease is present. In addition, differentiating between ADPKD and ARPKD has important implications for the genetic counseling of the affected families.

Alport Syndrome

Alport syndrome is a genetic defect of glomerular basement membranes that results in hematuria and can lead to ESKD. It is currently the second most common inherited cause of ESKD after PKD (Chertow et al., 2021). High-frequency sensorineural deafness and ocular defects are also associated with Alport syndrome. Because it is carried on the X chromosome, males have more severe disease than females, and although it usually progresses to ESKD in adulthood, it can occur during adolescence (Kashtan et al., 2018; Lau & Wyatt, 2005). In the CARDINAL trial (Chertow et al., 2021), a new therapy is currently being studied that may slow disease progression compared to the current treatment of ACEI/ARB therapy. The final outcome remains to be seen.

Congenital Anomalies of the Kidney and Urinary Tract

CAKUT can present as part of a syndrome or as an isolated diagnosis, and familial clustering suggests a genetic component to the etiology. However, monogenic causes account for only 10% to 15% of CAKUT diagnoses at the time of this publication. Renal morphology still seems to be the main predictor of prognosis over knowledge of a molecular defect (Knoers et al., 2022).

Pharmacogenetics

The role of genetics in pharmacotherapies is another exciting development to monitor. The use of pharmacogenetics in daily practice is closer than ever, thanks to our knowledge of pharmacokinetics and pharmacodynamics. Tailoring drug therapies for patients based on their pharmacogenetic profile has offered hope for patients with complex conditions, especially in the area of transplant immunosuppression. However, pharmacogenetics is an area that needs further study before implementing it into clinical practice (Waters & Lemaire, 2016).

The internet has made it possible for professionals and lay individuals to access education, peer consulting, continuing education sites for licensure and certification updates, and discussion groups (see Resources, later). Nutritional information and recipes can be downloaded, and dialysis and transplant medications can be researched. Electronic journals related to nephrology are available for professionals and interested individuals.

ASSOCIATED PROBLEMS OF CHRONIC KIDNEY DISEASE AND TREATMENT

CARDIOVASCULAR DISORDERS

Risk Factors and Morbidity/Mortality

The abnormal cardiac function associated with CKD can be attributed to hypertension, anemia, uremia, and vascular calcifications. Congestive heart failure can result from fluid overload, severe hypertension, or uremic myocardiopathy. Heart murmurs are common in children with CKD as a result of anemia, hypertension, and volume overload. Electrocardiographic abnormalities are associated with left ventricular hypertrophy and hyperkalemia. The presence of anemia and AV shunting (from vascular access) can increase cardiac workload and contribute to congestive heart failure (Borlaug et al., 2022). Excessive fluid removal during hemodialysis can lead to myocardial stunning (Hayes & Paglialonga, 2019). As with the general population, cardiovascular disease advances with age, but the risk for cardiovascular disease is significantly higher for individuals with ESKD than in the general population.

Associated Problems

Chronic Kidney Disease and Treatment

- Cardiovascular disorders
- Hypertension
- Neurologic complications
- Aluminum toxicity
- Uremic neuropathy
- Encephalopathy
- Chronic kidney disease–mineral bone disorder
- Urologic manifestations
- Dermatologic manifestations
- Gastrointestinal manifestations
- Intercurrent illness

Furthermore, cardiovascular disease is the leading cause of mortality in adulthood for patients with CKD, compounded by the childhood onset of kidney disease. Estimated mortality rates for children with kidney failure receiving dialysis are 30 times higher than those without kidney failure on dialysis (Mitsnefes et al., 2013; Quennelle et al., 2021), and this is especially true in children under 5 years of age (Mitsnefes et al., 2013). Still, most neonates and infants survive long enough to receive a kidney transplant (Chesnaye et al., 2018). Other comorbidities include obesity, failure to thrive, and short stature.

HYPERTENSION

Hypertension must be controlled to limit further complications of cardiovascular disease. Evidence suggests that intensive control that aims for blood pressures below the 50th percentile for sex, age, and height can slow the progression or even reverse end-organ damage (Flynn et al., 2017). This may be difficult to achieve due to the side effects and medication burden often required to accomplish this target. Certainly, aiming for blood pressures below the 90th percentile has benefits, albeit not as impactful on the long-term cardiovascular morbidity known to coexist for CKD patients compared with intensive control recommendations. ACEIs and ARBs are considered the optimal classes of medications to treat patients who have both CKD and hypertension (Flynn et al., 2017). While ACEIs and ARBs are considered first-line therapy because of the benefit of proteinuria and hypertension, very advanced CKD can cause hyperkalemia and elevations in serum creatinine levels (Warady et al., 2021). They are also considered teratogenic, so females of childbearing capacity should be counseled about contraception to prevent pregnancy. Although central alpha-agonists, beta-blockers, peripheral vasodilators, calcium channel blockers, ARBs, and ACEIs are groups of drugs available for CKD-associated hypertension, many of these are utilized off label (Gabriel & Koch Nogueria, 2019). As such, hypertension must be managed primarily by or in consultation with a pediatric nephrology team. Managing hypertension in children also includes nonpharmacologic interventions, such as exercise, reducing obesity, smoking cessation, restricting fluid and dietary salt, and excess fluid removal with dialysis.

NEUROLOGIC COMPLICATIONS

Neurologic manifestations are attributed to the retention of uremic toxins. Multiple studies have noted neuropsychological abnormalities in children with CKD. Such abnormalities include general developmental delays, cerebral atrophy, poor school performance, memory deficits, and impairment of language development (Al Hamed et al., 2019).

ALUMINUM TOXICITY

A syndrome of progressive neurologic deterioration in children with CKD has been linked to aluminum toxicity, which causes speech disorders, seizures, dementia, and a slow electroencephalogram. By 1990 avoiding aluminum-based phosphate binders and improvements in dialysis water purification significantly decreased exposure to aluminum and its resultant neurotoxic manifestations (Wesseling-Perry & Salusky, 2013). The use of nonaluminum-based binders is safer and more effective than their aluminum-based predecessors (see earlier).

UREMIC NEUROPATHY

Uremic neuropathy symmetrically affects the distal portions of the extremities, with the lower extremities more affected than the upper extremities. Signs of neuropathy caused by uremia include muscle weakness, a reduction in deep tendon reflexes, muscle wasting, and impaired vibration sense (Baluarte, 2017). Uremic neuropathy may be improved with adequate dialysis and relieved by successful transplantation.

ENCEPHALOPATHY

Encephalopathy may be seen in advanced renal failure. Children may exhibit early symptoms, including headache, depression, fatigue, and listlessness. Hiccups, myoclonic twitching, memory loss, decreased attention span, drowsiness, impaired speech, and psychosis appear as deterioration in renal function progresses (Baluarte, 2017). Rapid reduction of urea from the blood through highly efficient hemodialysis may cause cerebral edema, which results in the syndrome of dialysis disequilibrium. When a very high blood urea nitrogen (BUN) level is present, the rate of urea clearance must be reduced until control of BUN is obtained. Mannitol can be given through the dialysis circuit to minimize the osmotic changes and treat seizures caused by this syndrome (Borzych-Duzalka & Harvey, 2021).

CHRONIC KIDNEY DISEASE–MINERAL BONE DISORDER

As discussed, CKD-MBD is a significant problem for the child with CKD. Growth retardation, bony abnormalities (including rickets and slipped epiphysis), fractures, and extraskeletal classifications are often seen in later stages of CKD (Srivastava & Warady, 2021), although the initial changes may begin as early as stage 2, which emphasizes the importance of early identification and referral to a pediatric nephrologist for prompt management. Extraskeletal calcifications, including those occurring in the vascular spaces, exacerbate the risk for cardiovascular disease (Khouzam et al., 2015).

Treatment includes diet modifications with careful attention to DRI of calcium and phosphorus. Dietary phosphorus restriction in children with renal problems is difficult because it curtails the intake of many of their favorite foods, which include dairy products, processed foods, and meat. It is especially difficult to

provide adequate nutrition to infants with CKD because of dairy restrictions. Low-phosphorus formulas, such as Similac PM 60/40 (Abbott Nutrition) or RenaStart (Nestlé) for infants, dietary phosphorus restriction in older children, and use of nonaluminum-based phosphorus binders, such as calcium carbonate, calcium acetate, and sevelamer (Renagel), and for children with ESKD, routine peritoneal dialysis or hemodialysis, help keep the serum concentration of phosphorus within the normal range in an attempt to prevent bony deformities and normalize growth velocity (McAlister et al., 2020). Additionally, medication therapy with active vitamin D therapy, such as calcitriol (Rocaltrol), paricalcitol (Zemplar), or doxercalciferol (Hectorol), or inactive vitamin D therapy, such as cholecalciferol or ergocalciferol, is required. Additionally, calcimimetics, such as cinacalcet (Sensipar), have been introduced into the medication regimen for resistant cases of CKD-MBD. ROD (alterations in bone morphology due to abnormalities of bone turnover and mineralization; see earlier) is one component of CKD-MBD (Srivastava & Warady, 2021).

UROLOGIC ABNORMALITIES

Early and close monitoring of vesicoureteral reflux, including periodic urine cultures, voiding cystourethrograms to monitor the degree and any improvement of reflux, and renal scans to detect scarring, sometimes can prevent permanent damage. Renal deterioration and failure may be prevented with antibiotic prophylaxis to prevent recurrent UTIs; however, with the continued concerns over drug-resistant bacteria, studies are investigating whether reflux in children can be managed safely without antibiotic prophylaxis (Cornwell et al., 2020). Despite antibiotic prophylaxis, surgical intervention is indicated in some children with severe reflux and recurrent UTIs. Posterior urethral valves and urethral atresia can cause severe hydronephrosis in utero and may be detected by a prenatal sonogram. Percutaneous placement of a stent, while in utero or open fetal surgery, can be performed to decrease fetal hydronephrosis until surgical correction of valves can be accomplished. Still, stent placement carries high risks of shunt-related complications and thus is not a common intervention (Liu et al., 2014).

DERMATOLOGIC MANIFESTATIONS

CKD-associated pruritus is a common complaint, and its pathophysiologic mechanism is poorly understood. Symptoms can vary in severity from intermittent pruritus lasting a few minutes per day to symptoms that continue throughout the day; pruritus tends to be more severe at night (Verduzco & Shirazian, 2020). As a child's course progresses toward ESKD, calcium and phosphorus imbalances can lead to a rare but serious complication called calciphylaxis, which involves metastatic calcifications of the skin that can present as painful and poorly healing lesions that often blister and have superimposed infections (Nigwekar et al., 2015).

GASTROINTESTINAL MANIFESTATIONS

Uremic symptoms of anorexia, nausea, vomiting, stomatitis, and halitosis improve with the adequacy of dialysis and control of anemia. Furthermore, children who have received a kidney transplant will generally experience resolution of uremic symptoms due to an appropriately functioning kidney.

INTERCURRENT ILLNESS

The development of intercurrent illnesses in children with CKD must be thoroughly assessed and appropriately managed to prevent further complications and promote optimal health. Common bacterial and viral infections occur in children with CKD. UTIs are common in children with abnormal urinary tracts. Infection is a frequent and common complication, especially of the CVC and peritoneum. Heart failure, pericarditis, pulmonary edema, and GI disease may occur with uremia. Children treated with immunosuppressive therapy, either because they have received a renal transplant or have conditions such as lupus or nephrotic syndrome, are much more susceptible to infection (Simon & Levin, 2001).

PROGNOSIS

Of the most common causes of pediatric CKD (CAKUT and GN), those with CAKUT have the best survival probability. Conversely, poor survival is attributed to patients with secondary GN, systemic lupus erythematosus, and vasculitis. Patients experiencing growth failure have twice the mortality risk compared to peers of normal height and experience a lower health-related quality of life. Depression and anxiety plague many children with advanced stages of CKD due to concerns about body image, relationships, and achieving life goals. Failed kidney transplants due to nonadherence also put the patient at risk for longer wait times due to high levels of reactive antibodies against future donors.

Unknown etiology is responsible for approximately 24% of CKD in children less than 1 year of age and as much as 31% of CKD in children age 13 to 17 years (USRDS, 2021). Additionally, many children born with CAKUT had related anomalies in other organ systems due to the timing of embryonic development and gestational age when the abnormality occurred. Children with glomerular disease can quickly progress (Warady et al., 2015). Obtaining a timely diagnosis impacts the ability to identify proper treatment regimens, offer genetic counseling, provide surgical intervention (as early as in utero), plan for transplant, or minimize the length of time on dialysis. Prenatal imaging, genetic testing, and kidney biopsy are all possible ways to identify the cause(s) of CKD. Collaboration with a fetal health specialist, pediatric nephrologist, and geneticist is necessary to appropriately manage underlying diseases.

Cardiovascular complications and infections are the two most common causes of death in children on dialysis (Mitsnefes et al., 2013). As mentioned, estimated mortality rates for children with kidney failure receiving dialysis are 30 times higher than those without kidney failure on dialysis (Mitsnefes et al., 2013; Quennelle et al., 2021). A substantial decrease in mortality rates was appreciated for older children and adolescents who initiated dialysis between 1990 and 2010 (Chesnaye et al., 2018, Mitsnefes et al., 2013). Posttransplantation outcomes have also continued to improve significantly, with 1- and 5-year survival rates above 90% for deceased and living donor transplants (Chesnaye et al., 2018). Additionally, with the likelihood of some children requiring hemodialysis access throughout their lifetime, vein preservation in childhood has become a vital component of improving long-term prognosis. Limiting venipunctures, prioritizing distal-first approaches in the dominant extremity, and empowering patients and families to speak up about vein preservation are some of the ways pediatric providers can preserve vasculature for future use (Singh et al., 2021).

Attention has been given recently to social determinants of health and the impact on prognosis and outcomes for populations considered to be at high risk for complications. Reevaluations of social constructs have begun to identify flaws in our previous approaches to identifying at-risk individuals and confirm trends in health inequities among communities of low socioeconomic status (SES). Prior data from CKiD has suggested that low SES is independently associated with increased complications from CKD, poor ESKD management, and longer wait times for kidney transplantation for children with ESKD (Hidalgo et al., 2013). Black children have been more likely to progress to ESKD quickly, more likely to initiate dialysis vs. receiving a kidney transplant, and less likely to receive a transplant within 2 years of dialysis initiation compared to their White counterparts (Boynton et al., 2022). Similarly, Hispanic pediatric dialysis patients have a lower likelihood of transplantation compared to their White counterparts, which is also seen in the adult dialysis population (Laster et al., 2017).

In contrast to adults, Black pediatric dialysis patients have worse survival than their non-Hispanic White counterparts, whereas Hispanics have a similar to lower mortality risk than non-Hispanic White patients. Children from low SES households were also more likely to develop ESKD and less likely to be listed for a kidney transplant after dialysis initiation (Boynton et al., 2022). In another CKiD study, families with public health insurance were more likely to report suboptimal utilization of health care services across the spectrum of CKD (Molino et al., 2022). Further research is needed, but in areas with low SES, increased progression to ESKD does not seem to occur when corrected for patient characteristics (race, ethnicity, sex, family income). Unfortunately, hospitalization and emergent health care utilization are increased despite insurance coverage by either commercial or public means, demonstrating that perhaps there are other barriers to receiving care (i.e., low density of first-line providers, low health literacy rates, physical and geographic impediments) (Boynton et al., 2022).

Global pandemics can profoundly impact the child with CKD, especially those with advanced stages. Public health strategies that may require isolation from others can compound mental health issues for an already vulnerable patient population. Awaiting the development of therapeutics and vaccinations can be difficult and create uncertainty, especially for the pediatric patient and family, because many initial trials do not include children in their studies. Further recommendations from public health officials may include postponing or canceling diagnostic and surgical procedures, including transplants or kidney biopsies. Telehealth and telemedicine visits have become commonplace, offering a safe alternative for access to care during a pandemic. This also presents challenges for those without reliable internet service or access to smartphones, electronic tablets, or computers. Even so, as more information becomes available and public health and governmental policies, support, and recommendations change, recovering from a pandemic continues to be a challenge for those who are immunosuppressed or awaiting a transplant. Vaccines may not be available for certain age groups, or more doses are required to achieve adequate immunity. New therapies may interact with immunosuppression medications, and access to infusion centers for antibody therapies may be limited. The social response to public health recommendations may be limited, further isolating vulnerable populations. Vaccine hesitancy may delay herd immunity, and new variants of the contagion continue to evolve.

PRIMARY CARE MANAGEMENT

HEALTH CARE MAINTENANCE

Growth and Development

Incorporating developmental and behavioral assessments into primary health care evaluations can help identify deviations and promote early intervention. Children with renal disease may not have any clinical signs except stunted growth. Many children exhibit growth retardation at the time of referral to the pediatric nephrologist, but inadequate growth remains a problem for many individuals, including those undergoing dialysis or patients who

have prolonged exposure to steroids (Franke et al., 2015). Weight loss is most likely to occur when eGFR falls below 35 mL/min/m² (Ku et al., 2018a). Except for infancy, the next greatest physical growth stage is puberty. Inadequate growth, especially during these phases, should raise suspicion about CKD (Haffner, 2020). Children with CKD often have delayed linear growth and development of secondary sexual characteristics. Decreased estrogen and testosterone levels may occur. Estimating target height can be done using the Tanner staging formula for females and males or the Molinari formula, both of which have been shown to be more accurate even for children with CKD compared to other formulas (Drube et al., 2019).

The frequency of growth assessment in pediatric CKD depends on the child's age and CKD stage, with more frequent assessments performed in the very young or advanced CKD stage (Drube et al., 2019). Collaboration with a pediatric renal dietitian can be helpful. Updated growth charts should be utilized for plotting length (0–2 years) or height (age ≥2 years). A length board for children less than 2 years of age (or for those whose standing is difficult) and a stadiometer for those 2 years and older should be used to obtain accurate measurements. Shoes should be removed for both methods. Accurate and consistent methods of measuring length or height are imperative to monitor trends and calculate height velocity, performed using two measurements 6 months apart (Drube et al., 2019). Anecdotal experience suggests that children receiving GH may experience accelerated pubertal development, although no specific evidence supports this.

Nonetheless, pubertal assessment using the Tanner stages should be performed annually for children older than 10 years (Drube et al., 2019). Furthermore, radiography of the left wrist should be performed annually to assess for epiphyseal closure as part of the evaluation for initiation or continuation of GH. If the child is on GH, therapy should be stopped when (1) genetic target adult height is achieved, (2) epiphyses are closed, (3) SCFE occurs, (4) intracranial hypertension is found, (5) severe hyperparathyroidism is present, or (6) within the first year posttransplant (Drube et al., 2019).

Developmental assessment should be done with the onset of CKD and repeated at 2- to 9-month intervals, depending on a child's age and disease severity. Although the timing of milestones may be delayed, children with CKD have the same developmental needs as healthy children and must progress through the same developmental stages. The level of development attained must be assessed to assure that each child attains developmental milestones. Assessment tools are useful in obtaining objective data. The effect of the disease process on the child's psychological status, school attendance, intellectual performance, and social development should be assessed every 6 to 9 months.

Diet

As with their healthy counterparts, children with CKD are encouraged to eat a diet low in processed, high-sugar, or fast foods. As CKD progresses, the associated anorexia and decreased appetite negatively impact the quality of diet and nutrient intake. Although protein restriction may delay the progression of CKD, it is not acceptable in children (Chen et al., 2017). In addition to growth and developmental delay in children, poor nutrition—especially with low serum albumin levels—is associated with increased morbidity and mortality. Nutritional problems are manifested long before ESKD is reached and continue after RRT is initiated. Evaluation and regular follow-up with a registered dietitian with renal experience are essential to achieve and maintain optimal growth and development in a child with CKD (Kogon & Harshman, 2019). For children with CKD not yet on dialysis, energy and protein intake should provide approximately 100% of the daily estimated energy expenditure for chronologic age, activity level, and body size. For children on dialysis, protein requirements may be up to 140% of the DRI (Kogon & Harshman, 2019).

Children receiving peritoneal dialysis experience a feeling of fullness soon after eating small amounts because of abdominal distention from the volume of peritoneal fluid. This sensation often leads to the active refusal of meals or oral feeding and may exacerbate gastroesophageal reflux. Glucose absorption from the dialysate in both hemodialysis and peritoneal dialysis provides calories, occasionally resulting in obesity. Anemia control via rHuEPO injections results in increased appetite, energy level, and eventual weight gain, which helps reduce the incidence of malnutrition in children with CKD. Additionally, with adequate clearance from either dialysis modality, some children may find an improved appetite, decreased nausea, and subsequent weight gain, although the amount of weight gain is usually still inadequate.

Parents of infants and small children soon become frustrated with unsuccessful efforts to get children to eat the recommended calories and protein. Children with renal failure are often poor eaters, and more than 70% experience symptoms of gastroesophageal reflux. If energy requirements cannot be met with oral intake, supplemental tube feedings by orogastric, nasogastric, or gastrostomy tube or button may be required (KDOQI, 2009).

Dietary restrictions change with the ESKD modality. In hemodialysis, sodium, potassium, and phosphorus generally govern the dietary prescription. Greater dietary freedom is possible with peritoneal dialysis due to the daily nature of this modality, and protein may be increased. The posttransplant diet also has restrictions of no added salt, low fat, and low cholesterol to prevent hypertension and obesity. Because eating is a social custom in our society and not solely for sustenance, pizza may be the favorite food of a child with CKD, making dietary restrictions difficult. Phosphorus restriction limits dairy products, and most children get a majority of their energy and protein intake from milk (Chen et al., 2017). Potassium is also found in milk and often must be restricted in the child with ESKD. Fluid restriction depends on a child's urinary output volume and is calculated by intake volume allowed being equal to output plus insensible loss (400 mL/m^2). The primary care provider should obtain the dietary management plan from the nephrology team to reinforce family education.

Safety

Although children with CKD should be encouraged to pursue normal childhood activities, some considerations and limitations must be considered. Delays in cognitive and gross motor development may result in these children being academically and physically slower than their classmates and smaller in size. Children with CKD may become the brunt of jokes and unkind comments. Coping mechanisms must be reviewed and encouraged with the patient and caregivers, which is usually under the direction of social workers or child psychologists. Children taking immunosuppressive therapy are more at risk for infections, and their injuries heal more slowly. As mentioned previously, children with CKD are more prone to fractures, especially as CKD progresses. Physical activity, however, should be encouraged to promote physical and mental health. Group aerobic exercise programs, camping, group games at picnics, and other fun outings are excellent ways to promote controlled exercise, encourage independence, and help raise self-esteem.

Some children require special occupational and physical therapy programs to enhance their physical ability and improve their skills and stamina. Bike helmets and knee pads can be used to help prevent easy bruising. For children on dialysis, their dialysis access is truly their lifeline. Protecting the CVC, AVF, AVG, and peritoneal dialysis catheter from trauma or infection is imperative. Activities that may compromise circulation or cause rupture of the AVF should be avoided. Children and young adults are taught and encouraged to monitor the blood flow at least daily, avoid blood pressure measurement and venipuncture in the affected arm, and avoid sleeping on or wearing accessories and restrictive clothing, which can lead to venostasis and clotting. Submersion of catheters for hemodialysis and peritoneal dialysis should be avoided (Warady & Andrews, 2021), and swimming in fresh water or pools is prohibited. Swimming and showering with peritoneal dialysis catheters are controversial and require the nephrology team's specific clearance and direction regarding catheter and exit site care procedures. For those who have received a kidney transplant, activities that cause jarring and jolting (i.e., trampolines and roller coasters) are not advised, especially in the initial postoperative months. For other activities, a fitted kidney guard can offer protection. As the child grows, kidney guards must be resized. Many of these can be obtained through durable medical equipment or orthotic companies. Clearance for activities should be discussed with the nephrology and surgical teams. Children should be encouraged to wear a medical alert bracelet or necklace to notify other health care providers of their CKD status, medication needs, and other possible complications.

Immunizations

Routine immunizations should be given to children with CKD, except for a few specific disease conditions and therapies (Centers for Disease Control and Prevention, 2022). A reduced response or duration of immunity may occur in children with CKD or ESKD who receive immunizations (Massengil & Ferris, 2014). Immunosuppressive therapy is used not only with transplantation but also to treat some renal conditions, including GN, nephrotic syndrome, and lupus nephritis. Unfortunately, the associated therapies for many underlying causes of CKD contribute to delayed immunizations (Massengill & Ferris, 2014), which may impact the timeline to transplant for those with ESKD. The primary care provider should consult with the nephrology team to determine the safest approach to providing vaccines, especially if catchup doses are required.

Immunosuppression is a contraindication for live virus immunizations, including the measles-mumps-rubella and varicella vaccines, rotavirus, and live attenuated influenza vaccine (*ACIP contraindications guidelines for immunization, 2023*). Disease-specific immunoglobulins may be given after known exposure. Pneumococcal and inactivated influenza vaccines are recommended for children with CKD and active nephrotic syndrome because of their increased susceptibility to these respiratory infections (Massengil & Ferris, 2014). Vaccination against COVID-19 remains controversial despite Food and Drug Administration approval in 2022 for children as young as 6 months. For all recommended vaccines, hesitancy from parents continues to be a challenge.

Even though rHuEPO has decreased the need for blood transfusions in children with ESKD, the risk for hepatitis B still exists, especially for those who receive hemodialysis. If a child has never been vaccinated or has received previous vaccination but has negative titers for hepatitis B antigen, the hepatitis vaccine series should be started as soon as possible so the series can be completed before possible transplant. Compared to their healthy counterparts, children with CKD and on dialysis lose serologic

immunity at an increased rate and often need revaccination (Onder & Somers, 2021). These children can be given higher doses of vaccine and immunized on an accelerated schedule. If there is an inadequate response to two rounds of hepatitis B vaccination, no further attempts are recommended (Massengill & Ferris, 2014). As part of the transplant evaluation process, extensive immunologic screening is performed to determine exposure to a variety of infectious diseases, including HIV.

Screenings

Vision. A yearly eye examination by a pediatric ophthalmologist is recommended. The eyes should be examined for scleral calcification caused by hypercalcemia or uncontrolled hyperphosphatemia. The fundus should be examined for arterial narrowing, hemorrhages, exudates, and papilledema secondary to hypertension. Cataract assessment should be included for any child treated with steroid therapy. Other syndromes that impact the kidney, such as Alport syndrome and cystinosis, may also have ocular involvement and should have close follow-up with a pediatric ophthalmologist (Savige et al., 2015).

Hearing. An annual assessment by an audiologist is recommended. High-frequency sensorineural deafness is characteristic of Alport syndrome (Savige et al., 2015). Hearing loss can also result from the use of ototoxic drugs (e.g., furosemide, gentamicin).

Dental. Routine dental care (every 6 months) and vigilant oral hygiene are recommended for children with CKD. It is not uncommon for primary care providers to prescribe antibiotic prophylaxis for children receiving immunosuppressive medications and those who have indwelling catheters, grafts, or fistulas for dialysis. Data are insufficient to support this practice, however, and the American Heart Association (AHA) does not recommend antibiotic prophylaxis unless the child has a prior history of infective endocarditis (AHA, 2022).

Children with renal disease often have enamel defects. Poor nutritional intake may lead to poor mineralization of teeth. In an effort to improve nutrition, small children with CKD may be allowed to use a bottle for a longer time, resulting in deformities of the primary teeth. The use of oral iron for anemia may stain teeth; liquid preparations should be placed in the mouth beyond the teeth.

Drug-induced gingival hyperplasia may occur in children with CKD receiving drugs such as phenytoin (Dilantin) for seizures, calcium channel blockers (e.g., nifedipine [Procardia], amlodipine [Norvasc], or verapamil [Calan]) for hypertension, and cyclosporine (Neoral) for immunosuppression in transplant, lupus, and nephrotic syndrome treatment. Good dental and oral hygiene with mechanical stimulation by daily brushing and flossing, gingival massaging, and plaque control can contain gum growth to within acceptable limits.

Blood pressure. For a child without CKD, an annual blood pressure measurement must be obtained starting at age 3 years. For the child with CKD, blood pressures should be obtained at every clinic visit. Oscillometric blood pressure machines validated for use in children are appropriate for use in the clinic setting (Flynn et al., 2017). Manual blood pressure measurements should be considered when the oscillometric readings are in question (Ku et al., 2018b). Initiation and follow-up of antihypertensive therapy should be done in consultation with the pediatric nephrologist. Caffeine intake, anxiety, or white coat hypertension may explain higher blood pressure in clinics. Repeated blood pressures over the course of the visit often demonstrate a decrease in readings, although it may not be enough to change the classification (Flynn et al., 2017). For best practices on accurate blood pressure measurement in children, refer to the 2017 Clinical Practice Guideline for Screening and Management of High Blood Pressure in Children and Adolescents (Flynn et al., 2017). Ambulatory blood pressure monitors should be used for the confirmation of hypertension in children and adolescents with office blood pressure measurements in the elevated category for 1 year or more or with stage 1 hypertension over three clinic visits, but often require referral to a specialist and application by trained health care staff (Flynn et al., 2017). These monitors are worn for 24 hours and can give better insight into the true daily overall blood pressure at rest and during activity and facilitate ideal medical management (Ku et al., 2018b).

Hematocrit. Routine screening may be deferred if the other renal function tests include a recent complete blood count (CBC). Anemia is a chronic problem that is usually monitored by the nephrology team.

Urinalysis. Routine screening is not necessary because of the frequent urinalysis done by the nephrology team (Noone & Langlois, 2016). Some children with CKD have little to no urine output, so urinalysis is not indicated on a routine basis. If proteinuria is noted incidentally on a urinalysis, follow-up with a random UP/C ratio within 3 months is prudent, with subsequent consultation with pediatric nephrology for persistent UP/C ratio above 0.2 mg/mg.

Tuberculosis. Yearly screening is recommended.

Condition-Specific Screening
Lab work. The nephrology team regularly monitors the CBC, serum ferritin, iron, transferrin, folate, and reticulocyte counts to assess anemia management. Serum electrolytes, BUN, creatinine, calcium, phosphorus, alkaline phosphatase, protein, albumin, cholesterol, and liver function tests help monitor renal function and treatment efficacy. Metabolic acidosis must be promptly identified and treated to prevent bone demineralization and growth retardation. PTH levels should be monitored every 3 to 6 months and correlated with radiologic findings for prevention and/or management of CKD-MBD. Fasting blood levels are best for monitoring cholesterol and triglycerides, which is difficult in small children or infants. Viral titers for the varicella-zoster virus, cytomegalovirus, herpes simplex virus, Epstein-Barr virus, hepatitis profile (i.e., hepatitis A virus, hepatitis C virus, hepatitis B virus [HBV], antibody to HBV), rubella, rubeola, and HIV should initially be monitored as a baseline, then before transplant, and periodically as determined by the pediatric nephrologist.

Cardiac screening. A chest radiograph, baseline electrocardiogram, and echocardiogram should initially be performed and then again at 6- to 12-month intervals to assess the cardiovascular status of children with CKD for long-term management and prevention of end-organ damage, as well as preparation for the transplant.

Radiologic screening. Radiologic bone studies can show evidence of subperiosteal resorption of bone and the widening of the metaphyses in children with CKD-MBD, also known as rickets (Carpenter, 2021). Examination of the hands and knees should initially be obtained and then again at 6-month intervals to assess for improvement or worsening of ROD and compare bone age with chronological age to determine growth potential. Bone density studies and bone biopsies are helpful but less commonly used methods for assessing children's bone mineralization. For children taking GH, bone age films should be obtained yearly, as treatment should be discontinued when the epiphyses close (Mahan & Warady, 2006).

COMMON ILLNESS MANAGEMENT
Differential Diagnosis
Infections. Children with CKD may be at greater risk for routine infections and their sequelae because of a compromised immune system. Primary care providers should evaluate and manage routine pediatric problems (e.g., influenza, UTIs, GI infections, fever), consulting the pediatric nephrologist about a child's hydration status and residual renal function, as well as the antibiotic selection and dose related to a child's renal disease and residual function. Temporary alterations in a child's dialysis program or immunosuppression regimen for transplant may be necessary during illness. If other common benign causes of fever have been ruled out, the pediatric nephrologist should

manage fever related to a dialysis access infection or peritonitis.

Gastrointestinal symptoms. Nausea and vomiting are common symptoms in childhood. Decreasing renal function must be ruled out in children with mild renal failure, especially in the absence of associated fever. Diarrhea should be worked up for common causes. However, in some regions of the United States, the hemolytic uremic syndrome can be a complication of infection with a Shiga toxin–producing bacteria such as *Escherichia coli* that presents with AKI and often leads to kidney failure (Bitzan & Lapeyraque, 2016). Infection with *Clostridium difficile* should also be considered for the patient who is being treated with antibiotic therapy for frequent UTIs, dialysis-related infection, or other common childhood infections.

Headache. Uncontrolled hypertension should be ruled out in children with CKD who complain of frequent headache. Increased intracranial hypertension should be considered for the patient receiving rhGH. Medication side effects and worsening kidney function should also be considered.

Drug Dosing and Interactions

The most important factors to consider in pharmacokinetics are the extent to which the kidney excretes the drug, the degree of renal impairment, and the drug's interactions with various other medications needed in the ESKD treatment regimen.

Dosing recommendations for medications prescribed for pediatric patients with CKD are scant (Al-Khouja et al., 2020). Once the GFR drops below 50 mL/min/1.73 m², care must be taken to adjust the dosing of certain medications to avoid the accumulation of drug metabolites that could cause significant side effects or harm. Loading doses usually do not need to be adjusted, and in subsequent dosing the adjustment is usually made by either decreasing the dose, lengthening the interval between doses, or both (Matzke et al., 2011), especially for patients with hemodialysis or peritoneal dialysis. One study recently found that as many as 26% of pediatric patients with CKD were prescribed one or more potentially nephrotoxic medications compared with 15% of those without CKD by primary care providers. Indeed, primary care providers play an important role in protecting children with CKD from further injury to the kidneys (Lefebvre et al., 2020).

Children with anemia and CKD who receive a calcium-based phosphate binder given with food or within 30 minutes after eating should wait at least 1 hour before taking oral iron because of the likelihood of decreased iron absorption (Lexicomp, 2022). Depending on the specific medication, dosage calculations should be based on the weight, BSA, and/or pubertal stage of a child with CKD, not the chronologic age.

Medications that are removed by dialysis (i.e., vitamins, some antihypertensive medications, and aminoglycoside antibiotics) should be given after dialysis (i.e., at night with CAPD or in the morning with CCPD or NIPD). For patients receiving rhGH and who use the hemodialysis modality, injections should be timed for bedtime to limit the risk of bleeding complications due to the heparin used for anticoagulation during hemodialysis. The pediatric nephrologist should be consulted for appropriate medication selection and dosage adjustment.

Children with CKD may need to take up to 40 pills daily, which requires much determination and perseverance for both the child and the parents. Transplant medications can total up to six or seven different medications (and comprise 30 or 40 pills) and are critical to the life of the transplant. Identifying barriers such as but not limited to work and school schedules, size, formulation of medications (i.e., pill vs. liquid), and taste aversions may help the health care team work with the patient and family to find practical ways to increase adherence.

DEVELOPMENTAL ISSUES

Sleep Patterns

Sleep disturbances are common in children receiving dialysis. Complaints included sleep-disordered breathing, restless leg syndrome/periodic leg movements, and excessive daytime sleepiness (Stabouli et al., 2016). Children of all ages should be encouraged to utilize healthy sleep hygiene practices to achieve a normal sleep pattern at night. An increased need for sleep, lethargy, or depression may indicate increasing renal failure and should be reported to the pediatric nephrology team. Most children can sleep undisturbed with nocturnal CCPD/NIPD treatment, although frequent machine alarms may contribute to poor sleep quality. Restlessness, insomnia, or cramps may indicate the need for troubleshooting dialysis efficacy or physical activity to promote rest. It is not uncommon for children with CKD to require melatonin to aid with falling asleep. Other sleep aids may also be prescribed but should be done in consultation with the nephrology team.

Toileting

Children with CKD may be oliguric, anuric, or have normal urine output, as determined largely by the cause of the renal disorder. Congenital abnormalities, such as neuropathic bladder, posterior urethral valves, and vesicoureteral reflux, cause malformations of the lower urinary tract and often require consultation with a urologist along with surgical intervention and the creation of a urinary diversional system to preserve renal function or prepare for kidney transplantation (Chu et al., 2019). Adolescents with urinary stomas and appliances may have difficulty accepting and participating in peer activities and emotionally accepting the diversional system. Families and children need instruction in the care of the stoma and supportive care as indicated.

Even after corrective urologic surgery, some children may be unable to achieve urinary continence. Toilet training for urinary continence is often deferred until after the transplant if a child is capable of urinary continence. Female children and their parents should be taught to wipe properly to prevent UTIs. Bowel training should be initiated when a toddler is developmentally ready and may need collaboration with gastrointestinal or colorectal surgical specialists if coexisting abnormalities of the GI tract are present.

Discipline

Many parents are hesitant to set limits with their children because of anxiety, guilt, or ambivalence about their child's diagnosis. Children with chronic conditions need discipline—the same as any other child. Many parents eventually realize that one of the best things they can do is treat their children like any other child. All children need to develop self-discipline regardless of their health status. The primary care and nephrology teams should reinforce healthy parenting skills, with resources made available when needed.

Children may have difficulty coping with procedures related to their CKD management. For pain associated with procedures, management techniques (e.g., holding techniques, guided imagery, hypnosis, progressive muscle relaxation) can be taught to children and their parents. Topical anesthetics (e.g., eutectic mixture of lidocaine and prilocaine cream) are commonly used in many pediatric nephrology programs for children with AV fistulas or implanted port-a-catheters. The involvement of child life professionals to engage the child in play therapy helps children work through these difficult situations and lets parents or other caregivers know their unexpressed thoughts.

Children should be encouraged to participate in their care by performing achievable tasks and making decisions. It is acceptable to give children input on when and where to take their medications, including body sites for epogen or recombinant GH injections. Once a schedule is agreed on, it is important to stick to it. It can make it easier for children to cope with unpleasant tasks if they know when the unpleasantries are coming and will be completed. Conversely, if a schedule needs to be modified, this can be done in collaboration with the health care team.

Child Care

Children with CKD are not restricted from day care. Because children receiving immunosuppressive and corticosteroid therapy are more susceptible to infections, licensed home care or small-group child care is recommended. Day care and preschool settings provide stimulation for learning and sharing with other children and may be positive, especially if classes are small. When child care is used, the caregiver must be taught about the child's dietary restrictions, medications, and any special treatment regimens. Specific instructions should be given in writing, with a telephone contact in case of questions. The nephrology team should encourage children receiving CAPD and their parents to arrange the dialysis schedule around the child care hours when possible. If a child has vascular access, those entrusted as caregivers must be given instructions on potential emergencies and actions to be taken.

Schooling

School-age children must be encouraged to attend school full time, but academic success may be impacted by several variables associated with CKD, including but not limited to neurocognitive delays, hypertension, anemia, sleep quality, and interruptions from dialysis schedules (Johnson & Harshman, 2021). CAPD exchanges should be scheduled around school activities with the least possible interference; nocturnal CCPD/NIPD may be preferable for school-age children. Schedule changes to accommodate after-school activities can be discussed with the pediatric nephrology team. Pediatric hemodialysis centers should include a schoolteacher or tutor to help children with missed schoolwork. A dual school-home educational program may be established with both teachers communicating with each other for the continuity of the child's learning. Children with renal disease may need a note to be allowed extra trips to the bathroom because of a small bladder capacity or infection, to perform intermittent catheterization, to drink more/less fluids, or receive assistance with ureterostomy or CVC care. Some children need to be assigned to a school with a nurse in attendance daily, but this does not mean that the child needs to be in special education classes. The pediatric nephrology team may need to provide educational materials on specific CKD management and in-service presentations on a child's physical or emotional needs to school personnel, and participate in a child's individualized education plan (IEP) conference. Parents need to be informed about laws protecting their child's educational rights.

Poor school performance must be evaluated for contributing factors, including family disharmony. Cognitive deficits have been correlated with more advanced CKD and congenital etiologies. Additionally, the presence of attention-deficit/hyperactivity disorder was found to be higher in a CKiD sample (9%) compared to the general worldwide pediatric population (7.2%) (Harshman et al., 2019).

Adolescence can be a time of turbulence that is associated with transition, maturational crises, and adjustment. Tables 29.5–29.7 highlight some of the characteristics of adolescents with ESKD.

Sexuality

The onset of puberty and the pubertal growth spurt is delayed by approximately 2 to 2.5 years in children with ESKD (Haffner & Rees, 2016). Adolescent males with ESRD may show delayed development of genitalia, pubic hair, and testicular size and decreased sperm counts. A successful transplant usually returns hormonal function and fertility capability to normal. These are important issues in adolescent sexuality and preparation for adulthood, as well as for families of small children concerned about the ability of their child to have a normal life.

Adolescents with CKD must be counseled about birth control, sexually transmitted infections (STIs), and acquired immunodeficiency syndrome. Females with CKD may have delayed menarche, abnormal menstrual cycles, or decreased fertility. Many of these issues resolve after kidney transplants, putting them at increased risk for STIs (Chang et al., 2021). Females of childbearing potential with CKD and hypertension or coagulopathies should avoid estrogen-containing combined hormonal contraceptives (pills, patches, rings) because of the risk of worsening protein-uria, hypertension, and thromboembolism (Chang et al., 2021). Lastly, females of childbearing potential should be counseled on the teratogenic effects of anti-hypertensives, such as ACEI/ARBs, NSAIDs (indo-methacin), immunosuppressants (mycophenolate mofetil [CellCept]), and cocaine (Ismaili et al., 2016). Consultation with the nephrologist or primary care provider should be done as soon as pregnancy is suspected, as these pregnancies are considered high risk (Chang et al., 2021).

Some children and young adults may be exploring their gender identity and sexuality, which may differ from their assigned sex at birth or cultural norms. Treatments are available for patients who wish to undergo gender transition. Currently there is limited information on the impact of gender reassignment to determine eGFR, staging of kidney disease, or other gender-related considerations for CKD management. Careful collaboration between the primary, nephrology, and endocrine teams will need to occur to monitor for changes in kidney function as it relates to hormonal changes, body mass, and the impact on kidney function. There is a need for further studies to evaluate the impact gender reassignment will have on managing kidney disease in this population.

Transition and Transfer to Adulthood

Children with CKD are living, thriving, and becoming adults with CKD, which means they must be educated on the aspects of transition prior to their transfer to adult care. The goal of the transition is to provide

Table 29.5 Characteristics of Adolescents With End-Stage Renal Disease by Developmental Domain: Nutrition, Sleep, Activity

	N = 30	%
Children's Nutritional Habits		
Appetite loss:		
Yes	27	90
No	3	10
Number of meals/day:		
2	21	70
3	6	20
>3	3	10
Preferred restricted food:	20	66.7
Salty diet	9	30
Dairy products	2	6.67
Meat	3	10
Salty snacks	6	20
No preferred food	10	33.3
Type of food prepared for the child at home:		
Special diet	20	66.7
Family diet	10	33.3
Food intake:		
Limited	15	50
On demand	15	50
Children's Sleeping Pattern		
Place of sleep		
Alone	5	16.7
With other siblings	10	33,3
Beside mother	15	50
Number of hours of sleep/night:		
<8	21	70
8	6	20
>8	3	10
Nap frequency:		
Daily	0	0
On the day of dialysis	25	83.3
None	5	16.7
Sleep problems:		
Difficulty to sleep	10	33.3
Interrupted sleep	16	53.3
Normal sleep	4	13.3
Physical Exercise		
Practice of physical exercises:		
Yes	7	23.3
No	23	76.7
Where exercise:		
At home	3	10
At street	4	13.3
At school	0	0
Reasons for not exercising (n = 21):		
Not allowed because of health condition	3	10

Table 29.5 — Characteristics of Adolescents With End-Stage Renal Disease by Developmental Domain: Nutrition, Sleep, Activity—cont'd

	N = 30	%
Afraid of any accident to vascular access	18	60
Easy fatigability and dyspnea	2	6.7
School Achievement		
Irregular school attendance	30	100
School performance: (last year) failed	6	20
Have low marks	11	36.7
Have good marks	13	43.3

The majority (90%) of studied patients experienced appetite loss, and only one-third of the studied children were sharing the family diet, with half of patients receiving food and fluids on demand. Approximately half of the studied children (53.3%) experienced interrupted sleep, and approximately one-third of children experienced difficulty sleeping, with 70% of the studied children sleeping <8 hours per night. Physical activity within this studied population found that three-fourths of them engaged in no physical activity, claiming fear of injury, school restrictions, tiring easily, and dyspnea.
From El-Gamasy, M. A., & Eldeeb, M. M. (2017). Assessment of physical and psychosocial status of children with ESRD under regular hemodialysis, a single centre experience. *International Journal of Pediatrics and Adolescent Medicine*, 4(2), 81–86.

Table 29.6 — Characteristics of Adolescents With End-Stage Renal Disease by Developmental Domain: Emotions and Behaviors

VARIABLE	N = 30	%
Practice degree of religious obligation (regular prayer):		
Yes	12	40
No	18	60
Feeling that disease is a punishment from Allah:		
Yes	3	10
No	27	90
Sense of difference:		
Yes	19	63.3
No	11	36.7
Hiding from others:		
Yes	16	53.3
No	14	46.7
Planning for the future:		
Yes	7	23.3
No	23	76.7
Spiritual satisfaction:		
Yes	5	16.7
No	25	83.3

Of the studied children, 60% were not religiously active, and more than half felt a sense of difference from others, choosing to hide and not make plans for the future. The majority (83.3%) lacked spiritual satisfaction.
From El-Gamasy, M. A., & Eldeeb, M. M. (2017). Assessment of physical and psychosocial status of children with ESRD under regular hemodialysis, a single centre experience. *International Journal of Pediatrics and Adolescent Medicine*, 4(2), 81–86.

Table 29.7 — Characteristics of Adolescents With End-Stage Renal Disease by Developmental Domain: Social Relationships

SOCIAL RELATION	N = 30	%
Children-parent relationship:		
Overprotection	24	80
Preference for their siblings	3	10
Most requests are achieved	15	50
Children-sibling relationships:		
Violence (teasing)	3	10
Incongruent with each other	5	16.7
Children-peer relationships:		
Violence (teasing)	1	3.3
Incongruent with each other	3	10
Children-teacher relationships:		
Good	21	70
Bad	9	30
Visiting relatives:		
Yes	6	20
No	24	80
Prefer isolation from others:		
Yes	20	66.7
No	10	33.3
Seeking children with the same disease:		
Yes	18	60
No	12	40

Of the studied children, 80% felt parents were overprotective and that preferences for siblings came first for 10%. Complaints of violence (teasing) and incongruence with siblings were found in 16.7%. Overall, 70% of the studied children felt they had good sibling relationships.
From El-Gamasy, M. A., & Eldeeb, M. M. (2017). Assessment of physical and psychosocial status of children with ESRD under regular hemodialysis, a single centre experience. *International Journal of Pediatrics and Adolescent Medicine*, 4(2), 81–86.

coordinated, continuous health care, and it is recommended that a formal transition program occur by early adolescence, with a curriculum that provides education on a variety of self-management tasks (e.g., filling prescriptions and insurance) that are crucial to the successful preparation and transfer of the emerging adult. Active collaboration between the pediatric team and members of the adult nephrology team should be encouraged to allow for continued modification/improvement of the program (Warady et al., 2014). Brain development and maturation continue up to 25 years of age, and this may explain the substantial risks of nonadherence at the time of transfer from pediatric to adult care and among the cohort of patients younger than 25 years who are managed in adult care. This may account for the increased risk-taking, impulsive behavior, and nonadherence issues that are so common in this age group (Watson et al., 2011). The road to independence and career development begins before a child reaches adulthood, and patient feedback suggests that starting the transition process early is beneficial (Joslin et al., 2020). Individuals must be encouraged to eat a healthy diet and avoid drug, alcohol, and tobacco use. Chronic illness during childhood and adolescence can interfere with the natural maturation process. Collaboration between pediatric and adult programs occurs, but relationships can be difficult to establish between the two due to an imbalance of multidisciplinary resources and unfamiliarity with the causes of childhood CKD for adult providers (Watson et al., 2011). In addition, transition education that emphasizes self-care can help prepare teens for this stage. It should be emphasized that the transition process takes years to complete. Young adults should be encouraged that it is okay to have a family member, close friend, or significant other accompany them to clinic visits. The American Association of Kidney Patients (AAKP) can supply dozens of adult role models (see Resources, later).

Family Concerns

A child's CKD affects the entire family. Parents may have to deal with the following: feelings of shock and disbelief, anger, loss, guilt at causing renal failure, depression, fatigue and burnout associated with constant care and appointments, inadequacy at not being able to heal or fix the problem, frustration with the medical establishment for no cure, overprotection vs. being too lenient, marital stress, and financial worries. Frequent trips to the dialysis center or clinic, daily or nightly peritoneal dialysis treatments, and additional physical care interfere with family schedules, school, extracurricular activities, and outings.

Attention to family coping skills, dynamics, and the behaviors of the child with CKD are important in identifying those children and families in need of extra support and counseling. Health-related quality of life may differ between patients and caregivers, impacting adherence to the medical regimen, influencing family dynamics, and impacting school performance. Many children with CKD suffer from depression, which negatively impacts their quality of life (Kogon et al., 2016). Providing counseling and peer networking sessions is often helpful. Social support is important, particularly in adolescents, when many physical, social, and emotional changes occur. Child and family support can be provided by working in partnership with the child and family, strengthening positive informal social networks, and involving outside organizations to provide needed services. A variety of social support groups can be found through organizations such as the NKF, AAKP, and Transplant Families, as well as social media (see Resources, later). Families should be encouraged to continue normal activities (e.g., family outings, camps for children, vacations), proactively arranging transient dialysis scheduling at a pediatric dialysis center if necessary.

A family's belief system must be considered. Religious practices may prohibit blood transfusions, even in life-threatening situations, or challenge that healing by faith alone is all that is needed. The multicultural nature of the United States means the health care team is very likely to encounter patients with religious and cultural beliefs that differ from their own. A willingness to learn and understand more about the family's background, religious and cultural beliefs and practices, dietary beliefs and practices associated with health care, and identification of the primary leader of the family (e.g., a great-grandmother) are valuable to health care professionals when effective interventions require altering a child's or family's health care practices, and the effect it may have on adherence with the medical regimen. For instance, outcomes may be negatively impacted if medication adherence is not prioritized (McQuaid & Landier, 2018).

Quality-of-life issues and parental rights vs. minor children's rights are being discussed with no clear-cut answers (Watson, 2014). Some members of medical and legislative committees would argue that many children should not receive all ESKD services because of cost containment. Technologic advances in dialysis and transplant have improved the quality of life and increased life expectancy for thousands with ESKD while outpacing the resources. Even the smallest, very ill infant might be treated with life-sustaining dialysis—but at a high cost. The platform for CKRT, Cardio-Renal Pediatric Dialysis Emergency Machine (Carpediem; Bellco-Medtronic, Mirandola, Italy), is more widely performed today with positive results. Equipment, supplies, and professional expertise are more costly for infants with ESKD. Many of these infants have other congenital anomalies; morbidity and mortality are high in this early period. Children with severe developmental or intellectual delays are being successfully treated with dialysis and transplantation, but they require considerable comprehensive and long-term care. Families need support as they make decisions about their child's care that will have emotional, ethical, and financial implications.

As of August 13, 2022, there were 1096 children younger than age 18 listed on UNOS awaiting a kidney transplant (Organ Procurement and Transplant Network, 2022). Inflation-adjusted spending for ESKD care increased 13% from $45 billion in 2009 to $51 billion in 2019 (USRDS, 2021a). On July 1, 1973, the Social Security Act was amended to provide Medicare benefits for persons younger than 65 years who were certified to have chronic kidney failure and require dialysis or transplantation (HR-1, Public Law 92-603). Because the Medicare payment process becomes quite complicated, families should be referred to the nephrology social worker for assistance in accessing available services. Additional financial assistance information is available through the NKF affiliates, the American Kidney Fund, and the AAKP.

RESOURCES

American Association of Kidney Patients: https://aakp. org/center-for-patient-research-and-education/ pediatric-kidney-pals

American Kidney Fund (free educational materials and helpline): http://www.kidneyfund.org

American Nephrology Nurses Association: http:// anna.inurse.com

National Kidney Foundation (local chapters provide information on education assistance, summer camps, support groups, financial data): http:// www.kidney.org

Renal Physicians Association: www.renalmd.org

OTHER ONLINE RESOURCES

CKiD U25 eGFR calculator: https://ckid-gfrcalculator. shinyapps.io/eGFR/# (or in the QxMD calculator smartphone app)

National Kidney Foundation: Parents of Children with Kidney Disease: https://healthunlocked.com/nkf-parents

NKF Bedside Schwartz 2009 and CKiD cystatin-C 2012 eGFR calculators: https://www.kidney.org/ professionals/kdoqi/gfr_calculatorPed

NKF CKD-EPI 2021 eGFR calculator: https://www. kidney.org/professionals/kdoqi/gfr_calculator

Pediatric ESKD risk calculator: https://www.kidney. org/professionals/kdoqi/gfr_calculatorPedRiskCalc

PKD Foundation (for research of polycystic kidney disease): https://pkdcure.org

Transplant Families (for pediatric transplant families): https://www.transplantfamilies.org

TransWeb (for transplant and organ donation information): www.transweb.org

United Network for Organ Sharing: www.unos.org

US Renal Data System: www.usrds.org

 Summary

Primary Care Needs for the Child With Chronic Kidney Disease

HEALTH CARE MAINTENANCE

Growth and Development

- Despite advances in medical management, dialysis, and transplant, growth retardation is a major problem in children with CKD (most are ≥2 SDs below the mean height for their age).
- Accurate growth measurements should be taken at initial visit and every 3 to 4 months for children older than 2 years. Head circumference should be monitored every 3 to 4 months on all children between the ages of 2 and 3 years. Children younger than 2 years of age should be assessed monthly for changes in growth.
- Achievement of developmental milestones (all ages) is delayed; sexual maturation is delayed.
- Developmental assessment and Tanner staging should be monitored.
- Adolescent characteristics differ between early, middle, and late adolescence; areas of growth, cognition, identity, sexuality, emotionality, family, and peer relationships across the age span should be assessed.
- Ventilation of emotions; counseling, physical activity for emotional health, independence, and support groups should be encouraged.
- Aggressive nutrition, adequate dialysis efficiency, and GH injections may improve growth.

Diet

- Protein and caloric needs in children with CKD are greater than the normal recommended daily allowance to enhance growth and development and offset losses (protein in peritoneal dialysis). Glucose is absorbed in peritoneal dialysis.
- Supplemental oral, nasogastric, or gastrostomy tube feedings should be considered to improve nutrition.
- Dietary restrictions differ with change in ESKD modality.

Safety

- Children with CKD should be encouraged to live as normal and active lives as possible, with modifications as necessary. Occupational and physical therapy may improve skills and stamina.
- Medical alert bracelets are recommended.
- Immunosuppression and CKD-MBD increase risk of infection and fracture.
- Kidney guards are available for pediatric kidney transplant recipients.

Immunizations

- Routine immunizations are recommended. Live virus vaccines are prohibited in the immunosuppressed child.
- COVID, influenza, pneumococcal, varicella, and hepatitis vaccines are recommended. Immunoglobulin is given after known exposure to virus (i.e., hepatitis, varicella-zoster).

Screening

- *Vision.* Routine annual examinations by a pediatric ophthalmologist are recommended to assess for calcification, arterial hemorrhages, cataracts (if child is receiving steroid therapy), and vision testing.
- *Hearing.* Routine annual examinations are recommended; hearing should be monitored when a child is using ototoxic drugs.
- *Dental.* Routine dental care at 6-month intervals. Prophylactic antibiotics are no longer formally recommended for patients without a history of infective endocarditis, although some programs still utilize this practice.
  - Gingival hyperplasia, enamel defects, and poor mineralization should be monitored.
- *Blood pressure.* Blood pressure should be taken at all medical visits; frequency of measurement depends on the blood pressure value. Correct size cuff and process should be used. Antihypertensive therapy should be managed by the pediatric nephrologist. Goal is normal blood pressure.

Continued

- *Hematocrit.* Anemia is a chronic problem. CBC count is monitored by the pediatric nephrology team.
- *Urinalysis.* Routine screening is done by pediatric nephrology team if indicated. Proteinuria should be followed up with a UP/C ratio; persistent proteinuria warrants consultation with pediatric nephrology.
- *Tuberculosis.* Yearly screening is done.

Condition-Specific Screening

- *Bloodwork.* CBC and RBC indices, folate studies, electrolytes, BUN, creatinine, calcium, phosphorus, alkaline phosphatase, albumin, ferritin, PTH, and iron are monitored regularly. Cholesterol, triglycerides, and viral titers periodically.
- *Cardiac screening.* Monitor chest x-ray, electrocardiogram, and echocardiogram every 6 to 12 months.
- *Radiologic screening.* Monitor bone radiographs for skeletal growth and complications from CKD-MBD or GH treatment.

COMMON ILLNESS MANAGEMENT
Differential Diagnosis

- Routine pediatric care should be provided by a pediatric provider in collaboration with the pediatric nephrologist.
- Antibiotics should be discussed with the pediatric nephrology team to ensure the correct dosing or use of antifungal prophylaxis.
- Fever should always be assessed for etiology; fever related to a vascular access or peritoneal dialysis catheter infection or peritonitis should be managed by the pediatric nephrologist. GI symptoms should be assessed for decreasing renal function.
- Headache should be assessed for hypertension; blood pressure should be controlled to normal.

Drug Interactions

- For all medications in CKD management, the route of excretion, degree of renal impairment, and interaction with other medications in CKD management should be known.
- Dosage of all medications should be calculated by the child's weight, not age.
- Drugs excreted renally may require dosage adjustment.
- Antifungal prophylaxis may be warranted by nephrology team for peritoneal dialysis patients receiving antibiotics.
- Calcium-based—not aluminum-based—phosphate binders should be used.
- Acetaminophen should be used for pain or fever rather than aspirin or ibuprofen.
- Absolute medication compliance is the key to a successful kidney transplant; many graft losses are because of noncompliance, especially in adolescents.
- Medication teaching should be related to the child's developmental level.

DEVELOPMENTAL ISSUES
Sleep Patterns

- Increased fatigue and need for sleep may indicate decreasing renal failure.
- Restlessness, insomnia, or cramps may indicate need for increased dialysis time or more physical activity.

Toileting

- Children with CKD may have normal urine output, oliguria, or anuria. Urinary diversion may present greater difficulty for adolescents.

- Not all children can achieve urinary continence.
- Bowel training should begin when a child is developmentally ready.
- Proper wiping direction should be taught to female children and their parents.

Discipline

- Parents' own emotions may interfere with discipline of the child (e.g., overprotective or too lenient without discipline). Healthy parental coping skills should be encouraged.
- Agree on a plan for medications or procedures and stick to it.
- Nonadherence with plan of care is a source of conflict.
- Children with CKD should learn self-discipline and begin taking age-appropriate responsibility for self-care as soon as possible.

Child Care

- The child care provider must be taught about diet, medications, special treatment regimen, and emergency measures.
- The dialysis schedule should be arranged around child care hours.
- Children may be exposed to more infections in day care.

School

- School attendance, when possible, should be encouraged or an alternative (home school, tutor, teacher in dialysis) provided.
- Teachers should be instructed about the child's care plan and needs.
- Children may need additional school-based services to perform catheterizations, take medication, or deal with fatigue.
- An IEP should be established.
- Poor school performance should be evaluated for physical vs. psychological factors contributing to the cause.

Sexuality

- Delayed sexual development is common.
- Erectile dysfunction is common in males but may resolve with transplantation.
- Counseling on birth control, STIs, HIV exposure should be provided.
- Responsibility toward transition into adulthood should be promoted.

Transition to Adulthood

- CKD makes independence difficult, and brain maturation occurs until age 25 years.
- Transition programs that teach self-management should begin early.
- Collaboration with adult programs is vital to ensure a smooth transfer.

Family Concerns

- CKD affects the entire family; the goal is to strengthen the total family unit.
- Networking with the other families of children with CKD should be provided.
- Religious, ethnic, cultural, and racial factors affect adjustment to CKD and care.
- Ethical issues are closely related to economics and are highly controversial.
- Health care team should practice patient advocacy.
- Cost containment has an effect on care.

REFERENCES

Ahmed, O. F., Hamodat, O. M., Kakamad, F. H., Abduljabbar, R. S., Salih, A. M., Omar, D. A., Mustafa, M. Q., Hassan, M. N., Mohammed, S. H., Mikael, T. M., Najar, K. A., & Hussen D. A. (2021). Outcomes of arteriovenous fistula for hemodialysis in pediatric age group. *Annals of Medicine and Surgery (Lond), 72,* 103100. doi:10.1016/j.amsu.2021.103100.

Ainslie, G. R., Wolf, K. K., Li, Y., Connolly, E. A., Scarlett, Y. V., Hull, J. H., & Paine, M. F. (2014). Assessment of a candidate marker constituent predictive of a dietary substance-drug interaction: Case study with grapefruit juice and CYP3A4 drug substrates. *Journal of Pharmacology and Experimental Therapeutics, 351*(3), 576–584. doi:10.1124/jpet.114.216838.

Al Hamed, R., Bazarbachi, A. H., Malard, F., Harousseau, J. L., & Mohty, M. (2019). Current status of autologous stem cell transplantation for multiple myeloma. *Blood Cancer Journal, 9*(4), 44. doi:10.1038/s41408-019-0205-9.

Al-Khouja, A., Park, K., Anderson, D. J. C., Young, C., Wang, J., Huang, S. M., Khurana, M., & Burckart, G. J. (2020). Dosing recommendations for pediatric patients with renal impairment. *Journal of Clinical Pharmacology, 60*(12), 1551–1560. https://doi.org/10.1002/jcph.1676.

Almaani, S., Mear, A., & Rovin, B. H. (2017). Update on lupus nephritis. *CJASN, 12,* 825–835. https://doi.org/10.2215/CJN.05780616.

American Academy of Pediatrics, Section on Nephrology & American Society of Pediatric Nephrology. Choosing wisely: Five things physicians and patients should question. (2022). Available at: https://www.choosingwisely.org/societies/american-academy-of-pediatrics-section-on-nephrology-and-the-american-society-of-pediatric-nephrology/. Accessed July 24, 2022.

American Heart Association. Infective endocarditis. (2022). Retrieved on 8/14/2022 from: https://www.heart.org/en/health-topics/infective-endocarditis.

Atkinson, M. A., Ng, D. K., Warady, B. A., Furth, S. L., & Flynn, J. T. (2021). The CKiD study: Overview and summary of findings related to kidney disease progression. *Pediatric Nephrology (Berlin, Germany), 36*(3), 527–538. https://doi.org/10.1007/s00467-019-04458-6.

Atkinson, M. A., & Warady, B. A. (2018). Anemia in chronic kidney disease. *Pediatric Nephrology (Berlin, Germany), 33*(2), 227–238. https://doi.org/10.1007/s00467-017-3663-y.

Baluarte, J. H. (2017). Neurological complications of renal disease. *Seminars in Pediatric Neurology, 24*(1), 25–32. https://doi.org/10.1016/j.spen.2016.12.004.

Berns J. (2022). Diagnosis of iron deficiency in chronic kidney disease. *UpToDate.* Retrieved from https://www.uptodate.com/contents/diagnosis-of-iron-deficiency-in-chronic-kidney-disease#H9 on 7/24/2022.

Bitzan, M., & Lapeyraque, A. L. (2016). Post infectious hemolytic uremic syndrome. In Geary, D. F., & Schaefer, F. (Eds.), *Pediatric kidney disease* (2nd ed.). Springer-Verlag. doi:10.1007/978-3-662-52972-0_2.

Boehm, M., Chand, D. H., & Brandt, M. L. (2021). Hemodialysis Vascular Access in Children. In: Warady, B. A., Alexander, S. R., Schaefer, F. (eds) Pediatric Dialysis. *Springer, Cham.* https://doi.org/10.1007/978-3-030-66861-7_19.

Bökenkamp, A. (2020). Proteinuria—take a closer look! *Pediatric Nephrology, 35,* 533–541. https://doi.org/10.1007/s00467-019-04454-w.

Borlaug BA, Beathard GA, Golper TA. (2022). Evaluation and management of heart failure caused by hemodialysis arteriovenous access. *UpToDate.* Retrieved on 8/14/2022 from: https://www.uptodate.com/contents/evaluation-and-management-of-heart-failure-caused-by-hemodialysis-arteriovenous-access#H1501537144.

Borzych-Duzalka, D., & Harvey, E. (2021). Non-infectious complications of hemodialysis in children. In Warady, B. A.,

Alexander, S. R., & Schaefer, F. (Eds.), *Pediatric dialysis* (3rd ed.). Springer https://doi.org/10.1007/978-3-030-66861-7.

Boynton, S. A., Matheson, M. B., Ng, D. K., Hidalgo, G., Warady, B. A., Furth, S. L., & Atkinson, M. A. (2022). The relationship between neighborhood disadvantage and kidney disease progression in the Chronic Kidney Disease in Children (CKiD) Cohort. *American Journal of Kidney Diseases, 80*(2), 207–214. https://doi.org/10.1053/j.ajkd.2021.12.008.

Brophy, P. D, Muff-Luett, M. (2022). Pediatric acute kidney injury (AKI): Indications, timing, and choice of modality for kidney replacement therapy (KRT). *Up To Date.* Retrieved on 8/14/2022 from: https://www.uptodate.com/contents/pediatric-acute-kidney-injury-aki-indications-timing-and-choice-of-modality-for-kidney-replacement-therapy-krt?search=aki%20pediatrics&source=search_result&selectedTitle=4~150&usage_type=default&display_rank=4.

Brown, D. D., Roem, J., Ng, D. K., Reidy, K. J., Kumar, J., Abramowitz, M. K., Mak, R. H., Furth, S. L., Schwartz, G. J., Warady, B. A., Kaskel, F. J., & Melamed, M. L. (2020). Low Serum Bicarbonate and CKD Progression in Children. *Clinical Journal of the American Society of Nephrology: CJASN, 15*(6), 755–765. https://doi.org/10.2215/CJN.07060619.

Brown, D. D., Carroll, M., Ng, D. K., Levy, R. V., Greenbaum, L. A., Kaskel, F. J., Furth, S. L., Warady, B. A., Melamed, M. L., & Dauber, A. (2022). Longitudinal associations between low serum bicarbonate and linear growth in children with CKD. *Kidney360, 3*(4), 666–676. https://doi.org/10.34067/KID.0005402021.

Bukutu, C., & Vohra, S. (2016). Complementary and alternative treatments for renal diseases. In Geary, D. F., & Schaefer, F. (Eds.), *Pediatric kidney disease* (2nd ed.). Springer-Verlag. doi:10.1007/978-3-662-52972-0_2.

Carpenter T. Overview of rickets in children. (2021). *UpToDate.* Retrieved on 8/14/2022 from: https://www.uptodate.com/contents/overview-of-rickets-in-children?topicRef=6092&source=see_link#H2256742.

Center for Disease Control and Prevention. (2022). Vaccine recommendations and guidelines for the Advisory Council for Immunization Practice (ACIP). Retrieved on 8/4/22 from https://www.cdc.gov/vaccines/hcp/acip-recs/general-recs/contraindications.html.

Centers for Disease Control and Prevention. (2023). *ACIP contraindications guidelines for immunization.* Centers for Disease Control and Prevention. https://www.cdc.gov/vaccines/hcp/acip-recs/general-recs/contraindications.html.

Chadha, V., Schaefer, F. S., & Warady, B. A. (2010). Dialysis-associated peritonitis in children. *Pediatric Nephrology (Berlin, Germany), 25*(3), 425–440. https://doi.org/10.1007/s00467-008-1113-6.

Chang, D. H., Dumanski, S. M., & Ahmed, S. B. (2021). Female reproductive and gynecologic considerations in chronic kidney disease: Adolescence and young adulthood. *Kidney International Reports, 7*(2), 152–164. https://doi.org/10.1016/j.ekir.2021.11.003.

Chanu, P., Schaefer, F., Warady, B. A., Schmitt, C. P., Reigner, B., Schnetzler, G., Meyer Reigner, S., Eisner, M., Weichert, A., & Frey, N. (2020). Model-based approach for methoxy polyethylene glycol-epoetin beta drug development in paediatric patients with anaemia of chronic kidney disease. *British Journal of Clinical Pharmacology, 86*(4), 801–811. https://doi.org/10.1111/bcp.14186.

Chen, W., Ducharme-Smith, K., Davis, L., Hui, W. F., Warady, B. A., Furth, S. L., Abraham, A. G., & Betoko, A. (2017). Dietary sources of energy and nutrient intake among children and adolescents with chronic kidney disease. *Pediatric Nephrology (Berlin, Germany), 32*(7), 1233–1241. https://doi.org/10.1007/s00467-017-3580-0.

Chertow, G. M., Appel, G. B., & Andreoli, S. (2021). Study design and baseline characteristics of the CARDINAL trial: A phase 3 study of bardoxolone methyl in patients with Alport syndrome. *American Journal of Nephrology, 52*(3), 180–189. https://doi.org/10.1159/000513777.

Chesnaye, N. C., van Stralen, K. J., & Bonthuis, M. (2018). Survival in children requiring chronic renal replacement therapy. *Pediatric Nephrology (Berlin, Germany), 33*(4), 585–594. https://doi.org/10.1007/s00467-017-3681-9.

Chu, D. I., Abraham, A. G., Tasian, G. E., Denburg, M. R., Ross, M. E., Zderic, S. A., & Furth, S. L. (2019). Urologic care and progression to end-stage kidney disease: A Chronic Kidney Disease in Children (CKiD) nested case-control study. *Journal of Pediatric Urology, 15*(3), 266.e1–266.e7. https://doi.org/10.1016/j.jpurol.2019.03.008.

Cornwell, L. B., Riddell, J. V., & Mason, M. D. (2020). New-onset ESRD secondary to reflux nephropathy has decreased in incidence in the United States. *Journal of Pediatric Urology, 16*(5), 566.e1–566.e7. https://doi.org/10.1016/j.jpurol.2020.06.023.

Delgado, C., Baweja, M., Crews, D. C., Eneanya, N. D., Gadegbeku, C. A., Inker, L. A., Mendu, M. L., Miller, W. G., Moxey-Mims, M. M., Roberts, G. V., St Peter, W. L., Warfield, C., & Powe, N. R. (2022). A unifying approach for GFR estimation: Recommendations of the NKF-ASN Task Force on Reassessing the Inclusion of Race in Diagnosing Kidney Disease. *American Journal of Kidney Diseases, 79*(2), 268–288.e1. https://doi.org/10.1053/j.ajkd.2021.08.003.

Desloovere, A., Renken-Terhaerdt, J., Tuokkola, J., Shaw, V., Greenbaum, L. A., Haffner, D., Anderson, C., Nelms, C. L., Oosterveld, M. J. S., Paglialonga, F., Polderman, N., Qizalbash, L., Warady, B. A., Shroff, R., & Vande Walle, J. (2021). The dietary management of potassium in children with CKD stages 2-5 and on dialysis-clinical practice recommendations from the Pediatric Renal Nutrition Taskforce. *Pediatric Nephrology (Berlin, Germany), 36*(6), 1331–1346. https://doi.org/10.1007/s00467-021-04923-1.

Drube, J., Wan, M., Bonthuis, M., Wühl, E., Bacchetta, J., Santos, F., Grenda, R., Edefonti, A., Harambat, J., Shroff, R., Tönshoff, B., Haffner, D., & European Society for Paediatric Nephrology Chronic Kidney Disease Mineral and Bone Disorders, Dialysis, and Transplantation Working Groups (2019). Clinical practice recommendations for growth hormone treatment in children with chronic kidney disease. *Nature Reviews Nephrology, 15*(9), 577–589. https://doi.org/10.1038/s41581-019-0161-4.

Fernandez, H. E., & Foster, B. J. (2022). Long-term care of the pediatric kidney transplant recipient. *CJASN, 17*(2), 296–304. https://doi.org/10.2215/CJN.16891020.

Fervenza, F. C., Seth, i S. (2020). Focal segmental glomerulosclerosis: Epidemiology, classification, clinical features, and diagnosis. *UpToDate.* Obtained on 8/8/22 from Focal segmental glomerulosclerosis: Epidemiology, classification, clinical features, and diagnosis - UpToDate.

Flynn, J. T., Kaelber, D. C., Baker-Smith, C. M., Blowey, D., Carroll, A. E., Daniels, S. R., de Ferranti, S. D., Dionne, J. M., Falkner, B., Flinn, S. K., Gidding, S. S., Goodwin, C., Leu, M. G., Powers, M. E., Rea, C., Samuels, J., Simasek, M., Thaker, V. V., Urbina, E. M., & Subcommittee on Screening and Management of High Blood Pressure in Children (2017). Clinical practice guideline for screening and management of high blood pressure in children and adolescents. *Pediatrics, 140*(3), e20171904. https://doi.org/10.1542/peds.2017-1904.

Franke, D., Thomas, L., Steffens, R., Pavičić, L., Gellermann, J., Froede, K., Querfeld, U., Haffner, D., & Živičnjak, M. (2015). Patterns of growth after kidney transplantation among children with ESRD. *Clinical Journal of the American Society of Nephrology, 10*(1), 127–134. https://doi.org/10.2215/CJN.02180314.

Fuhrman, D. Y., Schneider, M. F., Dell, K. M., Blydt-Hansen, T. D., Mak, R., Saland, J. M., Furth, S. L., Warady, B. A., Moxey-Mims, M. M., & Schwartz, G. J. (2017). Albuminuria, proteinuria, and renal disease progression in children with CKD. *Clinical Journal of the American Society of Nephrology, 12*(6), 912–920. https://doi.org/10.2215/CJN.11971116.

Gabriel, M. M., & Koch Nogueria, P. C. (2019). Management of hypertension in CAKUT: Protective factor for CKD. *Frontiers in Pediatrics, 7*(222). https://doi.org/10.3389/fped.2019.00222.

Gbadegesin, R., Gibson, K. L., & Smoyer, W. E. (2016). Steroid resistant nephrotic syndrome. In Geary, D. F., & Schaefer, F. (Eds.), *Pediatric kidney disease* (2nd ed.). Springer-Verlag. doi:10.1007/978-3-662-52972-0 2.

Haffner, D., & Rees, L. (2016). Growth and puberty in chronic kidney disease. In Geary, D. F., & Schaefer, F. (Eds.), *Pediatric kidney disease* (2nd ed.). Springer-Verlag. doi:10.1007/978-3-662-52972-0_2.

Haffner, D. (2020). Strategies for optimizing growth in children with chronic kidney disease. *Frontiers in Pediatrics, 8*, 399. https://doi.org/10.3389/fped.2020.00399.

Harshman, L. A., Johnson, R. J., Matheson, M. B., Kogon, A. J., Shinnar, S., Gerson, A. C., Warady, B. A., Furth, S. L., & Hooper, S. R. (2019). Academic achievement in children with chronic kidney disease: A report from the CKiD cohort. *Pediatric Nephrology (Berlin, Germany), 34*(4), 689–696. https://doi.org/10.1007/s00467-018-4144-7.

Hayes, W., & Paglialonga, F. (2019). Assessment and management of fluid overload in children on dialysis. *Pediatric Nephrology (Berlin, Germany), 34*(2), 233–242. https://doi.org/10.1007/s00467-018-3916-4.

Hebert, S. A., Swinford, R. D., Hall, D. R., Au, J. K., & Bynon, J. S. (2017). Special considerations in pediatric kidney transplantation. *Advances in Chronic Kidney Disease, 24*(6), 398–404. https://doi.org/10.1053/j.ackd.2017.09.009.

Hidalgo, G., Ng, D. K., Moxey-Mims, M., Minnick, M. L., Blydt-Hansen, T., Warady, B. A., & Furth, S. L. (2013). Association of income level with kidney disease severity and progression among children and adolescents with CKD: A report from the Chronic Kidney Disease in Children (CKiD) Study. *American Journal of Kidney Diseases, 62*(6), 1087–1094. https://doi.org/10.1053/j.ajkd.2013.06.013.

Hoenig, M. P., & Hladik, G. A. (2022). Overview of kidney structure and function. In Gilbert, S. J., Weinger, D. E., Bomback, A. S., Perazella, M. A., & Rifkin, D. E. (Eds.), *National Kidney Foundation's primer on kidney diseases* (8th ed.). Elsevier.

Inker, L. A., Astor, B. C., & Fox, C. H. (2014). KDOQI US commentary on the 2012 KDIGO clinical practice guideline for the evaluation and management of CKD. *American Journal of Kidney Diseases, 63*(5), 713–735. https://doi.org/10.1053/j.ajkd.2014.01.416.

Inker, L. A., & Levey, A. S. (2023). Staging and management of kidney disease. In Gilbert, S. J., Weiner, D. E., Bobmack, A. S., Perazella, M. A., & Rifkin, D. E. (Eds.), *National Kidney Foundation's primer on kidney diseases* (8th ed.). Elsevier.

Ismaili, K., Cassart, M., Avni, F. E., & Hall, M. (2016). Antenatal assessment of morphology and function. In Geary, D. F., & Schaefer, F. (Eds.), *Pediatric kidney disease* (2nd ed.). Springer-Verlag. doi:10.1007/978-3-662-52972-0_2.

Johnson, R. J., & Harshman, L. A. (2021). Neurocognition in pediatric chronic kidney disease: A review of data from the Chronic Kidney Disease in Children (CKiD) study. *Seminars in Nephrology, 41*(5), 446–454. https://doi.org/10.1016/j.semnephrol.2021.09.007.

Joshi, S., McMacken, M., & Kalantar-Zadeh, K. (2021). Plant-based diets for kidney disease: A guide for clinicians. *American Journal of Kidney Diseases, 77*(2), 287–296. https://doi.org/10.1053/j.ajkd.2020.10.003.

Joslin, B., Langman, C., Nishi, L., & Ghossein, C. (2020). Assessing success in transitioning of young adults from pediatric to adult kidney practice. *BMC Nephrology, 21*(1), 8. https://doi.org/10.1186/s12882-019-1665-7.

Kallash, M., & Rheault, M. N. (2020). Approach to persistent microscopic hematuria in children. *Kidney, 1*(9), 1014–1020. *360.* https://doi.org/10.34067/KID.0003222020.

Kashtan, C. E., Ding, J., Garosi, G., Heidet, L., Massella, L., Nakanishi, K., Nozu, K., Renieri, A., Rheault, M., Wang, F., & Gross, O. (2018). Alport syndrome: A unified classification of genetic disorders of collagen IV α345: A position paper of the Alport Syndrome Classification Working Group. *Kidney International, 93*(5), 1045–1051. https://doi.org/10.1016/j.kint.2017.12.018.

KDOQI Work Group. (2009). KDOQI clinical practice guideline for nutrition in children with CKD: 2008 update. Executive summary. *American Journal of Kidney Diseases, 53*(3 Suppl 2), S11–S104. https://doi.org/10.1053/j.ajkd.2008.11.017.

Ketteler, M., Block, G. A., Evenepoel, P., Fukagawa, M., Herzog, C. A., McCann, L., Moe, S. M., Shroff, R., Tonelli, M. A., Toussaint, N. D., Vervloet, M. G., & Leonard, M. B. (2018). Diagnosis, evaluation, prevention, and treatment of chronic kidney disease-mineral and bone disorder: Synopsis of the kidney disease: Improving Global Outcomes 2017 Clinical Practice Guideline Update. *Annals of Internal Medicine, 168*(6), 422–430. https://doi.org/10.7326/M17-2640.

Khouzam, N. M., Wesseling-Perry, K., & Salusky, I. B. (2015). The role of bone in CKD-mediated mineral and vascular disease. *Pediatric Nephrology (Berlin, Germany), 30*(9), 1379–1388. https://doi.org/10.1007/s00467-014-2919-z.

Kirsztajn, G. M., Suassuna, J. H., & Bastos, M. G. (2009). Dividing stage 3 of chronic kidney disease (CKD): 3A and 3B. *Kidney International, 76*(4), 462–464. https://doi.org/10.1038/ki.2009.178.

Kleta, R., & Bockenhauer, D. (2018). Salt-losing tubulopathies in children: What's new, what's controversial? *JASN, 29*(3), 727–739. https://doi.org/10.1681/ASN.2017060600.

Knoers, N., Antignac, C., Bergmann, C., Dahan, K., Giglio, S., Heidet, L., Lipska-Ziętkiewicz, B. S., Noris, M., Remuzzi, G., Vargas-Poussou, R., & Schaefer, F. (2022). Genetic testing in the diagnosis of chronic kidney disease: recommendations for clinical practice. *Nephrology Dialysis Transplantation, 37*(2), 239–254. https://doi.org/10.1093/ndt/gfab218.

Kogon, A. J., Matheson, M. B., Flynn, J. T., Gerson, A. C., Warady, B. A., Furth, S. L., Hooper, S. R., & Chronic Kidney Disease in Children (CKiD) Study Group (2016). Depressive symptoms in children with chronic kidney disease. *The Journal of Pediatrics, 168,* 164–170.e1. https://doi.org/10.1016/j.jpeds.2015.09.040.

Kogon, A. J., & Harshman, L. A. (2019). Chronic kidney disease: Treatment of comorbidities I: Nutrition, growth, neurocognitive function, and mineral bone disease. *Current Treatment Options in Pediatrics, 5,* 78–92. https://doi.org/10.1007/s40746-019-00152-9.

Koury, M. J., & Haase, V. H. (2015). Anaemia in kidney disease: Harnessing hypoxia responses for therapy. *Nature Reviews Nephrology, 11*(7), 394–410. https://doi.org/10.1038/nrneph.2015.82.

Ku, E., Kopple, J. D., McCulloch, C. E., Warady, B. A., Furth, S. L., Mak, R. H., Grimes, B. A., & Mitsnefes, M. (2018a). Associations between weight loss, kidney function decline, and risk of ESRD in the Chronic Kidney Disease in Children (CKiD) cohort study. *American Journal of Kidney Diseases, 71*(5), 648–656. https://doi.org/10.1053/j.ajkd.2017.08.013.

Ku, E., Kopple, J. D., McCulloch, C. E., Warady, B. A., Furth, S. L., Mak, R. H., Grimes, B. A., & Mitsnefes, M. M. (2018b). Twenty-four-hour ambulatory blood pressure versus clinic blood pressure measurements and risk of adverse outcomes in children with CKD. *Clinical Journal of the American Society of Nephrology, 13*(3), 422–428. https://doi.org/10.2215/CJN.09630917.

Laster, M., Soohoo, M., Hall, C., Streja, E., Rhee, C. M., Ravel, V. A., Reddy, U., Norris, K. C., Salusky, I. B., & Kalantar-Zadeh, K. (2017). Racial-ethnic disparities in mortality and kidney transplant outcomes among pediatric dialysis patients. *Pediatric Nephrology (Berlin, Germany), 32*(4), 685–695. https://doi.org/10.1007/s00467-016-3530-2.

Lau, K., & Wyatt, R. (2005). Glomerulonephritis. *Adolescent Medicine Clinics, 16,* 67–85.

Lefebvre, C. E., Filion, K. B., Reynier, P., Platt, R. W., & Zappitelli, M. (2020). Primary care prescriptions of potentially nephrotoxic medications in children with CKD. *Clinical Journal of the American Society of Nephrology, 15*(1), 61–68. https://doi.org/10.2215/CJN.03550319.

Lexicomp. Drug interactions: Calcium carbonate, ferrous sulfate, sevelamer. 2022. Retrieved on 8/14/2022 from: https://online.lexi.com/lco/action/interact.

Liu, D. B., Armstrong, W. R., & Maizels, M. (2014). Hydronephrosis: Prenatal and postnatal evaluation and management. *Clinics in Perinatology, 41*(3), 661–678. https://doi.org/10.1016/j.clp.2014.05.013.

Mahan, J. D., & Warady, B. A. (2006). Consensus Committee. Assessment and treatment of short stature in pediatric patients with chronic kidney disease: A consensus statement. *Pediatric Nephrology (Berlin, Germany), 21*(7), 917–930. https://doi.org/10.1007/s00467-006-0020-y.

Massengill, S. F., & Ferris, M. (2014). Chronic kidney disease in children and adolescents. *Pediatrics in Review, 35*(1), 16–29. https://doi.org/10.1542/pir.35-1-16.

Matzke, G. R., Aronoff, G. R., Atkinson, A. J., Jr, Bennett, W. M., Decker, B. S., Eckardt, K. U., Golper, T., Grabe, D. W., Kasiske, B., Keller, F., Kielstein, J. T., Mehta, R., Mueller, B. A., Pasko, D. A., Schaefer, F., Sica, D. A., Inker, L. A., Umans, J. G., & Murray, P. (2011). Drug dosing consideration in patients with acute and chronic kidney disease-a clinical update from Kidney Disease: Improving Global Outcomes (KDIGO). *Kidney International, 80*(11), 1122–1137. https://doi.org/10.1038/ki.2011.322.

McAlister, L., Pugh, P., Greenbaum, L., Haffner, D., Rees, L., Anderson, C., Desloovere, A., Nelms, C., Oosterveld, M., Paglialonga, F., Polderman, N., Qizalbash, L., Renken-Terhaerdt, J., Tuokkola, J., Warady, B., Walle, J. V., Shaw, V., & Shroff, R. (2020). The dietary management of calcium and phosphate in children with CKD stages 2-5 and on dialysis-clinical practice recommendation from the Pediatric Renal Nutrition Taskforce. *Pediatric Nephrology (Berlin, Germany), 35*(3), 501–518. https://doi.org/10.1007/s00467-019-04370-z.

McQuaid, E. L., & Landier, W. (2018). Cultural issues in medication adherence: Disparities and directions. *Journal of General Internal Medicine, 33*(2), 200–206. https://doi.org/10.1007/s11606-017-4199-3.

Meyer, T. W., & Hostetter, T. H. (2014). Approaches to uremia. *JASN, 25*(10), 2151–2158. https://doi.org/10.1681/ASN.2013121264.

Mitsnefes, M. M., Laskin, B. L., Dahhou, M., Zhang, X., & Foster, B. J. (2013). Mortality risk among children initially treated with dialysis for end-stage kidney disease, 1990-2010. *JAMA, 309*(18), 1921–1929. https://doi.org/10.1001/jama.2013.4208.

Molino, A. R., Minnick, M. L. G., Jerry-Fluker, J., Karita Muiru, J., Boynton, S. A., Furth, S. L., Warady, B. A., Ng, D. K., & Chronic Kidney Disease in Children Study (2022). Health and dental insurance and health care utilization among children, adolescents, and young adults with CKD: Findings from the CKiD cohort study. *Kidney Medicine, 4*(5), 100455. https://doi.org/10.1016/j.xkme.2022.100455.

National Kidney Foundation. (2015). KDOQI clinical practice guideline for hemodialysis adequacy: 2015 update. *American Journal of Kidney Diseases, 66*(5), 884–930. https://doi.org/10.1053/j.ajkd.2015.07.015.

Nelson, M. V., van den Heuvel-Eibrink, M. M., Graf, N., & Dome, J. S. (2021). New approaches to risk stratification for Wilms tumor. *Current Opinion in Pediatrics, 33*(1), 40–48. https://doi.org/10.1097/MOP.0000000000000988.

Neu, A. M., Richardson, T., Lawlor, J., Stuart, J., Newland, J., McAfee, N., Warady, B. A., & SCOPE Collaborative Participants (2016).

Implementation of standardized follow-up care significantly reduces peritonitis in children on chronic peritoneal dialysis. *Kidney International, 89*(6), 1346–1354. https://doi.org/10.1016/j.kint.2016.02.015.

Ng, D. K., Xu, Y., Hogan, J., Saland, J. M., Greenbaum, L. A., Furth, S. L., Warady, B. A., & Wong, C. S. (2020). Timing of patient-reported renal replacement therapy planning discussions by disease severity among children and young adults with chronic kidney disease. *Pediatric Nephrology (Berlin, Germany), 35*(10), 1925–1933. https://doi.org/10.1007/s00467-020-04542-2.

Nigwekar, S. U., Kroshinsky, D., Nazarian, R. M., Goverman, J., Malhotra, R., Jackson, V. A., Kamdar, M. M., Steele, D. J., & Thadhani, R. I. (2015). Calciphylaxis: risk factors, diagnosis, and treatment. *American Journal of Kidney Diseases, 66*(1), 133–146. https://doi.org/10.1053/j.ajkd.2015.01.034.

Noone, D., & Langlois, V. (2016). Laboratory evaluation of renal disease in childhood. In Geary, D. F., & Schaefer, F. (Eds.), *Pediatric kidney disease* (2nd ed.). Springer-Verlag. doi:10.1007/978-3-662-52972-0_2.

North American Pediatric Renal Trials and Collaborative Studies. NAPRTCS 2014 annual transplant report. 2014. Retrieved on 8/13/2022 from: https://naprtcs.org/system/files/2014_Annual_Transplant_Report.pdf.

Onder, A. M., & Somers, M. J. G. (2021). Infectious complications of hemodialysis in children. In Warady, B. A., Alexander, S. R., & Schaefer, F. (Eds.), *Pediatric dialysis* (3rd ed.). Springer https://doi.org/10.1007/978-3-030-66861-7.

Organ Procurement and Transplant Network. (2022). Kidney competing risk median waiting time to deceased donor transplant for registrations listed: 2003-2014. Based on OPTN data as of August 5, 2022. Retrieved on 8/9/22 from: https://optn.transplant.hrsa.gov/data/view-data-reports/national-data/#.

Organ Procurement Transplant Network. (2022). National data, organ by age; current wait list. Retrieved on 8/13/2022 from: https://optn.transplant.hrsa.gov/data/view-data-reports/national-data/.

Pierce, C. B., Muñoz, A., Ng, D. K., Warady, B. A., Furth, S. L., & Schwartz, G. J. (2021). Age- and sex-dependent clinical equations to estimate glomerular filtration rates in children and young adults with chronic kidney disease. *Kidney International, 99*(4), 948–956. https://doi.org/10.1016/j.kint.2020.10.047.

Poliquin, P. G., Lagacé-Wiens, P., Verrelli, M., Allen, D. W., & Embil, J. M. (2015). Pasteurella species peritoneal dialysis-associated peritonitis: Household pets as a risk factor. *Canadian Journal of Infectious Diseases and Medical Microbiology, 26*(1), 52–55. doi:10.1155/2015/389467.

Quennelle, S., Ovaert, C., Cailliez, M., Garaix, F., Tsimaratos, M., & El Louali, F. (2021). Dilatation of the aorta in children with advanced chronic kidney disease. *Pediatric Nephrology (Berlin, Germany), 36*(7), 1825–1831. https://doi.org/10.1007/s00467-020-04887-8.

Savige, J., Sheth, S., Leys, A., Nicholson, A., Mack, H. G., & Colville, D. (2015). Ocular features in Alport syndrome: Pathogenesis and clinical significance. *Clinical Journal of the American Society of Nephrology, 10*(4), 703–709. https://doi.org/10.2215/CJN.10581014.

Sethna, C. B., Bryant, K., Munshi, R., Warady, B. A., Richardson, T., Lawlor, J., Newland, J. G., Neu, A., & SCOPE Investigators (2016). Risk factors for and outcomes of catheter-associated peritonitis in children: The SCOPE collaborative. *Clinical journal of the American Society of Nephrology, 11*(9), 1590–1596. https://doi.org/10.2215/CJN.02540316.

Sethna, C. B., & Gipson, D. S. (2014). Treatment of FSGS in children. *Advances in Chronic Kidney Disease, 21*(2), 194–199. https://doi.org/10.1053/j.ackd.2014.01.010.

Shroff, R., Wan, M., Nagler, E. V., Bakkaloglu, S., Fischer, D. C., Bishop, N., Cozzolino, M., Bacchetta, J., Edefonti, A., Stefanidis, C. J., Vande Walle, J., Haffner, D., Klaus, G., Schmitt, C. P., & European Society for Paediatric Nephrology Chronic Kidney

Disease Mineral and Bone Disorders and Dialysis Working Groups (2017). Clinical practice recommendations for native vitamin D therapy in children with chronic kidney disease Stages 2-5 and on dialysis. *Nephrology Dialysis Transplantation, 32*(7), 1098–1113. https://doi.org/10.1093/ndt/gfx065.

Simon, D. M., & Levin, S. (2001). Infectious complications of solid organ transplantation. *Infectious Disease Clinics of North America, 15*, 521–549.

Singh, N. S., Grimes, J., Gregg, G. K., Nau, A. E., Rivard, D. C., Fields, M., Flaucher, N., Sherman, A. K., Williams, M. U., Wiley, K. J., Kerwin, K., & Warady, B. A. (2021). "Save the Vein" Initiative in children with CKD: A quality improvement study. *American Journal of Kidney Diseases, 78*(1), 96-102.e1. doi:10.1053/j.ajkd.2020.11.016.

Srivastava T, Warady B. (2021). Pediatric chronic kidney disease-mineral and bone disorder (CKD-MBD) obtained on 7/28/22. https://www.uptodate.com/contents/pediatric-chronic-kidney-disease-mineral-and-bone-disorder-ckd-mbd.

Stabouli, S., Papadimitriou, E., Printza, N., Dotis, J., & Papachristou, F. (2016). Sleep disorders in pediatric chronic kidney disease patients. *Pediatric Nephrology (Berlin, Germany), 31*(8), 1221–1229. https://doi.org/10.1007/s00467-015-3237-9.

Swartz, S. J., & Paglialonga, F. (2021). Maintenance Hemodialysis During Infancy. In: Warady, B. A., Alexander, S. R., Schaefer, F. (eds) Pediatric Dialysis. Springer, Cham. https://doi.org/10.1007/978-3-030-66861-7_22.

Sweeney, W. E., Jr., & Avner, E. D. (2014). Pathophysiology of childhood polycystic kidney diseases: New insights into disease-specific therapy. *Pediatric Research, 75*(1-2), 148–157. https://doi.org/10.1038/pr.2013.191.

Talati, A. N., Webster, C. M., & Vora, N. L. (2019). Prenatal genetic considerations of congenital anomalies of the kidney and urinary tract (CAKUT). *Prenatal Diagnosis, 39*(9), 679–692. https://doi.org/10.1002/pd.5536.

Tambur, A. R. (2016). Hiding in plain sight—a new look at HLA epitopes: A case report. *American Journal of Transplantation, 16*(11), 3286–3291. https://doi.org/10.1111/ajt.13918.

Torra, R., Furlano, M., Ortiz, A., & Ars, E. (2021). Genetic kidney diseases as an underrecognized cause of chronic kidney disease: Tthe key role of international registry reports. *Clinical Kidney Journal, 14*(8), 1879–1885. https://doi.org/10.1093/ckj/sfab056.

Trautmann, A., Vivarelli, M., Samuel, S., Gipson, D., Sinha, A., Schaefer, F., Hui, N. K., Boyer, O., Saleem, M. A., Feltran, L., Müller-Deile, J., Becker, J. U., Cano, F., Xu, H., Lim, Y. N., Smoyer, W., Anochie, I., Nakanishi, K., Hodson, E., Haffner, D., … International Pediatric Nephrology Association (2020). IPNA clinical practice recommendations for the diagnosis and management of children with steroid-resistant nephrotic syndrome. *Pediatric Nephrology (Berlin, Germany), 35*(8), 1529–1561. https://doi.org/10.1007/s00467-020-04519-1.

United States Renal Data System. (2021a). *USRDS annual data report: Epidemiology of kidney disease in the United States.* Bethesda, MD: National Institutes of Health, National Institute of Diabetes and Digestive and Kidney Diseases.

United States Renal Data System. (2021b). *USRDS annual data report: Total spending for ESRD 2009-2019.* Bethesda, MD: National Institutes of Health, National Institute of Diabetes and Digestive and Kidney Disease. Retrieved on 8/14/22 from. https://adr.usrds.org/2021/end-stage-renal-disease/9-healthcare-expenditures-for-persons-with-esrd.

Verduzco, H. A., & Shirazian, S. (2020). CKD-associated pruritus: New insights into diagnosis, pathogenesis, and management. *Kidney International Reports, 5*(9), 1387–1402. https://doi.org/10.1016/j.ekir.2020.04.027.

Vogt, B., & Avner E. (2007). Renal failure. In: R. Kleigman, R. Behrman, H. Jensen et al., (Eds) *Nelson's Textbook of Pediatrics* (18th ed.) Philadelphia: Saunders.

Warady, B. A., Abraham, A. G., Schwartz, G. J., Wong, C. S., Muñoz, A., Betoko, A., Mitsnefes, M., Kaskel, F., Greenbaum,

L. A, Mak, R. H., Flynn, J., Moxey-Mims, M. M., & Furth, S. (2015). Predictors of rapid progression of glomerular and nonglomerular kidney disease in children and adolescents: The Chronic Kidney Disease in Children (CKiD) Cohort. *American Journal of Kidney Diseases, 65*(6), 878–888. doi:10.1053/j.ajkd.2015.01.008. Epub 2015 Mar 19.

Warady, B. A., & Andrews, W. S. (2021). Peritoneal access in children receiving dialysis. In Warady, B. A., Alexander, S. R., & Schaefer, F. (Eds.), *Pediatric dialysis* (3rd ed.). Springer https://doi.org/10.1007/978-3-030-66861-7.

Warady, B. A., Bakkaloglu, S., Newland, J., Cantwell, M., Verrina, E., Neu, A., Chadha, V., Yap, H. K., & Schaefer, F. (2012). Consensus guidelines for the prevention and treatment of catheter-related infections and peritonitis in pediatric patients receiving peritoneal dialysis: 2012 update. *Peritoneal Dialysis International, 32*(Suppl 2), S32–S86. https://doi.org/10.3747/pdi.2011.00091.

Warady, B. A., Neu, A. M., & Schaefer, F. (2014). Optimal care of the infant, child, and adolescent on dialysis: 2014 update. *American Journal of Kidney Diseases, 64*(1), 128–142. https://doi.org/10.1053/j.ajkd.2014.01.430.

Warady, B. A., Weidemann, D., Srivastava, T. (2021). Chronic kidney disease in children: Complications. *UpToDate.* Retrieved on 8/14/2022 from: https://www.uptodate.com/contents/chronic-kidney-disease-in-children-complications?sectionName=Hypertension&search=use-of-diuretics-in-patients-with-&topicRef=6131&anchor=H4280729683&source=see_link#H4280729683.

Waters, A., & Lemaire, M. (2016). Genetic diagnosis of renal diseases: Basic concepts and testing. In: Geary, D. F., & Schaefer, F. (Eds.), *Pediatric kidney disease* (2nd ed.). Springer-Verlag. doi:10.1007/978-3-662-52972-0_2.

Watson, A. R. (2014). Ethical issues and children with chronic kidney disease. *Paediatrics and Child Health, 24*(7), 317–320. https://doi.org/10.1016/j.paed.2014.04.007.

Watson, A. R., Harden, P. N., Ferris, M. E., Kerr, P. G., Mahan, J. D., Ramzy, M. F., & International Society of Nephrology; International Pediatric Nephrology Association (2011). Transition from pediatric to adult renal services: a consensus statement by the International Society of Nephrology (ISN) and the International Pediatric Nephrology Association (IPNA). *Kidney International, 80*(7), 704–707. https://doi.org/10.1038/ki.2011.209.

Wesseling-Perry, K., Pereira, R. C., Tseng, C. H., Elashoff, R., Zaritsky, J. J., Yadin, O., Sahney, S., Gales, B., Jüppner, H., & Salusky, I. B. (2012). Early skeletal and biochemical alterations in pediatric chronic kidney disease. *Clinical Journal of the American Society of Nephrology, 7*(1), 146–152. https://doi.org/10.2215/CJN.05940611.

Wesseling-Perry, K., & Salusky, I. B. (2013). Phosphate binders, vitamin D and calcimimetics in the management of chronic kidney disease-mineral bone disorders (CKD-MBD) in children. *Pediatric Nephrology (Berlin, Germany), 28*(4), 617–625. https://doi.org/10.1007/s00467-012-2381-8.

Wong, C. S., Kogon, A. J., Warady, B. A., Furth, S. L., Lantos, J. D., & Wilfond, B. S. (2019). Ethical and policy considerations for genomic testing in pediatric research: The path toward disclosing individual research results. *American Journal of Kidney Diseases, 73*(6), 837–845. https://doi.org/10.1053/j.ajkd.2019.01.020.

Zahr, R. S., Greenbaum, L. A., & Schaefer, F. (2021). The decision to initiate dialysis in children and adolescents. In: Warady, B. A., Alexander, S. R., & Schafer, F. (Eds.), *Pediatric dialysis* (3rd ed.). Springer https://doi.org/10.1007/978-3-030-66861-7.

30 Mood Disorders: Behavioral and Developmental Influences

Beth Heuer, Donna Hallas

The Centers for Disease Control and Prevention (CDC) gathers data from representative surveys from parents of children and adolescents about their children's mental, emotional, and behavioral well-being (CDC, 2022b). Mental health affects children in several ways, including how they view the world at home, in school, and during play activities, interactions with other children and adults, ways they handle stress, make friends, relate to family, and how to make choices as they grow (CDC, 2022a). Approximately 4.4% of children, or 2.7 million children in the United States between the ages of 3 and 17 years, were identified as depressed on parental surveys (Bitsko et al., 2022). For adolescents between the ages of 12 and 17 in 2018–19, 15.1% had a major depressive disorder (MDD) episode, 36.7% had persistent feelings of sadness or hopelessness, and 18.8% seriously considered attempting suicide, with 15.7% making a suicide plan (CDC, 2022). These data represent serious mental and behavioral health problems among pediatrics and adolescents throughout the United States. Advanced practice registered nurses (APRNs) have opportunities to make a difference in the lives of these patients and their families during primary care visits. By obtaining a comprehensive history, including screenings, assessments, and a physical exam, the APRN can identify mental, behavioral, social, and developmental problems early on and intervene. The APRN can then formulate an appropriate treatment plan to address the issues, which may include referrals to specialized psychiatric care to reduce the adverse effects of untreated mental, behavioral, and developmental problems.

Disorders of behavioral and developmental health and mood disorders in children and adolescents are not a single clinical entity with a clearly determined etiology or predictable lifetime course. Rather, these disorders are conditions characterized by prolonged, pervasive emotional and behavioral disturbance and are associated with increased risk of disability, self-harm, and mortality. Of note, the term *mood disorders* is no longer a specific category within the *Diagnostic and Statistical Manual of Mental Disorders* (5th ed., text revision [DSM-5-TR]) (American Psychiatric Association [APA], 2022). They are now categorized as (1) developmental depressive disorders, which include disruptive mood dysregulation disorder (DMDD), and (2) bipolar and related disorders.

This chapter presents content for APRNs caring for pediatric, adolescent, and young adults who present with symptoms and behaviors consistent with depression and/or mood disorders. The following topics are presented:

- Comprehensive approach to care management of mood disorders
- Overview of the disorder, incidence, and prevalence
- Presenting symptoms and behaviors
- Analysis of screening and assessment tools
- Diagnosis to establish primary and possible comorbid diagnoses
- Evidence-based treatment plans (including medication management)
- Treatments and modifications of plans to meet individual and family health care needs
- Primary care management of children, adolescents, and young adults with mood disorders (including DMDD and bipolar and related disorders)

DEVELOPMENTAL CONSIDERATIONS

Improving longitudinal data collection of mental and behavioral health conditions for infants, toddlers, preschoolers, children, adolescents, and young adults may result in an improved understanding of how these conditions change over time and across different developmental stages (Shim et al., 2022), thereby aiding in the development of targeted preventive interventions. Insults to normal growth and developmental patterns adversely affect brain development beginning in the antenatal period if the fetus is exposed to maternal depression or such insults as illicit drugs and/or alcohol. Insults to brain development may occur throughout the pediatric ages into adolescence and young adulthood based on emotional and environmental factors encountered during each of these developmental ages. Achieving developmental milestones at appropriate ages is a major goal for the pediatric and adolescent populations. Failure to achieve age-appropriate developmental milestones requires expert assessments and immediate interventions to prevent developmental delays and adverse childhood experiences (ACEs).

This chapter discusses developmental assessments of infants, preschoolers, school-age children, adolescents, and young adults for mood disorders with APRNs to identify variants from normal patterns, leading them to formulate differential diagnoses and establish a diagnosis to enable the patient to resume normal growth and developmental patterns. For example, developmental factors (e.g., difficulties in verbalizing mood symptoms and behaviors that can be misinterpreted as psychopathologic, such as grandiosity and elation) can make formulating a diagnosis more challenging in older adolescent and adult populations (Elhosary & Birmaher, 2022). APRNs who have developed a strong knowledge base in diagnostic reasoning using an analysis of presenting symptomatology and the known pathophysiologic basis underlying the disorders are key to preventing diagnostic errors and designing evidence-based treatment plans.

ROLE OF APRN IN CARING FOR PEDIATRIC/ADOLESCENT/YOUNG ADULTS WITH MOOD DISORDERS

Screening for behavioral and mental health problems to identify the diagnosis as early as possible in primary care settings is paramount to successful health care outcomes (Box 30.1) (Hallas, 2019b). The Bright Futures/American Academy of Pediatrics (AAP) Periodicity Schedule (AAP, 2022) recommends behavioral/social/emotional screening at every well-child visit. Depression and suicide risk screening begins yearly at age 12 at well-child visits but should be instituted at any visit where concerns are identified. Patients should be referred to developmental/behavioral specialists or psychiatry for any complex mental health concerns, although many pediatric practices and specialty clinics will manage a variety of diagnoses (Box 30.2).

Primary care APRNs, including pediatric nurse practitioners, family nurse practitioners, psychiatric mental health nurse practitioners, and psychiatric clinical nurse specialists, can obtain additional education and certification to improve their management of children/adolescents with mood disorders. APRN certification with the Pediatric Primary Care Mental Health Specialist (PMHS) credential has experience in early identification and intervention for developmental, behavioral, and mental health concerns (Pediatric Nursing Certification Board, n.d.). Providers with the PMHS certificate have demonstrated increased knowledge, skills, and abilities and have clinical experience in assessing, diagnosing, and managing these concerns. PMHS certification allows work in integrative practices such as a pediatric primary care setting that also diagnoses and treats children with developmental and behavioral health problems. APRNs who hold the PMHS provide behavioral health services such as play therapy for young children (Thomas et al., 2022), talk therapy, cognitive-behavioral therapy (American Psychological Association, 2023), and screening, brief intervention, and referral to treatment

| Box **30.1** | **ICD-10 Coding for Diagnoses and Therapy Services** |

DEPRESSION

F32.0: Major depressive disorder, single episode, mild
F32.A: Unspecified depressive disorder
F32.1: Major depressive disorder, single episode, moderate
F32.3: Major depressive disorder: single episode, severe without psychotic features
F32.4: Major depressive disorder, single episode, in partial remission
F32.5: Major depressive disorder, single episode, in full remission
F32.8: Other depressive episodes
F32.9: Major depressive disorder, single episode, unspecified
F33.1: Major depressive disorder, recurrent, moderate
F33.2: Major depressive disorder, recurrent, severe
F33.4: Major depressive disorder, in remission, unspecified
F33.9: Major depressive disorder, recurrent, unspecified
F34.1: Persistent depressive disorder (dysthymia)

DISRUPTIVE MOOD DYSREGULATION DISORDER

F34.81: Disruptive mood dysregulation disorder

BIPOLAR DISORDER

F31.0: Bipolar disorder, current episode hypomanic
F31.10: Bipolar disorder, current episode manic without psychotic features
F31.11: Bipolar disorder, current or most recent episode manic (mild)
F31.12: Bipolar disorder, current or most recent episode manic (moderate)
F31.12: Bipolar disorder, current or most recent episode manic (severe)
F31.2: Bipolar disorder, current episode manic severe with psychotic features
F31.3: Bipolar disorder, current episode depressed (mild severity)
F31.3: Bipolar disorder, current episode depressed (moderate severity)
F31.4: Bipolar disorder, current episode depressed, severe, without psychotic features
F31.5: Bipolar disorder, current episode depressed, severe, with psychotic features
F31.73: Bipolar disorder, in partial remission
F31.73: Bipolar disorder, in full remission
F31.81: Bipolar II disorder
F31.9: Bipolar disorder, unspecified

2024 ICD-10-CM codes F30-F39: Mood [affective] disorders. ICD10Data.com. (2023, October 1). https://www.icd10data.com/ICD10CM/Codes/F01-F99/F30-F39.

(US Department of Health and Human Services [HHS], 2022) for drug and alcohol use. APRNs with the PMHS may also serve as a bridge to patients and families awaiting referral for more specialized care (e.g., the management of children and adolescents with a diagnosis of major depression disorders). Additionally, PMHS providers collaborate and coordinate care with other professionals in both medical and educational settings (Hallas et al., 2022; Pediatric Nursing Certification Board, n.d.).

Box 30.2	When to Consider Consultation or Referral to a Higher Level of Care

- The diagnosis is not clear.
- The advanced practice registered nurse (APRN) believes further assessment is needed.
- The APRN believes medication may be needed but will not be prescribing it.
- The APRN has started medications and needs further psychopharmacologic consultation.
- Chronic medical regimen nonadherence has a risk of lethality.
- Individual, family, or group psychotherapy is needed.
- Psychotic symptoms (hallucinations, paranoia) are present.
- Bipolar disorder is suspected.
- Delirium is suspected.

SOCIAL DETERMINANTS OF HEALTH AND PSYCHOLOGICAL FACTORS

The social determinants of health (SDOH) are nonmedical factors that influence the health of individuals, families, and communities (CDC, 2022b). SDOH are the conditions in which people are born, grow, play, work, live, and age that shape day-to-day life and overall lifestyles. Numerous factors impact SDOH, including economic policies, social norms, social policies, racism, climate change, and political systems (CDC, 2022b). The CDC has made SDOH one of the top three priority items for HealthyPeople 2032 (CDC, 2022b).

SDOH are good predictors of the risk of developing a mood disorder over a lifetime. Those living in low-income areas with high crime rates and less positive influences in their lives typically have reduced access to care and more difficulty obtaining the skills to cope with trauma healthily (D'cruz & Chaturvedi, 2021; Shim et al., 2022). A 2022 review found that belonging to a cultural minority alone does not necessarily increase one's vulnerability to mood disorders and may even contribute to resilience (D'cruz & Chaturvedi, 2021).

ADVERSE CHILDHOOD EXPERIENCES

ACEs are traumatic events that a child experiences before the age of 18 years. ACEs include various stressful experiences in the home environment, such as parental substance abuse; sexual, emotional, and physical abuse; domestic violence; and incarceration of a parent. The original CDC-Kaiser ACE study found a graded relationship between the number of ACEs experienced by a parent and the prevalence of adverse health and social outcomes (About the CDC-Kaiser Ace Study | Violence prevention | injury Center | CDC 2021); HHS, n.d.). This graded relationship showed the adverse effects on the adults who experienced ACEs as a child. The adults reported substance use disorders, smoking, high-risk sexual activity, obesity, cardiovascular disorders, and depression (Fairbanks, 2019).

Thus parents who have experienced ACEs as a child and have symptoms or a clinical diagnosis of depression are transferring these emotional responses to their day-to-day interactions with their children, increasing the likelihood that they may also suffer from clinical depression (CDC, 2022b).

ACEs increase the vulnerability of youth to mood disorders and the tendency toward more severe episodes, poor response to treatment, and greater impairment of functioning. Recent studies have shown that children in the child welfare system have experienced at least one ACE event compared to the general population, these children have experienced at least four ACEs (HHS, n.d.).

DEPRESSIVE DISORDERS

Infants, toddlers, children, and adolescents experience many feelings throughout childhood. They experience joy, pleasure, happiness, fears, worries, and sadness and may experience more extreme feelings of hopelessness and depression (CDC, 2022a). Infants, toddlers, and preschoolers may display a variety of feelings directly related to interactions with parents who have been diagnosed with maternal or paternal depression or parents who display symptoms of depression but have not been diagnosed with depression. School-age children, adolescents, and young adults may display feelings of depression from encounters with parents, peers, teachers, or social gatherings related to stress or may have depression symptoms from individual perceptions of themselves or the pathophysiologic processes of depression. When the child's or adolescent's emotional state is primarily fear, worries, overwhelming sadness, or hopelessness, the feelings are out of the individual's control, and the individual may be diagnosed with the mood disorder called depression. Data has revealed that despite high rates of mental health conditions, there remain low rates of treatment in those living in poverty: 11.4% annually for White, 9.8% for Black, and 8.7% for Hispanic children (Bitsko et al., 2022).

The discussion in this section on depression focuses on one of the major classifications of mood disorders called unipolar or MDD, which may also be referred to as major depression or clinical depression (Takahashi, 2019). Unipolar depression appears in all pediatric age groups, including young children. Major depression, or clinical depression, is one of the most common mental health disorders in the United States (HHS, 2022). Major depression is defined as "a period of at least two weeks when a person experienced a depressed mood or loss of interest or pleasure in daily activities and had a majority of specified symptoms, such as problems with sleep, eating, energy, concentration, or self-worth" (APA, 2013; HHS, 2022, p. 1). In addition, for some children and adolescents with major depression, the symptoms prohibit them from carrying out routine day-to-day activities, as they may not be able to get out of bed, attend school, or work. In 2020, data from the National Survey on Drug Use and Health showed that 12% of adolescents age 12 to 17 in the United States had at least one major depressive episode with severe impairment in the past year. This statistic represents 2.9 million adolescents between 12 and 17 years of age (HHS, 2022). Psychiatric (or mental health) treatment for these adolescents ranged from 41.6% with a major depressive episode to 46.9% for those with a major depressive episode accompanied by severe impairment (HHS, 2022). These statistics are alarming, as over 50% of adolescents in this age range are not being treated according to clinical practice guidelines (American Psychological Association, 2021), thus having a greater potential to harm themselves (in particular, suicide ideation, suicide attempts, suicide plans, or suicide). To change the trajectory of major depression and the potential for personal harm, primary care nurse practitioners must consistently use evidence-based depression screening tools in clinical practice to assess and begin the diagnostic processes for treatment and management, including referral to treatment by psychiatric mental health specialists, (i.e., psychiatric mental health nurse practitioners, psychiatrists, psychologists, or pediatric primary care mental health specialists) (Hallas et al., 2022).

ETIOLOGY AND PATHOPHYSIOLOGY OF DEPRESSION

Genetics plays an important role in the etiology and pathophysiology of depression. For a unipolar disorder, studies have shown that monozygotic twins have a 62% and dizygotic twins have a 28% rate of genetic expression of the disorder. Adopted children with a biological family history of a mood disorder have a higher incidence of developing major depression when compared to adopted children with a negative family history (Takahashi, 2019).

There are several hypotheses for the explanation of the pathophysiology and symptoms of MDD. The monoamine hypothesis of depression supports a deficit in the brain concentrations of norepinephrine, dopamine, and/or serotonin as the underlying cause of the presenting symptoms. Drugs that increase the monoamine neurotransmitter levels within the brain synapses result in antidepressant effects (Takahashi, 2019). Another hypothesis is the dysregulation of the hypothalamic-pituitary-adrenal (HPA) system. Stress activates this system, increasing HPA hormone secretion. Another interesting hypothesis for major depression is the relationship between inflammation and triggering the onset of depression. A study of 73,131 Danish individuals revealed that elevated C-reactive protein (CRP) levels were associated with an increased risk of depression (Wium-Andersen et al., 2013).

INFANT-CHILD-ADOLESCENT DEVELOPMENT

MATERNAL DEPRESSION AND PATHOPHYSIOLOGY IN INFANT BRAIN DEVELOPMENT

A detailed family history for a newborn/infant may reveal a diagnosis of depression in the mother, another primary caregiver, or a first-degree relative who displays symptoms characteristic of depression. These individuals may or may not have a clinical diagnosis of depression but come to practice with their infant with symptoms suggestive of maternal depression. The role of the APRN in clinical practice is to ask the mother to respond to the Edinburgh Postnatal Depression Scale (EPDS). If the mother scores positive, the APRN should refer her to her obstetrician or primary care provider for further evaluation and mental health support (Negeri et al., 2020). For adolescents in the APRN's practice who are mothers of newborns, the EPDS should be administered and interpreted by the APRN, and referral to mental health treatment, if indicated, can be made directly by the APRN.

MATERNAL ANTENATAL DEPRESSION: EFFECTS ON INFANT BRAIN DEVELOPMENT

Researchers have identified a link between maternal depression during pregnancy and a risk for abnormal neurodevelopmental outcomes in the newborn/infant (Sethna et al., 2021). While the mechanisms for this relationship are unknown, researchers identified a possible relationship between clinically diagnosed maternal antenatal depression and an adverse impact on fetal and infant brain development (Schadt, 2019). Researchers compared a data set of magnetic resonance images of 3- to 6-month-old infants ($N = 31$) to a sample of infants born to women without a current or past psychiatric diagnosis ($N = 33$). Study findings revealed that infants born to mothers with clinically diagnosed antenatal depression and compared with infants born to mothers without a history or clinical diagnosis of antenatal depression had larger subcortical gray matter volumes and smaller midbrain volumes (Sethna et al., 2021). Researchers concluded that maternal antenatal depression is associated with differences in infant brain anatomy in early postnatal life compared to infants not exposed in utero to maternal depression (Sethna et al., 2021). Future long-term prospective studies need to be conducted to assess for any significant long-term effects of these antenatal brain anatomic changes as the infant grows and develops and any long-term effects, such as a clinical depression diagnosed in childhood and/or young adulthood (Sethna et al., 2021). However, even without further studies or more data, these anatomic changes in the newborn who antepartum were exposed to maternal depression strengthen the support for performing depression screenings during pregnancy and at the 1-, 2-, 4-, and 6-month-old infant well visits to identify and refer to treatment all mothers of newborns/infants who present with a possible diagnosis of clinical depression (Earls, 2019).

PATERNAL DEPRESSION

In mothers, antenatal and postnatal internalizing symptoms predict infant negative affectivity (NA) (Spry et al., 2020). In addition, studies have shown that fathers' postnatal internalizing symptoms also predict infant NA. Thus these findings suggest greater complexity involving the transmission of feelings from the father to the infant than just the biologic in utero effects alone or direct contact with the mother postnatally (Spry et al., 2020). NA involves numerous emotions that are harmful to an infant, including sadness and anger (Hallas, 2019b). Other emotions identified by researchers include fear, frustration, and slow recovery from distress and sadness (Spry et al., 2020). The APRN should screen and discuss concerns with fathers when present who have evidence of clinical depression and refer them for diagnosis and treatment as soon as the symptoms are identified in pediatric clinical practice.

INFANT DEPRESSION

Infant depression is not a diagnosis in the DSM-5TR. However, in addition to infants who may or may not have been exposed to maternal antenatal depression, research studies have shown that infants who are exposed to stress after birth (e.g., maternal depression, limited or no bonding opportunities) on a regular basis have an increased risk of experiencing lasting effects on the developing brain, including a greater risk of depression and anxiety in later childhood and adulthood (Hallas, 2019a; Murgatroyd et al., 2010).

Developmental assessment throughout infancy is a critical component of every well-infant visit to determine the attainment of physical, psychological, and psychosocial milestones. Infants as young as 2 months bond with the mother, father, siblings, and other immediate family members who are regularly present in the infant's daily routines. Infants who are 8 months old are capable of seven different emotions (Izard et al., 1980; Walle et al., 2020). These emotions include joy, contentment, anger, disgust, surprise, interest, and sadness. Of these seven emotions, anger, disgust, and sadness are negative emotions imprinting into the developing brain and may result in lifelong adverse effects, including developing behavioral and mental health disorders (Blair & Raver, 2016; Lipina & Columno, 2009). Granat et al., (2017) studied infant emotions of anger with the mother, anger with a stranger, joy with the mother, and joy with a stranger. Study results revealed that infants of depressed mothers looked less at their mothers than infants whose mothers did not have a diagnosis of depression. The authors identified these findings as evidence of social withdrawal in the infant who was consistently in contact with a mother diagnosed with depression. Mothers with evidence of or a diagnosis of depression should be referred for treatment to help the mother and reduce the impact on the

developing brain of negative imprinting (Feldman, 2016; Granat et al., 2017).

In summary, infants living with mothers diagnosed with antenatal and postpartum depression are at increased risk of adverse emotional outcomes. Infants deprived of a healthy mother–infant bonding experience, daily positive maternal–infant interactions, or poor social-emotional development are more apt to have a sad effect, make little to no eye contact, have excessive crying behaviors, experience altered sleep patterns, and have poor eating patterns. These infants are at high risk for the adverse effects of poor growth and development, continued poor social interactions, and depression (Hallas, 2019b).

Interventions for Infant Depression

The goal of treatment for infant depression is to provide support to the mother, father, and family as needed so that the infant can grow and meet developmental milestones. Parents are encouraged to play with their infants; it is helpful to demonstrate brief office-based interventions in which age-appropriate infant play activities that elicit positive infant responses are demonstrated for the parents, with returned parental demonstration. Asking the mother to video-record parent–infant interactions while at home is a useful strategy to further guide maternal–infant and paternal–infant bonding at home and for the clinician to make additional recommendations for the care of the infant (Hallas, 2019b).

In addition, office or telehealth visits provide numerous opportunities to demonstrate to the mother, father, significant other, or other primary caregivers ways to interact with the infant, including age-appropriate ways to engage the infant to interact with the APRN and family member. For example, the APRN may demonstrate object permanence with a 9-month-old by hiding a toy under a blanket and watching how the infant tries to find the object. Then the APRN would demonstrate emotional reactions by clapping and praising the infant and picking up the infant while talking in an excited voice.

DEPRESSION IN TODDLERS AND PRESCHOOL-AGE CHILDREN

Children as young as 3 years may display several clinical features of early childhood depression. Parental surveys analyzed by the CDC revealed that depression in children between the ages of 3 and 17 is approximately 4.4%, representing 2.7 million children/adolescents (Bitsko et al., 2022). The most common symptom parents identify as the reason for seeking medical and/or behavioral/mental health care for a child under age 6 years is intense irritability (Luby, 2009). Young children who present with intense irritability and symptoms or evidence of social withdrawal, anhedonia, and/or extremes of guilty feelings must have a diagnosis of clinical depression high on the list of differential diagnoses (Luby, 2009). Other symptoms a parent may not consider important to report include play activities, decreased social interest during preschool activities or play dates, changes in sleep patterns, and/or new onset of rigid rituals (Luby, 2009). In preschool children, childhood depression may also be obfuscated by somatic complaints (e.g., abdominal pain or fullness shortly after beginning a meal; "head hurts"), aggression, or disruptive behaviors at home, in preschool, and/or during play activities. Thus a detailed history and physical examination are essential to formulating a comprehensive differential diagnosis to avoid diagnostic errors with preschoolers. This includes screenings, assessment, and appropriate testing to establish whether somatic complaints are founded or are masking the actual diagnosis of clinical depression and whether the child has cooccurring medical or behavioral health diagnoses.

Evidence-Based Treatments for Toddler and Preschool Children

Parent and Child Interaction Therapy–Emotion Development (PCIT-ED) is an evidence-based dyadic psychotherapeutic approach to treatment. When it was first introduced, researchers were able to establish efficacy for the treatment of disruptive behaviors in preschoolers (Zisser & Eyberg, 2010). Beginning in 2009, the PCIT-ED was tested as the first- and second-line treatment for depression in preschoolers with the addition of an emotion development module using emotion education strategies (Luby, 2009; Zisser & Eyberg, 2010). The dyadic psychotherapeutic approach assesses and treats the parent and child together as a team (dyad), which was designed to reflect the developmental level of preschoolers who are socially and emotionally dependent upon the parent or caregiver in their day-to-day encounters and interactions within the home/family unit, preschool environments, and play activities. The PCIT-ED is a 14-session evidence-based psychotherapeutic treatment. The primary caregiver is the critical link between the implementation of the treatment and the child, with the educated parent serving as the therapist's extension (Luby, 2009).

Luby et al., (2020) conducted a randomized controlled trial (RCT) using the PCIT and a novel emotion with unrecognized, untreated diagnosis of depression or unsuccessfully treated depression during the preschool years. Gudmundsen et al., (2019) studied the emergence of symptoms of anxiety and depression in school-age children. The researchers conducted a retrospective study asking 468 caregivers of seventh graders to identify symptoms of depression and anxiety in their children from kindergarten through sixth grade. Data analysis revealed that the caregivers identified 14 symptoms of depression and anxiety in this study sample of school-age children. Excessive guilt was identified in 20% of the children, while 50% experienced concentration problems during elementary school (Gudmundsen et al., 2019). Symptoms similar to

preschoolers included excessive guilt, anhedonia, and social withdrawal. Thus early recognition of symptoms and the formulation of differential diagnoses with an evidence-based treatment plan must be part of the treatment plan to reduce the onset of symptoms in the school-age years. Other symptoms school-age children presented with included sadness or depressed mood, low energy, and excessive worry. Early recognition of the symptoms during an annual or episodic history that is more prevalent in school-age populations is critical to the mental health of the child and adolescent. Establishing a diagnosis with an evidence-based treatment plan started earlier is more likely to prevent the onset of MDD in the adolescent population. In this study, researchers reported that older children (adolescents) who met the criteria for MDD had a significantly higher likelihood of displaying symptoms of depression or anxiety disorders in their elementary school years (Gudmundsen et al., 2019).

Emotion Development modules were designed to determine the efficacy for the treatment of early childhood depression. The ED module was designed with a child-directed and a parent-directed intervention. The RCT results revealed that the ED module demonstrated added efficacy for treating early childhood depression (Luby et al., 2020). Changes in the child's neural response to rewards and the parental response to the child's emotional expressions were directly correlated to the teaching-learning components of the ED module. Study findings demonstrated positive changes in the status of depression in preschool-age study participants (Zisser & Eyberg, 2010).

Playing with children is an important part of the day-to-day life of a parent and child. Toddlers and preschoolers who are emotionally stressed for any number of reasons (e.g., parental divorce, exposure to caregivers who are depressed) may benefit from referral to a therapist who performs play therapy.

DEPRESSION IN SCHOOL-AGE CHILDREN, ADOLESCENTS, AND YOUNG ADULTS

As children progress through the school-age and adolescent years, symptoms of anxiety and depression may emerge as new onset or may be a carryover from earlier years of development (CDC, 2022a). From a national sample of 1570 parents and guardians of children between the ages of 5 and 12 years, moderate-severe levels of depression were reported in 14.1% of the adult sample. Of importance to APRNs in clinical practice is that data showed adults with depression were higher for females, younger parents and guardians, and parents and guardians reporting lower household incomes (Sequeira et al., 2021). APRNs who include an annual review of parental and family history may be able to identify children at higher risk for depression if the parent reports depression symptoms or treatment for depression. The children of these parents should be screened using the Pediatric Symptom Checklist or the Patient Health Questionnaire

Patient health questionnaire-9 (PHQ-9)				
Over the <u>last 2 weeks</u>, how often have you been bothered by any of the following problems? *(Use "✓" to indicate your answer)*	Not at all	Several days	More than half the days	Nearly every day
1. Little interest or pleasure in doing things	0	1	2	3
2. Feeling down, depressed, or hopeless	0	1	2	3
3. Trouble falling or staying asleep, or sleeping too much	0	1	2	3
4. Feeling tired or having little energy	0	1	2	3
5. Poor appetite or overeating	0	1	2	3
6. Feeling bad about yourself — or that you are a failure or have let yourself or your family down	0	1	2	3
7. Trouble concentrating on things, such as reading the newspaper or watching television	0	1	2	3
8. Moving or speaking so slowly that other people could have noticed? Or the opposite — being so fidgety or restless that you have been moving around a lot more than usual	0	1	2	3
9. Thoughts that you would be better off dead or of hurting yourself in some way	0	1	2	3

For office coding ___0___ + _____ + _____ + _____

= Total score: _____

If you checked off <u>any</u> problems, how <u>difficult</u> have these problems made it for you to do your work, take care of things at home, or get along with other people?

Not difficult at all	Somewhat difficult	Very difficult	Extremely difficult
☐	☐	☐	☐

Fig. 30.1 **Patient Health Questionnaire-9.** (Courtesy Robert L. Spitzer, Janet B.W. Williams, Kurt Kroenke, and colleagues, with an educational grant from Pfizer Inc.)

9 (PHQ-9) (Fig. 30.1) based on the age of the child/young adolescent to identify the children as early as possible and refer them for treatment.

Additional considerations for the health and well-being of school-age children with a diagnosis of mental, emotional, developmental, or behavioral disorder are the data report these children are victims of bullying behaviors. Iyanda (2022) reported that children with depression had a 10.8% chance of being bullied (adjusted odds ratio: 2.688; 95% confidence interval: 2.031–3.557). Iyanda (2022) concluded that effective bullying prevention strategies could improve the quality of life for children with

depression. APRNs must identify children at risk of bullying by asking direct historical questions about bullying behaviors. Once identified, the APRN can assist in developing a treatment plan for the child.

Adolescent depression is a major concern, along with ideas of suicide ideation. Ho et al., (2022) reported on a study of multilevel predictors of depression symptoms in relation to adolescent brain cognitive development (ABDC study), with 7995 participants. The authors reported three factors that were predictors of adolescent depression: parental history of depression, greater family conflict, and shorter sleep duration.

Table 30.1   FDA Approvals for Antidepressant Medications Used in Children

		ANTIDEPRESSANTS
MEDICATION CLASS	MEDICATION NAME	FDA INDICATIONS
SSRI	Fluoxetine	**MDD**: >8 yr: 10–20 mg PO every day, initially; start at 10 mg/day in lower weight children, may gradually increase dose after 1 wk; not to exceed 20 mg/day
SSRI	Escitalopram	**MDD**: ≥12 yr: 10 mg PO every day; may increase dose after at least 3 wk; not to exceed 20 mg/day
TCA	Amitriptyline	**Depression**: adolescents; initial: 25–50 mg/day PO in divided doses; increase gradually to 100 mg/day in divided doses

FDA, US Food and Drug Administration; *MDD*, major depressive disorder; *PO*, oral (per os); *SSRI*, selective serotonin reuptake inhibitor; *TCA*, tricyclic antidepressant.
From Medscape. (n.d.). Psychiatrics. http://reference.medscape.com/drugs/psychiatrics.

Hawes et al., (2022) studied the effects of the COVID-19 pandemic on adolescents. They reported increased depression related to school and home confinement because of the pandemic, and these factors were independently related to changes in symptoms. For APRNs working with adolescents, as they enter young adulthood, considerable thought and treatment planning must be part of each health care visit to assess the risk of adverse mental health effects related to the sudden abrupt stoppage of normal growth and developmental patterns during adolescence.

Suicidal ideation and attempted suicide are major concerns for adolescents with a diagnosis of depression. Athey et al., (2022) reported on a study of 158 depressed adolescents who experienced exposure to friends' and family members' suicidal behaviors. Of importance to APRNs in the care of depressed adolescents were the findings that showed adolescents exposed to suicidal behaviors reported experiencing physical and sexual abuse and suicide attempts (Athey et al., 2022). For every annual and episodic health care visit, the APRN must assess the adolescent for depression, care management plan, medication management, and suicidal ideation with or without a plan (Table 30.1). These are sensitive conversations to have with the adolescent privately; however, the conversation is essential to the health and well-being of the adolescent and is a key factor in suicide prevention.

Tools for Assessment of Depression
The US Preventive Services Task Force has concluded with moderate certainty that screening for MDD in adolescents age 12 to 18 years has a moderate net benefit. Evidence was insufficient for screening for MDD in children younger than 11 years. Additionally, there was insufficient evidence about the benefits and harms of screening for suicide risk in children and adolescents (Mangione et al., 2022).

DISRUPTIVE MOOD DYSREGULATION DISORDER (ICD-10 F34.81)

DMDD is a childhood-onset depressive disorder characterized by persistent irritable or angry mood

interspersed with frequent, excessively severe temper outbursts (Findling et al., 2021). Irritability refers to a heightened proneness to anger relative to that of peers (Mürner-Lavanchy et al., 2021). In 2013, the APA added DMDD as a specific disease entity, addressing the concern that children with persistent irritability were being inappropriately diagnosed with bipolar disorder (BPD) and prescribed antipsychotic medications (APA, 2013). The pervasive irritability of DMDD occurs in different settings (at home, at school, and with peers) for most of the day, almost every day. DMDD is diagnosed in children older than 6 years of age, and onset must be observed by the age of 10 years, with a minimum symptom duration of 1 year (APA, 2022).

DMDD is associated with impairment in relationships, activities, and self-regulation. Youth with DMDD are more likely to have learning difficulties, impairment in activities of daily living, self-injurious behavior, and suicidal ideation when compared to youth with at least one psychiatric diagnosis other than DMDD (Bruno et al., 2019).

INCIDENCE AND PREVALENCE
DMDD is now diagnosed in a substantial number of youth who, prior to 2013, may have instead received a diagnosis of BPD. The prevalence of DMDD ranges from 0.8% to 3.3%, and rates of diagnosis are rising. Current estimates indicate the prevalence of 2% to 3% in preschool children, 1% to 3% in 9- to 12-year-olds, and 0% to 0.12% in adolescents, showing that DMDD seems to decrease with age (Bruno et al., 2019; Findling et al., 2021; Mürner-Lavanchy et al., 2021).

In general, risk factors for disruptive behaviors include early life trauma (e.g., physical, emotional, or sexual abuse), recent family stressors, family history (e.g., maternal and postpartum depression, psychiatric diagnoses, substance abuse), and malnutrition or vitamin deficiencies (Bruno et al., 2019).

DMDD has high rates of comorbidity with other pediatric psychiatric disorders. Its main clinical manifestations overlap with attention-deficit/hyperactivity disorder (ADHD), oppositional defiant disorder, and conduct disorder, but other related disorders include intermittent explosive disorder, obsessive-compulsive disorder, posttraumatic stress disorder, and substance use disorder (Bruno et al., 2019; Disruptive Mood Dysregulation Disorder, 2022).

TOOLS FOR ASSESSMENT OF DMDD

In a systematic review (Mürner-Lavanchy et al., 2021), the most frequently used rating scale to assess DMDD was the Kiddie Schedule for Affective Disorders and Schizophrenia Present and Lifetime Version (K-SADS-PL) supplement for depressive and bipolar-related disorders (Kaufman et al., 2016). The K-SADS-PL is a semistructured interview to diagnose mental disorders in children age 6 to 18 years. The supplement for depressive and bipolar-related disorders is a DMDD module focusing on irritability and recurrent temper outbursts. Additional assessment tools with irritability measures include the Affective Reactivity Index, used in ages 7 to 18 years, and the Aberrant Behavior Checklist, used in ages 5 to adult.

BRIEF OVERVIEW OF THE TREATMENT OF DMDD

Evidence-based treatment for all disruptive behavior disorders (including oppositional defiant disorder and conduct disorder) emphasizes the role of psychosocial interventions (Sukhodolsky et al., 2016). Behavioral therapy and parent training interventions are considered a cornerstone in DMDD treatment (Bruno et al., 2019). Treatment modalities include PCIT or family-based therapy. Parents receive coaching to make clear and direct requests of their child, explain commands, provide immediate positive feedback, and use time-outs effectively. This includes ignoring questions or bad behavior that occurs during a time-out.

CURRENT EVIDENCE FOR PSYCHOPHARMACOLOGIC TREATMENT OF DMDD

There is a paucity of research on effective medication therapy for this mood disorder. Since its introduction as a diagnosis in 2013, DMDD has been associated with increased antipsychotic and polypharmacy prescriptions as well as higher rates of comorbidity and inpatient hospitalization compared to youth with a BPD diagnosis (Findling et al., 2021). Antipsychotic medications (specifically, second-generation antipsychotics [SGAs]) are the only class of medications with a US Food and Drug Administration (FDA)–approved indication for the core symptom of DMDD: irritability. There is concern that the DMDD diagnosis has led to treating providers' overuse of these medications (Havens et al., 2022; Hendrickson et al., 2019).

Current treatment for DMDD trends toward the use of psychostimulants and antidepressants. Bruno et al., (2019) note that antidepressants, mainly selective serotonin reuptake inhibitors (SSRIs) and serotonin norepinephrine reuptake inhibitor (SNRIs), may be used for treating chronic and persistent irritability and anger in children and adolescents. Psychostimulants and alpha-agonists (guanfacine and clonidine) are used in ADHD because of their positive effect on aggressive behaviors and impulsivity. There are currently no medications that are FDA approved specifically for use in DMDD.

BIPOLAR AND RELATED DISORDERS

In the DSM-5-TR, bipolar and related disorders include bipolar I disorder (BPD-I), bipolar II disorder (BPD-II), cyclothymic disorder, substance/medication-induced bipolar and related disorder, a bipolar and related disorder due to another medical condition, other specified bipolar and related disorder, and unspecified bipolar and related disorder (APA, 2022).

As a whole, BPDs are characterized by manic, hypomanic, depressive, or mixed-mood episodes. They are chronic disorders despite being episodic, with exacerbations of symptoms followed by periods of remission. Many children experience a depressed mood as a primary feature of the disorder. Children and adolescents with BPD are at much higher risk for adverse outcomes, including psychiatric hospitalizations, substance use disorders, and suicidality (Yule et al., 2019).

The subtypes of BPD are characterized by manic, hypomanic, depressed, and unspecified episodes. Symptoms for current or most recent manic or depressed episodes can be mild, moderate, or severe. Patients may also present with psychotic features. Children often present with deficits in cognitive control, memory, and attention. Changes in activity/energy (e.g., fatigue, hyperactivity) and depressed mood are the most prominent mood symptoms among adolescents with bipolar spectrum disorders (Weintraub et al., 2020). A meta-analysis by Van Meter et al., (2016) examined the clinical characteristics of pediatric BPD. The frequency rates of manic symptoms were as follows: increased energy (79%), irritability (77%), mood lability (76%), distractibility (74%), goal-directed activity (72%), euphoria/elated mood (64%), pressured speech (63%), hyperactivity (62%), racing thoughts (61%), poor judgment (61%), grandiosity (57%), inappropriate laughter (57%), decreased need for sleep (56%), and flight of ideas (54%). There is an overlap with symptoms of other psychiatric disorders, especially ADHD. BPD is differentiated through the presence of specific symptoms (e.g., elation, episodic high energy, hypersexualized behaviors, and a need for less sleep) and the clinical course (Table 30.2).

Incidence and Prevalence

The worldwide prevalence of pediatric BPD-I is estimated at 1 in 200, but the rate of subthreshold symptoms of BPD, at 4.3%, is much higher (Findling et al., 2018). Rates in the United States are estimated at 1.8%. Although the National Survey for Children's Health examines the prevalence of depression, anxiety, and

Table 30.2   Clinical Presentation for Bipolar Disorder and Attention-Deficit/Hyperactivity Disorder (ADHD)

CLINICAL PRESENTATION	BIPOLAR DISORDER: MANIA	ADHD
Decreased need for sleep	Yes	No
Destruction of property	Deliberate	Due to inattention
Disrupted sleep/late insomnia	Yes	No
Early insomnia	Reduced need for sleep	Bedtime resistance
Euphoria/elation	Yes	No
Forgetfulness	No	Yes
Hyperactivity	Fluctuations in activity levels day/night	All day worsens when on-task behavior or prolonged attention required
Hypersexuality	Yes	No
Impulsivity	Yes	Yes
Inattention	Yes	Yes
Incompletion of tasks	No	Yes
Irritability	Infrequent; more noted with withdrawal from stimulants	Very frequent, especially with morning arousal
Mood shifts	Frequent rapid mood shifts	Not frequent; may worsen with stimulant withdrawal
Physical aggression	Deliberate	Rare
Pressured speech	Difficult to stop and focus	Can be redirected and focused
Psychotic symptoms	Yes	No
Racing/crowded thoughts	Yes	No
Self-esteem	Generally inflated	Usually worsens over time
Sleep difficulty	Difficulty falling asleep; awakening during night	No
Suicidal thoughts/ideation	Yes	No
Verbal aggression	Deliberate	Due to frustration

From Marangoni, C. (2018). ADHD, bipolar disorder, or borderline personality disorder: Getting to the right diagnosis. *Psychiatric Times, 35*(10), 18.

other more common pediatric mental health diagnoses, it does not measure the prevalence of BPD in children. A 2019 meta-analysis of epidemiologic studies of pediatric BPDs indicates that rates of diagnosis for these diagnoses are not increasing over time and are not higher in the United States than in other Western countries (Van Meter et al., 2019).

Etiology and Pathophysiology of BPD
The pathophysiology of BPD is multifactorial and seen as a complex interaction between genetics and environment. Disrupted energy metabolism and mitochondrial dysfunction have been proposed as factors associated with the development of BPD (Selvaraj et al., 2020). There appears to be a significant component of immune dysregulation and inflammation, as noted earlier with depression. During active phases of BPD (marked by mania or depression), there are increased levels or activity of proinflammatory cytokines, including CRP, interferon-gamma, interleukin-6, and tumor necrosis factor-alpha. These cytokines then partially or completely normalize during periods of euthymia (Magioncalda & Martino, 2021).

Neuroimaging changes are noted in BPD, including abnormalities in the prefrontal cortex, decreases in amygdala volume, and increased rates of deep white matter hyperintensities. There are indications that these changes have a key role in emotional dysregulation (Selvaraj et al., 2020; Elhosary & Birmaher, 2022).

Genetic Factors
There is a strong genetic predisposition to BPD, with some twin studies showing heritability around 90% (APA, 2022). One tool for assessing BPD's genetic impact is using a polygenic risk score (PRS). PRS is the weighted average of single nucleotide polymorphisms, which are single base pair variations in a DNA sequence. In genetic studies assessing PRS within families where BPD is present within families, there was a 59% increase in the risk of the offspring developing BPD (Birmaher et al., 2022). Additionally, a familial relationship is noted between subtypes of lithium-responsive patients compared with those who are lithium unresponsive. Males have a higher predisposition for developing BPD.

Tools for Assessment of BPD
There are multiple assessment tools for symptoms of depression, aggression, risk-taking behaviors, attention deficit, social problems, and hyperactivity behaviors in children, including the Child Behavior Checklist (CBCL). There is a high correlation between specific CBCL findings and BPD-I symptoms (Yule et al., 2019).

This profile (termed the *CBCL-BP profile*) consists of elevations in attention, anxiety/depression, and aggression subscales (>2 SD above the norm) combined with a structured interview to formulate the BPD diagnosis. Findings suggest that this CBCL-BP profile may be an efficient tool to help identify children who are very likely to suffer from BPD-I (Yule et al., 2019).

Other standardized assessment tools used to assess for BPD-I–specific symptoms include the Young Mania Rating Scale, the Child Mania Rating Scale, and the Children's Depression Rating Scale, Revised. These are not administered in the primary care setting, but it can help to be familiar with how the diagnosis is made when these patients are seen in practice.

BIPOLAR I DISORDER

To meet the criteria for diagnosis of BPD-I it is necessary to have had a manic episode, either preceded by or possibly followed by a hypomanic or major depressive episode (APA, 2022). It is characterized by one or more manic episodes with or without depression.

BIPOLAR II DISORDER

BPD-II is characterized by one or more major depressive episodes and one or more hypomanic episodes. The average age of onset of BPD-II is the mid-20s, although youth may present with this diagnosis in later adolescence. Patients diagnosed with BPD-II have experienced a manic episode. Additionally, the hypomanic and major depressive episodes cannot be better explained by schizoaffective disorder and cannot be superimposed on schizophreniform disorder, schizophrenia, delusional disorder, or other specified or unspecified schizophrenia spectrum and other psychotic disorders (APA, 2022). Patients with BPD-II typically present to their provider during an episode of major depression. The hypomanic episodes do not cause impairment in this patient group, and they may not recognize the symptoms (or may find them desirable). According to the APA, (2022), many individuals have experienced several episodes of major depression prior to recognizing a hypomanic episode. There may be a 10-year lag time between illness onset and BPD-II diagnosis.

CYCLOTHYMIC DISORDER

Cyclothymic disorders typically emerge during adolescence or early adulthood and are characterized by chronic, fluctuating mood disturbance. Most young persons who are diagnosed with cyclothymic disorder display mood disorder symptoms prior to age 10 years. To meet the criteria for a diagnosis of cyclothymic disorder, children must experience at least 12 months of combined hypomanic and depressive periods but never fulfill the criteria for an episode of hypomania, mania, or major depression. During this 12-month period, symptoms must have been present for at least half the time without a remission period lasting 2 months or longer. This diagnosis is made only if the criteria for major depressive, manic, or hypomanic episodes have never been met. As with other disorders in the DSM-5-TR, symptoms cannot be better explained by another disorder or attributable to the physiologic effects of a substance (e.g., prescribed medication, illicit substance) or another medical condition.

Individuals with cyclothymic disorder may subsequently develop BPD-I or BPD-II. The conversion rate is between 15% and 50%. Care must be taken to differentiate this diagnosis from BPD, depressive disorder, and borderline personality disorder.

BRIEF OVERVIEW OF THE TREATMENT OF BPD IN CHILDREN AND ADOLESCENTS

BPD is a complex disorder typically managed in collaboration with a psychiatrist or psychiatric mental health nurse practitioner. The initial assessment includes the determination of the severity of the presenting episode, characteristics of prior episodes, and the patient's current safety level. Severe episodes can be complicated by depression (leading to suicidal ideation and/or suicide attempts), manic episodes (resulting in high-risk behaviors), and psychosis. Inpatient hospitalization may be required. The recommendation for the treatment of childhood/adolescent BPD is a combination of psychoeducation, psychopharmacologic management, and psychosocial interventions (Findling et al., 2018).

Current Evidence for Psychotherapy Treatment of Pediatric BPD

Psychotherapy is an essential component of treating BPD in children and adolescents. In RCTs comparing psychoeducation to family-focused therapy (FFT), patients receiving FFT showed improvements in family cohesion, longer periods between depressive episodes and without suicidal ideation, and better rates of recovery from baseline depressive symptoms (Hobbs et al., 2022) (Table 30.3).

Table 30.3 Psychotherapy for Bipolar Disorder in Children and Adolescents

FEATURES COMMON TO EFFECTIVE THERAPIES	BENEFITS OF PSYCHOTHERAPY
• Family focused • May include family-focused treatment and age-appropriate cognitive-behavioral therapy techniques	• Supports overall psychosocial development • Addresses comorbid symptoms • Improves treatment adherence • Reduces relapses • Improves overall functioning

From Findling, R.L., Stepanova, E., Youngstrom, E.A., & Young, A.S. (2018). Progress in diagnosis and treatment of bipolar disorder among children and adolescents: An international perspective. *Evidence-Based Mental Health, 21*(4), 177–181.

Current Evidence for Psychopharmacologic Treatment of Pediatric BPD

An expert review of the literature was conducted to determine areas of consensus regarding pharmacologic treatment for BPD in children (Goldstein et al., 2017). The key takeaways were: (1) SGAs are effective in mitigating symptoms; (2) youth tend to be highly sensitive to metabolic side effects of SGAs; (3) mood stabilizers are less efficacious than in adults; and (4) stimulants for comorbid ADHD, in conjunction with a mood stabilizer, are typically safe and effective.

There are currently five FDA-approved SGAs (aripiprazole, asenapine, olanzapine, quetiapine, risperidone) for the treatment of manic/mixed episodes (Tables 30.4 & 30.5). Two additional medications (lurasidone and olanzapine-fluoxetine combination) are approved for the treatment of major depressive episodes. Two antiepileptic drugs (AEDs), divalproex sodium and oxcarbazepine, have been studied in pediatric RCTs but have failed to separate from a placebo (Hobbs et al., 2022). Lamotrigine is another AED that has been trialed as an add-on medication for maintenance/relapse prevention and has shown efficacy in delaying the recurrence of depressed episodes in BPD (Findling et al., 2015). Lithium carbonate and aripiprazole are the only two medications with an FDA indication for the maintenance treatment of pediatric BPD.

Adverse effects and monitoring. For depression symptoms, the combination of olanzapine-fluoxetine is associated with weight gain, somnolence, hyperlipidemia, elevated hepatic enzymes, elevated prolactin, and QT prolongation (Hobbs et al., 2022). SGAs are associated with multiple adverse effects and require close monitoring. Sedation, anticholinergic effects (e.g., dry mouth, constipation), and mild tremors are relatively common side effects. More severe adverse effects include weight gain, elevated glucose, insulin resistance, elevated cholesterol and triglyceride levels, gynecomastia, galactorrhea, and irreversible involuntary movements (tardive dyskinesia).

There are consensus guidelines regarding regular monitoring for cardiometabolic risk factors associated with these medications (American Diabetes Association et al., 2004). Screening and monitoring measures include family and/or personal history of cardiovascular disease, diabetes, hypertension, and dyslipidemia; weight and height for body mass index (BMI) calculation; waist circumference; blood pressure; hemoglobin A1c (HbA1c) (previously measured as fasting plasma glucose [FPG]); and fasting lipid profile (American Diabetes Association et al., 2004). The frequency of assessment of each measure is as follows:

1. Family and/or personal history of risk factors to be assessed at baseline and annually
2. BMI assessed at baseline, then weeks 4, 8, 12, and then quarterly
3. Waist circumference to be assessed at baseline, then annually
4. Blood pressure assessed at baseline, at week 12, then annually
5. FPG at baseline, at week 12, then annually. (This guideline was updated in 2010 to measure HbA1c instead.)
6. Fasting lipid profile at baseline, week 12, then every 5 years if no significant abnormalities are present. If abnormalities are noted at baseline or at week 12, monitor annually.

The American Academy of Child and Adolescent Psychiatry (AACAP) recommended that patients on SGAs be assessed for movement disorders using a structured measure such as the Abnormal Involuntary Movement Scale or the Barnes Akathisia Rating Scale, at baseline and regular intervals (AACAP, 2011; Riddle, 2019). Coordination of monitoring between the psychiatric prescriber and the primary care provider is essential. Primary care APRNs have an important role in monitoring weight gain and metabolic effects, as they typically have ready access to phlebotomy and clinical labs, compared with psychiatric prescribers (Romba & Perez-Reisler, 2020).

Patients who are prescribed lithium carbonate require additional monitoring. Each exam should include history focused on adverse effects (baseline and at each follow-up visit); physical examination focused on adverse effects, central nervous system, thyroid (baseline and at each follow-up visit); vital

Table 30.4 FDA-Recommended Dosing for Mania in Bipolar Disorder Used in Children

MEDICATION	AGES (YR)	INITIAL DOSE (MG)	RECOMMENDED DOSE (MG)	MAXIMUM DOSE (MG)
Aripiprazole	10–17	2	10	30
Asenapine	10–17	2.5 SL every 12 hr initially; may increase to 5 mg SL every 12 hr after 3 days and to 10 mg SL every 12 hr after 3 additional days		20
Olanzapine	13–17	2.5–5	10	NA
Quetiapine	10–17	25 twice a day	400–800	600
Risperidone	10–17	0.5	1–2.5	6

FDA, US Food and Drug Administration; *NA,* not applicable; *SL,* sublingual.

| Table 30.5 | FDA Approvals for Antipsychotic Medications Used in Children | |

MEDICATION CLASS	MEDICATION NAME	FDA INDICATIONS
Antimanic agent, second-generation antipsychotic (SGA)	Aripiprazole	**Bipolar mania:** acute manic or mixed episodes, either as monotherapy or as an adjunct to lithium or valproate Age 10–17 yr: 2 mg/day PO initially; increased to 5 mg/day after 2 days; increased to recommended dosage of 10 mg/day after additional 2 days; may subsequently be increased by 5 mg/day; maintenance: 10–30 mg/day
SGA	Asenapine	**Bipolar disorder:** indicated as monotherapy for acute treatment of manic or mixed episodes associated with bipolar I disorder Age <10 yr: safety and efficacy not established; 10–17 yr: 2.5 SL every 12 hr initially; may increase to 5 mg SL every 12 hr after 3 days and to 10 mg SL every 12 hr after 3 additional days
SGA	Olanzapine	**Bipolar I disorder (manic or mixed episodes):** Age <13 yr: safety and efficacy not established; 13–17 yr: 2.5–5 mg/day PO initially; target dosage 10 mg/day; adjust by increments/decrements of 2.5–5 mg; dosage range, 2.5–20 mg/day **Schizophrenia:** Age <13 yr: safety and efficacy not established; 13–17 yr: 2.5–5 mg/day PO initially; target dosage 10 mg/day; adjust by increments/decrements of 2.5–5 mg; dosage range, 2.5–20 mg/day
SGA, antimanic agent	Quetiapine	**Bipolar I disorder, mania:** Age <10 yr: safety and efficacy not established; >10 yr (monotherapy, immediate release): day 1: 50 mg/day PO divided every 12 hr, day 2: 100 mg/day PO divided every 12 hr, day 3: 200 mg/day PO divided every 12 hr, day 4: 300 mg/day PO divided every 12 hr, day 5: 400 mg/day PO divided every 12 hr; further adjustments should be in increments ≤100 mg/day; dosage range: 400–600 mg/day, depending on response and tolerance, daily dose may be divided every 8 hr; age >10 years (monotherapy, extended release): day 1: 50 mg/day PO once daily, day 2: 100 mg/day PO once daily, day 3: 200 mg/day PO once daily, day 4: 300 mg/day PO once daily, day 5: 400 mg/day PO once daily; further adjustments should be in increments ≤100 mg/day; dosage range: 400–600 mg once daily
SGA, antimanic agent	Risperidone	**Bipolar mania:** Age <10 yr: safety and efficacy not established; >10 yr: 0.5 mg/day PO in morning or evening initially; may be increased in increments of 0.5–1 mg/day at intervals ≥24 hr to recommended dosage of 2.5 mg/day; dosage range: 0.5–6 mg/day (dosages >2.5 mg/day have not proven to be more effective and are associated with increased incidence of adverse effects); if persistent somnolence occurs, daily dose may be divided every 12 hr

FDA, US Food and Drug Administration; *PO*, oral (per os); *SL*, sublingual.
From Medscape. (n.d.). Psychiatrics. http://reference.medscape.com/drugs/psychiatrics.

signs (baseline, 3 months, 6 months, then annually): height, weight, blood pressure, and pulse (Table 30.6). The target lithium therapeutic level for bipolar disorder is typically in the 0.8 to 1.2 mEq/L range.

PRIMARY CARE MANAGEMENT

In general, depression, DMDD, and BPD are not associated with specific alterations in normal physical growth and development, although there can be individual variations. At all ages, routine screenings are completed per the AAP Periodicity Schedule (AAP, 2022). Routine immunizations should be given as recommended by the CDC.

DIET

Patients and parents may note changes in eating patterns with mood disorders. Symptoms can include increased or increased appetite and changes in food preferences. During hypomanic or manic episodes, children and adolescents may be too distracted to stop for a meal.

Diet and weight monitoring are essential in youth on psychotropic medications. SSRIs, tricyclic antidepressants, mood stabilizers, and antipsychotic medications frequently cause weight gain. Youth are considered more vulnerable to weight gain than adults when taking antipsychotic medication (Almandil et al., 2013). Nutritional counseling and psychoeducation are

Table **30.6**	Lithium Monitoring in Pediatric Populations	
LAB TEST	**FREQUENCY**	
Lithium level (12-hr serum trough level after ≥5 days on stable dose)	Baseline, during dose escalation, then every 3 mo	
Complete blood count	Baseline, then annually	
Thyroid-stimulating hormone	Baseline, 6 mo, 12 mo, then annually	
Electrolytes, blood urea nitrogen, creatinine	Baseline, 3 mo, 6 mo, 12 mo, then annually	
Human chorionic gonadotropin test	Baseline as indicated	
Electrocardiogram	Baseline, 3 mo, 12 mo, then annually	

From Riddle, M. (2019). *Pediatric psychopharmacology for primary care* (2nd ed.). American Academy of Pediatrics.

important components of care to ensure that youth are adherent due to worries about weight gain.

SLEEP

Mood disorders can cause sleep disturbances, including insomnia, hypersomnia, vivid dreams, and nightmares. The primary care provider must obtain a good sleep history and initiate psychoeducation regarding sleep hygiene. Ongoing monitoring is essential, as medication therapy can also impact sleep negatively. Some providers suggest a bedtime dose of melatonin to help facilitate sleep onset for those with sleep onset disturbance.

MEDICATION ADHERENCE AND SAFETY

Follow-up appointments should include monitoring for adherence to the prescribed medication regimen and assessment for side effects of psychotropic medications (even if the primary care provider is not the prescriber). Treatment adherence is essential in many youth experiencing mood disorders, and medication education should be reviewed at every visit. Educational goals include understanding the medication's purpose, desired effects, dosage, and timing; related tests and monitoring; potential adverse effects; risk for overdose; possible drug–drug and drug–food interactions; and anticipated time frame for treatment.

Remind patients and families to keep psychotropic medications secure and to use them as directed. Youth with depressive disorders, DMDD, and bipolar and related disorders are at risk for suicidal ideation and self-injurious behaviors. Further, the black box warnings for SSRIs and SNRIs include the possibility of suicidal behavior in children and adolescents. Assess for warning signs of suicidal ideation at each visit

using screening tools such as the HEADSS (Home, Education, Drugs, Sexuality, Safety), the SSHADESS (Strengths, School, Home, Activities, Drugs, Emotions, Sexuality, Safety), and/or the PHQ-9 (see Fig. 30.1). Patients and families should have the National Suicide Hotline number (988), local crisis intervention, and emergency primary care provider contact information available at all times.

SOCIAL DEVELOPMENT

Impairments in social development and interaction can contribute to mood disorders. Additionally, the symptoms related to these disorders can create or exacerbate social difficulty. The primary care nurse practitioner must ask about function at home, school, and social settings.

SCHOOL PERFORMANCE

Children and youth with mood disorders may experience significant changes in school performance. Psychoeducational or neuropsychological testing may be indicated. Schools may require verification of diagnosis to provide accommodations such as an individualized education plan (through the Individuals with Disabilities Education Act) or a 504 plan.

SUBSTANCE ABUSE

Youth with mood disorders may attempt to self-medicate by using alcohol and street drugs. Substance use can mask mood disorder symptoms and places youth at risk for overdose, accidents, impulsive sexual behavior, acts of aggression, and illegal activity. Although assessing substance use among children, adolescents, and young adults is always an important component of primary care, ongoing evaluation is essential whenever a youth has a mood disorder.

TRANSITION TO ADULTHOOD

Primary care providers are critical to transition planning in children and youth with chronic health conditions. There has been a lack of substantial evidence for the role of primary care in transition care for children with severe mental health disorders (Toulany et al., 2019). More recent research indicates that primary care involvement in transitional care may moderate or improve long-term health outcomes (including reduced mental health hospitalizations) for youth with mental illness (Toulany et al., 2019).

RESOURCES

NATIONAL FEDERATION OF FAMILIES FOR CHILDREN'S MENTAL HEALTH

9605 Medical Center Dr.
Rockville, MD 20850
(240) 403-1901; Fax: (240) 403-1909

Email: ffcmh@ffcmh.org
Website: www.ffcmh.org

National Institute of Mental Health Bipolar Disorder in Children and Teens
Website: https://www.nimh.nih.gov/health/
    publications/bipolar-disorder-in-children-and-teens

INTERNET RESOURCES

The Bipolar Child
Website: www.bipolarchild.com
Pendulum Resources
Website: www.pendulum.org

Organizations
Brain & Behavior Research Foundation
747 Third Avenue, 33rd Floor
New York, NY 10017
646-681-4888/800-829-8289
Website: https://bbrfoundation.org/

Juvenile Bipolar Research Foundation
17595 Harvard Ave. | Suite C-616 | Irvine, CA 96214
Website: www.jbrf.org/

Mental Health America
500 Montgomery Street,
Suite 820
Alexandria, VA. 22314
Phone (703) 684.7722
Toll Free (800) 969.6642
Website: www.nmha.org

National Alliance for the Mentally Ill (NAMI)
Colonial Place Three
2107 Wilson Blvd., Suite 300
Arlington, VA 22201-3042
(703) 524-7600; (800) 950-NAMI (6264); Fax (703) 524-9094
Website: www.nami.org

 Summary

Primary Care Needs for the Child or Adolescent With a Mood Disorder

HEALTH CARE MAINTENANCE
Growth and Development
- Failure to achieve expected weight gains, weight loss without dieting, and increases or decreases in appetite require additional evaluation.
- Psychopharmacotherapy may cause appetite and weight changes.
- Failure to reach academic standards and poor social integration may threaten the psychosocial development of affected youth.
  - Evaluate information about functioning at home, in school, and in social settings.

Diet
- Decreased or increased appetite, hoarding, binge eating, and changes in food preferences can occur.
- During mania, children and adolescents may become "too busy" to stop for meals.
- Poor nutrition results from binge eating, filling up on junk food and sweets, or inadequate intake of calories and nutrients during mania.
- Increased risk for the development of a coexisting eating disorder requires careful monitoring throughout the treatment and recovery phases.
- Psychotropic medications can cause changes in appetite and weight.
  - Monitor diet and weight and educate about the side effects of medications.

Safety
- Suicidal thoughts, threats, or gestures always must be taken seriously; children and adolescents with mood disorders are considered to be at high risk for self-harm.
- When a hypomanic or manic episode is suspected or evident, assess the potential for self-injury because of poor judgment and risk-taking behavior.

- Risk of overdose, particularly with tricyclic antidepressants (TCAs), and potential for serious adverse reactions necessitate intensive education of affected youths and their parents at the initiation of treatment and follow-up education at every health care visit.
- Medication and dietary interactions with the use of MAOIs pose special risks.

Immunizations
- No changes in the routine schedule of immunizations are needed.

Screening
- Vision. Routine age-related screening for vision is recommended.
  - Ensure that symptoms of withdrawal, low self-esteem, distractibility, irritability, and impaired attention are not caused in part by impaired sight by conducting vision screening when assessing for a mood disorder.
- Hearing. Routine age-related screening for hearing is recommended.
  - Ensure that symptoms of withdrawal, low self-esteem, distractibility, irritability, and impaired attention are not caused in by impaired hearing. Conduct a hearing screening when assessing for a mood disorder.
- Dental. Routine screening is recommended.
- Blood Pressure. Routine screening is recommended.
  - Baseline blood pressure assessment and regular monitoring should be done during the first several weeks of medication treatment if TCAs, MAOIs, or atypical antipsychotics are prescribed; monitoring should be every few months thereafter.
  - If MAOIs are in use, the risk of hypertensive crisis is serious if the required diet is not followed carefully or if drug interactions occur. Education is essential to prevent this type of crisis.

- Hematocrit. Routine screening is recommended.
- Urinalysis. Routine screening is recommended.
- Tuberculosis. Routine screening is recommended.

Condition-Specific Screening

- Speech and language. If speech and language do not normalize after treatment is implemented, additional evaluation is needed.
- Cardiac function. Children taking TCAs and antipsychotics are at risk for cardiac effects, including tachycardia, prolonged QTc interval, and orthostatic hypotension.
  - Obtaining baseline blood pressure, complete blood count (CBC), and an electrocardiogram (ECG) is recommended.
  - If a dosage is changed, blood pressure, CBC, and ECG should be repeated.
  - Lowering the dose is warranted when the PR interval reaches 0.22 seconds, or QRS reaches 130% of baseline, heart rate is >140 beats/min, or blood pressure is >140/90 mm Hg.
- Drug toxicity. Monitor for safety and follow specific recommendations for each class of drugs.

COMMON ILLNESS MANAGEMENT

Differential Diagnosis

- Overlap in symptoms with several other psychiatric disorders and common childhood illnesses requires evaluation of diagnostic DSM-V-TR criteria and an assessment of physical symptoms.
- The clinician must determine which symptoms are occurring in isolation and which appear to be associated with or caused by another physical or psychological ailment.
- A detailed and thorough history from the youth and parent or other caregivers is often the best strategy to help the clinician create an accurate timeline of the onset of symptoms.
- The most common psychiatric disorders to be considered as differential diagnoses include: adjustment disorder, posttraumatic stress disorder (PTSD), anxiety disorders, attention-deficit/hyperactivity disorder (ADHD), eating disorders, and substance use disorders.
- Discerning between a symptom of a known mood disorder and a symptom that may represent another problem is difficult at times.
  - To determine the most accurate diagnosis, careful observations are required, sometimes over an extended period.
  - Routine common illness management with attention to potential drug interactions is needed.

Drug Interactions

- Combination therapy increases the risk of drug interactions.
- Changing from one class of drugs to another can produce interactions.
- Selective serotonin reuptake inhibitors (SSRIs) in combination with MAOIs, designer drugs of abuse, and other medications can produce a potentially lethal interaction: serotonin syndrome.
  - Follow guidelines carefully if changing from MAOI to SSRI and vice versa.
- SSRIs, particularly fluoxetine, are inhibitors of their own metabolism and can inhibit the metabolism of other medications.

- Lithium is cleared by the kidneys with an approximate half-life of 14 to 30 hours.
- Young people tend to have a faster lithium clearance rate than older adults.
- Safe treatment requires regular monitoring of lithium serum levels.
- Toxic effects from lithium typically occur with serum levels >1.5 mEq/L, and levels >2.0 mEq/L are associated with life-threatening side effects.
- Changes in hydration, renal function, and sodium levels will alter lithium serum levels.
- Valproate is metabolized by the liver and is highly protein-bound; therefore, interactions may occur with other metabolized or protein-bound medications.
  - Valproate's weak inhibition of drug oxidation results in increased serum concentrations of drugs that undergo oxidative metabolism.
- Co-administration of many other medications can decrease or increase serum concentrations of valproate, requiring careful evaluation of all medications administered.
  - Valproate toxicity can result from co-administration with other protein-bound medications.
- Carbamazepine decreases plasma levels of many other medications, including TCAs, thyroid hormones, hormonal contraceptives, and neuroleptics.
- Drugs that inhibit carbamazepine metabolism, including erythromycin, calcium channel blockers diltiazem and verapamil, and SSRIs, will increase serum levels.
- Topiramate (Topamax) may decrease phenytoin (Dilantin) and valproate levels, as well as levels of combined hormonal contraceptives.
- Quetiapine can prolong the QTc interval and may interact with other QT interval prolongers, such as macrolide antibiotics.
- Aripiprazole is metabolized on CYP 2D6 pathway and could interact with both fluoxetine and quetiapine.

DEVELOPMENTAL ISSUES

Sleep Patterns

- Change in sleep patterns may be an early sign of a mood disorder. Excessive sleeping, too little sleep, disrupted sleep, and poor quality of sleep are common symptoms.
- Abnormal sleep contributes to irritability, poor school performance, and fatigue or agitation.
- In bipolar disorder, the affected youths may alternate between periods of very little sleep and hyperactivity to periods of utter exhaustion during which the child may want to sleep all day.
- Sedating effects of many medications must be considered when evaluating sleep.
- Eliciting an account of recent sleep patterns helps identify signs of a mood disorder.
- Keeping a sleep diary helps track patterns and monitor response to treatment.
- Implementing good sleep habits, including a regular bedtime, avoidance of caffeine in the evening, and relaxing routines before sleep, helps normalize sleep patterns.

Toileting

- Mood disorders generally are not associated with significant difficulties in toileting.
  - Problems with bedwetting and soiling sometimes occur with bipolar disorder.

Continued

Discipline
- Parents and teachers may interpret withdrawal or irritibility as a lack of cooperation or respect. Children wit bipolar disorder are prone to aggressive behavior and disruptive and alienating outbursts.
- Consistent limits and clear explanations of behavioral contingencies are appropriate discipline strategies. Enforcing rules regarding safety also is essential for purposes of protection.

Child Care
- Children frequently have trouble relating to peers. Irritability makes them difficult to be around and tends to push others away.
- Children with symptoms or diagnosis of bipolar disorder typically have periods of disruptive behavior that can cause safety problems and interfere with group activities.
- A lack of pleasure or interest limits engagement in social activities.
- Regular schedules and placement in small family settings or centers with high staff/child ratios and stable personnel are ideal.

Schooling
- A downward slide in grades, difficulty managing school-related activities, and behavior problems in the classroom can indicate a mood disorder.
- Poor concentration, irritability, disorganization, lack of self-confidence or grandiosity, and withdrawal or fighting interfere with academic work.
- School-related problems can escalate and lead to academic failure and dropping out.
- In severe cases, hospitalization and residential placement may need to substitute for usual school attendance.

- Children often require special accommodations, and an Individualized Educational Plan (IEP) may assist affected students to function in the classroom.

Sexuality
- Interest and performance ability may lessen among adolescents.
- Difficulty establishing close relationships may interfere with the development of healthy sexuality.
- Bipolar disorders are associated with poor judgment during manic episodes that could lead to promiscuous behavior and related risks for unwanted pregnancy and sexually transmitted diseases (STDs).

Transition to Adulthood
- Mood disorders interfere with being able to relate to peers, develop intimate relationships, and manage responsibilities.
- Appropriate adjunctive therapeutic approaches include social skills training, academic and occupational counseling, and education in life skills.

Family Concerns
- Mood disorders take a toll on the family. "Well" siblings may harbor feelings of resentment as the "ill" child gets special accommodations based on the condition.
- The child with bipolar disorder also may embarrass family members with angry public outbursts of rage.
- Concerns about possible genetic transmission can create feelings of guilt, anger, and anxiety about future generations.
- Difficulty obtaining adequate health care coverage for long-term psychiatric conditions creates a real financial burden and stress for families.
- National organizations, local support groups, and informational websites are available resources for families.

REFERENCES

Almandil, N., Liu, Y., Murray, M., Besag, F., Aitchison, K., & Wong, I. (2013). Weight gain and other metabolic adverse effects associated with the atypical antipsychotic treatment of children and adolescents: A systematic review and meta-analysis. *Pediatric Drugs, 15*(2), 139–150. https://doi.org/10.1007/s40272-013-0016-6.

American Academy of Pediatrics. (2022). 2022 recommendations for preventive pediatric health care. *Pediatrics, 150*(1), e2022058044. https://doi.org/10.1542/peds.2022-058044.

American Academy of Child and Adolescent Psychiatry (AACAP). Practice parameter for the use of atypical antipsychotic medications in children and adolescents. 2011. Accessed from https://www.aacap.org/App_Themes/AACAP/docs/practice_parameters/Atypical_Antipsychotic_Medications_Web.pdf.

American Diabetes Association. (2004). American Psychological Association, American Association of Clinical Endocrinologists, & North American Association for the Study of Obesity. Consensus development conference in antipsychotic drugs and obesity and diabetes. *Diabetes Care, 27*(2), 596–601. https://doi.org/10.2337/diacare.27.2.596.

American Psychiatric Association. (2013). *Diagnostic and statistical manual of mental disorders* (5th ed.). American Psychiatric Association.

American Psychiatric Association. (2022). *Diagnostic and statistical manual of mental disorders* (5th ed., text rev.). American Psychiatric Association.

American Psychological Association. Decision-making within evidence-based practice in psychology using the APA clinical practice guideline for the treatment of depression in children and adolescents. 2021. Retrieved from https://www.apa.org/depression-guideline/decision-aid-children-adolescents.pdf.

American Psychological Association. Clinical practice guideline for the treatment of posttraumatic stress syndrome. Cognitive behavioral therapy. 2023. https://www.apa.org/ptsd-guideline/patients-and-families/cognitive-behavioral.

Athey, A., Overholser, J. C., & Beale, E. E. (2022). Depressed adolescents' exposure to suicide attempts and suicide loss. *Death Studies, 46*(8), 1862–1869. doi:10.1080/07481187.2020.1864063. Epub 2021 Jan 13.

Birmaher, B., Hafeman, D., Merranko, J., Zwicker, A., Goldstein, B., Goldstein, T., Axelson, D., Monk, K., Hickey, M. B., Sakolsky, D., Iyengar, S., Diler, R., Nimgaonkar, V., & Uher, R. (2022). Role of polygenic risk score in the familial transmission of bipolar disorder in youth. *JAMA Psychiatry, 79*(2), 160–168. doi:10.1001/jamapsychiatry.2021.3700. Erratum in: JAMA Psychiatry. 2022;79(6):632.

Bitsko, R. H., Claussen, A. H., Lichstein, J., Black, L. I., Jones, S. E., Danielson, M. L., Hoenig, J. M., Davis Jack, S. P., Brody, D. J., Gyawali, S., Maenner, M. J., Warner, M., Holland, K. M., Perou, R., Crosby, A. E., Blumberg, S. J., Avenevoli, S., Kaminski, J. W., Ghandour, R. M., & Contributor (2022). Mental health surveillance among children—United States, 2013–2019. *MMWR Supplements, 71*(2), 1–42. https://doi.org/10.15585/mmwr.su7102a1.

Blair, C., & Raver, C. C. (2016). Poverty, stress, and brain development: new directions for prevention and intervention. *Academic Pediatrics, 16*(3 Suppl), S30–36. doi:10.1080/07481187.2020.1864063.

Bruno, A., Celebre, L., Torre, G., Pandolfo, G., Mento, C., Cedro, C., Zoccali, R. A., & Muscatello, M. R. A. (2019). Focus on disruptive mood dysregulation disorder: A review of the literature. *Psychiatry Research, 279,* 323–330. https://doi.org/10.1016/j.psychres.2019.05.043.

Centers for Disease Control and Prevention. (2021, April 6). *About the CDC-Kaiser Ace Study | Violence prevention | injury Center | CDC.* Centers for Disease Control and Prevention. https://www.cdc.gov/violenceprevention/aces/about.html.

Centers for Disease Control and Prevention. National Center on Birth Defects and Developmental Disabilities. Data and statistics on children's mental health. 2022. https://www.cdc.gov/childrensmentalhealth/data.html.

Centers for Disease Control and Prevention. Children's mental health: Anxiety and depression in children. National Center on Birth Defects and Developmental Disabilities. 2022a. https://www.cdc.gov/childrensmentalhealth/depression.html.

Centers for Disease Control and Prevention. Children's mental health: Mental health of children and parents—a strong connection. 2022b. https://www.cdc.gov/childrensmentalhealth/features/mental-health-children-and-parents.html.

D'cruz, M. M., & Chaturvedi, S. K. (2021). Sociodemographic and cultural determinants of mood disorders. *Current Opinion in Psychiatry, 35*(1), 38–44. https://doi.org/10.1097/yco.0000000000000766.

Disruptive mood dysregulation disorder. *Archives of Disease in Childhood, 107*(4), 358. https://doi.org/10.1136/archdischild-2022-324063.

Earls, M. (2019). Screening new parents for depression helps mother, child and the whole family. *American Academy of Pediatrics, AAP Voices Blog.* Retrieved from https://www.aap.org/en/news-room/aap-voices/screening-new-parents-for-depression/.

Elhosary, M., & Birmaher, B. (2022). Pediatric bipolar disorder—misinformation with unintended negative consequences for children and adolescents. *European Journal of Neuropsychopharmacology, 59,* 4–6. https://doi.org/10.1016/j.euroneuro.2022.02.011.

Fairbanks, H. (2019). Toxic Stress. In Hallas, D. (Ed.), *Behavioral pediatric healthcare for nurse practitioners: A growth and developmental approach to intercepting abnormal behaviors* (pp. 429–441). Springer Publishing Company.

Feldman, R. (2016). The neurobiology of mammalian parenting and the biosocial context of human caregiving. *Hormones and Behavior, 77,* 3–17. https://doi.org/10.1016/j.yhbeh.2015.10.001.

Findling, R. L., Chang, K., Robb, A., Foster, V. J., Horrigan, J., Krishen, A., Wamil, A., Kraus, J. E., & DelBello, M. (2015). Adjunctive maintenance lamotrigine for pediatric bipolar I disorder: A placebo-controlled, randomized withdrawal study. *Journal of the American Academy of Child and Adolescent Psychiatry, 54*(12), 1020–1031. e3. https://doi.org/10.1016/j.jaac.2015.09.017.

Findling, R. L., Stepanova, E., Youngstrom, E. A., & Young, A. S. (2018). Progress in diagnosis and treatment of bipolar disorder among children and adolescents: An international perspective. *Evidence-Based Mental Health, 21*(4), 177–181. https://doi.org/10.1136/eb-2018-102912.

Findling, R. L., Zhou, X., George, P., & Chappell, P. B. (2021). Diagnostic trends and prescription patterns in disruptive mood dysregulation disorder and bipolar disorder. *Journal of the American Academy of Child and Adolescent Psychiatry, 61*(3), 434–445. https://doi.org/10.1016/j.jaac.2021.05.016.

Goldstein, B. I., Birmaher, B., Carlson, G. A., DelBello, M. P., Findling, R. L., Fristad, M., Kowatch, R. A., Miklowitz, D. J.,

Nery, F. G., Perez-Algorta, G., Van Meter, A., Zeni, C. P., Correll, C. U., Kim, H. W., Wozniak, J., Chang, K. D., Hillegers, M., & Youngstrom, E. A. (2017). The International Society for Bipolar Disorders Task Force report on pediatric bipolar disorder: Knowledge to date and directions for future research. *Bipolar Disorders, 19*(7), 524–543. https://doi.org/10.1111/bdi.12556.

Granat, A., Gadassi, R., Gilboa-Schechtman, E., & Feldman, B. (2017). Maternal depression and anxiety, social synchrony, and infant regulation of negative and positive emotions. *Emotion, 1,* 11–27. https://doi.org/10.1037/emo0000204.

Gudmundsen, G. R., Rhew, I. C., McCauley, E., Kim, J., & Stoep, AV. (2019). Emergence of depressive symptoms from kindergarten to sixth grade. *Journal of Clinical Child & Adolescent Psychology, 48,* 501–515. https://doi.org/10.1080/15374416.2017.141082.

Hallas, D. (2019a). Infant depression. In Hallas, D. (Ed.), *Behavioral pediatric healthcare for nurse practitioners: A growth and developmental approach to intercepting abnormal behaviors* (pp. 83–89). Springer Publishing Company.

Hallas, D. (2019b). Intercepting behavioral health problems: A conceptual model. In Hallas, D. (Ed.), *Behavioral pediatric healthcare for nurse practitioners: A growth and developmental approach to intercepting abnormal behaviors* (pp. 3–16). Springer Publishing Company.

Hallas, D., Heuer, B., Sesay-Tuffour, S., & Foerster, A. (2022). Pediatric primary care mental health specialist examination: Job task analysis. *Journal for Nurse Practitioners, 19*(2), 104441. https://doi.org/10.1016/j.nurpra.2022.08.024.

Havens, J. F., Marr, M. C., & Hirsch, E. (2022). Editorial: From bipolar disorder to disruptive mood dysregulation disorder: Challenges to diagnostic and treatment specificity in traumatized youths. *Journal of the American Academy of Child and Adolescent Psychiatry, 61*(3), 364–365. https://doi.org/10.1016/j.jaac.2021.07.012.

Hawes, M. T., Szenczy, A. K., Kein, D. N., Hajcak, G., & Nelson, B. D. (2022). Increases in depression and anxiety symptoms in adolescents and young adults during the COVID-19 pandemic. *Psychological Medicine, 52,* 3222–3230. https://doi.10.1017/S0033291720005358.

Hendrickson, B., Girma, M., & Miller, L. (2019). Review of the clinical approach to the treatment of disruptive mood dysregulation disorder. *International Review of Psychiatry, 32*(3), 1–10. https://doi.org/10.1080/09540261.2019.1688260.

Ho, T. C., Shah, R., Mishra, J., May, A. C., & Tapert, S. F. (2022). Multi-level predictors of depression symptoms in the adolescent brain cognitive development (ABCD) study. *Journal of Child Psychology and Psychiatry, 63,* 1523–1533. https://doi.10.1111/jcpp.13608.

Hobbs, E., Reed, R., Lorberg, B., Robb, A. S., & Dorfman, J. (2022). Psychopharmacological treatment algorithms of manic/mixed and depressed episodes in pediatric bipolar disorder. *Journal of Child and Adolescent Psychopharmacology, 32*(10), 507–521. https://doi.org/10.1089/cap.2022.0035.

Iyanda, A. E. (2022). Bullying victimization of children with mental, emotional, and developmental or behavioral (MEDB) disorders in the United States. *Journal of Child and Adolescent Trauma, 15,* 221–223. https://doi.10.1007/s40653-021-00368-8.

Izard, C. E., Huebner, R. R., Risser, D., McGinnes, G., & Dougherty, L. (1980). The young infant's ability to produce discrete emotional expressions. *Developmental Psychology, 16,* 132–140. https://doi.org/10.1037/0012-1649.16.2.132.

Kaufman, J., Birmaher, B., Axelson, D., Perepletchikova, F., Brent, D., Ryan, N. (2016). K-SADS-PL DSM-5. Supplement 1: Depressive and bipolar related disorders. 2016. Retrieved from https://www.pediatricbipolar.pitt.edu/sites/default/files/KSADS_DSM_5_SCREEN_Final.pdf.

Lipina, S. J., & Columno, J. A. (2009). *Poverty and brain development during childhood: An approach from cognitive psychology and neuroscience.* American Psychology Association.

Luby, J. L. (2009). Early childhood depression. *American Journal of Psychiatry, 166*(9), 974–979. https://doi:10.1176/appi.ajp.2009.08111709.

Luby, J., Gilbert, K., Whalen, D., Tillman, R., & Barch, D. M. (2020). The differential contribution of the components of parent-child interaction therapy emotion development for treatment of preschool depression. *Journal of American Child and Adolescent Psychiatry, 59*(7), 868–879. https://doi:10.1016/jaac.2019.07.937.

Magioncalda, P., & Martino, M. (2021). A unified model of the pathophysiology of bipolar disorder. *Molecular Psychiatry, 2022*(7), 202–211. https://doi.org/10.1038/s41380-021-01091-4.

Mangione, C. M., Barry, M. J., Nicholson, W. K., Cabana, M., Chelmow, D., Coker, T. R., Davidson, K. W., Davis, E. M., Donahue, K. E., Jaén, C. R., Kubik, M., Li, L., Ogedegbe, G., Pbert, L., Ruiz, J. M., Silverstein, M., Stevermer, J., & Wong, J. B. (2022). Screening for depression and suicide risk in children and adolescents: US Preventive Services Task Force Recommendation Statement. *JAMA, 328*(15), 1534–1542. https://doi.org/10.1001/jama.2022.16946.

Marangoni, C. (2018). ADHD, bipolar disorder, or borderline personality disorder: Getting to the right diagnosis. *Psychiatric Times, 35*(10), 18+.

Murgatroyd, C., Wu, Y., Bockmuhl, Y., & Spengler, D. (2010). Genes learn from stress. *Epigenetics, 5,* 194–199. https://doi:10.4161/epi.5.3.11375.

Mürner-Lavanchy, I., Kaess, M., & Koenig, J. (2021). Diagnostic instruments for the assessment of disruptive mood dysregulation disorder: A systematic review of the literature. *European Child and Adolescent Psychiatry.* https://doi.org/10.1007/s00787-021-01840-4.

Negeri, Z., Sun, Y., Benedetti, A., & Thomas, B. D. (2020). Accuracy of the Edinburgh postnatal depression scale (DPDS) for screening to detect major depression among pregnant and postpartum women: Systematic review and meta-analysis of individual participant data. *BMJ, 371.* https://doi.org/10.1136/bmj.m4022.

Pediatric Nursing Certification Board (n.d.). *The PMHS role.* Retrieved from: https://www.pncb.org/pmhs-role.

Riddle, M. (2019). *Pediatric psychopharmacology for primary care* (2nd ed.). American Academy of Pediatrics.

Romba, C., & Perez-Reisler, M. (2020). Management of adverse effects of psychotropic medications. *Pediatric Annals, 49*(10), e431–e435. https://doi.org/10.3928/19382359-20200922-03.

Schadt, E. (2019). Brain development and compelling outcomes of ineffective parent child bonding. In Hallas, D. (Ed.), *Behavioral pediatric healthcare for nurse practitioners: A growth and developmental approach to intercepting abnormal behaviors* (pp. 17–23). Springer Publishing Company.

Selvaraj, S., Brambilla, P., & Soares, J. C. (2020). *Mood disorders.* Cambridge University Press.

Sequeira, S. L., Morrow, K. E., Silk, J. S., Kolko, D. J., Pilkonis, P. A., & Lindhiem, O. (2021). National norms and correlates of the PHQ-8 and GAD-7 in parents of School-age children. *Journal of Child Family Studies, 30*(9), 2303–2314. https://doi.org/10.1007/s10826-021-02026-x.

Sethna, V., Siew, J., Gudbrandsen, M., Pote, I., Wang, S., Daly, E., Deprez, M., Pariante, C. M., Seneviratne, G., Murphy, D. G. M., Craig, M. C., & McAlonan, G. (2021). Maternal depression during pregnancy alters infant subcortical and midbrain volumes. *Journal of Affective Disorders, 291,* 163–170. https://10.1016/j.jad.2021.05.008.

Shim, R., Szilagyi, M., & Perrin, J. M. (2022). Epidemic rates of child and adolescent mental health disorders require an urgent response. *Pediatrics, 149*(5), e2022056611. https://doi.org/10.1542/peds.2022-056611.

Spry, E. A., Aarsman, S. R., Youssef, G. J., Patton, G., Macdonald, J., Sanson, A., Thomson, K., Hutchinson, D., Letcher, P., & Olsson, C. (2020). Maternal and paternal depression and anxiety and offspring infant negative affectivity: A systematic review and meta-analysis. *Developmental Review, 58*(1). https://doi.10.1016/j.dr.2020.100934.

Sukhodolsky, D. G., Smith, S. D., McCauley, S. A., Ibrahim, K., & Piasecka, J. B. (2016). Behavioral interventions for anger, irritability, and aggression in children and adolescents. *Journal of Child and Adolescent Psychopharmacology, 26*(1), 58–64. https://doi.org/10.1089/cap.2015.0120.

Takahashi, L. K. (2019). Neurobiology of schizophrenia, mood disorders, anxiety disorders, and obsessive-compulsive disorder. In McCance, K. L., & Huether, S. E. (Eds.), *Pathophysiology: The biological basis for disease in adults and children* (8th ed., chap. 19). Elsevier.

Thomas, S., White, V., Ryan, N., & Byren, L. (2022). Effectiveness of play therapy in enhancing psychosocial outcomes in children with chronic illness: A systematic review. *Journal of Pediatric Nursing, 63,* e72–e81. https://doi.org/10.1016/j.pedn.2021.10.009.

Toulany, A., Stukel, T., Kurdyak, P., Fu, L., & Guttmann, A. (2019). Association of primary care continuity with outcomes following transition to adult care for adolescents with severe mental illness. *JAMA Network Open, 2*(8), e198415. https://doi.org/10.1001/jamanetworkopen.2019.8415.

US Department of Health and Human Services. Children's Bureau. Child Welfare Information Gateway. (n.d.). Adverse childhood experiences (ACEs). https://www.childwelfare.gov/topics/preventing/overview/framework/aces/.

US Department of Health and Human Services, National Institutes of Health, National Institute of Mental Health. *Bipolar disorder in children and adolescents* (NIH Publication No. 20-MH-8081). 2020. Retrieved from https://www.nimh.nih.gov/health/publications/bipolar-disorder-in-children-and-teens.

US Department of Health and Human Services. Substance Abuse and Mental Health Services Administration [SAMHSA]. Screening, brief intervention, and referral to treatment (SBIRT). 2022. https://www.samhsa.gov/sbirt.

Van Meter, A. R., Burke, C., Kowatch, R. A., Findling, R. L., & Youngstrom, E. A. (2016). Ten-year updated meta-analysis of the clinical characteristics of pediatric mania and hypomania. *Bipolar Disorders, 18*(1), 19–32. https://doi.org/10.1111/bdi.12358.

Van Meter, A., Moreira, A. L. R., & Youngstrom, E. (2019). Updated meta-analysis of epidemiologic studies of pediatric bipolar disorder. *Journal of Clinical Psychiatry, 80*(3). https://doi.org/10.4088/jcp.18r12180.

Walle, E. A., & Lopez, L. D. (2020). Emotion recognition and understanding in infancy and early childhood. *Encyclopedia of Infant and Early Childhood Development,* 537–545. https://doi.org/10.1016/b978-0-12-809324-5.23567-0.

Weintraub, M. J., Schneck, C. D., Axelson, D. A., Birmaher, B., Kowatch, R. A., & Miklowitz D. J. (2020). Classifying mood symptom trajectories in adolescents with bipolar disorder. *Journal of the American Academy of Child & Adolescent Psychiatry, 59*(3), 381–390. doi:10.1016/j.jaac.2019.04.028.

Wium-Andersen, M. K. (2013). Elevated C-RP levels, psychological distress, and depression in 73131 individuals. *JAMA Psychiatry, 70,* 176–184.

Yule, A., Fitzgerald, M., Wilens, T., Wozniak, J., Woodworth, K. Y., Pulli, A., Uchida, M., Faraone, S. V., & Biederman, J. (2019). Further evidence of the diagnostic utility of the child behavior checklist for identifying pediatric bipolar I disorder. *Scandinavian Journal of Child and Adolescent Psychiatry and Psychology, 7*(1), 29–36. https://doi.org/10.21307/sjcapp-2019-006.

Zisser, A., & Eyberg, S. M. (2010). Parent-child interaction therapy and the treatment of disruptive behavior disorders. In Weisz, J. R., & Kazdin, A. E. (Eds.), *Evidence-based psychotherapies for children and adolescents* (pp. 179–193). The Guilford Press.

Muscular Dystrophy, Duchenne

Alison Ballard

ETIOLOGY

Muscular dystrophy (MD) is a group of genetically inherited degenerative muscle disorders characterized by hypotonia, progressive muscle weakness, and dystrophic or myopathic features on muscle biopsy. Historically, diagnoses were based on clinical features and histopathology. However, in the era of rapid expansion and accessibility of genetic testing, we are gaining a better understanding of phenotypic variability and overlap between congenital muscular dystrophies and congenital myopathies (Butterfield, 2019). The most common types of MD include dystrophinopathies (Duchenne [DMD] and Becker [BMD]), congenital muscular dystrophies, limb-girdle muscular dystrophy, Emery-Dreifuss muscular dystrophy, facioscapulohumeral muscular dystrophy, myotonic dystrophy, and oculopharyngeal muscular dystrophy. Table 31.1 summarizes the inheritance pattern, age of onset, type of muscle affected, and rate of progression for each of the most common types of MD (Muscular Dystrophy Association [MDA], 2022). Although this chapter focuses on males with DMD, much of the diagnostic process, treatment, and primary care are similar across types of MD.

DMD, the most common form in children, is named after a French neurologist who first described it in 1868 (Duchenne de Boulogne, 1973). DMD is primarily a disease of the skeletal, heart, and respiratory muscles but can also affect cognition. DMD is X-linked recessive and thus primarily affects males; although female carriers can be affected and may be referred to as symptomatic carriers, there is no consensus on proper nomenclature (Gruber et al., 2022). DMD is a chronic, progressive, and life-limiting disorder, with children appearing normal at birth, followed by progressive weakness throughout childhood. With advances in therapies and supportive care, particularly respiratory and cardiac care, many patients with DMD can expect to live into their fourth decade (Landfeldt et al., 2020).

DMD is caused by a genetic change in the dystrophin gene at position Xp21 (Monaco et al., 1986). It is one of the largest genes in the human genome, with 79 exons (Stockley et al., 2006), having a high proclivity for mutations. Approximately 60% to 70% of males with DMD have deletions, 5% to 15% with duplications, and the other 20% have point mutations, small

deletions, or insertions (Duan et al., 2021). Deletions may occur at any point along the dystrophin gene, with most occurring in two hot-spot regions within the gene, located at exons 45 to 55 (47%) and 3 to 9 (7%) (Duan et al., 2021). These genetic changes disrupt essential functional domains of the dystrophin molecule resulting in a truncated and unstable dystrophin protein with impaired function (Yiu & Kornberg, 2015).

In muscles, dystrophin is part of a protein complex and acts as a link between the cytoskeleton and the extracellular matrix (Yiu & Kornberg, 2015). Dystrophin-deficient muscle fibers are susceptible to degeneration of muscle fibers that are replaced by fat and connective tissue, which give the muscle the appearance of pseudohypertrophy and a firm, rubbery feel. The exact mechanism of muscle degeneration due absence of dystrophin is unknown but involves cytoskeleton disruption, sarcolemma instability, and abnormal calcium homeostasis (Yiu & Kornberg, 2015) The dystrophin protein is nearly absent in the muscles of males with DMD (Hoffman, 2020) and partially absent in those with BMD, a milder form of MD. The gene also codes for protein products that localize to other tissue types, including the brain, and the absence of these products is associated with brain-related comorbidities, including cognitive deficits, behavioral concerns, and epilepsy (Hoogland et al., 2019).

INCIDENCE AND PREVALENCE

DMD is the most common genetically determined neuromuscular disease of childhood and shows no predilection for race or ethnic group. It occurs in 1 in 3600 to 5000 live male births (Gruber et al., 2022). It is an X-linked recessive disorder, and there is a 50% chance that a male child will be affected with DMD and a 50% chance that a female child will be a carrier with each pregnancy if the mother carries the pathogenic variant (Basta & Pandya, 2022). Although females typically are asymptomatic (<1 per million DMD females), the importance of carrier testing and the need for ongoing cardiac surveillance beginning in the third decade of life is necessary due to many female carriers having findings of cardiac fibrosis on cardiovascular magnetic resonance imaging (CMR) (Mah et al., 2020).

Table 31.1   Seven Major Types of Muscular Dystrophy (MD) That Affect Children and Young Adults

TYPE	AGE OF ONSET	SEX MOST AFFECTED	MUSCLES AFFECTED	PROBLEMS ASSOCIATED WITH THIS TYPE
Duchenne (DMD)	The most common form of MD in children. Duchenne typically starts at age 2 or 3 years, with children being wheelchair dependent wheelchair by age 9 to 10 years.	Male	Begins with muscle weakness in the trunk and spreads to the arms and legs	• Heart and lung • Abnormal curvature of the spine • Mental health problems
Becker (BMD)	Similar to DMD but less common, with milder symptoms and slower progression.	Male	Begins with muscle weakness in the trunk and spreads to the arms and legs	• Heart and lung • Abnormal curvature of the spine • Mental health problems
Myotonic (MMD or Steinert disease)	Infancy, childhood, teen years, or adulthood	Male and female	Face, arms, and leg muscles	• Muscular pain • Heart, eyes, brain, and sexual organs • Breathing and swallowing issues • Stomach pain, diarrhea, and/or constipation • Cataracts • Thyroid disorders • Diabetes
Limb-girdle	Early in childhood (typically 8 to 15 years of age) or later in life. Usually wheelchair dependent by age 30 years.	Male and female	Shoulders and hips	• Heart • Contractures with limited movement of certain joints
Facioscapulohumeral (FSHD or Landouzy-Dejerine)	Typically begins at age 10 to 20 years or younger.	Male and female	Severe weakness of facial muscles, sometimes affecting the legs, shoulders, and upper arms. Unlike other dystrophies, FSHD is commonly asymmetric.	• Pain • Hearing • Heart • Mental health problems
Congenital	At birth	Male and female	"Floppy baby"; moderate hypotonia with many weak muscles	• Contractures with limited movement of certain joints
Emery-Dreifuss	Rare form of MD that typically begins in early childhood to age 20 years or older.	Male and female	Weakness typically starts in the arms and later affects the legs, with facial weakness.	• Life-threatening heart • Contractures with limited movement of certain joints

Modified from Liaqat, S. T., Akram, F., Waseem, R., Akram, A., Altaf, M. Z., Haider, B., Zulfiqar, N., & Arif, A. (2023). Overview of muscular dystrophy, its types, symptoms, management and possible treatment. *Pure and Applied Biology, 12*(1), 261–273.

DIAGNOSTIC CRITERIA

DMD is a well-characterized inherited disorder with a strong genotype-phenotype relationship (Lim et al., 2020). Recent advances in molecular diagnoses have made it possible to identify precise mutations in up to 93% to 96% of individuals with a DMD phenotype (Thomas et al., 2022), thus allowing for more accurate genetic diagnoses.

LABORATORY TESTING: CREATINE KINASE

If DMD is suspected, a serum creatine kinase (CK) level can be obtained as a screening tool. CK is an enzyme concentrated in muscle and is released into the blood with muscle damage. CK levels can be markedly elevated in individuals with DMD, reaching 10 to 20 times the upper limit of normal (Yiu & Kornberg, 2015). However, serum CK elevations alone do not confirm the diagnosis of DMD, and confirmatory genetic testing is warranted in patients with an elevated CK level. Other causes for an elevated CK include other congenital muscular dystrophies, birth trauma, and nonneuromuscular disorders. In DMD, serum CK is highest at birth in those with DMD and then gradually declines as muscle mass decreases throughout the course of the disease (Zygmunt et al., 2023). Alanine aminotransferase (ALT) and aspartate aminotransferase (AST) are also released from damaged muscle (McMillan et al., 2011). This may inadvertently be considered a sign of liver disease. Therefore a CK level should be checked in individuals with elevated ALT and AST and no other hepatic symptoms (McMillan et al., 2011).

MUSCLE BIOPSY

Immunohistochemistry analysis of the biopsied muscle shows an absence of dystrophin in DMD (Ohlendieck & Swandulle, 2021). Currently, muscle biopsy is mainly used to confirm a diagnosis of Duchenne BMD when genetic testing is unable to confirm the suspected diagnosis and should be interpreted by an experienced neuromuscular pathologist. Muscle biopsies can be anxiety provoking and typically require anesthesia in children; hence they should be avoided when possible (Mendell et al., 2001).

ELECTROMYOGRAPHY

Electromyography and nerve conduction studies are often obtained as part of the evaluation of a suspected underlying neuromuscular disorder. However, these studies are not indicated in the assessment of DMD, according to expert panels (Bushby et al., 2010).

NEWBORN SCREENING, TESTING, AND FAMILY PLANNING

Newborn screening has several potential benefits and risks in DMD. Benefits include providing families access to emerging therapies, avoiding the potentially difficult and time-consuming process of establishing a diagnosis, enabling families to become knowledgeable and develop strategies for managing complex health care needs in advance, and informing future reproductive planning (Chung et al., 2022). Historically, DMD has not met the health screening criteria to be included on the Recommended Uniform Screening Panel (RUSP) as it does not present in infancy and lacks effective treatment (Ross et al., 2017). However, with emerging DMD therapies, Parent Project Muscular Dystrophy (PPMD), in conjunction with the MDA, recently submitted a nomination package to add Duchenne to the RUSP, which will initiate the review process through the Advisory Committee on Heritable Disorders in Newborns and Children, which advises the US Department of Health and Human Services about which conditions should be considered for newborn screening. Several pilot studies have completed screening for DMD because of potential benefits beyond medical treatment (Gruber et al., 2022).

Females with a familial history of DMD can undergo carrier testing to make informed reproductive choices. Pre- and posttest counseling are recommended, and reproductive options may need to be discussed, including pregnancy with or without prenatal testing, preimplantation diagnosis, pregnancy by egg or sperm donation, parenting by adoption, or remaining childless (Pagon et al., 2001).

CLINICAL MANIFESTATIONS AT TIME OF DIAGNOSIS

Presenting symptoms typically become evident between 2 and 3 years of age and include gross motor milestone delays, gait abnormalities, difficulty climbing stairs, getting up from the floor, keeping up with peers, and frequent falls (Duan et al., 2021). Around 2 to 3 years of age, males with DMD may appear to be somewhat clumsy, and by age 3 to 5 years, they often have difficulty keeping up with their peers on the playground (Yiu & Kornberg, 2015). Presenting symptoms include proximal weakness progressing at different rates but consistent in pattern, proximal muscle weakness before distal, lower extremity weakness before upper extremity, and extensors weakening before flexors (McDonald et al., 1995). Initially, individuals have difficulty running, jumping from a standing position, and climbing stairs; and they may experience frequent falls (Leigh et al., 2018).

◎ Clinical Manifestations at Time of Diagnosis

SLOW ACQUISITION OF MOTOR MILESTONES
- 18 mo: start walking
- Age 2–3 yr: somewhat clumsy appearance
- Age 3–5 yr: difficulty keeping up with peers

CONSISTENT PATTERN OF WEAKNESS THAT VARIES IN RATE
- Proximal muscles weaken before distal muscles
- Legs weaken before arms
- Extensors weaken before flexors

PHYSICAL PRESENTATION
- Difficulty running, jumping from a standing position, climbing stairs
- Frequent falls
- Toe walking
- Calf and forearm pseudohypertrophy
- Positive Gowers maneuver
- Lumbar lordosis

As weakness progresses, the Achilles tendons become contracted, causing individuals to shift their weight onto the balls of their feet, a compensatory mechanism known as toe walking (Williams, 2007). Often this is associated with exaggerated lumbar lordosis. Muscles have a firm, rubbery consistency, and calf muscles appear larger (calf pseudohypertrophy) (Thangarajh et al., 2019). When asked to get up from a sitting position on the floor, males will typically get into a knee-elbow position, extend their elbows and knees, bring their hands and feet as close together as possible, and then raise their rears in the air and, using their arms as support, will "walk" their hands up their legs to get into a standing position; this movement is known as the Gowers maneuver (Thangarajh et al., 2019). If the diagnosis of DMD is suspected by the primary care provider, simple tests can be performed during the physical examination to detect proximal weakness, such as asking the child to walk on the heels, jump, run, climb stairs, and get up from the floor. Early subtle signs of weakness may also include antigravity neck weakness and preserved neck flexion strength, as seen in BMD (Suthar & Sankhyan, 2018).

TREATMENT

While there is no cure for DMD today, therapies and treatments are available to slow progression. Treatment and management plans should be individualized so that each patient may take advantage of current disease-modifying therapies, emerging therapies, and access to the standard of care. The goals of treatment for males with DMD should be consistent with optimizing the performance of daily activities, which may include the use of assistive devices to achieve independent function, maintain mobility, maintain range of motion, maximize muscle strength, and optimize cardiac and pulmonary function. The males' developmental and functional needs should determine the treatment plan. Anticipatory treatment, interventions, and recommended assessments should be considered using the five stages of Duchenne:

Stage 1: Diagnosis
Stage 2: Early ambulatory
Stage 3: Late ambulatory
Stage 4: Early nonambulatory
Stage 5: Late nonambulatory

Goals of care should be centered on a multidisciplinary approach, including specialists from the following areas: genetics, neurology, pulmonology, cardiology, nutrition, rehabilitation medicine, physical therapy, orthopedics, and neuropsychology (Birnkrant et al., 2018a).

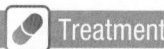 **Treatment**

THERAPIES
Physical
Occupational
Recreational
Aqua
Speech

ADAPTIVE EQUIPMENT
Orthotic devices
Customized mobility and seating

SURGERY
Achilles tendon release surgery
Posterior spinal fusion
Sedation and anesthesia precautions

RESPIRATORY DEVICES
Noninvasive positive pressure ventilation
Mechanical insufflator-exsufflator
Suction machine

PHARMACOLOGIC THERAPY
Angiotensin-converting enzyme inhibitors, beta-blockers, diuretics, digoxin to treat progressive cardiac abnormalities
Corticosteroid therapy to increase strength, performance, pulmonary function, and progression of weakness
Benefits vs. risks

THERAPIES

Physical, Occupational, Recreational, and Aqua Therapies

Because of the progressive nature of DMD, it is important for rehabilitation specialists to proactively determine ways to maximize the independence and quality of life of males with DMD (Birnkrant et al., 2018a). Physical therapy aims at maintaining the range of motion, minimizing contractures, and preserving muscle function while minimizing muscle damage. It also plays an important role in pain management (Birnkrant et al., 2018a). Stretching and passive range-of-motion exercises are often recommended; however, there is little evidence to document the exact type of physiotherapy that is most advantageous (Bushby & Straub, 2005). Proper selection of adaptive equipment optimizes independent function, minimizes complications such as skin breakdown and musculoskeletal pain, and improves the quality of life for males and their caregivers (Birnkrant et al., 2018a; Landfeldt et al., 2018).

Males with DMD should be encouraged to participate in adapted activities that enhance their quality of life and minimize muscle damage, such as adaptive sports, gardening (Birnkrant et al., 2018b), arts and crafts, chess, card games, and computer activities. Playing music, especially small wind instruments that can be held, such as the clarinet, may improve their respiratory function. Aqua therapy is especially helpful as being in water may relieve pressure on the joints and make exercises easier to perform, allowing males with DMD to move their extremities much farther and more often.

Speech Therapy

Early treatment of DMD typically includes speech therapy, as children with DMD have significantly higher rates of speech and developmental delay (Birnkrant et al., 2018a). Early initiation of speech therapy helps improve the quality of life for young children with DMD (Hinton et al., 2006; Ong et al., 2018).

ADAPTIVE EQUIPMENT

Orthotic Devices

The use of resting ankle night splints assists with providing a gentle stretch to maintain ankle range of motion and alignment, and contracture prevention is recommended to be initiated at diagnosis or early ambulatory phase. Most devices are lightweight and custom to be used overnight or while seated. These are not recommended to be worn during walking activities. In the nonambulatory phase, males may still wear braces to help maintain foot alignment and prevent contractures. As males grow and their needs for support progress, these devices will require modification to maintain proper function and fit. Most orthotic devices are recommended by a physical therapist, prescribed by a physiatrist, primary care provider, or other specialist (e.g., neurologist), and fitted for by an orthotist. Resting hand splints are considered when signs of finger or wrist tightness are noted, generally in older children or adolescents. They are custom molded by an experienced occupational therapist, physical therapist, or orthotist to provide a gentle stretch and support hand, wrist, and fingers in a neutral and flat position when at rest. They are not recommended when hands and fingers are fixed in a fisted position (PPMD, 2020).

Standing Devices

Standers can be considered in individuals who are unable to stand by themselves, have difficulty standing independently, or with loss of ambulation. There are several standing device options, including sit-to-stand, supine standers, and wheelchairs that transition to standing (PPMD, 2020). Active standing may help with bone health, but caution must be taken if muscles and joints are in poor alignment (PPMD, 2020).

Customized Mobility and Seating

By the late ambulatory phase, most males with DMD are chronically fatigued and become fully wheelchair dependent. Manual wheelchairs may be used initially, but as males become increasingly dependent, a motorized wheelchair is needed (Birnkrant et al., 2018a) and should be custom fit for each child. Motorized chairs are controlled electronically, typically by a joystick that is located near the child's dominant hand; if muscle strength in the upper extremities becomes affected, adaptations can be made for other ways to control chair movement. Wait time for a custom-built chair can be lengthy, and the process should be started as soon as the need is anticipated and before the use of a chair becomes necessary. The physical therapist and physiatrist can assist in ordering the chair and with follow-up to ensure timely delivery.

Pain should be monitored and evaluated using a multidisciplinary team approach, including physical therapy, postural correction, wheelchair modifications, and adjustments to sleeping surfaces to allow independent mobility and pressure relief (Birnkrant et al., 2018a).

SURGERY

Achilles Tendon Release Surgery

Although historically used in the 1970s (Spencer & Vignos, 1962), Achilles tendon release surgery is sometimes still performed to assist in managing contractures. If done, it needs to be considered with caution in males with DMD and combined with the use of ankle-foot orthoses. It may extend the ambulatory period by approximately 2 years, although factors such as remaining strength, motivation, and residual walking ability also play a role (Stevens, 2006). If the male is weak in ambulation with early evidence of distal muscle weakness and contractures, surgery may lead to overlengthening of the tendon and result in a further weakness (Do, 2002). With the use of standardized strength and functional outcome measures, hopefully these will help guide informative decisions of candidacy and timing of the surgical procedure.

Posterior Spinal Fusion

Posterior spinal fusion (PSF) for scoliosis in DMD has been highly effective in stabilizing the spine and maintaining seating balance and comfort. However, it does not reduce the rate of respiratory decline (Alexander et al., 2013). Corrective surgery may be considered when curves are above 35 degrees, as the likelihood of progression is high. As curves progress and function decreases, the complication rates increase, and recovery is more difficult. Growth-friendly surgical approaches have promise in young patients with larger curves but typically require a definitive PSF later and are not without complications. The uncertainty of benefits and potential risks should be discussed with families. Quality of life, functional status, respiratory function, and life expectancy should be considered when considering surgery.

Sedation and Anesthesia Precautions

A consensus statement by the American College of Chest Physicians states that males with DMD have an increased risk for complications when undergoing sedation or general anesthesia, which include potentially fatal reactions to inhaled anesthetics and certain muscle relaxants, upper airway obstruction, hypoventilation, atelectasis, congestive heart failure, cardiac dysrhythmias, respiratory failure, and difficulty weaning from mechanical ventilation (Birnkrant, 2009). A plan, including a preoperative pulmonary and cardiac evaluation, should be tailored to meet the specific needs of the patient and the surgery. Respiratory complications can occur during the postoperative period (Bushby et al., 2010), and aggressive airway clearance and extubation to positive pressure ventilation should be used to help reduce the frequency and severity of these complications.

RESPIRATORY DEVICES

Respiratory complications are common as DMD progresses, and implementation of respiratory care considerations and guidelines requires a multidisciplinary team approach. Pulmonary function testing (PFT) should begin at 5 years of age and be monitored every 6 to 12 months. Sleep studies can also aid in respiratory monitoring, especially in individuals unable to perform PFTs and monitor for sleep-disordered breathing (Birnkrant et al., 2018b).

The need for respiratory support typically occurs after loss of ambulation (Birnkrant et al., 2018b). Individuals with DMD develop an ineffective or weak cough compromising airway clearance and are at increased risk for atelectasis, pneumonia, and recurrent respiratory tract infections. A peak cough flow of less than 270 L/min and forced vital capacity (FVC) below 60% of predicted generally indicate a weak cough, with treatment consisting of mechanically assisted coughing (Birnkrant et al., 2018b). A mechanical insufflator-exsufflator device can be used when FVC is 60% predicted or less to preserve lung compliance and aid in lung volume recruitment by providing deep lung inflation once or twice daily (Birnkrant et al., 2018b). This in turn may help prevent the onset of respiratory infections such as pneumonia.

It is important to monitor for symptoms of sleep-disordered breathing, including fatigue, morning headaches, frequent nighttime awakenings, difficulty with arousal, and poor concentration. Symptoms of respiratory weakness usually begin at nighttime and are initially supported with the nocturnal use of non-invasive positive pressure ventilation (NIPPV), which allows for the entry of more air into the lungs, reduces hypoventilation, rests chronically fatigued muscles, may reduce daytime hypercapnia, allowing for recovery of inspiratory muscles. Nocturnal NIPPV should be considered when a patient's FVC approaches less than 50% predicted (Birnkrant et al., 2018b) and/or findings of sleep-disordered breathing. In DMD, hypoxemia is usually a sign of hypoventilation, and use of oxygen should be in junction with NIPPV and close monitoring of CO_2 levels (Birnkrant et al., 2018b). With disease progression, the use of NIPPV extends to the daytime. Mouthpiece ventilation (MPV) can be an option for daytime ventilatory support and can be mounted directly to a powered wheelchair. However, this can be a safety concern if the individual has limited function to independently access MPV. The use of noninvasive methods for assisted ventilation is preferred; however, indications for tracheostomy include patient preference, inability to use noninvasive ventilation effectively or failure to prevent recurrent aspiration/pneumonia, and inability to extubate (Birnkrant et al., 2018b).

Ideally, a pulmonologist should manage the respiratory complications of DMD, although in some instances the primary care provider may be involved and should be knowledgeable about commonly used devices. The settings of respiratory equipment should be monitored by a respiratory therapist who is knowledgeable in neuromuscular diseases and can educate families on the proper use of these devices.

PHARMACOLOGIC THERAPY

Cardiac

Electrocardiogram (ECG) and echocardiogram should be performed regularly to check for evidence of cardiomyopathy. CMR is the noninvasive imaging of choice but may not be feasible for younger individuals (Birnkrant et al., 2018b). A National Heart, Lung, and Blood Institute expert working group recommended the use of angiotensin-converting enzyme inhibitors (ACEIs) or angiotensin receptor blockers in DMD by 10 years of age, barring contraindications (McNally et al., 2015). Early treatment with an ACEI in asymptomatic patients with normal left ventricular systolic

function can improve long-term cardiac outcomes (Birnkrant et al., 2018b). Regardless of age, if abnormal cardiac findings occur, including myocardial fibrosis, depressed left ventricular function, or abnormal imaging studies (CMR or echocardiogram), pharmacologic therapy should be initiated (Birnkrant et al., 2018b). In general, treatment strategies are similar to traditional heart failure management due to the lack of dystrophin-targeted cardiac therapies (Birnkrant et al., 2018b). There is some evidence a mineralocorticoid receptor antagonist (eplerenone) reduced circumferential strain (Birnkrant et al., 2018b). However, further studies are warranted to evaluate the effectiveness (Birnkrant et al., 2018b).

CORTICOSTEROID THERAPY

Prednisone and deflazacort are both corticosteroids used in the treatment of DMD to reduce muscle inflammation and slow disease progression, reduce the risk of scoliosis, and potentially slow the decline of pulmonary and cardiac function (Bushby et al., 2010). Practice parameters regarding corticosteroid treatment of DMD set forth by a subcommittee of the American Academy of Neurology suggest that daily corticosteroid treatment with prednisone should be offered to improve muscle strength and pulmonary function, reduce the need for scoliosis surgery, and delay the onset of cardiomyopathy onset by 18 years of age. The preferred dosing regimen of prednisone is 0.75 mg/kg/day, with a risk of significant side effects, including excessive weight gain, hirsutism, and cushingoid appearance. Although no long-term data exist, over a 12-month period, prednisone 10 mg/kg/weekend is equally effective (Gloss et al., 2016). Both prednisone (0.75 mg/kg/day) and deflazacort (0.9 mg/kg/day) significantly slow the disease process and functional loss in males with DMD (Fox et al., 2020). Deflazacort may be associated with an increased risk of developing cataracts than prednisone (Gloss et al., 2016). Deflazacort received US Food and Drug Administration (FDA) approval for the treatment of DMD in 2016 (Hoffman, 2020). Several comparison studies have demonstrated the superiority of deflazacort vs. prednisone, including a slower functional decline over a 48-week period in patients treated with deflazacort compared to prednisone (McDonald et al., 2020). However, insurance will often not approve the use of deflazacort without a demonstrated failure to prednisone, including excessive weight gain and intolerable behavioral concerns.

Steroid treatment is not without side effects. Males with DMD on long-term corticosteroid therapy have a significantly decreased risk of scoliosis and an increase of 3 or more years of independent ambulation, yet they are also at an increased risk of vertebral and lower limb fractures (Fox et al., 2020). The primary care provider must monitor males receiving steroid therapy carefully for weight gain, growth suppression, hypertension, cushingoid appearance, skin changes (e.g., acne, hirsutism, hyperpigmentation, skin thinning, striae), altered behavior, osteoporosis leading to vertebral fracture, and cataracts (Guglieri et al., 2017). Many parents and health care providers believe that the benefits of corticosteroid treatment outweigh the adverse effects.

EXON SKIPPING THERAPIES

The first approved exon skipping therapy was approved by the FDA in September 2016, targeting 13% of males with DMD who have a genetic change in the dystrophin gene that is amenable to exon 51 skipping (Birnkrant et al., 2018a). Exon skipping is disease-modifying therapy that converts out-of-frame to in-frame deletions to produce a shortened or truncated partially functional dystrophin protein rather than a nonfunctional one. In an in-frame deletion, the reading frame is preserved, allowing for production of a partially functional dystrophin protein, although it may be shorter than normal, producing a milder phenotype (Becker MD). An out-of-frame deletion disrupts the reading frame completely and does not allow for dystrophin production resulting in a more severe phenotype (DMD). It is important to note there are always exceptions to the reading frame rule, and sometimes frame deletions can cause a more severe phenotype. Exon skipping therapies are mutation-specific therapies.

Ataluren is approved in the European Union and Brazil for the treatment of DMD in ambulatory males age 2 years and older with a nonsense mutation in the dystrophin gene. It is aimed at producing a full-length, functional dystrophin protein, targeting 11% of males with DMD having a nonsense mutation, which serves to prematurely stop the translation of the dystrophin gene. This treatment allows the ribosome to read through stop-codon and produce dystrophin yet still obey normal signals to stop translation. The FDA has rejected the drug approval, pending further data. The advantage of this treatment is that it is a small molecule that can be easily swallowed in pill form, and there is a large margin between an effective and toxic dose, allowing for the feasible delivery of a safe and effective dose.

COMPLEMENTARY AND ALTERNATIVE MEDICINE

Complementary and alternative medicine (CAM) use is common in the management of Duchenne and Becker muscular dystrophies, noted in Muscular Dystrophy Surveillance, Tracking and Research Network (MD STARnet), with an estimated reported use of 80% of families using CAM for their children (Zhu et al., 2014). The most frequently reported uses of CAM therapies include aqua therapy, prayer and/or blessing, special diet, and massage, with aqua therapy and special diet being the most recommended by health care providers. Additional reported uses of CAM therapies include supplemental vitamins, massage, chiropractic manipulation, hippotherapy, companion animals, acupuncture, and homeopathy (Zhu et al., 2014).

ANTICIPATED ADVANCES IN DIAGNOSIS AND MANAGEMENT

The most current and updated clinical trial treatments for DMD are available at ClinicalTrials.gov. Strategies under development include drugs targeting restoring or replacing dystrophin (gene therapy, GalGT2, Dup2, CRISPR/Cas9), exon skipping (second-generation antisense oligonucleotides), and nonsense mutation read-through (small molecules) (McNally et al., 2015). There are also several therapies looking at the treatment of downstream effects due to a lack of dystrophin, including combatting fibrosis, reducing inflammation, regulating calcium balance, improving muscle growth and protection, restoring cell energy, and improving pulmonary and cardiac function (McNally et al., 2015).

A potential challenge in finding a cure is the fact that not all affected individuals have the same mutation, and thus the same strategies may not be beneficial for everyone. Despite these challenges, it is reasonable to expect that the next decade will see great advances in the field of treatment for DMD.

ASSOCIATED PROBLEMS OF DUCHENNE MUSCULAR DYSTROPHY AND TREATMENT

Secondary problems associated with DMD usually result from increasing muscle weakness as males grow older and the disease progresses.

Associated Problems
Duchenne Muscular Dystrophy and Treatment

- Pulmonary effects
- Weakened cough
- Respiratory insufficiency
- Respiratory tract infections
- Sleep-related disturbances
- Cardiac dysfunction
- Cardiomyopathy
- Cognitive impairments
- Lower than average IQ
- Deficient immediate verbal memory skills
- Language impairments
- Motor impairment
- Contractures and gait changes
- Scoliosis
- Osteoporosis and fractures
- Feeding and swallowing difficulties
- Obesity
- Weight gain caused by limited movement or corticosteroid therapy
- Constipation
- Decubitus ulcers
- Psychosocial and behavioral issues
- Distractibility and poor attention span
- Low frustration threshold
- Features of obsessive-compulsive behavior
- Anxiety
- Depression

PULMONARY EFFECTS

Pulmonary complications are a major cause of morbidity and mortality in patients with DMD (Birnkrant et al., 2018b). Common complications include diaphragmatic muscle weakness, mucous plugging, atelectasis, pneumonia, and chronic and acute respiratory failure (Birnkrant et al., 2018b). An anticipatory approach to the monitoring of respiratory muscle function using the stages of Duchenne can be a helpful approach to the management of pulmonary care (Birnkrant et al., 2018b). In the ambulatory stage, serial monitoring of pulmonary function, starting at age 5 to 6 years, is imperative for pulmonary care (Birnkrant et al., 2018b). Generally, the FVC rises with growth until the patient becomes nonambulatory, followed by a plateau and then a decline over time (Birnkrant et al., 2018b). An earlier loss of ambulation is associated with a lower peak FVC and a more rapid decline in FVC compared with a later loss of ambulation (Birnkrant et al., 2018b). Sleep studies should be considered during this stage if they are unable to perform spirometry or if symptoms develop concerning sleep-disordered breathing (Birnkrant et al., 2018b) with the loss of ambulation, vital capacity decreases development of stiff, noncompliant chest walls, and lung volume restriction. Mechanical insufflation-exsufflation is recommended to provide deep lung inflation as FVC approaches 60% predicted or less (Birnkrant et al., 2018b). In the late nonambulatory stage, assisted ventilation is needed and should be initiated with signs or symptoms of hypoventilation or sleep-disordered breathing. Some individuals remained asymptomatic in the presence of hypoventilation, and assisted ventilation should be considered when a patient's FVC is less than 50% (Birnkrant et al., 2018b). Hypoxemia in DMD is often due to hypoventilation, atelectasis, or pneumonia, and supplemental oxygen should be used in conjunction with assisted ventilation and assisted coughing (Birnkrant et al., 2018b). Assisted ventilation is often extended to daytime use in individuals experiencing symptoms of hypoventilation, including dyspnea, fatigue, and difficulty concentrating (Birnkrant et al., 2018b). Patients on continuous ventilation that provides life support should have a backup ventilator in case of malfunction of the primary ventilator (Birnkrant et al., 2018b).

CARDIAC DYSFUNCTION

Cardiac complications are a leading cause of morbidity and mortality in patients with DMD due to a lack of dystrophin in the heart and are characterized by progressive dilated cardiomyopathy, leading to heart failure, cardiac insufficiency, cardiac fibrosis, conduction abnormalities, and sudden cardiac death (Duan et al., 2021). Certain data suggest glucocorticoids slow the development of cardiomyopathy (Annexstad et al., 2014). In the ambulatory and early nonambulatory stages, patients should have annual cardiac assessments, including ECG and noninvasive imaging. CMR is the noninvasive imaging modality of choice in patients who do not require anesthesia (Birnkrant et al., 2018b). Echocardiography is recommended until age 6 to 7 years or until CMR can be done without anesthesia. The risk of left ventricular dysfunction increases after the age of 10 years and is often asymptomatic. In the late nonambulatory stage, myocardial fibrosis leads to ventricular dysfunction and may require more frequent monitoring. Common symptoms of heart failure, including fatigue, weight loss, vomiting, abdominal pain, sleep disturbance, and inability to tolerate daily activities, are often unrecognized due to immobility (Birnkrant et al., 2018b). Annual Holter monitoring has been recommended in patients with abnormal ventricular function or myocardial fibrosis (Birnkrant et al., 2018b).

COGNITIVE IMPAIRMENTS

Approximately one-third of males with DMD have a nonprogressive cognitive impairment (Annexstad et al., 2014). The average intelligence quotient (IQ) of males with DMD falls approximately 1 SD lower than the population means (Annexstad et al., 2014). Cognitive profiles in DMD demonstrate an increased risk of attention-deficit/hyperactivity disorder (ADHD), autism spectrum disorders, obsessive-compulsive traits, epilepsy, and specific reading, language, and learning disabilities (Annexstad et al., 2014). There is increasing interest in genotype-phenotype correlations and neurodevelopmental disorders, and the role disruption of different dystrophin isoforms may play in brain development and function (Ricotti et al., 2016). Deletions affecting the expression of either the Dp140 or Dp71 isoforms of the dystrophin gene that may be related to cognitive impairment vs. those that spared disruption of the Dp140 isoform demonstrated higher cognitive and language comprehension (Connolly et al., 2013).

MOTOR IMPAIRMENT

As outlined previously, there are five stages of Duchenne; these stages characterize the well-known pattern of progressive weakness and corresponding management needs. Standardized functional assessments specific to DMD and other neuromuscular conditions should be used to monitor clinical progression, assist with the prediction of upcoming strength and functional changes to help guide proactive care, and assess response to treatment therapies (Birnkrant et al., 2018b). During the late ambulatory, early nonambulatory, and late nonambulatory phases, males with DMD lose skeletal muscle strength, function, and endurance and develop multifocal contractures (Ohlendieck and Sawndulla, 2021). Males with DMD begin using a waddling (Trendelenburg) gait (Birnkrant et al., 2018b). Waddling caused by weakness of the gluteus media and maximus and subsequent inability to support a single leg stance and weakness of the quadriceps requires that forward motion be propagated by circumducting each leg and leaning forward toward the opposite side to maintain balance (Do, 2002). With disease progression, contractures of the hip flexors, knee flexors, and plantar flexors will develop (Stevens, 2006). Daily stretching exercises and proper bracing should be utilized (Birnkrant et al., 2018b).

SCOLIOSIS

Inspection of the spine should be included at each clinical visit. Spine radiographs should be obtained every 6 months in patients who are skeletally immature once a curve is detected and annually in skeletally mature individuals. A referral should be placed to an orthopedic surgeon for all curves measuring 20 degrees or more (Birnkrant et al., 2018b). A PSF is recommended in nonambulatory patients who have a spinal curve measuring greater than 20 to 30 degrees, are steroid naïve due to a high risk of progression, and have not reached puberty (Birnkrant et al., 2018b). Steroid-treated patients can also develop scoliosis with more variable progression and should be monitored closely for clear evidence of progression (Birnkrant et al., 2018b). PSF can improve sitting tolerance, reduce pain, and improve quality of life (Birnkrant et al., 2018b).

OSTEOPOROSIS AND FRACTURES

Vertebral compression fractures are frequent manifestations of osteoporosis, and those treated with long-term corticosteroid therapy should receive regular spinal imaging regardless of symptoms (Birnkrant et al., 2018b). Patients with the earliest signs of bone fragility should be referred to endocrinology for bone health management (Birnkrant et al., 2018b). It is important to ensure adequate intake of calcium and vitamin D supplementation.

FEEDING AND SWALLOWING DIFFICULTIES

Swallowing dysfunction (dysphagia) is common, particularly during the advanced stages of the disease related to muscle weakness, and anticipatory assessments should be done routinely (Birnkrant et al., 2018a). Individuals with concerns of dysphagia on screening should be referred to a speech-language pathologist, an occupational therapist, or a swallowing team for a clinical feeding and swallowing evaluation. A videofluoroscopic swallowing study or fiberoptic evaluation of swallowing to assist in the diagnosis and management should be performed (Birnkrant et al., 2018a). Unintentional weight loss may be a sign of respiratory insufficiency, cardiomyopathy, or dysphagia.

OBESITY

Excessive weight gain in children with neuromuscular conditions can be multifactorial and include excessive caloric intake, reduced energy expenditure in the setting of a child with limited mobility, and corticosteroid related in patients with DMD. A proactive, comprehensive nutritional plan discussed at each visit should include recommendations for the required intake of fluids, calories, proteins, and micronutrients. Subsequent close monitoring following the initiation of corticosteroids is recommended. The impact of obesity in DMD impacts clinical outcomes, including the risk of fractures and obstructive sleep apnea (OSA) at a younger age (Billich et al., 2022).

CONSTIPATION

Constipation, defined as hard stools or reduced frequency of bowel movements, is a common gastrointestinal (GI) complication in this population of children. Reduced fluid and/or fiber intake, immobility, and slowed intestinal motility are potential causes of constipation. Management of constipation may include modifying the diet, increasing water intake, and the use of medications such as osmotic laxatives or stimulants.

DECUBITUS ULCERS

Skin problems may arise when bony prominences rub against surfaces because of positioning in chairs or beds. Decubitus ulcers can occur quickly, and vigilant skin management is necessary. Frequent repositioning, especially at nighttime, should be done to prophylactically prevent the development of pressure sores, and bony prominences should be protected with soft coverings. Medical attention should be sought as soon as any skin breakdown is detected.

PSYCHOSOCIAL CARE

Psychosocial support should be provided by a mental health clinician throughout the lifespan of patients and family members due to the increased risk of depression and anxiety, particularly at major transition points in the progression of their disease (Birnkrant et al., 2018a). Mental health screening, addressing suicidality, and quality of life should be monitored at each neuromuscular clinic visit (Birnkrant et al., 2018a). Standard evidence-based care guidelines should be followed in the treatment of psychological disorders (Birnkrant et al., 2018a). Individuals with DMD should have a comprehensive neuropsychological assessment to evaluate the following domains: cognition, attention, executive functions, memory, academic achievement, language skills, fine motor skills, visual-motor integration, visual processing, emotional and behavioral functions, and adaptive functions. Determining neuropsychological strengths and needs can help with daily planning and educational planning and provide beneficial information to patients and family members.

PROGNOSIS

Advances in supportive care, corticoid steroid use, and emerging disease-modifying therapies have changed the natural history of the disease, with most individuals with DMD surviving into adulthood (Thangarajh et al., 2019). This further highlights the need for high-quality, coordinated multidisciplinary neuromuscular care in individuals with DMD. Most affected individuals eventually succumb to respiratory complications or cardiopulmonary issues. Palliative care can be beneficial throughout the lifespan to aid in medical decision making and support.

PRIMARY CARE MANAGEMENT

HEALTH CARE MAINTENANCE

Growth and Development

Most individuals with DMD experience normal growth and development in the early ambulatory stage, but the rate of growth likely will be altered as males become increasingly limited in physical activity, after the initiation of corticosteroid therapy, and as muscle mass declines with disease progression into the late ambulatory and early nonambulatory stages of DMD. There have been several studies demonstrating that regardless of steroid therapy, males with DMD are shorter compared to a typical male child, with distal deletions of the dystrophin gene being more frequently associated with short stature (Salera et al., 2017). Good nutritional status is defined as weight for length or body mass index (BMI) that falls between the 10th and 85th percentiles (Birnkrant et al., 2018a). The use of standardized growth charts can be misleading due to individuals with DMD having altered body composition (Birnkrant et al., 2018a). Primary care providers should monitor linear growth at every visit with the appropriate measurement devices and plot weight, length or height, head circumference, and weight-for-length or BMI (when appropriate). Standing height should be used in ambulatory males and plotted on a standardized growth curve (Birnkrant et al., 2018a). Assessment of height in nonambulatory individuals can include using ulnar length, segmental height, or arm span, which requires specialized training and has not been validated in DMD. Impaired growth is considered if there is a downward crossing of height percentiles, height velocity of less than 4 cm/year, or height below the 3rd percentile and should be referred to an endocrinologist (Birnkrant et al., 2018a).

It is important that anthropomorphic measurements be assessed as accurately as possible, especially as the disease progresses. In the rare instance that an infant or small male presents with DMD, weight should be measured using an electronic digital infant scale. During the early and late ambulatory stages, from ages 2 to 10 years, males should stand on a scale to be weighed if they are able to stand independently. For males who are unable to stand independently

but can easily be held by a caregiver, the caregiver's weight should be subtracted from the total. Starting at age 10 to 12 years, in the early nonambulatory stage, when a male with DMD becomes fully dependent on a wheelchair, he should be weighed in his chair by rolling onto the platform of a digital electronic scale. The first time this is done, the male should be weighed in his chair and then safely transferred onto a stationary chair while the wheelchair is weighed independently; the weight of the chair should then be subtracted from the total weight. The chair weight should be recorded in the male's chart for future use. The provider should remove any excess baggage or cushions from the chair and should ask if any modifications have been made to the chair at every visit.

Delayed puberty and hypogonadism are potential complications of glucocorticoid therapy and can often cause physiologic distress and impair quality of life (Birnkrant et al., 2018a). Physical assessment of pubertal status should be performed every 6 months, starting at 9 years of age (Birnkrant et al., 2018a). A referral to an endocrinologist should be made if there is an absence of pubertal development by 14 years of age (Birnkrant et al., 2018a).

Diet

A decrease in energy expenditure should be considered when calculating the daily caloric needs of males with DMD in the late ambulatory and nonambulatory stages. Males with DMD require fewer calories compared with typical male children (80% of the recommended caloric intake for healthy children in ambulatory males and 70% in nonambulatory males) (Bianchi et al., 2011). Therefore caloric intake recommendations should be individualized based on physical activity and ambulation status (Bianchi et al., 2011). The greatest risk of excessive weight gain occurs during the preteen and teenage years, late ambulatory and early nonambulatory stages, with weight loss and undernourishment being more prevalent in the late nonambulatory stage (Salera et al., 2017). A dietitian should be involved in the routine care of males with DMD. The following can be used to estimate energy needs:

- For infants: Recommended dietary allowance (RDA) range for age is generally appropriate.
  Begin with an estimate at the low end of RDA for age and adjust as needed based on feeding history and growth parameters.
- To predict resting energy expenditure (REE) in steroid-treated ambulatory males with DMD (age 10–14 years): Schofield weight equation (1985), $REE = 17.7 \times wt + 657$ (multiply by the activity factor [AF] to determine energy needs) (Schofield, 1985). Predicting resting energy expenditure in males with DMD (Elliott et al., 2012).
- To predict REE in nonambulatory males with DMD: $(REE \times 0.8) \times AF$.

Primary care providers should use clinical judgment in determining caloric needs and helping patients maintain a healthy weight and should consult with a nutritionist when necessary. Healthy food choices, portion control, limiting calorie-containing drinks, and selecting low-sodium foods should also be part of nutritional planning, and adjustments should then be tailored to meet individual nutritional needs throughout the course of the disease.

Safety
Young individuals with DMD initially may not be restricted in physical activity but should be adequately supervised, and normal safety precautions should be taken. As muscle weakness progresses and gait changes ensue, individuals with DMD may experience unexpected falls. Thus extra precautions should be taken regarding bath and playground safety. Both the home and school environment should be kept safe and clear from objects on the floor and sharp edges and corners to safeguard against injurious falls. When an individual becomes wheelchair dependent, the home and school environment should be made wheelchair accessible. An adapted car seat with additional neck support or a wheelchair-accessible vehicle with tie-downs will become necessary to ensure safety while traveling. Home and school emergency plans should be made to accommodate a wheelchair, and local police and fire departments should be alerted to facilitate safety during an emergency.

Immunizations
Unless specifically contraindicated, immunizations for healthy children, as recommended by the American Academy of Pediatrics (AAP), should be given to children with chronic conditions (AAP, 2021), such as DMD. Intramuscular (IM) injections should be given in the locations normally recommended for age, using a needle long enough to reach the muscle when possible. In males with DMD with decreased muscle mass, IM injections should be given in the best available muscle, according to AAP guidelines.

Males with DMD have cardiorespiratory involvement and are at increased risk for complications of influenza, varicella, COVID-19, and pneumococcal infection. Annual immunization with inactivated influenza vaccine is recommended for males with DMD 6 months of age and older, following the Centers for Disease Control and Prevention (CDC) guidelines (AAP, 2021). Primary care providers should also encourage all family members and household contacts to be immunized as well. Given the risk for pulmonary disease, males should be immunized with 13-valent pneumococcal conjugate (PCV-13) before age 2 years, and males age 2 years and older should receive a 23-valent pneumococcal polysaccharide vaccine (PPSV-23) as recommended for age and immunization status (AAP, 2021).

Prior to the start of corticosteroid treatment, live attenuated vaccine series should be completed. For younger children receiving systemic corticosteroid therapy, 2 mg/kg/day or more of prednisone or 2.4 mg/kg/day or more of deflazacort are immunosuppressed. Older children receiving 20 mg/day or more of prednisone or 24 mg/day or more of deflazacort are considered immunosuppressed and should not receive live attenuated vaccines (McNally et al., 2015). Additionally, those on chronic steroids who are considered immunosuppressed should follow the CDC recommendations for moderate or severely immunocompromised COVID-19 vaccine schedule, including boosters, as recommendations differ.

Screening Considerations
Vision. Routine screening is recommended for males with DMD. Males on steroid therapy should be monitored annually by a pediatric ophthalmologist due to a higher risk of developing cataracts and proliferative retinopathy (Birnkrant et al., 2018a).

Hearing. Standardized hearing screening is recommended (Birnkrant et al., 2018a).

Dental. Early and routine dental screening is recommended (Birnkrant et al., 2018a). DMD affects orofacial function, structure, and risk of development of malocclusion (Papaefthymiou et al., 2022). Macroglossia is also a common finding among individuals with DMD and can lead to the development of an open bite and interferences between the posterior dentition (Papaefthymiou et al., 2022). An enlarged tongue can also contribute to worsening dental malocclusion, changing the appearance of the face, and causing more difficulties with chewing (PPMD, 2020).

Cardiovascular risk factors. Blood pressure should be measured at every visit because of possible hypertension resulting from corticosteroid therapy; family history should be updated annually, and screening for hypercholesterolemia (Birnkrant et al., 2018b).

Transition
With the emergence of disease-modifying therapies and advances in cardiorespiratory and supportive care, males with DMD are living into adulthood. It is imperative to implement a well-coordinated transition program to help navigate complex health care needs, improve health-related outcomes, and ensure a successful transition into adulthood. Utilizing the DMD transition toolkit will assist in assessing transition readiness, tracking longitudinal progress and transition goals, and ensuring all components of transition are addressed (Trout et al., 2018).

Condition-Specific Screening
For a summary of comprehensive care of individuals with DMD, see Fig. 31.1.

	Stage 1: At diagnosis	Stage 2: Early ambulatory	Stage 3: Late ambulatory	Stage 4: Early non-ambulatory	Stage 5: Late non-ambulatory
Neuromuscular management	Lead the multidisciplinary clinic; advise on new therapies; provide patient and family support, education, and genetic counselling				
	Ensure immunisation schedule is complete	Assess function, strength, and range of movement at least every 6 months to define stage of disease			
	Discuss use of glucocorticosteroids	Initiate and manage use of glucocorticosteroids			
	Refer female carriers to cardiologist				Help navigate end-of-life care
Rehabilitation management	Provide comprehensive multidisciplinary assessments, including standardised assessments, at least every 6 months				
	Provide direct treatment by physical and occupational therapists, and speech-language pathologists, based on assessments and individualised to the patient				
	Assist in prevention of contracture or deformity, overexertion, and falls; promote energy conservation and appropriate exercise or activity; provide orthoses, equipment, and learning support		Continue all previous measures; provide mobility devices, seating, supported standing devices, and assistive technology; assist in pain and fracture prevention or management; advocate for funding, access, participation, and self-actualisation into adulthood		
Endocrine management	Measure standing height every 6 months				
	Assess non-standing growth every 6 months				
		Assess pubertal status every 6 months starting by age 9 years			
		Provide family education and stress dose steroid prescription if on glucocorticosteroids			
Gastrointestinal and nutritional management	Include assessment by registered dietitian nutritionist at clinic visits (every 6 months); initiate obesity prevention strategies; monitor for overweight and underweight, especially during critical transition periods				
	Provide annual assessments of serum 25-hydroxyvitamin D and calcium intake				
		Assess swallowing dysfunction, constipation, gastro-oesophageal reflux disease, and gastroparesis every 6 months			
		Initiate annual discussion of gastrostomy tube as part of usual care			
Respiratory management		Provide spirometry teaching and sleep studies as needed (low risk of problems)		Assess respiratory function at least every 6 months	
	Ensure immunisations are up to date: pneumococcal vaccines and yearly inactivated influenza vaccine				
				Initiate use of lung volume recruitment	
				Begin assisted cough and nocturnal ventilation	
					Add daytime ventilation
Cardiac management	Consult cardiologist; assess with electrocardiogram and echocardiogram* or cardiac MRI†	Assess cardiac function annually; initiate ACE inhibitors or angiotensin receptor blockers by age 10 years	Assess cardiac function at least annually, more often if symptoms or abnormal imaging are present; monitor for rhythm abnormalities		
			Use standard heart failure interventions with deterioration of function		
Bone health management		Assess with lateral spine x-rays (patients on glucocorticosteroids: every 1-2 years; patients not on glucocorticosteroids: every 2-3 years)			
		Refer to bone health expert at the earliest sign of fracture (Genant grade 1 or higher vertebral fracture or first long-bone fracture)			
Orthopaedic management	Assess range of motion at least every 6 months				
		Monitor for scoliosis annually		Monitor for scoliosis every 6 months	
	Refer for orthopaedic surgery if needed (rarely necessary)	Refer for surgery on foot and Achilles tendon to improve gait in selected situations		Consider intervention for foot position for wheelchair positioning; initiate intervention with posterior spinal fusion in defined situations	
Psychosocial management	Assess mental health of patient and family at every clinic visit and provide ongoing support				
	Provide neuropsychological evaluation/interventions for learning, emotional, and behavioural problems				
		Assess educational needs and available resources (individualised education programme, 504 plan); assess vocational support needs for adults			
		Promote age-appropriate independence and social development			
Transitions	Engage in optimistic discussions about the future, expecting life into adulthood	Foster goal setting and future expectations for adult life; assess readiness for transition (by age 12 years)	Initiate transition planning for health care, education, employment, and adult living (by age 13–14 years); monitor progress at least annually; enlist care coordinator or social worker for guidance and monitoring		
			Provide transition support and anticipatory guidance about health changes		

Fig. 31.1 **Summary of comprehensive care of individuals with Duchenne muscular dystrophy.** (From Birnkrant, D.J., Bushby, K., Bann, C.M., Apkon, S.D., Blackwell, A., Brumbaugh, D., Case, L.E., Clemens, P.R., Hadjiyannakis, S., Pandya, S., Street, N., Tomezsko, J., Wagner, K.R., Ward, L.M., Weber, D.R., DMD Care Considerations Working Group. [2018]. Diagnosis and management of Duchenne muscular dystrophy, part 1: Diagnosis, and neuromuscular, rehabilitation, endocrine, and gastrointestinal and nutritional management. *Lancet Neurology*, 17(3), 251–267.)

Pulmonary function testing. Spirometry to measure FVC should be part of the regular assessment of all individuals with DMD, starting at age 5 to 6 years (Birnkrant et al., 2018b). Additional measures should include maximum inspiratory pressure/maximum expiratory pressure (MIP/MEP), peak cough flow (PCF), saturation of peripheral oxygen (SpO_2), and partial pressure of end-tidal carbon dioxide ($PetCO_2$)/transcutaneous carbon dioxide partial pressure ($PtcCO_2$). An anticipatory approach to management should be implemented to help guide interventions with the possibility that therapy may be started at an earlier age (Birnkrant et al., 2018b). In the ambulatory phase, spirometry should be measured at least annually and twice yearly in the early nonambulatory and late nonambulatory stages (Birnkrant et al., 2018b).

Polysomnography. Sleep studies with capnography should be performed at any stage with symptoms of sleep-disordered breathing and as often as annually in the nonambulatory stage. It may also be helpful in patients with cognitive impairment who are unable to perform reliable PFT or for preoperative surgical planning (Birnkrant et al., 2018a).

Cardiac. In the ambulatory and early nonambulatory stages, the cardiac assessment includes noninvasive cardiac imaging, with CMR being the imaging modality of choice in individuals who can cooperate (Birnkrant et al., 2018b). Therefore echocardiography should be performed until age 6 to 7 years or until CMR can be performed without anesthesia (Birnkrant et al., 2018b). Cardiac assessments, including ECG and noninvasive imaging, should be performed at least annually and prior to major surgical procedures, with an increase in the frequency of assessments at the discretion of the cardiologist when abnormalities are identified (Birnkrant et al., 2018b).

Endocrine. Lateral thoracolumbar spine radiograph is recommended every 1 to 2 years on steroids and every 2 to 3 years not on steroids to evaluate for vertebral compression fractures (Birnkrant et al., 2018a).

Orthopedic. A spine radiograph is recommended at the loss of ambulation or if a visual inspection is unhelpful. Spine radiographs every 6 months in skeletally immature once the curve has been identified and annually in skeletally mature individuals (Birnkrant et al., 2018b).

Gastrointestinal problems. GI symptoms in males with DMD are thought to be caused by the malfunction of the smooth muscle lining in the GI tract (Salera et al., 2017). Caregivers should carefully monitor the frequency and consistency of stools, straining efforts associated with bowel movements, and evidence of abdominal distention associated with constipation. Constipation can be managed by the primary care provider or a gastroenterologist knowledgeable in neuromuscular disorders either nutritionally or pharmacologically (or both). The development of complications from chronic constipation, such as urinary symptoms, fecal impaction, hemorrhoids, and colonic dysmotility, should be carefully assessed by the primary care provider, and a referral to a gastroenterologist should be made if the provider suspects a GI complication. Common GI complications are delayed gastric emptying, gastroesophageal reflux, chronic constipation, and gastric and intestinal dilation from air swallowing due to chronic ventilation (i.e., gastric bloat) (Salera et al., 2017).

PAIN MANAGEMENT

Pain management is an important aspect of care for individuals with DMD because it has an impact on mobility, school performance, recreational activities, and overall quality of life. Common injury-related pain occurs from exercise sprains or falls; condition-related pain is caused by abnormal posture or gait, injury secondary to instability due to severe weakness, muscle cramping and contractures, possible nerve impingement, or pressure areas resulting from prolonged use of wheelchair. Pain is usually effectively managed by the primary care provider, but if it becomes severe or seemingly unmanageable, then referral to a pain management team may be warranted.

The primary care provider should offer a medical home that is accessible, family centered, continuous, comprehensive, coordinated, compassionate, and culturally sensitive for individuals with DMD (Birnkrant et al., 2018a). The goal of the primary care provider is to offer primary care for individuals with DMD, including immunizations, nutrition management, dental care, safety counseling, monitoring of adrenal insufficiency, psychosocial care, and anticipatory guidance of potential interventions before acute medical crises (Birnkrant et al., 2018a).

EMERGENCY MANAGEMENT

Respiratory Status

Individuals with DMD are at high risk for acute respiratory complications when nonambulatory and have a baseline FVC less than 50% predicted. Sparing cardiac findings, hypoxemia is often related to mucous plugging and/or hypoventilation due to impaired cough and restrictive lung physiology (Birnkrant et al., 2018b). Treatment should be focused on treating the underlying cause, including frequent use of assisted cough therapy, noninvasive ventilation, and suction (Birnkrant et al., 2018b). Hypoxemia should not be treated with oxygen alone due to the risk of hypercapnia (Birnkrant et al., 2018b). A chest x-ray should be obtained to evaluate for aspiration, atelectasis, and/or pneumonia (Birnkrant et al., 2018b).

Cardiac

Cardiomyopathy is the leading cause of death in individuals with DMD and is more common in the second decade of life, often presenting with subtle symptoms due to immobility (Birnkrant et al., 2018b). Common symptoms may include tachycardia, abdominal pain, a history of decreased appetite, edema, orthopnea, and unexplained weight loss (Birnkrant et al., 2018b). Patients with DMD presenting to the emergency department with acute chest pain, elevated cardiac

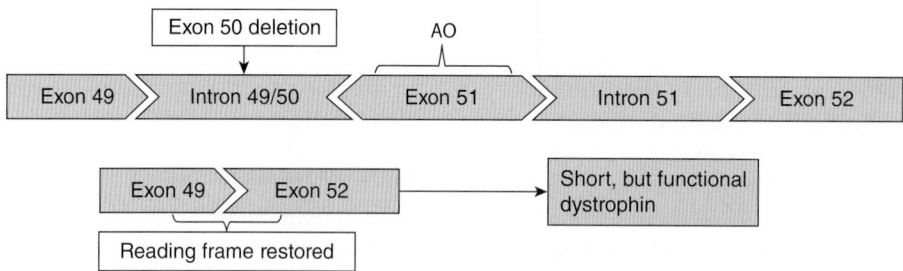

Fig. 31.2 Specialists involved in multidisciplinary care.

biomarkers, and ECG changes consistent with myocardial ischemia and reduced left ventricular systolic function by echocardiogram may be due to cardiomyopathy disease progression (Al Hajri et al., 2022).

Orthopedic

Individuals with DMD who present with respiratory distress, hypoxemia, and a history of recent long bone fracture, orthopedic surgery, or significant soft tissue injury, fat embolism syndrome should be considered (Birnkrant et al., 2018b).

Endocrine

Individuals treated with chronic use of systemic steroids should not stop medication therapy abruptly and should receive stress dose steroids during periods of illness, concerns of fracture, and surgery procedures due to the risk for adrenal insufficiency. Stress steroid dosing should be given. Treatment with hydrocortisone in a dose of 50 mg intravenous (IV)/IM for children younger than 2 years and 100 mg IV/IM for children/adults 2 years and older. Stress dosing with hydrocortisone should be continued at a dose of 50 to 100 mg/m² of body surface area/day divided every 4 to 6 hours until the illness has resolved. The PJ Nicholoff Steroid Protocol provides a protocol for managing adrenal suppression, including symptoms of acute adrenal crisis, prevention with stress dose regimens, corticosteroid dose equivalences, and how to taper doses after emergency care (Kinnett & Noritz, 2017).

Gastrointestinal

Complaints of abdominal pain are a common presenting illness to the emergency department in individuals with DMD. It is important to be able to differentiate between symptoms related to heart failure vs. fecal impaction, colonic dysmotility, gastroesophageal reflux disease, or other potential etiologies.

Anesthesia

Individuals with DMD are at risk for potential rhabdomyolysis and fatal hyperkalemia (Birnkrant et al., 2018). Succinylcholine is contraindicated, and a total IV technique should be used; also avoid inhalational anesthetics (Birnkrant et al., 2018a). Nitrous oxide

used during dental procedures is considered safe by an observant dentist (PPMD, 2020). Individuals with DMD are at risk for hypoventilation and apnea during anesthesia, and the use of assisted ventilation may be warranted in selected individuals during induction, maintenance, and recovery from sedation and anesthesia (Birnkrant et al., 2018a) (Fig. 31.2).

Drug Interactions

There are no specific pharmaceutical contraindications for corticosteroids; however, immunosuppression can occur with larger doses. Precautions should be taken when administering live virus vaccinations (see Immunizations, earlier). ACEIs are cleared by the kidneys, and individuals with DMD should avoid nonsteroidal antiinflammatory medications while on ACEIs to avoid the chance for renal compromise, as those medications are cleared by the kidneys as well. Tylenol would be a safe choice for pain or fever.

EDUCATION

PPMD has developed "Education Matters," a comprehensive guide for parents and teachers to optimize the learning environment for children, teens, and adults living with DMD (Poysky, 2011). Learning and behavioral challenges are prevalent in DMD and may be related to dystrophin disruption in the brain (Poysky, 2011). Cognitive skills may be affected, with those individuals with DMD having a below-average IQ compared with the general population. Language development may be impacted, resulting in an increased risk of language-based disabilities (dyslexia and dysgraphia). Weaknesses in executive functioning, as well as socioemotional and behavioral issues (ADHD, obsessive-compulsive disorder, anxiety, depression, autism spectrum disorder) that impact the school setting, are also common (Poysky, 2011). It is important to establish an individualized education plan (IEP) or 504 plan for students with DMD. Accommodation considerations include physical and occupational therapy, adapted physical education, an emergency evacuation plan, and safe access to field trips and/or school events. The Individuals with Disabilities Education Act, a US federally mandated legislation, mandates access to special education accommodations and services that require a formal IEP/504 plan. The IEP/504 plan should be updated annually to reflect a child's changing needs and developmental progress (Birnkrant et al., 2018a).

SEXUALITY

By the time most individuals reach the appropriate age for the development of intimate relationships, they are in the nonambulatory phase and dependent on activities of daily living. As a result, many young individuals are unable to function independently and may not experience intimate sexual relationships. Adolescents with DMD do, however, go through regular pubertal development and have sexual desires, sometimes expressed through masturbation. This behavior should not be discouraged and should be handled appropriately, as with any adolescent in this developmental stage. Adolescents with DMD should be educated regarding sexual development and healthy and safe sex practices. This may also be beneficial in fostering healthy self-esteem. Sexual education should be initiated by the primary care provider when appropriate to foster healthy sexual relationships. This is an important time for individuals to meet with a genetic counselor to discuss inheritance risk and ensure an understanding of their genetic diagnosis.

TRANSITION TO ADULTHOOD

It is important to recognize the care of DMD extends into adulthood, and primary care providers should be knowledgeable in transition planning for individuals with complex multidisciplinary health care needs. Independence should be stressed, and adolescents should have a role in decision making as much as possible. The transition to adult medicine can be a challenging time as families become comfortable with pediatric providers who have cared for their children from a very young age. Primary care providers should facilitate transition conversations starting at an early age.

A transition toolkit for individuals with DMD was developed to better assess transition readiness, track progress toward transition goals, and provide a template for documenting key elements of medical care, medical equipment, and services over a continuum (Trout et al., 2018). Transition efforts should begin at age 13 to 14 years with dedicated time alone with a health care provider (Trout et al., 2018). Transition planning has been organized into the following domains: (1) health care, (2) education and employment, (3) housing, (4) assistance with activities of daily living, (5) transportation, and (6) relationships (Trout et al., 2018). These topics have been incorporated into a transition checklist to track progress over time and assess readiness for transition entry into adulthood (Trout et al., 2018).

The commonly accepted age of maturity for adult decision making is age 18 years (Trout et al., 2018).

However, many factors may affect an individual's ability to make a medical decision, including cognitive functioning and intellectual disability, and may require decision-making support, which could include having a medical durable power of attorney or a guardian or conservator (Trout et al., 2018). A comprehensive neuropsychological evaluation should be performed to determine the level of support needed (Trout et al., 2018).

Palliative care can begin as early as the time of diagnosis and is comprised of a multidisciplinary team of health care providers to assist patients and family members with medical decision making grounded in goals of care, advance care planning, and maximizing quality of life (Veerapandiyan & Rao, 2022). These services are often underutilized in DMD care (Veerapandiyan & Rao, 2022). "Visions of Hope" curriculum takes principles of pediatric palliative care that can be integrated into the care of individuals with DMD (Birnkrant et al., 2018a). As the illness progresses, the level of psychosocial and emotional stress for the family living with DMD rises, providing the opportunity to develop a palliative care plan tailored specifically to the family's individual needs and communication style. The early introduction of a palliative care team allows a relationship of trust to develop and serves as the foundation for the interventions necessary to meet the needs that arise during the care of a child with a chronic illness such as DMD (Veerapandiyan & Rao, 2022).

FAMILY CONCERNS

The care of males with DMD presents many complex issues and should be focused on the entire family, especially considering that more than one child is commonly affected within a family. Supportive care, based on palliative principles, should be provided throughout the course of the disease. The primary care provider should also provide suitable anticipatory guidance throughout the disease course and should facilitate decision making regarding transitions of care. The primary care provider must be aware of psychosocial needs and should make referrals for individual, family, and genetic counseling as an essential early intervention for DMD.

Caring for individuals with DMD can be overwhelming. A systematic review of the literature demonstrated caring for a person with DMD may have a substantial impact on a wide variety of aspects of mental and physical health, as well as activities of daily living and work life (Landfeldt et al., 2018). Targeting anticipatory interventions and providing support and education during challenging periods associated with peak stress can promote adaptation and build resilience among caregivers (Porteous et al., 2021). It is proposed that more effectively supporting the parent(s) will potentially have positive effects on family functioning (Porteous et al., 2021).

Further research is needed to better understand the clinical implications of caregiving in DMD (Landfeldt et al., 2018). The primary care provider should provide families of individuals with DMD an array of resources from the time of diagnosis and throughout the progression of the disease. Some of these are summarized in the Resources section (later).

RESOURCES

WEBSITES

American Occupational Therapy Association: www.aota.org

American Physical Therapy Association: www.apta.org

Information and Technical Assistance on the Americans with Disabilities Act: ada.gov

The Arc: https://futureplanning.thearc.org

ADA National Network: www.adata.org

Centers for Disease Control and Prevention: www.cdc.gov

Coalition Duchenne: coalitionduchenne.org

Cure Congenital Muscular Dystrophy: www.curecmd.org

Cure Duchenne: www.cureduchenne.org

Duchenne Therapy Network: www.duchennetherapynetwork.com

Got Transition: gottransition.org

Jett Foundation: jettfoundation.org

Laughing At My Nightmare: laughingatmynighmare.com

Muscular Dystrophy Association: www.mda.org

National Institute of Child Health and Human Development, National Institutes of Health: www.nichd.nih.gov

Parent Project Muscular Dystrophy: www.parentprojectmd.org

Society for Accessible Travel and Hospitality: www.sath.org

Treat-NMD Neuromuscular Network: www.treatnmd.org

World Duchenne: worldduchenne.org

BOOKS FOR YOUNGER CHILDREN

Kurth, A., & Kurth, O. (2021). *Zac's mighty wheels and the giant problem*. Greenhouse Press.

Yasmeh, J. (2016). *Dan and DMD*. Create Space Independent Publishing Platform.

BOOKS FOR FAMILY MEMBERS AND SIBLINGS OF CHILDREN WITH SPECIAL NEEDS

Draper, S.M. (2010). *Out of my mind*. Atheneum Books.

Meyer, D., & Holl, E. (2014). *The sibling survival guide: Indispensable information for brothers and sisters of adults with disabilities*. Woodbine House.

Siegel, I.M. (1999). *Muscular dystrophy in children: A guide for families*. Demos Health.

Stacy, E.J. (2021). *A small if: The inspiring story of a 17-year-old with a fatal disease—and a mission to cure it*. Lioncrest Publishing.

FILMS

Burnett, R. (Director). (2016). *The fundamentals of caring*. Levantine, in association with Worldwide Pants.

Jayasuriya, C. (2015). Dusty's trail: Summit of Borneo. Present Moment Yogi and Dreamquest Productions.

PODCASTS

Once upon a gene (siblings edition). https://apple.co/2TxHDWC

PROFESSIONAL DEVELOPMENT AND EDUCATION

Parent Project Muscular Dystrophy. (n.d.). Duchenne professional masterclass. A comprehensive curriculum covering the basics through advanced concepts for the Duchenne professional community. masterclass.parentprojectmd.org

---

 Summary

Primary Care Needs for the Child With Duchenne Muscular Dystrophy

HEALTH CARE MAINTENANCE
Growth and Development
- Close surveillance of growth is necessary, adapting measurement techniques is necessary as disease progresses.
- Monitor growth parameters at every visit with the appropriate measurement and plotting of weight, length or height, head circumference, and BMI.
- Monitor the development and need for adaptive equipment.

Diet
- Encourage individuals to remain as active as possible and to maintain a healthy weight by making healthy food choices.

- Closely monitor weight gain with decreasing mobility and exercise and corticosteroid use.
- Consider a decrease in energy expenditure when calculating daily caloric needs using an appropriate formula.
- Consider calcium and vitamin D supplementation when on corticosteroid therapy.
- Diet modifications and adaptive equipment needed with disease progression.

Safety
- Instruct families in keeping both the home and school environment safe and clear from objects on the floor and sharp edges and corners. An evacuation plan is in place at school in case of fire.

- Assist in arranging a home evaluation to assess for accessibility.
- Suggest adaptations to ensure safety.
- Assist in relocation to accessible housing or an apartment building with an elevator when necessary.
- Instruct families to notify local police and fire departments to facilitate safety during an emergency.

Immunizations
- Routine immunizations should be given on schedule.
- All family members should be immunized against influenza on an annual basis and COVID-19.
- Administer PCV-13 before age 2 years, and males age 2 years and older should receive PPSV-23 as recommended for age and immunization status.
- Systemic corticosteroid therapy can cause immunosuppression. Empiric guidelines recommend that children receiving 2 mg/kg/day or more of prednisone or 2.4 mg/kg/day or more of deflazacort are immunosuppressed. Older children receiving 20 mg/day or more of prednisone or 24 mg/day or more of deflazacort are considered immunosuppressed and should not receive live attenuated vaccines.

Screening
- *Vision.* Routine screening is recommended. Annual pediatric ophthalmologist referral is needed for males on steroid therapy to monitor for cataracts.
  - Mild color blindness may be present.
- *Hearing.* Routine screening is recommended.
- *Dental.* Routine screening and early referral to a dentist is recommended.
- *Blood pressure.* Screen at every visit after start of corticosteroid treatment.

Condition-Specific Screening
- PFTs; chest radiograph if wheelchair-dependent; oxyhemoglobin saturation by pulse oximetry; spirometric measurements of FVC, forced expiratory volume of 1 second, and maximal midexpiratory flow rate; maximum inspiratory and expiratory pressures; peak cough flow; noninvasive cardiac evaluation; pulmonary and cardiac evaluations before any type of surgery; evaluation for obstructive sleep apnea, oropharyngeal aspiration, gastroesophageal reflux, and asthma as indicated and anthropomorphic measurements reflective of nutritional status are routinely assessed at multidisciplinary care settings.

COMMON ILLNESS MANAGEMENT
- *Respiratory tract infections.* Distinguish between common viral or bacterial illness vs. respiratory tract infection resulting from impaired respiratory muscle function and treat appropriately. Be aware of frequent upper or lower respiratory tract infections and assess for aspiration, atelectasis, or pneumonia caused by prolonged cough, chest congestion, or influenza complicated by respiratory muscle weakness.
- *Pain management.* Treat condition-related pain caused by abnormal posture or gait; injury secondary to instability due to severe weakness; muscle cramping and contractures; possible nerve impingement; or pressure areas resulting from prolonged use of wheelchair with proper analgesics.
- *GI problems.* Assess for complications due to malfunction of smooth muscle lining in the GI tract and refer to a gastroenterologist if necessary. Treat complications of chronic constipation resulting from immobility.

DEVELOPMENTAL ISSUES
Sleep Patterns
- Instruct in repositioning to prevent the development of pressure sores and to maintain comfort.
- Assess for early signs of sleep-disordered breathing, namely obstructive sleep apnea and sleep hypoventilation, and order overnight sleep studies.
- Initiate the use of NIPPV when appropriate.

Toileting
- Encourage age-appropriate toilet training.
- Obtain input from occupational/physical therapists regarding adaptive equipment.
- Develop toileting plans for both home and school that include designated individuals to assist with toileting.

Discipline
- Encourage caregivers to remain consistent when disciplining all children using developmentally appropriate techniques.
- Routinely assess for and report any signs of abuse and neglect.

Child Care
- Child care can be provided in traditional or specialized settings.

Schooling
- Individuals should be challenged to achieve their maximum potential in school and should be placed in an intellectually appropriate classroom setting.
- Early intervention services, an IEP or 504 plan, and special education may be required.
- Therapeutic interventions may be provided in school, and frequent classroom interruptions should be weighed.
- A baseline comprehensive neuropsychiatric evaluation should be obtained prior to starting elementary school to assess cognitive, academic, and socioemotional measures.
- Discuss vocational, technologic, or college preparation programs.
- Assist in finding appropriate after-school programs and respite programs (that are accessible with adequate adaptations).

Sexuality
- Meet with genetic counselor.
- Educate regarding sexual development and healthy and safe sex practices when appropriate.
- Initiate discussion in a comfortable environment to address any concerns around intimacy. Individuals with more advanced cardiorespiratory disease and bone fragility may be concerned about changes in heart rate, blood pressure, respiration, and injury in the context of acts of intimacy.

Transition to Adulthood
- Transition discussions should begin early, by age 13 to 14 years.
- Independence should be maintained as long as possible.
- Referral to vocational rehab, community support, and employment opportunities is recommended.
- Consider guardianship before age 18 years, if warranted.
- Assist with exploring personal care attendants and standardize training, mentors, and respite care.
- Regularly assess for quality of life, advance care planning.

Continued

Family Concerns
- Care presents many complex and evolving issues and should focus on the entire family.
- Provide anticipatory guidance.
- Advocate and provide support regarding separation and loss; experiencing and expressing emotions;

and changing values, expectations, roles, and responsibilities.
- Be aware of psychosocial needs and refer for counseling services as needed.
- Initiate and participate in palliative care plans with familial input.

REFERENCES

Alexander, W. M., Smith, M., Freeman, B. J., Sutherland, L. M., Kennedy, J. D., & Cundy, P. J. (2013). The effect of posterior spinal fusion on respiratory function in Duchenne muscular dystrophy. *European Spine Journal, 22*(2), 411–416. doi:10.1007/s00586-012-2585-4.

American Academy of Pediatrics. (2021). *Red book: 2021 report of the Committee on Infectious Diseases* (32nd ed.). Author.

Annexstad, E. J., Lund-Petersen, I., & Rasmussen, M. (2014). Duchenne muscular dystrophy. *Tidsskr Nor Laegeforen, 134*(14), 1361–1364. https://doi.org/10.4045/tidsskr.13.0836.

Basta, M., & Pandya, A. M. (2022). Genetics, X-linked inheritance. StatPearls Publishing.

Bianchi, M. L., Biggar, D., Bushby, K., Rogol, A. D., Rutter, M. M., & Tseng, B. (2011). Endocrine aspect of Duchenne muscular dystrophy. *Neuromuscular Disorders, 21*, 298–303.

Billich, N., Adams, J., Carroll, K., Truby, H., Evans, M., Ryan, M. M., & Davidson, Z. E. (2022). The relationship between obesity and clinical outcomes in young people with duchenne muscular dystrophy. *Nutrients, 14*(16), 3304. https://doi.org/10.3390/nu14163304.

Birnkrant, D. J. (2009). The American College of Chest Physicians consensus statement on therespiratory and related management of patients with Duchenne musculardystrophy undergoing anesthesia or sedation. *Pediatrics, 123*(Suppl 4), S242–244. doi:10.1542/peds.2008-2952J.

Birnkrant, D. J., Bushby, K., Bann, C. M., Apkon, S. D., Blackwell, A., Brumbaugh, D., Case, L. E., Clemens, P. R., Hadjiyannakis, S., Pandya, S., Street, N., Tomezsko, J., Wagner, K. R., Ward, L. M., Weber, D. R., & DMD Care Considerations Working Group (2018a). Diagnosis and management of Duchenne muscular dystrophy, part 1: Diagnosis, and neuromuscular, rehabilitation, endocrine, and gastrointestinal and nutritional management. *Lancet Neurology, 17*(3), 251–267. doi:10.1016/S1474-4422(18)30024-3. Epub 2018 Feb 3. Erratum in: Lancet Neurol. 2018 Apr 4.

Birnkrant, D. J., Bushby, K., Bann, C. M., Alman, B. A., Apkon, S. D., Blackwell, A., Case, L. E., Cripe, L., Hadjiyannakis, S., Olson, A. K., Sheehan, D. W., Bolen, J., Weber, D. R., Ward, L. M., & DMD Care Considerations Working Group (2018b). Diagnosis and management of Duchenne muscular dystrophy, part 2: Respiratory, cardiac, bone health, and orthopaedic management. *Lancet Neurology, 17*(4), 347–361. doi:10.1016/S1474-4422(18)30025-5. Epub 2018 Feb 3.

Bushby, K., & Straub, V. (2005). Nonmolecular treatment for muscular dystrophies. *Current Opinion in Neurology, 18*, 511–518.

Bushby, K., Finkel, R., Birnkrant, D. J., Case, L. E., Clemens, P. R., Cripe, L., Kaul, A., Kinnett, K., McDonald, C., Pandya, S., Poysky, J., Shapiro, F., Tomezsko, J., Constantin, C., & DMD Care Considerations Working Group (2010). Diagnosis and management of Duchenne muscular dystrophy, part 1: Diagnosis, and pharmacological and psychosocial management. *Lancet Neurology, 9*(1), 77–93. doi:10.1016/S1474-4422(09)70271-6. Epub 2009 Nov 27. PMID:19945913.

Butterfield, R. J. (2019). Congenital muscular dystrophy and congenital myopathy. *Continuum (Minneapolis, MN), 25*(6),

1640–1661. doi:10.1212/CON.0000000000000792. PMID: 31794464.

Chung, W. K., Berg, J. S., Botkin, J. R., Brenner, S. E., Brosco, J. P., Brothers, K. B., Currier, R. J., Gaviglio, A., Kowtoniuk, W. E., Olson, C., Lloyd-Puryear, M., Saarinen, A., Sahin, M., Shen, Y., Sherr, E. H., Watson, M. S., & Hu, Z. (2022). Newborn screening for neurodevelopmental diseases: Are we there yet? *American Journal of Medical Genetics Part C: Seminars in Medical Genetics, 190*(2), 222–230. doi:10.1002/ajmg.c.31988. Epub 2022 Jul 15.

Connolly, A. M., Florence, J. M., Cradock, M. M., Malkus, E. C., Schierbecker, J. R., Siener, C. A., Wulf, C. O., Anand, P., Golumbek, P. T., Zaidman, C. M., Philip Miller, J., Lowes, L. P., Alfano, L. N., Viollet-Callendret, L., Flanigan, K. M., Mendell, J. R., McDonald, C. M., Goude, E., Johnson, L., … MDA DMD Clinical Research Network (2013). Motor and cognitive assessment of infants and young boys with Duchenne muscular dystrophy: Results from the Muscular Dystrophy Association DMD Clinical Research Network. *Neuromuscular Disorders, 23*(7), 529–539. doi:10.1016/j.nmd.2013.04.005. Epub 2013 May 28. PMID: 23726376; PMCID: PMC3743677.

Do, T. (2002). Orthopedic management of the muscular dystrophies. *Current Opinion in Pediatrics, 14*, 50–53.

Duan, D., Goemans, N., Takeda, S., Mercuri, E., & Aartsma-Rus, A. (2021). Duchenne muscular dystrophy. *Nature Reviews Disease Primers, 7*(1), 13. https://doi.org/10.1038/s41572-021-00248-3.

Duchenne de Boulogne, G. B. A. (1973). *Recherches sur la paralysie musculaire pseudohypertrophique, ou paralysie myo-sclerosique* (Studies on pseudohypertrophic muscular paralysis or myosclerotic paralysis). In Wilkins, R. H., & Brody, I. A. (Eds.), *Neurological classics*. Johnson Reprint.

Elliott, S. A., Davidson, Z. E., Davies, P. S., & Truby, H. (2012). Predicting resting energy expenditure inboys with Duchenne muscular dystrophy. *European Journal of Paediatric Neurology, 16*(6), 631–635. doi:10.1016/j.ejpn.2012.02.011.

Fox, H., Millington, L., Mahabeer, I., & van Ruiten, H. (2020). Duchenne muscular dystrophy. *British Medical Journal, 368*, l7012. doi:10.1136/bmj.l7012. PMID: 31974125.

Gloss, D., Moxley, R. T. 3rd, Ashwai, S., & Oskoui, M. (2016). Practice guideline update summary: Corticosteroid treatment of Duchenne muscular dystrophy: Report of the Guideline Development Subcommittee of the American Academy of Neurology. *Neurology, 86*(5), 465–472.

Gruber, D., Lloyd-Puryear, M., Armstrong, N., Scavina, M., Tavakoli, N. P., Brower, A. M., Caggana, M., & Chung, W. K. (2022). Newborn screening for Duchenne muscular dystrophy— early detection and diagnostic algorithm for female carriers of Duchenne muscular dystrophy. *American Journal of Medical Genetics Part C: Seminars in Medical Genetics, 190*(2), 197–205. doi:10.1002/ajmg.c.32000. Epub 2022 Sep 24.

Guglieri, M., Bushby, K., McDermott, M. P., Hart, K. A., Tawil, R., Martens, W. B., Herr, B. E., McColl, E., Wilkinson, J., Kirschner, J., King, W. M., Eagle, M., Brown, M. W., Willis, T., Hirtz, D., Shieh, P. B., Straub, V., Childs, A. M., Ciafaloni, E., … Griggs, R. C., (2017). Developing standardized corticosteroid treatment for Duchenne muscular dystrophy. *Contemporary Clinical Trials, 58*, 34–39. doi:10.1016/j.cct.2017.04.008. Epub 2017 Apr 24. PMID: 28450193; PMCID: PMC6279424.

Al Hajri, H. S., El Husseiny, E. M., & Qayyum, H. (2022). Chest pain and electrocardiographic changes in a child with Duchenne muscular dystrophy. *Cureus, 14*(6), e26105. doi:10.7759/cureus.26105. PMID: 35747106; PMCID: PMC9207991.

Hinton, V. J., Nereo, N. E., Fee, R. J., & Cyrulnik, S. E. (2006). Social behavior problems in boys with Duchenne muscular dystrophy. *Developmental and Behavioral Pediatrics, 27*(6), 470–476. https://doi.org/10.1097/00004703-200612000-00003.

Hoffman, E. P. (2020). The discovery of dystrophin, the protein product of the Duchenne muscular dystrophy gene. *FEBS Journal, 287*(18), 3879–3887. doi:10.1111/febs.15466. Epub 2020 Jul 21.

Hoffman, E. P. (2020). Pharmacotherapy of Duchenne muscular dystrophy. *Handbook of Experimental Pharmacology, 261*, 25–37. doi:10.1007/164_2019_256. PMID: 31375923.

Hoogland, G., Hendriksen, R. G. F., Slegers, R. J., Hendriks, M. P. H., Schijns, O. E. M. G., Aalbers, M. W., & Vles, J. S. H. (2019). The expression of the distal dystrophin isoforms Dp140 and Dp71 in the human epileptic hippocampus in relation to cognitive functioning. *Hippocampus, 29*(2), 102–110. doi:10.1002/hipo.23015. Epub 2018 Dec 6.

Kinnett, K., & Noritz, G. (2017). The PJ Nicholoff Steroid Protocol for Duchenne and Becker muscular dystrophy and adrenal suppression. *PLoS Currents. 9*:ecurrents.md.d18deef7dac96ed135e0dc8739917b6e. doi:10.1371/currents.md.d18deef7dac96ed135e0dc8739917b6e. PMID:28744411; PMCID: PMC5505768.

Landfeldt, E., Edström, J., Buccella, F., Kirschner, J., & Lochmüller, H. (2018). Duchenne muscular dystrophy and caregiver burden: A systematic review. *Developmental Medicine & Child Neurology, 60*(10), 987–996. doi:10.1111/dmcn.13934. Epub 2018 Jun 14. PMID: 29904912.

Landfeldt, E., Thompson, R., Sejersen, T., McMillan, H. J., Kirschner, J., & Lochmuller, H. (2020). Life expectancy at birth in Duchenne muscular dystrophy: A systematic review and meta-analysis. *European Journal of Epidemiology, 35*, 643–653.

Lim, K. R. Q., Nguyen, Q., & Yokota, T. (2020). Genotype-phenotype correlations in Duchenne and Becker muscular dystrophy patients from the Canadian Neuromuscular Disease Registry. *Journal of Personalized Medicine, 10*(4), 241. doi:10.3390/jpm10040241.

Leigh, F., Ferlini, A., Biggar, D., Bushby, K., Finkel, R., Morgenroth, L. P., & Wagner, K. R. (2018). Neurology care, diagnostics, and emerging therapies of the patient with Duchenne muscular dystrophy. *Pediatrics, 142*(Suppl 2), S5–S16. doi:10.1542/peds.2018-0333C. PMID: 30275245.

Mah, M. L., Cripe, L., Slawinski, M. K., Al-Zaidy, S. A., Camino, E., Lehman, K. J., Jackson, J. L., Iammarino, M., Miller, N., Mendell, J. R., & Hor, K. N. (2020). Duchenne and Becker muscular dystrophy carriers: Evidence of cardiomyopathy by exercise and cardiac MRI testing. *International Journal of Cardiology, 316*, 257–265. https://doi.org/10.1016/j.ijcard.2020.05.052.

McDonald, C. M., Abresch, R. T., Carter, G. T., Fowler, W. M., Jr, Johnson, E. R., Kilmer, D. D., & Sigford, B. J. (1995). Profiles of neuromuscular diseases: Duchenne muscular dystrophy. *American Journal of Physical Medicine and Rehabilitation, 74*(Suppl5), S70–S92. https://doi.org/10.1097/00002060-199509001-00003.

McDonald, C. M., Sajeev, G., Yao, Z., McDonnell, E., Elfring, G., Souza, M., Peltz, S. W., Darras, B. T., Shieh, P. B., Cox, D. A., Landry, J., Signorovitch, J., & ACT DMD Study Group and the Tadalafil DMD Study Group (2020). Deflazacort vs prednisone treatment for Duchenne muscular dystrophy: A meta-analysis of disease progression rates in recent multicenter clinical trials. *Muscle Nerve, 61*(1), 26–35.

doi:10.1002/mus.26736. Epub 2019 Nov 7. PMID: 31599456; PMCID: PMC6973289.

McMillan, H. J., Gregas, M., Darras, B. T., & Kang, P. B. (2011). Serum transaminase levels in boys with Duchenne and Becker muscular dystrophy. *Pediatrics, 127*(1), e132–e136. doi:10.1542/peds.2010-0929. Epub 2010 Dec 13. PMID: 21149430.

McNally, E. M., Kaltman, J. R., Benson, D. W., Canter, C. E., Cripe, L. H., Duan, D., Finder, J. D., Groh, W. J., Hoffman, E. P., Judge, D. P., Kertesz, N., Kinnett, K., Kirsch, R., Metzger, J. M., Pearson, G. D., Rafael-Fortney, J. A., Raman, S. V., Spurney, C. F., Targum, S. L., … Parent Project Muscular Dystrophy (2015). Contemporary cardiac issues in Duchenne muscular dystrophy. Working Group of the National Heart, Lung and Blood Institute in collaboration with Parent Project Muscular Dystrophy. *Circulation, 131*(18), 1590–1598. doi:10.1161/CIRCULATIONAHA.114.015151. Erratum in: Circulation. 2015 Jun 23;131(25):e539. Groh, William J [added].

Mendell, J. R., Buzin, C. H., Feng, J., Yan, J., Serrano, C., Sangani, D. S., Wall, C., Prior, T. W., & Sommer, S. S. (2001). Diagnosis of Duchenne dystrophy by enhanced detection of small mutations. *Neurology, 57*, 645–650. https://doi.org/10.1212/wnl.57.4.645.

Monaco, A. P., Neve, R. L., Colletti-Feener, C., Bertelson, C. J., Kurnit, D. M., & Kunkel, L. M. (1986). Isolation ofcandidate cDNAs for portions of the Duchenne muscular dystrophy gene. *Nature, 323*(6089), 646–650. doi: 10.1038/323646a0.

Muscular Dystrophy Association. (MDA). *Diseases in the MDA program, master list.* 2022. Available at https://www.mda.org/disease/list. Retrieved June 15, 2022.

Ohlendieck, K., & Swandulla, D. (2021). Complexity of skeletal muscle degeneration: Multi-systems pathophysiology and organ crosstalk in dystrophinopathy. *Pflugers Archiv: European Journal of Physiology, 473*(12), 1813–1839. doi:10.1007/s00424-021-02623-1. Epub 2021 Sep 22. PMID: 34553265; PMCID: PMC8599371.

Ong, K. S., Kinnett, K., Soelaeman, R., Webb, L., Bain, J. S., Martin, A. S., Westfield, C., Bolen, J., & Street, N. (2018). Evaluating implementation of the updated care considerations for Duchenne muscular dystrophy. *Pediatrics, 142*(Suppl 2), S118–S128. https://doi.org/10.1542/peds.2018-0333N.

Pagon, R. A., Hanson, N. B., Neufeld-Kaiser, W., & Covington, M. L. (2001). Genetic consultation. *Western Journal of Emergency Medicine, 174*(6), 397–399. https://doi.org/10.1136/ewjm.174.6.397.

Papaefthymiou, P., Kekou, K., & Özdemir, F. (2022). Orofacial manifestations associated with muscular dystrophies: A review. *Turkish Journal of Orthodontics, 35*(1), 67–73. doi:10.5152/TurkJOrthod.2021.21021. PMID: 35370136; PMCID: PMC9128359.

Parent Project Muscular Dystrophy (PPMD). (2020). Range of motion management in Duchenne muscular dystrophy—treatment options. Available https://www.parentprojectmd.org/wpcontent/uploads/2020/05/Range_of_motion_guidelines_download.pdf. Retrieved August 28, 2022.

Porteous, D., Davies, B., English, C., & Atkinson, J. (2021). An integrative review exploring psycho-social impacts and therapeutic interventions for parent caregivers of young people living with Duchenne's muscular dystrophy. *Children (Basel), 8*(3), 212. doi:10.3390/children8030212. PMID: 33799499; PMCID: PMC7999999.

Poysky James T. Education matters. 2011. https://www.parentprojectmd.org/care/for-families/classroom-resources-for-teaching-about-duchenne/.

Ricotti, V., Mandy, W. P., Scoto, M., Pane, M., Deconinck, N., Messina, S., Mercuri, E., Skuse, D. H., & Muntoni, F. (2016). Neurodevelopmental, emotional, and behavioural problems in Duchenne muscular dystrophy in relation to underlying dystrophin gene mutations. *Developmental Medicine & Child*

Neurology, 58(1), 77–84. doi:10.1111/dmcn.12922. Epub 2015 Sep 14. PMID: 26365034.

Ross, L. F., & Clarke, A. J. (2017). A historical and current review of newborn screening for neuromuscular disorders from around the world: Lessons for the United States. *Pediatric Neurology, 77*, 12–22. doi:10.1016/j.pediatrneurol.2017.08.012. Epub 2017 Aug 25. PMID: 29079012.

Salera, S., Menni, F., Moggio, M., Guez, S., Sciacco, M., & Esposito, S. (2017). Nutritional challenges in duchenne muscular dystrophy. *Nutrients, 9*(6), 594. doi: 10.3390/nu9060594.

Schofield, W. N. (1985). Predicting basal metabolic, new standards and review of previouswork. *Human Nutrition. Clinical Nutrition, 39C*(Suppl 1), 5–41.

Spencer, G. E., & Vignos, P. J. (1962). Bracing for ambulation in childhood progressive muscular dystrophy. *Journal of Bone and Joint Surgery, 44*, 234–242.

Stevens, P. M. (2006). Lower limb orthotic management of Duchenne muscular dystrophy: A literature review. *Journal of Prosthetics and Orthotics, 18*(4), 111–119.

Stockley, T. L., Akber, S., Bulgin, N., & Ray, P. N. (2006). Strategy for comprehensive molecular testing for Duchenne and Becker muscular dystrophies. *Genetic Testing, 10*(4), 229–243. https://doi.org/10.1089/gte.2006.10.229.

Suthar, R., & Sankhyan, N. (2018). Duchenne muscular dystrophy: A practice update. *Indian Journal of Pediatrics, 85*(4), 276–281. doi:10.1007/s12098-017-2397-y. Epub 2017 Jun 27. PMID: 28653137.

Thangarajh, M., Kaat, A. J., Bibat, G., Mansour, J., Summerton, K., Gioia, A., Berger, C., Hardy, K. K., & Wagner, K. R. (2019). The NIH Toolbox for cognitive surveillance in Duchenne musculardystrophy. *Annals of Clinical and Translational Neurology, 6*(9), 1696–1706. doi: 10.1002/acn3.50867. Epub 2019 Aug 31. Erratum in: Ann Clin Transl Neurol. 2019 Dec;6(12):2609.

Thomas, S., Conway, K. M., Fapo, O., Street, N., Mathews, K. D., Mann, J. R., Romitti, P. A., Soim, A., Westfield, C., Fox, D. J., Ciafaloni, E., & Muscular Dystrophy Surveillance, Tracking, and Research Network (MD STARnet) (2022). Time to diagnosis of Duchenne muscular dystrophy remains unchanged: Findings from the Muscular Dystrophy Surveillance, Tracking, and Research Network, 2000–2015. *Muscle Nerve, 66*(2), 193–197. doi:10.1002/mus.27532. Epub 2022 Apr 11. PMID: 35312090; PMCID: PMC9308714.

Trout, C. J., Case, L. E., Clemens, P. R., McArthur, A., Noritz, G., Ritzo, M., Wagner, K. R., Vroom, E., & Kennedy, A. (2018). A transition toolkit for Duchenne muscular dystrophy. *Pediatrics, 142*(Suppl 2), S110–S117. https://doi.org/10.1542/peds.2018-0333M.

Veerapandiyan, A., & Rao, V. K. (2022). Palliative care in Duchenne muscular dystrophy: Goals of care discussions and beyond. *Muscle Nerve, 65*(6), 627–629. doi:10.1002/mus.27544. Epub 2022 Apr 13. PMID: 35362613.

Williams, O. (2007). Diseases of muscle. In Brust, J. M. C. (Ed.), *Current diagnosis and treatment in neurology*. McGraw-Hill.

Yiu, E. M., & Kornberg, A. J. (2015). Duchenne muscular dystrophy. *Journal of Paediatrics and Child Health, 51*(8), 759–764. https://doi.org/10.1111/jpc.12868.

Zhu, Y., Romitti, P. A., Conway, K. M., Andrews, J., Liu, K., Meaney, F. J., Street, N., Puzhankara, S., Druschel, C. M., & Matthews D. J. (2014). Complementary and alternative medicine for Duchenne and Becker muscular dystrophies: characteristics of users and caregivers. *Pediatric Neurology, 51*(1), 71–77. doi: 10.1016/j.pediatrneurol.2014.02.003.

Zygmunt, A. M., Wong, B. L., Horn, P. S., Lambert, J., Bange, J. E., Rybalsky, I., Chouteau, W., & Tian, C. (2023). A longitudinal study of creatine kinase and creatinine levels in Duchenne muscular dystrophy. *Muscle Nerve, 67*(2), 138–145. doi:10.1002/mus.27760. Epub 2022 Dec 5.

Renée L. Davis, Michele Polfuss

ETIOLOGY

Obesity is a significant public health problem that is both complex and multifactorial in origin. Ultimately, obesity is the result of a positive energy balance that in the past has been oversimplified as an excess in energy intake from food compared to energy expenditure in physical activity. While not incorrect, a deeper understanding of multiple factors contributing to this positive energy balance, including energy intake, expenditure, and storage, is needed. Furthermore, these components of energy balance are not isolated and are influenced by the interaction of biologic, environmental, and behavioral factors (Kadouh & Acosta, 2017).

Biologic factors can include genetics, brain-gut axis, intrauterine or prenatal determinants, medical conditions, medications, disability, and the gut microbiome (Kadouh & Acosta, 2017). The study of the link between genetics and obesity has increased as new technology and analytic approaches become available. Genetics is notable for playing a major role in both the occurrence and extent of obesity in any individual (Loos & Yeo, 2022). The variation in body weight or heritability of obesity is reported to be between 40% and 70% based on twin, family, and adoption studies (Loos & Yeo, 2022; Riveros-McKay et al., 2019). Overweight and obesity in the child are highly associated with a parent being overweight or obese, which may be a combination of genetics and environmental factors (Lee et al., 2022).

Genome-wide association studies and sequencing are constantly identifying new biology and pathways associated with obesity, but causal determination and a deeper understanding are needed. Childhood obesity is a feature of several genetic conditions, including Down syndrome, Prader-Willi, Bardet-Biedl, Klinefelter, Turner, and fragile X (Butler et al., 2019). As collaborations and data sharing expand in studies that focus on genetics, sample sizes will increase, and findings will further our insight into the biology of obesity and support the advancement of precision medicine with an individualized approach to the prevention and treatment of obesity (Butler, 2016; Loos & Yeo, 2022).

The regulation of food intake is partially explained by the brain-gut axis. The brain-gut axis is a complex system that is influenced by neural and hormonal substances and nutrients and regulates hunger by impacting satiation, gastric capacity and emptying, and associated behavioral factors (e.g., food-seeking behavior, decision making, palatability) (Kadouh & Acosta, 2017). An oversimplified example of the brain-gut axis is that prior to the consumption of food, initial steps occur that influence an individual's hunger and satiety. Through an individual's senses (taste, smell, sight), gastrointestinal signals are activated and interact with hormones such as ghrelin (hunger stimulating) and leptin (appetite suppressing) as well as other signaling pathways to regulate appetite (Kansra et al., 2020).

Prenatal or intrauterine factors have been identified as being an influence or related to obesity in children. Examples that have been associated with childhood obesity include the mother being overweight or obese prior to pregnancy, having a high weight gain during pregnancy, or having gestational diabetes and smoking during pregnancy (Katzmarzyk et al., 2014; Page et al., 2019; Schnurr et al., 2022). Gestational diabetes or maternal obesity may affect the child's hypothalamic response to glucose and have a subsequent impact on the child's development of obesity (Page et al., 2019).

Medical conditions and medications have been associated with overweight or obesity. Exemplary conditions include Cushing syndrome, hypothyroidism, and polycystic ovary syndrome (PCOS) (Kadouh & Acosta, 2017). Classes of medications that have been associated with weight gain include antidepressants, antidiabetics, antiepileptics, antihistamines, antihypertensives, antipsychotics, steroids, and contraceptives (Kadouh & Acosta, 2017). Disabilities that have intellectual and physical components have been associated with a higher prevalence of obesity (Centers for Disease Control and Prevention [CDC], 2019). Prevalence rates for individuals with these disabilities may be underreported as a body mass index (BMI), the most commonly used screening tool for obesity, may be inaccurate for individuals with less lean muscle mass or if challenges with obtaining an inaccurate height are present (e.g., spinal cord injury, spina bifida) (Calcaterra et al., 2019; CDC, 2019; Polfuss et al., 2021). Depending on the condition, the etiology of obesity will vary but can be a combination of factors such as mobility issues that may alter participation in physical activity, which can be further exacerbated by the environment, hormonal imbalances, decreased basal energy expenditure, dietary factors, or medications used in their treatment regimen (Must et al., 2014).

The gut microbiome is made up of all microbes that are present in the intestinal tract. An individual's gut microbiome is involved with energy homeostasis and inflammation, making it an important determinant of obesity. The microbiome may be influenced by behaviors that occur during pregnancy (e.g., mode of delivery) and early childhood years (e.g., early antibiotic exposure and breastfeeding). Specific examples of work include examining the use of prebiotic and probiotics to influence the metabolic pathways and return the microbiota to its original state (Petraroli et al., 2021). Further research is needed to better understand the role of the gut microbiota in obesity and to explore potential mechanisms to positively alter it or prevent or treat obesity (Petraroli et al., 2021).

The burden of obesity in the population is expected to grow along with the rates of obesity and severe obesity. The CDC in 2019 reported the estimated annual medical cost of obesity was nearly $173 billion (CDC, 2022a). Obesity prevalence is elevated in certain racial and ethnic groups (American Indian/Native Alaskan, non-Hispanic Black, and Hispanic), as well as certain characteristics associated with lower socioeconomic status (SES) (Isong et al., 2018). Variables associated with SES (e.g., household income, parental education, occupation) have been reported to contribute to obesity in the child (CDC, 2022a; Ogden et al., 2018; Williams et al., 2018). One potential contributing factor to the association of obesity with lower SES may be food insecurity, which has a higher likelihood of occurring in families with lower income (St. Pierre et al., 2022). Multiple rationales for this relationship between food insecurity and obesity have been proposed. Possible explanations include the barriers to nutritious foods due to lack of resources or access to healthier options leading to increased reliance on low-cost processed foods with added sugars or refined grains (Kral et al., 2017). Another suggestion is that food insecurity may alter eating patterns due to the need to skip meals due to the availability of food or as a mechanism to work with a decreased food budget (Kral et al., 2017). Understanding that the association is present between obesity and lower SES and challenges that can occur with less financial means supports the need to consider and address families' available resources and potential stressors that may accompany the lack of resources in the prevention and treatment of obesity.

Treatment of obesity cannot necessarily reverse the underlying long-term health effects of being overweight, particularly when it begins in childhood. This represents a significant challenge to health professionals and health care organizations to design strategies to identify children at risk for being overweight and to implement programs for children and adolescents with sedentary lifestyles. Prevention makes economic sense for both public and private health care payers and leads to better health outcomes throughout the lifespan.

OBESOGENIC ENVIRONMENT

The prevalence of child overweight and obesity has increased in our society since the 1970s at a rate that cannot be fully attributable to genetics. While genetics may predispose an individual to obesity, the person's environment and behaviors will need to cooccur or interact to trigger/facilitate the weight gain to occur (Jackson et al., 2020). Coinciding with the increased prevalence of obesity, significant changes have occurred within our society leading to an obesogenic environment, which is the "sum of the influences that the surroundings, opportunities or conditions of life have on promoting obesity in individuals and populations" (Mei et al., 2021, p. 1). The interaction of these influences is often supported by a socioecologic framework based on the ecologic systems theory by Urie Bronfenbrenner, which allows a systematic approach to understanding and visualizing these influences (Pereira et al., 2019). The application of this framework necessitates considering not only individuals and their own biologic makeup, knowledge, attitudes, and behaviors but also how individuals are impacted by their interpersonal relationships (peers, family, social networks), institutions, organizations (schools, child care, workplace, rules, regulations), the community (built environment, geographic locations). and local, state, and federal policies that impact each of these contexts, with a specific focus on those that regulate/support healthy actions (Fig. 32.1) (Pereira et al., 2019). Understanding the complexity of these interactions provides further support that prevention and treatment cannot be focused on only one factor and cannot rely on a one-size-fits-all approach.

The availability and decreased cost of foods that have poor nutritional quality has increased as our nation has become more industrialized, disrupting our relationship with food. The advancements made in the food industry have increased the production and marketing of convenience foods that are highly processed and may promote increased consumption (Hall, 2018). These foods often are energy dense yet have low nutritional value with high amounts of salt, sugar, fat, and flavor additives that may prompt overconsumption. As these foods are made from inexpensive agricultural ingredients (e.g., high-fructose corn syrup), they can be sold at a lower cost and can have a longer shelf life, allowing them to be sold in locations that individuals have easy access to, such as gas stations. Similarly, fast-food restaurants, which consumers often rely upon

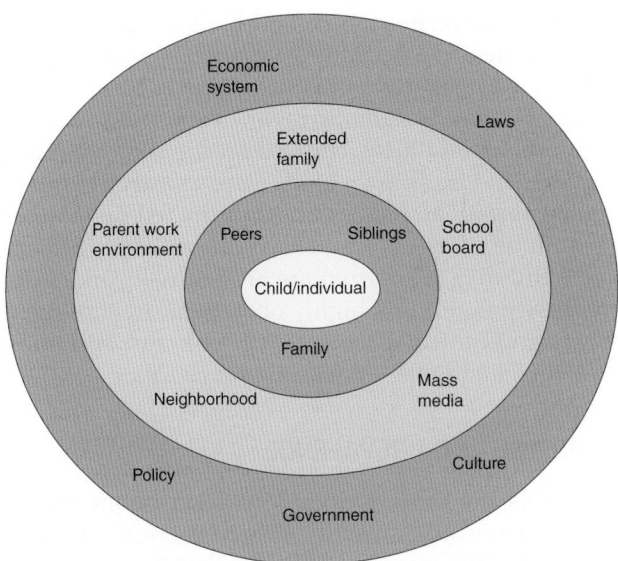

Fig. 32.1 Socioecologic framework of childhood obesity. (From Pereira, M., Padez, C.M.P., & Nogueira, H. [2019]. Describing studies on childhood obesity determinants by socio-ecological model level: A scoping review to identify gaps and provide guidance for future research. *International Journal of Obesity [London]*, *43*(10), 1883–1890.)

because of convenience and ready availability, often promote the intake of sweetened beverages and ultra-processed foods at higher portion sizes (Singh et al., 2021).

While food may be generally available, access to healthy, high-quality, nutritious foods can still be a challenge for some, referred to as a food desert, and is often measured as the distance between a person's residence and the nearest supermarket (Cooksey-Stowers et al., 2017). The marketing of food can further influence a person's attitudes, preferences, and consumption of food; unfortunately, marketing techniques are often focused on foods that have low nutritional value. Marketing can occur through multiple venues such as television, websites, and games and be connected with businesses and schools (Smith et al., 2019). In addition, most people living in our industrialized, modern nation do not expend a high number of calories through daily activities. This is reinforced by the lack of individuals who engage in hard physical labor or even walk from one place to another. As our lives have become busier and technology has advanced, we have become more reliant on computers and the use of screens for work or recreation. This has only further promoted sedentary everyday lifestyles. Busy schedules and fast-paced lives prompt reliance on efficient processes that promote convenience, such as fast food and less eating within the home environment as a family or eating foods prepared in the home. Whereas human environments and lifestyles have changed dramatically in the last century, our genetic makeup has not. The human body remains programmed for the conversion of excess energy intake into fat cells for the days of starvation and high energy demand that are no

longer a reality, hence contributing to the higher prevalence of obesity in society.

The built environment refers to the physical infrastructure in which individuals live. Due to the influence that it has on an individual's behaviors, ability, and choice to engage in physical activity and sedentary activity, it is an important aspect when discussing the etiology of obesity (Malacarne et al., 2022). Factors related to the built environment include neighborhood walkability, safety, and availability/accessibility of parks, playgrounds, and recreation centers, as well as environmental factors such as traffic noise and air pollution, each of which can influence the opportunity to engage in physical activity or promote sedentary activity (Malacarne et al., 2022). As opportunities to engage in activity become limited, new habits develop that often neither include nor promote physical activity.

The role of the family is instrumental in the development of a child's habits surrounding physical activity and nutrition (Notara et al., 2020). It has been well documented that if the parent or caregiver is overweight or obese, it increases the odds of having a child who is overweight or obese (Notara et al., 2020). The child's diet and food preferences are influenced by the parent's own diet, preferences, and options available to them on a regular basis. The family is a key factor in deciding what is available and how often the child is exposed to food. Early on, parental feeding style can play an important role in how food is introduced or provided to a child. Similar to parenting styles, there can be authoritarian practices that are seen as unfavorable and include strict restrictions on foods labeled unhealthy or the use of a "clean your plate" mentality. This feeding style has been associated with an increased desire for unhealthy food choices and a higher weight for the child (Sahoo et al., 2015). In addition, the family structure and routine can determine if foods are made within or prepared outside the home, processed or fresh, or eaten with family members at a table or in front of a screen. It has been reported that eating meals in front of a screen and not eating meals at a table with family are associated with higher weight in children (Hayes et al., 2020). In addition, family responsibilities, demands, composition, marital status, and employment may impact the development of health habits in the child by affecting the time and resources that the caregiver is able to provide (Hayes et al., 2020). Concurrently, the lack of time or increased responsibilities can hinder the ability of the caregiver to provide self-care and engage in healthy habits, which can then be role-modeled for the child.

Day care and school environments also affect childhood obesity. It is estimated that 12.5 million children (i.e., 3 of every 5 children age 0–5 years), spend time in child care outside of the home (CDC, 2022c). Acknowledging the time spent during these formative years, it is important to consider how healthy habits can be supported in this early care and educational (ECE) setting. The CDC suggests that ECEs adopt and implement standards that support healthy eating, increase physical activity, limit screen time, and support breastfeeding. To assist this effort, the CDC (2022c) provides a guide to assist ECEs in meeting national obesity prevention standards by integrating these changes at the state level (see Resources, later).

The school environment plays a key role in influencing the child's quality of nutrition, activity level, and mental health (Totura et al., 2015). Children spend extended periods of time within the school environment and may even depend on the school for the provision of one or more of their daily meals and snacks. Similar to ECEs, schools can adopt policies that promote a safe and healthy environment for all students and can assist students in eating more fruit and vegetables. This takes away access to processed foods and increases the opportunity to engage in physical activity through curriculum offerings, sports programs, or even by partnering with community organizations and allowing the use of its facilities for programs that promote activity (CDC, 2022d). Committing to all children having the opportunity to engage in high-quality activity during class and recess, promoting healthy food options, decreasing the availability of marketing for unhealthy food, and engaging with the community can create an environment that may decrease the likelihood of childhood obesity.

Similar to the influential role that parents have on their children, teachers can also be role models, so including wellness activities and promoting health for students and faculty can be a benefit (Harvard, 2022). While in theory these efforts make sense, they are not always easy to implement. A multipronged approach with the engagement of school administrators, faculty, health care providers, school nurses, and family members can collaborate and leverage effort in pursuing change at the local and state levels, which is often needed to make sustainable change.

Culture influences the onset of obesity in multiple ways. Ethnic foods and their traditional preparation are important ways for group members to preserve and celebrate their heritage. Culture determines the acceptable foods for its members and their most desirable preparation. Culture also dictates the acceptable types of physical activity by sex, generally supporting sports participation for males more than females. Gene-environment interactions are an aspect of culture as well. The timing of immigration, particularly at earlier ages, to the obesogenic environment in the United States has been reported to contribute to an initial rapid weight gain (Chatham & Mixer, 2020). Previously, an increased emphasis was placed on the acculturation of the practices of individuals living in the United States being a primary contributor to weight gain. This is still a factor but has diminished for certain subgroups as the prevalence of child obesity has increased globally,

with Mexico having the second-highest rate after the United States, so a decreased variation is evident when moving to the United States (Chatham & Mixer, 2020). In a qualitative systematic review conducted by Chatham and Mixer (2020), cultural practices such as family meals and traditional foods were a protective factor against obesity and should be encouraged by families to continue when living in the United States. Similar to US children, if children are at high risk genetically for obesity, entering a highly obesogenic environment may significantly increase their risk for becoming overweight and obese (Jackson et al., 2020).

INCIDENCE AND PREVALENCE

Obesity is the most serious long-term public health risk of the century currently facing America's children (World Health Organization [WHO], 2020). The problem is most prominent among developed countries, and the United States has the highest prevalence of children and adolescents who are overweight in the world. From 1999–2000 to 2017–2018, the percentage of US school-age children and adolescents who are obese (defined as a BMI ≥95th percentile on the CDC growth charts) has increased from 13.9% to 19.3%, and severe obesity (BMI ≥120% of the 95th percentile for age and sex on CDC growth charts) in US children and adolescents has increased from 3.6% to 6.1% (National Center for Health Statistics, 2020).

The National Health and Nutrition Examination Survey reports the prevalence of obesity among children and adolescents who reached the obese level age was 19.7% for ages 2 to 19 years (Stierman et al., 2021). Obesity rates among preschool-age children ages 2 to 5 years were 12.7% and increased to 20.7% for ages 6 to 11 and 22.2% for ages 12 to 19 years (Stierman et al., 2021). This segment of children and adolescents represents those at greatest risk for the cardiovascular and metabolic complications of obesity.

Most concerning in the current epidemic of overweight and obesity is the overrepresentation of children living in low-income families, particularly children who are racially and ethnically diverse (Stierman et al., 2021). The obesity rate is 24.8% for non-Hispanic Black children ages 2 to 19 years and highest in Hispanic or Latino youth at 26.2% (Stierman et al., 2021). A national study found that the prevalence of obesity in childhood is additionally multifaceted in socioeconomic influences and varies by level of education attained by the head of household, race of Hispanic or Latino origin, and income levels and sex (Ogden et al., 2018).

DIAGNOSTIC CRITERIA

Accurate growth measurements are important to track growth and to screen for and monitor weight status. In a clinical environment, these assessment measures must be able to be performed efficiently and be cost effective. While many measures to determine body composition are available, they may not be standardized or feasible to perform in the clinic. Examples of these include bioelectrical impedance analysis, skinfold measures, and waist-to-hip ratio. Currently, a calculated BMI is recommended for children 2 years of age and older. BMI values are not standardized for children less than 2 years of age because younger children normally have greater amounts of adipose tissue. The American Academy of Pediatrics (AAP), CDC, and WHO recommend the use of weight-for-length value to describe body fat in infants and young toddlers (Krebs et al., 2007; Kuczmarski et al., 2002; Styne et al., 2017). A weight-for-length value above the 97.7th percentile in this age group defines obese (Styne et al., 2017). Accurate plotting on standard growth charts is essential (available at http://www.cdc.gov/growthcharts).

BMI is a measure of body weight adjusted for height and sex, and the data on this chart are used to define overweight and obesity. BMI is calculated by dividing the individual's weight in kilograms by the square of height in meters. Although BMI does not measure body fat directly and fails to account for other factors affecting the risks of overweight and obesity, such as fat distribution, muscle mass, genetics, and level of physical fitness, it is a clinically useful tool for assessing the degree of body fat and the recommended measure for identifying overweight and obesity in both children and adults (Kuczmarski et al., 2002; Styne et al., 2017; US Preventive Services Task Force [USPSTF], 2017; WHO, 2021). BMI alone is insufficient for identifying the child's or adolescent's full degree of risk from excessive weight gain. It is important for the practitioner to interpret the child's risk within the context of the family health history, the child's growth pattern over time, and all relevant clinical information in assigning the degree of risk in relation to BMI and body fat.

The AAP Expert Committee (Barlow & Expert Committee, 2007) defines overweight as having a BMI for age and sex between the 85th and 94th percentiles, and the term *obese* applies to children and adolescents having a BMI above the 95th percentile for age and sex (Barlow & Expert Committee, 2007; Styne et al., 2017; USPSTF, 2017). For older adolescents, obesity is defined as a BMI of 30 kg/m^2, which utilizes the adult obesity cutoff. Recommendations are for at least annual determination of BMI for children and adolescents beginning at 2 years of age and every 3 to 6 months if the child meets the criteria for overweight or obesity. This valid and clinically acceptable tool has the added benefit of continuity with the recommended standard measurement for monitoring adult weight (Krebs et al., 2007).

There has been a recognized need for additional stratification since the last guidelines were published by the AAP in 2007 to identify and more accurately classify the child and adolescents with severe obesity,

which replaces the term *morbid obesity*. Concerns that BMI z scores are not as accurate for severe obesity, the CDC recommends using a relatively calculated BMI to describe severe obesity by division of severe obesity into three classes. Class I obesity has a BMI at or above the 95 percentile, class II is a BMI at or above 120% of the 95th percentile, and class III is any BMI at or above 140% of the 95th percentile (Skinner et al., 2018; Styne et al., 2017). Consequently, experts have agreed that children and adolescents who have severe obesity, especially class II and III, should receive priority for the most intensive level of intervention because they have a higher risk for metabolic and cardiovascular comorbidities (Skinner et al., 2018).

TERMINOLOGY AND UNCONSCIOUS BEHAVIOR

Terms and behaviors used when discussing overweight and obesity and the physical clinical environment can have a significant impact on the patient and, if not thoughtfully approached, can negatively affect the person's self-concept and erode the provider-patient relationship. The AAP and The Obesity Society published a joint statement focusing on the bias and stigma of obesity (Pont et al., 2017). Important points raised with overweight and obesity are the use of person-first language, unbiased language, and behaviors that fosters a respectful clinical environment. The person-first language would be stating a child with overweight vs. an overweight child. Unbiased language would include the use of neutral terms such as *weight* or *BMI* vs. *fat* or *morbidly obese* (Kaufman et al., 2020). Bias can be implicit or explicit and can be exhibited through body language. Examining one's own attitudes and beliefs surrounding obesity is recommended because this can be unconsciously translated through words and actions. The physical environment should be inclusive and inviting for people of all sizes. Confirming that appropriately sized equipment such as exam tables, scales, blood pressure cuffs, and chairs in the exam rooms and waiting area are available is a foundational step. Any form of weight bias or stigma in health care environments or by any office personnel can deter the person from seeking care and negate the building of a patient-centered practice (Haqq et al., 2021; Pont et al., 2017).

CLINICAL MANIFESTATIONS

Common findings at the time of diagnosis include excessive truncal adipose tissue, although providers may not recognize early overweight or obesity simply through visual inspection. The child or adolescent with severe obesity may also have tachypnea on exertion, such as climbing onto the examination surface, and may become pale and sweaty even in a cool examination room. A waddling gait or limp during ambulation, bowed legs, or apparently painful feet may also mark

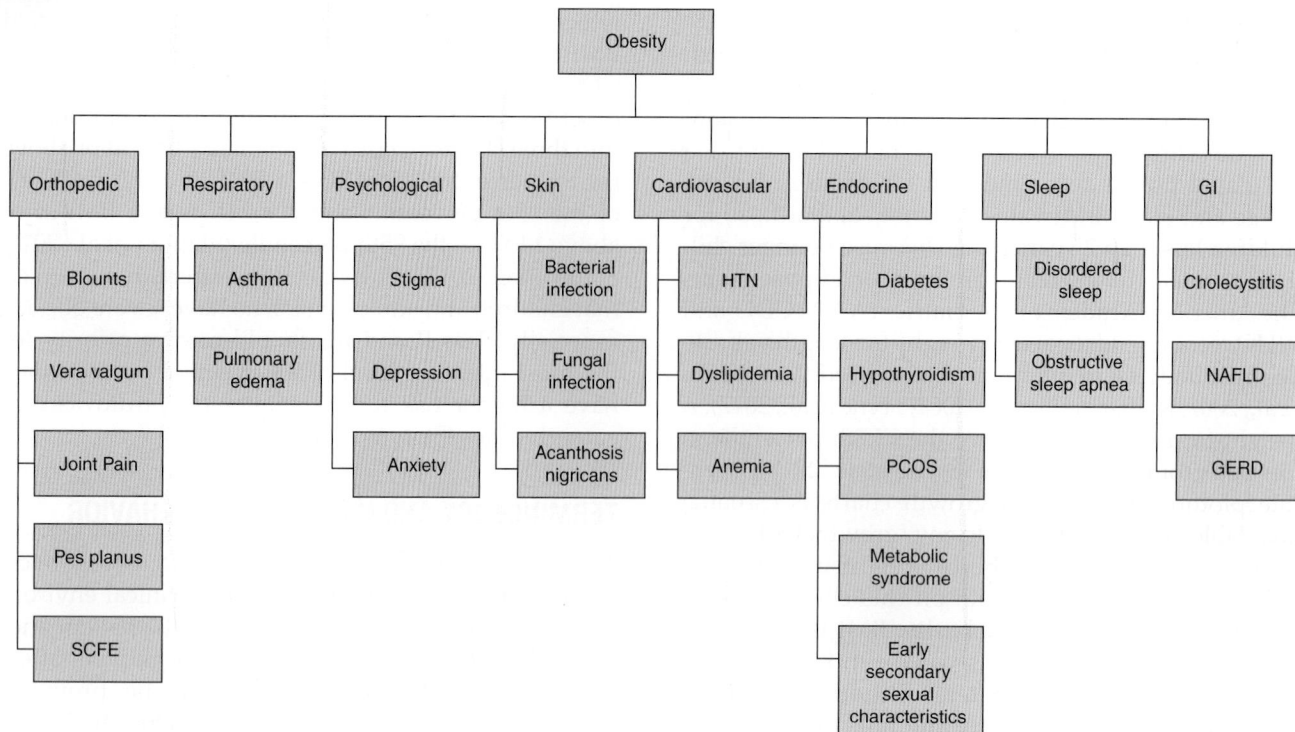

Fig. 32.2 **Clinical manifestations and associated concerns related to obesity.** *GERD*, Gastroesophageal reflux disease; *GI*, gastrointestinal; *HTN*, hypertension, *NAFLD*, nonalcoholic fatty liver disease; *PCOS*, polycystic ovary syndrome; *SCFE*, slipped capital femoral epiphysis. (From Armstrong, S., Lazorick, S., Hampl, S., Skelton, J.A., Wood, C., Collier, D., & Perrin, E.M. [2016]. Physical examination findings among children and adolescents with obesity: An evidence-based review. *Pediatrics, 137*(2), e20151766.)

the obese child's presentation. Pubertal females may have severe acne and fine hair over the face and parts of the body.

Children who have overweight and obesity require a thorough physical examination. This is necessary to identify the extent of the excessive weight gain, to identify all associated problems, and plan treatment that addresses all their health care needs (Fig. 32.2) (Styne et al., 2017).

The development of secondary sexual characteristics before age 8 years for White females, before age 7 years in Black females, and before age 9 years in males signals early-onset puberty. The occurrence of earlier secondary sexual characteristics can be more frequent among children with overweight and obesity (Alderman et al., 2019; Brix et al., 2020). Distinguishing between adipose tissue and the true glandular enlargement or thelarche in females and gynecomastia in males can be challenging. In females, darkening of the areola and prominence of the nipple indicate the onset of true thelarche. Adipose tissue also may cause the examiner to falsely identify micropenis in males. In males, true micropenis and undescended testes, along with truncal obesity, suggest the possibility of Prader-Willi syndrome.

Acanthosis nigricans, a velvety, hyperpigmented plaque, occurs more often in darker-skinned and overweight children. It occurs most often in the axillae, groin, and body folds, over the dorsal neck surface,

and over joint surfaces. Its presence has been thought to be a strong indication of hyperinsulinemia; however, recent data suggest it may not be a strong predictor of the presence of metabolic abnormalities (Brady & Rawla, 2022).

TREATMENT

Obesity affects almost all body systems and contributes to the development of a variety of medical conditions. The primary care provider's goal is to achieve a BMI at or below the 85th percentile for sex, age, and height (Daniels et al., 2015; Spear et al., 2007; Styne et al., 2017). Methods to accomplish this include working with the child and family throughout the child's life to develop and maintain healthy habits related to nutrition and physical activity and to monitor weight status to observe for any concerning trends in weight gain that are not in alignment with the child's growth and development.

PREVENTING CHILDHOOD OVERWEIGHT: ESTABLISHING ENERGY BALANCE

Prevention of overweight and obesity remains the most important strategy for stemming the epidemic of childhood obesity. Once obesity is established, it is difficult to reverse because it is multifaceted and is impacted by every aspect of a child's or adolescent's life and reinforced by habits. Obesity prevention strategies focus

Box 32.1 Preventative Guidance

PREVENTION
- At least annual growth measurements
- At least annual body mass index determination and plotting
- Explanation of growth to parents
- At least annual nutrition review and education
- At least annual physical activity review and education
- At least annual review of screen time and education

RECOMMENDED DAILY DIETARY INTAKE
- Half the plate should be fruits and vegetables
- Fat-free or low-fat milk or equivalent dairy foods
- At least half of grain servings should be from whole grain
- Lean meats, fish, or vegetable protein
- Water as supplemental beverage
- Avoid all sweetened beverages
- Avoid trans fats
- Emphasize monounsaturated and polyunsaturated fat sources
- Limit saturated fat intake

RECOMMENDED SLEEP
- Infants (age 4–12 mo): 12–16 h, including naps
- Children (age 1–2 yr): 11–14 h, including naps
- Children (age 3–5 yr): 10–13 h, including naps
- Children (age 6–12 yr): 9–12 h
- Adolescents (age 13–18 yr): 8–10 h

RECOMMENDED PHYSICAL ACTIVITY
- At least 60 min/day of moderate-vigorous physical activity to maintain weight
- At least 90 min/day of moderate-vigorous physical activity to lose weight
- No more than 2 h/day of screen time

Box 32.2 Health Care Maintenance Guidance

GROWTH AND DEVELOPMENT
- Regular measures of growth and their plotting are key to alerting the clinician and family about changes in the growth pattern presaging the onset or the worsening of overweight and obesity.
- Measure height and weight at each visit and plot them on the 2000 Centers for Disease Control and Prevention growth charts.
- Calculate the body mass index (BMI) and plot it on the growth chart for all children age ≥2 yr.
- Plot weight-for-length for infants and toddlers age ≤2 yr.
- Review the growth chart with the parent, older child, and adolescent, explaining meaning.
- Alert parents, older children, and adolescents to excessive weight gain.
- Review daily nutrition, physical activity level, and amount of screen time when upward changes become evident across weight and BMI percentiles.

DIET
- Educate parents, older children, and adolescents about the need to balance energy intake from food with energy output in physical activity.
- Provide regular nutritional counseling at every well-child visit in literacy-friendly ways, adapting advice to the family's culture.
- Encourage and support new mothers to choose breastfeeding.
- Encourage cue-based feeding throughout infancy at home and in child care.
- Instruct parents to avoid using food as a reward, eating for comfort, and negative or coercive feeding practices that promote excessive weight gain.
- Set a regular schedule for meals, including daily breakfast and snacks, and provide only healthful foods.
- Allow the child to determine whether to eat and how much to eat at mealtime.
- Serve meals at the family table as often as possible.
- Serve a low-fat diet rich in fruits, vegetables, whole grains, sources of calcium, and lean meat, fish, or vegetable protein.

SLEEP HYGIENE
- Set a consistent bedtime and routine.
- Keep room dark, quiet, and relaxing at bedtime.
- Remove screens and electronics from bedroom.
- Avoid large meals, caffeine, and alcohol before bedtime.
- Regular exercise is beneficial to sleep patterns.

SAFETY
- Assist the family in securing a safety seat system for their vehicle that best protects the child because many seats have weight limits.
- Prepare the family and child with anticipatory guidance about best ways to manage bullying and teasing about the child's weight.
- Promote local school policies that ensure a violence-free environment for all children.

on improving the quality and quantity of nutrient intake, ensuring effective levels of physical activity to balance energy intake, and limiting inactivity through education, lifestyle counseling, and motivational interventions by a team of health professionals (Box 32.1).

Individuals achieve their best health when there is a daily balance between energy intake from food and energy expenditure in growth and activity, in conjunction with other areas that are developmentally appropriate to consider (Box 32.2). Assessment of the individual and family patterns related to nutrition, activity, and inactivity provides the basis for interventions regarding family history of risk factors for obesity and cardiovascular disease. Assessments of the family's and child's or adolescent's readiness to change, as well as their treatment preferences, guide practitioners in supporting changes in these fundamental aspects of daily life (Styne et al., 2017).

Recommended Dietary Intake

Energy intake through healthful nutrition is one-half of the equation for obtaining and maintaining the best health at every age. Education needs to be sufficiently detailed to be useful, conveyed in literacy-friendly

Table 32.1 — Calories per Day by Sex, Age, and Activity Level

AGE (YR)	SEDENTARY	MODERATELY ACTIVE	ACTIVE
Male			
2–3	1000	1000–1400	1000–1400
4–8	1400	1400–1600	1600–2000
9–13	1800	1800–2200	2000–2600
14–18	2200	2400–2800	2800–3200
19–30	2400	2600–2800	3000
Female			
2–3	1000	1000–1200	1000–1400
4–8	1200	1400–1600	1400–1800
9–13	1600	1600–2000	1800–2200
14–18	1800	2000	2400
19–30	2000	2000–2200	2400

From US Department of Agriculture. (2020). *Dietary guidelines for healthy Americans, 2020–2025*. https://www.dietaryguidelines.gov/sites/default/files/2020-12/Dietary_Guidelines_for_Americans_2020-2025.pdf.

Table 32.2 — MyPlate Fruit and Vegetable Intake Recommendations by Age and Sex

AGE (YR)	MALES[a] FRUIT (CUPS)	MALES[a] VEGETABLE (CUPS)	FEMALES[a] FRUIT (CUPS)	FEMALES[a] VEGETABLE (CUPS)
2–3	1	1–1.5	1	1–1.5
4–8	1–1.5	1.5–2.5	1–1.5	1.5–2.5
9–13	1.5–2	2.5–3.5	1.5	2–3
14–18	2–2.5	3–4	1.5–2	2.5–3

[a]Less active children should be toward the lower end of recommended serving ranges.
From US Department of Agriculture. (n.d.). *MyPlate*. https://www.myplate.gov/; US Department of Health and Human Services. (2020). *Dietary guidelines for Americans, 2020–2025*. https://www.dietaryguidelines.gov/resources/2020-2025-dietary-guidelines-online-materials.

ways, and tailored to the cultural preferences of the family (Stormacq et al., 2020).

The US Department of Agriculture (USDA) has set the standards for a high-quality diet for Americans of all age groups in the 2020-2025 *Dietary Guidelines for Americans* recommendations (US Department of Health and Human Services [HHS], 2020). These guidelines recommend a diet rich in fruits, vegetables, dairy, protein, and whole-grain foods for optimal health, with calorie recommendations based on sex, age, and activity level (Table 32.1). Resources are available through their sites, in addition to MyPlate, which allows for personalization of dietary portions and servings per day; recommendations are given once age, sex, height, weight, and activity are entered (Tables 32.2 and 32.3) (USDA, n.d.).

Food groups each have important components to help children and adolescents grow and stay healthy. Half of the plate should be fruits and vegetables, and sizes are recommended by sex and age (see Table 32.2) (USDA, n.d.). Fruits and vegetables are high in micronutrients and fiber but low in calories when fat and fat-containing products are not added. Due to 100% fruit

juice being rich in natural fructose sugars, the AAP recommends no juice for those under 1 year of age (Heyman et al., 2017; Schneider et al., 2018).

Grain products should be consumed daily, at least half of which should be from whole-grain products. The recommended servings vary based on the age and activity level of the child or adolescent (see Table 32.3). Whole-grain products contain more vitamins and fiber than nonenriched, refined grain products. The additional fiber in fruits, vegetables, and whole-grain products creates greater feelings of satiety, thus limiting food and calorie intake. Fiber also removes fat from the digestive tract, limiting its absorption and promoting digestive function.

The intake of fat deserves particular attention. Pediatric experts recommend a low-fat diet but not a fat-free diet for children. Fat is a necessary part of the diet to meet the active, growing child's energy requirements. However, fats are energy rich (9 calories/g) compared with carbohydrates and proteins (4 calories/g). Fat intake should ideally be no more than 20% to 35% of daily calorie intake depending on age group, with less than 10% of fat from saturated fat sources if older than age 2 years. Additionally, none to minimal amounts of fat should be from trans fat, with the remainder of fat sources from polyunsaturated and monounsaturated fat sources (HHS, 2020).

Protein is a critical element in the daily diet and includes lean meats, seafood, poultry, and eggs, as well

Table 32.3 — MyPlate Protein, Grain, and Dairy Intake Recommendations by Age and Sex

AGE (YR)	MALES PROTEIN (OZ)	MALES GRAIN (OZ)	MALES DAIRY (CUPS)	FEMALES PROTEIN (OZ)	FEMALES GRAIN (OZ)	FEMALES DAIRY (CUPS)
2–4	2–5	3–5	2–2.5	2–5	3–5	2–2.5
5–8	3–5.5	4–6	2.5	3–5.5	4–6	2.5
9–13	5–6.5	5–9	3	4–6	5–7	3
14–18	5.5–7	6–10	3	5–6.5	6–8	3

From US Department of Agriculture. (n.d.). *MyPlate*. https://www.myplate.gov/; US Department of Health and Human Services. (2020). *Dietary guidelines for Americans, 2020–2025*. https://www.dietaryguidelines.gov/resources/2020-2025-dietary-guidelines-online-materials; Kansra, A.R., Lakkunarajah, S., & Jay, M.S. (2020). Childhood and adolescent obesity: A review. *Frontiers in Pediatrics, 8*, 581461.

as plant protein sources such as nuts, seeds, soy, and legumes. Dairy foods are the richest and most bioavailable source of calcium. Calcium sources and meeting the recommended servings per day are important parts of the diet for growing children who need to build the foundation of maximal bone density by the end of adolescence (see Table 32.3) (Golden & Abrams, 2014). Because of the energy density of milk fat, low-fat or nonfat dairy products are better choices than products with full milk fat content. Whole fat milk is recommended for 12 to 24 months of age due to the fat needed for growth and brain development. If after 24 months with good weight gain trends, recommend transitioning to low-fat milk (Muth et al., 2019). Nonfat products are best for those adolescents who have completed puberty and entered the phase of weight maintenance.

An important strategy in maintaining a healthy weight is raising parent awareness of the average daily calorie needs for sex, age, and level of activity (see Table 32.1), the number of servings of each macronutrient group per day, and serving sizes appropriate to the child's age and activity level. Portion size or serving is the age-appropriate amount of food typically eaten at one sitting and is unique to the age of the child or adolescent. Serving sizes vary with the age of the child and are not one-size-fits-all portions (e.g., a serving of cooked vegetables for a 9-month-old is 1 tablespoon vs. a serving for a 7-year-old is 0.5 cup). In general, the amounts of food eaten are underestimated, and the amounts of physical activity are overestimated (Verduci et al., 2021). Serving a larger portion of food results in greater food consumption by individuals 5 years of age and older and is associated with an increased BMI (Verduci et al., 2021). Discussion and education with families on portion sizes and options could positively impact the child and family.

Another strategy for maintaining a healthy weight is by encouraging family meals, regular mealtimes, and not skipping meals, especially breakfast, which are nutritional interventions that can be encouraged during regular wellness visits (Stiglic & Viner, 2019; Verduci et al., 2021). Parents should focus on providing only healthful choices in foods and beverages, which includes offering varied, low-fat diets rich in fruits, vegetables, and whole grains, and should avoid food battles by allowing the child to decide when and how much to eat. Family mealtimes promote the intake of more nutritious foods while supporting positive mental health (Verduci et al., 2021). One potential positive of the COVID-19 pandemic is many families were having more meals at home than previously, and providers should leverage and encourage this for positive changes in home nutrition (Sanders et al., 2021).

During infancy, research also demonstrates that excessive early rapid weight gain in the first 9 months of life significantly increases the risk of later childhood overweight (Isong et al., 2018). Contributing factors can be feeding and parenting practices. The weight gain patterns of breastfed infants demonstrate a slower rate of weight gain compared with that of bottle-fed infants during infancy and beyond (Flores-Barrantes et al., 2020; Styne et al., 2017). Therefore education regarding information about the infant's changing hunger and satiation cues and encouragement with knowledgeable support of breastfeeding are first components in teaching (Polfuss et al., 2020; Styne et al., 2017; USPSTF, 2017). Thus parents who are formula feeding their infant, even partially, need instruction in recognizing the feeding cues of their infant because inadequate bottle-feeding practices or use of a bottle to soothe can negatively contribute to greater intake than metabolically needed (AAP, 2021b). Other key skills for infant feeding include the use of a pacifier or rocking and holding vs feeding an infant when crying, growth patterns and weight expectations, delaying solid foods until the second 6 months of life, and the value of play and tummy time in promoting infant activity.

For school-age children through adolescence, anticipatory guidance focuses on understanding growth patterns during the prepubertal and pubertal years, supporting healthy choices in eating and physical activity, providing family mealtimes, limiting screen time, and ensuring adequate sleep (USPSTF, 2017). Excessive parental control of access to food and eating also increases the risk of overweight and obesity by blunting the child's responsiveness to sensations of hunger and satiety and by increasing the desirability of energy-dense, forbidden foods. When these forbidden foods become available, children tend to overeat those, fostering overweight. Learned behaviors that should be avoided are eating in the absence of hunger, using food as a reward for good behavior, or using food as a stress reliever.

Culturally mediated attitudes related to foods and eating practices must be discussed before addressing any changes in feeding practices so that the parent and child feel that their concerns are heard by the clinician, and their culture is respected. Changes recommended without this consideration are less likely to be successful or adopted (Marshall et al., 2022).

Likewise, addressing parental and child behaviors around feeding practices, food choices, and mealtimes is important. Increased parental stressors are inversely related to the number of family meals a week; healthy food availability and information on healthy routines could improve outcomes for improved diet choices and availability (Fulkerson et al., 2019).

Physical Activity

Current guidelines recommend that children 6 years old and older and adolescents participate in 60 minutes or more of daily moderate-vigorous intensity physical activity, which includes aerobic, muscle strengthening, and bone strengthening activities as appropriate by age and development (HHS, 2018). Muscle strengthening activities involve muscles doing more than their daily tasks, and bone strengthening activities include weightbearing events, including running and jumping, and both should be 3 days/week within aerobic activities. Preschool children should be active physically throughout the day with varied activities (HHS, 2018). The activities should be geared toward options that are varied, ones that the child or adolescent enjoys, and that use large muscle groups. Additionally, if family participation in activities or family sports are available, there are positive results for the child's or adolescent's weight as well (Yang et al., 2022). Negative comments should be avoided on performance or ability.

A desirable workout pattern includes a 5- to 10-minute warmup period, stretching, the workout, a cooldown period, and more stretching. Children who have been inactive or are overweight or obese should start with shorter periods of moderate-vigorous physical activity with a gradual increase to recommended levels over time to avoid injury and build strength (HHS, 2018). If good supervision is available, weight training is also valuable (Stricker et al., 2020). Strength sports such as football, wrestling, javelin, hammer, and discus throwing are all good choices.

Energy intake must be balanced with energy expenditure to achieve energy balance. Energy expenditure includes the balance of physical activity and avoidance of sedentary behavior. Physical activity is the positive side of energy expenditure; relative physical inactivity during sedentary activities leads to energy conservation due to low metabolic demand. Activities that are associated with large amounts of inactivity, such as screen time (e.g., video games, smartphone time) should be decreased to allow time for physical activity. The AAP and WHO recommend no screen time for children under the age of 2 years and less than 1 hour up to age 5 years (Council on Communications Media et al., 2016; Guideline Development Panel for Treatment of Obesity & American Psychological Association [APA], 2020; WHO, 2019). Children and adolescents should have a maximum 2 hours of screen time if over 2 years of age, with less time recommended in younger age groups. Research has found as the number of hours of screen time increases, an association between a higher BMI and poorer cardiorespiratory fitness exists (Stiglic & Viner, 2019).

In addition to the physiologic benefits of physical activity, moderate and intense levels of activity are also associated with improved mood and attention (Stiglic & Viner, 2019). Other studies indicate that regular moderate-vigorous physical activity reduces cardiovascular risk factors regardless if the person loses weight.

Sleep

According to the American Academy of Sleep Medicine and Paruthi et al. (2016), recommendations on the duration of sleep in a 24-hour period vary by age group:

- Infants (age 4–12 months): 12 to 16 hours, including naps
- Children (age 1–2 years): 11 to 14 hours, including naps
- Children (age 3–5 years): 10 to 13 hours, including naps
- Children (age 6–12 years): 9 to 12 hours
- Adolescents (age 13–18 years): 8 to 10 hours

When examining a child's sleep, it is important to focus not only on sleep duration but also on the quality, efficiency, and timing or patterns of sleep (Morrissey et al., 2020). Inadequate sleep or not consistently meeting the recommended sleep duration has been associated with behavior and learning problems, hypertension, obesity, diabetes, and depression (Paruthi et al., 2016).

Positive sleep hygiene recommendations include having a consistent sleep and wake cycle, including weekdays and weekends. The sleep environment should be quiet, dark, and kept at a comfortable temperature. Prior to going to bed, restricting large meals or caffeine intake, not using any electronics (e.g., television, computers, smartphones), and removing electronics from the bedroom are recommended (Pacheco & Sleep Foundation, 2022). Finally, engagement in physical activity during the day can promote better sleep at night (CDC, 2016).

Strong evidence supports the inverse relationship between sleep duration of the primary school-aged child and the child's weight status (Morrissey et al., 2020). Of the 112 studies on sleep duration, 83% reported a significant negative association between sleep duration and weight status, with shorter duration associated with poorer weight status, and this was further supported in 19 of 22 studies that were longitudinal in nature with a cross-sectional relationship present in the remaining three longitudinal studies (Morrissey et al., 2020). A lesser number of studies focused on sleep timing, but of the 19 studies that reported on a child's bedtime, 12 reported a later sleep onset or going to bed as associated with poorer weight status. An additional 12 studies examined sleep efficiency, defined as either efficiency of falling asleep or maintaining sleep based on wake episodes. Seven of 12 studies examined time spent asleep, with 4 studies reporting a significant negative association between higher sleep efficiency scores and poorer anthropometric measures in the children. Two studies reported more night awakenings occur in a higher proportion of children who are overweight or obese (Morrissey et al., 2020). Further study is recommended, but the importance of sleep in relation to obesity is supported.

Table **32.4**	Staged Approach to Obesity Treatment
COMPONENTS	**IMPLEMENTATION**
Stage 1: Prevention Plus	
≥5 servings of fruits and vegetables per day ≤2 h television per day No television in bedroom Decrease sugar-sweetened beverages Portion control Daily breakfast Decrease eating out Family meals At least 60 min moderate-vigorous physical activity per day	Setting: primary care provider (PCP) office Personnel: PCP or staff Visits: based on readiness to change and severity of condition Advance stage based on progress, medical condition, risks, length of time, and readiness to change
Stage 2: Structured Weight Management	
In addition to above: Balanced macronutrient diet Limit energy-dense foods High protein Self/parent monitoring Medical screening: laboratory tests Mental health referral for parenting skills, family conflict, motivation (as needed)	Setting: PCP office + registered dietitian (RD) Personnel: PCP + RD Visits: monthly tailored and based on readiness to change and severity of condition Advance to next stage based on progress, age, medical condition, risks, length of time, and readiness to change
Stage 3: Comprehensive, Multidisciplinary Treatment	
In addition to above: Referral to community weight management center or specially trained staff with comprehensive, intense behavioral interventions with >26 contact hours More frequent visits (monthly) with assessment of measures Multidisciplinary approach (dietitian, psychiatrist, physical therapist, medical doctor, nurse practitioner [NP], physician's assistant) Behavioral modification training for parents Strong parental involvement initially Group sessions may be helpful	Setting: PCP coordinates care Community weight management program: pediatric weight center, commercial programs Personnel: interdisciplinary team: behavior, RD, PCP Visits: weekly; include nutrition, exercise, and behavioral counseling Advance depending on response, age, health risk, and motivation
Stage 4: Tertiary Care Treatment	
Pediatric weight management center	Multidisciplinary team Personnel: behavioral counselor, medical social worker, psychologist, RN, NP, RD, mental health care provider, exercise specialist, may involve surgeon Visits: according to protocol

Modified from Barlow, S.E., & Expert Committee. (2007). Expert Committee recommendations regarding the prevention, assessment, and treatment of child and adolescent overweight and obesity: Summary report. *Pediatrics, 120*(4), S164–S192; Guideline Development Panel for Treatment of Obesity, American Psychological Association. (2020). Summary of the clinical practice guideline for multicomponent behavioral treatment of obesity and overweight in children and adolescents. *American Psychologist, 75*(2), 178–188; and US Preventive Services Task Force. (2017). Screening for obesity in children and adolescents: US Preventive Services Task Force recommendation statement. *JAMA, 317*(23), 2417–2426.

Psychological Assessment

Decreased psychosocial functioning has been associated with overweight and obesity. Children and adolescents with overweight and obesity may experience discrimination, social isolation, and bullying, which can lead to negative consequences such as the individual developing a poor body image, having depressive symptoms, or having low self-esteem (Sagar & Gupta, 2018). The primary care provider should be aware of the psychosocial risks and perform baseline assessments during visits, examining if there have been changes in the child's behavior that may include irritability, sadness,

aggressiveness, anxiety, or a decline in academic attendance or performance (Pont et al., 2017; Sagar & Gupta, 2018). Questioning if children have experienced teasing or bullying, body dissatisfaction, or implementing unhealthy eating practices could be red flags that would benefit from further exploration and possibly consultation with a mental health provider.

STAGED TREATMENT FOR OBESITY

Expert Committee recommendations (Barlow & Expert Committee, 2007) suggest a staged approach to treatment (Table 32.4). Although evidence supports the components of these stages, additional considerations and recommended include the following:

1. The program should be specifically designed for children and adolescents.
2. Behavior modification emphasizes cultural sensitivity, positive reinforcement, and sensitivity to body image issues; incorporates family; and requires frequent visits.
3. Nutrition and exercise components are conducted by trained professionals.
4. Cost of the program is affordable to the family.
5. Culturally appropriate interventions are used.
6. Outcomes of intervention are monitored.
7. Attrition rate is low.
8. Evidence-based alternative and complementary methods are used, and the use of over-the-counter medications is avoided.

Stage 1: Prevention Plus

The prevention plus stage is an appropriate place to start for all children and adolescents who are overweight or obese. The goal of this stage is for the child's BMI to move toward the 85th percentile. It may take 3 to 6 months for the recommended changes in this stage to produce a noticeable change in BMI. Advancement to stage 2 may be recommended if the child is not making adequate progress, the BMI has increased, comorbidities have developed or worsened, or the child and family indicate readiness for more aggressive management.

Stage 2: Structured Weight Management

The second stage of treatment focuses on the same behavioral changes as stage 1 (improving nutrition quality, increasing physical activity, and decreasing inactivity), as well as offering additional behavioral counseling. This stage requires staff with special training in behavior change and involves more frequent weight management visits, greater intervention structure, and close monitoring of progress toward behavior change goals. In stage 2, the nutrition plan includes education regarding a balanced-macronutrient diet, limitation of energy-dense foods, provision of structured daily meals and snacks, increased behavior monitoring to ensure meeting of recommendations, and positive reinforcement strategies. Regular meetings with a registered dietitian who has pediatric obesity experience are desirable. Weight loss should not exceed 1 lb/month for children age 2 to 11 years or 2 lb (0.907 kg)/month for adolescents age 12 years and older. Weight maintenance in youth who are continuing to grow in height is an indication of adequate progress. Monthly follow-up is recommended. Indications of failure to make progress at this stage are the same as for stage 1: an increase in BMI, appearance of new comorbidities or worsening of existing comorbidities, and child and family readiness for more intensive treatment.

Stage 3: Comprehensive, Multidisciplinary Intervention

The components of treatment at this stage include all the strategies in stages 1 and 2, with an increase in the intensity of behavior change strategies, more frequent weight management visits, and specialty referral as available. Negative energy balance is the goal at this stage. Structured behavioral modification to alter diet and physical activity and systematic evaluation of body measurements, dietary intake, and physical activity mark this stage. Weight loss goals remain the same as those outlined previously. Providers may also refer the individual to a commercial weight loss program that meets the criteria for safety and appropriateness for children and adolescents.

Stage 4: Tertiary Care Intervention

Stage 4 treatment involves referral to a specialized pediatric obesity center. Youth with severe obesity who are unable to decrease their degree of adiposity and mitigate their health risks through lifestyle interventions and who meet the criteria receive this level of care. Criteria for this most intensive level of care include attempted weight loss at stage 3; the maturity to understand the possible risks associated with stage 4 interventions; and willingness to maintain physical activity, followed by a prescribed diet, and to participate in behavior modification. Treatment strategies may include meal replacement, a very-low-energy diet, pharmacotherapy, or bariatric surgery.

Additional updated recommendations from the USPSTF (2017) and the AAP (2022) include that children and adolescents age 6 years and older with obesity should be offered and referred to a comprehensive, intensive behavioral intervention with greater than 26 contact hours; this intervention shows improvements in weight status (Guideline Development Panel for Treatment of Obesity & APA, 2020; Llabre et al., 2018).

PHARMACOLOGIC THERAPY

Weight loss medications are available and commonly used for the management of weight in adults. Caution related to the absence of a scientific evaluation of their effectiveness and the unknown, long-term effects of these substances on the growth and development of children has limited their use. Few guidelines are available for the safe use of weight loss medications in the pediatric population, and a stepwise approach focused on lifestyle modification remains the preferred treatment (Singhal et al., 2021). However, weak evidence exists for a reduction in BMI for children and adolescents who rely on lifestyle modifications focused on nutrition, physical activity, and behavior modifications, particularly for severe obesity (Singhal et al., 2021). Currently there are three medications approved by the US Food and Drug Administration

(FDA) for use in children, with the third (liraglutide) only recently approved in 2020.

Orlistat is FDA approved for use in adolescents age 12 years and older as a reversible lipase inhibitor that blocks the action of pancreatic and gastric lipase, preventing the breakup and absorption of fat in the lumen of the stomach and intestine, decreasing lipid absorption (Singhal et al., 2021). The unabsorbed fat is excreted in the stool. Side effects include abdominal cramping, flatus, and oily bowel movements. Orlistat is available as a prescription drug at a dose of 120 mg three times a day, taken with meals. There is a 60-mg version (Alli) available over the counter. It is intended for use along with a low-calorie and low-fat diet and regular physical activity. Because it blocks fat absorption, it increases the risk for fat-soluble vitamin deficiencies. Vitamin supplements are recommended to decrease this risk. It is contraindicated in chronic malabsorption, cholestasis, and pregnancy.

Phentermine is an appetite suppressant preventing the reuptake of serotonin, norepinephrine, and dopamine. It is currently approved for use in adolescents age 16 years or older (Singhal et al., 2021). The prescribed dose can vary between 15 mg, 30 mg, and 37.5 mg, taken once per day for a short duration of 12 weeks. Side effects can include insomnia, mood alteration, dry mouth, dizziness, headache, increased heart rate and blood pressure, and gastrointestinal side effects. It is not recommended for individuals who have cardiovascular disease, hyperthyroidism, glaucoma, or concurrent use of monoamine oxidase inhibitors (Singhal et al., 2021).

The newest drug approved for chronic weight management in adolescents age 12 years and older and obese is liraglutide. This drug is provided as a 3-mg injection once per day for adolescents who are a minimum of 60 kg and have an initial BMI (based on age and sex) that corresponds to 30 kg/m² or greater for adults. Liraglutide is a glucagon-like peptide 1 (GLP-1) receptor agonist that is used along with a reduced-calorie diet and increased physical activity. It is effective in enhancing insulin secretion and increasing satiety by slowing gastric emptying and effecting the acuate nucleus of the hypothalamus, limbic/reward system in the amygdala, and cortex (Singhal et al., 2021). According to the product information site, liraglutide is contraindicated in individuals with a personal or family history of medullary thyroid carcinoma or multiple endocrine neoplasia syndrome type 2, having a serious hypersensitivity to liraglutide, or pregnancy (NovoMEDLINK, 2022). Warning and precautions are noted if individuals have a risk of thyroid C-cell tumor, acute pancreatitis, acute gallbladder disease, hypoglycemia, increased heart rate, renal impairment, or suicidal behavior or ideation. The most common adverse reactions include nausea, diarrhea, constipation, vomiting, reaction at the injection site, headache, fatigue, dizziness, gastroenteritis, abdominal pain, and gastroenteritis.

Off-label use of FDA approved medications in adults for weight management have been implemented with caution in adolescents. Examples of these include topiramate, phentermine/topiramate extended-release combination, metformin, bupropion/naltrexone combination, and lisdexamfetamine (Singhal et al., 2021). In a systematic review of randomized controlled trials, metformin was reported to have modest but favorable effects on weight and insulin resistance, along with acceptable safety when used by children with obesity (Masarwa et al., 2021).

METABOLIC AND BARIATRIC SURGERY

Metabolic and bariatric surgery (MBS) has been determined as a safe and effective treatment modality to be used with a multidisciplinary approach in children with severe obesity. Adolescents who meet the definition of class II severe obesity (120% of the 95th percentile) based on the CDC age and sex-matched growth charts and a comorbidity or class III obesity (140% of the 95th percentile) may be considered as a candidate for MBS. When MBS has been used, in addition to significant weight loss, there are improvements in cardiovascular risk factors (e.g., dyslipidemia, elevated blood pressure), systemic inflammation, elevated insulin levels and insulin resistance, type 2 diabetes, obstructive sleep apnea, nonalcoholic steatohepatitis (NASH), reflux, and outcomes related to orthopedic disease (e.g., Blount disease, slipped capital femoral epiphysis). Beyond medical comorbidities, MBS has been associated with improved quality of life in adolescents who were treated (Pratt et al., 2018). Concurrent findings need to be acknowledged as they may support or negate success following MBS. This can include dysfunctional family relationships, a history of childhood maltreatment, a higher risk of substance use behaviors, and disordered eating. When working with a child who is severely obese, MBS should be considered a viable option that can be further reviewed by tertiary care with an early referral to an MBS center (Pratt et al., 2018). A large, prospective, multicenter trial starting in 2006 evaluated the effects of bariatric surgery on adolescents. Initial results from 240 adolescents reported that the teens lost 26% of their body weight and had better results than adults who underwent MBS in regard to better blood glucose control without the use of medication to have normalized blood pressure and not needing to take blood pressure medications. Risks reported from the trial included an increased need for additional abdominal surgery, such as gallbladder removal, and to have low iron and vitamin D levels (National Institute of Diabetes and Digestive and Kidney Diseases, 2022).

COMPLEMENTARY AND ALTERNATIVE THERAPIES

The National Center for Complementary and Alternative Medicine defines complementary and alternative medicine (CAM) as "a group of varied medical and healthcare systems, practices, and products that are not considered to be part of any current Western health care system" (Esteghamati et al., 2015, p. 1). There are no studies of CAM therapies addressing the management of obesity in children. When treating obesity there is a preponderance of CAM options that are available and that have been used in adults, including herbal supplements, acupuncture, and body sculpting. Despite the increased use and availability, there is a lack of testing and evidence to support the use of CAM in any population. Until rigorous studies and clinical trials are employed, the use of CAM to address the management of obesity in children and adolescents is not supported.

PARENTING CONSIDERATIONS

Studies of obesity treatment in children and adolescents have demonstrated the importance of parental participation in weight control (Llabre et al., 2018). Parents serve as role models for healthy lifestyle choices for their children when they provide healthy foods within the home and monitor the eating and physical activity patterns of their children (Box 32.3) (Blanchette et al., 2019; Coto et al., 2019). In a study of 86 children age 5 to 7 years that examined the association between fruit and vegetable intake, the children of parents who consumed the recommended intake of fruit and vegetables were 10 times more likely to also consume the recommended

---

| Box 32.3 | Developmental Considerations in Children and Adolescents With Obesity |

SLEEP PATTERNS
- Many children and adolescents who are overweight have disordered sleep patterns, hypoventilation syndrome, and obstructive sleep apnea. Adequacy of sleep and the presence of symptoms such as snoring should be assessed for at each wellness visit. Referrals may be necessary for sleep studies or evaluation for tonsillectomy and adenoidectomy.
- Poor quality of sleep is associated with problems in memory and behavior. Sleep disorders should be considered with reports of school failure or behavior problems.

DISCIPLINE
- Parents of children who are overweight need detailed counseling on reasonable limits on food and beverage purchases and choices, as well as limiting the child's amount of screen time.
- Advise parents to monitor and support 60 minutes of daily active play and moderate to vigorous physical activity. Being active together as a family is important.
- Advise parents to avoid the use of food or sedentary time as rewards. Recommend family activities, stickers, or just special time with the parents as appropriate rewards.
- Help identify parents' concerns regarding needed family lifestyle changes and barriers to change.

CHILD CARE
- Advise parents to carefully evaluate feeding and activity practices in child care and preschool settings, selecting providers who respect infant cues for feeding, offer only healthful food and snacks, and ensure regular active play throughout the day.
- In preschool, providers should be alerted to recognizing and effectively dealing with teasing or exclusion of overweight peers from play groups.

SCHOOLING
- Children who are overweight or obese are at increased risk for poor academic performance possibly as a consequence of impaired sleep.
- Children who are overweight or obese are also frequently the victims of bullying and teasing that damages self-esteem. Children and parents need counseling and support to address these difficult situations.

- Many children who are overweight or obese are embarrassed to participate in physical education classes and sports. It is important to work with schools to include children of all levels of ability and skill in physical education and sports.

SEXUALITY
- Adolescents who are overweight or obese of either sex are less likely to view themselves as attractive and seldom have the social and dating experiences they desire to have.
- Effective contraception may be more difficult to achieve for females who are obese because some contraceptives are less effective in females who are overweight, and many hormone-based options promote weight gain.
- Early pubarche is common, especially in females. They require sensitive education and guidance about the care of their changing bodies and handling social pressures.
- Gynecomastia is a concerning and embarrassing problem for many males who are obese.

TRANSITION TO ADULTHOOD
- Clinicians should assist the adolescent in finding an adult health care provider with expertise in the care of young adults who are overweight and obese.
- Young adults need to be assisted in assuming responsibility for independent self-management of a healthful diet and physically active lifestyle, as well as the management of any comorbid conditions.
- Primary care providers need to develop a ready list of community resources to support healthful nutrition, cooking and shopping skills, and physical activity.

FAMILY SUPPORT
- A collaborative partnership with the family is the most effective way to approach significant lifestyle change to improve child health.
- Cultural barriers and family concerns must be explored, and plans of care adapted to the concerns, needs, and preferences of each family and child.
- Families should be active partners in developing the plan of care for lifestyle change at home.

servings of fruit and vegetables as compared to the children of parents who did not meet the recommendations (Coto et al., 2019). Clinicians can indirectly influence children's health behaviors by teaching and supporting parents in their important family leadership roles by providing age-appropriate anticipatory guidance (Barlow & Expert Committee, 2007).

Motivational interviewing (MI) is a technique for establishing a collaborative relationship with children and their families that reflects the value of partnership with families (Suire et al., 2020). Strategies recognize that making healthier lifestyle choices is really in the hands of the family and the individual; providers cannot instill the motivation to change or make needed changes happen. The role of the provider is to support the family and individual in moving forward in readiness to change, increasing family and individual confidence in effectively making change, and facilitating the development of workable plans to make changes and overcome barriers to change (Kaufman et al., 2020). MI has effectively been used as a strategy to facilitate decision making specific to health behaviors. Due to its accepting and nonjudgmental approach to collaborative communication, it can facilitate autonomous decision making and goal setting and increase self-efficacy in health behavior change. In a systematic review specific to childhood obesity, MI supported the positive effects of a parent's influence on a child's anthropometric measures when compared to usual care (Suire et al., 2020).

Discipline and age-appropriate limit setting are beneficial to all children. In the context of childhood obesity, limit setting, supervision, and role modeling by parents for their children are critical in managing overweight and obesity.

For children of most ages, parents and child care providers are in charge of food selection, purchase, preparation, and the determination of eating times for family members. If unhealthful foods are not brought into the home or offered to children as a choice, children will eat more healthful diets. Serving only nutritious foods will also avoid the use of restrictive practices such as withholding preferred, calorie-dense foods from overweight children. This strategy enhances the desirability of low-nutrient, energy-dense foods and often results in the overeating of these foods when access is obtained.

A more helpful message is that there really are no bad foods, but there is a need to limit calorie intake to match calorie output in physical activity. When parents monitor their children's activity, encourage active play often each day, and limit television and other forms of screen time, their children have more discretionary calories to devote to highly palatable, energy-dense foods. It is also important to discuss the impact of food advertising on child food requests and preferences; less television viewing decreases the child's exposure to advertising.

Positive reinforcement is the best strategy to use in building good dietary and physical activity habits. The use of inexpensive nonfood reinforcements such as stickers and the award of special time with parents to do whatever the child prefers are effective ways to value the child's healthful food and activity choices. The use of food as a reward is potentially harmful; therefore it is important to counsel parents to avoid this behavior. This is a particular issue for low-income parents for whom the purchase of a candy bar as a reward is affordable, whereas the purchase of a new book as a reward may not be affordable.

Parents of children who have overweight and obesity often have heightened concerns about how best to address the need to make healthful changes in the family's diet and worry about the child perceiving them as behaving in a mean manner. Parents of younger children may be quelled by tantrums over demands for unhealthful foods and are often tempted to give in to their child because they feel helpless or too stressed to deal not only with dietary changes for the family but also with the child's protests, which can be embarrassing in public. When counseling, the clinician needs to dispel the parents' perception that the child will view them as being mean when they refuse to purchase and prepare unhealthful foods or reduce the frequency of such food. It sets a critically important example for lifelong good health for their child and sends a strong message of caring concern to the child. Although it is important to acknowledge the difficulty of taking on this challenge, it is also important to offer concrete help to the parent in developing specific strategies for implementing a healthier diet for the family and overcoming the barriers they anticipate.

SAFETY CONSIDERATIONS

Car and Booster Seat

Age-appropriate car safety concerns should be addressed with parents. The AAP recommends that children should remain rear facing until 2 years of age and in a car seat until they outgrow it before transitioning into a booster seat (AAP, 2021a). The AAP recommends a child to be 57 in. or taller before transitioning out of a booster seat. Parents of children who are overweight or obese may experience significant difficulty in finding appropriate car seats to accommodate their weight, height, and age (AAP, 2019). Though the child who is overweight and obese may outgrow the weight limits of the individual seat earlier than the height requirements, the child may not be tall enough to fit in a car with only the seat belt safely. Infant and toddler car seats have weight and height restrictions for tested safety effectiveness. Conversations regarding when it is safe to transition to a seat belt alone are imperative.

CHILD CARE CONSIDERATIONS

It is estimated the 61% of preschool-age children are enrolled in child care outside of the home and that 80%

of these children may spend an average of 40 hours a week. This leads to the child having as much as 67% of their dietary intake while in child care (Hassink, 2017). When choosing a child care setting, parents must consider many factors, including the quality of nutrition and the opportunities to engage or encourage safe and vigorous physical activity. The child care provider should avoid the use of food for distraction, comfort, or reward; offer only healthful foods in appropriate serving sizes on a predictable schedule; and be skillful in engaging the more sedentary child in active, physical play in at least 10-minute bouts throughout the day, both indoors and outdoors.

As weight stigmatization has increased, it is important for all child care facilities to monitor and promote an antibullying environment. Reports of negative weight-based stereotypes toward children can occur as early as 3 years of age (Pont et al., 2017). It is essential that child care providers be watchful for any teasing or avoidance of play and social time with the overweight child and that they know how to handle these situations skillfully.

SCHOOLING CONSIDERATIONS

Academic success is linked to long-term positive social and economic outcomes (Carey et al., 2015). Research suggests that increased weight status is associated with poorer educational outcomes. When compared to children who are of normal weight, children who have obesity will more often repeat a grade or have increased absenteeism and decreased cognitive abilities or executive functioning later in adolescence (Carey et al., 2015; Martin et al., 2017). The issues surrounding the educational environment are not always a direct outcome of the child's or adolescent's abnormal weight status. The physical or mental health outcomes associated with being overweight and obese can lead to missed school days or psychosocial distress secondary to teasing or isolation, poor sleep secondary to disordered breathing, low levels of physical activity or fitness, or poor quality of nutritional intake (Martin et al., 2017). Clinicians should inquire about the child's or adolescent's engagement and success with academics. In addition, it is imperative to ask if the child has been the victim of bullying or teasing and have appropriate mental health resources available to recommend if needed.

Children who are overweight or obese may be less likely to perform well in team sports and physical education classes. They may experience peer rejection and ridicule, as well as negative comments from peers, coaches, and teachers, which can lead to social distancing. Negative feedback has a powerful, damaging impact on the time spent in physical activity, not only exacerbating the extent and persistence of overweight or obesity but also promoting problems in psychological and emotional well-being among obese children and adolescents (Ievers-Landis et al., 2019).

Schools are the natural environment for children. Primary care providers should attempt to influence community school programs to establish physical education programs to address the activity capabilities and needs of all children and adolescents, including those who are overweight and obese.

CLINICAL CHALLENGES OF WEIGHT MANAGEMENT

In addition to the regularly recommended health screenings and assessments recommended by the AAP in their "Recommendations for Preventative Pediatric Health Care" table and routine immunizations recommended by the CDC, primary care health care providers have an important role in the prevention and treatment of childhood obesity through assessment, screenings, and education (AAP, 2022; CDC, 2022b). The primary care provider has the opportunity to build a relationship with the family, monitor a child's weight and observe trends over time, and provide anticipatory guidance related to the child's weight and weight-related behaviors (e.g., nutrition, activity, sleep). However, weight management within the primary care clinic has multiple barriers associated with it.

Clinicians have reported a lack of knowledge, inadequate training, or decreased confidence about how to talk to and counsel families regarding obesity management and practice-based issues such as lack of time and resources (Rhee et al., 2018). Concurrently, parents are not always aware that their child has overweight or obese, which can decrease receptiveness to guidance or interventions provided. Parents' lack of awareness of a child's abnormal weight status can be compounded by beliefs that they will outgrow the excess weight. If the child does not have immediate health issues, it may not seem to be a concern, or the child may not fit the picture that society uses to identify overweight, which often includes a child with severe obesity (Ruiter et al., 2020). Building a trusting relationship early on that can provide education and awareness of a child's weight status in a sensitive manner is an important first step. To assist the clinician at the system level having documents of existing treatment options and community resources available, having complementary resources such as a clinical educator or nutritionist, and leveraging the use of the electronic medical record (EMR) is suggested. The EMR can streamline best practices and provide links to online resources and evidence-based handouts in addition to mechanisms to aid documentation that includes templates, dropdown menus, and smart phrases (Rhee et al., 2018).

The clinician must collaborate with parents and their children to develop an action plan that will provide them with a sense of empowerment (Turer et al., 2015). First, it must be determined if the parents recognize lifestyle factors that place their child at risk of being overweight or obese and the potential long-term health risks. Families with multiple family members who are overweight may also not recognize the health risks but attribute their size to family physical characteristics instead of lifestyle patterns. The clinician may encounter resistance from parents who do not believe that the BMI standards used to determine overweight are appropriate standards for their child (Jones et al., 2018).

Parents may be more motivated to seek healthier eating practices and to provide increased opportunities for physical activity for their children when they realize not only the health consequences but also the negative social consequences for the child who is overweight or obese. Interestingly, parents and children often express more concerns about the visible signs of obesity, such as acanthosis nigricans and striae, and want to know more about how they can remove these unsightly skin markings than they do about the long-term health consequences.

Making significant changes in lifestyle is a complex process. Recognition that there is a problem requiring change is the first step in this process. At every health visit, primary care providers should offer support and encouragement to take action and assist the family and child in exploring barriers to action, build confidence in taking action, and work with them on a concrete plan for action that works in their lives once they are ready to move forward.

Uncovering parental perceptions and concerns about what would be required to change to more healthful nutrition and increased physical activity facilitates the change process (Turer et al., 2015). Many parents and children believe a radical diet will be imposed, making them always feel hungry, or that the changes will mark them as different from other children.

Children with overweight or obesity may be resistant to counseling about physical activity and the adoption of more healthful food choices. Adolescents often have more opportunities to make independent decisions related to their nutritional intake and participation in an activity that adds another layer of complexity when suggesting change. Recommendations for increased physical activity are often thought to mean doing strenuous exercise they may feel incapable of doing. It is important to discuss acceptable types of enjoyable physical activity that appeal to them with a gradual but planned increase in daily physical activity and a decrease in sedentary or screen time. The most successful solutions and choices come from the parents and children themselves.

In a qualitative study, parents reported that the primary care provider's role in weight management for their child included monitoring the child's weight, being sensitive when discussing health risks and lifestyle changes, and providing consistent follow-up to address not only weight but changes in behaviors. Related to nutrition, the preference was for suggestions on healthy dietary practices that are easy to follow, with examples of focusing on servings vs. a strict calorie-counting diet (Turer et al., 2015).

Unfortunately, there are no easy solutions for preventing and treating overweight in today's society. The primary care provider's challenge is to skillfully support parents and children in building the confidence and competence to take effective action for the best health of all family members.

PRIMARY CARE MANAGEMENT

HEALTH CARE MAINTENANCE

Obesity affects all spheres of the child's or adolescent's life. Psychological and physical variations are common (see Fig. 32.2). Primary care providers are responsible for screening, assessment, diagnosis, and management of obesity and should work with families to make positive changes in their lives and health (Box 32.4).

Growth and Development

Primary prevention of childhood obesity is critical. Each well visit from birth through young adulthood offers the opportunity for primary care providers to measure and plot the individual's growth parameters, as well as interpret the child's growth for parents and child (Rhee et al., 2018). Each health care maintenance visit is an opportunity for education regarding diet and exercises appropriate for the child's age and identification of excessive weight gain and additional concurrent risk factors (Brown et al., 2015).

Growth measurements, including BMI and BMI percentiles, should be obtained and plotted. Discussion of these values and their interpretation with older children, adolescents, and parents is an important strategy for enlisting and retaining the family commitment to making healthier lifestyle choices. Changes in growth patterns also alert providers to the need to alter the plan of care to a higher stage of intensity with continued gains in weight or increase in BMI percentiles, as well as to provide the opportunity for positive reinforcement for effective efforts in weight maintenance or weight loss (Brown et al., 2015).

At all ages, decreases in physical activity are associated with increased obesity (Brown et al., 2015). Decreased engagement in physical activity in early childhood can lead to delays in physical skill development and peer socialization (Carson et al., 2019). Conversely, participation in physical activity, including physical education and sports, has been associated with improved coping skills, decision making, goal setting, communication, and overall socialization (Opstoel et al., 2020). Limiting screen time, which includes video game use, television, and nonhomework computer use, can vary by the child's age. For younger children, increased screen time at 24 and 36 months was associated with poorer performance on behavioral, cognitive, and social development

---

Box 32.4   Overview Screening and Condition-Specific Screening for Children and Adolescents With Obesity

SCREENING

- *Overall screening:* Follow AAP Screening Preventative Services recommendations.
- *Blood pressure.* Obtain reading at least annually, preferably at every health visit.
  - Blood pressure should be compared to norms established by National Heart, Lung, and Blood Institute (NHLBI) for sex, age, and height for both diastolic and systolic pressure.
  - If blood pressure is at or above the 90th percentile, two more pressures should be obtained at 10- to 15-minute intervals during the visit.
  - If the child receives the diagnosis of elevated blood pressure or hypertension, offer counseling on weight loss, nutrition quality, and increased physical activity.
  - If 6 months of diet and activity therapy fail to result in weight loss and a drop in blood pressure below the 90th percentile, refer the child for specialist care.
- *Anemia.* Routine screening is not recommended. Complete nutritional history to assess risk.
  - Screen more often if the nutrition history indicates a diet low in iron sources, the child is on a severely restricted diet, or the child has had bariatric surgery.
- *Urinalysis.* Routine screening is not recommended without risk factors.
  - For children 10 years of age or older who are obese with a positive family history of type 2 diabetes, urine screens are warranted.
  - More frequent urine screening is also appropriate for obese children with family history or symptoms of diabetes.

CONDITION-SPECIFIC SCREENING

- *Lipids.* Serum lipid screening is recommended for children who are overweight or obese with a positive family history

of dyslipidemia, high cholesterol, early heart disease requiring a palliative procedure, or early death from heart disease, before age 55 years in males and age 65 years in females.
  - If the random screen reveals lipid abnormalities, a fasting serum lipid panel should be obtained.
  - If the fasting lipid panel reveals elevated triglycerides and low-density lipoprotein (LDL) cholesterol or a low high-density lipoprotein (HDL) cholesterol value, evaluate the child's diet and activity patterns. Instruct the family and child on needed changes because weight loss and increased physical activity are often effective treatments for dyslipidemias.
  - If values remain elevated, refer to a lipid specialist for management.
- *Glucose and insulin testing.* Fasting serum glucose and glucose tolerance testing should be obtained for the child who is overweight or obese with a positive family history for type 2 diabetes, or if the child has acanthosis nigricans, tachycardia and excessive sweating at rest, or polydipsia and polyuria.
  - For the child who is overweight or obese with a negative family history for type 2 diabetes and in the absence of the signs and symptoms listed above, fasting glucose levels and oral glucose tolerance testing should begin at 10 years of age and be repeated every 2 years or sooner with a change in family history or the child's presentation.
  - Insulin levels are not established for children of varying ages and sex; therefore insulin levels are not recommended at this time.
- *Thyroid function tests.* Routine thyroid tests are not recommended for children who are overweight and obese in the absence of signs and symptoms of hypothyroidism.

---

screening tests (Madigan et al., 2019). As technology and the use of social media have increased, an individualized approach to screening or media recommendations for school-age children and adolescents has become paramount. Recognition of benefits and risks have been identified, such as use for social facilitation and support and opportunities for learning as compared to risks related to negative associations with weight and sleep, security and privacy issues, and access to negative or inaccurate information. Based on this, the AAP recommends that the family and provider develop a family media use plan that takes the child's developmental stage into consideration and promotes a balance in the child's daily life (Council on Communications and Media, 2016). With a focus on weight management and the association between time spent viewing and obesity, less screen time is recommended. The associated factors for this concern include increased mindless eating while watching a screen, exposure to marketing of high-calorie, low-quality nutrition, and competition for sleep (Robinson et al., 2017). Team sports and physical education classes are important opportunities not only for

weight control but also for socialization with peers, fun, and skill building (Opstoel et al., 2020).

Sexuality

Teens who are overweight or obese often face additional challenges related to their developing concept of personal sexuality. Adolescents who have obesity have been reported to be less likely to initiate or engage in a romantic relationship or to have sexual intercourse (Walsh et al., 2022). Of those who are sexually active, they may be more likely to engage in risky sexual behaviors (Walsh et al., 2022). For the adolescent who is considering or is sexually active, the selection of a contraceptive for an adolescent female who is obese should take into consideration the potential of some contraceptives for added weight gain or decreased efficacy in overweight women.

Being overweight or obese has been linked with earlier secondary sexual development in females and males, although less evidence is present for males (Wagner et al., 2012). Changes in body image brought on by the emergence of early sexual maturation in females can be a source of anxiety for these children and result in increased teasing. Similarly, gynecomastia, a benign proliferation of breast tissue in males, is associated with obesity and often is viewed as an embarrassment for the overweight adolescent male. Males with this problem are commonly self-conscious and reluctant to go without a heavy shirt to cover their chest (Kipling et al., 2014).

CARDIOVASCULAR SYSTEM–ASSOCIATED ASSESSMENT AND CONDITIONS

Children and adolescents with obesity are at an increased risk of cardiovascular conditions or comorbidities. A thorough family history and physical assessment is warranted. A three-generation family genogram is helpful in identifying the extent of heritable cardiovascular and cardiometabolic risks such as hypertension and hyperlipidemia. Beginning with the biological grandparents, a detailed history of obesity and cardiovascular conditions should be obtained. This should include overweight and obesity in all family members, diabetes mellitus, hypertension, stroke, hypercholesterolemia, atherosclerosis, and sudden death of a grandparent or parent under 55 years of age for males and under 65 years of age for females (Flynn et al., 2017; Krebs et al., 2007; Styne et al., 2017).

Assessment of the cardiovascular system includes measuring resting pulse rate and blood pressure, auscultating heart tones, palpating pulses, and evaluating capillary refill. Heart rate is an important vital sign for an overweight and obese child. An increased resting pulse rate often reflects a lack of physical fitness, whereas a low pulse rate may suggest hypothyroidism.

Hypertension

Blood pressure elevation frequently accompanies overweight and obesity in children and adolescents because of the associated increase in blood volume servicing the adipose tissue. Blood pressure monitoring should occur at least annually for healthy children starting at age 3 years and preferably at each health encounter for those with obesity, renal disease, diabetes, congenital cardiac malformations, and if taking certain medications (Flynn et al., 2017). Care needs to be taken to ensure an accurate blood pressure measurement with a cuff that covers at least 80% of the upper right arm circumference and at least 40% of the width. Blood pressure measurements should be compared with standards for the child's sex, height, and age (Flynn et al., 2017). Regular and accurate measurements are necessary and beneficial as the higher the blood pressure is in childhood, the greater the correlation of high blood pressure in adulthood (Flynn et al., 2017).

Hypertension is common among children who are overweight and obese, with a reported range of prevalence of 3.8% to 24.8% (Flynn et al., 2017). Obesity and hypertension in youth are associated with being accompanied by additional risk factors for other cardiometabolic disorders. For children under age 13 years, blood pressure measurements are classified by percentiles according to age, sex, and height. For children over the age of 13 years, simpler measurements are utilized for the diagnosis of hypertension. An additional blood pressure measurement should be taken by auscultation and then averaged for a child under age 13 years if systolic or diastolic blood pressure measures are at or above the 90th percentile, and for a child over 13 years for a systolic at or above 120 mm Hg or diastolic at or above 80 mm Hg. If the measurement remains at or above the 90th percentile or at or above 120 mm Hg systolic and/or above 80 mm Hg diastolic, respectively, utilize the AAP charts for classification of blood pressure to diagnosis.

Newer child and adolescent blood pressure classifications now include normal blood pressure, elevated blood pressure, stage 1 hypertension, and stage 2 hypertension (Flynn et al., 2017). Treatment for hypertension should follow the NHLBI recommendations in addition to treatment to reduce BMI (Flynn et al., 2017). Lifestyle interventions, including physical activity, healthy diet, and sleep, should be discussed with the classification of elevated blood pressure, and referral to a nutritionist or weight management should be considered. If hypertension remains after 6 months of treatment, additional blood pressure measurements of upper and lower extremities (both arms and one leg) with additional lifestyle interventions should be reviewed. If it remains elevated at 12 months, consider referral to a specialist, and additional testing can be considered, including laboratory testing (urinalysis, chemistry panel, liver testing, etc.) based on assessment findings.

A child or adolescent who has stage 1 hypertension should have repeat measurements in 1 to 2 weeks in upper and lower extremities (both arms and one leg) and then at 3 months with lifestyle intervention teaching. For those with stage 2 hypertension, repeat the measurement and then refer to specialty care within 1 week (Flynn et al., 2017; NHLBI, 2011).

Dyslipidemia

Lipid profile abnormalities are one of the most common obesity-related comorbidities. Children and adolescents who are overweight or obese are at increased risk for dyslipidemia, particularly if dyslipidemia and early cardiovascular disease are in the family history. The provider should review and update the family history for risk factors and obtain a detailed assessment of both the child's typical daily food intake with a particular emphasis on sources of fat and the child's daily and weekly activity and inactivity patterns (NHLBI, 2011; Stewart et al., 2020). A review of cardiovascular risk factors should be completed annually, while lipid panel screening should be completed once universally between ages 9 and 11 years and again between ages 17 and 21 years. The universal screening can be completed as nonfasting (NHLBI, 2011). Because lipid values fluctuate during puberty, particularly after the child reaches a sexual maturity rating of 3, no routine screening is recommended between 12 and 16 years of age unless there are positive risk factors. Risk factors that warrant targeted lipid screening between 2 and 8 or 12 and 16 years of age, taking into account calculation of the non-HDL level, include (1) having a parent, grandparent, aunt/uncle, or sibling with premature atherosclerotic cardiovascular disease, (2) having a parent with total cholesterol at or above 240 mg/dL, or (3) if the child or adolescent has diabetes, hypertension with obesity, smokes cigarettes or is exposed to second-hand smoke, has chronic kidney disease or a cardiac transplant, chronic inflammatory disease, or Kawasaki disease with current or previous coronary aneurysms (NHLBI, 2011; Stewart et al., 2020). A fasting lipid profile should also be obtained when the child's BMI is at or above the 85th percentile, even in the absence of other risk factors (Stewart et al., 2020).

Normal lipid panel results include a total cholesterol less than 170 mg/dL, while 170 to 199 mg/dL is in the borderline category, and 200 mg/dL and above is considered elevated (NHLBI, 2011; Stewart et al., 2020). LDL cholesterol levels of less than 110 mg/dL are acceptable; levels of 110 to 129 mg/dL are classified as borderline, and levels of 130 mg/dL and above are elevated. Non-HDL is calculated by subtracting the HDL cholesterol value from the total cholesterol value. A non-LDL cholesterol level greater than 145 mg/dL or an HDL cholesterol value under 40 mg/dL indicates dyslipidemia.

Acceptable triglyceride levels vary on age. Desired triglyceride levels for children 9 years and younger should be less than 75 mg/dL; if 10 to 19 years of age, levels should be less than 90 mg/dL (Stewart et al., 2020). For children age 0 to 9 years, borderline levels are 75 to 99 mg/dL, and high levels are 100 mg/dL and above. Elevated triglyceride levels considered to be borderline include 90 to 129 mg/dL, whereas levels at or above 130 mg/dL are considered high for children and adolescents age 10 to 19 years.

Abnormal serum triglyceride levels (>110 mg/dL) and low HDL levels (≤40 mg/dL) respond well to increased physical activity. It is critical, then, that clinicians develop skills in forming effective partnerships with families and children to improve both the level of physical activity and their diet by reducing fat and cholesterol. A 6-month trial of a low-fat diet, increase in physical activity, and limitation of screen time to 1 hour or less per day should be initiated. A fasting lipid profile should then be obtained (Stewart et al., 2020). If the lipid profile has normalized, maintain the dietary and lifestyle changes and reassess the child every 6 to 12 months. If the levels are highly elevated (such as triglycerides level ≥500 mg/dL) and do not respond to dietary changes, the child should be referred to a pediatric cardiologist or lipid specialist for assessment

of the benefits and risks of medication to normalize serum lipids because these have been proven safe and effective in children.

Anemia

Routine risk assessment for anemia with follow-up screening as needed is recommended per the AAP recommendations on the Preventative Care/Periodicity Schedule, which is updated annually (AAP, 2022). The incidence of anemia has been reported to be higher in those who are overweight or obese (Alshwaiyat et al., 2021). Therefore if diet history reflects a low or marginal intake of foods rich in iron, the clinician should obtain a screening for hematocrit/hemoglobin. Additionally, children being treated for extreme obesity with extremely low-calorie diets or bariatric surgery, as well as those with high-risk conditions associated with obesity, should have bloodwork done regularly by the tertiary treatment center. These children should be managed in conjunction with specialty care providers.

ENDOCRINE DISORDERS

Type 2 Diabetes Mellitus

Type 2 diabetes mellitus is a significant complication of obesity that has increased prevalence in adolescents. Features most predictive of type 2 diabetes include a slow onset that is often asymptomatic, presence of obesity, a strong family history of type 2 diabetes, ethnic minority group membership, acanthosis nigricans, and the absence of autoimmune disorders (American Diabetes Association [ADA], 2022; Arslanian et al., 2018).

Children with overweight or obesity who are 10 years of age and older or postonset puberty (depending on which occurs earlier) who exhibit one or more risk factors for type 2 diabetes should be screened (ADA, 2022; Arslanian et al., 2018). Additional risk factors include a maternal history of diabetes or gestational diabetes, a family history of type 2 diabetes in a first- or second-degree relative, and signs of insulin resistance or a condition associated with insulin resistance. Furthermore, ethnicities such as Native American, African, Latino, Asian, or Pacific Islander are at greater risk for developing type 2 diabetes mellitus (ADA, 2022; Arslanian et al., 2018). Screening should start before puberty in high-risk children and be repeated every 3 years at a minimum but more frequently if BMI percentiles are increasing. Fasting glucose of 126 mg/dL or higher or a hemoglobin A1c at or above 6.5% indicates diabetes and requires referral to a pediatric endocrinologist (ADA Professional Practice Committee, 2021). Fasting glucose levels of 100 to 125 mg/dL or hemoglobin A1c of 5.7% to 6.4% are considered prediabetes.

Routine urinalysis screening without a diabetes diagnosis is not recommended. However, in the presence of obesity and a positive family history of diabetes mellitus, a urine screen for ketones and glucose should be obtained at least annually, particularly in children 10 years of age or older who are at greatest risk for the onset of type 2 diabetes mellitus (ADA, 2022; Arslanian et al., 2018). If the parent notes or the child complains of excessive thirst and frequent urination, a urinalysis should also be obtained. Constipation with concomitant urinary tract infections may also occur due to a lack of physical activity and diets low in fiber.

Experts recommend aggressive management with weight loss and exercise in addition to medications. The three medications approved for type 2 diabetes mellitus in youth include insulin, metformin, and GLP-1 receptor agonists. If the A1c is less than 8.5% and there are no signs of acidosis or ketosis with normal renal function, then metformin should be initiated and titrated up to a maximum dose of 2000 mg/day as tolerated for children and adolescents in addition to recommendations for weight loss and exercise (ADA, 2022; Medscape, 2022). The pediatric health care provider should educate on the side effects of metformin, which can be substantial and include nausea, vomiting, and diarrhea. If the hemoglobin A1c is 8.5% or higher with no signs of acidosis or ketosis, basal insulin should be initiated and titrated based on blood glucose monitoring results and guidelines while initiating and titrating the metformin dose similarly to those with hemoglobin A1c under 8.5%. If showing signs of acidosis and/or diabetic ketoacidosis, emergent care is needed for management.

The microvascular consequences of diabetes are accelerated in children with type 2 diabetes compared with type 1 diabetes (ADA, 2022). Yearly monitoring of kidney function via testing for urine albumin/creatinine ratio and for eye disease with an ophthalmologic evaluation is critical (ADA, 2022; Arslanian et al., 2018).

Polycystic Ovary Syndrome

PCOS occurs more frequently in adolescents and young females who are obese. Infrequent menstrual cycles and/or oligomenorrhea and biochemical or clinical evidence of hyperandrogenism (i.e., oily skin, facial acne, hirsutism) are the required features for diagnosis (Trent & Gordon, 2020). Laboratory assessment may reveal insulin resistance, type 2 diabetes, or metabolic syndrome. Diagnosis is based on reproductive hormone laboratory tests and physical assessment. Monitoring and management by an endocrinologist, a gynecologist, or an adolescent specialist are indicated to protect fertility.

Metabolic Syndrome

Metabolic syndrome is a multisystem abnormality associated with obesity, type 2 diabetes, and cardiovascular disease. Important risk factors or characteristics in addition to being overweight include acanthosis nigricans, abnormal glucose metabolism, hypertension, and dyslipidemia (Kansra et al., 2020). Additional disorders associated with metabolic syndrome include NASH, PCOS, and proinflammatory states (Al-Hamad & Raman, 2017). Criteria to diagnose metabolic syndrome in children are not well defined, with inconsistency in the cutoff points (Al-Hamad & Raman, 2017). In adults, having three of the following five symptoms is sufficient for diagnosis: increased waist circumference, hypertension, hyperglycemia and hypertriglyceridemia, and decreased HDL levels (Kansra et al., 2020).

When obesity is present, the metabolic syndrome should be considered. Assessment for the clinical features of obesity, dyslipidemia, hypertension, glucose intolerance or type 2 diabetes, nonalcoholic fatty liver disease (NAFLD), PCOS, and elevated inflammatory markers such as interleukin-6, tumor necrosis factor-alpha, and C-reactive protein would warrant consideration for further assessment (Al-Hamad & Raman, 2017). The screening will overlap with the necessary testing that occurs with obesity-related comorbidities, including obstructive sleep apnea, liver disease, cardiovascular disease, hypertension, and insulin resistance or type 2 diabetes, as indicated per their respective guidelines.

Hypothyroidism

Hypothyroidism should be ruled out in cases of obesity with stunted linear growth, fatigue, and decline in academic performance (American Thyroid Association, n.d.). Symptoms may include a goiter, otherwise known as an enlarged goiter. Thyroid function and thyroid autoantibody tests are not indicated in youth with normal linear growth and the absence of symptoms other than obesity. They are often done as part of the initial workup for obesity to reassure the family that hypothyroidism is not the cause of the child's increased weight.

Primary Cushing Syndrome

Primary Cushing syndrome is extremely rare and involves stunted linear growth, moon facies, fine downy hair, and violaceous striae (Lodish et al., 2018). Referral to an endocrinologist is indicated if Cushing syndrome is suspected.

RESPIRATORY DISORDERS

Respiratory disorders pose a special challenge to children who are overweight and obese. Because of the frequent comorbidity of asthma, the common cold and other respiratory triggers may provoke exacerbations. It is critical that these children have a current and effective asthma plan, that they have adequate supplies of medications and administration equipment at home and at school, and that both parents and children are skilled and knowledgeable in their use.

Wheezing and shortness of breath on exertion are common among overweight and obese children. Evidence supports a positive association between BMI and asthma or asthma-like symptoms. Moderating factors for this relationship include age, sex, ethnicity, age of onset, and duration of obesity (Lu et al., 2016). While there is a risk of someone with asthma having decreased engagement in physical activity and thus the diagnosis contributes to weight gain, longitudinal studies have documented that obesity is present prior to the asthma diagnosis (Lu et al., 2016).

In a large retrospective cohort study that examined electronic medical record data over 6 years in 507,496 patients age 2 to 17 years, baseline characteristics were statistically different based on if the child had a normal BMI or overweight or obese BMI. Patient characteristics identified included age, sex, race, ethnicity, health insurance status, and institution. Additional comorbidities associated with the BMI group included esophageal reflux, eczema urticaria, food allergy, and allergic rhinitis (Lang et al., 2018). Similar to obesity, asthma has underlying genetic and environmental factors that can be triggered by a person's biology or environment (e.g., smoking and exposure to allergens). Specific factors that may influence the development of asthma include a low-grade systemic inflammation related to obesity, which may affect the pulmonary epithelium and increase an individual's susceptibility to asthma.

There is a common underlying feature of inflammation in both obesity and asthma (Lu et al., 2016). Children who have shortness of breath or exercise intolerance should receive pulmonary function testing to identify reversible airway obstruction and an appropriate asthma management plan (Calogero et al., 2018). Weight loss improves asthma symptoms in children as well. Because increased physical activity is helpful in controlling weight gain and facilitating weight loss, pediatric professionals should provide counseling on strategies to minimize asthma symptoms that interfere with physical activity.

Wheezing and coarse rales may also indicate pulmonary edema from the additional stress placed on the cardiovascular system. An elevated respiratory rate at rest and dyspnea in the prone position also suggest possible pulmonary edema. Pulmonary edema is more likely to occur among overweight children who were preterm infants and who have residual chronic lung disease. It is also more likely to happen among overweight children with special health care needs accompanied by limited mobility and impaired cardiac or respiratory function.

ORTHOPEDIC DISORDERS

The unique features of children's bones place children who are overweight or obese at greater risk for orthopedic disorders. Overweight and obese children experience more fractures and musculoskeletal discomfort than children with normal weight (Smith et al., 2014). Excessive weight places tremendous stress on growth plates, increasing the risk for displacement and deformity. Because pain and frequent injuries interfere with much needed physical activity, early intervention, including physical therapy, is recommended.

Slipped Capital Femoral Epiphysis

Slipped capital femoral epiphysis can occur in children of any weight but is seen more frequently in children age 9 to 16 years who are obese. Its presentation includes knee and hip pain and a limp with walking. On physical assessment there is a limited range of motion of the hip, and diagnosis is made via frog-leg, lateral radiographic imaging of the hips. Treatment is an immediate referral to orthopedic surgery for pinning of the femoral epiphysis.

Genu Valgum and Tibia Vara

Genu valgum and tibia vara (bowing of the lower extremity; Blount disease) occur more often in children who are obese than in children with normal weight (Mandel et al., 2021; Walker et al., 2019). Diagnosis is made by anteroposterior radiographic views of the affected knee taken while the child is standing for tibia vara but can be made by clinical diagnosis or radiographic views of the affected knee(s) for genu valgum. Management includes referral to an orthopedic surgeon for evaluation and treatment.

Pes Planus

Pes planus (flat feet) has an increased prevalence in children and adolescents with overweight and obesity (Stolzman et al., 2015). It is important for the provider to determine if the pes planus is flexible or rigid, as rigid pes planus is more concerning for underlying pathology (Armstrong et al., 2016). Typically, rigid pes planus will be noted during both weightbearing and nonweightbearing, whereas flexible pes planus is more common with weightbearing only (Armstrong et al., 2016). Treatment options range from conservative options (e.g., orthoses [custom made or over the counter], nonsteroidal antiinflammatory drugs, physical activity modifications) to surgical options (Stolzman et al., 2015).

Gastrointestinal and Genitourinary Disorders

Cholelithiasis (gallstones) are more prevalent in children who are obese (Heida et al., 2014). Rapid weight loss increases the risk of developing this condition. Classic symptoms include intermittent episodes of intense, colicky pain in the right upper quadrant (RUQ) of the abdomen (Armstrong et al., 2019). However, milder pain and epigastric pain may be the initial symptoms. Physical examination reveals RUQ tenderness. Abdominal ultrasound evaluation reveals the presence of gallstones and cholecystitis.

NAFLD is a condition consisting of steatosis, steatohepatitis, fibrosis, and cirrhosis resulting from a fatty liver. NAFLD causes no symptoms in most individuals (Sweeny & Lee, 2021). Some children have RUQ abdominal pain and demonstrate tenderness to palpation or mild hepatomegaly during abdominal palpation. Serum alanine aminotransferase (ALT) and aspartate aminotransferase (AST) levels may be elevated and are good screening tests for the presence of this condition. ALT and AST levels twice the normal level should prompt referral to a hepatologist. Ultrasonography reveals changes consistent with NAFLD; however, it cannot determine the degree of inflammation or fibrosis. Liver biopsy is the standard method for diagnosis. Weight loss through lifestyle changes related to diet and activity leads to improvement in the condition (Sweeny & Lee, 2021).

Gastroesophageal reflux and constipation increase in severity with obesity. Treatment for these conditions is the same as for children of normal weight; however, the clinician should be aware of the increased likelihood of the conditions with obesity and treat the overweight condition as well.

SLEEP DISORDERS

Sleep-disordered breathing can include obstructive sleep apnea and obesity hypoventilation syndrome and have a direct association with obesity (Ryan et al., 2014). When obesity is present, the upper respiratory tract can become narrow secondary to the fat that sits in the area resulting in decreased muscle activity and leading to hypoxic and apneic episodes (Jehan et al., 2017). The lack of available oxygen for the body causes tissue hypoxia that contributes to atherosclerosis and subsequent cardiovascular disease (Jehan et al., 2017). In addition, increased inflammation and abnormal hormone levels (e.g., melatonin, leptin, insulin, ghrelin) are associated with obstructive sleep apnea (Jehan et al., 2017).

When concerns of a sleep disorder are present, a complete sleep history from the parent and child (if developmentally appropriate) is indicated. The history should include patterns, schedules, habits, and routines with consideration of the sleep environment and potential stressors (Srivastava et al., 2018). Age-specific screening tools are available and should be available within the clinic. Confirmatory diagnosis of obstructive sleep apnea is made through polysomnography. Treatment recommendations include weight loss, increasing physical activity, and dietary changes, along with the conventional treatment of continuous positive airway pressure (Jehan et al., 2017).

NEUROLOGIC DISORDERS

Pseudotumor cerebri (idiopathic intracranial hypertension) is a very rare condition, but there is an increased incidence in children who are obese (Barmherzig & Szperka, 2019). Symptoms include severe headache with photophobia, diplopia, and blurred vision. During the examination, papilledema may be present. Papilledema refers to the swelling of the optic disc and may appear as blurring of the discs during the fundoscopic examination. The patient will require an urgent referral to an ophthalmologist and likely a lumbar puncture (Armstrong et al., 2019).

PSYCHOLOGICAL CONSIDERATIONS

Research consistently shows that overweight and obesity carry a negative stigma that often damages the self-esteem and social development of children (Haqq et al., 2021). Children who are overweight experience an increased prevalence of psychiatric disorders (Rankin et al., 2016).

Stigma related to obesity often begins from negative personal attitudes or beliefs of individuals with obesity (Haqq et al., 2021). Obesity-related stigma most often is manifested as victimization, teasing, and bullying and can occur in multiple environments, and is perpetuated by a variety of individuals (Haqq et al., 2021; Pont et al., 2017). The person who is stigmatized often internalizes the negative beliefs and attitudes and facilitates a self-devaluation of oneself (Haqq et al., 2021). The stigma may be secondary to the belief that obesity is due to the individual making poor choices regarding eating and activity and that obesity is self-inflicted. Other reasons for stigma can be the belief that blaming or shaming the person will motivate the person to lose weight (Haqq et al., 2021).

For children and adolescents, peers are common perpetrators of harassment secondary to an individual's weight. The awareness of differences in body shapes and the application of negative stereotypes or characteristics have been reported as early as preschool years, and this can continue with adolescents reporting that the primary reason that they are teased is due to their weight (Pont et al., 2017). As technology has advanced, stigmatization does not always occur in person but can be conducted through social media and online game systems (Roberts et al., 2021). Beyond peers, weight-based victimization and stigma have been reported by educators and family members. Research has demonstrated that teachers will have a lower expectation of a student with obesity-related physical, social, and academic abilities and inhibit negative weight-related stereotypes (Pont et al., 2017). Adolescents have identified parents as teasing or bullying them about their weight. In a study of adolescents with severe obesity, the teasing or victimization from family members was exacerbated when the time was split between two households that had inconsistent levels of support (Roberts et al., 2021). The media play a key role in demonstrating the stigma related to obesity. In a study of children's media, characters who are overweight or obese were negatively depicted the majority of the time (Pont et al., 2017). As exposure to social media by youth increases, this continues to reinforce negative beliefs and stereotypes about obesity.

The health care environment has been a source of weight stigma. This can include all health care professionals, and it has been documented through self-report studies that there is a negative bias or prejudice toward individuals who are overweight or obese. Associated beliefs have been reported that individuals with obesity are lazy, noncompliant, lack self-control, or not as intelligent (Pont et al., 2017). These negative experiences have led to decreased quality of care provided and to families avoiding the health care environment by not seeking prevention or treatment or delaying interactions (Haqq et al., 2021; Pont et al., 2017; Roberts et al., 2021).

Anxiety and Depression

The negative effects of obesity are immense and lead to psychological manifestations. Children and adolescents who have experienced stigmatization have been documented as having increased psychological manifestations such as depression, anxiety, negative mood states, poor self-esteem, unhealthy eating practices, and a decreased health-related quality of life (Pont et al., 2017; Rankin et al., 2016). To cope, the child or adolescent often increases social isolation and further reduces physical activity or poor nutritional choices, thus furthering the obesity (Haqq et al., 2021; Pont et al., 2017; Rankin et al., 2016). Early screening and identification of psychological manifestations with the availability of providing resources are essential. In addition, being aware of the provider's own biases and assessing the clinical environment and staff are crucial to providing a safe and supportive environment.

SKIN CONDITIONS

Children who are overweight and obese are at greater risk for skin breakdown and infections in the intertriginous skin areas. Common infections include *Candida* infections in skinfolds of the neck, groin, and axillae, as well as the vagina in females. Repeated *Candida* infections should prompt the primary care provider to evaluate for the onset of type 2 diabetes.

Staphylococcal skin infections, especially abscesses such as pilonidal cysts, are more common among children who are overweight and obese. These children may often find it more difficult to maintain good skin hygiene. They also tend to perspire, experience more friction between skin surfaces, and have clothing that fits snugly, all of which contribute to skin breakdown and infection.

TRANSITION TO ADULTHOOD

Many of the principles on transitioning to adult services for the adolescent with a chronic health condition are applicable to one who is overweight or obese. The adolescent who is obese may have chronic health care issues that are likely to continue and often worsen during adulthood if excessive weight gain continues. Finding an adult primary health care provider who is willing and able to work effectively with adolescents or young adults who are overweight or obese is challenging. With age and advancing weight, coexisting physical health conditions such as increased cholesterol levels, hypertension, type 2 diabetes, orthopedic conditions that impair mobility, and a host of other problems may either emerge or become more severe, requiring more medical interventions and care by specialists. The pediatric primary health care provider should assist the family in selecting an adult primary care provider who enjoys working with young adults and has a reputation for effectively working with those who are overweight or obese.

The pediatric primary health care provider should also help the adolescent understand the steps and processes to transition to an adult health care provider. Providers can utilize National Alliance to Advance Adolescent Health (2022) resources, including its *Six Core Elements,* to guide the transition. The key to transition planning for adolescents who are overweight or obese is the provision of education about the need for a lifelong commitment to obtaining and maintaining an appropriate weight through healthy diet patterns and eating behaviors, and daily physical activity. The pediatric primary health care provider should strive to establish an effective relationship with adolescents that supports their engagement in learning about the risks accompanying obesity and their crucial role in making the commitment to important lifestyle changes for their best health (Alderman et al., 2019). Both parents and the clinician should ensure their adolescents' knowledge of their own health history and family health history, and health record. Adolescents should also be provided with and encouraged to maintain and understand their health records, including growth charts, blood pressure readings, and diagnostic tests and results. Self-management, no restrictions, or requirements of others should be emphasized.

RESOURCES

PARENTS, CHILDREN, AND ADOLESCENT RESOURCES

Baylor University Nutritional Research Center (offers calculators for child and adult BMI, healthy eating calculator, kids energy calculator, and a weblink to the popular Portion Distortion Quiz): www.bcm.edu/cnrc

Centers for Disease Control and Prevention:

Early Child Care (early child care and education under obesity): https://www.cdc.gov/obesity/strategies/childcareece.html

Fruits and Vegetables (information on fruits and vegetables, recipes, and helpful ideas on increasing their consumption): https://www.cdc.gov/healthyweight/healthy_eating/fruits_vegetables.html

Physical Activity (information about understanding the need for daily physical activity and ways to ensure that you are expending enough calories each day safely; includes many interactive features): www.cdc.gov/nccdphp/dnpa/physical/measuring

Healthy Schools: Parents for Healthy Schools (information for Healthy Schools' framework and parent engagement): https://www.cdc.gov/healthyschools/parentsforhealthyschools/p4hs.htm?CDC_AA_refVal=https%3A%2F%2Fwww.cdc.gov%2Fhealthyschools%2Fparentengagement%2Fparentsforhealthyschools.htm

Healthy Weight, Nutrition and Physical Activity (tips for parents on healthy weight, nutrition, and physical activity): https://www.cdc.gov/healthyweight/children/index.html

KidsHealth (parent site includes fact sheets and helpful suggestions for parents about this problem): https://www.kidshealth.org/en/parents/nutrition-center

MyPlate (includes recipes, information, and activities for children): www.myplate.org

Nutrition.gov (tips on shopping, meal planning, and recipes): https://www.nutrition.gov/topics

Parents Action for Children (offers parents information about raising healthy children): https://parents.actionforchildren.org.uk/nutrition-and-healthy-eating

US Department of Agriculture Food and Nutrition Service (for parents and caregivers to provide information on healthy eating, being more physically active and acting as a role model for children; includes *Dietary Guidelines for Americans, 2020–2025* and resources): www.usda.gov; https://www.fns.usda.gov/tn/nutrition-education-materials

US Department of Health and Human Services (contains *Physical Activity Guidelines for Americans*): https://health.gov/sites/default/files/2019-09/Physical_Activity_Guidelines_2nd_edition.pdf

We Can (information and interactive features about childhood overweight and prevention of obesity; many practical tips and resources): https://www.nhlbi.nih.gov/health/educational/wecan/index.htm

Zero to Three (provides practical information for parents about health, nutrition, and physical activity): https://www.zerotothree.org/issue-areas/physical-health-nutrition

CLINICIAN RESOURCES

Access to Child and Teen BMI Calculator (information about nutrition, physical activity, and obesity): www.cdc.gov/nccdphp/dnpa/obesity/childhood

Action for Healthy Kids (nonprofit organization dedicated to addressing the epidemic of overweight, undernourished, and sedentary youth): www.actionforhealthykids.org

American Academy of Pediatrics, Overweight and Obesity (contains family, community, and professional resources): https://www.aap.org/en/patient-care/institute-for-healthy-childhood-weight/aap-policy-statements-on-obesity

American Psychological Association (clinical practice guideline information and 50 resources based on topic of behavior change, nutrition, and activity): https://www.apa.org/obesity-guideline/for-clinicians

American School Food Service Association/School Nutrition Association (lists many key articles and resources related to overweight in schoolchildren): https://schoolnutrition.org

Centers for Disease Control and Prevention:

Healthy Schools: Obesity (information about prevalence, science-based strategies, policy guidance, and national, state, local programs and addressing in schools): https://www.cdc.gov/healthyschools/obesity/index.htm

School Health Guidelines: https://www.cdc.gov/healthyschools/npao/strategies.htm

School Nutrition: https://www.cdc.gov/healthyschools/npao/strategies.htm

Physical Education and Physical Activity: https://www.cdc.gov/healthyschools/physicalactivity/index.htm

Local School Wellness Policy: https://www.cdc.gov/healthyschools/nutrition/wellness.htm?CDC_AA_refVal=https%3A%2F%2Fwww.cdc.gov%2Fhealthyschools%2Fnpao%2Fwellness.htm

"Childhood Obesity: Evidence-Based Guidelines for Clinical Practice—Part Two" (includes a toolkit for childhood obesity for health care providers and parents; Davis, R. L., Quinn, M., Thompson, M. E., Kilanowski, J. F., Polfuss, M. L., & Duderstadt, K. G. [2021]. Childhood obesity: Evidence-based guidelines for clinical practice—part two. *Journal of Pediatric Health Care*, 35[1], 120–131. https://doi.org/10.1016/j.pedhc.2020.07.011)

National Alliance to Advance Adolescent Health: Got Transition (resources and guidance on transition to adult care with the Six Core Elements): https://www.gottransition.org

US Department of Health and Human Services (National Institutes of Health), Weight-Control Information Network (provides resources on the topics of overweight, physical activity, and weight control for health professionals and the general public): https://www.niddk.nih.gov

Summary

Primary Care Needs for the Child With Obesity

HEALTH CARE MAINTENANCE
Growth and Development
- Regular measures of growth and their plotting are key to alerting the clinician and family about changes in the growth pattern presaging the onset or the worsening of overweight and obesity.
- Measure height and weight at each visit and plot them on the most up-to-date CDC growth charts.
- Calculate the BMI and plot it on the growth chart for all children 2 years of age and older.
- Plot weight-for-length for infants and toddlers ≤ 2 years of age.
- Review the growth chart with the parent, older child, and adolescent, explaining the meaning.
- Alert parents, older children, and adolescents to excessive weight gain.
- Review daily nutrition, physical activity level, and amount of screen time when upward changes become evident across weight and BMI percentiles.

Diet
- Educate parents, older children, and adolescents about the need to balance energy intake from food with energy output in physical activity.
- Provide regular nutritional counseling at every well-child visit in literacy-friendly ways, adapting advice to the family's culture.
- Encourage and support new mothers to choose breastfeeding.
- Encourage cue-based feeding throughout infancy at home and in child care.
- Instruct parents to avoid using food as a reward, eating for comfort, and negative or coercive feeding practices that promote excessive weight gain.
- Set a regular schedule for meals, including daily breakfast and snacks, and provide only healthful foods.
- Allow the child to determine whether or not to eat and how much to eat if he or she is eating.
- Serve meals at the family table as often as possible.
- Serve a low-fat diet rich in fruits, vegetables, whole grains, sources of calcium, and lean meat, fish, or vegetable protein.

Safety
- Assist the family in securing a safety seat system for their vehicle that best protects the child because many seats have weight limits.
- Prepare the family and child with anticipatory guidance about best ways to handle bullying and teasing about the child's weight.
- Promote local school policies that ensure a violence-free environment for all children.

Immunizations
- Routine immunizations are recommended.

Screening
- *Vision.* Routine screening is recommended for children without type 2 diabetes.
  - Thorough ophthalmologic evaluation is recommended at least annually for children with type 2 diabetes and more often with changes in vision.
- Hearing. Routine screening is recommended.

- Dental. Routine screening is recommended.
  - Caries may be more prevalent among overweight children with a high sugar intake.
- Blood pressure. Blood pressure should be obtained at least annually, preferably at every health visit.
  - Blood pressure should be compared to norms established by NHLBI for sex, age, and height for both diastolic and systolic pressure.
  - If the blood pressure is ≥ the 90th percentile, two more pressures should be obtained at 10- to 15-minute intervals during the visit. If the blood pressure remains elevated, the child should return weekly for 3 weeks for blood pressure measurement to establish the diagnosis of hypertension.
  - If the child receives the diagnosis of hypertension, offer counseling on weight loss, nutrition quality, and increased physical activity. Recheck the blood pressure in a month.
  - If 6 months of diet and activity therapy fail to result in weight loss and a drop in blood pressure below the 90th percentile, refer the child for specialist care.
- Hematocrit. Routine screening is recommended.
  - Screen more often if the nutrition history indicates a diet low in iron sources, the child is on a severely restricted diet, or the child has had bariatric surgery.
- Urinalysis. Routine screening is recommended.
  - For children 10 years of age or older who are obese with a positive family history of type 2 diabetes, annual urine screens for ketones and glucose are warranted.
  - More frequent urine screening is also appropriate for obese children with constipation, enuresis, or encopresis.
- Tuberculosis. Routine screening is recommended.

Condition-Specific Screening
- Lipids. Serum lipid screening is recommended for children who are overweight or obese with a positive family history of dyslipidemia, high cholesterol, early heart disease requiring a palliative procedure, or early death from heart disease, before age 55 in men and age 65 in women.
  - If the random screen reveals lipid abnormalities, a fasting serum lipid panel should be obtained.
  - If the fasting lipid panel reveals elevated triglycerides and LDL cholesterol or a low HDL cholesterol value, evaluate the child's diet and activity patterns. Instruct the family and child on needed changes, because weight loss and increased physical activity are often effective treatments for dyslipidemias.
  - If values remain elevated, refer to a lipid specialist for management.
- Glucose and insulin testing. Fasting serum glucose and glucose tolerance testing should be obtained for the child who is overweight or obese with a positive family history for type 2 diabetes, or if the child has acanthosis nigricans, tachycardia and excessive sweating at rest, or polydipsia and polyuria.
  - For the overweight or obese child with a negative family history for type 2 diabetes and in the absence

of the signs and symptoms listed above, fasting glucose levels and oral glucose tolerance testing should begin at 10 years of age and be repeated every 2 years or sooner with a change in family history or the child's presentation.

- Insulin levels are not established for children of varying ages and different sexes; therefore insulin levels are not recommended at this time.
- Thyroid function tests. Routine thyroid tests are not recommended for children who are overweight and obese in the absence of signs and symptoms of hypothyroidism such as bradycardia, thyroid enlargement, impaired linear growth, and a BMI ≥ the 97th percentile.

COMMON ILLNESS MANAGEMENT
Differential Diagnosis
- Respiratory disorders. Viral infections of the upper respiratory tract may provoke asthma exacerbations. Primary care providers should annually update the overweight and obese asthmatic child's asthma care plan and assess child and parent knowledge and skill in the use of medications and delivery systems. Assure rescue inhalers are available at home and school and that they have not expired.
  - Overweight and obese children with asthma should receive the flu vaccine annually.
- Skin rashes. Children who are overweight and obese children are prone to both fungal and staphylococcal skin infections.
  - It is important to culture wound drainage to identify MRSA-positive skin infections to ensure effective treatment.

Drug Interactions
- Sibutramine should not be combined with selective serotonin reuptake inhibitors (SSRIs) or monoamine oxidase inhibitor (MAOI) drugs because this may provoke suicidal ideation, suicide, or serotonin storm.
  - Over-the-counter cough and cold medications containing decongestants should be avoided when taking sibutramine because they may augment the vasoconstrictive and hypertensive effects of sibutramine.
  - Caution should also be used in prescribing migraine medications and opiates for children using sibutramine.
- Metformin serum levels are increased by 40% when cimetidine is taken concomitantly.
- Hyperglycemia occurs when sulfonylurea drugs are taken with estrogen-containing medications, antibiotics, antihypertensives, rifampin, MAOI drugs, Dilantin, thiazide and phenothiazine diuretics, prednisone, and thyroid supplements.
- Hypoglycemia occurs when sulfonylurea drugs are taken with alcohol or oral miconazole.

DEVELOPMENTAL ISSUES
Sleep Patterns & Hygiene
- Many children and adolescents who are overweight have disordered sleep patterns, hypoventilation syndrome, and obstructive sleep apnea. Adequacy of sleep and the presence of symptoms such as snoring should be assessed at each wellness visit. Referrals may be necessary for sleep studies or evaluation for tonsillectomy and adenoidectomy.

- Poor quality of sleep is associated with problems in memory and behavior. Sleep disorders should be considered with reports of school failure or behavior problems.
  - Set a consistent bedtime and routine.
  - Keep the room dark, quiet, and relaxing at bedtime.
  - Remove screens and electronics from the bedroom.
  - Avoid large meals, caffeine, and alcohol before bedtime.
  - Regular exercise is beneficial to sleep patterns.

Toileting
- Constipation is more common among overweight and obese children who lack adequate levels of physical activity and fiber in the diet.
- Enuresis and encopresis, as well as bladder infections, are more common among children with constipation.

Discipline
- Parents of children who are overweight need detailed counseling on reasonable limits on food and beverage purchases and choices, as well as limiting the child's amount of screen time.
- Advise parents to monitor and support 60 minutes of daily active play and moderate to vigorous physical activity. Being active together as a family is important.
- Advise parents to avoid the use of food or sedentary time as rewards. Recommend family activities, stickers, or just special time with the parents as appropriate rewards.
- Help identify parents' concerns regarding needed family lifestyle changes and barriers to change.

Child Care
- Advise parents to carefully evaluate feeding and activity practices in child care and preschool settings, selecting providers who respect infant cues for feeding, offer only healthful food and snacks, and ensure regular active play throughout the day.
- In preschool, providers should be alerted to recognizing and effectively dealing with teasing or exclusion of overweight peers from play groups.

Schooling
- Overweight and obese children are at increased risk for poor academic performance, possibly as a consequence of impaired sleep.
- Overweight and obese children are also frequently the victims of bullying and teasing that damage self-esteem. Children and parents need counseling and support to address these difficult situations.
- Many children who are overweight or obese are embarrassed to participate in physical education classes and sports. It is important to work with schools to include children of all levels of ability and skill in physical education and sports.

Sexuality
- Overweight and obese adolescents of both sexes are less likely to view themselves as attractive and seldom have the social and dating experiences they desire to have.
- Effective contraception may be more difficult to achieve for females who are obese because some contraceptives are less effective in overweight females and many hormone-based options promote weight gain.

Continued

- Early pubarche is common, especially in girls. They require sensitive education and guidance about the care of their changing bodies and handling social pressures.
- Gynecomastia is a concerning and embarrassing problem for many obese males.

Transition to Adulthood

- Clinicians should assist the adolescent in finding an adult health care provider with expertise in the care of overweight and obese young adults.
- Young adults need to be assisted in assuming responsibility for independent self-management of a healthful diet and physically active lifestyle, as well as the management of any comorbid conditions.

- Primary care providers need to develop a ready list of community resources to support healthful nutrition, cooking and shopping skills, and physical activity.

FAMILY CONCERNS

- A collaborative partnership with the family is the most effective way to approach significant lifestyle change to improve child health.
- Cultural barriers and family concerns must be explored and plans of care must be adapted to the concerns, needs, and preferences of each family and child.
- Families should be active partners in developing the plan of care for lifestyle change at home.

REFERENCES

Al-Hamad, D., & Raman, V. (2017). Metabolic syndrome in children and adolescents. *Translational Pediatrics, 6*(4), 397–407. https://doi.org/10.21037/tp.2017.10.02.

Alderman, E. M., & Breuner, C. C., Committee on Adolescence. (2019). Unique needs of the adolescent. *Pediatrics, 144*(6). https://doi.org/10.1542/peds.2019-3150.

Alshwaiyat, N. M., Ahmad, A., Wan Hassan, W. M. R., & Al-Jamal, H. A. N. (2021). Association between obesity and iron deficiency (review). *Experimental and Therapeutic Medicine, 22*(5), 1268. https://doi.org/10.3892/etm.2021.10703.

American Academy of Pediatrics. (2019). *Car seats for children who are overweight or obese: Suggestions for parents.* HealthyChildren.org. Retrieved 09/11/2022 from https://www.healthychildren.org/English/safety-prevention/on-the-go/Pages/Car-Safety-Seats-and-Obese-Children-Suggestions-for-Parents.aspx.

American Academy of Pediatrics. (2021a). *Car seats: Information for families.* HealthyChildren.org. Retrieved 09/11/2022 from https://www.healthychildren.org/English/safety-prevention/on-the-go/Pages/Car-Safety-Seats-and-Obese-Children-Suggestions-for-Parents.aspx.

American Academy of Pediatrics. (2021b). *Infant food and feeding.* Retrieved September 4 from https://www.aap.org/en/patient-care/healthy-active-living-for-families/infant-food-and-feeding/.

American Academy of Pediatrics. (2022). 2022 recommendations for preventive pediatric health care. *Pediatrics, 150*(1). https://doi.org/10.1542/peds.2022-058044.

American Diabetes Association Professional Practice Committee. (2021). Classification and diagnosis of diabetes: Standards of medical care in diabetes—2022. *Diabetes Care, 45*(Supplement_1), S17–S38. doi:10.2337/dc22-S002.

American Diabetes Association. (2022). Standards of medical care in diabetes—2022 abridged for primary care providers. *Clinical Diabetes, 40*(1), 10–38. doi:10.2337/cd22-as01.

American Thyroid Association. (n.d.). *Hypothyroidism in children and adolescents FAQs.* Retrieved 09/04/2022 from https://www.thyroid.org/hypothyroidism-children-adolescents/.

Armstrong, S., Lazorick, S., Hampl, S., Skelton, J. A., Wood, C., Collier, D., & Perrin, E. M. (2016). Physical examination findings among children and adolescents with obesity: An evidence-based review. *Pediatrics, 137*(2), e20151766. https://doi.org/10.1542/peds.2015-1766.

Armstrong, S. C., Bolling, C. F., Michalsky, M. P., Reichard, K. W., & Section on Obesity, Section on Surgery (2019). Pediatric metabolic and bariatric surgery: Evidence, barriers, and best practices. *Pediatrics, 144*(6). https://doi.org/10.1542/peds.2019-3223.

Arslanian, S., Bacha, F., Grey, M., Marcus, M. D., White, N. H., & Zeitler, P. (2018). Evaluation and management of youth-onset type 2 diabetes: A position statement by the American Diabetes Association. *Diabetes Care, 41*(12), 2648–2668. https://doi.org/10.2337/dci18-0052.

Barlow, S. E., & Expert Committee. (2007). Expert Committee recommendations regarding the prevention, assessment, and treatment of child and adolescent overweight and obesity: Summary report. *Pediatrics, 120*(Supplement_4), S164–S192. https://doi.org/10.1542/peds.2007-2329C.

Barmherzig, R., & Szperka, C. L. (2019). Pseudotumor cerebri syndrome in children. *Current Pain and Headache Reports, 23*(8), 58. https://doi.org/10.1007/s11916-019-0795-8.

Blanchette, S., Lemoyne, J., & Trudeau, F. (2019). Tackling childhood overweight: Parental perceptions of stakeholders' roles in a community-based intervention. *Global Pediatric Health, 6.* 2333794x19833733. https://doi.org/10.1177/2333794x19833733.

Brady, M., & Rawla, P. (2022). *Acanthosis nigricans.* StatPearls. Retrieved from https://www.ncbi.nlm.nih.gov/books/NBK431057/.

Brix, N., Ernst, A., Lauridsen, L. L. B., Parner, E. T., Arah, O. P., Olsen, J., Henriksen, T. B., & Ramlau-Hansena, C. H. (2020). Childhood overweight and obesity and timing of puberty in boys and girls: Cohort and sibling-matched analyses. *International Journal of Epidemiology, 49*(3), 834–844. doi:10.1093/ije/dyaa056. Erratum in: Int J Epidemiol. 2021 Jul 9;50(3):1047.

Brown, C. L., Halvorson, E. E., Cohen, G. M., Lazorick, S., & Skelton, J. A. (2015). Addressing childhood obesity: Opportunities for prevention. *Pediatric Clinics of North America, 62*(5), 1241–1261. https://doi.org/10.1016/j.pcl.2015.05.013.

Butler, M. G. (2016). Single gene and syndromic causes of obesity: Illustrative examples. *Progress in Molecular Biology and Translational Science, 140,* 1–45. https://doi.org/10.1016/bs.pmbts.2015.12.003.

Butler, M. G., Miller, J. L., & Forster, J. L. (2019). Prader-Willi syndrome—clinical genetics, diagnosis and treatment approaches: An update. *Current Pediatric Reviews, 15*(4), 207–244. https://doi.org/10.2174/1573396315666190716120925.

Calcaterra, V., Pelizzo, G., & Cena, H. (2019). BMI is a poor predictor of nutritional status in disabled children. What is the most recommended method for body composition assessment in this pediatric population? *Frontiers in Pediatrics, 7,* 226. https://doi.org/10.3389/fped.2019.00226.

Calogero, C., Fenu, G., & Lombardi, E. (2018). Measuring airway obstruction in severe asthma in children. *Frontiers in Pediatrics, 6,* 189. https://doi.org/10.3389/fped.2018.00189.

Carey, F. R., Singh, G. K., Brown, H. S., 3rd, & Wilkinson, A. V. (2015). Educational outcomes associated with childhood obesity in the United States: Cross-sectional results from the 2011–2012 National Survey of Children's Health. *International Journal of Behavioral Nutrition and Physical Activity, 12*(Suppl 1(Suppl 1)), S3. https://doi.org/10.1186/1479-5868-12-s1-s3.

Carson, V., Lee, E. Y., Hesketh, K. D., Hunter, S., Kuzik, N., Predy, M., Rhodes, R. E., Rinaldi, C. M., Spence, J. C., & Hinkley, T. (2019). Physical activity and sedentary behavior across three time-points and associations with social skills in early childhood. *BMC Public Health, 19*(1), 27. https://doi.org/10.1186/s12889-018-6381-x.

Centers for Disease Control and Prevention. Tips for better sleep. (2016). Retrieved 09/18/2022 from https://www.cdc.gov/sleep/about_sleep/sleep_hygiene.html.

Centers for Disease Control and Prevention. Adult obesity facts. (2022a). Retrieved 09/07/2022 from https://www.cdc.gov/obesity/data/adult.html.

Centers for Disease Control and Prevention. Child and adolescent immunization schedule: Recommendations for ages 18 years and younger, United States. (2022b). https://www.cdc.gov/vaccines/schedules/hcp/imz/child-adolescent.html.

Centers for Disease Control and Prevention. Early care and education (ECE). (2022c). Retrieved 09/04/2022 from https://www.cdc.gov/obesity/strategies/childcareece.html.

Centers for Disease Control and Prevention. Obesity. (2022d). Retrieved 09/05/2022 from https://www.cdc.gov/healthy-schools/obesity/index.htm.

Centers for Disease Control and Prevention. Disability and obesity. (2019). Center for Disease Control and Prevention. https://www.cdc.gov/ncbddd/disabilityandhealth/obesity.html.

Chatham, R. E., & Mixer, S. J. (2020). Cultural influences on childhood obesity in ethnic minorities: A qualitative systematic review. *Journal of Transcultural Nursing, 31*(1), 87–99. https://doi.org/10.1177/1043659619869428.

Cooksey-Stowers, K., Schwartz, M. B., & Brownell, K. D. (2017). Food swamps predict obesity rates better than food deserts in the United States. *International Journal of Environmental Research and Public Health, 14*(11). https://doi.org/10.3390/ijerph14111366.

Coto, J., Pulgaron, E. R., Graziano, P. A., Bagner, D. M., Villa, M., Malik, J. A., & Delamater, A. M. (2019). Parents as role models: Associations between parent and young children's weight, dietary intake, and physical activity in a minority sample. *Maternal and Child Health Journal, 23*(7), 943–950. https://doi.org/10.1007/s10995-018-02722-z.

Council on Communications and Media. (2016). Media use in school-aged children and adolescents. *Pediatrics, 138*(5). https://doi.org/10.1542/peds.2016-2592.

Council on Communications and Media, Hill, D., Ameenuddin, N., Reid Chassiakos, Y., Cross, C., Hutchinson, J., & Swanson, W. S. (2016). Media and young minds. *Pediatrics, 138*(5). https://doi.org/10.1542/peds.2016-2591.

Daniels, S. R., & Hassink, S. G. Council on Nutrition. (2015). The role of the pediatrician in primary prevention of obesity. *Pediatrics, 136*(1), e275–e292. https://doi.org/10.1542/peds.2015-1558.

Esteghamati, A., Mazaheri, T., Vahidi Rad, M., & Noshad, S. (2015). Complementary and alternative medicine for the treatment of obesity: A critical review. *International Journal of Endocrinology and Metabolism, 13*(2), e19678. https://doi.org/10.5812/ijem.19678.

Flores-Barrantes, P., Iguacel, I., Iglesia-Altaba, I., Moreno, L. A., & Rodríguez, G. (2020). Rapid weight gain, infant feeding practices, and subsequent body mass index trajectories: The CALINA study. *Nutrients, 12*(10), 3178. https://www.mdpi.com/2072-6643/12/10/3178.

Flynn, J. T., Kaelber, D. C., Baker-Smith, C. M., Blowey, D., Carroll, A. E., Daniels, S. R., de Ferranti, S. D., Dionne, J. M., Falkner, B., Flinn, S. K., Gidding, S. S., Goodwin, C., Leu, M. G., Powers, M. E., Rea, C., Samuels, J., Simasek, M., Thaker, V. V., Urbina, E. M., & Subcommittee on Screening and Management of High Blood Pressure in Children (2017). Clinical practice guideline for screening and management of high blood pressure in children and adolescents. *Pediatrics, 140*(3), e20171904. https://doi.org/10.1542/peds.2017-1904.

Fulkerson, J. A., Telke, S., Larson, N., Berge, J., Sherwood, N. E., & Neumark-Sztainer, D. (2019). A healthful home food environment: Is it possible amidst household chaos and parental stress? *Appetite, 142*, 104391. https://doi.org/10.1016/j.appet.2019.104391.

Golden, N. H., & Abrams, S. A. (2014). Optimizing bone health in children and adolescents. *Pediatrics, 134*(4), e1229–e1243. https://doi.org/10.1542/peds.2014-2173.

Guideline Development Panel for Treatment of Obesity, American Psychological Association. (2020). Summary of the clinical practice guideline for multicomponent behavioral treatment of obesity and overweight in children and adolescents. *American Psychologist, 75*(2), 178–188. https://doi.org/10.1037/amp0000530.

Hall, K. D. (2018). Did the food environment cause the obesity epidemic? *Obesity (Silver Spring), 26*(1), 11–13. https://doi.org/10.1002/oby.22073.

Haqq, A. M., Kebbe, M., Tan, Q., Manco, M., & Salas, X. R. (2021). Complexity and stigma of pediatric obesity. *Childhood Obesity, 17*(4), 229–240. https://doi.org/10.1089/chi.2021.0003.

Harvard School of Public Health. School obesity prevention recommendations complete list. Retrieved 09/04/2022 from https://www.hsph.harvard.edu/obesity-prevention-source/obesity-prevention/schools/school-obesity-prevention-recommendations-read-and-print/.

Hassink, S. G. (2017). Early child care and education: A key component of obesity prevention in infancy. *Pediatrics, 140*(6). https://doi.org/10.1542/peds.2017-2846.

Hayes, K., Williams, S. G., Fruh, S., Graves, R. J., Minchew, L. A., & Hall, H. R. (2020). Sleep, screen time, and family meal frequency in preschool children: A pilot study. *Nurse Practitioner, 45*(8), 35–41. https://doi.org/10.1097/01.Npr.0000681788.13417.56.

Heida, A., Koot, B. G., vd Baan-Slootweg, O. H., Pels Rijcken, T. H., Seidell, J. C., Makkes, S., Jansen, P. L., & Benninga, M. A. (2014). Gallstone disease in severely obese children participating in a lifestyle intervention program: Incidence and risk factors. *International Journal of Obesity (London), 38*(7), 950–953. https://doi.org/10.1038/ijo.2014.12.

Heyman, M. B., Abrams, S. A. Section on Gastroenterology, Heptology, and Nutrition, Committee on Nutrition, Heitlinger, L. A., & Schwarzenberg, S. J. (2017). Fruit juice in infants, children, and adolescents: Current recommendations. *Pediatrics, 139*(6). https://doi.org/10.1542/peds.2017-0967.

Ievers-Landis, C. E., Dykstra, C., Uli, N., & O'Riordan, M. A. (2019). Weight-related teasing of adolescents who are primarily obese: Roles of sociocultural attitudes towards appearance and physical activity self-efficacy. *International Journal of Environmental Research and Public Health, 16*(9). https://doi.org/10.3390/ijerph16091540.

Isong, I. A., Rao, S. R., Bind, M. A., Avendaño, M., Kawachi, I., & Richmond, T. K. (2018). Racial and ethnic disparities in early childhood obesity. *Pediatrics, 141*(1). https://doi.org/10.1542/peds.2017-0865.

Jackson, S. E., Llewellyn, C. H., & Smith, L. (2020). The obesity epidemic—nature via nurture: A narrative review of high-income countries. *SAGE Open Medicine, 8*, 2050312120918265. https://doi.org/10.1177/2050312120918265.

Jehan, S., Zizi, F., Pandi-Perumal, S. R., Wall, S., Auguste, E., Myers, A. K., Jean-Louis, G., & McFarlane, S. I. (2017). Obstructive sleep apnea and obesity: Implications for public health. *Journal of Sleep Medicine and Disorders, 1*(4), 00019.

Jones, M., Huffer, C., Adams, T., Jones, L., & Church, B. (2018). BMI health report cards: Parents' perceptions and reactions. *Health Promotion Practice, 19*(6), 896–904. https://doi.org/10.1177/1524839917749489.

Kadouh, H. C., & Acosta, A. (2017). Current paradigms in the etiology of obesity. *Techniques in Gastrointestinal Endoscopy, 19*(1), 2–11. https://doi.org/10.1016/j.tgie.2016.12.001.

Kansra, A. R., Lakkunarajah, S., & Jay, M. S. (2020). Childhood and adolescent obesity: A review. *Frontiers in Pediatrics, 8*, 581461. https://doi.org/10.3389/fped.2020.581461.

Katzmarzyk, P. T., Barlow, S., Bouchard, C., Catalano, P. M., Hsia, D. S., Inge, T. H., Lovelady, C., Raynor, H., Redman, L. M., Staiano, A. E., Spruijt-Metz, D., Symonds, M. E., Vickers, M., Wilfley, D., & Yanovski, J. A. (2014). An evolving scientific basis for the prevention and treatment of pediatric obesity. *International Journal of Obesity (London), 38*(7), 887–905. https://doi.org/10.1038/ijo.2014.49.

Kaufman, T. K., Lynch, B. A., & Wilkinson, J. M. (2020). Childhood obesity: An evidence-based approach to family-centered advice and support. *Journal of Primary Care in Community Health, 11*, 2150132720926279. https://doi.org/10.1177/2150132720926279.

Kipling, M., Ralph, J. E., & Callanan, K. (2014). Psychological impact of male breast disorders: Literature review and survey results. *Breast Care (Basel), 9*(1), 29–33. https://doi.org/10.1159/000358751.

Kral, T. V. E., Chittams, J., & Moore, R. H. (2017). Relationship between food insecurity, child weight status, and parent-reported child eating and snacking behaviors. *Journal for Specialists in Pediatric Nursing, 22*(2). https://doi.org/10.1111/jspn.12177.

Krebs, N. F., Himes, J. H., Jacobson, D., Nicklas, T. A., Guilday, P., & Styne, D. (2007). Assessment of child and adolescent overweight and obesity. *Pediatrics, 120*(Supplement_4), S193–S228. https://doi.org/10.1542/peds.2007-2329D.

Kuczmarski, R. J., Ogden, C. L., Guo, S. S., Grummer-Strawn, L. M., Flegal, K. M., Mei, Z., Wei, R., Curtin, L. R., Roche, A. F., & Johnson, C. L. (2002). 2000 CDC Growth Charts for the United States: Methods and development. *Vital Health Stat, 11*(246), 1–190. PMID: 12043359.

Lang, J. E., Bunnell, H. T., Hossain, M. J., Wysocki, T., Lima, J. J., Finkel, T. H., Bacharier, L., Dempsey, A., Sarzynski, L., Test, M., & Forrest, C. B. (2018). Being overweight or obese and the development of asthma. *Pediatrics, 142*(6), e20182119. https://doi.org/10.1542/peds.2018-2119.

Lee, J. S., Jin, M. H., & Lee, H. J. (2022). Global relationship between parent and child obesity: A systematic review and meta-analysis. *Clinical and Experimental Pediatrics, 65*(1), 35–46. https://doi.org/10.3345/cep.2020.01620.

Llabre, M. M., Gray, J., Ard, J., Nece, P., Bennett, G., Polfuss, M., Brantley, P., Raynor, H., Fiese, B., West, D., & Wilfley, D. (2018). *Clinical practice guideline for multicomponent behavioral treatment of obesity and overweight in children and adolescents: Current state of the evidence and research needs.* American Psychological Association. https://www.apa.org/about/offices/directorates/guidelines/obesity-clinical-practice-guideline.pdf.

Lodish, M. B., Keil, M. F., & Stratakis, C. A. (2018). Cushing's syndrome in pediatrics: An update. *Endocrinology and Metabolism Clinics of North America, 47*(2), 451–462. https://doi.org/10.1016/j.ecl.2018.02.008.

Loos, R. J. F., & Yeo, G. S. H. (2022). The genetics of obesity: From discovery to biology. *Nature Reviews Genetics, 23*(2), 120–133. https://doi.org/10.1038/s41576-021-00414-z.

Lu, K. D., Manoukian, K., Radom-Aizik, S., Cooper, D. M., & Galant, S. P. (2016). Obesity, asthma, and exercise in child and adolescent health. *Pediatric Exercise Science, 28*(2), 264–274. https://doi.org/10.1123/pes.2015-0122.

Madigan, S., Browne, D., Racine, N., Mori, C., & Tough, S. (2019). Association between screen time and children's performance on a developmental screening test. *JAMA Pediatrics, 173*(3), 244–250. https://doi.org/10.1001/jamapediatrics.2018.5056.

Malacarne, D., Handakas, E., Robinson, O., Pineda, E., Saez, M., Chatzi, L., & Fecht, D. (2022). The built environment as determinant of childhood obesity: A systematic literature review. *Obesity Review, 23*(Suppl 1), e13385. https://doi.org/10.1111/obr.13385.

Mandel, M., & Seeley, M., American Board of Orthopedic Surgery, Fellowship Trained in Pediatric Orthopedics. (2021). Genu valgum and obesity in the pediatric patient. *Pediatrics, 147*(3_MeetingAbstract), 833–834. https://doi.org/10.1542/peds.147.3MA9.833.

Marshall, S., Taki, S., Laird, Y., Love, P., Wen, L. M., & Rissel, C. (2022). Cultural adaptations of obesity-related behavioral prevention interventions in early childhood: A systematic review. *Obesity Reviews, 23*(4), e13402. https://doi.org/10.1111/obr.13402.

Martin, A., Booth, J. N., McGeown, S., Niven, A., Sproule, J., Saunders, D. H., & Reilly, J. J. (2017). Longitudinal associations between childhood obesity and academic achievement: Systematic review with focus group data. *Current Obesity Reports, 6*(3), 297–313. https://doi.org/10.1007/s13679-017-0272-9.

Masarwa, R., Brunetti, V. C., Aloe, S., Henderson, M., Platt, R. W., & Filion, K. B. (2021). Efficacy and safety of metformin for obesity: A systematic review. *Pediatrics, 147*(3). https://doi.org/10.1542/peds.2020-1610.

Medscape. Metformin (Rx): Pediatric dosing and uses. (2022). Retrieved 09/10/2022 from https://reference.medscape.com/drug/glucophage-metformin-342717.

Mei, K., Huang, H., Xia, F., Hong, A., Chen, X., Zhang, C., Qiu, G., Chen, G., Wang, Z., Wang, C., Yang, B., Xiao, Q., & Jia, P. (2021). State-of-the-art of measures of the obesogenic environment for children. *Obesity Reviews, 22*(S1), e13093. https://doi.org/10.1111/obr.13093.

Morrissey, B., Taveras, E., Allender, S., & Strugnell, C. (2020). Sleep and obesity among children: A systematic review of multiple sleep dimensions. *Pediatric Obesity, 15*(4), e12619. https://doi.org/10.1111/ijpo.12619.

Must, A., Curtin, C., Hubbard, K., Sikich, L., Bedford, J., & Bandini, L. (2014). Obesity prevention for children with developmental disabilities. *Current Obesity Reports, 3*(2), 156–170. https://doi.org/10.1007/s13679-014-0098-7.

Muth, N. D., Dietz, W. H., Magge, S. N., & Johnson, R. K., American Academy of Pediatrics; Section on Obesity; Committee on Nutrition; American Heart Association (2019). Public policies to reduce sugary drink consumption in children and adolescents. *Pediatrics, 143*(4), e20190282. https://doi.org/10.1542/peds.2019-0282.

National Alliance to Advance Adolescent Health. *Got transition.* (2022). Retrieved 09/11/2022 from https://www.gottransition.org/

National Center for Health Statistics. (2020). QuickStats: Prevalence of obesity and severe obesity among persons aged 2–19 years—National Health and Nutrition Examination Survey, 1999–2000 through 2017–2018. *MMWR, 69*(13), 390. https://doi.org/10.15585/mmwr.mm6913a6.

National Heart, Lung, and Blood Institute. (2011). Expert panel on integrated guidelines for cardiovascular health and risk reduction in children and adolescents: Summary report. *Pediatrics, 128*(Supplement_5), S213–S256.

National Institute of Diabetes and Digestive and Kidney Diseases. *Bariatric surgery for teens with severe obesity study: Teen-LABS.* 2022. Retrieved 09/05/2022 from https://www.niddk.nih.gov/about-niddk/research-areas/obesity/bariatric-surgery-teens-severe-obesity-study-teen-labs.

Notara, V., Giannakopoulou, S. P., Sakellari, E., & Panagiotakos, D. B. (2020). Family-related characteristics and childhood obesity: A systematic literature review. *International Journal of Caring Sciences, 13*(1), 61–72.

NovoMEDLINK. Saxenda. (2022). Retrieved 09/05/2022 from https://www.novomedlink.com/obesity/products/treatments/saxenda/about/for-adolescents.html.

Ogden, C. L., Carroll, M. D., Fakhouri, T. H., Hales, C. M., Fryar, C. D., Li, X., & Freedman, D. S. (2018). Prevalence of obesity among youths by household income and education level of head of household—United States 2011–2014. *MMWR. Morbidity and Mortality Weekly Report, 67*(6), 186–189. https://doi.org/10.15585/mmwr.mm6706a3.

Opstoel K., Chapelle L., Prins, F. J., De Meester A.., Haerens L.., van Tartwijk J., & De Martelaer, K. (2020). Personal and social development in physical education and sports: A review study. *European Physical Education Review, 26*(4), 797–813. https://doi.org/10.1177/1356336x19882054.

Pacheco D., Sleep Foundation. Sleep strategies for kids. (2022). Retrieved 09/18/2022 from https://www.sleepfoundation.org/children-and-sleep/sleep-strategies-kids.

Page, K. A., Luo, S., Wang, X., Chow, T., Alves, J., Buchanan, T. A., & Xiang, A. H. (2019). Children exposed to maternal obesity or gestational diabetes mellitus during early fetal development have hypothalamic alterations that predict future weight gain. *Diabetes Care, 42*(8), 1473–1480. https://doi.org/10.2337/dc18-2581.

Paruthi, S., Brooks, L. J., D'Ambrosio, C., Hall, W. A., Kotagal, S., Lloyd, R. M., Malow, B. A., Maski, K., Nichols, C., Quan, S. F., Rosen, C. L., Troester, M. M., & Wise, M. S. (2016). Recommended amount of sleep for pediatric populations: A consensus statement of the American Academy of Sleep Medicine. *Journal of Clinical Sleep Medicine, 12*(6), 785–786. https://doi.org/10.5664/jcsm.5866.

Pereira, M., Padez, C. M. P., & Nogueira, H. (2019). Describing studies on childhood obesity determinants by socio-ecological model level: A scoping review to identify gaps and provide guidance for future research. *International Journal of Obesity (London), 43*(10), 1883–1890. https://doi.org/10.1038/s41366-019-0411-3.

Petraroli, M., Castellone, E., Patianna, V., & Esposito, S. (2021). Gut microbiota and obesity in adults and children: The state of the art. *Frontiers in Pediatrics, 9*, 657020. https://doi.org/10.3389/fped.2021.657020.

Polfuss, M., Forseth, B., Schoeller, D. A., Huang, C. C., Moosreiner, A., Papanek, P. E., Sawin, K. J., Zvara, K., & Bandini, L. (2021). Accuracy of body mass index in categorizing weight status in children with intellectual and developmental disabilities. *Journal of Pediatric Rehabilitation Medicine, 14*(4), 621–629. https://doi.org/10.3233/prm-200727.

Polfuss, M. L., Duderstadt, K. G., Kilanowski, J. F., Thompson, M. E., Davis, R. L., & Quinn, M. (2020). Childhood obesity: Evidence-based guidelines for clinical practice—part one. *Journal of Pediatric Health Care, 34*(3), 283–290. https://doi.org/10.1016/j.pedhc.2019.12.003.

Pont, S. J., Puhl, R., Cook, S. R., & Slusser, W. (2017). Stigma experienced by children and adolescents with obesity. *Pediatrics, 140*(6). https://doi.org/10.1542/peds.2017-3034.

Pratt, J. S. A., Browne, A., Browne, N. T., Bruzoni, M., Cohen, M., Desai, A., Inge, T., Linden, B. C., Mattar, S. G., Michalsky, M., Podkameni, D., Reichard, K. W., Stanford, F. C., Zeller, M. H., & Zitsman, J. (2018). ASMBS pediatric metabolic and bariatric surgery guidelines. *Surgery for Obesity and Related Diseases, 14*(7), 882–901. https://doi.org/10.1016/j.soard.2018.03.019.

Rankin, J., Matthews, L., Cobley, S., Han, A., Sanders, R., Wiltshire, H. D., & Baker, J. S. (2016). Psychological consequences of childhood obesity: Psychiatric comorbidity and prevention. *Adolescent Health, Medicine and Therapeutics, 7*, 125–146. https://doi.org/10.2147/ahmt.S101631.

Rhee, K. E., Kessl, S., Lindback, S., Littman, M., & El-Kareh, R. E. (2018). Provider views on childhood obesity management in primary care settings: A mixed methods analysis. *BMC Health Services Research, 18*(1), 55. https://doi.org/10.1186/s12913-018-2870-y.

Riveros-McKay, F., Mistry, V., Bounds, R., Hendricks, A., Keogh, J. M., Thomas, H., Henning, E., Corbin, L. J., Understanding Society Scientific Group, O'Rahilly, S., Zeggini, E., Wheeler, E., Barroso, I., & Farooqi, I. S. (2019). Genetic architecture of human thinness compared to severe obesity. *PLoS Genetics, 15*(1), e1007603. https://doi.org/10.1371/journal.pgen.1007603.

Roberts, K. J., Polfuss, M. L., Marston, E. C., & Davis, R. L. (2021). Experiences of weight stigma in adolescents with severe obesity and their families. *Journal of Advanced Nursing, 77*(10), 4184–4194.

Robinson, T. N., Banda, J. A., Hale, L., Lu, A. S., Fleming-Milici, F., Calvert, S. L., & Wartella, E. (2017). Screen media exposure and obesity in children and adolescents. *Pediatrics, 140*(Suppl 2), S97–S101. https://doi.org/10.1542/peds.2016-1758K.

Ruiter, E. L. M., Saat, J. J. E. H., Molleman, G. R. M., Fransen, G. A. J., van der Velden, K., van Jaarsveld, C. H. M., Engels, R. C. M. E., & Assendelft, W. J. J. (2020). Parents' underestimation of their child's weight status. Moderating factors and change over time: A cross-sectional study. *PLoS One, 15*(1), e0227761. https://doi.org/10.1371/journal.pone.0227761.

Ryan, S., Crinion, S. J., & McNicholas, W. T. (2014). Obesity and sleep-disordered breathing—when two 'bad guys' meet. *QJM, 107*(12), 949–954. https://doi.org/10.1093/qjmed/hcu029.

Sagar, R., & Gupta, T. (2018). Psychological aspects of obesity in children and adolescents. *Indian Journal of Pediatrics, 85*(7), 554–559. https://doi.org/10.1007/s12098-017-2539-2.

Sahoo, K., Sahoo, B., Choudhury, A. K., Sofi, N. Y., Kumar, R., & Bhadoria, A. S. (2015). Childhood obesity: Causes and consequences. *Journal of Family Medicine and Primary Care, 4*(2), 187–192. https://doi.org/10.4103/2249-4863.154628.

Sanders, L. M., Allen, J. C., Blankenship, J., Decker, E. A., Christ-Erwin, M., Hentges, E. J., Jones, J. M., Mohamedshah, F. Y., Ohlhorst, S. D., Ruff, J., & Wegner, J. (2021). Implementing the 2020–2025 dietary guidelines for Americans: Recommendations for a path forward. *Journal of Food Science, 86*(12), 5087–5099. https://doi.org/10.1111/1750-3841.15969.

Schneider, M. B., & Benjamin, H. J., Committee on Nutrition, Council on Sport Medicine and Fitness. (2018). Sports drinks and energy drinks for children and adolescents: Are they appropriate? *Pediatrics, 141*(3), e20174173. https://doi.org/10.1542/peds.2017-4173.

Schnurr, T. M., Ängquist, L., Nøhr, E. A., Hansen, T., Sørensen, T. I. A., & Morgen, C. S. (2022). Smoking during pregnancy is associated with child overweight independent of maternal pre-pregnancy BMI and genetic predisposition to adiposity. *Science Reports, 12*(1), 3135. https://doi.org/10.1038/s41598-022-07122-6.

Singh, S. A., Dhanasekaran, D., Ganamurali, N. L. P., & Sabarathinam, S. (2021). Junk food-induced obesity—a growing threat to youngsters during the pandemic. *Obesity Medicine, 26*, 100364. https://doi.org/10.1016/j.obmed.2021.100364.

Singhal, V., Sella, A. C., & Malhotra, S. (2021). Pharmacotherapy in pediatric obesity: Current evidence and landscape. *Current Opinion in Endocrinology, Diabetes and Obesity, 28*(1), 55–63. https://doi.org/10.1097/med.0000000000000587.

Skinner, A. C., Ravanbakht, S. N., Skelton, J. A., Perrin, E. M., & Armstrong, S. C. (2018). Prevalence of obesity and severe obesity in US children, 1999–2016. *Pediatrics, 141*(3). https://doi.org/10.1542/peds.2017-3459.

Smith, R., Kelly, B., Yeatman, H., & Boyland, E. (2019). Food marketing influences children's attitudes, preferences and consumption: A systematic critical review. *Nutrients, 11*(4). https://doi.org/10.3390/nu11040875.

Smith, S. M., Sumar, B., & Dixon, K. A. (2014). Musculoskeletal pain in overweight and obese children. *International Journal of Obesity (London), 38*(1), 11–15. https://doi.org/10.1038/ijo.2013.187.

Spear, B. A., Barlow, S. E., Ervin, C., Ludwig, D. S., Saelens, B. E., Schetzina, K. E., & Taveras, E. M. (2007). Recommendations for treatment of child and adolescent overweight and obesity. *Pediatrics, 120*(Supplement_4), S254–S288. https://doi.org/10.1542/peds.2007-2329F.

Srivastava, G., O'Hara, V., & Browne, N. (2018). Sleep disturbance as a contributor to pediatric obesity: Implications and screening. *Journal of Sleep Disorder Management, 4*, 19.

St Pierre, C., Ver Ploeg, M., Dietz, W. H., Pryor, S., Jakazi, C. S., Layman, E., Noymer, D., Coughtrey-Davenport, T., & Sacheck, J. M. (2022). Food insecurity and childhood obesity: A systematic review. *Pediatrics, 150*(1), e2021055571. https://doi.org/10.1542/peds.2021-055571.

Stewart, J., McCallin, T., Martinez, J., Chacko, S., & Yusuf, S. (2020). Hyperlipidemia. *Pediatrics in Review, 41*(8), 393–402. https://doi.org/10.1542/pir.2019-0053.

Stierman, B., Afful, J., Carroll, M. D., Te-Ching, C., Orlando, D., Fink, S., Fryar, C., Qiuping, G., Hales, C., Hughes, J., Ostchega, Y., Storandt, R., & Akinbami, L. (2021). *National health and nutrition examination survey 2017–March 2020 prepandemic data files development of files and prevalence estimates for selected health outcomes* [journal issue]. National Health Statistics Reports. https://stacks.cdc.gov/view/cdc/106273.

Stiglic, N., & Viner, R. M. (2019). Effects of screentime on the health and well-being of children and adolescents: A systematic review of reviews. *BMJ Open, 9*(1), e023191. https://doi.org/10.1136/bmjopen-2018-023191.

Stolzman, S., Irby, M. B., Callahan, A. B., & Skelton, J. A. (2015). Pes planus and paediatric obesity: A systematic review of the literature. *Clinical Obesity, 5*(2), 52–59. https://doi.org/10.1111/cob.12091.

Stormacq, C., Wosinski, J., Boillat, E., & Van den Broucke, S. (2020). Effects of health literacy interventions on health-related outcomes in socioeconomically disadvantaged adults living in the community: A systematic review. *JBI Evidence Synthesis, 18*(7), 1389–1469. https://doi.org/10.11124/jbisrir-d-18-00023.

Stricker, P. R., Faigenbaum, A. D., McCambridge, T. M., & Council on Sports Medicine and Fitness (2020). Resistance training for children and adolescents. *Pediatrics, 145*(6), e20201011. https://doi.org/10.1542/peds.2020-1011.

Styne, D. M., Arslanian, S. A., Connor, E. L., Farooqi, I. S., Murad, M. H., Silverstein, J. H., & Yanovski, J. A. (2017). Pediatric obesity—assessment, treatment, and prevention: An Endocrine Society clinical practice guideline. *Journal of Clinical Endocrinology & Metabolism, 102*(3), 709–757. https://doi.org/10.1210/jc.2016-2573.

Suire, K. B., Kavookjian, J., & Wadsworth, D. D. (2020). Motivational interviewing for overweight children: A systematic review. *Pediatrics, 146*(5). https://doi.org/10.1542/peds.2020-0193.

Sweeny, K. F., & Lee, C. K. (2021). Nonalcoholic fatty liver disease in children. *Gastroenterology and Hepatology (New York), 17*(12), 579–587.

Totura, C. M., Figueroa, H. L., Wharton, C., & Marsiglia, F. F. (2015). Assessing implementation of evidence-based childhood obesity prevention strategies in schools. *Preventive Medicine Reports, 2*, 347–354. https://doi.org/10.1016/j.pmedr.2015.04.008.

Trent, M., & Gordon, C. M. (2020). Diagnosis and management of polycystic ovary syndrome in adolescents. *Pediatrics, 145*(Supplement_2), S210–S218. https://doi.org/10.1542/peds.2019-2056J.

Turer, C. B., Mehta, M., Durante, R., Wazni, F., & Flores, G. (2015). Parental perspectives regarding primary-care weight-management strategies for school-age children. *Maternal and Child Nutrition, 12*(2), 326–338. https://doi.org/10.1111/mcn.12131.

US Department of Agriculture. (n.d.). *MyPlate*. Retrieved September 1 from https://health.gov.

US Department of Health and Human Services. (2018). *Physical activity guidelines for Americans* https://health.gov/our-work/nutrition-physical-activity/physical-activity-guidelines.

US Department of Health and Human Services. (2020). *Dietary guidelines for Americans, 2020–2025*. Retrieved from https://www.dietaryguidelines.gov/resources/2020-2025-dietary-guidelines-online-materials.

US Preventive Services Task Force. (2017). Screening for obesity in children and adolescents: US Preventive Services Task Force recommendation statement. *JAMA, 317*(23), 2417–2426. https://doi.org/10.1001/jama.2017.6803.

Verduci, E., Bronsky, J., Embleton, N., Gerasimidis, K., Indrio, F., Köglmeier, J., de Koning, B., Lapillonne, A., Moltu, S. J., Norsa, L., Domellöf, M., & ESPGHAN Committee on Nutrition (2021). Role of dietary factors, food habits, and lifestyle in childhood obesity development: A position paper from the European Society for Paediatric Gastroenterology, Hepatology and Nutrition Committee on Nutrition. *Journal of Pediatric Gastroenterology and Nutrition, 72*(5), 769–783. https://doi.org/10.1097/mpg.0000000000003075.

Wagner, I. V., Sabin, M. A., Pfäffle, R. W., Hiemisch, A., Sergeyev, E., Körner, A., & Kiess, W. (2012). Effects of obesity on human sexual development. *Nature Reviews Endocrinology, 8*(4), 246–254. https://doi.org/10.1038/nrendo.2011.241.

Walker, J. L., Hosseinzadeh, P., White, H., Murr, K., Milbrandt, T. A., Talwalkar, V. J., Iwinski, H., & Muchow, R. (2019). Idiopathic genu valgum and its association with obesity in children and adolescents. *Journal of Pediatric Orthopedics, 39*(7), 347–352. https://doi.org/10.1097/bpo.0000000000000971.

Walsh, Ó., Dettmer, E., Regina, A., Dentakos, S., Christian, J., Hamilton, J., & Toulany, A. (2022). 'Teenagers are into perfect-looking things': Dating, sexual attitudes and experiences of adolescents with severe obesity. *Child: Care, Health and Development, 48*(3), 406–414. https://doi.org/10.1111/cch.12940.

Williams, A. S., Ge, B., Petroski, G., Kruse, R. L., McElroy, J. A., & Koopman, R. J. (2018). Socioeconomic status and other factors associated with childhood obesity. *Journal of the American Board of Family Medicine, 31*(4), 514–521. https://doi.org/10.3122/jabfm.2018.04.170261.

World Health Organization. (2019). *Guidelines on physical activity, sedentary behaviour and sleep for children under 5 years of age*. https://apps.who.int/iris/handle/10665/311664.

World Health Organization. (2020). *Noncommunicable diseases: Childhood overweight and obesity*. Retrieved September 4 from https://www.who.int/news-room/questions-and-answers/item/noncommunicable-diseases-childhood-overweight-and-obesity.

World Health Organization. (2021). *WHO guideline: Management of adolescents 10–19 years of age with obesity for improved health, functioning and reduced disability: A primary health care approach*. Retrieved 09/05/2022 from https://www.who.int/news-room/events/detail/2021/09/28/default-calendar/2nd-GDG-meeting-management-of-adolescents-10-19-years-of-age-with-obesity-for-improved-health-functioning-and-reduced-disability-a-primary-health-care-approach.

Yang, L., Liang, C., Yu, Y., Xiao, Q., Xi, M., & Tang, L. (2022). Family sports interventions for the treatment of obesity in childhood: A meta-analysis. *Journal of Health, Population and Nutrition, 41*(1), 40. https://doi.org/10.1186/s41043-022-00317-7.

Organ Transplantation

33

Stacia Marie Hays

Pediatric solid organ transplantation is the only curative therapeutic procedure for various end-stage organ diseases; it is now a standard and effective treatment. The purpose of transplantation is to positively impact children's health and quality of life (Jara et al., 2020). The goals of transplantation include preventing rejection of the organ (graft), minimizing long-term sequelae of medications, and aiding recipients to lead healthy and normal lives. As pediatric organ transplants become more prevalent, it is essential that primary care providers are aware of the specialized needs, complications, and follow-up required for optimal outcomes in this population. Collaborative, multidisciplinary care is at the forefront of management. This complex surgical procedure is followed by intensive surgical and medical management to promote stable organ function. Routine postoperative monitoring is required to maintain graft function while minimizing medical, surgical, and developmental complications. The liver, kidney, and heart are the most commonly transplanted solid organs in the pediatric population. Less common are lung, heart, lung-heart combination, and intestinal transplants. The Organ Procurement and Transplantation Network (OPTN) reported 1890 solid organ transplants in children less than 1 year of age through age 17 years performed in the United States in 2021 (OPTN, 2022a). Since 1988, more than 52,000 children have received a kidney, liver, or heart transplant with 5-year patient survival rates of 75% to 88% (Table 33.1) (OPTN, 2022b).

As the science of transplantation evolves, indications for liver, kidney, heart, lung, and intestine transplantation continue to expand (Table 33.2). However not all pediatric patients with indications for transplant qualify. These include a patient not experiencing significant impact from the organ disease, has an active infection(s), or is too sick to tolerate the surgery. Psychosocial concerns may also prevent transplantation concerns regarding family support, and those with severe disabilities and crippling conditions where transplantation may extend suffering may not be good candidates for transplantation (Prüfe, 2022).

This chapter will discuss the most common solid organ transplants performed in children and guide the pediatric-focused provider in supporting the transplant recipient and family. Understanding the pre-, intra-, and postoperative transplant processes, identifying primary care needs and possible transplant complications, and providing guidance in regard to contacting the transplant center and coordinator for direction related to the care of the child before and after transplantation help promote successful transplantation outcomes.

SOLID ORGAN TRANSPLANTATION

RENAL

Renal transplantation was first introduced in 1954 and is the gold-standard treatment in those with end-stage renal disease (ESRD) because it increases survival and improves the quality of life (Dirix et al., 2022). In 2021, there were 710 renal transplants in children age 1 to 17 years, and 66% (472) were in children age 7 to 11 years (OPTN, 2022a). In recent years adolescents have had the highest number of renal transplants. Historically, common causes of renal failure resulting in pediatric ESRD requiring transplantation are aplastic/hypoplastic/dysplastic kidneys, obstructive uropathy, and focal segmental glomerulosclerosis (FSGS) (North American Pediatric Renal Trials and Collaborative Studies [NAPRTCS], 2014). Several renal conditions have genetic etiologies that can lead to chronic and end-stage renal disease. Genetic etiologies include Alport syndrome, FSGS, Wilms tumor, familial juvenile nephronophthisis, and polycystic kidney disease (which can be either autosomal dominant or autosomal recessive).

Gene therapy for the treatment of chronic kidney disease (CKD) has gained momentum over the past few years. Gene therapy could provide a way to deliver genes that slow or reverse cell damage that leads to CKD. Researchers are working to develop ways to identify the genes that cause inherited kidney diseases and treat conditions in transplanted organs (Sauerwein, 2018). The hope is that this research will provide new technology to diagnose, treat, and possibly prevent renal failure in children.

LIVER

As an established curative treatment for pediatric patients with acute or chronic end-stage liver disease (ESLD) and failure, liver transplantation remains the most common solid organ transplant in this population. Biliary atresia, an obstructive biliary tract condition,

787

Table 33.1　Survival Rates of Pediatric Solid Organ Transplant Recipients by Organ

	1-YR SURVIVAL (%)	3-YR SURVIVAL (%)	5-YR SURVIVAL (%)
Kidney	>95	90–94	78–88
Liver	87–93	83–88	79–88
Heart	87–97	84–92	75–84
Lung	74–100	60–76	43–66

From Katz, D. T., Torees, N. S., Chatani, B., Gonzalez, I. A., Chandar, J., Miloh, T., Rusconi, P., Garcia, J. (2020). Care of pediatric solid organ transplant recipients: An overview for primary care providers. *Pediatrics, 146*(6), e20200696.

Table 33.2　Comparative Indications for Transplantation in Children by Organ[a]

RENAL	LIVER	CARDIAC	LUNG AND DUAL TRANSPLANT
Congenital Condition	**Cholestatic Disease**	**Cardiomyopathy**	**Lung**
Congenital nephrotic syndrome	Alagille syndrome	Dilated	Cystic fibrosis
Eagle-Barrett syndrome	Byler syndrome	Hypertrophic	Primary pulmonary
Renal dysplasia	Biliary atresia	Restrictive	Hypertension
Renal hypoplasia/aplasia	Familial cholestasis	**Congenital Heart Defects**	Pulmonary arterial hypertension
Wilms tumor	**Parenchymal Disease**	Hypoplastic left	Obliterative bronchiolitis
Obstructive uropathy	Budd-Chiari syndrome	heart syndrome	Interstitial lung disease
Reflux nephropathy	Congenital hepatic fibrosis	Tetralogy of Fallot	**Heart and Liver**
Acquired Disease	Cystic fibrosis	Transposition of the	Familial hypercholesterolemia
Chronic pyelonephritis	Neonatal hepatitis	great vessels	with ischemic cardiomyopathy
Focal segmental glomerulosclerosis	Acute fulminant hepatic failure	Ebstein anomaly	Intrahepatic biliary atresia and dilated cardiomyopathy
Glomerulonephritis	Hepatitis B		**Liver and Kidney**
Hemolytic-uremic syndrome	Hepatitis C		Cystinosis
Henoch-Schönlein purpura	**Metabolic Disorders**		Oxalosis
Immunoglobulin A nephropathy	Alpha$_1$-antitrypsin deficiency		**Heart and Lung**
Lupus nephritis	Glycogen storage disease, types I, III, IV		Congenital heart defects with elevated pulmonary vascular resistance (e.g., Eisenmenger syndrome)
Membranoproliferative glomerulonephritis, types I, II	Tyrosinemia		
Renal infarct	Wilson disease		
Sickle cell nephropathy	Crigler-Najjar syndrome		
Hereditary Condition	Urea cycle disorders		
Alport syndrome	Hepatomas		
Juvenile nephronophthisis	Hepatoblastoma		
Polycystic kidney disease	Hepatocellular carcinoma		
Metabolic Disorders			
Cystinosis			
Oxalosis			

[a]Includes the most common indications for pediatric transplant and is not all inclusive.

accounts for approximately 50% of pediatric liver transplants performed (Elisofon et al., 2020). A surgical procedure known as a Kasai portoenterostomy may result in improved bile drainage if performed within an infant's first 120 days of life. After that time, progressive liver disease and mortality risk increase significantly, requiring transplantation before the age of 2 years. Metabolic conditions that may require transplantation include Wilson disease, alpha$_1$-antitrypsin deficiency, glycogen storage disease, hemochromatosis, maple syrup urine disease, cystic fibrosis, and phenylketonuria (Sanad et al., 2021). Causes of acute liver failure include a variety of etiologies depending on age group. In younger children, infections, such as viral hepatitis and metabolic disorders, are the most common causes; in children

and adolescents, toxic ingestions, including medications such as acetaminophen, are a significant cause (Shanmugam & Dhawan, 2018).

Several etiologies of liver disease requiring transplantation have a genetic predisposition. These include familial cholestasis, Alagille syndrome, Byler syndrome, Wilson disease, and alpha$_1$-antitrypsin deficiency. In addition, some children with cystic fibrosis, an autosomal recessive disorder, may have secondary liver disease requiring transplantation. Research continues for the prevention and treatment of diseases causing ESLD.

CARDIAC

The first human-to-human cardiac transplant was performed in 1968. Since then, cardiac transplants have become a standard of care for children with end-stage cardiac failure. Cardiomyopathy and congenital heart diseases (CHD) are the leading indications for heart transplantation in children. In infants, the major cause for transplantation is due to CHD, while adolescents have an increased incidence of myopathies requiring transplantation (Bock & Chinnock, 2022; National Organization for Rare Disorders [NORD], 2019). The etiologies of cardiomyopathy are varied. Factors include genetic, familial, or secondary causes such as infection, systemic disease, exposure to toxins, or malnutrition (CDC, 2023).

LUNG

Lung transplantation has grown into an accepted therapeutic alternative for children with end-stage lung disease. Although 1-year survival rates have improved, long-term outcomes and survival remain less than other organ transplants (Faro & Visner, 2019). Cystic fibrosis and pulmonary hypertension most commonly lead to end-stage lung disease requiring lung transplantation, with cystic fibrosis being the most frequent pretransplant diagnosis in children age 1 to 10 years (Faro & Visner, 2019). In infants, CHD, surfactant dysfunction syndromes, and idiopathic pulmonary hypertension are the most common causes. Pediatric heart-lung transplantation is rare, especially in infants, mainly due to the limited availability of organs and poor 1-year survival rates of only 27% (Carvajal et al., 2022).

PREVALENCE OF SOLID ORGAN TRANSPLANTATION

The number of pediatric solid organ transplants increases yearly compared to the previous year (OPTN, 2022b). As of November 25, 2022, the OPTN reported that nearly 105.327 children age less than 1 year to 17 years were listed for solid organ transplantation (OPTN, 2022a).

Table 33.3 demonstrates the number of total pediatric organ transplantations in 2022 by age and organ. Nearly 2000 children received a solid organ transplant; the most common was renal transplant, followed in descending order by liver, cardiac, and lung (OPTN, 2022b).

DIAGNOSTIC CRITERIA

Referral for transplant is a multidisciplinary and complex process. In general, it should be considered when the benefit of transplantation outweighs the risk of living with the failing organ. When possible, referral should begin before the need for transplantation becomes urgent (Table 33.4). This allows an opportunity to address barriers to transplant, such as social support, malnutrition, and vaccine requirements, and provide education regarding the pretransplant, perioperative, and posttransplant periods.

Preemptive transplantation is recommended to improve outcomes in renal transplantation. Recent studies have identified a negative relationship between time spent on dialysis and patient and/or graft survival (Haller et al., 2017). Assessment of the glomerular filtration rate (GFR) is the most important test for determining kidney function. GFR is a good indicator of CKD. In children, the Schwartz formula is used to determine GFR, which is expressed in mL/min/1.73 m^2. This formula considers the child's age and weight in addition to the serum creatinine level. In North America, the pediatric end-stage liver disease (PELD) score and the model for end-stage liver disease (MELD) score were developed to accurately measure the severity of liver disease and better predict the risk of dying or moving to an intensive care unit for 3 months posttransplant. The PELD score takes into consideration the international normalized ratio (INR), total bilirubin, serum albumin, age less than 1 year, and height less than 2 SD from the mean for age and gender; however, its accuracy is a subject of debate. The MELD score for those age 12 years and older is based on bilirubin, INR, and serum creatinine and has been recognized as more accurate than PELD in older children (United Network for Organ Sharing [UNOS], 2008).

There are few published objective criteria for being placed on a list for pediatric heart transplantation. One such indicator is decreased exercise tolerance with peak oxygen consumption less than 50% for predicted age and sex (Canter et al., 2007). Other indications include heart failure with ventricular dysfunctions, near sudden death episodes, reactive pulmonary hypertension, and severe cyanosis (Thrush & Hoffman, 2014). In the absence of clear objective criteria, expected survival of

Table **33.3**	US National Data: 2022 Transplants by Age and Organ				
AGE	**NUMBER TRANSPLANTED**	**KIDNEY TRANSPLANT**	**LIVER TRANSPLANT**	**HEART**	**LUNG**
<1 yr	263	1	145	114	1
1–5 yr	434	148	170	97	3
6–10 yr	263	122	67	66	1
11–17 yr	834	432	144	214	13
Total	1777	703	526	298	18

From Organ Procurement and Transplant Network. (2022b). National data. https://optn.transplant.hrsa.gov/data/view-data-reports/national-data/.

Table 33.4   **Indicators of Organ Dysfunction**

RENAL	LIVER	CARDIAC	LUNG
Anemia	Ascites	Abdominal pain, indigestion	Dyspnea, even while resting
Dysgeusia (taste distortion)	Coagulopathy	Cardiomegaly	Exercise intolerance
Edema	Elevated hepatic enzymes	Color change with feeding	Feeding intolerance/poor
Hypertension	(ALT, AST, bilirubin, GGTP)	(pallor or dusky)	feeding/appetite
Fatigue	Cholangitis	Dyspnea, even while resting	Fatigue
Growth failure, failure to	Encephalopathy	Edema	Frequent infections
thrive	Fatigue	Exercise intolerance	Growth failure, failure to
Hypophosphatemia	Hepatomegaly	Growth failure, failure to	thrive
Malnutrition, muscle wasting	Hyperammonemia	thrive	Persistent cough
Poor feeding	Hypoalbuminemia,	Fatigue	Poor oxygen saturation
Recurrent emesis	hypoproteinemia	Growth failure, failure to	Weight loss
Rickets	Jaundice	thrive	Persistent wheezing
	Malnutrition, muscle wasting	Feeding intolerance/poor	
	Pruritis	feeding/appetite	
	Rickets, fractures (inabil-	Nonspecific ST segment,	
	ity to absorb fat-soluble	T-wave changes	
	vitamins)	Pallor	
	Splenomegaly	Recurrent vomiting	
	Variceal bleeding	Syncope (older child)	
	Xanthomas	Tachycardia	
	Growth failure, failure to thrive	Weight loss	

ALT, alanine aminotransferase; *AST*, aspartate aminotransferase; *GGTP*, Gamma-Glutamyl Transpeptidase.

less than 2 years and quality of life without transplant are important considerations.

Expected survival and quality of life are key considerations for potential lung transplant recipients. The current criteria for being placed on a listing for a lung transplant are for patients with greater than a 50% chance of death from lung disease (International Society for Heart & Lung Transplant [ISHLT], 2021). Diagnostic criteria include forced expiratory volume in 1 second (FEV_1) of less than 30%, the accepted threshold for lung transplantation assessment, and below 50% for those with cystic fibrosis (ISHLT, 2021).

CLINICAL MANIFESTATIONS FOR TRANSPLANTATION CONSIDERATION

The symptoms and severity of illness in children with end-stage organ disease vary according to the specific condition and affected organ, length of illness, age of the child, and effectiveness of treatments. Table 33.5 identifies common clinical manifestations at the time of transplant consideration.

RENAL

Children with ESRD exhibit symptoms related to fluid and electrolyte imbalances, hypertension, fatigue, feeding intolerance, recurrent emesis, growth failure, edema, anemia, and rickets (National Institute of Diabetes and Digestive Kidney Diseases, 2022).

LIVER

Children with liver disease may have an acute or chronic course of illness depending on the etiology

and severity of the liver condition. Some children may remain stable for several years with appropriate medical management, and others may have a moderate to rapid decline in hepatic function, requiring more emergent transplantation. Depending on the cause of liver disease, ESLD can rapidly progress to liver failure in a few weeks. Symptoms of liver dysfunction may include jaundice, hepatomegaly, splenomegaly, ascites, pruritus, xanthomas, and variceal bleeding. Hepatic enzymes, bilirubin, gamma-glutamyl transpeptidase phosphate (GGTP), and ammonia levels are elevated. Albumin and total protein levels will be low due to the inability to process fats and fat-soluble vitamins; bruising due to decreased clotting abilities may be noted. Children who have biliary atresia or a Kasai portoenterostomy are also at risk for cholangitis with symptoms of abdominal pain and fever. Other symptoms associated with liver failure may include delayed growth, malnutrition, rickets, and osteomalacia with fractures. With the progression of hepatic dysfunction, cerebral edema increases, causing intracranial hypertension, which can lead to irreversible neurologic damage, uncal herniation, and death (American Liver Foundation, 2022).

CARDIAC

Complex CHD and cardiomyopathies requiring transplantation may have similar initial symptoms. Symptoms of cardiomyopathy vary depending on the child's age at onset of the illness and the type of cardiomyopathy. The clinical manifestations of dilated cardiomyopathy include signs and symptoms of congestive heart failure as a result of decreasing

Table 33.5   Clinical Manifestations at Time of Transplant Consideration

RENAL	LIVER	CARDIAC	LUNG
Anemia	Ascites	Arrhythmias	Exercise intolerance
Congestive heart failure	Coagulopathies	Cardiac murmurs	Growth retardation
Edema/hypervolemia	Encephalopathy	Congestive heart failure	Malnutrition
Elevated blood urea nitrogen and creatinine	Hepatomegaly	Growth retardation	Respiratory distress
Growth retardation	Hormone imbalance	Respiratory distress	
Hyperkalemia	Hyperammonemia	ST- and T-wave abnormalities	
Hyperlipidemia	Hypercholesterolemia	Tachypnea	
Hyperphosphatemia	Hypoalbuminemia		
Hypertension	Hypoglycemia		
Metabolic acidosis	Jaundice		
Pericarditis	Malnutrition		
Peripheral neuropathy	Portal hypertension		
Renal osteodystrophy	Splenomegaly		
Secondary hyperparathyroidism			

myocardial contractility. These include an enlarged heart on chest radiography, nonspecific ST segment and T-wave changes, sinus tachycardia on electrocardiography (ECG), and gallop rhythm on auscultation. Nonspecific symptoms are common and include fever, vomiting, weight loss, poor feeding, or failure to thrive (NORD, 2019), which are often first identified by the primary care provider. A cardiac defect should be suspected when a cluster of nonspecific signs and symptoms are identified.

Most children discovered to have hypertrophic cardiomyopathy do not have prominent cardiac symptoms since the thickening of the left ventricular wall may remain stable or progress slowly. Children and young adults are at risk for episodes of syncope and sudden death during exercise when the left ventricular demand increases and obstruction to the outflow tract occurs. This diagnosis is sometimes first made on autopsy.

LUNG

Lung transplant candidates have evidence of advanced chronic lung disease no longer alleviated by medical therapy, predicted survival of less than 50%, an FEV_1 less than 30%, poor tolerance on a 6-minute walk test demonstrated by poor arterial oxygen saturation, declining nutritional status, and poor quality of life (Leard et al., 2021; Weill et al., 2015). However, quality of life occasionally does not mirror the child's clinical condition and must be assessed independently.

MANAGEMENT AND TREATMENT

PRETRANSPLANT MANAGEMENT

Management of the patient requiring transplantation requires a multidisciplinary team approach (Box 33.1). This includes the transplant team, dietitian, physical therapist, occupational therapist, and (most importantly) transplant coordinator, who is the main point of contact for those outside of the transplant team. The primary care provider is an important member of this team because families may contact the provider before reaching out to the transplant team. The relationship between the transplant coordinator and primary care provider is vital to maintaining the child's growth, development, and overall health in the pretransplant phase.

Renal. Conservative therapy for CKD involves managing fluid, electrolyte, metabolic imbalances, hypertension, and anemia. Conservative therapy is not always an option in cases of acute renal failure or CKD. Transplantation is the treatment choice for children with ESRD to maximize survival, growth and development, and overall quality of life (Ghelichi-Ghojogh et al., 2022).

Liver. Children with chronic liver disease may be followed on an outpatient basis with medical management designed to optimize and stabilize hepatic function. To meet nutritional requirements, these children may require enteral supplementation, administration of fat-soluble vitamins, and/or total parenteral nutrition. Synthetic function of the liver, coagulation times, ammonia levels, electrolytes, fluid balance, and renal function must be frequently monitored to assess for changes that may impact listing for transplant.

Medications may provide symptomatic relief to mitigate the effects of hepatic dysfunction. For those with coagulopathy, vitamin K is taken daily. Ursodeoxycholic acid may help decrease cholestasis. Cholestatic pruritus may be lessened with single or combination therapy, including bile acid sequestrants (i.e., cholestyramine), rifampicin, and antihistamines such as hydroxyzine, naltrexone, and sertraline (Dull & Kremer, 2020; Kriegermeier & Green, 2020). Elevated

Box 33.1   Peri- and Pretransplant Management

RENAL
Conservative therapy for renal condition
Manage fluid balance
Treat metabolic disturbance
Manage hypertension
Treat anemia
Dialysis

LIVER
Medical management to stabilize hepatic function
Management of coagulopathy
Prevention of bleeding from esophageal and gastric varices
Enteral supplementation
Fat-soluble vitamin replacement
Pharmacologic treatment for symptoms

CARDIAC
Maximize cardiac function and controlling symptoms of congestive heart failure
Surgical intervention as necessary
Management of arrhythmias
Management of pulmonary hypertension
Ventricular assist device for bridge to transplantation

LUNG
Management of pulmonary hypertension
Management of hypoxemia
Enteral supplementation
Extracorporeal life/lung support

EVALUATION FOR TRANSPLANTATION (ALL ORGANS)
Multidisciplinary evaluation
Pretransplant surgical procedures
Laboratory assessment

POSTTRANSPLANTATION (ALL ORGANS)
Immunosuppressive management
Infection prophylaxis
Graft evaluation
Ancillary therapies to improve function and quality of life

---

ammonia levels may be improved by lactulose, neomycin, and/or metronidazole (Liu et al., 2018).

Acute and recurrent cholangitis are common complications in children with a history of the Kasai procedure. Caused by biliary stasis and bacterial contamination, symptoms include a fever greater than 38°C (100.4°F), abdominal pain, worsening jaundice with increased serum bilirubin concentration, and an elevated white blood cell count (Calinescu et al., 2022). Diagnosis is confirmed primarily through positive blood cultures. Treatment includes an appropriately sensitive intravenous antibiotic. Long-term prophylaxis with trimethoprim-sulfamethoxazole-metronidazole or ciprofloxacin hydrochloride remains controversial due to the potential for antibiotic resistance (Calinescu et al., 2022).

In children, bleeding episodes from esophageal and gastric varices caused by portal hypertension can be temporized by sclerotherapy (Chiu et al., 2019). Band

ligation is not recommended for small children. Sclerotherapy consists of the injection of a sclerosing agent into the varix with the goal of obliterating the targeted vessel. In the event of massive bleeding, refractory to sclerotherapy transjugular intrahepatic portosystemic shunting may be required. Although this procedure may help stabilize a child during the waiting period, it is accompanied by a higher risk of hepatic encephalopathy (Chiu et al., 2019).

Cardiac. Medical management of children with cardiomyopathy differs depending on the specific symptoms and type. Management of dilated cardiomyopathy consists of managing the symptoms of congestive heart failure. This is done by maximizing cardiac output through decreasing fluid retention and therefore workload. Digoxin and diuretics are the most common medications used. Vasodilators, such as angiotensin-converting enzyme (ACE) inhibitors, are used for afterload reduction. Antiarrhythmics may also be required. Anticoagulation therapy may help prevent thrombus formation in a dilated and poorly contracting heart (NORD, 2019).

In contrast, symptoms of hypertrophic cardiomyopathy vary widely (NORD, 2019). Some may experience shortness of breath upon exertion, fatigue, excessive diaphoresis, poor appetite, and growth failure. As affected children grow, they mare experience syncope and pulmonary edema. Affected individuals can be at high risk for cardiac arrest and sudden death. Medical management for hypertrophic cardiomyopathy consists of maintaining a normal preload and afterload while reducing ventricular contractility. Typical treatment includes calcium channel blockers and/or beta-blockers to decrease the septal muscle from obstructing the left ventricular outflow tract. Antiarrhythmics may be needed for ventricular arrhythmias. The use of implanted cardioverter-defibrillator devices in children waiting for a heart transplant has been an ongoing debate over the past decade (Vandenberk et al., 2018). Due to the long wait times on the transplant list, it is becoming more common in children with hypertrophic cardiomyopathy to prevent sudden death.

Management of children with CHD who develop ventricular dysfunction, lethal arrhythmias, and/or irreversible pulmonary hypertension is similar to that of dilated cardiomyopathy. Still, it may vary slightly depending on the type of CHD and previous operative or palliative procedures (Centers for Disease Control and Prevention [CDC], 2023). Some children and adolescents with cyanotic heart defects may have additional management issues related to polycythemia, hypoxemia, and central nervous system (CNS) sequelae.

In some instances, a ventricular assist device (VAD) can be utilized as a bridge to transplantation. A revolutionary VAD for children is the Berlin Heart, a relatively compact and mobile unit allowing children to participate in activities such as physical therapy, the playroom, or resume some independent activities of daily living (Berlin Heart, 2020). Studies demonstrate children with VAD have better renal function. VAD complications include infection, bleeding, and neurologic issues (Morales et al., 2019). However, the proportion of patients successfully bridged to transplant approaches 80% (Morales et al., 2019).

Lung. As with other transplant candidates, optimizing the clinical condition is the primary aim for children before lung transplantation (Leard et al., 2021). This includes maximizing nutritional status, maintaining and improving physical endurance through preoperative pulmonary rehabilitation, and providing respiratory support (e.g., with supplemental oxygen) as necessary. Prompt identification and treatment of pulmonary infections are crucial, especially in a patient with cystic fibrosis, so eligibility on the transplant waitlist can be maintained.

Evaluation for Transplantation

Evaluation for organ transplantation requires a multidisciplinary approach that includes medical, surgical, nutritional, and psychosocial assessments with multiple diagnostic tests, laboratory data, radiologic testing, and consultant evaluations (OPTN, n.d.). The evaluation process is organ and institution specific. Consultations are completed by the transplant team comprised of the surgeon, specialty physician, nursing support, social workers, transplant coordinators, financial coordinators, nutritional therapists, and behavioral and psychological specialties. Additional specialty medical services may include those impacted by transplant and ancillary services (e.g., nephrology for liver transplant, anesthesiology, interventional radiology, physical and occupational therapists) (Tan et al., 2019). Transplant coordinators, who are registered nurses, nurse practitioners, or physician assistants, maintain communication with the family and patient throughout the process. Although not involved in direct care, financial counselors assist families with insurance and billing questions. Evaluations are usually scheduled on an outpatient basis in specialty clinics, with routine outpatient follow-up facilitated by the transplant coordinator during the waiting period. Children with more advanced diseases may be hospitalized during the evaluation and/or require long-term hospitalization while awaiting transplantation. In some cases, pretransplant surgical procedures may be necessary to provide corrective or palliative repairs to prepare or stabilize a child for transplantation. For example, a preemptive bilateral nephrectomy may be done to decrease proteinuria and procoagulant state that may cause a thrombus in the new kidney (Gunawardena et al., 2021).

Laboratory data commonly obtained for all children awaiting organ transplant include a complete blood count; blood type and crossmatch; a full chemistry profile to assess electrolytes, renal function, and nutritional status; and prothrombin and partial thromboplastin times. Serologic testing is also completed to diagnose previous infections with hepatitis (A, B, and C), cytomegalovirus (CMV), Epstein-Barr virus (EBV), human immunodeficiency virus (HIV), herpes, and varicella-zoster virus. Organ-specific laboratory data may include autoimmune markers, human leukocyte antigens (HLA), ECG, echocardiogram, ultrasound, and pulmonary testing, among others., A child's immunization record is reviewed, and every attempt is made to administer delayed or missing vaccines if the child is well enough to tolerate a vaccination. Live vaccines, such as the measles, mumps, rubella (MMR) vaccine and varicella virus vaccine, should be administered at least 6 weeks prior to transplant if possible. Typically, these are not administered after transplantation because of the increased risk of acquiring the virus from a live vaccine when the immune system is suppressed; however, some centers are now administering live vaccines to select patients based on research (Kemme et al., 2021).

Blood typing is required for kidney, liver, lung, and heart transplants to achieve ABO-matched organs. In addition, HLA tissue typing, antibody crossmatch compatibility, and percent panel reactive antibody are necessary. The transplant candidate with preexisting anti-HLA antibodies presents a significant challenge as anti-HLA antibodies increase the chance of antibody-mediated organ rejection (Kardol-Hoefnagel & Otten, 2021).

For the past several years many strategies have been recommended to prevent and mitigate HLA sensitization. Some pretransplant strategies include limiting blood transfusions; induction using immunosuppression with rituximab, belatacept, azathioprine, and mycophenolate mofetil (MMF) and/or tacrolimus; intravenous immunoglobulin; and plasmapheresis (Claeys & Vermeir, 2019). The results of these interventions are variable, and management protocols differ between transplant centers and organ groups.

Exclusion Criteria

Although most children with end-stage organ disease are suitable candidates for transplantation, there are some exclusion criteria. These criteria have decreased significantly over the past 2 decades because of innovations in care and advances in surgical techniques. Exclusion criteria vary by institution, but most centers agree that children with systemic sepsis, multisystem organ failure, and metastatic disease are not appropriate candidates. Individuals who are HIV positive were once considered an absolute contraindication to transplantation but are now receiving transplants at many centers. Children with cystic fibrosis colonized with *Burkholderia cepacia* have poorer posttransplant outcomes and higher mortality and are not considered transplant candidates at many centers (Weill, 2018). A history of medical nonadherence and poor social support may place the transplant recipient at increased risk for graft failure (Killian et al., 2018). A referral to the local child and family services department may be necessary if a family cannot or unwillingly provide appropriate care to the child before or after the transplant.

Transplantation Waitlist

Following acceptance as a transplant candidate, a child is listed with UNOS according to organ-specific criteria. While waiting at home or in a community hospital for transplantation, the child is medically managed by the primary care provider, who is in frequent communication with the transplant center typically through the transplant coordinator. The primary care provider should update the transplant coordinator regularly of any changes, deterioration, or complications in the child's medical status. Because the primary care provider may also have developed a supportive relationship with the child and family during the diagnosis of the illness and pretransplant care, this provider may be best able to assess the child's and family's coping abilities, responses to stress, level of understanding, and adaptability. This assessment should be communicated to the transplant team to help build on the family's strengths as the family learns to cope with and adapt to the various stressors of the transplant process. The waiting period is variable, depending on the organ(s) needed and the child's blood type, weight, and medical status. Waiting for a cadaveric organ may range from a few days to months and possibly years. It is a highly stressful time for family members as they hope for an organ before their child's condition deteriorates.

Once the evaluation process is complete, the candidate is presented to a medical review board consisting of the transplant team and additional services as appropriate. Once approved, the child is listed for transplant in the UNOS database. UNOS is a nonprofit organization under contract with the federal government to manage the national transplant waiting list, match donors, maintain a transplant database for all organ transplant events that occur in the United States, monitor to ensure transplant policies are followed, and provide education to families and transplant professionals. UNOS has also developed scoring systems for all solid organs to fairly allocate organs to those who need them most and to those who have a higher likelihood of favorable transplant outcomes.

AFTER TRANSPLANT

The primary care provider has a unique and vital opportunity to support optimal health after transplantation. Early recognition of complications, including rejection and infection, promotes optimal growth and development through frequent assessments, and timely referrals are key to minimizing morbidity. Medication adherence can be greatly improved through reinforcement at every encounter, particularly among adolescents. Frequent adjustments to posttransplant medications and dosing by the transplant team are typical during the first 6 months after transplant. Reviewing the current medication schedule with the patient and family should be done at each visit. This may prevent unintended medication interactions should the primary care provider need to prescribe a new medication. Primary care providers also play an important role in the transition of transplant recipients to adult providers (Katz et al., 2020). As for other children with chronic illnesses, the concept of a medical home for transplant recipients is gaining traction. This model provides patient- and family-centered care, care coordination and planning, and team-based care, as well as transition to adult care within the realm of the primary care provider (White & Cooley, 2018).

Immunosuppressive Management

In organ transplantation, immunosuppressive therapy aims to prevent organ rejection while minimizing drug side effects. A careful balance is maintained to prevent organ rejection while limiting the risks of cancer and infection due to overimmunosuppression (Tönshoff, 2019). Table 33.6 provides an overview of immunosuppressive side effects. Immunosuppression is highest immediately after transplantation, then is decreased over the first year posttransplant as the immune system adapts to the graft. The most common posttransplant immunosuppressive medications used alone or in combination therapy are tacrolimus, corticosteroids, sirolimus, and MMF (Nelson et al., 2022). There is no standardized approach to immunosuppression, and it is often transplant center specific. Therapeutic levels and doses vary according to the organ transplanted, the length of time posttransplant, the presence of infection, and/or risk rejection.

Tacrolimus, a calcineurin inhibitor (CNI), has been the mainstay of solid organ transplantation since its introduction in 1994. CNIs prevent T-cell activation and transcription factors involved in proinflammatory cytokines such as interleukin-2 (IL-2), IL-4, and IL-5 (Nelson et al., 2022). CNIs have a narrow therapeutic window with wide pharmacokinetic activity, so drug monitoring is mandatory. Tacrolimus is typically monitored with a 12-hour trough level. CNIs have a variety of significant side effects. The severity of side effects may be decreased or eliminated after transplantation as levels are decreased over time. The most significant are nephro- and neurotoxicities (Nelson et al., 2022). Nephrotoxicity can be acute or chronic and is not always reversible. Individuals on CNIs have higher

Table 33.6	Immunosuppressive Medication Side Effects		
CALCINEURIN INHIBITORS	**CORTICOSTEROIDS**	**MYCOPHENOLATE MOFETIL**	**SIROLIMUS**
Common to all: increased risk for infections; cancers, especially skin, cervical; gastrointestinal irritation; sun sensitivity Prevents T-cell activation, impacts cytokines, interleukin-2 (IL-2), IL-4, IL-5 Diabetes Hand tremors Headaches Hyperkalemia, hyponatremia, hypomagnesemia Insomnia Nephrotoxicities, even at low dose Neurotoxicities, even at low dose Paresthesias Vison changes	Broad antiinflammatory effects on cell-mediated immunity Acne Cataracts/glaucoma Cushingoid facies Elevated glucose/ diabetes Hypertension Mood swings Muscle wasting Polyphagia (persistent hunger) Osteoporosis, increased fracture risk	Decreases B- and T-cell lymphocytes Bone marrow suppression (anemia, leukopenia, neutropenia)	Prevents progression of the cell cycle; suppresses T-lymphocyte activation Delayed wound healing Hypercholesterolemia Nausea Oral ulcers

rates of posttransplant diabetes mellitus, particularly when used in conjunction with corticosteroids. Posttransplant lymphoproliferative disease (PTLD), particularly when associated with primary EBV infection, has been associated with tacrolimus use (Nelson et al., 2022). Neurotoxicities, particularly hand tremors, are associated with tacrolimus use, though their severity can be improved with dose reductions. Other neurotoxic side effects include headaches, insomnia, and paresthesias (Nelson et al., 2022).

Other common, potentially significant side effects of CNIs are hyperkalemia, hyponatremia, and metabolic acidosis; hypomagnesemia may also occur. Elevated levels of tacrolimus during the early postoperative period may result in hyperkalemia, hypophosphatemia, hypomagnesemia, or metabolic acidosis. Common signs and symptoms of elevated levels of tacrolimus include shaking hands (jitteriness), hypertension, headache, changes in vision or behavior, and feelings of nervousness or anxiety (Astellas Cares, 2021).

Hypertension is common, especially when given in combination with high-dose corticosteroids, but is usually responsive to antihypertensive therapy with calcium channel blockers, amlodipine, or beta-adrenergic blockers. Calcium channel blockers, especially diltiazem, are often preferred due to their protection of vascular flow, especially in liver and heart recipients. Beta-adrenergic blockers may exacerbate chronotropic incompetence in children with heart transplants and are generally not used as first-line therapy. ACE inhibitors should be avoided in people with marginal renal function or hyperkalemia. Although nephrotoxicity is a concern in all transplant recipients, it may be more critical in those with renal transplants because renal dysfunction may reflect CNI toxicity, rejection, and acute tubular necrosis.

Corticosteroids are part of the immunosuppressive regimen at most transplant centers. They have broad antiinflammatory effects on cell-mediated immunity while leaving humoral immunity relatively intact (Nelson et al., 2022). The antiinflammatory effects of steroids may play a large role in protecting the transplanted organ. Depending on the dose and length of treatment, steroids produce a variety of mild to severe side effects. Stomach irritation, cushingoid facies, mood swings, acne, swelling and weight gain, hypertension, and insomnia are most commonly seen. Side effects of higher, long-term doses may include cataracts, glaucoma, hyperglycemia, delayed growth, osteoporosis, and muscle weakness. Several transplant centers have been utilizing steroid-sparing and/or rapid steroid withdrawal. The ability to wean and withdraw steroids from transplant recipients benefits posttransplant health, growth, and development. With steroid withdrawal, side effects from long-term high-dose steroids (e.g., cushingoid facies, growth failure, osteoporosis, cataract formation, hypertension, diabetes, and an increased risk of infection) can be minimized or eliminated.

MMF was approved by the US Food and Drug Administration (FDA) in 1995 for the prevention of acute rejection in renal transplantation and has replaced azathioprine as part of the standard triple therapy. MMF is an antimetabolite agent that decreases the number of functional B and T lymphocytes and inhibits the response of human lymphocytes to antigen tolerance (Nelson et al., 2022). Its main side effects are gastrointestinal (GI) distress and hematologic side effects such as anemia, leukopenia, and neutropenia, which can be life threatening if not identified early.

Sirolimus, approved in 1999 for the prevention of organ transplant rejection in patients older than 13 years of age, was originally found in soil samples from Easter Island and was developed into an immunosuppressant. Sirolimus inhibits the activation of the mammalian target of rapamycin (mTOR), which prevents the progression of the cell cycle, suppressing T-lymphocyte activation and proliferation and antibody production. Sirolimus alone appears to cause less nephrotoxicity, neurotoxicity, and hypertension as compared with CNIs; however, it delays wound healing, so it is not used in the immediate posttransplant period (Nelson et al., 2022). The addition of sirolimus for immunosuppression allows decreased doses of tacrolimus in the hopes of minimizing their nephrotoxic side effects. Side effects of sirolimus include hypercholesterolemia, nausea, and oral ulcers (Nelson et al., 2022).

In renal transplantation, combination therapy protocols are frequently used, with nearly 65% of recipients on tacrolimus/MMF/prednisone 1 year after transplant (Nelson et al., 2022).

Infection Prophylaxis

The risk of opportunistic infections related to the use of immunosuppressive medications is a posttransplant concern. Prophylactic medications, including antibiotics (trimethoprim-sulfamethoxazole), antivirals, and antifungals, are used to prevent infectious complications, particularly in the early posttransplant period.

Graft Evaluation

For the first several months posttransplant, the recipient is seen frequently at the transplant center for additional lab monitoring. Once graft function has stabilized, most transplant centers prefer that pediatric transplant recipients return to the transplant center for an annual evaluation of the graft. Bloodwork and organ-specific testing are completed as indicated and may include an abdominal ultrasound, echocardiogram, chest x-ray, or renal flow scan. Biopsies of the transplanted organ are not routinely obtained unless clinically significant concerns exist.

Although follow-up varies by center, the majority of transplant centers prefer to manage the recipient's immunosuppressive therapy. The child's primary care provider will continue to see the child for routine childhood illnesses and examinations, with any fevers or illnesses reported to the transplant center as well. Although the child may have what appears to be a community virus, it is also important to assess the child for posttransplant viral infections, such as CMV or EBV. Laboratory results are sent to the transplant center, where the team will develop a plan for treatment complications indicated by the results.

Herbal Therapies

Herbal dietary supplements are commonly used to support the immune system; however, because of interactions with immunosuppressants and other posttransplant medications, herbal remedies are not recommended in children awaiting transplants or after transplantation. Any herbal or natural supplement

affecting the activity of cytochrome P-450 (CYP450) 3A4, a major drug-metabolizing enzyme, can affect the metabolism of CNIs. For example, St. John's wort induces the CYP450 3A4 pathway, increasing the metabolism of immunosuppressant and thereby reducing the serum concentration of tacrolimus. This results in decreased levels of immunosuppression, placing the child at risk for rejection and allograft loss (Miedziaszczyk et al., 2022). Other medication-herb interactions include ma huang (ephedra) and ginseng, which interact with antihypertensives and increase blood pressure; aloe vera, which can decrease the effectiveness of diuretics; and echinacea, which stimulates the immune system, interfering with the effects of immunosuppressants (UpToDate, n.d.). Additionally, herbs such as kava, ma huang (found in many weight loss preparations), and black cohosh have been associated with hepatic toxicity requiring transplantation (Stournaras & Tziomalos, 2015). As part of the medication review at each primary care visit, it is important to inquire about herbal therapies and supplements. If these have been initiated, the primary care provider should discuss them with the transplant coordinator and team.

ADVANCES IN DIAGNOSIS AND MANAGEMENT

Recipient and graft survival has improved significantly over the past 3 decades because of advances in immunosuppression, surgical techniques, organ preservation, and monitoring for infections, as well as a better understanding of postoperative management and intensive care medicine. New approaches to standard immunosuppressive protocols that result in optimum graft function with minimal side effects are being explored. Ongoing research focuses on immunosuppressive medications that, more specifically, inhibit the immune system and decrease the incidence of rejection, placing a child at less risk for long-term infection and nephrotoxicity. Steroid-free regimens, induction therapies, and weaning trials are innovative immunosuppressive protocols that are being investigated with the goal of inducing tolerance of the transplanted organ.

Induction therapy with antilymphocyte globulin and/or tacrolimus is being administered preoperatively or intraoperatively to decrease rejection and decrease the dosage of CNIs to prevent adverse drug effects (Nelson et al., 2022). Induction therapy is becoming a more accepted treatment with promising early outcomes; however, the advantages of this type of immunosuppression must be balanced with the risk of infection and recurrent disease.

CHIMERISM AND TOLERANCE

Tolerance is the absence of a harmful alloimmune response to transplanted tissue in the absence of immunosuppression (Scandling et al., 2019). Complete chimerism is a form of tolerance in which all cells in the recipient are of donor origin (Scandling et al., 2019). Research continues to develop protocols and identify patients most likely to develop tolerance and/or chimerism after transplant. One study demonstrated the stability of tolerance more than 12 years after transplantation and maintaining graft function after complete withdrawal of immunosuppression (Scandling et al., 2019).

XENOTRANSPLANTATION

An average of 10 people die each day in the United States while waiting on the transplant list (FDA, 2021). Cadaveric and living donor organ donations have been unable to meet the demands of the increasing numbers of individuals requiring organ transplantation. Xenotransplantation is the transplantation of animal sources of cells, tissues, or organs into humans. It is being researched as one option to supply the growing demand for organs. Animal-to-human xenotransplantation has been done experimentally: Pig and baboon livers were transplanted into individuals with fulminant hepatic failure, but none had long-term success (FDA, 2021). Pig neural tissue has been implanted in some people with Parkinson disease, and the graft was maintained for many months on cyclosporine alone. Although successful xenotransplantation may provide an increased source of organs, concern about transmitting infections from the animal source to the recipient and immunologic interactions between the recipient's immune system with the graft have deterred the progress of this strategy (FDA, 2021).

ABO-INCOMPATIBLE HEART TRANSPLANTATION

Matching donor and recipient blood groups have been the standard for organ matching. This often contributes to an extended pretransplant waiting time until a blood group–matched donor is available (Urschel et al., 2021). A progressively accepted therapy in young children awaiting heart transplants is the use of previously ABO-incompatible (ABOI), or mismatched, blood types in pediatric cardiac transplants for those under the age of 2 years. It has proven to be a clinically safe approach with similar rates of survival, rejection, and other known posttransplant complications (Urschel et al., 2021). The infant immune system is immature, B-cell memory is not fully developed, and ABH blood group antigens are reduced or absent in the first 6 to 24 months of life. This is postulated to allow acceptance of the incompatible blood group heart without rejection (Urschel & West, 2016). ABOI heart transplant recipients have specialized requirements regarding the transfusion of blood products so that antibody against the recipient or donor blood group is not introduced (Urschel & West, 2016). Primary care providers should be aware

of these requirements if they have an ABOI transplant recipient in their care. In addition, the primary care provider may be involved in facilitating routine blood tests to monitor isohemagglutinin titers.

LIVING DONOR LUNG TRANSPLANTATION

Living-related donor lobar transplantation has been performed for more than 20 years and involves the donation of a lower lobe from two separate living donors (Date, 2017). This procedure addresses the issue of deceased donor shortages but is controversial because it places two donors at risk (Date, 2017). With the recent changes to lung allocation guidelines, the need for living donor lung transplants has decreased significantly, as waitlist times have decreased, and fewer children are dying while awaiting transplants (Hong et al., 2021). This is not a common transplant procedure in the United States, but Japan utilizes living donor transplants for many of its pediatric lung transplant recipients (Hong et al., 2021). Living lung donors face similar potential complications to lung lobectomy for other indications, including pain, bleeding, infection, and other problems. Living lung donors can expect to have lung function return to approximately 90% of preoperative value 1 year after lobectomy (Date, 2017).

COMPLICATIONS OF SOLID ORGAN TRANSPLANTATION AND MANAGEMENT

The goals of immunosuppression in solid organ transplantation are to prevent rejection while minimizing side effects and poor outcomes (Tönshoff, 2019). This requires serial monitoring and dose adjustments of immunosuppressive levels to maintain a therapeutic range. Immunosuppressive medications in transplant alter the immune response mechanisms but are not immunologically specific, so this careful balance is important to identify the dose that prevents rejection and minimizes risks of overimmunosuppression leading to rejection, infection, and cancer.

REJECTION

Rejection is an inflammatory response by the immune system in which the transplanted tissue is recognized as foreign. This can lead to organ dysfunction and loss (Crowther, 2019). Acute cellular rejection occurs during the first 6 months after transplantation. This type of rejection is a T-cell–mediated event and is usually reversible by increasing the level of immunosuppression. Chronic rejection develops over a longer time and is a combination of cellular and humoral immune responses. Increased immunosuppressive therapies may not resolve chronic rejection, and the graft may be lost. Rejection and infection have similar signs and symptoms. These include fever, pain at the organ site,

Table 33.7 Clinical Signs of Organ Rejection

LIVER	RENAL	CARDIAC	LUNG
Abdominal tenderness	Anorexia, oliguria, hypertension	Abdominal pain, vomiting	Decreased exercise tolerance
Acholic stools and bile-stained urine	Edema (particularly of lower extremities)	Cardiomegaly	Decrease in FEV$_1$ from baseline
Ascites	Elevated BUN and creatinine	Elevated liver enzymes	Malaise
Edema	Fever	Fever	
Fever	Lethargy, fatigue, malaise, irritability	Heart failure	
Elevated LFTs	Tenderness at the graft site	Hepatomegaly	
Jaundice	Weight gain	Poor feeding and irritability (infants)	
Lethargy, fatigue, malaise, irritability		Sudden change in blood pressure	

BUN, Blood urea nitrogen; *FEV$_1$*, forced expiratory volume in 1 sec; *LFTs*, liver function tests.

organ enlargement, and changes in lab values. It is important for the primary care provider to contact the transplant coordinator and center when infection is suspected. Collaboratively, diagnostics can be ordered, and differentials can be ruled out.

Acute rejection is characterized by graft inflammation and injury due to recipient T cells activating donor antigens. Fever, lethargy, and/or abdominal pain may be the first signs of rejection (Table 33.7). It may be reversed if detected early and treated promptly. Acute rejection is a major cause of chronic allograft dysfunction, and multiple episodes of acute rejection can lead to poorer long-term outcomes (Clayton et al., 2019). Treatment varies by center, organ, and severity but usually involves an increased level of baseline immunosuppression, increased corticosteroids, the addition of an adjunctive immunosuppressant (azathioprine, MMF, sirolimus), and/or conversion of immunosuppression from one CNI to another. Muromonab-CD3, a monoclonal antibody, or antilymphocyte globulin or antithymocyte globulin, may be used to treat rejection that is refractory to steroids and/or increased baseline immunosuppression (Crowther, 2019). Repeat biopsies may be performed to evaluate the effectiveness of treatment and determine changes needed for immunosuppression.

Liver Rejection

Symptoms of liver rejection include fever, elevated liver function tests, abdominal tenderness, irritability, and fatigue (see Table 33.7). If left untreated, rejection may progress from mild to moderate symptoms to those of hepatic dysfunction: ascites, jaundice, acholic stools, bile-stained urine, pruritus, encephalopathy, decreased synthetic function, and renal dysfunction. A percutaneous liver biopsy may be performed to definitively diagnose rejection since elevated enzymes and fever may also be seen with infectious processes, biliary tract complications, or hepatic artery thrombosis. Chronic rejection occurs in 3% to 17% of all liver transplants and is defined by the progressive disappearance of bile ducts with subsequent cholestasis and liver failure (i.e., vanishing bile duct syndrome). This

may result in retransplantation or death (Choudhary et al., 2017).

Renal Rejection

Advances in immunosuppressive therapy have significantly decreased the risk of both acute and chronic rejection. Of children who received a renal transplant from 2005 to 2013, acute rejection occurred in 39% of cases (NAPRTCS, 2014). Careful assessment is key because low-grade fever and hypertension may be the only signs of early acute rejection. Other symptoms of rejection may include irritability, malaise, oliguria, increased blood urea nitrogen (BUN) and creatinine levels, weight gain from fluid retention, swelling, tenderness at the graft site, edema of the lower extremities, and anorexia. Rejection is confirmed definitively through percutaneous renal biopsy and renal flow scan. Treatment varies based on center-specific immunosuppressive protocols and severity of rejection but usually involves an increased level of baseline immunosuppression, increased corticosteroids, and the possible addition of an adjunctive immunosuppressant. Antibody therapy with antilymphocyte globulin or basiliximab may also be used to reduce the immune response. Repeat biopsies may be performed to evaluate the effectiveness of treatment.

Acute and chronic rejection causes nearly half of all graft losses in renal transplantation (NAPRTCS, 2014). Chronic rejection is a slow process in which the transplant recipient progressively loses renal function, resulting in graft loss in approximately 35% of all renal allograft failures (NAPRTCS, 2014).

Cardiac Rejection

Unlike acute rejection of the liver or kidney, children with heart transplants usually do not develop symptoms until rejection is severe. It is a significant issue as it is associated with a mortality rate as high as 30% to 50% (Kim, 2021). Most acute rejection is identified by echocardiogram, biomarkers, or surveillance cardiac biopsy before the child is symptomatic. Severe rejection results in graft dysfunction that manifests as heart failure with tachycardia, tachypnea, arrhythmia, gallop rhythm, hepatomegaly, and cardiomegaly. Other symptoms may include shortness of breath, increased respiratory rate, edema and/or sudden weight gain, and changes in blood pressure. Nonspecific findings may include fever, irritability, and poor feeding, particularly in infants. Abdominal pain and vomiting secondary to decreased cardiac output and perfusion to the GI tract may also be seen. Rejection is diagnosed through clinical assessment and echocardiography and confirmed by cardiac biopsy. Depending on the transplant center protocol, surveillance biopsies may be performed more frequently in the early postoperative period and then less often as the risk of rejection decreases. However, numerous consecutive biopsies can lead to serious complications such as fistulae (Kim, 2021).

Chronic heart allograft rejection is also known as transplant coronary artery vasculopathy (CAV). This progressive condition usually occurs over many years, resulting in graft loss. It is characterized by circumferential narrowing of the coronary artery and thickening of the intima and is detected by arteriography and dobutamine stress echocardiography. However, 60% of pediatric patients are free of CAV 11 years after transplant (Kim, 2021). Retransplantation is the primary treatment for chronic rejection. Unfortunately, syncope or sudden death may be the first clinical sign of chronic rejection.

Lung Rejection

Acute rejection in the lung transplant recipient presents in the same manner as patients with infections, including cough, fever, decreased lung function, and radiographic changes (Faro & Visner, 2019). Transplant recipients are instructed to perform regular home spirometry to identify early changes in lung function. To differentiate rejection from infection, bronchoscopy with lavage and transbronchial biopsy are required to identify changes.

Chronic rejection in lung transplantation is known as bronchiolitis obliterans syndrome (BOS) and manifests as progressive shortness of breath and decreased exercise tolerance with decreasing FEV_1 well below the posttransplant baseline (Faro & Visner, 2019). BOS is the most common cause of death in lung transplant recipients more than 2 years after the transplant, and nearly half of pediatric lung transplant recipients will have some evidence of BOS by 5 years after the transplant (Faro & Visner, 2019).

INFECTION

The dilemma of transplantation is that an adequately suppressed immune system to prevent rejection must be balanced with one that is also competent in resisting infection. This delicate equilibrium can be easily disturbed when immunosuppression is increased to treat or avoid rejection. The common result is an infection, which is a significant cause of morbidity and mortality following transplantation.

Immunocompromised individuals must take extra precautions around certain animals. Reptiles, poultry, rodents, and exotic pets are more likely to carry diseases that can make one sick and therefore are considered high risk (CDC, 2022d). It is also important to avoid cleaning litter boxes due to the risk of toxoplasmosis.

The period when the child is at the highest risk for infections is within the first 6 months after the transplant when immunosuppression is at its peak (van Delden et al., 2020). During the first 30 days of the postoperative period, infections related to surgical complications, nosocomial, and donor-derived infections are most common (UNOS, 2023). The most common nosocomial infections are wound or line infections, pneumonia, and urinary tract infections (UTIs) (van Delden et al., 2020). Donor-derived infections may be CMV, EBV, BK polyomaviruses, hepatitis B and C, toxoplasma, and *Clostridium difficile* infection (Timsit et al., 2019).

During months 1 through 6 after transplant, the most common infections are opportunistic, such as *Pneumocystis jirovecii* (PCJ; formerly *P. carinii*), polyomavirus, and adenovirus. CMV- and EBV-associated lymphoproliferative disorders are also seen during this time (UNOS, 2023; van Delden et al., 2020). Six months after transplant, those recipients who have satisfactory graft function are on maintenance immunosuppression. Infections in this group are most commonly community acquired and other opportunistic infections such as pneumonia, rhinovirus, and influenza (UNOS, 2023; van Delden et al., 2020).

Cytomegalovirus

CMV is a common viral infection following transplantation and is a significant source of morbidity and mortality in pediatric transplant recipients. CMV usually occurs within the first several months after the transplant (van Delden et al., 2020). Children who are CMV seronegative before transplant and receive a seropositive organ are at greater risk of developing the primary disease. Additional risk factors include the intensity and duration of immunosuppression, particularly antilymphocyte and antithymocyte therapies, and acute rejection. CMV disease is manifested frequently as fever and cytopenia; however, other signs include lymphadenopathy, thrombocytopenia, and tissue invasive diseases, such as pneumonitis, hepatitis, colitis, and chorioretinitis (Mombelli & Manuel, 2022; Timsit et al., 2019). Diagnosis is based on clinical presentation, CMV polymerase chain reaction (PCR)–based assays, and serology, including newer assays such as PP65 tegument protein, a CMV antigenemia assay, and histopathology (Mombelli & Manuel, 2022).

Treatment protocols differ between transplant centers for the prevention and treatment of CMV;

however, intravenous (IV) ganciclovir or oral valganciclovir is widely used due to its potent ability to inhibit viral DNA replication of the human herpesviruses. In pediatrics, IV ganciclovir is preferred due to the erratic absorption of an oral preparation in children with varied eating habits and concomitant medications. The duration of antiviral therapy is based on the CMV viral load, level of immunosuppression, coinfection(s), and institution protocols (Åsberg et al., 2016; Bock & Chinnock, 2022).

Lymphoproliferative Disorders

PTLDs are a consequence of immunosuppression in transplant recipients. It may range from a self-limiting mononucleosis to malignant monoclonal lymphoma, including non-Hodgkin lymphoma. EBV infection has been demonstrated in 10% to 15% of immunosuppressed recipients of solid organ transplantation and accounts for more than half of posttransplantation malignancies in pediatric transplant recipients (Asleh et al., 2022; Lau et al., 2021). Survival rates of PTLD are reported at 50% to 80% (Chiou et al., 2018; Lau et al., 2021).

Risk factors for EBV infection include young age, EBV seromismatch or primary infection, and exposure to antilymphocyte antiserum and other T-cell depletion strategies (Asleh et al., 2022). The most common symptoms are fever and lymphadenopathies; however, symptoms may include malaise, tonsillitis, pharyngitis, abdominal mass, oral lesions, CNS disease, or GI disturbances. Tumorlike infiltrations and ulcerations of the GI tract with abdominal pain and bleeding are seen in invasive diseases (Ashrafi et al., 2021).

Early diagnosis is vital to recovery and is based on clinical presentation, histopathology, laboratory studies, and radiographic findings. A biopsy is often performed on an accessible node, and a computed tomography scan is obtained to assess the chest and abdomen for enlarged nodes or disseminated disease. EBV-PCR and EBV-DNA quantification testing are sensitive tools that help monitor viral load and are used to track disease progression in transplant recipients (Kimura & Kwong, 2019).

Treatment and management of EBV and PTLD are typically multimodal: decreasing immunosuppression and anti-CD20 antibodies such as rituximab and chemotherapy. Other treatments include the use of antiviral agents and irradiation (Vergote et al., 2022).

Pneumocystis jirovecii Pneumonia

Children who are immunosuppressed are at risk for PCJ pneumonia, a rare but serious pulmonary infection. Trimethoprim-sulfamethoxazole is widely accepted as effective prophylaxis. Most cases occur within 1 to 6 months posttransplant. If a transplant recipient has a fever and a lower respiratory tract infection and is not receiving prophylaxis, the primary care provider should place PCJ pneumonia as a primary differential diagnosis, especially in the early posttransplant period.

Varicella-Zoster Virus

Varicella-zoster virus is a highly contagious childhood disease that can be potentially severe in an immunocompromised child (CDC, 2022c). In the first 6 months posttransplant, prophylaxis against varicella-zoster is recommended if seropositive prior to transplantation (Wang et al., 2018). Postexposure prophylaxis with varicella-zoster immunoglobulin is no longer recommended due to the lack of demonstrated impact on the clinical outcome of the disease (Wang et al., 2018). Recommended management of varicella-zoster infection is with decreased oral antiviral therapy with acyclovir or valacyclovir (Wang et al., 2018). Graft function should be monitored closely for rejection for several weeks in the setting of reduced baseline immunosuppression. Following exposure to or outbreak of the disease, transplant recipients should be tested for immunity to the varicella-zoster virus to determine whether precautions need to be taken with future exposures.

The varicella-zoster vaccine is routinely administered to children at 1 and 4 years of age who are immunocompetent; however, because this vaccine is a live virus, it is not recommended for use in a child who is immunocompromised. If the child awaiting transplant is otherwise medically stable, the transplant is not imminent; the vaccine should be administered before transplant and as early as 9 months of age (Infectious Disease Advisor, 2019). Families of those on the transplant list or recipients should be fully immunized before transplantation.

Fungal Infections

Fungal infections usually occur during the early postoperative period. Infections with *Candida* species cause the majority of posttransplant fungal infections, although *Aspergillus* can be seen more commonly in lung transplant recipients (CDC, 2020). Fungal infections are usually opportunistic and manifest as noninvasive infections of the oropharynx, esophagus, or genitalia caused by high immunosuppressive levels. Noninvasive *Candida* appears as plaques on the oral mucosa or as a papular rash of the genitalia. Treatment with an oral swish and swallow solution of nystatin or mycostatin troche usually resolves a noninvasive infection. Invasive disease (fungemia) can develop related to surgical complications, steroid administration, broad-spectrum antibiotics, prolonged operative time, repeat laparotomies, retransplantation, and renal or respiratory compromise. The invasive disease causes fever, irritability, malaise, decreased appetite, or an erythematous central catheter site and is confirmed by blood, urine, throat, or wound cultures. Fungemia is treated with an IV antifungal agent with close monitoring of renal function (Papon et al., 2021).

Polyomavirus

Human polyomaviruses, composed of subgroups BK virus (BKV), JC virus (JCV), and simian virus 40, are DNA viruses. BKV has been associated with polyomavirus-associated nephropathy (PVAN) and JCV with progressive multifocal leukoencephalopathy. On average, each individual is infected with nine different human polyomaviruses (Kamminga et al., 2021), and most children become seropositive by age 10 years. Approximately 2% to 8% of children with renal transplants are diagnosed with PVAN, which often precedes renal allograft dysfunction. Though not fully understood, the transmission of BKV is thought to occur by oral-enteric or respiratory routes. Risk factors for PVAN include BKV-seropositive donors and BKV-negative recipients, age less than 5 years, reduced BKV-specific cellular immunity, and positive BKV viruria. Infection, typically asymptomatic in persons with an intact immune system, can cause hemorrhagic cystitis, interstitial nephritis, and ureteral stenosis in renal transplant recipients (Kamminga et al., 2021). Interstitial nephritis can mimic the symptoms of rejection, making the identification of BKV important when making treatment decisions. A renal biopsy is the current gold standard of diagnosis, though serum and urine assays using PCR are being used to assess response to therapy. Whereas intensified immunosuppression is used for rejection, a reduction of immunosuppression is appropriate for the treatment of BKV.

RENAL DYSFUNCTION

The development of renal dysfunction and CKD after nonrenal transplantation remains a common complication after a solid organ transplant. Its cause and prevention have gained attention, and research over the past 2 decades shows slight changes in renal function are associated with adverse outcomes (Kowalewski et al., 2021). According to the ISHLT, 13% of pediatric heart recipients require renal replacement therapy by 13 years after transplantation. Long-term follow-up of pediatric liver transplant recipients identifies up to 33% of children have CKD (Elisofon et al., 2020; Kowalewski et al., 2021). Contributors to renal dysfunction include the use of CNIs, pretransplant renal disease, perioperative hemodynamic instability, hypertension, and diabetes. Vigilant monitoring of the GFR, decreasing exposure to nephrotoxic medications, weaning of CNIs, and strict control and management of hypertension and proteinuria are crucial to maximizing renal function after solid organ transplantation (Jain & Mattoo, 2016).

RECURRENT DISEASE

In select causes of renal failure there is a risk of posttransplant recurrence. Hyperoxaluria and FSGS can recur rapidly in the transplanted allograft. Recurrence rates of FSGS vary from 30% to 60% (Uffing et al., 2021). Membranous nephropathy, immunoglobulin A nephropathy, Henoch-Schönlein purpura, and hemolytic uremic syndrome are other renal diseases that may recur following transplantation. Treatment for both FSGS and membranous nephropathy is rituximab and plasmapheresis.

There are particular liver diseases that can recur after transplant, such as autoimmune diseases such as autoimmune hepatitis and primary sclerosing cholangitis. Viral infections such as hepatitis B or C can be reactivated, and Budd-Chiari syndromes can all recur but may not cause as significant a disease as prior to transplant because of posttransplant allograft dysfunction (Lim & Lake, 2020).

THE FUTURE OF PEDIATRIC TRANSPLANTATION

During the last 4 decades, pediatric transplant recipients' life span and quality of life have continued to increase. The development and improvement of surgical techniques, posttransplant care, and new immunosuppressive strategies have decreased complications, increased graft survival rate, and improved outcomes (Jara et al., 2020). The longest living transplant recipient celebrated her 80th birthday in 2022, 38 years after receiving a liver transplant; kidney recipients have lived as long as 50 years after transplantation (Sanada, 2021).

Excessive doses and long-term use of CNIs and other immunosuppression continue to place transplant recipients at high risk for declining renal function, recurrent infections, and malignancies (Leww et al., 2022). The use of genomics to evaluate the response to immunosuppressive medication and the risk of rejection are being researched (Bock & Chinnock, 2022). Cohort studies across the United States and Canada are working to personalize immunosuppression for liver transplant recipients, including extensive weaning and prolonged-release tacrolimus. Tolerance and chimerism continue to be the ultimate transplant goals. Utilizing noninvasive biomarkers and imaging, the goal is to identify candidates who may be able to tolerate these modifications in immunosuppression without compromising graft function (Friman et al., 2021; Papaz et al., 2018).

Innovative technology is increasingly utilized in health care. Smartphones, personal wearable devices to monitor health, and artificial intelligence are being investigated for use in transplantation. Addressing medication adherence, vaccine and visit reminders, telehealth visits, and transplant education are situations where technology can be leveraged to improve outcomes. Health information systems have positively impacted aspects of transplant care, including timeliness of care, medication management, and reduction of medication errors (Niazkhani et al., 2017).

PRIMARY CARE MANAGEMENT

HEALTH CARE MAINTENANCE

Prior to any solid organ transplantation surgery, pediatric patients may experience signs and symptoms of end-stage organ dysfunction. Most common are malnutrition, anorexia, anemia, loss of muscle mass, and fatigue, among others. These are often present for several months after transplantation. The pediatric-focused primary care provider plays an important role in transplant recipients achieving and maintaining optimum growth and development. It is important for primary care providers to be aware of issues specific to those required or who have received a solid organ transplant, including common long-term medication side effects, immunosuppression status, and drugs that interact with common posttransplant medications.

Growth and Development

The primary goals of pediatric organ transplantation are the attainment of target terminal adult height as well as normal neurologic and physical development with improved quality of life. Growth restriction is seen in all children prior to solid organ transplants for end-stage organ failure. Growth improves during the first 18 months of the posttransplant period, but the child may not achieve full adult height. This is likely due to posttransplant issues such as anemia, age and z score at transplantation, primary diagnosis, and effect of high-dose corticosteroids on initial immunosuppression (Aull, 2019). Studies also demonstrate the impact of social determinants of health on transplant outcomes for all organs (Rea et al., 2023). Outpatient therapies, such as physical and occupational, may continue to be needed during this initial posttransplant period. The primary care provider has an essential role in monitoring the child's long-term growth and development. Height, weight, and body mass index (BMI) should be routinely documented on standardized growth charts and evaluated, and concerns should be quickly addressed with the transplant team.

Transplant candidates exhibit symptoms and effects of chronic diseases such as anorexia, vomiting, malnutrition, anemia, and bone problems, which affect growth and development, as well as neurologic and behavioral potential. Although transplantation may resolve some of these complications, aggressive nutritional support and minimization or discontinuation of steroids will contribute to catchup growth. Increased or intensified nutritional support or growth hormone therapy may be required in some cases of growth retardation (Aull, 2019). Neurologic complications after transplant occur in 15% to 35% of children and typically occur soon after transplant due to high-dose immunosuppressant with tacrolimus and posttransplant neurologic complications (Gungor et al., 2017).

The average child awaiting renal transplant is nearly 2 SD below the mean for height (NAPTRCS, 2014) at the time of transplantation. Growth after renal transplantation is affected by age at transplant, antihypertensive medication, renal osteodystrophy, graft function, and immunosuppressive medications (Aull, 2019; NAPTRCS, 2014). Of children transplanted before the age of 15 years, at least 40% remain below the 3rd percentile for height as adults (NAPRTCS, 2014). Catchup growth has been seen primarily in children who were under 6 years of age at the time of transplant, with children under 2 years of age showing the most improvement (NAPRTCS, 2014).

Growth restriction in children with liver transplants is a result of malnutrition secondary to anorexia, vomiting, malabsorption of fat and fat-soluble vitamins, decreased hepatic protein synthesis, and increased energy demands with decreased oral intake (Aull, 2019). The Studies of Pediatric Liver Transplantation (SPLiT), a cooperative research network of pediatric liver transplantation centers in the United States and Canada, reports that the pediatric liver transplant candidate is an average 1.4 SD below the age- and gender-adjusted height level (SPLiT Research Group, 2001). Early catchup growth occurs during the first 2 years after transplantation, with a plateau at year 7 posttransplantation (Loeb et al., 2018). Younger children (age <5 years) have even greater height deficits, although they experience the best catchup growth within 18 months after transplant. Approximately 69% of all liver transplant recipients remain below the 50th percentile for height and 23% below the 10th percentile after 10 years (SPLiT Research Group, 2001).

Children with chronic conditions, including transplants, have almost double the risk for mental health issues than children without chronic conditions (Stein, 2022). This may be attributed to a variety of causes, including neurodevelopmental abnormalities; disruptions that occur in education because of illness, appointments, or hospitalizations; limited social experiences; and changes in function caused by the chronic condition and its treatment (Stein, 2022). The primary care provider should perform frequent screenings for depression, suicide, and risky behaviors. Routine developmental screening should also occur; screenings are encouraged outside of the standard well-visit schedule.

Cerebral atrophy has been seen in 12% to 23% of children with ESRD. Children with congenital nephrotic syndrome, cystinosis, and Lowe syndrome are at higher risk. Most children with mild-moderate CKD exhibit average to slightly low-average intelligence and deficits related to attention regulation, working memory, and school achievement (Harshman & Hooper, 2020). Those on dialysis had the lowest IQ scores. Studies have demonstrated significant improvement in IQ scores after transplantation (Chen et al., 2018).

Recent studies report preserved health-related quality of life for children after liver transplantation by both parents and children when compared to children with other chronic conditions (Duvant et al., 2021; Lazor et al., 2017).

Many children with heart failure experience inadequate growth. Heart transplantation helps optimize linear growth and weight gain in this patient population. Many pediatric heart transplant recipients can achieve appropriate growth and development (Bock & Chinnock, 2022). Factors such as age at the time of transplant and length of steroid use after transplant can affect optimal growth. As with all children, close observation of weight gain in the context of linear growth is important to ensure an appropriate BMI. After heart transplantation, most children return to school, participate in sports and age-appropriate activities, and have no activity restrictions. However, many are not able to meet the American Academy of Pediatrics (AAP) adolescent physical activity recommendations due to low exercise capacity (Arora et al., 2019). Studies identify approximately 38% of children after heart transplants have abnormal motor development (Sprong et al., 2021). Intellectual impairments in CHD are a known complication, with degree and trajectory depending on the subtype and severity of the illness (Feldman et al., 2021). One study identified up to 50% of pediatric heart transplant recipients with cognitive performance issues after transplantation (Gold et al., 2020). Although many children achieve good psychological outcomes after transplant, ongoing attention to this area of development is essential.

Information regarding growth and development after lung transplant is limited. Many children with cystic fibrosis are at risk for poor nutritional status and low BMI. There is emerging evidence that BMI improvement after transplant may depend on pretransplant BMI: Low preoperative BMI was less likely to have a BMI recovery; however, those with higher pretransplant BMI were likely to improve their BMI after the transplant, reflecting improved growth and nutrition (Pryor et al., 2022). Once stable, most children do not have required activity limitations after lung transplantation (Wickerson et al., 2016).

Diet

Attention to nutritional management for children both before and after transplantation is crucial in achieving optimal wound healing, catchup growth, and ultimately normal growth and development. After the transplant, a child's diet is usually liberalized. Renal recipients may have mild-moderate sodium intake restrictions, and cardiac recipients are encouraged to maintain healthy eating habits and avoid excessive intake of foods high in sodium and cholesterol. In addition, medication side effects may cause hyperkalemia, hypertension, hypomagnesemia, hypophosphatemia,

hyperglycemia, or hyperlipidemia, requiring a respective dietary restriction or additives. Hyperlipidemia not controlled by diet and exercise, particularly in cardiac recipients, is often treated with lipid-lowering agents (Bock & Chinnock, 2022).

Just as herbal therapies and supplements may cause fluctuations in immunosuppressant levels, many foods also interact with these medications. Some may cause medication levels to become subtherapeutic, while others may cause toxicity leading to long-term adverse effects. For example, spinach, grapefruit, and drinks made with grapefruit juice may cause toxic levels of CNIs. High-fat foods taken with CNIs may decrease drug levels, which may cause organ rejection. High-potassium foods such as bananas, oranges, and potatoes should be limited or avoided completely, as many of the immunosuppressants cause hyperkalemia. Additionally, unpasteurized foods, raw eggs, seafood, rare meat, and oysters should be avoided due to the weakened immune system and increased risk of infection (US Department of Agriculture, 2020).

Some transplant recipients may require temporary tube feedings after transplant for several weeks or months to achieve their established BMI goal (Shah et al., 2021). Children with unique nutritional requirements, such as those with cystic fibrosis, may need individualized nutritional therapy, including enteral tube feedings. Most children are eventually weaned from these therapies.

Safety

As with all routine pediatric visits, counseling about safety issues (e.g., the proper use of car seats, seat belts, and bicycle helmets; childproofing the home) at a child's age and developmental level is necessary for all families with a child who has had an organ transplant. Because most children have good graft function and are prescribed maintenance doses of immunosuppression, good hand-washing techniques and avoidance of others with obvious infections are sound guidelines to decrease the risk of infection.

Activity

In children with a heart or heart-lung transplant, it is important to understand that the incisions in the heart sever the sympathetic and parasympathetic nerves, which ordinarily regulate heart rate. This lack of neural connections is known as denervation. Without direct control of the CNS, the transplanted heart will beat faster in a resting state. This faster-than-normal rate is associated with normal cardiac function and the capability of sustaining vigorous physical activity. The transplanted heart depends on circulating adrenalin and related hormones produced by the adrenal gland instead of a direct impulse from the brain to change its rate. The transplanted heart may take up to 10 minutes before an increase in heart rate is seen in response to exercise, and up to 1 hour may pass after stopping exercise before a decrease in rate is seen (McCalmont & Velleca, 2017). Another effect of denervation is that chest pain or angina pectoris cannot be perceived if coronary artery disease develops; however, some recipients may regrow these nerves and will experience the typical symptoms of coronary artery blockage if it develops. Consequently, coronary arteriograms and dobutamine stress echocardiograms are obtained to assess evidence of vasculopathy.

Pediatric heart recipients are activity restricted for the first 6 to 8 weeks after surgery to allow the sternum to heal. Recipients should avoid bicycling, climbing, situps, pushups, roller skating, and contact sports and should refrain from lifting, pushing, or pulling heavy objects during this period. After 8 weeks, all activities and physical education classes at school may be resumed. Teens who are licensed drivers may also resume driving 2 months after the transplant. A physical therapist should instruct children on an exercise program before discharge from the hospital. This program consists of a 5-minute warmup and cooldown period before and after peak physical activity. The cooldown period should begin if a child shows increased shortness of breath or fatigue. Physical education teachers should be informed of the heart recipient's additional exercise considerations.

Children who have received liver or kidney transplants are encouraged to resume previous activities, although there are some limitations in the early postoperative period. Pushups or situps and activities that stretch or put pressure on the abdomen and incision are to be avoided for 3 to 6 months. Recipients should avoid heavy lifting for at least 6 months. Although some centers discourage contact sports, most children can participate in age-appropriate activities as they develop greater endurance and fitness, such as soccer, softball, basketball, bicycling, skating, swimming, dancing, and gymnastics.

Some transplant centers prefer that families notify the transplant coordinator when they plan to travel for an extended time or to a foreign country. This notification is particularly important for children awaiting an organ transplant so that a means of communication is available in case an organ becomes available. Medication doses and schedules should always be maintained while a child is on vacation, and an adequate supply of medication should be taken with the child. Medications should be carried onto airplanes rather than being checked with luggage. Parents are encouraged to obtain medical alert bracelets for their child to identify the child as a transplant recipient and provide the name and telephone number of the transplant center in case of an emergency. In addition, infectious disease precautions need to be taken with foreign travel to certain areas where immunizations may not be available for all children and adults.

Immunizations

Because of the inconsistent rates of serologic conversion of many vaccines after transplant, care should be taken to complete the schedule for routine immunizations before transplantation when possible (Danziger-Isakov & Kumar, 2019). Children who have been previously immunized should have serologic testing for antibodies to vaccine-preventable diseases prior to transplantation. Those children who are susceptible should be reimmunized (CDC, 2022a).

Because children are more highly immunosuppressed in the early posttransplant period, they may be unable to mount an immunologic response to the vaccine, and no immunizations should be given during this time. The immunization schedule for immunosuppressed children should commence once the recipient receives maintenance immunosuppression. This time frame can vary by transplant center and organ group but is usually 3 to 12 months after the transplant. If a child is receiving augmented immunosuppression to treat rejection, any scheduled immunizations should be postponed for at least 1 to 3 months. Live virus vaccines after transplant remain contraindicated by most transplant centers and should not be undertaken by the primary care provider.

After transplant, primary care providers should follow the guidelines established for children who are immunosuppressed (CDC, 2022a). Live vaccines are generally contraindicated in this population, and only inactivated vaccines (e.g., the inactivated polio and flu vaccines) should be administered. Siblings of the transplant recipient should receive the MMR and varicella vaccines before transplant.

In children who are immunosuppressed, some vaccines are recommended outside of routine age groups (CDC, 2022a). Pneumococcal vaccines (PCV13, PPSV23) are recommended. The meningococcal vaccine series can be administered between the age of 2 and 23 months. Meningococcal serogroup B vaccines can be administered as early as 10 years of age.

The influenza vaccine should be administered annually to children with organ transplants who are 3 months or more posttransplant. All family members living within the household should also receive the vaccine. In 2014, the AAP released its recommendation for the prevention of respiratory syncytial virus (RSV) with palivizumab (Synagis) immunization for children 12 months and under with hemodynamically significant CHD (American Academy of Pediatrics Committee on Infectious Diseases, & American Academy of Pediatrics Bronchiolitis Guidelines Committee, 2014). There is no specific recommendation for the RSV vaccine in children who are immunocompromised, but potential benefits in certain circumstances are acknowledged.

Hepatitis B is an infrequent but significant cause of decreased graft survival, morbidity, and mortality. Children awaiting transplants, including those with ESRD receiving dialysis, should be vaccinated against hepatitis B. Children whose hepatitis B vaccine is not up to date may receive it 3 to 12 months after transplantation following posttransplant guidelines. It is recommended that siblings, caretakers, and household contacts also be immunized.

Transplant recipients have an increased risk of cancer as compared to the general population. The human papillomavirus (HPV) vaccine is the only cancer-preventing immunization to date and is recommended for those age 9 to 26 years (CDC, 2021b). If age appropriate, the HPV vaccine should be administered either prior to or 6 months after transplantation. The dosing for transplant recipients is three doses regardless of age (Nailescu et al., 2022). The primary care provider should contact the transplant center for specific immunization guidelines for the child and family. Administration and maintenance of routine childhood vaccinations after transplant are important roles of the primary care provider with this patient population.

PRIMARY CARE SCREENING AND ASSESSMENT

Depression

While there is a positive association between receiving a transplant and quality of life, many studies have identified that recipients experience poor mental health after transplantation (Penner et al., 2022). Some studies demonstrate that pediatric transplant recipients are at least four times more likely to meet the criteria for posttraumatic stress disorder (PTSD) and anxiety than the general population. It is important for the primary care provider to perform routine depression and trauma screening to better understand the impact of transplantation on children's mental health.

Vision

Routine screening is recommended. Because cataracts, glaucoma, and pseudotumor cerebri may be side effects of long-term steroid use, an annual ophthalmologic examination should be performed on children at risk for these conditions. Infection with CMV and a history of infection with toxoplasmosis require ophthalmologic follow-up for 6 months after infection or until resolution (Schwenk et al., 2021).

Hearing

Routine screening is recommended. In addition, transplant recipients who received IV ototoxic medications (i.e., gentamicin, vancomycin) frequently before and after transplant are at risk for hearing deficits and should be referred to an audiologist for screening. Audiograms are recommended to determine the extent of hearing loss and to recommend interventions.

Dental

Biannual dental visits and good oral hygiene practices are recommended for children following organ transplantation. Gingival hyperplasia is commonly seen in children receiving cyclosporine or CNIs. Good dental and oral hygiene with mechanical stimulation by daily brushing and flossing, gingival massaging, and plaque control can contain gum growth to within acceptable limits. Although the American Heart Association does not recommend antibiotic prophylaxis prior to dental procedures as standard for all transplant patients, the primary care provider should discuss with the transplant team whether prophylaxis is requested. For example, heart transplant recipients who have developed cardiac valvulopathy or those recipients who have had a previous case of infective endocarditis may require prophylaxis (American Dental Association, 2022; National Institute of Dental and Craniofacial Research, 2011).

Blood Pressure

Because hypertension is a common side effect of some immunosuppressants, blood pressure measurement should be a part of all discharge teaching plans. If antihypertensive medications are prescribed, parents are instructed to measure the child's blood pressure before administering these medications. Administration guidelines based on blood pressure parameters should be clearly delineated for the child and family. Parents may be advised to maintain a record of blood pressure readings and administer antihypertensive medications so that the primary care provider and transplant team can monitor treatment and adjust medications. Antihypertensive medications are usually not required long term after transplant if the child is steroid free or if immunosuppressive levels are maintained at a low level.

A trend in nighttime hypertension in people with heart transplants has been noted. It is suspected that denervation of the transplanted heart plays a role in this as a result of decreased parasympathetic tone, which would normally contribute to lower blood pressure at night. Consequently, a single daytime blood pressure measurement may not accurately reflect the blood pressure profile, and occasional 24-hour blood pressure monitoring is recommended (Bennett & Ventura, 2017).

Hematocrit

The hematocrit is obtained with routine laboratory tests as recommended by the transplant center during the early postoperative period and through the primary care provider if the child is discharged from the transplant area. Laboratory tests are obtained frequently, up to weekly or twice weekly, during the first 3 months after the transplant and then with decreasing frequency over time. Children with renal transplants may develop anemia secondary to progressive renal dysfunction from recurrent disease or chronic rejection.

Urinalysis

Nephrotoxicity is a well-recognized complication of both tacrolimus and cyclosporine immunosuppressive therapy in all solid organ transplantation and can be detected in urine and blood specimens. BUN, creatinine, and GFR are monitored to assess kidney function. Additionally, urine samples are obtained for urinalysis and culture in renal transplant recipients as part of posttransplant management. Routine monitoring of the serum creatinine and total protein and urinalysis is essential to screen for recurrent renal diseases, such as FSGS or membranoproliferative glomerulonephritis.

In children with liver and heart transplantation, urinalysis is obtained to monitor for nephrotoxicity resulting from immunosuppressive therapies. Otherwise, a urinalysis is obtained only if the child is symptomatic or as part of an evaluation of fever. Fever in the posttransplant period is usually diagnostic of rejection or infection. If the rejection is ruled out, infection is likely, and cultures of urine, blood, stool, and sputum should be obtained.

Tuberculosis

Immunosuppressed individuals are at high risk of latent tuberculosis (TB) infection. Many transplant centers recommend QuantiFERON-TB Gold Plus or the T-SPOT test to screen for TB rather than Mantoux purified protein derivative (PPD) before and with presumed exposure after transplantation (Hasan et al., 2018). Treatment is with isoniazid or rifampin; both can cause hepatotoxicity, so close monitoring of hepatic enzymes during treatment is warranted (Hasan et al., 2018).

Malignancy

Malignancies are more prevalent after transplant than in the general population due to immunosuppression. Skin, oral, anogenital, and lung cancers are at least double that of the age- and sex-matched general population. Smoking cessation and sunscreen application (sun protection factor ≥30) must be reinforced topics. Regular skin cancer screening should be performed on all transplant recipients, regardless of age. HPV vaccination is vital in this population, and regular cancer screenings (in some situations) are more intensive than in the general population (Berk & Volk, 2021; CDC, 2021b).

CONDITION-SPECIFIC SCREENING

Posttransplant Blood Tests

Laboratory blood testing is usually obtained at weekly to biweekly clinic visits after discharge from the hospital. Laboratory tests vary depending on the organ transplanted, length of time after transplant, current complications, and center-specific protocols. Leukopenia and neutropenia can be side effects of immunosuppressant or antiviral medications, and an adjustment of those medications may be required to avoid over-immunosuppression and decrease the risk of post-transplant infections. The most commonly obtained laboratory tests include a complete blood cell count with differential and a full chemistry profile, including glucose, BUN, creatinine, magnesium, phosphorus, bicarbonate, uric acid, aspartate aminotransferase, alanine aminotransferase, GGTP, lactic dehydrogenase, creatine phosphokinase, cholesterol, and triglycerides.

Medication Levels

Trough levels of tacrolimus or sirolimus are usually obtained with these routine tests. In addition, fasting lipids and glycated hemoglobin A1c are done periodically to screen for hyperlipidemia and diabetes.

Maintenance Laboratory Testing

Laboratory testing decreases over time. By 6 months after transplant, most children have stable graft function and require monthly laboratory testing. Long-term survivors commonly have laboratory testing completed every 2 to 3 months; however, laboratory tests may be required more frequently during episodes of infection or rejection.

COMMON ILLNESS MANAGEMENT

Differential Diagnosis

Fever. Children are more highly immunosuppressed for the first 3 to 6 months after transplantation and consequently are at greater risk for infection. As discussed, bacterial infections are most commonly seen in the early period related to a preexisting chronic condition, surgical complications, or nosocomial infections. Viruses and opportunistic infections are more common in the intermediate and late periods following transplantation. Fever demands a thorough assessment, especially in the first 3 months after the transplant. The differential diagnoses of rejection or infection must be investigated with each febrile episode, particularly in the early postoperative period. The primary care provider and the transplant specialist work cooperatively to evaluate and manage febrile episodes, treating the cause promptly with appropriate intervention. If seen in the primary care office, the provider should notify the transplant coordinator of the fever and any additional presenting signs and symptoms.

Abdominal symptoms. Abdominal pain in children with liver transplants during the early postoperative period most commonly indicates a surgical complication, including a postoperative ileus, hepatic artery thrombosis, or portal vein thrombosis. Biliary complications may also cause abdominal pain and may occur in the early postoperative period as well as weeks to months after the transplant. Acute rejection of the liver may also cause abdominal pain.

Abdominal pain in renal transplant recipients and tenderness in the kidney area may be a symptom of UTI, acute pyelonephritis, posttransplant lymphoproliferative disease, CMV infection, or rejection.

Although abdominal pain and vomiting in the child with a heart transplant may be a viral illness, this clinical presentation warrants an echocardiogram to evaluate for the possibility of rejection secondary to decreased cardiac output and decreased perfusion to the GI tract.

As with the general pediatric population, the differential diagnoses of abdominal pain may also include intestinal obstruction, peptic ulcer disease, appendicitis, or viral or bacterial gastroenteritis. A definitive diagnosis is determined through clinical presentation, laboratory testing, and radiologic testing. If the diagnosis is unclear, the primary care provider should notify the transplant coordinator and discuss differentials and diagnostics.

Vomiting and diarrhea. The incidence of viral gastroenteritis in transplant recipients is higher than in those without transplants and has an increased mortality rate (Abbas et al., 2021). Prolonged vomiting or diarrhea caused by a community-acquired virus may result in altered absorption of immunosuppressant medications leading to toxic or subtherapeutic blood levels that may place the child at risk. Parents should contact the transplant coordinator if the child is unable to retain the immunosuppressive medication. The primary care provider will facilitate the transplant center's immunosuppression recommendations and supervise the medical management of fluids and electrolytes. A protracted course of vomiting or diarrhea may result in hospitalization for IV administration of tacrolimus, fluid management, and any indicated workup for infection.

Metabolic abnormalities. Children with stable graft function receiving maintenance immunosuppression usually do not experience metabolic abnormalities. Elevated levels of tacrolimus during the early postoperative period may result in hyperkalemia, hypophosphatemia, hypomagnesemia, or metabolic acidosis. Common signs and symptoms of elevated levels of tacrolimus include shaking hands (jitteriness), hypertension, headache, changes in vision or behavior, and feelings of nervousness or anxiety (Astellas Cares, 2021).

Drug interactions. Tacrolimus is metabolized in the liver by the cytochrome P450 III system (Gaston, 2006). Metabolism of tacrolimus depends on liver function and other agents that induce or inhibit this enzyme system, subsequently affecting blood levels. Because primary care providers often prescribe medications for a variety of acute and chronic childhood illnesses, it is important that the family or health care provider contact the transplant center to discuss possible drug interactions. Drugs that interact with tacrolimus disrupt an otherwise stable level, which may result in

drug-related neuro- and nephrotoxicities. Fluctuating levels may also increase the risk of rejection or infection.

Differential Diagnosis

Fever: Common childhood conditions vs. rejection
Abdominal symptoms: Common childhood conditions vs. obstruction in the common bile duct, ulcers, small bowel obstruction, peritonitis, or rejection
Vomiting and diarrhea: May result in altered absorption of medications
Metabolic abnormalities: Hyperkalemia, hyperglycemia, and low CO_2 levels may be related to immunosuppressant medications
Neurologic symptoms: Lethargy, irritability, and tremors may be related to elevated levels of calcineurin inhibitors

DEVELOPMENTAL ISSUES

Sleep Patterns

Sleep disturbances in children with end-stage organ disease are common and may be caused by the existing chronic condition, symptoms of organ deterioration (e.g., severe pruritus from liver disease), emotional distress, and psychological effects of extended hospitalization. In addition, tacrolimus, cyclosporine A, and steroids are reported to cause insomnia. During periods of rejection, when the child is treated with increased immunosuppression with tacrolimus and high-dose oral steroids or IV methylprednisolone, sleep patterns may be significantly altered, and insomnia and irritability are common. Healthy sleep supports healthy brain development, and research demonstrates that childhood sleep disturbances are associated with behavioral, mood, and cognitive disturbances, as well as poor school performance and absenteeism (Svingos et al., 2018).

Parents may find it helpful to maintain home routines and rituals to the fullest extent possible while the child is hospitalized. Strategies to improve sleep include maintaining an organized sleep-wake cycle, avoiding late-afternoon napping, and minimizing evening television watching and caffeine intake (CDC, 2022b). In some cases, professional counseling may help the child and family.

Toileting

Regression in toileting habits is expected in toddlers and preschool-age children during and after hospitalization. Care providers should be aware of this temporary regression and support children in regaining their toileting skills. Pediatric renal transplant recipients may have specific concerns and issues related to toileting and the establishment or reestablishment of urinary flow and continence.

The initiation of urine flow for a child following renal transplantation is often a time of great excitement for the child and family. However, the child may have periods of incontinence while learning to recognize the body cues that signal the need to urinate and to control the urine flow.

Some heart and renal transplant recipients may require diuretic therapy, which may contribute to increased incontinence, consequently affecting toileting routines and new behaviors. When possible, diuretics should be administered early in the day to decrease nighttime incontinence, frequency of nightly urination, and sleep disruption. Incontinence and enuresis are common occurrences in the early post-transplant period, and parents should be counseled about the implications of the child's medical management on daily routines, the need for emotional support for their child, and consistency of home routines.

Discipline

A child's chronic condition affects the entire family, its system of functioning, and the roles within it. As a child with end-stage organ disease improves significantly after transplantation, former coping mechanisms used by the family, parental roles, and family dynamics may no longer be successful. It is often difficult for families to make the transition from parenting a sick child to parenting a healthier one. Many parents continue to overprotect their children and now have additional concerns about infection and rejection. Parents may have difficulty encouraging children to develop independence and peer relationships and are often reticent to integrate the child into school and community activities. In contrast, other parents may have trouble setting limits on inappropriate behavior and may overindulge the child.

The primary care provider plays an essential role in evaluating family dynamics and the parents' ability to appropriately discipline and nurture a child after transplantation. The caregiver can help parents achieve a balance between establishing age-appropriate and consistent limits and allowing the child some control in decision making. Encouraging independence helps promote confidence and positive self-esteem. Family counseling can be a highly effective method to help families cope with the ongoing stressors of the transplant process.

Child Care

Attendance at day care centers is generally not recommended by most transplant centers for 1 to 3 months following transplantation due to high levels of immunosuppression during that time with a greater risk for infection. As immunosuppressive levels are decreased, routine social contact and participation in group activities and day care programs may be resumed. Community-acquired viruses are usually tolerated well by children who are receiving lower-dose maintenance immunosuppression. However, parents should be informed by the primary care provider or day care staff of any outbreaks of varicella or measles in the community or day care center, as these viruses could be potentially serious for the child with a transplant even if immunized prior to transplantation.

Schooling

Children are encouraged to return to school as soon as possible after transplantation to resume a normal routine, continue class work, and interact with peers. Although most children can return to the classroom within 3 months after transplantation, some children benefit from gradually increasing school attendance from a few hours daily to a full schedule as tolerated. As provided by the school district, tutoring at home may be an ideal option when children have had an extended absence from school and are significantly behind in class content. An individualized education plan (IEP) may be needed to allow the child to adjust to a school schedule and workload while healing from a long-term illness and significant surgery.

Parents are often hesitant to return their children to school due to concerns about exposure to infections, their perception of the child's fragility and increased demands on the child, and peer influences. Primary care providers should encourage the resumption of routine childhood activities and school while emphasizing the benefits of developmentally appropriate play, social interactions, and instruction. Teachers also have an important role in normalizing the child's school experience by accommodating medical absences and encouraging optimal academic performance.

The child's medication schedule should be organized to accommodate the school day with minimal interruptions. Medications prescribed daily or twice daily are easily adaptable to the child's schedule. Frequent visits to the health office for medications or having a parent visit daily to administer medications is disruptive to the child's school routine and may emphasize the child's different needs. Children may be particularly sensitive to these intrusions during adolescence.

Sexuality and Pregnancy

Most children experience significant physical appearance improvements following successful solid organ transplantation. Older school-age children and adolescents are very aware of these dramatically positive physical changes: increased energy and strength, a natural skin color following the resolution of jaundice or cyanosis, a normal body shape in the absence of ascites or peripheral edema, increased growth and maturation, and the absence of appliances such as central venous lines, gastrostomy tubes, oxygen cannulas, or dialysis catheters. In addition, daily care routines, laboratory testing, clinic visits, and medical routines may be considerably minimized with stable graft function.

Recipients may also experience some negative effects on appearance and body image. The physical stigmata of immunosuppressive therapy and steroids include hirsutism, cushingoid facies, gingival hyperplasia, obesity, and short stature. Steroids may also intensify outbreaks of acne in adolescents and cause mood swings. Physical stigmata as a result of immunosuppressive therapy with tacrolimus is very rare, although a small percentage of children experience transient alopecia. Scarring from multiple surgeries, invasive lines, catheters, and other procedures is unavoidable. Parents and children are advised about skin care issues as they recuperate from surgery. Some adolescents are interested in minimizing scarring and any keloid formations and may benefit from a plastic surgery consultation. Professional counseling and support groups are also encouraged for this population because these children may be at risk for depression, nonadherence, or increased risk-taking behaviors.

Transplant education for adolescents should include information about puberty, sexual development, sexual activity/abstinence, birth control, and sexually transmitted diseases. The HPV vaccine should be initiated as soon as it clears through the transplant center if not received prior to transplantation (CDC, 2021b). Adolescents with chronic organ disease often experience delayed pubertal development. Typically, when stable graft function is achieved, there is often subsequent initiation or resumption of menses, progression of puberty, and return of libido (Transplant Australia, 2019). Pretransplant and posttransplant counseling and education will help the adolescent prepare for and adapt to these sudden changes. Adolescent females should be referred to their primary care provider, teen clinic, or gynecology practitioner for birth control counseling and gynecologic examinations as indicated.

Sexual activity may resume at 6 to 8 weeks after transplantation. Sexually active adolescents can choose from any of the standard options for adolescent contraception, including hormonal contraception and emergency contraception after unprotected sex; however, estrogen- and progesterone-containing contraceptives interact with posttransplant immunosuppressive medications and may increase levels of corticosteroids, tacrolimus, and sirolimus. Blood levels and signs of increased side effects should be monitored during the first few weeks of initiation of these contraceptive medications. Azathioprine can cause liver toxicity, and MMF can cause diarrhea, which may affect the absorption or metabolism of contraceptive medications. Blood pressure control is important in these children because hypertension is a contraindication for estrogen- and progesterone-containing contraceptives. Bone density should be monitored in those adolescents who choose to use depot medroxyprogesterone acetate (Flinn, 2015). The risks and benefits of contraception, side effects, and pregnancy must be considered before deciding on a method of contraception.

With increased long-term survival and a significantly improved physical status, pregnancy is now a more frequent occurrence for females with solid organ transplants. Successful pregnancies in solid organ transplant recipients are possible but not without certain risks and complications. Recommendations for planning a pregnancy may include discontinuation of teratogenic medications at least 3 months before suspending birth control, achievement of stable graft function with low levels of immunosuppression, and genetic counseling for recipients with an inherited etiology of organ disease. The pregnancy should be carefully monitored with a close assessment of graft function and fetal development. In addition to routine prenatal care, pregnant females require frequent monitoring to assess immunosuppressive levels and specific laboratory tests to evaluate for rejection caused by the physiologic changes of pregnancy. These females are at higher risk for spontaneous abortions, intrauterine growth retardation, preeclampsia, or worsening of preexisting hypertension. Premature deliveries and low birth weight in infants are also risks for females with transplants (Transplant Pregnancy Registry International, 2023).

Transition to Adulthood

Adolescence is a vulnerable time of development, which may lead to struggles with maintaining a consistent medication regimen (Florida State University College of Social Work, 2022). Adolescent and young adult transplant recipients have the highest rates of graft loss among all transplant recipients (Wurm et al., 2022). Adolescents after transplant struggle with the same issues of identity, developing independence, sexuality, and social life but within the context of adapting to complex illnesses, medication schedules, and demanding medical follow-up (Wurm et al., 2022). Due to a suppressed immune system, the transplant recipient is more likely to develop sexually transmitted diseases if safe sex practices are not followed. Drugs, alcohol, cigarette smoking, and vaping affect transplanted organs and may interfere with metabolism of immunosuppressive medications. Tattoos and body piercings, which are popular among this age group, also place transplant recipients at risk for infection. Deviation from prescribed medication and care routines is most often reported in adolescents and can jeopardize the graft, resulting in rejection and ultimately graft loss and death. Providing support to adolescent transplant recipients, engaging them in care decisions, and individualizing immunosuppression regimens and follow-up testing can help these adolescents incorporate necessary treatments into daily life activities.

Securing employment and obtaining insurance are significant concerns for the late adolescent entering college or the job force. An employer may be fearful of possible physical limitations and potential absences from work. Young adults eventually lose their parents' insurance coverage and must find health insurance through a private carrier or apply for medical assistance. Private insurance may be difficult to obtain because of a preexisting condition or employment issues. During the first year posttransplant, recipients may qualify for government disability depending on the level of illness persisting. Although the expenses of transplantation decrease in the long term, an ongoing financial obligation remains for the recipient's lifetime. Medications, laboratory tests, and physical examinations are routinely required. Additional invasive testing and hospitalization may be necessary if the individual acquires an infection or has an episode of acute rejection. Transplant financial counselors and social workers from the transplant center offer counseling about insurance options, medication programs, and grants. Additionally, support groups and websites established by a variety of foundations, pharmaceutical companies, private individuals, and community groups provide information about the transplant process and resources (see Resources, later).

Supporting adolescents during the transition to adulthood may be difficult for parents as they help their child achieve the developmental tasks of adolescence and as the adolescent assumes greater responsibility for routine care. Individual and family counseling is recommended and encouraged. Consistent and routine communication with the transplant center may also help provide parents with strategies and advice in working through these complex issues within the context of transplantation. In addition, as the adolescent progresses chronologically and developmentally into adulthood, a gradual transition to an adult transplant center should be planned to better meet the needs of an adult transplant recipient.

Transition to adult care. Navigating the health care system as an adult requires skills and practice. Scheduling appointments, filling prescriptions, and understanding insurance coverage is complicated, and even more so for those dealing with a chronic condition such as an organ transplant. Studies show that failure to plan for the transition to adult care for an adolescent with a chronic illness leads to poor health outcomes and increased mortality and morbidity (White & Cooley, 2018). Transition to adult care includes the entire process of teaching health care independence for young adults, preparing for transfer, and ensuring its completion. It is not a single event of switching from pediatric to adult-based care (Got Transition, 2020). Formal planning for the eventual transfer to adult care should start as early as age 12 years. However, teaching younger children how to call the pharmacy for refills, utilize timers for medications, and knowing the names of medications, for example, can be initiated earlier as developmentally appropriate.

Additionally, the provider should include the younger child in discussions during the health care visit by asking questions and for input directly from the child while confirming the responses with parents or caretakers. Parents and providers play an important role in guiding young adults in managing their health care. Pediatric primary care providers are encouraged to have a plan for transitioning their transplant patients to adult care. Including the adolescent and family is important for success. Several resources are available, most notably the website Got Transition (see Resources, later), which provides a process guide utilizing six core elements for a successful transition to adult care (Got Transition, 2020).

Family Concerns

Transplantation is an exchange of end-stage organ disease for the chronic condition of transplantation. Although most families and recipients believe this is an acceptable trade-off, anxiety and apprehensions about the future may be ongoing. Long-term survival, the child's transition into adulthood, nonadherence with care, fear of rejection, late infections, need for possible retransplantation, and the child's future employment and quality of life are major concerns.

Medication nonadherence is a major cause of late rejection and other complications in solid organ transplantation. Because nonadherence is such a significant problem following transplantation, adherence to medication and care routines should be discussed with the child and family throughout the transplant process, from the pretransplant evaluation through chronic care follow-up. Nonadherence rates are reported to be up to 36% in renal transplant recipients and up to 15% of all other organ recipients (Sandal et al., 2021). Pediatric transplant recipients have nonadherence rates as high as 60% during adolescence, leading to many hospitalizations, organ rejections, and death (Killian et al., 2018). Medication is just one aspect of the posttransplant regimen. Follow-up testing, frequent appointments with the transplant center, diet, exercise, and other lifestyle elements can be a challenge for the child and family to incorporate into their daily lives.

Adherence. Nonadherence should always be considered in the differential diagnosis of rejection, particularly if the child is an adolescent and a long-term survivor. Psychosocial risk factors for nonadherence include adolescents, racial/ethnic minority status, and the presence of mental health issues. Familial predictors included single-parent households, lower socioeconomic status, lower family cohesion, presence of family conflict, and poor family communication (Killian et al., 2018). The transplant team must work closely with the adolescent to ensure that the outcome and consequences of poor adherence to medical routines are understood. Repeated education about medications, rejection, infection, and chronic care requirements is essential and must be reinforced during visits with the pediatric provider and transplant providers. Counseling with a psychologist or medical social worker may help the adolescent recognize the underlying causes of nonadherence and lead to changes to increase adherence. The transplant team should also make every effort to help by minimizing medication requirements and the number of daily dosages while working with the child to create a schedule that is supported by the child's daily routine, is easy to adhere to, and does not interfere with other activities. A system for routinely obtaining laboratory tests and communicating with the transplant coordinator is also imperative. In repeated cases of nonadherence, a contract may be helpful to delineate the responsibilities of the child and the transplant center, the adherence plan, and the consequences of breaking the contract. Ultimately, some extreme cases may require a referral to family services.

The financial impact of transplantation may be another significant concern for families. The transplant surgery and initial hospitalization, possible repeat admissions, an array of medications, living expenses while at the transplant center, and ongoing expenses at home amass an enormous financial burden for many families. Financial support can come from third-party health insurance payers, community fundraising, state funding, or the family's own resources.

Ongoing communication, updated information, and emotional support from the transplant team and primary care providers will help families cope with their fears and uncertainty about their child's future as they progress and adapt to life after transplantation.

RESOURCES

Alpha-1-Antitrypsin Disease: www.alpha1.org
American Association of Kidney Patients: www.aakp.org

American Heart Association: www.americanheart.org
American Liver Foundation: www.liverfoundation.org
Children's Liver Association for Support Services: www.classkids.org
Children's Organ Transplant Association: www.cota.org
Donate Life America: www.donatelife.net
Got Transition: www.gottransition.org
International Pediatric Transplant Association: www.iptaonline.org
International Society for Heart and Lung Transplantation: www.ishlt.org
International Transplant Nurses Society: www.itns.org
Minority Organ Tissue Transplant Education Program: www.nationalmottep.org
National Foundation for Transplant: www.transplants.org
National Kidney Foundation, Inc.: www.kidney.org
National Organization for Rare Disorders: https://rarediseases.org
National Transplant Assistance Fund and Catastrophic Injury Program: https://helphopelive.org
North American Transplant Coordinators' Organization: www.natco1.org
Thomas Starzl Transplant Institute: https://stiresearch.health.pitt.edu
Transplant Lyfe: www.transplantlyfe.com
Transplant Recipients' International Organization: www.trioweb.org
Transplant Pregnancy Registry International: www.transplantpregnancyregistry.org
Transweb: www.transweb.org
United Network for Organ Sharing: www.unos.org
Wilson Disease Association: www.wilsonsdisease.org

 Summary

Primary Care Needs for the Child With Solid Organ Transplant

HEALTH CARE MAINTENANCE
Growth and Development
- Measure height and weight at each visit.
- Measure head circumference for children under age 3 years at each visit.
- Linear growth may be compromised by the long-term use of corticosteroids.
- Catchup growth may be attained after transplantation.
- Growth hormone may be advised for children under age 1 year before renal transplantation and for children over age 1 year following renal transplantation.
- Improved physical development after transplantation has a positive effect on psychosocial development.
- Cognitive functioning should be monitored at regular intervals.
- Screening for depressive symptoms related to body image changes, side effects of medications, and adaptation to the chronic condition may be advisable.

Diet
- A regular oral diet without restrictions is common following stable graft function, although renal recipients may have sodium restrictions.
- Enteral supplements may be needed to meet caloric requirements for catchup growth and wound healing, particularly in younger children.
- Dietary restrictions are instituted when indicated for electrolyte imbalances or hyperglycemia.
- Children with heart transplants are on a heart-healthy diet.

Safety
- Good hand washing and avoidance of people with infection are recommended to decrease the risk of toxoplasmosis and other potential infections.
- Medical alert bracelets are recommended.
- The transplant center should be contacted before traveling outside the United States or to report extended travel arrangements to give contact information.

Continued

- Activity and exercise are usually restricted for 6 to 8 weeks after the transplant. Age-appropriate safety issues should be addressed as in the healthy pediatric population: seat belts, helmets, Mr. Yuk stickers, electrical outlet covers, etc.

Immunizations

- All recommended immunizations should be administered at least 1 month before the transplant when possible.
- Interrupted immunization schedules can usually be resumed 3 to 6 months after transplantation.
- Live virus vaccines are contraindicated in transplant recipients; they should receive inactivated vaccines when available.
- All routine childhood immunizations, including inactivated poliovirus, MMR, and varicella vaccines, should be given to siblings and other close contacts. HPV should be administered as early as possible.
- Transplant recipients and family members within the household should get the annual inactivated influenza vaccine.

Screenings

- *Depression.* Routine screening is recommended. Pediatric transplant recipients are at high risk for depression, PTSD, and lower quality of life.
- *Vision.* Routine screening is recommended. Pediatric transplant recipients receiving high-dose long-term steroid therapy are at risk for developing glaucoma and cataracts and may require more frequent examinations. Children with chronic CMV infection should be screened for infection-related retinitis.
- *Hearing.* Audiograms should be obtained to evaluate hearing loss in children who have received ototoxic drugs.
- *Dental.* Routine screening is recommended.
  - CSA may cause gingival hyperplasia. Antibiotic prophylaxis is indicated only for cardiac transplant recipients with valvular disease.
- *Blood pressure.* Measurement should be obtained at each sick and well visit.
  - If antihypertensive medications are prescribed, blood pressure should be checked and recorded before administration of each dose. A record of blood pressure results should be kept and assessed at each sick and well visit. Further evaluation may be required for long-term hypertension.
- *Hematocrit.* Screening should be done per the transplant center routine.
  - Anemia may occur because of renal dysfunction or recurrent disease.
- *Urinalysis.* Nephrotoxicity is a complication of cyclosporine and tacrolimus.
  - Additional screening is necessary for children with kidney transplants.
  - Immunosuppression may mask symptoms of UTI. Urinalysis should be obtained in children with fever and possible UTI.
- *Tuberculosis.* Screening with a PPD and anergy panel is recommended. Chest radiography is obtained if indicated. A lifetime course of isoniazid is recommended in patients with positive PPD and chest films.

Condition-Specific Screening

- *Bloodwork.* Routine laboratory testing is obtained at regular intervals, usually weekly to monthly, depending on the time after the transplant and any current episodes of infection or rejection.
- Tacrolimus, cyclosporine A, and/or sirolimus levels are also monitored regularly and adjusted as indicated per transplant center protocols.

COMMON ILLNESS MANAGEMENT

Differential Diagnosis

- *Fever.* The risk of bacterial, fungal, and viral infections is highest during the first 3 months after a transplant and when immunosuppression is maximized.
  - Immunosuppression may mask symptoms, so careful assessment of any fever is very important.
  - Normal childhood illnesses should be ruled out.
  - Fever may indicate organ rejection or infection.
- *Abdominal symptoms.* Abdominal pain should be investigated to rule out appendicitis, intestinal obstruction, ulcers, peritonitis, rejection, or PTLD.
  - Abdominal pain in liver transplant recipients may be a sign of rejection or surgical complications.
  - Abdominal pain or vomiting may be a sign of rejection in heart transplant recipients.
  - Vomiting and diarrhea may lower therapeutic blood levels of immunosuppressant drugs.
- *Metabolic abnormalities.* Hyperkalemia can result from drug therapy.
  - Hyperglycemia may result from immunosuppressant medications.

Drug Interactions

- Cyclosporine A and tacrolimus absorption is altered by phenytoin, phenobarbital, ketoconazole, fluconazole, erythromycin, diltiazem, and other drugs.
- When administered with anticonvulsants, higher doses of cyclosporine A may be needed to achieve a therapeutic range.
- Acetaminophen should be used instead of aspirin or ibuprofen.
- If the child is hypertensive, decongestants should be avoided.
- It is important for the primary care provider to contact the transplant center before prescribing any medication.

DEVELOPMENTAL ISSUES

Sleep Patterns

- End-stage organ disease, hospitalization, or drugs may alter sleep patterns.
- Familiar routines and rituals should be maintained when possible.

Toileting

- Regression in toddlers and preschoolers is to be expected.
- Children with renal transplantation may need to relearn body cues to achieve toilet training.
- Children taking diuretics may have difficulty with urinary continence and training.
- Emotional support is required as children learn skills.

Discipline

- Parental overprotectiveness is likely; parents may need help to promote independence in their children.
- Family counseling may be helpful.

Child Care

- Children may attend day care 3 months after surgery if immunosuppression requirements have been reduced.

- Precautions should be taken to limit exposure to communicable diseases.

Schooling
- Normal schooling should be resumed 1 to 3 months after transplantation.
- Additional academic help may be needed to attain grade-level skills because of time lost.
- An IEP should be initiated if school problems develop.

Sexuality
- The transplant experience may affect body image and self-esteem.
- Barrier methods of birth control are recommended.
- Childbearing is possible after transplantation.
- Physiologic strain on the maternal system must be monitored.

- Effects of immunosuppression on the fetus must be monitored.

Transition to Adulthood
- Many individuals have difficulty attaining independence.
- Body image and intimacy may be negatively affected.
- Concerns about employment and health insurance develop.
- Planning and preparation for the eventual transition to adult primary and transplant care are important.

FAMILY CONCERNS
- Family concerns include the fear of rejection, the search for a new organ, organ donor issues, and finances.
- Securing employment and continued health insurance may be difficult.
- Adolescents are at high risk for nonadherence.

REFERENCES

Abbas, A., Zimmer, A. J., & Florescu, D. (2021). Viral enteritis in solid-organ transplantation. *Viruses, 13*(10). https://doi:10.3390/v13102019.

American Academy of Pediatrics Committee on Infectious Diseases, & American Academy of Pediatrics Bronchiolitis Guidelines Committee (2014). Updated guidance for palivizumab prophylaxis among infants and young children at increased risk of hospitalization for respiratory syncytial virus infection. *Pediatrics, 134*(2), e620–e638. https://doi.org/10.1542/peds.2014-1666.

American Dental Association. (2022, January 5). Antibiotic prophylaxis prior to dental procedures. https://www.ada.org/resources/research/science-and-research-institute/oral-health-topics/antibiotic-prophylaxis.

American Liver Foundation. (2022, July 20). *Diagnosing hepatic encephalopathy.* https://liverfoundation.org/liver-diseases/complications-of-liver-disease/hepatic-encephalopathy/diagnosing-hepatic-encephalopathy/.

Arora, N., De Souza, A., Galvin, C., Sueyoshi, T., Lui, S., Cole, A., Human, D., & Armstrong, K. (2019). Physical activity, exercise capacity and quality of life in adolescent heart transplant patients. *Journal of Heart and Lung Transplantation, 38*(4), S471. https://doi.org/10.1016/j.healun.2019.01.1198.

Åsberg, A., Humar, A., Rollag, H., Jardine, A. G., Kumar, D., Aukrust, P., Ueland, T., Bignamini, A. A., & Hartmann, A. (2016). Lessons learned from a randomized study of oral valganciclovir versus parenteral ganciclovir treatment of cytomegalovirus disease in solid organ transplant recipients: The VICTOR trial. *Clinical Infectious Diseases, 62*(9), 1154–1160. https://doi.org/10.1093/cid/ciw084.

Ashrafi, F., Shahidi, S., Mehrzad, V., Mortazavi, M., & Hosseini, S. F. (2021). Survival of post-transplant lymphoproliferative disorder after kidney transplantation in patients under rapamycin treatment. *International Journal of Hematology-Oncology and Stem Cell Research, 15*(4), 239–248. doi:10.18502/ijhoscr.v15i4.7479.

Asleh, R., Alnsasra, H., Haberman, T. M., Briasoulis, A., & Kushwaha, S. S. (2022). Post-transplant lymphoproliferative disorder following cardiac transplantation. *Frontiers in Cardiovascular Medicine, 23.* https://doi.org/10.3389/fcvm.2022.787975.

Astellas Cares. (2021, August). Prograf. https://www.prograf.com/side-effects.

Aull, M. J. (2019). Growth and development after transplantation. *Medscape.* https://emedicine.medscape.com/article/1014599-overview#a5.

Bennett, A. L., & Ventura, H. O. (2017). Hypertension in patients with cardiac transplantation. *Medical Clinics of North America, 101*(1), 53–64. https://doi.org/10.1016/j.mcna.2016.08.011.

Berk, C., & Volk, M. L. (2021). Preventive care in adult liver transplant recipients. *Clinical Liver Disease, 18*(1), 14–17. https://doi.org/10.1002/cld.1086.

Berlin heart. Medical Professionals EXCOR Pediatric. (2020). https://www.berlinheart.de/en/medical-professionals/excorr-pediatric/.

Bock, M., & Chinnock, R. E. (2022). Pediatric heart transplantation. *Medscape.* https://emedicine.medscape.com/article/1011927-medication#2.

Calinescu, A. M., Madadi-Sanjani, O., Mack, C., Schreiber, R. A., Superina, R., Kelly, D., Petersen, C., & Wildhaber, B. E. (2022). Cholangitis definition and treatment after Kasai hepatoportoenterostomy for biliary atresia: A Delphi process and international expert panel. *Journal of Clinical Medicine, 11*(3), 494. https://doi.org/10.3390/jcm11030494. Published 2022 Jan 19.

Canter, C. E., Shaddy, R. E., Bernstein, D., Hsu, D. T., Chrisant, M. R., Kirklin, J. K., Kanter, K. R., Higgins, R. S., Blume, E. D., Rosenthal, D. N., Boucek, M. M., Uzark, K. C., Friedman, A. H., Young, J. K., American Heart Association Council on Cardiovascular Disease in the Young, American Heart Association Council on Clinical Cardiology, American Heart Association Council on Cardiovascular Nursing, American Heart Association Council on Cardiovascular Surgery and Anesthesia, & Quality of Care and Outcomes Research Interdisciplinary Working Group (2007). Indications for heart transplantation in pediatric heart disease: A scientific statement from the American Heart Association Council on Cardiovascular Disease in the Young; the Councils on Clinical Cardiology, Cardiovascular Nursing, and Cardiovascular Surgery and Anesthesia; and the Quality of Care and Outcomes Research Interdisciplinary Working Group. *Circulation, 115*(5), 658–676. https://doi.org/10.1161/CIRCULATIONAHA.106.180449. [published correction appears in Circulation. 2007 Apr 3;115(13):e385. Friedman, Allen H [corrected to Friedman, Alan H]].

Carvajal, H. G., Costello, J. P., Miller, J. R., Eghtesady, P., & Nath, D. S. (2022). Pediatric heart-lung transplantation: Technique and special considerations. *Journal of Heart and Lung Transplantation, 41*(3), 271–278. doi:10.1016/j.healun.2021.12.002.

Centers for Disease Control and Prevention. Organ transplant patients and fungal disease. (2020). https://www.cdc.gov/fungal/infections/organ-transplant.html#:~:text=Some%20types%20of%20fungal%20infections,fungal%20infections%20are%20also%20possible.&text=For%20lung%20transplant%20patients%2C%20aspergillosis%20is%20most%20common.

Centers for Disease Control and Prevention. People with weakened immune systems. (2021a). https://www.cdc.gov/healthypets/specific-groups/high-risk/organ-transplant-patients.html?CDC_AA_refVal=https%3A%2F%2Fwww.cdc.gov%2Fhealthypets%2Fspecific-groups%2Forgan-transplant-patients.html.

Centers for Disease Control and Prevention. HPV vaccine. (2021b). https://www.cdc.gov/hpv/parents/vaccine-for-hpv.html.

Centers for Disease Control and Prevention. Altered immunocompetence. (2022a). https://www.cdc.gov/vaccines/hcp/acip-recs/general-recs/immunocompetence.html.

Centers for Disease Control and Prevention. Tips for better sleep. (2022b). https://www.cdc.gov/sleep/about_sleep/sleep_hygiene.html.

Centers for Disease Control and Prevention. Chickenpox (varicella). (2022c). https://www.cdc.gov/chickenpox/hcp/index.html#:~:text=Second%20occurrence%20of%20varicella%20may,causing%20illness%20or%20detectable%20viremia.

Centers for Disease Control and Prevention. Healthy pets, healthy people: Keeping pets healthy keeps people healthy too!. (2022d). https://www.cdc.gov/healthypets/index.html.

Centers for Disease Control and Prevention. (2023). Cardiomyopathy. https://www.cdc.gov/heartdisease/cardiomyopathy.htm.

Chen, K., Didsbury, M., van Zwieten, A., Howell, M., Kim, S., Tong, A., Howard, K., Nassar, N., Barton, B., Lah, S., Lorenzo, J., Strippoli, G., Palmer, S., Teixeira-Pinto, A., Mackie, F., McTaggart, S., Walker, A., Kara, T., Craig, J. C., & Wong, G. (2018). Neurocognitive and educational outcomes in children and adolescents with CKD: A systematic review and meta-analysis. *Clinical Journal of the American Society of Nephrology*, 13(3), 387–397. https://doi.org/10.2215/CJN.09650917.

Chiou, F. K., Sharif, K., Perera, T., Nuiesan, P., Vickers, M., Beath, S., Morland, B., Mirza, D., & Gupte, G. (2018). Poorer long-term survival associated with monomorphic post-transplant lymphoproliferative disorder after solid organ transplantation in children. *Transplant*, 102, s457–s458. https://doi.org/10.1097/01.tp.0000543252.38543.d1.

Chiu, K. W., Lin, T. L., Yong, C. C., Lin, C. C., Cheng, Y. F., & Chen, C. L. (2019). Endoscopic injection sclerotherapy for pediatric bleeding esophageal varices complicated by gastric vein, main portal vein, splenic mesenteric junction, and splenic vein occlusion: A case report. *BMC Gastroenterology*, 19(1), 37. doi:10.1186/s12876-019-0955-7. Published 2019 Feb 28.

Choudhary, N. S., Saigal, S., Bansal, R. K., Saraf, N., Gautam, D., & Soin, A. S. (2017). Acute and chronic rejection after liver transplantation: What a clinician needs to know. *Journal of Clinical and Experimental Hepatology*, 7(4), 358–366. doi:10.1016/j.jceh.2017.10.003.

Claeys, E., & Vermeir, K. (2019). Immunosuppressive drugs in organ transplantation to prevent allograft rejection: Mode of action and side effects. *Journal of Immunology Science*, 3(4), 14–21. https://doi.org/10.29245/2578-3009/2019/4.1178.

Clayton, P. A., McDonald, S. P., Russ, G. R., & Chadban, S. J. (2019). Long-term outcomes after acute rejection in kidney transplant recipients: An ANZDATA analysis. *Journal of the American Society of Nephrology*, 30(9), 1697–1707. https://doi.org/10.1681/ASN.2018111101.

Crowther, B. (2019). Immunosuppression in pediatric SOT. *PedSAP. Book 2: Transplantation*. https://www.accp.com/docs/bookstore/pedsap/ped2019b2_sample.pdf.

Danziger-Isakov, L., & Kumar, D. (2019). Vaccination of solid organ transplant candidates and recipients: Guidelines from the American Society of Transplantation Infectious Diseases Community of Practice. *Clinical Transplantation*, 33(9), e13563. https://doi.org/10.1111/ctr.13563.

Date, H. (2017). Living-related lung transplantation. *Journal of Thoracic Disease*, 9(9), 3362–3371. https://doi.org/10.21037/jtd.2017.08.152.

Dirix, M., Philipse, E., Vleut, R., Hartman, V., Bracke, B., Chapelle, T., Roeyen, G., Ysebaert, D., Van Beeumen, G., Snelders, E., Massart, A., Leyssens, K., Couttenye, M. M., Abramowicz, D., & Hellemans, R. (2022). Timing of the pre-transplant workup for renal transplantation: Is there room for improvement?

Clinical Kidney Journal, 15(6), 1100–1108. https://doi.org/10.1093/ckj/sfac006.

Dull, M. M., & Kremer, A. E. (2020). Newer approaches to the management of pruritus in cholestatic liver disease. *Current Hepatology Reports*, 19, 86–95. https://doi.org/10.1007/s11901-020-00517-x.

Duvant, P., Fillat, M., Garaix, F., Roquelaure, B., Ovaert, C., Fouilloux, V., Tsimaratos, M., Auquier, P., Fabre, A., & Baumstarck, K. (2021). Quality of life of transplanted children and their parents: A cross-sectional study. *Orphanet Journal of Rare Diseases*, 16(1), 364. doi:https://doi.org/10.1186/s13023-021-01987-y. Published 2021 Aug 17.

Elisofon, S. A., Magee, J. C., Ng, V. L., Horslen, S. P., Fioravanti, V., Economides, J., Erinjeri, J., Anand, R., Mazariegos, G. V., & Society of Pediatric Liver Transplantation Research Group (2020). Society of Pediatric Liver Transplantation: Current registry status 2011-2018. *Pediatric Transplantation*, 24, e13605. https://doi.org/10.1111/petr.13605.

Faro, A., & Visner, G. (2019). Pediatric lung transplantation: Overview of pediatric lung transplantation. *Medscape*. https://emedicine.medscape.com/article/1013065-overview.

Feldmann, M., Bataillard, C., Ehrler, M., Ullrich, C., Knirsch, W., Gosteli-Peter, M. A., Held, U., & Latal, B. (2021). Cognitive and executive function in congenital heart disease: A meta-analysis. *Pediatrics*, 148(4), e2021050875. https://doi.org/10.1542/peds.2021-050875.

Flinn, S. K. (2015). *Health facts: Depo Provera and bone mineral density*. National Women's Health Network. https://nwhn.org/depo-provera-and-bone-mineral-density/.

Florida State University College of Social Work. Study on digital adherence programs improves pediatric transplant health outcomes. (2022). https://csw.fsu.edu/article/study-digital-adherence-program-improves-pediatric-transplant-health-outcomes.

Friman, S., Tisone, G., Nevens, F., Lehner, F., Santaniello, W., Bechstein, W. O., Zhuvarel, S. V., Isoniemi, H., Rummo, O. O., Klempnauer, J., Anaokar, S., Hurst, M., Kazeem, G., Undre, N., & Trunečka, P. (2021). Long-term prolonged-release tacrolimus-based immunosuppression in de novo liver transplant recipients: 5-year prospective follow-up of patients in the DIAMOND Study. *Transplantation Direct*, 7(8), e722. https://doi.org/10.1097/TXD.0000000000001166.

Gaston, R. S. (2006). Current and evolving immunosuppressive regimens in kidney transplantation. *American Journal of Kidney Diseases*, 47(4 Suppl 2), S3–21. doi:10.1053/j.ajkd.2005.12.047.

Ghelichi-Ghojogh, M., Mohammadizadeh, F., Jafari, F., Vali, M., Jahanian, S., Mohammadi, M., Jafari, A., Khezri, R., Nikbakht, H. A., Daliri, M., & Rajabi, A. (2022). The global survival rate of graft and patient in kidney transplantation of children: A systematic review and meta-analysis. *BMC Pediatrics*, 22(1), 503. doi:10.1186/s12887-022-03545-2. Published 2022 Aug 24.

Gold, A., Bondi, B. C., Ashkanase, J., & Dipchand, A. I. (2020). Early school-age cognitive performance post-pediatric heart transplantation. *Pediatric Transplantation*, 24(8), e13832. https://doi.org/10.1111/petr.13832.

Got Transition. The six core elements of healthcare transition 3.0. 2020. https://www.gottransition.org/6ce/?side-by-side.

Gunawardena, T., Sharma, H., Sharma, A. J., & Mehra, S. (2021). Surgical considerations in paediatric kidney transplantation: An update. *Renal Replacement Therapy*, 7(54). https://doi.org/10.1186/s41100-021-00373-5.

Gungor, S., Kilic, B., Arslan, M., Selimoglu, M. A., Karabiber, H., & Yilmaz, S. (2017). Early and late neurological complications of liver transplantation in pediatric patients. *Pediatric Transplantation*, 21(3). doi:10.1111/petr.12872. https://pubmed.ncbi.nlm.nih.gov/28042689/.

Haller, M. C., Kainz, A., Baer, H., & Oberbauer, R. (2017). Dialysis vintage and outcomes after kidney transplantation: A retrospective cohort study. *Clinical Journal of the American Society of Nephrology, 12*(1), 122–130. doi:10.2215/CJN.04120416.

Harshman, L. A., & Hooper, S. R. (2020). The brain in pediatric chronic kidney disease: The intersection of cognition, neuroimaging, and clinical biomarkers. *Pediatric Nephrology, 35*(12), 2221–2229. https://doi.org/10.1007/s00467-019-04417-1.

Hasan, T., Au, E., Chen, S., Tong, A., & Wong, G. (2018). Screening and prevention for latent tuberculosis in immunosuppressed patients at risk for tuberculosis: A systematic review of clinical practice guidelines. *BMJ Open, 8*(9), e022445. https://doi.org/10.1136/bmjopen-2018-022445.

Hong, B. A., Schuller, D., Yusen, R. D., & Barr, M. L. (2021). Pediatric living donor lung transplant candidates: Psychiatric status of utilized and non-utilized donors. *Journal of Clinical Psychology in Medical Settings, 29*(1), 62 70. https://doi.org/10.1007/s10880-021-09777-1. Epub 2021 Apr 21.

Infectious Disease Advisor. Updated AST IDCOP guidelines for vaccination of organ transplant recipients. (2019). https://www.infectiousdiseaseadvisor.com/home/topics/prevention/updated-ast-idcop-guidelines-for-vaccination-of-organ-transplant-recipients/#:~:text=In%20pediatric%20patients%20requiring%20a%20transplant%2C%20the%20varicella%20vaccine%20may,of%204%20weeks%20is%20acceptable.

International Society for Heart & Lung Transplantation – professional guidelines and consensus documents. ISHLT. (2021). https://ishlt.org/publications-resources/professional-resources/standards-guidelines/professional-guidelines-and-consensus-documents.

Jain, A., & Mattoo, T. K. (2016). Late renal dysfunction after pediatric heart transplant. *Progress in Pediatric Cardiology, 41,* 41–45. https://doi.org/10.1016/j.ppedcard.2015.12.004.

Jara, P., Baker, A., Baumann, U., Borobia, A. M., Branchereu, S., Candusso, M., Carcas, A. J., Chardot, C., Cobas, J., D'Antiga, L., Ferreras, C., Fitzpatrick, E., Frauca, E., Hernández-Oliveros, F., Kaliciński, P., Lindemans, C., Lopes, M. F., López-Granados, E., de Magnée, C., … ERN TransplantChild (2020). Cross-cutting view of current challenges in paediatric solid organ and haematopoietic stem cell transplantation in Europe: The European Reference Network Transplant Child. *Orphanet Journal of Rare Diseases, 15*(1), 16. https://doi.org/10.1186/s13023-020-1293-0. Published 2020 Jan 15.

Kamminga, S., van Rijn, A. L., de Brouwer, C. S., Rotmans, J. I., Zaaijer, H. L., & Feltkamp, M. C. W. (2021). JC and Human polyomavirus 9 after kidney transplantation: An exploratory serological cohort study. *Journal of Clinical Virology, 143,* 104944. doi:10.1016/j.jcv.2021.104944.

Kardol-Hoefnagel, T., & Otten, H. G. (2021). A comprehensive overview of the clinical relevance and treatment options for antibody-mediated rejection associated with non-HLA antibodies. *Transplantation, 105*(7), 1459–1470. https://doi.org/10.1097/TP.0000000000003551.

Katz, D. T., Torres, N. S., Chatani, B., Gonzalez, I. A., Chandar, J., Miloh, T., Rusconi, P., & Garcia, J. (2020). Care of Pediatric Solid Organ Transplant Recipients: An Overview for Primary Care Providers. *Pediatrics, 146*(6), e20200696. doi:10.1542/peds.2020-0696.

Kemme, S., Kohut, T. J., Boster, J. M., Diamond, T., Rand, E. B., & Feldman, A. G. (2021). Live vaccines in pediatric liver transplant recipients: To give or not to give. *Clinical Liver Disease (Hoboken), 18*(4), 204–210. doi:10.1002/cld.1123. Published 2021 Oct 27.

Killian, M. O., Schuman, D. L., Mayersohn, G. S., & Triplett, K. N. (2018). Psychosocial predictors of medication nonadherence in pediatric organ transplantation: A systemic review. *Pediatric Transplantation, 22*(4), el3188. https://doi.org/10.1111/petr.13188.

Kim, Y. H. (2021). Pediatric heart transplantation: How to manage problems affecting long-term outcomes? *Clinical and Experimental Pediatrics, 64*(2), 49–59. https://doi.org/10.3345/cep.2019.01417.

Kimura, H., & Kwong, Y. L. (2019). EBV viral loads in diagnosis, monitoring, and response assessment. *Frontiers in Oncology, 9,* 62. doi:10.3389/fonc.2019.00062. Published 2019 Feb 12.

Kowalewski, G., Kaliciński, P., Stefanowicz, M., Grenda, R., Czubkowski, P., & Szymczak, M. (2021). Long-term follow-up of renal function in children after liver transplantation—a single center retrospective study. *Children (Basel), 8*(8), 633. doi:10.3390/children8080633. Published 2021 Jul 25.

Kriegermeier, A., & Green, R. (2020). Pediatric cholestatic liver disease: Review of bile acid metabolism and discussion of current and emerging therapies. *Frontiers in Medicine (Lausanne), 7,* 149. doi:10.3389/fmed.2020.00149. Published 2020 May 5.

Lau, E., Moyers, J. T., Wang, B. C., Jeong, I. S. D., Lee, J., Liu, L., Kim, M., Villicana, R., Kim, B., Mitchell, J., Kamal, M. O., Chen, C. S., Liu, Y., Wang, J., Chinnock, R., & Cao, H. (2021). Analysis of post-transplant lymphoproliferative disorder (PTLD) outcomes with Epstein-Barr Virus (EBV) assessments—a single tertiary referral center experience and review of literature. *Cancers (Basel), 13*(4), 899. https://doi.org/10.3390/cancers13040899. Published 2021 Feb 21.

Lazor, T., Grasemann, H., Solomon, M., & Anthony, S. (2017). Impact of pediatric lung transplant on quality-of-life outcomes. *American Journal of Transplantation, 52*(11), 1495–1504. https://doi.org/10.1002/ppul.23788.

Leard, L. E., Holm, A. M., Valapour, M., Glanville, A. R., Attawar, S., Aversa, M., Campos, S. V., Christon, L. M., Cypel, M., Dellgren, G., Hartwig, M. G., Kapnadak, S. G., Kolaitis, N. A., Kotloff, R. M., Patterson, C. M., Shlobin, O. A., Smith, P. J., Solé, A., Solomon, M., … Ramos, K. J. (2021). Consensus document for the selection of lung transplant candidates: An update from the International Society for Heart and Lung Transplantation. *Journal of Heart and Lung Transplantation, 40*(11), 1349–1379. doi:10.1016/j.healun.2021.07.005. https://www.jhltonline.org/article/S1053-2498(21)02407-4/fulltext.

Leww, J., Perito, E. R., & Feng, S. (2022). We asked the experts: Toward personalized immunosuppression for liver transplant recipients. *Editorial World Journal of Surgery, 46,* 876–877. https://doi.org/10.1007/s00268-021-06417-5.

Lim, N., & Lake, J. (2020). Recurrent disease after liver transplantation. *Current Hepatology Reports, 19,* 54–62. https://doi.org/10.1007/s11901-020-00507-z.

Liu, J., Lkhagva, E., Chung, H. J., Kim, H. J., & Hong, S. T. (2018). The pharmabiotic approach to treat hyperammonemia. *Nutrients, 10*(2), 140. doi:10.3390/nu10020140. Published 2018 Jan 28.

Loeb, N., Owens, J. S., Strom, M., Farassati, F., Van Roestel, K., Chambers, K., Kean, P., Ng, V. L., Avitzur, Y., Carricato, M., Wales, P. W., & Courtney-Martin, G. (2018). Long-term follow-up after pediatric liver transplantation: Predictors of growth. *Journal of Pediatric Gastroenterology and Nutrition, 66*(4), 670–675. https://doi.org/10.1097/MPG.0000000000001815.

McCalmont, V., & Velleca, A. (2017). Heart transplantation. In Cupples, S. A., Lerret, S., McCalmont, V., & Ohler, L. (Eds.), *Core curriculum for transplant nurses* (2nd ed., pp. 307–412). Elsevier.

Miedziaszczyk, M., Bajon, A., Jakielska, E., Primke, M., Sikora, J., Skowrońska, D., & Idasiak-Piechocka, I. (2022). Controversial interactions of tacrolimus with dietary supplements, herbs and food. *Pharmaceutics, 14*(10), 2154. https://doi.org/10.3390/pharmaceutics14102154. Published 2022 Oct 10.

Mombelli, M., & Manuel, O. (2022). Cytomegalovirus Infection. *BMJ Best Practices.* https://bestpractice.bmj.com/topics/en-us/560.

Morales, D. L. S., Rossano, J. W., VanderPluym, C., Lorts, A., Cantor, R., St Louis, J. D., Koeh, D., Sutcliffe, D. L., Adachi, I., Kirklin, J. K., Rosenthal, D. N., Blume, E. D., & Pedimacs Investigators (2019). Third annual pediatric interagency registry for mechanical circulatory support (Pedimacs) report: Preimplant characteristics and outcomes. *Annals of Thoracic Surgery, 107*(4), 993–1004. https://doi.org/10.1016/j.athoracsur.2019.01.038.

Nailescu, C., Ermal, A. C., & Shew, M. L. (2022). Human papillomavirus-related cancer risk for solid organ transplant recipients during adult life and early prevention strategies during childhood and adolescence. *Pediatric Transplantation, 26*(7), e14341. https://doi.org/10.1111/petr.14341.

National Institute of Dental and Craniofacial Research. (2011). Dental management of the organ transplant patient. https://www.in.gov/health/files/OrganTransplantProf.pdf.

National Institute of Diabetes and Digestive and Kidney Diseases (2022, August). Kidney disease in children. https://www.niddk.nih.gov/health-information/kidney-disease/children.

National Organization for Rare Disorders (NORD). (2019). Pediatric cardiomyopathy. https://rarediseases.org/rare-diseases/pediatric-cardiomyopathy/.

Nelson, J., Alvey, N., Bowman, L., Schulte, J., Segovia, M. C., McDermott, J., Te, H. S., Kapila, N., Levine, D. J., Gottlieb, R. L., Oberholzer, J., & Campara, M. (2022). Consensus recommendations for use of maintenance immunosuppression in solid organ transplantation: Endorsed by the American College of Clinical Pharmacy, American Society of Transplantation, and International Society for Heart and Lung Transplantation: An executive summary. *Pharmacotherapy, 42*(8), 594–598. https://doi.org/10.1002/phar.2718.

Niazkhani, Z., Pirnejad, H., & Khazaee, P. R. (2017). The impact of health information technology on organ care: A systematic review. *International Journal of Medical information, 100,* 95–107. https://doi.org/10.1016/j.ijmedinf.2017.01.015.

North American Pediatric Renal Trials and Collaborative Studies. 2014. NAPRTCS 2014 annual transplant report. https://naprtcs.org/system/files/2014_Annual_Transplant_Report.pdf.

Organ Procurement and Transplant Network. (2022a). Transplants in the US by recipient age. Retrieved December 20, 2022.

Organ Procurement and Transplant Network. (2022b). National data. https://optn.transplant.hrsa.gov/data/view-data-reports/national-data/. Retrieved December 20, 2022.

Organ Procurement and Transplant Network. (n.d.). Pediatric transplants: A guide when your child needs a transplant. Retrieved December 20, 2022. https://optn.transplant.hrsa.gov/patients/about-transplantation/pediatric-tranplants/#:~:text=Your%20transplant%20team%20will%20order,psychological%20readiness%20and%20social%20support.

Papaz, T., Allen, U., Blydt-Hansen, T., Birk, P. E., Min, S., Hamiwka, L., Phan, V., Schechter, T., Wall, D. A., Urschel, S., Foster, B. J., & Mital, S. (2018). Pediatric outcomes in transplant: PersOnaliSing Immunosuppression To ImproVe Efficacy (POSITIVE Study): The collaboration and design of a national transplant precision medicine program. *Transplantation direct, 4*(12), e410. https://doi.org/10.1097/TXD.0000000000000842.

Papon, N., Nevez, G., Le Gal, S., Vigneau, C., Robert-Gangneux, F., Bouchara, J. P., Cornely, O. A., Denning, D. W., & Gangneux, J. P. (2021). Fungal infections in transplant recipients: Pros and cons of immunosuppressive and antimicrobial treatment. *The Lancet Microbe, 2*(1), e6–e8. https://doi.org/10.1016/S2666-5247(20)30199-3.

Penner, E. K., Walker, H., Moon, E., Slavec, J., Hind, T., & Blydt-Hansen, T. D. (2022). The mental health profiles of pediatric organ transplant recipients. *Pediatric Transplantation, 26*(1), e14151. doi:10.1111/petr.14151.

Prüfe, J. (2022). Decision making in the context of paediatric solid organ transplantation medicine. *Transplant International, 35,* 10625. doi:10.3389/ti.2022.10625. Published 2022 Jul 14.

Pryor, J. B., Bradford, M. C., Jennerich, A. L., Wai, T. Y. H., Pilewski, J. M., Kapnadak, S. G., Aitken, M. L., Goss, C. H., & Ramos, K. J. (2022). Body mass index recovery after lung transplant for cystic fibrosis. *Annals of the American Thoracic Society, 19*(7), 1130–1138. https://doi.org/10.1513/AnnalsATS.202108-969OC.

Rea, K. E., West, K. B., Dorste, A., Christofferson, E. S., Lefkowitz, D., Mudd, E., Schneider, L., Smith, C., Triplett, K. N., & McKenna, K. (2023). A systematic review of social determinants of health in pediatric organ transplant outcomes. *Pediatric Transplantation, 27*(1), e14418. https://doi.org/10.1111/petr.14418.

Sanada, Y., Sakuma, Y., Onishi, Y., Okada, N., Yamada, N., Hirata, Y., Miyahara, G., Katano, T., Horiuchi, T., Omameuda, T., Lefor, A. K., & Sata, N. (2021). Outcomes after living donor liver transplantation in pediatric patients with inherited metabolic diseases. *Annals of Transplantation, 26,* e932994. https://doi.org/10.12659/AOT.932994. Published 2021 Oct 1. https://www.ncbi.nlm.nih.gov/pmc/articles/PMC8491557/pdf/anntransplant-26-e932994.pdf.

Sandal, S., Chen, T., & Cantarovich, M. (2021). Evaluation of transplant candidates with a history of nonadherence: An opinion piece. *Canadian Journal of Kidney Health and Disease, 8,* 2054358121990137. doi:10.1177/2054358121990137 Published 2021 Jan 27.

Sauerwein, K. (2018). *Gene therapy method developed to target damaged kidney cells.* Washington University School of Medicine. https://medicine.wustl.edu/news/gene-therapy-method-developed-to-target-damaged-kidney-cells/.

Scandling, J. D., Busque, S., Lowsky, R., Shizuru, J., Shori, A., Engleman, E., Jensen, K., & Strober, S. (2018). Macrochimerism and clinical transplant tolerance. *Human Immunology, 79*(5), 266–271. https://doi.org/10.1016/j.humimm.2018.01.002.

Schwenk, H. T., Khan, A., Kohlman, K., Bertaina, A., Cho, S., Montoya, J. G., & Contopoulos-Ioannidis, D. G. (2021). Toxoplasmosis in pediatric hematopoietic stem cell transplantation patients. *Transplantation and Cellular Therapy, 27*(4), 292–300. https://doi.org/10.1016/j.jtct.2020.11.003.

Shah, P., Lowery, E., Chaparro, C., Visner, G., Hempstead, S. E., Abraham, J., Bhakta, Z., Carroll, M., Christon, L., Danziger-Isakov, L., Diamond, J. M., Lease, E., Leonard, J., Litvin, M., Poole, R., Vlahos, F., Werchan, C., Murray, M. A., Tallarico, E., … Hachem, R. R. (2021). Cystic fibrosis foundation consensus statements for the care of cystic fibrosis lung transplant recipients. *Transplantation and Cellular Therapy, 40*(7), 539–556. https://doi.org/10.1016/j.healun.2021.04.011.

Shanmugam, N., & Dhawan, A. (2018). Acute liver failure in children. *Pediatric Hepatology and Liver Transplantation,* 145–153. doi:10.1007/978-3-319-96400-3_8. Published 2018 Oct 16.

SPLIT Research Group, (2001). Studies of Pediatric Liver Transplantation (SPLIT). *Transplantation, 72*(3), 463–476.

Sprong, M. C. A., Broeders, W., van der Net, J., Breur, J. M. P. J., de Vries, L. S., Slieker, M. G., & van Brussel, M. (2021). Motor developmental delay after cardiac surgery in children with a critical congenital heart defect: A systematic literature review and meta-analysis. *Pediatric Physical Therapy, 33*(4), 186–197. https://doi.org/10.1097/PEP.0000000000000827.

Stein, R. E. (2022). Mental health concerns and childhood chronic physical health conditions: A narrative review. *Pediatric Medicine, 5*(5). http://dx.doi.org/10.21037/pm-20-107.

Stournaras, E., & Tziomalos, K. (2015). Herbal medicine-related hepatotoxicity. *World Journal of Hepatology, 7*(19), 2189–2193. https://doi.org/10.4254/wjh.v7.i19.2189.

Svingos, A., Grief, S., Bailey, B., & Heaton, S. (2018). The relationship between sleep and cognition in children referred to neuropsychological evaluation: A latent modeling approach. *Children, 5*(3), 33. https://doi.org/10.3390/children5030033.

Tan, L., Yang, Y., Ma, G., Zhu, T., Yang, J., Liu, H., & Zhang, W. (2019). Early acute kidney injury after liver transplantation in patients with normal preoperative renal function. *Clinics and Research in Hepatology and Gastroenterology, 43*(4), 475–482. https://doi.org/10.1016/j.clinre.2018.07.009.

Thrush, P. T., & Hoffman, T. M. (2014). Pediatric heart transplantation—indications and outcomes in the current era. *Journal of Thoracic Diseases, 6*(8), 1080–1096. http://dx.doi.org/10.3978/j.issn.2072-1439.2014.06.16.

Timsit, J. F., Sonneville, R., Kalil, A. C., Bassetti, M., Ferrer, R., Jaber, S., Lanternier, F., Luyt, C. E., Machado, F., Mikulska, M., Papazian, L., Pène, F., Poulakou, G., Viscoli, C., Wolff, M., Zafrani, L., & Van Delden, C. (2019). Diagnostic and therapeutic approach to infectious diseases in solid organ transplant recipients. *Intensive Care Medicine, 45*(5), 573–591. https://doi.org/10.1007/s00134-019-05597-y.

Tönshoff, B. (2019). Immunosuppressants in organ transplantation. In Kiess, W., Schwab, M., & van den Anker, J. (Eds.), *Pediatric pharmacotherapy. Handbook of experimental pharmacology* (pp. p. 261). Springer https://doi.org/10.1007/164_2019_331.

Transplant Australia. Lifestyle and sex after transplant. (2019). https://transplant.org.au/living-with-your-transplant/self-care/lifestyle-and-sex-after-transplant/#:~:text=Fertility%20and%20libido%20returns%20quickly,their%20body%20after%20the%20transplant.

Transplant Pregnancy Registry International – Gift of Life Institute. Transplant Pregnancy Registry International – A registry for transplant patients and research related to effects of medications on fertility and pregnancy. (2023). https://www.transplantpregnancyregistry.org/.

Uffing, A., Hullekes, F., Riella, L. V., & Hogan, J. J. (2021). Recurrent glomerular disease after kidney transplantation: Diagnostic and management dilemmas. *Clinical Journal of the American Society of Nephrology, 16*(11), 1730–1742. doi:10.2215/CJN.00280121.

United Network for Organ Sharing. (2008, March) Talking about transplantation: Questions and answers for transplant candidates about MELD and PELD. https://unos.org/wp-content/uploads/MELD_PELD.pdf.

United Network for Organ Sharing (2023). Transplant living. https://transplantliving.org/after-the-transplant/preventing-rejection/infections-and-immunity/.

UpToDate. (n.d.) Lexicomp drug interactions. Retrieved December 20, 2022. https://doctorabad.com/UpToDate/d/di.htm.

US Food and Drug Administration. (2021, March 3). Xeno-transplantation. https://www.fda.gov/vaccines-blood-biologics/xenotransplantation.

United States Department of Agriculture. (2020). Food safety: A need-to-know guide for those at risk. https://www.fsis.usda.gov/sites/default/files/media_file/2021-04/at-risk-booklet.pdf.

Urschel, S., Ballweg, J. A., Cantor, R. S., Koehl, D. A., Reinhardt, Z., Zuckerman, W. A., Dipchand, A. I., Kanter, K. R., Sparks, J., McCoy, M., Kirklin, J. K., & Carlo, W. F. (2021). Clinical outcomes of children receiving ABO-incompatible versus ABO-compatible heart transplantation: A multicentre cohort study. *Lancet, 5*(5), 341–349. https://doi.org/10.1016/S2352-4642(21)00023-7.

Urschel, S., & West, L. J. (2016). ABO-incompatible heart transplantation. *Current Opinion in Pediatrics, 28*(5), 613–619. doi:10.1097/MOP.0000000000000398.

van Delden, C., Stampf, S., Hirsch, H. H., Manuel, O., Meylan, P., Cusini, A., Hirzel, C., Khanna, N., Weisser, M., Garzoni, C., Boggian, K., Berger, C., Nadal, D., Koller, M., Saccilotto, R., Mueller, N. J., & Swiss Transplant Cohort Study (2020). Burden and timeline of infectious diseases in the first year after solid organ transplantation in the Swiss Transplant Cohort Study. *Clinical Infectious Diseases, 71*(7), e159–e169. https://doi.org/10.1093/cid/ciz1113.

Vandenberk, B., Vandael, E., Robyns, T., Vandenberghe, J., Garweg, C., Foulon, V., Ector, J., & Willems, R. (2018). QT correction across the heart rate spectrum, in atrial fibrillation and ventricular conduction defects. *Pacing and Clinical Electrophysiology, 41*(9), 1101–1108. doi:10.1111/pace.13423. Epub 2018 Jul 12.

Vergote, V. K. J., Deroose, C. M., Fieuws, S., Laleman, W., Sprangers, B., Uyttebroeck, A., Van Cleemput, J., Verhoef, G., Vos, R., Tousseyn, T., & Dierickx, D. (2022). Characteristics and outcome of post-transplant lymphoproliferative disorders after solid organ transplantation: A single center experience of 196 patients over 30 years. *Transplant International, 35*, 10707. https://doi.org/10.3389/ti.2022.10707. Published 2022 Dec 14.

Wang, L., Verschuuren, E. A. M., van Leer-Buter, C. C., Bakker, S. J. L., de Joode, A. A. E., Westra, J., & Bos, N. A. (2018). Herpes zoster and immunogenicity and safety of zoster vaccines in transplant patients: A narrative review of the literature. *Frontiers in Immunology, 9*, 1632. https://doi.org/10.3389/fimmu.2018.01632. Published 2018 Jul 16.

Weill, D. (2018). Lung transplantation: Indications and contraindications. *Journal of Thoracic Disease, 10*(7), 4574–4587. https://doi.org/10.21037/jtd.2018.06.141.

Weill, D., Benden, C., Corris, P. A., Dark, J. H., Davis, R. D., Keshavjee, S., Lederer, D. J., Mulligan, M. J., Patterson, G. A., Singer, L. G., Snell, G. I., Verleden, G. M., Zamora, M. R., & Glanville, A. R. (2015). A consensus document for the selection of lung transplant candidates: 2014-An update from the Pulmonary Transplantation Council of the International Society for Heart and Lung Transplantation. *Journal of Heart and Lung Transplantation, 34*(1), 1–15. https://doi.org/10.1016/j.healun.2014.06.014.

White, P. H., & Cooley, W. C. (2018). Transition from adolescent to adulthood in the medical home. *Pediatrics, 142*(5), e20182587. https://www.floridahats.org/wp-content/uploads/2018/10/peds.2018-2587.full_.pdf.

Wickerson, L., Rozenberg, D., Janaudis-Ferreira, T., Deliva, R., Lo, V., Beauchamp, G., Helm, D., Gottesman, C., Mendes, P., Vieira, L., Herridge, M., Singer, L. G., & Mathur, S. (2016). Physical rehabilitation for lung transplant candidates and recipients: An evidence-informed clinical approach. *World Journal of Transplantation, 6*(3), 517–531. https://doi.org/10.5500/wjt.v6.i3.517.

Wurm, F., McKeaveney, C., Corr, M., Wilson, A., & Noble, H. (2022). The psychosocial needs of adolescent and young adult kidney transplant recipients, and associated interventions: A scoping review. *BMC Psychology, 10*(1), 186. doi:10.1186/s40359-022-00893-7. Published 2022 Jul 29.

34

Phenylketonuria

Pamela Harris Bryant

ETIOLOGY

Phenylketonuria (PKU) is an autosomal recessive inborn error of metabolism where there is a deficiency in the hepatic enzyme phenylalanine hydroxylase (PAH) (Elhawary et al., 2022). Delayed diagnosis can lead to progressive, irreversible neurologic impairment (Chen et al., 2019; Mainka et al., 2021). High levels of phenylalanine (Phe) are toxic to the nervous system, particularly during development, and untreated individuals experience intellectual disability and other complications, including microcephaly, seizures, skin disease (eczematous rash, light pigmentation), and behavioral and psychiatric problems (Bodamer, 2022). PKU is caused by a mutation of the *PAH* gene on chromosome 12 and exposure to dietary Phe, an essential amino acid found in most protein foods. The absence or deficiency of *PAH* halts the conversion of Phe to tyrosine (Tyr) and results in hyperphenylalaninemia (HPA).

More than 1000 mutations (allelic variations) in the human *PAH* gene have been described and compiled in the *PAH* mutation database (www.biopku. org). Mutations result from a variety of mechanisms, including insertions, deletions, missense and nonsense mutations, and DNA splicing defects; missense mutations in *PAH* are the most commonly seen. Mutations change the DNA code for *PAH*, which is believed to have a deleterious effect on enzyme function secondary to misfolding and resultant enzyme instability (Danecka et al., 2015). PKU is an autosomal recessive disorder; therefore individuals with PKU have mutations on both copies of their *PAH* alleles, typically inheriting one from each parent. An individual with one normal allele and one mutant allele will produce adequate functional *PAH* and be an asymptomatic carrier of the disease.

Most cases of PKU result from allelic heterogeneity, whereby a different mutation is inherited from each parent, making the affected individual a compound heterozygote. Significant variations in specific *PAH* mutations are seen in different geographic areas and ethnic populations. Fig. 34.1 depicts a family pedigree in which the affected child inherited one allele for mild HPA and one allele for classic PKU.

The degree of HPA in an affected child cannot be accurately predicted from genotype information at the current time. Correlation of genotype with biochemical and metabolic phenotype has been established for some common genotypes, and this information is available in the *PAH* mutation database (www.biopku. org), but allelic heterogeneity complicates the analysis. Identifying genotype-phenotype correlations is a major area of interest because some new treatments for HPA may be, at least in part, genotype based (Danecka et al., 2015). There are many challenges in this body of research related to the number of known mutations and the probable influence of modifier genes and environmental factors. For example, variations in the transport of Phe into the brain may explain the existence of siblings with the same genotype at the *PAH* locus who exhibit different clinical phenotypes and the existence of the rare individuals with PKU who experience no neurologic damage (Vockley et al., 2014).

The metabolic pathway for Phe is predominantly in the liver. Phe not used for new protein synthesis is converted to Tyr for use in the biosynthesis of protein, melanin, thyroxine, and catecholamines. Loss of *PAH* activity in PKU increases the serum concentration of Phe relative to that of Tyr and subsequently causes an accumulation of Phe metabolites such as phenylpyruvic acid, phenylacetic acid, and others. A high level of Phe inhibits the transport of large neutral amino acids (LNAAs) into the brain, disrupting the synthesis of essential substances such as myelin, neurotransmitters, and other proteins. These deficiencies all contribute to the neuropathology of PKU, although the exact mechanisms of neurologic damage remain poorly understood and remain an important area of research (Anderson et al., 2004, 2007; Channon et al., 2004; Regier & Greene, 2000; Van Spronsen et al., 2021; VanZutphen et al., 2007).

The Phe hydroxylation system is a complex biochemical reaction that requires the presence of oxygen, active site bound Fe^{2+}, and the cofactor tetrahydrobiopterin (BH4; see discussion later). A deficiency in any enzyme involved in the synthesis or regeneration of BH4 will result in HPA. BH4 disorders, found in approximately 1% to 2% of individuals with HPA, are phenotypically and genotypically distinct from PKU, require different modes of therapy, and have a different prognosis. Testing for BH4 disorders should be done in all newborns with HPA and in any child with microcephaly, intellectual disability, seizure disorder,

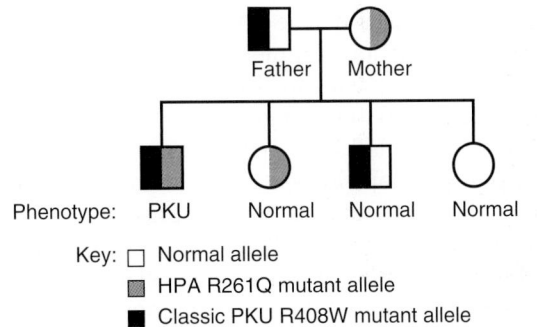

Phenotype: PKU   Normal   Normal   Normal

Key: ☐ Normal allele
      ▨ HPA R261Q mutant allele
      ■ Classic PKU R408W mutant allele

Fig. 34.1 Hypothetical family pedigree showing segregation of mutant phenylketonuria *(PKU)* and mutant hyperphenylalaninemia *(HPA)* alleles with haplotype.

developmental delay, disturbance of tone and posture, hyperreflexia, movement disorder, hyperpyrexia, or other unexplained neurologic findings (Acosta & Yannicelli, 2001; Regier & Greene, 2000).

Offspring of females with PKU, who generally do not have PKU themselves, may be exposed to toxic levels of Phe in utero and experience the effects of maternal PKU (MPKU) syndrome (Clarke, 2003). MPKU syndrome is becoming an increasing cause for concern because many healthy young females with PKU are now reaching childbearing age. Despite the recommendation that all individuals with PKU follow a Phe-restricted diet for life, nonadherence during adolescence is common. The success of dietary therapy in arresting the neurologic deficits caused by PKU has resulted in an increasing number of offspring with intellectual disabilities with MPKU syndrome.

INCIDENCE AND PREVALENCE

In the United States the incidence of PKU is approximately 1 in 15,000 births; it is 1 in 10,000 births in the United Kingdom, 1 in 2600 births in Turkey, and less than 1 in 100,000 births in Japan (Mei et al., 2013). This incidence is greater in White and Native American populations and decreased in Black, Hispanic, and Asian populations (Stone et al., 2023). There are no sex differences, although there is significant racial and ethnic variability, with an increased incidence in certain European White and Native American populations and a decreased incidence in Black, Hispanic, and Asian individuals (Hardelid et al., 2008; National Institutes of Health [NIH], 2000). For autosomal recessive disorders, carrier (heterozygote) frequency is calculated from PKU incidence (Nussbaum et al., 2001); consequently, the incidence of carrier frequency for PKU also varies among populations. For a population with a PKU incidence of 1 in 10,000, the carrier frequency is calculated to be 2%; 1 in 50 people possesses one copy of the mutated *PAH* gene. The nonuniform distribution of cases of PKU and its major alleles may be explained by migration, genetic drift, recurrent

mutation, and intragenic recombination over the past 100,000 years (Scriver, 2007).

The incidence of PKU is calculated from data collected through mandated newborn screening programs. An NIH consensus development panel on PKU (NIH, 2000) reviewed the Council of Regional Networks for Genetic Services National Newborn Screening Report (Newborn Screening Committee, 1999) and found several factors that confound incidence estimates of PKU: States do not uniformly report the number of infants born, the number of infants screened, the sex or race of the infant, or data about non-PKU HPA. In addition, there are variations in the blood Phe levels considered diagnostic of PKU and HPA (e.g., in most states, classic PKU is defined as blood Phe >20 mg/dL, compared with four states that use 10 mg/dL as the cutoff value Waisbren et al., 2007b). Such discrepancies alter estimates of PKU incidence and lead to state-to-state differences in referrals for follow-up testing and treatment.

DIAGNOSTIC CRITERIA

Individuals with HPA caused by deficient *PAH* are historically classified as having classic PKU if their untreated Phe levels are consistently greater than 1200 μmol/L (20 mg/dL) without treatment, moderate PKU between 900 and 1200 μmol/L, mild PKU (Phe levels between 600 μmol/L [10 mg/dL] and 900 μmol/L [20 mg/dL]), or mild HPA for Phe levels between 360 and 600 μmol/L (10 mg/dL) (Camp et al., 2014; Weglage et al., 2001). There is variation in this terminology, however, and in some settings the term *non-PKU HPA* is used to refer to all individuals whose Phe levels are greater than 120 μmol/L (2 mg/dL) but less than 1200 μmol/L (20 mg/dL) (Camp et al., 2014).

Screening of newborn infants for PKU is conducted in all US states, the District of Columbia, the Commonwealth of Puerto Rico, the Virgin Islands, Guam, all provinces in Canada, among other countries. Guthrie's method of detecting elevated Phe in a blood spot on a piece of filter paper became widely used in the 1960s. Applications of the method have changed over the years, including the Guthrie bacterial inhibition assay, automated fluorometric analysis, and high-performance liquid chromatography. States now use tandem mass spectrometry (TMS) to screen newborn blood spots. TMS allows the detection of elevated Phe and a large number of other metabolic disorders simultaneously, and it has been shown to reduce the incidence of false-positive results (NIH, 2000; Rinaldo et al., 2004; Vockley et al., 2014)

Screening refers to efforts to distinguish persons who have a condition from those who do not. The concepts of positive and negative predictive values may help explain why newborns with positive newborn screening tests for PKU may not have PKU (Umberger et al, 2017). Newborns with positive newborn screening tests for PKU may or may not actually have PKU;

further testing is always required to make a diagnosis of PKU. An infant with a positive screening test should be referred to a metabolic specialty center for a diagnostic workup as soon as possible. This evaluation will reveal false-positive results or confirm the diagnosis of HPA, allowing treatment to be initiated immediately. False-positive results can be seen in PKU newborn screening; however, these results may occur for a variety of reasons, most commonly due to the administration of supplemental nutrition (i.e., total parenteral nutrition [TPN]), early specimen collection, or a result of poorly controlled PKU in the mother. To address this issue of false-positive results in PKU newborn screening, many programs now utilize a Phe-to-Tyr ratio, which has greatly improved specificity and positive predictive value for PKU newborn screen.

Blood levels of Phe and Tyr will be checked on all babies with a positive newborn screen for PKU to make this distinction. Parents of a newborn with a positive screening test are notified in various ways, depending on the policy of the regional screening laboratory. Dietary treatment of the child with PKU should ideally start within the first week of life with blood Phe levels within the treatment range of 2 weeks, and therefore every effort must be made to avoid delays in the diagnostic process (NIH, 2000; Vockley et al., 2014).

Although 98% to 99% of cases of HPA result from *PAH* deficiency, it is essential to rule out defects in the biopterin synthase group of enzymes, dihydropterin reductase (DHPR) deficiency, or *PAH* with decreased affinity for BH4 because these require different therapies. Pterin metabolites in the urine and DHPR in the blood will be evaluated in all babies with HPA (Acosta & Yannicelli, 2001; American College of Medical Genetics, 2006; Vockley et al., 2014; Walter et al., 2006; Wilcox & Cederbaum, 2002). It is important to be cognizant of the finding that false-positive newborn screening results are not benign and have long-term effects on parental stress, as well as objective indices such as the number of hospital visits during the first year of life. Premature infants are known to have a high incidence of false-positive newborn screening results, with TPN being a factor (Kamleh et al., 2021).

The PKU specialty center may suggest DNA analysis to determine the specific PKU mutation. Direct DNA analysis of the *PAH* gene can be performed to determine the specific mutation present in a child with HPA. Currently, this information is not required for routine diagnostic or therapeutic decisions, but it may be useful for genetic counseling. For fetal diagnosis in families with a known history of HPA, the mode of testing depends on whether the mutations of the original proband are known. If the mutant alleles are known, chorionic villus sampling or amniocentesis can be used to identify the carrier status of the fetus. If the mutant alleles are not known, identification of polymorphisms in the *PAH* gene is usually necessary. All individuals have identifiable normal variations in the DNA surrounding the *PAH* locus on chromosome 12, called restriction fragment length polymorphisms (RFLPs). Because specific RFLPs segregate with the PKU mutation on the *PAH* gene, they act as markers for PKU and are called PKU haplotypes (haps). Analysis of the parental haps in association with the *PAH* mutation enables prenatal genetic counseling (Edwards et al., 2015; Scriver et al., 2008).

Despite screening efforts, some cases of PKU and HPA are diagnosed late or undiagnosed. False-negative screening results may occur if the blood is collected before the infant is 24 hours old. Early discharge of newborns from the hospital necessitates a second test, although there is a lack of uniformity in state policies related to repeat testing. Others at risk for a missed diagnosis of PKU include premature infants who are transferred to neonatal intensive care units shortly after birth, those whose parents refuse the screening test, or those born outside of a health care institution or who immigrate to the United States at a young age. Primary care providers should be alert to the possibility of PKU in any of these situations or when the child has unexplained signs and symptoms associated with untreated PKU. In addition, MPKU syndrome should be suspected in a child with unexplained microcephaly, cardiac defects, or other dysmorphology or developmental delay because some females have undiagnosed mild forms of PKU or HPA.

CLINICAL MANIFESTATIONS AT TIME OF DIAGNOSIS

UNTREATED PHENYLKETONURIA

For more than 50 years newborn screening has successfully prevented clinical manifestations in children with PKU in the United States. Nevertheless, many persons still experience the consequences of misdiagnosis, late diagnosis, or lack of metabolic control. Infants with PKU generally appear normal at birth but may have feeding difficulties, vomiting, and irritability soon after birth. Approximately one-third of infants with untreated PKU demonstrate a lack of increase in head circumference and infantile spasms with hypsarrhythmia or other abnormalities on electroencephalogram (EEG) after the first few months of life (Nyhan et al., 2005; Sadek et al., 2013; Walter et al., 2006). Infantile spasms (West syndrome) often occur as one of the clinical signs of untreated PKU (Pavone et al., 2020; Zhongshu et al., 2001).

As the infant ages there are noticeable developmental delays and an unpleasant mousy or musty odor of the body or urine from the excretion of phenylacetic acid, a metabolite of the accumulated Phe. Intellectual disability is generally severe, with a drop in developmental quotient to 50 points by 1 year of age and to 30 points by 3 years of age (Ashe et al., 2019; Koch & Wenz, 1987). Neurologic features may include seizures (25%), EEG abnormalities (50%), tremors, tics, abnormalities of gait and posturing, and hypertonicity with hyperactive deep tendon reflexes (Rezvani, 2000). Excitability, autism, schizophrenia-like behaviors, and self-destructiveness have also been described in untreated individuals with PKU (Sadek et al., 2013; Walter et al., 2006).

Children with untreated PKU have lighter skin, eyes, and hair than their unaffected siblings because of impaired melanin synthesis in the absence of sufficient levels of Tyr. In children of ethnic backgrounds where black hair is expected, this feature will be expressed as hair that is brown or even reddish (Blenda, 2022). Other physical manifestations of untreated PKU include eczema (20–40%), prominent maxilla with widely spaced teeth, enamel hypoplasia, and growth retardation that is more evident in males (Nyhan et al., 2005; Rezvani, 2000; Rush, 2022; Sadek, et al., 2013; Walter et al., 2006).

MATERNAL PHENYLKETONURIA SYNDROME

Children of females with PKU are obligatory heterozygotes who can only have PKU if they inherit a second mutation; thus the vast majority do not have PKU. The greatest risk to these infants is prenatal exposure to high levels of Phe in the mother's blood. Until the 1980s it was common to discontinue the diet in middle childhood, and presently lack of adherence to the recommended diet remains problematic. It is highly recommended that females with PKU who plan to become pregnant maintain a strict diet. It is important to identify those things helpful for females with PKU to restart a low-Phe diet before conception and during pregnancy (Rohde et al., 2021).

Infants born to females with PKU who do not adhere to a low-Phe diet before and during pregnancy have a high incidence of intellectual disability, microcephaly, and heart defects (Elhawary et al., 2022; Feillet et al., 2010; Rohde et al., 2021). Other features of MPKU syndrome include intrauterine and postnatal growth delay and dysmorphic facial features that resemble fetal alcohol syndrome. There is also a higher incidence of other birth defects in infants with MPKU syndrome, including dysgenesis of the corpus callosum (Manganaro et al., 2017; Nissenkorn et al., 2001) and tracheoesophageal fistula (Koch et al., 2003; Regier & Greene, 2000; Vockley et al., 2014). Other congenital malformations have been reported, such as bowel malrotation, bladder exstrophy, orofacial clefting, and eye abnormalities such as coloboma and cataracts (Walter et al., 2006).

In a pregnant female with PKU, a transplacental gradient that favors the fetus results in a fetal-maternal ratio of Phe of about 1.5, although that ratio may be as high as 2.9 (Scriver et al., 2008); thus studies of MPKU rely on maternal Phe levels, and these may not be valid indicators of the fetal level. Many studies document a dose-dependent teratogenic effect of maternal Phe on a developing fetus, which is more pronounced in the early weeks of pregnancy. Rouse et al. (1997) determined that at maternal Phe levels of 900 μmol/L (15 mg/dL), 85% of infants had microcephaly, 51% had postnatal growth retardation, and 26% had intrauterine growth retardation, compared with 6%, 4%, and 0%, respectively, if the maternal Phe level was less than 360 μmol/L (6 mg/dL). Levy et al. (2001) found that a basal maternal Phe level above 900 μmol/L (15 mg/dL) may be the threshold for congenital heart disease in the fetus and that a level above 1800 μmol/L (30 mg/dL) poses a significant risk of congenital heart disease.

According to Koch et al. (2003), in the Maternal Phenylketonuria Collaborative Study, infants who were born with congenital heart defects (CHD) were born to mothers who, in the first 8 weeks of pregnancy, had Phe levels greater than 600 μmol/L (10 mg/dL). Infants were also found to have an increased risk of CHD when their mothers had inadequate protein, vitamin B_{12}, and fat intake. Phe levels of 120 μmol/L and 360 μmol/L (2–6 mg/dL) have been shown to pose a relatively low risk of fetal anomalies and developmental disabilities, which is the goal advised for most females (Koch et al., 2003). A review of the maternal PKU registry in the United Kingdom confirmed that initiating dietary restriction before conception significantly improved outcomes (Cleary & Skeath, 2019; Lee et al., 2005). A review of the MPKU registry in the United Kingdom confirmed that initiating dietary restriction before conception significantly improved outcomes (Cleary & Skeath, 2019; Lee et al., 2005).

TREATMENT

Dietary modification is the primary treatment for PKU and the prevention of MPKU syndrome. It is well established that a Phe-restricted diet can prevent the severe neurologic consequences associated with untreated PKU. However, metabolic control in PKU may be difficult to achieve in practice; it requires frequent monitoring of blood Phe levels, maintaining a highly restrictive diet, careful monitoring of food intake, frequent visits to a PKU clinic, and supplementation with a formula that many persons find unpalatable.

The NIH (2000) consensus statement on the management of PKU recommends that treatment of the neonate with PKU be initiated as soon as possible but no later than 7 to 10 days after birth. Blood Phe levels should be maintained between 120 μmol/L (2 mg/dL) and 360 μmol/L (6 mg/dL) (Singh et al., 2014; Vockley et al., 2014) throughout the life span. For females of childbearing age, a Phe level between 120 μmol/L (2 mg/dL) and 360 μmol/L (6 mg/dL) should be achieved at least 3 months before conception and maintained throughout the pregnancy. Individuals with mild HPA whose Phe levels remain below 360 μmol/L (6 mg/dL) may remain on a natural protein diet.

The diet for PKU is far more involved than simple restriction of Phe. Since whole proteins in food contain

Phe, whole protein sources need to be restricted. This also restricts other nutrients. Therefore supplements are required to ensure adequate nutrient intake for optimum growth and development. The PKU treatment center team continually monitors the child's Phe tolerance and prescribes the diet. An individual's Phe and other nutrient requirements depend on many factors, including *PAH* activity, age, growth rate, adequacy of energy and protein intake, and state of health. The precise tolerance for Phe varies, but for most individuals with PKU it is between 250 and 600 mg/day (Camp et al., 2014). Phe tolerance may change over time, so careful and continuous monitoring of individuals whose Phe intake is restricted is necessary to avoid both elevations and deficiencies of Phe. Long-term deficiencies of Phe from excessive restriction are also associated with adverse outcomes, including poor growth and development and, in some cases when treatment for PKU was first initiated, death (Acosta & Yannicelli, 2001; Scriver et al., 2008; Seashore, 2008).

In the neonate, breast milk supplemented with Phe-free formula is recommended. If the infant is formula fed, one of the commercially available Phe-free elemental medical foods (EMFs) should be used in conjunction with the family's standard baby formula. These products are modified protein hydrolysates in which Phe is removed or mixtures of free amino acids that do not contain Phe. EMFs provide the essential amino acids in suitable proportions for the given age of the individual. As the infant begins to eat solid foods, the Phe content must be calculated and the amount of EMF adjusted to ensure that all nutrients are ingested in proper amounts, and the desired blood Phe level is maintained. Parents invariably require the assistance of a dietitian to accomplish these goals.

There is much controversy over the need for supplementation of certain nutrients for individuals on Phe-restricted diets. Tyr deficiency is a consequence of inadequate Phe metabolism in PKU, and it has been postulated that low Tyr levels may be responsible for learning difficulties in well-treated individuals with PKU. EMFs are enriched with Tyr; however, additional Tyr supplementation in PKU has not been found to improve neuropsychological function in studies, and this is thought to be related to nonsustained plasma Tyr elevations after ingestion of the supplement with inadequate levels reaching the brain (Kalsner et al., 2001; Van Wegberg et al., 2017). The potential dangers of fluctuating Tyr levels have prompted some researchers to recommend against additional supplementation and advocate reduction of the Tyr content in EMFs and the development of slow-release Tyr dietary compounds (Van Spronsen et al., 2001; Van Wegberg et al., 2017).

Long-chain polyunsaturated fatty acids, including docosahexaenoic acid (DHA) and arachidonic acid (AA), may be reduced in the blood of individuals treated for PKU, and blood lipid monitoring with supplementation of DHA and AA in deficient individuals is recommended (Camp et al., 2014; Moseley et al., 2002). There is also evidence that supplementation with omega-3 long-chain polyunsaturated fatty acids from fish oil improves visually evoked potentials and motor function in children with treated PKU (Beblo et al., 2001, 2007). Other dietary components commonly monitored and supplemented in individuals with PKU include vitamin B_{12}, folic acid, calcium, zinc, iron, phosphate, and selenium (NIH, 2000; Van Bakel et al., 2000; Van Wegberg et al., 2017).

Individuals with late diagnosed PKU should also be placed on the Phe-restricted diet no matter how late they are identified. Improvements in behavior and neurologic status have been seen in individuals with severe intellectual disability who had untreated PKU (Ashe et al., 2019; Baumeister & Baumeister, 1998; Fitzgerald et al., 2000; Grosse, 2010). In a study of 57 people with a late diagnosis and a mean intelligence quotient (IQ) of 44 at the time of diagnosis, the institution of the Phe-restricted diet improved their mean IQ to 73 (Koch et al., 1999). In addition, return to diet for adults with PKU who have discontinued it has been shown to improve a variety of conditions, including brain magnetic resonance imaging (MRI) changes, agoraphobia, panic attacks, and recurrent headache (Anderson & Leuzzi, 2010; Koch et al., 1999). Another study revealed that 60% of individuals reported improved quality of life after resumption or initiation of the diet, though only 47% of those in this research group maintained dietary compliance (Gassió et al., 2003).

In late 2007, the US Food and Drug Administration (FDA) approved a new medication that has been an important adjuvant to dietary treatment in some individuals with PKU (Hydery & Coppenrath, 2019; Pollack, 2007). BH4 is a cofactor in the *PAH* system and has been shown to reduce Phe levels by 20% to 30% or greater in up to 50% of individuals with HPA (Vockley et al., 2014). BioMarin Pharmaceuticals has developed and is now marketing BH4 as Kuvan (sapropterin dihydrochloride). It had originally been postulated that it would be possible to predetermine a person's response to BH4 based on genotype-phenotype correlation, but the research is inconsistent, and therefore the current recommendation is for all persons with PKU over 1 month of age who are interested in having a trial with Kuvan to determine their responder status (Vockley et al., 2014; Zurflüh et al., 2008). The usual maintenance dosing range is 5 to 20 mg/kg/day, and different clinics will be using different algorithms to start children and adults on Kuvan and determine the appropriate dosage (Levy et al., 2007). The definition of responders also varies, but most providers would expect a responder to achieve a 20% to 30% decrease in plasma Phe level with the appropriate dose of Kuvan and no dietary change. This could allow for significant liberalization of the diet in these individuals. Of note, utilization of Kuvan may be limited by the prohibitive cost, which can be up to $200,000 per year for large adults, though people who are insured should have at least part of this cost covered (Pollack, 2007).

The effects of long-term use of BH4 are currently unknown, but at least one European study has attempted long-term treatment with no significant ill effects (Longo et al., 2015; Trefz et al., 2005). This same team has used BH4 without dietary treatment in a small group of infants with mild PKU diagnosed on newborn screening. They have thus far witnessed no significant side effects and normal somatic and psychomotor development in this limited study. They note that further studies are necessary before offering medication alone as a clinical treatment for all infants with mild PKU.

In 2018, the US Department of Agriculture (USDA) approved a new enzyme replacement therapy, Palynziq (pegvaliase), produced by BioMarin. This therapy involves taking a subcutaneous injection titrated up daily for some with a maximum dose of 60 mg/day. The Palynziq dosage is titrated in a stepwise manner, based on tolerability, over at least 5 weeks; not all patients require the maximum dose. The goal is to achieve a serum Phe concentration of less than or equal to 600 μmol/L. An epinephrine autoinjector should also be prescribed because of black box warnings for anaphylaxis related to medication administration. Also, consider premedication with antihistamines (i.e., H1 receptor antagonist, H2 receptor antagonist), and/or antipyretic to prevent hypersensitivity reactions (based on patient tolerability). The patient should be monitored for at least 60 minutes (or more) following first injection (Lexicomp, 2023).

COMPLEMENTARY AND ALTERNATIVE THERAPIES

Complementary therapies for PKU must be administered in conjunction with conventional dietary treatment. A person with PKU should not take dietary supplements or herbal remedies without the approval of the metabolic practitioner because many of these contain high amounts of protein or aspartame. However, affected children and their families may derive significant benefits from relaxation training, spirituality, imagery, and therapies involving art, music, and touch. PKU, like any chronic condition requiring constant care and vigilance, places enormous stress on all involved. Online and local support groups and email mailing lists for families with PKU may provide practical information and act as a resource for relevant complementary therapy programs.

ANTICIPATED ADVANCES IN DIAGNOSIS AND MANAGEMENT

Although diet therapy is an effective treatment for PKU, some individuals have difficulty adhering to the strict regimen and experience poor outcomes. Potential alternative treatments that are being investigated include gene therapy, which is continuing to progress with clinical trials.

Although liver transplants are unlikely to become standard therapy for a condition treatable by diet therapy, Phe tolerance was restored to a 10-year-old male with PKU who received a liver transplant for concurrent active cirrhosis (Scriver et al., 2008). Hepatocyte transplantation is under consideration for PKU; in this scenario, the person's own liver cells are removed, the normal *PAH* gene is inserted into the cells, and the cells are then reinserted into the person. Techniques for insertion of the *PAH* gene into the skin, lymphocytes, or other human cells may eventually be able to restore normal Phe metabolism in people with PKU, but at the present time there are many obstacles to overcome in the field of gene therapy; some animal studies have been promising, but gene therapy for humans with metabolic disorders likely continues to be a long way off (Harding et al., 2006; Scriver et al., 2008; Spirito et al., 2001).

Research on foods and supplements also shows promise for improving the lives of those affected by PKU. Glycomacropeptide (GMP) is a whey protein and the only known protein free of Phe; researchers have successfully created foods from GMP that were met with positive reviews by people with PKU who tried them. Some GMP foods and formulas are available and may prove to be a useful adjunct to the current low-protein food options (Cleary & Skeath, 2019; Etzel, 2002; Lim et al., 2007; Ney et al., 2008; Van Calcar & Ney, 2012).

There is some evidence that LNAAs lower the brain Phe level by competing with Phe for transport across the blood-brain barrier (Pietz et al., 1999). It was once thought that brain Phe levels and low brain Tyr levels could be measured, but traditional magnetic resonance spectroscopy could not adequately measure either (Waisbren et al., 2017). Recent studies in Australia indicate that LNAAs are unlikely to benefit individuals who are compliant with the consumption of their EMF and diet but may improve functioning and decrease plasma Phe in people unable to maintain good control. Further studies are needed to refine our understanding of the utility of LNAAs (Giovannini et al., 2007; Schindeler et al., 2007).

Regular blood Phe monitoring is an important aspect of care in PKU. Home monitoring devices are being developed (PKU News, 2022), and the possibility of a noninvasive monitoring device is being investigated (PKU News, 2022). Current at-home Phe monitoring consists of placing dry blood spots on special filter paper collection devices, which are mailed in per the Metabolic Clinic instructions. Such technologies would give the individual greater autonomy and potentially improve Phe control (Bilginsoy et al., 2005). Researchers are also working to create a test to monitor Phe levels through urine samples, potentially improving compliance with testing frequency (Langenbeck et al., 2005).

ASSOCIATED PROBLEMS OF PHENYLKETONURIA AND TREATMENT

Although dietary treatment has largely eliminated the severe problems associated with untreated PKU, questions remain about subtle abnormalities people with PKU may have with neurologic function, cognitive development, behavioral adjustment, school achievement, and physical health (NIH, 2000). Unfortunately, it is difficult to determine precisely what factors account for impairments; high Phe levels are presumed to cause pathophysiologic changes in body systems, but low Tyr levels, low fatty acid levels, or imbalances in other substances may also play a role. A systematic review revealed that patients with early-treated PKU appear to have a higher prevalence of behavior problems and psychological disturbance than controls. The range of problems reported include excessive sadness, fear, and anxiety; a sense of isolation and poor self-image; and lack of autonomy and drive (Smith & Knowles, 2000). However, based on all the available evidence, it is generally agreed that early and consistent Phe control is associated with better outcomes in all domains.

 Associated Problems

Phenylketonuria and Treatment

- Consistent dietary treatment reduces severe problems
- Neurologic changes
- Cognitive deficits
  - Poorer performance on IQ tests
  - Cognitive difficulties related to planning, problem solving, self-regulation
- Behavioral manifestations
  - Tendency toward depression, anxiety, phobias
  - Attention-deficient/hyperactivity disorder
- Dermatitis
- Decreased bone mineral density

Neurologic Manifestations

Abnormal findings in cerebral white matter on MRI have been observed in some individuals with PKU, which are likely related to a myelin defect secondary to elevated Phe and decreased Tyr. The clinical significance of white matter abnormalities remains unclear, and the severity of signs and symptoms may not consistently reflect the degree of visualized abnormality; people with more extensive white matter abnormalities, particularly those extending into frontal and subcortical regions, appear to have the most significant impairments in executive functioning and cognition. Reversal of cerebral white matter change has been observed when Phe restriction is resumed (Anderson et al., 2007). Studies have shown that MRI changes are reversible when blood PHE levels are lowered within approximately 2 months (Cleary & Skeath, 2019). Abnormal visual and auditory evoked potentials have

been identified in some individuals with treated PKU. Other signs of impaired nerve conduction found in some individuals who relax their dietary Phe restriction include hyperactive tendon reflexes, intention tremors, and abnormal EEG findings (NIH, 2000; Walter et al., 2006; Welsh & Pennington, 2000).

Cognitive Deficits

Dietary discontinuation before age 8 years is associated with poorer performance on IQ tests; adults and adolescents on relaxed diets have stable IQ scores but may have poorer performance on measures of attention and speed of processing. Adults whose diet has been consistently maintained continue to show subtle deficits compared with unaffected controls in executive function, memory, and learning tasks. However, these deficits were not consistent across all tasks performed in the study—in some, the adults with PKU performed as well as control subjects—and the researchers posited that perhaps these deficits represent slowed information processing (Channon et al., 2004). The variation in severity of disease and metabolic control at different ages make it difficult to generalize these studies to an individual. However, it is clear that adolescence is the stage at which many children begin to discontinue their diet, and an increase in deficits of executive functioning corresponding with an increase in Phe has been found in multiple studies (VanZutphen et al., 2007).

The NIH (2000) Consensus Panel also reviewed 37 studies reporting outcomes that involved school achievement, behavioral adjustment, or cognitive functions other than IQ tests. Poorer performance among persons with PKU was found in 29 of these studies, with the most prominent findings being diminished school achievement and greater difficulty on achievement tests. Cognitive difficulties reported include executive functions (planning, problem solving, self-regulation) and attention. The panel noted that many of these studies were limited by small sample sizes and inconsistent use of comparison groups, but they concluded that levels of Phe show moderate relationships to performance on measures of cognitive function and the presence of behavioral difficulties.

Evaluation of the relationship between various Phe levels and cognitive functioning remains an active area of research. Weglage et al. (2001) reported normal intellectual and educational outcomes in 31 adolescent subjects with mild HPA (persistent Phe levels between 360 and 600 μmol/L) when compared with unaffected controls. Griffiths et al. (2000) found that verbal intelligence in the primary school years tends to normalize if blood Phe is maintained below 360 μmol/L in infancy, but spatial intelligence may remain poor. Huijbregts et al. (2002) found that people with PKU with Phe levels above 360 μmol/L exhibited lower speed of information processing, less ability to inhibit task-induced cognitive interference, less consistent performance, and a stronger decrease in performance level over time compared with control subjects. A recent large-scale literature review and meta-analysis confirmed that IQ and executive function are inversely influenced when the diet is discontinued, and thus Phe increased during childhood (Waisbren et al., 2007a). Some of these neuropsychological changes can be mitigated by close adherence to the diet, and it is crucial to discuss these research findings with all families, particularly those whose children are in poor control.

Behavioral Manifestations
Both anecdotal evidence and scientific evidence support the conclusion that certain neuropsychiatric and psychological deficits are more frequent in persons with PKU and that these may sometimes be relieved by a return to a strict diet. Anxiety, depression, anorexia, and agoraphobia may be associated with high blood Phe levels that decrease dopamine and serotonin in the brain. A link between PKU and autism has also been noted, especially in late-treated individuals (NIH, 2000). Smith and Knowles (2000) reviewed 34 studies related to behavioral problems in people with treated PKU and found evidence that affected individuals are more prone to depression, anxiety, phobic tendencies, and isolation from peers; the authors suggested that these findings are related to a combination of the stress of maintaining the diet and the degree of neurobiologic impairment.

Attention-deficit/hyperactivity disorder (ADHD) is more common in children with early-treated PKU than in the general population (Antshel, 2001; Burton et al., 2015; Welsh & Pennington, 2000). One study of 38 children with PKU found that 26% were using a stimulant to control symptoms of ADHD, compared with a matched control group and the population norm, in which 6.5% and 5% of children, respectively, were using stimulants; the plasma Phe of the children receiving stimulants was significantly higher than those not reporting problems with attention (Arnold et al., 2004). One explanation for some of the attention deficits noted in children with early-treated PKU was posited by Banich et al. (2000), who found that interhemispheric interaction is compromised in the brains of these children as compared with normal controls.

Dermatitis
Scaling eczematous dermatitis is more prevalent in children with PKU presumably because of the toxic effects of Phe and its metabolites. Skin and muscle indurations resembling scleroderma have been reported, especially on the arms and buttocks of young children with PKU. These skin manifestations have been noted to improve with better dietary control (NIH, 2000; Nyhan et al., 2005).

Decreased Bone Mineral Density
Decreased total bone mineral density and spine bone mineral density may occur in prepubertal children and adults with treated PKU; these changes are associated with an increased incidence of fractures (Modan-Moses et al., 2007). Whether a nutrient deficiency causes this in the diet or a pathophysiology inherent in the disease remains unclear. Poor linear growth has also been seen in some children with PKU, and there is still debate as to whether this correlates with protein deficiency (Dobbelaere et al., 2003; Nyhan et al., 2005).

PROGNOSIS
Individuals treated early for PKU may be expected to grow and develop normally. Several factors affect the prognosis for PKU, including age at the time of diagnosis and Phe restriction, degree of metabolic control, and the specific mutation responsible. Adherence to the treatment regimen, a primary predictor of overall health in PKU, is undoubtedly affected by psychosocial factors.

PRIMARY CARE MANAGEMENT
HEALTH CARE MAINTENANCE
Growth and Development
Growth is normal for children with early-treated PKU on a controlled Phe-restricted diet. Careful monitoring of height, weight, and head circumference on growth charts, as well as body mass index, is an especially important aspect of primary care of a child with PKU because efforts to limit Phe may result in inadequate protein or calorie intake. Head circumference, weight, and length should be measured at scheduled monthly intervals for the first year, every 3 months until after the prepubertal growth spurt, and then every 6 months throughout adolescence to monitor the adequacy of the diet.

Cognitive deficits and learning difficulties may be present in children with good dietary management. Development should be monitored in primary care in conjunction with the specialty provider. Referral to the PKU treatment center or neurology for psychological testing and developmental assessment is recommended. Young children with evidence of delay should be referred to early intervention programs (e.g., Birth to Three).

Diet
The goals of diet therapy are to maintain blood Phe levels in the safe range and provide adequate amounts of all other nutrients to support growth and prevent protein catabolism. The requirements for the PKU diet vary among individuals and throughout their lifetimes, and Phe levels must be monitored on a regular basis.

Consultation with a dietitian experienced with PKU is essential to care. Dietary management of PKU is

Table 34.1 Recommended Daily Nutrient Intakes (Ranges) for Infants, Children, and Adults With Phenylketonuria

AGE	PHE (MG/KG)	TYR (MG/KG)	PROTEIN (G/KG)	ENERGY (KCAL/KG)	FLUID (ML/KG)
Infants					
0–3 mo	25–70	300–350	3.5–3	120 (95–145)	160–135
3–6 mo	20–45	300–350	3.5–3	120 (95–145)	160–130
6–9 mo	15–35	250–300	3–2.5	110 (80–135)	145–125
9–12 mo	10–35	250–300	3–2.5	105 (80–135)	135–120
Children					
1–4 yr	200–400	1.72–3	>30	1300 (900–1800)	900–1800
4–7 yr	210–450	2.25–3.5	>35	1700 (1300–2300)	1300–2300
7–11 yr	220–500	2.55–4	>40	2400 (1650–3300)	1650–3300
Adolescent and Adult Females					
11–15 yr	250–750	3.45–5	>50	2200 (1500–3000)	1500–3000
15–19 yr	230–700	3.45–5	>55	2100 (1200–3000)	1200–3000
>19 yr	220–700	3.75–5	>60	2100 (1400–2500)	2100–2500
Adolescent and Adult Males					
11–15 yr	225–900	3.38–5.5	>55	2700 (2000–3700)	2000–3700
15–19 yr	295–1100	4.42–6.5	>65	2800 (2100–3900)	2100–3900
>19 yr	290–1200	4.35–6.5	>70	2900 (2000–3300)	2000–3300

From Acosta, P.B., & Yannicelli, S. (Eds.). (2001). *The Ross metabolic formula system: Nutrition support protocols* (4th ed.). Ross Products Division/Abbott Laboratories.

simple in theory but very difficult in reality. Parents are often overwhelmed to learn that their child has PKU, yet they must begin to make modifications immediately. Most parents have never heard of PKU at the time their newborn is diagnosed, so they have numerous concerns about the implications of having a genetic condition in the family, the child's prognosis, and details of the treatment. It takes time for parents to adjust to the diagnosis and the knowledge that this condition will require lifelong attention and management.

Although the decision to breastfeed is personal, clinicians should inform mothers of the advantages of human breastmilk for a newborn with PKU. Mature human breastmilk has a mean Phe content of 48 mg/dL, which is lower than the mean Phe content of cow's milk (164 mg/dL) and common infant formulas such as Isomil (88 mg/dL) and Similac (59 mg/dL) (Acosta & Yannicelli, 2001; Banta-Wright et al., 2014). Formula-fed infants generally accept one of the commercially available Phe-free infant formulas. Since some Phe is essential in the diet, infants are also given a prescribed amount of a Phe-containing formula. Table 34.1 gives the recommended daily nutrient intakes for persons with PKU; these values provide general guidelines but cannot substitute for monitoring Phe levels and nutritional indices. Frequent diet adjustments are necessary throughout life but especially in periods of rapid growth. PKU treatment centers have knowledgeable dietitians to assist families.

Solid foods should be introduced to infants with PKU as they would be for any infant, but parents must monitor and adjust the child's Phe intake. In general, protein foods are high in Phe, so foods to avoid include cheese, eggs, meat, milk, poultry, nuts, dried beans and peas, most breads, seeds, and peanut butter. Foods that are low in protein include fruits, fats, vegetables, sweets, and some cereals. Special low-protein breads, pasta, and cereal should be encouraged because they will become an important part of the lifelong diet. Such products are commercially available, although many families prefer to prepare their own.

One common method for calculating Phe intake involves the use of exchanges, where one exchange is equal to 15 mg of Phe. Other practitioners prefer to instruct parents to calculate milligrams of Phe and to maintain a daily intake that will keep their blood level in the desired range. Some clinics recommend using a gram scale or standard scoops and household measures.

Detailed lists of the Phe content in foods are available from https://metabolicpro.org, https://howmuchphe.org, medical food companies, the dietitian at the metabolic clinic, or the National PKU News website (see Resources, later). Parents may be asked to weigh or measure and record all the food the child eats for 3 days before the clinic visit and blood test. This diet record allows the dietitian to calculate necessary adjustments.

All persons with PKU require some Phe-free EMF to maintain proper nutrition. A typical individual requires three servings of EMF daily, which accompanies regular meals. In any case, optimal growth and Phe homeostasis are best maintained by distributing the protein intake throughout the day. The EMF products look and taste very different from the milk, and many individuals find them unpalatable.

EMF ingestion is critical for the health of the child with PKU because it contains both supplemental Phe-free protein and vitamins and minerals the children might lack secondary to the restricted diet; therefore parents and significant others need to be very careful not to communicate any distaste for the product. Most children readily accept the EMF if it is started early and if the family has a positive attitude about it. The use of straws and sippy cups often facilitates EMF ingestion. Some children prefer flavorings added to the formula, such as Tang, Kool-Aid mixes, chocolate syrup, concentrated fruit juice, or flavor packets available from the EMF Company. The dietitian must approve such flavorings, and great care must be taken to avoid any product containing aspartame, which is converted to Phe in the gastrointestinal tract. Older children may choose to take their EMF in the form of a capsule or bar; however, more than 100 capsules per day may be required and are not widely used. Many states require that insurance companies or state agencies provide formula and/or low-protein foods for individuals with PKU (www.pkunews.org).

Parents should follow the instructions supplied by the manufacturer when preparing EMF products. The amount of powder to be ingested should be carefully measured, although the volume of liquid to be used may be adjusted according to individual preferences. Some children prefer a more concentrated mixture so they have to drink less. All the powder must be ingested, which may necessitate further dilution of any remaining sludge in the bottom of the container. Most people prefer to mix a 24-hour supply of the EMF and store it in the refrigerator for use the following day. These products should not be heated beyond 130.1°F (54.5°C) to avoid a chemical reaction that alters their protein structure. The shelf life of EMF products is limited, and parents should note the expiration date on the can.

Many children exhibit feeding problems at some point in their development, and children with PKU are no different. However, parents may be more concerned about such problems when they know their child's health depends on adherence to a strict diet. Parents may be reassured that 1 or 2 days of poor intake will not harm the child, nor will occasional nonsustained elevations in Phe. As with any child, parents should not force feed. It is often useful to offer smaller portions; the child can always ask for more but may feel overwhelmed by large helpings. The EMF should be served first. Giving the child choices in the selection of foods and having large amounts of "free" foods available are also useful strategies. In an older child, extra protein-free foods may be necessary to meet calorie and energy requirements. However, these should be monitored carefully because they often contain large amounts of sugar and fat and may lead to obesity if used in excess.

There are anecdotal reports of increased incidence of eating disorders in children with PKU. The idea of a young child being on a "diet" may cause confusion or abnormal perceptions about the meaning of food. As one young adult with PKU so aptly put it, "My main advice for parents of children with PKU is to try not to make PKU a big deal or a central issue in the child's life. What you eat is not even remotely close to being the most important aspect of life" (Beck, 1999).

Because diet for life is the primary treatment for PKU, it is important to initiate self-management at an early age. The child must be taught to make low-Phe food choices and to understand the importance of doing so. At the same time, great care must be taken not to make the child feel stigmatized by different eating habits. Overemphasizing the restrictions may instill undue fear or guilt in a young child. Establishing a balance between a healthy Phe-restricted diet and making the child feel normal takes tremendous effort and sensitivity on the part of parents and caregivers.

Safety

The only safety concerns particular to PKU are related to nutritional imbalances. Overrestriction resulting in long-term Phe deficiency may lead to aminoaciduria, hypoproteinemia, bone changes, decreased growth, anemia, intellectual disability, and hair loss (Acosta & Yannicelli, 2001). Ingestion of Phe that exceeds the individual's tolerance leads to complications associated with HPA. Occasional ingestion of a high-Phe substance such as aspartame is less deleterious than chronic lapses of the restricted diet. Teaching the child and significant others about the importance of a Phe-restricted diet is the best prevention against this hazard.

Immunizations

Routine immunizations are recommended.

Screenings

Vision. Routine screening is recommended.

Hearing. Routine screening is recommended.

Dental. The diet for PKU includes a high proportion of carbohydrates to meet the daily requirement for calories. Dietary sugars are known to increase the risk for dental caries, although one study found no greater incidence of tooth decay in children with PKU (Lucas et al., 2001). To promote dental health, parents should be cautioned not to put the baby to bed with a bottle. Wean the infant to a cup as early as 6 months of age; offer foods such as fruits in place of more retentive forms of refined sugars and liquid forms of carbohydrates that promote oral clearance. Fluoride supplementation is recommended if it is not added to the local water supply. Oral hygiene and dentist visits should be implemented soon after the teeth erupt. Children with

PKU who were diagnosed late may require specialized dental care if they have enamel hypoplasia or abnormal tooth spacing.

Blood pressure. Routine screening is recommended.

Hematocrit. Children on protein-restricted semisynthetic diets are at risk for inadequate intake of iron and other trace elements, though EMFs are supplemented with vitamins and minerals that children on restricted diets often lack. Hematocrit monitoring and related tests are part of the biochemical and nutritional assessment done at the metabolic clinic. Primary care practitioners should communicate with the metabolic practitioner to determine the need for additional tests.

Urinalysis. Routine screening is recommended.

Tuberculosis. Routine screening is recommended.

Condition-Specific Screening
Newborns who test positive, blood Phe and Tyr, and nutritional indices (Box 34.1).

Blood Phe monitoring. Plasma Phe and Tyr levels are evaluated twice weekly in newborns with PKU until concentrations are stabilized, and approximate dietary Phe and Tyr requirements are known. Blood Phe is evaluated weekly until age 1 year, twice monthly until age 12 years, monthly after age 12 years, and twice weekly for pregnant females (NIH, 2000; Vockley et al., 2014). Parents may be taught to collect the capillary blood samples on filter paper at home and return them to the metabolic clinic or another laboratory. The PKU treatment center team evaluates these results, making dietary adjustments as needed.

Nutritional indices monitoring. Nutrient intake is evaluated for Phe, Tyr, protein, and energy intake by the nutritionist on the PKU treatment team. Protein status is evaluated by plasma transthyretin, albumin, or prealbumin

levels every 3 months in infants and every 6 months in children and adolescents. The metabolic treatment team also monitors for insufficient intake of iron, folate, vitamin B_{12}, and other nutrients (Acosta & Yannicelli, 2001).

COMMON ILLNESS MANAGEMENT
Differential Diagnosis
Differential diagnoses occur at routine visits when conditions are suspected or emerge (Box 34.2).

Well-nourished children with PKU respond to infection and trauma in the same way as any child. Children with chronically elevated Phe levels may exhibit the associated signs and symptoms of PKU, including eczematous skin lesions, musty body odor, and cognitive and neurologic sequelae.

Management During Illness and Surgery
Minor uncomplicated surgery with general anesthesia does not cause a major alteration in the blood Phe level. Febrile illness and trauma are normally accompanied by protein catabolism, which may elevate plasma Phe concentrations. These elevations are generally transient and do not require additional Phe monitoring. Supportive measures should be undertaken to limit protein catabolism; liberal volumes of fruit juices, liquid gelatin, caffeine-free soft drinks, or electrolyte formulas (e.g., Pedialyte) without aspartame should be allowed. Polycose powder or liquid or a Phe-free additive recommended by the medical food company may be mixed with the fluids. Acetaminophen, ibuprofen, antibiotics, or other medications may be recommended or prescribed for any child, but the Phe content of these substances must be taken into consideration. EMFs are reinstituted as soon as possible, initially at half strength. If parenteral amino acid solutions are indicated for any reason, the involvement of a specialist familiar with PKU is essential (Acosta & Yannicelli, 2001).

Drug Interactions
Aspartame. Aspartame (L-aspartyl-L-phenylalanine methyl ester) is contraindicated in individuals with PKU because it is converted to Phe in the gastrointestinal tract. It is an artificial sweetener, and 56% of it is converted to free Phe; therefore it should be excluded from a low-Phe diet (MacDonald et al., 2020). Currently marketed under the brand names NutraSweet, Equal, or Canderel, aspartame must be identified on the label

---

Box 34.1 Condition-Specific Screening

NEWBORNS WITH POSITIVE SCREENING TEST
- Quantitative tests for Phe and Tyr
- Pterin metabolites in urine
- Dihydropterin reductase in blood

BLOOD PHE AND TYR
- Twice weekly with Tyr levels until stable
- Weekly until age 1 yr
- Twice monthly until age 12 yr
- Monthly after age 12 yr
- Weekly or twice weekly in pregnant women

NUTRITIONAL INDICES MONITORING
- Plasma transthyretin, albumin, or prealbumin every 3 mo in infants, every 6 mo in children and adolescents
- Iron, folate, vitamin B_{12} levels per nutritionist

Box 34.2 Inborn Errors of Metabolism

CEREBRAL PALSY

Inherited neurotransmitter disorders
Seizures (epilepsy)
Tetrahydrobiopterin
Developmental delays
Musky or mouselike body odor
Irritability
Dry, scaly skin (eczema)

Table **34.2**	Phe Content of Selected Medications[a]
PRODUCT	**PHE CONTENT**
Amoxicillin 250 mg chew tabs (Warner Chilcott)	2 mg/tablet
Amoxil 200 mg chewable tablet	1.82 mg/tablet
Benadryl Allery chewable	4.2 mg/tablet
Children's Advil chewable tablets 50 mg grape flavor	2.1 mg/tablet
Dramamine chewable tablets	1.5 mg/tablet
Flintstones Complete chewable tablets	2 mg/tablet
Pedialyte freezer pops	0 mg (updated January 2020)
Triaminic soft chews cough and sore throat	28.1 mg/tablet

[a]https://www.pkunews.org/drug-products-containing-phenylalanine/ (last updated in 2007). This is not an exhaustive list but rather examples. Formulations change regularly, so please refer to the manufacturer.

of all products with the statement "Phenylketonurics: Contains phenylalanine." This artificial sweetener can be found in soft drinks, chewing gum, jelly desserts, and other sweeteners (MacDonald et al., 2020). A quart of aspartame-sweetened fruit drink contains 280 mg of Phe, more than one-half the daily allowance for a child with PKU (Scriver et al., 2008).

Parents should be cautioned about aspartame in over-the-counter medications, vitamins, or any product labeled "sugar-free." The exact amount of Phe in medications must be calculated as part of a child's daily Phe intake. A variety of resources are available for information about the Phe content of medications, including the manufacturer, the product information, a pharmacist, and the *Physicians' Desk Reference*. The National PKU News website has a frequently updated list of the Phe content of over-the-counter and prescription medications (see Resources); a few of the common ones are listed in Table 34.2.

DEVELOPMENTAL ISSUES

Sleep Patterns
There are no particular sleep disturbances associated with PKU. Routine counseling about establishing and maintaining healthy sleep habits is recommended. Children who have behaviors consistent with ADHD may have an increase in sleep problems.

Toileting
Children with PKU achieve bowel and bladder control at the same age as children without PKU. If Phe levels are chronically elevated, the child may be more prone to eczematous skin lesions that are associated with an increased risk for diaper rash. There is a characteristic musty smell to urine containing Phe metabolites, but this does not occur in children with well-treated PKU.

Discipline
Parenting strategies for a child with PKU are the same as for any child. Positive reinforcement of good behavior is always more effective than negative reinforcement of undesirable behavior. Limit setting and consistent expectations are essential, even if the parent has ambivalent feelings because the child has a chronic condition.

Food is an important social factor in any child's life, and how it is managed from the very beginning by parents can determine the success of the therapy. A major pitfall in disciplining children with PKU is to use food as a reward system and the need for blood tests as punishment. It is critical to establish healthy habits when the child is very young because the child must begin to make the right food choices independently once school age is reached.

Child Care
All individuals in the child's home environment should be knowledgeable about the Phe-restricted diet and the preparation of EMF products. Grandparents and other caregivers play an essential role in supporting the diet and should be included in educational sessions at the metabolic clinic or in primary care. Everyone who spends time with the child must support the parents' efforts to provide the diet and resist the temptation to treat the child to ice cream or other restricted foods. Most day care providers will feed the child whatever the parents send but will need to be educated about the importance of dietary restrictions and the potential hazards of sharing protein foods with other children at day care. Parents devise creative ways to make their child feel normal, such as preparing low-Phe look-alike treats to take to birthday parties or other food-related activities. As the child's primary advocates, parents find themselves teaching others in the community about PKU on a constant basis.

Schooling
Children with PKU are likely to progress in school just like other children. Although there is some evidence of an increased risk for ADHD or mild cognitive dysfunction, most experts agree that these may be minimized with good control of Phe. If a child needs to be evaluated for an individualized education program, the primary care or metabolic care provider may

be involved in reviewing the plan or communicating information about the child. Children with PKU may undergo psychological testing at the PKU treatment center, including developmental assessments, language development tests, intelligence tests, and tests of executive functioning or attention. Ideally, testing is initiated at 6 months of age, continued every 6 months until 2 years, and done at annual or 3-year intervals thereafter. For optimal performance it is important that the child's blood Phe level be in the maintenance range on the day of testing.

School personnel may have little or no knowledge of or experience with PKU. It is often necessary for the professionals at the metabolic clinic, primary care practice, or parents to educate teachers, cafeteria personnel, and school administrators about the child's special needs. The school nurse may be enlisted to assist with these efforts. A useful publication, "A Teacher's Guide to PKU," is available through the Texas Department of Health (see Resources, later). This booklet explains PKU and gives teachers specific guidelines related to dietary restrictions.

Because the diet is the primary aspect of life affected by PKU, cafeteria personnel can be of great help in preventing the child from feeling different. Many parents report that their children have positive experiences with school meals thanks to the willingness of the personnel to provide detailed information about weekly cafeteria menus, heat meals sent from home, weigh portions, or give the child specially prepared items. Open and frequent communication between the family and the school is essential.

Sexuality

Sexual development and curiosity are no different for children with PKU than for any other child. Females with PKU must be educated from an early age about strict Phe control before and throughout pregnancy. The best approach to preventing MPKU is always to foster adherence to diet. Numerous educational materials are available for parents and adolescents related to sexuality and PKU. These may be obtained from the metabolic center or through online resources available to families. Discussions of contraception and the implications of being a female with PKU should be individualized and approached with sensitivity. PKU peer support groups, online chat rooms, and written materials and videos designed specifically for adolescents with PKU are available.

Transition to Adulthood

All adolescents face the challenges of peer pressure, a desire for independence from authority figures, and social and emotional change. Adolescents with conditions such as PKU or diabetes need much support to adhere to a restricted diet and to take their medical foods. Parents' influence often makes it easy for these children to adhere to the PKU diet. However, adherence usually decreases during adolescence likely due to their sense of independence from parental and peer influence (Cazzorla et al., 2018). Pediatric metabolic clinics may not routinely follow individuals with PKU after the age of 18 years. It is not unusual for persons in this age group to abandon routine medical care for a variety of reasons. Every effort must be made to ensure that individuals with PKU receive continuing primary care and metabolic follow-up, given the recent compelling evidence of the benefits of lifelong therapy and the need to prevent the growing problem of MPKU syndrome.

Before the 1980s, most adults with PKU relaxed or discontinued Phe restriction. Consequently, many adults with PKU are currently attempting to reinstitute the diet. This has proved very difficult, and individuals may benefit from the guidance of professionals who can promote adherence, primary care providers, family counseling, and peer support mechanisms. Previously untreated adults with PKU may show improvement in behavior, neurologic status, and IQ (Koch et al., 1999) after the institution of a low-Phe diet. Specific protocols are available (Acosta & Yannicelli, 1997; Dolan et al., 2000).

The transition is helped if children start assisting in calculating their daily intake and mixing their formula at an early age. It is also important for adolescents to be reminded that high levels of Phe can be found in all types of food and drink, including alcohol, and all of these must be considered in planning their daily intake.

Special concerns of females of childbearing age. Contact with a metabolic clinic is often lost in adulthood, so primary care providers have an essential role in preventing MPKU syndrome. Females of childbearing age must prevent pregnancy or maintain Phe levels between 120 μmol/L (2 mg/dL) and 360 μmol/L (6 mg/dL) before conception to prevent birth defects in the fetus and potential developmental and behavioral disabilities in their offspring. Practitioners who care for adolescent and adult females with PKU or HPA should reinforce this at every opportunity and counsel those of childbearing age with PKU or HPA to have their blood levels checked and to achieve metabolic control of Phe before becoming pregnant. However, primary care providers should also be prepared to give guidance regarding the significant barriers to good metabolic control. Returning to control after going off diet can be very difficult. Also, obtaining insurance coverage for EMF can be challenging, and the cost of formula and low-protein foods can be prohibitive for some people. Many obstetric providers are unfamiliar with the management of PKU, so ensuring that females with PKU who are of childbearing age continue to be followed by a metabolic provider familiar with PKU is of the utmost importance. Ideally, a care provider familiar with

PKU or one who is in close association with such an expert will provide prenatal care.

Pregnancy in females with PKU is a medical challenge. Phe must be restricted, but adequate Tyr, vitamins, and other nutrients must be supplied. Special EMF products and detailed guidelines for nutrition management are available (Acosta & Yannicelli, 2001). Currently, sapropterin is classified as a Class C drug. Patients should discuss with their metabolic provider the risks and benefits of taking sapropterin during pregnancy. BioMarin has created a pregnancy registry, and it is hoped that more will be understood about the benefits and risks of using BH4 during pregnancy in the future.

Several factors affect a female's adherence to a Phe-restricted diet in pregnancy, including age, socioeconomic status, and social support. Females with higher intellectual levels are more likely to follow dietary guidelines; thus females with late-diagnosed or inadequately treated PKU are at greater risk of having affected offspring. In one study, young age and economic factors were the two most significant barriers to good control before and during pregnancy (Brown et al., 2002). Strategies that have improved dietary adherence in pregnant women include the use of specially trained resource mothers and MPKU camps. Researchers and providers involved in the maternal PKU project continue to investigate strategies to prevent MPKU (Clarke, 2003).

Phenylketonuria in males. Although much emphasis has been placed on adherence to diet in females with PKU owing to the grave effects of Phe on the fetus, young males should also be counseled about the importance of diet for life and supported in this endeavor by their primary care provider. The benefits of Phe level maintenance include decreased depression, agitation, and aggressiveness and improved attention span, concentration, and skin condition. Males with PKU and their partners may also wish to have genetic counseling to discuss the risks of having a child with PKU before conceiving.

Family Concerns

Families often have difficulty adjusting to the frequent clinic visits, blood draws, and rigid diet control required to care for a child with PKU. As with any new chronic condition diagnosis, each family will react differently, and some may have more difficulty during this time than others. Cultural practices have an impact on the family's acceptance and management of PKU. Beliefs about disease causality, customs related to parenting, and dietary preferences are just some of the factors a practitioner must consider to provide comprehensive care.

Successful treatment of a child with PKU requires the support and commitment of everyone involved with the child. More than one individual in the home should be knowledgeable about the Phe-restricted diet,

preparation of EMF products, and obtaining blood samples. It is not necessary or advisable for the entire family to adopt the eating habits of the child with PKU, although children in vegetarian families may have less difficulty adhering to the protein-restricted PKU diet. The focus of mealtime discussions should be on topics other than food.

Raising a child with PKU can be very expensive. The financial burden of PKU is variable, owing to inconsistent policies on the part of third-party payers, Medicare/Medicaid, and other entities regarding funding for medical and supportive care, formula, and low-protein foods. A list of state laws and policies related to reimbursement for formula and foods is posted on the National PKU News website (see Resources), and the regional metabolic center should be able to provide this information. Although most states require coverage for infant formula, many do not cover the cost of food. The primary care provider may need to intercede on behalf of the parents in negotiating coverage of the expenses of EMF, low-protein medical foods, and blood Phe monitoring.

The diagnosis of PKU has implications for the blood relatives of the affected child. Parents with a child with PKU are obligate carriers of the disorder and have a 25% chance of recurrence in subsequent pregnancies. Other children in the family, grandparents, and the child's aunts and uncles may also be carriers. A metabolic specialist, genetic counselor, genetics trained nurse, social worker, psychologist, or other providers can offer genetic counseling. Carrier testing is available for families whose mutations are known, although some individuals prefer not to know because there is some psychological burden associated with knowledge of one's own or one's family member's genetic information. Different family planning options are available to parents of a child with PKU. Some families choose to have additional pregnancies without additional testing or interventions. Other parents may choose to prevent another affected pregnancy through contraception, prenatal diagnosis with pregnancy termination, or preimplantation genetic diagnosis (Raz et al., 2019). Factors shown to have the greatest impact on the reproductive decisions of parents with a child with a metabolic disorder include stress, worry about the child's future, difficulty meeting the child's needs, and lower functional level of the child (Read, 2002).

RESOURCES

Children's PKU Network (nonprofit that aims to address special needs and concerns of children and families with PKU): http://www.pkunetwork.org

National PKU News (nonprofit that provides information to families and professionals): http://www.pkunews.org

National PKU Alliance: https://www.npkua.org

NATIONAL PKU NEWS

National PKU News
P.O. Box 43552
Montclair, NJ 07043 USA
Phone: (973) 619-9160
Email: sarah@pkunews.org
Website: http://www.pkunews.org

CHILDREN'S PKU NETWORK

Children's PKU Network
3306 Bumann Rd
Encinitas, CA 92024
(858) 775-9978; (800) 377-6677
Fax: (858) 509-0768
Email: pkunetwork@aol.com
Website: http://www.pkunetwork.org

OTHER WEBSITES

BIOPKU (hosts pediatric neurotransmitter disorders databases, including the locus-specific database of *PAH* variants and the BIOPKU genotypes database): http://www.biopku.org/home/home.asp

Texas Department of Health (provides "A Teacher's Guide to PKU" that explains PKU and gives teachers specific guidelines related to dietary restrictions): www.dshs.state.tx.us/newborn/teachpku/shtm

University of Washington (provides "A Babysitters' Guide to PKU" that explains the basic principles of PKU and the special diet that must be followed): https://depts.washington.edu/pku/pdfs/Babysitters_Guide_03.pdf

US Department of Agriculture Nutrient Database (provides detailed lists of Phe content in foods): www.nal.usda.gov/fnic/cgi-bin/nut_search.pl

US National Library of Medicine (provides a brief review of many genetic conditions, including PKU, and is especially useful for families awaiting the follow-up results of a positive newborn screen): https://medlineplus.gov/genetics/condition/phenylketonuria

 Summary

Primary Care Needs for the Child With Phenylketonuria

HEALTH CARE MAINTENANCE

Growth and Development
- Growth should be normal on a Phe-restricted diet.
- Careful monitoring of growth charts is necessary to ensure adequate nutrient intake and to avoid obesity from high-carbohydrate, high-fat foods.
- Development should be monitored with psychological and behavioral testing.

Diet
- Breastfeeding is recommended for infants.
- Involvement of a professional nutritionist is essential.
- Phe-restricted diet is for life.
- Dietary modifications are dictated by blood Phe and Tyr levels.
- Self-management of a Phe-restricted diet should be initiated early in childhood.
- Elemental medical food (EMF) products should be prepared as prescribed and taken with meals.
- Avoid overemphasis on the diet as the central issue in the child's life.

Safety
- Only individuals with a diagnosis of PKU should ingest EMF products as prescribed.
- Occasional high Phe levels are unlikely to be detrimental.

Immunizations
- Routine immunizations are recommended.

Screening
- *Vision.* Routine screening is recommended.
- *Hearing.* Routine screening is recommended.
- *Dental.* Early evaluation is recommended because of the high-carbohydrate diet.
- *Blood pressure.* Routine screening is recommended.
- *Hematocrit.* Hematocrit is part of the nutritional assessment at metabolic clinic; routine screening is not usually required.
- *Urinalysis.* Routine screening is recommended.
- *Tuberculosis.* Routine screening is recommended.

Condition-Specific Screening
- Blood Phe monitoring
- Nutritional indices monitoring

COMMON ILLNESS MANAGEMENT
- Catabolic state related to common childhood illnesses should be prevented with adequate hydration and caloric intake. Transient Phe increases during periods of illness are expected. Analgesics, antipyretics, and antibiotics should be used for any child, but formulations with the lowest Phe content should be sought.

Drug Interactions
- Aspartame ingestion is contraindicated.
- Check Phe content of all medications.

DEVELOPMENTAL ISSUES

Sleep Patterns
- Routine counseling is recommended.

Toileting
- Routine counseling is recommended.

Discipline
- Expectations are normal based on age and developmental level.
- Avoid use of food as a reward system and blood tests as punishment.

Child Care
- All care providers must be aware of dietary modifications.

Schooling
- Children with good Phe control generally progress normally.
- Developmental testing should be done as indicated and educational support given as needed.
- School personnel must be made aware of child's dietary restrictions.

- School cafeteria personnel should be aware of child's dietary restrictions and instructed on preparation of Phe-restricted meals.

Sexuality

- Young women with PKU should be educated about the risks of maternal PKU syndrome and the need to adhere to Phe-restricted diet before conception and throughout pregnancy.

Transition to Adulthood

- All individuals should remain on a Phe-restricted diet for life. There are no special considerations related to alcohol consumption, although types of alcohol have varying amounts of Phe and adolescents should be reminded that this must be included in their calculations of daily Phe intake.
- Participation in PKU support groups and professional counseling as needed are recommended for adults with PKU and their families. Some metabolic clinics have special programs that help transition adolescents from pediatric to adult care. Other clinics provide metabolic care throughout the life span and are equipped to handle the changing issues and concerns that arise as children with PKU transition to self-management.

FAMILY CONCERNS

- Many barriers exist that prevent persons with PKU from adhering to the diet, including complexity and inconvenience, poor palatability and cost of the foods, and psychosocial factors.
- Multiple supports are available and should be promoted by the practitioner.
- Genetic counseling for all family members is advisable.

REFERENCES

Acosta, P. B., & Yannicelli, S. (1997). *Ross metabolic formula system: Nutrition support protocol for previously untreated adults with phenylketonuria.* Ross Products Division/Abbott Laboratories.

Acosta, P. B., & Yannicelli, S. (Eds.). (2001). *Ross metabolic formula system: Nutrition support protocols* (4th ed.). Ross Products Division/Abbott Laboratories.

American College of Medical Genetics. Newborn screening ACT sheet [increased phenylalanine] phenylketonuria (PKU). (2006). Available at www.acmg.net/resources/policies/ACT/ACT-sheet_Phenylalanine_5-2-06_ljo.pdf. Retrieved December 4, 2007.

Anderson, P. J., Wood, S. J., Francis, D. E., Coleman, L., Warwick, L., Casanelia, S., Anderson, V. A., & Boneh, A. (2004). Neuropsychological functioning in children with early-treated phenylketonuria: Impact of white matter abnormalities. *Developmental Medicine & Child Neurology, 46*(4), 230–238. doi:10.1017/s0012162204000386.

Anderson, P. J., Wood, S. J., Francis, D. E., Coleman, L., Anderson, V., & Boneh, A. (2007). Are neuropsychological impairments in children with early-treated phenylketonuria (PKU) related to white matter abnormalities or elevated phenylalanine levels? *Developmental Neuropsychology, 32*(2), 645–668. https://doi.org/10.1080/87565640701375963.

Anderson, P. J., & Leuzzi, V. (2010). White matter pathology in phenylketonuria. *Molecular Genetics and Metabolism, 99*(Suppl 1), S3–S9.

Antshel, K. (2001). ADHD and PKU. *National PKU News, 13*(2), 3.

Arnold, G. L., Vladutiu, C. J., Orlowski, C. C., Blakely, E. M., & DeLuca, J. (2004). Prevalence of stimulant use for attentional dysfunction in children with phenylketonuria. *Journal of Inherited Metabolic Disease, 27*(2), 137–143. https://doi.org/10.1023/B:BOLI.0000028725.37345.62.

Ashe, K., Kelso, W., Farrand, S., Panetta, J., Fazio, T., De Jong, G., & Walterfang, M. (2019). Psychiatric and cognitive aspects of phenylketonuria: The limitations of diet and promise of new treatments. *Frontiers in Psychiatry, 10*, 561. https://doi.org/10.3389/fpsyt.2019.00561.

Banich, M. T., Passarotti, A. M., White, D. A., Nortz, M. J., & Steiner, R. D. (2000). Interhemispheric interaction during childhood: II. Children with early-treated phenylketonuria. *Developmental Neuropsychology, 18*(1), 53–71. https://doi.org/10.1207/S15326942DN1801_4.

Banta-Wright, S. A., Press, N., Knafl, K. A., Steiner, R. D., & Houck, G. M. (2014). Breastfeeding infants with phenylketonuria in the United States and Canada. *Breastfeeding Medicine: The Official Journal of the Academy of Breastfeeding Medicine, 9*(3), 142–148. https://doi.org/10.1089/bfm.2013.0092.

Baumeister, A., & Baumeister, A. (1998). Dietary treatment of destructive behavior associated with hyperphenylalaninemia. *Clinical Neuropharmacology, 21*(1), 18–27.

Beblo, S., Reinhardt, H., Demmelmair, H., Muntau, A. C., & Koletzko, B. (2007). Effect of fish oil supplementation on fatty acid status, coordination, and fine motor skills in children with phenylketonuria. *Journal of Pediatrics, 150*(5), 479–484. https://doi.org/10.1016/j.jpeds.2006.12.011.

Beblo, S., Reinhardt, H., Muntau, A. C., Mueller-Felber, W., Roscher, A. A., & Koletzko, B. (2001). Fish oil supplementation improves visual evoked potentials in children with phenylketonuria. *Neurology, 57*(8), 1488–1491. https://doi.org/10.1212/wnl.57.8.1488.

Beck, T. (1999). My life with PKU. *National PKU News, 10*(3), 11–12. Available at. www.astro.sunysb.edu/tracy/mystory.html. Retrieved January 16, 2009.

Bilginsoy, C., Waitzman, N., Leonard, C. O., & Ernst, S. L. (2005). Living with phenylketonuria: perspectives of patients and their families. *Journal of Inherited Metabolic Disease, 28*(5), 639–649. https://doi.org/10.1007/s10545-005-4478-8.

Blenda, A. V. (2022). BH4 deficiency (tetrahydrobiopterin deficiency). *Background, Pathophysiology, Epidemiology.* https://emedicine.medscape.com/article/949470-overview.

Bodamer, O. A. (2022). Overview of phenylketonuria. *UpToDate.* Retrieved March 7, 2023, from https://www.uptodate.com/contents/overview-of-phenylketonuria.

Brown, A. S., Fernhoff, P. M., Waisbren, S. E., Frazier, D. M., Singh, R., Rohr, F., Morris, J. M., Kenneson, A., MacDonald, P., Gwinn, M., Honein, M., & Rasmussen, S. A. (2002). Barriers to successful dietary control among pregnant women with phenylketonuria. *Genetics in Medicine, 4*(2), 84–89. https://doi.org/10.1097/00125817-200203000-00006.

Burton, B., Grant, M., Feigenbaum, A., Singh, R., Hendren, R., Siriwardena, K., Phillips, J., 3rd, Sanchez-Valle, A., Waisbren, S., Gillis, J., Prasad, S., Merilainen, M., Lang, W., Zhang, C., Yu, S., & Stahl, S. (2015). A randomized, placebo-controlled, double-blind study of sapropterin to treat ADHD symptoms and executive function impairment in children and adults with sapropterin-responsive phenylketonuria. *Molecular Genetics and Metabolism, 114*(3), 415–424. https://doi.org/10.1016/j.ymgme.2014.11.011.

Camp, K. M., Parisi, M. A., & Acosta, P. B. (2014). Phenylketonuria scientific review conference: State of the science and future research needs. *Molecular Genetics and Metabolism, 112*(2), 87–122.

Cazzorla, C., Bensi, G., Biasucci, G., Leuzzi, V., Manti, F., Musumeci, A., Papadia, F., Stoppioni, V., Tummolo, A., Vendemiale, M., Polo, G., & Burlina, A. (2018). Living with phenylketonuria in adulthood: The PKU ATTITUDE study. *Molecular Genetics* and Metabolism Reports, 16, 39–45. https://doi.org/10.1016/j.ymgmr.2018.06.007.

Channon, S., German, E., Cassina, C., & Lee, P. (2004). Executive functioning, memory, and learning in phenylketonuria. Neuropsychology, 18(4), 613–620. https://doi.org/10.1037/0894-4105.18.4.613.

Chen, S., Zhu, M., Hao, Y., Feng, J., & Zhang, Y. (2019). Effect of delayed diagnosis of phenylketonuria with imaging findings of bilateral diffuse symmetric white matter lesions: A case report and literature review. Front Neurol, 10, 1040. doi: 10.3389/fneur.2019.01040.

Clarke, J. T. (2003). The maternal phenylketonuria project: A summary of progress and challenges for the future. Pediatrics, 112(6 pt 2), 1584–1587.

Cleary, M. A., & Skeath, R. (2019). Phenylketonuria. Pediatric and Child Health, 29(3), 111–115.

Danecka, M. K., Woidy, M., Zschocke, J., Feillet, F., Muntau, A. C., & Gersting, S. W. (2015). Mapping the functional landscape of frequent phenylalanine hydroxylase (PAH) genotypes promotes personalised medicine in phenylketonuria. Journal of Medical Genetics, 52(3), 175–185. https://doi.org/10.1136/jmedgenet-2014-102621.

Dobbelaere, D., Michaud, L., Debrabander, A., Vanderbecken, S., Gottrand, F., Turck, D., & Farriaux, J. P. (2003). Evaluation of nutritional status and pathophysiology of growth retardation in patients with phenylketonuria. Journal of Inherited Metabolic Disease, 26(1), 1–11. https://doi.org/10.1023/a:1024063726046.

Dolan, B. E., Koch, R., Bekins, C., & Schuett V. (2000). Diet intervention guidelines for adults with untreated PKU. Available at www.pkunews.org/adults/guide.htm. Retrieved February 12, 2008.

Edwards, J. G., Feldman, G., Goldberg, J., Gregg, A. R., Norton, M. E., Rose, N. C., Schneider, A., Stoll, K., Wapner, R., & Watson, M. S. (2015). Expanded carrier screening in reproductive medicine—points to consider: A joint statement of the American College of Medical Genetics and Genomics, American College of Obstetricians and Gynecologists, National Society of Genetic Counselors, Perinatal Quality Foundation, and Society for Maternal-Fetal Medicine. Obstetrics and Gynecology, 125(3), 653–662. https://doi.org/10.1097/AOG.0000000000000666.

Elhawary, N. A., AlJahdali, I. A., Abumansour, I. S., Elhawary, E. N., Gaboon, N., Dandini, M., Madkhali, A., Alosaimi, W., Alzahrani, A., Aljohani, F., Melibary, E. M., & Kensara, O. A. (2022). Genetic etiology and clinical challenges of phenylketonuria. Human Genomics, 16(1), 22. https://doi.org/10.1186/s40246-022-00398-9.

Etzel, M. R. (2002). Glycomacropeptide (GMP) update. National PKU News, 14(1), 2.

Feillet, F., van Spronsen, F. J., MacDonald, A., Trefz, F. K., Demirkol, M., Giovannini, M., Bélanger-Quintana, A., & Blau, N. (2010). Challenges and pitfalls in the management of phenylketonuria. Pediatrics, 126(2), 333–341. doi:10.1542/peds.2009-3584. Epub 2010 Jul 12.

Fitzgerald, B., Morgan, J., Keene, N., Rollinson, R., Hodgson, A., & Dalrymple-Smith, J. (2000). An investigation into diet treatment for adults with previously untreated phenylketonuria and severe intellectual disability. Journal of Intellectual Disability Research, 44(Pt 1), 53–59. https://doi.org/10.1046/j.1365-2788.2000.00260.x.

Gassió, R., Campistol, J., Vilaseca, M. A., Lambruschini, N., Cambra, F. J., & Fusté, E. (2003). Do adult patients with phenylketonuria improve their quality of life after introduction/resumption of a phenylalanine-restricted diet? Acta Paediatrica (Oslo, Norway: 1992), 92(12), 1474–1478.

Giovannini, M., Verduci, E., Salvatici, E., Fiori, L., & Riva, E. (2007). Phenylketonuria: Dietary and therapeutic challenges. Journal of Inherited Metabolic Disease, 30(2), 145–152. https://doi.org/10.1007/s10545-007-0552-8.

Griffiths, P. V., Demellweek, C., Fay, N., Robinson, P. H., & Davidson, D. C. (2000). Wechsler subscale IQ and subtest profile in early treated phenylketonuria. Archives of Disease

In Childhood, 82(3), 209–215. https://doi.org/10.1136/adc.82.3.209.

Griffiths, P. Y., Demellweek, C., Fay, N., Robinson, P. H., & Davidson, D. C. (2000). Wechsler subscale IQ and subtest profile in early treated phenylketonuria. Archives of Disease in Childhood, 82(3), 209–215. https://doi.org/10.1136/adc.82.3.209.

Grosse, S. D. (2010). Late-treated phenylketonuria and partial reversibility of intellectual impairment. Child Development, 81(1), 200–211.

Hardelid, P., Cortina-Borja, M., Munro, A., Jones, H., Cleary, M., Champion, M. P., Foo, Y., Scriver, C. R., & Dezateux, C. (2008). The birth prevalence of PKU in populations of European, South Asian and sub-Saharan African ancestry living in South East England. Annals of Human Genetics, 72(Pt 1), 65–71. https://doi.org/10.1111/j.1469-1809.2007.00389.x.

Harding, C. O., Gillingham, M. B., Hamman, K., Clark, H., Goebel-Daghighi, E., Bird, A., & Koeberl, D. D. (2006). Complete correction of hyperphenylalaninemia following liver-directed, recombinant AAV2/8 vector-mediated gene therapy in murine phenylketonuria. Gene Therapy, 13(5), 457–462. https://doi.org/10.1038/sj.gt.3302678.

Huijbregts, S. C., de Sonneville, L. M., Licht, R., van Spronsen, F. J., Verkerk, P. H., & Sergeant, J. A. (2002). Sustained attention and inhibition of cognitive interference in treated phenylketonuria: Associations with concurrent and lifetime phenylalanine concentrations. Neuropsychologia, 40(1), 7–15. https://doi.org/10.1016/s0028-3932(01)00078-1.

Hydery, T., & Coppenrath, V. A. (2019). A comprehensive review of pegvaliase, an enzyme substitution therapy for the treatment of phenylketonuria. Drug Target Insights. 13:1177392819857089. https://doi.org/10.1177/1177392819857089.

Kalsner, L. R., Rohr, F. J., Strauss, K. A., Korson, M. S., & Levy, H. L. (2001). Tyrosine supplementation in phenylketonuria: Diurnal blood tyrosine levels and presumptive brain influx of tyrosine and other large neutral amino acids. Journal of Pediatrics, 139(3), 421–427. https://doi.org/10.1067/mpd.2001.117576.

Kamleh, M., Williamson, J. M., Casas, K., & Mohamed, M. (2021). Reduction in newborn screening false positive results following a new collection protocol: A quality improvement project. Journal of Pediatric Pharmacology and Therapeutics, 26(7), 723–727.

Koch, R., Hanley, W., Levy, H., Matalon, K., Matalon, R., Rouse, B., Trefz, F., Güttler, F., Azen, C., Platt, L., Waisbren, S., Widaman, K., Ning, J., Friedman, E. G., & de la Cruz, F. (2003). The maternal phenylketonuria international study: 1984-2002. Pediatrics, 112(6 Pt 2), 1523–1529.

Koch, R., Moseley, K., Ning, J., Romstad, A., Guldberg, P., & Guttler, F. (1999). Long-term beneficial effects of the phenylalanine-restricted diet in late-diagnosed individuals with phenylketonuria. Molecular Genetics and Metabolism, 67(2), 148–155. https://doi.org/10.1006/mgme.1999.2863.

Koch, R., & Wenz, E. (1987). Phenylketonuria. Annual Review of Nutrition, 7, 117–135.

Langenbeck, U., Baum, F., Mench-Hoinowski, A., Luthe, H., & Behbehani, A. W. (2005). Predicting the phenylalanine blood concentration from urine analyses. An approach to noninvasive monitoring of patients with phenylketonuria. Journal of Inherited Metabolic Disease, 28(6), 855–861. https://doi.org/10.1007/s10545-005-0160-4.

Lee, P. J., Ridout, D., Walter, J. H., & Cockburn, F. (2005). Maternal phenylketonuria: Report from the United Kingdom Registry 1978-97. Archives of Disease in Childhood, 90(2), 143–146. https://doi.org/10.1136/adc.2003.037762.

Levy, H., Burton, B., Cederbaum, S., & Scriver, C. (2007). Recommendations for evaluation of responsiveness to tetrahydrobiopterin (BH(4)) in phenylketonuria and its use in treatment. Molecular Genetics and Metabolism, 92(4), 287–291. https://doi.org/10.1016/j.ymgme.2007.09.017.

Levy, H. L., Guldberg, P., Güttler, F., Hanley, W. B., Matalon, R., Rouse, B. M., Trefz, F., Azen, C., Allred, E. N., de la

Cruz, F., & Koch, R. (2001). Congenital heart disease in maternal phenylketonuria: Report from the Maternal PKU Collaborative Study. *Pediatric Research, 49*(5), 636–642. https://doi.org/10.1203/00006450-200105000-00005.

Lexicomp. Pegvaliase: Drug information. (2023). *UpToDate.* Retrieved March 7, 2023 from https://www-uptodate-com.proxy.hsl.ucdenver.edu/contents/pegvaliase-drug-information?search=Palynziq%20&source=panel_search_result&selectedTitle=1~2&usage_type=panel&kp_tab=drug_general&display_rank=1#F55353047.

Lim, K., van Calcar, S. C., Nelson, K. L., Gleason, S. T., & Ney, D. M. (2007). Acceptable low-phenylalanine foods and beverages can be made with glycomacropeptide from cheese whey for individuals with PKU. *Molecular Genetics and Metabolism, 92*(1-2), 176–178. https://doi.org/10.1016/j.ymgme.2007.06.004.

Longo, N., Arnold, G. L., Pridjian, G., Enns, G. M., Ficicioglu, C., Parker, S., Cohen-Pfeffer, J. L., & Phenylketonuria Demographics, Outcomes and Safety Registry. (2015). Long-term safety and efficacy of sapropterin: The PKUDOS registry experience. *Molecular Genetics and Metabolism, 114*(4), 557–563. https://doi.org/10.1016/j.ymgme.2015.02.003.

Lucas, V. S., Contreras, A., Loukissa, M., & Roberts, G. J. (2001). Dental disease indices and caries related oral microflora in children with phenylketonuria. *ASDC Journal of Dentistry for Children, 68*(4), 263–229.

MacDonald, A., van Wegberg, A. M. J., Ahring, K., Beblo, S., Bélanger-Quintana, A., Burlina, A., Campistol, J., Coşkun, T., Feillet, F., Giżewska, M., Huijbregts, S. C., Leuzzi, V., Maillot, F., Muntau, A. C., Rocha, J. C., Romani, C., Trefz, F., & van Sponsen, F. J. (2020). PKU dietary handbook to accompany PKU guidelines. *Orphanet Journal of Rare Diseases, 15*(1), 171. https://doi.org/10.1186/s13023-020-01391-y.

Mainka, T., Fischer, J. F., Huebl, J., Jung, A., Lier, D., Mosejova, A., Skorvanek, M., de Koning, T. J., Kühn, A. A., Freisinger, P., Ziagaki, A., & Ganos, C. (2021). The neurological and neuropsychiatric spectrum of adults with late-treated phenylketonuria. *Parkinsonism & Related Disorders, 89*, 167–175. https://doi.org/10.1016/j.parkreldis.2021.06.011.

Manganaro, L., Bernardo, S., De Vito, C., Antonelli, A., Marchionni, E., Vinci, V., Saldari, M., Di Meglio, L., Giancotti, A., Silvestri, E., Catalano, C., & Pizzuti, A. (2017). Role of fetal MRI in the evaluation of isolated and non-isolated corpus callosum dysgenesis: Results of a cross-sectional study. *Prenatal Diagnosis, 37*(3), 244–252. https://doi.org/10.1002/pd.4990.

Mei, L., Song, P., Kokudo, N., Xu, L., & Tang, W. (2013). Current situation and prospects of newborn screening and treatment for Phenylketonuria in China – compared with the current situation in the United States, UK and Japan. *Intractable & Rare Diseases Research, 2*(4), 106–114. https://doi.org/10.5582/irdr.2013.v2.4.106.

Modan-Moses, D., Vered, I., Schwartz, G., Anikster, Y., Abraham, S., Segev, R., & Efrati, O. (2007). Peak bone mass in patients with phenylketonuria. *Journal of Inherited Metabolic Disease, 30*(2), 202–208. https://doi.org/10.1007/s10545-007-0462-9.

Moseley, K., Koch, R., & Moser, A. B. (2002). Lipid status and long-chain polyunsaturated fatty acid concentrations in adults and adolescents with phenylketonuria on phenylalanine-restricted diets. *Journal of Inherited Metabolic Disease, 25*(1), 56–64.

National Institutes of Health. (2000). Phenylketonuria (PKU): Screening and management. *NIH Consensus Statement, 17*(3). Available at www.nichd.nih.gov/publications/pubs/pku/index.htm. Retrieved December 4, 2007.

Newborn Screening Committee. (1999). *The Council of Regional Networks for Genetics Services (CORN). National newborn screening report—1994.* Atlanta: CORN.

Ney, D. M., Hull, A. K., van Calcar, S. C., Liu, X., & Etzel, M. R. (2008). Dietary glycomacropeptide supports growth and reduces the concentrations of phenylalanine in plasma and brain in a murine model of phenylketonuria. *Journal of Nutrition, 138*(2), 316–322. https://doi.org/10.1093/jn/138.2.316.

Nissenkorn, A., Michelson, M., Ben-Zeev, B., & Lerman-Sagie, T. (2001). Inborn errors of metabolism: A cause of abnormal brain development. *Neurology, 56*(10), 1265–1272. https://doi.org/10.1212/wnl.56.10.1265.

Nussbaum, R., McInnes, R., & Willard, H. (2001). *Thompson and Thompson genetics in medicine* (6th ed.). Saunders.

Nyhan, W. L., Barshop, B. A., & Ozand, P. T. (2005). *Atlas of metabolic diseases* (2nd ed.). Hodder Arnold.

Pavone, P., Polizzi, A., Marino, S. D., Corsello, G., Falsaperla, R., Marino, S., & Ruggieri, M. (2020). West syndrome: A comprehensive review. *Neurological Sciences, 41*(12), 3547–3562. https://doi.org/10.1007/s10072-020-04600-5.

Pietz, J., Kreis, R., Rupp, A., Mayatepek, E., Rating, D., Boesch, C., & Bremer, H. J. (1999). Large neutral amino acids block phenylalanine transport into brain tissue in patients with phenylketonuria. *Journal of Clinical Investigation, 103*(8), 1169–1178. https://doi.org/10.1172/JCI5017.

PKU News. (2022). Drug products containing phenylalanine. https://pkunews.org/drug-products-containing-phenylalanine/.

Pollack, A. (2007). Agency approves drug to treat genetic disorder that can lead to retardation. *New York Times.* http://www.nytimes.com/2007/12/14/health/14genetic.html?scp=2&sq=KUVAN&st=cse. Retrieved January 16, 2009.

Raz, A. E., Amano, Y., & Timmermans, S. (2019). Coming to terms with the imperfectly normal child: Attitudes of Israeli parents of screen-positive infants regarding subsequent prenatal diagnosis. *Journal of Community Genetics, 10*(1), 41–50.

Read, C. Y. (2002). Reproductive decisions of parents of children with metabolic disorders. *Clinical Genetics, 61*, 268–276.

Regier, D. S., & Greene, C. L. (2000). Phenylalanine hydroxylase deficiency. In: Adam, M. P., Everman, D. B., & Mirzaa, G. M. et al. (Eds.), *GeneReviews* (pp. 1993–2022). University of Washington–Seattle.

Rezvani, I. (2000). Defects in metabolism of amino acids: Phenylalanine. In: Behrman, R. E., Kliegman, R. M., & Jenson, H. B. (Eds.), *Nelson textbook of pediatrics* (16th ed.). Saunders.

Rinaldo, P., Tortorelli, S., & Matern, D. (2004). Recent developments and new applications of tandem mass spectrometry in newborn screening. *Current Opinions in Pediatrics, 16*(4), 427–433.

Rohde, C., Thiele, A. G., Baerwald, C., Ascherl, R. G., Lier, D., Och, U., Heller, C., Jung, A., Schönherr, K., Joerg-Streller, M., Luttat, S., Matzgen, S., Winkler, T., Rosenbaum-Fabian, S., Joos, O., & Beblo, S. (2021). Preventing maternal phenylketonuria (PKU) syndrome: Important factors to achieve good metabolic control throughout pregnancy. *Orphanet Journal of Rare Diseases, 16*(1), 477. doi:10.1186/s13023-021-02108-5.

Rouse, B., Azen, C., Koch, R., Matalon, R., Hanley, W., de la Cruz, F., Trefz, F., Friedman, E., & Shifrin, H. (1997). Maternal phenylketonuria collaborative study (MPKUCS) offspring: Facial anomalies, malformations, and early neurological sequelae. *American Journal of Medical Genetics, 69*(1), 89–95. https://onlinelibrary.wiley.com/doi/10.1002/(SICI)1096-8628(19970303)69:1%3C89::AID-AJMG17%3E3.0.CO;2-K.

Rush, M. (2022). *Phenylketonuria (PKU).* Practice Essentials, Background, Pathophysiology. https://emedicine.medscape.com/article/947781-overview.

Sadek, A. A., Emam, A., & Alhaggagy, M. Y. (2013). Clinicolaboratory profile of phenylketonuria (PKU) in Sohag University Hospital-Upper Egypt. *Egyptian Journal of Medical Human Genetics, 14*, 293–298.

Schindeler, S., Ghosh-Jerath, S., Thompson, S., Rocca, A., Joy, P., Kemp, A., Rae, C., Green, K., Wilcken, B., & Christodoulou, J. (2007). The effects of large neutral amino acid supplements in PKU: An MRS and neuropsychological study. *Molecular Genetics and Metabolism, 91*(1), 48–54. https://doi.org/10.1016/j.ymgme.2007.02.002.

Scriver, C. R. (2007). The PAH gene, phenylketonuria, and a paradigm shift. *Human Mutation, 28*(9), 831–845.

Scriver, C. R., Levy, H., & Donlon, J. (2008). Hyperphenylalaninemia: Phenylalanine hydroxylase deficiency. Online Metabolic and Molecular Bases of Inherited Disease. www.ommbid.com/OMMBID/the_online_metabolic_and_molecular_bases_of_inherited_disease/b/abstract/part8/ch77. Retrieved February 3, 2009.

Seashore, M. R. (2008). Personal communication.

Singh, R. H., Rohr, F., Frazier, D., Cunningham, A., Mofidi, S., Ogata, B., Splett, P. L., Moseley, K., Huntington, K., Acosta, P. B., Vockley, J., & Van Calcar, S. C. (2014). Recommendations for the nutrition management of phenylalanine hydroxylase deficiency. *Genetics in Medicine 16*(2), 121–131. https://doi.org/10.1038/gim.2013.179.

Smith, I., & Knowles, J. (2000). Behavior in early treated phenylketonuria: A systematic review. *European Journal of Pediatrics, 159*, S89–S93.

Spirito, F., Meneguzzi, G., Danos, O., & Mezzina, M. (2001). Cutaneous gene transfer and therapy: The present and the future. *The Journal of Gene Medicine, 3*(1), 21–31. https://onlinelibrary.wiley.com/doi/10.1002/1521-2254(2000)9999:9999%3C::AID-JGM156%3E3.0.CO;2-I.

Stone, W. L., Basit, H., & Los, E. Phenylketonuria. (2023). In: StatPearls [Internet]. Treasure Island (FL): StatPearls Publishing; 2023 Jan–.

Trefz, F. K., Scheible, D., Frauendienst-Egger, G., Korall, H., & Blau, N. (2005). Long-term treatment of patients with mild and classical phenylketonuria by tetrahydrobiopterin. *Molecular Genetics and Metabolism, 86*(Suppl 1), S75–S80. https://doi.org/10.1016/j.ymgme.2005.06.026.

Umberger, R. A., Hatfield, L. A., & Speck, P. M. (2017). Understanding negative predictive value of diagnostic tests used in clinical practice. *Dimensions of Critical Care Nursing, 36*(1), 22–29.

van Bakel, M. M., Printzen, G., Wermuth, B., & Wiesmann, U. N. (2000). Antioxidant and thyroid hormone status in selenium-deficient phenylketonuric and hyperphenylalaninemic patients. *American Journal of Clinical Nutrition, 72*(4), 976–981. https://doi.org/10.1093/ajcn/72.4.976.

Van Calcar, S. C., & Ney, D. M. (2012). Food products made with glycomacropeptide, a low-phenylalanine whey protein, provide a new alternative to amino acid-based medical foods for nutrition management of phenylketonuria. *Journal of the Academy of Nutrition and Diet, 112*(8), 1201–1210.

van Spronsen, F. J., Blau, N., Harding, C., Burlina, A., Longo, N., & Bosch, A. M. (2021). Phenylketonuria. *Nature Reviews Disease Primers, 7*(1), 36. https://doi.org/10.1038/s41572-021-00267-0.

van Spronsen, F. J., van Rijn, M., Bekhof, J., Koch, R., & Smit, P. G. (2001). Phenylketonuria: Tyrosine supplementation in phenylalanine-restricted diets. *American Journal of Clinical Nutrition, 73*(2), 153–157. https://doi.org/10.1093/ajcn/73.2.153.

Van Wegberg, A., MacDonald, A., & Ahring, K. (2017). The complete European guidelines on phenylketonuria: Diagnosis and treatment. *Orphanet Journal of Rare Diseases, 12*(1), 162.

VanZutphen, K., Packman, W., Sporri, L., Needham, M., Morgan, C., Weisiger, K., & Packman, S. (2007). Executive functioning in children and adolescents with phenylketonuria. *Clinical Genetics, 72*(1), 13–18. https://doi.org/10.1111/j.1399-0004.2007.00816.x.

Vockley, J., Andersson, H. C., Antshel, K. M., Braverman, N. E., Burton, B. K., Frazier, D. M., Mitchell, J., Smith, W. E., Thompson, B. H., Berry, S. A., & American College of Medical Genetics and Genomics Therapeutics Committee (2014). Phenylalanine hydroxylase deficiency: Diagnosis and management guideline. *Genetics in Medicine: Official Journal of the American College of Medical Genetics, 16*(2), 188–200. https://doi.org/10.1038/gim.2013.157.

Waisbren, S. E., Prabhu, S. P., Greenstein, P., Petty, C., Schomer, D., Anastasoaie, V., Charette, K., Rodriguez, D., Merugumala, S., & Lin, A. P. (2017). Improved measurement of brain phenylalanine and tyrosine related to neuropsychological functioning in phenylketonuria. *JIMD Reports, 34*, 77–86. https://doi.org/10.1007/8904_2016_11.

Waisbren, S. E., Albers, S., Amato, S., Ampola, M., Brewster, T. G., Demmer, L., Eaton, R. B., Greenstein, R., Korson, M., Larson, C., Marsden, D., Msall, M., Naylor, E. W., Pueschel, S., Seashore, M., Shih, V. E., & Levy, H. L. (2003). Effect of expanded newborn screening for biochemical genetic disorders on child outcomes and parental stress. *JAMA, 290*(19), 2564–2572. https://doi.org/10.1001/jama.290.19.2564.

Waisbren, S. E., Noel, K., Fahrbach, K., Cella, C., Frame, D., Dorenbaum, A., & Levy, H. (2007). Phenylalanine blood levels and clinical outcomes in phenylketonuria: A systematic literature review and meta-analysis. *Molecular Genetics and Metabolism, 92*(1–2), 63–70. https://doi.org/10.1016/j.ymgme.2007.05.006.

Walter, J., Lee, P., & Burgard, P. (2006). Hyperphenylalinemias. In: Fernandes, J., Saudubray, J. M., & Van den Berghe, G., et al. (Eds.), *Inborn metabolic disease: Diagnosis and treatment* (4th ed.). Springer.

Welsh, M. C., & Pennington, B. F. (2000). Phenylketonuria. In K. O. Yeats, D. Ris. & H. G. Taylor (Eds). *Pediatric Neuropsychology. Research, Theory, and Practice*. New York: Guilford Press.

Wilcox, W. R., & Cederbaum, S. D. (2002). Amino acid metabolism. In J. M. Connor, R. Pyeritz, B. Korf, (Eds.) (2002). Emery and Rimoin's Principles and Practice of Medical Genetics, (4th ed.). Philadelphia:Saunders.

Weglage, J., Pietsch, M., Feldmann, R., Koch, H. G., Zschocke, J., Hoffmann, G., Muntau-Heger, A., Denecke, J., Guldberg, P., Güttler, F., Möller, H., Wendel, U., Ullrich, K., & Harms, E. (2001). Normal clinical outcome in untreated subjects with mild hyperphenylalaninemia. *Pediatric Research, 49*(4), 532–536. https://doi.org/10.1203/00006450-200104000-00015.

Zhongshu, Z., Weiming, Y., & Ykio, F. (2001). Clinical analysis of West syndrome associated with phenylketonuria. *Brain Dev, 23*(7), 552–557.

Zurflüh, M. R., Zschocke, J., Lindner, M., Feillet, F., Chery, C., Burlina, A., Stevens, R. C., Thöny, B., & Blau, N. (2008). Molecular genetics of tetrahydrobiopterin-responsive phenylalanine hydroxylase deficiency. *Hum Mutat, 29*(1), 167–175. doi:10.1002/humu.20637.

35

Prematurity

Michelle M. Kelly

INCIDENCE AND PREVALENCE

Preterm birth is a global health challenge whose implications last from infancy through adulthood. Preterm birth is defined as birth before the completion of 37 weeks of gestation (World Health Organization, 2018), with the edge of viability at approximately 23 to 24 weeks of gestation (American College of Obstetricians and Gynecologists [ACOG] & Society for Maternal-Fetal Medicine, 2017). Globally preterm birth rates range from 5% to 18% (Synnes & Hicks, 2018), with 15 million infants born preterm, of which a staggering 1 million children die before age 5 years (Walani, 2020). The United States, India, China, Nigeria, Pakistan, and Indonesia account for 50% (~7.4 million) of all preterm births worldwide (Walani, 2020). Preterm birth is a significant focus of the United Nations Sustainable Development Goal 3, targeting preventable newborn and child deaths under 5 years of age by 2030 (United Nations, 2023). Despite this, survival rates can range from 90% to 95% in areas of the world with adequate access to advanced neonatal care and technology, such as prenatal steroids, exogenous surfactants, and advanced respiratory management (Raju et al., 2017). The American Academy of Pediatrics (AAP, 2004) provides neonatal terminology to help in understanding this discussion (Table 35.1).

Over the last several decades, the US preterm birth rate hovered just under 10% (Osterman et al., 2022). In the United States, 2.7% of preterm births occur less than 34 weeks of gestation, with the majority of preterm births (7.4%) occurring late preterm, or 34 to 36 weeks of gestation (Osterman et al., 2022). Multiple gestations increase the likelihood of preterm delivery, with 98.7% of triplets and 59.4% of twins delivering preterm compared to 8.42% of singleton deliveries (Osterman et al., 2022). Health care disparities in the United States may contribute to the variation in preterm birth rates in specific populations. For example, according to the National Vital Statistics Report on Births in 2020, the preterm birth rates across racial designations were as follows: 8.51% non-Hispanic Asian, 9.1% non-Hispanic White, 9.84% Hispanic, and 14.36% non-Hispanic Black (Osterman et al., 2022).

ACOG (2017) asserts that ultrasound measurement obtained prior to 14 weeks of gestation is the most accurate method to establish the estimated date of delivery and gestational age. Estimation based on the first day of the mother's last menstrual period (LMP) fails to consider cycle irregularities, variability in ovulation, and inaccurate recall of LMP (ACOG, 2017). Pregnancies resulting from assisted reproductive technology should have gestational age assigned using the age of the embryo and embryo transfer dates (ACOG, 2017). When neither early ultrasound nor LMP data are available, physical and neurologic findings during the first few hours of life can be used to provide a rough estimate of gestational age (Ballard et al., 1991; Dubowitz et al., 1970).

The most frequently cited estimation of the economic burden associated with preterm birth in the United States is proposed costs in excess of $26 billion annually (Behrman et al., 2007). This estimation includes the cost of complex care, caregiver costs, lost wages, and educational and support service costs for children up to 5 years of age. This estimation, however, did not include the costs connected with long-term comorbidities associated with preterm birth, such as asthma, learning disabilities, mental health, or behavioral conditions (Frey & Klebanoff, 2016). Health care costs associated with neonatal intensive care unit (NICU) admissions are highest for infants born at the lowest gestational ages; however, the largest percentage of infants born preterm are those born late preterm. Outcome research focusing on adolescents and adults born preterm highlights the ongoing health consequences in this population, regardless of gestational age (Kelly & Griffith, 2019; Raju et al., 2017).

PREVENTION

Worldwide, two-thirds of all preterm births occur without an identifiable cause (Ferrero et al., 2016). Risk factors of prematurity are believed to include a combination of medical, social, and environmental factors: stress, poverty, domestic violence, smoking, drug abuse, poor nutrition, inadequate prenatal care, short intrapartum intervals, lower levels of education, preeclampsia, prior preterm delivery, extremes of body mass (large or small), intrauterine infections, uteroplacental insufficiency, incompetent cervix, and multiple gestations (Ferrero et al., 2016). Prior preterm delivery and preeclampsia are the top risk factors worldwide

Table 35.1	Neonatal Terminology
TERM	**DEFINITION**
Gestational age	Time elapsed between first day of last menstrual period and day of delivery
Chronologic age	Time elapsed since birth
Corrected age	Chronologic age – number of weeks born before 40 wk
Postmenstrual age	Gestational age + chronologic age
Gestational Age Categories	
Previable	Born between 21 and 25 wk gestation
Extremely preterm	Born <28 wk gestation
Very preterm	Born between 28 and 32 wk gestation
Moderately preterm	Born between 32 and 34 wk gestation
Late preterm	Born between 34 and 37 wk gestation
Preterm	Born <37 wk gestation
Early term birth	Born between 37 and 39 wk gestation
Full term	Born between 39 and 40 wk gestation
Late term	Born between 41 and 42 wk gestation
Postterm	Born >42 wk gestation
Birth Weight Categories	
Low birth weight	<2500 g (5.5 lb)
Very low birth weight	<1500 g (3.3 lb)
Extremely low birth weight	<1000 g (2.2 lb)
Weight for Gestational Age	
Appropriate for gestational age	Birth weight between 10% and 90% for gestational age
Large for gestational age	Birth weight <90% for gestational age
Small for gestational age	Birth weight <10% gestational age

From Stewart, D.L., & Barfield, W.D. (2019). American Academy of Pediatrics Committee on Fetus and Newborn. Updates on an at-risk population: Late-preterm and early-term infants. *Pediatrics, 144*(5), e20192760.

(Ferrero et al., 2016). Effective methods for the prevention of prematurity and for prolonging pregnancy are elusive, as is the ability to predict which mother-fetal dyad will deliver prematurely.

Fetal fibronectin and transvaginal ultrasound measurements of cervical length are two assessments the obstetric provider makes to predict preterm delivery (Giouleka et al., 2022). Fetal fibronectin, a biochemical marker that is abnormal in the cervicovaginal mucus after 22 weeks, is more likely to be positive in those delivering preterm. A positive fetal fibronectin result equates to an increased risk of spontaneous preterm delivery and may be used in conjunction with the measurement of cervical length to determine the indication for tocolytics (Giouleka et al., 2022).

The use of vaginal progesterone, intramuscular 17-alpha-hydroxyprogesterone, and prophylactic cervical cerclage are considerations for preventing or delaying preterm delivery in females with a history of prior preterm birth and are most effective in singleton deliveries (Giouleka et al., 2022). Antenatal maternal corticosteroids (betamethasone) will accelerate fetal lung maturation, decrease the incidence and severity of respiratory distress syndrome, and decrease the incidence of some associated morbidities, including bronchopulmonary dysplasia (BPD), intraventricular

hemorrhage (IVH), and necrotizing enterocolitis (NEC) for infants born before 32 weeks of gestation. The use of maternal corticosteroids (two 12-mg doses of betamethasone given 24 h apart) is currently recommended for use in females 24 and 34 weeks of gestation with clinical indications of possible preterm delivery (Giouleka et al., 2022). Betamethasone is most effective when administered within 1 week of delivery. Outcome research underscores the importance of antenatal maternal corticosteroid administration even for threatened, moderately preterm delivery.

A 2021 systematic review and meta-analysis of preconception and periconception interventions failed to support the use of micronutrients in preventing preterm birth or low birth weight (LBW) delivery; however, the use of iron and folic acid supplementation decreased the incidence of small for gestational age delivery (Partap et al., 2022). Maternal bedrest, at home or in the hospital, is commonly prescribed to mothers with preterm labor; however, there is little evidence to either support or refute its efficacy in prolonging pregnancy. Prophylactic tocolytics are of no benefit, although tocolysis in the presence of preterm labor may prolong pregnancy to allow the administration of maternal corticosteroids. Interventions aimed at improving maternal health prior to conception, managing preexisting hypertension and diabetes, decreasing smoking during pregnancy, and maintaining adequate interpregnancy intervals may reduce preterm birth rates overall.

Some prenatal treatments are aimed not at stopping preterm delivery but improving the clinical condition of the fetus at delivery. When feasible, the mother-fetal dyad should be transferred to a center with expertise in managing preterm labor, high-risk deliveries, and care of high-risk newborns. This proactive transfer will improve infant outcomes and allow the mother and infant to be in the same location after delivery. Regardless of the delivery site there should be at least one person whose primary responsibility is the neonate and who is capable of initiating resuscitation. Either that person or someone else who is immediately available should have the skills required to perform a complete neonatal resuscitation (AAP & ACOG, 2017).

ASSOCIATED CONDITIONS OF THE PRETERM INFANT

The infant delivered very prematurely will appear distressed, smaller, and less able to transition from intrauterine to extrauterine life. Respiratory distress, poor skin integrity, hypothermia, hypoglycemia, and a lack of subcutaneous fat characterize the premature newborn.

ANEMIA

At birth, the relative increase in oxygen content and the increase in oxygen delivery to the tissues results in a decrease of erythropoietin (EPO) production and suppression of erythropoiesis. The subsequent physiologic anemia of infancy results in the full-term infant's hemoglobin falling to 11 g/dL by 8 to 12 weeks of age. In the preterm infant, this response occurs more rapidly and with a more significant decrease in hemoglobin, marked by a nadir of 7 to 8 g/dL at 4 to 6 weeks of age (Cibulskis et al., 2021). This situation is further aggravated by reduced iron stores, blood loss through repeat blood draws, and the infant's short erythrocyte survival time.

No single, specific definition for anemia exists in this population; hemoglobin level or hematocrit value must be considered in conjunction with the infant's age and clinical condition. Tachycardia, tachypnea, apnea, poor growth, feeding difficulties, increased oxygen requirement, and acidosis are nonspecific symptoms of anemia. In the preterm infant, comorbidities (including respiratory distress, chronic lung disease [CLD], LBW, congenital heart disease, and problematic apnea) may worsen the physiologic symptoms. Severe anemia, relative to the oxygen-carrying capacity of the blood, can result in white matter injury and may contribute to NEC (Cibulskis et al., 2021).

Management of neonatal anemia aims to optimize oxygen-carrying capacity and support the hemodynamically unstable patient. Delayed cord clamping at birth has become a standard for the increasing transfer of blood from the placenta, with the resulting decreased need for blood transfusion (Cibulskis et al., 2021). Minimizing blood loss through phlebotomy in the NICU is an important measure to reduce the need for blood transfusions. Supplementation of 2 to 4 mg/kg of elemental iron per day, increased to 6 mg/kg/day for infants receiving exogenous EPO, is standard care. Recombinant human EPO appears to increase erythropoiesis and reticulocyte count. Despite the variation in blood transfusion protocols, as many as 42% of very LBW (VLBW) and 80% of extremely LBW (ELBW) infants require blood transfusions (Cibulskis et al., 2021). Attempts to minimize blood loss, supplementation with iron and EPO, and utilization of split units of packed red blood cells may reduce donor exposures and overall blood transfusions.

APNEA

Apnea of prematurity is defined as sudden cessation of breathing that lasts for at least 20 seconds or is accompanied by bradycardia and oxygen desaturation in an infant less than 37 weeks of gestational age. Apnea can be categorized by its etiology: Central apnea occurs because of immature respiratory control mechanisms; obstructive apnea occurs due to the collapsibility of the chest wall and diaphragm; mixed apnea results when components of both types coexist. Apnea of prematurity and newborn periodic breathing patterns are consequences of an immature respiratory control system (Erickson et al., 2021). Apnea of prematurity is expected in infants born less than 28 weeks of gestation, while experienced by only 10% after 34 weeks postmenstrual age (PMA) (Erickson et al., 2021). Apnea of prematurity is believed to resolve by 37 weeks PMA but may persist to 43 to 44 weeks PMA, particularly in children born at less than 28 weeks of gestation. This prolonged incidence of apnea/bradycardia events in extremely premature infants may indicate that the central nervous system develops slower in these infants.

During the NICU stay, methylxanthines are the primary choice of pharmacologic treatment for apnea of prematurity (Erickson et al., 2021). Caffeine is preferred over theophylline owing to its wide therapeutic index, safety profile, and longer half-life (Erickson et al., 2021). The timing of caffeine discontinuation and NICU discharge varies by institution; however, most will observe the infant for 3 to 8 days after discontinuing caffeine (Erickson et al., 2021). The routine use of home cardiorespiratory monitors varies significantly by geographic and institutional preference and has not been shown to result in an earlier discharge (Erickson et al., 2021). Similarly, commercially available home pulse oximeters have not been studied for effectiveness, benefits, or ability to prevent potential life-threatening events.

BRONCHOPULMONARY DYSPLASIA/CHRONIC LUNG DISEASE

In the 1960s, neonatal lung injury and its radiographic findings were classified as BPD by Norway et al.

(1967). The terms BPD and CLD of prematurity are often used interchangeably in the medical literature. BPD is defined for infants born less than 32 weeks of gestation as the need for supplemental oxygen at 28 days of life. For infants born greater than 32 weeks of gestation, it is defined as the need for supplemental oxygen at 36 weeks of corrected age. Physiologic conditions associated with prematurity, including surfactant deficiency, pneumonia, sepsis, meconium aspiration, pulmonary hypoplasia, persistent pulmonary hypertension, and congenital anomalies, predispose the premature infant to respiratory difficulties.

The progression and treatments of respiratory distress in preterm infants have undergone many changes during the last 60 years. Ventilation strategies, the routine use of antenatal steroids, and exogenous surfactant therapy have increased the viability and reduced associated comorbidities in infants born preterm. CLD complicates all other aspects of care, increases the financial and social burden of the family, and contributes to adverse outcomes.

NECROTIZING ENTEROCOLITIS

Although many factors, including altered intestinal microbiota and enteral feedings, have been implicated as causative agents for NEC, the only clear predisposing condition for NEC is prematurity. NEC is a gastrointestinal emergency that may develop insidiously over days or acutely as a life-threatening event. Nonspecific symptoms include abdominal distention, feeding intolerance, gastric residuals, guaiac-positive stools, bilious vomiting, and lethargy. Early and aggressive treatment includes antibiotics, bowel rest, serial radiographic studies to evaluate the bowel, and supportive therapies for disseminated intravascular coagulation and shock (Rich & Dolgin, 2017). Pneumatosis intestinalis and portal vein gas are pathognomonic signs of NEC. Perforation of the bowel may lead to bowel necrosis and the need for surgical resection. Surgical intervention, ranging from open surgical resection to the placement of a peritoneal drain, occurs in 50% of cases (Rich & Dolgin, 2017).

NEC results in increased risk for all other complications of prematurity, including IVH, periventricular leukomalacia (PVL), BPD, retinopathy of prematurity (ROP), poor growth, and gastrointestinal-specific complications such as short bowel syndrome, dysmotility, and strictures (Bazacliu & Neu, 2019). Breastmilk feeding in the preterm infant has been shown to reduce the incidence of NEC (Rich & Dolgin, 2017). Probiotics have been advocated for the prevention of NEC; however, inconclusive evidence, coupled with unavailability of pharmaceutic grade products in the United States, necessitates that usage occurs only after careful conversations regarding risks and benefits (Poindexter & Committee on Fetus and Newborn, 2021). The economic burden of NEC because of prolonged hospitalization, resource utilization, surgeries, and associated comorbidities is estimated to range from $500 million to $1 billion in the United States annually (Bazacliu & Neu, 2019).

NEONATAL SEPSIS

Neonatal sepsis is classified based on the timing of symptom onset: early (vertical transmission from mother to infant presents between birth and 72 hours of age) or late (typically acquired horizontally from the environment but may be delayed vertical transmission, which presents >72 hours of life). Maternal factors such as lack of prenatal care, substance abuse, and chorioamnionitis (also called intraamniotic infection) may contribute to early delivery (Glaser et al., 2021).

Preterm infants are at increased risk for sepsis due to immaturity, invasive treatment devices, congenital anomalies, and delayed enteral feedings (Glaser et al., 2021). *Escherichia coli* is the most common cause of morbidity and mortality associated with early-onset sepsis, while less common pathogens include *Streptococcus pneumoniae, Staphylococcus aureus, Enterococcus* spp., gram-negative bacilli (*Enterobacter* spp. and *Haemophilus influenzae*), and *Listeria monocytogenes* (Glaser et al., 2021). Late-onset sepsis is most often caused by gram-positive bacteria (coagulase-negative staphylococci, group B strep [GBS], and *S. aureus*) but can also be caused by fungi, viruses, and gram-negative bacteria (*E. coli, Klebsiella pneumonia, Serratia marcescens, Enterobacter* spp., and *Pseudomonas aeruginosa*) (Glaser et al., 2021).

Prevention of infection is a critical goal in the care of the preterm infant; however, immunologic limitations, physiologic stress, inadequate nutrition, and nosocomial exposures in the NICU constantly challenge this goal. The preterm infant born before 32 weeks of gestation receives a limited quantity of the maternal antibody immunoglobulin G (IgG) that normally crosses the placenta in greater quantities late in the third trimester. In addition, the preterm infant has a limited ability to generate IgG, which, coupled with deficiencies in complement, neutrophil, and phagocytic function, places the preterm infant at greater risk for sepsis.

The 2019 AAP and ACOG recommendations include universal GBS screening of all females between 36 and 38 weeks of gestation and all females who present in preterm labor. Treatment with intrapartum antibiotics is recommended for females who are GBS positive and have had a previous child with GBS infection or whose GBS status is unknown. Risk-based assessment is advocated to balance the risks associated with empiric antibiotic therapy in the neonate (AAP & ACOG, 2017).

PATENT DUCTUS ARTERIOSUS

The ductus arteriosus is a fetal shunt that connects the pulmonary artery with the descending aorta and facilitates blood return to the placenta, typically closing in the first few days of life. In the preterm infant, the persistence of ductus arteriosus and the subsequent increased pulmonary blood flow can result in respiratory compromise, pulmonary edema, pulmonary hemorrhage, and decreased blood flow to other portions of the body (Hamrick et al., 2020). Clinical symptomatology includes a systolic murmur, bounding peripheral pulses, and pulmonary venous congestion by the third postnatal day. More than 50% of infants born less than 28 weeks of gestation will experience a patent ductus arteriosus (PDA). Infants with small, nonhemodynamically significant PDA may be discharged prior to ductal closures with recommendations for follow-up by primary care or cardiology as appropriate.

A ductal diameter greater than 1.5 mm, as measured on a transthoracic echocardiogram in the first hours of life, is predictive of a hemodynamically significant PDA, although no consensus exists for defining closure criteria (Hamrick et al., 2020). Pharmacologic closure with prostaglandin inhibitors has been the mainstay of nonsurgical treatment of a PDA, traditionally with intravenous indomethacin. Newer formulations of prostaglandin inhibitors, including oral ibuprofen, appear to have increased safety profiles and equivalent efficacy in treating PDA and may be the preferred choice for treating symptomatic infants with PDA over 6 days of age (Hamrick et al., 2020). Paracetamol appears less effective but may have a role in infants in which indomethacin or ibuprofen are ineffective or contraindicated (Hamrick et al., 2020). Alternative methods for closing the hemodynamically significant PDA include catheter-based closure and surgical ligation.

PERIVENTRICULAR/INTRAVENTRICULAR HEMORRHAGE

Periventricular/intraventricular hemorrhage (PIVH) results from bleeding in the germinal matrix, often within the first 3 days of life, with 95% occurring prior to day 7 (Mukerji et al., 2015). Gestational age at birth is inversely related to the occurrence of IVH; the younger the infant at birth, the more likely to develop an IVH, with an overall incidence of 25% (Hand et al., 2020). The classification used for IVH, described by Papile et al. (1978), includes the following: grade I, germinal matrix hemorrhage; grade II, IVH; grade III, IVH with dilation of the ventricle; and grade IV, IVH with the extension of bleeding into the brain parenchyma (Papile, 2002). Research suggests mild and severe PIVH contribute to adverse long-term outcomes compared to those without PIVH (Mukerji et al., 2015). The increasing severity of PIVH is associated with increasing disability, but it is important to recognize that mild PIVH is not benign (Mukerji et al., 2015). PVL is a disorder of the periventricular cerebral white matter, described as cystic or diffuse, that occurs most often in preterm infants less than 30 weeks of gestation (Hand et al., 2020). PVL is associated with significantly worse neurologic outcomes.

Neuroimaging recommendations for the preterm infant born less than 30 weeks of gestation include an initial cranial ultrasound within the first 7 days of life, a repeat between weeks 4 and 6, and a third ultrasound prior to discharge (Hand et al., 2020). Nonsedated magnetic resonance imaging may be considered based on clinical course, clinician, and family discussion. Infants born over 30 weeks og gestation who have a complicated clinical course or have additional risk factors may be included in the neuroimaging protocol. Treatment is supportive; however, it may include shunts if hydrocephalus develops.

RETINOPATHY OF PREMATURITY

ROP is a process of incomplete vascularization of the retina and the arresting of normal retinal development due to preterm birth. If untreated, this condition can lead to visual impairment and blindness (Fierson et al., 2018). ROP develops in phases and is classified by stages. Phase I occurs as the normal vascularization is interrupted by the hyperoxic extrauterine life, resulting in vascular injury and retinal avascularity. The second phase of abnormal neovascularization is a response to the increased demands of the developing retina and the relative hypoxia experienced from the vascular injury. Retinal examinations must be performed by an experienced and confident ophthalmologist with examinations of the preterm infant (Fierson et al., 2018). The 2018 AAP Section on Ophthalmology recommendations for screening include all infants with birth weights less than 1500 g, infants less than 30 weeks of gestation, select infants between 1500 and 2000 g, and those greater than 30 weeks of gestation with an unstable clinical course or those determined by the neonatal clinician to be at increased risk (Fierson et al., 2018). The 2018 guidelines acknowledge the use of digital image interpretation and evolving treatments such as bevacizumab and anti-VEGF treatments (Fierson et al., 2018). Follow-up examinations should continue, with the frequency determined by the ophthalmologist, until full vascularization is complete (Fierson et al., 2018).

NUTRITION IN THE NICU

PARENTERAL NUTRITION

Parenteral nutrition consisting of carbohydrates, lipids, amino acids, electrolytes, and other micronutrients is a lifesaving source of nutrition for premature infants. Nutrition for premature infants must balance caloric intake with the demands of comorbid conditions, immature metabolic and gastrointestinal systems, and risks of immunologic insufficiency. There is ongoing debate as to the ideal levels and formulations of protein and lipids in parenteral nutrition for preterm infants unable to tolerate enteral feedings. Complications of parenteral nutrition are mechanical, metabolic, or infectious in nature. Mechanical and infectious complications are related to the intravenous delivery catheter, central or peripheral, as a source of infection, infiltration, or other mechanical malfunction. Metabolic complications include cholestasis (defined as direct bilirubin >2 mg/dL in an infant receiving parenteral nutrition for >2 weeks), hyperglycemia or hypoglycemia, abnormal mineral or electrolyte levels, and elevated triglycerides.

ENTERAL FEEDING

The ultimate nutritional goal for any infant is tolerance of enteral feedings that supply adequate volume and calories for sustained and appropriate growth. Small-volume trophic feeds increase the production of gastric hormones, including gastrin and motilin, and support gut maturation. A 2019 review supports the introduction of trophic feeds for very preterm or VLBW infants in the first 48 hours of life, ideally with breastmilk with subsequent advancement of the feeding of greater than 24 mL/kg/day as tolerated (Kwok et al., 2019). Extremely preterm or ELBW infants may require a slower, more conservative advancement of feeds. Clinically stable, preterm infants above 30 weeks of gestation may be able to avoid parenteral nutrition with the institution of enteral feedings shortly after birth.

Early feedings are typically delivered via nasogastric or orogastric tube, in either a continuous or bolus feeding schedule. Some infants are thought to be mature enough to begin nutritive sucking with adequate respiratory control as early as 32 weeks of gestation; however, this develops between 34 and 36 weeks of gestation in most infants. Attainment of full enteral feedings is crucial to adequate growth and bone mineralization during the postnatal period. Poor nutrition and inadequate intakes of calcium and phosphorus place the preterm infant at risk of fractures and rickets.

Caloric requirements of preterm infants range from 100 to 120 kcal/kg/day for sustained growth of 15 to 25 g/day. Preterm infants with increased energy expenditure (e.g., those with CLD) may require 120 to 160 kcal/kg/day, necessitating manipulation of the caloric density of the feedings. Using commercially available formulas at 24, 27, or 30 kcal/oz with formula-fed infants may provide additional calories. Breastmilk, while the preferred enteral feeding for all infants, can be challenging to meet the increased caloric needs of the VLBW infants within the volumes tolerated (Parker et al., 2021). Mothers who have delivered a preterm infant will have breastmilk with higher protein concentrations for the first 10 to 12 weeks after birth; however, this is still less than what is recommended for preterm infants (Parker et al., 2021). Human milk fortification may be required to meet the preterm infant's caloric needs. Education and recommendations should be provided to caregivers regarding the safe usage of commercially available human milk fortifiers (Parker et al., 2021).

PRIMARY CARE MANAGEMENT

As a standard of care, premature infants are discharged from the NICU when they are physically mature. This state of physiologic stability is typically achieved when the infant is breathing without respiratory support, feeding orally (either by breast or bottle), maintaining adequate temperature, and showing a sustained pattern of growth, usually between 36 and 37 weeks of gestation (Velumula et al., 2020). Infants who are otherwise physically mature but have difficulty with respiratory stability or meeting nutritional demands may be discharged with medical technology support such as supplemental oxygen, ventilator, and enteral feeding pumps (Velumula et al., 2020).

Overall, infants born preterm represent a unique category of children with established or potential special health care needs that benefit from comprehensive follow-up and continued surveillance (Boone et al., 2019). Primary care providers report limited training or educational experience focused on children born preterm (Kelly & Dean, 2017). Outpatient collaborative care partnerships with neonatal or pediatric health care providers who have experience with medically complex premature infants' needs are ideal for facilitating a smooth transition to the home environment (Bowles et al., 2016). Unfortunately, these partnerships are not available in all geographic regions and are typically restricted to medically complex infants, leaving most infants born preterm in the care of typical primary care providers.

Children born preterm experience chronic conditions common to all children but experience them with increased frequency. Utilizing the National Survey of Children's Health data, researchers identified the six most frequently occurring chronic health conditions in children as attention-deficit/hyperactivity disorder (ADHD), anxiety, asthma, learning disability, speech problems, and developmental delay (Kelly, 2018). These conditions occurred with increased frequency in those born less than 37 weeks compared to term-born peers (Kelly, 2018). Because these conditions are not unique to children born preterm, the link between preterm birth and these conditions is often overlooked. However, this link is critical because recognizing risk provides an opportunity for primary care providers to modify the expression of that risk with early diagnosis, referral for services, and treatment.

The first comprehensive clinical practice recommendations for addressing preterm birth history across the life span were published in 2021 (Kelly et al., 2021). These evidence-based recommendations were developed based on existing research, with input from an interdisciplinary group of health care providers regarding agreement and feasibility. The recommendations address (1) assessment and diagnosis, (2) prevention and management, and (3) referral and treatment (Kelly et al., 2021). The recommendation and level of evidence support are identified in

Table **35.2**   Preterm Birth History Recommendations

ASSESSMENT/DIAGNOSIS	AGREEMENT	FEASIBILITY	SUPPORTING LITERATURE	AACN LEVEL OF EVIDENCE
Preterm birth history, of any gestation <37 wk, should be obtained for every new patient, at all ages, and be included in past medical history for all ages.	96%	96%	Crump et al., 2021 Kajantie et al., 2019 Raju et al., 2017	B C D C
Adult health care providers should elicit preterm birth history at initial and interval visits to incorporate:	93%	85%	Raju et al., 2017	D C
• Recognition of preterm birth as an additive and lifelong risk factor for pulmonary, cardiovascular, and metabolic conditions	96%	96%	Hovi et al., 2016 Islam et al., 2015 Raju et al., 2017	A C C
• Recognition of preterm birth history as an additive and lifelong risk factor for psychiatric and mental health conditions	100%	96%	Aarnoudse-Moens et al., 2009 Allotey et al., 2018 Burnett et al., 2011 Cassiano et al., 2016 Matthewson et al., 2017 Sømhovd et al., 2012	A A A C C A
The anticipatory guidance and education of families of children born preterm should emphasize:				
• The importance of all vaccinations, including yearly influenza vaccines	100%	100%	Kroger et al., 2020	D
• The vital role families play in supporting speech-language skills	100%	100%	Barre, et al., 2011 Moore et al., 2013 van Noort-van der Spek et al., 2012	A A A A
• Access to community support systems to support the family, reduce poverty	100%	100%	Kelly & Li, 2019 McGowan & Vohr, 2019 Moreira et al., 2014	C C C
• The importance of preparing the family and preterm adolescent for transition to adult care, including informing future providers of preterm birth history	96%	92%	Raju et al., 2017	C
• Preterm birth history, of any gestation <37 wk, should be considered a lifelong and additional cardiovascular risk factor, particularly for females and those with other family history and lifestyle risks	100%	100%	Hovi et al., 2016 Markopoulou et al., 2019 Raju et al., 2017	A A C
• Blood pressure screening, consistent with NHBPED 2004 and AAP 2017 guidelines should occur in all children born preterm at or before the 3-year-old routine health visit	96%	96%	deJong et al., 2012 Flynn et al., 2017 Hovi et al., 2016 Parkinson et al., 2013 Raju et al., 2017	A D A A C

Continued

Table 35.2	Preterm Birth History Recommendations—cont'd			
ASSESSMENT/DIAGNOSIS	**AGREEMENT**	**FEASIBILITY**	**SUPPORTING LITERATURE**	**AACN LEVEL OF EVIDENCE**
• Preterm birth history should be specifically considered at the 9- to 11-year-old routine health visits in conjunction with dyslipidemia screening and cardiovascular risk assessment	100%	100%	Parkinson et al., 2013	A
• Lifestyle modifications to combat cardiovascular risk and metabolic syndrome should be actively encouraged at every routine health visit for families and individuals with preterm birth history	100%	96%	deJong et al., 2012 Markopoulou et al., 2019 Parkinson et al., 2013	A A A
• Preterm birth history, of any gestation <37 wk, should be considered a lifelong and additional pulmonary risk factor	96%	100%	Been et al., 2014 Gough et al., 2012 Islam et al., 2015 Kotecha et al., 2018 Raju et al., 2017 Sonnenschein-van der Voort et al., 2014	C C C A C A
• Lifestyle modifications to combat pulmonary risk should be actively encouraged at every routine health visit for families and individuals with preterm birth history	100%	100%	Been et al., 2014 Collaco et al., 2018 den Dekker et al., 2016 Edwards et al., 2015 Kotecha et al., 2013 Kotecha et al., 2018	C C A A A A
• Specifically avoidance of smoking, secondhand smoke, and air pollution/environmental toxins	100%	100%	Kotecha et al., 2013 Kotecha et al., 2018	A A
• Preterm birth history, of any gestation <37 wk, should be considered a lifelong and additional metabolic syndrome risk factor	96%	95%	Markopoulou, 2019	A
• Monitor total body fat mass at annual visits	83%	95%	Markopoulou, 2019	A
• Fasting glucose, serum insulin levels, and lipid profile screening should occur	78%	95%	Markopoulou, 2019	A
Preterm birth history, of any gestation <37 wk, should be considered a lifelong and additional risk factor when considering referral for developmental delay, speech-language disorder, developmental coordination disorder.	100%	100%	Aarnoudse-Moens et al., 2009 Chan et al., 2016 Geldof et al., 2012 Moore et al., 2013	A A A A
Positive screening for developmental delay should result in referral for preventative/supportive services in patients of all ages.	100%	100%	Agrawal et al., 2018 Moore et al., 2013	A A
Positive screening for speech-language delay should result in a prompt referral to speech-language services.	100%	95%	Aarnoudse-Moens et al., 2009 Barre et al., 2011 van Noort-van der Spek et al., 2012	A A A

Table 35.2 Preterm Birth History Recommendations—cont'd

ASSESSMENT/DIAGNOSIS	AGREEMENT	FEASIBILITY	SUPPORTING LITERATURE	AACN LEVEL OF EVIDENCE
Positive screening for developmental coordination disorder should result in referral for preventative/supportive services in patients of all ages.	100%	91%	Allotey et al., 2018 de Kievet et al., 2009 Edwards et al., 2011 FitzGerald et al., 2018 Moreira et al., 2014	A A A A C
Children born preterm of any gestation <37 wk, should be screened at age 5 yr for motor delay and developmental coordination disorder.	96%	95%	de Kievet et al., 2009 FitzGerald et al., 2018	A A
Preterm birth history, of any gestation <37 wk, should be recognized as a lifelong and additional risk factor when determining eligibility for academic support services for children and adolescents.	87%	100%	Aarnoudse-Moens et al., 2009 Allotey et al., 2018 Chan et al., 2016 Kovatchy et al., 2015 Moreira et al., 2014 Raju et al., 2017	A A C A C C
Preterm birth history, of any gestation <37 wk, should be considered a lifelong and additional risk factor when considering referral for mental and behavioral health concerns.	91%	100%	Aarnoudse-Moens et al., 2009 Allotey et al., 2018 Burnett et al., 2011 Cassiano et al., 2016 Matthewson et al., 2017 Somhovd et al., 2012	A A A C C A
Positive screenings, family or teacher concerns for behavioral concerns should be referred to appropriate behavioral and family support services.	100%	100%	Agrawal et al., 2018 Kajantie et al., 2019 Matthewson et al., 2017	A A A

AACN, American Association of Colleges of Nursing; AAP, American Academy of Pediatrics; NHBPED, National High Blood Pressure Education Program.
From Kelly, M.M., Tobias, J., & Griffith, P. (2021). Addressing preterm birth history with clinical practice recommendations across the life course. *Journal of Pediatric Health Care, 35*(3), e5–e20.

Table 35.2. Consistent with several systematic and narrative reviews and the NIH Executive Summary, *Adults Born Preterm: Epidemiology and Biologic Basis for Adult Outcomes* (Raju et al., 2017), the recommendations advocate a paradigm shift relative to preterm birth history. Health care providers must consider the health implications of preterm birth history across the life span. This shift begins with consistent and continued documentation of preterm birth as a feature of past medical history requires an appreciation for the additive health risks and compels health care providers to take steps to mitigate those risks.

CONDITION-SPECIFIC CONCERNS

The Late Preterm Infant

In 2019, the AAP updated the clinical guidance for late preterm (born 34–37 weeks of gestation) and early-term infants (born 37–39 weeks of gestation), reinforcing the vulnerability of infants born even a little early (Stewart et al., 2019). Depending on the infant's condition at birth, the late preterm infant may be admitted to the NICU, special care nursery, or the well-baby nursery. The late preterm infant may appear to be of good weight and begin to transition appropriately but may fail to maintain this stability. Therefore those caring for late preterm infants in the well-baby nursery or after hospital discharge should appreciate the risk for respiratory distress, hypoglycemia associated with poor feeding, temperature instability, hyperbilirubinemia, and infection (Stewart et al., 2019). These conditions contribute to the two- to threefold increase in hospital readmission rates experienced by late preterm infants (Stewart et al., 2019).

In 2022, the AAP revised guidelines for the management of hyperbilirubinemia for infants born 35 to 40 weeks of gestation, with an emphasis on prevention, use of total serum bilirubin levels for treatment decisions, the need for a bilirubin measurement (serum or transcutaneous) prior to discharge, and a revision to the initiation of phototherapy graph (Kemper et al., 2022). The 2022 guidelines present gestational age and chronologic age thresholds for initiating phototherapy and exchange transfusion for infants without hyperbilirubinemia neurotoxicity risk factors and separate thresholds for infants with one or more risk factors (Kemper et al., 2022).

Respiratory

Infants with BPD should be followed routinely by pulmonology and cardiology, including coordination of supplemental oxygen, ventilatory support, and diuretics, as well as monitoring for pulmonary and systemic hypertension (Velumula et al., 2020). Weaning of oxygen support requires significant caregiver education and involvement, with the understanding that weaning requires balancing the infant's effort of breathing, pulse oximeter reading during strenuous activities (e.g., feeding or playing) and sleep, maintenance of adequate growth, and cardiovascular testing for those with pulmonary hypertension (Velumula et al., 2020).

Infants born preterm, with or without a BPD/CLD diagnosis, are at increased risk for rehospitalization for respiratory conditions in the first year after NICU discharge (Fierro et al., 2019). Systematic reviews of pulmonary outcomes suggest that school-age children born preterm experience wheezing and decreased respiratory function independent of a BPD/CLD diagnosis (Kelly & Griffith, 2020). Decreased pulmonary function, increased wheezing, and asthma diagnosis persists into adolescence and adulthood (Kelly & Griffith, 2019).

Cardiovascular

Preterm infants may be at risk for developing hypertension, possibly related to complications from umbilical artery catheters or other acute care interventions. Premature infants should have blood pressure measurements at all routine well examinations. Hypertension screening should be done several times in the first year of life and then routinely in childhood. Screening equipment should be of appropriate size and used consistently to track trends in measurement. Pediatric cardiac evaluations, including an echocardiogram, are indicated if hypertension is identified.

A significant increase in hypertension in adolescents and adults born preterm warrants an ongoing assessment. Children who were not initially hypertensive may begin to exhibit increased systolic blood pressure in adolescence. Lifestyle modifications and considerations of pharmacologic treatments should occur with the recognition of preterm birth history as an additive risk factor. Decreased physical activity and decreased pulmonary function may require creative approaches to increasing daily activity levels.

Gastroesophageal Reflux

Preterm infants almost universally experience some degree of gastroesophageal reflux (GER) as a function of transient lower esophageal sphincter relaxation (Eichenwald & Committee on Fetus and Newborn, 2018). This phenomenon is exacerbated by a liquid diet, positioning, nasogastric tube, and relative gastric distention (Eichenwald & Committee on Fetus and Newborn, 2018). Evaluation of GER in preterm infants is best accomplished using multichannel

intraesophageal impedance monitoring, with or without a pH sensor (Eichenwald & Committee on Fetus and Newborn, 2018). The use of pH monitoring alone is of little value due to the frequent feedings and higher baseline pH (Eichenwald & Committee on Fetus and Newborn, 2018). Clinical GER diagnoses include feeding intolerance, poor growth, apnea, desaturations, bradycardia, worsening pulmonary disease, and associated behavioral signs, including arching, irritability, and perceived discomfort.

Traditional recommendations for nonpharmacologic management, including head-up positioning, have shown minimal efficacy, with placement in a car seat exacerbating GER symptoms (Eichenwald & Committee on Fetus and Newborn, 2018). The risk for sudden infant death syndrome (SIDS) outweighs the GER benefit of lateral or prone positioning and should be avoided. Thickening feedings will reduce regurgitation episodes but not alter GER's acidic nature. Thickening agents, specifically xanthan gum, are associated with late-onset NEC in preterm infants (Eichenwald & Committee on Fetus and Newborn, 2018). Pharmacologic agents are regularly prescribed to preterm infants; however, their efficacy and safety in the preterm population are not established, and the AAP advocates for sparing use (Eichenwald & Committee on Fetus and Newborn, 2018).

HEALTH MAINTENANCE
Growth and Nutrition

Growth charts from the NICU should be part of the discharge summary and be incorporated into the medical chart in the primary care practice. Measurements for length, weight, and head circumference should be plotted according to corrected age, not chronologic age, until approximately age 2 years. Weight gain trends should be well established before NICU discharge and closely followed in the primary care setting, as the infant's feeding endurance may limit growth, coordination of oral feeds, energy expenditure, and caloric density of feeds. After discharge, human milk with fortification should be supported as appropriate to meet the caloric demands of continued growth. Formula-fed infants should continue to receive preterm formulas that contain increased protein, minerals, and trace elements until the infant reaches term (40 weeks) and may be continued for another 3 to 6 months.

Infants discharged with enteral feeding support, nasogastric tube, or gastrointestinal tube are at risk for conditions related to tube malfunction, dislodgement, displacement, and stoma infection (Velumula et al., 2020). Caregivers require ongoing device support, advancing oral feedings if appropriate, and coordination of in-home nursing support.

Of critical importance is reframing the message of healthy weight gain to caregivers of children born preterm. During the NICU stay, a large focus is on tolerating feedings and gaining weight. While weight gain remains essential, the focus must shift to healthy weight gain. Children born less than 32 weeks of gestation who gained excessive weight in the first year (defined as 700 g/month in the first year of life) experienced a 3.72-fold increase in the risk of wheezing in preschool and a 4.47-fold increased risk at school age (Kelly & Griffith, 2020). The first 1000 days are critical for developing and preventing obesity, especially in children born preterm (Ingol et al., 2021). Obesity is underdiagnosed in the preterm population, even in children with two or more BMI measurements at the 98th percentile (Ingol et al., 2021). Children born preterm are more likely to be born into families that experience food insecurity and decreased socioeconomic advantage, which may limit the availability of healthy food choices (Ingol et al., 2021).

Immunizations

The AAP recommends that all preterm and LBW infants receive recommended vaccines, at full doses, at the same chronologic age as their full-term peers, regardless of gestational age and birth weight (Advisory Committee on Immunization Practice [ACIP], 2022). Despite these recommendations, preterm and LBW infants are underimmunized (Nestander et al., 2018). This underimmunization has been associated with a gestational age of less than 32 weeks, CLD, missed health care supervision visits, and provider changes (Nestander et al., 2018). With twins and higher multiples, sibling immunizations should be coordinated when possible. Immunizations during the infant's NICU stay should be documented on the infant's discharge summary.

All 2-month immunizations may be given simultaneously in preterm and LBW infants (ACIP, 2022). Despite these recommendations, the injections may be spread out over a few days if the infant is still hospitalized when receiving the 2-month immunizations. This practice appears to be based on unit or provider tradition, aimed at mitigating potential cardiorespiratory instability associated with vaccinations (Gopal et al., 2018). Hospitalized infants should be observed for 48 hours after immunization prior to discharge.

Combination vaccines are appropriate for use in premature infants, but those containing hepatitis B components should be delayed until the baby is 6 weeks and over 2000 g (ACIP, 2022). If a mother's hepatitis B status is unknown, the preterm infant born less than 2000 g should receive a dose of the hepatitis B vaccine and hepatitis B immune globulin (HBIG) within 12 hours of birth. For the infant with less than 2000 g, this dose does not count in the regular series and should be repeated according to the immunization schedule. The HBIG may be delayed if the infant is over 2000 g for up to 7 days, pending the mother's hepatitis B surface antigen testing (ACIP, 2022).

Protective immunity is of paramount importance to premature infants. Family and caregivers should be vaccinated yearly for influenza. Caregivers should receive boosters for diseases that may have waning efficacy; most cases of pertussis occurring in children less than 12 months of age can be attributed to the waning immunity of these children's adult and adolescent caregivers. Parents and caregivers of preterm infants may benefit from a Tdap booster rather than a Td booster.

Respiratory syncytial virus (RSV) is a highly contagious respiratory virus that accounts for more than 3 million hospitalizations and 60,000 hospitalized deaths in children less than 5 years of age (Staebler & Blake, 2021). Infection with RSV does not confer immunity, and reinfections occur routinely within the same season. The most current AAP recommendations from 2014 and reaffirmed without change in 2019 limit the usage of palivizumab to preterm infants born less than 29 weeks of gestation and younger than 12 months of age at the start of RSV season (October–May in the United States) (Table 35.3). Infants with CLD or hemodynamically significant congenital heart disease have a slightly broader qualification range. While US Food and Drug Administration approved for wider usage (up to 24 months), monthly immunoprophylaxis with palivizumab is limited by the significant expense, ranging from $6000 to $20,000 per child per season (Staebler & Blake, 2021). Interestingly, following the COVID-19 pandemic, a significant interseasonal spread of RSV prompted the AAP to support the consideration of palivizumab outside the typical October to May season in the United States (AAP, 2021).

Table 35.3 AAP Guidelines for RSV Immunoprophylaxis With Palivizumab

CONDITION	PALIVIZUMAB GUIDELINES
Preterm infant	All infants born <29 wk gestation and <12 mo at start of RSV season
BPD/CLD	All infants born <32 wk gestation and requiring oxygen for at least the first 28 days postbirth All those age <12 mo at start of RSV season All those age 12–24 mo at start of RSV season requiring medications in the last 6 mo
HS-CHD	All those age <12 mo at start of RSV season

AAP, American Academy of Pediatrics; *BPD*, bronchopulmonary dysplasia; *CLD*, chronic lung disease; *HS-CHD*, hemodynamically significant congenital heart disease; *RSV*, respiratory syncytial virus.

From American Academy of Pediatrics Committee on Infectious Diseases & American Academy of Pediatrics Bronchiolitis Guidance Committee. (2014/2019). Updated guidelines for palivizumab prophylaxis among infants and young children at increased risk for hospitalization for respiratory syncytial virus infection. *Pediatrics, 134*(2), 415–420.

Safety

Preterm infants are at particular risk for cardiorespiratory events while seated in the semireclined position of an infant car seat. The AAP recommends that before hospital discharge, all infants less than 37 weeks of gestation should be observed in their own car safety seat to monitor for apnea, bradycardia, and desaturation (Bull et at., 2009). The car seat tolerance test should last for 90 to 120 minutes or the anticipated duration of travel, whichever is longer (Bull et at., 2009). A car bed may be considered for infants unable to maintain cardiorespiratory stability in a car seat. Car beds allow infants to be fully reclined and secured with an internal harness (Bull et at., 2009). When transitioning an infant from a car bed to a car seat, a car seat tolerance test should be conducted in the home or outpatient setting (Bull et at., 2009).

Infants born late preterm are of special consideration and should be included in car seat tolerance testing protocols (Magnarelli et al., 2020). Late preterm infants, with or without NICU stay, experience respiratory control center instability during the first days of transition to extrauterine life. Failure rates of late preterm infants were reported at just under 5%, with 24% of those infants failing repeat testing (Magnarelli et al., 2020).

A smaller, infant-only seat, with a distance from the lowest set of harness slots to the bottom of the seat that is short enough so that the harness is at or below the infant's shoulders, is preferred. The distance from the crotch strap to the back of the seat should be short enough so that the infant's bottom is held back against the seat and does not slide forward. Rolls may be placed laterally to center the infant in the seat; however, items should not be placed under or behind the infant (Fig. 35.1). Recommendations are summarized in Box 35.1. It is important to remember that as these children age, they may still be smaller than their peers and should use booster seats until they meet the recommended weight and height for adult seat belts. Families should be educated that other infant seating equipment, such as swings, backpacks, and slings, may result in the same degree of cardiorespiratory instability.

Travel with a preterm infant poses some challenges. Feedings require frequent stops, and an adult should ride in the back seat with the infant. For the infant home on oxygen and monitoring, traveling may be even more difficult. Monitoring equipment should have battery backup for at least twice the duration of the trip. All equipment should be secured to prevent them from becoming projectiles in an accident. Air travel is best avoided until the infant has developed mature respiratory control and is off supplemental oxygen.

Sleep

While in the NICU, preterm infants are often placed in the prone position to improve respiratory distress,

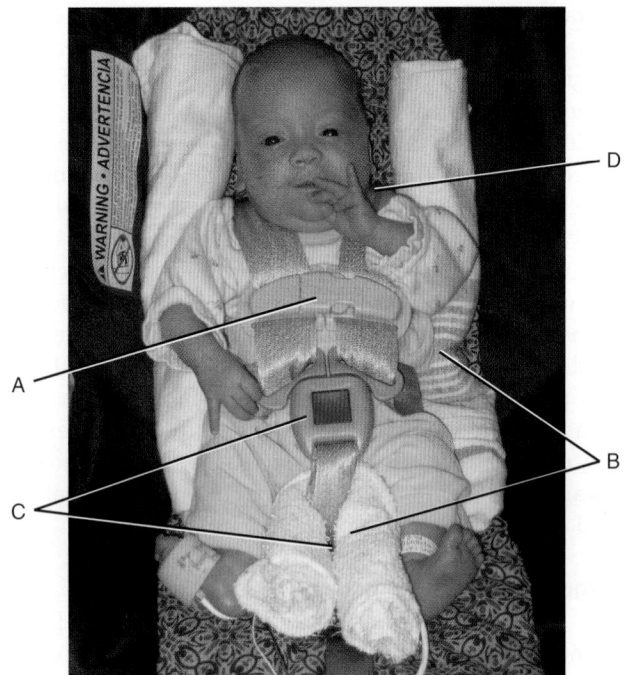

Fig. 35.1 Positioning of premature infant in car safety seat. (A) Retainer clip positioned on infant's chest. (B) Blanket rolls on both sides of trunk and between crotch strap and infant. (C) Distance from lowest set of harness slots to the bottom of the seat should allow the harness to be at or below infant's shoulders. (D) Distance from crotch strap to the back of the seat should be such that the infant's bottom is held back against the seat.

Box 35.1 Premature Infant–Specific Recommendations for Travel

1. Before hospital discharge infants born <37 wk gestation, or with suspected cardiorespiratory instability, should be observed in their own car seat for 90–120 min or the duration of anticipated travel.
2. Choose an infant-only rear-facing seat with a three- or five-point harness, with the shortest distances from crotch strap to seat back. A small cloth can be rolled between the infant and crotch strap to secure the infant.
3. The infant should be positioned with buttocks and back flat against the back of the car safety seat.
4. Avoid the use of aftermarket positioning devices that require the loosening of the harness. Rather use small cloths or blanket rolls to provide lateral support of the head and trunk.
5. Secure monitors or other equipment to prevent from becoming projectiles during travel.
6. Car beds may be indicated for infants unstable in a semireclined position.
7. When possible, an adult should ride in the back seat with the infant.

From Bull, M.J., Engle, W.A., Committee on Injury, Violence, and Poison Prevention, Committee on Fetus and Newborn, & American Academy of Pediatrics. (2009/2013). Safe transportation of preterm and low birth weight infants at hospital discharge. *Pediatrics, 123*(5), 1424–1429.

reduce GER episodes, facilitate developmentally appropriate care, and avoid positional plagiocephaly (Goodstein et al., 2021). This positioning is contrary to the recommendations for SIDS prevention in the home environment. The AAP advocates that education and behaviors should follow the safe home sleeping environment recommendations once the preterm infant is stable and ready to transition to an open crib (Goodstein et al., 2021).

Infants born preterm are at increased risk for brief resolved unexplained events (BRUE), previously defined as apparent life-threatening events (Erickson et al., 2021). The degree of risk is inversely related to gestational age, with the greatest risk seen in infants born at the youngest gestational age. Infants born preterm are also at increased risk for sleep-disordered breathing, which may contribute to the occurrence of BRUE.

Toileting

Toileting should begin when the child shows signs of readiness, as with any healthy child. A retrospective case-control study found that preterm children start toilet training later than full-term children, with no difference between term and preterm babies on the end date of toilet training (Yildiz et al., 2019). Gross and fine motor delays in preterm children may hamper independent toileting and should be taken into consideration.

Health and Developmental Surveillance

High-risk infants should be enrolled in developmental follow-up programs and early intervention; however, most children born preterm do not qualify for these services (Kelly & Griffith, 2020). Qualifications for early intervention vary by state but generally include infants born less than 30 weeks of gestation or those with complex NICU courses. This leaves the identification of concerns and delays to the family, primary care clinician, and educational system.

Behavioral/Mental Health

The incidence of autism spectrum disorder in the general population is reported to be 0.7% to 1.5%, compared to the 7% incidence reported in children born preterm; this increased risk persists despite excluding children with other disabilities from analysis (Kelly & Griffith, 2020). The risk of autism is inversely tied to gestational age, with each additional week of gestation reducing the risk of autism by 5% (Crump et al., 2021). While there is a significant hereditary association with autism spectrum disorder, inflammation and early life environmental exposures may contribute significantly to the increased prevalence of autism in the preterm population (Crump et al., 2021).

The preterm phenotype is described as exhibiting internalizing behaviors rather than externalizing behaviors. The severity of impairment increases with decreasing gestational age; however, no degree of prematurity is free from potential risk (Kelly & Griffith,

2020). Adolescents and young adults born preterm are statistically more likely to experience any psychiatric diagnosis, particularly anxiety, depression, and shyness, than their term peers (Kelly & Griffith, 2019). Conditions identified in childhood, such as ADHD, internalizing behaviors, and social difficulties, continue with increased frequency in adolescence and adulthood.

Dental

Prolonged orotracheal intubation affects the growing palate and may contribute to high arched palates, deep palatal grooves, and impaired future dentition. Nasal and mask continuous positive airway pressure devices may lead to nasal septum and upper lip or gum line deformities. Dental eruption may be delayed in premature infants and further delayed with poor growth or nutrition. Fluoride supplements should follow term infant recommendations. Referral to a pediatric dentist should occur as with any term infant or earlier if there is concern regarding dentition.

Hearing

All term and preterm infants should have automated auditory brainstem response screening before hospital discharge (Early Hearing Detection and Intervention [EHDI], 2019). If the infant fails screening in either ear, a referral should be made to an audiologist with expertise in hearing loss for rescreening and comprehensive evaluation for both ears before 3 months of age (EHDI, 2019). This guideline applies to all infants; however, many preterm infants may remain in the NICU at 3 months of age. Therefore preterm infants should undergo a diagnostic audiology exam prior to discharge from the NICU (EHDI, 2019). Appropriate support services should be implemented as soon as possible to support language development. Any concerns for auditory or communication skills delay should prompt a referral for evaluation and management.

Neurodevelopment

While the incidence of cerebral palsy has remained stable at approximately 2.11 per 1000 live births, the prevalence is highest in those born less than 28 weeks of gestation (Kelly & Griffith, 2020). The presence of motor or coordination impairment ranges from 7% to 72%, dependent on the assessment used, and impairments may persist through childhood into adolescence, increasing the risk of decreased daily activity (Kelly & Griffith, 2020).

A systematic review of school-age outcomes of children born preterm identified an increased risk of attention problems, internalizing behaviors, and executive function difficulties that impair academic performance (Kelly & Griffith, 2020). This is evidenced by the increased utilization of special health care services such as physical therapy, speech therapy, and occupational therapy that persist from childhood into adolescence (Kelly, 2018).

Vision

Premature infants at risk for vision loss due to ROP must have clearly defined follow-up plans with an ophthalmologist familiar with ROP before NICU discharge (Fierson et al., 2018). Primary care providers must verify that these appointments are scheduled and completed and that these infants have ongoing ophthalmologic evaluations (Fierson et al., 2018). Preterm infants, with or without ROP, are at risk of developing strabismus, cataracts, amblyopia, and glaucoma (Fierson et al., 2018). All preterm infants should have a routine ophthalmologic visit 4 to 6 months after NICU discharge, regardless of ROP status (Fierson et al., 2018). The long-term complications of ROP continue to evolve as generations of infants with ROP survive into adulthood.

Transition to Adulthood

Best practices for transition to adult health care providers should be implemented well in advance of the adolescent's targeted transition date. However, unique to this preterm population is that as the preterm birth survivors born after technologic advances of the 1990s reach adulthood, every health care provider, regardless of specialty, is caring for people who were born preterm. Unfortunately, regardless of specialty, health care providers rarely consider preterm birth a relevant part of past medical history for adolescents and young adults. The increased risk of common chronic health conditions persists into adulthood; therefore those who were preterms need to be educated to share their preterm birth history as a feature of their past medical history and may, at times, need to explain its significance to unfamiliar health care providers with the current research.

RESOURCES

Healthy Children:
- Car seat product listing (annually updated listing of commercially available car seats with weight and height parameters): https://www.healthychildren.org/English/safety-prevention/on-the-go/Pages/Car-Safety-Seats-Product-Listing.aspx
- Preemie (educational resources for caregivers and clinician resources): https://www.healthychildren.org/English/ages-stages/baby/preemie/Pages/default.aspx

March of Dimes (a leader in research, education, and advocacy to support healthy mothers and babies): https://www.marchofdimes.org/#

National Institute of Child Health and Human Development (provides resources for caregivers and health care providers regarding preterm birth): https://www.nichd.nih.gov/health/topics/factsheets/preterm

US Department of Transportation (lists car seat inspection centers): https://www.nhtsa.gov/equipment/car-seats-and-booster-seats

Zero to Three (a leader in public and private initiatives to support children from birth to 3 years of age): https://www.zerotothree.org

---

 Summary

Primary Care Needs for the Premature Infant

HEALTH CARE MAINTENANCE

Growth and Development
- Use corrected age to plot height, weight, and head circumference.
- All preterm infants, regardless of gestational age, are at risk for developmental delays.
- Use corrected age and a standardized developmental screening tool.
- Referrals to early intervention should occur as soon as a delay is suspected.

Diet
- Nasogastric tube feedings may be indicated after discharge if all other criteria for discharge are met.
- Breastfeeding is recommended.
- Fortification of breastmilk may be indicated if growth or laboratory values indicate the need.
- Multivitamins and iron supplementation are indicated for infants fed standard formula or unfortified breastmilk. Recommendations for vitamin D should be followed.
- Enriched transitional formula may be used for up to 1 year after hospital discharge.

- Introduction of additional foods should be delayed until the infant shows signs of readiness. Juice and water are not appropriate until after 6 months of corrected age.

Safety
- Home monitoring is not aimed at preventing SIDS but may be indicated as a tool to alert caregivers to prolonged apneic events.
- Infant-only car seats with smaller dimensions are recommended for preterm infants.
- Air travel should be delayed until the infant tolerates lower environmental oxygen concentrations.
- Anticipatory guidance is based on developmental age.

Immunizations
- Immunizations should be administered at the same chronologic ages recommended by the AAP for term infants.
- Preterm infants after 6 months of age and their caretakers should receive the influenza vaccine and COVID-19 vaccines as recommended by the AAP and Centers for Disease Control and Prevention.

- Family/caregivers of preterm infants should receive pertussis boosters.
- RSV prophylaxis should be administered to at-risk infants according to AAP guidelines.

Screening

- *Vision.* Assessment of fixation, alignment, and funduscopic examination is recommended. Ophthalmologic follow-up is necessary for infants with ROP and yearly for all preterm infants.
- *Hearing.* Screening is recommended for all infants before hospital discharge.
  - Prompt referral to audiology and otolaryngology is recommended if hearing loss is suspected.
- *Dental.* Prolonged intubation affects palate and dentition.
  - Tooth eruptions may be delayed, and teeth may be abnormally shaped or discolored.
  - Routine fluoride supplementation is recommended after 6 months of corrected age.
- *Blood pressure.* Hypertension screenings should be done at 1, 2, 6, 12, and 24 months of age and then routinely in childhood.
  - Children with consistently elevated blood pressure should be evaluated for etiology and management.
- *Hematocrit.* Hematocrit values should be evaluated routinely based on history, nutritional status, and symptoms.
- *Urinalysis.* Routine screening is recommended.
- *Tuberculosis.* Routine screening is recommended.

COMMON ILLNESS MANAGEMENT

Differential Diagnosis

- Risk of infection—particularly respiratory infection and bronchiolitis—is increased.
- RSV, herpes simplex virus, *Chlamydia,* group B strep, *S. aureus,* and *E. coli* must all be considered possible pathogens. The risk for *S. pneumoniae* and *H. influenzae* type b infections must be evaluated.

DEVELOPMENTAL ISSUES

Sleep Patterns

- Children may have disorganized sleep patterns.
- Premature infants with poor growth should be woken for feedings every 3 to 4 hours.
- Back to Sleep practices should be balanced with allowing time in the prone position when awake.
- Home monitors do not prevent SIDS.
- All infants should have independent sleep surfaces consistent with AAP recommendations.

Toileting

- Toileting readiness is based on developmental age.
- Gross motor delays may impede toilet training.

Discipline

- Children should be assessed for vulnerable child syndrome.
- Limits should be set as with any other child.
- Prematurity increases a child's risk of behavioral issues.
- Children born preterm are at higher risk for experiencing abuse than full-term children.

Child Care

- Home care or small day care programs are preferred over large day care centers to limit infectious exposures.
- All caregivers should be comfortable with the special needs of the premature child.

Schooling

- Early intervention services may be continued until the child is transitioned to school-based services.
- Education services are crucial for a child with the potential for developmental delays.
- Delayed school entry is not universally recommended and should be considered based on the needs of the individual.

Sexuality

- Adolescents who were born preterm should have normal pubertal sexual development.
- There is an increased incidence of preterm delivery with a family history of preterm delivery.

Transition to Adulthood

- Preexisting developmental or behavioral problems may become more exaggerated.
- Adolescents born preterm report a self-perception of a good quality of life.
- Concerns regarding medical consequences of prematurity, cosmetic deformities, parental overprotection, and communication should be addressed.

FAMILY CONCERNS

- Family concerns include guilt, grief, financial considerations, concerns about developmental outcomes, and attachment issues as a result of prolonged hospitalization.
- Symptoms of depression and intense emotional distress can affect parent-infant bonding and developmental outcomes.

REFERENCES

Aarnoudse-Moens, C. S. H., Weisglas-Kuperus, N., van Goudoever, J. B., & Oosterlaan, J. (2009). Meta-analysis of neurobehavioral outcomes in very preterm and/or very low birth weight children. *Pediatrics, 124*(2), 717–728. doi: 10.1542/peds.2008-2816.

Advisory Committee on Immunization Practice. (2022). General best practice guidelines for immunization: Special situations: Vaccination of preterm infants. Retrieved 8/23/2022 from https://www.cdc.gov/vaccines/hcp/acip-recs/general-recs/special-situations.html.

Agrawal, S., Rao, S. C., Bulsara, M. K., & Patole, S. K. (2018). Prevalence of autism spectrum disorder in preterm infants: A meta-analysis. *Pediatrics, 142*(3), 1–15. doi:10.1542/peds.2018-0134.

Allotey, J., Zamora, J., Cheong-See, F., Kalidindi, M., Arroyo-Manzano, D., Asztalos, E., van der Post, J., Mol, B. W., Moore, D., Birtles, D., Khan, K. S., & Thangaratinam, S. (2018). Cognitive, motor, behavioural and academic performances of children born preterm: A meta-analysis and systematic review involving 64 061 children. *British Journal of Obstetrics and Gynaecology, 125*(1), 16–25. doi:10.1111/1471-0528.14832.

American Academy of Pediatrics (AAP). (2004). Policy statement: Age terminology during the perinatal period. *Pediatrics, 114,* 1362–1364.

American Academy of Pediatrics Committee on Infectious Diseases & American Academy of Pediatrics Bronchiolitis Guidance Committee. (2014). Updated guidelines for palivizumab prophylaxis among infants and young children at increased risk for hospitalization for respiratory syncytial virus infection. *Pediatrics, 134*(2), 415–420.

Reaffirmed February 2019. https://doi.org/10.1542/peds.2014-1665.

American Academy of Pediatrics (AAP) & American College of Obstetricians and Gynecologists. (2017). Guidelines for perinatal care. Washington, DC.

American Academy of Pediatrics. Committee on Infectious Diseases. (2021). Updated guidance: Use of palivizumab prophylaxis to prevent hospitalization from severe respiratory syncytial virus during the 2022–2023 RSV season. In Kimberlin, D. W., Barnett, E. D., Lynfield, R., & Sawyer, M. H. (Eds.), Red book: 2021–2024 report of the Committee on Infectious Diseases. Elk Grove Village, IL: American Academy of Pediatrics. https://doi.org/10.1542/9781610025782.

American College of Obstetricians and Gynecologists (ACOG). (2017). Committee Opinion No 700: Methods for estimating the due date. Obstetrics and Gynecology, 129(5), e150–e154. https://doi.org/10.1097/AOG.0000000000002046.

American College of Obstetricians and Gynecologists (ACOG) & Society for Maternal-Fetal Medicine (SMFM). (2017). Obstetric care consensus No. 6: Periviable birth. Obstetrics and Gynecology, 130(4), e187–e199. https://doi.org/10.1097/AOG.0000000000002352.

Ballard, J. L., Khoury, J. C., Wedig, K., Wang, L., Eilers-Walsman, B. L., & Lipp, R. (1991). New Ballard score, expanded to include extremely premature infants. Journal of Pediatrics, 119(3), 417–423. https://doi.org/10.1016/s0022-3476(05)82056-6.

Barre, N., Morgan, A., Doyle, L. W., & Anderson, P. J. (2011). Language Abilities in Children Who Were Very Preterm and/or Very Low Birth Weight: A Meta-Analysis. The Journal of Pediatrics, 158(5), 766-774.e1. doi:10.1016/j.jpeds.2010.10.032.

Bazacliu, C., & Neu, J. (2019). Necrotizing enterocolitis: Long term complications. Current Pediatric Reviews, 15(2), 115–124. https://doi.org/10.2174/1573396315666190312093119.

Been, J. V., Lugtenberg, M. J., Smets, E., van Schayck, C. P., Kramer, B. W., Mommers, M., & Sheikh, A. (2014). Preterm birth and childhood wheezing disorders: A systematic review and meta-analysis. PLoS Medicine, 11(1), e1001596. doi:10.1371/journal.pmed.1001596.

Behrman, R. E., Butler, A. S., & Institute of Medicine (U.S.) Committee on Understanding Premature Birth and Assuring Healthy Outcomes (Eds.). (2007). Preterm birth: Causes, consequences, and prevention. (U.S.): National Academies Press.

Boone, K. M., Nelin, M. A., Chisolm, D. J., & Keim, S. A. (2019). Gaps and factors related to receipt of care within a medical home for toddles born preterm. Journal of Pediatrics, 207, 161–168. https://doi.org/10.1016/j.jpeds.2018.10.065.

Bowles, J. D., Jnah, A. J., Newberry, D. M., Hubbard, C. A., & Roberston, T. (2016). Infants with technology dependence: Facilitating the road to home. Advances in Neonatal Care, 16(6), 424–429. https://doi.org/10.1097/ANC.0000000000000310.

Bull, M. J., Engle, W. A., Committee on Injury, Violence, and Poison Prevention and Committee on Fetus and Newborn, & American Academy of Pediatrics. (2009). Safe transportation of preterm and low birth weight infants at hospital discharge. Pediatrics, 123(5), 1424–1429. Reaffirmed in 2013. https://doi.org/10.1542/peds.2009-0559.

Burnett, A. C., Anderson, P. J., Cheong, J., Doyle, L. W., Davey, C. G., & Wood, S. J. (2011). Prevalence of psychiatric diagnoses in preterm and full-term children, adolescents and young adults: A meta-analysis. Psychological Medicine, 41(12), 2463–2474. doi:10.1017/S003329171100081X.

Cassiano, R. G. M., Gaspardo, C. M., & Linhares, M. B. M. (2016). Prematurity, neonatal health status, and later child behavioral/emotional problems: A systematic review. Infant Mental Health Journal, 37(3), 274–288. doi:10.1002/imhj.21563.

Chan, E., Leong, P., Malouf, R., & Quigley, M. A. (2016). Long-term cognitive and school outcomes of late-preterm and early-term births: A systematic review. Child: Care, Health and Development, 42(3), 297–312. doi:10.1111/cch.12320.

Cibulskis, C. C., Maheshwari, A., Rao, R., & Mathur, A. M. (2021). Anemia of prematurity: How low is too low? Journal of Perinatology: Official Journal of the California Perinatal Association, 41(6), 1244–1257. https://doi.org/10.1038/s41372-021-00992-0.

Collaco, J. M., & McGrath-Morrow, S. A. (2018). Respiratory phenotypes for preterm infants, children, and adults: bronchopulmonary dysplasia and more. Annals of the American Thoracic Society, 15(5), 530–538.

Crump, C., Sundquist, J., & Sundquist, K. (2021). Preterm or early term birth and risk of autism. Pediatrics, 148(3), e2020032300. https://doi.org/10.1542/peds.2020-032300.

de Jong, F., Monuteaux, M., van Elburg, R., Gillman, M., & Belfort, M. (2012). Systematic review and meta-analysis of preterm birth and later systolic blood pressure. Hypertension, 59, 226–234. doi:10.1161/hypertensionaha.111.181784.

de Kieviet, J. F., Piek, J. P., Aarnoudse-Moens, C. S., & Oosterlaan, J. (2009). Motor development in very preterm and very low-birth-weight children from birth to adolescence: A meta-analysis. Journal of the American Medical Association, 302(20), 2235–2242. doi:10.1001/jama.2009.1708.

den Dekker, H. T., Sonnenschein-van der Voort, A. M. M., de Jongste, J. C., Anessi-Maesano, I., Arshad, S. H., Barros, H., Beardsmore, C. S., Bisgaard, H., Phar, S. C., Craig, L., Devereux, G., van der Ent, C. K., Esplugues, A., Fantini, M. P., Flexender, C., Frey, D., Forastiere, F., Gehring, U., Gorgi, D., van der Gugten, A., C., & Duijts, L. (2016). Early growth characteristics and the risk of reduced lung function and asthma: A meta-analysis of 25,000 children. The Journal of Allergy and Clinical Immunology, 137(4), 1026–1035. doi:10.1016/j.jaci.2015.08.050.

Dubowitz, L. M., Dubowitz, V., & Goldberg, C. (1970). Clinical assessment of gestational age in the newborn. Journal of Pediatrics, 77, 1–10.

Edwards, M. O., Kotecha, S. J., Lowe, J., Watkins, W. J., Henderson, A. J., & Kotecha, S. (2015). Effect of preterm birth on exercise capacity: A systematic review and meta-analysis. Pediatric Pulmonology, 50(3), 293–301. doi:10.1002/ppul.23117.

EHDI: Year 2019 position statement: Principles and guidelines for Early Hearing Detection and Intervention programs. Journal of Early Hearing Detection and Intervention, 4(2), 1–44. DOI: https://doi.org/10.15142/fptk-b748

Eichenwald, E. C., & Committee on Fetus and Newborn. (2018). Diagnosis and management of gastroesophageal reflux in preterm infants. Pediatrics, 142(1), e20181061. https://doi.org/10.1542/peds.2018-1061.

Erickson, G., Dobson, N. R., & Hunt, C. E. (2021). Immature control of breathing and apnea of prematurity: The known and unknown. Journal of Perinatology, 41, 2111–2123. https://doi.org/10.1038/s41372-021-01010-z.

Ferrero, D. M., Larson, J., Jacobsson, B., Di Renzo, G. C., Norman, J. E., Martin, J. N., Jr., D'Alton, M., Castelazo, E., Howson, C. P., Sengpiel, V., Bottai, M., Mayo, J. A., Shaw, G. M., Verdenik, I., Tul, N., Velebil, P., Cairns-Smith, S., Rushwan, H., Arulkumaran, S., … Simpson, J. L. (2016). Cross-country individual participant analysis of 4.1 million singleton births in 5 countries with very high human development index confirms known associations but provides no biologic explanation for 2/3 of all preterm births. PLoS ONE, 11(9), e0162506. https://doi.org/10.1371/journal.pone.0162506.

Fierro, J. L., Passarella, M., & Lorch, S. A. (2019). Prematurity as an independent risk factor for the development of pulmonary disease. Journal of Pediatrics, 213, 110–114. https://doi.org/10.1016/j.jpeds.2019.05.066.

Fierson, W. M., American Academy of Pediatrics Section on Ophthalmology, American Academy of Ophthalmology, American Association For Pediatric Ophthalmology and Strabismus, & American Association of Certified Orthoptists. (2018). Screening examination of premature infants for retinopathy of prematurity. *Pediatrics, 142*(6), e20183061. https://doi.org/10.1542/peds.2018-3061.

FitzGerald, T. L., Kwong, A. K. L., Cheong, J. L. Y., McGinley, J. L., Doyle, L. W., & Spittle, A. J. (2018). Body structure, function, activity, and participation in 3- to 6-year-old children born very preterm: An ICF-based systematic review and meta-analysis. *Physical Therapy, 98*(8), 691–704. doi:10.1093/ptj/pzy050.

Flynn, J. T., Kaelber, D. C., Baker-Smith, C. M., Blowey, D., Carroll, A. E., Daniels, S. R., de Ferranti, S. D., … Subcommittee on screening and management of high blood pressure in children (2017). Clinical practice guideline for screening and management of high blood pressure in children and adolescents. *Pediatrics* 140. doi:10.1542/peds.2017-1904.

Frey, H. A., & Klebanoff, M. A. (2016). The epidemiology, etiology, and costs of preterm birth. *Seminars in Fetal & Neonatal Medicine, 21*(2), 68–73. https://doi.org/10.1016/j.siny.2015.12.011.

Geldof, C. J. A., van Wassenaer, A. G., de Kieviet, J. F., Kok, J. H., & Oosterlaan, J. (2012). Visual perception and visual-motor integration in very preterm and/or very low birth weight children: A meta-analysis. *Research in Developmental Disabilities, 33*(2), 726–736. doi:10.1016/j.ridd.2011.08.025.

Giouleka, S., Tsakiridis, I., Kostakis, N., Koutsouki, G., Kalogiannidis, I., Mamopoulous, A., Athanasiadis, A., & Dagklis, T. (2022). Preterm labor: A comprehensive review of guidelines on diagnosis, management, prediction and prevention. *Obstetrical & Gynecological Survey, 77*(5), 302–317. https://doi.org/10.1097/OGX.0000000000001023.

Glaser, M. A., Hughes, L. M., Jnah, A., & Newberry, D. (2021). Neonatal sepsis: A review of pathophysiology and current management strategies. *Advances in Neonatal Care: Official Journal of the National Association of Neonatal Nurses, 21*(1), 49–60. https://doi.org/10.1097/ANC.0000000000000769.

Goodstein, M. H., Stewart, D. L., Keels, E. L., Moon, R. Y., Committee on Fetus and Newborn, & Task Force on Sudden Infant Death Syndrome. (2021). Transition to a safe home sleep environment for the NICU patient. *Pediatrics, 148*(1), e2021052045. https://doi.org/10.1542/peds.2021-052045.

Gopal, S. H., Edwards, K. M., Creech, B., & Weitkamp, J. H. (2018). Variability in immunization practices for preterm infants. *American Journal of Perinatology, 35*(14), 1394–1398. https://doi.org/10.1055/s-0038-1660453.

Hamrick, S., Sallmon, H., Rose, A. T., Porras, D., Shelton, E. L., Reese, J., & Hansmann, G. (2020). Patent ductus arteriosus of the preterm infant. *Pediatrics, 146*(5), e20201209. https://doi.org/10.1542/peds.2020-1209.

Hand, I. L., Shellhaas, R. A., Milla, S. S., & Committee on Fetus and Newborn, Section on Neurology, Section on Radiology. (2020). Routine neuroimaging of the preterm brain. *Pediatrics, 146*(5), e2020029082. https://doi.org/10.1542/peds.2020-029082.

Hovi, P., Vohr, B., Ment, L. R., Doyle, L. W., McGarvey, L., Morrison, K. M., Evensen, K. A., van der Pal S, Grunau R. E.; APIC Adults Born Preterm International Collaboration; Brubakk AM, Andersson S, Saigal S, & Kajantie E. (2016). Blood Pressure in Young Adults Born at Very Low Birth Weight: Adults Born Preterm International Collaboration. *Hypertension, 68*(4):880–887. doi:10.1161/HYPERTENSIONAHA.116.08167.

Ingol, T. T., Li, R., Ronau, R., Klebanoff, M. A., Oza-Frank, R., Rausch, J., Boone, K. M., & Keim, S. A. (2021). Underdiagnosis of obesity in pediatric clinical care settings among children born preterm: A retrospective cohort study. *International Journal of Obesity, 45*, 1717–1727. https://doi.org/10.1038/s41366-021-00834-1.

Islam, J. Y., Keller, R. L., Aschner, J. L., Hartert, T. V., & Moore, P. E. (2015). Understanding the short- and long-term respiratory outcomes of prematurity and bronchopulmonary dysplasia. *American Journal of Respiratory and Critical Care Medicine, 192*(2), 134–156. doi:10.1164/rccm.201412-2142PP.

Kajantie, E., Strang-Karlsson, S., Evensen, K. A. I., & Haaramo, P. (2019). Adult outcomes of being born late preterm or early term–What do we know? In *Seminars in Fetal and Neonatal Medicine* (Vol. 24, No. 1, pp. 66-83). WB Saunders.

Kelly, M. M. (2018). Health and educational implications of prematurity in the United States: National Survey of Children's Health 2011/2012 data. *Journal of American Association of Nurse Practitioners, 30*(3), 131–139. https://doi.org/10.1097/JXX0000000000000021.

Kelly, M. M., & Dean, S. (2017). Utilization of the premature birth knowledge scale to assess pediatric provider knowledge of neurodevelopmental outcomes. *Journal of Pediatric Health Care, 31*(4), 476–483. https://doi.org/10.1016/j.pedhc.2016.12.006.

Kelly, M. M., & Griffith, P. (2019). The influence of preterm birth beyond infancy: Umbrella review of outcomes of adolescents and adults born preterm. *Journal of American Association of Nurse Practitioners, 32*, 555–562. https://doi.org/10.1097/JXX.0000000000000248.

Kelly, M. M. & Li, K. (2019). Poverty, toxic stress and education in children born preterm. *Nursing Research, 48*. doi:10.1097/NNR.0000000000000360.

Kelly, M. M., & Griffith, P. (2020). Umbrella review of school age health outcomes of preterm birth survivors. *Journal of Pediatric Health Care, 34*, E59–E76. https://doi.org/10.1016/j.pedhc.2020.05.007.

Kelly, M. M., Tobias, J., & Griffith, P. (2021). Addressing preterm birth history with clinical practice recommendations across the life course. *Journal of Pediatric Health Care, 35*(3), e5–e20. https://doi.org/10.1016/j.pedhc.2020.12.0088.

Kemper, A. R., Newman, T. B., Slaughter, J. L., Maisels, M. J., Watchko, J. F., Downs, S. M., Grout, R. W., Bundy, D. G., Stark, A. R., Bogen, D. L., Holmes, A. V., Feldman-Winter, L. B., Bhutani, V. K., Brown, S. R., Maradiaga Panayotti, G. M., Okechukwu, K., Rappo, P. D., & Russell, T. L. (2022). Clinical practice guideline revision: Management of hyperbilirubinemia in the newborn infant 35 or more weeks of gestation. *Pediatrics*, e2022058859. Advance online publication. https://doi.org/10.1542/peds.2022-058859.

Kotecha, S. J., Edwards, M. O., Watkins, W. J., Henderson, A. J., Paranjothy, S., Dunstan, F. D., & Kotecha, S. (2013). Effect of preterm birth on later FEV1: A systematic review and meta-analysis. *Thorax, 68*(8), 760–766. doi:10.1136/thoraxjnl-2012-203079.

Kovatchy, V. N., Adams, J. N., Tamaresis, J. S., & Feldman, H. M. (2015). Reading abilities in school-aged preterm children: A review and meta-analysis. *Developmental Medicine & Child Neurology, 57*(5), 410–419. doi:10.1111/dmcn.12652.

Kwok, T. C., Dorling, J., & Gale, C. (2019). Early enteral feeding in preterm infants. *Seminars in Perinatology, 43*(7), 151159. https://doi.org/10.1053/j.semperi.2019.06.007.

Magnarelli, A., Shah Solanki, N., & Davis, N. L. (2020). Car seat tolerance screening for late-preterm infants. *Pediatrics, 145*(1), e20191703. https://doi.org/10.1542/peds.2019-1703.

Markopoulou, P., Papanikolaou, E., Analytis, A., Zoumakis, E., & Siahanidou, T. (2019). Preterm birth as a risk factor for metabolic syndrome and cardiovascular disease in adult life: a systematic review and meta-analysis. *The Journal of pediatrics, 210*, 69–80. doi:10.016/j.peds.2019.02.041.

Mathewson, K. J., Chow, C. H. T., Dobson, K. G., Pope, E. I., Schmidt, L. A., & Van Lieshout, R. J. (2017). Mental health of extremely low birth weight survivors: A systematic review and meta-analysis. *Psychological Bulletin, 143*(4), 347–383. doi:10.1037/bul0000091.

Moore, G. P., Lemyre, B., Barrowman, N., & Daboval, T. (2013). Neurodevelopmental outcomes at 4 to 8 years of children born at 22 to 25 weeks' gestational age: A meta-analysis. *JAMA Pediatrics, 167*(10), 967–974. doi:10.1001/jamapediatrics.2013.2395.

Moreira, R. S., Magalhães, L. C., & Alves, C. R. L. (2014). Effect of preterm birth on motor development, behavior, and school performance of school-age children: A systematic review. *Jornal De Pediatria, 90*(2),119–134. doi:10.1016/j.jped.2013.05.010.

Mukerji, A., Shah, V., & Shah, P. S. (2015). Periventricular/intraventricular hemorrhage and neurodevelopmental outcomes: A meta-analysis. *Pediatrics, 136*(6), 1132–1143. https://doi.org/10.1542/peds.2015-0944.

Nestander, M., Dintaman, J., Susi, A., Gorman, G., & Hisle-Gorman, E. (2018). Immunization completion in infants born at low birth weight. *Journal of the Pediatric Infectious Diseases Society, 7*(3), e58–e64. https://doi.org/10.1093/jpids/pix079.

Norway, W. H., Rosan, R. C., & Porter, D. Y. (1967). Pulmonary disease following respiratory therapy of hyaline-membrane disease: Bronchopulmonary dysplasia. *New England Journal of Medicine, 276*(7), 357–368.

Osterman, M. J. K., Hamilton, B. E., Martin, J. A., Driscoll, A. K., Valenzuela, C. P., & Division of Vital Statistics. (2022). *Births: Final data for 2020* (vol 70, no. 17). U.S. Department of Health and Human Services. https://www.cdc.gov/nchs/products/nvsr.htm.

Papile, L (2002). Intracranial hemorrhage. In Fanaroff, A. A., & Martin, R. J. (Eds.), *Neonatal-perinatal medicine* (7th ed.). St. Louis: Mosby.

Papile, L., Burstein, J., Burstein, R., & Koffler, H. (1978). Incidence and evolution of subependymal and intraventricular hemorrhages: A study of infants with birth weights less than 1500 grams. *Journal of Pediatrics, 92*(4), 529–534.

Parker, M. G., Stellwagen, L. M., Noble, L., Kim, J. H., Poindexter, B. B., Puopolo, K. M., & Section on Breastfeeding, Committee on Nutrition, Committee on Fetus and Newborn. (2021). Promoting human milk and breastfeeding for the very low birth weight infant. *Pediatrics, 148*(5), e2021054272. https://doi.org/10.1542/peds.2021-054272.

Parkinson, J. R. C., Hyde, M. J., Gale, C., Santhakumaran, S., & Modi, N. (2013). Preterm birth and the metabolic syndrome in adult life: A systematic review and meta-analysis. *Pediatrics, 131*(4), e1240-1263. doi:10.1542/peds.2012-2177.

Partap, U., Chowdhury, R., Taneja, S., Bhandari, N., De Costa, A., Bahl, R., & Fawzi, W. (2022). Preconception and periconception interventions to prevent low birth weight, small for gestational age and preterm birth: A systematic review. *BMJ Global Health, 7*, e007537. https://doi.org/10.1136/bmjgh-2021-007537.

Poindexter, B., & Committee on Fetus and Newborn. (2021). Use of probiotics in preterm infants. *Pediatrics, 147*(6), e2021051485. https://doi.org/10.1542/peds.2021-051485.

Raju, T. N. K., Pemberton, V. L., Saigal, S., Blaisdell, C. J., Moxey-Mims, M., & Buist, A. S. (2017). Long-term healthcare outcomes of preterm birth: An executive summary of a conference sponsored by the National Institute of Health. *Journal of Pediatrics, 181*, 309–318. https://doi.org/10.1016/j.jpeds.2016.10.015.

Rich, B. S., & Dolgin, S. E. (2017). Necrotizing enterocolitis. *Pediatrics in Review, 38*(12), 552–559. https://doi.org/10.1542/pir.2017-0002.

Somhovd, M. J., Hansen, B. M., Brok, J., Esbjorn, B. H., & Greisen, G. (2012). Anxiety in adolescents born preterm or with very low birth weight: A meta-analysis of case-control studies. *Developmental Medicine and Child Neurology, 54*(11), 988–994. doi:10.1111/j.1469-8749.2012.04407.x.

Staebler, S., & Blake, S. (2021). Respiratory syncytial virus disease: Immunoprophylaxis policy review and public health concerns in preterm and young infants. *Policy, Politics, & Nursing Practice, 22*(1), 41–50. https://doi.org/10.1177/1527154420965543.

Stewart, D. L., Barfield, W. D., & Committee on Fetus and Newborn. (2019). Updates on an at-risk population: Late-preterm and early-term infants. *Pediatrics, 144*(5), e20192760. https://doi.org/10.1542/peds.2019-2760.

Synnes, A., & Hicks, M. (2018). Neurodevelopmental Outcomes of Preterm Children at School Age and Beyond. *Clinics in Perinatology, 45*(3), 393–408. doi:10.1002/imhj.21563.

United Nations. (2023). Sustainable development goals: Goal 3: Ensure healthy lives and promote well-being for all at all ages. www.un.org/sustainabledevelopment/health.

Velumula, P., Jani, S., Kanike, N., & Chawla, S. (2020). Monitoring of infants discharged home with medical devices. *Pediatric Annals, 49*(2), e88–e92. https://doi.org/10.3928/19382359-20200121-01.

Walani, S. R. (2020). Global burden of preterm birth. *International Journal of Gynecology and Obstetrics, 150*(1), 31–33. https://doi.org/10.1002/ijgo.13195.

World Health Organization. (2018). Preterm birth fact sheets. Available at https://www.who.int/news-room/fact-sheets/detail/preterm-birth. Retrieved August 24, 2022.

Yildiz, D., Suluhan, D., Eren Fidanci, B., Mert, M., Tunc, T., & Altunkaynak, B. (2019). The differences between preterm and term birth affecting initiation and completion of toilet training among children: A retrospective case-control study. *Urology Journal, 16*(2), 180–185. doi:10.22037/uj.v0i0.4820.

Sickle Cell Disease

Julia Sabrick, Cheri Barber

ETIOLOGY

Sickle cell disease (SCD) is a term used to describe several inherited, sickling hemoglobinopathy syndromes, including sickle–beta-thalassemia (Hb S/β^0 thal or Hb S/β^+ thal), sickle-C disease (Hb S/C), and—most commonly—sickle cell anemia (Hb S/S) (Fig. 36.1 and Box 36.1). Adult hemoglobin contains two pairs of polypeptide chains, alpha and beta. Each of these hemoglobinopathy syndromes involves the mutated sickle hemoglobin (Hb S), which differs from normal hemoglobin (Hb A) by the substitution of a single amino acid, valine, for glutamic acid at the sixth position of the beta-globin chain (Ware et al., 2017).

SCD is a complex, chronic inflammatory condition characterized by hemolysis and vasoocclusion. Red blood cells (RBCs) that contain normal hemoglobin are pliable, biconcave discs with a life span of approximately 120 days. When deoxygenated, RBCs containing predominantly Hb S polymerize and form microtubules (i.e., rods) that distort the shape of the cell characteristically to a crescent or sickle shape (Brandow & Liem, 2020). In this form, the cell is rigid and friable, causing vasoocclusion in the small vessels of the circulatory system. Hypoxia and acidosis, which may be caused by fever, infection, dehydration, or other factors, are known to induce this change in shape (Fig. 36.2). Many times, however, the RBC changes shape without apparent provocation. To a limited degree, this change in shape is reversible, though not indefinitely. These cells eventually become irreversibly sickled cells with a life span of approximately 10 to 20 days. The fragility and shortened life span of these RBCs leads to chronic anemia, which serves as a stimulus for the bone marrow to create new RBCs, resulting in an elevated reticulocyte count. These stress reticulocytes have adhesion molecules that are expressed on their surfaces, contributing to adhesion to the vascular endothelium. This sets in motion a cycle of abnormal adhesion–inflammation–increased adhesion that is continually occurring (Kato et al., 2018). The vasoocclusion and hemolysis described previously are the hallmarks of SCD, contributing to the complications that can occur in multiple organs of the body.

Fetal hemoglobin (Hb F), a minor hemoglobin of normal adults, predominates from 10 weeks after conception through the remainder of gestation and normally begins to decline at 34 weeks. Hb F makes up 60% to 80% of the total hemoglobin at birth and declines to normal adult levels (1–2%) by 5 to 6 months of age (Inusa et al., 2019). The remaining 20% to 40% of hemoglobin found at birth has the adult electrophoresis forms, Hb A and Hb A_2 or Hb S, if found to be affected. Hb F does not sickle, so it is unusual to find clinical manifestations of the condition with significant amounts of Hb F. High Hb F is associated with reduced instances of painful leg ulcers and acute pain episodes (Steinberg, 2020). Because of this phenomenon, manifestations of SCD may not be clinically apparent until 4 to 6 months of age or later.

SCD has an autosomal recessive inheritance pattern. Both parents must carry some type of abnormal hemoglobin (i.e., one or both of them must carry sickle hemoglobin) for the condition to be manifested in their child. Carriers of SCD are described as having sickle cell trait (Hb A/S). When two individuals, each of whom has Hb A/S, elect to have a child, there is a 25% chance that they will have a child with Hb S/S. These individuals also have a 50% chance of having a child with Hb A/S and a 25% chance of having a child with entirely normal hemoglobin (Hb AA) with each pregnancy (Fig. 36.3). All states require newborn screening, and aside from two states, screening does not require parental consent. Testing methods and referral policies differ across states, but all newborn screening programs consist of education, screening, short-term follow-up, diagnosis, management, evaluation, and long-term follow-up (El-Haj & Hoppe, 2018). Most screening programs use isoelectric focusing of an Elute filter paper impregnated with blood that is used to screen for phenylketonuria, hypothyroidism, and other disorders, although some states rely on high-performance liquid chromatography or cellulose acetate electrophoresis. Many programs confirm the diagnosis by DNA analyses to detect hemoglobin variants, but this practice is not standardized across states (Kato et al., 2018). The diagnosis is confirmed using hemoglobin electrophoresis (Kavanagh et al., 2022). Major gaps in newborn screening practices occur in the variability of statewide educational programs (Kato et al., 2018). Emerging point-of-care tests may have the potential to overcome the need for follow-up appointments and other barriers because it is easy to use, inexpensive, and accurate (Kavanagh et al., 2022).

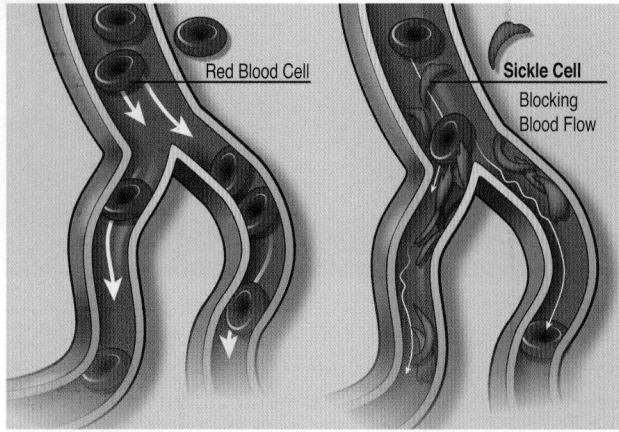

Fig. 36.1 Normal blood cells *(left)* and blood cells in sickle cell disease *(right)*, which do not flow through the circulatory system smoothly. (From MedlinePlus. [n.d.]. Sickle cell disease. https://medlineplus.gov/genetics/condition/sickle-cell-disease/. Courtesy Darryl Leia, National Human Genome Research Institute.)

Box **36.1** Overview of the Main Hemoglobinopathies

THALASSEMIA
- Alpha- and beta-thalassemia
- Delta-beta-thalassemia

ABNORMAL HEMOGLOBINS
- Anomalies of the beta-globin chain (Hb S, Hb E, Hb C)
- Anomalies of the alpha-globin chain (Hb Constant Spring)
- Fusion hemoglobins (Hb Lepore)

HEREDITARY PERSISTENCE OF FETAL HEMOGLOBIN

Various forms of hemoglobinopathies can also occur in combination (i.e., frequently encountered are a combination of alpha- with concurrent beta-thalassemia, as are thalassemias combined with abnormal hemoglobins, or the simultaneous presence of two abnormal hemoglobins [e.g., Hb S/C]).

From Busse, B., Tepedino, M.F., Rupprecht, W., & Klein, H.G. (2016). Stepwise diagnostics of hemoglobinopathies. *Laboratoriums Medizin, 39*(S1).

INCIDENCE AND PREVALENCE

SCD is one of the most common genetic conditions and is most often seen in individuals of African descent but is also found in other ethnic groups, including those from the Caribbean, Mediterranean, Arabian Peninsula, and India. It is the most common hemoglobinopathy, with about 300,000 new cases diagnosed globally every year (Darbari et al., 2020). In the United States, 1 in 12 Blacks is a carrier of the sickle cell gene, and 1 in 360 manifests the condition (Kato et al., 2018). The exact number of individuals living with SCD across the globe is unknown. In the United States, the population of SCD is about 100,000 and is likely to increase (Centers for Disease Control and Prevention [CDC], n.d.).

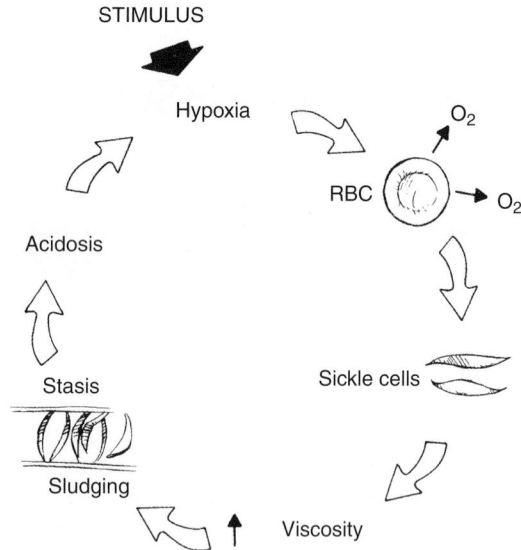

Fig. 36.2 Cycle causing vasoocclusive episodes in sickle cell anemia. *RBC*, Red blood cell. (From Hockenberry, M., & Coody, D. [Eds.]. [1986]. *Pediatric oncology and hematology: Perspectives on care.* Mosby.)

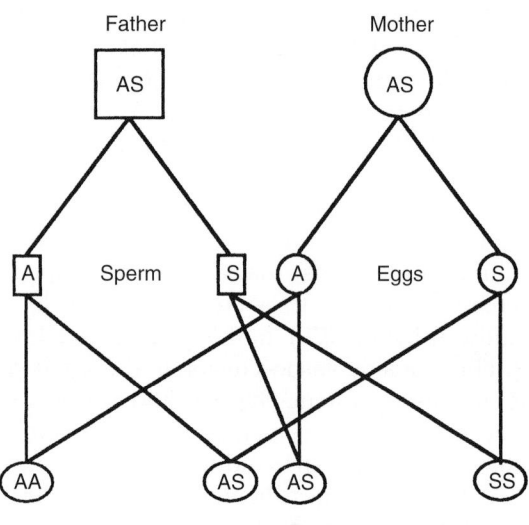

Possible offspring

Fig. 36.3 Genetics of sickle cell anemia. Both parents possess one gene for normal hemoglobin (*A*) and one for sickle hemoglobin (*S*). With each pregnancy, there is a 25% statistical chance that the child will have normal hemoglobin (*AA*) and a 25% chance that the child will have sickle cell anemia (*SS*); 50% of the children will have the sickle cell trait (*AS*). (From Miller, D., & Baehner, R. [Ed.]. [1990]. *Blood diseases of infancy and childhood* [6th ed.]. Mosby.)

DIAGNOSTIC CRITERIA

Prenatal diagnosis is available to couples known to be carriers of hemoglobinopathies. Diagnosis may be accomplished via chorionic villi sampling during the first trimester or amniocentesis during the second trimester. The method depends on the risks and benefits of the techniques involved; both are adequate to determine the diagnosis. Screening, follow-up, and diagnosis of SCD must be followed with prompt referral to knowledgeable providers of comprehensive care (Health Resources and Services Administration, n.d.).

The sickle prep (solubility testing) is often used to screen infants and children for SCD. This test is inexpensive and rapidly performed but is not very specific. A sickle prep result will be positive for Hb A/S, Hb S/S, and other sickle hemoglobinopathies but will not distinguish one from another (Kato et al., 2018). The definitive diagnosis of SCD is determined by performing a complete blood count (CBC), peripheral blood smear, and—most important—a quantitative hemoglobin electrophoresis. Measurement of hematologic indices is vitally important in the differential diagnoses of thalassemia syndromes and hemoglobinopathies. It is occasionally helpful to perform hematologic studies on a child's parents to confirm a diagnosis.

Clinical Manifestations at Time of Diagnosis

NEONATES
- Normal birth weight
- No evidence of hemolytic anemia
- Hemoglobin electrophoresis shows no evidence of hemoglobin A production
- Neonatal jaundice (when present) related to ABO hemolytic disease of the newborn, not to sickle cell disease

INFANTS AND TODDLERS
- Development of anemia
- Colic-like symptoms, often associated with feeding difficulties
- Generalized episodes of bone or abdomen pain preceded by acute, febrile infection
- Hand-foot syndrome associated with heat, pain, swelling, erythema
- Splenic hypofunction marked by the presence of Howell-Jolly bodies in the blood smear
- Autosplenectomy preceded by splenomegaly in 73% of infants, followed by a decrease in size
- Splenomegaly noted frequently during febrile episodes

EARLY CHILDHOOD
- Generalized vasoocclusive crisis (VOC) of bone or abdomen that may or may not be preceded by acute, febrile infection; seemingly triggered by emotional stress or abrupt weather changes
- Usually, nonpalpable spleen but sometimes retained in sickle-C disease
- Males may develop priapism
- Biliary colic caused by stasis and gallstones
- Development of cerebral vasculopathy with cerebral infarction

LATE CHILDHOOD
- Gallstones with or without symptoms
- Delayed pubescence
- Females may have an increased incidence of VOC with menses, presumably caused by hormonal changes
- Males may develop priapism
- Early signs of sickle retinopathy
- Early signs of sickle nephropathy

CLINICAL MANIFESTATIONS AT TIME OF DIAGNOSIS

As a result of current newborn screening programs for hemoglobinopathies, infants are now identified before the onset of acute symptoms (Table 36.1 and Fig. 36.4). The anemia from which Hb S/S derives its name is broadly characterized as uncompensated hemolytic anemia, in which a markedly shortened overall RBC survival (i.e., an increased rate of RBC destruction) is insufficiently balanced by the increase in production (i.e., erythropoiesis) to maintain normal levels of total RBC and hemoglobin.

Treatment
- Supportive symptomatic care
- Aggressive treatment of fever and infection
- Maintenance of optimal hydration
- Maintenance of body temperature
- Penicillin prophylaxis
- Pneumococcal immunization
- Drug therapy with hydroxyurea, crizanlizumab, voxelotor
- Selective use of transfusions
- Hematopoietic stem cell transplant in selected individuals

The "Natural History of Sickle Cell Disease," a hallmark study by Powars (1975), indicated that in the first two decades of life, Hb S/S is marked by periods of clinical quiescence and relative physical well-being, interspersed with episodes of acute illness. This classic study supports that these illnesses are treatable by state-of-the-art medical care and are often preventable. The expression of untreated Hb S/S is often characterized by septicemia or meningitis during infancy, followed by cerebral vasculopathy with cerebral infarction during early childhood. Splenic hypofunction is present in nearly 30% of infants with Hb S/S by their first birthday and in 90% by age 6 years, accounting for the high risk of sepsis by polysaccharide-encapsulated organisms (Brousse et al., 2014).

TREATMENT

SUPPORTIVE SYMPTOMATIC CARE

Stem cell (bone marrow) transplants are the only cure for SCD. Despite the thorough understanding that exists among researchers and clinicians about the inheritance, diagnosis, and pathophysiology of SCD, treatment is essentially supportive and symptomatic. This approach is aimed at aggressive treatment of the infection and maintenance of optimal hydration and body temperature to prevent hypoxia and acidosis. Standard care includes bedrest, hydration, transfusions, analgesics, penicillin prophylaxis, and monitoring with close follow-up by a medical team specializing in sickle cell care. Treatment has moved from care during specific crises to the prevention of sickling episodes. Compared to other similar genetic

Table 36.1   Differential Diagnosis of Common Hemoglobinopathies

	CLINICAL SEVERITY	HEMOGLOBIN (g/dL)	HEMATOCRIT (%)	MEAN CORPUSCULAR VOLUME (µm³)	% OF RETICULOCYTES	RBC MORPHOLOGY	SOLUBILITY TEST	ELECTROPHORESIS (%)	DISTRIBUTION OF FETAL HEMOGLOBIN
S/S	Moderate-severe	7.5 (6–11)	22 (18–30)	>80	11 (5–20)	Many ISCs, target cells, nucleated RBCs, normochromic H-J bodies	Positive	>90 s <10 F <3.6 A₂	Uneven
S/C	Mild-moderate	10 (10–15)	30 (26–40)	75–95	3 (5–10)	Many target cells, anisopoikilocytosis	Positive	50 S 50 C <5	Uneven
S/β⁰ THAL	Moderate-severe	8.1 (6–10)	25 (20–36)	<80	8 (5–20)	Marked hypochromia, microcytosis and target cells, variable ISCs	Positive	>80 S <20 F >3.5 A₂	Uneven
S/β⁺ THAL	Mild-moderate	11 (9–12)	32 (25–40)	<75	3 (5–10)	Mild microcytosis, hypochromia, rare ISCs	Positive	55–75 S 15–30 A <20 F >3.5 A₂	Uneven
S/HBFH	Asymptomatic	14 (12–14)	40 (32–48)	<80	1.5 (1–2)	No ISCs, occasional target cells, and mild hypochromia	Positive	<70 S >30 F <2.5 A₂	Even
A/S	Asymptomatic	Normal	Normal	Normal	Normal	Normal	Positive	38–45 S 60–55 A 1–3 A₂	Uneven

H-J, Howell-Jolly; *ISC*, irreversibly sickled cell; *RBC*, red blood cell; *S/HPFH*, sickle hereditary persistence of fetal hemoglobin.
From Charche, S., Lubin, B., & Reid, C. (1995). *Management and therapy of sickle cell disease.* NIH Publication No. 95–2117. US Government Printing Office.

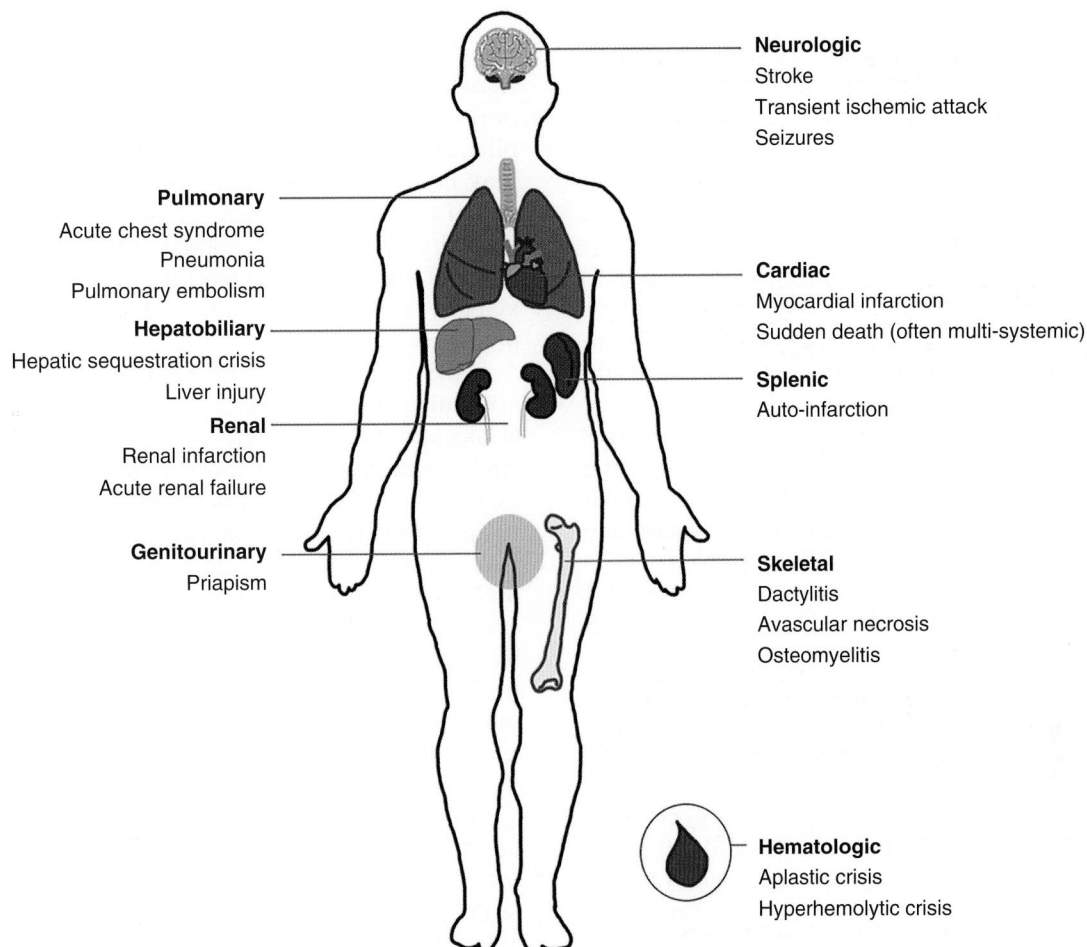

Fig. 36.4 Illustration showing that sickle cell disease may present with various clinical manifestations because the disease affects many organ systems. (From Al Farii, H., Zhou, S., & Albers, A. [2020]. Management of osteomyelitis in sickle cell disease: Review article. *JAAOS: Global Research and Reviews*, 4[9].)

diseases, SCD has lacked substantial research funding, inhibiting the availability of high-quality evidence for disease-modifying therapies (Kavanagh et al., 2022). A 2020 research study reported that US research funding for cystic fibrosis (US prevalence of about 30,000) was 10-fold greater than for SCD (US prevalence of about 100,000) (Farooq et al., 2020).

DRUG THERAPY WITH HYDROXYUREA

One current method induces the production of Hb F with hydroxyurea (HU), a ribonuclease reductase inhibitor that induces fetal hemoglobin production, which normally dissipates shortly after birth (Kavanagh et al., 2022). HU is the first US Food and Drug Administration (FDA)–approved medication for use in adults with SCD. For individuals with SCD, it increases the production of Hb F through mechanisms that remain unclear. Expression of Hb F, in combination with the native Hb S, forms a diluted pool of RBCs with Hb F and Hb S. This combination reduces both the polymerization of the cells and the rate of hemolysis and improves anemia. Other observers note that HU decreases the production of platelets and white blood cells (WBCs) and increases RBC survival time (Kavanagh et al., 2022). Additionally, HU decreases cellular adhesion to the endothelium and increases microvascular perfusion (Wang et al., 2011). Researchers recognize the complex interplay of sickle erythrocytes, leukocytes, vascular endothelium, platelets, plasma clotting factors, and certain mediators of inflammation in producing tissue ischemia and end-organ damage.

Pediatric trials of HU therapy have shown significant improvement in Hb F production, mean corpuscular volume, and a mild-moderate increase in hemoglobin, which in turn reduces the number of sickle cell crises (Wang et al., 2011). Among high-income countries, HU therapy reduces the incidence of vasoocclusive crises, hospitalizations, and mortality and has an excellent safety profile (Kato et al., 2018). Growth failure in children with SCD has long been identified, probably secondary to their hypermetabolic state. Treatment with HU decreases the resting energy expenditure, thus improving the hypermetabolic state with better growth parameters than expected (Thornburg et al., 2012). HU is considered a first-line treatment for all individuals with Hb S/S and Hb S/β^0 thal. These children should be started on HU at 9 months of age (Wang et al., 2011). Individuals with Hb S/C and Hb S/β⁺ thal who report frequent acute pain episodes, ACS, or hospitalizations should also be considered for HU therapy (Qureshi et al., 2018). Recent studies have shown that only 28% of eligible children were prescribed HU (Brousseau et al., 2019). Low HU usage is due to a lack of clinician expertise in SCD and mistrust from a patient population that has been historically mistreated and marginalized by the health care system (Lanzkron et al., 2008). Lack of response to HU therapy is most often due to poor adherence or pharmacogenomic reasons (Kato et al., 2018). They are generally started on 15 mg/kg of HU per day, with doses escalating by 5 mg/kg every 8 weeks if no signs or symptoms of toxicity are noted. The maximum dose is usually 30 mg/kg/day or the maximum tolerated dose as determined by the health care team (National Institutes of Health [NIH], 2002).

Clinical observations have not detected an increased rate of cancer in people with sickle cell treated with HU (Thornburg et al., 2012). The potential side effects of HU, such as myelosuppression of blood cells, particularly the WBCs, and platelets, mandate strict monitoring of blood counts. However, the benefits of HU appear to far outweigh the risks. A 2022 systematic review of nine randomized controlled trials evaluating the use of HU in individuals with SCD found that the treatment generally decreases the frequency of pain episodes and other acute complications and prevents life-threatening neurologic events. There is less evidence of the effectiveness of HU on individuals with SCD Hb S/C (Rankine-Mullings & Nevitt, 2022).

TRANSCRANIAL DOPPLER SCREENING AND TRANSFUSIONS

A hallmark study done within the Cooperative Study of Sickle Cell Disease (CSSCD), Stroke Prevention in Sickle Cell Anemia (STOP I), looked at genetic markers, laboratory and radiographic indicators, and clinical findings that were predictive of stroke in this population (Adams et al., 1998). Over 2000 children, between ages 2 and 16, with Hb S/S and Hb S/β⁰ thal were screened by transcranial Doppler (TCD) ultrasound. This noninvasive technique reliably demonstrates cerebral flow abnormalities by demonstrating that high velocities (i.e., 200 cm/sec) in either the distal intracerebral or middle cerebral arteries are associated with an increased risk of subsequent stroke.

In the STOP I study, those identified with abnormal velocities were randomized to receive either monthly transfusions or no transfusion at all. The risk of stroke, about 10% in SCD, was reduced by 90% in those children treated with transfusions (Adams, 2000). This dramatic finding caused the early termination of the study and a recommendation by the National Heart, Lung, and Blood Institute (NHLBI) that all children with Hb S/S and Hb S/β⁰ thal be screened with TCD (Adams et al., 1998).

STOP II, using the population identified with abnormal TCD findings, studied the length of time that transfusion therapy is needed to normalize and retain normalization of the TCD findings (Adams & Brambilla, 2005). It also sought to determine if transfusions may be stopped after some period of time when the risk of stroke has diminished (Abboud et al., 2011). The study by Adams and Brambilla (2005) found that there is a significant risk of reverting to an abnormal TCD velocity or experiencing an overt stroke if transfusions are discontinued.

Children identified with high velocities are offered scheduled transfusions as a means of preventing stroke and its subsequent consequences. Further studies have indicated that those children with abnormal TCD should also be screened with magnetic resonance imaging (MRI) and magnetic resonance angiography (MRA) (Bernaudin et al., 2016). Silent infarcts are seen on MRI in a substantial minority of children with SCD, even those with normal neurologic function. The combination of abnormal TCD and silent infarct on MRI further increases the risk of stroke or recurrent silent infarcts (Bernaudin et al., 2016). These children should be aggressively treated with scheduled transfusion therapy.

The landmark trial, TCD With Transfusions Changing to Hydroxyurea (TWiTCH), evaluated standard treatment of conditional TCD velocities in children with SCD (transfusion) vs alternative treatment (HU) (Ware et al., 2016). Results showed that for high-risk children with SCD and conditional TCD velocities who underwent at least 4 years of chronic transfusion therapy, HU therapy is a safe substitute to maintain TCD velocities to help prevent primary stroke (Ware et al., 2016).

In 1995, the CSSCD group completed another hallmark study evaluating the preoperative transfusion needs of children with SCD (Koshy et al., 1995). It is well known that general anesthesia places an individual with SCD at increased risk for stroke, acute chest syndrome (ACS), and painful vasoocclusive crisis (Kokoska et al., 2004). The standard protocol has been to transfuse individuals to a hemoglobin value of 10 to 12 g/dL with a Hb S level of less than 30% before surgery (Linder & Chou, 2021). Raising hemoglobin levels above 12 g/dL is avoided to limit the risk of hyperviscosity. Red cell transfusions are usually provided by the simple exchange for its convenience and use of lesser units. Red cell exchange (RCE) involves taking out a patient's RBCs and replacing them with donor cells via automated (apheresis machines) or manual method. Despite increased exposure to donors with the RCE method, studies have not shown increases in alloimmunization rates associated with RCE (Venkateswaran et al., 2011). RCE is recommended over simple transfusion for acute ischemic stroke, severe ACS, chronically transfused patients with significant iron overload, and patients with high baseline hematocrits requiring transfusion (Linder & Chou, 2021). The

American Society of Hematology suggests using automated RCE for patients with SCD who receive chronic transfusion therapy (Chou et al., 2020).

In the past, chelation treatment (removal of iron overload) has been very time intensive, and compliance has often been very difficult to maintain. Traditional therapy included overnight infusion of deferoxamine (Desferal) multiple nights per week. An oral chelation agent, deferasirox (Exjade), was approved by the FDA in November 2005 (Lindsey & Olin, 2007). Extra iron binds to the drug, which then facilitates its removal from the body's circulation. The iron is primarily excreted in the feces. Exjade should be taken on an empty stomach at least 30 minutes before food, preferably at the same time every day. Occasional auditory and ocular disturbances have been reported with Exjade; therefore hearing and vision screening and follow-up are recommended while this medication is in use.

HEMATOPOIETIC STEM CELL TRANSPLANT AND GENE THERAPIES

From a preventive point of view, providing genetic counseling for those individuals with Hb A/S, prenatal diagnosis for pregnant females who are at risk for delivering a child with SCD, and education for parents of newly diagnosed children is the standard of care. As awareness has grown regarding the benefits of umbilical cord blood salvage, large-scale banking has begun in Europe and the United States (Kavanagh et al., 2022). The Sibling Cord Blood Donor Program (www.chori.org/Services/Sibling_Donor_Cord_Blood_Program/indexcord.html) in Oakland, California, currently offers free storage of cord blood for families considering the option of cord blood transplant.

Currently, a hematopoietic stem cell transplant (HSCT) is the only intervention that can cure SCD (Kanter et al., 2021). As of 2021 there are no published randomized controlled trials for HSCT in individuals with SCD. This approach is limited because only 24% of individuals have a human leukocyte antigen (HLA)–matched donor sibling. The American Society of Hematology recommends the use of HLA identical sibling cord blood over bone marrow if HSCT is performed (Kanter et al., 2021). HSCT with a matched sibling donor is the standard of care for individuals with severe disease (Kavanagh et al., 2022). The National Marrow Donor Program (which operates Be The Match) has expanded its minority representation. Only about 10% of patients in the United States have matched related donors (Germino-Watnick et al., 2022). Eighty-eight percent of transplants are from HLA-matched sibling donors, and 84% are younger than 16 years of age at transplant; graft rejection occurred in 9% (Shenoy, 2007). Overall survival after HSCT is 93%. Eighty-five percent of those surviving are sickle cell free (Bhatia & Walters, 2008).

About 2000 individuals with SCD have undergone HSCTs, with a survival rate of 90% in US and European studies (Neumayr et al., 2019; Walters et al., 2016). Overall, HSCT is a time-intensive, rigorous, high-risk procedure that is used only when the benefits of a cure outweigh the procedure risks. Gene therapy has long been touted as a potential cure for SCD. Recent advances in genomic sequencing technology have increased researchers' understanding of hemoglobin (Hb) regulation and genome modification. Gene addition strategies, which use gene transfer vectors, have been trialed to increase the expression of normal globins; however, many barriers have prevented them from translating to clinical successes, including collecting enough stem cells, increasing the expression of transferred genes, and understanding the safety assessment (Abraham & Tisdale, 2021). There is a need for comprehensive psychosocial assessments and evaluation processes for pediatric patients with SCD (and their caregivers) undergoing HSCT (Schulz et al., 2018). When considering HSCT, it is crucial for multidisciplinary care teams to assess patients' and caregivers' facilitators and barriers, including measures related to comprehension, expectations, mental and behavioral health, family functioning, and social support (Annunziato et al., 2010).

SECOND-LINE THERAPIES

L-Glutamine

L-glutamine is an oral amino acid supplement that was approved by the FDA in 2017 to reduce SCD-related complications in patients older than 5 years of age. Evidence suggests that L-glutamine may improve the nicotinamide adenine dinucleotide redox potential of RBCs, preventing oxidative damage to RBCs. In a clinical trial of 230 patients who had at least two pain crises in the past year and who were all on a stable HU dose for 3 months, patients randomized to receive L-glutamine therapy had fewer pain crises, fewer hospitalizations for sickle cell pain, fewer cumulative days in the hospital, and fewer occurrences of ACS (Darbari et al., 2020; Niihara et al., 2018).

Voxelotor

Voxelotor, a 1500-mg once-daily medication approved for patients age 4 years and older, promotes the oxygenated state of hemoglobin by promoting Hb S binding to oxygen, which decreases Hb S polymerization and hemolysis (Kavanagh et al., 2022). In a phase III randomized controlled trial of patients age 12 to 65 years with severe or symptomatic anemia, voxelotor was found to increase hemoglobin by at least 1 g/dL vs patients randomized to placebo (Vichinsky et al., 2019). Voxelotor should be prescribed to patients with a hemoglobin between 5.5 and 10.5 g/dL and with more than one pain crisis per year despite HU therapy or for patients unable to tolerate HU therapy (Kavanagh et al., 2022).

Crizanlizumab

Approved by the FDA in 2019 for patients older than 16 years of age with SCD, crizanlizumab is a monoclonal antibody that binds to P-selectin to block its interaction with P-selectin glycoprotein ligand 1 and interactions between endothelial cells, platelets, RBCs, and leukocytes (Darbari et al., 2020). In phase II randomized, placebo-controlled, double-blind clinical trial with patients age 16 to 65 years (SUSTAIN), patients who were treated with high-dose (5 mg/kg) crizanlizumab therapy every 4 weeks experienced sickle cell pain crises at a rate of 45.3% less than compared to placebo. High-dose crizanlizumab therapy was also shown to increase the median times between the first and second crises. The trial showed that there were no differences in hemolysis between the two groups. Overall, crizanlizumab is associated with a low rate of adverse effects, with or without concomitant HU therapy (Ataga et al., 2017).

COMPLEMENTARY AND ALTERNATIVE THERAPIES

Complementary and alternative medicine (CAM) provides popular alternatives to traditional pain management medications (including opioids) that are first-line treatment during acute vasoocclusive episodes (Alsabri et al., 2023). A 2023 meta-analysis found that CAMs may potentially decrease sickle cell–related pain. Prayer and spiritual healing were found to be the most common CAM modalities. It is crucial that practitioners discuss CAMs with their patients, as it was also found that many patients do not disclose their CAMs due to perceived stigma. Acupuncture, massage, cognitive-behavioral therapy, and biofeedback delivered in outpatient settings significantly decreased pain reported by pediatrics with SCD (Alsabri et al., 2023).

ASSOCIATED PROBLEMS OF SICKLE CELL DISEASE AND TREATMENT

Associated problems (Table 36.2) are primarily caused by the following: (1) vasoocclusion, a blockage of small blood vessels secondary to the clumping of sickled RBCs and increased adhesion of other circulating cells that causes tissue ischemia; and (2) hemolytic anemia and the resulting chronic hemolysis. The consequences of this vasoocclusion and chronic hemolysis lead to a state of chronic vasculopathy affecting nearly every organ in the body (Fig. 36.5).

Associated Problems
Sickle Cell Disease and Treatment

- Functional asplenia
- Acute splenic sequestration
- Neurologic problems
- Vasoocclusive crisis
- Acute chest syndrome
- Transient red cell aplasia
- Hemolysis
- Renal problems
- Priapism
- Skeletal changes
- Ophthalmologic changes
- Audiologic problems
- Leg ulcers
- Preparation for anesthesia, contrast medium
- Cardiac problems
- Hepatobiliary problems
- Transfusion complications
- Formation of antibodies
- Iron overload
- Bloodborne pathogens

FUNCTIONAL ASPLENIA

The splenic function is normal at birth in infants with SCD, but by 6 months of age a state of splenic dysfunction develops from changes in RBC adherence and plastic and signaling properties (Brousse et al., 2014). By age 1 year, approximately 86% of children with SCD have a loss of splenic function (Kinger et al., 2021). Children with SCD are typically functionally asplenic by age 5 years (Gale et al., 2016). Palpation of the spleen on physical examination is not an indication of splenic function. The spleens of children with SCD can be clinically palpable or not and can be functional or not, with no relation to size and function. Rather, the presence of Howell-Jolly bodies (e.g., pocked/pitted cells) on blood smears confirms the condition of functional asplenia (Brousse et al., 2014).

Splenic malfunction and failure to make specific immunoglobulin G antibodies to polysaccharide antigens contribute to unusual susceptibility to infection. Without adequate splenic function, children with SCD are at high risk for infection from organisms such as *Streptococcus pneumoniae, Haemophilus influenzae,* and *Neisseria meningitides* (Driscoll, 2007). The advent of pneumococcal and *H. influenzae* immunizations has significantly reduced this risk (Ram et al., 2010). Less common causes of bacteremia include other streptococci, *Escherichia coli, Staphylococcus aureus,* and gram-negative bacteria such as *Klebsiella* spp., *Salmonella*

Table 36.2	Main Types of Sickle Cell Disorders
Hemoglobin S/S	The most severe form affects 65% of children with sickle cell disease. Most or all of the hemoglobin is abnormal, causing chronic anemia.
Hemoglobin S/C disease	Roughly 25% of children with sickle cell disease have this mild-moderate form of the disease. Symptoms generally develop later in childhood but may be as severe as in Hb S/S.
Sickle beta plus thalassemia	Affects around 8% of children with sickle cell disease. This is generally considered a mild form of sickle cell disease, but severity can vary greatly.
Sickle beta zero thalassemia	A severe but less common form, accounting for 2% of sickle cell disease. It is similar to Hb S/S.

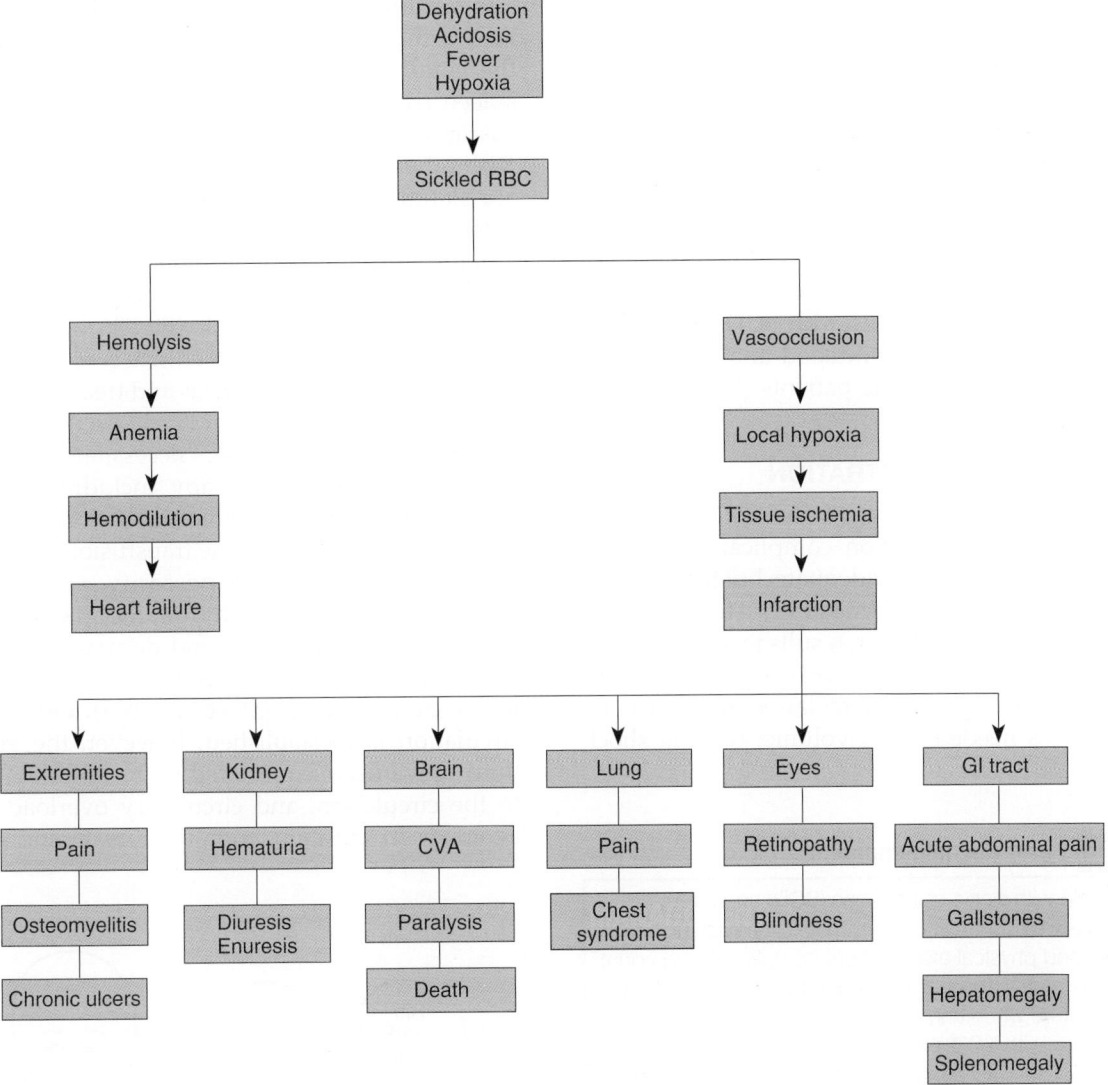

Fig. 36.5 Tissue effects of sickle cell anemia. *CVA,* Cerebrovascular accident; *GI,* gastrointestinal; *RBC,* red blood cell. (From Hockenberry, M, & Wilson, D. [2006]. *Nursing care of infants and children* [8th ed.]. Mosby.)

spp., and *Pseudomonas aeruginosa.* Other organisms associated with frequent infections in Hb S/S include *Mycoplasma* and *Chlamydia pneumoniae.*

Intervention should be threefold: (1) aggressive management of infectious episodes; (2) timely immunization, including the *H. influenzae* type B (Hib) and pneumococcal vaccines (Prevnar, Pneumovax); and (3) antibiotic prophylaxis. Penicillin prophylaxis is the standard of care for all young children with SCD and should be started at the time of diagnosis—beginning by 2 months of age and continuing until at least 5 years (American Academy of Pediatrics [AAP], 2021). The usual doses for penicillin V or G are 125 mg twice daily for children 2 months of age until less than 3 years and 250 mg twice daily for those over age 3 years. For children who are not adherent to oral antibiotic therapy at home, 1.2 million units of long-acting penicillin may be given intramuscularly every 3 weeks (AAP, 2021). If an individual is allergic to penicillin, erythromycin (20 mg/kg) may be substituted. Some experts have

recommended amoxicillin (20 mg/kg/day) or trimethoprim (TMP)–sulfamethoxazole (SMX) (4 mg/kg/day TMP to 20 mg/kg/day SMX) for children under age 5 years (AAP, 2021). As with other children taking antibiotics, the potential for fungal infections, gastrointestinal upset, and allergy exists.

The number of cases of penicillin-resistant invasive pneumococcal infections and the presence of nasopharyngeal carriage for those on penicillin prophylaxis may indicate that penicillin is no longer as effective at preventing invasive pneumococcal infections. The age at which prophylaxis should be discontinued is often an empirical decision, and currently there is no evidence-based recommendation available (Hirst & Owusu-Ofori, 2014). All children having surgical splenectomies or a history of pneumococcal sepsis must continue penicillin prophylaxis indefinitely. Parents must be counseled to always seek immediate medical assistance with all febrile episodes (McCavit et al., 2011).

FEVER

Children with SCD presenting with fever require a rapid assessment with a CBC, reticulocyte count, blood culture, and treatment with broad-spectrum antibiotics (Box 36.2). A reliable indicator of infection in children with SCD is a fever greater than or equal to 38.5°C, which is the point at which clinicians should treat more aggressively than they would with healthy children (Yawn et al., 2014). Primary care providers should encourage individuals with SCD to maintain appropriate adherence to childhood and adult vaccination schedules for asplenic patients (Brousse et al., 2014).

ACUTE SPLENIC SEQUESTRATION COMPLICATION

In acute splenic sequestration complication (ASSC), blood flow into the spleen is adequate, but the vascular outflow system from the spleen to the systemic circulation is occluded. This occlusion results in a large collection of blood pooling in the spleen, causing significant enlargement. The systemic circulation may then be deprived of its needed blood volume, causing shock and cardiovascular collapse. The acute illness is associated with a hemoglobin level of 2 g/dL or more below the child's baseline value with an acutely enlarged spleen (Beck et al., 2022). Children with Hb S/S are susceptible to this at an early age (i.e., <5 years). Those with other variants of the disease may continue to be at risk until their teenage years because they maintain splenic circulation longer than children with Hb S/S. Parents can be taught to palpate and measure their child's spleen using a simple measuring device such as a calibrated tongue blade (Fig. 36.6). Knowledge of the child's steady-state spleen size is essential in determining appropriate diagnosis and treatment during an acute event.

Management of ASSC necessitates hospitalization with immediate therapy, including transfusion. If shock is present, systemic circulation must be supported with fluids. After the transfusion, monitoring is needed to assess for hyperviscosity syndrome, where trapped RBCs are released from the spleen, increasing the circulating RBC mass and decreasing blood flow. This can lead to ischemic end-organ injury, especially in the brain (Kavanagh et al., 2022). Once adequate circulation is reestablished, however, the volume of fluid previously sequestered in the spleen is returned to the circulation, and circulatory overload must be avoided. In children with life-threatening episodes,

---

Box 36.2   Fever Recommendations

1. In people with sickle cell disease (SCD) and a temperature ≥101.3°F (38.5°C), immediately evaluate with history and physical examination, complete blood count with differential, reticulocyte count, blood culture, and urine culture when urinary tract infection is suspected.
2. In children with SCD and a temperature ≥101.3°F (38.5°C), promptly administer ongoing empiric parenteral antibiotics that provide coverage against *Streptococcus pneumoniae* and gram-negative enteric organisms. Subsequent outpatient management using an oral antibiotic is feasible in people who do not appear ill. Careful follow-up at primary care provider in 24 and 48 hours with an assurance of parental compliance is necessary for outpatient management.
3. Hospitalize people with SCD and a temperature ≥103.1°F (39.5°C) who appear ill for close observation and intravenous antibiotic therapy.
4. In people with SCD whose febrile illness is accompanied by shortness of breath, tachypnea, cough, and/or rales, manage according to the preceding recommendations and obtain an immediate chest x-ray to investigate for ACS.

Treatment consists of the prompt assessment of the child, followed by blood and urine cultures and administration of ceftriaxone or cefotaxime to all children. These cephalosporins have a half-life of 8 to 9 hours and are ideal antibacterial agents for most of the bacterial pathogens likely to be associated with septic episodes in SCD, including *S. pneumoniae*, *Haemophilus* sp., and *Salmonella* sp. Children who appear toxic, have an extremely high fever, and have an unreliable caretaker or to whom close outpatient follow-up is not possible should be hospitalized.

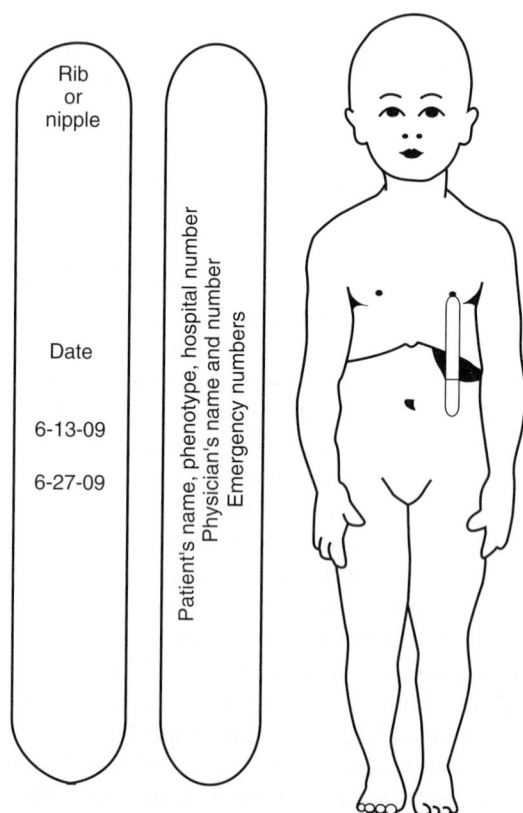

Fig. 36.6 **Measurement of spleen size with a spleen stick.** (From Eckman, J., & Platt, A. [1991]. *Problem oriented management of sickle syndromes.* NIH Sickle Cell Center.)

splenectomy is recommended, or else these children are placed on a chronic transfusion program (Kinger et al., 2021). In contrast to the acute episodes, some children develop chronic, massive splenomegaly. Splenectomy is indicated in these children when pressure or pain from the enlarged spleen is evident or accompanied by thrombocytopenia, neutropenia, or severe anemia. Patients should be assessed for delayed hemolytic transfusion reaction for 28 days after the last RBC transfusion (Chou et al., 2020).

NEUROLOGIC PROBLEMS

The vasculature of the brain is subject to vasoocclusive episodes in children with SCD. The estimated age of the first cerebrovascular accident (CVA) differs significantly for children with Hb S/S and Hb S/C. In the absence of prophylactic treatment, between 5% and 17% of SCD patients will experience a stroke in childhood or adolescence (Baker et al., 2015). Among this patient population, about 75% of strokes are ischemic, while the rest are hemorrhagic (Kirkham & Lagunju, 2021). Overall, about 2% of patients with SCD will experience a stroke (DeBaun et al., 2014).

A transient ischemic attack (TIA) occurs when a blood vessel is partially occluded by a small embolus or vessel spasm. The manifestations may be focal and last less than 24 hours without residual deficit. The general recommendation is that all children with recurrent TIAs receive the appropriate therapy for stroke prevention (i.e., chronic transfusion therapy).

When the affected vessel is completely occluded by thrombus or embolus—with or without narrowing of the vessel lining—a CVA occurs. Intracranial hemorrhage is a rare but usually fatal complication that occurs when blood vessel walls are thinned by intravascular sickling and then dilate and rupture. Computed tomography (CT), MRI, and MRA can show infarcts and areas of hemorrhage. MRI provides better detail of ischemia and can show the patchy white matter abnormal signals that are present in individuals with SCD—both with and without neurologic deficits—and are thought to be due to disease in penetrating arterioles. MRA may show large vessel occlusive disease or aneurysms. It also allows the detection of moyamoya disease, a severe form of cerebral artery stenosis that can occur in Hb S/S (Kauv et al., 2019). Symptoms include hemiparesis, aphasia, visual disturbances, seizures, altered sensation, alertness, and mentation.

Initial treatment consists of an exchange transfusion and hydration. The American Society of Hematology guidelines recommend children age 2 to 16 years with SCD Hb S/S or Hb S/β^0 thal receive an annual TCD screening. Children with Hb S/S or Hb S/β^0 thal with an abnormal TCD velocity should receive regular blood transfusions for at least 1 year with the goal of keeping maximum Hb S levels below 30%. After 1 year, these children should have HU treatment at the maximum tolerated dose to replace transfusion therapy (DeBaun et al., 2020).

Hyperthermia increases cerebral metabolism and therefore should be treated. Hypotension is treated to prevent further ischemia. Admission to an intensive care unit (ICU) facilitates the treatment and observation that these children require. Chronic transfusion (every 3–4 weeks) therapy is the standard of care to prevent recurrent stroke.

Studies have implicated SCD itself and the impact of silent infarcts in children with SCD with decreased neurocognitive development (Longoria et al., 2022). Silent cerebral infarct is associated with lower performance on measures of verbal and nonverbal reasoning, working memory, academics, and a lower full-scale intellectual quotient (IQ) (Gold et al., 2008). Assessment of neurocognitive development is warranted at an early age with ongoing evaluation of cerebral vessels by TCD for primary stroke prevention in children with Hb S/S or Hb S/β^0 thal.

VASOOCCLUSIVE CRISIS

Painful, vasoocclusive episodes are the most common cause of emergency department visits and hospital admissions for individuals with SCD. Vasoocclusion is a physiologic process, but the resultant pain is a complex biopsychosocial event. Physiologic factors combined with social considerations (e.g., developmental stage, pain history, family/child coping skills) contribute to the expression of vasoocclusion (Stinson & Naser, 2003). Each child exhibits an individualized pattern of duration, frequency, severity, and location of vasoocclusive crises. The hallmark of these crises is their unpredictability. There are two major kinds of assessment: (1) rapid assessment of the acute episode to focus on pain intensity, prompt treatment, and relief, and (2) a comprehensive assessment of chronic pain induced by boney changes (NIH, 2002).

Precipitation of painful episodes in SCD has been related to numerous factors, including weather changes (i.e., warm to cold), stress, and menstrual cycles in females. The frequency of painful episodes is indirectly related to the Hb F level, and numerous painful crises are a prognostic sign of further complications as a result of sickling. There are no laboratory values that can predict the acute onset of vasoocclusive crises, so clinicians are limited to the patient report. Clinicians should note the location, intensity, and duration of symptoms typical of the patient's pain crisis to determine whether to consider another diagnosis (Darbari et al., 2020).

Vasoocclusive crises typically affect the lower back, femur, hips, and knees, although any area in the body or organ is subject to sickling episodes (Brandow et al., 2020). In infants, the metatarsals and metacarpals can be involved resulting in dactylitis, a painful swelling of the hands and feet (Brandow et al., 2020). In long bones, infarcts are most common in the shaft and are usually confined to the medulla. Muscular infarcts occasionally occur with secondary hemorrhage and myonecrosis and are clearly seen on CT and MRI scans. Abdominal pain is often referred pain from other sites and could be mesenteric in origin. In adolescents, pain involving the vertebral bodies is often manifested.

The optimal treatment for vasoocclusive crises is multimodal and includes treating any antecedent causes, improving circulation, and providing analgesia (Brandow et al., 2020). History taking includes effective treatments at home, usual drugs, dosages, and side effects during acute pain, and medications and timing since the onset of acute pain. Primary care providers must be aware that an extraneous illness possibly precipitates a painful episode, and the child has two independent problems.

Hydration is an important part of improving circulation to the affected area. Children may be hydrated orally or intravenously with an electrolyte solution. Options for oral hydration include juice, bouillon, water, milk, sports drinks, Pedialyte, and Infalyte. As of 2020 the American Society of Hematology offers no recommendations related to intravenous fluids in conjunction with standard pharmacologic treatment (Brandow et al., 2020). Circulation to infarcted areas may also be improved by the local application of heat (e.g., heating pad, warm bath, whirlpool). Once comfort has been established, a passive range of motion and massage may be initiated. These children should be encouraged to be as active as possible.

Severe pain should be considered a medical emergency that prompts timely and aggressive management. Analgesia may take several forms, including nonpharmacologic agents, nonsteroidal antiinflammatory drugs (NSAIDs), and oral or parenteral narcotics. Multimodal therapy, which includes several of these approaches, is more effective than single agents because each agent increases analgesia (Brandow et al., 2020). NSAIDs act on peripheral inflammatory pain receptors, and narcotics act centrally. This combination therapy may also contravene the ceiling effect that occurs with nonsteroidal drugs and acetaminophen, and have a significant narcotic-sparing effect. The dose given should begin at a standard therapeutic dose or a dose known to be therapeutic for a given child and then be adjusted as needed. Placebos are never appropriate because they erode the trusting relationship between the health care provider and the child.

Many narcotics have very brief half-lives, and care must be taken to administer them often enough for analgesic effect. For example, when a medication with a 12-hour half-life is used, dosing should be approximately every 2 hours to maintain consistent pain relief (Ellison & Shaw, 2007). Early in the course of a vasoocclusive episode, the vascular occlusion is constant—not intermittent. Therefore early in the course of a painful episode, as-needed dosing is

inappropriate; scheduled doses of narcotics should be given over the first 24 hours after admission for vasoocclusive crisis. Later in the course, collateral circulation may develop, or the occlusion may have decreased, improving vascular circulation to the infarcted area. It is preferable to control a child's pain early in the course of the illness and maintain control by frequent reassessment. The first dose of parenteral opioid analgesia should be administered to the patient within 1 hour of arriving at the emergency department (Brandow et al., 2020).

It is inappropriate to administer intramuscular injections to children for pain relief because an injection alone can be quite painful unless it is for a single dose and a longer half-life is desired (e.g., for outpatient management) or if intravenous access has not been obtained. Intrathecal catheters have been suggested as a route for analgesic administration for children who are hospitalized with severe, intractable pain but should not be considered before an adequate trial of maximal doses of systemic opioid and adjuvant medications are given.

Because all pain episodes cannot be prevented, children and their families should be taught to manage mild pain and recognize symptoms that suggest serious problems. For mild pain, nonnarcotic medicines, including acetaminophen, aspirin (provided there is no concurrent viral process or other contraindication), ibuprofen, and ketorolac, are appropriate and may be given at the standard recommended dosages. Caution should be exercised with the use of NSAIDs in children with renal or liver complications. Optimal management requires adequate education of the child, family, and health care providers (Fig. 36.7).

When children become significantly uncomfortable, they experience anxiety and consequently a heightened perception of pain. They may ultimately develop dysfunctional illness behavior as a result of inadequately treated pain. It is important for the child, family, and health care providers to have realistically attainable goals related to pain control. The goal of pain management should be prompt pain relief to a functional level. Relief could be defined as a pain intensity reduction of at least 50% to 60% from the upper end of the pain scale. The alleviation of pain provided by narcotics must be balanced against known side effects such as pruritus, nausea, constipation, and respiratory depression. Hospitalized children are routinely started on stool softeners and laxatives at the onset of opioid therapy and given standing orders for antihistamines for pruritus and antinausea medications. Side effects, such as respiratory depression, should be closely monitored by scheduled visual observations and pulse oximetry.

Several classic studies have documented the low prevalence of drug addiction within this population (Ahmed et al., 2022). Despite these studies, health care providers continue to believe that drug addiction is

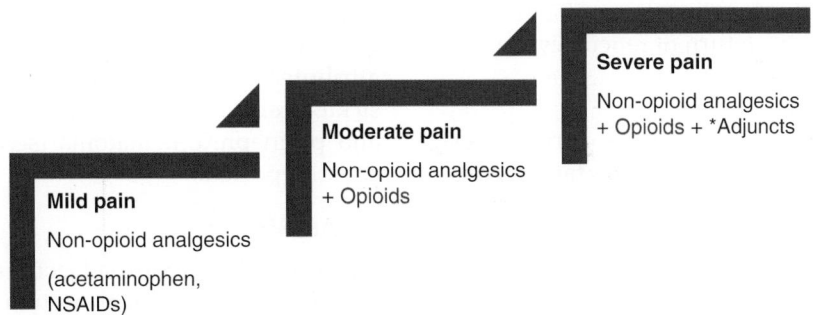

Fig. 36.7 **Pain treatment options.** *NSAID,* Nonsteroidal antiinflammatory drug. *Adjuncts include nonopioid analgesics such as ketamine, lidocaine, and gabapentinoids. (From Gai, N., Naser, B., Hanley, J., Peliowski, A., Hayes, J., Aoyama, K. (2020). A practical guide to acute pain management in children. *J Anesth, 34*(3), 421–433. doi:10.1007/s00540-020-02767-x.)

a major problem among people with SCD, which is unfortunate because this misperception can interfere with the provision of adequate health care. Tolerance and physical dependence are expected pharmacologic consequences of long-term opioid use and should not be confused with addiction (NIH, 2002).

ACUTE CHEST SYNDROME

ACS ranks second as a cause of hospitalization and is responsible for 25% of all deaths from SCD. ACS is an illness characterized by a new infiltrate on a chest x-ray accompanied by pain, leukocytosis, hypoxia, cough, or fever (Jain et al., 2017). ACS is a life-threatening complication that results from infection, pulmonary fat embolism, or pulmonary infarction (Jain et al., 2017). ACS can also be induced by respiratory depression caused by narcotics or general anesthesia. Twenty-five percent of individuals with SCD who undergo major surgery are shown to develop postoperative ACS (Jain et al., 2017).

Fever, cough, and tachypnea are often the only abnormal findings in children. ACS may be difficult to differentiate from and may be concurrent with pneumonia. Physical examination usually reveals tachypnea, but there may also be evidence of pulmonary consolidation, pleural effusion, a new pulmonary infiltrate, or pleural friction rub. Thirty-five percent of individuals with ACS will have a normal lung examination (Jain et al., 2017). Chest radiographic studies may be normal for the first few days, especially if a child is dehydrated.

ACS is often a fulminant process and may rapidly progress to pulmonary failure and death. Admission to the ICU may be necessary for close monitoring. Pulse oximetry and vital signs should be followed closely, and supplemental oxygen and further respiratory support should be provided as needed. All children should be encouraged to use scheduled incentive spirometry to fully aerate their lungs. Early transfusion may be necessary to prevent progressive problems because hypoxia will induce further sickling; partial or complete exchange transfusion may be needed (NIH, 2002). Pulmonary consultation is recommended to optimize early and aggressive treatment.

ACS is the most common cause of death in children with SCD. Pulmonary pressures increase during an episode of severe ACS, resulting in pulmonary hypertension (pHTN) (Jain et al., 2017). pHTN is detected by an echocardiogram (Jain et al., 2017), is associated with accelerated mortality rate, and is present in about 30% of adults with Hb S/S. The prevalence in children with SCD is largely unknown. A recent study indicated that in children with SCD, a history of sepsis, ACS, or obstructive lung disease was a factor associated with pHTN (Jain et al., 2017). In a cohort study, 30% of children (age ≥10 years) with SCD were found to have pHTN (Jain et al., 2017). Recent recommendations at many comprehensive sickle cell centers include obtaining an echocardiogram annually after age 10 years (Jain et al., 2017). Frequent episodes of ACS and painful events are associated with shorter life spans (NIH, 2002). A study by Quinn et al. (2007) showed that an episode of ACS in the first 3 years of life predicts recurrent ACS throughout childhood. Since ACS may be difficult to differentiate from pneumonia, primary care providers should empirically use antibiotics directed against *S. pneumoniae, H. influenzae, S. aureus,* and other pathogens commonly seen in community-acquired pneumonia.

TRANSIENT RED CELL APLASIA (FORMERLY APLASTIC CRISIS)

Periodically the bone marrow does not respond to a fall in hemoglobin and hematocrit values caused by the rapid turnover of RBCs. In this scenario, the hemoglobin and hematocrit values drop, and there is a lack of compensatory rise in the reticulocyte count that usually happens during or following a viral infection. Symptoms may include fever, more severe anemia than usual, headache, fatigue, and dyspnea, and the child may have signs of respiratory involvement or gastrointestinal involvement. Human parvovirus B19 has been implicated in 70% to 100% of episodes of transient red cell aplasia (NIH, 2002). Children being cared for during and shortly after a viral illness should be observed for unusual pallor or prolonged lethargy. Therapy includes slow transfusion to a hemoglobin level slightly above the baseline hemoglobin level. Recovery is indicated by a return of reticulocytosis.

HEMOLYSIS

Hemolysis in SCD is usually of only moderate severity. The symptoms of anemia (e.g., pallor, fatigue, dyspnea) are not the hallmarks of this disorder. Hemolysis is generally associated with clinical observations of scleral icterus, tea-colored urine, and elevated bilirubin and urobilinogen levels. One long-term consequence of hemolysis is the high prevalence of gallstones in children with SCD. Pigmented gallstones develop in approximately 30% of children with SCD by age 18 years (Wilson et al., 2003). Increased hemolysis may be triggered by bacterial infections, poisons, or glucose-6-phosphate dehydrogenase deficiency. Hemolysis accompanied by brisk reticulocytosis requires no treatment.

RENAL PROBLEMS

The environment within the renal medulla is characterized by low oxygen tension, acidosis, and hypertonicity. Therefore intravascular sickling occurs more rapidly in the kidney than in any other organ. Persistent proteinuria, beginning early in life, is the hallmark of sickle nephropathy that occurs in all forms of SCD and is associated with the severity of the disease (Fitzhugh et al., 2005). This intravascular sickling leaves the kidney with a relative inability to concentrate urine (i.e., hyposthenuria) or adequately acidify urine, which is an early sign of end-stage renal disease. The relative inability to concentrate urine often leads to enuresis or nocturia and also results in a relative inability to excrete potassium and uric acid. Of children with SCD, 16% experience microalbuminuria; an annual assessment is recommended beginning at 10 years of age (NHLBI, 2014). Patients with significant albuminuria should see a nephrologist for full evaluation (Liem et al., 2019).

Renal failure as a result of progressive sickle cell nephropathy affects 4% to 20% of adults with SCD (McKie et al., 2007). Early detection of proteinuria may indicate the need for therapy to prevent chronic, progressive renal insufficiency (Fitzhugh et al., 2005). Several studies have shown that the presence of microalbuminuria precedes proteinuria and serves as an early marker for glomerular injury in SCD (Fitzhugh et al., 2005; McKie et al., 2007). The use of enalapril has been shown to reduce urinary protein excretion and normalize serum albumin. Combination therapy with HU has been shown to further normalize the urine protein/creatinine ratio (Fitzhugh et al., 2005).

Gross hematuria may occur in children with SCD or sickle trait. Blood loss is usually minimal, resolving within 1 to 3 days with bedrest and hydration, and does not require transfusion. As with all individuals with gross hematuria, diagnoses of glomerulonephritis, tumor, renal stones, urinary tract infection, and bleeding disorders must be excluded. When other diagnoses have been eliminated, hematuria is often attributed to areas of ischemia or necrosis caused by sickled cells. Renal papillary necrosis, renal infarction, and perinephric hematoma (secondary to infarction) are all reported.

PRIAPISM

Males with Hb S/S are subject to episodes of priapism. Priapism occurs when an accumulation of sickled cells obstructs the venous drainage of the corpora cavernosa of the penis, causing a prolonged and exquisitely painful erection of the penis. Priapism is not associated with sexual desire or excitement (Wilson et al., 2003). In addition, micturition is often difficult, and urinary retention may occur. If left untreated, irreversible fibrosis and impotency may occur. MRI is useful in demonstrating corporal destruction with the development of intracorporeal fibrosis and hemosiderin deposition.

The mean age at manifestation is 12 years, and by age 20 years approximately 89% of all males with SCD will have experienced one or more episodes of priapism (Wilson et al., 2003). The following two general patterns of priapism are described:

1. Stuttering (recurrent) attacks lasting less than 3 hours that may precede a severe episode
2. Severe attacks lasting longer than 3 hours that may lead to impotence

At the onset, the child should be counseled to urinate (a full bladder aggravates priapism), drink extra fluids, walk, take a warm shower, and use oral analgesics (Kavanagh et al., 2022; Maples & Hageman, 2004). Treatment of severe episodes also begins with conservative measures and, after 3 hours, includes progression to hospitalization, hydration, transfusions, pain management, and urologic consultation. The application of ice is inappropriate because it promotes vasoconstriction. Surgical intervention is considered if there is no detumescence after 4 to 6 hours of conservative treatment (NIH, 2002). Surgical measures aim to reestablish adequate venous outflow and circulation of the corporal body via aspiration and—if not successful—placement of a shunt (Wilson et al., 2003).

Prophylactic regimens include the addition of vasodilatory drugs, including hydralazine and pseudoephedrine, alpha- and beta-agonists, and chronic transfusion programs (Wilson et al., 2003). Despite the intervention, impotence is a frequent complication of priapism. Research is currently looking into new pharmacologic agents, as well as improved surgical interventions, to address this troublesome complication (Maples & Hageman, 2004).

SKELETAL CHANGES

SCD involves both hematologic and osseous abnormalities because it affects the two major functions of bone tissue: hematopoiesis and osteogenesis. Skeletal changes, such as dactylitis (see earlier), occur because of the expansion of the bone marrow and recurrent infarction in children with SCD. Back pain is common in older children and is recognized on radiographs by fish-mouthed vertebrae, which have decreased vertical height and increased width (Mulligan, 2004).

Sudden infarction causes acute symptoms of pain and must be differentiated from those of bacterial origin. Osteomyelitis is the second most common infection in children with SCD, with *Salmonella* osteomyelitis occurring several hundred times more often in SCD as compared with the general pediatric population (Al Farii et al., 2020). Common sites include the long bones and vertebral bones. Common symptoms consist of pain, warmth, and swelling, as well as limitation of motion to the affected area.

The pathophysiology of bone erosions in Hb S/S results from necrosis produced by repeated microinfarction. Repeated infarction may lead to avascular necrosis. This pathology most commonly involves the head of the femur but may also occur in the head of the humerus or fibula. Treatment includes physical therapy (PT) and judicious use of local heat and analgesics for pain relief.

OPHTHALMOLOGIC CHANGES

Ophthalmologic complications are a direct result of the vasoocclusive process within the eye. Because early stages of eye disease do not result in visual symptoms, they may go undiagnosed unless an eye examination is performed by an ophthalmologist. Most screenings begin at age 8 or 9 years, when the child is able to cooperate, although most defects occur during the second decade of life (Menaa et al., 2017). The ophthalmologic examination should occur every year beginning at age 10 years (Thornburg et al., 2012). These complications include nonproliferative retinopathy, proliferative retinopathy, and elevated intraocular pressure. Sickle cell retinopathy most often occurs in individuals with SCD type S/C (de Melo, 2014).

Nonproliferative retinopathy may not affect visual acuity. Proliferative sickle retinopathy can cause vitreous hemorrhage and subsequent retinal detachment and blindness. The occurrence of proliferative sickle retinopathy depends on an individual's age and type of hemoglobinopathy and is progressive.

AUDIOLOGIC PROBLEMS

Vasoocclusive episodes within the circulation of the inner ear and the administration of ototoxic drugs may cause sensorineural hearing loss. This loss may be unilateral or bilateral but is generally manifested as a high-frequency deficit. As expected with hearing loss, speech screening should be implemented. Children with SCD typically have either an articulation disorder or a fluency disorder at a rate higher than expected.

LEG ULCERS

Leg ulcers are experienced by 8% to 10% of adults with SCD (Onimoe & Rotz, 2020). There is an increased risk in tropical regions, in males, and in those with low hematocrit. Trauma is believed to be a common cause of leg ulcers in SCD. Anemia, thrombocytosis, and venous incompetence are also thought to be contributing factors. Sickle cell ulcers classically appear as round, punched-out ulcers with raised margins, deep bases, and necrotic slough and can produce significant pain and limit movement (Minniti et al., 2010). Early, prompt treatment includes bedrest, elevation, and wound care with antibiotics for cellulitic areas, but skin grafting and transfusion therapy may also be needed. The specific type of wound care is controversial and should be directed by a competent plastic surgeon. Patients should be referred to a wound care clinic. There is no evidence that chronic transfusions are a suitable treatment (Minniti & Kato, 2016).

PREPARATION FOR ANESTHESIA OR CONTRAST MEDIUM (SURGERY OR RADIOLOGIC STUDIES)

General anesthesia and hyperosmolar contrast medium are both known to induce sickling (Kokoska et al., 2004). If an operative or diagnostic procedure using these agents is anticipated, most hematologists suggest that children with SCD receive transfusion to a hemoglobin level of 10 g/dL. Children with Hb S/C usually carry this hemoglobin value at baseline and most likely would not require a transfusion. Unusually high-risk children are the exception to this rule. All children undergoing tonsillectomies and adenoidectomies should be transfused because these surgeries appear to be more serious for the child with SCD as a result of associated blood loss, fluid loss, and inability to orally hydrate (Hirst & Williamson, 2012). Additional measures such as warming the operating room, warming the intravenous fluids, and placing the child on a warming blanket during surgery are warranted (Kokoska et al., 2004).

CARDIAC PROBLEMS

Over time the cardiovascular system accommodates chronic anemia with increased cardiac output (Sachdev et al., 2021). This chronic volume overload causes cardiac enlargement. Cardiac enlargement is often apparent on chest radiographs, the precordium is hyperactive, and a low-grade systolic ejection murmur may be heard in the second and third left intercostal spaces on examination. Cardiomegaly is an adaptation to anemia and alone should not be considered pathologic. Children with Hb S/S are subject to the same medical conditions as other children; therefore findings suggestive of congenital, rheumatic, or underlying heart disease should be investigated. In such cases, an echocardiogram and cardiac consultation are recommended. Machado et al. (2007) reported increased pulmonary pressures during exercise that may contribute to morbidity and mortality risk in individuals with SCD.

HEPATOBILIARY PROBLEMS

Biochemical and radiologic hepatic abnormalities are common in individuals with SCD. The ongoing elevated rate of RBC hemolysis generates an increase in serum bilirubin (Kyrana et al., 2021). Likewise, elevations of the serum alkaline phosphatase and lactic dehydrogenase levels as a result of bone metabolism and hemolysis are often seen. Elevation in the serum alkaline phosphatase is common, particularly during pain crises. Children who have right upper quadrant pain, increased jaundice, and fever need careful evaluation and management. Crisis pain involving the liver is often indistinguishable from acute cholecystitis. Transfused children are at risk for viral hepatitis and hepatic hemosiderosis, which can result in hepatic injury and fibrosis (Chou et al., 2020).

Gallstones of bile or calcium bilirubinate are a common finding and are easily seen via ultrasound. These gallstones are found in 14% to 30% of children with SCD and are most common in individuals with Hb S/S (Kyrana et al., 2021).

Surgeons should be aware of the finding that concomitant common bile duct stones have been reported in individuals with SCD and cholelithiasis. Both laparoscopic and open cholecystectomies are approved for individuals with SCD, given that appropriate preoperative preparation is addressed (Hirst & Williamson, 2012).

A hepatic crisis (sometimes known as right upper quadrant syndrome or acute sickle hepatic crisis) may be indistinguishable from acute cholecystitis. RBC sequestration in the liver causes hepatocellular dysfunction, which decreases bilirubin excretion. This syndrome is most often self-limited and resolves within 2 weeks with intravenous fluid hydration and analgesia, but hepatic failure resulting from massive sickling has also been reported (Friedman, 2007).

TRANSFUSION COMPLICATIONS

Individuals with SCD may need transfusions emergently, episodically, or chronically. Performing RBC phenotyping before transfusion avoids the problems associated with the development of RBC antibodies. Children requiring RBC transfusions should be given phenotypically matched units. Several centers have been successful in recruiting minority donors for extended matching for RBC antigens. This matching has markedly decreased the occurrence of alloimmunization and should be the standard for children needing chronic transfusions. The complications of transfusions include possible exposure to bloodborne infectious agents, formation of alloantibodies, and iron overload resulting from chronic or multiple transfusions. Individuals with iron overload experience progressive organ dysfunction, leading to iron-induced cardiac damage and death. Iron load is measured by serum ferritin levels and, more specifically, by liver biopsy.

PROGNOSIS

In a classic study done over 30 years ago (Powars, 1975), a group of adults and children were longitudinally followed to determine the natural history of SCD. The disease effects in the adults tended to be chronic and organ related, and the problems in the children were acute and often infectious. The predicted overall survival in one large cohort of individuals with Hb S/S and Hb S/β⁰ thal at age 18 years was found to be 86%. A study by Reed and Vichinsky (2001) indicated that the overall mortality rate (at least in some regions of the United States) has decreased to less than 2% by age 10 years. The average longevity in persons with the Hb S/S genotype is 42 years for males and 48 years for females, whereas males and females with the Hb S/C genotype live to age 60 and 68 years, respectively (Reed & Vichinsky, 2001). In the United States, the current life expectancy for individuals with SCD is 54 years, compared to 76 years for individuals without SCD (Lubeck et al., 2019). Young adults age 20 to 24 years with SCD experience increased mortality rates. This is thought to be due to loss of insurance coverage, discontinuity of care, worsening SCD complications, and increased reliance on emergency room care as opposed to primary and hematology clinicians (Mainous et al., 2019).

SCD is characterized by a highly variable phenotype within each genotype, leading to varying severity of disease among the population. The CSSCD identified the following factors as predictors of adverse outcomes: lower hemoglobin level, lower Hb F level, increased pain rate, and an increased steady-state WBC count (Quinn, 2016). This striking variability between genotypes provides another example of the variable presentation of symptoms and complications that must be considered by the primary care provider. Sickle thalassemia is reported to have lower rates of complications and mortality in children who inherit this genetic variant. The beta-globin gene cluster haplotypes further affect the severity of the disorder (Powars et al., 1994).

This information on genotypes assumes urgency in prenatal diagnosis and in making decisions about potentially life-threatening procedures (e.g., bone marrow transplant). The decision to continue a pregnancy can rest on the perceived future clinical course of a child. Factors determining the extremely variable clinical course include the following: (1) genetic factors (e.g., a thalassemia, beta-globin gene haplotypes, heterocellular hereditary, persistence of Hb F, and high total hemoglobin) and (2) adherence to suggested clinical guidelines (e.g., penicillin prophylaxis, pneumococcal vaccinations, adequate hydration, and early recognition of life-threatening complications) (Chui & Dover, 2001).

The incidence of invasive pneumococcal disease has decreased by 68% since the advent of the pneumococcal conjugate vaccine (Prevnar) (Adamkiewicz et al., 2008). Adherence to prophylactic penicillin administration is critical in the early years. Improving parental knowledge about SCD has proven to correlate with increased use of the appropriate and timely medical intervention. As early intervention decreases or eliminates deaths from sepsis, ACS, and splenic sequestration, the primary issue will be chronic organ damage—notably renal, neurologic, and pulmonary changes.

Intrinsic, sociocultural, health care, and structural factors all contribute to an individual's experience with SCD. Many individuals with SCD perceive health care as inadequate to their needs, which has been demonstrated through stigma, bias, bidirectional mistrust, lack of therapy options, and poor access to clinical trials (Lee et al., 2019).

PRIMARY CARE MANAGEMENT

Primary care providers play an important role in the care of these patients as the umbrella to the medical home, supporting the primary care office visits and coordinating care with the interdisciplinary team. The primary care provider must be familiar with the manifestations and management of SCD.

HEALTH CARE MAINTENANCE

Regular Office Visits

The aims of regular attendance at the primary care office include the following:

1. Facilitates partnership between the patient, family, health care providers, and medical staff of the specialty care clinics
2. Encourages adherence to treatment plans, particularly penicillin prophylaxis and immunization schedule
3. Continues to educate on the signs and symptoms to ensure early access to medical care when appropriate
4. Monitors general health, nutrition, and growth
5. Discusses treatments and screening tests and refers to appropriate specialists

Primary Care Office Visits

The following is a guide to what should be included in office visits for children diagnosed with SCD.

History should include the following:

- Review of current symptoms, painful episodes, illnesses, accidents, emergency attendances, or hospital admissions since the last visit
- A focused inquiry about symptoms (e.g., abdominal pain, pica, enuresis, priapism, headaches, snoring, other neurologic symptoms suggestive of ischemia)

- Adherence to penicillin prophylaxis and any other medications
- Adherence to the vaccination schedule
- A review of how pain and fever are managed at home
- School attendance and reasons for absence
- Outcome of developmental screening tests, school progress, and achievement in national tests (e.g., standard attainment tests, General Certificate of Secondary Education)
- Advance planning for travel, in particular, if involving air travel, which is associated with increased risk of complications (airlines will have their own regulations)

Examinations should include the following:

- An assessment of growth and development
- A general physical exam, noting any pallor, jaundice, spleen size, or presence of a murmur
- Blood pressure

Growth and Development

Classic studies by Modebe and Ifenu (1993) and Platt (1994) show that—starting at approximately 6 months of age and being clearly defined by the preschool years—children with Hb S/S and Hb S/β⁰ thal demonstrate a pattern of physical growth that is divergent from that of their unaffected peers. These children are shorter, weigh less, and have a smaller percentage of body fat and delayed bone age. However, their muscle mass and head circumference are comparable with those of their unaffected peers. Weight is affected more than height, and males are affected more than females. People with SCD develop slower because of anemia; sickle cells are unstable and burst prematurely, making the body unable to make enough RBCs causing anemia and delayed growth (Hoyt et al., 2022). Pubertal changes are also delayed for both males and females, with normal height typically being achieved by adulthood, but weight remains lower with SCD. Factors known to impact child development include socioeconomic status, parental education levels, nutrition, and sleep; frequent hospitalizations, school absences, and medication side effects (common with chronic illnesses); and brain injury, impaired cerebral perfusion, and chronic anemia specific to SCD (Lance et al., 2021).

Infants with SCD are typically of average size; by 2 to 5 years of age, their slower growth becomes apparent. Females may experience recovery of height and weight as they go through puberty, whereas males may continue delayed growth beyond their teen years (Lance et al., 2021).

These changes are coincident with the usual physiologic waning of Hb F levels. It has also been noted that the growth of children who, for unknown reasons, persist in producing Hb F is usually not as delayed as that of other children with SCD. Children receiving chronic transfusions, however, maintain age-appropriate growth parameters, which suggests that hemolytic anemia plays a major role in the growth delay in children with Hb S/S.

Physical growth parameters should be measured and plotted on standardized growth charts every 3 to 4 months for children with SCD. The pattern of growth of an individual child, however, is more important than the comparison with unaffected children.

There are many standardized screening tools for developmental delay: Ages and Stages Questionnaires, Battelle Developmental Inventory Screening Tool, Child Development Inventory, Parents' Evaluation of Developmental Status, among others. Children found to be at developmental risk should be referred for a more thorough developmental assessment and connected with developmental services. A consistent health care provider is invaluable for monitoring developmental progress in children with SCD.

Diet

A child's diet should be well balanced with a generous amount of fluid. Diet during illness or disease exacerbation may include whatever nutritive dense solid foods children desire with oral fluids at 1.5 times their usual fluid intake. Maintenance of daily fluid intake is essential in maintaining homeostasis in children with SCD. A fluid sheet outlining times to increase fluids and amounts of oral fluids should be given as a reference to parents.

Because of increased metabolic demands, children with SCD have a relative deficiency of energy, protein, and several micronutrients, so the recommended daily allowances for the normal population may not be applicable. Limited metabolic studies support the hypothesis that chronic hemolysis leads to a state of high protein turnover and increased metabolic requirements. Although reduced physical activity may allow the energy balance to be maintained in the short term, a persistent energy deficit leads to growth retardation.

Classically associated with iron deficiency and lead poisoning, pica (compulsively eating nonfood items) can also be an emotional response to the stressors associated with chronic or recurrent pain. Several studies show a high incidence of pica in children with SCD, especially those with low hemoglobin levels and high reticulocyte counts (Rodrigues et al., 2019). Children with SCD have an unusually high prevalence of pica. Pica is the repeated and compulsive ingestion of nonnutritive substances for at least 1 month. Classically, pica has been associated with iron deficiency anemia and lead encephalopathy; because of the independent association of SCD and pica, more frequent surveillance for both pica and blood lead levels in the SCD population is warranted (Jung & Peddinti, 2018).

Due to increased erythropoiesis with SCD, there is an increased risk for folate deficiency. Folic acid therapy is commonly recommended at 1 mg orally every day with documented reduced iron stores as measured by serum iron, serum ferritin, and iron binding capacity (Dixit et al., 2018).

Safety

Most children with Hb S/S regularly take oral medicines (e.g., folic acid, antibiotics, narcotics) at home. Ingestion of narcotics beyond the prescribed amount can lead to lethargy and respiratory depression or death. All medicines should be safely stored. Adolescents should be cautioned about driving a car or using machinery while taking narcotics and be counseled that alcohol may potentiate the depressant effects of narcotics. Alcohol should also be avoided because it can cause dehydration and subsequent sickling. Smoking is strongly discouraged because it leads to vasoconstriction and concomitant problems. Parents should be cautioned about allowing exposure to reptiles as pets because of the risk of salmonella exposure (CDC, 2022).

Guidance regarding the importance of supplementing routine hydration in hot temperatures and with viral illnesses is essential. Recreational activities that involve prolonged exposure to cold, prolonged exertion, or exposure to high altitudes (i.e., >10,000 feet) in an unpressurized aircraft should be avoided. Sports injuries should not be treated with ice because this can cause localized sickling. An awareness of each child's baseline spleen size is an important aspect of safety education when the child with sickle cell is engaging in physical activity.

Adolescents with SCD often demonstrate the same limit-testing and risk-taking behaviors as their unaffected peers. Parents must balance their child's need for safety with their child's need to become self-sufficient. An information card or medical alert bracelet is often helpful in emergency situations.

Immunizations

The current recommendation from the Advisory Committee on Immunization Practices (ACIP) is strict adherence to the recommended immunization schedule for asplenic patients (Infanti et al., 2020). The specific schedule recommended by the ACIP for patients with SCD includes the Hib vaccine, pneumococcal vaccines (PCV7, PCV13, PPSAV23), the meningococcal vaccines for serogroups A, C, W, and Y (MenACWY), and serogroup B (MenB) (Figs. 36.8, 36.9, 36.10, and 36.11).

Screenings

Guidelines recommend universal screenings for all patients in specialty and subspecialty clinics. The socioeconomic factors that influence health outcomes or social determinants of health (SDoH) are often noted in subspecialty clinics that require additional resources and are often limited for individuals who have a chronic illness and racial disparities. Health care providers can impact both the quality of life and the clinical outcomes for SCD patients by implementing screenings and referral programs that address SDoH (Power-Hays et al., 2019).

Blood pressure. Blood pressure should be measured at every visit due to the increased risk of cardiovascular disease in children and adolescents with SCD. Increased systolic blood pressure differed for males and females with SCD compared to the general population (Kupferman et al., 2022).

Dental. Routine screening is recommended. Providing children with special health care needs with high-quality dental care necessitates active liaisons with health care facilitators and requires work across professions to make certain that these children's oral health is prioritized. Guidelines for prophylaxis should be followed per specialists and AAP (2022b) recommendations.

Hearing. Routine audiologic evaluations are recommended to screen for hearing loss related to vasoocclusion or hyperviscosity in the inner ear. Any abnormal findings on routine school screenings should be followed up on immediately. Sensorineural hearing loss has been occasionally described in this population.

Hematocrit. Routine hematocrit screening is not necessary because of regular CBC monitoring, which should be done every 4 to 6 months at a sickle cell treatment center.

Mental health. Routine check-ins with the patient and family are recommended to see how they are

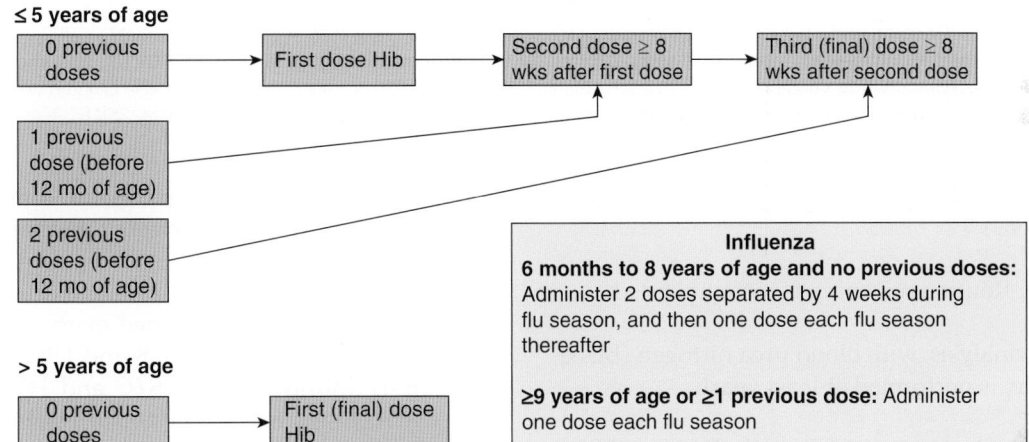

Fig. 36.8 Recommended immunization schedule for Hib in patients with sickle cell disease and those relevant for the purpose of this study. (From Infanti, L.M., et al. [2020]. Immunization adherence in children with sickle cell disease: A single institution experience. *Journal of Pediatric Pharmacology and Therapeutics, 25*[1], 39–46.)

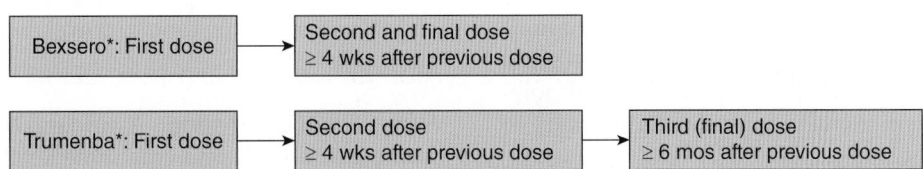

Fig. 36.9 Recommended immunization schedule for MenB in patients 10 years of age and older with sickle cell disease and those relevant for the purpose of this study. *Bexsero or Trumenba, not both. (From Infanti, L.M., et al. [2020]. Immunization adherence in children with sickle cell disease: A single institution experience. *Journal of Pediatric Pharmacology and Therapeutics, 25*[1], 39–46.)

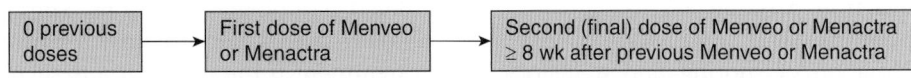

Note: Wait until at least 4 weeks after completed PCV series to administer.

Fig. 36.10 Recommended immunization schedule for meningococcal ACWY (MenACWY) in patients 2 years of age and older with sickle cell disease and those relevant for the purpose of this study. (From Infanti, L.M., et al. [2020]. Immunization adherence in children with sickle cell disease: A single institution experience. *Journal of Pediatric Pharmacology and Therapeutics, 25*[1], 39–46.)

2–5 years of age

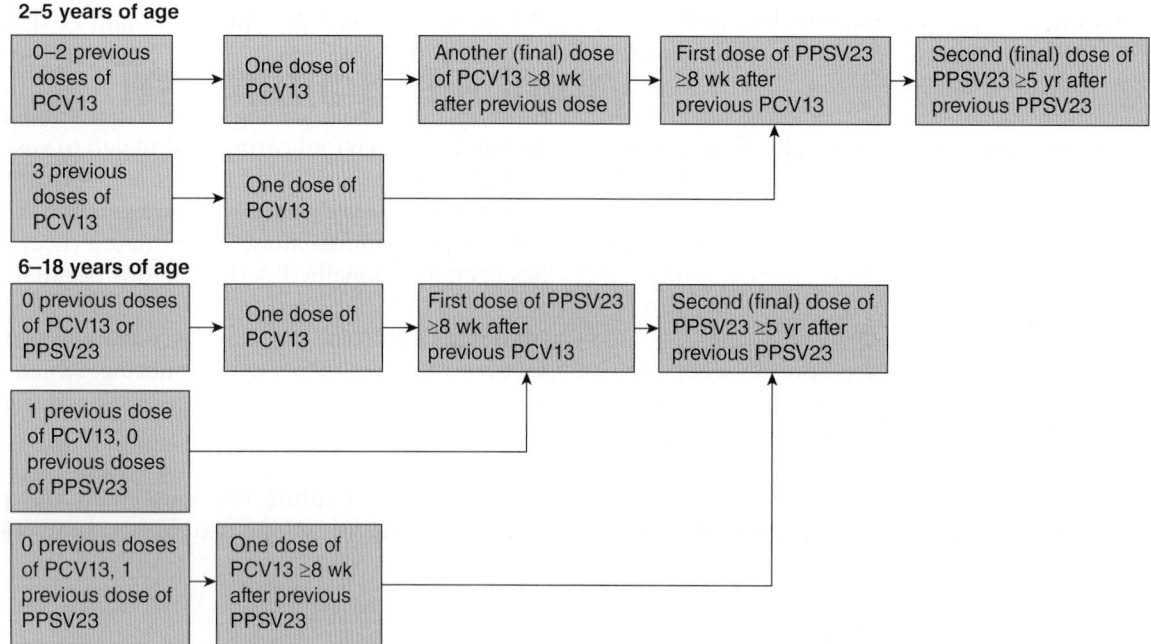

6–18 years of age

Fig. 36.11 Recommended immunization schedule for pneumococcal vaccines in patients with sickle cell disease and those relevant for the purpose of this study. Pneumococcal conjugate vaccine (PCV13), pneumococcal polysaccharide vaccine (PPSV23). (From Infanti, L.M., et al. [2020]. Immunization adherence in children with sickle cell disease: A single institution experience. *Journal of Pediatric Pharmacology and Therapeutics*, 25[1], 39–46.)

coping with the SCD (e.g., pain, fatigue, medical visits, hospitalizations).

Tuberculosis. Routine screening is recommended.

Urinalysis. Urinalysis, with blood urea nitrogen (BUN) and creatinine, is performed at least yearly.

Vision. Appropriate referral for screening should be made for children with SCD for routine screening. Based on the risk factors with SCD, the current recommendation by the AAP is for retinopathy screening of children by dilated fundoscopic examination with Hb S/S and Hb S/C beginning at age 10 years for baseline evaluation followed by appropriate eye examinations based on ocular findings (Pahl et al., 2017). If a child sustains any eye trauma, referral to an ophthalmologist for evaluation of increased intraocular pressure or retinal detachment is necessary.

Condition-Specific Screening

Pulse oximetry. Readings should be obtained at every visit, noting changes from baseline. Because children with SCD are susceptible to infections that may progress to ACS, a baseline reading is invaluable in determining divergence from baseline.

Sleep apnea. Notation of snoring and a history of restless sleep should be obtained at each visit, noting episodes of daytime sleepiness. Enlarged tonsils or adenoids may be the culprit in inducing episodes of sleep apnea, and if found in the sleep study, it is an indication

for surgical removal. Oxygen desaturation occurs during these episodes and is a trigger for sickling events.

Hematologic screening. CBC with differential and reticulocyte counts are obtained every 4 to 6 months (every 3–4 months for Hb S/S and Hb S/β0 thal and every 6–12 months for Hb S/C and Hb S/β+ thal). These screenings are important to establish baseline data and determine bone marrow function. Knowing the RBC phenotype of a well child who has not had a transfusion can expedite any future transfusions. Quantitative hemoglobin electrophoresis is obtained at 1 year of age to determine the presence of fetal hemoglobin. Some comprehensive sickle cell centers test children during this time to correlate Hb F levels with clinical severity.

Renal function testing. A urinalysis should be performed, and BUN and creatinine levels checked annually to monitor renal function. Commonly seen in children with SCD is the inability to concentrate or acidify urine, which will be evident in the urinalysis. Urobilinogen, a by-product of bilirubin metabolism, is also a frequent finding. Hematuria may be a manifestation of renal dysfunction secondary to SCD or other unrelated pathologic conditions. These children should be referred to a nephrologist for further evaluation and treatment if the hematuria is severe or casts are present in the urine. Proteinuria is the most common and early clinical manifestation of glomerular injury to the kidney. Follow-up requires a urine culture and sensitivity and—if negative—a 24-hour collection of urine for protein quantitation. An elevation requires referral to a nephrologist.

Lead poisoning. Bright Futures (AAP, 2022a) Periodicity Schedule 4 recommends risk assessments at well-child visits (age 6 months, 9 months, 12 months, 18 months, 24 months, 3 years, 4 years, 5 years, and 6 years) and, if positive, obtaining blood lead levels. Obtaining serum lead levels is the most appropriate test to facilitate a diagnosis of lead poisoning. Box 36.3 provides guidelines for targeted screening.

Scoliosis. Scoliosis screenings should be done through late adolescence because of the delayed growth spurts of children with SCD.

Cardiac function. Electrocardiography (ECG) and echocardiography (ECHO) may be performed every 1 to 2 years after age 5 years to evaluate the impact of chronic anemia on ventricular function. Efforts should be made to establish whether symptoms of chest pain, dyspnea, or decreased exercise tolerance have occurred, and significant symptoms should be evaluated with exercise testing. Functional murmurs are frequently heard in these children because of chronic anemia, and parents should be counseled as to their compensatory mechanism.

Liver function. Yearly liver function studies are helpful in evaluating RBC metabolism and liver function. Bilirubin is often elevated as a consequence of hemolysis, as well as liver disease. Bilirubin levels rise gradually until the third decade of life. Scleral icterus and tea-colored urine are indicative of bilirubin produced by chronic hemolysis and are frequently seen. Alkaline phosphatase levels fall after periods of rapid growth in adolescence and reach lower levels in females than in males. Children on chronic transfusion programs should be screened yearly for human immunodeficiency virus (HIV) and hepatitis C.

COMMON ILLNESS MANAGEMENT

Differential Diagnosis

Fever. As a result of functional asplenia, a bacterial infection is a significant cause of morbidity and mortality in children with SCD. The incidence of bacteremia in children with SCD is highest among those under 2 years of age and declines from age 2 to 6 years. Febrile patients under age 2 years in the past were admitted with fevers and SCD. Newer evidence-based research shows a pathway for clinical management of pediatric patients with SCD under age 2 years to safely decrease hospital admissions who meet low-risk criteria. Caregivers must be alert to these exceptions and closely monitor antibiotic effectiveness and compliance with penicillin prophylaxis (Freiermuth et al., 2023). The most common pathogen in children younger than 6 years is *S. pneumoniae*.

E. coli bacteremia is often associated with urinary tract infection and *Salmonella* sp. bacteremia with osteomyelitis. Capillary blockage by sickle cells may cause a gut infarction, which—combined with the defective function of the liver and spleen—allows for the invasion of *Salmonella* spp. Combined with expanded bone marrow and poor blood flow, this provides an ischemic focus for *Salmonella* spp. localization.

Fever is a common finding during vasoocclusive crisis, as well as during infectious episodes. There is no test or diagnostic tool to differentiate a fever of an infectious origin from a fever that results from inflammation secondary to infarction. Primary care providers must be aware of the fact that children may have two independent problems (e.g., infection and vasoocclusion), both of which require aggressive treatment and management. Some health care workers measure C-reactive protein, which might indicate an inflammatory reaction.

Children with SCD should be considered at risk for fatal sepsis regardless of whether they are on penicillin prophylaxis and have received pneumococcal vaccinations. An aggressive search for the cause of the fever should include a CBC, blood culture, urinalysis, urine culture, chest radiograph, and possibly sinus radiographs if symptoms are suggestive of infection. Lumbar puncture should be performed if meningitis is suspected. Health care providers are increasingly aware of the development of penicillin-resistant organisms, which contribute to the difficulty of treating a child with a fever. Bacterial meningitis, suspected or proven to be caused by *S. pneumoniae*, should be treated with combination therapy of vancomycin and cefotaxime or ceftriaxone on all children at least 1 month of age. Penicillin or ceftriaxone should be continued based on culture and sensitivity results, discontinuing vancomycin if not needed. Rifampin is only used if found to be sensitive to the identified organism (Taketomo, 2022).

Common infections, such as otitis media or sinusitis, may precipitate a vasoocclusive crisis if fluid intake is reduced and dehydration and acidosis result. During periods of illness, a child must be assessed frequently for early signs of crisis. Maintaining fluid intake and controlling fever is critical.

Box **36.3**	Targeted Screening Guidelines for Lead

1. Does your child live in or regularly visit a house with peeling or chipping paint built before 1960?
2. Does your child live in or regularly visit a house built before 1970 with recent or ongoing renovation or remodeling?
3. Does your child have a sibling or playmate being treated for lead poisoning?
4. Does your child live with an adult whose job or hobby involves exposure to lead?
5. Does your child live near an active lead smelter, battery recycling plant, or other industry likely to release lead?

Urinary tract infections. Asymptomatic bacteriuria, symptomatic urinary tract infection, and pyelonephritis occur more commonly in individuals with SCD than in the general population. A child with a urinary tract infection or pyelonephritis should have a blood culture obtained because bacteremia may be present in those children with SCD and a urinary tract infection. Appropriate antibiotic therapy should be instituted, and adequate follow-up, including a repeat culture, should be arranged. Further diagnostic studies (e.g., renal ultrasound or voiding cystourethrogram) should be done to exclude treatable conditions in children with pyelonephritis or recurrent urinary tract infection.

Orthopedic symptoms. Areas of bone infarction may be easily confused with osteomyelitis or rheumatologic disorders. It is important to differentiate areas of infarction from areas of infection because children with SCD have an increased incidence of osteomyelitis (Al Farii et al., 2020). With both pathologic processes, a child may have an elevated WBC count, fever, and equivocal radiographic findings. Osteomyelitis is most often associated with an increased number of immature granulocytes, bacteremia, and a purulent joint aspirate.

Acute gastroenteritis. Vomiting and diarrhea must be carefully evaluated and managed in children with SCD because they lack the ability to concentrate urine to compensate for decreased fluid intake or excess losses. Significant dehydration may quickly occur and lead to metabolic acidosis and increased sickling. If a child's oral fluid intake is less than that needed to maintain hydration, the child must receive intravenous hydration.

Abdominal pain. Episodes of infarction of the abdominal organs (e.g., liver, spleen, abdominal lymph nodes) occur and may be quite painful. These abdominal crises should be differentiated from problems that would require surgical intervention (e.g., appendicitis, cholecystitis). Abdominal pain and cramps found commonly in young children are possibly related to mesenteric ischemia. Normal bowel sounds with a lack of ileus support nonsurgical management with adequate pain control. The duration may last days to weeks, with fluctuations in the severity of pain. Abdominal pain triggered by constipation is a common complaint and may be treated with a combination of stool softeners and laxatives. The use of narcotics to treat vasoocclusive crisis increases the risk of constipation, and bowel prophylaxis should be concurrent with pain management efforts.

Paralytic ileus is common during acute abdominal pain, making the diagnosis problematic. Right upper quadrant pain creates further complications because intrahepatic sickling mimics cholecystitis. Neither ultrasound nor laboratory values aid in defining the process. Leukocytosis of 30,000 can be seen with both infarction and infection. Most children find that their sickle cell pain has a unique quality or character, and they can often report whether their pain is typical of vasoocclusive pain. Deviation from a characteristic pattern (i.e., lower abdominal pain with persistent local tenderness) with symptoms lasting several hours suggests a surgical problem.

Anemia. Virtually all children with SCD are anemic at baseline. A child with SCD may periodically have acute lethargy and pallor. CBC and reticulocyte count should be obtained. If these reveal a significant drop in the hemoglobin and hematocrit levels, a child is probably experiencing an aplastic crisis or splenic sequestration. A fall in the hemoglobin and hematocrit values is usually a stimulus to the bone marrow, which then produces new RBCs in the form of reticulocytes. If the reticulocyte count is low in the presence of low hemoglobin and hematocrit levels, a child is experiencing an aplastic crisis. If a child has an enlarged spleen, pallor, lethargy, and an associated drop in hemoglobin, then splenic sequestration is the likely cause. Regardless of the exact diagnosis, the child will require immediate hospitalization with close observation and transfusion.

Respiratory distress. Increased respiratory rate and effort, chest pain, fever, rales, and dullness to percussion may indicate pneumonia or ACS. Infiltrates on the chest radiograph may reflect either process. With ACS, the chest radiograph may be clear in the first few days, but a pleural effusion is often seen. These children should receive antibiotics, hydration, analgesics, and oxygen as needed. Transfusion or partial exchange transfusion may be indicated, depending on the degree of respiratory distress. ACS is a medical emergency and necessitates hospitalization.

Neurologic changes. A child who has a seizure, hemiparesis, blurred or double vision, or changes in speech, gait, or level of consciousness should have an expedient neurologic and radiologic evaluation for the presence of a stroke. These neurologic changes are a medical emergency and require an exchange transfusion as soon as possible.

Complementary and Alternative Therapies

Complementary and alternative medical therapies are a popular alternative to opioid and analgesic treatments for children with SCD. Inpatient therapies that have been studied are yoga, virtual reality, and acupuncture, whereas outpatient therapies include cognitive-behavioral therapy, massage therapy, and guided imagery. These therapies increased pain tolerability and decreased pain scale scores in the pediatric population (Alsabri et al., 2023).

Drug Interactions

Antihistamines and barbiturates given concurrently with narcotics may cause respiratory depression, hypoxia, and further sickling. Diuretics and some bronchodilators, which have a diuretic effect, may cause dehydration and sickling and should be used with caution in children with SCD. Children receiving narcotics for pain control should be given stool softeners and cautioned about the use of alcohol or other sedatives.

DEVELOPMENTAL ISSUES

Sleep Patterns

Because of chronic anemia, some children with SCD may fatigue more easily than their unaffected peers and may desire extra sleep. Parents often report that their child with SCD naps after coming home from school—a routine that can be encouraged. Snoring, in combination with daytime sleepiness, is an indication for a sleep study to determine if obstruction from enlarged tonsils or adenoids exists, particularly if pulse oximetry readings are below 90%.

Toileting

Toilet training should be initiated using the conventional guidelines to assess readiness for training. Bowel training usually progresses without difficulty. Bladder training progresses along normal developmental patterns in toddlers with SCD. Older children may have difficulty concentrating urine and thus produce a large volume of dilute urine. All children may need the opportunity to go to the toilet every 2 to 3 hours during the day. Primary enuresis often occurs in young children and commonly continues into the teenage years. It is especially troublesome when a child requires extra fluids during a vasoocclusive crisis. Some children who previously achieved nighttime continence may develop secondary enuresis as subtle insults to the kidney occur. A pattern of enuresis typically emerges as a child begins having more wet than dry nights. This pattern may reflect the gradual loss of the kidneys' ability to concentrate urine. Daytime continence is unaffected by these renal changes.

Routine counseling regarding enuresis should be offered. Young children may initially use diapers. By the time a child reaches preschool or school age, however, the use of diapers often adversely affects the child's self-esteem and sense of mastery. Many families choose to wake the child once or twice during the night to urinate, but the severe restriction of fluids is not wise because hydration needs must be met. Avoidance of caffeine ingestion during the evening hours may help prevent enuresis. Careful questioning by the primary care provider may point to a subclinical infectious process that can be treated. Parents need to be counseled regarding the physiology behind sickle cell enuresis in an effort to plan appropriate interventions aimed at preventing the loss of their child's self-esteem.

Discipline

Expectations for the behavior of children with SCD should vary little from those held for their unaffected siblings or peers. These expectations should be as clear and consistent as possible. Likewise, parents should strive to make discipline fair and consistent. Many parents are fearful of disciplining or setting limits for their child with SCD, especially because emotional stress is thought to possibly precipitate a VOC. Primary care providers can point out to parents that a lack of or inconsistency in setting limits may be more stressful to a child than consistently set limits. Parents and guardians should also be encouraged to note which behaviors their child consistently demonstrates when in pain (e.g., a certain pitch to a cry, a change in activity level, or changes in appetite) to help them discriminate episodes of pain from other behavior.

Child Care

Children with SCD can participate in normal day care centers, although small group or home-centered day care may be preferable because it provides less exposure to infections. Caregivers must be informed of a child's need for extra fluids and frequent need to void. They may also need to administer medications during day care hours and must be instructed in this regard. Caregivers must be able to contact a parent or quickly seek medical care for the child in the event of fever, painful vasoocclusive crisis, respiratory distress, or symptoms of stroke, all of which may be life threatening. It is commonly accepted that children attending day care centers are at higher risk for acquiring community-based resistant infections, so health care workers must take this into consideration when prescribing antibiotic coverage.

Schooling

Parents are encouraged to meet with school officials before the beginning of each school year to allow them to communicate about the usual symptoms their child has relative to SCD. A plan should be developed for absences, makeup work, intermittent homebound study (if necessary), and transfer of assignments from school to home. These children are frequently eligible for special education services.

Many primary care providers play an active role in educating school officials about the needs of children with SCD. Some visit schools and give presentations, and others provide written materials (see Resources, later). The need for adequate hydration, frequent bathroom breaks, rest, physical education, and appropriate dress are all subjects for discussion by the health care team. School officials, in turn, can provide information about learning abilities and behavior. This open exchange of information helps ensure a successful school year for the student. Knowing whom to call when parents cannot be reached reduces anxiety on the part of the school staff.

As previously discussed, some children with SCD and silent infarcts have declining IQs with increasing age. Children with SCD should be referred for eligibility for special education services. Repeated testing to identify impairments affecting education may be necessary because of the possible progression of symptoms, especially from recurrent TIAs or small strokes. Children with splenomegaly should be cautioned about the risks of injury with contact sports. Modified physical education classes should be offered to keep these children engaged in group activities, which are important to their overall adjustment and well-being. School personnel should be counseled about the needs of children affected with chronic orthopedic problems (e.g., osteomyelitis or avascular necrosis of the femoral head). These children may need additional time to get to classes or may need to obtain an elevator key during times of bone healing and/or physical discomfort with ambulation.

Sexuality

Children with SCD progress through the Tanner stages in an orderly and consistent manner but usually experience puberty several years later than their unaffected peers, which can have significant adverse effects on their self-concepts. Once sexual maturation has occurred, fertility and contraception are important issues that must be addressed by primary care providers. For males, impotence is often a problem after a major episode of priapism. For female adolescents, menarche is often delayed by 2 to 2.5 years, but fertility is normal. Decisions about contraception must take into account the attitudes, lifestyle, and maturity of the adolescent, as well as the hematologic ramifications of the method chosen. During pregnancy, close hematology follow-up is recommended for females with SCD.

Various contraceptive choices are available to adolescents with SCD, including all barrier forms of contraception (e.g., condoms for males and foam and diaphragms for females). Females may also use oral contraceptives, preferably those brands containing low levels of estrogen.

Progesterone-only pills are useful because progestins stabilize the red cell membrane. Medroxyprogesterone (Depo-Provera) has also been used in this population and is often the method of preference (American College of Obstetricians and Gynecologists, 2019). Adolescents with SCD should receive careful, repeated genetic counseling before puberty and during adolescence. They need to understand the pattern of transmission of SCD and the availability of testing for partners before conceiving a child.

Transition to Adulthood

Early vocational counseling should be offered to children and adolescents with SCD. Consideration should be directed toward the child's or adolescent's interests and intellectual abilities. Work in a climate-controlled environment is preferred over rigorous outdoor work, which might trigger a crisis. SCD excludes a person from military service, so technical and academic training is encouraged. Many community-based sickle cell organizations offer scholarships for skilled and academic work. The Sickle Cell Disease Association of America, Inc. (2021) can direct families to local resources.

Families should be counseled about the progressive organ damage that develops as a child ages. Continuity of care by a knowledgeable primary care provider will afford the best quality of life and should be encouraged.

Family Concerns

The families of children with SCD experience the same psychological ramifications as other families of children with chronic conditions, often in the context of limited resources. These families bear the additional burden of knowing that this disease is genetically transmitted. This knowledge can prompt feelings of overwhelming guilt and responsibility. Exacerbations of the condition often occur without provocation, prompting feelings of helplessness. Many manifestations of the condition are not objectively visible or measurable; therefore children with SCD can appear to be well when they are potentially extremely ill. Many parents are fearful that the therapeutic effects of narcotics and blood transfusions will be outweighed by their potentially deleterious effects.

Genetic counseling should be offered to the parents of a child with SCD at the time of the child's diagnosis and when subsequent pregnancies are contemplated. In addition to the Black population, permeations of sickle hemoglobinopathies are found in Hispanics, Central Americans, Greeks, Arabs, Asians, and Caribbean natives. Cultural considerations about health, coping, and wellness must be considered by all health care providers. Primary care providers must be mindful of the differences within and between cultures. Emphasis should focus on the different strengths families bring with them. For example, extended family support is a dominant feature in the US Black community and should play a role during crisis episodes.

Research shows that Black families prefer to use their family members as sources of support instead of using formal support groups. Close friends can be considered kin and fulfill some functions of extended family members within different cultures. When working with minority families, primary care providers need to explore and understand the effects of ethnicity on the family's daily life. Such understanding seeks out cultural practices (e.g., male and female roles and Black language, communication styles, and family rituals). Instructions should be delivered to the head of the household. In contrast to the matriarchal leadership found in many Black households, Muslim families center their decision making on the father or male head of the household. Strong church affiliations are often in place and offer consolation and hope, leading to greater acceptance and improved quality of life.

Individuals espousing the Jehovah's Witness faith will deny blood transfusions to their children, placing extra stress on the primary care provider. Sensitive, open communication and vigilant intensive care management may prevent the need for transfusions and thereby support the religious beliefs of the family. In all instances, members of a particular ethnic or minority group should be consulted when actions or choices conflict with those of the medical care team.

RESOURCES

American Academy of Family Physicians (tips for preventing a sickle cell crisis): https://www.aafp.org/pubs/afp/issues/2000/0301/p1363.html

American Sickle Cell Anemia Association (information and support groups): https://ascaa.org

ASH Sickle Cell Disease Initiative: https://www.hematology.org/advocacy/sickle-cell-disease-initiative

Be the Match for Siblings of SCD: https://bethematch.org/templates/displaypagecontent/?id=9924

Children's Hospital of Philadelphia Sickle Cell Center (sickle cell school outreach tools, educational and other excellent resources): https://www.chop.edu/centers-programs/sickle-cell-center

Children's Mercy Kansas City: https://www.childrensmercy.org/departments-and-clinics/division-of-pediatric-hematology-oncology-and-blood-and-marrow-transplantation/hematology/sickle-cell-disease-program

SCD CONDITIONS, RESEARCH, AND PATIENT STORIES

Evidence-Based Management of Sickle Cell Disease (Expert Panel Report, 2014: Guide to Recommendations for Providers): https://www.nhlbi.nih.gov/sites/default/files/media/docs/Evd-Bsd_SickleCellDis_Rep2014.pdf

Nationwide Children's Hospital: https://www.nationwidechildrens.org/specialties/sickle-cell-and-thalassemia-program

SICKLE CELL AND THALASSEMIA PROGRAM

NIH Management and of Sickle Cell Disease: https://www.nhlbi.nih.gov/health/sickle-cell-disease

Parent Guide to Sickle Cell Disease: https://www.sicklecellsociety.org/resource/parentsguide

Sickle Cell Disease Association of America: https://www.sicklecelldisease.org

Sickle Cell Disease and COVID-19: https://www.sicklecelldisease.org/2020/03/18/sickle-cell-disease-and-covid-19-provider-directory

Sickle Cell Fact Sheet for School: https://kidshealth.org/en/parents/sickle-cell-factsheet.html

Sickle Cell Information Center (information about SCD; resources for patients, families, and health care providers; research; clinical trials; news; and books): https://scinfo.org

Sickle Cell & School: https://drive.google.com/file/d/157vatJXjcnGTCBEJCdv2L7IVu2p89yD5/view

Super Sam vs. the Marrow Monsters (from Be The Match for children): https://www.youtube.com/watch?v=8cKXUd95XTc

Summary
Primary Care Needs for the Child With Sickle Cell Disease

HEALTH CARE MAINTENANCE
Growth and Development
- Children with SCD tend to weigh less and be shorter than their peers. Weight is affected more than height, and males are affected more than females. Weight and height should be checked and plotted every 3 to 4 months.
- Puberty is delayed for both sexes with Hb S/S.
- Developmental impairment varies. Cerebral microvascular occlusion or stroke outcome can have an impact on intellectual and motor development. Refer for neurologic testing if screening results or clinical assessment warrants.

Diet
- Diet should be well balanced with a generous amount of fluid; fluid intake should be increased during a febrile illness, times of increased activity, environmental heat, dehydration, traveling, or while experiencing a vasoocclusive crisis.
- Increased metabolic demands require additional protein, micronutrients, and food for energy.
- Pica is more common in children with sickle cell disease.
- Folic acid supplements are encouraged.

Safety
- Ingestion of narcotics beyond the prescribed amount can lead to respiratory depression.
- Alcohol may cause dehydration and potentiate narcotics.
- Narcotics may impair judgment while driving or the safe use of machinery.
- Smoking leads to vasoconstriction and is strongly discouraged.
- Recreational activities that involve prolonged exposure to cold, prolonged exertion, or exposure to high altitudes should be avoided.
- Dehydration should be avoided. Ice should never be used to treat injuries.
- A medical alert bracelet is recommended.

Immunizations
- Routine standard immunizations are recommended.
- The pneumococcal vaccine should be given at 24 months, with a single booster given at 5 years with another booster given 5 years after the second immunization. Prevnar should be given as scheduled.
- An annual influenza vaccine is strongly recommended.

Continued

- Hepatitis A vaccination should be a part of each child's routine immunization schedule.

Screening
- *Vision.* Routine screening is recommended. At 10 years of age, annual retinal examinations are recommended to rule out sickle retinopathy. If a child sustains eye trauma, then refer to an ophthalmologist to rule out increased intraocular pressure or retinal detachment.
- *Hearing.* Routine audiologic examination is recommended. More frequent evaluation is warranted if the clinical status indicates.
- *Dental.* Routine screening is recommended, as well as antibiotic prophylaxis prior to invasive procedures.
- *Blood pressure.* Measure at each visit. An increase in systolic pressure increases the risk of stroke. Children with high blood pressure should be evaluated for renal dysfunction.
- *Hematocrit.* Routine screening is deferred because of condition-specific screening.
- *Urinalysis.* Routine screening is deferred because of condition-specific screening.
- *Tuberculosis.* Routine screening is recommended.

Condition-Specific Screening
- *Pulse oximetry.* Reading should be obtained at each visit and compared to the baseline.
- *Sleep apnea.* Screen for snoring, restlessness, daytime sleepiness, or enlarged tonsils or adenoids; these may induce sleep apnea and subsequent oxygen desaturation.
- *Hematologic screening.* A CBC with differential platelet count, reticulocyte count, and RBC smear should be checked every 3 to 6 months.
- *Renal function screening.* BUN and creatinine levels should be checked routinely, and a urinalysis should be done yearly. A child should be referred to a urologist if severe hematuria is noted or casts are found in urine.
- *Lead poisoning.* Lead screening using the erythrocyte protoporphyrin (EP) level is unreliable; the serum lead level must be determined.
- *Scoliosis.* Screening should be extended to late teens because of delayed puberty.
- *Cardiac function.* Both ECG and ECHO are recommended every 1 to 2 years after age 10 years if clinically warranted.
- *Liver function.* Serum liver function tests should be done yearly. The gallbladder should be assessed via ultrasound if the child becomes symptomatic.
- Transfused children should be routinely screened for HIV and hepatitis C.

COMMON ILLNESS MANAGEMENT
Differential Diagnosis
- *Fever.* A child with a temperature above 101.2°F (38.3°C) must be evaluated immediately, cultures taken, and ceftriaxone administered intramuscularly or intravenously. Outpatient management may be considered if the source of the fever can be identified, appropriate antibiotics are given, and reliable follow-up and reassessment as needed are ensured.
- The child's age, past history, clinical condition, laboratory values, adherence to therapy, and ability to obtain follow-up care determine whether the child should receive inpatient care.
- *Urinary tract infections.* Asymptomatic bacteriuria, urinary tract infections, and pyelonephritis are more common with SCD.
  - Blood cultures should be done to rule out bacteremia if a urinary tract infection is diagnosed.
  - Treatment must cover cultured organisms, and follow-up is essential.
- *Orthopedic symptoms.* It is difficult to differentiate bone infarction from osteomyelitis or rheumatologic disorders. MRI studies are used to identify bone marrow infarction.
- *Acute gastroenteritis.* Significant dehydration may occur quickly and lead to acidosis and sickling. If oral intake is inadequate, intravenous hydration is needed.
- *Abdominal pain.* Abdominal pain crises may be differentiated from surgical problems by evaluating fever, hematologic changes, peristalsis, and response to symptomatic, supportive therapy.
- *Anemia.* Hemoglobin and hematocrit levels significantly lower than baseline may reflect an aplastic crisis, hyperhemolytic crisis, or splenic sequestration. Splenic sequestration and aplasia may be life-threatening conditions.
- *Respiratory distress.* It is important that individuals are evaluated for ACS, which may be fulminant and require exchange transfusion.
- *Neurologic changes.* Neurologic changes may indicate a stroke. A rapid, thorough evaluation is critical.
- Exchange transfusion should be performed as quickly as possible if a stroke occurs.

Drug Interactions
- Antihistamines, alcohol, and barbiturates may potentiate sedation with narcotics.
- Diuretics and bronchodilators (which may have diuretic effects) may cause dehydration and sickling.
- Stool softeners are useful while on narcotics.

DEVELOPMENTAL ISSUES
Sleep Patterns
- Routine care is recommended. Clinical assessment of obstructive sleep apnea requires thorough evaluation.

Toileting
- Enuresis is often a long-term issue because of the large volume of dilute urine in this population.
- Nocturia may persist.

Discipline
- Expectations should be consistent, fair, and similar to those of unaffected peers and siblings.

Child Care
- Caregivers must be mindful of fluid requirements, the importance of maintaining normal body temperature, and the critical importance of notifying parents of fever, signs of vasoocclusive crisis, or respiratory distress, and they must be able to administer medicines.

Schooling
- These children may have frequent, unpredictable absences.
- While at school, they need access to fluids and liberal bathroom privileges.
- They may participate in mainstream physical education as tolerated.

- Evaluation for special education services is warranted if the child is having difficulty with learning.

Sexuality
- Puberty may be delayed.
- Females usually have normal fertility patterns and may use all forms of birth control.
- Increased monitoring by a hematologist may be warranted during pregnancy.
- Males must be aware of the risk of impotency after multiple episodes of priapism.
- Genetic counseling is important.

Transition to Adulthood
- Early vocational counseling is recommended.
- Insurance problems may be encountered.

FAMILY CONCERNS
- Because SCD is genetically transmitted, there is a need for genetic counseling and ongoing support to process feelings of guilt and responsibility.
- Support for cultural beliefs and family structure are important components of long-term care.

REFERENCES

Abboud, M. R., Yim, E., Musallam, K. M., & Adams, R. J. (2011). Discontinuing prophylactic transfusions increases the risk of silent brain infarction in children with sickle cell disease: Data from STOP II. *Blood, 118*(4), 894–898. https://doi.org/10.1182/BLOOD-2010-12-326298.

Abraham, A. A., & Tisdale, J. F. (2021). Gene therapy for sickle cell disease: Moving from the bench to the bedside. *Blood, 138*(11), 932–941. https://doi.org/10.1182/BLOOD.2019003776.

Adamkiewicz, T. V., Silk, B. J., Howgate, J., Baughman, W., Strayhorn, G., Sullivan, K., & Farley, M. M. (2008). Effectiveness of the 7-valent pneumococcal conjugate vaccine in children with sickle cell disease in the first decade of life. *Pediatrics, 121*(3), 562–569. https://doi.org/10.1542/peds.2007-0018.

Adams, R. (2000). Lessons from the Stroke Prevention Trial in Sickle Cell Anemia (STOP) study. *Journal of Child Neurology, 15*(5), 344–349.

Adams, R., & Brambilla, D. (2005). Discontinuing prophylactic transfusions used to prevent stroke in sickle cell disease. *New England Journal of Medicine, 353*(26), 2769–2778.

Adams, R. J., McKie, V. C., Hsu, L., Files, B., Vichinsky, E., Pegelow, C., Abboud, M., Gallagher, D., Kutlar, A., Nichols, F. T., Bonds, D. R., & Brambilla, D. (1998). Prevention of a first stroke by transfusions in children with sickle cell anemia and abnormal results on transcranial Doppler ultrasonography. *The New England Journal of Medicine, 339*(1), 5–11. https://doi.org/10.1056/NEJM199807023390102

Ahmed, N., Okany, N., Singh, D., Rungkitwattanaku, D., & Weaver, S. B. (2022). Rates of opioid misuse amongst patients receiving pain management for sickle cell disease in an urban setting. *Journal of Pharmacy Practice.* https://doi.org/10.1177/08971900221128335.

Al Farii, H., Zhou, S., & Albers, A. (2020). Management of osteomyelitis in sickle cell disease: Review article. *JAAOS: Global Research and Reviews, 4*(9). https://doi.org/10.5435/jaaosglobal-d-20-00002.

Alsabri, M., Carfagnini, C., Amin, M., Castilo, F., Lewis, J., Ashkar, M., Hamzah, M., Mohamed, N., Saker, M., Mahgerefteh, J., St Victor, R., Peichev, M., Kupferman, F., & Viswanathan, K. (2023). Complementary and alternative medicine for children with sickle cell disease: A systematic review. *Blood Reviews*, 59, 101052. https://doi.org/10.1016/j.blre.2023.101052.

American Academy of Pediatrics (AAP). Committee on Infectious Diseases (L.K. Pickering, Ed.). (2021). Red Book: 2021 Report of the Committee on Infectious Diseases (32nd. ed.). Elk Grove Village, IL: American Academy of Pediatrics.

American Academy of Pediatrics. (2022a). Preventive care/periodicity schedule. Retrieved February 19, 2023, from https://publications.aap.org/pediatrics/article/150/1/e2022058044/188302/2022-Recommendations-for-Preventive-Pediatric.

American Academy of Pediatrics. (2022b). AAP updates recommendations on maintaining, improving children's oral health. Retrieved February 19, 2023, from https://www.aap.org/en/news-room/news-releases/aap/2022/american-academy-of-pediatrics-updates-recommendations-on-maintaining-improving-childrens-oral-health/.

American College of Obstetricians and Gynecologists. (2019). ACOG Practice Bulletin No. 206: Use of hormonal contraception in women with coexisting medical conditions. *Obstetrics & Gynecology, 133*(2). https://doi.org/10.1097/aog.0000000000003072.

Annunziato, R. A., Fisher, M. K., Jerson, B., Bochkanova, A., & Shaw, R. J. (2010). Psychosocial assessment prior to pediatric transplantation: A review and summary of key considerations. *Pediatric Transplantation, 14*(5), 565–574. https://doi.org/10.1111/J.1399-3046.2010.01353.X.

Ataga, K. I., Kutlar, A., Kanter, J., Liles, D., Cancado, R., Friedrisch, J., Guthrie, T. H., Knight-Madden, J., Alvarez, O. A., Gordeuk, V. R., Gualandro, S., Colella, M. P., Smith, W. R., Rollins, S. A., Stocker, J. W., & Rother, R. P. (2017). Crizanlizumab for the prevention of pain crises in sickle cell disease. *The New England Journal of Medicine, 376*(5), 429–439. https://doi.org/10.1056/NEJMoa1611770.

Baker, C., Grant, A. M., George, M. G., Grosse, S. D., & Adamkiewicz, T. V. (2015). Contribution of sickle cell disease to the pediatric stroke burden among hospital discharges of African-Americans—United States, 1997–2012. *Pediatric Blood & Cancer, 62*(12), 2076–2081. https://doi.org/10.1002/PBC.25655.

Beck, C. E., Trottier, E. D., Kirby-Allen, M., & Pastore, Y. (2022). Acute complications in children with sickle cell disease: Prevention and management. *Paediatrics & Child Health, 27*(1), 50. https://doi.org/10.1093/PCH/PXAB096.

Bernaudin, F., Verlhac, S., Arnaud, C., Kamdem, A., Hau, I., Leveillé, E., Vasile, M., Kasbi, F., Madhi, F., Fourmaux, C., Biscardi, S., Gluckman, E., Socié, G., Dalle, J. H., Epaud, R., & Pondarré, C. (2016). Long-term treatment follow-up of children with sickle cell disease monitored with abnormal transcranial Doppler velocities. *Blood, 127*(14), 1814–1822. https://doi.org/10.1182/blood-2015-10-675231

Bhatia, M., & Walters, M. (2008). Hematopoietic cell transplantation for thalassemia and sickle cell disease: Past, present and future. *Bone Marrow Transplant, 41*, 109–117.

Brandow, A. M., Carroll, C. P., Edwards-Elliott, R., Glassberg, J., Hurley, R. W., Kutlar, A., Seisa, M., Stinson, J., Strouse, J. J., Yusuf, F., Zempsky, W., & Lang, E. (2020). American Society of Hematology 2020 guidelines for sickle cell disease: Management of acute and chronic pain. *Blood Advances, 4*(12), 2656–2701. doi:10.1182/bloodadvances.2020001851.

Brandow, A. M., & Liem, R. I. (2020). Advances in the diagnosis and treatment of sickle cell disease. *Journal of Hematology & Oncology, 15*(1), 20. https://doi.org/10.1186/S13045-022-01237-Z.

Brousse, V., Buffet, P., & Rees, D. (2014). The spleen and sickle cell disease: the sick(led) spleen. *British Journal of Haematology, 166*(2), 165–176. https://doi.org/10.1111/BJH.12950.

Brousseau, D. C., Richardson, T., Hall, M., Ellison, A. M., Shah, S. S., Raphael, J. L., Bundy, D. G., & Arnold, S. (2019). Hydroxyurea use for sickle cell disease among Medicaid-enrolled children. *Pediatrics, 144*(1), e20183285. https://doi.org/10.1542/peds.2018-3285.

Busse, B., Tepedino, M. F., Rupprecht, W., & Klein, H. G. (2016). Stepwise diagnostics of hemoglobinopathies. *Laboratoriums Medizin, 39*(s1). https://doi.org/10.1515/labmed-2016-0009.

Centers for Disease Control and Prevention. (2022). Reptiles and amphibians. Retrieved February 12, 2023, from https://www.cdc.gov/healthypets/pets/reptiles.html#print.

Centers for Disease Control and Prevention. (n.d.). Data & statistics on sickle cell disease. Retrieved September 14, 2022, from https://www.cdc.gov/ncbddd/sicklecell/data.html.

Chou, S. T., Alsawas, M., Fasano, R. M., Field, J. J., Hendrickson, J. E., Howard, J., Kameka, M., Kwiatkowski, J. L., Pirenne, F., Shi, P. A., Stowell, S. R., Thein, S. L., Westhoff, C. M., Wong, T. E., & Akl, E. A. (2020). American Society of Hematology 2020 guidelines for sickle cell disease: Transfusion support. *Blood Advances, 4*(2), 327–355. https://doi.org/10.1182/bloodadvances.2019001143.

Chui, D., & Dover, G. (2001). Sickle cell disease: No longer a single gene disorder. *Current Opinion in Pediatrics, 13*, 23–37.

Darbari, D. S., Sheehan, V. A., & Ballas, S. K. (2020). The vaso-occlusive pain crisis in sickle cell disease: Definition, pathophysiology, and management. *European Journal of Haematology, 105*(3), 237–246. https://doi.org/10.1111/EJH.13430.

Davis, H., Schoendorf, K. C., Gergen, P. J., & Moore, R. M., Jr. (1997). National trends in the mortality of children with sickle cell disease, 1968 through 1992. *American Journal of Public Health, 87*(8), 1317–1322. https://doi.org/10.2105/ajph.87.8.1317.

DeBaun, M. R., Gordon, M., McKinstry, R. C., Noetzel, M. J., White, D. A., Sarnaik, S. A., Meier, E. R., Howard, T. H., Majumdar, S., Inusa, B. P., Telfer, P. T., Kirby-Allen, M., McCavit, T. L., Kamdem, A., Airewele, G., Woods, G. M., Berman, B., Panepinto, J. A., Fuh, B. R., Kwiatkowski, J. L., … Casella, J. F. (2014). Controlled trial of transfusions for silent cerebral infarcts in sickle cell anemia. *The New England Journal of Medicine, 371*(8), 699–710. https://doi.org/10.1056/NEJMoa1401731.

DeBaun, M. R., Jordan, L. C., King, A. A., Schatz, J., Vichinsky, E., Fox, C. K., McKinstry, R. C., Telfer, P., Kraut, M. A., Daraz, L., Kirkham, F. J., & Murad, M. H. (2020). American Society of Hematology 2020 guidelines for sickle cell disease: Prevention, diagnosis, and treatment of cerebrovascular disease in children and adults. *Blood Advances, 4*(8), 1554–1588. https://doi.org/10.1182/bloodadvances.2019001142.

de Melo, M. B. (2014). An eye on sickle cell retinopathy. *Revista Brasileira de Hematologia e Hemoterapia, 36*(5), 319–321. https://doi.org/10.1016/J.BJHH.2014.07.020.

Dixit, R., Nettem, S., Madan, S. S., Soe, H. H. K., Abas, A. B., Vance, L. D., & Stover, P. J. (2018). Folate supplementation in people with sickle cell disease. *The Cochrane Database of Systematic Reviews, 3*(3), CD011130. https://doi.org/10.1002/14651858.CD011130.pub3.

Driscoll, M. (2007). Sickle cell disease. *Pediatrics Review, 28*(7), 259–268.

El-Haj, N., & Hoppe, C. C. (2018). Newborn screening for SCD in the USA and Canada. *International Journal of Neonatal Screening, 4*(4). https://doi.org/10.3390/IJNS4040036.

Farooq, F., Mogayzel, P. J., Lanzkron, S., Haywood, C., & Strouse, J. J. (2020). Comparison of US federal and foundation funding of research for sickle cell disease and cystic fibrosis and factors associated with research productivity. *JAMA Network Open, 3*(3), e201737. https://doi.org/10.1001/JAMANETWORKOPEN.2020.1737.

Fitzhugh, C., Wigfall, D., & Ware, R. (2005). Enalapril and hydroxyurea therapy for children with sickle nephropathy. *Pediatr Blood Cancer, 45*(7), 982–985.

Freiermuth, C., Kavanagh, P., Bailey, L., & Brousseau, D. (2023). Sickle cell [sickle cell point-of-care tool]. *American College of Emergency Physicians*. Retrieved February 25, 2023, from https://www.acep.org/sickle-cell.

Friedman, L. (2007). Liver transplantation for sickle cell hepatopathy. *Liver Transplant, 13*(4), 483–485.

Gai, N., Naser, B., Hanley, J., Peliowski, A., Hayes, J., & Aoyama, K. (2020). A practical guide to acute pain management in children. *Journal of Anesthesia, 34*(3), 421–433. https://doi.org/10.1007/s00540-020-02767-x.

Gale, H. I., Bobbitt, C. A., Setty, B. N., Sprinz, P. G., Doros, G., Williams, D. D., Morrison, T. C., Kalajian, T. A., Tu, P., Mundluru, S. N., & Castro-Aragon, I. (2016). Expected sonographic appearance of the spleen in children and young adults with sickle cell disease: An update. *Journal of Ultrasound in Medicine, 35*(8), 1735–1745. https://doi.org/10.7863/ultra.15.09023.

Germino-Watnick, P., Hinds, M., Le, A., Chu, R., Liu, X., & Uchida, N. (2022). Hematopoietic stem cell gene-addition/editing therapy in sickle cell disease. *Cells, 11*(11). https://doi.org/10.3390/CELLS11111843.

Gold, J. I., Johnson, C. B., Treadwell, M. J., Hans, N., & Vichinsky, E. (2008). Detection and assessment of stroke in patients with sickle cell disease: Neuropsychological functioning and magnetic resonance imaging. *Pediatric Hematology and Oncology, 25*(5), 409–421. https://doi.org/10.1080/08880010802107497.

Health Resources and Services Administration. (n.d.). Advisory Committee on Heritable Disorders in Newborns and Children. Retrieved March 2, 2023, from https://www.hrsa.gov/advisory-committees/heritable-disorders.

Hirst, C., & Owusu-Ofori, S. (2014). Prophylactic antibiotics for preventing pneumococcal infection in children with sickle cell disease. *The Cochrane Database of Systematic Reviews, (11).* https://doi.org/10.1002/14651858.CD003427.PUB3.

Hirst, C., & Williamson, L. (2012). Preoperative blood transfusions for sickle cell disease. *The Cochrane Database of Systematic Reviews, 1.* https://doi.org/10.1002/14651858.CD003149.PUB2.

Hoyt, C. R., Varughese, T. E., Erickson, J., Haffner, N., Luo, L., L'Hotta, A. J., Yeager, L., & King, A. A. (2022). Developmental delay in infants and toddlers with sickle cell disease: A systematic review. *Developmental Medicine & Child Neurology, 64*(2), 168–175. https://doi.org/10.1111/dmcn.15048.

Infanti, L. M., Elder, J. J., Franco, K., Simms, S., Statler, V. A., & Raj, A. (2020). Immunization adherence in children with sickle cell disease: A single-institution experience. *The Journal of Pediatric Pharmacology and Therapeutics, 25*(1), 39–46. https://doi.org/10.5863/1551-6776-25.1.39.

Inusa, B. P. D., Hsu, L. L., Kohli, N., Patel, A., Ominu-Evbota, K., Anie, K. A., & Atoyebi, W. (2019). Sickle cell disease-genetics, pathophysiology, clinical presentation and treatment. *International Journal of Neonatal Screening, 5*(2), 20. https://doi.org/10.3390/ijns5020020.

Jain, S., Bakshi, N., & Krishnamurti, L. (2017). Acute chest syndrome in children with sickle cell disease. *Pediatr Allergy Immunol Pulmonol, 30*(4), 191–201. doi:10.1089/ped.2017.0814.

Jung, J. M., & Peddinti, R. (2018). Lead toxicity in the pediatric patient with sickle cell disease: Unique risks and management. *Pediatric Annals, 47*(1). https://doi.org/10.3928/19382359-20171218-01.

Kanter, J., Liem, R. I., Bernaudin, F., Bolaños-Meade, J., Fitzhugh, C. D., Hankins, J. S., Murad, M. H., Panepinto, J. A., Rondelli, D., Shenoy, S., Wagner, J., Walters, M. C., Woolford, T., Meerpohl, J. J., & Tisdale, J. (2021). American Society of

Hematology 2021 guidelines for sickle cell disease: Stem cell transplantation. *Blood Advances, 5*(18), 3668–3689. https://doi.org/10.1182/bloodadvances.2021004394C.

Kato, G. J., Piel, F. B., Reid, C. D., Gaston, M. H., Ohene-Frempong, K., Krishnamurti, L., Smith, W. R., Panepinto, J. A., Weatherall, D. J., Costa, F. F., & Vichinsky, E. P. (2018). Sickle cell disease. *Nature Reviews Disease Primers, 4*, 18010. https://doi.org/10.1038/nrdp.2018.10.

Kauv, P., Gaudré, N., Hodel, J., Tuilier, T., Habibi, A., Oppenheim, C., Edjlali, M., Hervé, D., Calvet, D., & Bartolucci, P. (2019). Characteristics of moyamoya syndrome in sickle-cell disease by magnetic resonance angiography: An adult-cohort study. *Frontiers in Neurology, 10.* https://doi.org/10.3389/fneur.2019.00015.

Kavanagh, P. L., Fasipe, T. A., & Wun, T. (2022). Sickle cell disease: A review. *The Journal of the American Medical Association, 328*(1), 57–68. https://doi.org/10.1001/JAMA.2022.10233.

Kinger, N. P., Moreno, C. C., Miller, F. H., & Mittal, P. K. (2021). Abdominal manifestations of sickle cell disease. *Current Problems in Diagnostic Radiology, 50*(2), 241–251. https://doi.org/10.1067/J.CPRADIOL.2020.05.012.

Kirkham, F. J., & Lagunju, I. A. (2021). Epidemiology of stroke in sickle cell disease. *Journal of Clinical Medicine, 10*(18), 4232. https://doi.org/10.3390/JCM10184232.

Kokoska, E. R., West, K. W., Carney, D. E., Engum, S. E., Heiny, M. E., & Rescorla, F. J. (2004). Risk factors for acute chest syndrome in children with sickle cell disease undergoing abdominal surgery. *Journal of Pediatric Surgery, 39*(6), 848–850. https://doi.org/10.1016/j.jpedsurg.2004.02.027.

Koshy, M., Weiner, S. J., Miller, S. T., Sleeper, L. A., Vichinsky, E., Brown, A. K., Khakoo, Y., & Kinney, T. R. (1995). Surgery and anesthesia in sickle cell disease. Cooperative study of sickle cell diseases. *Blood, 86*(10), 3676–3684.

Kupferman, J. C., Rosenbaum, J. E., Lande, M. B., Stabouli, S., Wang, Y., Forman, D., Zafeiriou, D. I., & Pavlakis, S. G. (2022). Blood pressure in children with sickle cell disease is higher than in the general pediatric population. *BMC Pediatrics, 22*(1), 549. https://doi.org/10.1186/s12887-022-03584-9.

Kyrana, E., Rees, D., Lacaille, F., Fitzpatrick, E., Davenport, M., Heaton, N., Height, S., Samyn, M., Mavilio, F., Brousse, V., Suddle, A., Chakravorty, S., Verma, A., Gupte, G., Velangi, M., Inusa, B., Drasar, E., Hadzic, N., Grammatikopoulos, T., Hind, J., … Dhawan, A. (2021). Clinical management of sickle cell liver disease in children and young adults. *Archives of Disease in Childhood, 106*(4), 315–320. https://doi.org/10.1136/archdischild-2020-319778.

Lance, E. I., Cannon, A. D., Shapiro, B. K., Lee, L. C., Johnston, M. V., & Casella, J. F. (2021). Co-occurrence of neurodevelopmental disorders in pediatric sickle cell disease. *Journal of Developmental & Behavioral Pediatrics, 42*(6), 463–471. https://doi.org/10.1097/dbp.0000000000000914.

Lanzkron, S., Haywood, C., Hassell, K. L., & Rand, C. (2008). Provider barriers to hydroxyurea use in adults with sickle cell disease: A survey of the Sickle Cell Disease Adult Provider Network. *Journal of the National Medical Association, 100*(8), 968. https://doi.org/10.1016/S0027-9684(15)31420-6.

Lee, L. T., Smith-Whitley, K., Banks, S., & Puckrein, G. (2019). Reducing health care disparities in sickle cell disease: A review. *Public Health Reports, 134*(6), 599–607. https://doi.org/10.1177/0033354919881438/ASSET/IMAGES/LARGE/10.1177_0033354919881438-FIG2.JPEG.

Liem, R. I., Lanzkron, S., D Coates, T., DeCastro, L., Desai, A. A., Ataga, K. I., Cohen, R. T., Haynes, J., Osunkwo, I., Lebensburger, J. D., Lash, J. P., Wun, T., Verhovsek, M., Ontala, E., Blaylark, R., Alahdab, F., Katabi, A., & Mustafa, R. A. (2019). American Society of Hematology 2019 guidelines for sickle cell disease: Cardiopulmonary and kidney disease. *Blood Advances, 3*(23), 3867–3897. https://doi.org/10.1182/bloodadvances.2019000916.

Linder, G. E., & Chou, S. T. (2021). Red cell transfusion and alloimmunization in sickle cell disease. *Haematologica, 106*(7), 1805. https://doi.org/10.3324/HAEMATOL.2020.270546.

Lindsey, W., & Olin, B. (2007). Deferasirox for transfusion-related iron overload: A clinical review. *Clinical Therapeutics, 29*(10), 2154–2166.

Longoria, J. N., Heitzer, A. M., Hankins, J. S., Trpchevska, A., & Porter, J. S. (2022). Neurocognitive risk in sickle cell disease: Utilizing neuropsychology services to manage cognitive symptoms and functional limitations. *British Journal of Haematology, 197*(3), 260–270. https://doi.org/10.1111/BJH.18041.

Lubeck, D., Agodoa, I., Bhakta, N., Danese, M., Pappu, K., Howard, R., Gleeson, M., Halperin, M., & Lanzkron, S. (2019). Estimated life expectancy and income of patients with sickle cell disease compared with those without sickle cell disease. *JAMA Network Open, 2*(11), e1915374. https://doi.org/10.1001/jamanetworkopen.2019.15374.

Machado, R. F., Mack, A. K., Martyr, S., Barnett, C., Macarthur, P., Sachdev, V., Ernst, I., Hunter, L. A., Coles, W. A., Nichols, J. P., Kato, G. J., & Gladwin, M. T. (2007). Severity of pulmonary hypertension during vaso-occlusive pain crisis and exercise in patients with sickle cell disease. *British Journal of Haematology, 136*(2), 319–325. https://doi.org/10.1111/j.1365-2141.2006.06417.x.

Mainous, A. G., Rooks, B., Tanner, R. J., Carek, P. J., Black, V., & Coates, T. D. (2019). Shared care for adults with sickle cell disease: An analysis of care from eight health systems. *Journal of Clinical Medicine, 8*(8), 1154. https://doi.org/10.3390/JCM8081154.

Maples, B., & Hageman, T. (2004). Treatment of priapism in pediatric patients with sickle cell disease. *American Journal of Health-System Pharmacy, 61*, 355–363.

McCavit, T. L., Quinn, C. T., Techasaensiri, C., & Rogers, Z. R. (2011). Increase in invasive *Streptococcus pneumoniae* infections in children with sickle cell disease since pneumococcal conjugate vaccine licensure. *The Journal of Pediatrics, 158*(3), 505–507. https://doi.org/10.1016/J.JPEDS.2010.11.025.

McKie, K. T., Hanevold, C. D., Hernandez, C., Waller, J. L., Ortiz, L., & McKie, K. M. (2007). Prevalence, prevention, and treatment of microalbuminuria and proteinuria in children with sickle cell disease. *Journal of Pediatric Hematology/Oncology, 29*(3), 140–144. https://doi.org/10.1097/MPH.0b013e3180335081.

Menaa, F., Khan, B. A., Uzair, B., & Menaa, A. (2017). Sickle cell retinopathy: Improving care with a multidisciplinary approach. *Journal of Multidisciplinary Healthcare, 10*, 335–346. https://doi.org/10.2147/JMDH.S90630.

Minniti, C. P., Eckman, J., Sebastiani, P., Steinberg, M. H., & Ballas, S. K. (2010). Leg ulcers in sickle cell disease. *American Journal of Hematology, 85*(10), 831–833. https://doi.org/10.1002/AJH.21838.

Minniti, C. P., & Kato, G. J. (2016). Critical reviews: How we treat sickle cell patients with leg ulcers. *American Journal of Hematology, 91*(1), 22–30. https://doi.org/10.1002/AJH.24134.

Modebe, O., & Ifenu, S. (1993). Growth retardation in homozygous sickle cell disease: Role of caloric intake and possible gender related differences. *American Journal of Hematology, 44*(3), 149–154.

Mulligan, M. (2004). Regarding "fish" or "fish mouth" vertebrae. *American Journal of Roentgenology, 182*(6), 1600.

National Heart, Lung, and Blood Institute. (2014). Evidence-based management of sickle cell disease: Expert panel. https://www.nhlbi.nih.gov/health/sickle-cell-disease.

National Institutes of Health (NIH), Division of Blood Diseases and Resources (2002). The Management of Sickle Cell Disease. (4th ed.). NIH Publication No. 02-2117 Washington, DC: U.S. Government Printing Office.

Neumayr, L. D., Hoppe, C. C., & Brown, B. (2019). Sickle cell disease: Current treatment and emerging therapies. PubMed. *American Journal of Managed Care,* S335–S343.

https://pubmed-ncbi-nlm-nih-gov.dartmouth.idm.oclc. org/31809007/.

Niihara, Y., Miller, S. T., Kanter, J., Lanzkron, S., Smith, W. R., Hsu, L. L., Gordeuk, V. R., Viswanathan, K., Sarnaik, S., Osunkwo, I., Guillaume, E., Sadanandan, S., Sieger, L., Lasky, J. L., Panosyan, E. H., Blake, O. A., New, T. N., Bellevue, R., Tran, L. T., Razon, R. L., … Investigators of the Phase 3 Trial of L-glutamine in Sickle Cell Disease (2018). A phase 3 trial of L-glutamine in sickle cell disease. *The New England Journal of Medicine, 379*(3), 226–235. https://doi.org/10.1056/ NEJMoa1715971.

Onimoe, G., & Rotz, S. (2020). Sickle cell disease: A primary care update. *Cleveland Clinic Journal of Medicine, 87*(1), 19–27. https://doi.org/10.3949/CCJM.87A.18051.

Pahl, D. A., Green, N. S., Bhatia, M., & Chen, R. W. S. (2017). New ways to detect pediatric sickle cell retinopathy: A comprehensive review. *Journal of Pediatric Hematology/ Oncology, 39*(8), 618–625. https://doi.org/10.1097/ mph.0000000000000919.

Platt, O. (1994). Mortality in sickle cell disease. *The New England Journal of Medicine, 330*, 1639–1644.

Powars, D. (1975). Natural history of sickle cell disease—the first 10 years. *Seminars in Hematology, 12*, 267–281.

Powars, D. R., Meiselman, H. J., Fisher, T. C., Hiti, A., & Johnson, C. (1994). Beta-S gene cluster haplotypes modulate hematologic and hemorheologic expression in sickle cell anemia. Use in predicting clinical severity. *The American Journal of Pediatric Hematology/Oncology, 16*(1), 55–61.

Power-Hays, A., Li, S., Mensah, A., & Sobota, A. (2019). Universal screening for social determinants of health in pediatric sickle cell disease: A quality-improvement initiative. *Pediatric Blood & Cancer, 67*(1). https://doi.org/10.1002/pbc.28006.

Quinn, C. T. (2016). Minireview: Clinical severity in sickle cell disease: the challenges of definition and prognostication. *Experimental Biology and Medicine (Maywood), 241*(7), 679–88. doi: 10.1177/1535370216640385. Epub 2016 Mar 23. PMID: 27013545; PMCID: PMC4871738.

Quinn, C. T., Shull, E. P., Ahmad, N., Lee, N. J., Rogers, Z. R., & Buchanan, G. R. (2007). Prognostic significance of early vaso-occlusive complications in children with sickle cell anemia. *Blood, 109*(1), 40–45. https://doi.org/10.1182/ blood-2006-02-005082.

Qureshi, A., Kaya, B., Pancham, S., Keenan, R., Anderson, J., Akanni, M., Howard, J., & British Society for Haematology (2018). Guidelines for the use of hydroxycarbamide in children and adults with sickle cell disease: A british society for haematology guideline. *British Journal of Haematology, 181*(4), 460–475. https://doi.org/10.1111/bjh.15235.

Ram, S., Lewis, L. A., & Rice, P. A. (2010). Infections of people with complement deficiencies and patients who have undergone splenectomy. *Clinical Microbiology Reviews, 23*(4), 740–780. https://doi.org/10.1128/CMR.00048-09.

Rankine-Mullings, A. E., & Nevitt, S. J. (2022). Hydroxyurea (hydroxycarbamide) for sickle cell disease. *Cochrane Database of Systematic Reviews, 9*(9), CD002202. doi:10.1002/14651858. CD002202.pub3.

Reed, W., & Vichinsky, E. (2001). Transfusion therapy: A coming-of-age treatment for patients with sickle cell disease. *Journal of Pediatric Hematology/Oncology, 23*(4), 197–201.

Rodrigues, N., Shih, S., & Cohen, L. L. (2019). Pica in pediatric sickle cell disease. *Journal of Clinical Psychology in Medical Settings, 28*(1), 6–15. https://doi.org/10.1007/ s10880-019-09671-x.

Sachdev, V., Rosing, D. R., & Thein, S. L. (2021). Cardiovascular complications of sickle cell disease. *Trends in Cardiovascular Medicine, 31*(3), 187. https://doi.org/10.1016/J. TCM.2020.02.002.

Schulz, G. L., Foster, R. H., Kennedy Lang, V., Towerman, A., Shenoy, S., Lauer, B. A., Molzon, E., & Holtmann, M.

(2018). Early identification of barriers and facilitators to self-management behaviors in pediatric patients with sickle cell disease to minimize hematopoietic cell transplantation complications. *Journal of Pediatric Oncology Nursing, 35*(3), 199–209. https://doi.org/10.1177/1043454218762703.

Shenoy, S. (2007). Has stem cell transplantation come of age in the treatment of sickle cell disease? *Bone Marrow Transplant, 40*(9), 813–821.

Sickle Cell Disease Association of America Inc. (2021). Website. Retrieved January 25, 2023, from https://www. sicklecelldisease.org/.

Steinberg, M. H. (2020). Fetal hemoglobin in sickle cell anemia. *Blood, 136*(21), 2392–2400. https://doi.org/10.1182/ BLOOD.2020007645.

Stinson, J., & Naser, B. (2003). Pain management in children with sickle cell disease. *Pediatric Drugs, 5*(4), 229–241.

Taketomo, C. (2022). *Pediatric & neonatal dosage handbook: An extensive resource for clinicians treating pediatric and neonatal patients.* Lexicomp/Wolters Kluwer 2022.

Thornburg, C. D., Files, B. A., Luo, Z., Miller, S. T., Kalpatthi, R., Iyer, R., Seaman, P., Lebensburger, J., Alvarez, O., Thompson, B., Ware, R. E., Wang, W. C; BABY HUG Investigators. (2012). Impact of hydroxyurea on clinical events in the BABY HUG trial. *Blood, 120*(22), 4304–4310. *Blood, 128*(24), 2869. https:// doi.org/10.1182/BLOOD-2016-10-748764.

Thornburg, C. D. Investigators for the BH, Files BA. (2012). Impact of hydroxyurea on clinical events in the BABY HUG trial. *Blood, 120*(22), 4304–4310. https://doi.org/10.1182/ BLOOD-2012-03-419879.

Venkateswaran, L., Teruya, J., Bustillos, C., Mahoney, D., & Mueller, B. U. (2011). Red cell exchange does not appear to increase the rate of allo- and auto-immunization in chronically transfused children with sickle cell disease. *Pediatric Blood & Cancer, 57*(2), 294–296. https://doi. org/10.1002/PBC.22985.

Vichinsky, E., Hoppe, C. C., Ataga, K. I., Ware, R. E., Nduba, V., El-Beshlawy, A., Hassab, H., Achebe, M. M., Alkindi, S., Brown, R. C., Diuguid, D. L., Telfer, P., Tsitsikas, D. A., Elghandour, A., Gordeuk, V. R., Kanter, J., Abboud, M. R., Lehrer-Graiwer, J., Tonda, M., Intondi, A., … HOPE Trial Investigators (2019). A phase 3 randomized trial of voxelotor in sickle cell disease. *The New England Journal of Medicine, 381*(6), 509–519. https:// doi.org/10.1056/NEJMoa1903212.

Walters, M. C., De Castro, L. M., Sullivan, K. M., Krishnamurti, L., Kamani, N., Bredeson, C., Neuberg, D., Hassell, K. L., Farnia, S., Campbell, A., & Petersdorf, E. (2016). Indications and results of HLA-identical sibling hematopoietic cell transplantation for sickle cell disease. *Biology of Blood and Marrow Transplantation, 22*(2), 207–211. https://doi. org/10.1016/j.bbmt.2015.10.017.

Wang, W. C., Ware, R. E., Miller, S. T., Iyer, R. V., Casella, J. F., Minniti, C. P., Rana, S., Thornburg, C. D., Rogers, Z. R., Kalpatthi, R. V., Barredo, J. C., Brown, R. C., Sarnaik, S. A., Howard, T. H., Wynn, L. W., Kutlar, A., Armstrong, F. D., Files, B. A., Goldsmith, J. C., Waclawiw, M. A., … BABY HUG Investigators (2011). Hydroxycarbamide in very young children with sickle-cell anaemia: A multicentre, randomised, controlled trial (BABY HUG). *Lancet (London, England), 377*(9778), 1663–1672. https://doi.org/10.1016/ S0140-6736(11)60355-3.

Ware, R. E., Davis, B. R., Schultz, W. H., Brown, R. C., Aygun, B., Sarnaik, S., Odame, I., Fuh, B., George, A., Owen, W., Luchtman-Jones, L., Rogers, Z. R., Hilliard, L., Gauger, C., Piccone, C., Lee, M. T., Kwiatkowski, J. L., Jackson, S., Miller, S. T., Roberts, C., … Adams, R. J. (2016). Hydroxycarbamide versus chronic transfusion for maintenance of transcranial doppler flow velocities in children with sickle cell anaemia-TCD with Transfusions Changing to Hydroxyurea (TWiTCH): a multicentre, open-label, phase 3, non-inferiority trial.

Lancet (London, England), 387(10019), 661–670. https://doi.org/10.1016/S0140-6736(15)01041-7.

Ware, R. E., de Montalembert, M., Tshilolo, L., & Abboud, M. R. (2017). Sickle cell disease. *The Lancet, 390*(10091), 311–323. https://doi.org/10.1016/S0140-6736(17)30193-9.

Wilson, R., Krishnamurti, L., & Kamat, D. (2003). Management of sickle cell disease in primary care. *Clinical Pediatrics, 42*(9), 753–761.

Yawn, B. P., Buchanan, G. R., Afenyi-Annan, A. N., Ballas, S. K., Hassell, K. L., James, A. H., Jordan, L., Lanzkron, S. M., Lottenberg, R., Savage, W. J., Tanabe, P. J., Ware, R. E., Murad, M. H., Goldsmith, J. C., Ortiz, E., Fulwood, R., Horton, A., & John-Sowah, J. (2014). Management of sickle cell disease: summary of the 2014 evidence-based report by expert panel members. *JAMA, 312*(10), 1033–1048. https://doi.org/10.1001/jama.2014.10517.

37 Spina Bifida

Lauren Mitchell

ETIOLOGY

Myelomeningocele, also termed *spina bifida, spina bifida aperta*, or *open neural tube defect*, is a medically complex condition resulting in a neural tube defect (NTD) from incomplete closure of the spinal cord during day 28 of development in the embryonic period (Le & Mukherjee, 2015). During that timeframe many females are unaware they are pregnant. Spina bifida is one of the most common congenital malformations, which impacts the central nervous system (CNS) leading to lifelong physical and neurodevelopmental disabilities.

Spina bifida aperta is a Latin term that means "split or open spine." Spinal cord involvement can result in an open or closed NTD. An open NTD consists of a spinal cord malformation without dura, skin, bone, or muscle present at the site requiring surgical repair to close the open NTD and prevent cerebral spinal fluid from leaking with the risk of infection. A closed NTD has a malformed spinal cord with intact skin and requires surgical intervention (Micu et al., 2018). Surgical intervention continues to develop, typically occurring prenatally or postnatally (see Treatment, later).

Spina bifida is characterized by a complex multisystem involvement of the brain, upper and lower extremities, motor and sensory deficits, bladder, bowels, and sexual dysfunction (Joyeuz et al., 2018). Despite the complex medical conditions children with spina bifida have to manage, they are living into adulthood as medicine continues to advance.

INCIDENCE AND PREVALENCE

Children with spina bifida are a diverse population with multiple ethnicities and various levels of cognitive and physical function. Spina bifida occurs in all ethnicities, with Hispanic females having the highest rate of occurrence at 3.3%, non-Hispanic White females at 3.1%, non-Hispanic Black females at 2.8%, and non-Hispanic Asian-Pacific Islander females with the lowest rate at 1% (Kirby et al., 2019). Geographically, spina bifida is included as one of the highest rated of the 27 most common birth defects (Kirby et al., 2019). Studies have revealed an incidence rate of 3.63 per 10,000 live births in the United States compared to 18.6 in 10,000 worldwide (Hassan et al., 2022).

Poor prenatal care and maternal nutritional deficiencies will affect the risk for birth defects. Deficient folate is known to cause pregnancies complicated by spina bifida. Folic acid fortification in enriched foods and grains became mandatory in the United States in 1998, resulting in declining pregnancies with NTDs (Mai et al., 2022). Folate-fortified foods do not provide enough folate to prevent NTDs, however, because food folate decreases with food processing and cooking (Kancherla et al., 2022); therefore it is recommended that females of childbearing age consume 400 µg of folic acid daily to prevent NTDs (Mai et al., 2022).

Genetics, medications, and maternal factors can contribute to spina bifida. Ongoing studies are evaluating the genetic component to identify the various loci involved in multiple genes, with roughly 250 genes being identified to cause NTDs (Hassan et al., 2022). Valproic acid (valproate) is an antiepileptic medication linked to NTDs, with recommendations to avoid valproic acid in childbearing individuals (Hassan et al., 2022). Other antiepileptic medications are being investigated to determine the risk of NTD. The maternal factor linked to an increased risk for NTD is diabetes and obesity related to hyperglycemia and hyperinsulinemia, contributing to cell death in the neural plate (Hassan et al., 2022).

DIAGNOSTIC CRITERIA

The purpose of prenatal diagnosis is to educate the parents on spina bifida and their options to continue or terminate the pregnancy. If the parents choose to continue the pregnancy, prenatal diagnosis provides the family and health care team the opportunity to prepare for the birth of the child physically and emotionally (Corroenne et al., 2021). Genetic counseling will also be offered to the family.

A prenatal ultrasound is the gold standard for diagnosing spina bifida (Micu et al., 2018; Trudell & Odibo, 2014). Open spina bifida is commonly diagnosed in the first trimester, whereas closed spina bifida is diagnosed in the second trimester or postnatally (Lioa et al., 2021). The CNS should be visualized on the ultrasound to include three planes: transthalamic, transcerebellar, and transventricular, to further assess the skull, falx, cavum septum pellucidum, cerebellum, cisterna magna, thalamus, and ventricles (Micu et al., 2018).

Spina bifida characteristics are further delineated with three-dimensional ultrasound or magnetic resonance imaging (MRI). The ultrasound markers utilized to detect spina bifida consists of intracranial translucency (an obliterated fourth ventricle), an obliterated cisterna magna, banana sign (an abnormal curved and thinned cerebellum), lemon sign (biconcave frontal bones), and distance of the brainstem to the occipital bone with Chiari II malformation (hindbrain herniation) (Bahlmann et al., 2015; Teegala & Vinayak, 2017).

Fetal MRI is also helpful in documenting the NTD lesion and level, the presence or absence of hydrocephalus or other cerebral anomalies, such as Chiari II malformation, and other neurologic or systemic anomalies, such as syringomyelia, diastematomyelia (split cord malformation), hydronephrosis, and hip dysplasia.

CLINICAL MANIFESTATIONS

Spina bifida is NTD with incomplete closure. The neural tube consists of the brain and the spinal cord, which is an embryo's CNS. The development of the CNS occurs between days 17 and 28 after fertilization, with completion of closure at 28 days after conception (Hassan et al., 2022). The neural tube closure process consists of sequential folding, elevation, closing, and fusing along the midline spine (Hassan et al., 2022). An abnormal closure process of the neural tube leads to NTD from the midbrain to the lower spine. Spina bifida can cause hydrocephalus, Chiari II malformation, bladder, bowel, and sexual dysfunction, motor dysfunction, and latex hypersensitivity (see Associated Problems of Spina Bifida and Treatment, later).

Studies have not found one specific cause of spina bifida. There are associated risk factors, including genetics, anticonvulsant medications, and maternal factors (e.g., diabetes, obesity, toxins, folate metabolism) (Iskander & Finnell, 2022).

TREATMENT

No single medical or surgical treatment can completely restructure or recover the symptoms and deficits associated with spina bifida. Family counseling occurs with the multidisciplinary team after the prenatal ultrasound and fetal MRI have confirmed spina bifida. The family is educated on the defect and counseled on the treatment options to help them determine how to proceed with the pregnancy. Several options are available for a pregnancy diagnosed with spina bifida, including intrauterine myelomeningocele closure for eligible patients, postnatal closure with a cesarean section delivery, and termination of the pregnancy (Hassan et al., 2022).

Repair of fetal spina bifida defects is the latest surgical technique, which led to the development of a randomized trial from 2003 to 2010 called Management of Myelomeningocele Study (MOMS) (Adzick et al., 2011; Hassan et al., 2022). The study aimed to evaluate the safety and efficacy of the intrauterine repair of myelomeningocele between 19 and 25 weeks of gestation compared to the postnatal myelomeningocele repair. This study was beneficial in evaluating the children at 12 months and at 30 months to assess the physical, neurologic, and developmental findings. The MOMS trial revealed prenatal surgery prior to 26 weeks of gestation had decreased the risk of fetal or neonatal death or need for cerebrospinal fluid shunting by 12 months of age, improved Chiari II malformation, decreased rates for brainstem kinking, and syringomyelia. Motor development is primarily focused on the ability to walk, which depends on the NTD level. The children in the prenatal closure group were 42% more likely to walk without orthotics or assistive devices than those in the postnatal group at 21%. Prenatal surgery has risks that include premature births, oligohydramnios, chorioamniotic separation, placental abruption, spontaneous membrane rupture, area of dehiscence at the surgical scar site for the mother, and thin prenatal uterine surgery scar when delivering (Adzick et al., 2011). Educating families about the risks and benefits of prenatal surgery and postnatal surgery helps families determine their thoughts on the pregnancy. Overall, surgical treatments help with the quality of life and decrease the risk of infection (Hassan et al., 2022).

ANTICIPATED ADVANCES IN DIAGNOSIS AND MANAGEMENT

The anticipated advances in spina bifida include genetic research to determine the precise gene to cause the defect, to help with treatment and a cure (Spina Bifida Association [SBA], 2018). Currently there is no cure for spina bifida, only literature to reduce risk factors.

In 2021, a clinical trial (Cellular Therapy for In Utero Repair of Myelomeningocele [CuRe Trial]) began and continues to evolve, which uses stem cells to advance surgical effectiveness and improve outcomes (Hassan et al., 2022; Tomiyoshi, 2022).

 Associated Problems

Spina Bifida and Treatment

- Hydrocephalus
- Chiari II malformation
- Bowel and bladder dysfunction
- Motor dysfunction
- Learning disabilities
- Latex allergy

ASSOCIATED PROBLEMS OF SPINA BIFIDA AND TREATMENT

HYDROCEPHALUS

Hydrocephalus is the most common problem associated with spina bifida. Head ultrasounds are commonly used to monitor ventricular size and serial head circumference measurements to assess for the development of hydrocephalus. Hydrocephalus can be treated with surgical intervention by neurosurgeons. Roughly 60% to 80% of individuals with spina bifida will develop hydrocephalus depending on if the spina bifida surgical repair was closed prenatally or postnatally (Blount et al., 2021). Treatment of hydrocephalus is based on macrocephaly, increasing ventricular size, spina bifida closure site leaking, or neurologic decline. The two types of surgical intervention include ventriculoperitoneal shunt (VPS) placement and endoscopic third ventriculostomy with choroid plexus cauterization (ETV-CPC). The success rate for ETV-CPC is 45% to 50%; VPS success rate is significantly higher (Blount et al., 2021). VPS failure is diagnosed with radiographic imaging and clinical exam. Untreated hydrocephalus can cause neurologic disability and death in children or adolescents (Iskander & Finnell, 2022).

CHIARI II MALFORMATION

Chiari II malformation, a caudal migration of the cerebellar vermis with the brainstem and fourth ventricle, which distorts the brainstem and causes dysfunction, is noted in the spina bifida population with a controversial posterior fossa decompression (Blount et al., 2020, 2021). Chiari II malformation symptoms include brainstem dysfunction, poor secretion control, and airway obstruction with inspiratory stridor in infancy (Blount et al., 2021). With high morbidity and mortality related to posterior fossa decompression, the primary intervention had been to treat hydrocephalus (Blount et al., 2021; Iskander & Finnell, 2022).

BOWEL AND BLADDER DYSFUNCTION

To assist with emptying the bladder, intermittent catheterization began to prevent kidney and ureter damage, which can occur with a neurogenic bladder consisting of urine retention, urinary tract infections (UTIs), and incontinence (Iskander & Finnell, 2022). Ultrasound and bladder catheterization are utilized to assess bladder and kidney function. The urologist manages the bladders of patients with spina bifida as it is imperative to maintain safe bladders with good capacity and low pressure secondary to routine evaluation (Clayton et al., 2010). Anticholinergic medications are utilized

to decrease bladder pressures and increase bladder capacity. If medications are unsuccessful, surgical reconstruction interventions may occur (Iskander & Finnell, 2022). UTIs can mimic symptoms concerning VPS failure. In the setting of headaches and lethargy, individuals with spina bifida should obtain a catheterized urine analysis with culture, then start antibiotics before exploring the VPS. If the headaches and lethargy are related to a UTI, antibiotics management will resolve symptoms (Blount et al., 2021).

MOTOR DYSFUNCTION

Individuals with spina bifida have motor dysfunction due to NTDs. Severity of the motor dysfunction is based on the level of the defect (Iskander & Finnell, 2022). Ambulation delays can occur due to leg length discrepancy, scoliosis, or other neurologic deficits. Fig. 37.1 indicates the findings correlated to the level of the NTD.

LEARNING DISABILITIES

Individuals with spina bifida vary in strengths and weaknesses, and their primary disabilities involve language and reading comprehension with fewer concerns in speech and language (Fletcher & Brei, 2010). Neuropsychological testing is beneficial, especially in school-age individuals with spina bifida, to help with growth and development. Learning disabilities can occur with cerebellar dysfunction, which is the cerebellar triad of dysmetria, ataxia, and dysarthria (Dennis et al., 2010).

LATEX ALLERGY

Individuals with spina bifida are known to have a mild-severe reaction to latex, which varies from skin irritation, rash, hives, itchy eyes, sneezing, coughing, periorbital edema, nausea, vomiting, and anaphylaxis (Meneses et al., 2020). Individuals with spina bifida are exposed to latex secondary to natural rubber products in stores, hospitals, schools, and homes (Meneses et al., 2020), as well as multiple surgical interventions, placement of hardware with latex, and catheterization supplies. The high risk of latex exposure increases the risk of a latex allergic reaction. Individuals with spina bifida should have medical alert identification (e.g., bracelet, smartphone app). Educating clinicians and

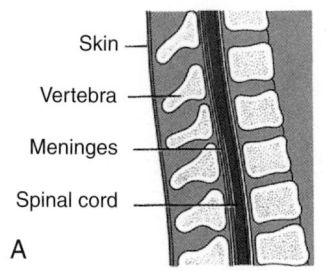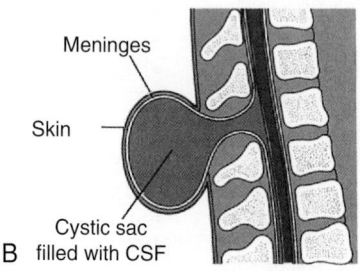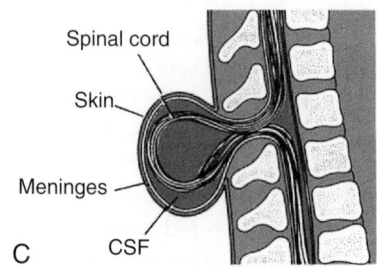

Fig. 37.1   Diagram showing section through (A) normal spine, (B) meningocele, and (C) myelomeningocele. *CSF,* Cerebrospinal fluid.

anyone involved in their care to make them aware of the latex allergy is beneficial to prevent latex allergy reactions, which can be life threatening (Meneses et al., 2020).

PROGNOSIS

Despite over 50 years of remarkable progress and a recent surge of new approaches to treatments, there still is no cure for spina bifida. Research continues to advance and supports the need for folate in all child-bearing women to help prevent NTDs. Folate is one way to decrease a pregnancy complicated by spina bifida, but it is far from a cure. New research is on the horizon for stem cells and chromosomal analysis to further assess which chromosome is linked to spina bifida.

Treatments and interventions will be necessary throughout the child's lifespan and are individualized to the child's needs and rendered when indicated by the clinical presentation, assessment, and evaluation. Life-threatening complications remain despite the vast improvement in treatment and management (Box 37.1). If untreated or not treated quickly enough, shunt malfunction can lead to brainstem herniation and death. Those with symptomatic Chiari malformations necessitating tracheostomies and feeding tubes are at risk of aspiration, pulmonary compromise, and arrest. Independent living and gainful employment are realistic goals directly affected by cognitive development, achievement of functional independence, good and consistent medical follow-up, and continued collaboration of the family, child, community, school resources, and medical team.

PRIMARY CARE MANAGEMENT

The optimal care of the infant, child, or youth with spina bifida is best provided by the primary health care provider and a multidisciplinary team collaborating to provide comprehensive and coordinated care to support the child and family. The goal of the care team is to meet the individual needs of each child and family by supporting, educating, and providing guidance.

HEALTH CARE MAINTENANCE
Growth and Development

The achievement of adequate nutrition and routine growth in children with spina bifida is the goal and a continual standard with the management of the primary care provider. The growth and development of a child with spina bifida are affected by the level of the defect, the motor and sensory impairment, and the presence of hydrocephalus. As with all children, monitoring growth by obtaining routine heights and weights during follow-up in a spina bifida clinic, as well as with the primary care provider, and plotting them on a standardized growth chart is crucial. Obtaining heights may be difficult, depending on the child's ability to stand. If necessary, the primary care provider should measure the full body length with the child supine or using an arm span. Short stature and precocious puberty are commonly seen in children with spina bifida. A referral to endocrinology to assess for growth hormone deficiency is indicated. The endocrine team will obtain bloodwork to determine if supplemental growth hormone is warranted.

Obesity is a common problem in children with spina bifida due to decreased activity levels based on the spinal defect level. Obesity can cause problems with skin breakdown and orthotic fitting. Obesity can interfere with the development of a positive self-image. Educating the family and child about healthy eating habits must begin early to establish healthy patterns.

Head circumference should be monitored closely by the primary care provider from infancy until 3 years of age to assess for any hydrocephalus-related concerns. If there is a progressive increase in head size or jumping multiple lines on the head circumference growth chart, a referral to a neurosurgeon and/or a spina bifida clinic should be made (see earlier).

Motor development may be affected and is directly related to lesion level (Table 37.1). The degree of weakness, paralysis, and decreased sensation varies. Early orthopedic and physical therapy assessment and intervention are important to prevent contractures, minimize deformities, and monitor muscle strength and flexibility. Surgical intervention is often recommended and sometimes required to achieve proper muscle balance and body alignment for problems common to this population (e.g., dislocated hips, scoliosis, kyphosis, clubfeet) that would limit the child's potential. Monitoring for orthotics, adaptive equipment, and mobility needs is ongoing throughout the child's life.

Promoting upright positioning and independent mobility is essential for the child's growth and development. As the child grows and develops, other adaptive equipment (i.e., braces, wheelchairs) increases mobility and independence. Each child's treatment

---

Box 37.1 Serious Complications of Spina Bifida

- Untreated hydrocephalus can cause neurologic disability and/or death in children or adolescents.
- Neurogenic bladder/bowels lead to poor control of kidneys and therefore chronic kidney disease.
- Abnormal sensation/paralysis can lead to skin breakdown, which puts the individual at risk for infection (sepsis, meningitis).
- Tethered spinal cord occurs in one-third of the spina bifida population. The symptoms prompting surgical intervention are related to motor decline, back or leg pain, bladder change, or (worse) orthotic deformities due to stretching of the spinal cord at the distal end.

From Dias, M. S., Wang, M., Rizk, E. B., et al. (2021). Tethered spinal cord among individuals with myelomeningocele: An analysis of the National Spina Bifida Patient Registry. *Journal of Neurosurgery, 28*(1), 21–27.

Table 37.1	Functional Alterations in Spina Bifida Related to Level of Lesion
LEVEL OF LESION	**FUNCTIONAL IMPLICATIONS**
Thoracic	Flaccid paralysis of lower extremities Variable weakness in abdominal trunk musculature High thoracic levels may have respiratory compromise Absence of bowel and bladder control
High lumbar	Voluntary hip flexion and adduction Flaccid paralysis of knees, ankles, and feet May walk with extensive braces and crutches Absence of bowel and bladder control
Midlumbar	Strong hip flexion and adduction Fair knee extension Flaccid paralysis of ankles and feet Absence of bowel and bladder control
Low lumbar	Strong hip flexion, extension and adduction, knee extension Weak ankle and toe mobility Absence of bowel and bladder control
Sacral	Normal function of lower extremities May have impaired bowel and bladder function

program varies because of differences in motivation of both the child and the family and access to and availability of resources.

The rate at which cognitive development and intellectual skills are acquired depends on a child's interaction with the environment, the defect's severity, and the presence of hydrocephalus. Infants should be considered at risk for cognitive and developmental delays, and early intervention services should be implemented in infancy. As part of a developmental approach to assessing children with spina bifida and hydrocephalus, baseline neuropsychological testing is critical in detecting cognitive function.

Diet

The goal of nutritional therapy in children with spina bifida is to promote normal growth and development. Nutrition is essential, especially for brain growth with a NTD. Any concerns for failure to thrive would prompt a referral specialist to evaluate the child for any swallowing concerns. Once cleared for swallowing concerns, the child will be monitored and followed by the pediatric primary care provider.

Early nutritional assessment and guidance are essential to care for children with spina bifida. Infancy is an excellent time to guide and educate parents on nutritional needs. It is important to teach parents early about the dangers of overfeeding, especially in children who are less mobile and have fewer caloric needs. Preventing obesity and avoiding the pattern of using food as a reward are primary goals in the nutritional management of children with spina bifida.

The child's diet should include plenty of fluids to lessen the chance of constipation and the incidence of UTIs. Dietary management is important in controlling the consistency of stools and in avoiding constipation. A diet high in fiber and low in constipating foods is usually recommended. Medications to soften stool or stimulate passage may be indicated. During infancy, problems related to a Chiari II malformation may cause feeding problems affecting growth. Compression on cranial nerve (CN) IX (glossopharyngeal), CN X (vagus), and CN XII (hypoglossal) can affect gagging and swallowing and increase the risk of aspiration, resulting in symptoms of failure to thrive, pneumonia, and respiratory compromise. Speech therapy should be consulted to complete a swallow evaluation. Children and adolescents may have increased difficulty swallowing, gagging with different textures, and choking. Videofluoroscopic swallowing study may be indicated to definitively assess and diagnose. A gastrostomy tube may be needed in children with severe Chiari II symptoms to prevent aspiration and malnutrition.

Children with known latex sensitivity or allergy should avoid plant products that contain the same allergy-producing proteins found in natural rubber latex because they may cause an allergic cross reaction. These include bananas, avocados, kiwis, plums, peaches, cherries, apricots, figs, papayas, tomatoes, potatoes, and chestnuts.

Safety

There are numerous safety issues specific to children with spina bifida. The congenital defect affects nerve function at and below the level of the defect on the spine, thus altering mobility and sensation of bone, muscle, and skin tissue below the level of the defect. This decreased sensation puts a child at greater risk for burns, fractures, and skin breakdown. Proper body positioning, frequent position changes, and assurance that adaptive equipment fits properly and is used correctly can reduce the risk of skin breakdown. Tepid water should be used for bathing to prevent burns. The condition of the child's skin should be checked at least twice daily for redness and irritation. As soon as children are competent to assume this responsibility, they should be taught how to perform a thorough skin check.

The potential for limited cognitive ability and altered judgment exists in these children. Awareness of limitations is essential to help these children with issues such as independence, decision making, self-care, and sexuality. Instructions on the proper use of equipment for mobility (e.g., wheelchairs, braces, crutches) should be appropriate to the child's developmental and cognitive abilities. In addition to age-appropriate anticipatory guidance about safety issues, primary care providers should emphasize the importance of wearing helmets for any activities that routinely require a helmet. A helmet is not needed on a day-to-day basis to protect the shunt. It is safe for the population with spina bifida to be active and participate in any activities, including wheelchair sports.

Parents of children with seizures should be instructed on how to intervene safely and appropriately during a seizure.

Latex allergy can be life threatening. Educating clinicians and anyone involved in their care to make them aware of the latex allergy is beneficial to prevent latex allergy reactions, which can be life threatening. The primary care provider must inform and educate the parents and individual about this potential sensitivity and the importance of avoiding contact with latex, observing signs, documenting the allergy, and prescribing EpiPen for home and school.

Immunizations

Routine immunizations are recommended for individuals with spina bifida to prevent diseases and infections. COVID-19 vaccine and yearly influenza vaccines are safe for individuals with spina bifida.

Screenings

Vision. Due to the high incidence of visual and perceptual deficits, ocular palsies, and astigmatism in children with spina bifida, practitioners should assess for these conditions during routine screenings with a referral to an ophthalmologist. At 6 months of age it is recommended for routine assessment or sooner, with yearly evaluations to follow unless positive findings are noted on previous exams.

Hearing. Routine screening is recommended. Children with spina bifida are commonly hypersensitive to loud noises. Awareness of this finding may alleviate parental concern.

Dental. Routine screening is recommended. Dentists should be notified of the increased risk of latex allergy. Information should be given for safe, alternative nonlatex products. Regarding antibiotic prophylaxis, the neurosurgeon of children with hydrocephalus and shunts undergoing dental procedures should be consulted. The American Academy of Pediatric Dentistry (AAPD) recommends antibiotic prophylaxis for children with a ventriculoatrial shunt (VAS). In contrast, the VPS does not involve vascular structures and does not require antibiotic protection (AAPD, 2022).

Blood pressure. Routine screening is recommended. Children with known renal problems such as urinary reflux or a history of hypertension should have a more frequent assessment. Nephrology manages some individuals with SB.

Urinalysis. Baseline urinalysis and urine cultures are obtained in newborns. If a UTI is suspected, a urine culture and sensitivity should be obtained by catheterization (bag specimens have been noted to have a higher chance of contamination). A positive urine culture should be reported to the child's urologist to determine if antibiotic treatment is warranted or if urine is routinely colonized with a particular bacteria based on past urine analysis results.

Condition-Specific Screening

Complete blood count. If an individual is receiving long-term antibiotic therapy (e.g., sulfonamides) for the prevention of UTIs, complete blood counts (CBCs) should be done approximately every 6 months to monitor changes.

Urine studies

Urinalysis and serum creatinine. Urinalysis, urine culture, and serum creatinine should be checked at birth and routinely to assess renal function and evaluate for UTIs and vesicoureteral reflux (Foster, 2020).

Renal ultrasound. Assess urinary tract, bladder capacity, and vesicoureteral reflex (Foster, 2020).

Urodynamic studies. Perform physiologic evaluation of urologic function, detrusor control, and sphincter function (Foster, 2020).

Psychometric screening. Assess cognitive dysfunction secondary to hydrocephalus, shunt revisions, infections, and CNS abnormalities. The psychometric screening will also assess intelligence, cognitive function, speech-language deficits, and academic skills (Foster, 2020).

Gait analysis evaluation. This screening tool will assess the child's functional status, including muscle innervation, strength, coordination, ambulation, need for bracing, and ability to live independently. A gait analysis is also a beneficial preoperative tool prior to surgeries, such as reducing dislocated hips and transfer of muscles (Foster, 2020).

X-rays. Screening for scoliosis, dislocated hips, and any limb abnormalities are helpful to assess routinely with x-rays. These images should be completed routinely during the first year of life and continue yearly throughout adolescence. The orthopedic team should manage these images.

Computed tomography/magnetic resonance imaging. These serial images should be completed routinely during the first year of life and continue yearly throughout adolescence. The neurosurgery team should manage these images. The images help evaluate hydrocephalus and monitor ventricular size. The MRIs are helpful prognostic tools as a baseline for any neurologic decline. MRI images are detailed to assess for brain or spinal cord malformations such as Chiari II, low-lying spinal cord, syrinx, or tethered spinal cord. All children with spina bifida have a tethered spinal cord radiographically (Foster, 2020).

Latex allergy. All children with spina bifida should be treated as latex sensitive from birth. Providers are responsible for educating children and their families about latex allergies and what to avoid. During routine visits, the provider should refill prescriptions for EpiPens, order medical alert bracelets, and/or review the use of medical alert mobile applications (see earlier).

COMMON ILLNESS MANAGEMENT

Differential Diagnosis

Chiari II malformation. Chiari malformation type II or Arnold-Chiari malformation consists of the cerebellar vermis and a portion of the brain stem descending below the level of the fourth cervical vertebrae, a common finding in individuals with spina bifida. The symptoms from the Chiari are commonly a concern during the neonatal and infant period. The symptoms consist of difficulty with swallowing, which results in poor feeding, weak cry, stridor, difficulty breathing, and spasticity to the upper extremities. The primary cause of death with spina bifida is due to a symptomatic Chiari. A brain and spine MRI is the test to complete to assess the Chiari and any other abnormalities noted in the brain and spine. A CO_2 breathing test is used to assess the somatosensory evoked response and the brainstem evoked response (SBA, n.d.).

Primary care providers must be cautious not to dismiss these findings as a simple upper respiratory infection but must consider the possibility that these symptoms result from pressure on the CN IX, X, or XII. A depressed or absent gag may be present, leading to possible aspiration pneumonia. Feeding difficulties, poor weight gain, and symptoms of failure to thrive may also be present. Treatment focuses on symptomatic relief of the presenting problems (e.g., gastrostomy tube and tracheostomy may be placed for absent gag and cough).

The primary importance of these symptoms is to assess the shunt first. The shunt-first approach ensures normal intracranial pressure is present prior to any surgical intervention on the Chiari. Most patients with spina bifida will have radiographic findings of a Chiari II, which does not require surgical intervention. Clinical indications for a surgical Chiari II decompression include severe symptoms related to brainstem dysfunction and CN dysfunction (SBA, n.d.).

Tethering of the spinal cord. Spina bifida is not a progressive condition; thus the primary care provider and the specialists should closely evaluate any signs of deterioration. Virtually all children with spina bifida have signs of spinal cord tethering on MRI as a result of the defect and subsequent surgical closure. Most children may only require one surgery

to untether the spinal cord. Roughly 10% to 20% of children will require repeat untethering spinal cord surgeries (SBA, n.d.). Signs and symptoms of the tethered spinal cord include decreased muscle strength, worsening gait, pain, spasticity, changes in bowel and bladder function, and scoliosis. The decision to intervene surgically requires careful assessment of the symptoms, the impact on the child's function, and the results of diagnostic studies, such as renal ultrasound, urodynamic studies, and spine MRI. Early detection and release of the tethered cord can stabilize or reverse the deterioration in most cases.

Hydrocephalus. Most individuals have an internal shunt system to treat hydrocephalus. The differential diagnosis of shunt malfunction and infection must be considered in the presence of lethargy, fever, visual changes, gastrointestinal distress, and headache (see earlier).

Urinary tract infections. UTIs are common among children with spina bifida. Fever associated with UTIs may be mild or severe. Other symptoms may include abdominal pain, vomiting, cloudy and malodorous urine, and increased voiding. These symptoms should alert the primary care provider to obtain a urine specimen by catheterization for culture. Frequency and burning may be masked because of decreased sensation.

A positive culture should be reported to the child's urologist, especially in cases with urinary reflux. Treatment of positive cultures may vary depending on the individual's urologist. Bacteriuria is found in many children with spina bifida, especially those who perform clean intermittent catheterization (CIC), and is termed *asymptomatic bacteriuria*. These children do not require antibiotic therapy or prophylactic suppression unless there is documented vesicoureteral reflux or symptoms such as fever, dysuria, or new-onset incontinence (SBA, 2018).

Fever. Fever is a symptom found in many common childhood illnesses with various causes. Individuals with spina bifida can have a fever related to shunt infection, UTI, skin breakdown, and cellulitis. Particular consideration must be given to the presence of fever because it may lower the seizure threshold in these children. A fever of unknown origin may be the result of an undetected fracture of an insensate extremity. Osteoporosis associated with paralysis, decreased weightbearing, and inactivity, especially after immobilization in a cast, may contribute to the occurrence of fractures. An undetected burn of insensate areas may also result in fever. The practitioner should carefully examine the area for swelling, redness, or abrasions. Obtaining a complete history from the individual and the parents may assist in determining if there has been recent trauma.

Gastrointestinal symptoms. Nausea, vomiting, and diarrhea are all common symptoms in children. In children with spina bifida, those symptoms are a concern for shunt malfunction and/or UTI. Children who have had a bladder augmentation and have referred pain to the shoulder should seek immediate medical attention because this could indicate a urinary leak into the peritoneum. A child with a neurogenic bowel may become impacted with stool, leading to gastrointestinal distress. The presence of diarrhea may be misleading because liquid stool passes around the impacted stool. A radiograph of the kidneys, ureters, and bladder may help differentiate diarrhea from impaction.

In children with a high lesion, practitioners should consider the possibility of appendicitis as a cause of nausea, vomiting, or fever; the classic symptom of pain may be altered due to decreased sensation.

Drug Interactions

Some children with spina bifida are on routine medication therapy. Potential interactions among these and other medications must be carefully considered when additional medications are prescribed. Commonly used drug categories are as follows:

1. Antibiotics are given for the treatment of UTIs or prophylaxis, including amoxicillin (Amoxil), trimethoprim-sulfamethoxazole (TMP-SMX), and nitrofurantoin (Furadantin). If a child requires other antibiotic therapy for common childhood illness, such as ear infections, the antibiotic for the UTI is discontinued during the needed course of treatment. Bladder irrigations can also contain antibiotics.
2. Anticholinergics are commonly used: oxybutynin chloride (Ditropan) and tolterodine (Detrol), which assist in urinary continence and reduce high bladder pressure. Oxybutynin chloride can cause heat prostration in the presence of high environmental temperatures.
3. Stool softeners and stimulants aid in the evacuation of stool. Many products are used for this purpose, and most are over-the-counter drugs. None of these should be administered in the presence of abdominal pain, nausea, vomiting, or diarrhea.
4. Anticonvulsants are given to control seizure activity and include phenobarbital, phenytoin sodium (Dilantin), and carbamazepine (Tegretol).

DEVELOPMENTAL ISSUES

Individuals with Chiari II malformation may experience sleep apnea, increased stridor, and snoring with sleep. These children are at increased risk for sudden respiratory arrest. Sleep studies help determine the severity of the sleep disorder and the need for positive airway pressure, such as bilevel positive airway pressure and continuous positive airway pressure. Parents must also be able to perform cardiopulmonary resuscitation in the event of an arrest. Alteration in the child's normal sleep pattern (e.g., longer naps, increased frequency of naps) may indicate increased intracranial pressure from a shunt malfunction. In addition, sleep may be interrupted if a child needs to be repositioned during the night to prevent pressure sores and skin breakdown from developing (see earlier).

Toileting

Bowel and bladder continence is essential in developing positive self-esteem and optimum functioning. A child's physical abilities and psychological readiness for toileting should be assessed. Children who are unable to sit without adaptive devices or unable to master self-dressing skills need special consideration when toileting is introduced. A physical or occupational therapist should be consulted about using bars or adaptive seats. Special clothing or underwear may be helpful to make access to the perineum easier.

Children should master self-care methods of toileting before entering school. Urinary and fecal incontinence can lead to difficulties socially, as well as issues with skin care. Bowel management should be monitored from birth to avoid constipation and impaction. At ages 2 to 3 years, the concept of toileting should be introduced to children. The goals of bowel management are to maintain soft, formed stools and develop a regular evacuation schedule on the toilet every 1 to 2 days to avoid impaction or soiling between bowel movements. These goals can be accomplished by having the child sit on the toilet at regular times, taking advantage of the gastrocolic reflex by toileting after meals, and increasing abdominal pressure by blowing bubbles, tickling the child to incite laughter, or placing the child's legs on a stool to increase pressure by hip flexion.

Miralax is often used to promote bowel movements and decrease the risk of constipation. Children should assume responsibility for timed evacuation and good perineal care as physical and cognitive development allows. Stool softeners, stimulants, lubricants, enemas, and glycerin suppositories are additional agents to utilize.

A Malone antegrade continence enema (MACE) is a surgical procedure to assist children with bowel management, including severe constipation or stool incontinence. This operative procedure benefits children who have failed aggressive bowel management programs. The MACE involves surgical placement of a continent stoma to the bowel that can be catheterized to administer enemas for predictable bowel movements. The ACE is flushed every day or every other day with various plans of care consisting of water, glycerin enemas, Miralax, or soap suds enemas through a catheter inserted into the stoma. It is a simple procedure with the goal of the child being able to manage the procedure independently. It is important to remember that the management program varies from child to child. A sympathetic manner in working with a child helps avoid feelings of guilt and blame for unavoidable accidents.

Self-catheterization (CIC) is a realistic goal for most children by early school age. An individualized approach accounting for the child's readiness is important in achieving this goal. Providing young children with an anatomically correct doll and catheter often helps in mastery of the skill. In children with limited cognitive abilities and poor manual dexterity, adaptation, such as an abdominal continent stoma, should be considered to enable independence for the child. Noncompliance with self-catheterization may become an issue in adolescence when catheterization is used as a focus in the fight for independence.

Discipline

There can be a wide range of emotional responses to having a child with a chronic disability, requiring some degree of psychological adjustment and family therapy (SBA, 2018). The feeling of the need to overprotect a child with a disability is not uncommon and can affect a child's independence and social adjustment. Children with such a complex long-term condition are at increased risk for experiencing psychosocial adjustment problems that may affect the parents' and family members' responses to discipline. Interventions are necessary at an early age to encourage independence in children with spina bifida (SBA, 2018).

Child Care

Primary care providers should be familiar with early intervention programs and child care placements available in the community because these programs for infants vary from state to state. Preschoolers are eligible for placement in public programs that meet their physical and educational needs. It is important that the day care or educational setting be notified in advance about a prospective student so that the staff can be educated regarding the child's abilities and medical care needs, and a smooth transition can be facilitated. The child's bladder and bowel program and procedures should be taught to the care provider, and education regarding medication administration while attending school. The school nurse and teachers should be educated on spina bifida, including CIC, medications, latex precautions, signs/symptoms of shunt malfunction, and UTIs.

Many children with spina bifida have adaptive equipment to aid in mobilization, maintain appropriate body alignment, prevent further deformity, and increase independence. Day care providers should be aware of the proper application and fit of the equipment. It is also important to communicate the child's motor and sensory capacity to prevent injury. Some children may need more time to transition between various classes around the school due to assistive devices. Schools should meet Americans with Disabilities Act (ADA) requirements to assist these children with getting around the school and attending classes. A list of emergency telephone numbers must accompany these children. If possible, primary care providers should be available to answer questions and concerns from child care staff.

Schooling

Learning disabilities are common in children with spina bifida. Problems may occur in perceptual-motor skills, comprehension, attention, activity, memory, organization, sequencing, and reasoning. In addition, attention problems are common and usually need to be treated, given the significant impact of such problems on functioning at home and school. Neuropsychology and psychological testing should be completed to help address the child's needs at school (SBA, 2018). Concerns regarding learning disabilities and attention disorders should be addressed early in the educational process so the identified needs may be met and adaptations made to minimize educational problems and frustrations for the child, family, and educators. Frequent absences can further compromise school performance as a result of illness or medical treatment. Federal laws protect the rights of children with disabilities to access appropriate education. Individualized education plans (IEPs) must be formulated to address each child's specific needs, including educational and physical requirements. The primary care provider, the child, and the family must actively collaborate with the school in this planning process. Each child's particular needs must be addressed in the IEP, including the necessity for catheterization; timed toileting; administration of medications; physical, occupational, and speech therapies; and individual counseling. These needs may require assistance from an aide.

School personnel should be aware of any adaptive equipment and its purpose and function and should involve the child's physical and occupational therapists in adapting the school environment for optimum functioning. Elevators may help a child get to classes on time and minimize fatigue. As children age, they may use a wheelchair for mobilization in school. This should be viewed as a means of increasing mobility and independence instead of decreasing independence. Ideally, the school should be free of structural barriers to enable the child to move freely and participate in all activities. Special provisions must be made for safe departure from the building in the event of an emergency and transportation to and from home (i.e., wheelchair van or bus). Individuals with a known latex allergy will need assistance identifying and avoiding latex in school. Common latex sources in the school environment include art supplies, pencil erasers, and gym mats or floors. The school nurse and allergists are possible resources to assist in this process.

Spina bifida and hydrocephalus affect the quality of life because of these conditions' chronicity and multisystem impact. Children with spina bifida may experience decreased opportunities for peer relationships, prolonged dependency on parents, and decreased community acceptance. Awareness of mental health and utilization of psychosocial services will help children be successful (SBA, 2018). Awareness of these potential problems is helpful for those working with children with spina bifida. Emotional independence is the foundation that supports the successful development of physical independence. Appropriate referrals for further psychological intervention and support may be advised. Primary care providers should encourage these children to be involved in extracurricular activities and find activities the child may enjoy, such as crafts, wheelchair sports, adaptive sports, journaling, fitness teams, cooking courses, among other areas of interest. Academic planning, career counseling, and independent living must be considered.

Sexuality

The issues of sexuality and reproduction are major areas of concern for children with spina bifida and their parents. Information regarding sexual function, intimacy, and reproduction should be discussed early and continued throughout childhood and adolescence. Developing good self-esteem and peer relationships is important in developing satisfying intimate relationships. As with all children, sex education should begin at home with information available through the educational system and further addressed by the spina bifida clinic team. If a primary care provider does not feel skilled in gynecologic care, the child should be referred to a sensitive specialist with experience examining individuals with disabilities.

Female health. Females with spina bifida are capable of normal fertility but have unique health care concerns related to body structure, including changes to the hips and spine during pregnancy (SBA, 2018). Females with spina bifida must be made aware of the risks of pregnancy, which consist of preterm birth and changes in bowel, bladder, and mobility (SBA, 2018). Birth control methods must be carefully evaluated on an individual basis. The importance of folic acid supplementation must be discussed and reinforced. The high incidence of latex allergies in this population prohibits the use of latex condoms and diaphragms; however, nonlatex condoms are available, and information should be made available by the primary care provider and the spina bifida team. Because of the increased risk for UTI with intercourse, females not taking routine antibiotics should take prophylactic antibiotics before and after intercourse. Females may benefit from using additional lubricating gels when attempting intercourse because vaginal lubrication in response to sexual arousal does not occur with lower spinal cord injury. Counseling regarding sexually transmitted diseases and pregnancy is essential, including use of nonlatex condoms.

Pregnancy in females with spina bifida is complicated by physical deformity, the presence of VPS, previous abdominal surgery for urologic and bowel management, varying degrees of impaired renal function, and hypertension. Early prenatal care is important, especially for screening the fetus for NTDs. Consult a high-risk obstetrician (OB) when planning for pregnancy, and the OB will continue with medical management during the pregnancy and afterward.

Male health. In males with spina bifida, the level of the spinal lesion will predict their capacity for erection and ejaculation. A thorough history regarding erections and ejaculations is important in determining potential sexual function. Infertility in males with spina bifida can be related to sperm transport or defects in spermatogenesis. Reproduction is greater with lower-level spina bifida lesions consistent with sacral reflexes and the absence of hydrocephalus. Sildenafil citrate is effective in maintaining erections in some males with spina bifida (Deng et al., 2018). Sperm retrieval followed by intracytoplasmic sperm injection may be a promising treatment option to help with infertility for males with ejaculatory dysfunction. Additional research is needed to assess infertility and the challenges males with spina bifida have encountered (Deng et al., 2018).

To review developmental guidelines by age from birth to +18 years of age, visit the SBA website (https://www.spinabifidaassociation.org/guidelines/guidelines-by-age).

Transition to Adulthood

Transitioning care from a pediatric to an adult practice is a process, not a single event requiring thorough preparation (Lestishock et al., 2018). Studies revealed that early discussion of transition allows the adolescent to feel comfortable answering the provider's questions independently without using a parent or guardian. When young adolescents are taught about their care and are interested in their health, they are likely to seek medical attention when experiencing abnormal symptoms related to their chronic medical health (Oswald et al., 2013). Increased autonomy occurs when providers educate the adolescents about their health at each clinic visit; designate a multidisciplinary team filled with case managers, social workers, and group leaders to help ease the transition process; and assess for feedback from adolescents and families on ways to enhance the autonomy toward transitioning care (Lestishock et al., 2018). Advanced practice providers are not used effectively to help adolescents with chronic illnesses meet the goal of independency to assist in transitioning care (Lestishock et al., 2018). To minimize delays with transitioning care, adolescents should receive adequate information and feel confident relaying the information back to the health care provider prior to transitioning care (Oswald et al., 2013).

A successful transition begins with early education with the child and their family. Motivation is key to the success of young adults and families transitioning to adult care facilities. Decision-making skills related to community living are necessary for a successful transition and must begin early. Development of a social support system, including peers, is needed to prevent social isolation that can lead to depression and loneliness, and an inability to access medical care (SBA, 2018).

The survival rate of individuals with spina bifida continues to increase. Coordinated care is of equal importance for adults, though, unfortunately, adult multidisciplinary clinics are rare, affecting the smooth transition process (SBA, 2018). Adults must learn to navigate the already complex medical system and piece together their care. The inadequate transition of care puts the adults at great risk for utilizing the emergency department as a routine medical home instead of establishing care with several health care providers and multiple clinic appointments. Primary health care should be provided by health professionals interested in and committed to working with this high-risk population. This necessary transition of care has been met with reluctance by many adult health care providers for a number of reasons, including a lack of familiarity with the complex needs of individuals with spina bifida. Access to health care insurance can be a challenge for individuals not on state-funded insurance.

Coordinated multidisciplinary care, education of health care providers and clients, costs, and promotion of client-directed care are issues that need to be addressed. A few adult programs have been developed in various parts of the United States. Individuals with spina bifida should contact a local adult neurosurgery clinic to assess multidisciplinary care clinics focusing on spina bifida.

Family Concerns

Families who deal with spina bifida have many special concerns, including shunt malfunctions, ambulation, and overall completing activities of daily living so their child can live independently. It is important for families and their children to attend a spina bifida multidisciplinary clinic to ask questions along the way. The journey will have moments of both frustration and reward. Providers must listen to families' concerns and worries to help address their needs.

Raising a child with spina bifida has greater parental stress in families than in the general population,

specifically with mothers, single parents, older parents, and disadvantaged or culturally diverse parents (SBA, 2018). These parents feel less satisfied and competent as parents; they are less optimistic, often feel isolated, and have a small network to socialize with (SBA, 2018).

The risk for sudden death as a result of a shunt malfunction or complications related to the Chiari II malformation is chronic and creates intense stress on the family system. This stress, in addition to the other complex needs of these children, often results in depression and posttraumatic stress disorder (SBA, 2018). Parents should be encouraged to treat their child as a member of the family, not the center of the family.

The multisystem involvement of this condition requires frequent hospitalizations, surgeries, outpatient services, and multidisciplinary care. These factors, in addition to items such as special equipment or medications that may be needed by these children, place a tremendous financial burden on parents. The health care system recognizes the many needs of children with spina bifida and their families and offers physical, emotional, spiritual, and social care. Nevertheless, no individual understands or feels the problems these children and families face in their day-to-day lives, as well as another child or family with the same disorder. Therefore support groups and opportunities available to provide this community support network are necessary and have proven to be a major factor in coping and adaptation for these families. Each region has its community-based network or local chapter. The primary care provider must be aware of available local resources.

RESOURCES

Centers for Disease Control and Prevention (topic information on living with spina bifida and clinical care guidance): https://www.cdc.gov/ncbddd/spinabifida

Children's Mercy Hospital–Kansas City (information on spina bifida: https://www.childrensmercy.org

Spina Bifida Association of America (provides up-to-date information for families on NICU experience, clinical care, genetics, urology, support groups, education, research, events, advocacy): spinabifidaassociation.org

 Summary

Primary Care Needs for the Children With Spina Bifida

HEALTH CARE MAINTENANCE
Growth and Development
- Height may be measured in the supine position.
- Both precocious puberty and short stature are reported.
- Obesity is common in these children due to a lack of motor activity.
- Head size may be enlarged if the child is diagnosed with hydrocephalus; measure head circumference at each visit until sutures are fused.

- Motor delays are common and depend on the level of the lesion. Surgical intervention for proper muscle balance may be necessary.
- Promoting upright positioning and independent mobility is a goal.
- Cognitive ability varies, and testing and early intervention are recommended.

Diet
- Caloric intake should be monitored to minimize the potential for obesity.

- Caution parents about using food as a reward.
- Diet should include increased fluids to lessen the chance of constipation and UTIs.
- Regurgitation, vomiting, and difficulties with gag reflex need to be evaluated for increased intracranial pressure and Chiari II malformation.
- Children with latex allergies may have allergic reactions to some foods.

Safety
- Increased risk of injuries (i.e., burns, fractures, skin breakdown) may occur with decreased sensation and mobility.
- Spina bifida population is at a high risk of wound breakdown and poor wound healing (lower extremities must be examined often for pressure ulcers).
- Skin integrity should be checked twice daily.
- Cognitive deficit may alter judgment regarding safety and use of equipment.
- Prolonged sitting in a wheelchair with bony prominences can cause lumbosacral pressure ulcers.
- Proper body positioning, frequent position changes, and proper fit of adaptive equipment are recommended.
- Education on emergency care of seizures is recommended.
- Increased risk for latex allergy. Educate on common sources of latex to avoid. Medical alert bracelets identifying allergies are recommended. EpiPens are necessary for severe reactions.

Immunizations
- Routine immunizations are recommended. Multidose vials may have latex tops and should be avoided.
- Immunizations are not contraindicated in children with seizures. Consultation with a pediatric neurologist is recommended for children with severe or poorly controlled seizures.

Screening
- *Vision.* These children have a high incidence of visual deficits such as ocular palsies, astigmatism, and visual-perceptual deficits. An ophthalmologist should evaluate children at 6 months of age and yearly after that.
- *Hearing.* Routine screening is recommended. Children may have hypersensitivity to loud noises if they have shunts. If children are exposed to aminoglycosides or have a history of CNS infection, their hearing should be evaluated by an audiologist.
- *Dental.* Routine care is recommended. Latex precautions are required. Antibiotic prophylaxis is not needed in children with VPS for hydrocephalus but is recommended for children with VAS.
- *Blood Pressure.* Routine monitoring is recommended.
- *Hematocrit.* Routine screening is recommended.
- *Urinalysis.* Baseline urinalysis and cultures should be obtained during the newborn period or when urologic concerns develop.
  - Bladder catheterization is recommended for obtaining urine for cultures.
  - Positive cultures should be reported to the urologist to determine treatment.
  - Children with renal problems may develop hypertension and should have more frequent monitoring of blood pressure. In rare cases, persistent hypertension may be a sign of shunt malfunction.

Condition-Specific Screening
- *Blood tests.* CBCs should be obtained frequently on children treated with sulphonamides for the prevention of UTI. Serum creatinine should be done on newborns and then as indicated when changes appear on renal ultrasound (i.e., hydronephrosis).
- *Head and spine CT/MRI.* Screening of hydrocephalus, ventricular size is recommended. VPS, Chiari II, or any other intracranial or spinal abnormalities are also of concern.
- *Latex allergies.* Latex precautions include monitoring signs and symptoms and educating the child, family, and other care providers. EpiPen is needed for severe reactions.
- *Renal ultrasound.* Routine screening of kidney and bladder with function is recommended.
- *Scoliosis.* Screening should be done yearly from birth through adolescence.

COMMON ILLNESS MANAGEMENT
Differential Diagnosis
- *Chiari II malformation.* Assess the shunt first before doing any surgical intervention to the Chiari. Symptoms may include respiratory difficulties, stridor, croupy cough, absent gag reflex, and headache. Refer to neurosurgery for evaluation.
- *Fevers.* Rule out shunt or CNS infection, UTI, and fracture or injury of the insensate area.
- *Gastrointestinal symptoms.* Rule out increased intracranial pressure with nausea and vomiting, UTI, fecal impaction, and appendicitis.
- *Shunt malfunction.* Vomiting, irritability, and sleepiness.
- *Tethered cord.* Symptoms may include scoliosis, altered gait pattern, changes in muscle strength and tone, disturbance in urinary and bowel patterns, and back pain.
- *UTI.* Fever, pain or burning when urinating or catheterizing, cloudy-looking and/or foul-smelling urine.

Drug Interactions
- No routine drug therapy exists, but children frequently take daily medications.
- Antibiotics may be given to prevent or treat UTIs.
- Anticholinergics are given to assist in urinary continence training.
- Stool softeners and bulking agents are used to prevent constipation.
- Anticonvulsants are used if seizures are present.
- Evaluate for possible drug interactions.

DEVELOPMENTAL ISSUES
Sleep Patterns
- Apnea, increased stridor, and snoring may occur in children with symptomatic Chiari II malformation. Sleep studies may be indicated.
- Lethargy may indicate increased intracranial pressure.
- Children may need to be repositioned during the night to prevent skin irritation resulting in fatigue.

Toileting
- Varies based on neurogenic bowel and bladder function.
- Some patients may begin with intermittent catheterization and a bowel regimen as early as infancy.
- Aggressive bowel and bladder management should begin early to avoid delayed incontinence.

Continued

- Independence should be encouraged when developmentally and physically appropriate.
- Parents should be trained in cardiopulmonary resuscitation.
- Bulking agents and stool softeners may be used daily to prevent constipation.
- Bowel regimens will vary. MACE is sometimes used.
- Intermittent catheterization is common, and compliance may be an issue during adolescence.

Discipline

- These children are at an increased risk of psychosocial adjustment problems.
- They need discipline and encouragement toward independence.
- They must develop coping strategies and attend spina bifida support groups. Parents need to learn the difficult balance between proper discipline and increasing their independence according to their abilities.

Child Care

- Choosing a day care or preschool setting that is familiar with this population is vital.
- Special medical care procedures must be taught to day care personnel.
- Care providers must be educated regarding signs and symptoms of shunt malfunction, UTIs, latex allergies, and precautions.
- Early intervention programs are ideal for infants and toddlers.
- Day care personnel must know how to use adaptive equipment and check for injury.
- Emergency contact information is necessary.

Schooling

- Learning disabilities and attention problems are common.
- Neuropsychological testing is recommended with IEPs.
- Educate the nurse and teacher on assistance with activities of daily living while at school.
- Frequent school absences may occur because of illness or medical treatments.

- Federal laws protect children with disabilities. Special physical needs must be tended to during school hours.
- Special provisions may be necessary for adaptive equipment, wheelchairs, transportation, accessibility, and safety in emergencies. Attend an ADA-criteria school.
- Latex items must be removed from the classrooms.
- Children may have adjustment problems because of low self-esteem and functional limitation. Participation in extracurricular activities may help with peer relationships.
- Families need assistance in IEP hearings.

Sexuality

- Sexuality and reproductive health should be introduced early and discussed by the primary care provider.
- Precocious puberty may occur.
- Sexual functioning may be altered because of sensory impairment.
- Females have normal fertility, so birth control is important when sexually active. Latex condoms and diaphragms must be avoided.
- Males may be unable to have an erection or ejaculation, depending on the level of spinal lesion.
- Genetic counseling is recommended.

Transition to Adulthood

- Primary health care needs, independent living, vocational training, and socialization must be addressed in transition planning.
- Social support systems are needed for independent living.
- Cognitive deficits and functional limitations must be evaluated for independent living.

Family Concerns

- Parents should be encouraged to treat their child as a member of the family, not the center of the family.
- Stress is related to frequent hospitalizations, surgeries, and the need for multidisciplinary care.
- Caring for these children can be a financial burden on families.

REFERENCES

American Academy of Pediatric Dentistry (AAPD). (2022). Antibiotic prophylaxis for dental patients at risk for infection. Retrieved from https://www.aapd.org/research/oral-health-policies–recommendations/antibiotic-prophylaxis-for-dental-patients-at-risk-for-infection/.

Adzick, N. S., Thom, E. A., Spong, C. Y., Brock, J. W. 3rd, Burrows, P. K., Johnson, M. P., Howell, L. J., Farrell, J. A., Dabrowiak, M. E., Sutton, L. N., Gupta, N., Tulipan, N. B., D'Alton, M. E., & Farmer, D. L.; MOMS Investigators. (2011). A randomized trial of prenatal versus postnatal repair of myelomeningocele. *New England Journal of Medicine, 364*(11), 993–1004. doi: 10.1056/NEJMoa1014379. Epub 2011 Feb 9.

Bahlmann, F., Reinhard, I., Schramm, T., Geipel, A., Gembruch, U., von Kaisenberg, C. S., Schmitz, R., Stupin, J., Chaoui, R., Karl, K., Kalache, K., Faschingbauer, F., Ponnath, M., Rempen, A., & Kozlowski, P. (2015). Cranial and cerebral signs in the diagnosis of spina bifida between 18 and 22 weeks of gestation: A German multicentre study. *Prenatal Diagnosis, 35*(3), 228–235. https://doi.org/10.1002/pd.4524.

Blount, J. P., Bowman, R., Dias, M. S., Hopson, B., Partington, M. D., & Rocque, B. G. (2020). Neurosurgery guidelines for the care of people with spina bifida. *Journal of Pediatric Rehabilitation Medicine, 13*(4), 467–477. https://doi.org/10.3233/PRM-200782.

Blount, J. P., Maleknia, P., & Hopson, B. D. (2021). Hydrocephalus in spina bifida. *Neurology India, 69*(8), 367–371.

Clayton, D. B., Brock, J. W., & Joseph, D. B. (2010). Urologic management of spina bifida. *Developmental Disabilities Research Reviews, 16*(1), 88–95.

Corroenne, R., Yepez, M., Pyarali, M., Johnson, R. M., Whitehead, W. E., Castillo, H. A., Castillo, J., Mehollin-Ray, A. R., Espinoza, J., Shamshirsaz, A. A., Nassr, A. A., Belfort, M. A., & Cortes, M. S. (2021). Prenatal predictors of motor function in children with open spina bifida: A retrospective cohort study. *BJOG, 128*(2), 384–391. https://doi.org/10.1111/1471-0528.16538.

Deng, N., Thirumavalavan, N., Beilan, J. A., Tatem, A. J., Hockenberry, M. S., Pastuszak, A. W., & Lipshultz, L. I. (2018). Sexual dysfunction and infertility in the male spina bifida patient. *Translational Andrology and Urology, 7*(6), 941–949. doi:10.21037/tau.2018.10.08. PMID: 30505732; PMCID: PMC6256049.

Dennis, M., Salman, M. S., Juranek, J., & Fletcher, J. M. (2010). Cerebellar motor function in spina bifida meningomyelocele.

Cerebellum, 9(4), 484–498. https://doi.org/10.1007/s12311-010-0191-8.

Dias, M. S., Wang, M., Rizk, E. B., Bowman, R., Partington, M. D., Blount, J. P., Rocque, B. G., Hopson, B., Ettinger, D., Lee, A., & Walker, W. O.; National Spina Bifida Patient Registry Group. (2021). Tethered spinal cord among individuals with myelomeningocele: An analysis of the National Spina Bifida Patient Registry. *Journal of Neurosurgery Pediatric, 28*(1), 21–27. doi: 10.3171/2020.12.PEDS20868.

Fletcher, J. M., & Brei, T. J. (2010). Introduction: Spina bifida—a multidisciplinary perspective. *Developmental Disabilities Research Reviews, 16*(1), 1–5.

Foster, M. R. (2020). Spina bifida workup. *Medscape.* Retrieved from https://emedicine.medscape.com/article/311113-workup.

Hassan, A. S., Du, Y. L., Lee, S. Y., Wang, A., & Farmer, D. L. (2022). Spina bifida: A review of the genetics, pathophysiology and emerging cellular therapies. *Journal of Developmental Biology, 10*(2), 22. https://doi.org/10.3390/jdb10020022.

Iskander, B. J., & Finnell, R. H. (2022). Spina bifida. *New England Journal of Medicine, 387*(5), 444–450.

Joyeux, L., Danzer, E., Flake, A. W., & Deprest, J. (2018). Fetal surgery for spina bifida aperta. *Archives of Disease in Childhood. Fetal and Neonatal Edition, 103*(6), F589–F595. https://doi.org/10.1136/archdischild-2018-315143.

Kancherla, V., Botto, L. D., Rowe, L. A., Shlobin, N. A., Caceres, A., Arynchyna-Smith, A., Zimmerman, K., Blount, J., Kibruyisfaw, Z., Ghotme, K. A., Karmarkar, S., Fieggen, G., Roozen, S., Oakley, G. P., Jr, Rosseau, G., & Berry, R. J. (2022). Preventing birth defects, saving lives, and promoting health equity: An urgent call to action for universal mandatory food fortification with folic acid. *Lancet Global Health, 10*(7), e1053–e1057. https://doi.org/10.1016/S2214-109X(22)00213-3.

Kirby, R. S., Mai, C. T., Wingate, M. S., Janevic, T., Copeland, G. E., Flood, T. J., Isenburg, J., Canfield, M. A., & National Birth Defects Prevention Network. (2019). Prevalence of selected birth defects by maternal nativity status, United States, 1999–2007. *Birth Defects Research, 111*(11), 630–639. https://doi.org/10.1002/bdr2.1489.

Le, J., & Mukherjee, S. (2015). Transition to adult care for patients with spina bifida. *Physical Medicine and Rehabilitation Clinics of North America, 26*(1), 29–38.

Lestishock, L., Daley, A. M., & White, P. (2018). Pediatric nurse practitioners' perspectives on health care transition from pediatric to adult care. *Journal of Pediatric Health Care, 32*(3), 263–272. doi:10.1016/j.pedhc.2017.11.005.

Liao, Y., Wen, H., Luo, G., Ouyang, S., Bi, J., Yuan, Y., Luo, D., Huang, Y., Zhang, K., Tian, X., & Li, S. (2021). Fetal open and closed spina bifida on a routine scan at 11 weeks to 13 weeks 6 days. *Journal of Ultrasound Medicine, 40*(2), 237–247. https://doi.org/10.1002/jum.15392.

Mai, C. T., Evans, J., Alverson, C. J., Yue, X., Flood, T., Arnold, K., Nestoridi, E., Denson, L., Adisa, O., Moore, C. A., Nance, A., Zielke, K., Rice, S., Shan, X., Dean, J. H., Ethen, M., Hansen, B., Isenburg, J., & Kirby, R. S. (2022). Changes in spina bifida lesion level after folic acid fortification in the US. *Journal of Pediatrics, 249*, 59–66.e1. https://doi.org/10.1016/j.jpeds.2022.06.023.

Meneses, V., Parenti, S., Burns, H., & Adams, R. (2020). Latex allergy guidelines for people with spina bifida. *Journal of Pediatric Rehabilitation Medicine, 13*(4), 601–609.

Micu, R., Chicea, A. L., Bratu, D. G., Nita, P., Nemeti, G., & Chicea, R. (2018). Ultrasound and magnetic resonance imaging in the prenatal diagnosis of open spina bifida. *Medical Ultrasonography, 20*(2), 221–227. https://doi.org/10.11152/mu-1325.

Oswald, D. P., Gilles, D. L., Cannady, M. S., Wenzel, D. B., Willis, J. H., & Bodurtha, J. N. (2013). Youth with special health care needs: Transition to adult health care services. *Maternal and Child Health Journal, 17*(10), 1744–1752. https://doi.org/10.1007/s10995-012-1192-7.

Spina Bifida Association. (n.d.). Symptomatic Chiari malformation. Retrieved from https://www.spinabifidaassociation.org/wp-content/uploads/Symptomatic-Chiari-Malformation1-final.pdf.

Spina Bifida Association. Guidelines for the care of people with spina bifida. (2018). Retrieved from https://www.spinabifidaassociation.org/wp-content/uploads/Guidelines-for-the-Care-of-People-with-Spina-Bifida-2018.pdf.

Teegala, A. L., & Vinayak, D. G. (2017). Intracranial translucency as a sonographic marker for detecting open spina bifida at 11-13+6 weeks scan: Our experience. *Indian Journal of Radiology and Imaging, 27*(4), 427–431.

Tomiyoshi, T. (2022). World's first stem cell treatment for spina bifida delivered during fetal surgery. *Children's Health.* Retrieved from https://health.ucdavis.edu/news/headlines/worlds-first-stem-cell-treatment-for-spina-bifida-delivered-during-fetal-surgery/2022/10#:~:text=Preliminary%20work%20by%20Farmer%20and,bifida%20walk%20without20noticeable%20disability.

Trudell, A. S., & Odibo A. O. (2014). Diagnosis of spina bifida on ultrasound: Always termination? *Best Practices and Research Clinical Obstetrics and Gynaecology, 28*(3), 367–377.

ETIOLOGY

Tourette syndrome (TS) is a heterogeneous disorder that affects individuals of all ages and does not have a cure. It is a neurobiologic condition characterized by vocal and motor tics that change over time and wax and wane in severity. Tics can be defined as a disturbance in the corticostriatal, mesolimbic circuitry, leading to the disinhibition of motor and limbic systems. There is an imbalance in dopaminergic neurotransmission and a decreased volume in the caudate nucleus and sensorimotor cortex. This volume depletion correlates with the severity of tics: More loss equals increased severity and has been found to decrease glucose in the basal ganglia; despite what has been previously thought, strep antibodies do not play a role (Rae et al., 2019) (Fig. 38.1). The etiology of TS is strongly familial, with the onset influenced by an interaction of genetics and environment, including perinatal factors and stressful life events. Infections are another potential cause that is being explored (Wolicki et al., 2019).

In 1885, neurologist Gilles de la Tourette (1857–1904) published the first paper on a rare disorder whose symptoms were described as sudden movements (tics) and shouting obscene language (coprolalia) (Walusinski, 2018). He was the first to describe nine individuals exhibiting unusual movements and sounds of the syndrome that bears his name (Lajonchere et al., 1996).

INCIDENCE AND PREVALENCE

TS is a movement and neurodevelopmental disorder that combines multiple motor and vocal tics that occur for over 1 year but not necessarily cooccurring in the same year, and they start prior to age 18 years. It is the most common hyperkinetic disorder in childhood (CDC, 2023C; Nikkhah et al., 2019). Tics are defined as sudden, rapid, recurrent, nonrhythmic motor movements or vocalizations generally preceded by an urge (Mederos & Sanford, 2022). Tics can include dystonic and tonic posturing or movements and are reproducible by the patient and can be described by the patient. Simple motor tics involve a single muscle group, such as grimacing, eye rolling, blinking, neck stretching, and nose wrinkling, whereas complex motor tics involve multiple muscle groups that last a little longer than simple motor tics, such as kicking, hitting, hopping, and jumping (Chou et al., 2023). Simple vocal/phonic tics involve one sound without meaning, such as sniffing, throat clearing, or clicking of the tongue. Complex vocal tics involve speech-language or a combination of multiple simple vocal tics, such as stuttering, shouting, slurring, and repeating phrases (echolalia). There can also be changes in pitch, emphasis, or volume. Like many neurologic disorders, illness, fatigue, and stress can make them more frequent or harder to conceal or exacerbated by anxiety, anger, or excitement (Singer, 2019). TS is autosomal dominant, without an isolated gene (Fig. 38.2). Predilection favors males over females (4:1), with it being more persistent in females (Chou et al., 2023). A misnomer among patients and families is that stimulants cause tics, in that they bring out tics or make them known in those already predisposed.

The only tic disorder that is included in the National Survey of Children's Health (NSCH) is TS. Data from the 2016–2019 NSCH indicate 0.3% of children and adolescents (age 3–17 years) received a diagnosis of TS and 0.2% of children and adolescents (age 3–17 years) were current with a diagnosis of TS (Table 38.1). The data showed the TS diagnosis was more common in males than females, with prevalence estimate comparable among various age groups, races/ethnicities (Hispanic and White), parent education levels, health insurance, household poverty level, and geographic classification.

Attention-deficit/hyperactivity disorder (ADHD) is a common comorbidity with those having TS; it sometimes leads to the diagnosis of TS. When a stimulant is used for the first time to treat ADHD, tics may surface, thereby uncovering the underlying disorder or comorbid diagnosis of tics. Tics may be more likely to increase with dextroamphetamine (Dexedrine, Adderall, Vyvanse, Procentra) compared to methylphenidate. The primary care provider must keep in mind that ADHD symptoms can potentially cause more difficulty than the tics in children with both conditions, so it is important to ensure that ADHD is adequately treated. Up to one-third of children with tics will have obsessive-compulsive disorder (OCD), and up to half will have ADHD (Piña-Garza et al., 2019). Most commonly, tics are worse and more frequent during puberty, and 50% of children are free from tics by age 18 years (Piña-Garza et al., 2019).

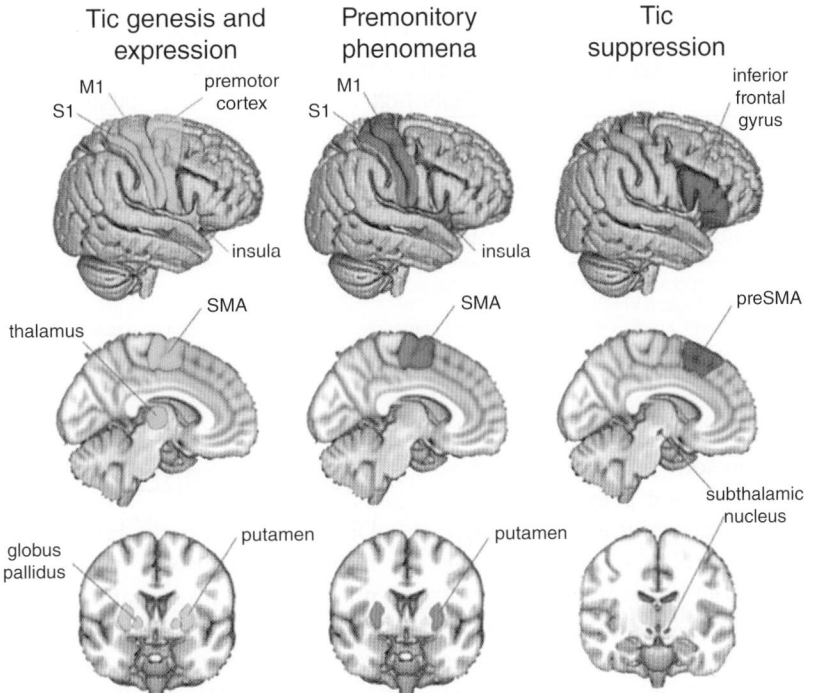

Fig. 38.1 Cortical and subcortical regions associated with the phenomenologic features of Tourette syndrome. Tic genesis and expression *(green)* is associated with the premotor cortex, SMA, insula, M1, S1, putamen, globus pallidus, and thalamus; premonitory sensations *(blue)* with the SMA, insula, M1, S1, and putamen; tic suppression *(red)* with the inferior frontal gyrus, preSMA, and subthalamic nucleus. *M1/S1*, Sensory motor cortex; *SMA*, supplementary motor area. (From Rae, C.L., Critchley, H.D., & Seth, A.K. [2019]. A Bayesian account of the sensory-motor interactions underlying symptoms of Tourette syndrome. *Frontiers in Psychiatry, 10*, 29.)

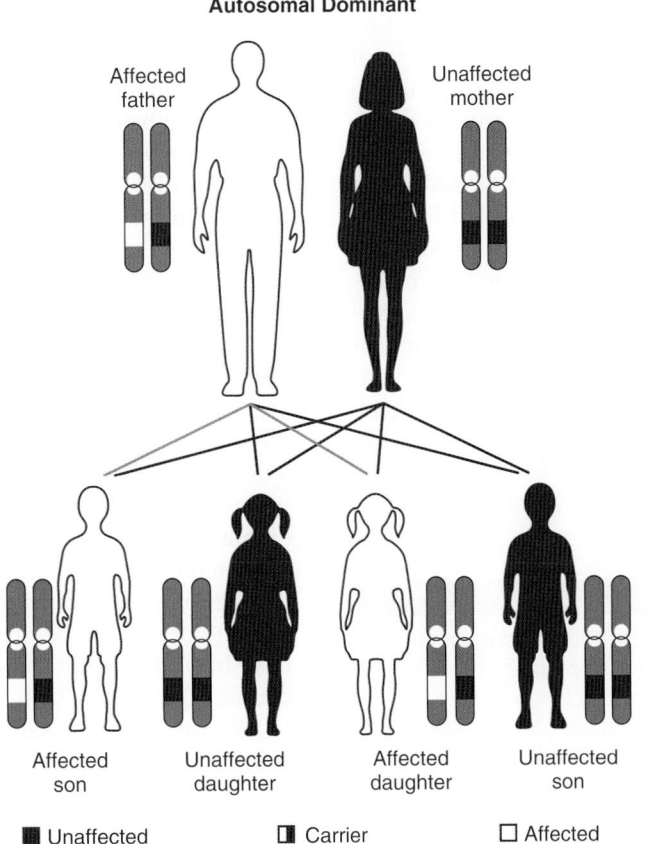

Fig. 38.2 Autosomal dominant inheritance. (From Norton, M.E., Scoutt, L.M., & Feldstein, V.A. [2017]. *Callen's ultrasonography in obstetrics and gynecology* [6th ed.]. Elsevier.)

Table 38.1	Does This Child Currently Have Tourette Syndrome, Age 3 to 17 Years?			
	CHILD DOES NOT HAVE THE CONDITION	CHILD DOES NOT CURRENTLY HAVE THE CONDITION	CHILD CURRENTLY HAS CONDITION	TOTAL %
%	99.8	0.0	0.2	100.0
CI	99.7–99.8	0.0–0.0	0.2–0.3	
Sample count	61,558	29	158	
Pop. est.	61,322,738	12,422	137,559	

Population estimates are weighted to represent child population in United States.
CI, 95% confidence interval; *pop. est.*, percentages and population estimates.
From Child and Adolescent Health Measurement Initiative. 2016–2017 National Survey of Children's Health (CSCH) data query. Data Resource Center for Child and Adolescent Health supported by the US Department of Health and Human Services, Health Resources and Services Administration (HRSA), Maternal and Child Health Bureau (MCHB). Retrieved November 2023 from www.childhealthdata.org.

Motor tics are usually present prior to vocal tics, and simple tics are usually present prior to complex tics. Transient/provisional tic disorder involves single or multiple motor and/or vocal tics within 1 year. Chronic tic disorder involves single or multiple motor or vocal tics (but not both) that wax and wane in frequency but have continued beyond 1 year. TS involves multiple motor and one or more vocal tics occurring not necessarily at the same time, but they may wax and wane in frequency, continuing for over 1 year since the first tic, with an age of onset prior to age 18 years; they are not attributed to physiologic effects of a substance or other medical condition. Adults typically tic less whether treated for them or not, and most patients will see a reduction in tic frequency over time into adulthood (American Psychiatric Association [APA], 2013).

The primary care provider must keep in mind several triggers for tics: injury to the basal ganglia, exposure to neurotoxins, autoimmune encephalopathy, and tics developing within 1 month of starting a new medication. Antipsychotics and antiemetics, which are dopamine-blocking drugs, can cause tics, and Dilantin, Lamictal, and Tegretol; stimulants do not cause tics but can bring them out in an already predisposed individual. According to the Centers for Disease Control and Prevention (CDC, 2023d), current research shows that genes play an important role in TS, showing that TS is inherited as a dominant gene with approximately a 50% chance of parents passing the gene on to their children. Other causative factors that are currently being researched are smoking during pregnancy, pregnancy complications, low birth weight, and infection (CDC, 2023d).

Key Points

Note the following key points about Tourette syndrome (TS):
- TS is a neurodevelopmental disorder characterized by involuntary, repetitive, and nonrhythmic motor and vocal tics.
- TS is a medical condition that usually begins in early childhood and persists throughout life.
- TS is characterized by the presence of multiple motor and vocal tics.
- Patients with TS commonly have behavioral problems that can be socially stigmatizing.
- TS can present very differently in each individual, ranging from mild to severe.

DIAGNOSTIC CRITERIA

Diagnosis is largely based on history and observation. The diagnosis can be challenging due to the many clinical presentations, suppressibility of tics, and fluctuating symptoms over time and under different conditions. There may be a genetic link in families, although no specific gene has been definitively identified; the *SLITRK1* gene has been found in a small number of people, with further research needed. In the last decade, whole genome/exome sequencing has been identified with several novel genetic mutations in patients with TS.

When clinically indicated, a thorough physical examination and neurologic evaluation by the primary care provider exclude other diseases in addition to the possibility of tics. Early diagnostic measures, such as imaging, blood, or cerebrospinal fluid biomarkers, have yet to be identified to enable the diagnosis before symptoms present themselves. Referrals to a neurologist or other specialist are warranted when exclusions with the initial history and exam are impossible. Increasing awareness of TS and its risk factors could support caregivers and help health care providers recognize tics and establish treatment plans early.

TS typically presents between 4 and 8 years of age, with frequency and severity that increases between 8 and 12 years of age (Quezada & Coffman, 2018). The APA *Diagnostic and Statistical Manual of Mental Disorders*, Fifth Edition (DSM-5) criteria to diagnose TS include the presence of tics before the age of 18 years (Table 38.2). The tics must be present for at least 1 year and include at least two motor tics and one phonic tic throughout the course of the disease. The different tics do not need to be present concurrently but should have been present at some point throughout the illness course (Quezada & Coffman, 2018).

Several rating scales can evaluate symptoms in children with TS (e.g., Yale Global Tic Severity Scale [YGTSS], TS Clinical Global Impression, Tourette Disorder Scale, Shapiro Tourette Syndrome Severity Scale, Premonitory Urges for Tics Scale). The most used tool to evaluate and determine the severity of tics is the YGTSS, where a score of 9 equates to an exacerbation of tics.

Table 38.2   DSM-5, With Comparison of ICD-10, ICD-11

	LABELS	PARENT CATEGORY	CRITERIA OF TS	CRITERIA OF CHRONIC/ PERSISTENT VOCAL AND/OR MOTOR TIC DISORDER	CRITERIA OF PROVISIONAL/ TRANSIENT TIC DISORDER
ICD-10	Combined vocal and multiple motor tic disorder (de la Tourette); chronic motor or vocal tic disorder; transient tic disorder; other tic disorders; tic disorder, unspecified	Behavioral and emotional disorders with onset usually occurring in childhood and adolescence	Multiple motor and one or more vocal tics, not necessarily occurring at the same time	One or more motor or vocal tics, but not both types Symptoms occur 12 mo	One or more motor and/or vocal tics Symptoms occur 12 mo
ICD-11	Tourette syndrome (combined vocal and motor tic disorder); persistent (chronic) motor or phonic tics; provisional tic disorder; substance-induced tic disorder; tic disorder due to general medical condition	Disorders of nervous system— primary; mental and behavioral disorders— secondary; obsessive-compulsive and related disorders; neurodevelopmental disorders	One or more motor and/or vocal tics occurring over the same period of time Symptoms occur 12 mo		
DSM-5	Tourette disorder; persistent (chronic) motor or vocal tic disorder provisional tic disorder; other specified tic disorder; unspecified tic disorder	Neurodevelopmental disorders	Multiple motor and one or more vocal tics at some point in illness May wax and wane, but have persisted 1 yr since onset Onset before 18 yr Not caused by substance or other condition	One or more motor or vocal tics present at some point, not both motor and vocal symptoms May wax and wane, but have persisted 1 yr since onset Onset before 18 yr Not caused by substance or other condition No history of TS Specify if motor tics only, vocal tics only	One or more motor and/or vocal tics Tics present for 1 yr since onset Onset before 18 yr Not caused by substance or other condition No history of TS or persistent tic disorder

DSM-5, Diagnostic and Statistical Manual of Mental Disorders, Fifth Edition; *ICD-10*, International Classification of Diseases, Tenth Edition; *ICD-11*, International Classification of Diseases, Eleventh Edition; *TS*, Tourette syndrome.

From Szejko, N., Robinson, S., Hartmann, A., Ganos, C., Debes, NM., Skov, L., Haas, M., Rizzo, R., Stern, J., Münchau, A., Czernecki, V., Dietrich, A., Murphy, T. L., Martino, D., Tarnok, Z., Hedderly, T., Müller-Vahl, KR., & Cath, D. C. (2022). European clinical guidelines for Tourette syndrome and other tic disorders-version 2.0. Part I: assessment. *Eur Child Adolesc Psychiatry*, 31(3), 383–402. doi:10.1007/s00787-021-01842-2. Epub 2021 Oct 18.

The following tests may be necessary to rule out other conditions. During bloodwork obtain a lead level in a child who shows developmental delay, Lyme titers if there is a tick history or the patient lives in an endemic area, thyroid studies, hemoglobin A1c, and comprehensive metabolic panel may be useful especially if the child is tremulous to rule out thyroid disorder or low glucose. An electroencephalogram (EEG) will rule out focal seizures or absence epilepsy, and magnetic resonance imaging of the brain is helpful if the EEG is abnormal or there is a concern for a tumor in the basal ganglia.

The primary care provider is the umbrella to the medical home; once the patient is diagnosed with TS, the primary care provider will ensure that the appropriate referrals are made to specialists. Specialists may include a pediatric ophthalmologist for notable tics involving eye movements such as blinking, rolling, or deviation, and a neuropsychologist for an evaluation that may elicit useful findings to uncover other diagnoses and learning disabilities contributing to stress and tics.

When taking the history, the primary care provider will need to assess for the other comorbidities commonly associated with tics and TS, as 85% of patients will have one or more (Box 38.1). ADHD is the most common comorbidity at 50% to 60% and can be assessed with the Vanderbilt scale or other

Box 38.1   **Common Comorbidities With Tourette Syndrome**

Attention-deficit hyperactivity disorder
Autism spectrum disorder
Childhood conduct disorder
Obsessive-compulsive disorder
Oppositional defiant disorder
Anxiety disorder
Depressive disorder

available tools. ADHD is typically diagnosed a few years prior to tic expression, whereas OCD occurs a few years after a tic diagnosis. Other comorbidities are learning disabilities and sleep disturbances (Fig. 38.3). Two useful screening tools that can be given while a patient is waiting to be seen are the Patient Health Questionnaire–9 and Generalized Anxiety Disorder–7. These two questionnaires are completed as self-assessments for depression and anxiety (Piña-Garza et al., 2019).

CLINICAL MANIFESTATIONS AT TIME OF DIAGNOSIS

TS is characterized by the onset of tics, which come in different forms; simple or complex motor tics and simple or complex vocal tics may cause marked distress or significant impairment in social skills (Table 38.3).

TREATMENT

As patients age, they can develop compulsions, repetitive behaviors, and impulsive behaviors that are not tics. Continue to listen to parents and patients when tics or movements change (e.g., Is the patient's quality of life affected? Is the patient unable to concentrate in school?). Consider intervention, too. There are nonpharmacologic,

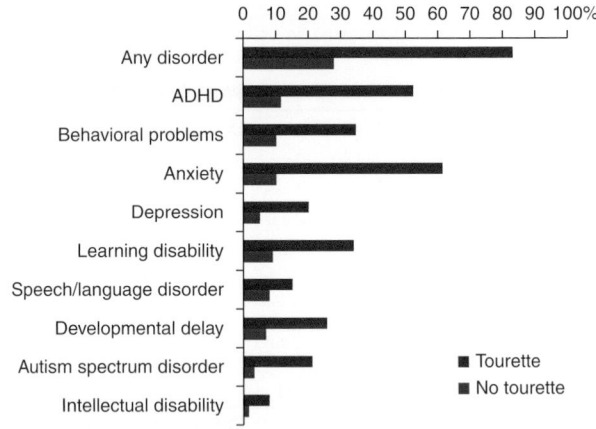

Percentage of children with and without Tourette syndrome and another mental, behavioral, or developmental disorder

Data on 51,001 US children aged 6–17 years from the 2016–2017 National Survey of Children's Health

Fig. 38.3 **Percentage of children with and without Tourette syndrome and another mental, behavioral, or developmental disorder.** (Data on 51,001 US children age 6 to 17 years from the 2016–2017 National Survey of Children's Health.) Child and Adolescent Health Measurement Initiative (CAHMI) (2019). 2016-2017 National Survey of Children's Health (2 Years Combined Data Set): Child and Family Health Measures, National Performance and Outcome Measures, and Subgroups, SPSS Codebook, Version 1.0, Data Resource Center for Child and Adolescent Health supported by Cooperative Agreement U59MC27866 from the U.S. Department of Health and Human Services, Health Resources and Services Administration (HRSA), Maternal and Child Health Bureau (MCHB). Retrieved [March 7, 2023] from www.childhealthdata.org.

pharmacologic, and surgical interventions available. In pediatrics, treatment is most often either nonpharmacologic and pharmacologic (Pringsheim et al., 2019). This chapter will focus on those modalities.

Treatment options should be individualized, and the choice should be the result of a collaborative decision among the patient, the caregiver, and the health care provider (Pringsheim et al., 2019). It is important to remember that treatment does not change the

Table 38.3   **Manifestations and Different Types of Tics and Their Characteristics at Time of Diagnosis of Tourette Syndrome**

TYPE OF TIC	TYPICAL FEATURES
Motor	Arise in the voluntary musculature and involve discrete muscles or muscle groups
Vocal	Consist of any noise produced by movement of air through the nose, mouth, pharynx
Stimulus bound	Occur in response to internal or external stimuli (visual, phonic, tactile, mental)
Blocking	Motor or vocal tics that interrupt the voluntary action without alteration of consciousness (dysfluency of speech or gait)
Simple	Are restricted to one muscle or a single muscle group (e.g., eye blinking, nose twitching, tongue protrusion), simple, meaningless sounds (e.g., grunting, throat clearing, coughing, sniffing, barking)
Complex	Involvement of more muscle groups (e.g., repetitive touching of objects or people, repetitive obscene movements [copropraxia], mimicking others [echopraxia], complex vocal tics that are words or phrases, expressing obscenities [coprolalia], repeating others [echolalia], or repeating oneself [palilalia])
Clonic	Last <100 ms
Dystonic	Last >300 ms; repetitively abnormal posture of a kind that one may see in dystonia
Tonic	Last >300 ms; relatively long duration of the contraction (e.g., in back muscles) without exhibiting abnormal postures

natural history or course of the disorder. The goals are reducing tics and improving daily life, not elimination. If symptoms are mild, watchful waiting is a good first step. Education is key at every visit. Teach families and caregivers that commenting on the patient's tics or drawing attention to them typically makes them worse. Accepting patients for who they are helps teach those close to them to ignore the tics. During well visits, the primary care provider must discuss the importance of diet, exercise, sleep, and stress reduction.

There is compelling evidence that nonpharmacologic treatment is highly effective for treating TS, consisting of cognitive-behavioral intervention for tics (CBIT) and habit reversal therapy (HRT). HRT focuses on teaching the patient how to recognize the urge and to perform a competing or opposite movement or noise that is less noticeable. The patient must be aware of the tics, the early signs preceding a tic, and the urge. CBIT should be considered the first therapeutic option, focusing on removing the patient from situations or activities causing increased tics or having a safe space to "tic out" (Quezada & Coffman, 2018). It also utilizes relaxation techniques. CBIT can be more difficult as the patient must remove oneself from situations that could contribute to more tics being expressed, such as in a crowd or during a presentation, which can be unrealistic. Some patients can release their tics and attend a stressful event, but others may not. Both therapies depend on the patient's age and understanding, as well as patient/parent buy-in, as both need to be practiced often to maintain. Due to a lack of providers for these two types of therapies, wait lists tend to be long.

Tichelper.com is an online treatment program for tics that specializes in patients over age 8 years. Other non-pharmacologic treatments include traditional cognitive-behavioral therapy, especially in patients with other common comorbidities, biofeedback, meditation, and the use of deep breathing exercises (PsycTech, 2014).

When CBIT is not appropriate, ineffective, or unavailable, then pharmacotherapy should be considered. Other reasons for pharmacologic treatment for tics are when they are causing social problems (e.g., bullying), emotional problems (e.g., low self-esteem, depression, anxiety), discomfort (e.g., physical pain or injuries), or decreased academic performance or sleep disruption (Quezada & Coffman, 2018). When initiating medication, it is important to educate the patient and family that medication may not completely eliminate tics, and by sharing this information the primary care provider can avoid disappointment and frustration. Like most medications, start low and titrate up based on the patient's response. Educate patients and families that medication works best when taken daily. After 2 weeks at the same dose, the primary care provider will reevaluate and may consider increasing for more benefit. Providers should give the medication a minimum of 2 weeks (allowing for a reduction in side effects, etc.) before considering a change.

Pharmacologic treatment options include alpha$_2$-agonists, also known as alpha-adrenergic receptor agonists, dopamine receptor blocking agents such as antipsychotics and neuroleptics, dopamine-depleting agents, antiepileptic drugs, serotonergic drugs, cannabinoids, and botulinum toxin injections (Gilbert & Jankovic, 2014). Alpha-adrenergic receptor agonists reduce sympathetic nerve impulses and inhibit norepinephrine at the frontal lobe, decreasing vasomotor tone and heart rate (Tables 38.4 and 38.5).

As tics naturally wax and wane it is also important when prescribing to remember that occasionally weaning off medication may be useful, particularly in the summer months when school is not in session (less school stress). The gold standard for a child with tics and ADHD is a combination of clonidine and a stimulant. Many other emerging or experimental treatment approaches may eventually be incorporated into the pediatric toolbox for the treatment of TS, including Botox and cannabidiol (CBD) (Quezada & Coffman, 2018). Surgical interventions include deep brain stimulation, but this too is reserved for refractory tics and is used mostly in adults. There is experimental evidence to suggest targeting the vagal nerve, such as in a vagal nerve stimulation device, which may decrease tic frequency (Piña-Garza et al., 2019).

The goal of medication is tic reduction, not elimination, as elimination is likely improbable. The pitfalls of pharmaceuticals include trial-and-error results and side effects. If side effects outweigh the benefit of tic reduction, it should be weaned off. Other medications, such as muscle relaxants, may be helpful for tic reduction.

COMPLEMENTARY AND ALTERNATIVE THERAPIES

The use of complementary and alternative medicine (CAM) in pediatric patients with TS is popular as providers and caregivers seek nonpharmacologic treatments. Although most CAM therapies appear to be benign when considering side effects, there is a need for more rigorous evidence-based research to support CAM therapies in this population (Patel et al., 2020). Common CAM modalities in pediatrics are included in Table 38.6.

ANTICIPATED ADVANCES IN DIAGNOSIS AND MANAGEMENT

Brain-gut axis (BGA) is an area of research currently getting a lot of attention. The relationship between gut microbiota and TS began to be deeply studied in the past 5 years. This important research shows how the brain can regulate gastrointestinal and homeostasis and how the intestines can affect mood, sleep, and even the development and repair of the nervous system. Another area of focus due to BGA and based on the existence of abnormal intestinal microorganisms in children with TS is whether oral probiotics can relieve tic symptoms in animal experiments and current clinical trials (Geng et al., 2023).

Table 38.4   Drugs for Use in Treating Tourette Syndrome

DRUG CLASS	DRUG NAME	USES	SIDE EFFECTS	DOSAGE
Alpha-adrenergic	Clonidine Guanfacine	Blood pressure lowering, attention-deficit/hyperactivity disorder (ADHD)	Sedation, weight gain, low blood pressure, low heart rate, headache, irritability, dry mouth	0.05 mg (<45 kg) or 0.1 mg (>45 kg) to start depending on patient age and weight. Max daily dose 0.4 mg. Usually given nightly and in extended-release form if patient can swallow small pills. Can also come in patches but is typically less tolerated in childhood. If the patient cannot swallow pills, may crush the regular release form and give it twice daily. 0.5–1 mg depending on age and weight. Max daily dose 4 mg. Again, see above for twice daily or once daily dosing depending on if patient can swallow pills yet.
Nonstimulant	Atomoxetine (Strattera)	ADHD	Nausea, dry mouth, dizziness, mood changes	0.5 mg/kg/day to start
Antiepileptic/antiseizure	Topiramate	Seizures, bipolar disorder, other mood disorders, migraines	Nausea, decreased appetite, paresthesia (many more at higher doses)	15–25 mg to start depending on age and weight. Twice daily dosing for better control. Using the extended-release form nightly depends on the patient's ability to swallow pills. If unable to swallow pills, 15 mg capsules can be opened onto food or put in a drink twice daily.
Atypical antipsychotics and neuroleptics (dopamine receptor blockers)	Aripiprazole (Abilify), haloperidol (Haldol), pimozide (Orap), risperidone (Risperdal), fluphenazine, ziprasidone	Hyperactivity, aggression, impulsivity, obsessive-compulsive disorder (OCD)	Sedation, irritability, weight gain, depression. Serious side effects include akathisia, tardive dyskinesia, tardive dystonia. Gynecomastia, QT prolongation, impaired concentration, metabolic side effects can also occur. May consider referral to psychiatrist if needing to go to this drug class.	Each drug is different. Refer to the formulary for dosing.
Serotonin-selective reuptake inhibitors	Fluoxetine (Prozac), escitalopram (Lexapro), sertraline (Zoloft)	Anxiety, OCD	Weight gain or loss, sexual uninterest, black box warning for increased suicidality in children and young adults	Each drug is different. Refer to the formulary for dosing.
Dopamine depleting	Tetrabenazine (Xenazine)	Hyperkinetic disorders	Sedation, suicidality, sadness/depression, akathisia, parkinsonism	Adult dosing: 12.5 mg every morning to start

OUTCOMES FROM THE PANDEMIC

Tics and TS are largely male-dominated disorders, but during the COVID-19 pandemic there was an increase in adolescent female referrals due to tics, which has largely been attributed to TikTok (Cleveland Clinic, 2021; Frey et al., 2022). As children were home learning virtually and having increased anxiety due to the pandemic, there was more time for social media and a change to their normal routines. These tics are different from your typical tics as the presentation is acute without premonitory urge or embarrassment. Underlying the increase were emotional disorders, stress, and likely neurodevelopmental disorders already present before the pandemic that expressed themselves in the way of tics.

Table 38.5	Titration of Medications for Tic Suppression

Alpha₂-Adrenergic Agonists—Tier 1	
Clonidine 0.1 mg tabs or in patch form	0.05 mg (½ tab) at bedtime for 3 days, then increase every 3–7 days by 0.05 mg to target dose of 0.05–0.1 mg three times per day
Guanfacine 1 mg tabs	0.5 mg by mouth (1/2 tab) at bedtime for 3 days, then increase every 3–7 days by 0.5 mg to target dose of 0.5–2 mg two times per day
Other Agents—Tier 2	
Topiramate	25 mg at bedtime for 1 week, then increase weekly by 25 mg to target dose of 50–75 mg two times per day
Baclofen	10 mg at bedtime for 3 days, then increase every 3–7 days by 10 mg to target dose of 10–30 mg two to three times per day
Benzodiazepines	Various agents (clonazepam, diazepam) are sometimes used for severe exacerbations or chronic treatment of tics with anxiety.
Ropinirole	Several studies suggest a modest benefit of low doses of dopamine agonists, conceptually similar to treating restless legs syndrome.
Botulinum toxin	Injections for focal or dystonic tics
Antipsychotics—Tier 3	
Fluphenazine, haloperidol, pimozide, risperidone	1 mg at bedtime for 1 week. Increase as needed every 3–7 days to target dose of 1–4 mg daily. Can divide the dose.
Ziprasidone	20 mg at bedtime for 1 week. Increase as needed weekly by 20 mg to a target dose of 20–100 mg daily. Can divide dose.
Aripiprazole	2 mg at bedtime for 1 week. Increase as needed weekly by 2–5 mg to target dose of 2–30 mg daily. Can divide dose.
Tetrabenazine	12.5 mg at bedtime for 1 week. Increase weekly by 12.5–25 mg to a target dose of 25–150 mg daily. Can divide dose.

From Gilbert, D. L., & Jankovic, J. (2014). Pharmacological treatment of Tourette syndrome. *Journal of Obsessive-Compulsive and Related Disorders*, 3(4), 407–414.

Table 38.6	Complementary and Alternative Medicine Therapies	
MODALITY		**FREQUENCY (%)**
Stress management		49
Herbal medicine		20
Homeopathy		14
Meditation		10
Chiropractic care		8
Prayer		5
Aromatherapy		5
Megavitamin		4
Yoga		2
Reduced exposure to screen time		1
Reflexology		1
School breaks		1
School sensory room		1
Suppression		1
Talk therapy		1
Pet therapy		1
Extraneous physical activity		1
Transfer energy into something else		1

home virtually. During the pandemic, patients could have been experiencing sleep disturbances, obsessive behaviors, social isolation, and stress or anxiety, which could explain the increase. There is more information that will follow with studies that come from the pandemic (Dayasiri & Anand, 2021; Heyman et al., 2021).

PRIMARY CARE MANAGEMENT

HEALTH CARE MAINTENANCE

Growth and Development
Children with TS are generally thought to achieve normal growth and developmental milestones unless they have additional conditions, such as pervasive developmental disorder or psychosis. Some medications used for TS may stimulate appetite, especially neuroleptics (such as haloperidol, pimozide, or risperidone) or alpha-adrenergic agonists (such as clonidine), and some selective serotonin reuptake inhibitors (SSRIs) are associated with weight gain.

Children and adolescents with TS have similar levels of intelligence to those without TS and are more likely to have learning differences, disabilities, or developmental delays that affect their ability to learn.

Diet
Food-avoidant behaviors are common concerns for children and adolescents with TS. Current evidence-based research shows that this population exhibits more food approaches and avoidant behaviors (Smith & Ludlow, 2022), with abrupt changes in dietary preferences being a part of their

A United Kingdom study found that from March 2020 to March 2021 there was a fourfold increase in the diagnosis of tics and a threefold increase in the diagnosis of TS. The study found some of these patients were watching videos of tics on TikTok. Another study in August 2021 found a 1% to 35% increase in sudden unexplained tics. Some other reasonable explanation for this could be that children no longer had to suppress tics all day while at school since they were development. It is reported that children with TS have higher levels of food selectivity and sensory sensitivity (Smith et al., 2019). As with all patients, pediatric primary care providers should pay close attention to the growth and body mass index charts of children with TS. Any failure to make or maintain expected gains in height and weight, failure to progress through puberty, or secondary amenorrhea in the absence of pregnancy should prompt a more careful history, examination, and referral to the appropriate specialists (Smith & Ludlow, 2022).

In looking for alternatives to allopathic medications, parents sometimes try elimination diets or restrict the intake of foods thought to trigger tics symptoms. Working with the family to ensure adequate caloric and nutritional intake is important in these situations.

Safety

Self-injurious behavior (SIB) is a poorly misunderstood manifestation of TS. SIB is a deliberate, repetitive, persistent self-harm unrelated to sexual arousal or a suicidal attempt. SIB in patients with TS is related not only to the tics but also to other cooccurring symptoms. The prevalence is reported to be 14% to 66% of those with TS (Baizabal-Carvallo et al., 2021). Some children with TS have impaired impulse control and risk-taking behaviors and feel compelled to self-cut, touch hot surfaces, and head hit. Some individuals with TS may have suicidal thoughts related to complex tics and compulsions (Baizabal-Carvallo et al., 2021).

Like other adolescents with chronic conditions, adolescents with TS may be more likely than their nonaffected peers to engage in risky behavior. Although parents may not be able to prevent all risky behavior or SIB in older children and adolescents, they should be alert to the possibility of such behaviors and seek guidance from professionals with expertise in TS if they occur. Treating SIB can be difficult, depending on whether the behavior is a complex tic or a compulsion (Baizabal-Carvallo et al., 2021).

Research continues to develop about whether CBD influences or decreases tic frequency or whether there are short-term benefits of cannabinoids with TS, which can lead to compelling motivation for experimentation (Artukoglu et al., 2019; Gorberg, 2021).

COMMON ILLNESS MANAGEMENT

Differential Diagnosis

Several conditions mirror symptoms that can resemble tics of TS. Some children with undiagnosed tic disorders have sniffing and coughing tics that may be misdiagnosed as symptoms of an upper respiratory infection or allergies. Symptoms of TS can increase during fevers, viral illnesses, and allergy flareups.

Changes in skin condition and musculoskeletal complaints may be due to bruising from tics, holding unusual positions as part of a tic, or SIB.

Differential Diagnosis

- Sniffing, coughing, throat clearing
  - Allergy
  - Upper respiratory infection
  - Vocal tics
- Pharyngitis
  - Streptococcal infection (observe for an increase in tics)
  - Vocal tics (cough, throat clearing)
- Headache
  - Medication side effects (e.g., clonidine)
  - Somatic preoccupation or obsession
- Abdominal pain
  - Muscle tics (abdominal muscles)
  - Constipation related to medication side effects
  - Somatic preoccupation or obsession
- Skin-mucosa changes
  - Bruising from tics
  - Self-injurious behavior
  - Nail biting
  - Trichotillomania
- Musculoskeletal complaints
  - Tics (muscle tightness, holding unusual positions)
  - Injury incurred during tic
- Other hyperkinetic movement disorders
  - Chorea
  - Dystonia
  - Athetosis
  - Myoclonus
  - Stereotypies
  - Tics
  - Tremor

Drug Interactions

Erythromycin and other macrolide antibiotics can interact with medications such as pimozide or aripiprazole (dopamine blockers) to prolong the QT interval (Taketomo et al., 2022). Dextromethorphan, a cough suppressant commonly found in over-the-counter medications and sometimes taken in high doses by adolescents for its psychoactive properties, may interact with fluoxetine to cause increased sedation, hallucinations, muscle dystonia, and hyperthermia, known as central serotonin syndrome. Many children with intrinsically slow or quicker metabolisms will affect the interaction between medications such as fluoxetine and codeine, preventing its breakdown and diminishing its analgesic properties (Taketomo et al., 2022). These examples should alert the provider to keep an accurate list of current medications and updated information about drug–drug interactions, ensuring that parents and adolescents are also aware of them. With the plethora of vitamins, supplements, CAMs available to families of children with TS, providers should engage in an open dialog with the child and family about possible drug interactions with any alternative treatments.

DEVELOPMENTAL ISSUES

Sleep Patterns
Children with TS commonly have sleep complaints and comorbid sleep disorders, including insomnia, excessive daytime sleepiness, disorders of arousal (e.g., sleepwalking, sleeptalking, sleep terrors, enuresis), and bruxism (Jankovic, 2022). Children can have difficulty falling or staying asleep if tics increase as they relax, or the bedclothes do not "feel right." Warm baths or massages can temporarily diminish the tics.

Toileting
Most children with TS are not diagnosed until school age when toilet training is no longer an issue. Comorbidities often noted with TS can interfere with toilet training and the establishment of ongoing continence.

Discipline
The typical cycle of withholding or releasing tics in TS can lead to confusion and misguided attempts by parents and teachers to use discipline or conditioning to stop the tics (Klass & Costello, 2021). Families adjusting to a TS diagnosis often have difficulty understanding and interpreting their child's unusual behavior (Klass & Costello, 2021). Families and caregivers of children and adolescents with TS will benefit from support groups and contact with parents of children with TS. Discussing with the primary care provider, specialists, and others regarding the appropriateness of behavior, fairness to siblings, and consequences for behavior that is only partially under the child's control are complex and will help support the outcomes and improve the family dynamics with a better understanding of the condition. In addition to developing increased flexibility for acceptable behavior standards, parents may have to adjust their systems of consequences and rewards.

Child Care
The combination of structure and flexibility is important for children with TS. Although children may not be formally diagnosed during the preschool years, they may have increased problems with adaptability and peer relationships, and child care providers can offer important information to parents who have concerns about their child's intellectual and social development.

Schooling
Children with TS are more likely to need additional educational support than children without TS. A careful assessment of cognitive functioning and school achievement must be performed for all children with TS. Tics may not be directly related to learning disabilities, but many interfere with school functioning: Arm tics may interfere with handwritten work, and eye tics or head movements may interfere with reading. The tics and the effort to suppress them may internally distract the child enough to limit the ability to concentrate in the classroom, and fatigue and irritability increase as the day progresses.

Children with TS can have dysgraphia and visual-motor integration problems, affecting all handwritten work and tasks that involve copying from the blackboard or a test booklet to an answer sheet. Educators and other school personnel can support children with TS and their families by learning more about the condition, knowing that tics may be disruptive to the class, and ways to handle the situation in a manner that is beneficial for all. By becoming more informed and educated about the condition, teachers can help students with TS reach their full potential.

A student with TS has educational rights and accommodations available. Two levels of educational support are available, a 504 plan and an individualized education plan (IEP), both of which are written plans to provide access to educational programs/protection from discrimination and special education services (Tourette Association of America, 2023). All children with TS can qualify for Section 504 protection, including preferential seating, parent input into teacher selection, allowing a child to stop an activity if "stuck," permission to leave the classroom to release tics, extra time on tests, and homework modification. It is important to have an IEP and create alliances with teachers and school personnel when possible (CDC, 2023b).

Children with TS acknowledge more behavioral difficulties and dysphoric moods than children without TS, which increase with symptom severity. Studies tend to show more difficulties with peer relations for all children with TS and social adjustment issues, which warrants an active collaboration with the school to ensure appropriate classroom management, curricular planning, strength building, and education with the teachers and community about TS.

Sexuality
Unless affected by other conditions, physical and sexual development and progression through puberty in children with TS are normal. However, the psychosocial aspects of sexuality in children with TS can be affected in several ways. In some individuals with TS, tics can be set off by touch or may increase during sexual activity. As with many medications, those used for TS, most notably SSRIs, have some effect on libido and sexual functioning (Taketomo et al., 2022), which may be distressing for adolescents and may affect adherence to medications.

Adolescents with TS may feel uncomfortable discussing sexuality with their parents and may be reluctant to raise the issue with a health care provider. To prevent teen pregnancy and sexually transmitted diseases, providers need to avoid reducing sexuality to intercourse and reproduction. Sexuality involves how one feels about one's body, touch, and caring—difficult issues for any teen and even more so for teens with tics and/or compulsions. It is the health care provider's responsibility to discuss sexuality with all adolescents offering guidance and education.

Transition to Adulthood

Virtually all colleges receive federal assistance and are required by law to provide services for students with disabilities. Although services vary from school to school, families who have struggled with public school systems for accommodations for their child with TS may find college disability services surprisingly easy to access. Parents should ensure that adolescents with either an IEP or a 504 plan have help when contacting college disability services and preparing documentation for submission, but the responsibility for using college disability services rests with the young adult. Adolescents with TS find that their tics dramatically decrease by adulthood.

Individuals with TS may experience discrimination in education or employment, including in the military and some areas of law enforcement. Parents, caregivers, and adolescents may benefit from hiring a case manager or working with their school's vocational rehabilitation services team to address the transition to adulthood and independent living issues (CDC, 2023b).

Family Concerns

Research suggests that parents and caregivers of a child with TS have lower self-concepts, higher caregiver burdens, and more difficulties within the home (Robinson et al., 2013). The stress of parenting a child with TS is best supported by receiving appropriate education and social support. The child's adjustment after a diagnosis of TS may be related to parenting style and family functioning in general. The child and parents or caregivers could benefit from the parents receiving emotional support after their child has been diagnosed with TS.

Parents and siblings of children with TS and its comorbidities experience stress in accommodating the child's behaviors and rituals. Siblings may feel ashamed of the child's bizarre behavior at school. Educate parents on methods to explain TS as a medical condition to the child's siblings and to validate the feelings of unfairness or possible embarrassment at their sibling's outbursts. Family meetings with the child's therapist to work out fair house rules may be helpful. Neuropsychiatric conditions have historically been associated with stigma and are difficult for family members to explain to friends, relatives, and school personnel (Robinson et al., 2013). Parents may not be used to advocating for their child and may be unsure whether to disclose the diagnosis of TS. Families can benefit from sympathetic guidance from their primary care providers and referral to the appropriate organizations and resources.

RESOURCES

ORGANIZATION

Tourette Association of America (provides educators' guide): https://tourette.org

BOOKS FOR ADULTS, FRIENDS, AND FAMILY

Dina, C. Z., & Porta, M. (2020). *Understanding Tourette syndrome: A guide to symptoms, management and treatment*. Routledge.

Handler, L. (2004). *Twitch and shout: A Touretter's tale*. University of Minnesota Press.

Kutscher, M. L., Attwood, T., & Wolff, R. R. (2014). *Kids in the syndrome mix of ADHD, LD, autism spectrum, Tourette's, anxiety and more!: The one-stop guide for parents, teachers and other professionals*. Jessica Kingsley Publishers.

Leicester, M., Apsley, & Collier, J. (2014). *Can I tell you about Tourette syndrome?: A guide for friends, family and professionals*. Jessica Kingsley Publishers.

Marsh, T.L. (Ed.). (2007). *Children with Tourette syndrome: A parents' guide* (2nd ed.). Woodbine House.

Radcliffe, S. (2021). *No more tics! Help for tic disorders, Tourette syndrome, TikTok tics and more*. Independently Published.

BOOKS FOR HEALTH CARE PROVIDERS

Kurlan, R. (Ed.). (2019). *Handbook of Tourette's syndrome and related tic and behavioral disorders (neurological disease and therapy)*. CRC Press.

Martino, D., & Leckman, J. (Eds.). (2022). *Tourette syndrome* (2nd ed.). Oxford University Press.

McGuire, J.F., Murphy, T.K., et al. (Eds.). (2018). *The clinician's guide to treatment and management of youth with Tourette syndrome and tic disorders*. Academic Press.

BOOKS FOR CHILDREN

Chowdhury, U., & Robertson, M. (2006). *Why do you do that? A book about Tourette syndrome for children and young people*. Jessica Kingsley Publishers.

Lesha, T. (2022). *Penelope Plum: A children's story on Tourette syndrome (colorful classroom)*. Tamika Lesha Books.

Mederos, M., & Sanford, A. (2022). *Tic & twitch: A story about Tourette syndrome*. Millennial Publishing Co.

Peters, D. (2007). *Tic talk: Living with Tourette syndrome. A 9-year-old boy's story in his own words*. Little Five Store.

WEBSITES

Centers for Disease Control and Prevention: At a Glance: Tourette Syndrome: https://www.cdc.gov/ncbddd/tourette/documents/tourette-overview-fact-sheet-508.pdf

Child Mind Institute: https://childmind.org/about-us

Challenging Kids, Inc. (Find a way or make a way): https://www.challengingkids.com/about

National Center for Complementary and Alternative Medicine: http://nccam.nih.gov

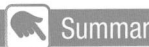

Summary

Primary Care Needs for the Child With Tourette Syndrome

HEALTH CARE MAINTENANCE
Growth and Development
- Growth is generally normal, although there are concerns about children's growth on long-term medication, such as SSRIs.
  - Consideration for a possible eating disorder if growth slows or weight falls in older children/adolescents.
  - Development is generally normal.
  - Some parents report decreased flexibility and increased difficulties with regulation, even before the emergence of specific symptoms.

Diet
- Abrupt changes in dietary preference may be due to comorbidities with TS, especially around contamination.
  - Parents may restrict intake to eliminate triggers from foods or food additives.

Safety
- Excessive risk taking is sometimes associated with tic behavior.
  - SIB
  - Adolescents may self-medicate with alcohol and/or recreational drugs for symptom relief or to take the focus off of their tics.

Immunizations
- Children with TS should be vaccinated following the schedule recommended by the American Academy of Pediatrics (Pannaraj, 2023) and the Centers for Disease Control and Prevention (2023a).

Screening
- *Vision.* Routine screening is recommended.
- *Hearing.* Routine screening is recommended.
- *Dental.* Routine screening is recommended. Clean teeth by hand if vibrations set off tics.
- *Blood pressure.* Routine screening is recommended. Children taking certain medications may need more frequent screening.
- *Hematocrit.* Routine screening is recommended. Additional frequency if taking atypical neuroleptics.
- *Urinalysis.* Routine screening is recommended.
- *Tuberculosis.* Routine screening is recommended.

Condition-Specific Screening
- Electrocardiogram if taking pimozide, other atypical neuroleptics, tricyclic antidepressants.
  - More frequent monitoring of blood and liver function for some atypical neuroleptic medications.
- Careful observation for signs of SIB.

COMMON ILLNESS MANAGEMENT
Differential Diagnosis
- *Sniffing, coughing, throat clearing*: Assess for allergy, upper respiratory infection, vocal tics.
- *Pharyngitis.* Streptococcal infection (observe for tics), vocal tics (cough, throat clearing).
- *Headache.* Medication side effects (e.g., clonidine), somatic preoccupation or obsession.
- *Abdominal pain.* Muscle tics (abdominal muscles), constipation related to toileting issues, medication side effects, somatic preoccupation or obsession.
- *Skin-mucosa changes.* Bruising from tics, SIB, nail-biting, trichotillomania.

- *Musculoskeletal complaints.* Tics (muscle tightness, holding unusual positions), an injury incurred during a tic.

Other Hyperkinetic Movement Disorders
- Chorea
- Dystonia
- Athetosis
- Myoclonus
- Stereotypies
- Tics
- Tremor

Drug Interactions
- Pimozide and aripiprazole interact with macrolide antibiotics to prolong the QT interval.
  - Dextromethorphan and club drugs such as Ecstasy interact with fluoxetine to increase the risk of central serotonin syndrome.
  - SSRIs reduce the effectiveness of codeine for analgesia.
  - St. John's wort and other supplements interact with SSRIs.

DEVELOPMENTAL ISSUES
Sleep Patterns
- Tics can increase as children relax, making falling asleep more difficult.
  - Bedtime rituals can delay sleep for several hours; parents may not be aware of the extent of rituals.

Toileting
- Primary care providers need to be mindful of comorbidities of TS and how those affect toileting.
- Be aware of obsessions and rituals that may affect toileting.
- Be aware of medications that may increase constipation.
- Be aware that avoidance of public toilets may lead to constipation and encopresis.

Discipline
- It may be difficult to distinguish between tics and more voluntary behaviors.
- Flexibility needed to accept unusual behavior may be difficult for parents.
- Timeouts may not be effective for children with rage attacks.

Child Care
- A combination of structure and flexibility is needed.
- Day care providers can give valuable feedback about socialization skills.

Schooling
- Tics and obsessions can interfere with concentration and written work.
- TS is associated with dysgraphia, visual-motor integration problems, and written expressive language.
- TS may be disruptive to the class.
- All children are eligible for Section 504 accommodations and IEPs.
- Peer relations may be impaired.
- Give a safe space for patients to "tic out."
- Tics should be considered part of the 504 plan as explained in CBIT treatment.

Sexuality
- Tics may increase with touch or during sexual activity.

Continued

- Adolescents may avoid touch due to contamination fears.
- Sexual obsessions may interfere with relationships.
- Some medications may decrease sexual desire and function.

Transition to Adulthood

- Tics often diminish significantly in adulthood.
- Individuals with TS and without other conditions have few behavioral problems but may experience educational, employment, and housing discrimination.

- TS may limit educational, work, and independent living options.

FAMILY CONCERNS

- Decisions about the disclosure of TS can be difficult.
- Siblings may feel that child's behavior is embarrassing, and families may need professional help to work out fair house rules.

REFERENCES

American Psychiatric Association. (2013). *Diagnostic and statistical manual of mental disorders: DSM-5* (Vol. 5, No. 5). American Psychiatric Association.

Artukoglu, B. B., & Bloch, M. H. (2019). The potential of cannabinoid-based treatments in Tourette syndrome. *CNS Drugs, 33*(5), 417–430. https://doi.org/10.1007/s40263-019-00627-1.

Baizabal-Carvallo, J. F., Alonso-Juarez, M., & Jankovic, J. (2021). Self-injurious behavior in Tourette syndrome. *Journal of Neurology, 269*(5), 2453–2459. https://doi.org/10.1007/s00415-021-10822-0.

Centers for Disease Control and Prevention. (2023a). Birth-18 years immunization schedule – healthcare providers. https://www.cdc.gov/vaccines/schedules/hcp/imz/child-adolescent.html.

Centers for Disease Control and Prevention. (2023b). Information about Tourette syndrome for education professionals. https://www.cdc.gov/ncbddd/tourette/educators.html#:~:text=Tourette%20Syndrome%20(TS)%20can%20affect,or%20rejected%20by%20other%20kids.

Centers for Disease Control and Prevention. (2023c). Learn about Tourette syndrome. Retrieved March 7, 2023, from https://www.cdc.gov/ncbddd/tourette/index.html.

Centers for Disease Control and Prevention. (2023d). Risk factors and causes for Tourette syndrome. https://www.cdc.gov/ncbddd/tourette/riskfactors.html.

Chou, C.-Y., Agin-Liebes, J., & Kuo, S.-H. (2023). Emerging therapies and recent advances for Tourette syndrome. *Heliyon, 9*(1). https://doi.org/10.1016/j.heliyon.2023.e12874.

Cleveland Clinic. (2021). Is TikTok causing tics in teen girls? What parents need to know. Retrieved from https://health.clevelandclinic.org/tiktok-causing-tics-in-teen-girls/.

Dayasiri, K., & Anand, G. (2021). 862 tics and the COVID pandemic-observation from a tertiary care seizure clinic. *Abstracts, 106*(1). https://doi.org/10.1136/archdischild-2021-rcpch.242.

Frey, J., Black, K. J., & Malaty, I. A. (2022). TikTok Tourette's: Are we witnessing a rise in functional tic-like behavior driven by adolescent social media use? *Psychology Research and Behavior Management, 15*, 3575–3585. https://doi.org/10.2147/prbm.s359977.

Geng, J., Liu, C., Xu, J., Wang, X., & Li, X. (2023). Potential relationship between Tourette syndrome and gut microbiome. *Jornal de Pediatria, 99*(1), 11–16. https://doi.org/10.1016/j.jped.2022.06.002.

Gilbert, D. L., & Jankovic, J. (2014). Pharmacological treatment of Tourette syndrome. *Journal of Obsessive-Compulsive and Related Disorders, 3*(4), 407–414. https://doi.org/10.1016/j.jocrd.2014.04.006.

Gorberg, V. (2021). *Effects of cannabinoids on motor-like and vocal-like tics in mouse models of Tourette syndrome*. University of Aberdeen.

Heyman, I., Liang, H., & Hedderly, T. (2021). COVID-19 related increase in childhood tics and tic-like attacks. *Archives of Disease in Childhood, 106*(5), 420–421.

Immunizations. Publications.aap.org. (2023). https://publications.aap.org/redbook/pages/Immunization-Schedules?autologincheck=redirected.

Jankovic, J. (2022). *Tourette syndrome: Pathogenesis, clinical features, and diagnosis*. UpToDate. https://www.uptodate.com/contents/tourette-syndrome-pathogenesis-clinical-features-and-diagnosis.

Klass, P., & Costello, E. (2021). *Quirky kids: Understanding and supporting your child with developmental differences*. American Academy of Pediatrics.

Lajonchere, C., Nortz, M., & Finger, S. (1996). Gilles de la Tourette and the discovery of Tourette syndrome. Includes a translation of his 1884 article. *Archives in Neurology, 53*, 567–574.

Mederos, M., & Sanford, A. (2022). *Tic & twitch: A story about Tourette syndrome*. Millennial Publishing Co.

Nikkhah, A., Karimzadeh, P., Taghdiri, M. M., Nasehi, M. M., Javadzadeh, M., & Khari, E. (2019). Hyperkinetic movement disorders in children: A brief review. *Iranian Journal of Child Neurology, 13*(2), 7–16.

Pannaraj, P. (2023). Immunization schedule updated for 2023; COVID vaccine added. Publications.aap.org. https://publications.aap.org/aapnews/news/23293/Immunization-schedule-updated-for-2023-COVID?autologincheck=redirected.

Patel, H., Nguyen, K. H., Lehman, E., Mainali, G., Duda, L., Byler, D., & Kumar, A. (2020). Use of complementary and alternative medicine in children with Tourette syndrome. *Journal of Child Neurology, 35*(8), 512–516. https://doi.org/10.1177/0883073820913670.

Piña-Garza, J. Eric, James, K. C., & Fenichel, G. M. (2019). *Fenichel's clinical pediatric neurology: A signs and symptoms approach*. Elsevier.

Pringsheim, T., Okun, M. S., Müller-Vahl, K., Martino, D., Jankovic, J., Cavanna, A. E., Woods, D. W., Robinson, M., Jarvie, E., Roessner, V., Oskoui, M., Holler-Managan, Y., & Piacentini, J. (2019). Practice guideline recommendations summary: Treatment of tics in people with Tourette syndrome and chronic tic disorders. *Neurology, 92*(19), 896–906. https://doi.org/10.1212/wnl.0000000000007466.

PsycTech, Ltd., (2014). *An online intervention for children with tic disorders*. TicHelper. Retrieved March 22, 2023, from https://www.tichelper.com/.

Quezada, J., & Coffman, K. A. (2018). Current approaches and new developments in the pharmacological management of Tourette syndrome. *CNS Drugs, 32*(1), 33–45. https://doi.org/10.1007/s40263-017-0486-0.

Rae, C. L., Critchley, H. D., & Seth, A. K. (2019). A Bayesian account of the sensory-motor interactions underlying symptoms of Tourette syndrome. *Frontiers in Psychiatry, 10*, 29.

Robinson, L. R., Bitsko, R. H., Schieve, L. A., & Visser, S. N. (2013). Tourette syndrome, parenting aggravation, and the contribution of co-occurring conditions among a nationally representative sample. *Disability and Health Journal, 6*(1), 26–35. https://doi.org/10.1016/j.dhjo.2012.10.002.

Singer, H. S. (2019). Tics and Tourette syndrome. *CONTINUUM: Lifelong Learning in Neurology, 25*(4), 936–958. https://doi.org/10.1212/con.0000000000000752.

Smith, B. L., & Ludlow, A. K. (2022). An exploration of eating behaviours and caregiver mealtime actions of children with Tourette syndrome. *Frontiers in Pediatrics, 10.* https://doi.org/10.3389/fped.2022.933154.

Smith, B., Rogers, S. L., Blissett, J., & Ludlow, A. K. (2019). The role of sensory sensitivity in predicting food selectivity and food preferences in children with Tourette syndrome. *Appetite, 135,* 131–136. https://doi.org/10.1016/j.appet.2019.01.003.

Taketomo, C. K., Hodding, J. H. H., & Pharm, D. H. (2022). *Pediatric & neonatal dosage handbook: An extensive resource for clinicians treating pediatric and neonatal patients.* Lexicomp/Wolters Kluwer.

Tourette Association of America. (2023). https://tourette.org/about-tourette/overview/what-is-tourette/.

Walusinski, O. (2018). Gilles de la Tourette syndrome. *Georges Gilles De La Tourette,* 145–212. https://doi.org/10.1093/med/9780190636036.003.0009.

Wolicki, S. B., Bitsko, R. H., Danielson, M. L., Holbrook, J. R., Zablotsky, B., Walkup, J. T., Woods, D. W., & Mink, J. W. (2019). Children with Tourette syndrome in the United States: Parent-reported diagnosis, co-occurring disorders, severity, and influence of activities on tics. *Journal of Developmental & Behavioral Pediatrics, 40*(6), 407–414. https://doi.org/10.1097/dbp.0000000000000667.

39 | Traumatic Brain Injury

Roni Lynn Robinson

ETIOLOGY

Traumatic brain injury (TBI) is the leading cause of death and disability in children. TBI is a broad term that describes a vast array of injuries that occur to the scalp, skull, brain, and underlying tissue and blood vessels in the child's head. It occurs from a wide range of mechanisms, including a bump, blow, jolt to the head or body, or penetrating head injury. These injuries disrupt the brain's normal function and can potentially alter the development of the growing brain (Lu et al., 2022). TBI has been widely referred to as the silent epidemic by several entities because of its heterogenous presentation, its high incidence, and the often externally invisible presentation (Dewan et al., 2018).

It is important to note that TBI in children has unique characteristics that differ from TBI in adults. One of the main differences is that children are more susceptible to head trauma than adults because the size of a child's head is proportionally larger than that of an adult. An infant's head is approximately 18% of the total body surface area in infancy; this will decrease to roughly 9% by adulthood (McGrath & Taylor, 2022). This heavier head mass and weak neck muscles are the main reasons children are more susceptible to head injury. The pathophysiology of children and how the injuries are managed are also important to note because of the age-related structural differences, mechanisms of injuries based on the physicality of a child, and difficulty in performing a neurologic evaluation in a child with a brain injury (Araki et al., 2017; Serpa et al., 2021). Another consideration in children suffering from TBI is the consequence of brain injury on a developing brain.

Within the umbrella of TBI there are both primary and secondary injuries to the brain that can occur. A primary injury occurs immediately when the trauma happens. A secondary injury occurs due to the sequela of the primary injury. These injuries produce an array of complications, ranging from obvious physical disability to less visible and sometimes incapacitating neuropsychological impairment (Babl et al., 2017a). Advances in aggressive acute management and intensive rehabilitation have greatly improved outcomes by preventing long-term impairments associated with the poor cognitive and psychological aftermath of TBI.

These injuries are further characterized as mild, moderate, and severe injuries. Mild TBI (mTBI) traditionally

has no structural abnormality; however, with the accessibility of neuroimaging to these patients, clinically insignificant structural brain injury is now more commonly observed. Moderate-severe TBI can be either focal or diffuse (Wang et al., 2018). Focal injuries are most associated with a direct blow to the head and generally result in cerebral contusions or hematomas. Examples of primary focal brain injuries include epidural, subdural, subarachnoid, and intracerebral bleeds. Primary injury induces an acute response from the brain, in which a cascade of biochemical and physiologic events can cause both direct neuronal damage and secondary brain injury (Lazaridis et al., 2019). Diffuse injuries are the result of inertial forces causing microtrauma to nerves and blood vessels. The most common example of this is diffuse axonal injury (DAI), the result of the violent motion of the brain inside the skull, as is experienced in a high-velocity mechanism (Angelova et al., 2021).

Secondary injuries are seen in moderate-severe TBI and are generally understood as the resulting hypoxemia, acidosis, and chemical or metabolic response to the cellular injury that occurs with the initial impact of TBI. The secondary injury cascade results in poor perfusion of the brain from systemic hypotension, intracranial hypertension, cerebral edema, or cerebral hemorrhage. There may also be hypoxemia, seizures, hypercapnia, or infection. These secondary conditions significantly increase morbidity and mortality rates for children with TBI (CDC, 2023). These secondary responses and the resulting injury to the brain are most amenable to medical and pharmacologic intervention and thus can affect the outcome. Although the damage from secondary complications is more diffuse in children than adults, it is also more likely to resolve during recovery and rehabilitation due to the neuroplasticity of the child's brain. This is the ability of the brain to adapt, change, or heal after injury (Hussain, 2018).

PHYSICAL MECHANISMS OF INJURY

The physical mechanisms of TBI are the result of primary injuries, such as a penetrating object or forces of deceleration, acceleration, coup-contrecoup, or rotational trauma (Fig. 39.1). Deceleration occurs when the head strikes an immovable object and suddenly stops; acceleration forces occur when a moving object strikes the head. A coup injury occurs when the brain strikes

914

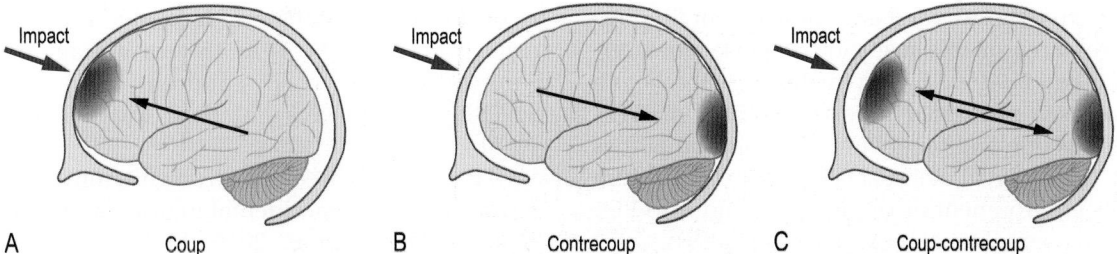

Fig. 39.1 Coup, contrecoup and coup-contrecoup head injury following blunt trauma. (A) Coup injury: impact against object. Site of impact and direct trauma to brain *(a)*. Shearing of subdural veins *(b)*. Trauma to base of brain *(c)*. (B) Contrecoup injury: impact within skull. Site of impact from brain hitting opposite side of skull *(a)*. Shearing forces through brain *(b)*. (C) These injuries occur in one continuous motion—the head strikes the wall (coup), then rebounds (contrecoup). (From Abduelmenem, A., & Soames, R. W. (2024). *Anatomy & Physiology for Paramedical Practice.* Elsevier Ltd.)

the cranium on the side of impact, and a contrecoup injury occurs when the brain rebounds and strikes the cranium on the contralateral side. Contrecoup injuries are considered more severe, and the size of the impact area affects the injury's severity. The smaller the area of impact, the greater the severity of the injury because of the concentration of force in a smaller area. Rotational trauma is a twisting of the brain during deceleration or acceleration. This can occur in combination with coup-contrecoup injuries, resulting in shearing of the tissues or as a complication of abusive head trauma (AHT; from shaking) to children under age 2 years (Christian, 2015).

ABUSIVE HEAD TRAUMA

ETIOLOGY

AHT, also known as nonaccidental injury, is an umbrella term that represents a spectrum of craniocerebral and craniospinal injuries caused by blunt trauma, shaking (including shaken baby syndrome), or a combination of these forces (CDC, 2018; Chevignard et al., 2020; Sidpra et al., 2021).

INCIDENCE AND PREVALENCE

AHT remains the leading cause of morbidity and mortality in infants and young children less than 2 years old with TBI (Duhaime & Christian, 2019). The incidence of AHT is estimated at 20 to 30 per 100,000 children, with victims' median age being 4 months, highlighting the vulnerability of young infants. More than 2000 hospitalized children are assigned diagnoses of AHT annually in the United States using code-based definitions (Duhaime & Christian, 2019).

PROGNOSIS

The prognosis of children with inflicted AHT is poor, with a mortality of 15% to 25%, and significantly more chronic neurologic sequelae that are associated with accidental head trauma (Sidpra et al., 2021).

CLINICAL MANIFESTATIONS

Children often present because of concerns of increased fussiness, vomiting, or changes in mental status. Other presenting features along with head and spine trauma include death, less severe trauma with an unexplained mechanism, and unsuspected findings on imaging or assessment for macrocephaly, developmental delay, seizures, or other neurologic concerns (Choudhary et al., 2018). Often clinical manifestations or abnormal physical findings are not consistent with the history provided by the caregivers, or there is a delay in presentation after the reported injury occurred (Kontos et al., 2020b).

DIAGNOSTIC FINDINGS

When AHT is a concern at presentation, neuroimaging is an integral part of the workup with computed tomography (CT) and/or magnetic resonance imaging. Subdural hematoma is the most common finding with neuroimaging, but children can present with an intracranial bleed in any area of the brain. Skull fractures are also one of the more common findings on neuroimaging. Skeletal surveys, whole-body x-ray imaging, should be performed to rule out occult skeletal fractures in children less than 2 years of age (Narang et al., 2020). Serum laboratory values should be included in the workup as clinically indicated to assess for anemia and abdominal/peritoneal trauma. When there are positive findings on neuroimaging suggesting AHT, an ophthalmologic exam should be performed as part of the workup. Ocular findings include retinal hemorrhage, orbital and lid ecchymosis, subconjunctival hemorrhage, anisocoria, and deconjugated eye movements (Ip et al., 2020). Retinal hemorrhage is the most important ocular finding consistent with AHT. Further evaluations should be performed and directed by a dedicated child abuse team where a comprehensive and multidisciplinary workup is completed to fully assess for other injuries and to rule out medical causes of abnormalities found (Chen et al., 2022).

TREATMENT AND LEGAL INTERVENTIONS

Consultation by the clinically indicated subspecialty surgical and medical teams is required based on the abnormalities found on imaging or as part of the workup. Treatments are administered as clinically necessary. Social workers are a part of this process to help determine the patient's safety and assist with decisions that must be made to report the injuries to child protective services and law enforcement. Reporting requires a reasonable suspicion of abuse, not a certainty, and can be done by any member of the health care team as a mandated reporter. Victims of AHT require protection and family intervention, sometimes requiring the removal of a suspected perpetrator from the child's environment or placing the child into kinship or foster care (Duhaime & Christian, 2019).

INCIDENCE AND PREVALENCE

TBI in children represents a significant public health burden in the United States as it is the leading cause of death and disability among children and adolescents (Centers for Disease Control and Prevention [CDC], 2015).

Data from a sample year period suggested that in children age 0 to 17 years, there were 16,070 TBI-related hospitalizations and 2774 TBI-related deaths annually (CDC, 2022). At least 29,000 children experience permanent neurologic symptoms, and another 7000 are fatally injured from head injuries each year. The two pediatric age groups at the highest risk for moderate-severe TBI are 0- to 4-year-olds and 15- to 19-year-olds, respectively (Yue et al., 2020).

These numbers, generated from the emergency department (ED) and inpatient sources, often do not account for the large number of children who sustain mTBIs, estimated to be about 80% of all TBIs in children. These mTBIs often do not require acute interventions; however, they can result in possible long-term impairment if not addressed properly (Graves et al., 2015). ED estimates of pediatric TBI most likely underestimate the public health burden; one study reported only 12% of pediatric mTBI patients presented to the health care system through the ED, with 82% initially visiting primary care providers and 5% presenting to specialty providers (Arbogast et al., 2016). Thus the actual rate and cost of all TBIs and their long-term consequences in children remain unknown.

While anyone can be at risk for TBI, certain qualities may increase a child's risk for TBI, including age, sex, psychological history, and socioeconomic factors (Listo et al., 2021). Males are more often affected than females, as high as 2:1 during adolescence. Attention-deficit/hyperactivity disorder (ADHD) or mood disturbances constitute behavioral risk factors for TBI (Johnson & Ivarsson, 2011; Liou et al., 2018). These conditions may have a genetic component and are a frequent premorbid element of the pattern of risk-taking behaviors noted in children with TBI. There is an increased incidence in low socioeconomic classes and increased incidence in spring and summer (Listo et al., 2021). Peak occurrence is during evenings, nights, weekends, and holidays when children are outside playing, swimming, bicycling, traveling in cars, or becoming victims of gunshot wounds. One novel study looked at the incidence of repeat mTBI in the 5- to 15-year-old age group and found that one in six children sustained a repeat mTBI within 2 years of their index injury (Curry et al., 2019).

TBIs in children commonly result from motor vehicle crashes, falls, nonaccidental injuries, and sport-related injuries (Dewan et al., 2016). In 2- to 4-year-olds, falls are the main cause of head injury. In older children, bicycle, vehicle, and recreational accidents are the main causes of head injury. Of TBIs in children, 20 are moderate or severe, and 5% are fatal (Dewan et al., 2016).

As TBIs continue to rise (most of which are mild), an important aspect of TBI epidemiology is prevention. The CDC has made extensive efforts to educate parents, coaches, and medical care providers through the Heads Up program, which provides recommendations on TBI prevention and general safety tips: (1) Use a seat belt or child safety seat for every car ride, (2) never drink or use drugs and then drive, (3) use appropriate sports helmets and protective equipment, and (4) childproof all living and playground areas (CDC, 2019).

DIAGNOSTIC CRITERIA

TRAUMATIC BRAIN INJURY CLASSIFICATION

Severity

Head injuries are classified by the severity of response (mild, moderate, severe) during the immediate postinjury period and use an established classification system known as the Glasgow Coma Scale (GCS), first published in 1974. The GCS remains the gold standard and most reliable indicator of injury severity and short-term deterioration or improvement (Table 39.1) (Gelineau-Morel et al., 2019). mTBIs are typically associated with a GCS score of 13 to 15. Moderate head injuries are typically associated with a GCS score of 9 to 12 (Table 39.2). Severe head injuries are associated with a GCS score of 8 or less and have significant potential for long-term morbidity or mortality risks (Gelineau-Morel et al., 2019). Because of limitations of the GCS for use in infants and preverbal children, individuals with a preinjury deficit (e.g., hemiparesis, cognitive deficit) or individuals who are intubated, a Children's Coma Scale (CCS) or Modified GCS was developed (Table 39.3) (Kirschen et al., 2019). This modified scale is not used as commonly as the original GCS.

Blunt Versus Penetrating

Most pediatric head injuries are blunt or closed in nature, without outward signs of increased intracranial pressure (ICP) (Birg et al., 2021). These injuries tend to result in cerebral contusion, hematoma, or concussion. Penetrating head injuries are rare and result in direct injury to the skull, brain tissue, and blood vessels; fatality occurs in about 40% of cases (Drosos et al., 2018).

Table 39.1 Glasgow Coma Scale

	CHILD AGE >2 YR OR ADULT		CHILD AGE <2 YR OR DEVELOPMENTALLY DELAYED	
Best eye-opening response	Spontaneously	4	Spontaneously	4
	To verbal command	3	Verbal command	3
	To pain	2	To pain	2
	No response	1	No response	1
Best verbal response	Oriented, converses	5	Coos, babbles	5
	Disoriented, converses	4	Irritable cry	4
	Inappropriate words	3	Cries to pain	3
	Incomprehensible sounds	2	Moans to pain	2
	No response	1	None	1
Best motor response	Obeys	6	Spontaneous	6
To verbal command	Localizes pain	5	Withdraws from touch	5
To painful stimulus	Flexion—withdrawal	4	Withdraws to pain	4
	Flexion—decorticate	3	Abnormal flexion	3
	Extension-decerebrate	2	Abnormal extension	2
	No response	1	None	1
Total		(3–15)		(3–15)

Table 39.2 Classification System for Traumatic Brain Injury

CLASSIFICATION	GLASGOW COMA SCALE	LOSS OF CONSCIOUSNESS	POSTTRAUMATIC AMNESIA
Mild	13–15	0–30 min	0–1 day
Moderate	9–12	>30 min and <24 hr	>1 day and <7 days
Severe	3–8	>24 hr	>7 days

From Assistant Secretary of Defense (2015). *Traumatic Brain Injury: Updated Definition and Reporting*. Washington, DC: Department of Defense.

TYPES OF CRANIAL INJURY

Skull Fracture

Skull fractures in pediatric patients are a significant clinical finding as they are a risk factor for intracranial injury, which can worsen neurologic outcomes (Adepoju & Adamo, 2017). Skull fractures are often caused by a fall, but other causes include motor vehicle crashes, sports-related injuries, or other direct blows to the head. Occasionally, newborns can sustain a depressed ping-pong fracture as a result of childbirth. Skull fractures can be nonaccidental injuries and are important for clinicians to identify in children who present with a head injury and subsequent skull fracture. This is particularly important in the nonmobile infant (McGrath & Taylor, 2022).

The incidence of skull fracture is higher in children than in adults, especially in children younger than 2 years, where the skull is thinner and more pliable, thus providing less protection to the brain (Arrey et al., 2015). Several types of skull fractures exist, including linear, depressed, open, diastatic, and growing (McGrath & Taylor, 2022). Depressed skull fractures can result in injury to the scalp and the underlying structures of the brain and can be a neurosurgical emergency (Köksal et al., 2020).

TYPES OF INTRACRANIAL INJURY

Concussion

The term *concussion* has historically been used interchangeably with mTBI, and concussion is now thought to more accurately describe a milder type of brain injury on the spectrum of brain injuries (Kazl & Torres, 2019). Over the last decade there has been an increase in concussion awareness (both in the lay and medical community), thus the prevalence of concussion diagnosis has also increased. With this heightened attention there is emerging evidence demonstrating that these increasingly more common injuries can lead to poor neurologic outcomes and functional disabilities that adversely affect academic, behavioral, and emotional aspects of quality of life (Russell et al., 2019). A concussion can also produce deficits in multiple domains, such as memory, concentration, sleep, processing speed, and visual and vestibular function. These outcomes often negatively impact the psychological and emotional functioning of concussed youth (Kazl & Torres, 2019).

Despite the increased attention that concussion has received, confusion and controversy over diagnosis and management still exist.

Several working definitions of concussion, along with position statements on concussion management,

Table 39.3 | Modified Pediatric Glasgow Coma Scale

RATING	CRITERION	GLASGOW COMA SCALE RATING	
		≥2 YR	<2 YR
Eye Opening			
4	Open before stimulus	Spontaneous	Spontaneous
3	After spoken or shouted request	To sound	To sound
2	After physical stimulation	To pressure	To pressure
1	No opening at any time, no interfering factor	None	None
NT	Closed by interfering factor	NT	NT
Verbal Response			
5	Correctly gives name, place date; or produces words or phrases normal for chronologic age	Oriented; words/phrases—normal for chronologic age	Babbles, coos; words/phrases—normal for chronologic age
4	Not oriented, but communicating coherently; or produces some words or phrases, but not normal for chronological age	Confused; some words/phrases—not normal for chronologic age	Some words/phrases—not normal for chronologic age
3	Intelligible single words	Words	Inconsolable crying
2	Only moans or groans	Sounds	Sounds
1	No audible response, no interfering factor	None	None
NT	Factor interfering with verbal communication	NT	NT
Motor Response			
6	Obeys two-part request or request appropriate for chronologic age	Obeys commands	Normal spontaneous movement
5	Bring hands above clavicle to stimulus on head or neck	Localizing	Rapidly withdraws extremity to stimulation
4	Bends arm at elbow rapidly, but features not predominantly abnormal	Normal flexion	Normal flexion
3	Bends arm at elbow, features clearly predominantly abnormal	Abnormal flexion	Abnormal flexion
2	Extends arm at elbow	Extension	Extension
1	No movement in arms/legs, no interfering factor	None	None
NT	Paralyzed or other interfering factor	NT	NT

NT, Nontestable.
From Kirschen, M. P., Snyder, M., Smith, K., et al. (2019). Inter-rater reliability between critical care nurses performing a pediatric modification to the Glasgow coma scale. *Pediatric Critical Care Medicine, 20*(7), 660–666.

can be found in the literature, and as the science of concussion continues to evolve so does the understanding of what a concussion is and how it is best managed. In 2004, the World Health Organization, American Congress of Rehabilitation Medicine, and CDC created a working group to further define concussion. Their definition described concussion as (Lumba-Brown et al., 2018):

An acute brain injury resulting from mechanical energy to the head from external physical forces including (1) One or more of the following: confusion or disorientation, loss of consciousness for 30 minutes or less, post-traumatic amnesia for less than 24 hours, and/or other transient neurological abnormalities such as focal signs, symptoms, or seizure; (2) Glasgow Coma Scale score of 13–15 after 30 minutes post-injury or later upon presentation for healthcare.

The disturbance in brain function associated with a concussion is thought to be more related to the disruption of brain metabolism than to any specific structural damage in the brain (Giza & Hovda, 2001). As such, concussion is a functional injury not seen on standard neuroimaging. Currently there are no evidence-based diagnostic biomarkers (neuroimaging, visual, tissue/saliva, or blood) available to diagnose or assess the severity of concussion, thus it remains a clinical diagnosis. Imaging is not recommended unless clinically indicated due to a concern of more severe injury (Lumba-Brown et al., 2018).

Complicated Versus Uncomplicated Mild Traumatic Brain Injury

To further clarify mTBI, some researchers and clinicians have categorized the injury as either complicated or uncomplicated. Complicated mTBI has a GCS between 13 and 15 with positive traumatic intracranial findings on CT at the time of presentation. Uncomplicated mTBI has a GCS between 13 and 15 without neuroimaging findings on CT. Those with complicated mTBI may have more prolonged symptoms after an injury, but there is conflicting evidence to support this (Panenka et al., 2015; Voormolen et al., 2019).

Cerebral Contusion
Cerebral contusions result from the brain moving within the skull, causing bruises along the brain's surface. Cerebral contusions can occur at the site of impact (coup) and/or opposite the site of impact (contrecoup), but less rare contusions are the most frequently seen lesions in older children following a head injury. Lesions tend to occur mostly in the frontal and temporal lobes, where the irregular surface of the cranial vault exists (Araki et al., 2017).

Cerebral Lacerations
Lacerations involve the tearing of the cortical surface of the brain with damage to the surrounding tissues. They may also occur along with contusions due to a penetrating head injury or depressed skull fracture (Arrey et al., 2015).

Cerebral Hemorrhage
Cerebral hemorrhage or hematoma is bleeding in the brain. The type of bleed is categorized by where it is located in the intracranial vault: epidural, subdural, intracerebral, or subarachnoid (Fig. 39.2). Severe bleeding can result in a mass lesion effect that causes shifts in the intracranial tissues and elevated ICP. Among individuals with TBI, approximately 3% develop epidural hematoma (Cremonini et al., 2020). These rare hemorrhages occur between the dura and the skull and are due to a bleeding blood vessel, most often an artery in the epidural space. Subdural hematomas occur in about 30% of children with severe head injuries (Taşkapılıoğlu et al., 2019). Blood collects between the dura and arachnoid meninges layer. Subdural hematomas are classified as acute (occurred in the past 48 hours), subacute (occurred in the past 2–14 days), and chronic (occurred >14 days ago). Intracerebral hemorrhage produces mass lesions primarily in the frontal and temporal lobes. Subarachnoid hemorrhage occurs when blood accumulates under the arachnoid layer of the membranous covering of the brain (meninges). These hemorrhages occur mainly in the presence of moderate-severe head injuries, such as significant blows to the head or depressed skull fractures (Griswold et al., 2022). Surgical evacuation of an intracerebral hemorrhage is necessary when medical therapies fail to decrease ICP.

Diffuse Axonal Injury
DAI usually occurs after blunt head trauma from a high mechanism injury such as a motor vehicle crash.

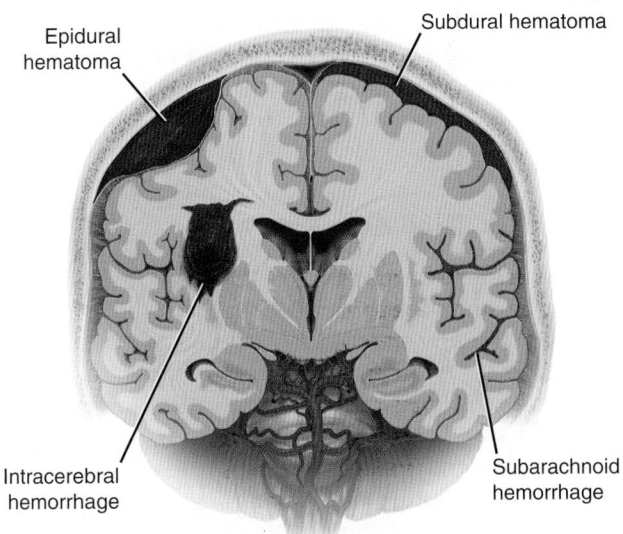

Fig. 39.2 Different types of posttraumatic intracranial hematoma. Epidural hematoma: a collection of blood between the skull and the outer membrane covering the brain (dura mater). Subdural hematoma: a collection of blood located underneath the dura mater, generally associated with bruising of the underlying brain tissue (contusions). Hemorrhagic contusion and intracerebral hematoma: lesions that reflect similar underlying pathologies, ranging from local bruising lesions that reflect similar underlying pathologies, ranging from local bruising (contusions) to bleeding into the brain tissue (hematoma). Subarachnoid hemorrhage: blood accumulates under the arachnoid layer of the membranous covering of the brain (meninges) (From Rengachary, S. S., Ellenbogen, R. G. (2005). *Principles of Neurosurgery* (2nd ed.). Edinburgh, Mosby Ltd.)

There is widespread axonal white matter shearing and tearing, along with diffuse cerebral swelling at the time of the impact. DAI often causes global neurologic dysfunction in the pediatric brain because of the relatively decreased myelin content and higher water content in the pediatric brain (Lang et al., 2021).

Cerebral Edema
Cerebral edema, either focal or diffuse, results from an increase in brain volume from the intracellular or extracellular fluid (Zusman et al., 2020). Peak occurrence for cerebral edema usually is up to 72 hours after a neurologic insult. It gradually resolves over 2 to 3 weeks. Cerebral edema may be caused by either the primary injury to the neuronal tissue or secondary injury in response to the biochemical, cellular injury cascade that causes hypoxia, hypercarbia, or cerebral ischemia. The Monro-Kellie hypothesis describes the relationship between volumes of the brain, cerebrospinal fluid (CSF), and blood within the fixed cranial vault (Zusman et al., 2020). When cerebral edema occurs, it increases brain volume, causing the other intracranial components (blood, CSF) to be forced out of the relatively closed space of the cranium. Left untreated or poorly controlled,

cerebral edema can have a devastating effect, resulting in intracranial hypertension and impaired cerebral perfusion. These can lead to neuronal tissue hypoxia, ischemia, cerebral herniation, and death (Jha & Kochanek, 2018).

DIAGNOSTIC IMAGING

Most children experiencing blunt head trauma have clinically insignificant injuries and do not require imaging; however, clinicians are tasked with identifying those with clinically important TBIs without unnecessarily irradiating those at lower risk. The gold standard for identifying TBIs is CT of the head; however, it is costly and exposes the child to the risks of radiation-induced malignancy. Children are at more risk of the effects of radiation due to their small body size and high rate of cell growth and division (Pennell et al., 2020). To standardize radiation exposure and be mindful of health care costs, the American Academy of Pediatrics (AAP), in collaboration with the American Academy of Family Physicians (AAFP), published a practice parameter for evaluating and managing minor closed head injury (AAP & AAFP, 1999; Gambacorta et al., 2022). They commented on the relative risk for intracranial injury and devised an algorithm for appropriate diagnostic imaging studies to safely clarify injury severity and guide acute intervention (Fig. 39.3). Since that time, several pediatric head imaging guidelines have been developed. The most widely used is from the Pediatric Emergency Care Applied Research Network, which created an age-based head injury decision rule. The rule was published in 2009 and provided further guidelines for children younger than and older than age 2 years by assisting in identifying those at low risk for clinically significant TBI to safely avoid CT scans (Kuppermann et al., 2009). It is currently used in many countries for the emergency management of children with closed head injuries (Gambacorta et al., 2022; Mastrangelo & Midulla, 2017) (Table 39.4).

CLINICAL MANIFESTATIONS AT TIME OF DIAGNOSIS AND TREATMENT

Clinical manifestations at the time of diagnosis vary, depending on the primary brain injury and the extent and involvement of secondary injury. Children who sustain TBI have varying degrees of alertness and responsiveness. Their presentation is influenced by the degree of increased ICP and other metabolic factors. If the extent of secondary responses progresses, clinical symptoms may worsen in the hours after an injury. For all head injuries, established pediatric guidelines for imaging should be followed (AAP, 1999; Kuppermann et al., 2009).

⊚ Clinical Manifestations at Time of Diagnosis

- Varying degrees of alertness and responsiveness determined by degree of intracranial pressure (see Table 39.2)
- Loss of consciousness
- Headache
- Seizures
- Vomiting
- Hemiparesis
- Fixed dilated pupils
- Brainstem herniation

MANIFESTATIONS OF MILD TRAUMATIC BRAIN INJURY
- Asymptomatic
- Confusion
- Loss of consciousness for <1 min
- Headache
- Vomiting
- Lethargy

ACUTE: MILD TRAUMATIC BRAIN INJURY/ CONCUSSION

Accurate identification of a TBI in children younger than age 2 years can be challenging. In the setting of mTBI, a child may initially be asymptomatic despite having a TBI. Therefore ongoing vigilance is essential when monitoring behavioral and neurologic changes following a head injury.

Diagnosing a concussion in the acute setting can pose challenges due to the transient nature of symptoms after the injury (Marklund et al., 2019). The best practice, once an injury occurs where there is a concern for a TBI due to reported or observed signs or symptoms (Box 39.1), is to ensure the child is no longer at risk of repeat head injury (removal from play or any high-risk activity for repeat injury if applicable). The next step is a proper assessment by a clinician educated in emergency care to rule out more serious injuries (Joseph & Paul, 2021). Concussion remains a clinical diagnosis, and several assessment strategies should be used to obtain an accurate diagnosis. These strategies include obtaining a thorough history, performing a concussion-specific examination (including the visio-vestibular exam), and using a validated post-concussion symptom checklist (Corwin et al., 2019; Master et al., 2022; McCrory et al., 2017) (Box 39.2). There are several tools in the literature that have been developed for this purpose, but best practice on which tool to use continues to evolve based on age and practice setting. Such tools include the Acute Concussion Assessment, Sports Concussion Assessment Tool 5, and Concussion Clinical Profiles Screening Tool (Babl et al., 2017b; Kontos et al., 2020a).

It is important to note that grading scales to describe concussion severity are no longer used because it is difficult to assess concussion severity based on the presentation of symptoms. Current recommendations are to diagnose a concussion without mild, moderate, or severe labels and use current consensus protocols

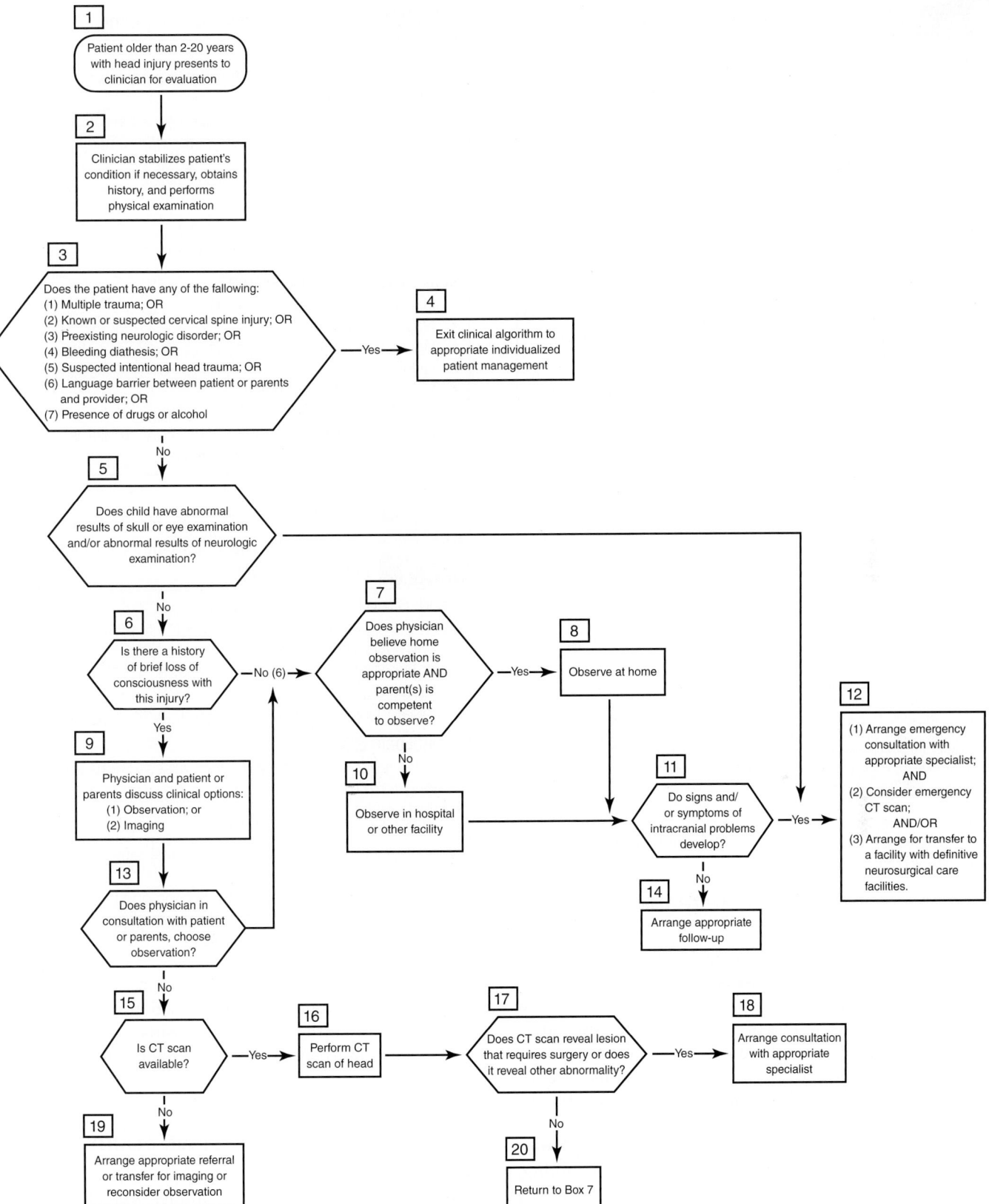

Fig. 39.3 Evaluation and triage of children and adolescents with minor head trauma. (From Committee on Quality Improvement, American Academy of Pediatrics and Commission on Clinical Policies and Research, American Academy of Family Physicians. (1999). The management of minor closed head injury in children. *Pediatrics, 106*(6), 1407–1415.)

Table 39.4	Indications for Computed Tomography Scan in Pediatric Trauma Patients Based on PECARN Guidelines	
CHILDREN AGE <2 YR	**CHILDREN AGE >2 YR**	
Age <3 mo	GCS <14 or any signs of altered mental status	
Palpable skull fracture		
GCS <14 or any signs of altered mental status	Signs of basilar skull fracture	
Agitation/irritability	Battle sign—ecchymosis of the mastoid process	
Somnolence		
Slow response to verbal communication	Raccoon eyes—periorbital ecchymosis	
Occipital, parietal, or temporal scalp hematoma (any nonfrontal hematoma)	CSF otorrhea or rhinorrhea	
	Loss of consciousness	
Loss of consciousness >5 s	Vomiting	
Not acting appropriately per parent	Severe headache	
	Severe mechanism	
Severe mechanism	Falls >3 ft	
Falls >3 ft	MVC with passenger ejection, rollover, or death of another passenger	
MVC with passenger ejection, rollover, or death of another passenger		
	Pedestrian or bicycle passenger unhelmeted and hit by a motor vehicle	
Pedestrian or bicycle passenger unhelmeted and hit by a motor vehicle		
Struck in head by a high-impact object		

CSF, Cerebrospinal fluid; *GCS,* Glasgow Coma Scale; *MVC,* motor vehicle collision; *PECARN,* Pediatric Emergency Care Applied Research Network.
From Kenefake, M. E., Swarm, M., & Walthall, J. (2013). Nuances in pediatric trauma. *Emergency Medical Clinics of North America, 31*(3), 627–652; Jaffe, D., & Wesson, D. (1991). Emergency management of blunt trauma in children. *New England Journal of Medicine, 324*(21), 1477–1482.

Box 39.1 Concussion Signs and Symptoms

CONCUSSION SIGNS OBSERVED
- Cannot recall events prior to or after a hit or fall
- Appears dazed or stunned
- Forgets an instruction, is confused about an assignment or position, or is unsure of the game, score, or opponent
- Moves clumsily
- Answers questions slowly
- Loses consciousness (even briefly)
- Shows mood, behavior, or personality changes

CONCUSSION SYMPTOMS REPORTED
- Headache or pressure in head
- Nausea or vomiting
- Balance problems or dizziness, or double or blurry vision
- Bothered by light or noise
- Feeling sluggish, hazy, foggy, or groggy
- Confusion, or concentration or memory problems
- Just not feeling right or feeling down

Box 39.2 Physical Exam Essentials for the Primary Care Provider After Head Injury—Quick Reference Guide

Head: Scalp hematoma, bleeding
Eyes: Pupil size and symmetry, nystagmus, periorbital ecchymosis (racoon eyes)
Ears: Hemotympanum, otorrhea, mastoid ecchymosis (Battle sign)
Associated injuries: Orthopedic, facial, trunk/abdomen

NEUROLOGIC EXAM

Cognition: Have patient give history, assess short- and long-term memory
Cranial nerves: Extraocular movements, pupil size and symmetry, facial symmetry
Motor (upper): Finger to nose, rapidly alternating movements, drift
Motor (lower): Gait, tandem walk, hop on one foot

Modified from American Academy of Pediatrics, Project ECHO. https://www.aap.org/en/practice-management/project-echo/.

to guide treatment and return to activities (Halstead et al., 2018).

ACUTE: MODERATE-SEVERE TRAUMATIC BRAIN INJURY

A child with a moderate-severe TBI with an intracranial injury can exhibit fluctuating clinical manifestations of a lucid period of wakefulness, deteriorating neurologic status, to loss of consciousness. Other signs and symptoms may include headache, seizure, vomiting, hemiparesis, and fixed and dilated pupils. Prompt identification and surgical management of life-threatening injuries favor a positive outcome.

Cerebral edema can cause increased ICP. Symptoms include irritability, lethargy, nausea and vomiting, headache, photophobia, pupillary changes, abnormal reflexes, seizures, widening pulse pressure, bradycardia, and apnea. If this persists, cerebral herniation can ensue (O'Brien et al., 2018). Clinical manifestations of herniation are changes in the level of consciousness, abnormal respiratory patterns, loss of protective reflexes (e.g., gag or corneal), changes in blood pressure and pulse pressure with bradycardia, pupillary dysfunction, papilledema, changes in motor function or posturing, nausea and projectile vomiting, a positive Babinski sign, and visual disturbances (Kochanek et al., 2019).

TREATMENT

ACUTE: MILD TRAUMATIC BRAIN INJURY/CONCUSSION

Traditionally, treatment for the milder type of mTBI or concussion has been thought to require minimal clinical management beyond watchful waiting and rest. Recent data in the literature have demonstrated that about 20% to 30% of those who sustain a concussion have prolonged symptoms lasting more than 4 weeks, which then causes significant disability (Lima et al., 2021). In response to this research, there is mounting evidence developing that active recovery, including supervised fitness, can promote the resolution of symptoms (Leddy et al., 2019; Lumba-Brown et al., 2018).

> ### 💊 Treatment
>
> - Prehospital ("in the field") stabilization and evaluation
> - Early treatment determined by severity of traumatic brain injury
> - Control of hypoxia, increased cerebral CO_2, and brain edema
> - Surgical intervention, if needed, for bleeding, trauma, or cerebral edema
> - Coma recovery to follow predictable patterns with variable time sequence
> - Rehabilitation program and family involvement both keys to long-term recovery

Initial treatment no longer includes sitting in a dark room and resting until symptoms resolve, as this step has been demonstrated to promote prolonged recovery (Strelzik et al., 2017). Rest after injury should be brief, minimizing metabolic demand for about 24 to 48 hours, followed by gradual advancement back to usual activities (sports, physical activity, and school) in small amounts of time (Thomas et al., 2015). The brief period of rest may include limited electronics, screen time, schoolwork, and physical activity, but the exact amount and type of limitations are still under question (Macnow et al., 2021). There are several published recommendations for returning to school after a concussion but no formal guidelines (McAvoy et al., 2020). Returning to school does not require formal clearance, but providing academic adjustments to support the student's return to school can help support recovery. A formal clearance for return to recreational and organized sports is recommended and required throughout the United States. Several iterations of return-to-play protocols have been developed to guide this process, the most recent from the Fifth International Conference on Concussion in Sport (Table 39.5) (McCrory et al., 2017).

Clinicians should also provide education to the child and family that includes the following (Lumba-Brown et al., 2018):
- Warning signs of more serious injury
- Description of injury and expected course of symptoms and recovery
- Instructions on how to monitor postconcussive symptoms

Table 39.5 Return-to-Sport Strategy—Each Step Typically Takes 24 Hours Minimum

STEP	EXERCISE STRATEGY	ACTIVITY AT EACH STEP	GOAL
1	Symptom-limited activity	Daily activities that do not exacerbate symptoms (e.g., walking)	Gradual reintroduction of work/school
2	Aerobic exercise **2A—Light** (up to ~55% maxHR) then **2B—Moderate** (up to ~70% maxHR)	Stationary cycling or walking at slow-medium pace. May start light resistance training that does not result in more than mild and brief exacerbation[a] of concussion symptoms.	Increase heart rate
3	Individual sport-specific exercise Note: If sport-specific training involves any risk of inadvertent head impact, medical clearance should occur prior to step 3	Sport-specific training away from the team environment (e.g., running, change of direction and/or individual training drills away from the team environment). No activities at risk of head impact.	Add movement, change of direction
Steps 4–6 should begin after the resolution of any symptoms, abnormalities in cognitive function, and any other clinical findings related to the current concussion, including with and after physical exertion.			
4	Noncontact training drills	Exercise to high intensity, including more challenging training drills (e.g., passing drills, multiplayer training) can integrate into a team environment.	Resume usual intensity of exercise, coordination, and increased thinking
5	Full contact practice	Participate in normal training activities.	Restore confidence and assess functional skills by coaching staff
6	Return to sport	Normal game play.	

[a]Mild and brief exacerbation of symptoms (i.e., an increase of no more than 2 points on a 0–10-point scale for <1 hour when compared with the baseline value reported prior to physical activity). Athletes may begin step 1 (i.e., symptom-limited activity) within 24 hours of injury, with progression through each subsequent step typically taking a minimum of 24 hours. If more than mild exacerbation of symptoms (i.e., >2 points on a 0–10 scale) occurs during steps 1–3, the athlete should stop and attempt to exercise the next day. Athletes experiencing concussion-related symptoms during steps 4–6 should return to step 3 to establish full resolution of symptoms with exertion before engaging in at-risk activities. Written determination of readiness to return to sport (RTS) should be provided by a health care provider before unrestricted RTS as directed by local laws and/or sporting regulations.
maxHR, Predicted maximal heart rate according to age (i.e., 220 – age).
From Patricios, J. S., Schneider, K. J., Dvorak, J., Ahmed, O. H., Blauwet, C., Cantu, R. C., Davis, G. A., Echemendia, R. J., Makdissi, M., McNamee, M., Broglio, S., Emery, C. A., Feddermann-Demont, N., Fuller, G. W., Giza, C. C., Guskiewicz, K. M., Hainline, B., Iverson, G. L., Kutcher, J. S., Leddy J. J., et al. (2022, October). Consensus statement on concussion in sport: The 6th International Conference on Concussion in Sport-Amsterdam. https://bjsm.bmj.com/content/57/11/695.

- Prevention of further injury
- Management of cognitive and physical activity/rest
- Instructions regarding return to play/recreation and school
- Clear clinician follow-up instructions

It is estimated that almost 80% of those with prolonged recovery after concussion have vision or vestibular deficits (Master et al., 2016). These symptoms can provoke significant disability and impede recovery. Vestibular rehabilitation in children with a concussion is associated with symptoms and visio-vestibular performance improvement (Storey et al., 2018). In patients with ongoing vision disorders, vision therapy in the form of vision rehabilitation has been demonstrated to be extremely effective in promoting recovery and optimal functional outcomes (Gallaway et al., 2017).

More research has surfaced describing the overall treatment of concussion to include healthy lifestyle practices such as optimizing sleep, optimizing hydration and nutrition, integrating daily noncontact fitness, and optimizing mental wellness as important factors in concussion treatment (Gerald et al., 2022; Markovic et al., 2021).

Early referral (within 7 days of injury) from primary care providers to a concussion specialist has been shown to decrease prolonged recovery after a concussion (Kontos et al., 2020b; Pratile et al., 2022).

ACUTE: MODERATE-SEVERE TRAUMATIC BRAIN INJURY

The first goal of acute injury management after TBI is to promote neuroprotection and cerebral perfusion (Kochanek et al., 2019). Treatment is focused on stabilizing the effects of the primary injury and preventing secondary injuries caused by hypoxia, hypercarbia, acidosis, free radicals, cerebral edema, seizures, infection, and aspiration, and surgically treating correctable intracranial lesions (O'Brien et al., 2015). Initial treatment at the scene of an injury begins with cervical stabilization and support of the airway, breathing, and circulation (Hansen et al., 2018). Successful medical management immediately at the scene of the injury is an important predictor of outcome.

Children who have sustained a severe TBI are best managed at a trauma center with multidisciplinary neurologic and neurosurgical services and a high-level pediatric intensive care program. To minimize secondary injuries, treatment includes intubation, ventilation, fluid resuscitation, diuretics, and blood pressure monitoring (Taşkapılıoğlu et al., 2019). Maintaining adequate cerebral perfusion pressure (CPP) in children has a goal of 40 to 50 mm Hg to maximize perfusion and avoid cerebral ischemia (Woods et al., 2021). In recent years there has been significant progress in various multimodal methods that can guide the treatment of children with severe TBI and monitor CPP, including a combination of neuroimaging, continuous pressure, cerebral autoregulation, and brain tissue oxygenation monitoring (Young et al., 2018).

Management of severe TBI can be divided into acute medical stabilization and intensive acute rehabilitation phases (Carney et al., 2017). These phases may flow together as children stabilize and become more tolerant of the stimulation and demands of the acute rehabilitation phase of care. The goals of treatment in children with TBI are to minimize complications and disability and to maximize the ability to function independently. An important goal within the acute inpatient rehabilitation setting is to plan the child's transition to the next level of care in the community, including outpatient medical care and therapies, and return to school.

Rehabilitation and Long-Term Management for Moderate-Severe Traumatic Brain Injury

Rehabilitation goals include maximizing the child's functional independence and neurocognitive abilities in developmentally age-appropriate activities of daily living. Goals are established upon admission and reevaluated throughout the recovery period (Popernack et al., 2015). Rehabilitation can hasten and maximize the restoration of lost functions, promote adaptation to disabilities, and aid in age-appropriate independence with reintegration into family and school life. Rehabilitation can enhance the quality of life for both children with TBI and their families.

Most children with brain injuries undergo some spontaneous recovery in the first 6 months after injury. Deficits remaining after this period typically are more permanent (Guilliams & Wainwright, 2016). There are several tools used to predict functional outcomes after TBI. Those most widely used in pediatrics are the GCS, Glasgow Outcome Scale (GOS), GOS-Extended Peds (GOS-E Peds), and Rancho Los Amigos Scale (RLAS) (Beers et al., 2012; Reuter-Rice et al., 2018). Both the GOS and GOS-E Peds scores help predict rehabilitation outcomes based on four categories: mild, moderate, severe, and vegetative state. GOS-E Peds provides valid outcome measures in infants, toddlers, school-age children, and adolescents through age 16 years and is sensitive to the severity of the injury and is associated with changes in TBI sequelae over time (Beers et al., 2012, Evans et al., 2020). The RLAS is a widely accepted medical scale used to describe cognitive and behavioral patterns in brain injury patients as they recover from injury. The eight-level behavior/response scale evaluates the patient's interaction with environmental stimulation as an indication of the stage of recovery from injury. The scale ranges from level I (unresponsive to stimuli) to VIII (purposeful and appropriate response to stimuli) (Lin & Wroten, 2022; Popernack et al., 2015).

A broad range of residual sequela persists after TBI, and they are manifestations of the location and severity of the primary and secondary injuries. These include muscle movement and tone abnormalities with associated orthopedic problems, seizures, visual deficits, cognitive and behavioral deficits, and sleep disorders.

Management of these symptoms requires an interdisciplinary approach to develop and implement an individualized treatment plan by a physical medicine and rehabilitation physician specializing in pediatric rehabilitation (Eapen et al., 2015). To date, a comprehensive and formal guideline for the care of children needing TBI rehabilitation does not exist, allowing for significant variability in their care and outcomes (Reuter-Rice et al., 2018).

Physical therapists work to optimize range of motion, strength, posture, and mobility. They use several modalities, including passive range of motion, strengthening exercises, limb splinting and bracing, and proper support and positioning. These approaches prevent physical deformities (e.g., joint contractures) that can result from prolonged immobilization and the effects of unbalanced muscle tone on a joint.

Occupational therapists help patients relearn or improve activities of daily living, such as eating, getting dressed, and bathing. They also work on sensory integration, fine motor skills such as writing, appropriate play skills, and environmental adaptation such as returning to school and home.

Speech-language pathologists address feeding, communication, and some cognitive areas; early in the course, they ensure readiness and safety for oral feeding. As children move to higher levels of cognitive function, speech-language pathologists work closely with the psychology and educational staff to identify and address orientation and memory weaknesses that may affect recovery (Caliendo et al., 2021).

Neuropsychologists and psychologists play a critical role in the rehabilitation process for the child after TBI. Neuropsychologists administer tests that can provide objective information to clarify how an injury has altered the brain's ability to process information and explain specific changes in behavior, which can then help guide treatment.

The psychologist can provide ongoing behavioral and emotional support for the complex needs of the child with a TBI and the family. The neuropsychologist and psychologist work together to provide valuable information regarding the behavioral, cognitive, and emotional difficulties that are frequently encountered by this population, and they can assist with treatment planning and discharge considerations (Johnson-Green, 2018).

This multidisciplinary team of specialists guides the challenging emotional, social, and behavioral aspects of a child's recovery (Zamani et al., 2019). The parents and family are essential members of the rehabilitation team as well. They contribute prior knowledge of the child's behavioral style and capabilities and an understanding of the culture and community to which the child will return.

The primary care provider must be incorporated into the rehabilitation process. The primary care provider should be updated on the child's medical conditions and functional capabilities, the team of subspecialists providing services, and the types of therapy and equipment necessary after hospital discharge. Together, the primary care provider and the rehabilitation team evaluate the community resources and services to activate the support necessary for the child and family upon returning home.

The process of recovery does not stop when a child is discharged from an inpatient unit. The decision to discharge a child from an inpatient rehabilitation program should be considered when reasonable safety has been achieved and when the child can tolerate a transition to a less intense and more community-based level of care. There is strong evidence that training family members to provide cognitive and motor therapy at home brings about more powerful improvements in cognitive and motor scores compared with clinician-delivered therapy alone (Durish et al., 2018). Ongoing medical, emotional, physical, and educational support for the child and family is essential, especially as the child moves forward and encounters the continuing developmental challenges common to all children.

INTEGRATIVE COMPLEMENTARY AND ALTERNATIVE MEDICINE IN TRAUMATIC BRAIN INJURY

Integrated complementary and alternative medicine (ICAM) goes beyond conventional medicine and is not regulated by the US Food and Drug Administration. Though not all therapies are proven treatments, research suggests that some of these approaches may help control ongoing sequela after TBI. *Integrative medicine* combines conventional medicine with other forms of medicine that, through research, are proven to be safe and potentially effective. An example of integrative medicine is acupuncture. Like integrative medicine, *complementary medicine* is used alongside conventional medicine. Examples of complementary medicine include meditation, therapeutic massages, and relaxation techniques (Wopker et al., 2020).

Until recently, most research in TBI treatment focused on the prevention of secondary injury; however, the ongoing failure of clinical trials for TBI treatment has instigated a step toward trialing ICAM therapies to treat ongoing TBI symptoms (Lucke-Wold et al., 2018). These novel therapies are slowly coming to the forefront to help prevent the cascade of events that can occur from secondary injuries, such as progressive neurodegeneration and further disease burden (Acabchuk et al., 2021). These effects include oxidative stress, endoplasmic reticulum stress, mitochondrial dysfunction, and neuroinflammation (Wang et al., 2019). Research is starting to demonstrate that therapies such as music therapy, acupuncture, acupressure, and mind-body practices such as tai chi, yoga, and mindfulness (Lucke-Wold et al., 2018; Siponkoski et al., 2020) may be useful tools in the management of TBI.

ICAM therapies may also help treat neuropsychiatric symptoms such as depression and anxiety that can be associated with TBI (Roddis & Tanner, 2020). Nutritional interventions such as eating and using nutritional or dietary supplements are currently being evaluated to treat prolonged TBI symptoms. Most TBI studies with these interventions are still using only animal models but may hold promise when done in humans in the future. Ways of eating, such as fasting or ketogenic diets, after TBI have been discussed in the literature and have demonstrated efficacy after TBI by improving cerebral metabolism, cognitive performance, and behavioral or emotional outcomes (Cao et al., 2022; McDougall et al., 2018). It is important to note that most studies have been on animal subjects; however, studies with human models in this area of research are on the rise. Some nutritional or dietary supplements that are in preclinical trials or have been studied in animal models include branched chain amino acids, choline, and dehydroepiandrosterone (Elkind et al., 2015, Lucke-Wold et al., 2018). Magnesium supplementation by mouth has demonstrated promising results in treating posttraumatic headaches in one study of human subjects (Standiford et al., 2021). This list of dietary and nutritional supplements is certainly not exhaustive and will likely continue to grow as research progresses.

Moving forward, it will be imperative to understand how these complementary and alternative therapies can be used with traditional clinical practices early in treatment to improve outcomes after TBI.

ANTICIPATED ADVANCES IN DIAGNOSIS AND MANAGEMENT

Despite the explosion of research in medical literature related to concussions, there continues to be confusion and controversy over methods of assessment, diagnosis, and treatment for several reasons. First, there are numerous consensus statements from different governing bodies and medical organizations regarding concussion care. Second, the science behind the pathophysiology and the lack of evidence-based data contribute to this dilemma. Lastly, published literature includes numerous working definitions of concussion and often presents an inconsistent use of terminology (e.g., concussion vs mTBI vs head injury) (Lumba-Brown et al., 2018). The term *persistent postconcussive symptom* (PPCS) is now preferred when describing protracted recovery versus postconcussion syndrome (PCS) (Leddy et al., 2021). These differences pose significant challenges to the understanding of concussions in both the medical and the lay communities. As science continues to evolve, researchers are working on methods to diagnose mTBI more objectively using various biomarkers. Ongoing research looks at neuroimaging biomarkers, tissue, saliva, blood, and visual biomarkers that can objectively provide diagnosis and guide treatment (Dadas et al., 2018; Master et al., 2020; Saliman et al., 2021; Wang et al., 2018). More research

needs to take place until we can use these methods on the sideline and in clinical practice.

Other research interests in the acute management of children with TBI involve preventing or treating secondary responses and secondary injuries. One promising theory holds that calcium influx is a major perpetrator of cellular damage, causing secondary injury. Research using calcium channel antagonists has demonstrated efficacy in preventing cerebral ischemia after intracranial hemorrhage; however, uncertainty remains regarding the exact mechanism of action and dosing (Carlson et al., 2020).

Another promising area of research in negating the ill effects of severe TBI is the use of stem cell–based therapies that have various mechanisms of action, some of which include treating neuroinflammation and promoting neurogenesis (Lengel et al., 2020). These treatments are still evolving as researchers continue to understand more of the pathophysiology of pediatric TBI in more detail.

ASSOCIATED PROBLEMS OF TRAUMATIC BRAIN INJURY

MILD TRAUMATIC BRAIN INJURY

mTBI can cause a range of problems, from the more common PPCS to the rare but serious and controversial second impact syndrome (SIS). Although symptoms from concussion and mTBI are known to be temporary, there is still great concern about experiencing protracted recovery and possible long-term outcomes. Historically it was thought that concussions usually resolved in about 7 to 10 days; however, more recent data in the literature suggest it can take up to 30 days for neurocognitive recovery (Kamins et al., 2017; Kent et al., 2020; Tamura et al., 2020). mTBI can affect many different systems in the body, including vision, vestibular, autonomic function, sleep, and emotional regulation. Each of these symptoms can recover at different rates, so being symptom free does not indicate recovery from mTBI or concussion.

Persistent Postconcussive Symptoms

PPCS (no longer PCS) is thought to occur when concussion symptoms last more than 4 weeks (Martin et al., 2020). There is research that supports various concussion profiles seen in people with PPCS. The symptoms can be broken down into categories, including dysautonomia, cognitive deficits, emotional changes, and vestibular/oculomotor dysfunction (Gornall et al., 2020; Master et al., 2016; McCrory et al., 2017; Miranda et al., 2018; Scheiman et al., 2021). Common symptoms include headaches, irritability, anxiety, behavioral disturbances, dizziness, fatigue, impaired concentration, forgetfulness, blurred vision, visual fatigue, nausea, sleep disturbances, and noise sensitivity. Treatment for PPCS includes an active recovery, including guided aerobic activity, vestibular and oculomotor rehabilitation, and vision rehabilitation (Fox et al., 2019; Leddy et al., 2021; Lumba-Brown et al., 2018; Storey et al., 2018). Initiation of these therapies remains in question, but some clinicians will start within the first week after injury.

It is important to note that part of concussion assessment is understanding preinjury or baseline symptoms and comorbidities. Those with a larger preinjury symptom burden or with significant comorbidities may be at risk for PPCS (McCrory et al., 2017). Recent pediatric guidelines endorsed by the CDC have compiled the following as risk factors for PPCS: history of prior TBI, lower cognitive ability (for children with intracranial lesion), neurologic or psychiatric disorders, learning difficulties, increased preinjury symptoms (i.e., postconcussive), and family or social stressors (Lumba-Brown et al., 2018). These preinjury risk factors can cause a greater symptom burden postinjury, worse cognitive functioning, and prolonged recovery (Kent et al., 2020; Terry et al., 2021).

Although various medications have been used in the setting of mTBI to treat headache, mental fogginess, and sleep disorders, no studies have demonstrated their efficacy in concussion. Treatment should shift from medication management to treating the cause of the symptoms with rehabilitation and cognitive-behavioral therapy. Mood disorders should be treated by an appropriate mental health professional.

Second Impact Syndrome
SIS is a rare but catastrophic event following a relatively mild head trauma. It is most often described in the male adolescent athlete, sustained after an initial and recent unresolved concussion (May et al., 2022). SIS is thought to be characterized by acute brain swelling and/or subdural hematoma, which in turn causes an increase in ICP, cerebral herniation, and then neurologic collapse (Engelhardt et al., 2021). It is believed to have originated from cerebral autoregulation. Athletes at risk are those who have sustained a recent concussion and then return to play when they have not recovered. Reports of SIS are few, and some argue that it is simply diffuse cerebral swelling unrelated to the first concussion (McLendon et al., 2016). The concern for SIS following head injury supports the recommendation that athletes should not return to play until a sport-related concussion has been ruled out or until they have recovered from the concussion, including completing a formal return to play protocol (McCrory et al., 2017).

MODERATE-SEVERE TRAUMATIC BRAIN INJURY
Neurologic Dysfunction
Posttraumatic hydrocephalus. Posttraumatic hydrocephalus occurs in a small number of individuals after brain injury, most commonly in those who have suffered a subarachnoid hemorrhage. This may occur weeks or months after TBI. In children with a severe injury, cerebral ventriculomegaly may be due to cerebral atrophy rather than true hydrocephalus. If a diagnosis of hydrocephalus is made, treatment may consist of the placement of a valve-regulating shunt. Surgical management via a shunt relieves acute symptoms of increased ICP.

Posttraumatic seizures. The incidence of posttraumatic seizures in children is about 10% (Elsamadicy et al., 2021). These seizures are classified as early (i.e., occurring within 7 days of injury) or late (i.e., occurring within 7 days after injury) (Pingue et al., 2021). Prophylactic administration of anticonvulsants given for 7 days after TBI reduces the incidence of early seizure. However, extended use of anticonvulsants does not reduce the incidence of late seizures. The onset of late seizures varies greatly, from soon after the initial injury to 2 years following the injury. Chronic seizures are usually well controlled with anticonvulsant medications.

Abnormal Motor and Sensory Function
There is significant heterogenicity of residual deficits after TBI. Common motor and sensory disabilities for children following moderate-severe TBI include spasticity/elevated muscle tone, movement problems (i.e., ataxia), contractures, paralysis, speech impairments, dysphagia, and dyspraxia (Popernack et al., 2015). Hearing and visual deficits may also occur after TBI. Rehabilitation therapies provided at regular intervals by physical and occupational therapists and speech-language pathologists can optimize outcomes. Ideally, these specialists work with the child and primary caregivers to help the child gain as much independence as possible, often providing recommendations for adaptive equipment such as crutches, walkers, wheelchairs, and lifts.

Speech/Communication Deficits
Methods of communication, both in expressive and receptive language, can be affected after TBI due to their interaction with cognitive, linguistic, emotional, physical, and contextual factors related to the TBI (Laane & Cooke, 2020). Common deficits are seen in memory, word retrieval, labeling, and verbal organization. It is imperative to understand any preexisting speech, language, and/or cognitive deficits in the child, as this can affect TBI outcomes. Such disorders would include ADHD, learning disorders, autism spectrum disorder, childhood apraxia of speech, learning disabilities, speech sound disorders, spoken language disorders, and written language disorders (American Speech-Language Hearing Association, 2022). Early assessment and intervention are key to promoting recovery.

Impaired Respiratory Function
Impairments in respiratory function can occur after TBI. Damage to the brain's respiratory centers may affect the ability to breathe independently, necessitating tracheostomy or mechanical ventilation; these may be temporary or permanent supports. Neurologic impairments can

affect posture by causing neuromuscular scoliosis. These can interfere with normal lung capacity and function.

Endocrine Dysfunction

After severe TBI, children may experience an array of endocrine disruptions, including hyperphagia, hypothyroidism, precocious puberty, amenorrhea, or growth failure (Krahulik et al., 2017). There may be signs of antidiuretic dysfunction such as (1) diabetes insipidus, which manifests as hypernatremia, polyphagia, polydipsia, and polyuria, or (2) syndrome of inappropriate secretion of antidiuretic hormone (SIADH), which manifests as hyponatremia and decreased urinary output. These conditions usually resolve after the acute posttraumatic phase but may become a lifelong issue for some. Precocious puberty may be associated with head trauma due to potential disruption of the normal hypothalamus and pituitary function. Premature sexual characteristics can include isolated breast, axillary, or pubic hair development. If any of these endocrine changes are present, the child should be referred to a pediatric endocrinologist for more in-depth assessment and long-term management (Dassa et al., 2019).

Altered Cognitive and Neuropsychological Function

Alterations in cognitive ability and neuropsychological function are common and critically important areas of postinjury dysfunction. Deficits may occur in memory, word retrieval, naming, verbal organization, comprehension of verbal information, comprehension of verbal abstractions, verbal learning, and effective conversation. Difficulties in attention and concentration, poor judgment, and impulsivity may occur. For those children with prior problems in these areas, such as children with ADHD, these deficits may become more severe. Neuropsychological testing can identify deficits. Special education designation is often helpful in providing essential school-based support. Severe TBI can also affect major milestone attainment or cause milestone regression. Developmental progress should be monitored closely, and referrals to community services should be made as needed for physical and occupational therapy, speech-language pathology, and academic specialists.

Psychiatric and Psychosocial Deficits

There is a risk for psychological sequelae after TBI (Ewing-Cobb et al., 2021), and many youth report behavioral health changes, including disturbed sleep, difficulty adhering to activity recommendations, pain, anxiety, and depression. Emotional or behavioral difficulties that predate the brain injury may be exacerbated and exaggerated, or new behavioral symptoms may occur. The most common pattern of psychiatric disorder among children who have sustained a severe TBI results from injury to the frontal lobes, which causes affective (mood) instability, aggression, impaired social judgment, and occasionally apathy or paranoia (Max et al., 2022). Despite commonality of these deficits after TBI, psychiatric and psychosocial needs often remain unmet after release from medical care. Reasons for this include a lack of identification of need, access to services, and social stigma around mental health (Donnelly et al., 2021).

PROGNOSIS

A TBI is a life-altering event that can have devastating and long-term disability (Kuehn, 2018). Most patients return to functional levels of activity within 2 years postinjury (McCrea et al., 2021). Several studies have evaluated functional outcomes after TBI; however, few have prospectively tracked long-term recovery from the acute through the chronic phase. The heterogenous and complex nature of TBI can make predicting recovery challenging at best.

There is an overall survival rate of over 90% for children who sustain TBI, most of which are mild in severity (Dewan et al., 2016). Of the children who sustain a severe injury, survival decreases to 50% to 60% (McCrea et al., 2021). The best predictor of good neurologic outcome is the maintenance of CPP between 40 and 50 mm Hg (Woods et al., 2021). Risk factors for worse outcomes include focal lesions in addition to DAI, significant associated injuries or polytrauma, and related problems of hypoxia and hypotension (Lazaridis et al., 2019). Important negative prognostic indicators include increased length of coma, lower postresuscitation GCS score, deterioration in GCS score in the first 24 hours, increasing age (up to 14 years), longer duration of posttraumatic amnesia, pathologic neurologic reflexes, posttraumatic seizures, CT scan mass findings, and lack of availability of rehabilitation services (Kochanek et al., 2019).

Lastly, keeping in mind the biopsychosocial ideology of healing after injury, it is imperative that mental health be assessed and supported to promote overall well-being after all severities of TBI (Howlett et al., 2022; Register-Mihalik et al., 2020).

PRIMARY CARE MANAGEMENT

HEALTH CARE MAINTENANCE AND ANTICIPATORY GUIDANCE

Primary care management after TBI should initially focus on routine general primary care assessments based on AAP recommendations for preventative health care, then narrow the assessments based on high-risk health care changes that can occur after TBI (Box 39.3).

Growth and Development

After TBI there is a high risk of alteration in nutritional intake. Growth parameters of weight and height should be followed routinely and plotted on a growth

Box 39.3 Associated Problems of Traumatic Brain Injury

MILD TRAUMATIC BRAIN INJURY
- Persistent postconcussive symptoms
- Confusion, disorientation
- Autonomic dysfunction
- Difficulty with schoolwork
- Balance and coordination problems
- Emotional lability
- Sleep disturbance
- Visual changes
- Vestibular dysfunction

MODERATE-SEVERE TRAUMATIC BRAIN INJURY
- Neurologic dysfunction
- Posttraumatic hydrocephalus
- Posttraumatic seizures
- Abnormal motor and sensory function
- Impaired respiratory function
- Endocrine dysfunction
- Altered cognitive and neuropsychological functions
- Speech/communication deficits
- Psychiatric and psychosocial deficits

ADDITIONAL ASSOCIATED PROBLEMS
- Focal neurologic deficits
  - Neurogenic pulmonary edema
  - Pneumonia
  - Gastrointestinal hemorrhage
  - Cardiac dysrhythmias
  - Disseminated intravascular coagulation
  - Pulmonary emboli
  - Heterotopic ossification
  - Increased muscle tone
  - Joint contractures
  - Aspiration
  - Hypertension
  - Disturbances of respiratory control
  - Hypopituitarism
  - Impaired nutritional status
  - Bladder incontinence
  - Bowel incontinence
  - Hyperphagia

From Chipps, E. M., Clanin, N. J., & Campbell, V. G. (1992). *Neurologic disorders.* Mosby.

chart at each health visit. Increasing head circumference in children under 24 months of age might indicate hydrocephalus; however, this is not a reliable indicator of hydrocephalus after the fontanels are closed.

Precocious puberty may be associated with head trauma due to potential disruption of the hypothalamus and pituitary function. Premature sexual characteristics can include isolated breast, axillary, or pubic hair development. Referral to pediatric endocrinology is recommended for more in-depth management.

Severe TBI may affect major milestone attainment or cause regression. Therefore developmental progress should be monitored and community services obtained for physical therapy, occupational therapy, and speech therapy as needed and available.

Nutritional Intake

A child's ability to eat is often an area of focus for a family because of the emotional, social, and cultural values surrounding feeding and nutrition. After severe TBI, children may experience feeding or swallowing difficulties because of oral-motor incoordination, dysphagia, or as the result of posture and upper extremity limitations. These can lead to aspiration or poor weight gain. Placement of a gastrostomy tube with fundoplication if there is significant gastroesophageal reflux may be considered for long-term nutritional management (Jackson et al., 2022). Placing an immobile child in a side-lying position during and after meals can minimize the potential for aspiration or gastroesophageal reflux. Referrals to a gastroenterologist, nutritionist, or psychotherapist may be helpful. A registered dietitian can help guide fluid balance, appropriate caloric intake, and adequate nutrition for growth and wellness. The primary care provider can help a family balance oral and nonoral feedings to simultaneously support nutritional goals.

Safety

As with all pediatric visits, counseling about safety practices and injury prevention for the child's age and developmental level is appropriate. Although it is impossible to prevent all head injuries, it is important to review ways to reduce the risk of TBI. The CDC (2022) discusses interventions such as using appropriate motor vehicle passenger seat restraints; using helmets appropriate for recreational or competitive sports; and childproofing the home, school, and community playgrounds.

Children with a history of TBI are at an increased risk for future injury caused by neuropsychological and neurobehavioral deficits resulting in overactivity, poor judgment, impulsivity, aggression, and perceptual deficits, like children with ADHD. Referrals to an appropriate professional who can effectively manage these behaviors with cognitive-behavioral therapy and psychopharmacologic agents as needed can be effective in keeping these children safe.

Immunizations

Routine immunizations are recommended after TBI. Immunizations can be given when the child's neurologic situation is stabilized. The risk of contracting preventable diseases and immunization side effects should be discussed with the family. Supplemental pneumococcal vaccines (PPV23) should be considered for children under 5 years of age if their respiratory status is significantly compromised (AAP, 2021). Postimmunization fever management with antipyretics is recommended in children with a known seizure history as they may be more susceptible to febrile seizures following the administration of diphtheria, tetanus, and acellular pertussis (AAP, 2021).

Differential Diagnosis

- Alterations in cognition or level of consciousness: Know child's current baseline neurologic status.
  - Alteration in mood: Be proactive in assessing and supporting mental health changes.
- Fever may increase potential for seizures in children with post-TBI seizures.
- Nausea and vomiting may indicate shunt malfunction in children with posttraumatic hydrocephalus. Prolonged or severe vomiting may require aggressive rehydration in children with poor nutritional intake or limited oral-motor skills.
- Respiratory infections pose risk of pneumonia and aspiration in the compromised child.
- Headaches are common after TBI. Headache diaries may help determine frequency, intensity, and efficacy of medication management.

Screenings

Vision. Vision can be adversely affected after a TBI. Children may experience symptoms of double vision, movement of fixed objects such as walls, eyestrain, visual fatigue, conversion insufficiency, accommodative amplitude deficits, and loss of peripheral vision (Master et al., 2016; Storey et al., 2017). A visio-vestibular exam should be performed if a concussion is suspected (Table 39.6). If visual deficits are suspected, a referral to a pediatric ophthalmologist or developmental optometrist should be made. Yearly screening for vision problems is recommended even if deficits are not determined in the immediate postinjury period.

Hearing. Hearing deficits can occur after TBI; the most common sequelae are tinnitus, vestibular dysfunction, intolerance to loud/sudden noises, and sensorineural hearing impairment (Chen et al., 2018; Hwang et al., 2022). A referral to an audiologist should be made if there is a suspicion of a hearing deficit. Routine periodic hearing screening is recommended even if deficits are not determined immediately.

Dental. Routine dental care is recommended. Children with head injuries may have fractured or missing teeth secondary to facial trauma, and a pediatric orthodontist referral would be necessary. Anticonvulsant drugs may cause gingival hyperplasia.

Blood pressure. Routine screening is recommended. Persistently elevated blood pressure should be carefully evaluated, particularly in the presence of an intracranial shunt.

Hematocrit. Routine screening is recommended.

Urinalysis. Routine screening is recommended. Low urine specific gravity may indicate diabetes insipidus, and high specific gravity may suggest SIADH.

Tuberculosis. Routine screening is recommended. If prophylactic medications are needed, evaluate potential drug interactions if the child is taking other medications.

Table 39.6	Visio-Vestibular Exam After Suspected Concussion	
TEST	**DESCRIPTION**	
Pursuit eye movements	Pursuit is examined by holding a near visual stimulus at 1–2 ft from the patient. Move the stimulus back and forth in a slow and steady fashion, horizontally about 160 degrees (from patient's ear to ear) and vertically about 120 degrees (from patient's forehead to chin). Both eyes should follow the stimulus symmetrically and smoothly.	
Saccadic eye movements	Saccades are tested with two near stimuli as above, one in each hand. Hold them about 2 ft apart, 1–2 ft in front of the patient, horizontally then vertically. Ask the patient to refixate between the two stimuli on your command several times horizontally then vertically. The eyes should move quickly and symmetrically and end accurately on the stimulus.	
Vestibulo-ocular reflex (VOR)	VOR is examined while holding the stimulus at 1–2 ft directly in front of the nose. The patient rotates the head horizontally for about 160 degrees (shaking head from side to side) and then vertically for about 120 degrees (nodding head up and down). The eyes should remain on the near stimulus throughout the head movement.	
Near point of convergence	Convergence testing is accomplished by holding a visual stimulus about 2 ft in front of the patient and bringing the stimulus toward the face until the eyes stop converging. The eyes should continue to converge on the stimulus until about 6 cm (~2 in.) from the forehead.	
Accommodative amplitude	Accommodation testing is performed monocularly using a standard reading card. After patching one eye, ask the patient to fixate on the smallest readable letter at about 2 ft away, move the card toward the eye until the patient reports blurring of that same letter, then measure that distance in centimeters. Most children will be able to see the letter clearly until 10 cm (~4 in.) from the eye.	
Strabismus	While the patient fixates on a distant target, the monocular cover-uncover test is performed by covering and uncovering each eye (right eye, then left eye), with the examiner watching carefully for any movement in the opposite, noncovered eye; such movement indicates the possible presence of strabismus.	

From Master, C. L., Bacal, D., Grady, M. F., Hertle, R., Shah, A. S., Strominger, M., Whitecross, S., Bradford, G. E., Lum, F., Donahue, S. P., AAP Section on Ophthalmology, American Academy of Ophthalmology, American Association for Pediatric Ophthalmology and Strabismus, & American Association of Certified Orthoptists. (2022). Vision and concussion: Symptoms, signs, evaluation, and treatment. *Pediatrics, 150*(2), e2021056047.

Condition-Specific Screening

Posttraumatic seizures. Family members and care providers should be knowledgeable about seizure precautions and seizure first aid. For children on anticonvulsant medication, periodic blood testing is necessary to determine medication blood levels and to test for hematologic side effects and liver dysfunction. These tests should be ordered in consultation with the child's neurologist.

Movement and postural problems. A motor evaluation, including assessment for scoliosis, contractures, weakness, and spasticity, should be conducted soon after discharge and annually, especially during periods of rapid height growth. Equipment and subspecialty evaluation might be indicated.

Skin integrity. For children with impaired mobility, sensation, nutrition, or cognitive status, frequent skin checks should be incorporated into daily care and should be included in visits to the primary care provider. It is essential to monitor for pressure areas, intertriginous infection, and skin breakdown. Appropriate equipment and proper fit and maintenance of equipment should also be ensured. This includes equipment used for mobility and items such as gastrostomy tubes, tracheostomies, and urine and stool drainage systems.

COMMON ILLNESS MANAGEMENT

Differential Diagnosis

Like any other child, children with TBI are susceptible to common childhood illnesses; however, the management of these illnesses may differ depending on individual factors.

Alterations in cognition or level of consciousness. Knowledge of the child's baseline neurologic status and behavior is key to accurate assessment. A significant change or deterioration in cognitive function should be viewed as pathologic and assessed further. Trauma, infections, tumors, and metabolic imbalances may cause alterations in arousal or cognition. Their onset may be sudden, subacute over a period of several days, or gradual over several weeks to months.

Alterations in mood. Changes in mood are very common after TBI, and it is imperative to assess and follow each child's psychosocial functioning. There is an emerging body of evidence suggesting that the sequela of TBI in the child comes with a multitude of emotions.

Psychiatric and behavioral problems. This is seen more so in the pediatric population, where childhood brain insult occurs during periods of significant reorganization of neural networks and the development of cognitive function, language, relationships, and social skills (Wearne et al., 2020). It is well known that symptoms of mood changes such as depression and anxiety can mimic other disorders such as headaches, gastrointestinal upset, and sleep disturbances.

Fevers. Fevers are a common occurrence in the presence of viral and bacterial illnesses. Routine fever management is appropriate. In children with a history of seizures, the risk of seizures may increase during a febrile illness.

Nausea and vomiting. Routine management of nausea and vomiting is advised. However, persistent vomiting or development of lethargy should be evaluated urgently in the child with an intracranial shunt.

Respiratory infections. Children with severe neurologic or motor deficits are more prone to pneumonia or chronic aspiration complications. They require early and frequent assessment of respiratory function during periods of acute illness.

Headaches. Posttraumatic headaches can be concerning to the family. A headache diary can be valuable in recording onset, frequency, and associated symptoms. Over-the-counter medications for headaches are generally not recommended due to concerns of rebound headaches. Nonpharmacologic treatment is directed toward the etiology of the headache as a form of treatment. If headaches persist in frequency and severity, further evaluation is recommended by a headache specialist (Dwyer, 2018).

Drug interactions. After a TBI, a child may receive a variety of medications, including antiepileptics, stimulants for behavior, headache prophylaxis, and muscle relaxants for spasticity. If additional medications such as antibiotics are necessary, it is important to consider potential drug interactions. There are several sources for this information, ranging from the pharmacist to the *Physicians' Desk Reference* to online resources such as Epocrates (https://online.epocrates.com).

DEVELOPMENTAL ISSUES

Sleep Patterns

Alterations in sleep patterns can be a challenge after TBI. Sleep disruption can be compounded by multiple stressors that can occur after TBI. Treatment should start with proper sleep hygiene, including a regular bedtime routine that promotes an evening winddown and a sleep period appropriate for age. Other important interventions that can enhance sleep include regular daily exercise, a soothing evening bath or shower to increase relaxation, a dark cool room with no electronics, and adjusting the timing of medication doses to promote sleep. Actions that can inhibit healthy sleep patterns include caffeine (in coffee, tea, or soft drinks), especially in the evening, late-evening exercise, and napping during the day. Cognitive-behavioral therapy may also promote healthy sleep patterns (Ludwig et al., 2020).

Toileting

Bowel and bladder continence may be disrupted after moderate-severe brain injury. These can generally be managed in conjunction with the rehabilitation team. Frequent toileting can help reregulate bowel and bladder control. The first goal is bowel and bladder control during the waking hours, with subsequent training in nighttime continence. Fluid intake should be limited to 2 hours before bedtime. If behavioral strategies are unsuccessful, consider the possibility of kidney disease, damage to the sacral nerves, or deficits in urine concentrating ability (Torelli et al., 2015).

The child who is immobile is prone to constipation and can benefit from anticipatory guidance regarding its prevention and management. These children may require a routine bowel regimen that includes the use of natural or medicated stool softeners, glycerin suppositories, or additional fluid and fiber intake for assisted elimination. It is most helpful to establish a predictable pattern for bowel elimination, such as a warm drink and a sitting period on a commode after the evening meal.

Discipline

Behavior and personality alterations should be anticipated following brain injury. Although it may be difficult to determine how TBI contributes to a child's behavior, the effects of a brain injury should always be included in the differential diagnosis. Behavioral changes commonly seen after brain injury are anger, apathy, anxiety, depression, disinhibition, emotional lability, impaired judgment, and impulsivity (Wearne et al., 2020).

Caregivers should be encouraged to be consistent with discipline and to reinforce normal household rules. Caregivers may have difficulty reinstating previous behavioral expectations after a catastrophic illness or injury. They may require support and encouragement around this area of perceived vulnerability. Persistent behavioral difficulties at home, altered family and peer relationships, disruption of academics, or issues in the use of leisure time can generalize into other settings such as school and the community. This can then interrupt learning and socialization.

More extreme difficulties with behavior and discipline may respond to behavioral therapy techniques. Clear and simple expectations, explained at an appropriate cognitive level, need to consider possible weaknesses in short-term memory and lack of impulse control. Caregivers need to be consistent in their style of discipline and behavior management. As with any behavioral intervention, avoid giving mixed or imprecise descriptions of desired behavior. The parents, care providers, and other family members should model desirable behavior. Pharmacologic management with

stimulants or other psychotropic medications may be considered. These medications are best used in conjunction with cognitive-behavioral therapy.

Child Care

Children who are mildly disabled may be appropriately cared for in a day care or home setting. For children in a day care or preschool setting, an individualized health plan can be useful in communicating medical information with early childhood educators.

Children who are severely disabled and technology dependent may require assisted nursing care in the home or other natural settings. Federal funds from Title XX of the Social Security Act, also known as the Social Services Block Grant (SSBG), are available for respite services, homemaker services, and foster home care. These funds enable each state to meet the needs of its residents through locally relevant social services. SSBGs support programs that allow families to achieve or maintain economic self-sufficiency to prevent, reduce, or eliminate dependency on social services.

Schooling

TBI of any severity can threaten a child's future ability to learn and perform in school. Children who experience a TBI before the age of 3 years are eligible for early intervention services under the Birth to Three Program, which is mandated in the Individuals with Disabilities Education Act (IDEA) of 2004. Early intervention programs are helpful in determining age-appropriate and developmentally enhancing activities. Other aspects of intervention include parent support, education, and training to create an environment that fosters the child's ability to work independently. IDEA also mandates preschool services, which include appropriate therapies for children with TBI if the resulting impairments affect the child's ability to learn.

The return to school represents a critical phase in recovery for all children with TBI. Successful school reentry entails ensuring the student receives the appropriate level of academic support and, if applicable, the student understands what that academic plan entails. Home-based academic tutoring or part-time attendance may initially support the transition back to a school program, especially if there is limited cognitive or physical endurance.

Recommended school reentry support includes (1) establishing communication among all persons caring for the child; (2) initiating an evaluation process, which may include neuropsychological testing; (3) integrating information in an interdisciplinary forum; (4) adapting education programs based on neuropsychological test results to meet the child's needs; (5) preparing the child for transitions; and (6) providing ongoing monitoring for possible late-developing problems. Some states have school reentry programs, such as Pennsylvania's Brain-STEPS. This state-funded program acts as a liaison between the school and the child to ensure the child has the appropriate support structures in place to optimize academic outcomes (Gioia et al., 2016).

Depending on the depth and breadth of persistent deficits, children with TBI can receive rehabilitative services in school. They may be eligible for physical therapy, occupational therapy, and speech-language pathology services for ongoing impairments, behavior management, and counseling as components of an individualized education program (IEP).

Sexuality

Individuals who have sustained a TBI may have altered inhibition or may make socially inappropriate sexualized comments and gestures. These need to be addressed in the broader context of appropriate social behavior. Impairment in motor and sensory function or impaired communication may alter sexual functioning. Social isolation can diminish self-esteem and may contribute to inappropriate sexual behaviors. The onset of precocious puberty may further complicate sexuality.

Concerns about sexuality expressed by the child or adolescent, family, and significant others should be addressed directly and calmly. Weaknesses in impulse control and short-term memory may necessitate repeated conversations about these issues and require emphasis from more than one individual in the child's life, such as caregivers, teachers, counselors, or peer coaches.

Transition to Adulthood

TBI can have a major effect on the subsequent education, vocational development, independent living skills, and future productivity of affected individuals. Supported living programs, supervised housing, shared services, or foster care should be evaluated with respect to the level of assistance required for activities of daily living. Supervised work experiences may be necessary to develop appropriate skills and work habits to succeed in gainful employment and contribute to the community. Health care insurance coverage and financial assistance programs should also be addressed as adolescents enter adulthood.

Family Concerns

The stress of TBI can negatively affect the mental health of the caregivers and undermine parent-child and family relationships. Emerging data in the literature suggest that family dynamics and environmental factors (especially those predating the injury) play a critical role in modeling recovery outcomes after pediatric TBI (Fischer et al., 2022). Parents confront fears about immediate survival, current condition, and long-term needs. While caring for a child with TBI, parents may feel guilty about the incident that caused the TBI and their need to focus time and attention on the injured child, feeling neglectful of the child's siblings. Siblings can experience emotional disturbances, school problems, and aggression, as well as a sense of guilt about experiencing a sense of relief that the injury happened to their brother or sister and not to them. It is helpful for all family members to become actively involved in the day-to-day care of the injured child; this will reduce their sense of helplessness and support the growth of the family unit (Fischer et al., 2022). TBI support groups for parents and siblings can offer reassurance and support to enhance coping.

Significant financial issues due to medical bills, changes in employment status due to care responsibilities, or conflict related to the parents' return to work may arise, adding to a family's stress. There might be anger if one parent was present at the time of the injury, such as driving the car in a motor vehicle crash (MVC). Additionally, there may be disability or death of a parent as a result of the MVC. Long-term family support and counseling can be extremely helpful. Families who seek support and work to cope with the situation may experience less stress and family dysfunction over time (Fischer et al., 2022).

Caregivers of children with the most severe sequela and the greatest unmet needs report the most significant family burden (Erlick et al., 2021). To help these families overcome such challenges, including significant financial and emotional burdens, a collaborative effort is necessary to help facilitate the transition seamlessly from acute care through long-term rehabilitation (Popernack et al., 2015). This collaboration starts with the acute care providers, transitions to the rehab providers, and continues to the primary care providers, who often play a key role in helping locate comprehensive care services that are congruent with the child and family's needs. Primary care providers can facilitate the family's coping with the injury and help in setting attainable goals for recovery (Erlick et al., 2021).

Caring for a child with TBI is a complex task because of the physical, cognitive, and psychosocial concerns that must be addressed. A multidisciplinary team is the best practice to address all the complexities these patients need. The nurse practitioner needs to know the resources available to support these needs (Peacock & Hernandez, 2020) (see Resources, later).

RESOURCES

American Association of Neurologic Surgeons: http://www.aans.org

American Congress of Rehabilitation Medicine: http://www.acrm.org

Association of Rehabilitation Nurses: http://www.rehabnurse.org

Brain Injury Association of America: https://www.biausa.org

Centers for Disease Control and Prevention: http://www.cdc.gov/TraumaticBrainInjury/data/index.html

Family Caregiver Alliance: http://www.caregiver.org

National Center on Shaken Baby Syndrome: http://www.dontshake.org

Rancho Los Amigos Scale: https://www.neuroskills.com/education-and-resources/rancho-los-amigos-revised

Summary

Primary Care Needs for the Child With a Traumatic Brain Injury

HEALTH CARE MAINTENANCE
Growth and Development

- Height and weight should be measured and plotted on growth charts for all children. Head circumference should be monitored at each visit until the fontanels are closed, at approximately 2 years of age.
- Monitor for pubertal development and for signs of precocious puberty and short stature.
- Screen and assess developmental, cognitive, and motor skills regularly. Monitor therapy intervention programs.
- Evaluate school and social functioning.

Nutritional Intake

- Eating and feeding problems can contribute to poor growth patterns.
- Decreased physical activity and immobility may lead to excessive weight gain. Tailor intake to meet the child's nutritional needs.
- Decreased physical activity and immobility may contribute to loss of bone calcium and osteopenia. Monitor dietary calcium intake and encourage weightbearing in physical therapy and recreational activities.
- Monitor protective reflexes (i.e., gag) to minimize risk of aspiration.
- Occupational therapy or speech therapy can assist with safe and optimal feeding programs.

Safety

- Increased risk of falls is present because of instability, poor coordination, potential seizures, and delays in motor skill acquisition.
- Provide anticipatory guidance on general safety precautions.
- Review emergency seizure procedures.
- Evaluate desirability of participating in risk-taking sports and activities. Ensure the use of proper protective equipment.
- Evaluate adolescents' cognition, attention, and neuromuscular status. Counsel on driving or use of motorized vehicles.

Immunizations

- Routine immunizations are recommended.
- Children with posttraumatic seizures may be at increased seizure risk.
- Fever prophylaxis with acetaminophen or ibuprofen is recommended.

Mental Health

- TBI is a significant risk factor for alterations in mood.
- Cognitive-behavioral therapy and counseling can help optimize neuropsychological outcomes.
- Routine screening by the primary care provider is recommended.

Screening

- *Vision.* Complete postinjury evaluation during the recovery period, with correction of minor deficits. Yearly screening is recommended.
- *Hearing.* Complete postinjury evaluation for hearing and vestibular deficits during the recovery period. Refer for correction of minor deficits.
- *Dental.* Routine screening.
  - Evaluate for possible dental trauma after a head injury.
  - More frequent evaluations may be necessary for children on seizure medications.
- *Blood pressure.* Monitor with each visit.
- *Hematocrit.* Routine screening is recommended.
- *Urinalysis.* Routine screening is recommended, including specific gravity for diabetes insipidus and SIADH.
- *Tuberculosis.* Routine screening is recommended. If prophylactic medications are needed, evaluate potential drug interactions in children receiving other medications.

Condition-Specific Screening

- *Posttraumatic seizure therapy.* Monitor complete blood count and chemistry panels along with anticonvulsant levels for the first 6 months after injury and periodically thereafter.
- *Movement and postural problems.* Assess for scoliosis, contractures, weakness, and spasticity, especially during growth spurts.
  - Ensure access to appropriate assistive devices.
- *Skin integrity.* Examine skin for pressure areas, breakdown, and signs of superficial infection.

LONG-TERM CARE MANAGEMENT
Differential Diagnosis

- A thorough knowledge of baseline neurologic status and behavior is key in assessing significance of deviations.
- Risk of seizures is increased with acute illness and fever.
- Consider the potential for increased ICP in the presence of an intracranial shunt with signs of nausea and vomiting.
- Evaluation of headaches requires careful history, neurologic examination, and symptom management.

Drug Interactions

- Potential drug interactions can occur if the child is taking epileptic drugs, stimulants for behavior, headache prophylaxis, and/or muscle relaxants for spasticity. Careful monitoring is required.

DEVELOPMENTAL ISSUES
Sleep Patterns

- Disruption in sleep patterns may occur. A structured sleep hygiene routine is recommended.

Toileting

- Bowel and bladder continence may be delayed in younger children or disrupted in older children who previously had voluntary control. A progressive training program with positive reinforcement will help reestablish control as cognition improves.
- Monitor for and manage chronic constipation.

Discipline

- Anticipate alterations in behavior and personality and institute early support and guidance. Recommend standard developmentally appropriate discipline with reinforcement of usual household rules.
- Manage persistent difficulties with behavior modification and discipline. Evaluation by a behavior specialist may be warranted.
- Anxiety, depression, and emotional lability may require mental health referral.

Child Care

- Assistance in identifying and accessing community respite care services for children with severe TBI is a priority area.

Schooling

- Birth to Three Program referral for assessment and intervention is recommended.
- Cognitive changes may persist from weeks to many months following head trauma.
- Fully assess learning needs and individualize approaches as soon as feasible after the injury.

- Children with significant TBI sequelae are eligible for special education. Families may require assistance with the IEP process.
- If formal neuropsychological and school performance testing is needed, the local school district must provide it.

Sexuality

- Monitor for precocious or delayed puberty. Refer to endocrinologist if these are present.
- Impairment in communication, motor, and sensory function or impaired behavioral self-regulation may alter sexual functioning. Anticipatory guidance in counselling is advised.

Transition to Adulthood

- TBI can have a major effect on the future education, vocational development, and independent living skills of the affected adolescent. School guidance and vocational counseling are essential.
- Establish working relationships with local adult primary care providers and subspecialists.

Family Concerns

- Severe stresses on the family unit arise following a head injury. Support groups or family counseling for parents and siblings may be helpful.
- Comprehensive care that is congruent with and respectful toward the child's and family's cultural background is a key element for successful coping.

REFERENCES

Acabchuk, R. L., Brisson, J. M., Park, C. L., Babbott-Bryan, N., Parmelee, O. A., & Johnson, B. T. (2021). Therapeutic effects of meditation, yoga, and mindfulness-based interventions for chronic symptoms of mild traumatic brain injury: A systematic review and meta-analysis. *Applied Psychology: Health and Well-Being, 13*(1), 34–62. doi: 10.1111/aphw.12244.

Adepoju, A., & Adamo, M. A. (2017). Posttraumatic complications in pediatric skull fracture: Dural sinus thrombosis, arterial dissection, and cerebrospinal fluid leakage. *Journal of Neurosurgery: Pediatrics, 20*(6), 598–603.

Angelova, P., Kehayov, I., Davarski, A., & Kitov, B. (2021). Contemporary insight into diffuse axonal injury. *Folia Medica, 63*(2), 163–170. https://doi.org/10.3897/folmed.63.e53709.

American Academy of Pediatrics. (2021). *Red book report of the Committee on Infectious Diseases* (32nd ed.). Author.

American Academy of Pediatrics & American Academy of Family Physicians. (1999). The management of minor closed head injury in children. *Pediatrics, 104*(6), 1407–1415.

American Speech-Language Hearing Association. Pediatric traumatic brain injury (Practice Portal). Available at: https://www.asha.org/PRPSpecificTopic.aspx?folderid=85 89942939&section=Treatment#Treatment_Options. Accessed December 26, 2022.

Araki, T., Yokota, H., & Morita, A. (2017). Pediatric traumatic brain injury: Characteristic features, diagnosis, and management. *Neurologia Medico-Chirurgica (Tokyo), 57*(2), 82–93.

Arbogast, K. B., Curry, A. E., Pfeiffer, M. R., Zonfrillo, M. R., Haarbauer-Krupa, J., Breiding, M. J., Coronado, V. G., & Master, C. L. (2016). Point of health care entry for youth with concussion within a large pediatric care network. *JAMA Pediatrics, 170*(7), e160294. https://doi.org/10.1001/jamapediatrics.2016.0294.

Arrey, E. N., Kerr, M. L., Fletcher, S., Cox, C. S., Jr, & Sandberg, D. I. (2015). Linear nondisplaced skull fractures in children: who should be observed or admitted? *Journal of Neurosurgery:*

Pediatrics, 16(6), 703–708. https://doi.org/10.3171/2015.4.PEDS1545.

Babl, F. E., Borland, M. L., Phillips, N., Kochar, A., Dalton, S., McCaskill, M., Cheek, J. A., Gilhotra, Y., Furyk, J., Neutze, J., Lyttle, M. D., Bressan, S., Donath, S., Molesworth, C., Jachno, K., Ward, B., Williams, A., Baylis, A., Crowe, L., Oakley, E., ... Paediatric Research in Emergency Departments International Collaborative (PREDICT) (2017a). Accuracy of PECARN, CATCH, and CHALICE head injury decision rules in children: a prospective cohort study. *Lancet, 389*(10087), 2393–2402. https://doi.org/10.1016/S0140-6736(17)30555-X.

Babl, F. E., Dionisio, D., Davenport, L., Baylis, A., Hearps, S. J. C., Bressan, S., Thompson, E. J., Anderson, V., Oakley, E., & Davis, G. A. (2017b). Accuracy of Components of SCAT to Identify Children With Concussion. *Pediatrics, 140*(2), e20163258. https://doi.org/10.1542/peds.2016-3258.

Beers, S. R., Wisniewski, S. R., Garcia-Filion, P., Tian, Y., Hahner, T., Berger, R. P., Bell, M. J., & Adelson, P. D. (2012). Validity of a pediatric version of the Glasgow Outcome Scale-Extended. *Journal of Neurotrauma, 29*(6), 1126–1139. https://doi.org/10.1089/neu.2011.2272.

Birg, T., Ortolano, F., Wiegers, E. J. A., Smielewski, P., Savchenko, Y., Ianosi, B. A., Helbok, R., Rossi, S., Carbonara, M., Zoerle, T., & Stocchetti, N.; CENTER-TBI Investigators and Participants. (2021). Brain temperature influences intracranial pressure and cerebral perfusion pressure after traumatic brain injury: A CENTER-TBI study. *Neurocritical Care, 35*(3), 651–661.

Caliendo, E. T., Kim, N., Edasery, D., Askin, G., Nowak, S., Gerber, L. M., Baum, K. T., Blackwell, L. S., Koterba, C. H., Hoskinson, K. R., Kurowski, B. G., McLaughlin, M., Tlustos, S. J., Watson, W. D., Niogi, S. N., Suskauer, S. J., & Shah, S. A. (2021). Acute imaging findings predict recovery of cognitive and motor function after inpatient rehabilitation for pediatric traumatic brain injury: A pediatric brain injury consortium study. *Journal of Neurotrauma, 38*(14), 1961–1968. https://doi.org/10.1089/neu.2020.7437.

Cao, S., Li, M., Sun, Y., Wu, P., Yang, W., Dai, H., Guo, Y., Ye, Y., Wang, Z., Xie, X., Chen, X., & Liang, W. (2022). Intermittent fasting enhances hippocampal NPY expression to promote neurogenesis after traumatic brain injury. *Nutrition, 97,* 111621. https://doi.org/10.1016/j.nut.2022.111621.

Carlson, A. P., Hänggi, D., Macdonald, R. L., & Shuttleworth, C. W. (2020). Nimodipine reappraised: An old drug with a future. *Current Neuropharmacology, 18*(1), 65–82.

Carney, N., Totten, A. M., O'Reilly, C., Ullman, J. S., Hawryluk, G. W., Bell, M. J., Bratton, S. L., Chesnut, R., Harris, O. A., Kissoon, N., Rubiano, A. M., Shutter, L., Tasker, R. C., Vavilala, M. S., Wilberger, J., Wright, D. W., & Ghajar, J. (2017). Guidelines for the management of severe traumatic brain injury, fourth edition. *Neurosurgery, 80*(1), 6–15. https://doi.org/10.1227/NEU.0000000000001432.

Centers for Disease Control and Prevention, National Center for Injury Prevention and Control. (2015). *Report to Congress on traumatic brain injury in the United States: Epidemiology and rehabilitation.* Author.

Centers for Disease Control and Prevention, National Center for Injury Prevention and Control. (2019). Heads Up. Accessed 2022, https://www.cdc.gov/headsup/basics/concussion_symptoms.html.

Centers for Disease Control and Prevention. National Center for Health Statistics. (2023). Mortality data on CDC WONDER. Accessed 2022, https://wonder.cdc.gov/mcd.html.

Centers for Disease Control and Prevention. (2018). Report to Congress: The management of traumatic brain injury in children, National Center for Injury Prevention and Control; Division of Unintentional Injury Prevention. Atlanta, GA.

Chen, I. C., Duh, M. C., Jaw, T. S., Liu, Y. C., Wu, Y. H., Yin, H. L., & Hsu, J. H. (2022). Experience with outreach services of a multidisciplinary team for child abuse identification. *Journal of the Formosan Medical Association, 121*(6), 1111–1116. https://doi.org/10.1016/j.jfma.2021.08.026.

Chen, J. X., Lindeborg, M., Herman, S. D., Ishai, R., Knoll, R. M., Remenschneider, A., Jung, D. H., & Kozin, E. D. (2018). Systematic review of hearing loss after traumatic brain injury without associated temporal bone fracture. *American Journal of Otolaryngology, 39*(3), 338–344. https://doi.org/10.1016/j.amjoto.2018.01.018.

Chevignard, M., Câmara-Costa, H., & Dellatolas, G. (2020). Pediatric traumatic brain injury and abusive head trauma. *Handbook of Clinical Neurology, 173,* 451–484.

Choudhary, A. K., Servaes, S., Slovis, T. L., Palusci, V. J., Hedlund, G. L., Narang, S. K., Moreno, J. A., Dias, M. S., Christian, C. W., Nelson, M. D., Jr Silvera, V. M., Palasis, S., Raissaki, M., Rossi, A., & Offiah, A. C. (2018). Consensus statement on abusive head trauma in infants and young children. *Pediatric Radiology, 48*(8), 1048–1065. https://doi.org/10.1007/s00247-018-4149-1.

Christian, C. W. Committee on Child Abuse and Neglect, American Academy of Pediatrics. (2015). The evaluation of suspected child physical abuse. *Pediatrics, 135*(5), e1337–e1354.

Corwin, D. J., Propert, K. J., Zorc, J. J., Zonfrillo, M. R., & Wiebe, D. J. (2019). Use of the vestibular and oculomotor examination for concussion in a pediatric emergency department. *The American Journal of Emergency Medicine, 37*(7), 1219–1223. https://doi.org/10.1016/j.ajem.2018.09.008.

Cremonini, C., Lewis, M., Wong, M. D., et al. (2020). Traumatic epidural hematomas in the pediatric population: Clinical characteristics and diagnostic pitfalls. *Journal of Pediatric Surgery, 55*(9), 1773–1778.

Curry, A. E., Arbogast, K. B., Metzger, K. B., Kessler, R. S., Breiding, M. J., Haarbauer-Krupa, J., DePadilla, L., Greenspan, A., & Master, C. L. (2019). Risk of repeat concussion among patients diagnosed at a pediatric care network. *Journal of Pediatrics, 210,* 13–19.

Dadas, A., Washington, J., Diaz-Arrastia, R., & Janigro, D. (2018). Biomarkers in traumatic brain injury (TBI): A review. *Neuropsychiatric Disease and Treatment, 14,* 2989–3000. https://doi.org/10.2147/NDT.S125620.

Dassa, Y., Crosnier, H., Chevignard, M., Viaud, M., Personnier, C., Flechtner, I., Meyer, P., Puget, S., Boddaert, N., Breton, S., & Polak, M. (2019). Pituitary deficiency and precocious puberty after childhood severe traumatic brain injury: A long-term follow-up prospective study. *European Journal of Endocrinology, 180*(5), 281–290. https://doi.org/10.1001/jamapediatrics.2016.0294.

Dewan, M. C., Mummareddy, N., Wellons, J. C., 3rd, & Bonfield, C. M. (2016). Epidemiology of global pediatric traumatic brain injury: Qualitative review. *World Neurosurgery, 91,* 497–509.e1. https://doi.org/10.1016/j.wneu.2016.03.045.

Dewan, M. C., Rattani, A., Gupta, S., Baticulon, R. E., Hung, Y. C., Punchak, M., Agrawal, A., Adeleye, A. O., Shrime, M. G., Rubiano, A. M., Rosenfeld, J. V., & Park, K. B. (2018). Estimating the global incidence of traumatic brain injury. *Journal of Neurosurgery, 130*(4), 1080–1097. https://doi.org/10.3171/2017.10.JNS17352.

Donnelly, K. Z., Baker, K., Pierce, R., St Ivany, A. R., Barr, P. J., & Bruce, M. L. (2021). A retrospective study on the acceptability, feasibility, and effectiveness of LoveYourBrain Yoga for people with traumatic brain injury and caregivers. *Disability and Rehabilitation, 43*(12), 1764–1775. https://doi.org/10.1080/09638288.2019.1672109.

Drosos, E., Giakoumettis, D., Blionas, A., Mitsios, A., Sfakianos, G., & Themistocleous, M. (2018). Pediatric nonmissile penetrating head injury: Case series and literature review. *World Neurosurgery, 110,* 193–205. doi: 10.1016/j.wneu.2017.11.037.

Dwyer, B. (2018). Posttraumatic headache. *Seminars in Neurology, 38*(6), 619–626.

Duhaime, A. C., & Christian, CW. (2019). Abusive head trauma: Evidence, obfuscation, and informed management. *Journal of Neurosurgery: Pediatrics, 24*(5), 481–488.

Durish, C. L., Yeates, K. O., Stancin, T., Taylor, H. G., Walz, N. C., & Wade, S. L. (2018). Home environment as a predictor of long-term executive functioning following early childhood traumatic brain injury. *Journal of the International Neuropsychological Society, 24*(1), 11–21. https://doi.org/10.1017/S1355617717000595.

Eapen, B. C., Allred, D. B., O'Rourke, J., & Cifu, D. X. (2015). Rehabilitation of moderate-to-severe traumatic brain injury. *Seminars in Neurology, 35*(1), e1–e3.

Elkind, J. A., Lim, M. M., Johnson, B. N., Palmer, C. P., Putnam, B. J., Kirschen, M. P., & Cohen, A. S. (2015). Efficacy, dosage, and duration of action of branched chain amino Acid therapy for traumatic brain injury. *Frontiers in Neurology, 6,* 73. https://doi.org/10.3389/fneur.2015.00073.

Elsamadicy, A. A., Koo, A. B., David, W. B., Lee, V., Zogg, C. K., Kundishora, A. J., Hong, C., Reeves, B. C., Sarkozy, M., Kahle, K. T., & DiLuna, M. (2021). Post-traumatic seizures following pediatric traumatic brain injury. *Clinical Neurology and Neurosurgery, 203,* 106556. https://doi.org/10.1016/j.clineuro.2021.106556.

Engelhardt, J., Brauge, D., & Loiseau, H. (2021). Second impact syndrome. Myth or reality? *Neurochirurgie, 67*(3), 265–275.

Erlick, M. R., Vavilala, M. S., Jaffe, K. M., Blayney, C. B., & Moore, M. (2021). Provider perspectives on early psychosocial interventions after pediatric severe traumatic brain injury: An implementation framework. *Journal of Neurotrauma, 38*(4), 513–518. https://doi.org/10.1089/neu.2020.7323.

Evans, E., Cook, N. E., Iverson, G. L., Townsend, E. L., Duhaime, A. C., & TRACK-TBI Investigators (2020). Monitoring outcome after hospital-presenting milder spectrum pediatric traumatic brain injury using the glasgow outcome scale-extended, pediatric revision. *Journal of Neurotrauma, 37*(14), 1627–1636. https://doi.org/10.1089/neu.2019.6893.

Ewing-Cobbs, L., Montroy, J. J., & Clark, A. E. (2021). As time goes by: Understanding child and family factors shaping behavioral outcomes after traumatic brain injury. *Frontiers in Neurology, 12*, 687740.

Fischer, J. T., Bickart, K. C., Giza, C., & Babikian, T. (2022). A review of family environment and neurobehavioral outcomes following pediatric traumatic brain injury: Implications of early adverse experiences, family stress, and limbic development. *Biological Psychiatry, 91*(5), 488–497. https://doi.org/10.1016/j.biopsych.2021.08.012.

Fox, S. M., Koons, P., & Dang, SH. (2019). Vision rehabilitation after traumatic brain injury. *Physical Medicine and Rehabilitation Clinics of North America, 30*(1), 171–188.

Gallaway, M., Scheiman, M., & Mitchell, GL. (2017). Vision therapy for post-concussion vision disorders. *Optometry and Vision Science, 94*(1), 68–73.

Gambacorta, A., Moro, M., Curatola, A., Brancato, F., Covino, M., Chiaretti, A., & Gatto, A. (2022). PECARN Rule in diagnostic process of pediatric patients with minor head trauma in emergency department. *European Journal of Pediatrics, 181*(5), 2147–2154. https://doi.org/10.1007/s00431-022-04424-9.

Gelineau-Morel, R. N., Zinkus, T. P., & Le Pichon, J. B. (2019). Pediatric head trauma: A review and update. *Pediatrics Reviews, 40*(9), 468–481.

Gerald, B., Ortiz, J. B., Green, T. R. F., Brown, S. D., Adelson, P. D., Murphy, S. M., & Rowe, R. K. (2022). Traumatic brain injury characteristics predictive of subsequent sleep-wake disturbances in pediatric patients. *Biology, 11*(4), 600. https://doi.org/10.3390/biology11040600.

Gioia, G. A., Glang, A. E., Hooper, S. R., & Brown, BE. (2016). Building statewide infrastructure for the academic support of students with mild traumatic brain injury. *Journal of Head Trauma Rehabilitation, 31*(6), 397–406.

Giza, C., & Hovda, D. (2001). The neurometabolic cascade of concussion. *Journal of Athletic Training, 36*(3), 228–235.

Gornall, A., Takagi, M., Clarke, C., Babl, F. E., Davis, G. A., Dunne, K., Anderson, N., Hearps, S. J. C., Demaneuf, T., Rausa, V., & Anderson, V. (2020). Behavioral and emotional difficulties after pediatric concussion. *Journal of Neurotrauma, 37*(1), 163–169. https://doi.org/10.1089/neu.2018.6235.

Graves, J. M., Rivara, F. P., & Vavilala, MS. (2015). Health care costs 1 year after pediatric traumatic brain injury. *American Journal of Public Health, 105*(10), e35–e41.

Griswold, D. P., Fernandez, L., & Rubiano, AM. (2022). Traumatic subarachnoid hemorrhage: A scoping review. *Journal of Neurotrauma, 39*(1-2), 35–48. doi:10.1089/neu.2021.0007.

Guilliams, K., & Wainwright, MS. (2016). Pathophysiology and management of moderate and severe traumatic brain injury in children. *Journal of Child Neurology, 31*(1), 35–45.

Halstead, M. E., Walter, K. D., & Moffatt, K. (2018). Sport-related concussion in children and adolescents. *Pediatrics, 142*(6), e20183074.

Hansen, G., McDonald, P. J., Martin, D., & Vallance, JK. (2018). Pre-trauma center management of intracranial pressure in severe pediatric traumatic brain injury. *Pediatric Emergency Care, 34*(5), 330–333.

Howlett, J. R., Nelson, L. D., & Stein, MB. (2022). Mental health consequences of traumatic brain injury. *Biological Psychiatry, 91*(5), 413–420.

Hussain, E. (2018). Traumatic brain injury in the pediatric intensive care unit. *Pediatric Annals, 47*(7), e274–e279.

Hwang, P. H., Nelson, L. D., & Sharon, J. D. TRACK-TBI Investigators. (2022). Association between TBI-related hearing impairment and cognition: A TRACK-TBI study. *Journal of Head Trauma Rehabilitation, 37*(5), E327–E335.

Ip, S. S., Zafar, S., Liu, T. Y. A., Srikumaran, D., Repka, M. X., Goldstein, M. A., & Woreta, F. A. (2020). Nonaccidental trauma in pediatric patients: evidence-based screening criteria for ophthalmologic examination. *Journal of American Association for Pediatric Ophthalmology and Strabismus, 24*(4), 226.e1–226.e5. https://doi.org/10.1016/j.jaapos.2020.03.012.

Jackson, J. E., Theodorou, C. M., Vukcevich, O., Brown, E. G., & Beres, A. L. (2022). Patient selection for pediatric gastrostomy tubes: Are we placing tubes that are not being used? *Journal of Pediatric Surgery, 57*(3), 532–537. https://doi.org/10.1016/j.jpedsurg.2021.06.001.

Jha, R. M., & Kochanek, PM. (2018). A precision medicine approach to cerebral edema and intracranial hypertension after severe traumatic brain injury: Quo vadis? *Current Neurology and Neuroscience Reports, 18*(12), 105.

Johnson-Greene, D. (2018). Clinical neuropsychology in integrated rehabilitation care teams. *Archives of Clinical Neuropsychology, 33*(3), 310–318.

Johnson, U., & Ivarsson, A. (2011). Psychological predictors of sport injuries among junior soccer players. *Scandinavian Journal of Medicine & Science in Sports, 21*(1), 129–36. doi:10.1111/j.1600-0838.2009.01057.x.

Joseph, M., & Paul, A. (2021). Emergency department assessment and management of pediatric acute mild traumatic brain injury and concussion. *Pediatric Emergency Medicine Practice, 18*(6), 1–28.

Kamins, J., Bigler, E., Covassin, T., Henry, L., Kemp, S., Leddy, J. J., Mayer, A., McCrea, M., Prins, M., Schneider, K. J., Valovich McLeod, T. C., Zemek, R., & Giza, C. C. (2017). What is the physiological time to recovery after concussion? A systematic review. *British Journal of Sports Medicine, 51*(12), 935–940. https://doi.org/10.1136/bjsports-2016-097464.

Kazl, C., & Torres, A. (2019). Definition, classification, and epidemiology of concussion. *Seminars in Pediatric Neurology, 30*, 9–13.

Kent, M., Brilliant, A., Erickson, K., Meehan, W., & Howell, D. (2020). Symptom presentation after concussion and pre-existing anxiety among youth athletes. *International Journal of Sports Medicine, 41*(10), 682–687. https://doi.org/10.1055/a-1107-3025.

Kirschen, M. P., Snyder, M., Smith, K., Lourie, K., Agarwal, K., DiDonato, P., Doll, A., Zhang, B., Mensinger, J., Ichord, R., Shea, J. A., Berg, R. A., Nadkarni, V., & Topjian, A. (2019). Inter-rater reliability between critical care nurses performing a pediatric modification to the glasgow coma scale. *Pediatric Critical Care Medicine, 20*(7), 660–666. https://doi.org/10.1097/PCC.0000000000001938.

Kochanek, P. M., Tasker, R. C., Bell, M. J., Adelson, P. D., Carney, N., Vavilala, M. S., Selden, N. R., Bratton, S. L., Grant, G. A., Kissoon, N., Reuter-Rice, K. E., & Wainwright, M. S. (2019). Management of pediatric severe traumatic brain injury: 2019 consensus and guidelines-based algorithm for first and second tier therapies. *Pediatric Critical Care Medicine, 20*(3), 269–279. https://doi.org/10.1097/PCC.0000000000001737.

Köksal, V., Karkucak, A., & Yalçinkaya, M. (2020). Surgical treatment of a child with acute cortical blindness caused by depressed skull fracture. *Journal of Craniofacial Surgery, 31*(7), e732–e735.

Kontos, A. P., Elbin, R. J., Trbovich, A., Womble, M., Said, A., Sumrok, V. F., French, J., Kegel, N., Puskar, A., Sherry, N., Holland, C., & Collins, M. (2020a). Concussion clinical profiles screening (cp screen) tool: Preliminary evidence to inform a multidisciplinary approach. *Neurosurgery, 87*(2), 348–356. https://doi.org/10.1093/neuros/nyz545.

Kontos, A. P., Jorgensen-Wagers, K., Trbovich, A. M., Ernst, N., Emami, K., Gillie, B., French, J., Holland, C., Elbin, R. J., & Collins, M. W. (2020b). Association of time since injury to the first clinic visit with recovery following concussion. *JAMA Neurology, 77*(4), 435–440. https://doi.org/10.1001/jamaneurol.2019.4552.

Krahulik, D., Aleksijevic, D., Smolka, V., Klaskova, E., Venhacova, P., Vaverka, M., Mihal, V., & Zapletalova, J. (2017). Prospective study of hypothalamo-hypophyseal dysfunction in children and adolescents following traumatic brain injury. *Biomedical Papers of the Medical Faculty of the University Palacky, Olomouc, Czechoslovakia, 161*(1), 80–85. https://doi.org/10.5507/bp.2016.047.

Kuehn, B. (2018). Lasting effects of childhood TBI. *JAMA, 319*(14), 1428. doi:10.1001/jama.2018.3167.

Kuppermann, N., Holmes, J. F., Dayan, P. S., Hoyle, J. D., Jr, Atabaki, S. M., Holubkov, R., Nadel, F. M., Monroe, D., Stanley, R. M., Borgialli, D. A., Badawy, M. K., Schunk, J. E., Quayle, K. S., Mahajan, P., Lichenstein, R., Lillis, K. A., Tunik, M. G., Jacobs, E. S., Callahan, J. M., Gorelick, M. H., … Pediatric Emergency Care Applied Research Network (PECARN) (2009). Identification of children at very low risk of clinically-important brain injuries after head trauma: A prospective cohort study. *Lancet, 374*(9696), 1160–1170. https://doi.org/10.1016/S0140-6736(09)61558-0.

Laane, S. A., & Cook, LG. (2020). Cognitive-communication interventions for youth with traumatic brain injury. *Seminars in Speech and Language, 41*(2), 183–194.

Lang, S. S., Kilbaugh, T., Friess, S., Sotardi, S., Kim, C. T., Mazandi, V., Zhang, B., Storm, P. B., Heuer, G. G., Tucker, A., Ampah, S. B., Griffis, H., Raghupathi, R., & Huh, J. W. (2021). Trajectory of long-term outcome in severe pediatric diffuse axonal injury: An exploratory study. *Frontiers in Neurology, 12*, 704576. https://doi.org/10.3389/fneur.2021.704576.

Lazaridis, C., Rusin, C. G., & Robertson, CS. (2019). Secondary brain injury: Predicting and preventing insults. *Neuropharmacology, 145*(Pt B), 145–152.

Lengel, D., Sevilla, C., Romm, Z. L., Huh, J. W., & Raghupathi, R. (2020). Stem cell therapy for pediatric traumatic brain injury. *Frontiers in Neurology, 11*, 601286.

Leddy, J. J., Haider, M. N., Ellis, M. J., Mannix, R., Darling, S. R., Freitas, M. S., Suffoletto, H. N., Leiter, J., Cordingley, D. M., & Willer, B. (2019). Early subthreshold aerobic exercise for sport-related concussion: A randomized clinical trial. *JAMA Pediatrics, 173*(4), 319–325. https://doi.org/10.1001/jamapediatrics.2018.4397.

Leddy, J. J., Haider, M. N., Noble, J. M., Rieger, B., Flanagan, S., McPherson, J. I., Shubin-Stein, K., Saleem, G. T., Corsaro, L., & Willer, B. (2021). Management of concussion and persistent post-concussive symptoms for neurologists. *Current Neurology and Neuroscience Reports, 21*(12), 72. https://doi.org/10.1007/s11910-021-01160-9.

Lima Santos, J. P., Kontos, A. P., Mailliard, S., Eagle, S. R., Holland, C. L., Suss, S. J., Jr, Abdul-Waalee, H., Stiffler, R. S., Bitzer, H. B., Blaney, N. A., Colorito, A. T., Santucci, C. G., Brown, A., Kim, T., Iyengar, S., Skeba, A., Diler, R. S., Ladouceur, C. D., Phillips, M. L., Brent, D., … Versace, A. (2021). White matter abnormalities associated with prolonged recovery in adolescents following concussion. *Frontiers in Neurology, 12*, 681467. https://doi.org/10.3389/fneur.2021.681467.

Lin, K., & Wroten, M. (2022). *Ranchos Los Amigos*. StatPearls Publishing.

Liou, Y. J., Wei, H. T., Chen, M. H., Hsu, J. W., Huang, K. L., Bai, Y. M., Su, T. P., Li, C. T., Yang, A. C., Tsai, S. J., Lin, W. C., & Chen, TJ. (2018). Risk of traumatic brain injury among children, adolescents, and young adults with attention-deficit hyperactivity disorder in Taiwan. *Journal of Adolescent Health, 63*(2), 233–238.

Listo, I., Salmi, H., Hästbacka, M., Lääperi, M., Oulasvirta, J., Etelälahti, T., Kuisma, M., & Harve-Rytsälä, H. (2021). Pediatric traumas and neighborhood socioeconomic characteristics: A population based study. *Journal of Pediatric Surgery, 56*(4), 760–767. https://doi.org/10.1016/j.jpedsurg.2020.05.040.

Lu, V. M., Hernandez, N., & Wang, S. (2022). National characteristics, etiology, and inpatient outcomes of pediatric traumatic brain injury: A KID study. *Child's Nervous System.*

Lucke-Wold, B. P., Logsdon, A. F., Nguyen, L., Eltanahay, A., Turner, R. C., Bonasso, P., Knotts, C., Moeck, A., Maroon, J. C., Bailes, J. E., & Rosen, C. L. (2018). Supplements, nutrition, and alternative therapies for the treatment of traumatic brain injury. *Nutritional Neuroscience, 21*(2), 79–91. https://doi.org/10.1080/1028415X.2016.1236174.

Ludwig, R., Vaduvathiriyan, P., & Siengsukon, C. (2020). Does cognitive-behavioral therapy improve sleep outcomes in individuals with traumatic brain injury: A scoping review. *Brain Injury, 34*(12), 1569–1578.

Lumba-Brown, A., Yeates, K. O., Sarmiento, K., Breiding, M. J., Haegerich, T. M., Gioia, G. A., Turner, M., Benzel, E. C., Suskauer, S. J., Giza, C. C., Joseph, M., Broomand, C., Weissman, B., Gordon, W., Wright, D. W., Moser, R. S., McAvoy, K., Ewing-Cobbs, L., Duhaime, A. C., Putukian, M., … Timmons, S. D. (2018). Centers for Disease Control and Prevention Guideline on the diagnosis and management of mild traumatic brain injury among children. *JAMA Pediatrics, 172*(11), e182853. https://doi.org/10.1001/jamapediatrics.2018.2853.

Macnow, T., Curran, T., Tolliday, C., Martin, K., McCarthy, M., Ayturk, D., Babu, K. M., & Mannix, R. (2021). Effect of screen time on recovery from concussion: A randomized clinical trial. *JAMA Pediatrics, 175*(11), 1124–1131. https://doi.org/10.1001/jamapediatrics.2021.2782.

Marklund, N., Bellander, B. M., Godbolt, A. K., Levin, H., McCrory, P., & Thelin, E. P. (2019). Treatments and rehabilitation in the acute and chronic state of traumatic brain injury. *Journal of Internal Medicine, 285*(6), 608–623. https://doi.org/10.1111/joim.12900.

Markovic, S. J., Fitzgerald, M., Peiffer, J. J., Scott, B. R., Rainey-Smith, S. R., Sohrabi, H. R., & Brown, B. M. (2021). The impact of exercise, sleep, and diet on neurocognitive recovery from mild traumatic brain injury in older adults: A narrative review. *Ageing Research Reviews, 68*, 101322. https://doi.org/10.1016/j.arr.2021.101322.

Martin, A. K., Petersen, A. J., Sesma, H. W., Koolmo, M. B., Ingram, K. M., Slifko, K. B., Nguyen, V. N., Doss, R. C., & Linabery, A. M. (2020). Concussion symptomology and recovery in children and adolescents with pre-existing anxiety. *Journal of Neurology, Neurosurgery, and Psychiatry, 91*(10), 1060–1066. https://doi.org/10.1136/jnnp-2020-323137.

Master, C. L., Bacal, D., & Grady, M. F. AAP Section on Ophthalmology; American Academy of Ophthalmology; American Association for Pediatric Ophthalmology and Strabismus; and American Association of Certified Orthoptists. (2022). Evaluation of the visual system by the primary care provider following concussion. *Pediatrics, 150*(2), e2021056048.

Master, C. L., Podolak, O. E., Ciuffreda, K. J., Metzger, K. B., Joshi, N. R., McDonald, C. C., Margulies, S. S., Grady, M. F., & Arbogast, K. B. (2020). Utility of pupillary light reflex metrics as a physiologic biomarker for adolescent sport-related concussion. *JAMA Ophthalmology, 138*(11), 1135–1141. https://doi.org/10.1001/jamaophthalmol.2020.3466.

Master, C. L., Scheiman, M., Gallaway, M., Goodman, A., Robinson, R. L., Master, S. R., & Grady, M. F. (2016). Vision diagnoses are common after concussion in adolescents. *Clinical Pediatrics, 55*(3), 260–267. https://doi.org/10.1177/0009922815594367.

Mastrangelo, M., & Midulla, F. (2017). Minor head trauma in the pediatric emergency department: Decision making nodes. *Current Pediatric Reviews, 13*(2), 92–99.

Max, J. E., Drake, I., Vaida, F., Hesselink, J. R., Ewing-Cobbs, L., Schachar, R. J., Chapman, S. B., Bigler, E. D., Wilde, E. A., Saunders, A. E., Yang, T. T., Tymofiyeva, O., & Levin, HS. (2022). Novel psychiatric disorder 6 months after traumatic brain injury in children and adolescents. *Journal of Neuropsychiatry and Clinical Neuroscience, 35*(2), 141–150.

May, T., Foris, L. A., & Donnally, C. J., III (2022). *Second impact syndrome*. StatPearls Publishing.

McAvoy, K., Eagan-Johnson, B., Dymacek, R., Hooper, S., McCart, M., & Tyler, J. (2020). Establishing consensus for essential elements in returning to learn following a concussion. *The Journal of School Health, 90*(11), 849–858. https://doi.org/10.1111/josh.12949.

McCrea, M. A., Giacino, J. T., Barber, J., Temkin, N. R., Nelson, L. D., Levin, H. S., Dikmen, S., Stein, M., Bodien, Y. G., Boase, K., Taylor, S. R., Vassar, M., Mukherjee, P., Robertson, C., Diaz-Arrastia, R., Okonkwo, D. O., Markowitz, A. J., Manley, G. T., TRACK-TBI Investigators, Adeoye, O., … Zafonte, R. (2021). Functional outcomes over the first year after moderate to severe traumatic brain injury in the prospective, longitudinal TRACK-TBI study. *JAMA Neurology, 78*(8), 982–992. https://doi.org/10.1001/jamaneurol.2021.2043.

McCrory, P., Meeuwisse, W., Dvořák, J., Aubry, M., Bailes, J., Broglio, S., Cantu, R. C., Cassidy, D., Echemendia, R. J., Castellani, R. J., Davis, G. A., Ellenbogen, R., Emery, C., Engebretsen, L., Feddermann-Demont, N., Giza, C. C., Guskiewicz, K. M., Herring, S., Iverson, G. L., Johnston, K. M., … Vos, P. E. (2017). Consensus statement on concussion in sport-the 5th international conference on concussion in sport held in Berlin, October 2016. *British Journal of Sports Medicine, 51*(11), 838–847. https://doi.org/10.1136/bjsports-2017-097699.

McDougall, A., Bayley, M., & Munce, SE. (2018). The ketogenic diet as a treatment for traumatic brain injury: A scoping review. *Brain Injury, 32*(4), 416–422.

McGrath, A., & Taylor, RS. (2022). *Pediatric skull fractures.* StatPearls Publishing.

McLendon, L. A., Kralik, S. F., Grayson, P. A., et al. (2016). The controversial second impact syndrome: A review of the literature. *Pediatric Neurology, 62,* 9–17.

Miranda, N. A., Boris, J. R., Kouvel, K. M., & Stiles, L. (2018). Activity and exercise intolerance after concussion: Identification and management of postural orthostatic tachycardia syndrome. *Journal of Neurologic Physical Therapy, 42*(3), 163–171. https://doi.org/10.1097/NPT.0000000000000231.

Narang, S. K., Fingarson, A., & Lukefahr, J. Council on Child Abuse and Neglect. (2020). Abusive head trauma in infants and children. *Pediatrics, 145*(4), e20200203.

O'Brien, N. F., Maa, T., & Reuter-Rice, K. (2015). Noninvasive screening for intracranial hypertension in children with acute, severe traumatic brain injury. *Journal of Neurosurgery: Pediatrics, 16*(4), 420–425.

O'Brien Sr, W. T., Caré, M. M., & Leach, JL. (2018). Pediatric emergencies: Imaging of pediatric head trauma. *Seminars in Ultrasound, CT, and MRI, 39*(5), 495–514.

Panenka, W. J., Lange, R. T., Bouix, S., Shewchuk, J. R., Heran, M. K., Brubacher, J. R., Eckbo, R., Shenton, M. E., & Iverson, G. L. (2015). Neuropsychological outcome and diffusion tensor imaging in complicated versus uncomplicated mild traumatic brain injury. *PloS One, 10*(4), e0122746. https://doi.org/10.1371/journal.pone.0122746.

Peacock, M., & Hernandez, E. (2020). A concept analysis of nurse practitioner autonomy. *Journal of the American Association of Nurse Practitioners, 32*(2), 113–119.

Pennell, C., Wilson, T., Bruce, M., Dykie, A., Arthur, L. G., Lindholm, E., & Ciullo, S. (2020). Adherence to PECARN criteria in children transferred to a pediatric trauma center: An opportunity for improvement? *The American Journal of Emergency Medicine, 38*(7), 1546.e1–1546.e4. https://doi.org/10.1016/j.ajem.2020.04.042.

Pingue, V., Mele, C., & Nardone, A. (2021). Post-traumatic seizures and antiepileptic therapy as predictors of the functional outcome in patients with traumatic brain injury. *Science Reports, 11*(1), 4708.

Popernack, M. L., Gray, N., & Reuter-Rice, K. (2015). Moderate-to-severe traumatic brain injury in children: Complications and rehabilitation strategies. *Journal of Pediatric Health Care, 29*(3), e1–e7.

Pratile, T., Marshall, C., & DeMatteo, C. (2022). Examining how time from sport-related concussion to initial assessment predicts return-to-play clearance. *Physician and Sportsmedicine, 50*(2), 132–140.

Register-Mihalik, J. K., DeFreese, J. D., Callahan, C. E., & Carneiro, K. (2020). Utilizing the biopsychosocial model in concussion treatment: Post-traumatic headache and beyond. *Current Pain Headache Reports, 24*(8), 44.

Reuter-Rice, K., Eads, J. K., Berndt, S., & Doser, K. (2018). The initiation of rehabilitation therapies and observed outcomes in pediatric traumatic brain injury. *Rehabilitation Nurse, 43*(6), 327–334.

Roddis, J. K., & Tanner, M. (2020). Music therapy for depression. *Research in Nursing & Health, 43*(1), 134–136.

Russell, K., Selci, E., Black, B., & Ellis, M. J. (2019). Health-related quality of life following adolescent sports-related concussion or fracture: A prospective cohort study. *Journal of Neurosurgery: Pediatrics, 23*(4), 455–464. https://doi.org/10.3171/2018.8.PEDS18356.

Saliman, N. H., Belli, A., & Blanch, RJ. (2021). Afferent visual manifestations of traumatic brain injury. *Journal of Neurotrauma, 38*(20), 2778–2789.

Scheiman, M., Grady, M. F., Jenewein, E., Shoge, R., Podolak, O. E., Howell, D. H., & Master, C. L. (2021). Frequency of oculomotor disorders in adolescents 11 to 17 years of age with concussion, 4 to 12 weeks post injury. *Vision Research, 183,* 73–80. https://doi.org/10.1016/j.visres.2020.09.011.

Serpa, R. O., Ferguson, L., Larson, C., Bailard, J., Cooke, S., Greco, T., & Prins, M. L. (2021). Pathophysiology of pediatric traumatic brain injury. *Frontiers in Neurology, 12,* 696510. https://doi.org/10.3389/fneur.2021.696510.

Sidpra, J., Chhabda, S., Oates, A. J., Bhatia, A., Blaser, S. I., & Mankad, K. (2021). Abusive head trauma: Neuroimaging mimics and diagnostic complexities. *Pediatric Radiology, 51*(6), 947–965. https://doi.org/10.1007/s00247-020-04940-6.

Siponkoski, S. T., Martínez-Molina, N., Kuusela, L., Laitinen, S., Holma, M., Ahlfors, M., Jordan-Kilkki, P., Ala-Kauhaluoma, K., Melkas, S., Pekkola, J., Rodriguez-Fornells, A., Laine, M., Ylinen, A., Rantanen, P., Koskinen, S., Lipsanen, J., & Särkämö, T. (2020). Music therapy enhances executive functions and prefrontal structural neuroplasticity after traumatic brain injury: Evidence from a randomized controlled trial. *Journal of Neurotrauma, 37*(4), 618–634. https://doi.org/10.1089/neu.2019.6413.

Standiford, L., O'Daniel, M., Hysell, M., & Trigger, C. (2021). A randomized cohort study of the efficacy of PO magnesium in the treatment of acute concussions in adolescents. *The American Journal of Emergency Medicine, 44,* 419–422. https://doi.org/10.1016/j.ajem.2020.05.010.

Storey, E. P., Master, S. R., Lockyer, J. E., Podolak, O. E., Grady, M. F., & Master, C. L. (2017). Near point of convergence after concussion in children. *Optometry and Vision Science, 94*(1), 96–100. https://doi.org/10.1097/OPX.0000000000000910.

Storey, E. P., Wiebe, D. J., D'Alonzo, B. A., Nixon-Cave, K., Jackson-Coty, J., Goodman, A. M., Grady, M. F., & Master, C. L. (2018). Vestibular rehabilitation is associated with visuovestibular improvement in pediatric concussion. *Journal of Neurologic Physical Therapy, 42*(3), 134–141. https://doi.org/10.1097/NPT.0000000000000228.

Strelzik, J., & Langdon, R. (2017). The role of active recovery and "rest" after concussion. *Pediatric Annals, 46*(4), e139–e144.

Tamura, K., Furutani, T., Oshiro, R., Oba, Y., Ling, A., & Murata, N. (2020). Concussion recovery timeline of high school athletes using a stepwise return-to-play protocol: Age and sex effects. *Journal of Athletic Training, 55*(1), 6–10. https://doi.org/10.4085/1062-6050-452-18.

Taşkapılıoğlu, M. Ö., Özmarasalı, A. İ., & Ocakoğlu, G. (2019). Retrospective analysis of decompressive craniectomy performed in pediatric patients with subdural hematoma. *Turkish Journal of Trauma and Emergency Surgery, 25*(4), 383–388.

Terry, D. P., Reddi, P. J., Cook, N. E., Seifert, T., Maxwell, B. A., Zafonte, R., Berkner, P. D., & Iverson, G. L. (2021). Acute effects of concussion in youth with pre-existing migraines. *Clinical Journal of Sport Medicine, 31*(5), 430–437. https://doi.org/10.1097/JSM.0000000000000791.

Thomas, D. G., Apps, J. N., Hoffmann, R. G., McCrea, M., & Hammeke, T. (2015). Benefits of strict rest after acute concussion: A randomized controlled trial. *Pediatrics, 135*(2), 213–223. https://doi.org/10.1542/peds.2014-0966.

Torelli, F., Terragni, E., Blanco, S., Di Bella, N., Grasso, M., & Bonaiuti, D. (2015). Lower urinary tract symptoms associated with neurological conditions: Observations on a clinical sample of outpatients neurorehabilitation service. *Archivio Italiano di Urologia e Andrologia, 87*(2), 154–157. https://doi.org/10.4081/aiua.2015.2.154.

Voormolen, D. C., Haagsma, J. A., Polinder, S., Maas, A. I. R., Steyerberg, E. W., Vuleković, P., Sewalt, C. A., Gravesteijn, B. Y., Covic, A., Andelic, N., Plass, A. M., & von Steinbuechel, N. (2019). Post-concussion symptoms in complicated vs. uncomplicated mild traumatic brain injury patients at three and six months post-injury: Results from the CENTER-TBI study. *Journal of Clinical Medicine, 8*(11), 1921. https://doi.org/10.3390/jcm8111921.

Wang, K. K., Yang, Z., Zhu, T., Shi, Y., Rubenstein, R., Tyndall, J. A., & Manley, G. T. (2018). An update on diagnostic and prognostic biomarkers for traumatic brain injury. *Expert Review of Molecular Diagnostics, 18*(2), 165–180. https://doi.org/10.1080/14737159.2018.1428089.

Wang, C. F., Zhao, C. C., He, Y., Li, Z. Y., Liu, W. L., Huang, X. J., Deng, Y. F., & Li, W. P. (2019). Mild hypothermia reduces endoplasmic reticulum stress-induced apoptosis and improves neuronal functions after severe traumatic brain injury. *Brain and Behavior, 9*(4), e01248. https://doi.org/10.1002/brb3.1248.

Wearne, T., Anderson, V., Catroppa, C., Morgan, A., Ponsford, J., Tate, R., Ownsworth, T., Togher, L., Fleming, J., Douglas, J., Docking, K., Sigmundsdottir, L., Francis, H., Honan, C., & McDonald, S. (2020). Psychosocial functioning following moderate-to-severe pediatric traumatic brain injury: Recommended outcome instruments for research and remediation studies. *Neuropsychological Rehabilitation, 30*(5), 973–987. https://doi.org/10.1080/09602011.2018.1531768.

Woods, K. S., Horvat, C. M., Kantawala, S., Simon, D. W., Rakkar, J., Kochanek, P. M., Clark, R. S. B., & Au, A. K. (2021). Intracranial and cerebral perfusion pressure thresholds associated with inhospital mortality across pediatric neurocritical care. *Pediatric Critical Care Medicine, 22*(2), 135–146. https://doi.org/10.1097/PCC.0000000000002618.

Wopker, P. M., Schwermer, M., Sommer, S., Längler, A., Fetz, K., Ostermann, T., & Zuzak, T. J. (2020). Complementary and alternative medicine in the treatment of acute bronchitis in children: A systematic review. *Complementary Therapies in Medicine, 49*, 102217. https://doi.org/10.1016/j.ctim.2019.102217.

Young, A. M. H., Guilfoyle, M. R., Donnelly, J., Smielewski, P., Agarwal, S., Czosnyka, M., & Hutchinson, P. J. (2018). Multimodality neuromonitoring in severe pediatric traumatic brain injury. *Pediatric Research, 83*(1-1), 41–49. https://doi.org/10.1038/pr.2017.215.

Yue, J. K., Upadhyayula, P. S., Avalos, L. N., & Cage, T. A. (2020). Pediatric traumatic brain injury in the United States: Rural-urban disparities and considerations. *Brain Sciences, 10*(3), 135. https://doi.org/10.3390/brainsci10030135.

Zamani, A., Mychasiuk, R., & Semple, BD. (2019). Determinants of social behavior deficits and recovery after pediatric traumatic brain injury. *Experimental Neurology, 314*, 34–45.

Zusman, B. E., Kochanek, P. M., & Jha, RM. (2020). Cerebral edema in traumatic brain injury: A historical framework for current therapy. *Current Treatment Options in Neurology, 22*(3), 9.

Index

Note: Page numbers followed by "*f*" indicate figures, "*t*" indicate tables, and "*b*" indicate boxes.

A

ABO-incompatible heart transplantation, 797
Abusive head trauma
  clinical manifestations, 915
  computed tomography, 915
  diagnostic findings, 915
  etiology, 915
  incidence, 915
  legal interventions, 915
  prevalence, 915
  prognosis, 915
  treatment, 915
Acanthosis nigricans, 502, 760
Achenbach system of empirically based assessment, 182–183
Achilles tendon release surgery, 739
Acidosis, 855
Acquired hemophilia, 238
Acquired hydrocephalus, 620
Acquired immunodeficiency syndrome, 600
  prognosis, 605
  related death, 605*f*
Acquired von Willebrand syndrome, 255
  prevalence of developing, 255
Acute adrenal insufficiency, 409
  signs and symptoms of, 408*b*
Acute chest syndrome, 867
Acute concussion assessment, 920
Acute injury management, 924
Acute rejection, 798
Acute sickle hepatic crisis, 870
Acute viral rhinitis, 149–150
Adalimumab, 672
Adaptive equipment, 738
  orthotic devices, 738
  respiratory devices, 739
Adenovirus, 292
ADHD rating scale-IV preschool version, 182
Adolescence transition to adulthood, 97–98
  biologic and psychosocial changes, 74
  cognitive and psychosocial development, 74
  coordination of transition planning, 84–85
    Got Transition program, 84–85
    pediatric primary care provider, role of, 84–85
    readiness assessment phase, 84–85
  developmental stages and transition planning, 76

Adolescence transition to adulthood *(Continued)*
  assessment and guidance on self-care skills, 76
  concerns of adjustments, 76
  protection of privacy and confidentiality, 76
  skills checklist, 77*t*
  factors moderating
    adolescent's attitudes, beliefs, and perceptions, 75
    cognitive development, 74
    health care autonomy, 75
    limbic and paralimbic structures, 74
    problem solving, 75
    psychosocial development, 74–75
    pubertal maturation, 74
    secondary sexual characteristics, 74
    sexuality, 75–76
    social interaction and friendships, 75
  linkage to insurance, 82–83, 82*t*
  obstacles, 73
  postsecondary education, 83–84
  primary goal of, 74
  in school system, 83
  timing of change, 74
  vocational rehabilitation services and job training, 84
  youth with chronic health conditions, 73
Adolescents with chronic conditions, developmental task for, 28
  delayed puberty, 28
  issue of social isolation, 28
  psychological difficulties, 28
  vulnerability to sexual exploitation, 28
Adrenal steroid pathway, 395, 396*f*
Advanced practice registered nurses, 59, 61
Advisory Committee on Immunization Practices, 872
Affordable Care Act, 13–15, 82
Ages and Stages Questionnaires, 213
Allergic asthma, 123
  immunoglobulin E, production of, 123
  type 2 T-helper cells, production of, 123
Allergies
  allergic conjunctivitis or ocular allergy, 145
  allergic rhinitis, 145*f*, 145
  anaphylactic reactions, 146
  as an immunologically based acquired change, 140

Allergies *(Continued)*
  associated problems of, 151
    asthma, 152
    atopic dermatitis (eczema), 152
    dental malocclusion, 152
    eustachian tube obstruction, 152
    sleep apnea, 152
    upper respiratory infections, 152
  classification of adverse food reactions, 142*f*
  condition-specific screening, 154–155
  developmental issues
    behavioral manifestations, 156
    child care, 156
    discipline, 155
    EpiPen, use of, 156–157
    schooling, 157
    sexuality, 158
    sleep-related problems, 155
    toileting, 155
    transition to adulthood, 158
  diagnostic criteria, 144
    blood testing, 144
    component resolved diagnostics, 144
    ELISA testing, 144
    oral challenges, 144–145
    in vitro testing, 144
    in vivo skin testing, 144
  diet for, 153
  differential diagnosis, 145*b*
    acute sinusitis, pharyngitis, and conjunctivitis, 150
    acute viral rhinitis, 149–150
    gastroenteritis, 150
    rhinitis medicamentosa, 150
    vasomotor rhinitis, 150
  eating in restaurants and, 148
  education regarding, 148
  etiology, 140, 142*f*
  family concerns, 159
  food, 143
    diagnosis, 144*f*
    milk, 153
    role of early diet diversification, 144
  Food Allergen Labeling and Consumer Protection Act of 2004, 148
  health care maintenance, 159*b*–160*b*
  immunizations, 154
  impact on growth and development, 152–153
  incidence and prevalence, 140–143
  Learning Early About Peanut trial, 143–144

Allergies (Continued)
  precautionary advisory labeling, 148
  production of antigen-specific
      mediators, 140
  routine screening, 154
  school safety against, 148
  symptoms, 145
      features of adenoid facies, 145
  theories related to, 143–144
      climate changes, 143
      dietary changes, 143
      lifestyle factors, 143
  treatment
      for allergic conjunctivitis, 147
      of allergic rhinoconjunctivitis, 141t
      avoidance of allergens at
          home, 146b
      complementary and alternative
          medicine therapies, 147
      early introduction of allergenic
          foods, 148
      emergency food allergy plan, 148,
          149f
      epicutaneous immunotherapy, 148
      epinephrine, 148, 154
      of food allergies, 147–148
      hydrolyzed formulas, 148
      immunotherapy, 147
      intranasal antihistamines, 147
      intranasal steroids, 146–147
      oral immunotherapy, 148
      pharmacologic therapy, 146
      sublingual immunotherapy, 148
Alpha-adrenergic receptor agonists, 905
Alport syndrome, 696
Altered cognitive function, 928
Alternative diets, 675
American Academy of Child and
      Adolescent Psychiatry
      (AACAP), 727–728
American Academy of Family
      Physicians, 79
American Academy of Pediatric
      Dentistry, 891
American College of Physicians, 79
American Society for Transplantation
      and Cellular Therapy, 271–272
American Society of Blood and
      Marrow Transplantation, 277
American Society of Hematology,
      SCD treatment suggestion
      by, 860–861, 865
Americans with Disabilities Act, 84,
      92–93, 112
Amoxicillin, 893
Amphetamine, 186–187, 187t
  extended release, 189t
ANA-positive arthritis, 676
Anemia, 686, 703, 839
  symptoms of, 868
Angelman syndrome, 218
Angiotensin-converting enzyme
      inhibitors, 792
Anomalous pulmonary venous
      return, 427
Anorexia nervosa, 536
  atypical, 542
  clinical manifestations, 540–542
  diagnostic criteria, 539

Anorexia nervosa (Continued)
  psychopharmacologic interventions,
      543–544
  psychotherapy, 543
  subtypes, 539
Anticholinergic medications, 888
Antidiuretic dysfunction, 928
Antinuclear antibody, 669
Anxieties, 164t
  in children, 163
  symptoms of, 163
Anxiety disorders
  assessment in clinical setting, 166
  in Diagnostic and Statistical Manual,
      163–164
  diagnostic interview, 167
      DSM-5 criteria, 167
  incidence and prevalence, 163
  psychometric assessment tools for
      diagnosis of, 167–168, 169t
      Children's Yale-Brown Obsessive-
          Compulsive Scale, 168
      Multidimensional Anxiety Scale
          for Children, Second Edition,
          168
      Revised Children's Manifest
          Anxiety Scale, Second
          Edition, 168
      Screen for Anxiety-Related
          Disorders, 168
  treatment of
      cognitive-behavioral therapy, 169,
          170b
      Coping Cat program, 169–170
      pharmacologic interventions
          for, 170
      psychotherapeutic
          interventions, 169
Aortic stenosis, 424–425, 429t–433t
Apheresis, 277
Aplastic crisis, 867
Apnea of prematurity, 839
ARCH National Respite Network and
      Resource Center, 199
Aretaeus of Cappadocia, 341
Aripiprazole (dopamine blockers), 908
Arrhythmias, 434–435, 442
  clinical manifestation, 435
  conduction abnormalities, 435
Asplenia, 875
Asthma, 152
  action plan, 129, 134f
  allergic, 123
  comorbidities and associated
      problems with
      allergies, 139, 140b
      gastroesophageal reflux, 139
      illness and sinusitis, 139
      sensitivity to aspirin and
          nonsteroidal antiinflammatory
          drugs, 139
      swallowing disorders, 140
  complications with influenza, 154
  conditions causing cough and
      wheeze, 139
  condition-specific screening, 154–155
  control scores, 138–139
      ACQ, 139
      ACT, 138

Asthma (Continued)
  C-ACT, 138–139
  TRACK, 139
  definition, 123
  developmental issues
      behavioral manifestations, 155
      child care, 156
      schooling, 157
      sexuality, 158
      sleep-related problems, 155
      toileting, 155
      transition to adulthood, 158
  diagnosis, 125, 139
      importance of clinical
          history, 125–126
      in infants and children, 126
      severity, 127
  diet for, 153
  etiology, 123
  factors contributing to development
      of, 123–124
      environmental, 124
      genetics, 123–124
      innate immunity, 123
  family concerns, 158
      smoking habits of family
          members, 158
  health care maintenance, 159b–160b
  immunizations, 154
  impact on growth and
      development, 152
  incidence and prevalence, 125
      in children, 125
      gender differences, 125
  inflammatory triggers, 124
  mortality rate, 125
  nonallergic, 123
  noninflammatory triggers, 124
  pathway, 124f
  phenotypes, 123
  response to triggers, 124f, 124–125
  routine screening, 154
  safety, 153
  severity of, 124, 127
  symptoms, 124, 126b, 126
      day/nighttime, 127–128
  testing for, 137–138
  treatment, 125–127, 129f
      anticholinergic agents, 136
      biologics, 136, 137t
      classification of therapy, 127f, 127
      components of asthma
          management, 126–127
      delivery of medicine with and
          without an aerochamber, 132, 134f
      dry powder inhalers, 132
      environmental remediations, 137
      HPA suppressive effects, 136
      immunotherapy, 137
      inhaled corticosteroids, 127–128,
          132–133, 135t
      leukotriene receptor antagonists, 136
      list of combination inhalers, 135t
      long-acting beta$_2$-agonists, 133
      metered-dose inhaler with a
          spacer, 129, 132
      NHLBI guidelines, 127
      quick relief or rescue
          medications, 129

Asthma (Continued)
    SABA medication, 129
    short-acting rescue medication, 126–127
    single maintenance and reliever therapy, 133
    step-down therapy, 127–128
    systemic corticosteroid, 136
    Xopenex, 129
Asthma Control Questionnaire, 138–139
Asymptomatic bacteriuria, 876
Ataluren, 741
Ataxia, 352
Atopic dermatitis, 152
    biologics for, 136
Atrial septal defect, 423, 429t–433t
Attention-deficit/hyperactivity disorder, 179, 217–218, 573, 900, 916
    associated problems, 191b, 192
        anxiety, 193
        conduct problems, 193
        drug and alcohol abuse/tobacco use, 193–194
        learning disabilities, 193
        ODD, 193
        speech and language impairments, 193
        video game addiction, 193
    association with genetic syndromes, 179
    attention and executive functioning deficits associated, 228–229
    behavioral, educational, environmental strategies for, 201b
    behavioral inhibition in, 180
    child care setting for, 199
    clinical manifestations, 183–184, 184b
    combined presentation, 180
    complications during pregnancy, 179
    definition, 181
    delayed brain maturation and, 180
    developmental issues
        discipline, 198–199
        sexual and reproductive health, 200
        sleep problems, 198, 199t
        toileting, 198
        transition of adulthood, 200–202
    diagnosis, 180
        changes from DSM-IV-TR to the DSM-5, 182, 182t
        DSM-5-TR criteria, 180, 181b
        neuropsychological testing, 183
        rating scales, 182–183, 183t
    environmental role in development of, 179
    evaluation to determine DSM-5 criteria, 182
    family concerns, 202
    genetic factors, 179
    genome-wide association studies, 179
    health care maintenance
        dietary restrictions, 195
        growth and development, 195
        immunizations, 196
        safety issues, 195–196
    impaired family and social relationships, 194

Attention-deficit/hyperactivity disorder (Continued)
    incidence and prevalence
        across stages of development, 180
        based on age, 180
        gender differences, 180
        worldwide estimate, 180
    as a multifactorial disorder, 192
    names, 179
    neuroimaging studies, 192
    neurologic factors, 179
    in older adolescents and adults, 184
    pathophysiology of, 180
    predominantly hyperactive-impulsive presentation, 180
    predominately inattention presentation, 180
    in preschool children, 184
    prognosis, 194
    psychosocial and health-related sequelae, 194
    risk factors of developing, 179
    school-based behavioral interventions, 199–200
    screening and management of problems, 184
        blood pressure, 196
        condition-specific, 196
        dental, 196
        hearing, 196
        hemotocrit, 196
        lead, 196
        learning disabilities, 196
        psychological and psychiatric conditions, 196
        tuberculosis, 196
        vision, 196
    symptoms of, 179
    teacher education regarding, 200
    treatment, 181
        AAP ADHD Clinical Practice Guidelines, 186
        behavioral classroom management, 185
        behavioral parent training, 185
        behavioral peer interventions, 185–186
        behavior therapy, 184–185, 185b
        cognitive training, 192
        complementary and alternative medicine, 191
        external trigeminal nerve stimulation, 192
        FDA-approved medications, 184
        goals of, 186
        intermediate and long-acting (extended-release) formulations, 187–188, 188t
        monitoring of, 191
        with nonstimulants, 190–191, 190t
        nutritional supplements, 191–192
        pharmacotherapy, 186
        prodrugs, 188
        psychosocial, 186
        short-acting/immediate-release formulations, 187
        with stimulants, 186–190, 189b, 197
        third-line medications, 191

Attention-deficit/hyperactivity disorder (Continued)
    training interventions, 186
    video game therapy, 192
Autism, 210
Autism and Developmental Disabilities Monitoring Network, 211
Autism Diagnostic Interview-Revised, 215–216
Autism Diagnostic Observation Schedule, 216–217
Autism spectrum disorder, 514–515
    adverse experiences, 225–226
        accidental drowning, 226
        bullying, 226
        deaths reported in children with, 226
        extremism and criminal conduct, 226
        law enforcement interaction, 226
        social camouflaging, 226
        unintentional injury, 226
    allied health and educational supports, 228
    coaching the family, 228
    behavioral characteristics of, 219
    biomarker-based diagnostic assessment, 219
    clinical and community identification of, 211–212
    common medical conditions with
        epilepsy and seizure disorders, 228
        feeding and eating problems, 227–228
        gastrointestinal and toileting problems, 227
        risk for obesity, 227–228
        sleep problems, 227
    complementary and alternative approaches, 228, 229b
    connection between gender/sexual identity diversity and, 230
    cooccurring psychiatric/developmental conditions, 217
    developmental surveillance for, 212
    diagnostic criteria for, 211, 215, 216b, 217
        applied behavioral analysis, 217
        developmental delay, 217
    diagnostic tools, 215–216
    etiology of, 210–211
        environmental factors, 210–211
        genetic factors, 210
        immune factors, 211
    health care maintenance, 220
        ABA-based interventions, 221, 225
        common psychosocial condition management, 221
        communication training, 221, 225
        functional communication training, 221–225
        growth and development, 220–221
        healthy lifestyle recommendations, 222t–224t
        immunization schedule, 221
        in school settings, 225
        techniques for care interactions, 220t

Autism spectrum disorder *(Continued)*
health disparities, 215
holistic family support, 229
incidence and prevalence
determining new-onset, 211
male-to-female sex ratio, 212
present estimates, 211
increasing diagnostic access, 218–219
language development, 212–213
medical and genetic evaluation, 218
nonpharmacologic approach, 228–229
pediatric primary care providers
and, 230
pharmacologic supports, 225
common psychological symptom
targets, 226t
prevalence estimates, 217t
prognosis, 219
risk factors for patients, 218
risk of sexual victimization
and inappropriate sexual
behaviors, 229
screening, 212, 213f
wait-and-see approaches, 215
self-injurious behavior, 218
severity levels, 212t
special education support, 230
telehealth diagnostic approaches, 219
transition planning, 230
universal developmental
screening, 213
Autologous transplants, 269–270

B
Bayley Scales of Infant
Development, 523–524
BEARS Sleep Screening Tool, 227
Behavior Disorder Rating Scale, 183
Beta-globin gene cluster haplotypes, 870
Bilateral sagittal split osteotomy, 381
Binge eating disorder
clinical manifestations, 542
diagnostic criteria, 539
interpersonal therapy, 543
psychopharmacologic
interventions, 544
psychotherapy, 543
Biochemical hepatic abnormalities, 870
Biometrics, 105
Bipolar disorders, 724, 726t
Bleeding disorders, 237
differential diagnosis, 260b
drug interactions/medication
management, 263
factor VIII, IV level tests, 263
HIV antibody testing, 262
liver function studies, 262
primary care management
abuse concerns, 261
child care, 261
diet, 260
discipline, 261
financial concerns, 261
growth and development, 260
health disparities and cultural
influences, 261–262
immunizations, 260
physical activity, 260–261
safety, 261

Bleeding disorders *(Continued)*
schooling, 262
support network, 262
screening recommendations
blood pressure, 262
dental evaluations, 262
ferritin, 262
hearing, 262
hematocrit, 262
hemoglobin, 262
urinalysis, 262
vision, 262
sexuality and sexual interactions,
263
transition to adulthood, 263
Blood clot formation process, 238f
Blunt *versus* penetrating, 916
Bone marrow transplantation, 269
BOSns syndrome, 293, 301
Botox, 905
Botulinum toxin injections, 905
Brain-gut axis, 905
Bronchial provocation tests, 138
Bronchodilation with short-
acting beta-agonist (SABA)
medications, 124–125
Bronfenbrenner's ecological systems
theory, 20f
Bulimia nervosa, 536
associated problems and treatment
of, 545
clinical manifestations, 542
physical effects of repetitive
purging, 542
diagnostic criteria, 539
psychopharmacologic
interventions, 544
fluoxetine, 544
monoamine oxidase inhibitors, 544
tricyclic drugs, 544
psychotherapy, 543
severity of, 539
Bullying, 226

C
CAM modalities, 862
Cancer
associated problems and
treatment, 325b
death, 326
development of late effects, 326,
327t–332t
long-term effects of therapy, 326
relapse, 326
vascular access, 326
clinical manifestations, 318–322
common illness management
drug interactions, 335–336
fever, 334–335
gastrointestinal symptoms, 335
headache pain, 335
pain, 335
common sites, 318
complementary therapies, 325
developmental issues
child care, 336
discipline, 336
family concerns, 337
fertility, 336–337

Cancer *(Continued)*
financial burden, 337
individualized education program
for, 336
participation of school activities, 336
secondary sexual characteristics
and amenorrhea, 337
sleep problems, 336
toileting, 336
transition to adulthood, 337
diagnosis, 318
etiology, 318
genetic predispositions in
developing, 318
health care maintenance
diet, 333
growth patterns, 333
immunizations, 333
intellectual development, 333
safety issues, 333
steroids, 333
incidence and prevalence, 318
in childhood, 318
participation in clinical trials, 318, 322
screenings
blood pressure, 334
dental, 334
hearing, 334
hemoglobin/hematocrit, 334
vision, 334
supportive care, 324
for alopecia, 325
for anorexia and weight loss, 324
antiemetics, 324
bone marrow suppression, 324–325
chemotherapeutic regimen, 324
epoetin alfa, 325
for fatigue, 325
granulocyte colony-stimulating
factor, 324–325
hand-washing techniques, 325
nutrition, 324
personal hygiene, 325
platelet transfusions, 325
for toxic effects of
chemotherapy, 325
survival rates, 318
treatment, 322
biotherapy, 323–324
checkpoint inhibitors, 323
chemotherapy, 322
child's treatment protocol, 322
hematopoietic stem cell
transplantation, 324
immunomodulators, 323
immunotherapy, 323
monoclonal antibodies, 323–324
oncolytic viruses, 323
radiation therapy, 323
surgery, 322
targeted therapies, 323–324
tyrosine kinase inhibitors, 323–324
vaccines, 323
Cannabidiol, 905
Carbamazepine, 893
Cardiac
catheterization, 436
dysfunction, 742
enlargement, 869–870

Cardiac physiology, 422
Cardiomegaly, 869–870
Cardiomyopathy, 747
Cardiopulmonary resuscitation, 893
Caregiver strain/burden, 11–12
    Modified Caregiver Strain Index, 11b
    negative impact, 11–12
Celiac disease, 341
    associated problems of, 345
    association of human leukocyte
        antigen with, 341
    capsule endoscopy for, 345
    CELIAC mnemonic, 346b
    clinical manifestations, 343, 345
        abdominal distention, 343
        diarrhea, 343
        extraintestinal, 343
        failure to thrive, 343
        neurologic and psychiatric
            syndromes, 343
    common illness management
        abdominal pain, 348
        chronic diarrhea, 348
        failure to thrive, 348
    developmental issues
        child care, 349
        development of sexuality, 349
        discipline, 348–349
        family concerns, 349
        school performance, 349
        sleep patterns, 348
        toileting, 348
        transition to adulthood, 349
    in diabetes mellitus, 500
    diagnostic criteria for, 341–342
        algorithm, 343f
        antigliadin IgG and IgA, 342
        DGP IgG, 342
        genetic typing, 342
        gold standard, 342
        intestinal biopsy, 342f, 342–343
        measurement of IgA and IgG,
            341–342
        4/5 rule, 342–343
        subtypes, 342–343
        TTG sensitivity, 342
    in Down syndrome, 517–518, 529
    environmental triggers of, 341
    etiology, 341
    genetic predisposition in, 341
    gluten-free diet, 344b, 344–346, 349
    gluten-free diet for, 341
    health care maintenance
        diet, 346
        growth and development, 346
        immunizations, 347
        safety, 346–347
    high-risk groups, 345b
    in IBD, 345
    immune cell-targeted therapy
        vaccinations for, 345
    iron deficiency in, 347
    nonresponsive, 343
    nutritional problems and, 347
    potential, 343
    prevalence among first-degree
        relatives, 341
    prognosis, 345–346
    refractory, 343

Celiac disease (Continued)
    screenings
        bone health, 347
        endocrine-associated disorders, 347
        hematology, 347
        liver and celiac disease, 347
        techniques, 345
    seronegative, 343
    signs and symptoms of a celiac
        crisis, 343–344
    testing and monitoring, 347
        with IgA anti-TTG antibodies, 347
        NASPGHAN guidelines, 347
    type I and type II refractory, 345–346
Center for International Blood
    and Marrow Transplant
    Research, 271
Centers for Disease Control and
    Prevention, 716
Central nervous system, 886
Cerebral artery stenosis, 865
Cerebral atrophy, 802
Cerebral edema, 919
Cerebral hemorrhage, 919f, 919
Cerebral lacerations, 919
Cerebral palsy, 352
    antecedents and consequences, 352
    associated problems and
        management, 359
        behavioral and mental health
            disorders, 362
        bladder control and urinary
            retention, 361
        cognitive impairments, 359b,
            359–360
        constipation, 361
        dental problems, 361, 362f
        epilepsy, 360
        feeding and eating difficulties, 361
        hearing impairment, 360
        latex allergy, 362
        motor impairments, 360–361
        perceptual problems and
            inattention, 360
        pulmonary effects, 361–362
        scoliosis, 361
        sensory deficits, 360
        skin problems, 362
        speech impairments, 360
        subluxation and dislocation of
            hip, 361
        vision impairment, 360
    ataxic, 352
    classification, 352, 353b
        ataxia, 352
        dyskinetic, 352
        motor dysfunction group, 352
        spastic, 352
        topographic, 353b
    definition, 352
    developmental considerations
        child care, 366
        discipline, 366
        family considerations, 367–368
        schooling, 366–367
        sexual and reproductive health,
            367
        sleep patterns, 365–366, 366t
        toileting, 366

Cerebral palsy (Continued)
        transition to adulthood, 367, 368f
    diagnosis, 355–356
        assessment of tone in infants, 357b
        evaluations/instruments
            used, 357b
        history or clinical findings, 356b
    dyskinetic, 352
    etiology and risk factors, 354–355,
        355t
    health maintenance
        diet and method of feeding, 363
        growth and development, 362–363
        nutrition, 363
        safety, 363–364
    incidence and prevalence, 354
    mixed, 352
    motor disorders, 352
    prognosis, 362
    screenings
        blood pressure, 364
        dental, 364
        hearing, 364
        hematocrit, 364
        malocclusions, 364
        motor and movement problems, 364
        urinalysis, 364
        vision, 364
    severity, 353
    spastic, 352
    treatments, 356–357, 357b
        complementary and alternative
            medicine, 359
        goals, 356–357
        multidisciplinary approach to
            care, 356b
        pain management, 359
        pharmacologic therapy, 358–359
        physical and occupational
            therapy, 357–358
        recreational therapy, 358
        selective dorsal rhizotomy, 359
        speech therapy, 358
        surgeries, 359
        use of orthotic devices, 358
Cerebrospinal fluid, 619
Child and Adolescent Health
    Measurement Initiative, 6
Child care in school
    allergies, 157
    asthma, 157
    bleeding disorders, 262
    cerebral palsy, 366–367
    cleft lip and cleft palate, 388–389
    congenital adrenal
        hyperplasia, 410–411
    congenital heart disease, 454
    cystic fibrosis, 481
    diabetes mellitus, 503–504
    congenital adrenal
        hyperplasia, 410–411
    Down syndrome, 530
    eating disorders, 552
    epilepsy, 576
    fragile X syndrome, 591
    hematopoietic stem cell
        transplantation, 307–308
    human immunodeficiency virus
        infections, 613

Child care in school (*Continued*)
  hydrocephalus, 633
  inflammatory bowel disease, 660
Child health, in United States, 1
Childhood Autism Rating Scale, 215–216
Childhood infections, 1
Children and youth with special health
    care needs, 5b, 13
  access to services for, 12–13
    challenges, 13–15
  Blueprint for Change, 12–13, 14f
  Care for Chronic Conditions
    Framework, 19f, 19
  chronic and disabling conditions, 5–6
  comprehensive, coordinated systems
    of care for, 18, 19f
  cultural appropriateness of services
    for, 10–11
  data collection, 6
  financial burden and unmet
    needs, 6, 8
  health-related quality of life, 12
  insurance coverage, 13, 15, 14f–15f
  MCHB definition, 6
  most prevalent conditions, 5t
  oral health care and dental caries, 8–9
  screener, 6, 7b–8b, 8
  service sectors, 13
  standards for systems of care, 15
Children with chronic conditions
  achieving developmental skill, 27
  attention-deficit/hyperactivity
    disorder, 26
  cooccurring conditions, 29f
  correlation between physiologic
    severity/persistence and
    developmental attainment, 25
  developmental iatrogeny, 26–27
  developmental limitations, 26
  developmental milestones, 27
    adolescence, 28
    behavioral regression, 27
    infants, 27
    preschoolers, 27–28
    school-age children, 28
    toddlerhood, 27
  developmental perspectives, 29–30
    understanding of body, 30–31
  individual characteristics, 28–29
  laws on education, 49
  life expectancies, 26
  multisystem involvement and
    neurologic impairment, 25–26
  pathophysiology, 25
    changes, 26
  prognosis, 26
    developmental lags, 26
    predicting, 26
  risk for coexisting psychiatric
    conditions, 29
  risk of developmental delay, 26
  stigmatization of, 26
  visibility of, 26
    Down syndrome, 26
Children with complex health
    conditions or disabilities, 1
Chimeric antigen receptor T-cell, 269
Chlamydia pneumoniae, 862–863
Cholestatic pruritus, 791–792

Chronic conditions in children, 5–6
Chronic disease
  anemia of, 674
Chronic heart allograft rejection, 799
Chronic hemolysis, 862
Chronic idiopathic urticaria
  biologics for, 136
Chronic kidney disease, 683
  associated hypertension, 697
  associated pruritus, 698–699
  mineral bone disorder, 698
Chronic rheumatic disease, 668
Chronic tic disorder, 902
Chronic transfusion therapy, 865
Clean intermittent catheterization, 892
Cleft lip and cleft palate, 372, 374f
  advances in diagnosis and
    management, 382–383
  associated problems and
    treatment, 383b
    abnormal hearing, 383
    dental and orthodontic
      problems, 384
    eustachian tube dysfunction, 383
    hearing loss, 383
    long-term psychosocial
      management, 384
    psychosocial functioning, 384–385
    speech articulation
      problems, 383–384
    underdevelopment of palatal
      musculature, 383
  association with cardiac
    malformation and
    developmental delay, 372–373
  classification, 373–374
    LAHSHAL, 373–374
    Veau, 373–374, 374f
  clinical manifestations, 374–375, 375b
    child with SMCP, 375–376
  common illness management
    fever, 387
  developmental issues
    child care, 388
    discipline, 388
    family concerns, 389–390
    reproductive issues, 389
    schooling, 388–389
    sleep patterns, 387–388
    toileting, 388
    transition to adulthood, 389
  diagnostic criteria, 373
  diet, 386
  environmental factors, 372
  genetically predisposition, 372–373
  genetic etiology for, 373
  growth and development, 385
    of infant with Pierre Robin
      sequence, 385
  imaging of, 374
  immunizations, 386–387
  incidence and prevalence, 373
    among Asian/Pacific Islander, 373
    among Hispanic Americans, 373
    among Indigenous Americans, 373
    left-sided, 373f, 373
    right-sided, 373
    in United States, 373
  nasal regurgitation, 386

Cleft lip and cleft palate (*Continued*)
  nonsyndromic and
    syndromic, 372–373
  prognosis, 385
  safety, 386
  screenings
    blood pressure, 387
    condition specific, 387
    dental, 387
    hearing, 387
    hematocrit, 387
    tuberculosis, 387
    urinalysis, 387
    vision, 387
  sequence, 372–373
    Pierre Robin sequence, 375b,
      372–373, 375, 376f, 378
  submucous cleft palate, 373–374
  treatment and team care, 376b, 376
    airway management, 378
    audiology and speech pathology
      management, 382
    automated auditory brainstem
      response screening, 383
    cleft orthodontic treatment, 380b
    complementary and alternative
      therapies, 382
    dental care and orthodontic
      treatment, 382
    Dr. Brown's Specialty Bottle
      system, 377
    enhanced recovery after
      surgery, 381
    evaluation of response to
      feeding, 377–378
    goal of feeding, 376
    initial management of a
      newborn, 376
    Lamb nipple, 377
    for maxillary retrusion, 381
    Mead Johnson Cleft Lip and
      Palate Nurser, 377f, 377
    nasoalveolar molding, 379b
    nutritional requirements, 376
    obturator, 378
    orthodontic nipple, 377
    orthognathic surgery, 381f, 381
    otolaryngology management,
      381–382
    Pigeon nipple, 377f, 377
    Ross cleft palate nipple, 377
    special-needs feeder, 377f, 377
    surgical reconstructive
      management, 378, 380
    tonsillectomy and superior
      (partial) adenoidectomy, 382
Cleft Outcomes Registry/Research
    Network, 382–383
Clotting factors, 237
Coagulation cascade, 237
Coarctation of aorta, 425, 429t–433t
Cognitive-behavioral intervention
    for tics, 905
Cognitive-behavioral therapy, 931–932
  binge eating disorder, 543
  bulimia nervosa, 543
Colony-stimulating factors, 269
Common motor disabilities, 927
Communicating hydrocephalus, 619

Complementary and alternative
     medicine, 90–91, 672–673
  allergies, 147
  attention-deficit/hyperactivity
     disorder, 191
  cerebral palsy, 359
  congenital adrenal hyperplasia, 404
  congenital heart disease, 437
  diabetes mellitus, 493–494
  Down syndrome, 515
  eating disorders, 544
  fragile X syndrome, 586
  hematopoietic stem cell
     transplantation, 282–283
  human immunodeficiency virus
     infections, 603
Complementary and alternative
     therapies, SCD treatment, 862
Complete atrioventricular canal
     (endocardial cushion defect),
     424, 429t–433t
Computed tomography, 865
Congenital abnormalities, 683
Congenital adrenal hyperplasia
  associated problems and treatment,
     405b, 405
     congenital anomalies, 405
     fertility, 405
     precocious puberty, 405
     prognosis, 405
  brain and, 405
  classification, 395
  clinical manifestations, 399b, 399
     classic salt-wasting congenital
        adrenal hyperplasia, 399
     classic simple virilizing, 399, 400f
     fertility, 401
     growth, 401
     nonclassic congenital adrenal
        hyperplasia, 400
     pubertal development, 401
  common illness management, 408
     drug interactions, 409b, 409
     fever, 408
     injuries, 409
     known or suspected bacterial
        illness, 408
     upper respiratory infections and
        allergies, 408
     varicella-zoster virus
        (chickenpox), 409
     vomiting, 408–409
  developmental issues
     changes in requirements for
        adolescent, 412
     child care, 410
     discipline, 410
     family concerns, 412–413
     schooling, 410–411
     sexual and reproductive
        development, 411
     sleep patterns, 409
     toileting, 409–410
     transition to adulthood, 411–412
     vaginal voiding, 409–410
  diagnosis, 397, 398b, 401t
     ACTH stimulation test, 398
     adrenal steroids, 398
     electrolytes, 398

Congenital adrenal hyperplasia
     (Continued)
     genotype-phenotype
        correlations, 398
     karyotype, 398
     molecular genetic analysis, 398
     newborn screening, 399
     17-OHP levels, 398
     plasma renin activity, 398
  etiology, 395
     examples, 397f
  genetic etiology, 395–397
     at-risk sibling, 397
     nonclassic form of 21-OHD
        CAH, 397
  health care maintenance
     development, 406
     diet, 406
     growth, 405–406
     immunizations, 407
     safety, 406–407
  incidence and prevalence
     classic CAH, 397
     nonclassic 21-OHD CAH, 397
  offspring of an affected
     individual, 397
  screenings, 407
     bone age, 408
     plasma renin activity, 407
     serum 17-OHP level, 407
  treatment, 401b
     androgen/estrogen antagonists
        and synthesis inhibitors, 404
     bilateral adrenalectomy, 404
     of classic 21-OHD CAH, 401–403
     complementary and alternative
        therapies, 404
     gender role assignments, 403
     gene therapy, 405
     genital surgery, 402–403
     glucocorticoid therapy, 401–402,
        404, 412
     growth hormone and
        gonadotropin-releasing
        hormone inhibitor, 404
     management of pregnant women
        with CAH, 403–404
     mineralocorticoids, 412
     mineralocorticoids and sodium
        chloride replacement, 402
     monitoring of, 402
     of nonclassic 21-OHD CAH, 403
     prenatal therapy, 404
     psychological assessment and
        support, 403
     stress therapy, 402
Congenital heart disease
  associated problems, 438b
     arrhythmias, 442
     central nervous system
        complications, 441–442
     conduction abnormalities, 442
     failure to thrive, 442–443
     heart block, 442
     hematologic problems, 439
     infections, 439–440
     infective endocarditis, 440–441,
        441b
     obesity, 443

Congenital heart disease (Continued)
     slow development, 443–444
     ventricular rhythm
        disturbances, 442
     vulnerable child syndrome, 444
  clinical manifestations, 428
  common illness management
     acquired heart disease, 452
     chest pain, 451b, 451–452
     drug interactions, 452
     fever, 449
     gastrointestinal symptoms, 450
     infective endocarditis, 449–450
     inflammatory reaction, 449
     neurologic symptoms, 450
     operative infection, 449
     respiratory compromise, 450
     syncope, 452
  cyanotic lesions
     anomalous pulmonary venous
        return, 427
     hypoplastic left heart
        syndrome, 427–428
     Tetralogy of Fallot, 426
     transposition of great
        arteries, 425–426
     tricuspid atresia, 426
     truncus arteriosus, 426
  developmental issues
     child care, 453–454
     contraceptive counseling, 454–455
     discipline, 453
     risk for adverse events during
        pregnancy and delivery, 455
     schooling, 454
     sexuality, 454
     sleep problems, 453
     toileting, 453
     transition to adulthood, 455–456
  diagnosis, 422
     criteria, 428
  environmental factors, 417, 420t–422t
  etiology, 417
     link between genetics and, 417
  family concerns, 456
  fertility procedures and, 417
  genetic syndrome and gene variants
     of, 418t–420t
  health care maintenance
     air travel, 447
     breastfeeding, 445
     diet, 445–446
     growth and development, 444–445
     immunization, 447–448
     nutrition, 446
     safety, 446–447
     surgery and procedures, 447
  incidence and prevalence, 417, 422t
     risk of recurrence, 417
     sex-based, 417
  information material available
     to family and health care
     providers, 457
  intracardiac shunting lesions in, 422
  left-to-right shunts
     atrial septal defect, 423
     complete atrioventricular
        canal (endocardial cushion
        defect), 424

Congenital heart disease *(Continued)*
　patent ductus arteriosus, 423
　ventricular septal defect, 423
　maternal prenatal risk factors, 417,
　　420t–422t
　obstructive lesions
　　aortic stenosis, 424–425
　　coarctation of aorta, 425
　　pulmonary stenosis, 424
　　right ventricular outflow tract
　　　obstructive lesions, 424
　parental concerns, 456
　parent support groups for, 456–457
　pathophysiology, 422
　physical examination findings,
　　429t–433t
　prognosis, 444
　screenings, 448
　　blood pressure, 448
　　dental, 448
　　drugs and electrolytes, 449
　　hearing, 448
　　hemoglobin/hematocrit, 448
　　lipid panel, 448
　　psychosocial, 448
　　tuberculosis, 448
　　urinalysis, 448
　　vision, 448
　survivors of, 417
　treatment
　　anticipated advancements, 437–438
　　cardiac catheterization, 436
　　complementary and alternative
　　　medicine, 437
　　electrophysiology procedures, 436
　　goal of, 435
　　postoperative management, 436
　　prevention of pulmonary
　　　hypertension, 437
　　staged repair, 435–436
　　surgery, 435
Congenital heart failure, 433
　clinical and physical findings, 434t
　clinical manifestation, 433
　control of, 436–437
　in infants and children, 433
Congenital hydrocephalus, 619–620
Connors Early Childhood Rating
　Scale, 182
Consolidated Omnibus Budget
　Reconciliation Act, 83
Constipation, 743
Continuous ambulatory peritoneal
　dialysis, 691
Contrecoup injury, 914–915
Coprolalia, 900
Corticosteroids, 795
Corticosteroid therapy, 740
Coup injury, 914–915, 915f
COVID-19 vaccine, 891
COX-2 Inhibitor, 671t
Cranial nerve IX
　(glossopharyngeal), 890
Cranial nerve X (vagus), 890
Cranial nerve XII (hypoglossal), 890
Crohn disease, 639–641
　characteristics of pediatric, 640, 644t
　clinical manifestations, 644
　infertility rates, 660

Crohn disease *(Continued)*
　lactose intolerance in, 657
　predictive considerations for
　　surgery, 656–657
　visual findings, 640
Cultural appropriateness of
　services, 10–11
　culturally sensitive intervention, 10–11
　ideal organization characteristics, 10
　linguistic services, 10
Cultural sensitivity, 10–11
Cushing syndrome, 755–756
Cyanosis, 434
Cyclothymic disorders, 725t, 726
Cystic fibrosis
　associated problems and treatment
　　abnormal behavioral eating
　　　patterns, 474
　　anxiety and depression, 473
　　chronic rhinosinusitis, 473
　　distal intestinal obstruction
　　　syndrome, 472, 476–479
　　gastroesophageal reflux
　　　disease, 476–479
　　infection prevention and
　　　control, 475–476
　　liver disease, 472–473
　　meconium ileus, 472
　　morbidity, 473
　　osteoporosis and bone disease, 473
　　pancreatic insufficiency, 472
　　rectal prolapse, 472
　　related diabetes, 473
　　urinary incontinence, 480
　　weight loss or weight gain,
　　　474–475, 475f
　clinical care schedule for
　　newborns, 477t
　clinical manifestation, 465–466
　　recurrent respiratory
　　　infections, 466
　common illness management
　　chest pain, 479
　　cough, 479
　　fever, 479
　　gastrointestinal symptoms,
　　　476–479
　　pediatric illnesses, 476
　　wheezing, 479
　developmental issues
　　child care, 481
　　discipline, 480–481
　　family concerns, 482
　　mentoring for support, 482
　　schooling, 481
　　sexual function, 481–482
　　sleep problems, 479–480
　　toileting, 480
　　transition to adulthood, 482
　diagnostic screening
　　CFTR-related abnormality, 464–465
　　CRMS/CFSPID, 464–465
　　diagnostic criteria, 464, 465f
　　IRT/IRT screening
　　　algorithm, 463–464
　　oral glucose tolerance test, 473
　　sweat testing, 464
　etiology, 463
　gene, 463

Cystic fibrosis *(Continued)*
　genetic mutations, 463
　health care maintenance
　　diet, 474–475
　　growth and development, 473–474
　　HEADSS assessment, 474
　　immunizations, 476
　incidence and prevalence, 463
　insurance coverage, 482
　life expectancy, 482
　mucous secretions, 463
　newborn screening for, 463–465
　pregnancy, 482
　prognosis, 473
　screenings
　　blood pressure, 476
　　condition-specific, 476
　　dental, 476
　　hearing, 476
　　hematocrit, 476
　　tuberculosis, 476
　　vision, 476
　serious complications, 474b
　survival rate, 464f
　symptoms, 464b, 466
　treatment
　　airway clearance and exercise, 468,
　　　470b
　　antibiotic therapy, 470–471, 471f
　　antiinflammatory therapy, 471–472
　　CFTR modulators, 468, 470t
　　chronic pulmonary therapies, 469t
　　DNase, 470
　　high-calorie diet, 467
　　inhaled saline, 470
　　lung transplantation, 472
　　mucolytics, 470
　　nutritional management, 466
　　pancreatic enzyme replacement
　　　therapy, 467, 467t
　　respiratory management, 468
　　vitamin, mineral, and sodium
　　　supplementation, 467–468
　　weight-for-stature assessment, 466
Cystic fibrosis transmembrane
　conductance regulator, 463
Cytomegalovirus, 292, 799
　surveillance for, 292

D
Dactylitis, 865–866
Decision making
　autonomy (self-determination), 91
　beneficence, 89
　　Baby Doe regulations, 89
　　individualized care outcomes, 89
　dealing with conflicts, 99–100
　ethical issues, 87, 88b
　informed consent, 92
　justice, 92
　　beneficence and, 93
　　ethical obligations of, 92–93
　　macroallocation of, 93
　minors' role in treatment, 95–96
　　importance of self-determination
　　　and well-being, 96
　　legal viewpoint on, 96–97
　　standards for determining, 96
　moral framework, 88b, 88–89

Decision making (Continued)
nonmaleficence, 89–90
  maltreatment, 91
  medical harms, 90
  new therapies, 90–91
  pain assessment and
    management, 90
parental role in treatment, 94–95
  for infants and children, 95
  limits on authority, 95
  in well-being, 95
respect for persons, 91–92
shared, 94b, 94, 97
  authentic, 97
  endorsement of model, 94
strategies for ethical
  genetic testing, 99
  knowledge of legal, public, and
    professional policies, 98
  proactive dialogue, assessment,
    and planning, 98–99
veracity and fidelity, 92
Decubitus ulcers, 743
deep poverty, 1–3
Deflazacort, 740
Dental malocclusion, 152
Dermatitis, 825
Desmopressin acetate, 246t, 257–258
Developmental milestones, 27
Dexrazoxane, 325
Dextromethorphan, 908
Diabetes mellitus
  anticipated advances in
    treatment, 494
    dipeptidyl peptidase 4 inhibitor
      (sitagliptin), 494
    insulin delivery and glucose
      sensor technology, 494
    islet-cell transplantation, 494
    pancreas transplantation, 494
    sodium-glucose transport protein
      2 inhibitor, 494
    transplantation of beta cells, 494
  associated problems
    cardiovascular complications, 496
    diabetic ketoacidosis, 494–495
    hyperglycemia, 495b, 495–496
    hyperlipidemia, 496
    hypertension, 496
    hypoglycemia, 495b, 495–496
    monilial vaginitis, 496
    nonalcoholic fatty liver disease, 496
    polycystic ovary syndrome, 496–497
  cause of, 487
  clinical manifestations, 488b, 488
    hepatic gluconeogenesis, 488–489
    obesity and acanthosis nigricans,
      488–489
    osmotic diuresis, 488
    peripheral insulin resistance,
      488–489
  common illness management
    hirsutism, 502
    ketone levels, 501
    maintaining hydration, 501
    medications and antibiotics, 502
    skin manifestations, 502
    vaginal discharge, 501
    vomiting and diarrhea, 501

Diabetes mellitus (Continued)
  weight loss, 502
  comparison of T1D and T2D, 488t
  developmental issues and family
    concerns
    child care, 503
    discipline, 502–503
    individualized 504 plan, 503
    nighttime hypoglycemia, 502
    schooling, 503–504
    sexual development, 504
    sleep patterns, 502
    social determinants of health, 505
    toileting, 502
    transition to adulthood, 504
    weight gain or loss, 504
  diagnostic criteria, 488, 489b
    glucose monitoring, 490, 492
    glycosylated hemoglobin test,
      488–489, 492–493
  etiology, 487
    associated with autoimmunity, 510
    associated with polycystic ovary
      syndrome, 487
    genetic and pathologic
      processes, 487
    human leukocyte antigen
      genes, 510
    peripheral insulin resistance, 487
  health care maintenance
    dietary plan, 498–499
    growth and development, 498
    immunizations, 499
    obesity, 498
    onset and progression of
      puberty, 498
    physical activity, 499
    safety, 499
  incidence and prevalence, 487–488
  long-term complications, 497
    blindness, 497
    cardiovascular disease, 497
    hypertension, 497
    microvascular disease, 497
    painful neuropathies, 497
    renal failure, 497
  from lower SES, 505
  psychosocial complications, 497
    anxiety, 497
    depression, 497
    disordered eating, 497
    freedom and independence, 497
    SEARCH for Diabetes in Youth
      Study, 497
    suicidal/death ideation, 497
  screenings, 499
    celiac disease, 500
    dental caries, 500
    depression, 500
    dyslipidemia, 499
    hypertension, 499
    nephropathy, 500
    neuropathy, 500
    nonalcoholic fatty liver disease, 500
    obstructive sleep apnea, 500
    polycystic ovary syndrome, 500
    by primary care provider, 501b
    retinopathy, 500
    urine testing, 502

Diabetes mellitus (Continued)
  signs and symptoms, 488, 489f
  support organizations
    American Diabetes
      Association, 505
    Beyond Type 1, 505
    Juvenile Diabetes Research
      Foundation, 505
  treatment for type 1, 490b
    in ambulatory setting, 490–491
    complementary and alternative
      therapies, 493–494
    Diabetes Control and
      Complications Trial, 490
    dietary therapy, 492
    glucose monitoring, 492
    injection of quick-acting
      insulin, 490–491
    insulin pump therapy, 490–491
    insulin replacement, 490
    Omnipod system, 491
    pump devices, 491
  treatment for type 2
    basal insulin therapy, 493
    complementary and alternative
      therapies, 494
    GLP-1 agonist, 493
    initial treatment, 492–493
    lifestyle intervention, 493
    Metformin therapy, 493
    pharmacologic treatment, 493
Diabetic ketoacidosis, 494–495
Diffuse axonal injury, 914, 919
DiGeorge syndrome, 372–373
Disease-modifying antirheumatic
  drugs, 670
Disruptive Behavior Disorder Rating
  Scale, 182
Disruptive mood dysregulation
  disorder, 723
DNA banking, 405
Donor lymphocyte infusions, 282
Do-not-attempt-resuscitation
  orders, 68–69, 69b
  Committee on School Health and
    Committee on Bioethics policy
    statement, 69
  in individual states, 69
  National Education Association
    guidelines, 69
Dopamine receptor blocking agents, 905
Down syndrome, 218
  age-specific risks, 512f, 512
  anticipated advances in diagnosis
    and management, 515
  associated problems with, 515b
    altered respiratory function, 517
    atlantoaxial instability, 516
    behavior disorders, 515
    cardiac defects, 515–516
    celiac disease, 517–518
    constipation, 530
    dental changes, 518
    frequency of seizure disorders, 518
    gastrointestinal tract anomalies, 516
    growth abnormalities, 517
    hearing loss, 516–517
    immune system deficits, 516
    intellectual capabilities, 515

Down syndrome (Continued)
  musculoskeletal and motor
    abilities, 516
  preleukemic and leukemia, risk
    for, 517
  respiratory syncytial virus
    bronchiolitis, 517
  skin conditions, 518
  sleep-disordered breathing, 518
  subluxation or dislocation, 516
  thyroid dysfunction, 517
  tumors, risk for, 517
  vision problems, 516
 cause of, 510
 clinical manifestations, 512
 common illness management
  behavioral changes, 529
  drug interactions, 529
  gastrointestinal symptoms, 529
  immune dysfunction, 529
  leukemia, 529
  upper respiratory tract
    infections, 529
 congenital anomalies, 518
 developmental issues
  child care, 530
  discipline, 530
  family concerns, 531–532
  premature aging, 531
  pubertal changes, 530–531
  schooling, 530
  self-care skills, 530–531
  sibling adjustments, 531
  sleep patterns, 529–530
  toileting, 530
  transition to adulthood, 531
  vocational choices, 531
 diagnosis, 512
 etiology, 510
 genetic counseling, 513b–514b, 513–514
 health care maintenance
  breastfeeding, 525–526
  diet plan, 524–526
  early intervention program, 523–524
  growth and development, 518,
    520, 524
  growth charts, 520, 520f–525f
  guidelines for health
    supervision, 519t, 526t, 527b
  immunizations, 527
  intellectual and developmental
    disability, 521–523
  safety, 526
 incidence and prevalence, 512
 informational materials for, 532
 nondisjunction, 510, 511f, 512
 numerous anatomic and physiologic
    aberrations, 518
 phenotype for, 510
 prenatal screening, 512
 prognosis, 518
 risk for autism spectrum
    disorders, 514–515
 risk of low bone mineral density, 515
 screenings
  atlantoaxial instability, 528
  celiac disease, 529
  dental, 528
  hearing, 527–528

Down syndrome (Continued)
  hip dislocation, 528
  mitral valve prolapse, 529
  vision, 527
 Supplemental Security Income
    for, 532
 by translocation, 510, 512
  balanced, 510
  recurrence risk for a second
    child, 510, 511f
  Robertsonian translocations, 510
  unbalanced, 510
 treatments, 512–513, 514b
  complementary and alternative
    therapies, 515
  early cardiac surgery, 516
  early interventions, 514–515
  individualized education
    program, 515
  preschool programs, 515
  of secondary conditions, 514
  surgery, 514
Drug-herb interactions, 695
Drug interactions, 173, 677b
Dry powder inhalers, 132
Duchenne muscular dystrophy, 746f
Ductus arteriosus, 840–841
Dyskinetic cerebral palsy, 352
Dyslipidemia, 499, 773
Dystrophin, 735

E
Eating disorders, 536
 advances in diagnoses and
    treatment, 544
 anorexia nervosa, 536
 associated problems and treatment
    of, 545
  amenorrhea, 546
  cardiac issues, 546
  constipation, 545–546
  dehydration from chronic
    purging, 546
  diarrhea with fever, 546
  diffuse abdominal pain, 546
  edema, 546
  endocrine problems, 546
  gastroesophageal reflux and
    disease, 545
  gastroparesis, 545
  osteopenia, 546
  osteoporosis, 546
  phosphorus and thiamine
    supplementation, 546–547
  refeeding syndrome, 546–547
  superior mesenteric artery
    syndrome, 546
  vomiting, 546
 binging episodes, 536
 bulimia nervosa, 536
 categories, 536
 clinical manifestations, 540, 541t, 542
 common illness management, 551
 developmental issues
  child care, 552
  discipline, 552
  family concerns, 553
  school adjustment, 552
  sexuality, 552–553

Eating disorders (Continued)
  sleep patterns, 551
  toileting, 551
  transition to adulthood, 553
 diagnostic criteria
  anorexia nervosa, 539
  avoidant/restrictive food intake
    disorder, 539–540
  binge eating disorder, 539
  bulimia nervosa, 539
 differential diagnosis, 552b
 etiology, 536
  association with COVID-19
    pandemic, 537
  biologic theories, 538
  family theories, 537
  psychological theories, 536–537
  role of subcultures, 537
  sexual orientation and gender
    identity, 537
  sociocultural theories, 537
  Western beauty standards and
    antifatness, 537
 health care maintenance, 549
  age-related safety and anticipatory
    guidance, 550
  growth and development, 549
  immunization schedule, 550
  nutrition, 549–550
  weight gain or loss, 549
 impact of, 536
 incidence and prevalence, 538
  in ethnoracial groups, 538–539
 physical exam, 542–543
 prevention of, 548
  consultation with specialist, 548
 primary care management, 547
  indications supporting
    hospitalization, 549b
  laboratory evaluation, 549b
  screening tools and targeted
    questions, 547–548, 548b
  targeted review of symptoms/
    systems, 548b, 548
 prognosis, 547
 psychosocial distress or impairment
    and, 536
 at risk group, 550
 screenings
  blood pressure, 550
  cardiac exam, 551
  condition-specific, 551
  dental, 550
  endocrine system, 551
  hearing, 550
  laboratory tests, 551
  metabolic profile, 551
  urinalysis, 551
  vision, 550
 signs and symptoms of, 536
 treatment, 543
  complementary and alternative
    therapies, 544
  psychopharmacologic
    interventions, 543–544
  psychotherapy, 543
Echocardiogram, 740
Echocardiography, 875
Echolalia, 900

E-consults, 107–108
Electrocardiogram (ECG), 740
Electrocardiography, 875
Electromyography, 737
Encephalopathy, 698
Endocrine dysfunction, 928
End-of-life management, 45–46
Endoscopic third ventriculostomy with choroid plexus cauterization, 887–888
End-stage liver disease, 787–788
Engraftment syndrome, 290
    diagnostic criteria, 290
    pathophysiology, 290
    symptoms, 290
Enhanced recovery after surgery, 381
Enthesitis-related arthritis, 669
Eosinophilic esophagitis, 151
    biologics for, 136
    Dupilumab (Dupixent), 151
    empiric elimination diet for, 151
    proton pump inhibitors, 151
    swallowed corticosteroids, 151
Epidural hematoma, 919
Epilepsy, 360
    in children undergoing gender-affirming hormone therapy, 577
    comorbidities with, 572
        anxiety, 573, 574t
        attention-deficit/hyperactivity disorder, 573
        depression and anxiety, 572–573
        functional neurologic disorder, 574–575
        functional seizures, 574–575
        injuries, 575
        mental health, 572
        neurodevelopmental disorders, 575
        sleep problems, 575
        sudden unexpected death in epilepsy, 572
    definition, 560
    diagnosis, 561–562
        EEGs, 562–563, 563b
        genetic testing, 564
        history, 562b, 562
        MRI, 563–564
        physical examination, 562, 563t
        provoking factors, 562
    differential diagnosis for seizures, 562
    etiology, 560
    in females, 577
    health care maintenance
        academic needs and support, 576
        bone density, 576
        diet, 575
        drug interactions, 576
        growth and development, 575
        immunizations, 576
        mental health comorbidities, 576
        seizure action plans, 576
        seizure restrictions, 576
    incidence of, 560
        febrile seizures, 560
    ketogenic diet, 571–572
    pathophysiology, 560
    recurrence of seizures, 564–565
    referral to neurologists, 577
    seizure classification, 560, 561t

Epilepsy (Continued)
    associated clinical features, 561
    febrile, 561
    focal, 560–561
    generalized, 561
    with unknown onset, 561
    Stevens-Johnson syndrome, risk of, 564
    suicidal thoughts and behaviors, risk of, 564
    treatment, 564–565
        cognitive-behavioral therapy, 573
        daily medication, 566t–568t
        deep brain stimulation, 571
        medication for rescue therapy, 569, 569t
        responsive nerve stimulation, 570
        surgery, 569–571
Epilepsy syndromes, 564, 565t
EPO-stimulating agent, 688–689
Epstein-Barr virus infection, 292
    asymptomatic, 292
    EBV posttransplant lymphoproliferative disease (EBV-PTLD), 292
    PCR monitoring, 292
Erythrocyte sedimentation rate, 669
Erythromycin, 908
Escherichia coli, 862–863
Estimated glomerular filtration rate, 683
Estrogen-based oral contraceptives, 677
Ethics, 87
    of care, 94
        values and expectations, 94
    ethical course of action, 87
    ethical decision making, 88b
    ethical deliberation, 87
    ethical dimensions of an issue or quandary, 87
    ethical questions, 87
    ethical theories and principles, 87–88, 88t, 94
    ethical thinking, 87
    genetic testing, 99
Eustachian tube obstruction, 152
Excessive fluid removal, 697
Exercise-induced bronchospasms, 126
    treatment, 136–137

F
Failure to thrive, 442–443
Family Educational Rights and Privacy Act, 59
Fetal hemoglobin, 855
Fetal spina bifida defects, repair of, 887
Fisap insulin, 494
Focal segmental glomerular sclerosis, 683
Focal segmental glomerulosclerosis, 696
Folate-fortified foods, 886
Food security status of a household, 3
Foreign-born population in United States, 9
Foundation for Accountability, 6
Fractional exhaled nitric oxide measures, 138
Fragile X syndrome, 179, 218, 582f
    associated problems of, 587b

Fragile X syndrome (Continued)
    autistic-like tendencies, 588
    cardiac problems, 587
    connective tissue problems, 587
    oral problems, 587
    psychiatric manifestations, 588
    seizures, 587
    sensory integration difficulties, 588
    speech and language difficulties, 587
    strabismus, 587
    vision problems, 587
    checklist, 582, 582t
    clinical manifestations, 583b
        aggression in childhood or adolescence, 585
        cognitive and physical features, 582–584, 583f
        enlarged testicles, 583
        in females, 584f, 584
        language skills, 583
        in males, 582–584, 584f
    common illness management
        connective tissue problems, 590, 592
        drug interactions, 590
        otitis media, 590
    developmental issues and treatment
        child care, 591
        computers for learning enhancement, use of, 591
        discipline, 590–591
        family concerns, 592–593
        schooling, 591
        sexual and reproduction health, 591–592
        sleep patterns, 590
        speech, language, and occupational therapy, 591
        toileting, 590
        transitioning to adulthood, 592
    diagnostic, 582, 590b
    family stress of individuals affected by, 586f
    fragile X-associated neuropsychiatric disorders, 581
    fragile X-associated primary ovarian insufficiency, 581
    fragile X-associated tremor/ataxia syndrome, 581
    genetics, 581
        fragile X messenger ribonucleoprotein 1 gene, 581
        role of X chromosome, 581
    health care maintenance
        diet, 588–589
        growth and development, 588
        immunizations, 589
        safety, 589
    incidence and prevalence, 581–582
    prognosis, 588
    psychological characteristics, 582
    screenings, 589b
        blood pressure, 589
        connective tissue evaluation, 590
        dental, 589
        hearing, 589
        hematocrit, 589
        mitral valve prolapse, 589

Fragile X syndrome *(Continued)*
  seizures, 590
  speech-language evaluation, 590
  tuberculosis, 589
  urinalysis, 589
  vision, 589
  treatment, 585*b*, 585
    clonidine (Catapres), 585
    complementary and alternative
      treatments, 586
    educational intervention, 585–586
    genetic counseling, 586
    metabotropic glutamate 5
      system, 586–587
    pharmacologic therapy, 585
    phosphodiesterase
      inhibitor, 586–587
    selective serotonin reuptake
      inhibitor, 585
    sensory integration therapy, 586
Free and appropriate public
  education, 51–52
Fungal infections, 800

G
Gastroesophageal reflux, 846
Gastrointestinal disorders, 776
Gastrostomy tube, 890
Generalized anxiety disorder, 165
  clinical manifestation of, 166
  cognitive-behavioral therapy, 169
  diagnostic criteria for, 165–166
Generalized Anxiety Disorder
  Questionnaire, 903–904
Gene therapy, 284, 861
Genetic Information
  Nondiscrimination Act, 2008, 99
Genitourinary disorders, 776
Genome modification, 861
Genome-wide association studies, 755
Genu valgum, 776
Gingival hyperplasia, 930
Glasgow Outcome Scale, 924
Glasgow Coma Scale, 916, 917*t*
  moderate head injuries, 916
  severe head injuries, 916
  complicated mTBI, 918–919
  uncomplicated mTBI, 918–919
Glomerulonephritis, 683
Gluten-free diet, 344–346, 349
  common pitfall to, 344*b*, 344–345
  excluded foods, 344
  grains and flours, 344*b*
  oats, 344
Got Transition program, 84–85
Gowers maneuver, 737–738
Graft *versus* host disease, 269
  acute, 286
    clinical signs, 286
    pathogenesis, 286
  chronic
    clinical manifestations, 305*t*
    manifestations, 287
    pathogenesis of, 287
    severe forms of, 287
  of gut, 301
  of oral mucosa, 300
  prevention and treatment of, 288
    calcineurin inhibitor, 289

Graft *versus* host disease *(Continued)*
    immunosuppressive therapies, 288
    nonpharmacologic approach, 289
    prophylactic approaches
      for, 288–289
    systemic steroids
      (methylprednisolone/
      prednisone), 289
    targeted topical therapies, 289
  risk factors for, 288
  target organ staging, 287*t*
Graft *versus* leukemia effect, 269
Granulocyte CSF, 277
Gross Motor Function Classification
  System, 353*t*
Growth failure, 687

H
Habit reversal therapy, 905
Haemophilus influenzae, 607–608,
  862–863, 867
Hashimoto thyroiditis, 500
Health care networks, 105–106
Health care transition, 73
  access to health care as an adult, 80–81
  adult care integration, 73
  to adult care services, 73
  barriers to, 76–78, 78*b*, 81–82
    adult and pediatric clinician
      transition, 79*b*
    care coordination, 78
    fear of lack of confidentiality, 78
    inadequate preparedness, 78
    insufficient self-management
      skills, 78
    judgment of health care
      providers, 78
    lack of resources, 78
    mistrust of health care
      providers, 78
    poor communication, 78
    stigma, 78
    system-level barriers, 78
  factors moderating transition, 78
    level of care, coordination, and
      frequent consultation, 78
    social determinants of health, 79,
      81*f*
    survival rates, 78–79
  learning health management skills, 74
  pediatric to adult-based, 79
  planning, 79, 80*b*
  proactive approach, 73
  self-management, 73–74
  six core elements of, 79–80, 81*t*
  structured transition interventions, 74
  team works, 74
  transfer, 73
  transition preparation, 73
Health equity, 12
Health insurance, 82–83, 82*t*
Health Insurance Portability and
  Accountability Act of 1996, 59, 99
Healthy childhood development
  developmentally appropriate
    information needs, 41
  family and social networks, role
    of, 29
    caregivers, 29

Healthy childhood development
  (Continued)
  multisensory approach, 41–42
  primary care provider's role, 31
    advocacy, 43
    anticipatory guidance, 40–41
    assessment and management,
      31–32, 33*t*–39*t*
    counseling, 43–44
    developmental surveillance, 32
    dying and hospice care, 45–46
    emergency care, 43
    fostering psychosocial health, 40*b*, 40
    hospitalization, 44–45
    integration of mental health into
      primary care, 43, 44*b*
    palliative care, 45
    patient and family-centered care, 31
    patient-centered health care
      home, 31
    person-centered language, use
      of, 32–40
    primary prevention, 44
    providing a label, 32
    referrals, 32
    secondary prevention, 44
    sports participation, support
      for, 41*b*
    therapeutic adherence, promoting,
      42*b*, 42–43
    youth transition to adult care, 41*b*
HEEADSSS screening process, 230
Hematocrit, 676, 805
Hematopoiesis, 868–869
Hematopoietic engraftment, 281
Hematopoietic stem cell transplant,
  269, 861
  adoptive immunotherapy/chimeric
    antigen receptor t-cell therapy,
    282
  allogeneic, 269–270, 270*b*
    indications for, 270–271
  antifungals during, 278–280
  autologous, 270*b*, 270, 281
    apheresis in, 277
    conditioning regimens for, 278
  in cancer treatment, 324
  chemotherapy or radiation
    therapy, 271
  chimerism testing, 282
  clinical manifestations in, 273
  common concerns following, 271
    medication administration/
      adherence/drug interactions,
      306–307
  common illness management
    children who are
      immunocompromised, 303
    fever management, 303–306
    gastrointestinal symptoms, 306
    headache, 306
    immunosuppressive
      medications, 303, 306
    pain, 306
    rashes and/or skin changes, 306
  complementary and alternative
    medicine, 282–283
  conditions commonly treated with,
    273, 274*t*–276*t*

Hematopoietic stem cell transplant (Continued)
consolidative radiation therapy and chemotherapy, 282
consolidative therapies following, 284
criteria for transplant eligibility
donor workup, 272–273
human leukocyte antigen typing, 272
identified risks for donors, 273
matching guidelines, 272
pretransplant evaluation, 272
recommendations regarding minor sibling donation, 273
referral and consultation, 271–272
specific comorbidity index, 272
transplant workup, 272
developmental issues
child care, 307
delayed pubertal development, 308
discipline, 307
education and future employment, 309
effects on self-image, 308
family concerns, 309
infertility, 308
schooling, 307–308
sleep patterns, 307
toileting, 307
transition to adulthood, 308–309
diagnosis and management, 283–284
diet and nutrition support, 297–298, 297t
calcium and vitamin D supplements, 298
tips for safe food storage, 298
differences between solid organ transplantation and, 271
donor compatibility/matching, 270
early development, 269
follow-up and surveillance testing, 295
growth disturbances
endocrine complications, 296
gonadal dysfunction and infertility, 296
hypothyroidism, 296
ovarian dysfunction, 296
standard deviations, 296
testicular failure, 296
thyroid dysfunction, 296
hematopoietic engraftment, 281
immunizations, 299, 299t
live virus vaccines, 299
reimmunization, 299
immunosuppressive regimens, 278, 280–281, 279t–280t
calcineurin inhibitor, 278–280, 288b, 288
posttransplant cyclophosphamide, 280–281
incidence and prevalence, 271
infection prevention, 281–282
palliative care, 283
peritransplant phase
conditioning regimens, 278
total body irradiation, 278
physical and occupational health, 299

Hematopoietic stem cell transplant (Continued)
posttransplant phase
acute and chronic GvHD, prevention and treatment of, 286–289, 287t–288t
anemia, 285
bacterial infections, 291
BK virus infection, 293
candida infections and aspergillosis, 294
Clostridioides difficile infection, 294
CMV infection, 292
community-acquired respiratory virus infections, 293
COVID-19 virus infection, 293
early complications posttransplantation, 284b, 284
engraftment syndrome, 290
Epstein-Barr virus infection, 292
fever with neutropenia, 291–292
fungal disease, 293–294
graft failure and graft rejection, 289
herpes simplex virus infection, 292
infections, 290–291, 291f
issue of poor graft function, 289
late effects, 294
mucositis, 285–286
myelosuppression, 284
neutropenia, risk for, 284
nutritional support, 286
Pneumocystis jirovecii pneumonia, 294
postengraftment infections, 292
respiratory syncytial virus infections, 293
risks of multidrug-resistant organisms, 291
sinusoidal obstructive syndrome/ venoocclusive disease, risk of, 290
thrombocytopenia, 284–285
transfusion-related GvHD, 285
varicella zoster virus infection, 293
primary care management, 295–296
prognosis, 295
recipient's immune system and, 271
risk for CMV retinitis, 299–300
safety guidelines, 298–299
screening recommendations
BMD evaluation, 301
bone health, 301
cardiovascular complications, 300
condition-specific screening/ monitoring, 302–303
dental evaluation, 300
gastrointestinal complications, 301
hearing, 300
infectious complications, 301
late complications, 303, 303t–304t
lymphoma or lymphoproliferative disorder, 302
neurocognitive effects, 302
pulmonary complications, 300–301
renal complications, 301
secondary leukemia, 302
secondary malignancies, 302
skin, 301
vision, 299

Hematopoietic stem cell transplant (Continued)
stem cell collection
from bone marrow, 273
from peripheral blood, 277
stem cell manipulation, 277
from umbilical cord and placenta, 277–278
stem cell sources, 269
success of, 295
survivors, 295–296
tandem transplants, 278
timeline, 281, 281t
transplant-related mortality rate, 270–271
Hematuria, 687, 868
Hemodialysis, 692
Hemoglobin regulation, 861
Hemolysis, 868
Hemolytic anemia, 862
Hemophilia, 259
acquired/inheritance, 237–238, 239f
clinical manifestations, 238
signs of bleeding, 239
hemophilia A (factor VIII deficiency), 237
hemophilia B (factor IX deficiency), 237
misconceptions, 239
severity of, 238t
testing for, 239
diagnosis of variants hemophilia A and B, 241
laboratory tests, 241
severity, 241
treatment
aminocaproic acid, 247
antifibrinolytic agents, 242, 247
bypassing agents, 242, 250
comparison of, 250f
core team for, 241
desmopressin acetate, 242, 246t, 247
emicizumab-kxwh (Hemlibra), 242, 247
hormonal therapy, 247–248
immune tolerance induction therapy, 251
with inhibitors, 249–250, 250b
interdisciplinary comprehensive evaluations, counseling and support services, 241
of joint bleeding, 249
of minor bleeding, 249
pain management, 251–252
in patients with acute bleeding, 248
pharmacologic, 242, 243t–244t
physical therapy, 251
prophylaxis, 243t–244t, 248
standard of care, 241
tranexamic acid (Lysteda), 247
treatment centers, 241–242
Hemostasis, 237
Hepatic crisis, 870
Hepatitis A vaccine, 609
Hepatitis B vaccine, 607
Herbal dietary supplements, 796
Herpes simplex virus infection, 292
Heterogeneous disorder, 900

Hib vaccine, 872, 873f
Hispanic pediatric dialysis, 699
Holistic understanding of a child's
    life, 89
Holoprosencephaly, 372–373
Household Food Security Scale, 4–5
Howell-Jolly bodies, 862
Human immunodeficiency virus
    clinical manifestations, 600–601
    common illness management
        fever, 610
        incidence of varicella, 611
        otitis media, 611
        respiratory distress, 611
        sinusitis, 611
    conditions associated with, 603
        failure to thrive, 603–604
        fungal infections, 605
        gastrointestinal problems, 604
        neurologic manifestations, 604
        opportunistic infections, 604
        pancytopenia, 605
        prenatal and perinatal substance
            use exposure, 605
        pulmonary disease, 604–605
    developmental issues
        child care, 612–613
        discipline, 612
        family concerns, 614
        schooling, 613
        sexual and reproductive health, 613
        sleep patterns, 612
        toileting, 612
        transition to adulthood, 613–614
    diagnosis, 597, 598f, 599
        antibody and antigen/antibody
            tests, 599–600
        dual-target total DNA/RNA
            test, 599
        maternal HIV testing, 599–600
        recommendations and timing, 599,
            600t
        use of IV intrapartum zidovudine,
            599–600
    drug interactions
        antiretroviral medications, 611, 612b
        intravenous immunoglobulin, 612
    epidemiology, 597
    health care maintenance, 606
        diet, 606–607
        growth and development, 606
        immunizations, 607–609, 608f
        safety precautions, 607
    pathogenesis and
        transmission, 598f–599f
    male-to-male sexual
        transmission, 597
    pathogenesis and transmission, 597
    reverse transcription, 597–598
    seroconversion, 599
    through maternal-to-child
        transmission, 598–599
    prognosis, 605
    in adolescents, 606
    screenings
        antiretroviral medication
            adherence assessment, 610
        blood count, 610
        blood pressure, 609

Human immunodeficiency virus
    (Continued)
        dental, 609
        hearing, 609
        hematocrit, 609
        HIV RNA viral load, 610
        immunologic markers, 610
        pulmonary function testing, 610
        recommendations, 597
        routine serum chemistry
            panels, 610
        tuberculosis, 609
        urinalysis, 609
        vision, 609
        vital signs, 610
    treatment, 601–602
        antiretroviral therapy regimens,
            597, 601b, 602t, 603
        complementary and alternative
            medicine, 603
        corticosteroids, 604–605
        dosages of medication, 603
        goals for, 602
        in infants, 601–602
        multidisciplinary team
            approach, 603
        panel's recommendations for
            intrapartum care, 601b
        preexposure prophylaxis, 603
        trimethoprim/
            sulfamethoxazole, 604–605
        virologic and immunologic
            principles for ART, 602–603
Human leukocyte antigen, 269, 861
Human papillomavirus vaccine, 609,
    805
Human parvovirus B19, 867–868
Human-to-human cardiac
    transplant, 788–789
Hurler syndrome, 273
Hydrocephalus
    acquired, 620
    associated problems and treatment
        intellectual deficits, 626–627
        motor disabilities, 627
        ocular abnormalities, 627
        seizures, 627
    cerebrospinal fluid production, 619
    clinical manifestations, 621b
        in children, 622
        in infancy, 621–622
        macrocephaly, 622
    common illness management
        fever, 631
        gastrointestinal symptoms, 631–632
        headaches, 632
        mood swings and temporary
            behavior changes, 632
        nausea and vomiting, 631
        pneumonia, 631
        scalp infections, 632f, 632
        shunt malfunction or infection
            symptoms, 630
        urinary tract infection, 631
    communicating and
        noncommunicating, 619–620
    congenital, 619–620
    developmental issues
        child care, 633

Hydrocephalus (Continued)
        discipline, 633
        family concerns, 634
        magnetic field interference, 635
        schooling, 633
        sexuality, 633–634
        sleep, 632
        toileting, 632–633
        transition to adulthood, 634
    diagnostic criteria, 621
        CT scans, 621
        fetal anomalies, 626
        MRI scans, 621
    etiology, 619
    external, 619
    health care maintenance
        diet, 628–629
        endocrine abnormalities, 628
        growth and development, 628
        immunizations, 629
        motor delays, 628
        safety, 629
    internal, 619
    with myelomeningocele, 620–621
    prognosis, 627
    screenings
        blood pressure, 630
        dental, 630
        head circumference
            measurements, 630
        hearing, 630
        hematocrit, 630
        tuberculosis, 630
        urinalysis, 630
        vision, 629
    treatment, 622b. See also Shunt
        catheters for CSF
        choroid plexus cauterization, 624
        complications from surgical, 624
        endoscopic third
            ventriculostomy, 624, 625f
        intrauterine closure of a
            myelomeningocele, 626
        nutritional guidelines, 626
        pharmacologic therapy, 622
        shunt catheters for, 623f, 623–624
        surgery, 622–623
Hyperglycemia, 495b, 495–496
Hyperkalemia, 685
Hyperkinetic disorder, 900
Hyperlipidemia, 496
Hyperosmolar contrast medium, 869
Hypertension, 496–497, 499, 697, 773
Hyperviscosity syndrome, 864–865
Hypoglycemia, 495b, 495–496
Hypoplastic left heart syndrome,
    427–428, 429t–433t
Hyposplenism, 345–346
Hyposthenuria, 868
Hypothyroidism, 755–756
Hypoxemia, 434
Hypoxia, 855

I
Idiopathic pneumonia
    syndrome, 300–301
Immunizations, 745
Immunosuppressive medication, 795t
Impaired respiratory function, 927

Increased intracranial pressure, 916
Individualized Education Program, 44, 52–53, 53b, 57, 894, 909
  content, 53, 54b
  eligibility assessment, 53
    questions to ask, 58b
    recommendations, 57–58
    special education assessment, 57
  evaluation process for eligibility, 53
Individualized health plan, 60
Individual Plan for Employment, 84
Individuals with Disabilities Education Act, 49–52, 57, 83, 92–93, 226, 932
  child's rights under, 57
  content, 54b
  development of IEP, 52–53, 53b, 58b
  disabilities entitled to special education, 55b
  eligibility, 53, 56f
  evaluation process, 53
  identifying and locating children with disabilities, 52
  inclusion, 53
  nondiscriminatory testing, 52
  parentally placed private school children, eligibility of, 54
  parental participation, 52
  parts, 52
  race and ethnicity receiving services under, 54
Individuals with Disabilities Education Improvement Act, 195, 514–515
Induction therapy, 796
inequalities in child health
  based on race, ethnicity, and family/ social complexities, 12
Infant mortality rates in United States, 10f, 10
Infants born preterm, 846
Inflammatory bowel disease, 639. See also Crohn disease; Ulcerative colitis; Very early onset IBD
  associated problems
    anemia, 655
    bone health, 653
    cholelithiasis and gallstones, 654
    fulminant colitis or toxic megacolon, 655
    glomerulonephritis, 654
    growth failure and delayed puberty, 652–653
    hepatobiliary complications, 653–654
    hypercoagulopathy, 655
    malignancy, 655–656
    morbidity and mortality, 654–656
    non-Hodgkin lymphoma and hepatosplenic T-cell lymphoma, 655
    osteopenia, 653
    PSC-IBD, 654
    psychosocial issues, 656
    renal complications, 654
    tubulointerstitial nephritis, 654–655
    vitamin D levels, 653
  categories of disease types, 639
  characteristics in Black and non- Black patients, 640
  clinical manifestations, 643

Inflammatory bowel disease (Continued)
  common illness management, 659
    diarrhea, 659
    osteoporosis, 659
    vomiting, 659
  condition, 639
  dermatologic manifestations, 645
  developmental concerns
    behavioral expectations for children, 660
    child care, 660
    family concerns, 660–661
    schooling, 660
    sexual and reproductive health, 660
    sleep patterns, 659–660
    toileting, 660
    transition to adulthood, 660–661
  diagnostic evaluation, 641
    colonoscopy, 643
    C-reactive protein, 642–643
    endoscopy and small bowel imaging, 643
    erythrocyte sedimentation rate, 642–643
    fecal calprotectin testing, 643
    head-to-toe physical examination, 642
    history, 641–642
    laboratory evaluation, 642–643, 643t
    signs of immunologic or genetic disorders associated, 642
    of symptoms, 642
  environmental exposures, 639
  etiology, 639
  extraintestinal manifestations, 645
  genetic influences on, 639
  health care maintenance
    diet and nutritional concerns, 657–658
    growth and development, 657
    immunizations, 658
    safety, 658
  incidence and prevalence, 639–640
  musculoskeletal manifestations, 645
  pathogenesis, 639
  prognosis, 656–657
  pyoderma gangrenosum in, 645
  risks of immunosuppression, 658
  screenings
    blood pressure, 659
    condition specific, 659
    dental, 659
    drug interactions, 659
    hearing, 658
    laboratory assessment, 659
    tuberculosis, 659
    vision, 658
  skin manifestations, 645
  treatment
    anti-TNF therapy, 646
    biologic therapy, 646
    biosimilars, 646
    complementary and alternative medicine, 652
    immunosuppressive therapy, 646, 649
    nutritional therapy, 649–651
    pharmacologic therapy, 646, 647t–651t

Inflammatory bowel disease (Continued)
    regimens, 646
    surgery, 649, 652t
Influenza vaccine, 608, 891
Inhaled corticosteroids (ICS), 127–128, 132–133, 135t
Innovative technology, 801
Integrated complementary and alternative medicine, 925
Integrated palliative care outcome scale, 482
Integrative medicine, 925
International Society for Peritoneal Dialysis, 690
Interprofessional Education Collaborative, 58–59
  core competencies
    interprofessional communication, 59
    roles and responsibilities, 59
    teams and teamwork, 59
    values and ethics, 59
Intracerebral hemorrhage, 919
Intracranial hemorrhage, 865
Intracranial ventricles, 620f
Invasive pneumococcal disease, 871
Ipratropium bromide, 136
Ischemic end-organ injury, 864–865
Islet cell antibodies, 487

J
Juvenile idiopathic arthritis, 668, 673–674
  inflammation in, 668
  pharmacologic therapy for, 671t
  systemic, 674

K
Karyotyping of fetal cells, 512
Kidney Disease Outcomes Quality Initiative guidelines, 684–685
Kidney transplantation, 693

L
Laws on education, 49
  Americans with Disabilities Act of 1990, 49–50, 55
    transition of students into employment positions, 55–56
  comparison of civil rights laws, 50t
  Elementary and Secondary Education Act, 51, 56
  elimination of using R-word, 50
  free public elementary and secondary education, 49
  Individuals with Disabilities Education Act, 49–52, 57
    child's rights under, 57
    content, 54b
    development of IEP, 52–53, 53b, 57
    disabilities entitled to special education, 55b
    eligibility, 53, 56f
    evaluation process, 53
    FAPE, 52
    identifying and locating children with disabilities, 52
    inclusion, 53
    intent of, 57
    LRE, 52

Laws on education (*Continued*)
  No Child Left Behind Act, 56–57
  nondiscriminatory testing, 52
  procedural due process, 52
  Rehabilitation Act, 50
    accommodation plans, 51
    definition of person with a
      disability, 50–51
    gender distribution, 51
    removal of barriers to education, 50
  related services, definition, 54
  Rosa's law, 50
  school-age students served under, 53
  special education, definition, 53
  student enrollment, 53
  zero reject, 52
Leucovorin, 325
Leukemia, 318–322
Leukopenia, 324–325
Lipid profile abnormalities, 767
Liver rejection, 798
Long-chain polyunsaturated fatty
  acids, 822
Lowe syndrome, 802
Lung transplantation, 789
Lyme titers, 903
Lymphomas, 318–322
Lymphoproliferative disorders, 800

M
Macrolide antibiotics, 908
Macroorchidism, 583
Magnetic resonance angiography
  (MRA), 860, 865
Magnetic resonance imaging (MRI),
  860, 865
Maladaptive health behaviors, 43
Malone antegrade continence
  enema, 893
Mandibular distraction
  osteogenesis, 380
Manual Abilities Classification
  System, 353, 354*f*
Maternal and Child Health Bureau, 6
Maternal phenylketonuria
  syndrome, 821
Measles-mumps-rubella, 211, 608–609,
  675–676
Medicaid, 13–15
Meningococcal B vaccine, 609
Meningococcal vaccine, 609
Mesna, 325
Mesosystem level of care for
  CYSHCN, 20
Metabolic acidosis, 688
Metabolic and bariatric surgery, 767
Metabolic syndrome, 775
Methylphenidate, 186, 187*t*
Metoclopramide, 545
Micrognathia, 372–373
Miralax, 893
Model for Effective Chronic Illness
  Care, 18
Model for end-stage liver disease
  score, 789
Moderate-severe TBI, 914, 927
  abnormal motor and sensory
    function, 927
  altered cognitive function, 928

Moderate-severe TBI (*Continued*)
  endocrine dysfunction, 928
  impaired respiratory function, 927
  neurologic dysfunction, 927
    posttraumatic hydrocephalus, 927
    posttraumatic seizures, 927
  neuropsychological function, 928
  psychiatric deficits, 928
  psychosocial deficits, 928
  speech/communication deficits, 927
Monilial vaginitis, 496
Monro-Kellie hypothesis, 919–920
Mood disorders, 729
Motor vehicle crash, 933
Moyamoya disease, 865
MPKU syndrome, 821
Mucormycosis, 294
Multidimensional Anxiety Scale for
  Children, Second Edition, 168
Muscular dystrophy, 735
  diagnostic criteria, 736
  incidence, 735
  prevalence, 735
  types of, 736*t*
Mycoplasma, 862–863
Myelodysplastic syndrome, 300–301
Myelomeningocele, 886
Myelosuppression, 284

N
Nasal reconstructive surgery, 380
Nasoalveolar molding, 379*b*
National Association of Pediatric
  Nurse Practitioners, 40–41
National Committee for Quality
  Assurance, 6
National Comprehensive Cancer
  Network, 271–272
National Fragile X
  Foundation, 592–593
National Healthcare Quality and
  Disparities Report, 80
National Marrow Donor Program, 269,
  271–272
National Survey of Children with
  Special Health Care Needs, 6
Naturalistic developmental behavioral
  interventions, 225
Neisseria meningitides, 862–863
Neonatal sepsis, 840
Nephropathy, 500
Neural tube defect, 886, 888*f*
Neurologic dysfunction, 927
Neurologic impairments, 927
Neuropsychological function, 888, 928
Neutropenia, 284
Newborn screening, 737
Next-generation DNA sequencing, 639
Nitrofurantoin (Furadantin), 893
Nonaccidental injury, 915
Nonallergic asthma, 123
Noncommunicating
  hydrocephalus, 619–620
Nondisjunction of chromosome 21,
  510, 511*f*
Nonpharmacologic agents, 866
Nonproliferative retinopathy, 869
Nonsteroidal antiinflammatory drugs,
  670, 866

O
Obesity, 443, 743
  clinical manifestations, 759
  diagnostic criteria, 758
  etiology, 755
  incidence and prevalence, 758
  treatment, 760, 765*t*
  treatment of, 756
Obsessive-compulsive disorder,
  163–164, 164*t*, 166, 900
  cognitive-behavioral therapy, 170–171,
    171*b*
  compulsive behaviors, 166
  developmental issues
    aspects of sexuality, 174–175
    child care, 174
    discipline, 173–174
    schooling, 174
    sleep patterns, 173
    toileting, 173
    transition to adulthood, 175
  family concerns, 175
  health care maintenance
    dietary preferences, 172
    growth and development, 172
    immunization, 172
  levels of educational support for, 174
  pharmacologic interventions for, 171
    clomipramine, 171
    fluoxetine, 171
    fluvoxamine, 171
    sertraline, 171
    SSRIs, 171
  psychotherapeutic interventions,
    170*b*, 170
  risky or self-injurious behaviors in,
    172*b*, 172
  screenings, 173
  self-injurious behavior in, 172
  suicidal ideation in, 172
  themes of, 167*b*
Obstructive sleep apnea
  syndrome, 152, 500
Oligoarthritis, 669
Olmstead decision 1999, 98
Omalizumab, 136
Open neural tube defect, 886
Oppositional defiant disorder, 180, 193
Oral allergy syndrome, 151
Oral antibiotic therapy, 863
Oral health care of CYSHCN, 8–9
  dental home for, 9
  financial and structural barriers, 9
  for gingivitis, 9
  goal for, 9
  for periodontal disease, 9
Orthognathic surgery, 381*f*, 381
Orthopedic disorders, 776
Osteogenesis, 868–869
Osteomyelitis, 869
Osteopenia, 653
Osteoporosis, 653, 743
Ototoxic drugs, 869
Oxybutynin chloride (Ditropan), 893

P
Pancreatic enzyme replacement
  therapy, 467, 467*t*
Pancytopenia, 324–325

Parent and Child Interaction Therapy-Emotion Development, 721
Parents' Evaluation of Developmental Status, 213
Patent ductus arteriosus, 423, 429t–433t
Patient and family-centered care, 31
Patient-centered health care home, 31
Patient Protection, 13–15
Patient Self-Determination Act, 97
Pediatric cancer
　common, 319t–321t
　symptoms, 322b
Pediatric end-stage liver disease score, 789
Pediatric head injuries, 916
Pediatric nephrology teams, 689
Pediatric Primary Care Mental Health Specialist, 717
Pediatric solid organ transplantation, 787
Pediatric Symptom Checklist, 182–183
PEERS for young adults, Sexuality Education for Youth on the Autism Spectrum, and Tackling Teenage programs, 229–230
Penetrating head injuries, 916
Penicillin prophylaxis, 863
Peripheral blood stem cells, 269
Peripherally inserted central catheters, 326
Peritoneal dialysis, 692
Periventricular/intraventricular hemorrhage, 841
Phenobarbital, 893
Phenylketonuria, 818
　diagnostic criteria, 819
　incidence, 819
　prevalence, 819
　primary care management, 825
　prognosis, 825
Photosensitive skin reactions, 675–676
Pica, 228
Pimozide, 908
Pneumococcal conjugate vaccine, 608
Polyarthritis, 669
Polyethylene glycol, 546
Polysomnography, 747
Posterior spinal fusion, 739
Postimmunization fever management, 929–930
Postsecondary education, 83–84
Posttraumatic headaches, 931
Posttraumatic hydrocephalus, 927
Posttraumatic seizures, 927
Posttraumatic stress disorder, 163–164
Poverty
　assistance programs for dealing, 1–3
　deep, 1–3
　racial disparities and, 1–3
　SPM for childhood poverty rates, 1–3
Pramlintide, 494
Precocious puberty, 929
Prednisone, 740
Premonitory Urges for Tics Scale, 902
Preschoolers with chronic conditions, developmental task for
　difficulties, 27–28
　egocentricity and naive reasoning processes, 27–28

Preschool Pediatric Symptom Checklist, 183
Primary care management
　AAP recommendations, 15
　medical home model, 16
　role of primary care provider, 15–16
　　level of intervention, 16, 18, 17b–18b
Project ECHO (Extension for Community Healthcare Outcomes), 106–107
Prophylactic administration of anticonvulsants, 927
Proteinuria, 687, 689, 868
Pruning of gray matter, 74
Pseudomonas aeruginosa, 862–863
Psoriatic arthritis, 669
Psychiatric deficits, 928
Psychosocial deficits, 928
Pulmonary stenosis, 424, 429t–433t
Pyelonephritis, 876
Pyoderma gangrenosum, 645

R
Radiologic hepatic abnormalities, 870
Reconstructive surgery of clefts, 378
　of alveolar cleft, 380
　of cleft lip, 378
　of cleft palate, 379
　cleft rhinoplasty, 380
　jaw, 380
Red blood cells, 855, 870
Rehabilitation Act, 50, 84
　accommodation plans, 51
　definition of person with a disability, 50–51
　gender distribution, 51
　removal of barriers to education, 50
Remote education, 106
Renal
　dysfunction, 801
　osteodystrophy, 686
　replacement therapy, 689
　transplantation, 787
Resources for pediatric health care providers and families, 46, 21t–22t
　attention-deficit/hyperactivity disorder, 202–203
　autism spectrum disorder, 230–231
　bleeding disorders, 263
　cancer, 337–338
　celiac disease, 349
　cerebral palsy, 368
　cleft lip and cleft palate, 390–391
　congenital heart disease, 457
　cystic fibrosis, 482
　diabetes mellitus, 505
　Down syndrome, 532
　epilepsy, 577
　fragile X syndrome, 593
　health care transition, 85
　hematopoietic stem cell transplantation, 309
　hydrocephalus, 635
　inflammatory bowel disease, 661
　management of asthma and allergies, 159
　obsessive-compulsive disorder, 175–176

Respiratory devices, 739
Respiratory disorders, 775
Retinal hemorrhage, 915
Retinal tumors, 318–322
Retinopathy, 500
Retinopathy of prematurity, 841
Rett syndrome, 218
Rhinitis medicamentosa, 150
Ribonuclease reductase inhibitor, 859
Rifampin, 875
Right upper quadrant syndrome, 870
Right ventricular outflow tract obstructive lesions, 424
Rosa's law, 50
Rotational trauma, 914–915
Rotavirus vaccine, 607
Routine urinalysis screening, 774–775

S
Salmonella osteomyelitis, 869
Salmonella spp., 862–863, 875
SARS-CoV-2 vaccine, 609
School systems
　academic experience for children with chronic illness
　　absenteeism, 62–64
　　academic performance, 62
　　accommodations for facilitating, 63–64
　　child's perceived sense of safety, 63
　　fatigue, 64–65
　　interpersonal school experiences, 63
　　medications and treatments, 65
　　mobility concerns, 64
　　peer relationships, 63
　　poorer engagement, 63
　　school reintegration, 67
　　specific conditions-related accommodation, 65
　academic success for children with chronic illness, factors impacting, 61–62
　based clinics, 57
　　using telehealth, 109
　influential role in children's development, 49
　Maternal and Child Health Bureau Title V services in, 57
　Medicaid fee-for-service in, 57
　primary care provider's role in, 57–58
　　knowledge base of medical consultant, 59b
　　nurses and advanced practice registered nurses, 59–61
　　school medical consultant, 59
　safety in, 66
　　for participation in intramural and varsity athletics, 67
　　provisions for transporting during emergencies, 67
　social and emotional needs, 65–66
　state children's insurance plans in school setting, 57
　terminally ill students and, 68
　　do-not-attempt-resuscitation orders, 68–69, 69b
　　successful school experience, 68
　　transition between hospital and, 67–68

Scoliosis, 743
Screen for Anxiety-Related Disorders, 168
Screening for Disordered Eating, 547
Screenings, SCD growth and
    development, 872
  blood pressure, 873
  condition-specific, 874
    cardiac function, 875
    hematologic screening, 874
    lead poisoning, 875, 875b
    liver function, 875
    pulse oximetry, 874
    renal function testing, 874
    scoliosis, 875
    sleep apnea, 874
  dental, 873
  hearing, 873
  hematocrit, 873
  mental health, 873
  tuberculosis, 874
  urinalysis, 874
  vision, 874
Second impact syndrome, 927
Secretion of antidiuretic hormone, 928
Selective norepinephrine reuptake
    inhibitors
  adverse effects, 190–191
  attention-deficit/hyperactivity
    disorder, 186
Selective serotonin reuptake inhibitor
    fragile X syndrome, 585
Selective serotonin reuptake inhibitors
  anxiety disorders, 170
  for binge eating disorder, 544
Sensory disabilities, 927
Separation anxiety disorder, 164
  age of onset, 164
  clinical manifestation of
    difficulties in daily adaptive
      functioning, 165
    in young adults and adults, 164–165
    in younger children and older
      children, 164
  cognitive-behavioral therapy, 169
  diagnosis, 164
  in DSM-5, 164
  lifetime prevalence for adults, 164
  12-month prevalence for adults, 164
Serotonin-norepinephrine reuptake
    inhibitors
  anxiety disorders, 170
Severe combined immunodeficiency, 269
Sexual maturation, 678–679
Shaken baby syndrome, 915
Shapiro Tourette Syndrome Severity
    Scale, 902
Shunt, 422–423
Shunt catheters for CSF, 623f, 623–624
  differential pressure valves, 624
  evaluation of function, 625
  flow regulation, 624
  impact of contact sports, 629
  lumboperitoneal shunts, 624
  magnetic field interference, 635
  overdrainage of CSF, 625
  prevention of infection, 626
  programming valve, 624f, 624
  shunt failure, 624
  shunt infection, 625–626

Shunt catheters for CSF (Continued)
  shunt malfunction or infection
    symptoms, management of, 630
  shunt occlusion, 625
  signs and symptoms of illness, 630b
  siphon-resisting valves, 624
Sickle cell disease (SCD), 855
  alternative therapies, 876
  carriers of, 855, 856f
  common illness management, 875
  complementary therapies, 876
  diagnosis, 856–857, 859f
  developmental issues, 877
    child care, 877
    discipline, 877
    family concerns, 878
    schooling, 877
    sexuality, 878
    sleep patterns, 877
    toileting, 877
    transition to adulthood, 878
  differential diagnosis, 875
    abdominal pain, 876
    acute gastroenteritis, 876
    anemia, 876
    fever, 875
    neurologic changes, 876
    orthopedic symptoms, 876
    respiratory distress, 876
    urinary tract infections, 876
  drug interactions, 876
  fluid requirements for, 876
  health care maintenance, 871
    primary care office visits, 871
    regular office visits, 871
  incidence, 856
  inheritance pattern cause, 855
  prevalence, 856
  primary care management, 871
  prognosis, 870
  standard care, 857–859
  treatment, 857
    associated problems of, 862
    complementary and alternative
      medicine, 862
    drug therapy with
      hydroxyurea, 859
    gene therapies, 861
    hematopoietic stem cell
      transplant, 861
    second-line therapies, 861
    supportive symptomatic care, 857
    transcranial doppler screening, 860
    transfusions, 860
  types of, 862t
Sickle cell retinopathy, 869
Sickle hemoglobin, 855, 856f
Sickle thalassemia, 870
Silent cerebral infarct, 865
Single maintenance and reliever
    therapy, 133
Sinusoidal obstructive syndrome/
    venoocclusive disease, risk of, 290
  clinical presentation, 290
  diagnosis, 290
  prophylaxis and treatment
    strategies, 290
    defibrotide, 290
    ursodiol, 290

Sleep apnea, 152, 893
Sleep-disordered breathing
    problems, 518
Sleep disorders, 777
Sleep disturbances, 704
Sleep problems
  allergies, 155
  asthma, 155
  attention-deficit/hyperactivity
    disorder, 198, 199t
  autism spectrum disorder, 227
  cancer, 336
  celiac disease, 348
  cerebral palsy, 365–366, 366t
  cleft lip and cleft palate, 387–388
  congenital adrenal hyperplasia, 409
  congenital heart disease, 453
  cystic fibrosis, 479–480
  diabetes mellitus, 502
  Down syndrome, 529–530
  eating disorders, 551
  epilepsy, 575
  fragile X syndrome, 590
  hematopoietic stem cell
    transplantation, 307
  human immunodeficiency virus
    infections, 612
  hydrocephalus, 632
  inflammatory bowel disease, 659–660
  obsessive-compulsive disorder, 173
Sleep-related screening tools, 199t
Slipped capital femoral epiphysis, 776
Social anxiety disorder (social
    phobia), 165
  clinical manifestations of, 165
    in adults, 165
    in children, 165
  cognitive-behavioral therapy, 169
  in context of dating, 165
  diagnostic criteria for, 165
  in DSM-5, 165
  lifetime prevalence of, 165
  median age of onset of, 165
Social camouflaging, 226
Social determinants of health, 4–5, 105,
    108
Social determinants of health, 718
  impact on glycemic control for
    children with diabetes, 505
  of teenagers living with HIV, 613
Social determinants of health, 872–873
Social Responsiveness Scale, 215–216
Social Security Disability Insurance, 83
Social Services Block Grant, 932
Solid organ transplants, 787, 789
Solubility testing, 857
Spastic cerebral palsy, 352
Spasticity, 352
Special Supplemental Nutrition
    Program for Women, Infants,
    and Children, 5
Spirometry, 137–138, 138f
  common terminology of, 138
Spina bifida, 886
  associated problems, 887
  clinical manifestations, 887
  common illness management, 892
  condition-specific screening, 891
  developmental issues, 893

Spina bifida (*Continued*)
  chiari II malformation, 892
  tethering of the spinal cord, 892
  hydrocephalus, 892
  urinary tract infections, 892
  gastrointestinal symptoms, 893
  diagnosis, 886–887, 892
  drug interactions, 893
  etiology, 886
  health care maintenance, 889
  immunizations, 891
  incidence, 886
  level of lesion, functional alterations
    to, 890t
  management, advances in, 887
  prenatal ultrasound, 886–887
  prevalence, 886
  primary care management, 889
  prognosis, 889
  risk factors, 887
  screenings, 891
  serious complications of, 889b
  treatment, 887
Spina bifida screenings, 891
  blood pressure, 891
  dental, 891
  condition-specific, 891
    complete blood count, 891
    computed tomography/magnetic
      resonance imaging, 891
    gait analysis evaluation, 891
    latex allergy, 892
    psychometric screening, 891
    urine studies, 891
    x-rays, 891
  hearing, 891
  urinalysis, 891
  vision, 891
Splenic hypofunction, 857
Splenic malfunction, 862–863
Spondyloarthropathy, 670
Standardizing Care to Optimize
    Pediatric End Stage Kidney
    Disease, 690
Staphylococcus aureus, 862–863
Stickler syndrome, 372–373
Streptococcus pneumoniae, 862–863
Stress steroid dosing, 748
Subdural hematoma, 919
Subglottic stenosis, 514
Sulfasalazine, 660
Supplemental nutrition assistance
    program, 1–3, 5
Supraventricular tachycardia, 435
Survey of Well-being in Young
    Children, 213
Swallowing dysfunction
    (dysphagia), 743
Symptomatic urinary tract
    infection, 876
Systemic arthritis, 669–670

T
Tacrolimus, 794–795, 807
Tdap vaccine, 609
Teleconsultation, 107–108
Tele-education, 106
Telehealth, 103
  accessibility and, 112

Telehealth (*Continued*)
  advantages, 103–104
  ambulatory modality, 103
  application, 105
  case study, 116
  certification and credentialing, 114
  challenges
    policies and funding, 104–105
    regulations, 104–105
    in terms of equity, 105
    types of payment programs, 104–105
  connectivity for, 105f, 105–106
  consultative model, 103–104
  during COVID-19 pandemic, 103,
    106, 112
  etiquette, 110–111
    environment, 111
    PEP model, 111–112
    privacy and security
      considerations, 111–112
    provider's performance, 111
  as a follow-up to in-person care, 103
  guidelines for, 110
  health equity and, 112
  hospital-to-hospital (facility-to-
    facility) modality, 103
  legal and regulatory
    considerations, 112–113, 113f
    APRN practice
      requirements, 113–114
    Center for Connected Health
      Policy, 113
    CMS legislation and
      regulation, 112–113
    HIPAA requirements, 111–113
    interstate licensure compacts, 113–114
    originating site (patient location),
      importance of, 113
    state laws and regulations, 113
  limitations of, 110
  malpractice coverage for, 114
  in pediatric chronic care
    management, 106–108
    children with developmental
      disabilities and complex
      health, 108–109
    implementation of essential care
      elements, 109
  in pediatrics, 104t
  research agenda, 115
  research collaboratives, 104
  in school setting, 109
    for chronic care management for
      pediatric asthma, 109
    effectiveness of virtual speech-
      language services, 109
  sign language or spoken language
    interpreters, use of, 112
  standard of care, 110f, 110
  successful implementation and
    sustainability of, 109–111
  support to patients from prenatal
    development through
    adulthood, 103
  technical innovations in, 114, 115f
  techniques for effective
    communication, 111b, 111
  technology and types of services
    in, 103

Telemedicine, 103
Telementoring, 106–107
Telepractice, 108
Temporomandibular joint, 674
Tepid water, 890
Tetanus immunoglobulin vaccine, 607
Tetralogy of Fallot, 426, 429t–433t
Thrombocytopenia, 284–285
Thyroid dysfunction
  in Down syndrome, 517
  hematopoietic stem cell
    transplantation, 296
Tibia vara, 776
Toileting issues with chronic illness, 173
  allergies, 155
  asthma, 155
  attention-deficit/hyperactivity
    disorder, 198
  celiac disease, 348
  cerebral palsy, 366
  cleft lip and cleft palate, 388
  congenital adrenal
    hyperplasia, 409–410
  congenital heart disease, 453
  cystic fibrosis, 480
  diabetes mellitus, 502
  Down syndrome, 530
  eating disorders, 551
  fragile X syndrome, 590
  hematopoietic stem cell
    transplantation, 307
  human immunodeficiency virus
    infections, 612
  hydrocephalus, 632–633
  obsessive-compulsive disorder, 173
Tolterodine (Detrol), 893
Total anomalous pulmonary venous
    return, 429t–433t
Tourette disorder scale, 902
Tourette syndrome, 900, 902b
  autosomal dominant inheritance, 901f
  CAM modalities, 905
  clinical manifestations, 904, 904t
  common illness management, 908
  comorbidities with, 903–904, 904b,
    904f
  complementary and alternative
    therapies, 905, 907t
  covid-19 pandemic outcomes, 906
  developmental issues, 909
  diagnosis, 900, 902t, 905, 908
  drug interactions, 908
  DSM-5 diagnose, 902
    with comparison of ICD-10,
      ICD-11, 903t
  electroencephalogram, 903
  etiology, 900
  growth and development, 907
    diet, 907
    safety, 908
  health care maintenance, 907
  incidence, 900
  management, advances in, 905
  prevalence, 900
  primary care management, 907
  with phenomenologic features
    of, cortical and subcortical
    regions, 901f
  self-injurious behavior, 908

Tourette syndrome *(Continued)*
   treatment, 904
      nonpharmacologic, 905
      pharmacologic, 905, 906t–907t
Transcranial Doppler, 860
Transfusion complications, 870
Transfusion refractory
         thrombocytopenia, 290
Transient ischemic attack, 865
Transient red cell aplasia, 867
Transition to adulthood
   allergies, 158
   asthma, 158
   attention-deficit/hyperactivity
         disorder, 200–202
   autism spectrum disorder, 230
   cancer, 337
   celiac disease, 349
   cerebral palsy, 367, 368f
   cleft lip and cleft palate, 389
   congenital adrenal
         hyperplasia, 411–412
   congenital heart disease, 455–456
   cystic fibrosis, 482
   diabetes mellitus, 504
   down syndrome, 531
   eating disorders, 553
   fragile X syndrome, 592
   hematopoietic stem cell
         transplantation, 308–309
   human immunodeficiency virus
         infections, 613–614
   hydrocephalus, 634
   inflammatory bowel disease, 660–661
   obsessive-compulsive disorder, 175
   obstacles, 73
   youth with chronic health
         conditions, 73
   youth with special health care
         needs, 73
Transposition of great arteries, 425–426,
         429t–433t
Trauma and stress-related
         disorders, 164t
Traumatic brain injury, 914
   anticipatory guidance, 928
   associated problems of, 926, 929b
   classification, 916, 917t
   common illness management, 931
   cranial injury, types of, 917
   developmental issues, 931
   diagnosis, 920, 926, 930–931
   diagnostic imaging, 920, 921f, 922t
   drug interactions, 931
   etiology, 914
   growth and development, 928
      nutritional intake, 929
      safety, 929
      immunizations, 929
   health care maintenance, 928

Traumatic brain injury *(Continued)*
   incidence, 916
   integrated complementary and
         alternative medicine, 925
   intracranial injury, types of, 917
   management, advances in, 926
   physical mechanisms of, 914, 915f
   prevalence, 916
   primary care management, 928
   primary injury, 914
   school reentry support, 932–933
   screenings, 930
   secondary injury, 914
   treatment, 920, 922
Traumatic brain injuries, 179
Tricuspid atresia, 426, 429t–433t
Trimethoprim-sulfamethoxazole, 800,
         893
Truncus arteriosus, 426, 429t–433t
Tuberous sclerosis, 179, 218

U
Ulcerative colitis, 639, 641
   characteristics of pediatric, 644t
   clinical manifestations, 644
   fertility rates in females, 660
   lactose intolerance in, 657
   risk factors for malignancy for, 656
Umbilical cord blood, 269
Uncontrolled hypertension, 704
Uncorrected metabolic acidosis, 685
Upper respiratory infections, 152
Uremia, 686–687, 687t
Uremic neuropathy, 698
Urologic abnormalities, 698
Urticaria, 151
US Hemophilia Treatment Center
         Network, 237
US Renal Data System, 683
Uveitis, 673

V
Vanderbilt, Connors, Impairment
         Rating Scale, 182
Vanderbilt ADHD Parent Diagnostic
         Rating Scale, 183
Vanderbilt scale, 903–904
Van der Woude syndrome, 372–373
Varicella vaccine, 609
Varicella zoster virus, 293, 800
Vasoconstriction, 237
Vasomotor rhinitis, 150
Vasoocclusion, 865
Velocardiofacial, 179
Ventricular rhythm disturbances, 442
Ventricular septal defect, 423,
         429t–433t
Ventriculoatrial shunt, 891
Ventriculoperitoneal shunt, 887–888
Very early onset IBD, 639, 641

Very early onset IBD *(Continued)*
   health care maintenance
      growth and development, 657
      malignancy rates, 655–656
Videofluoroscopic swallowing study, 890
Villous atrophy of duodenum, 342
Vinca alkaloids, 335
Virtual education, 106
Visio-vestibular exam, 930, 930t
Visual deficits, 927
Vitamin D deficiency, 468
Vocational rehabilitation services and
         job training, 84
Von Willebrand disease, 237
   acquired/inheritance, 254, 254f–255f
      type 1, 254f, 254
      type 2, 254f
      type 3, 254–255, 255f
   bleeding management
      for acute major bleeding and
         major surgery, 258
      antifibrinolytic agents, 258
      DDAVP, 258
      minor, 257–258
   clinical manifestations of, 255–256
   diagnosis, 252, 253f
   diagnostic testing, 256
   future treatment options for
         bleeding disorder, 259
      antitissue factor pathway
         inhibitor, 259
   incidence and prevalence, 253
   OB-GYN delivery, 259
      monitoring factor VIII activity, 259
   pharmacologic therapy, 257, 258t
      desmopressin acetate, 257
      hormonal therapy, 257
      oral antifibrinolytic agents, 257
      prophylactic therapy, 257
      von Willebrand factor replacement
         products, 257
   testing/diagnostic criteria, 256–257
      laboratory tests, 256
   types, 252t
Vulnerable child syndrome, 444

W
Wechsler Intelligence Scale for
         Children-Revised, 523–524
Williams syndrome, 179
Wilms tumor, 696
Workforce Innovation and
         Opportunity Act, 84

X
Xenotransplantation, 797
Xerostomia, 300

Y
Yale Global Tic Severity Scale, 902